198.95

HANDBOOK OF PHYSIOLOGY

Section 2: The Cardiovascular System
Volume I: The Heart

HANDBOOK OF PHYSIOLOGY

A critical, comprehensive presentation of physiological knowledge and concepts

Section 2: The Cardiovascular System

VOLUME I: The Heart

Edited by

ERNEST PAGE
Department of Medicine
University of Chicago
Chicago, Illinois

HARRY A. FOZZARD
Department of Medicine
University of Illinois
Chicago, Illinois

R. JOHN SOLARO
Department of Physiology and Biophysics
University of Illinois at Chicago College of Medicine
Chicago, Illinois

Published for the American Physiological Society by
OXFORD
UNIVERSITY PRESS
2002

OXFORD
UNIVERSITY PRESS

Oxford New York
Athens Auckland Bangkok Bogota
Bombay Buenos Aires Calcutta Cape Town
Dar es Salaam Delhi Florence Hong Kong Istanbul
Karachi Kuala Lumpur Madras Madrid
Melbourne Mexico City Nairobi Paris Shanghai
Singapore Taipei Tokyo Toronto

and associated companies in
Berlin Ibadan

Copyright © 2002 by the American Physiological Society

Published by Oxford University Press, Inc.
198 Madison Avenue, New York, New York 10016

Oxford is a registered trademark of Oxford University Press

All rights reserved. No part of this publication may be reproduced,
stored in a retrieval system, or transmitted, in any form or by any means,
electronic, mechanical, photocopying, recording, or otherwise,
without the prior permission of Oxford University Press.

Library of Congress Cataloging-in-Publication Data
The cardiovascular system / edited by Ernest Page, Harry A. Fozzard, R. John Solaro.
p. cm. — (Handbook of physiology ; section 2)
Includes bibliographical references and index.
ISBN 0-19-509886-2
Contents: v. 1. The heart
1. Heart—Physiology.
I. Page, Ernest. II. Fozzard, Harry A. (Harry Allen), 1931– III. Solaro, R. John.
IV. American Physiological Society (1887–)
V. Handbook of physiology (Bethesda, Md.) ; section 2.
[DNLM: 1. Heart—physiology. 2. Heart Diseases—physiopathology.
QT 104 H2361
QP6.H25 [QP111.4] 571 s—dc21 [612.1'7] 00-050142

9 8 7 6 5 4 3 2 1

Printed in the United States of America
on acid-free paper

Preface

This book represents the third stage of a long tradition of publishing critical essays on mechanisms underlying normal and abnormal physiology of the heart, beginning with the first volume on the heart in 1962, and continuing with the second volume in 1979. These earlier volumes continue to serve as invaluable resources for tracing the origins and evolution of modern physiological thought, but since 1979 there has been a revolution in scientific methods, greatly expanding our understanding of cardiac function. With the extraordinary growth of biological science that overlaps the heart, the boundaries between physiology and other biological disciplines has diminished or vanished. Realizing this, we chose to cover three areas in this volume: cardiac structure, cardiac muscle contraction, and cardiac electrophysiology. Studies in these three areas have made seminal contributions to science broadly, yet they remain critical properties of the heart. The distinguished scientists who have contributed to this volume lead the way into the new millennium of physiological research. Our great opportunity is to resolve the function of the protein products of our 30,000 genes, and that promises extraordinary advances in the understanding of normal and pathological physiology of the heart.

Contraction is the central function of the heart as a pump. Three great advances in our study of cardiac contraction have been the cloning, and in some cases the structural determination, of the contractile proteins and the regulators of intracellular calcium; optical methods to monitor intracellular calcium; and single-molecule studies of the biophysics of molecular motors. This splendid field is developed in six chapters by Walker, Solaro, Bers, Hryshko, Moss and Buck, and Tada and Toyofuko, extending from the molecular events in chemical-mechanical transduction to intracellular calcium cycling. Because the contractile system represents prime targets for therapeutic approaches to heart failure, two additional chapters by Covell and Ross and by Katz integrate the contractile system into whole heart function in health and disease.

Cardiac electrophysiology has also flourished in the new era of molecular science, benefitting from single-channel recording and the cloning and transgenic knockout of many important ion channels, which in several instances were first discovered in heart muscle. Stimulated by the recent discovery of ion channel defects in several genetic arrhythmic syndromes, we examine the electrical system in nine chapters. Spray, Suadicani, Srinivas, Gutstein, and Fishman, Heath, Gingrich and Kass, Nerbonne, Hiraoka, Antzelevitch and Dumaine, and Hanck, Martin, Tytgat and Ulens present the structure and function of the full array of cardiac ion channels, their modulation, and their cardiac expression patterns, including gap junctions, sodium, calcium, and potassium channels, and the recently cloned T-type calcium channels and pacemaker channels. A complete model of the interaction of these channels in the action potential is presented by Rudy. The electrical processes underlying normal and abnormal conduction and arrhythmias are elegantly discussed by Kléber, Janse and Fast and by Makielski and Fozzard. This field continues to provide leadership to electrophysiology in general, and it is finally becoming central to our understanding of arrhythmogenesis and to rational drug design.

Cardiac function is uniquely determined by cardiac structure and development. Four chapters by Goldstein and Schroeter, Anversa and Olivetti, Spyer, and Page, Iida and Doyle describe in detail cardiac ultrastructure, cardiac development, vagal nerves in the heart and their function, and the remarkable structures called caveolae.

Through the preparation of this volume we have focused on biology that is unique to the heart, while also placing the work in its full biological context. We chose distinguished authors who have a long history of special interest in cardiac function. To accompany their chapters, they have selected references that can lead the reader back to more general biology or on to more specialized cardiac science. The chapters are directed to the graduate student and postdoctoral fellow, as well as to the mature scientist interested in the heart. They will also undoubtedly be of interest to those presently working in this field.

The editors thank the Publications Committee of the American Physiological Society and the staff of Oxford University Press for their patience and continued support during the development of this book. We give special thanks to the authors of these chapters for their long hours of work in preparing their manuscripts.

Chicago, Illinois   E. P.
     H. A. F.
     R. J. S.

Contents

Contributors   ix

1. Ultrastructure of the Heart   3
   Margaret Ann Goldstein and John P. Schroeter

2. Cellular Basis of Physiological and Pathological Myocardial Growth   75
   Piero Anversa and Giorgio Olivetti

3. Cell Physiology and Cell Biology of Mycardial Cell Caveolae   145
   Ernest Page, Hiroshi Iida, and Donald D. Doyle

4. Gap Junctions in the Cardiovascular System   169
   David C. Spray, Sylvia O. Suadicani, Miduturu Srinivas, David E. Gutstein, and Glenn I. Fishman

5. Vagal Preganglionic Neurons Innervating the Heart   213
   K. Michael Spyer

6. Kinetics of the Actin-Myosin Interaction   240
   Jeffery W. Walker

7. Modulation of Cardiac Myofilament Activity by Protein Phosphorylation   264
   R. John Solaro

8. Cardiac Sarcoplasmic Reticulum Ca^{2+}-ATPase   301
   Michihiko Tada and Toshihiko Toyofuku

9. Regulation of Cellular Calcium in Cardiac Myocytes   335
   Donald M. Bers

10. The Cardiac Na^+-Ca^{2+} Exchanger   388
    Larry V. Hryshko

11. Regulation of Cardiac Contraction by Calcium   420
    Richard L. Moss and Scott H. Buck

12. Normal and Abnormal Conduction in the Heart   455
    André G. Kléber, Michiel J. Janse, and Vladimir G. Fast

13. The Cardiac Ventricular Action Potential   531
    Yoram Rudy

14. Ion Channels in the Heart: Cellular and Molecular Properties of Cardiac Na, Ca, and K Channels   548
    Bronagh Heath, Kevin Gingrich, and Robert S. Kass

15. Molecular Analysis of Voltage-Gated K$^+$ Channel Diversity and
    Functioning in the Mammalian Heart   568
    Jeanne M. Nerbonne

16. Modulation of Electrical Properties by Ions, Hormones, and Drugs   595
    Masayasu Hiraoka

17. Electrical Heterogeneity in the Heart: Physiological, Pharmacological,
    and Clinical Implications   654
    Charles Antzelevitch and Robert Dumaine

18. Newly Cloned Threshold Channels   693
    Dorothy A. Hanck, Ruth L. Martin, Jan Tytgat, and Chris Ulens

19. Ion Channels and Cardiac Arrhythmia in Heart Disease   709
    Jonathan C. Makielski and Harry A. Fozzard

20. Systolic and Diastolic Function (Mechanics) of the Intact Heart   741
    James W. Covell and John Ross, Jr.

21. A Modern View of Heart Failure: Practical Applications of Cardiovascular Physiology   786
    Arnold M. Katz

Index   805

Contributors

Charles Antzelevitch, Ph.D.
Masonic Medical Research Laboratory
Utica, New York

Piero Anversa, M.D.
Department of Medicine
New York Medical College
Valhalla, New York

Donald M. Bers, Ph.D.
Department of Physiology
Loyola University Chicago
Maywood, Illinois

Scott H. Buck, M.D.
Department of Pediatrics
Cardiovascular Research Center
University of Wisconsin Medical School
Madison, Wisconsin

James W. Covell, M.D.
School of Medicine
University of California San Diego
San Diego, California

Donald D. Doyle, Ph.D.
Department of Medicine
University of Chicago
Chicago, Illinois

Robert Dumaine, Ph.D.
Masonic Medical Research Laboratory
Utica, New York

Vladimir G. Fast, Ph.D.
Department of Physiology
University of Bern
Bern
Switzerland

Glenn I. Fishman, M.D., Ph.D.
Departments of Medicine, Physiology and Biophysics,
 and Biochemistry and Molecular Biology
Mount Sinai School of Medicine
New York, New York

Harry A. Fozzard, M.D.
Department of Medicine
University of Chicago
Chicago, Illinois

Kevin Gingrich, M.D.
Department of Anesthesiology
University of Rochester School of Medicine and Dentistry
Rochester, New York

Margaret Ann Goldstein, Ph.D.
Department of Medicine
Section of Cardiovascular Sciences
Baylor College of Medicine
Houston, Texas

David E. Gutstein, M.D.
Department of Medicine
Mount Sinai School of Medicine
New York, New York

Dorothy A. Hanck, Ph.D.
Cardiac Electrophysiology Laboratories
University of Chicago
Chicago, Illinois

Bronagh Heath, Ph.D.
Department of Pharmacology
College of Physicians and Surgeons
Columbia University
New York, New York

Masayasu Hiraoka, M.D., Ph.D.
Department of Cardiovascular Diseases
Medical Research Institute
Tokyo Medical and Dental University
Tokyo
Japan

Larry V. Hryshko, Ph.D.
Institute of Cardiovascular Sciences
University of Manitoba
Winnipeg, Manitoba
Canada

Hiroshi Iida, M.D.
Department of Agriculture
University of Kyushu
Kyushu, Japan

Michiel J. Janse, M.D., Ph.D.
Laboratory for Experimental Cardiology
University of Amsterdam
Amsterdam
The Netherlands

CONTRIBUTORS

Robert S. Kass, Ph.D.
College of Physicians and Surgeons
Columbia University
New York, New York

Arnold M. Katz, M.D.
Cardiology Division
University of Connecticut Health Center
Farmington, Connecticut

André G. Kléber, M.D.
Department of Physiology
University of Bern
Bern
Switzerland

Jonathan C. Makielski, M.D.
Departments of Medicine and Physiology
University of Wisconsin
Madison, Wisconsin

Ruth L. Martin, Ph.D.
Cardiac Electrophysiology Laboratories
University of Chicago
Chicago, Illinois

Richard L. Moss, Ph.D.
Department of Physiology
Cardiovascular Research Center
University of Wisconsin Medical School
Madison, Wisconsin

Jeanne M. Nerbonne, Ph.D.
Department of Molecular Biology and Pharmacology
Washington University Medical School
St. Louis, Missouri

Giorgio Olivetti, M.D.
Department of Medicine
New York Medical College
Valhalla, New York

Ernest Page, M.D.
Department of Medicine
University of Chicago
Chicago, Illinois

John Ross, Jr., M.D.
School of Medicine and Institute of Molecular Medicine
University of California San Diego
San Diego, California

Yorum Rudy, Ph.D.
Departments of Biomedical Engineering, Physiology and Biophysics, and Medicine
Cardiac Bioelectricity Research and Training Center
Case Western Reserve University
Cleveland, Ohio

John P. Schroeter, Ph.D.
Department of Medicine
Section of Cardiovascular Sciences
Rice University
Houston, Texas

R. John Solaro, Ph.D.
Department of Physiology and Biophysics
Program of Cadiovascular Sciences
College of Medicine
University of Illinois at Chicago
Chicago, Illinois

David C. Spray, Ph.D.
Department of Neuroscience
Albert Einstein College of Medicine
Bronx, New York

K. Michael Spyer, M.D., DSc., FMedSci.
Royal Free and University College Medical School
University College London
London
United Kingdom

Miduturu Srinivas, Ph.D.
Department of Neuroscience
Albert Einstein College of Medicine
Bronx, New York

Sylvia O. Suadicani, Ph.D.
Department of Neuroscience
Universidade São Judas Tadeu
São Paulo
Brazil

Michihiko Tada, M.D., Ph.D.
Department of Medicine and Pathophysiology
Osaka University Graduate School of Medicine
Suita, Osaka
Japan

Toshihiko Toyofuku, M.D., Ph.D.
Department of Internal Medicine and Therapeutics
Osaka University Graduate School of Medicine
Suita, Osaka
Japan

Jan Tytgat, Pharm. D., Ph.D.
Laboratory of Toxicology
Faculty of Pharmaceutical Sciences
University of Leuven
Leuven
Belgium

Chris Ulens, Pharm. D.
Laboratory of Toxicology
Faculty of Pharmaceutical Sciences
University of Leuven
Leuven
Belgium

Jeffery W. Walker, Ph.D.
Department of Physiology
University of Wisconsin
Madison, Wisconsin

HANDBOOK OF PHYSIOLOGY

Section 2: The Cardiovascular System
Volume I: The Heart

1. Ultrastructure of the heart

MARGARET ANN GOLDSTEIN — Department of Medicine, Section of Cardiovascular Sciences, and Department of Molecular and Cellular Biology, Baylor College of Medicine, Houston, Texas

JOHN P. SCHROETER — Department of Medicine, Section of Cardiovascular Sciences, Baylor College of Medicine, and Department of Ecology and Evolutionary Biology, Rice University, Houston, Texas

CHAPTER CONTENTS

Shape, Motion, and Force Vectors
The Extracellular Matrix
    Collagen weave
    Transverse (T)-tubules
Interior Supporting Network
    Microtubules
    Intermediate filament network
    Sarcolemmal associations
    Titin filament network
The Myofilament Bundles and Associated Structures
The Dynamic Z-Band Lattice
    Contractile and elastic components in relation to the Z-band
    Protein composition
    Perturbed states of the Z-band
    Functional states of the Z-band
Summary
Appendix: Imaging and Analyzing Cardiac Ultrastructure

THE DOMAIN OF ULTRASTRUCTURE TODAY is the three-dimensional world at or below the nanometer level. Coexisting is an emerging new world of light microscopy where cell structures are shown three-dimensionally in color and in real time. Our interpretation of cardiac morphological data is influenced by knowledge integrated from whole animal physiology, subcellular physiology, biochemistry, and molecular biology.

Previous reviews have shown general features of cardiac muscle cells and separated contractile and noncontractile components (71, 96, 101, 283, 284). Some have emphasized muscle membrane systems, viewing the muscle cells as a series of compartments with boundaries delineated by tracers (234, 283, 284). The sarcomere with its surrounding membranes and related other structures was considered a model subunit of muscle function. This approach is one way to manage the raw data from biochemistry, cytochemistry, and physiology concerning the detailed structures within each of the sarcomere components.

As techniques for ultrastructural analysis have advanced, a flood of new information has become available. High-voltage electron micrographs provide views of longer range ordering. Fast freezing interrupts processes occurring in the millisecond range. With the advent of interventions made possible by molecular biology, it became clear that a complex system like muscle is influenced at all levels by events at any level. The newer analysis techniques reveal the limitations of a reductionist approach. Muscles are affected by microgravity, applied mechanical forces, repeated electrical stimulation, and structural deletions at the molecular level.

This chapter takes a systems approach to the three-dimensional structures involved in the generation and modulation of contractile and elastic forces in muscle. The particular form of these structures and of the interactions between them must satisfy functional constraints such as efficient use of metabolic energy, a long functional life span, resistance to fatigue, and resistance to disease. These constraints result in the unique temporal and spatial integration of the structural network of the muscle. Both generation of tension and gross movement are constant features of the living heart. The job of the morphologist is to identify structural features and their variations to understand the role that these may play in heart muscle cell function.

At each level from the whole heart down to the molecular level there are patterns of organization that reflect the mechanical function peculiar to the heart. To appreciate the diversity of structural patterns is to understand the possible range of functional states. The electron micrographs presented in this chapter show a single moment in a sequence of changes in such features as sarcomere length, crossbridge position, and Z-band filament arrangement, among others. These patterns are most easily demonstrated in comparisons between cardiac muscle and slow skeletal muscle. The anatomical situation in the body, the physiological constraints put upon the muscle, and the mechanical functions performed are quite different. Yet the major proteins are very similar and most of the individual proteins are highly conserved in both muscle types.

The purpose of this chapter is to help cardiac specialists in other disciplines understand a morphologist's approach at the start of the new millennium. The literature is too vast for an exhaustive list of references. With the advent of computer searches, we have taken an alternative approach, listing some key names associated with major concepts and important reviews to allow the reader to use these bibliographies in turn for a more thorough search where interest is keen. We have cited the names of people most active in the field both now and in the past, to give persons new to the field a sense of the progression of ideas. The following key words were useful in our computer searches: heart, cardiac, muscle, muscles, ultrastructure, actin, myosin, tropomyosin, alpha-actinin, desmin, talin, titin, intermediate filaments, elastic filaments, Z-band, Z-disk, Z-line, and various combinations of these to limit searches of the Medline database back to 1966. References to skeletal muscle have been included because of the emphasis on properties of striated muscle and because some of the leading edge research, especially at the nanometer level, is done on skeletal muscle.

In this review, we acquaint the reader with the interconnectedness of multiple systems within the cell and between cells of the heart. We illustrate the extreme specialization required to extract detailed knowledge below the nanometer level and show how model systems influence study choices. Observations of other cell types that have features common to cardiac cells have been useful: the cytoskeleton in nonmuscle cells, general cell functions in smooth muscle cells, and the contractile apparatus in slow skeletal muscle cells.

For years, muscle research has been a multidisciplinary effort. For example, at the time of the last *Handbook* devoted to the heart, review of ultrastructure, quantitative pathology, and the study of mutants (e.g. axolotl heart) were useful approaches. Big changes to the whole heart resulted from a specific repertory of responses by the heart cells. Another popular model was the skinned fiber. Structural data were compared to those of normal cells. We were able to describe the differences in general terms. Now with the advent of specific deletions from DNA coding, transgenic animals, and nuclear transfer cloning, subcellular response to perturbations at the molecular level are possible. Not only in biology but in scientific research as a whole, we are in a position to understand the behavior of complex systems. We have the use of powerful computers to keep track of masses of data and to plot the input and outcome of complex variables.

We still rely a great deal on two-dimensional images for analysis and display. Recorded views of muscle continue to be limited by the very nature of the imaging process, and we have obscured some features from view by limitations of the preparations (thus allowing degradation by enzymes or contaminants), by removing components (as in skinned fibers), or by overlooking components (as in superposition or in a sampling error). Nevertheless, we have discovered new structures and will continue to do so. Color images in stereo are now available on the Internet and in video form.

This chapter has three parts. The first deals with structural factors outside the individual heart muscle cells. The second part deals with the organization and interaction between various intracellular components in two categories: the interior supporting networks and the myofilament bundle and associated structures. The third part highlights the dynamic Z-band lattice. (An appendix on imaging cardiac muscle is included at the end of this chapter for the convenience of the reader.)

SHAPE, MOTION, AND FORCE VECTORS

The shape of heart muscle cells is influenced by the larger context of the arrangement of muscle layers and the motion of various components, both inside and outside the cell. At the level of the sarcomeres, the repeating subunits that give the striated appearance to the heart muscle cell, the force generated is transmitted along the axis of the myofilament bundle. The complex squeezing motion required at the gross level for the function of the heart as a pump is the result of the side-to-side and end-on-end arrangement of individual sarcomeres within myocardial cells, the joining of cardiac cells at the intercalated disks, and, finally, the stacking of cells of different orientation to form multiple layers of these cardiac cells. The three-dimensional structural information emerging at the molecular level must be interpreted in the context of the three dimensional arrangement of multiple repeats of the sarcomeres. With each level of organization there are increasing possibilities for complex arrangement and function.

The broader view of the heart muscle cell as part of a mechanical pump must also take into account the structural dynamics of cycling. Structural cycling occurs both in a temporal context and in a spatial context. The duration of the cycle varies as a function of heart rate, with recovery from an occasional missing or irregular beat briefly superimposed on the regular alternation between contracting and resting states. Spatially, the contractile state must be coordinated along a contractile filament, as well as throughout each sarcomere, throughout each cell, and between disparate cells in the myocardium.

While it is widely believed that mechanical parameters are most important for the organization of cellular components and intracellular components in heart, specific developmental constraints should also be considered. The heart develops from a simple tube consisting of a muscle layer sandwiched between endothelial and epithelial coverings. Asymmetrical growth and the proper migration of cells result in a twisting tube that then begins to take on the complicated arrangement of muscle layers seen in the adult heart. Once the mature heart is in place, a myriad of lines of force development have been determined. Cineangiograms of intact beating hearts suggest the best analogy is that of a squeezing, rotating fist. There is a delicate balance between an even amount of functional participation for the stacks of muscle layers, and for each cell group needed to bring about this complex motion. Recent work on sarcomeric domains within cardiac myocytes suggests a mechanism for nonuniform distribution of stress and strain (227).

As seen in scanning electron micrographs, isolated cardiac muscle cells are flattened cylinders with irregular ends (286). Intact cardiac cells have similar surface features but are more nearly cylindrical. Their size is intermediate between that of smooth muscle cells and skeletal muscle cells. Measured with the light microscope, adult cells are about 80 µm long (range 35–130 µm) and 10–15 µm in average width (28, 90, 129, 291, 312). Heart cell diameters of neonates are half that value and hypertrophied cells can be twice that value. The shapes of intact mammalian cardiac fibers do not conform to any simple geometries. On at least one side, a consistent distance (20–22 nm) is maintained between cells over long distances.

As shown in Figure 1–1, myocardial cells have a single long axis. The cells are joined at intercalated disks where the cell borders interdigitate (interlock) in rectangular steps of irregular width and length (see Fig. 1–2). In general, mammalian ventricular cells are loosely packed. They are separated by frequent capillaries and bundles of collagen as well as by occasional fibroblasts. A fairly even distribution of the capillaries and collagen bundles is assured by their size and by an appropriate adjustment of capillary number and collagen bundle size relative to the variations in muscle cell size, surface area, and the overall dimensions of the intercalated disk. An overall impression of the variations in cell size and in the complexity of cellular arrangement is seen by comparing mammalian hearts of the different-sized animals used for experimental or pathological studies: mouse (71, 284), rat (see Figs. 1–25, 1–36, 1–37, 1–68, 1–69), guinea pig (Figs. 1–5, 1–23, 1–24), ferret (71), rabbit (284), opossum (284), cat (see Figs. 1–32, 1–58), dog (see Figs. 1–1 through 1–3, 1–6, 1–17 through 1–22, 1–26 through 1–30, 1–33 through 1–35, 1–38 through 1–40), monkey (71, 284), sheep (284), and human (see Fig. 1–55). Hearts of lower vertebrates have narrow cells, cell bundles tightly packed, and junctional complexes arranged in the intercalated disk in a manner similar to that in mammals but lacking the appearance of steep steps (284).

Like cells of skeletal and smooth muscles, heart muscle cells are elongated in the direction of force generated by the muscle. A supporting network of intermediate filaments and microtubules maintains the nuclei of cardiac muscle cells at a set position near the center of the cell (see Figs. 1–23 through 1–26). However, the nuclei also undergo shape changes in response to contractile waves from surrounding myofilament bundles (see Fig. 1–26). The Golgi components, the remnants of the ribosome-studded endoplasmic reticulum, and some mitochondria and glycogen accumulate at the ends of the nuclei (see Figs. 1–23, 1–24).

Cardiac muscle cells and slow skeletal muscle cells have numerous myofilament bundles and mitochondria all very closely packed (see Figs. 1–1 through 1–6). The large myofilament bundle size and the abundance of mitochondria found in both is characteristic of muscle cells that must support the demands of a continual load and also be resistant to fatigue. Compressible elements like the large nuclei and numerous mitochondria occupy a significant volume within the cardiomyocytes and probably modulate contractile force in ways as yet unknown.

The nature of the attachments between adjacent cells in cardiac muscle also influences the organization of various components within the cells. The intercalated disk, a conglomerate of three different junctional complexes (desmosome, intermediate junction, and gap junction), plays an extremely important role in defining unique features of cardiac muscle cells. The desmosomes (see Figs. 1–23 and 1–32) provide the mechanical stability and are the functional equivalent of the myotendinous junction in skeletal muscle. The papillary muscles, so widely used for structural and mechanical studies of individual sarcomeres, are interesting in this regard because they have a tendinous attachment to the valve leaflet at one end of the muscle. At the other end, the cells form typical cell-to-cell attachments, as in the rest of the ventricular wall. The fasciae adherentes (intermediate junctions) are specialized regions for attachment and insertion of the thin filaments from each longitudinal myofilament bundle. These junctions alternate with the desmosomes in the intercalated disk regions, which are oriented perpendicular to the myofibril axis. The gap junctions (see Figs. 1–23 and 1–32) are usually oriented parallel to the long axis of the myofilaments and occupy most or all of the longitudinal faces of the rectangular steps within the intercalated disk.

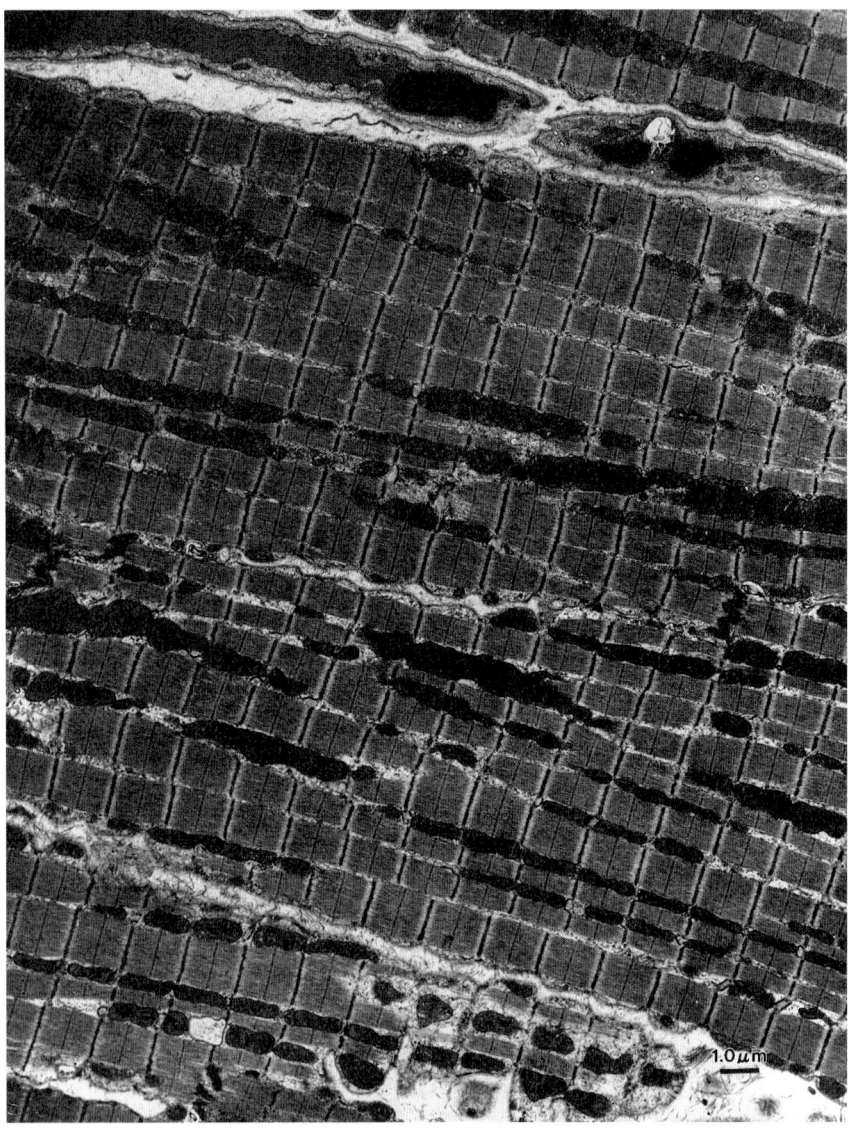

FIG. 1–1. Regularly repeating array of myofibrils and mitochondria in two cells and portions of two intercalated disks of dog papillary muscle fixed at rest length by immersion in glutaraldehyde–formaldehyde and postfixed with osmium tetroxide.

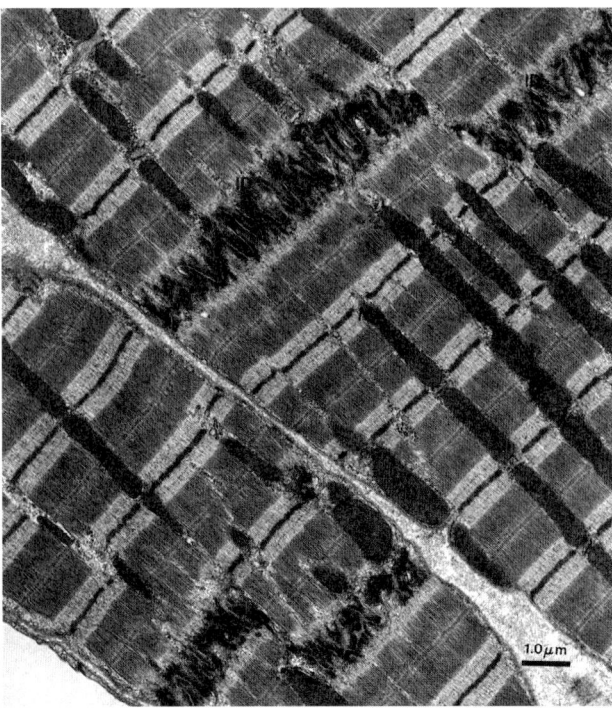

FIG. 1–2. Portions of two cardiac cells showing mitochondria (Mi) and stair step configurations of intercalated disks (ID) in longitudinal sections of dog papillary muscle.

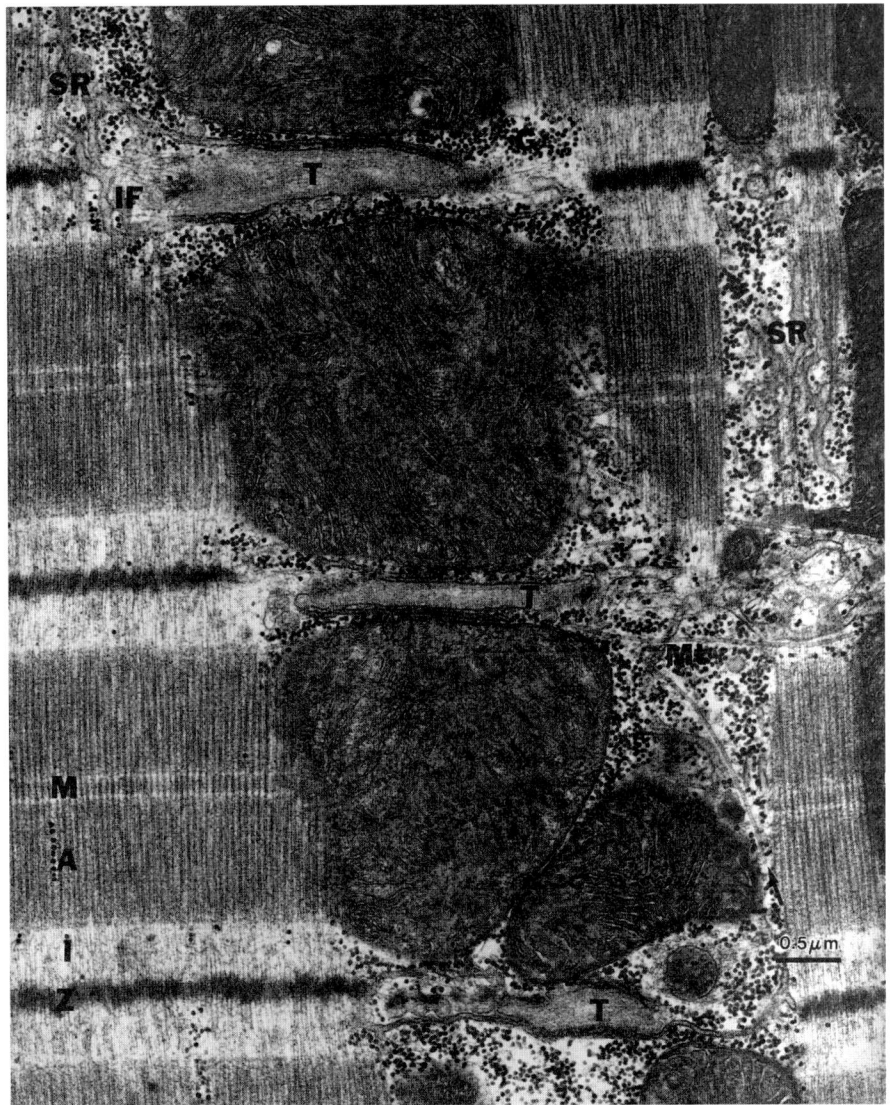

FIG. 1–3. Longitudinal section of a normal dog papillary muscle cell reveals most of the repeating sarcomere structures. Thick and thin filaments exhibit typical banding pattern (A, I, Z, M). Large mitochondria with tightly packed cristae are found along and between the usually large myofilament bundles. Microtubules (Mt), glycogen (G) and profiles of sarcoplasmic reticulum (SR) are visible in the planes between myofibrils. T-tubules (T) and terminal sacs of sarcoplasmic reticulum form triads. Intermediate filaments (IF) oriented transverse to the myofibril axis are visible near T-tubules. Note portion of mitochondrion tracking along the microtubule (*arrow*) (98). (Reprinted by permission of Rockefeller University Press.)

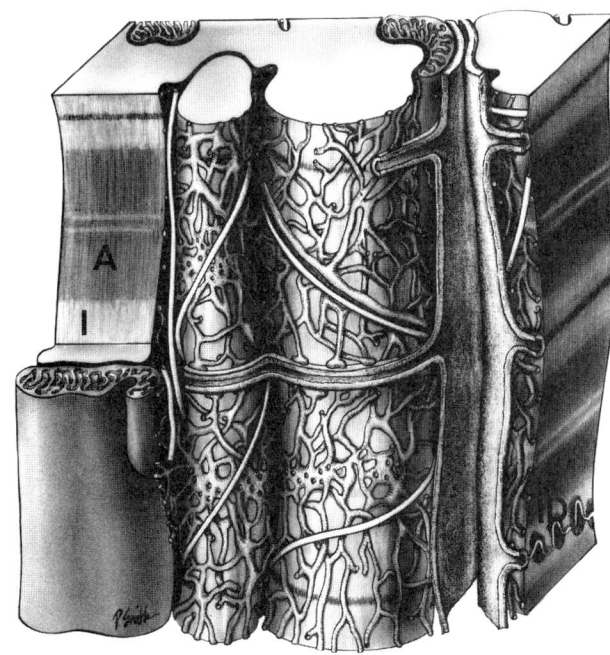

FIG. 1–4. Artist's sketch of cardiac muscle showing cut-away three-dimensional view of several sarcomeres. A = A-band; I = I-band; ID = intercalated disc (98). (Reprinted by permission of Rockefeller University Press.)

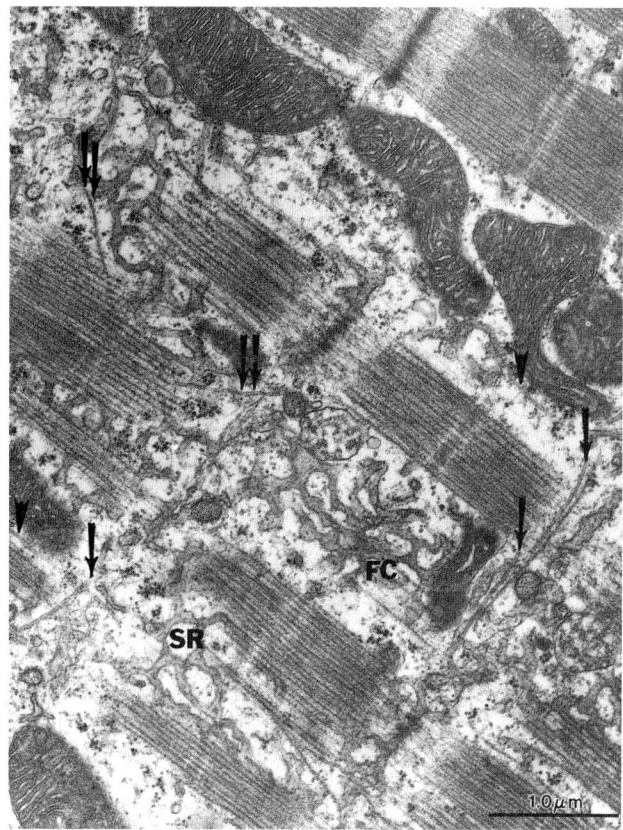

FIG. 1–5. Guinea pig papillary muscle in thin longitudinal section. Microtubules (*arrows*), intermediate filaments and sarcoplasmic reticulum (SR) profiles are visible around the myofilament bundles and the fenestrated collar (FC) of the SR.

FIG. 1–6. Longitudinal section of normal dog cardiac muscle cell. Thick and thin filaments of A-band hexagonal lattice are shown in two different orientations (A) with respect to this longitudinal plane of section through the middle of a myofibril. Mitochondrial profiles appear flattened in this view (refer to diagram in Figure 1–4). Note variation in Z-width (*arrows*) and the change in orientation of Z-lattice with respect to the plane of section.

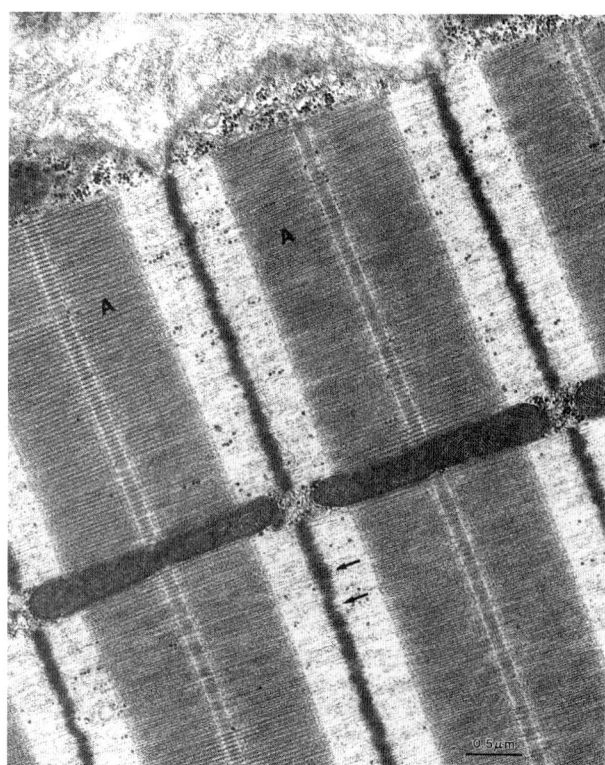

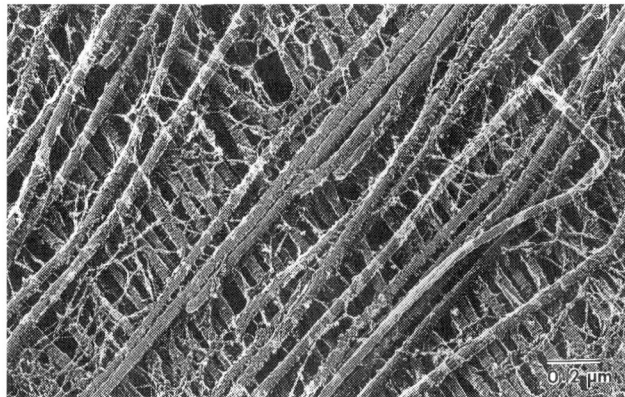

FIG. 1–7. Interstitial area between rabbit myocytes, ultrarapidly frozen, freeze-fractured, and then etched. The banded collagen fibrils are abundant and fill the interstitial space. With etching, the microthread network is evident as an extensive weave connecting collagen fibril to fibril. (347) (Reprinted by permission of Academic Press.)

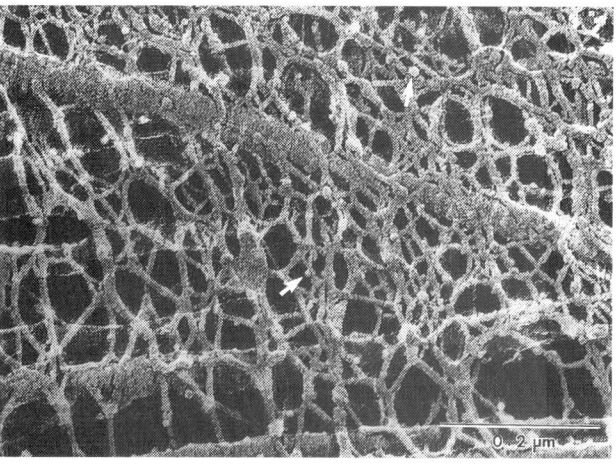

FIG. 1–8. High-magnification micrograph of deep-etched replica showing the collagen fibril microthread meshwork. The intertangled network that bridges and wraps around the collagen fibrils is visible in three-dimensional array. Granules of ~8–10 nm diameter are apparent at branch points of the microfibril–microthread lattice (*arrow*) (347). (Reprinted by permission of Academic Press.)

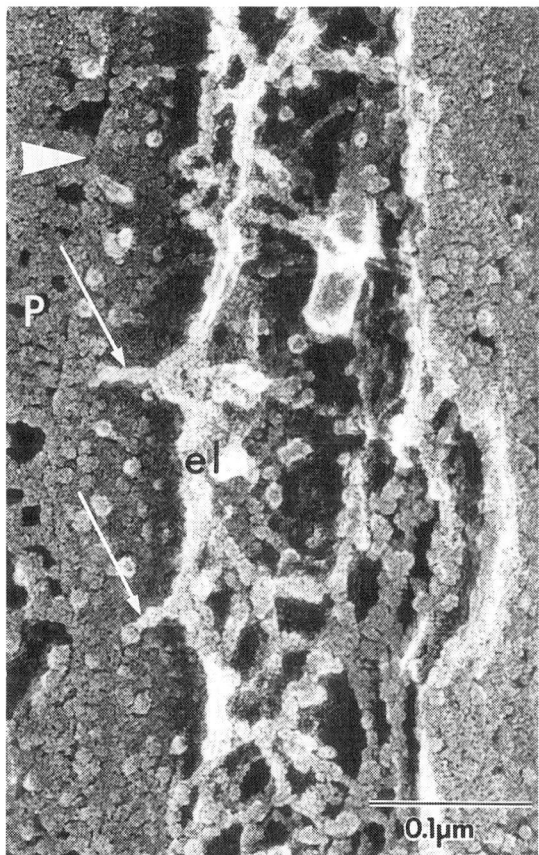

FIG. 1–9. Freeze-fractured, deep-etched replica from unfixed ultrarapidly frozen rabbit heart exposed to 0-Ca perfusion. The external lamina (el) is seen pulled back from the surface of the myocyte sarcolemma. The attachment of the external lamina is maintained at several sites by trabeculae (*arrows*). The demarcation between the bilayer surface of the cell and the fractured P face of the membrane is clearly visible (*arrowhead*) (347). (Reprinted by permission of Academic Press.)

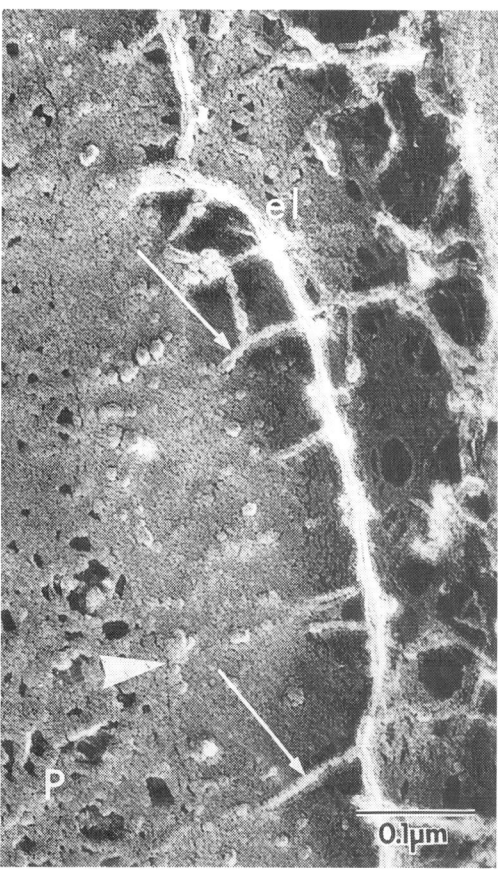

FIG. 1–10. Freeze-fractured, deep-etched replica from unfixed ultrarapidly frozen rabbit heart exposed to 0-Ca perfusion. This lower magnification micrograph should be compared to Figure 1–10. As in that figure, the external lamina (el) is pulled away from the sarcolemma but attached by trabeculae (*arrows*). *Arrowhead* indicates the demarcation between the bilayer cell surface and the fractured P face of the membrane (347). (Reprinted by permission of Academic Press.)

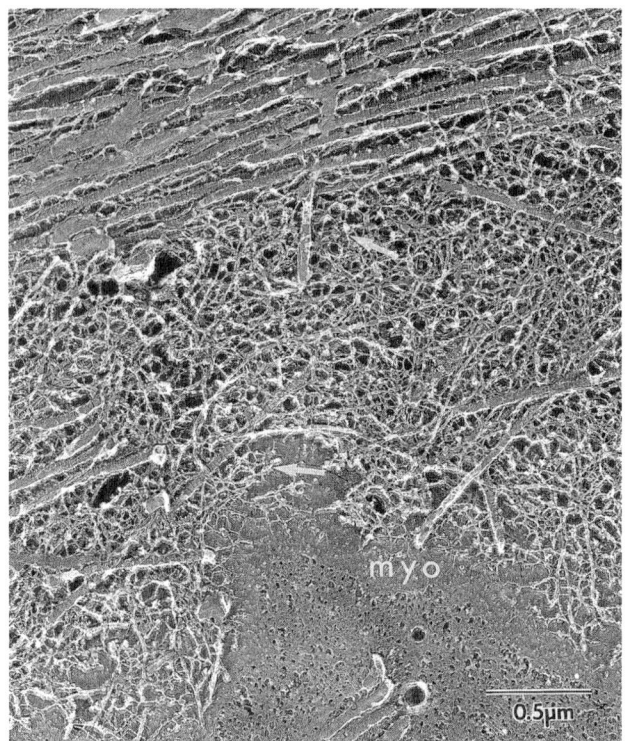

FIG. 1–11. Freeze-etch micrograph of unfixed ultrarapidly frozen rabbit papillary muscle. At this magnification, the connecting matrix of fine fibrils in between and connecting the collagen and the muscle surface is visible (*arrows*). In addition to the collagen bundle fibrils, individual 54 nm diameter collagen fibrils are visible at the myocyte cell surface (myo) (75). (Reprinted by permission of S. Karger.)

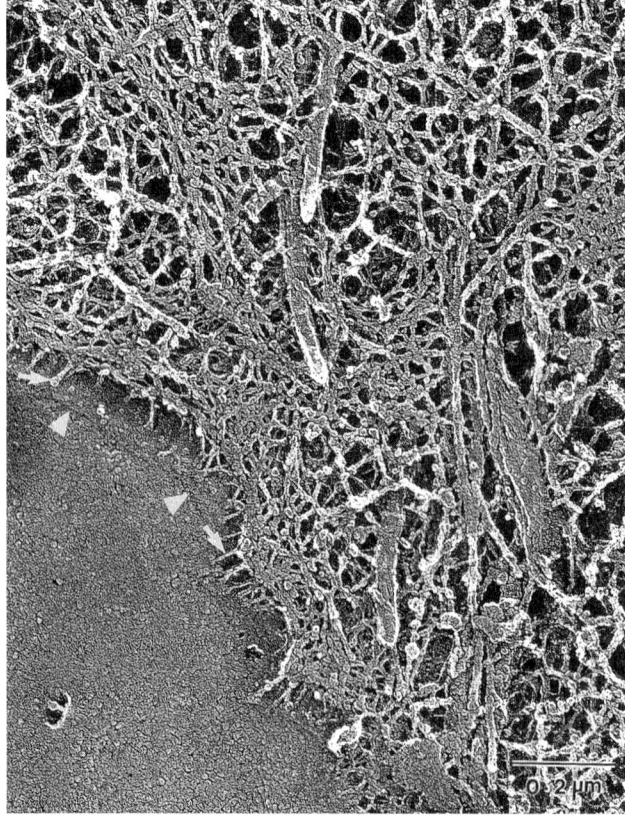

FIG. 1–12. Another view of unfixed ultrarapidly frozen rabbit papillary muscle. The regularly arranged trabeculae of the external lamina of the myocyte appear to insert directly into the bilayer. The series of linkages from collagen to myocyte membrane is visible. External lamina trabeculae of 'posts' (*arrow*) insert or attach to the bilayer. A fine line marks the boundary between the outer surface and the P face of the bilayer (*arrowheads*) (75). (Reprinted by permission of S. Karger.)

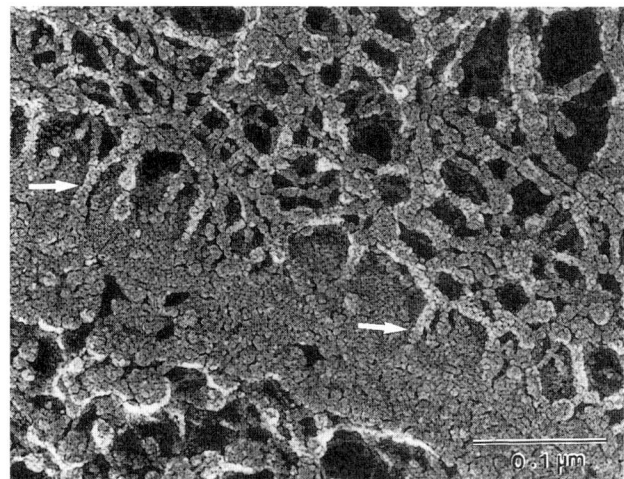

FIG. 1–13. Freeze-etch electron micrograph of 4 day-old rat myocyte. This high-magnification micrograph shows that by 4 days the cell surface and extracellular matrix fibrils are similar in density and organization to the adult. The trabeculae that link the external lamina into the bilayer are clearly visible (*arrows*) (75). (Reprinted by permission of S. Karger.)

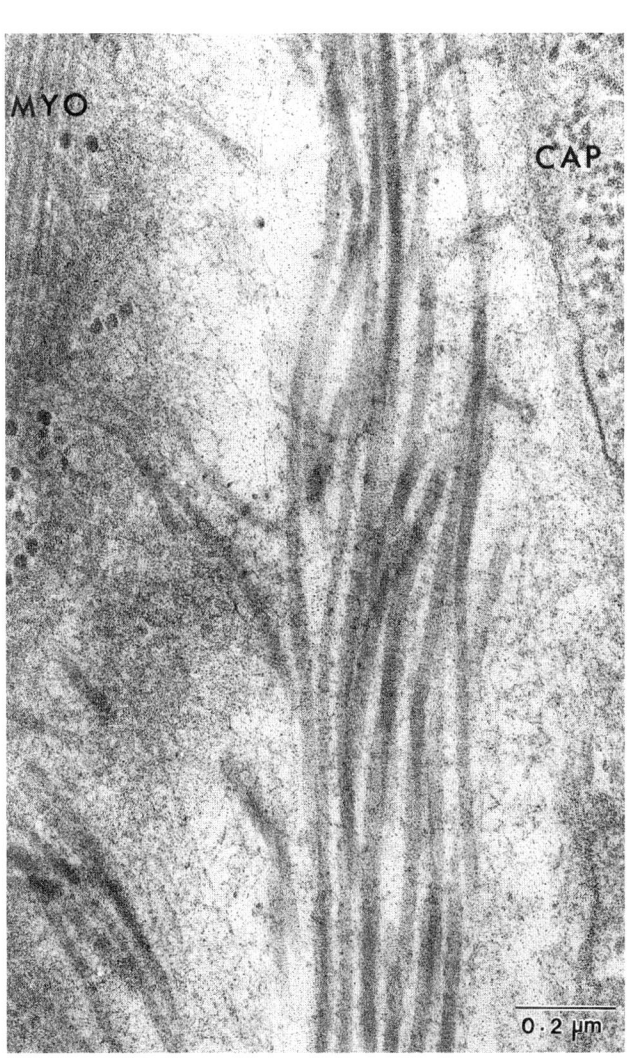

FIG. 1–14. Conventionally prepared (2% tannic acid present) thin-section electron micrograph shows the interstitial space between a rabbit myocyte (MYO) on the left and a capillary (CAP) on the right. The collagen fibrils run parallel to the long axis of the myocyte, with some collagen fibrils branching laterally to link with the myocyte cell surface and, on the other side, to the capillary. The individual structures involved in the linkages are not clearly visible in this type of preparation (75). (Reprinted by permission of S. Karger.)

THE EXTRACELLULAR MATRIX

The extracellular matrix (compartment) includes (1) the connective tissue that surrounds the cardiac muscle cells, the fibroblasts, and blood vessel cells; (2) the narrow intercellular spaces within bundles of closely packed cardiac fibers; and (3) the extracellular space along the surface, of individual cardiac muscle cells and in the invaginations of the cell surface, which form the transverse tubular system. Blood vessels occupy over half of this compartment, and connective tissue cells, collagen, and numerous protein substances fill the rest (162).

Capillaries are numerous in mammalian cardiac muscle because of the high metabolic demands. It has been estimated that one-third of the circumference of each myocardial cell is within 200 nm of a capillary (73). Capillaries have an internal diameter of approximately 7 µm and are spanned in cross section by two endothelial cells. These endothelial cells have a typical basal lamina as well as numerous caveolae. Transcapillary movement of large molecules is through vesicular transport, and that of small molecules is through intercellular junctions of predominantly the tight junction or zonula occludens variety. Permeability is also regulated by zonula adherentes, regions of cytoskeletal actin insertion in capillary cells.

The arterioles, arteries, and veins have a layer of smooth muscle cells, and their ultrastructure is typical of blood vessels found throughout the body. The lymph vessels are sparsely distributed within mammalian hearts, and ultrastructurally they are similar to capillaries. Unmyelinated autonomic nerve fibers are plentiful in cardiac muscle, especially in the regions of the right atrium. Fibroblasts are polymorphous cells with long, thin processes, and they play an active role in secreting the specific collagen proteins and other substances of the extracellular matrix (see Fig. 1–21).

From the metabolic standpoint, the capillaries and fibroblasts are important components of the extracellular space. These components vary in size and number in situations of hypertrophy and atrophy of the cardiac muscle cells. From a mechanical standpoint the collagen and elastin distribution is the most interesting component of the extracellular space (for a review of elastic fibers, see ref. 253).

Collagen Weave

The complex morphology of the extracellular matrix surrounding the interconnecting myocardial cells has been reviewed by Robinson et al. (256, 257). The matrix includes the thick 120–150 nm collagen bundles described with scanning electron microscopy by Caulfield and Borg (33). There is also a more extensive network of finer collagen fibrils 30–70 nm in diameter, as well as unbanded 8–10 nm microfibrils and even finer fibrils, the so-called microthreads, of 3–7 nm diameter (255–258). The collagen bundles vary in diameter and length with varying degrees of overlap (see Figs. 1–7 through 1–21). In some cases the bundles of collagen are cable-like, and in others they resemble spindles with a variable overlap pattern reminiscent of skeletal muscle cell overlap. These larger and smaller collagen bundles oriented along the myofiber axis are connected at regular intervals by small collagen cables forming struts that run at angles between the large and small bundles of collagen fibrils. In the myocardium the struts contain both collagen types I and III. The struts that are close to the cell surface are directed at regular intervals toward the cardiac muscle cells and appear to end right at the cell surface, always in the region of Z-bands. Until quite recently our knowledge of these structures of the extracellular matrix has come from studies using scanning electron microscopy and conventional and high-voltage transmission electron microscopy. Such studies have shown that the collagen that wraps around groups of myocytes is organized in a weave pattern. It is to these woven, undulating strands of collagen that the collagen struts attach, forming bridges between myocytes and between myocytes and capillaries. The fine struts that interconnect the lateral surfaces of cardiac myocytes and the rather narrow spaces between individual cardiac myocytes have been studied by Robinson and coworkers (258). They have identified microfibrils 8–10 nm and microthreads 3–7 nm in diameter using both conventional and high-voltage microscopy (75). Most recently these morphological details have been re-examined with ultrarapid freezing, freeze-fracture, and replication (75). Low-magnification comparisons of micrographs of fixed freeze-substituted thin sections with similar areas in micrographs of an unfixed freeze-etched preparation demonstrate the new information available with freeze-etch techniques. In the micrograph of a thin section of freeze-substituted muscle there is little indication of background material connecting collagen fibrils to each other or to the myocardial surface. The micrograph of the freeze-etch preparation, although at a low magnification (Fig. 1–7), suggests the complex nature of this extracellular matrix. A similar comparison at higher magnification reveals the small microfibrils and microthreads (Fig. 1–8). The collagen fibrils run parallel to the long axis of the myocytes, with some collagen fibrils branching laterally to link with the myocyte cell surface and to the opposing surface of the capillary. Collagen bundles can be routinely seen in tissue conventionally prepared for electron microscopy (see Figs. 1–18 and 1–19). Ultrarapidly frozen muscle (74, 75, 347) shows, in addition, the attachments made by 11 nm microfibrils connecting the collagen to the external lamina of the myocyte cell surface (Figs. 1–9 through 1–13). The mat-like arrangement of the external lamina is quite clear. In these preparations, the regularly arranged trabeculae of the external lamina of the myocyte are seen to insert directly into the bilayer (75).

Both light and electron micrographs of cardiac muscles consistently reveal collagen bundles oriented parallel to the myocyte long axis, consistent with the direction of force alignment in the muscles. In electron micrographs of papillary muscles the collagen struts, which appear to orient in a direction transverse to the long axis of the myocytes, are seen less frequently than in the ventricular working cells, where the lines of force may be more complicated, depending on orientation of particular cell layers. Regardless of the method of preparation or the particular muscle, the collagen displays some form of cross-banding of the fibrils, including the major (67 nm) periodicity (75) (Fig. 1–14). Etching unfixed collagen reveals transverse belts of material on the surface of collagen fibrils. In preparations of intact muscle the periodically spaced, raised cuffs of material, that contribute to the characteristic crossbanding, are visible (Fig. 1–8). Microthreads that range in diameter between 3 and 10 nm appear to attach to the transverse cuffs linking the collagen fibrils to each other. In freeze-etch preparations granules are prominent along the collagen fibrils at the junction between the microthreads and the collagen fibrils (Fig. 1–8). These granules have also been noted in stained and conventionally fixed thin sections. The elaborate network of fine threads, regular insertions into the cell surface, interconnections between the collagen fibrils, small groups of the collagen fibrils, and the larger collagen bundles provide a mechanical framework that ensures stability (Figs. 1–15 and 1–16). This extensive network (51) also allows for the flexible redistribution of forces generated within the muscle cells.

The concept of the extracellular matrix now encompasses the entire extracellular compartment. The emerging picture of this complex interactive system is that there are specific molecules released by fibroblasts and blood cells. These molecules find precise receptors with unique geometry at the cell surface and within the plasma membrane itself, both of the cells of the matrix (23) and of the muscle cells. An interactive system where influences occur at multiple levels is formed.

Changes in models of the cell membrane will continue to influence our thinking about the cardiac sarcolemma (144). The fluid mosaic model has characterized the cell membrane for 20 years as a two dimensional oriented solution of integral proteins while keeping the idea of a viscous phospholipid bilayer. These concepts have been revised to include complex diffusion on a nanometer scale, restricted mobility, tethered domains, transport complexes (as in gap junctions and ion exchanges), and membrane proteins propelled by cytoskeletal motors. The sarcolemma can be regarded as a programmable barrier.

In cardiac myocytes, cell adhesion receptors for cadherins and neutral cell adhesion molecules (NCAMs), as well as nutrient and growth factor receptors, are confined to small domains in the membrane, where they are associated with the spectrin meshwork of the cytoskeleton. Connexin43, the major protein of the cardiac gap junction, was one of the first molecules unique to cardiac sarcolemma shown to be in a specific ordered array spanning opposing membranes in the gap junction. Gap junctions have a particular distribution and arrangement relative to the regions of "desmosome-like" attachment and regions of insertion of actin filaments. The distribution of the Na–Ca exchange protein in mammalian cardiac myocytes has been demonstrated in the sarcolemma, and in the T-tubule system in adult guinea pigs and rabbits (76) and in developing rabbit myocardium (34). This protein is the main efflux mechanism for Ca^{2+} in cardiac myocytes. The protein is confined to the sarcolemma in very early development, but it moves into the T-tubules as development progresses. Thus segments of the cardiac sarcolemma are tethered, some remain relatively unchanged once mature, and some move freely, e.g. caveolae. Through cycles of normal turnover, of damage and repair, the relative orientation of membrane segments in relation to one another and to structures within the cell is preserved. The caveolae (shown in Figures 1–17 and 1–22) are a prominent feature of the cardiac sarcolemma that is discussed in detail elsewhere in this *Handbook* (see Chapter 3).

Transverse (T)-Tubules

The other equally important part of the extracellular space is the transverse tubular system (71, 284). The T-tubule system in a single muscle cell is a linked series of elaborate tubular networks that are invaginations of the sarcolemma (see Figs. 1–20 through 1–22). The networks extend transversely through the entire cross-section of the fiber at every Z-region. Some tubules run a straight course from the initial invagination in a given transverse plane up to 5 or 6 µm into the interior of the cell. Others show numerous outpocketings and branch in a longitudinal direction, occasionally connecting with a transversely oriented T-tubule at the Z-band in the next sarcomere along the myofibril axis. Some longitudinal connecting branches of the T-tubule system can bridge several sarcomeres. High-voltage studies of both cardiac and skeletal muscle reveal a long-range ordering of transverse tubules as a spiraling arrangement over distances of 10–15 sarcomeres. An outstanding feature of T-tubules in cardiac muscle is their large diameter compared to T-tubules of skeletal muscle (Figs. 1–18 through 1–22). Furthermore, the high degree of variation in the transverse tubular lumen diameter suggests a passive deformation or even a pulsatile wave extending along the tubule (Figs. 1–20 through 1–22). Typically the longitudinal branches of the transverse tubules have relatively small and rather uniform diameters, as opposed to the configurations of the transverse tubules at the Z-bands. Bristle-coated vesicles are immediately adjacent or still partially attached to transversely oriented T-tubules (Fig. 1–22). In cardiac muscle as in skeletal muscle, the T-system is formed by the sequential fusion of plasmalemmal caveolae. The elaborate transverse tubular network of mammalian hearts is typical of that of cardiac cells larger than 8 µm in diameter. The large diameter of the T-tubules in cardiac muscle indicates a large capacity of these structures, consistent with the significant amount of calcium that must move from the extracellular space to the interior of the cell with each and every beat. The variation in diameter and the movement of the transverse T-tubule components relative to the longitudinal components are consistent with the strong mechanical forces applied to the cell. The forces are transmitted in part by the ordered array of collagen fibrils that connect to the myocyte at the Z-band regions where the T-system invaginations occur. It is likely that coordinated movement of the T-tubules facilitates transport and transfer along and across the tubule walls.

INTERIOR SUPPORTING NETWORKS

Just as the myocardium has individual myocardial cells embedded in an elaborate meshwork of elastin and collagen fibrils and various protein substrates, so the cardiac myocyte itself has an interior supporting framework. The concept of a cytoskeleton in muscle cells is fairly new, but it becomes important (178, 281) as we seek to understand cardiac disease (273), the regulation of myofibril size (influenced by hypertrophy and atrophy), the development of muscle (influenced by genetic defects and congenital abnormalities), and the transmission of mechanical force over macroscopic distances. Targeted protein synthesis requires components of the cytoskeleton (127). In all eukaryotic cells the major components of the cytoskeleton are microtubules, intermediate filaments, and bundles of actin microfilaments (163). In striated muscle cells, the actin filaments contain a muscle type actin, co-polymerized with tropomyosin and other proteins to form a specialized contractile thin filament. The F-actin–containing thin filament array is arranged in the sarcomere and supported by a network of titin filaments that span the entire sarcomeric half-width. The non-muscle-type actin found early in development is believed to persist in some measure at the intercalated disks and just beneath the sarcolemma.

Microtubules

Light microscope images of muscle stained for tubulin, the protein building block of microtubules, show predominant localization in the longitudinal direction, between the myofilament bundles (247). Electron microscopy shows a complex array of microtubules with profiles curving along the surface of the myofilament bundles (see Fig. 1–4; 98). Microtubules oriented in a longitudinal direction form a loose cage around the myocardial cell nucleus at the center of the cell (Figs. 1–23 through 1–26). The microtubules are found in close association with both mitochondria and profiles of the sarcoplasmic reticulum in the narrow space between the edge of the myofilament bundle and the surface of the adjacent mitochondria (Figs. 1–27 through 1–30). These microtubules, although consistently present in large enough numbers to be of importance, are difficult to observe in low-magnification images of longitudinal sections of cardiac muscle. Since the microtubules course through a very narrow plane in longitudinal orientation, they are most often seen as round profiles in cross sections (Figs. 1–28 and 1–29).

Microtubules are more predominant when the cardiac cell is in the process of development (30, 247) or during hypertrophy when new myofibrils are being laid down. The microtubules are believed to play a role in orienting the new myofilament bundles to conform to the proper architecture of the muscle cell. Profiles of microtubules that bend in and out of the plane of the surface of the myofibril and microtubule profiles that course for considerable distances closely parallel to profiles of the sarcoplasmic reticulum suggest some long-range ordering. This ordering may have a role in transport as well as serving as a flexible strut for the interior of the cell.

Intermediate Filament Network

Two noncontractile filamentous systems in muscle have been identified: the intermediate filament lattice, called an *exosarcomeric* lattice, and the titin-nebulin lattice, which has been called an *endosarcomeric* lattice (328). Both of these lattices are linked to the Z-band lattices of the myofibrillar contractile apparatus (Fig. 1–31).

The 10 nm diameter intermediate filaments are composed of proteins that are specific to the muscle type (cardiac, smooth, or skeletal). These muscle-specific proteins belong to a larger family of filamentous proteins expressed in higher eukaryotic cells (244). The intermediate filament (exosarcomeric) lattice in cardiac muscle is linked to the cell membrane and forms a network throughout the cytoplasm (Figs. 1–32 through 1–35). The distribution of intermediate filaments has been studied in the Purkinje cells of the heart and in skeletal muscle (reviewed in refs. 242 and 300). The conducting cells of the Purkinje system were seen to contain particularly large numbers of intermediate filaments (300). The intermediate filament array between organelles and membranes was first described in contractile cardiac cells by Ferrans and Roberts (66), who showed that intermediate filaments are attached to nuclear pores and to the cardiac muscle cell nucleus. More recently it has been shown in other cell types that the nuclear matrix contains intermediate filament-type protein filaments. Therefore, it is thought that the intermediate filaments may continue through the nuclear pores, possibly by anchorage to lamina B. The intermediate filaments thus not only provide a three-dimensional supporting network from cell surface to nuclear membrane but they also link organelles.

During development and elongation of the assembling myofibrils along the longitudinal axis of the cell about 60% of the intermediate filaments become oriented parallel to the myofibrils, reflecting the similarly developing longitudinal distribution of the microtubules. The intermediate filaments that become associated with developing myofibrils are at this time composed of alternating domains of polymeric desmin and vimentin, as demonstrated by Tokuyasu and colleagues (306). Vimentin is eventually completely replaced, yielding the structure of desmin homopolymers that prevails in mature cardiac and skeletal muscle. There is some species variation, but by and large intermediate filaments in mature human striated muscle are primarily composed of desmin. Desmin comprises 2% of the total protein of cardiac muscle but only 0.35% of that of skeletal muscle.

The intermediate filaments form a three-dimensional network of longitudinal and transverse elements encircling and linking the peripheral regions of Z-bands of individual myofibrils, and also connect to adjacent myofibrils (Figs. 1–31 through 1–35). Both transverse and longitudinal elements of this network are anchored at the Z-band periphery. Intermediate filaments are subjacent to the large T-tubules at the level of the Z band in the space where the terminal sacs of the sarcoplasmic reticulum are not closely apposed to the T-system.

Since the cardiac intermediate filament network is so linked with other cellular structures, it is surprising that transgenic mice lacking desmin are viable (164, 205). It is possible that one of the other intermediate filament proteins such as vimentin, nestin, or synemin may substitute in vivo for desmin during prenatal development. However, muscles from desmin-negative mice show progressively greater structural abnormalities with age. The ultrastructural abnormalities include increasing myofibrillar misregistration, disrupted myofibrils near the intercalated disk, detachment from the sarcolemma, and swollen and disintegrating mitochondria. These abnormalities are most severe in the heart, suggesting that the continual cardiac work load exacerbates the damage (205).

Anti-desmin antibodies have been localized at a discrete distance from the electron-dense Z-band. Spectrin and anchorin are co-distributed with desmin, both at the Z-bands and in faint longitudinal arrays, suggesting that these proteins are associated with elements of the intermediate filament network. Spectrin and anchorin may therefore serve to bind the intermediate filaments to the periphery of the Z-bands.

The transversely oriented intermediate filaments that surround and link the adjacent Z-bands are seen more readily than the longitudinally oriented filaments because they are more densely packed in a regularly repeating fashion. They are easily demonstrated in electron micrographs of both longitudinal sections and cross sections of cardiac muscle. Numerous conventional electron microscopic studies of both cross sections and longitudinal sections reveal small bundles of 3–20 transverse intermediate filaments circling Z-bands and linking adjacent myofibrils at the Z-band level. Correlative immunofluorescence and immunoelectron microscopy have also demonstrated the transverse Z-to-Z intermediate filaments in chicken muscle. Thus, the exosarcomeric lattice in cardiac muscle is important for the lateral registration of myofibrils across the diameter of myocytes. Transverse intermediate filaments are attached to densities on the T-tubules in vertebrate cardiac muscle and link some myofibrils to mitochondria (305).

Sarcolemmal Associations

Cytoskeletal–sarcolemmal associations function to transfer general messages back and forth between the contractile apparatus and the extracellular environment.

The costamere is the site at which the Z-bands of the outermost myofibrils in the muscle cell contact the sarcolemma. Costameres are also the sites of lateral cytoskeletal to extracellular matrix attachment (230), and are likely to play an important mechanical role. Skelemin, a cytoskeletal protein at the M-disk, binds to myosin and to desmin (243). Integrins, a superfamily of heterodimeric cell surface glycoproteins, are likely candidates to mediate the myofibrillar–sarcolemmal association in the heart, because they participate in this type of linkage in other cell types, for example, in

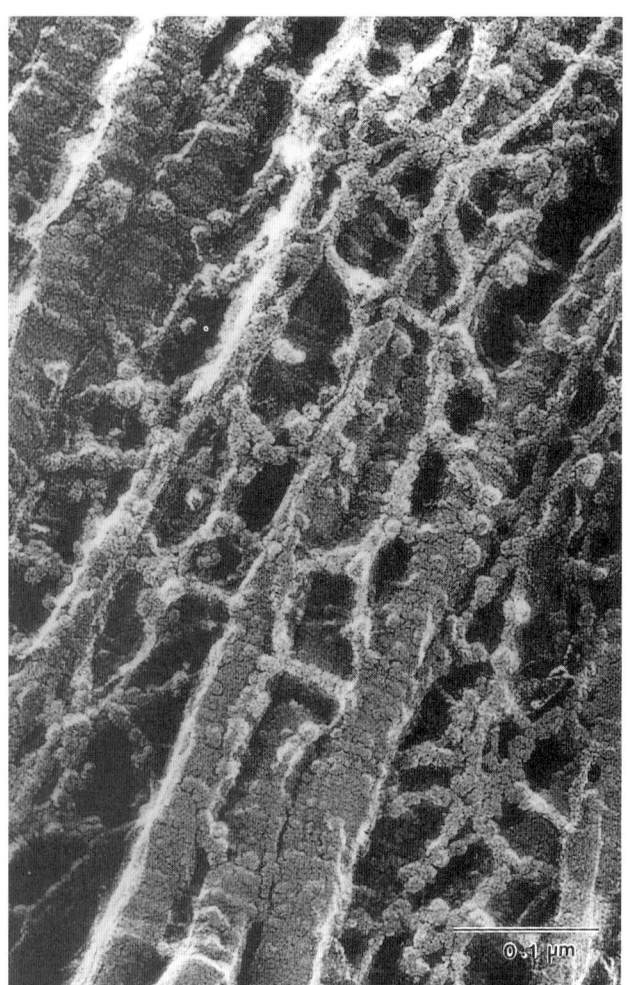

FIG. 1–15. High-magnification freeze-etch micrograph depicting collagen fibrils from adult rat heart. Compare to neonatal material shown in Figure 1–16 (75). (Reprinted by permission of S. Karger.)

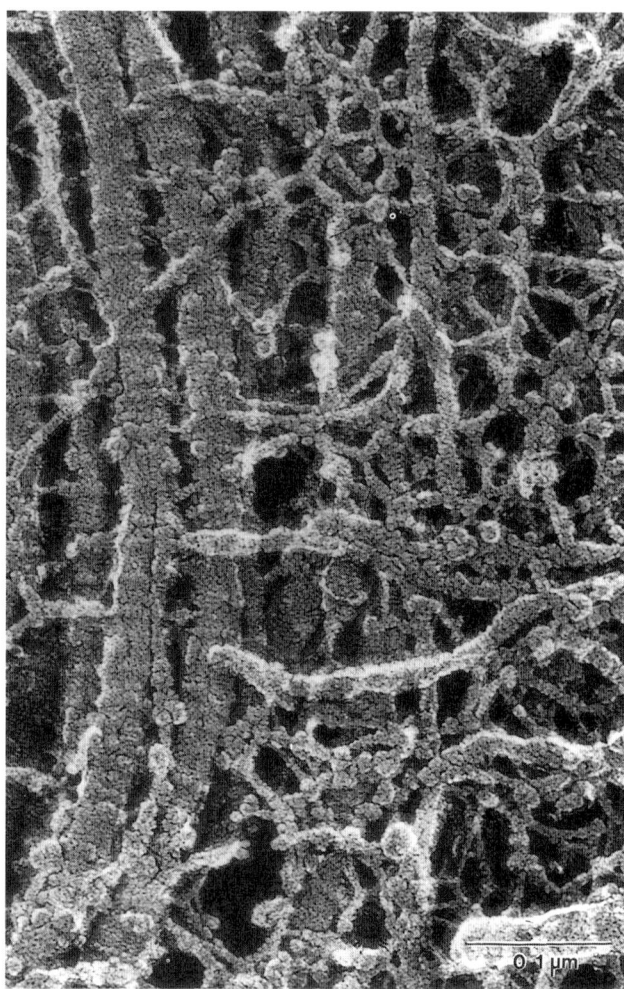

FIG. 1–16. High-magnification freeze-etch micrograph depicting collagen fibrils from 4 day-old neonatal rat heart. The collagen fibrils and the extensive connections linking them, microthreads, microfibrils, and granules, appear similar to that in the adult shown in Figure 1–15 (75). (Reprinted by permission of S. Karger.)

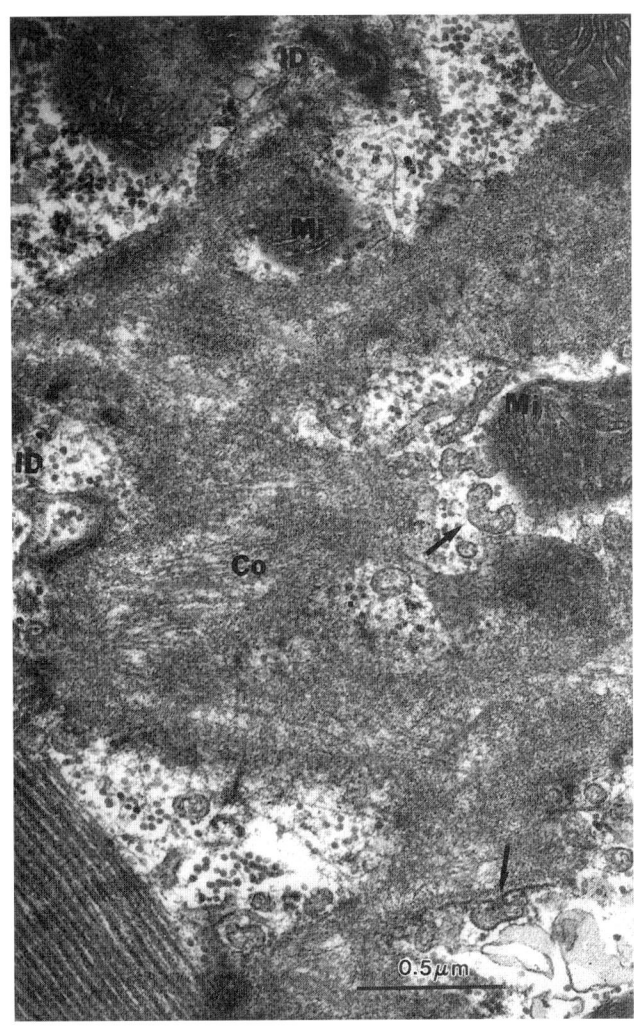

FIG. 1–17. Grazing profiles of cell membrane (intercalated disk = ID, calveolae = *arrows*) of dog papillary muscle showing relation of extracellular components (collagen = Co) to intracellular features (mitochondria = Mi) at the cell surface.

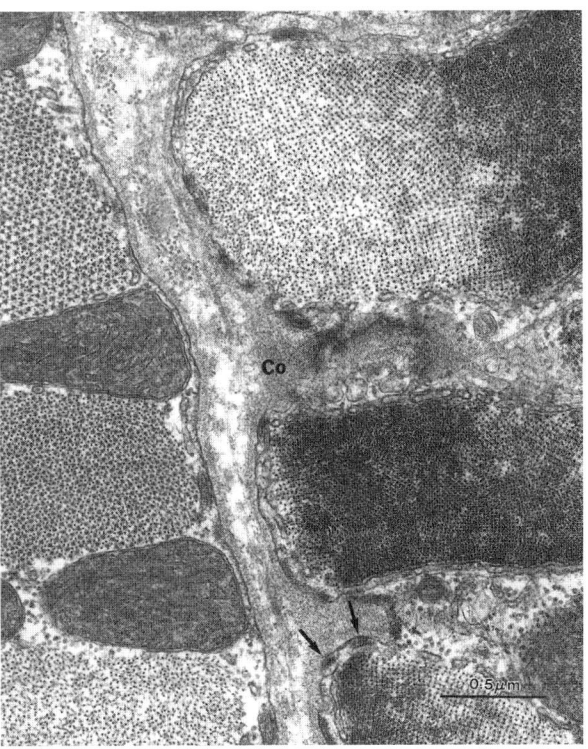

FIG. 1–18. Cross section of dog papillary muscle showing cross-cut collagen (Co) within extracellular matrix. Appearance of clear spaces is due to extraction during chemical fixation and an artifact of preparation. Note tufts of dense material just beneath the sarcolemma in cell at level of Z-bands (*arrows*).

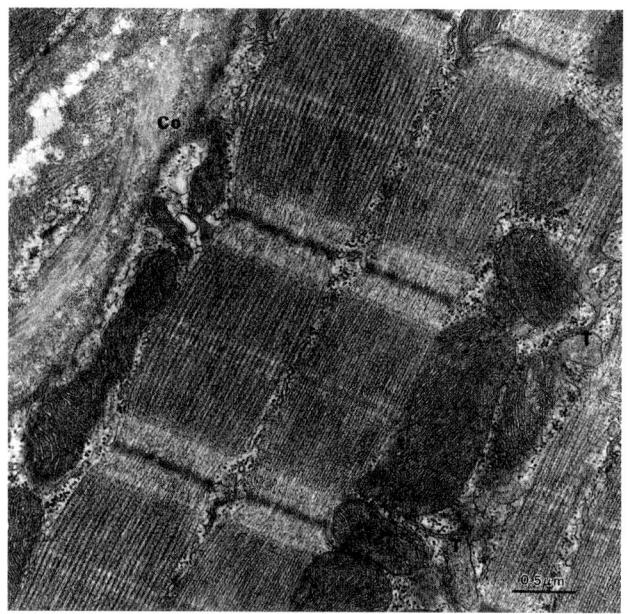

FIG. 1–19. Longitudinal section of dog papillary muscle showing cross-cut profiles of T-tubules (T) with lumen contents the same density as the extracellular matrix (collagen = Co) at the cell surface.

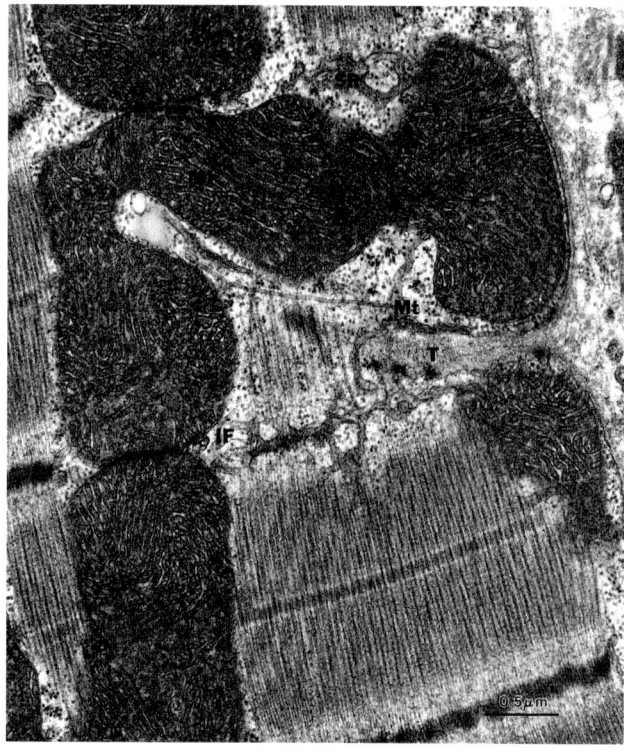

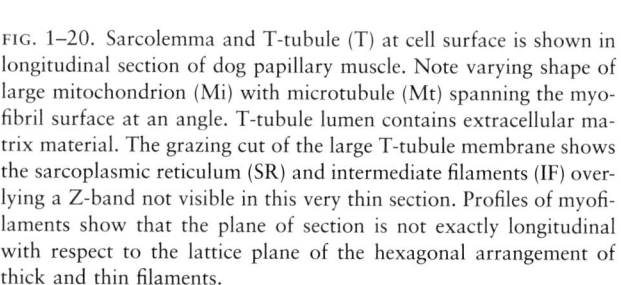

FIG. 1–20. Sarcolemma and T-tubule (T) at cell surface is shown in longitudinal section of dog papillary muscle. Note varying shape of large mitochondrion (Mi) with microtubule (Mt) spanning the myofibril surface at an angle. T-tubule lumen contains extracellular matrix material. The grazing cut of the large T-tubule membrane shows the sarcoplasmic reticulum (SR) and intermediate filaments (IF) overlying a Z-band not visible in this very thin section. Profiles of myofilaments show that the plane of section is not exactly longitudinal with respect to the lattice plane of the hexagonal arrangement of thick and thin filaments.

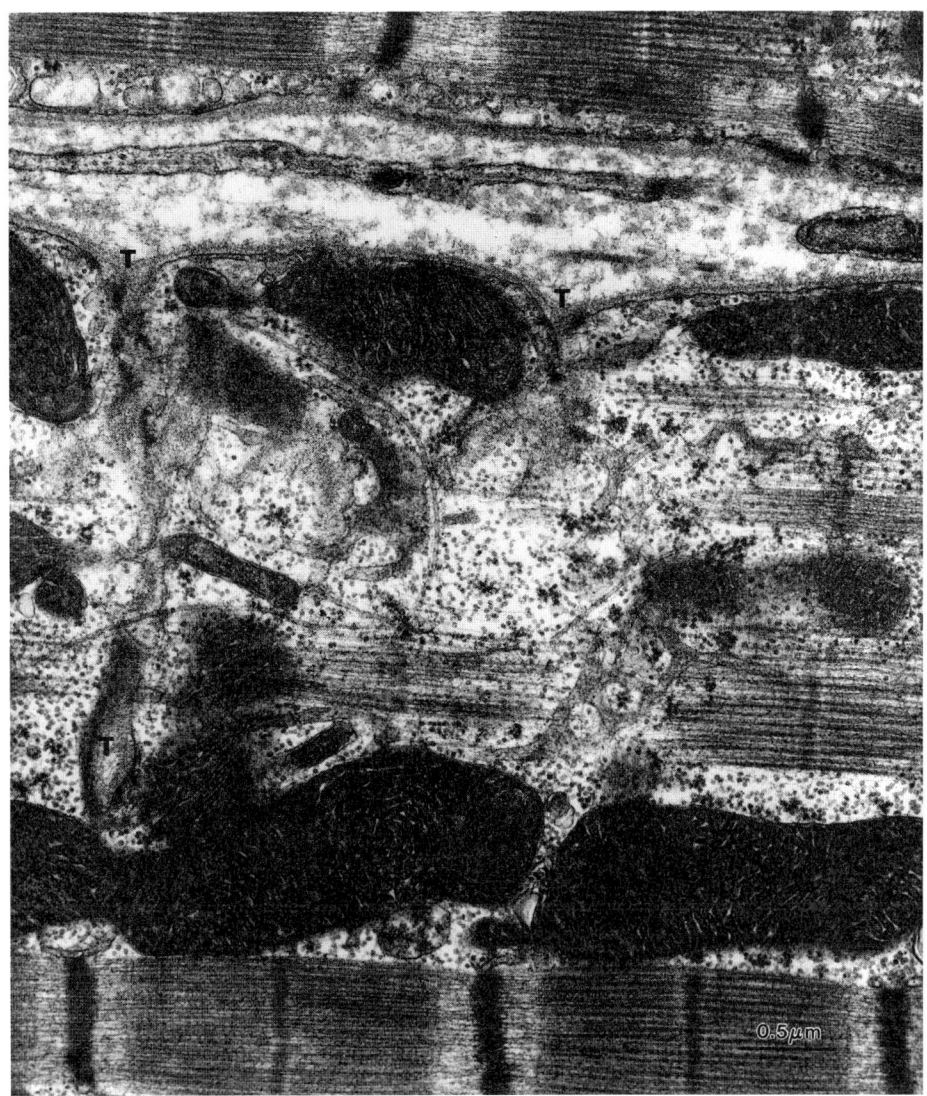

FIG. 1–21. A longitudinal section at same magnification as in Figure 1–20 shows fibroblast enmeshed in extracellular matrix. Indentations of the sarcolemma of this muscle cell indicate T-tubules (T), but the section plane is not through the middle of the tubule to show the full extent of the lumen.

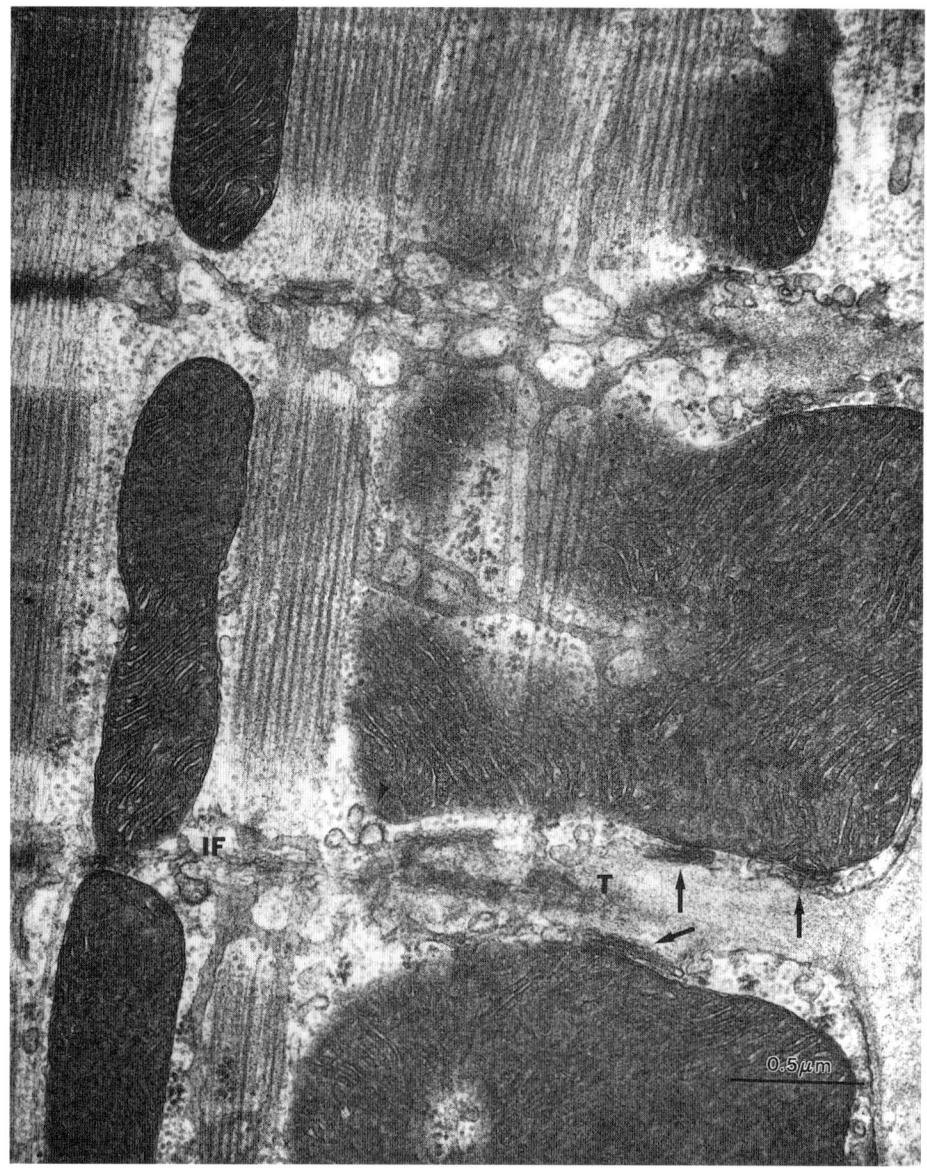

FIG. 1–22. A longitudinal section of dog papillary muscle at higher magnification than Figures 1–20 and 1–21 partly through the middle of the T-tubule (T) shows invagination of the sarcolemma, the extracellular matrix material, the diads and triads (*arrows*) formed with adjacent sarcoplasmic reticulum (SR), the outpocketing of the T-tubule membrane, a bristle-coated vesicle emerging (*arrowhead*) and the subjacent SR and intermediate filaments (IF). Note the good alignment with the Z-bands in the adjacent myofilament bundle and how the mitochondria conform to the space between adjacent T-tubules.

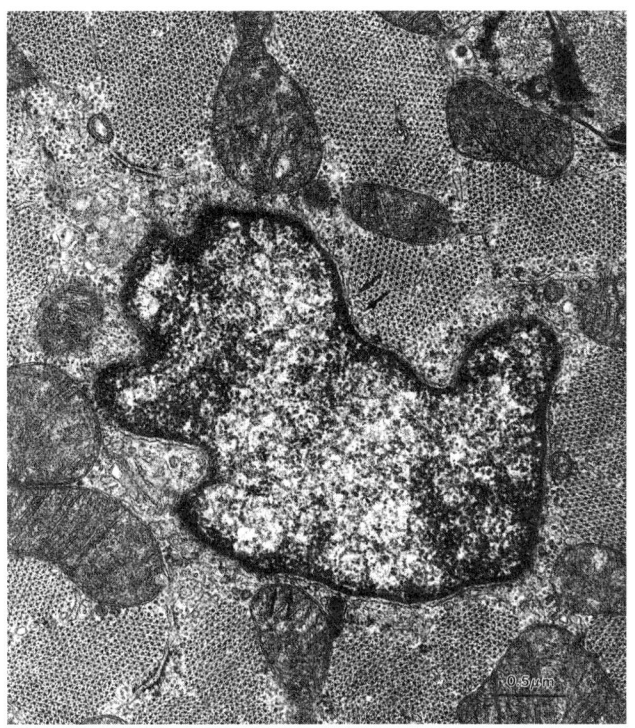

FIG. 1–23. Cross section of guinea pig papillary muscle showing cross-cut microtubules (*arrows*) distributed around the surface of the nucleus as well as between myofilament bundles.

FIG. 1–24. Longitudinal section of guinea pig papillary muscle showing longitudinal profiles of microtubules (*arrows*) near the nucleus.

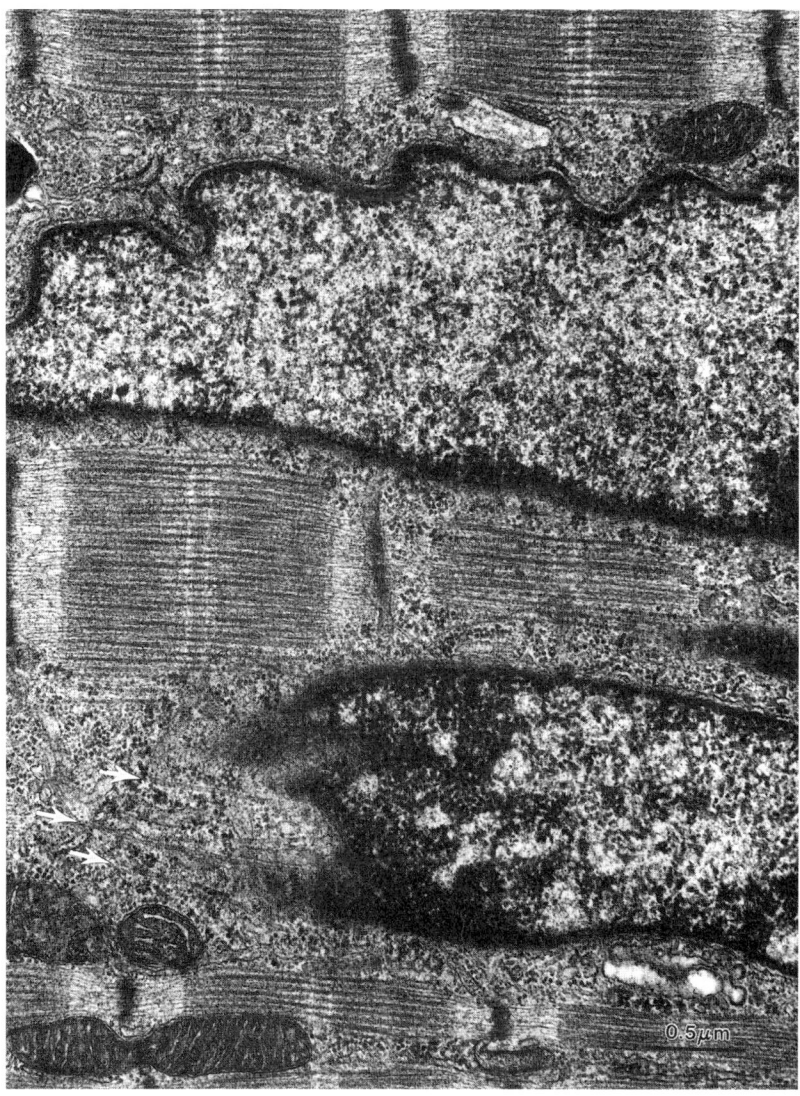

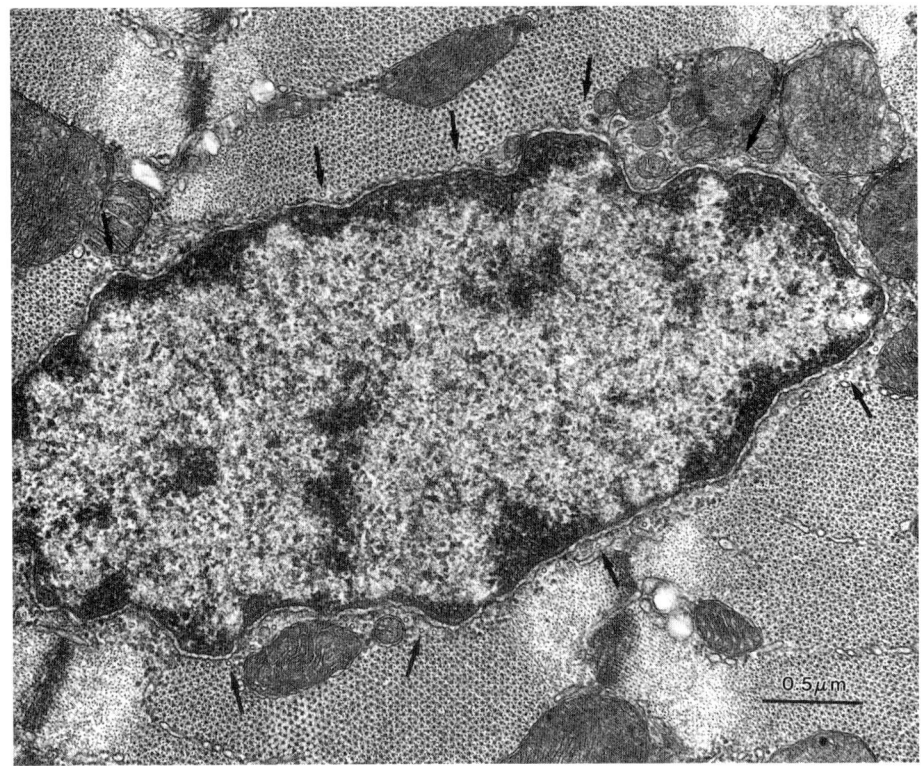

FIG. 1–25. Cross section of rat papillary muscle showing microtubules around the nucleus (*arrows*). This muscle has been stretched in a relaxing solution. Note how many microtubules (27) can be seen when they are aligned perpendicular to the plane of section.

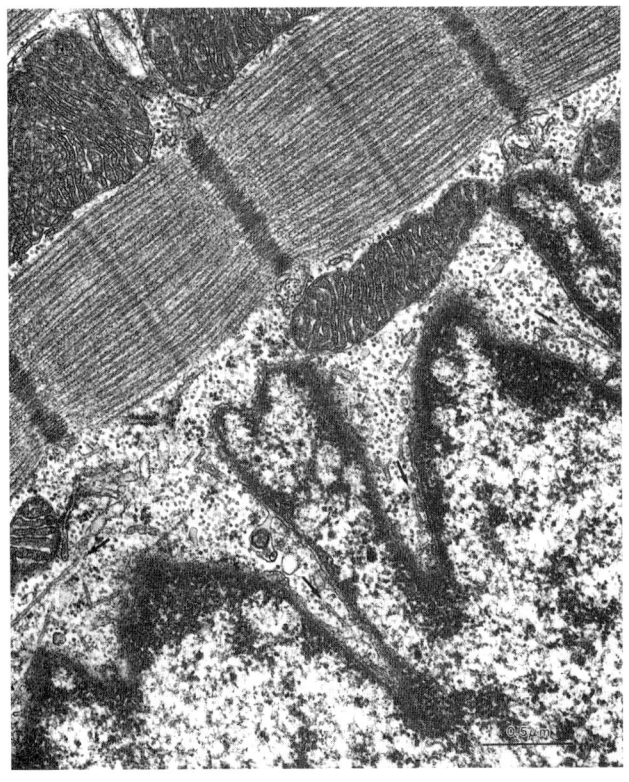

FIG. 1–26. Longitudinal section of contracted dog papillary muscle showing longitudinal profiles of microtubules (*arrows*) coming in and out of the plane of section near convoluted nucleus (98). (Reprinted by permission of Rockefeller University Press.)

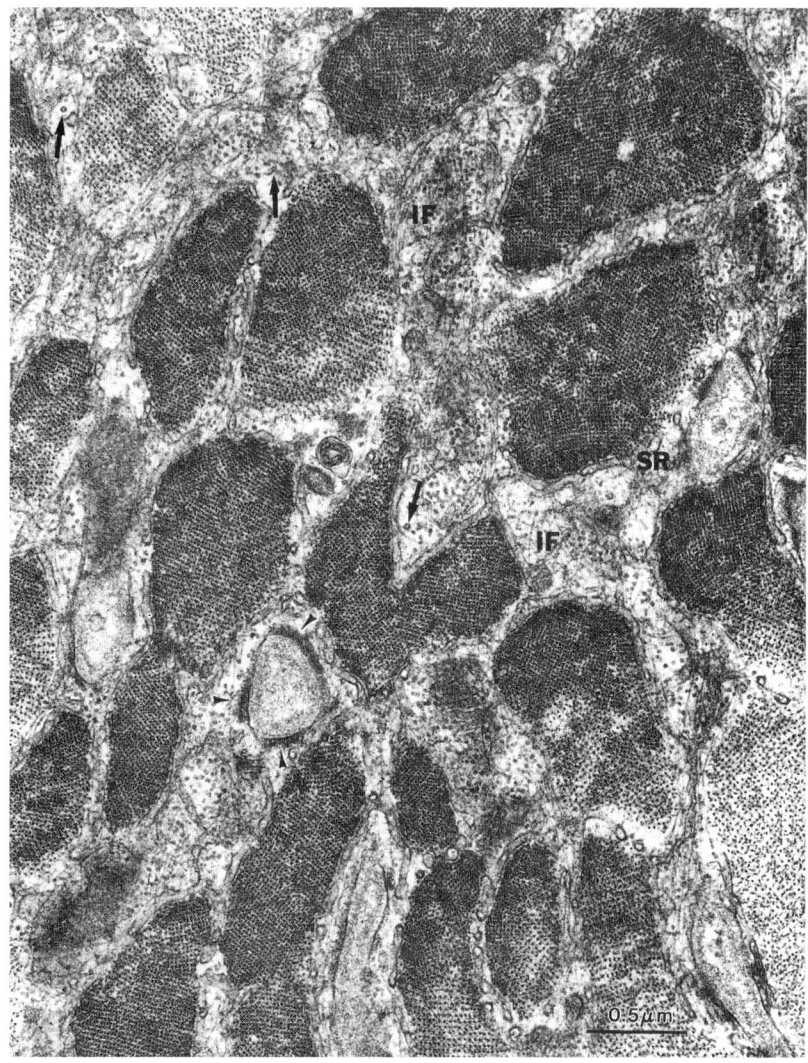

FIG. 1–27. Cross section of dog papillary muscle at level of Z-band showing cross-sectional profiles of microtubules (*arrows*), longitudinal profiles of intermediate filaments (IF), sarcoplasmic reticulum (SR) adhering to myofilament bundles with specialized regions of SR forming a complex with the T-tubule (*arrowheads*), and glycogen.

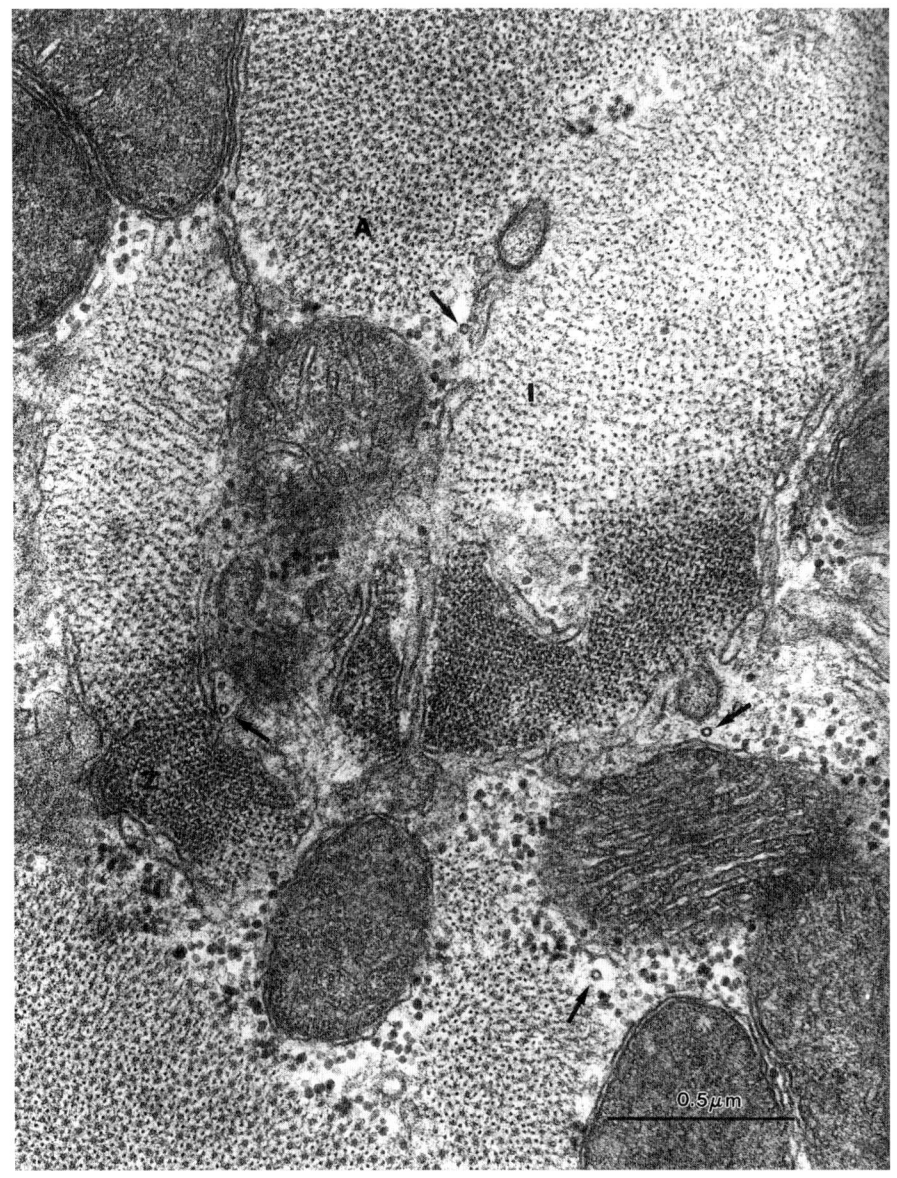

FIG. 1–28. Cross-sectional profiles of microtubules (*arrows*) in rat papillary muscle at higher magnification showing their location next to mitochondria (Mi) and just outside the profiles of the Sarcoplasmic reticulum at the level of the Z-bands and at the A–I junction.

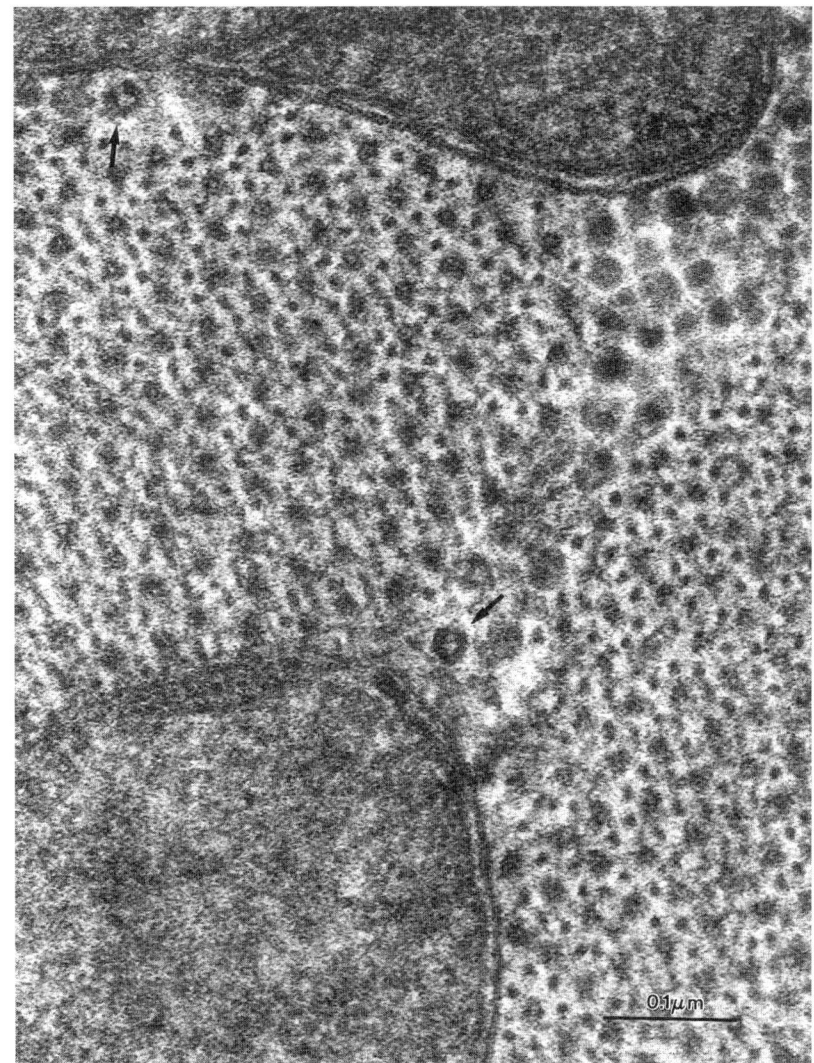

FIG. 1–29. Cross section of dog papillary myofilament bundles at the level of the A-band showing microtubule profiles (*arrows*) near mitochondria. The microtubules and membranes of the mitochondria are enhanced by treatment of muscle with 8% tannic acid before post-fixation with osmium tetroxide.

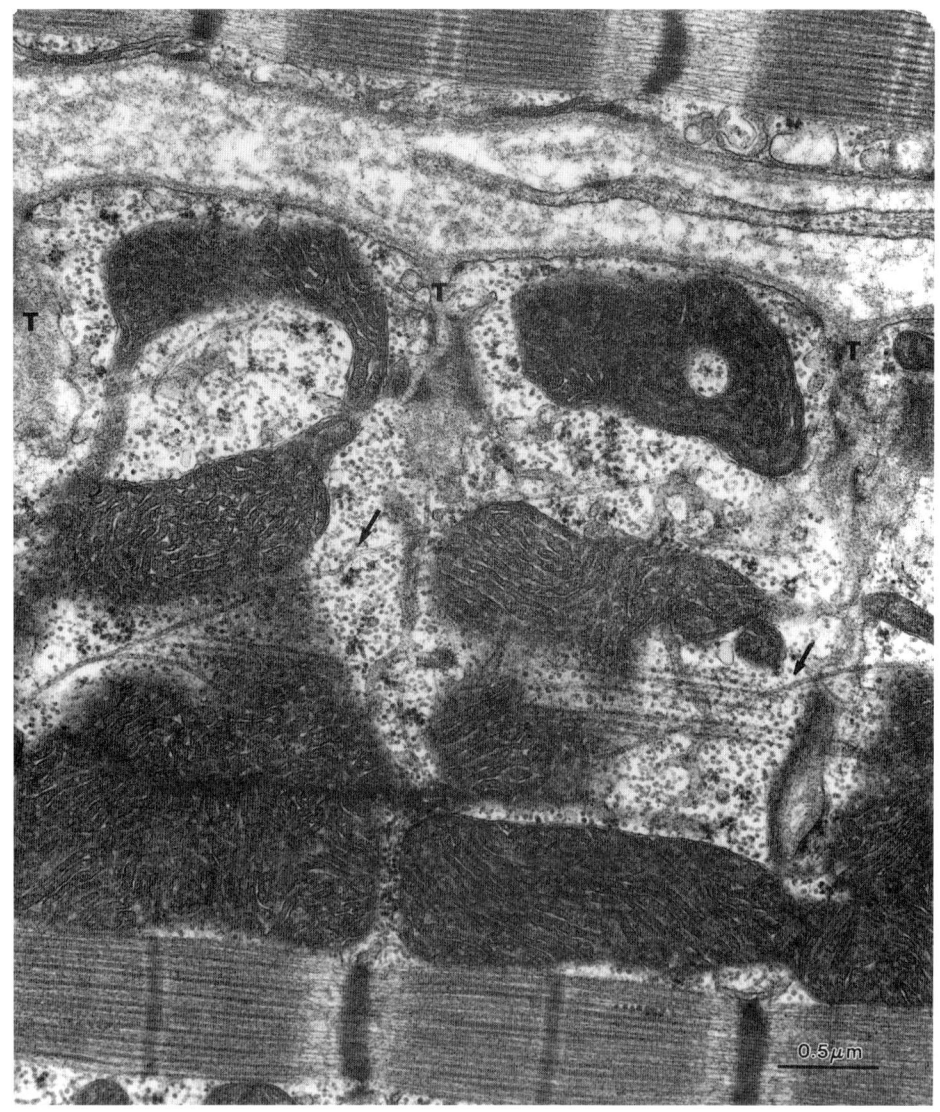

FIG. 1–30. Longitudinal section of dog papillary muscle showing microtubules (*arrows*) at cell surface. Three T-tubule profiles are evident (T). Microtubules arch across the surface of the myofilament bundles. Note also varying shapes of mitochondrial profiles. Portion of fibroblast is visible between two cells.

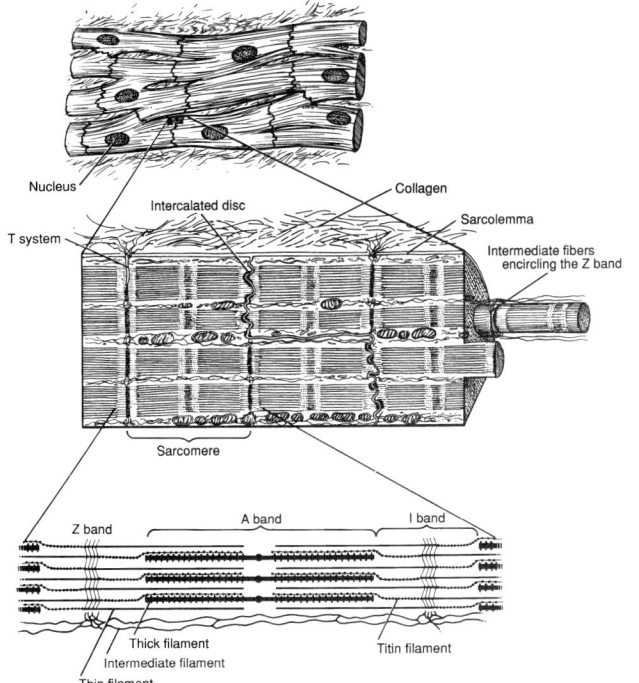

FIG. 1–31. Structure of myocardial cells at the level of light and electron microscopy is portrayed. *Top*: A portion of ventricular myocardium with branching muscle cells enmeshed in collagen. Nuclei are centrally placed and intercalated disks contain sites for end-to-end attachment of cells. *Middle*: Ultrastructure of portions of two cells in a cutaway view displaying the arrangement of myofibrils. A network of intermediate filaments, which surrounds the myofibrils like a cage, is periodically anchored to cell membrane plaques at the Z-bands and at transverse regions of the intercalated disks. Bottom: Within the sarcomeres, the contractile units of the muscle delimited at each end by a Z-band consist of three sets of filaments. Thick filaments containing primarily myosin are located in the A-band; thin filaments containing actin, tropomyosin, and troponin, and thin elastic filaments of titin extend from each Z-band toward the middle of the sarcomere. The thick and thin filaments interdigitate regularly to form a hexagonal array seen in cross section. The titin filaments attach periodically along the thick filament. The Z-band is a lattice of axial and cross-connecting Z-filaments. In the Z-band, the ends of the thin filaments from adjacent sarcomeres overlap and interdigitate in a centered tetragonal array and are held together periodically by cross-connecting Z-filaments (104). (Reprinted by permission of the American Physiological Society.)

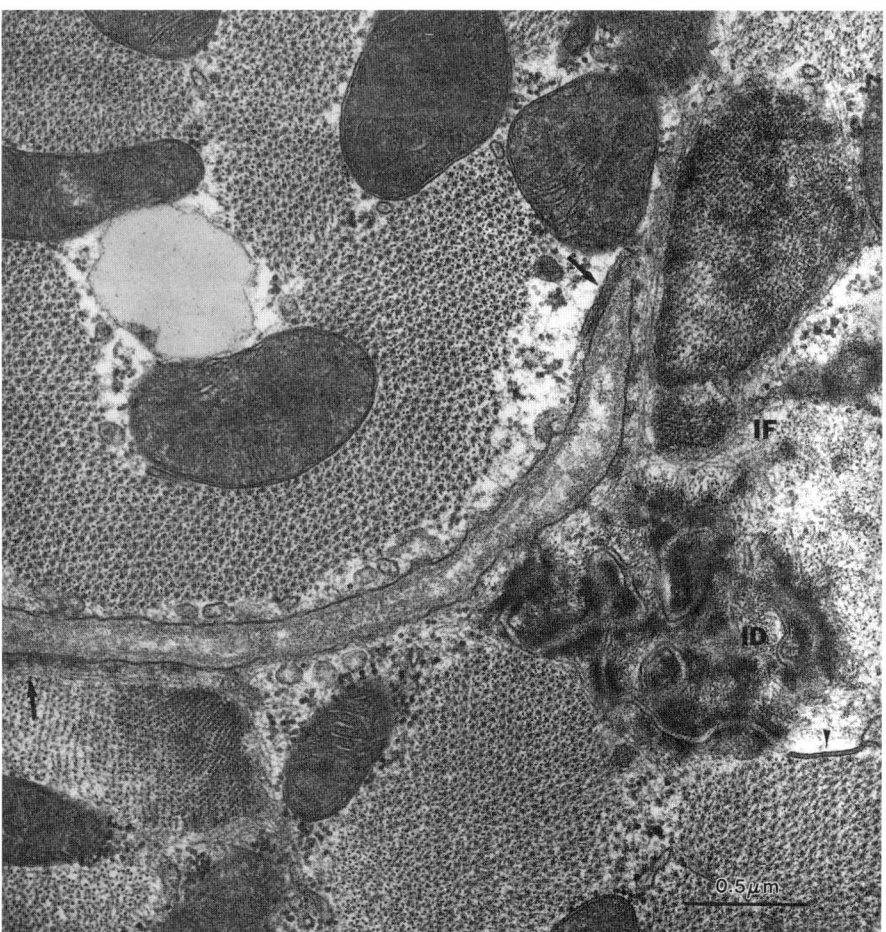

FIG. 1–32. Cross section of cat papillary muscle showing longitudinal profile of intermediate filaments (IF) near Z-bands and intercalated disk (ID). Long profile of T-tubule with portions of two diads (one at each end, *arrows*) near the intercalated disk (see diagram in Figure 1–4 for orientation). Note gap junction at lower right (*arrowhead*).

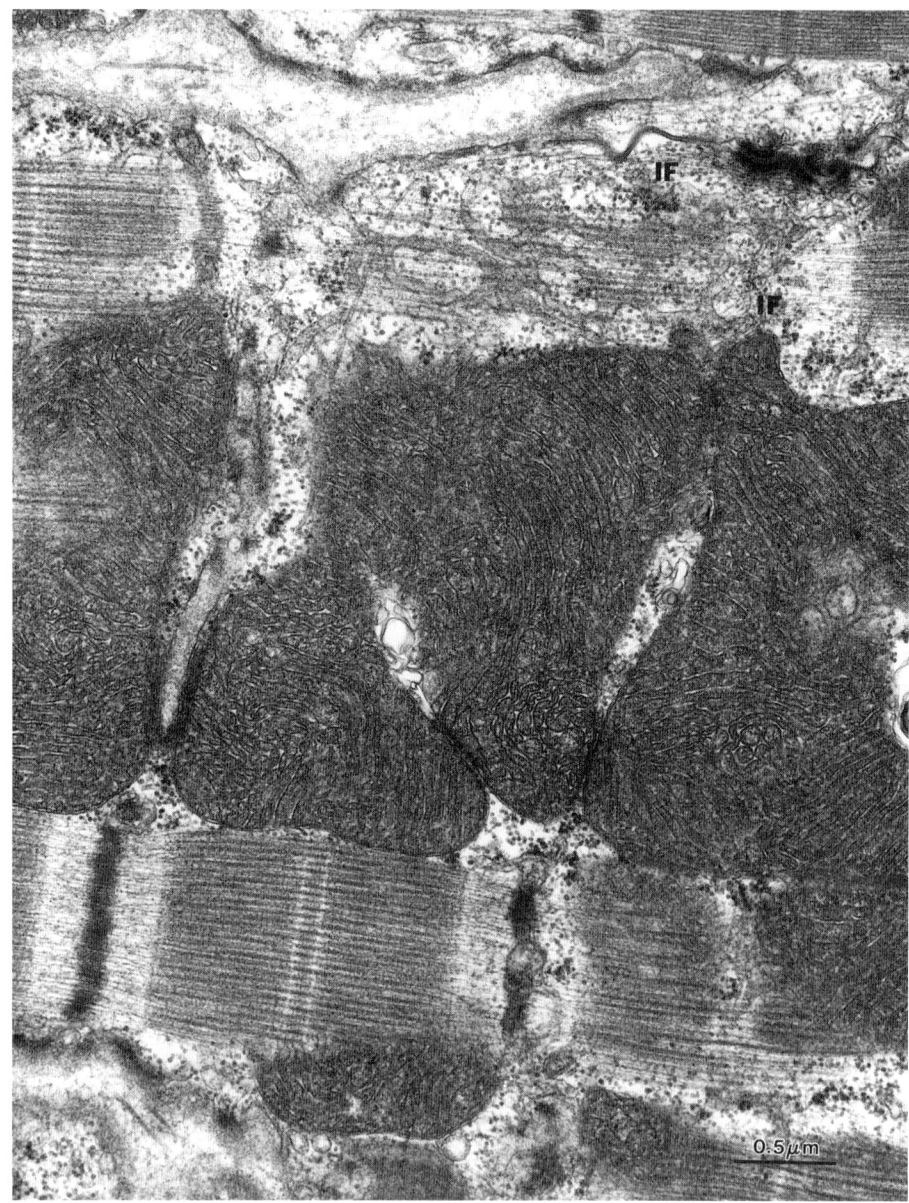

FIG. 1–33. Longitudinal section of dog papillary muscle showing intermediate filament bundles (IF) near cell surface at desmosome-like regions extending across the surface of the myofilaments at the Z band level and intermediate filament bundles at three other Z-bands.

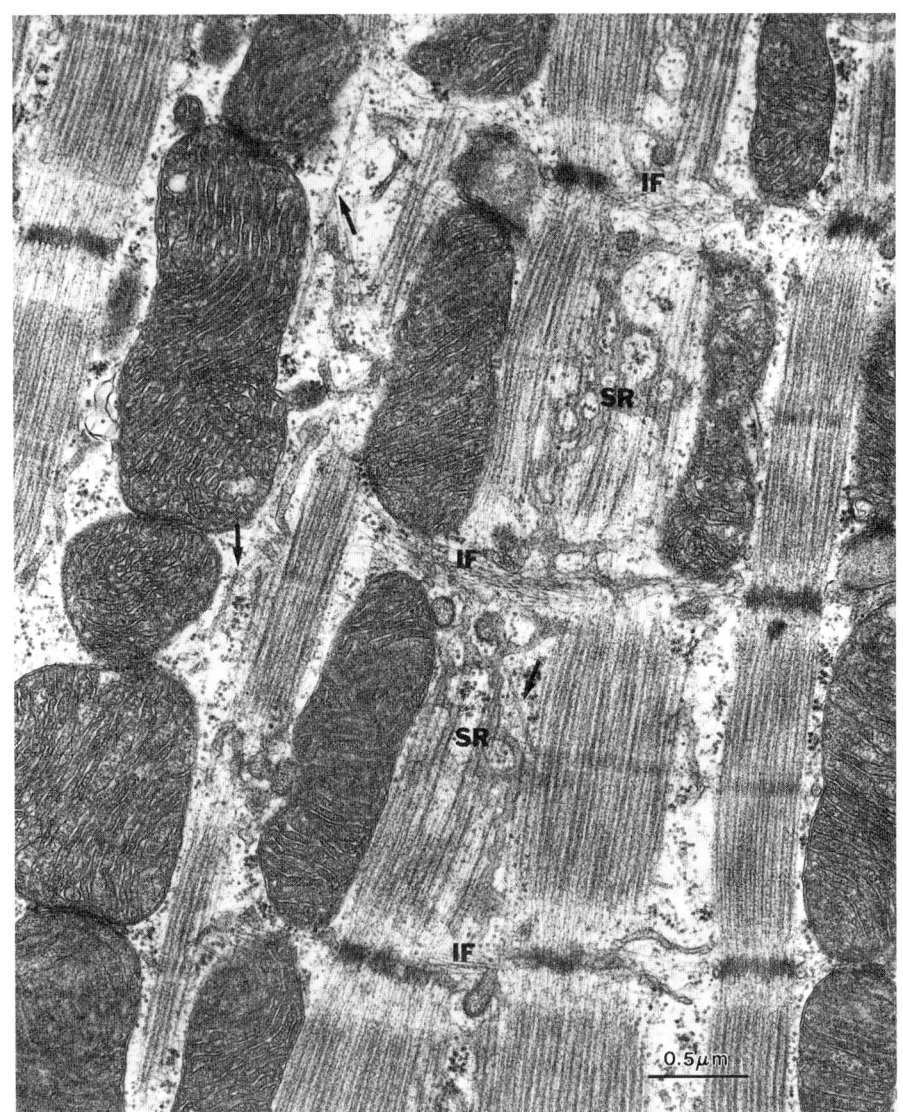

FIG. 1–34. Longitudinal section of dog papillary muscle showing intermediate filament bundles (IF) at three different Z-band levels spanning several myofilament bundles. Note profiles of sarcoplasmic reticulum (SR) and microtubules (*arrows*).

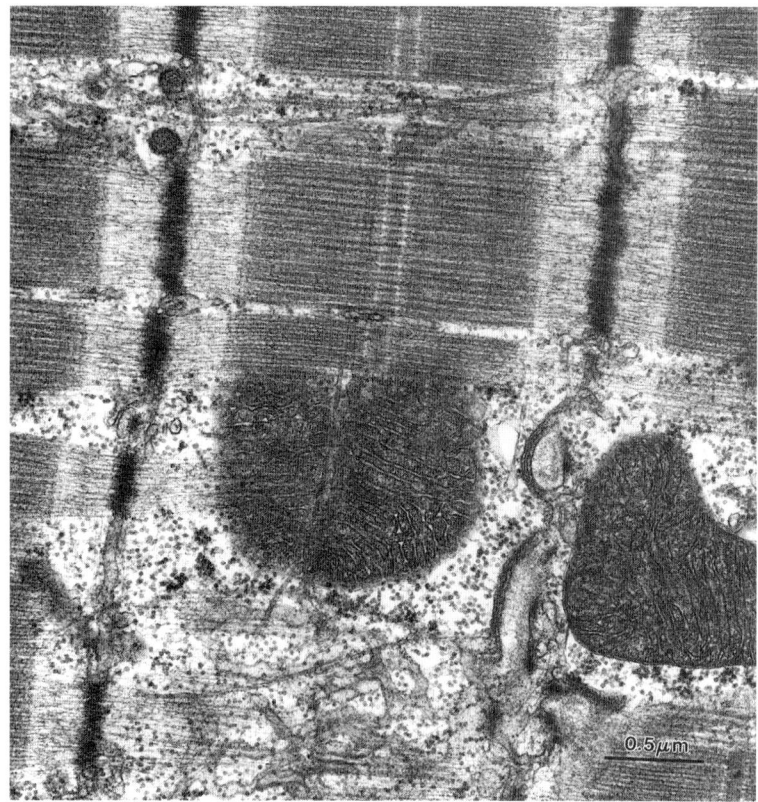

FIG. 1-35. Longitudinal section of dog papillary muscle showing intermediate filaments and microtubules.

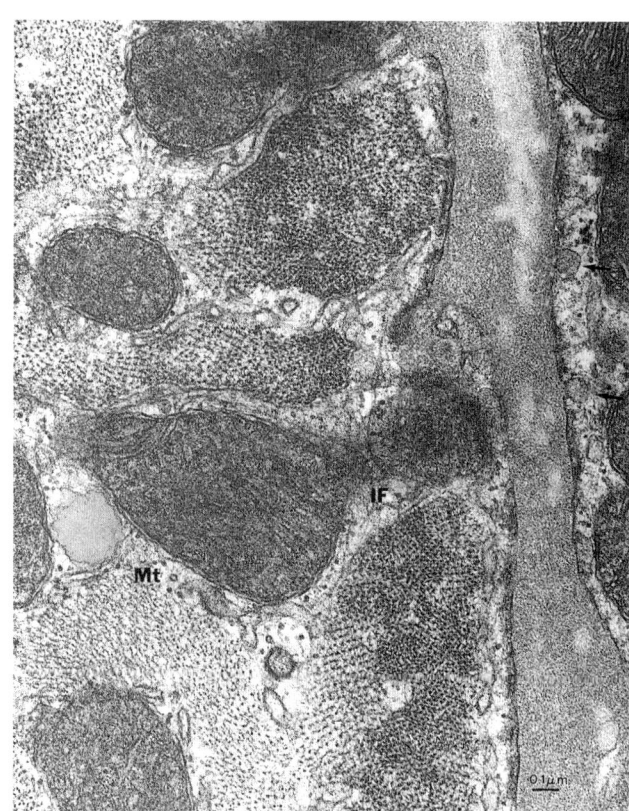

FIG. 1-36. Cross section of rat papillary muscle showing mitochondria and myofilament bundles, the two most prominent features of the cardiac sarcomere, together with two cytoskeletal components—cross-cut profiles of microtubules (Mt) and longitudinal profiles of intermediate filaments (IF). Note caveolae of sarcolemma of adjacent cell (*arrows*).

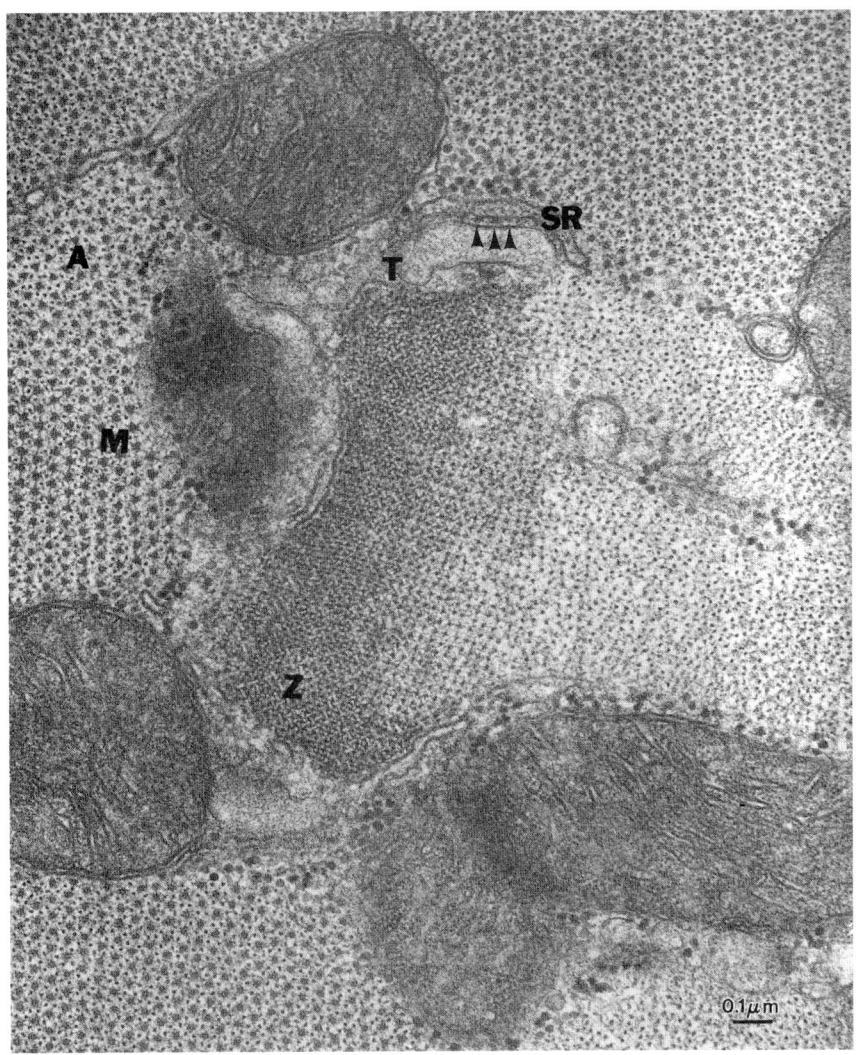

FIG. 1–37. Cross section of rat papillary muscle in interior of cell showing hexagonal arrangement of thick and thin contractile filaments in M-band and A-band. A T-tubule profile (T) at the level of the Z-band shows the region of contact with the sarcoplasmic reticulum specialized for excitation–contraction coupling and the "feet" structures (*arrowheads*).

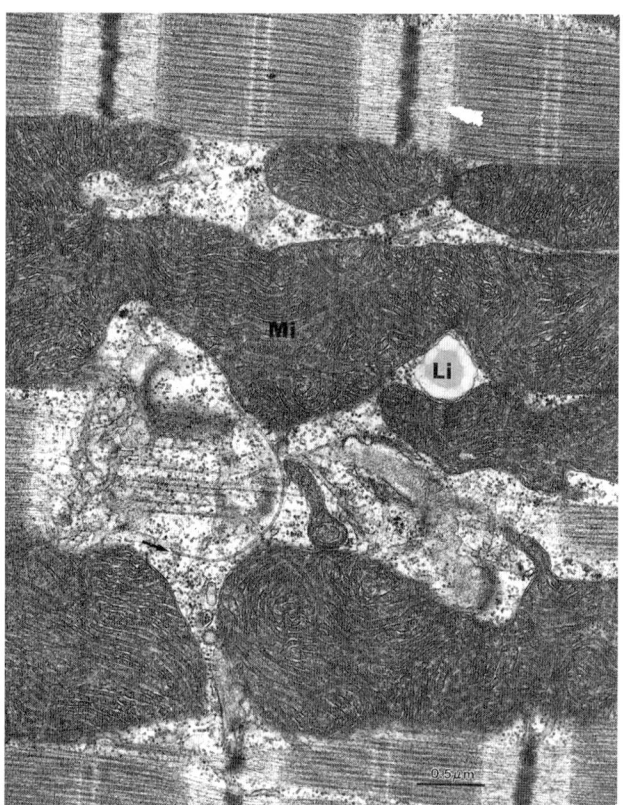

FIG. 1–38. Longitudinal section of dog papillary muscle showing long mitochondrial profile (Mi) spanning three sarcomeres. Note bowing profile of microtubule (*arrow*) aligning with surfaces of three different mitochondrial profiles and the partially extracted lipid droplet (Li) between two mitochondrial profiles.

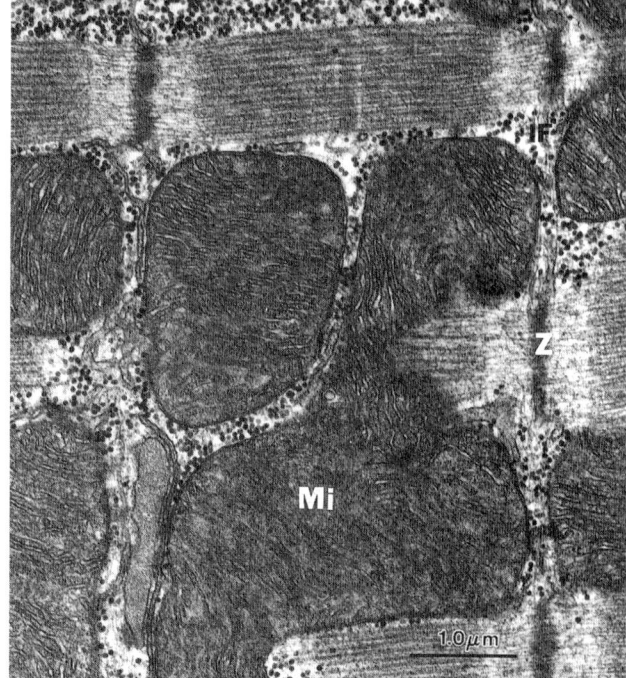

FIG. 1–39. Longitudinal section of dog papillary muscle showing relationship between varying shapes of mitochondrial profiles (Mi) and the intermediate filament (IF) bundles that maintain registration between adjacent Z-bands perpendicular to the myofibril axis. Note that the myofilament bundles are not aligned exactly in the longitudinal plane of section.

fibroblasts. The fibroblast focal adhesion, where the actin stress fibers terminate at the cell surface, is connected through integrin with the extracellular matrix. Additionally, the β1-subunit of integrin is found in all major myofibril–sarcolemmal junction areas in vertebrate skeletal muscle, including the costamere, the myotendinous junction, and the sarcolemma. Thus the costameres and the myotendinous junction in vertebrate skeletal muscles represent the primary interactive sites between the myofibrils and the cell membrane. The skeletal myotendinous junction is the functional analogue of the cardiac intermediate junction, where the actin filaments insert into the specialized regions of the intercalated disks. Developmental considerations lead to the conclusions that heart muscle cells should express the same integrin subunit types as those of fibroblasts, endothelial cells, and smooth muscle, whereas vertebrate skeletal muscle integrin represents a more specialized end point.

The απ integrin subunit is a prominent component of the costamere. Other subunits, such as the α3-subunit are transiently associated with myofibrils during myofibrillogenesis. As the myofibrils become striated, α3 integrin dissociates from the localized pattern along the myofibrils and the distribution becomes more diffuse (198). Such observations suggest that integrins may participate in the organization and stabilization of myofibrils, together with other components of the cytoskeleton, such as the microtubules and the actin stress fibers.

It is clear that integrins in different muscle types have different ligand specificities and tissue distributions. For example, skeletal muscle expresses β1-integrin in a number of structures involved in cytoskeletal–sarcolemmal linkages. β1-integrins in smooth muscle are confined to the dense plaques that anchor actin to the sarcolemma. In mature striated muscle cells the filamentous material that spans the exosarcomeric space between the peripheral Z-bands and the costameres has traditionally been thought to consist of desmin intermediate filaments, but it may also contain γ-actin (4, 41, 326), which could provide interaction sites for other actin-binding proteins.

One protein involved in the myofibril-sarcolemmal association is talin, which was first identified in adhesion plaques (25, 26). Talin has been isolated in skeletal (301), cardiac(11), and smooth muscle (209). Talin has been shown to bind actin (154, 188), vinculin (24), and integrin (137) at sites on its ~200 kDa C-terminal portion; it also aids actin polymerization (93). The 47 kDa N-terminal fragment of talin interacts with liposomes (93, 217), suggesting a mediating role for talin between myofibrillar proteins and the plasma membrane. Immunofluorescence studies show that talin occurs in the cardiac intercalated disk as well as in the costameres of both cardiac and skeletal muscle, where it co-localizes with vinculin near the sarcolemmal membrane (11). Talin does not localize on myofibrils within the cell, suggesting that, with vinculin (224), it is involved in the myofibril–membrane attachment. Talin has also been found in papillary muscle myotendinous junctions, where it co-localizes with integrin (302). With electron microscopy, the talin molecule, at physiological strength, appears as a series of 10–12 globular domains connected by apparently elastic links (335). Thus, talin may contribute to the passive elastic force of the muscle as well as serve as a connecting component between the myofibrils and extracellular integrin-bound structures.

Each junction of the cytoskeletal apparatus to the extracellular matrix through the cell surface appears to have a unique function and location within muscle cells. There is a clear role for β1-integrins in the assembly of alpha-actinin into myofibrils, but it is also clear that other mechanisms play a role in the assembly of α-actinin into myofibrils. Dystrophin and its associated linkage complex have recently been shown to bind both F-actin and laminin (61). These dystrophin-associated proteins, like the αV are costameric linkages with the extracellular matrix.

In cardiac myocytes, dystrophin (218, 222, 336) is localized at the peripheral sarcolemma and T-tubule membranes, but it is absent from the intercalated disk (77). In contrast to skeletal muscle, dystrophin in cardiac muscle is not exclusively a component of the costamere (288). Dystrophin appears with cytoskeletal proteins in normal human hearts of fetuses at 8 weeks (213). Recent evidence for phosphorylation sites at C-terminal regions, cysteine-rich binding sites for calmodulin and some associated kinases, suggests that dystrophin may be actively involved in transducing signals across the sarcolemma.

Titin Filament Network

Two giant elastic filament proteins have been identified in striated muscle (195, 308). Titin (3–4 MDa) is found in cardiac and skeletal muscle, while nebulin (0.6–0.9 MDa) is found only in skeletal muscle (337). Titin filaments are found within the sarcomere (333) and extend parallel to the myofibril axis and along the periphery of myosin filaments (166, 328). These long, thin filaments extend from a Z-band attachment site to the M-band (155). An inextensible portion adheres closely to the surface of the myosin-containing thick filaments, while an extensible portion interdigitates between the thin filaments in the I-band (88, 327). Titin is the largest known protein monomer to date and each titin filament contains one titin polypeptide (308). This is confirmed by the linear nonrepetitive arrangement of different epitopes identified by monoclonal antibodies. Titin molecules are flexible and slender with a beaded-string appearance and one globular head, and thus they form a polar structure. Since the titin molecules are calculated to be about 1.2 μm long, they are approximately half a sarcomere in length.

Isolated titin molecules are quite elastic along their length, but the assembled titin filaments in myofibril preparations are not uniformly extensible along the entire length (310). The extensible or elastic domain is in the I-band between the end of the A-band and the Z-band, while the far larger domain (about 80% of the total filament) is closely associated with individual myosin filaments in a ratio of six titin molecules per myosin half-filament (176a, 308). Periodic anchorage into the myosin in the A-band region of titin accounts for this inextensibility (86, 138). The link between titin filaments and the Z-band lattice has been demonstrated in skinned muscle fiber preparations by digestion of the actin filaments by gelsolin (84, 85). Electron micrographs show filaments 4 nm in diameter, about the size of titin filaments, extending from the myosin filaments in the A-bands to the remaining Z-band material. Additionally, the N-terminal end of titin has recently been shown to bind α-actinin, a known Z-band component (223, 344). The size, distribution, and measured elastic properties of the titin filaments (146a, 175a, 308, 309, 311, 311a) suggest that they can account for a significant portion of the intracellular passive series elastic property described by muscle biophysicists and attributed to the "third filament" (109).

Titin is expressed early in myofibrillogenesis (10), immediately preceding the detection of the first cardiac myofibril and coincident with the presence of the first organized skeletal myosin filaments. This early expression of titin suggests its importance in myofibril assembly. Titin and α-actinin are among the earliest proteins to exhibit periodic localization (81, 330). Myosin appears in striations at about the same time as titin or shortly thereafter (143). The intermediate filament protein desmin localizes at Z-bands several days after α-actinin and titin (317). Studies of these various cytoskeletal proteins and their interactions with the contractile proteins of the sarcomeres in development suggest that there are a number of redundancies in the system. The correct sequence of protein distribution, the alignment of polymers and co-polymers in individual filaments, and the correct placement of filaments into symmetrical arrays in the development of myofibrils is assured.

The binding properties of titin are of interest. The titin globular head is anchored at the M band and contains a myomesin binding site (220, 221, 319). Titin is also highly phosphorylated in vivo with approximately 12 moles of phosphate incorporated per mole of titin. The titin myofibrillar repeating unit consists of approximately six pairs of titin molecules linked to either side and spanning the Z-band (110, 344) then extending parallel with actin and myosin to within 0.2 μm of the M-disk. Thus the opposite ends of each myosin thick filament are linked to opposite Z-bands by two sets of six titin molecules with opposite polarity. Pulling on one end of a thick filament then stretches the I-band domain of the set of titin filaments attached to the opposite Z-band (136). The titin lattice, therefore, appears to restore myosin filaments to the center of the sarcomere on relaxation.

The titin lattice provides continuity throughout a myofibril during overstretch, when the thick and thin filaments do not overlap (136). This situation is much more likely to occur in skeletal muscle than in cardiac muscle, since skeletal muscle normally operates over a wide range of sarcomere lengths including some that are quite long. Cardiac muscle, on the other hand, has a number of features to ensure that the sarcomere length is very closely regulated to values around rest length (109). In cardiac muscle, the overstretch phenomenon most often occurs in cases of early pathological conditions such as ischemia, anoxia, and adaptation to scarring, which may necessitate a more stretched sarcomere in neighboring cells.

Recent work suggests that titin is an integral part of the thick filament. Partial sequences of titin show two types of motifs that repeat in a pattern leading to a super-repeat. Antibody studies and modeling based on the known inter-domain spacing of 4 nm suggests a super repeat distance of 44 nm. This is very close to the 43 nm repeat distance of the helix that describes the myosin geometry in the filaments. Direct evidence of a 43 nm periodicity in A-band titin is provided by monoclonal antibody studies (328).

Studies of the interaction of titin and myosin suggest a binding to the light meromyosin region of the tail of myosin, which forms the thick filament shaft. Binding to C-protein along the thin filament at a similar periodicity has also been reported. The myosin heads themselves emerge from the thick filament at roughly one-third of this distance, namely 14.3 nm. There is a kinase-like domain of titin located near the central M1-band at the center of the sarcomere (220). The globular C-terminal head of titin has been localized at the M-line in situ. The kinase-like domain is approximately 100 nm away from this head, and resembles myosin light chain kinase.

Another similarly large, thin, and flexible molecule of high molecular weight is nebulin, which is found only in skeletal muscle and not in cardiac muscle (308). Nebulin is most closely associated with the thin filaments, and the individual molecules probably span the length of individual thin filaments. The nebulin molecule follows the long pitch helical structure of the filament in much the same way as tropomyosin. The sevenfold character of the nebulin super-repeat suggests that successive discrete α-helical domains in the nebulin molecule may bind to successive actin subunits in the thin filament. Assuming a continuous a-helix, this arrangement would be compatible with the estimated chain weight of nebulin. Furthermore, a completely α-helical molecule of this size would span about 1 µm, comparable to the length of the vertebrate skeletal muscle thin filament (328). An attractive hypothesis is that nebulin functions as a protein rule to regulate the length of the thin filament in skeletal muscle. In this model, skeletal muscle actin, tropomyosin, and troponin molecules would assemble along the length of the nebulin template until the end of the molecule is reached. Thus, in muscles where thin filament length is exactly specified, the size of the nebulin molecule should correlate with the length value. Chicken, rabbit, and beef muscles have been analyzed and have thin filament lengths of 1.05, 1.1 and 1.3 µm, respectively. The mobility of the muscle-specific nebulin band on gels was seen to vary roughly in inverse proportion to these values (211, 328).

In cardiac muscle, which does not have nebulin, the thin filament lengths are not exactly specified and can vary by as much as 30%. Cardiac muscle does contain a nebulin homologue known as *nebulette,* which has been shown to localize at the Z-band (203, 210, 212). However, the nebulette molecule is much smaller than nebulin and extends only about 25% of the length of the cardiac thin filament. Thus, regulation of thin filament length must proceed by a somewhat different mechanism in cardiac muscle than in skeletal muscle.

THE MYOFILAMENT BUNDLES AND ASSOCIATED STRUCTURES

The sarcomere is the repeating unit of structure along the longitudinal axis of the cardiac myocyte. The energy-producing components—the mitochondria, lipid droplets, and glycogen granules, the energy-consuming contractile apparatus, and the modulators of these processes—the sarcoplasmic reticulum, the T-system network, and the cytoskeleton—are all a part of this repeating pattern. About 40% of the volume of the cardiac cell is occupied by the mitochondria, and more than 50% of the volume of the cell is occupied by the cardiac myofilaments themselves (Figs. 1–36, and 1–37).

The mitochondria are noted for their numerous tightly packed cristae (Figs. 1–38 and 1–39). The varying shapes and sizes of the mitochondrial profiles in longitudinal and cross sections of cardiac muscle are an indication of their movement, plasticity, and selective degradation (119). Rows of mitochondrial profiles one sarcomere in length are seen between the myofibrils, but profiles two to three sarcomeres in length and even at times giant mitochondria six to seven sarcomeres in length can be seen (Figs. 1–38 through 1–40). The significance of this variation in surface membranes to interior cristae membrane ratio is not known. Mitochondria in the nerve cell, another elongated polarized cell type, track along microtubule and intermediate filament pathways. Microtubules also play a role in selective degradation of cardiac mitochondria (119). Therefore, mitochondria may be propelled along the myofibrils as well as squeezed into place by the accompanying movement of the contractile filament lattices.

The sarcoplasmic reticulum has been studied in great detail because the transport of calcium into and out of the myofilament bundles and the coupling of excitation and contraction are essential to understanding the cardiac contraction–relaxation cycle. The micrographs included in this chapter show the important features at the sarcomere level (see Figs. 1–3 through 1–5, 1–18 through 1–22, 1–30, 1–32 through 1–34, and 1–36 through 1–43). The reader should consult other references (70, 82, 100) for the unique geometry and protein composition of the membranes of particular regions of the sarcoplasmic reticulum (SR) and of the T–SR junctions.

The purpose of sarcomere structure is to allow for interaction between the contractile proteins and to ensure that the contractile force is distributed in the direction of muscle shortening. Cardiac muscle cells within the myocardium must conform to the anatomical shape of the heart as well as to multidirectional mechanical forces. Hence, the bundles of myofilaments in cardiac muscle vary in width and are not always separated by surrounding membrane profiles along their entire length (Figs. 1–41 and 1–42). Nevertheless most of the time they appear as myofibrils, the end-on-end arrangement of sarcomeres. The myofibrils are attached at each end of the cell to the cell membrane in specific regions of the intercalated disk, as previously discussed. The mechanical force from individual cardiac cells is transmitted to neighboring cells via these regions.

In micrographs the alternating dark and light bands of the sarcomeres are in fairly good axial register so that adjacent myofibrils give the muscle cell its striated appearance (Figs. 1–1 through 1–3, 1–24, 1–26, 1–34, 1–35, and 1–40). The Z-band is located in the center of adjacent I-bands, and successive Z-bands mark the limit of each sarcomere (Fig. 1–43). The longitudinal separation between adjacent Z-bands in the same myofibril is termed the *sarcomere length,* and this distance is reduced by a proportionate amount when the muscle shortens.

The cardiac sarcomere can be defined at three levels of organization: (1) the banding pattern seen in the light microscope and in the electron microscope, (2) the three-dimensional ordering of filament arrays, and (3) the filaments and their substructure. At all three levels it is possible to relate structural information to physiological properties. For instance, at the first level, the length of the sarcomeres, and thus the length of the myofibril bundle, is related to the width of the I-band, which decreases on muscle shortening (see Figs. 1–26 and 1–30). According to the sliding filament model of contraction, the A-band width remains essentially constant with variations in sarcomere length, though some investigators have disputed this conclusion by evidence of A-band shortening (240, 241). It is currently believed that the Z-band remains centered between the I–A junctions of neighboring sarcomeres during muscle shortening. The Z-band centering forces would be provided by both the endosarcomeric and exosarcomeric lattices. Such forces would provide for a relatively uniform distribution of sarcomere length, so that neighboring sarcomeres are at similar points on their length–tension curve (104, 296). The centering forces would operate longitudinally as well as transversely, that is, in three dimensions, so that successive sarcomeres in a single myofibril maintain similar lengths. The width of the Z-band (265) and the number of M-lines in the M-band (231, 316a) are related to the particular speed of contraction and type of the muscle, and are thought to remain essentially unchanged in striated muscle during normal function.

At the next structural level, the changing three-dimensional structure of the sarcomeric filament arrays directly reflects the physiological (functional) state of the muscle. The amount of force generated by the cardiac sarcomere is related to the degree of interdigitation of the thick and thin filaments in the A-band (254). In the A-band, cross-cut thick and thin filaments interdigitate in a hexagonal array, with a thick filament occupying the center of a hexagon of thin filament profiles as shown both by electron microscopy (Figs. 1–44 and 1–45) and by X-ray diffraction of living muscle (139, 196, 346). The cross-sectional thick filament array in mammalian skeletal and cardiac muscle forms a statistical super-lattice, which manifests intrinsic disorder (179). The crossbridge interconnections between the thick and thin filaments cycle rapidly, with the number and state of binding directly related to force generation as well as to sarcomere length (130). The A-band d_{10} (transverse) lattice spacing is modulated by the crossbridges and other passive elastic forces so that it decreases with increasing sarcomere length (57) and expands during contraction at normal osmolarity (142). At the central bare region, the thick filaments are anchored together at the M-band by several transverse layers of connecting M-bridges exhibiting a threefold symmetry (43, 44; Figs. 1–43 and 1–46). Two other sets of interconnections, the M-filaments and secondary M-bridges, have been postulated to aid in the maintenance of thick filament ordering (180). Since the M disk has a twofold symmetry in the longitudinal direction, the overall symmetry observed in both cardiac and skeletal M-bands is 3,2 (231). The prominence of the M1-line may be related to disorder in the A-band lattice, suggesting that the M-band plays a definitive role in the arrangement of the thick filaments (231). Vertebrate cardiac muscle has four or five M-lines; the number may be related to heart rate (231). The I-band lattice appears rather disordered in electron micrographs of cross sections and longitudinal sections (Fig. 1–47); however, several transverse striations, the N-lines, are recognized (343; Fig. 1–43). The N1- and N2-lines are associated with specific titin epitopes (84, 88, 194, 295, 310). Finally, the Z-band in vertebrate muscle exhibits projected fourfold symmetry in cross section (63, 97; Fig. 1–48). In normal cardiac muscle 2–4 longitudinal repeating units are observed (97). Thin filaments in slow skeletal muscle exhibit "four nearest-neighbor" filament ordering throughout the I-band, but they assume a tetragonal arrangement near the edge of the Z-band (307). The vertebrate Z-band lattice has at least two structural states that are related to the contractile state, as discussed in the next section.

At the third or macromolecular level the structure of muscle is described in terms of the structure of individual proteins, protein polymers, and their assembly into working filaments and connecting scaffolds permeated with more amorphously distributed proteins. At this level, the organization seen in electron micrographs represents a two-dimensional projection of a still life of the interaction between individual muscle proteins. Biochemical studies of various combinations of these proteins under conditions that mimic those of the cell have contributed to our understanding of the details of these interactions.

The major proteins in the thick and thin filaments are actin and myosin. The thick filament is composed primarily of myosin, helically arranged in a polar fashion (112) so that myosin heads (248, 249) have opposing orientations in neighboring A-bands, with a "bare" region at the location of the M-band. The thin filament is a copolymer of actin and

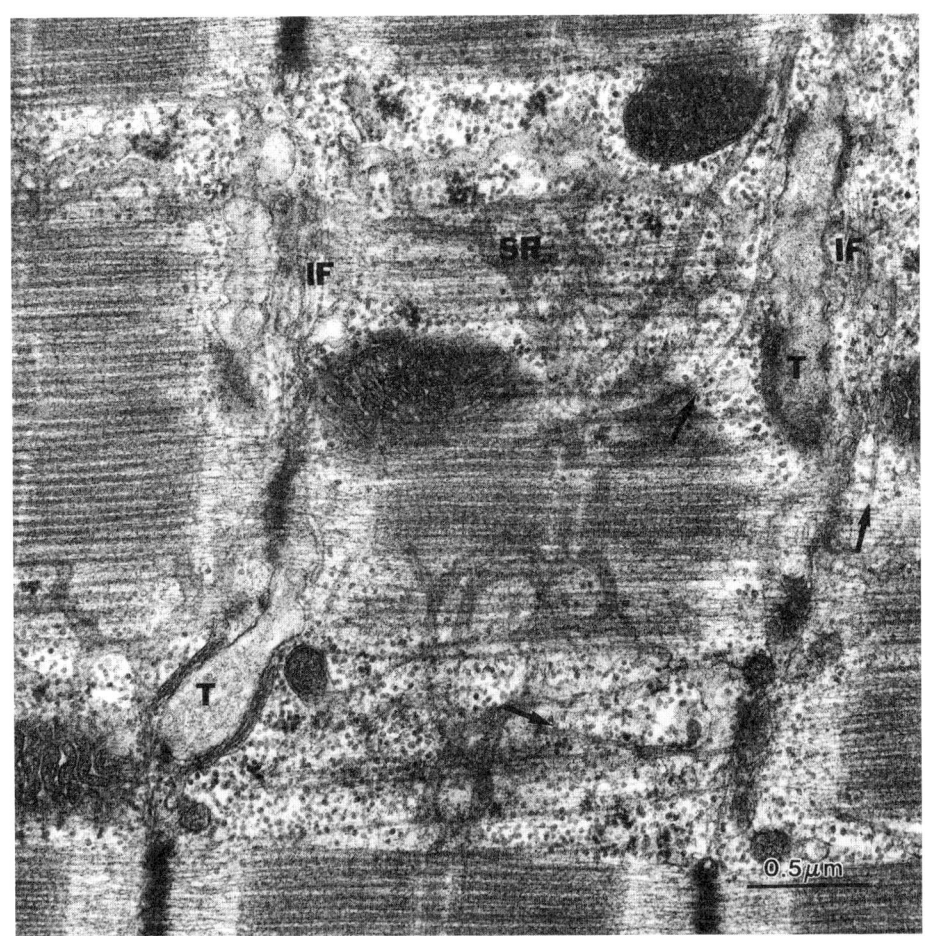

FIG. 1-40. Longitudinal section of dog papillary muscle showing the relationship between longitudinal profiles of microtubules (*arrows*), sarcoplasmic reticulum, T-tubules (T), intermediate filaments (IF) and adjacent myofilament bundles. (98) (Reprinted by permission of Rockefeller University Press)

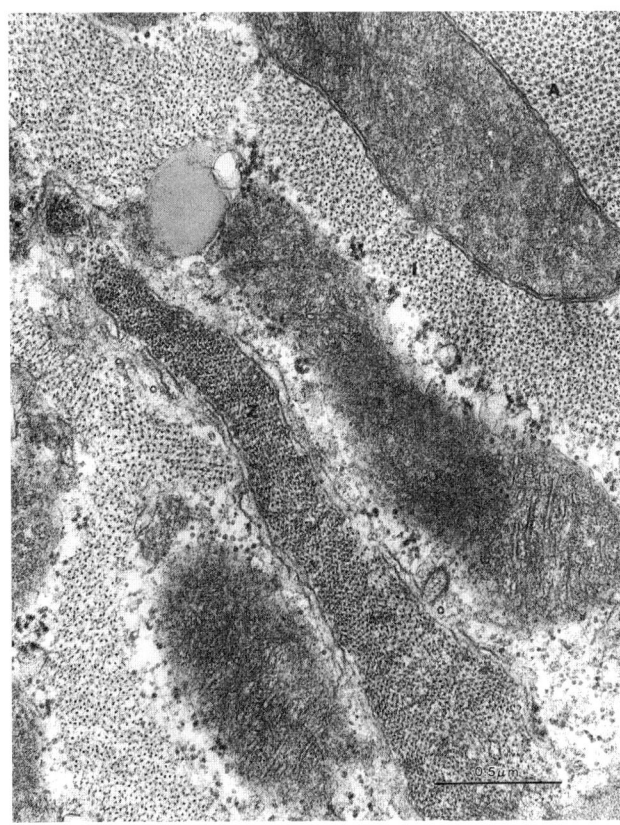

FIG. 1-41. Cross section of myofilament bundles from papillary muscle showing A, I and Z-bands. Compare with Figure 1-6 to see corresponding appearance in a longitudinal section of papillary muscle.

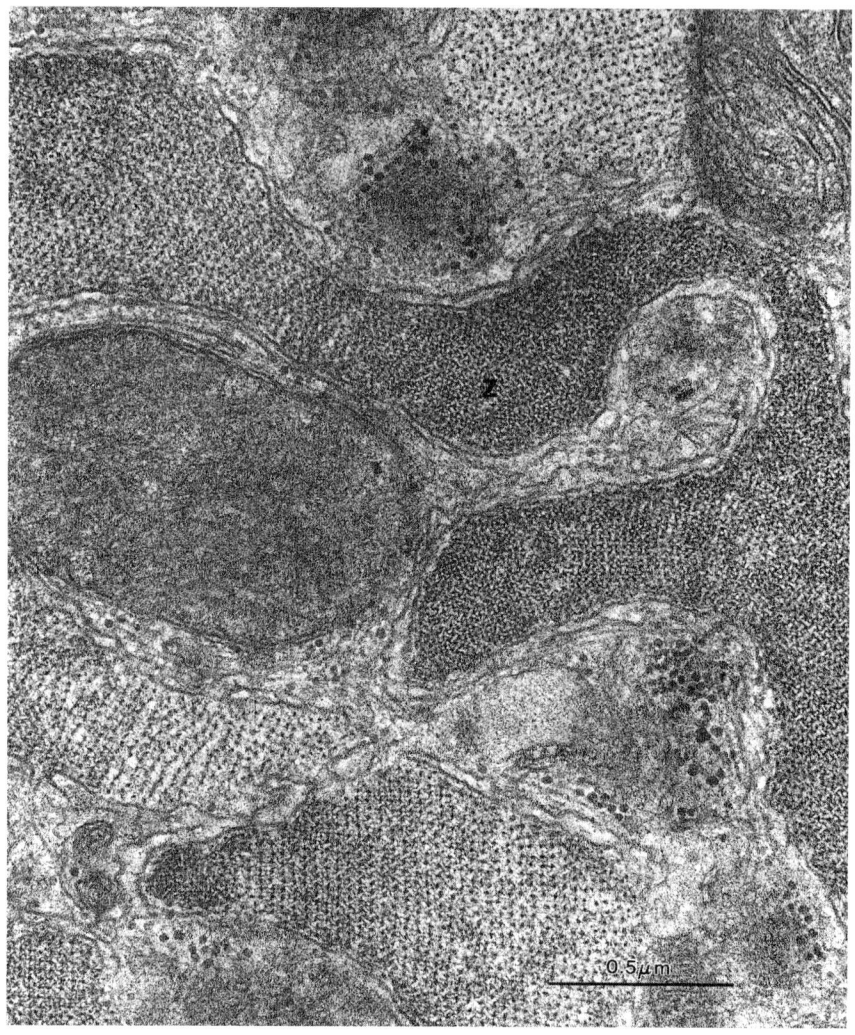

FIG. 1–42. Cross section of rat papillary myofilament bundle at level of Z-band showing one of the unusual myofibril shapes.

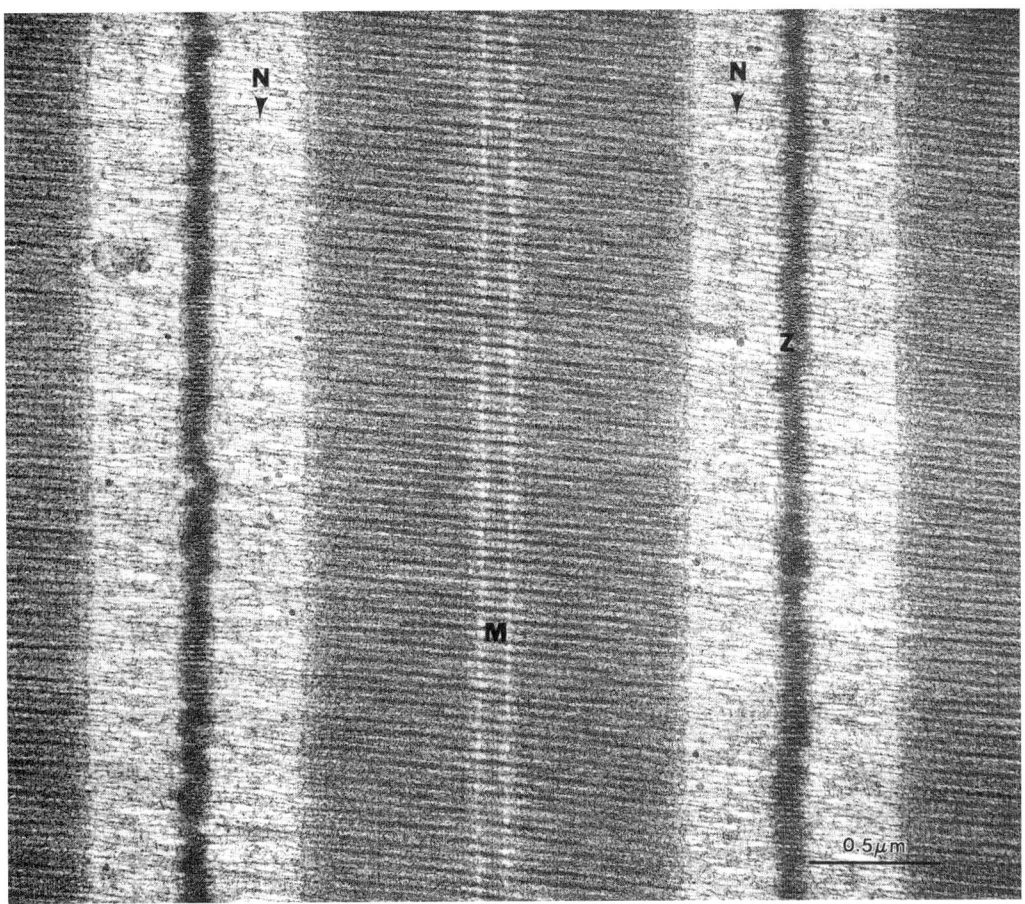

FIG. 1–43. Thin longitudinal section of dog papillary myofibril. Periodicities along thick and thin filaments can be seen by viewing figure from above at 45 degrees. Striations within M-band and Z-lattices can be seen at this magnification. Note N-lines (*arrowheads*).

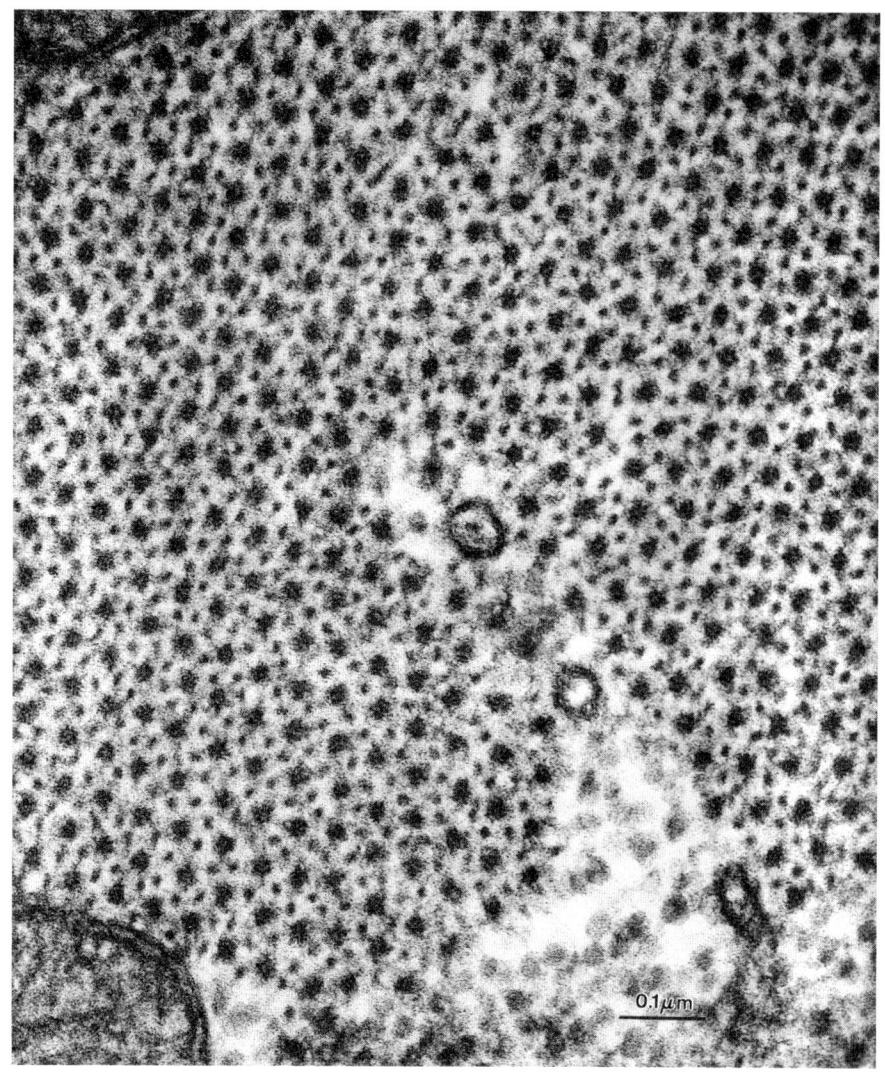

FIG. 1–44. Thick and thin filaments in hexagonal array in cross section of A-band can be seen by viewing the figure from above at 45 degrees. Try rotating the figure as you view to get best perspective.

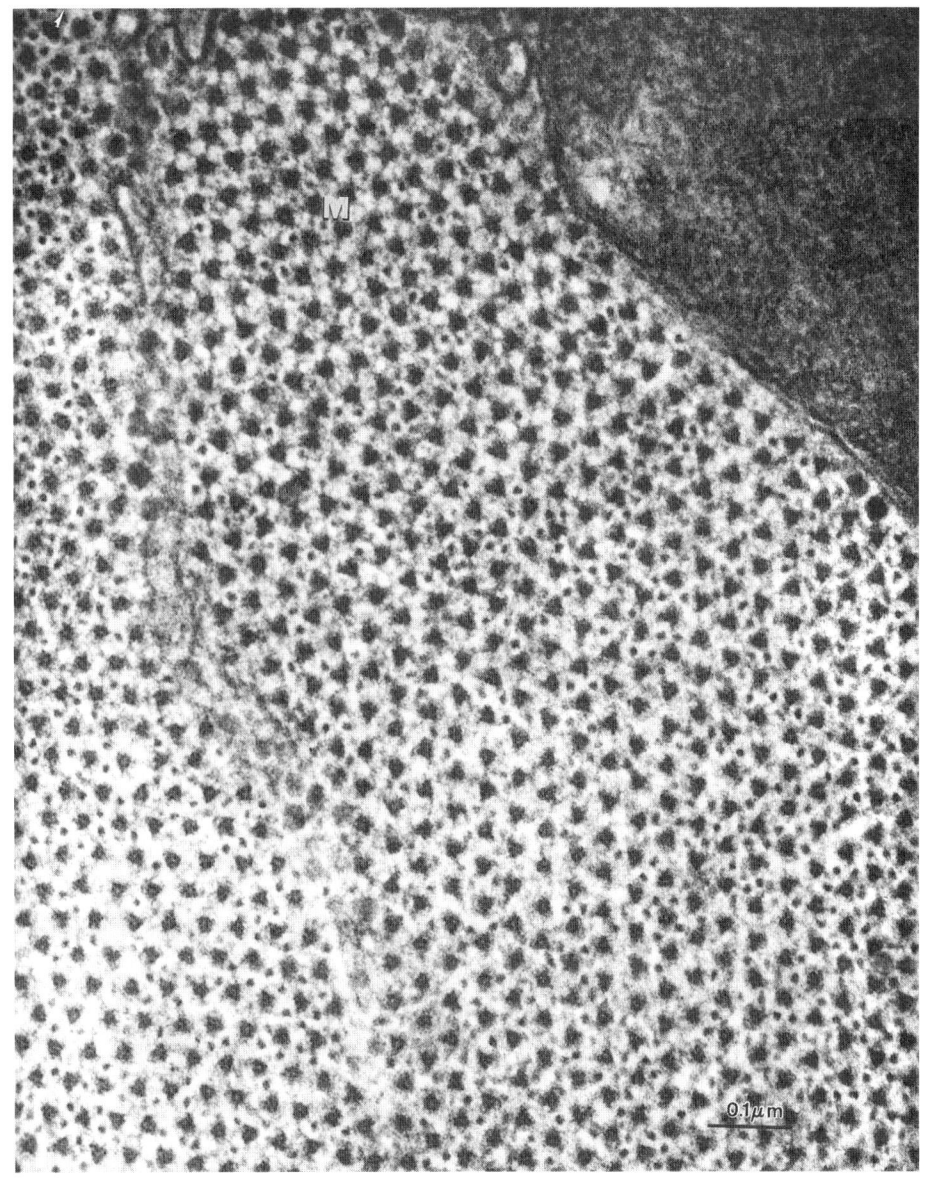

FIG. 1–45. Cross section of dog papillary myofibril at level of M-band and edge of A-band. Note distinct triangular appearance of cross-cut thick filaments and the filaments connecting all six thick filaments and a central thick filament in several arrays in middle of M-band. Some thin filaments penetrate into the H-zone because some are much longer than others.

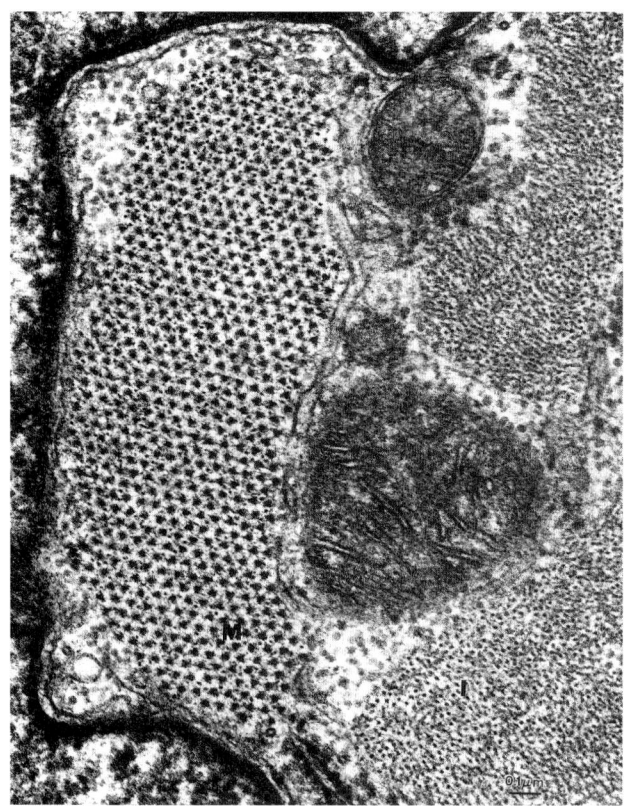

FIG. 1–46. Cross section of sarcomere near nucleus exhibits M-band ordering of thick filaments. Adjacent myofilament bundles are at I-band level. Not all myofibrils are in exact register across the cell in cardiac muscle.

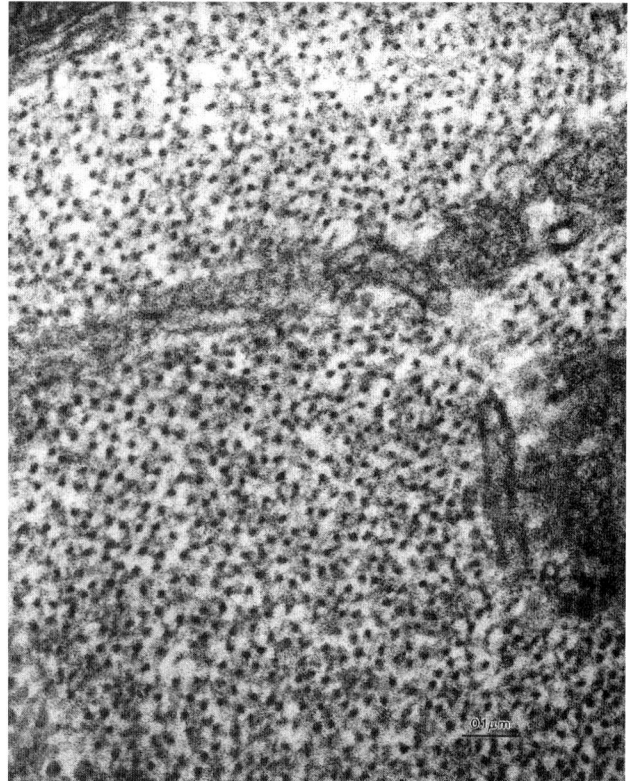

FIG. 1–47. Thin filaments in I-band lack precise symmetry, are not random, but exhibit nearest-neighbor ordering. Note connections between some pairs of thin filaments in this cross section of dog papillary muscle.

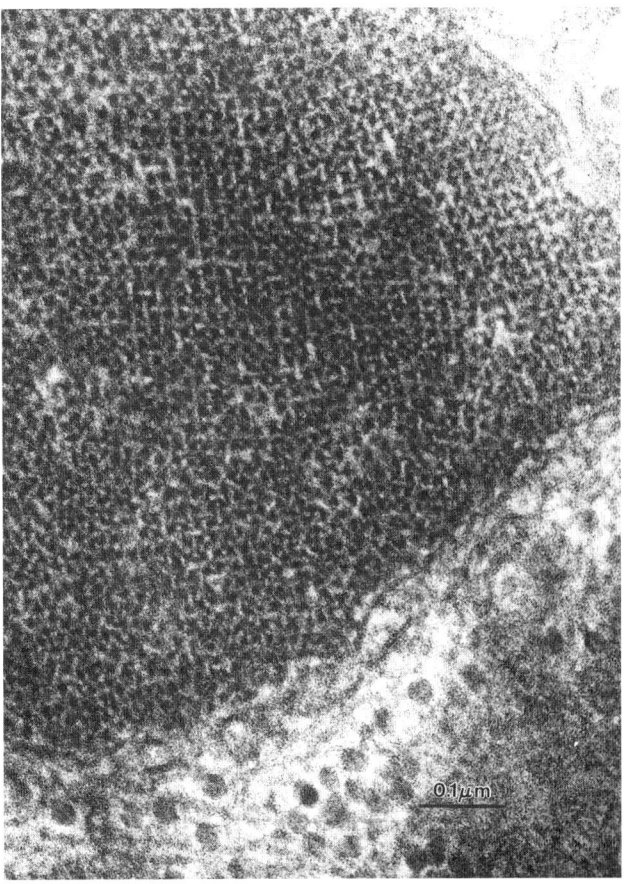

FIG. 1–48. Cross section of Z-band lattice of a single sarcomere. The basket weave, or bw, lattice appearance predominates in this unstimulated cardiac muscle.

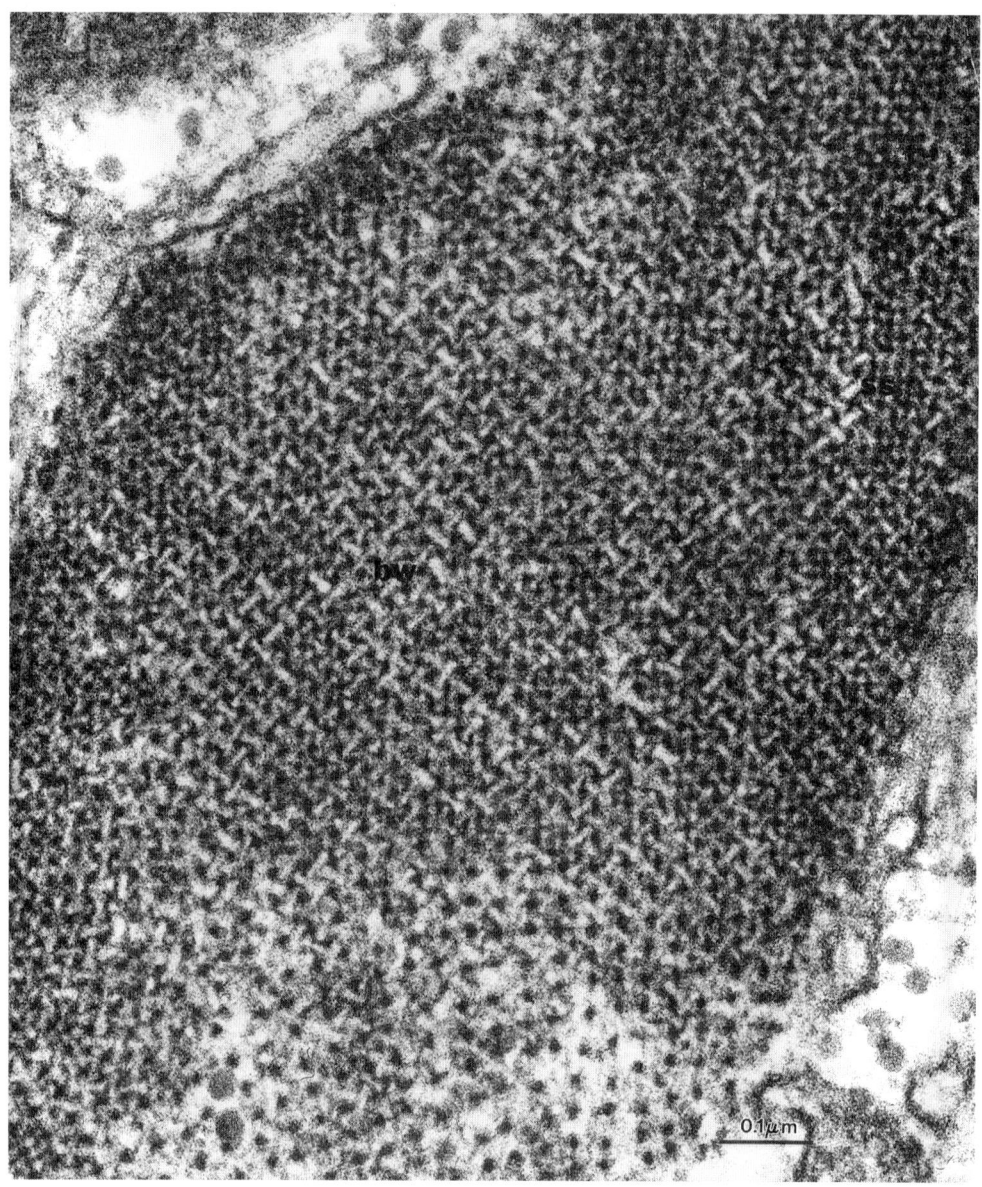

FIG. 1–49. Cross section of unstimulated dog papillary muscle showing portion of Z-band exhibiting two different lattice appearances: the basket weave pattern (bw) predominates, but a small region of small square pattern (ss) is visible at far right.

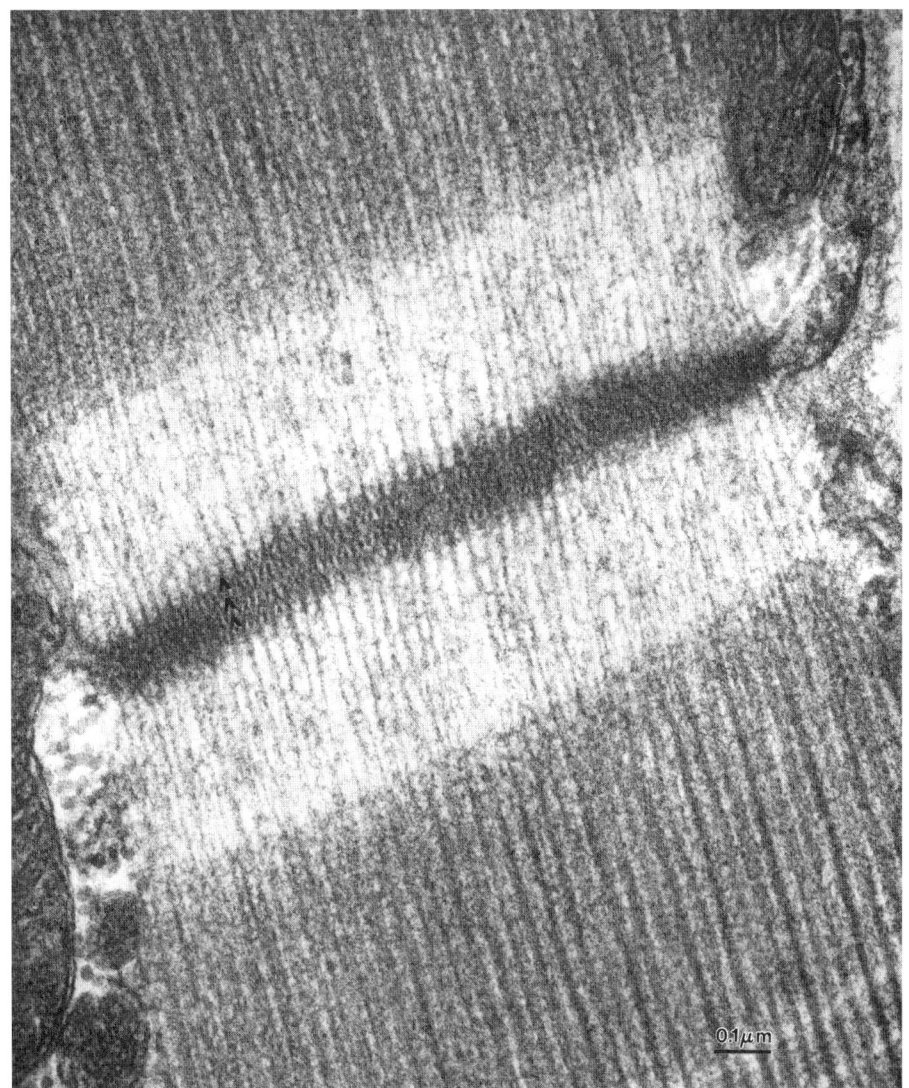

FIG. 1–50. Longitudinal section of Z-band anchored near the sarcolemma. The chevron pattern typical of this 24 nm (1,0) orientation of the Z-lattice is shown. Thin filaments of adjacent sarcomeres interdigitate and the distance between adjacent thin filaments from the same sarcomere is 24 nm.

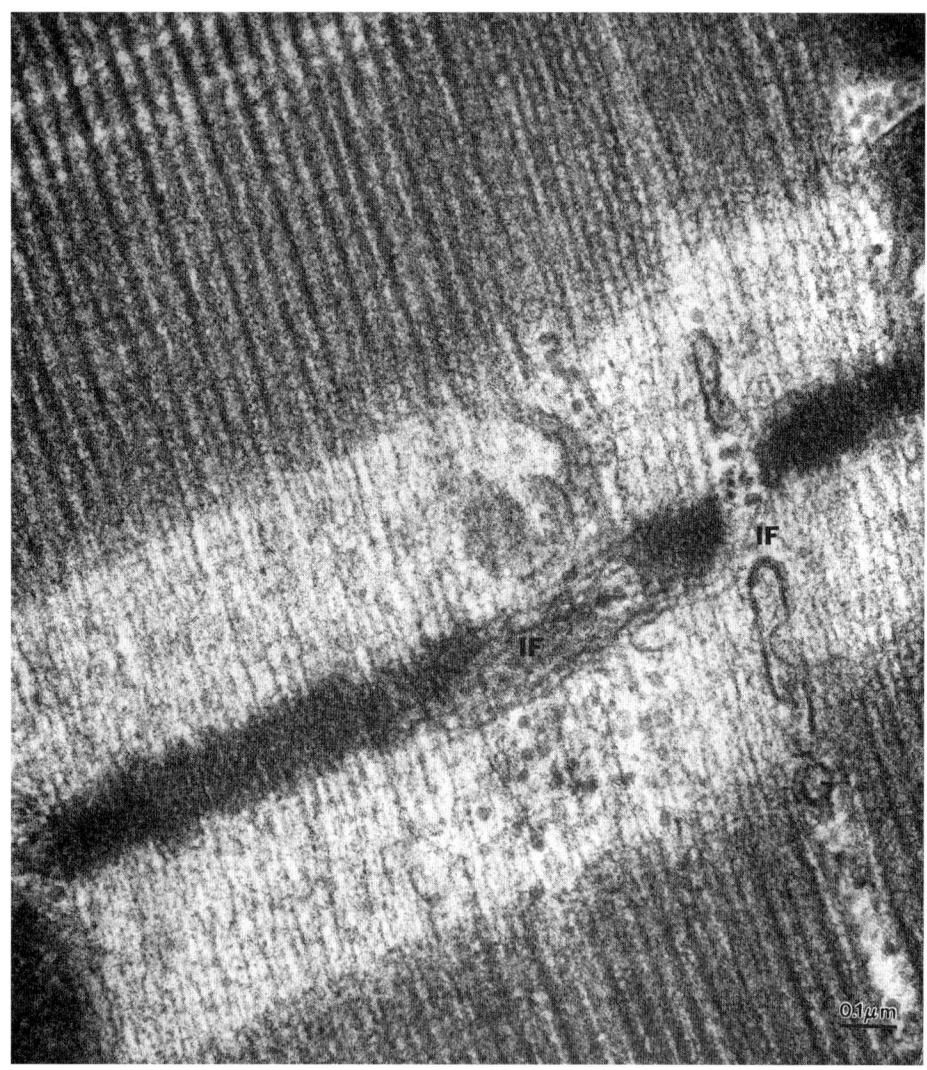

FIG. 1–51. Longitudinal section of Z-band showing intermediate filaments (IF) going between adjacent Z-bands and around periphery of Z-lattice.

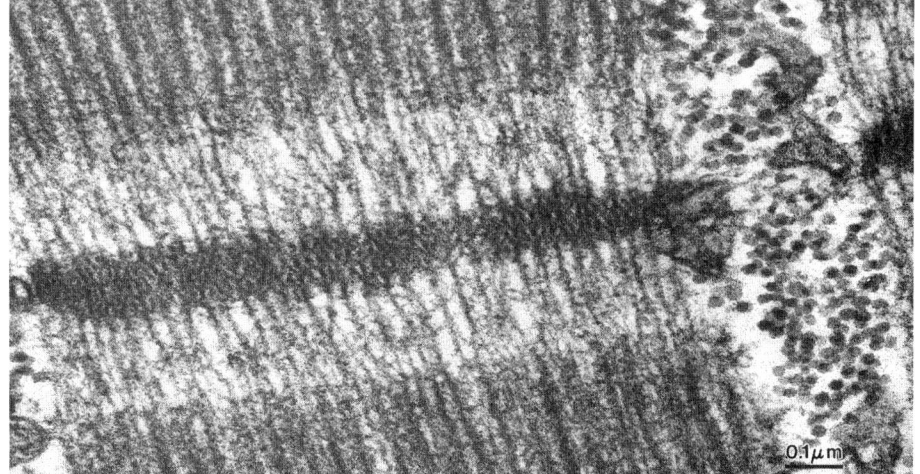

FIG. 1–52. Longitudinal section of Z-band lattice exhibiting chevron appearance typical of the 24 nm (1,0) orientation. This Z lattice is especially uniform with respect to the plane of section, yet there are 3–4 subunits visible at the left, whereas at the bottom only two are visible. This is seen most easily if viewed at an angle of 45 degrees.

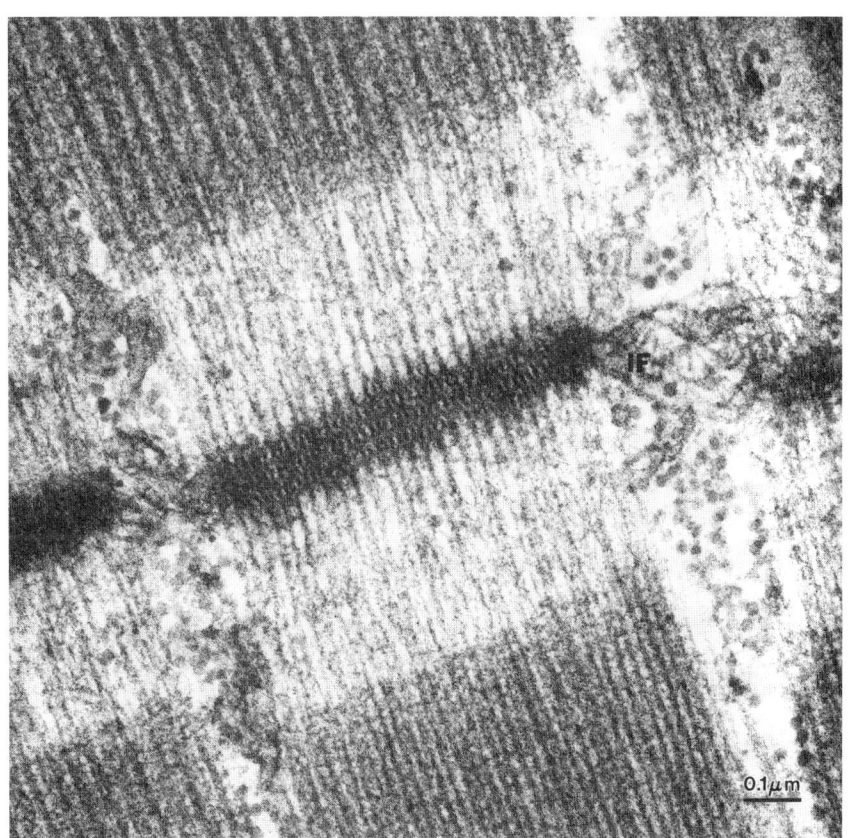

FIG. 1–53. Longitudinal section of Z-band in same orientation as Figure 1–52, but the sarcomere is longer. The appearance of the Z-lattice is the same. Experimental evidence shows that passive stretch does not induce a change in lattice appearance or spacing. Intermediate filaments (IF) are visible between adjacent Z-bands.

tropomyosin, with troponin and other proteins arranged in a complex helical structure (69, 204, 238). Successive myosin head binding sites arranged with helical symmetry provide the regions for the crossbridge attachment associated with contraction (132, 303). Numerous actin-binding proteins such as CapZ (272), nebulin (328), tropomodulin (72), and others (293) are involved in actin regulation in the muscle thin filament. For a detailed discussion of the structure and function of the thick and thin filaments, see the related chapters in this *Handbook*. Some passive elastic forces can be directly related to the structure of the titin filament and its interactions with myosin, as previously discussed; however, both the thick (120, 139) and thin (140, 322) filaments exhibit modest elastic compliance. In the M-band, three protein constituents are recognized: creatine kinase, myomesin, and M-protein. Creatine kinase has been shown to be a component of the M-bridges at the M4-line in skeletal muscle, where it may act as a structural link as well as serving its function in ATP regeneration (220, 325). It has been suggested that M-protein may be a component of the M1-line (29, 220), since muscle fibers devoid of M-protein show no M1-lines. Myomesin, the third M-band protein, is thought to traverse the M-band (220, 319). Both myomesin and M-protein bind the C-terminal region of titin (216, 221, 319). Myomesin has been shown to bind myosin (220, 221) Both myomesin and M-protein associate with myosin in solid phase binding assays (316a).

The cross-connecting Z-filaments of the Z-band lattice are primarily α-actinin, an actin-binding protein. The substructure of this lattice, of its protein components, and of their role in contraction are discussed in detail in the next section.

The three-dimensional structure of the cardiac myofibril is thus dependent on the composition and interaction of thin and thick filaments to form the Z, I, A, and M-band lattices, the arrangement of these lattices to form sarcomeres, and the end-to-end and side-to-side registration of the sarcomeres within the context of the cytoskeleton and other components. Thus, modifications of individual proteins at the lowest structural level may profoundly affect structure and function at the level of the sarcomeric lattices, of the myofilament bundles, and finally, of the whole muscle.

THE DYNAMIC Z-BAND LATTICE

Contractile and Elastic Components in Relation to the Z-Band

The interaction of contractile and elastic components in striated muscle continues to intrigue morphologists and physiologists (104, 153, 318). To understand the pivotal role of the Z-band in the cardiac sarcomere, it is important to compare the mechanical properties of skeletal and cardiac muscle. Skeletal muscle cells are mechanically as well as anatomically arranged in parallel. They can function independently, with the total force generated equal to the sum of the forces from each one. Additionally, skeletal muscle cells are normally relaxed and recruited to generate force and movement (13). Cardiac muscle cells are significantly smaller in length and diameter (65, 71, 283) and are connected in series with one another, as well as in parallel. In the ventricle, the cardiac muscle cells form a continuous sheet in a twisted figure-eight configuration. The cells are mechanically interdependent since pressures are transmitted outward from the ventricular cavity and contractions of some cells necessarily alter the load on other cells. The Z-band represents the physical link between the forces inside the cell—between sarcomeres, between myofibrils—and the forces outside the cell.

The following observed mechanical properties of cardiac muscle are important in relation to ultrastructural features of the Z-band (104): (*1*) higher resting tension than skeletal muscle, (*2*) tension development over a very narrow range of sarcomere lengths, and (*3*) exponential rise in tension at lengths greater than 85% of L_{max}. This tension is generated by crosslinks between myosin and actin. In cardiac muscle, the crossbridges themselves are an elastic component, and the variable length of the thin filaments provides for variation in myofilament overlap and sarcomere nonuniformity. The Z-band is a participant in these internal forces. The amount and type of collagen and elastin in the extracellular matrix and the amount of sarcolemma are all determining factors in the elastic properties of cardiac muscle, and they represent the forces outside the cell. They impinge on the Z-band, as mentioned before.

The cooperative movement of contractile and elastic components thus occurs at several structural levels in cardiac muscle, all of which eventually impinge on the Z-band (104, 318). At the level of the whole muscle, individual contractile cells are enmeshed in an ordered array of collagen and elastic filaments (16, 33) and are attached to adjacent cells (71) by side-to-side struts at the Z-bands (74, 258, 347). The ends of the muscle fiber are inserted into collagenous tendons at the terminal Z-bands (55). At the cellular level, the contractile myofilament bundles or myofibrils are enmeshed in a cytoskeleton of microtubules (98, 247) and intermediate filaments (171) attaching at Z-bands. The myofibrils are also attached to the cell surface through a filamentous network connecting laterally to the Z-band surface (278; see Fig. 1–50) and longitudinally to terminal Z-bands (242). At the sarcomere level, the hexagonal array of thick and thin filaments is interspersed with the endosarcomeric lattice. The interconnections between opposing thin filaments and between opposing titin filaments both occur at the Z-band. At all these levels the Z-band is involved in stabilizing against lateral forces and in facilitating axial forces.

In cardiac muscle, two sets of filaments—thin filaments and titin filaments—extend from the Z-band into the A-band to interact with myosin in the thick filaments. In the Z-band, the thin filaments connect to a complex filamentous lattice of which α-actinin is the primary component. The N-terminal tail of titin has been localized to this Z-band lattice (223, 309). Titin binds to the rod domain of α-actinin at the edge of the Z-lattice, and central titin Z-repeats interact with the α-actinin C-terminal domain (110, 344, 344a). Active and passive tension generated at the crossbridge level and transmitted via the thin and titin filaments may then be modulated by corresponding changes within the Z-band lattice (310). Passive tension is alternately or simultaneously transmitted via the titin filaments to attachment points at the Z-lattice.

In the Z-band the thin filaments from adjacent sarcomeres overlap and interdigitate in an array with approximate four-fold symmetry in cross section (103, 161; Fig. 1–49). The opposite polarity of thin filaments from opposite sarcomeres required for the crossbridge attachment of the contractile mechanism is maintained in the Z-band so that nearest-neighbor thin filaments have opposite polarity (251, 339). Cross-connecting Z-filaments attach periodically and hold the ends of the thin filaments together in a three-dimensional lattice in such a regular manner that the Z-lattice can be detected by X-ray diffraction in living muscle (118, 344, 345) and by optical diffraction of electron micrographs of fixed muscle (97; (Figs. 1–50 through 1–54, 1–60 through 1–62). Minimal and maximal separation distances (Z-spacing) of the ends of the thin filaments are limited by these cross-connecting Z-filaments. The approximately tetragonal symmetry of the vertebrate cardiac and skeletal Z-band is maintained in the lattice of longitudinal repeating units. This longitudinal maintenance of four-fold symmetry occurs despite its incommensurability with the symmetry of α-actinin binding sites along the actin in the axial filament. It is likely that other proteins affect the apparent symmetry of the cross-connecting Z-filaments (107), and it is possible that Z-band lattice disorder serves to obscure the symmetry of the actin-binding sites (276). Interestingly, Z-bands from insect muscle, though of a similar protein composition (318), exhibit a threefold symmetry quite different from that seen in vertebrate muscle (2, 35, 48, 267).

Protein Composition

Filamentous actin is found in Z-bands in vertebrate and invertebrate cardiac and skeletal muscle. The axial filament extensions of the thin filaments of the I-band, when treated with a Ca^{2+}-activated neutral protease, can be decorated with myosin subfragments to show the overlap of opposing actin-containing filaments (338–340). Tropomyosin, also at the Z-band, may remain associated with the extensions of the thin (axial) filaments, but it is not necessarily a part of the cross-connecting Z-filament lattice (274, 292).

Alpha-actinin is the best characterized of the Z-band–specific proteins and is an essential component of the cross-connecting Z-filaments (250, 318). Alpha-actinin is an anti-parallel homodimer of molecular weight 94–103. The N-terminal region is a highly conserved actin-binding domain and the C-terminal region contains an Ef-hand calcium-binding domain (15). Its actin-binding properties point to an important role in axial filament interconnection in the Z-band (107, 199, 298). Anti–alpha-actinin has been localized at the Z-band at the light microscopic level (36, 268, 274) and at the electron microscopic level (304, 324, 349). The dimensions of the cross-connecting Z-filaments are compatible with the molecular dimensions of α-actinin. However, anti–alpha-actinin Fab fragments have been found to be distributed evenly throughout the Z-lattice, both along the axial filaments and around the cross-connecting filaments (349). Multiple isoforms of α-actinin exist, and in skeletal muscle the expression of different isoforms is correlated with Z-band width and troponin T/tropomyosin isoforms (270, 277)

CapZ, a heterodimeric protein of molecular weight 32–36 was first isolated from skeletal muscle (31) and occurs as well in nonmuscle cells in both vertebrates and invertebrates. In skeletal and cardiac muscle, it is localized at the Z-band (32, 271). CapZ binds α-actinin and forms an anchoring complex for both the thin filaments and titin (229). CapZ binds with high affinity to the barbed ends of actin filaments, and appears at an early stage in the formation of I-Z-I brushes during myofibrillogenesis. CapZ prevents the addition or loss of monomers of actin from the barbed end of the filament (27, 72, 318).

Nebulin has been localized to the Z-band of skeletal muscle and is thought to play a role in regulation of thin filament length. Although it is not found in cardiac muscle, a related but much smaller homolog, called *nebulette* has been localized at the cardiac muscle Z-band (203, 210, 212). Both nebulin and nebulette bind α-actinin, and there is a 70% homology between nebulette and the C-terminal end of nebulin (212). Nebulette is co-localized with α-actinin in early stages of cardiac myofibrillogenesis (212).

There is evidence for several other proteins associated with the Z-lattice. Zeugmatin is a high molecular weight heterodimer with a subunit size and mobility between nebulin and titin (189). However, it is now considered to be a fragment of titin (3, 313, 314). It has not been observed in nonmuscle cells. Of particular interest is the appearance of this protein in cultured muscle cells before α-actinin and dense bodies are seen, suggesting that it may be a titin precursor (318).

Amorphin, an 85 kDa protein (36) is so similar to glycogen phosphorylase that it is believed to be the same. It may be a particular isoform important for Z-lattice activity. Amorphin may be extracted from the Z-band without disturbing the cross-connecting Z-filaments, and so is thought to be a component of the amorphous Z-band density.

At least nine other Z-band proteins have been described in vertebrate striated muscle (64, 89, 318, 329). Three of these have been identified in cardiac muscle. Annexin V has recently been shown to co-localize with α-actinin in cardiac myocytes. It does not bind F-actin in vitro, and its role in Z-band structure is uncertain (329). Gamma-filamin/ABP-L, an isoform of filamin, has been localized to the Z-band in mammalian cardiac and skeletal muscle. The protein appears in Z-bands in the first stages of formation, suggesting that it may have a role in development (316). Eu-actinin, a 42 kDa protein, binds to actin and α-actinin in vitro, and is localized exclusively in the Z-band (165). Eu-actinin has been shown to speed actin filament nucleation in vitro, and so could have a function in I-Z-I assembly.

Perturbed States of the Z-Band

Damage to the sarcomere is often seen first in the Z-band. Changes in Z-band appearance are used as a standard to estimate preservation of myofibrillar structure in stress and disease states, as well as during fast freezing and other preparative routines. Z-band abnormalities are associated with various disease states and states characteristic of perturbed muscle (Figs. 1–55 through 1–59). Z-crystals or Z-rods are extremely widened Z-bands that may contain ten or more longitudinal repeating units, sometimes enough to reach completely through the sarcomere to the opposing Z-band (Figs. 1–56 through 1–59). These structures are observed in senescence (152, 297; Fig. 1–58), in development (174), in various myopathies (99, 279), and in hypertrophy in both cardiac (14, 191) and skeletal muscle (158). Z-band width is also affected by overexpression of calmodulin in cardiomyocytes (111) and in Z-band streaming, which is associated with muscle damage from eccentric contraction (121) and disease states (191). Widened Z-bands represent a change in the Z-band width regulatory mechanism (Fig. 1–57). This mechanism is not well understood, and it operates in mature muscle as well as during development. For example, Z-band width may change when the speed of a skeletal muscle is transformed (56, 253, 299), or in cases of regression of Z-rods (122). Schachat and co-workers (270) have shown a correlation between Z-band width and α-actinin isoform, which may be part of the regulatory mechanism. Titin and nebulette seem to be involved in Z-band width regulation (110, 203, 229, 344).

Models of the Z-band structure usually explain differing Z-band widths on the basis of different number of longitudinal repeating units (63, 95, 97, 341) or layers of cross-connecting Z-filaments (103, 156, 157, 185). However, three-dimensional reconstructions of muscle indicate that the detailed structure of the thinnest Z-bands may differ from that seen in unstimulated mammalian skeletal muscle and in Z-rods (182, 184, 185, 214, 276). These reconstructions validate the notion that two different structural states exist at a variety of Z-band widths.

The cardiac Z-band is affected by exposure of the whole animal to microgravity and to hypergravity. Upon exposure to microgravity, cardiac muscle myofibrils atrophy, and the disk radius of the Z-band shrinks along with the myofibril (105). Conversely, with the modest cardiac hypertrophy observed upon exposure of rats to 2G for 14 days, the Z-bands were seen to expand in total cross-sectional area along with the myofibrils, but they show no other apparent ultrastructural changes (106). In skeletal muscle, multi-G induced hypertrophy is associated with a transformation of fast muscle fibers to slow muscle, with a concomitant increase in the width (longitudinal extent) of the Z-band (usually in the range of 1–2 to 3–4 longitudinal subunits) (193).

Functional States of the Z-Band

The Z-band in both cardiac and skeletal muscle can exhibit two different structural appearances in cross section. One lattice pattern is called small square (ss) and the other is called basket weave (bw). Each lattice form has a characteristic optical diffraction pattern (103). Evidence from electron microscopy of vertebrate fixed muscle shows that the two states can occur at a variety of Z-band lattice spacings in different muscles (47, 63, 95, 97, 118, 169, 185, 341). However, a correlation between Z-band lattice form and Z-spacing has been observed in electron micrographs of fixed vertebrate skeletal and cardiac muscles in differing functional states (54, 103, 275). In each case in mammalian muscle there is an expansion of the Z-lattice perpendicular to the myofibril axis when the bw lattice pattern is observed. A similar percentage change in Z-spacing has been observed in X-ray diffraction of living frog skeletal muscle upon activation (142).

Unstimulated cardiac muscle Z-bands from rat show predominantly the bw pattern (102; see Figs. 1–49 and 63), with a measured Z-spacing of 24.04 ± 0.4 nm. The same lattice pattern (Z-spacing = 24.31 ± 0.21 nm) is seen in tetanized mammalian slow skeletal muscle (Fig. 1–64). However, unstimulated mammalian skeletal muscle predominantly exhibits the ss pattern with a smaller Z-spacing of 19.55 ± 0.19 nm (103). The bw pattern in the tetanized skeletal muscle is observed at a variety of sarcomere lengths and is not induced by forces resulting from a passive stretch (Figs. 1–65 through 1–67). In frog muscle, which exhibits bw in the unstimulated state, passive stretch beyond sarcomere lengths of ~2.4 μm (beyond lengths seen in normal cardiac muscle) induces the transition to the ss pattern (342).

In cardiac muscle, the bw pattern predominates, but patches of the ss lattice are occasionally observed (see Fig. 1–49), suggesting that the unstimulated cardiac Z-band is not wholly in an "activated" state. When treated with a Ca^{2+} chelating agent, EGTA, cardiac muscle predominately exhibits the ss pattern in the Z-band, with a reduction in the Z-spacing to 20.30 ± 0.20 nm (Figs. 1–68 and 1–69). This suggests that the bw Z-band observed in unstimulated cardiac muscle is correlated with calcium concentration, the high resting tension (i.e. crossbridge binding in the A-band), or both (102). In mammalian skeletal muscle prepared in a calcium-free state of rigor, the A-band crossbridges are uniformly bound to the thin filament, and the Z-band exhibits the bw form and dimensions. This suggests that the cardiac bw state may also be associated with crossbridge binding. In tetanized and rigor mammalian skeletal muscle, A-bands are characterized by crossbridge attachment. In the case of the reversible tetanized condition, crossbridge cycling is occurring, so that it is not surprising that some regions of the myofibrils would appear momentarily relaxed. In the case of the rigor condition, the crossbridges are firmly attached, and uniform myofibril lattice appearances are observed. Correspondingly, the Z-band lattice shows a more uniform bw appearance in the rigor state (54).

As in mammalian skeletal muscle (Figs. 1–63 through 1–65), passive stretch of either the unstimulated or EGTA-treated cardiac muscle has little effect on Z-band form or dimensions (102). Interestingly, the Z-crystal seen in muscle hypertrophy and in various pathological states has been shown to exhibit the ss form. Sarcomeres containing Z-crystals are functionally impaired and may not develop normal tension (95, 99).

The Z-band may function as an elastic component by storing or releasing energy during the ss to bw transition in skeletal muscle. The reversibility of the transition has been shown in tetanized mammalian skeletal muscle (103) and in frog muscle in response to osmotic changes (342). Earlier Z-band models of this transition (97, 315, 341) explained the structural change as a straightening of the crossconnecting Z-filaments resulting from a variation in longitudinal and/or cross-sectional dimension of the repeating unit (see Fig. 1–53). Three-dimensional reconstructions of the Z-rod (214) and of the Z-band in unstimulated skeletal muscle (276; Figs. 1–70 and 1–71; Plate 1) suggest that the transition is more complex. Both of these reconstructions show a connecting body containing a filamentous "Z-RIB" structure, which lies between and parallels the axial filaments. This structure is missing in two-dimensional cross-sectional projections of the bw lattice (Fig. 1–72), and in three-dimensional reconstructions of a bw Z-band in fish muscle (185). Hence, the ss to bw transition in skeletal muscle requires some mechanism for elimination of the Z-RIB.

In cardiac muscle, computerized image enhancement of two-dimensional cross-sectional projections of the bw and ss lattices show a detailed structural difference that suggests a mechanism for the transition. In these images, the apparent diameter of the cross-cut axial filament was observed to be much larger in the bw form of the lattice than in the ss from (275). These results are confirmed in a preliminary three dimensional reconstruction of the unstimulated cardiac Z-band (Fig. 1–73 and 1–74). This hints that protein in the Z-RIB and crossconnecting Z-filaments may wrap around or otherwise bind more closely to the axial filaments in the bw Z-band (145a). Such a mechanism could provide a continuum of states for cardiac Z-band activation. Labeling of the cardiac Z-band with anti–alpha-actinin results in a dose-dependent decrease in the spontaneous oscillation amplitude of isolated cardiac myofibrils (175). This suggests that the Z-band plays a dynamic role in contraction for cardiac muscle as well as for skeletal muscle.

SUMMARY

At each level from the whole heart down to the molecular level there are patterns of organization that reflect the mechanical function peculiar to the heart. In this review we have emphasized the cytoskeleton and the Z-band and included recent discoveries of structure and function for titin, intermediate filament proteins, microtubules, and the Z-band. We have suggested how contractile and elastic forces are

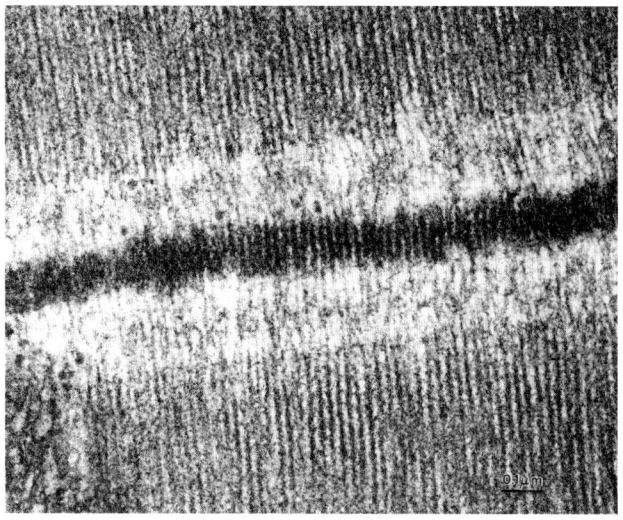

FIG. 1–54. Longitudinal section of Z-band in 17 nm (1,1) orientation (17 is half-diagonal of a 24 nm square). Thin filaments appear to go straight through the Z-band, when in fact the overlapping ends of the thin filaments form a centered square arrangement.

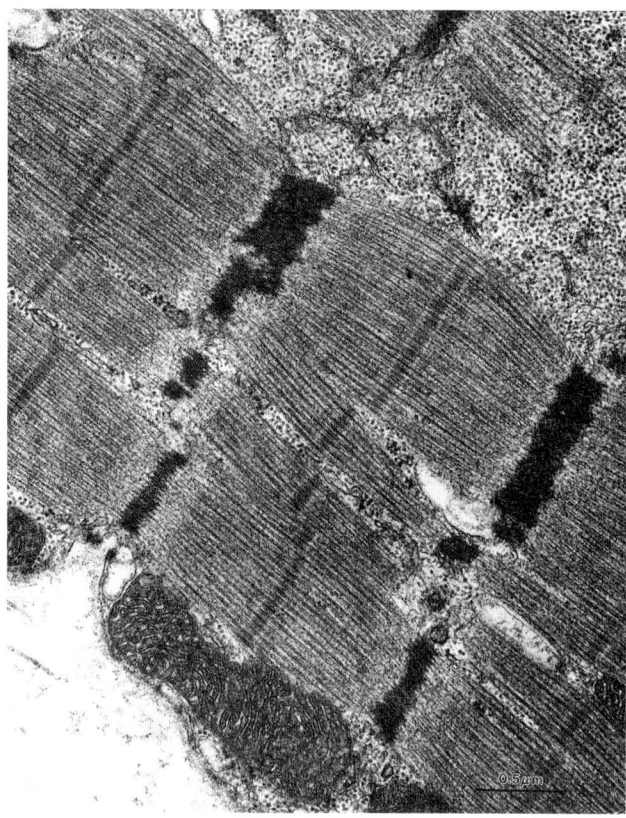

FIG. 1–56. Longitudinal section of normal dog cardiac sarcomeres showing Z-bands of different widths. The Z-band at the bottom left has the usual appearance, is well centered in the I-band, and the M-bands of adjacent sarcomeres are in register. The widened Z-band in the next sarcomere of the same myofilament bundle is taking up more of the I-band. The two widest Z-bands flanking a barrel-shaped A-band take up most of the I-band.

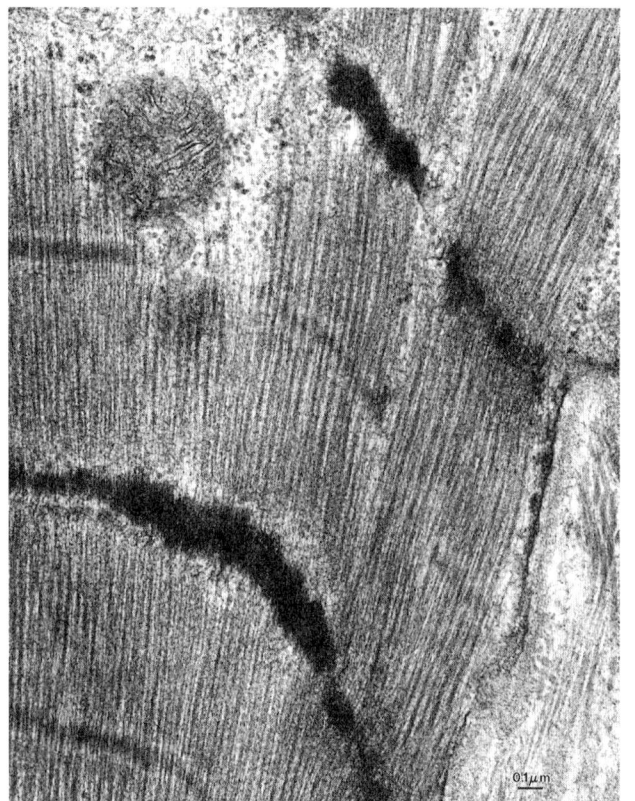

FIG. 1–55. Longitudinal section from human atrial biopsy showing widening of several Z-bands. Note loss of exact registration of thick and thin filaments within the sarcomeres. Edges of I, A, and M-bands are uneven.

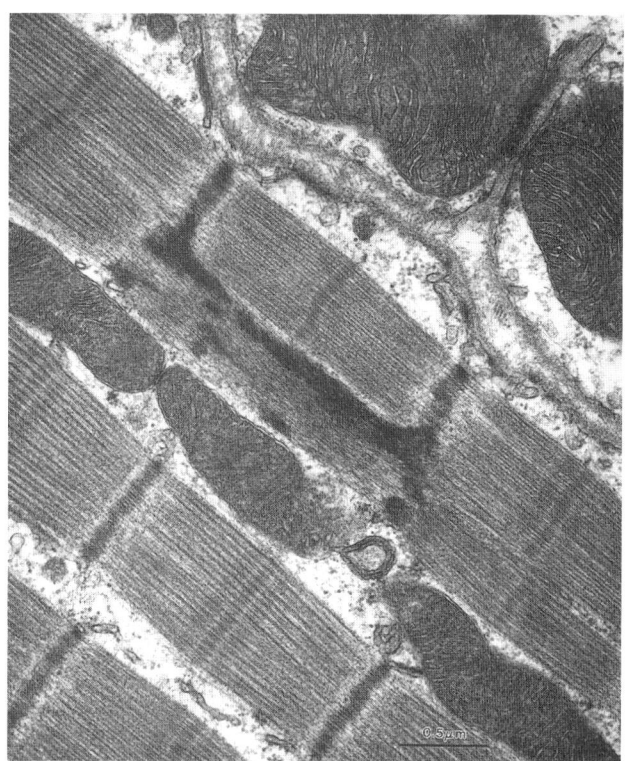

FIG. 1–57. Longitudinal section of papillary muscle taken from another normal dog showing the profile of Z-band material spanning the entire sarcomere length and maintaining continuity with adjacent sarcomeres both in the same myofilament bundle and in the adjacent myofilament bundle.

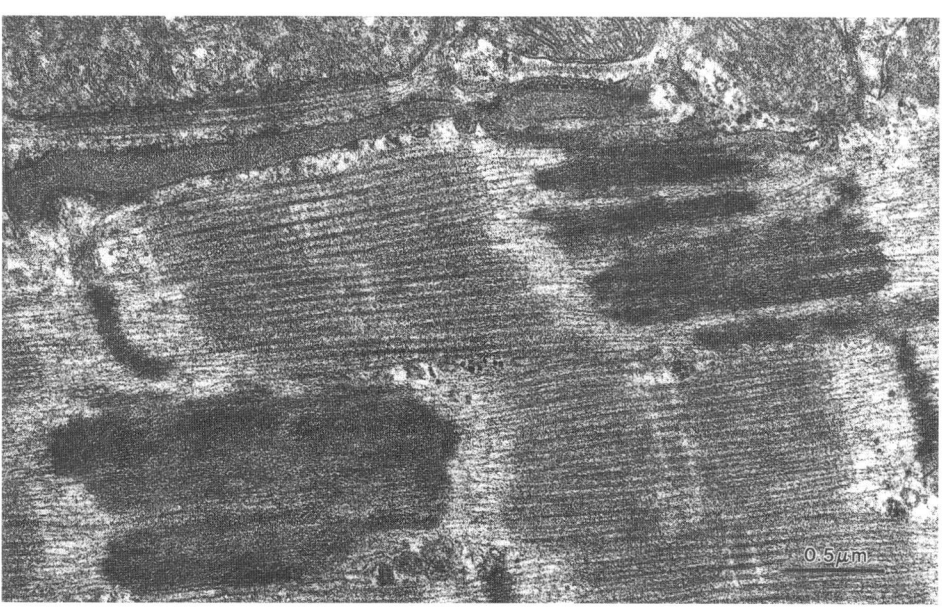

FIG. 1–58. Z-crystals in aged cat myocardium in several different orientations with respect to plane of section. All are aligned along the myofibril axis and all have thin filaments emerging into normal-looking A-bands with normal Z-bands at the opposite ends of these sarcomeres.

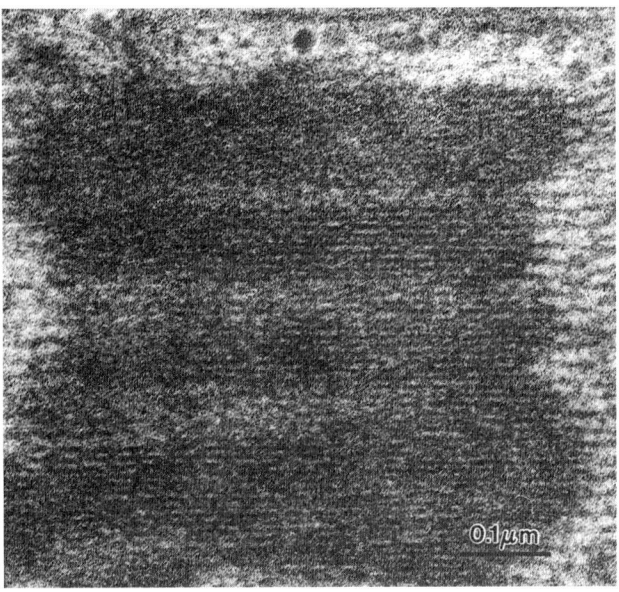

FIG. 1–59. Longitudinal section of Z-crystal or rod in normal dog papillary muscle. Note continuity of axial filaments with thin filaments in the adjacent I-band and chevron pattern of normal Z-band. The three-dimensional reconstructions of Z-rod and normal Z-band are very similar.

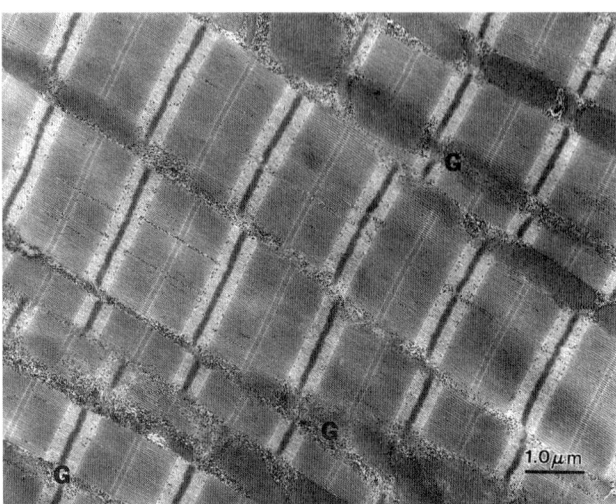

FIG. 1–61. High-voltage electron micrograph of half-micron section of dog cardiac muscle. The exact alignment of thick and thin filaments within each sarcomere gives reinforcement of the banding patterns, Z, I, A, M, but registration of adjacent myofilament bundles is not exact. Compare to high-magnification cross sections of thin sections of myofilaments shown in Figures 1–37, 1–41, and 1–46. Note the abundance of glycogen granules (G) in these thick sections.

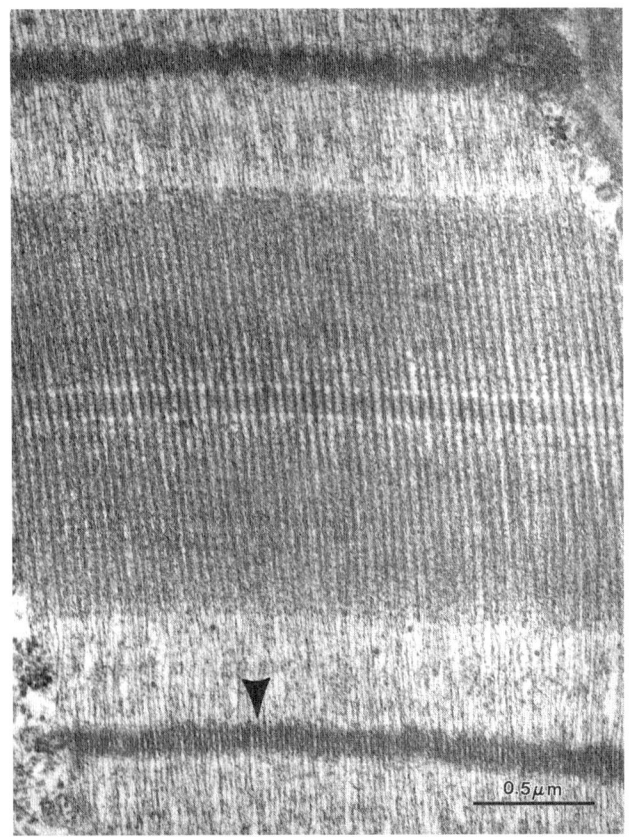

FIG. 1–60. Typical sarcomere seen in normal myofibers adjacent to dog heart cell containing Z-crystal shown in Figure 1–59. The A-band length is 1.56 µm. The 17 nm (1,1) orientation of the Z-band (*arrowhead*) where the thin filaments appear to pass through the Z-band lattice is one of the two orientations of the tetragonal Z-lattice that gives maximal reinforcement to the axial filaments.

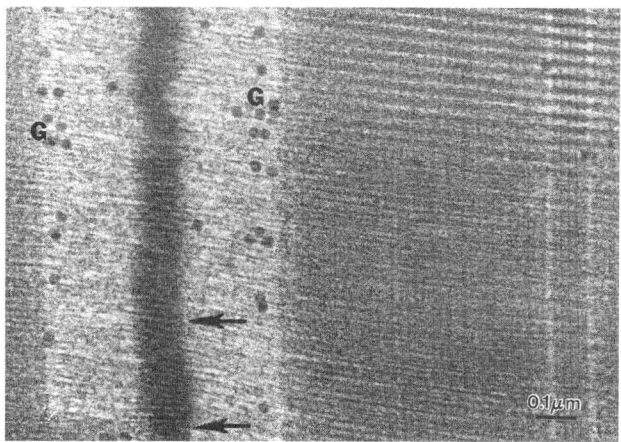

FIG. 1–62. High-voltage electron micrograph of half-micron section of cardiac muscle. Note the variation in Z-band width (i.e. number of lattice subunits in axial direction) occurring within a region of the same lattice orientation (*arrows*) and occurring in a region of changing orientation toward the top of the figure. The periodicities within the I, A, and M-bands are clearly visible. The glycogen granules (G) appear as black dots, mostly in I-band but also one or two in M-band.

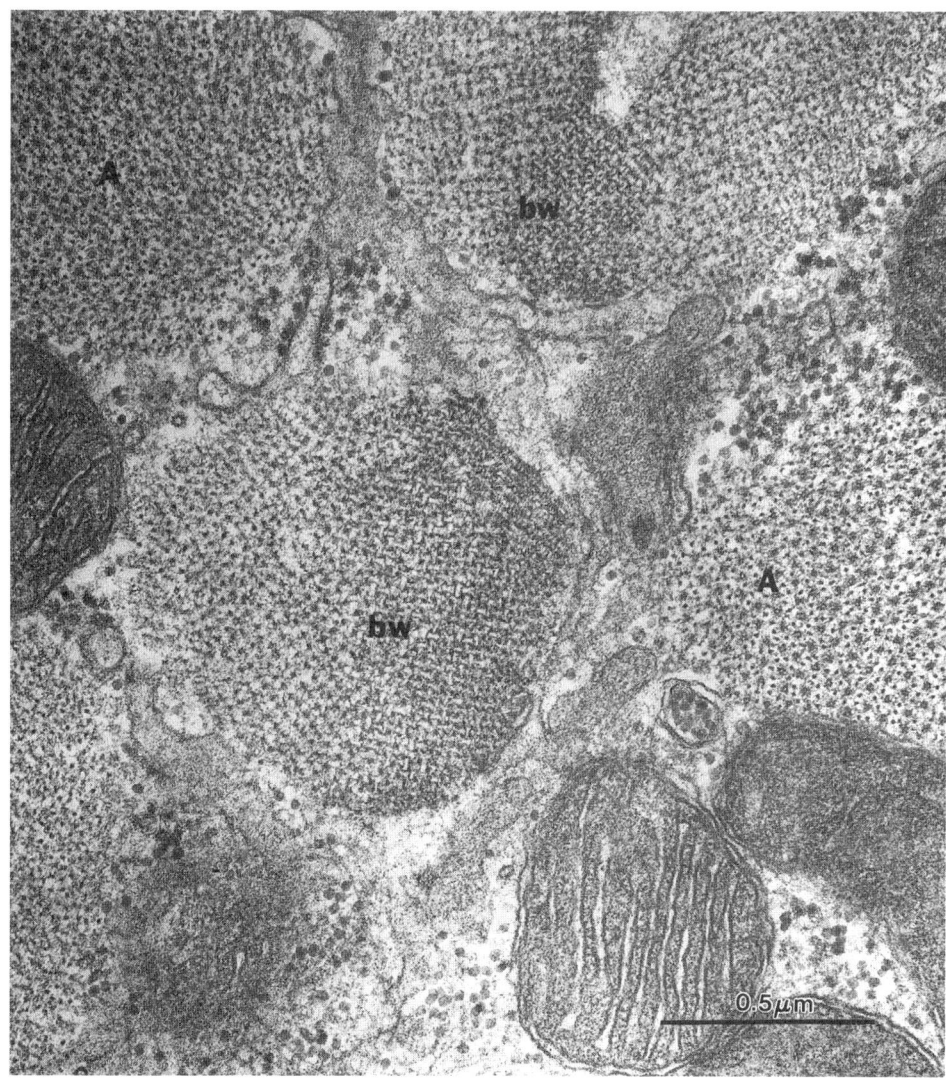

FIG. 1–63. Electron micrograph of unstimulated cardiac muscle in cross section showing the Z band in the bw form and the adjacent A-bands.

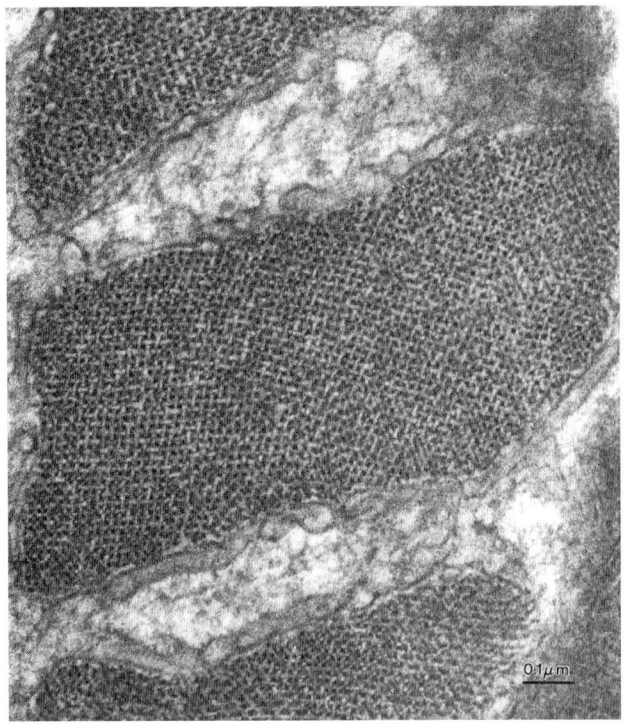

FIG. 1–64. Electron micrograph of a cross section of soleus perfusion-fixed during a tetanic contraction in situ. The bw form of the Z-lattice is predominant. (103) (Reprinted by permission of Kluwer Academic and Lippencott-Raven Publishers.)

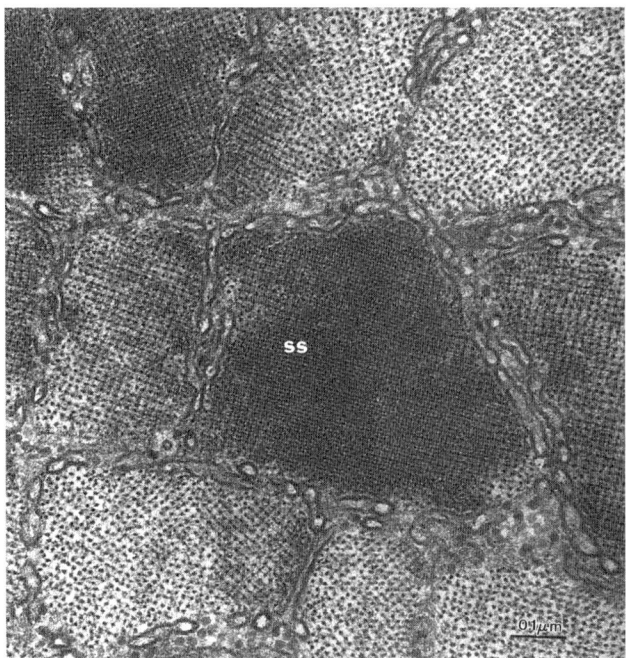

FIG. 1–66. Cross section of rat soleus muscle stretched in a muscle myograph in 100 mM PIPES buffer by applying a load of 6 g, adjusting for stress relaxation, and fixing at the final length achieved after 30 min at 6 g load. The average sarcomere length of this muscle preparation was 2.5 μm. The Z-band exhibits the small square (ss) lattice pattern.

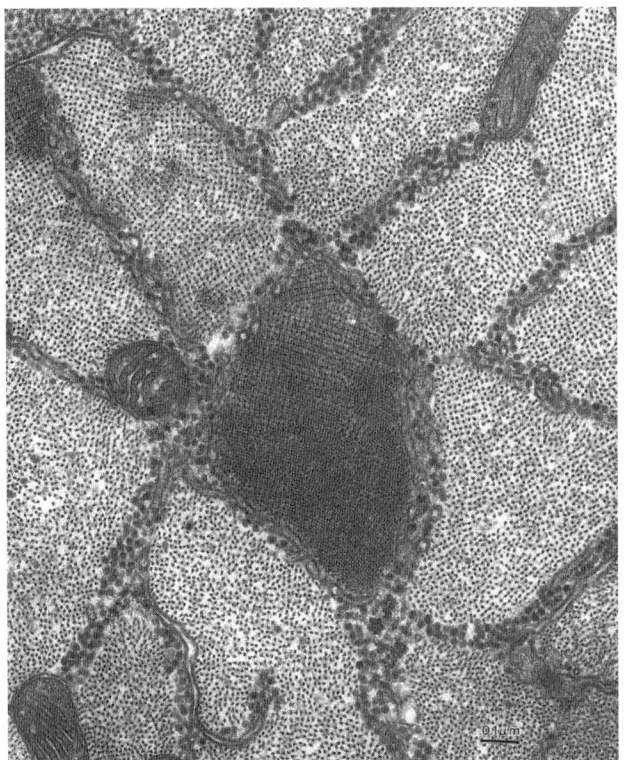

FIG. 1–65. Electron micrograph of a cross section of rat soleus muscle stretched in a muscle myograph in 100 mM PIPES buffer by applying a load of 3 g, adjusting for stress relaxation and fixing at the final length achieved after 30 min at 3 g load. The Z-lattice exhibits the small square (ss) pattern.

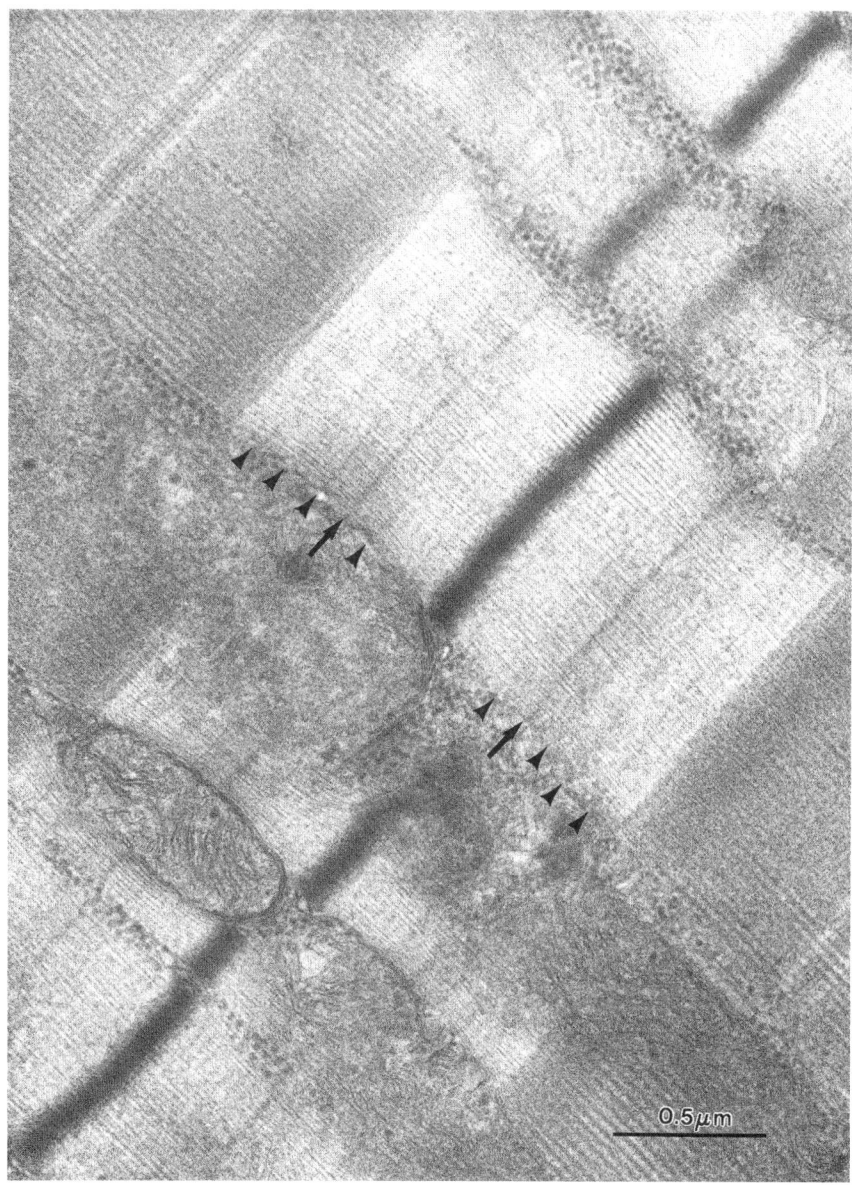

FIG. 1–67. Longitudinal section of adult rat soleus muscle stretched by a 6 g load in a bath containing 5 mM EGTA in 100 mM PIPES buffer, pH 7.2. At least five distinct stripes (*arrowheads*) are present in the I-band on either side of the Z-band, four of which are within a region of increased electron density as well as the N_2 line (*arrow*). Sarcomere lengths in this section average 3.35. Section is 200 nm thick, stained with uranyl acetate and Sato's lead stain, and photographed at 200 kV.

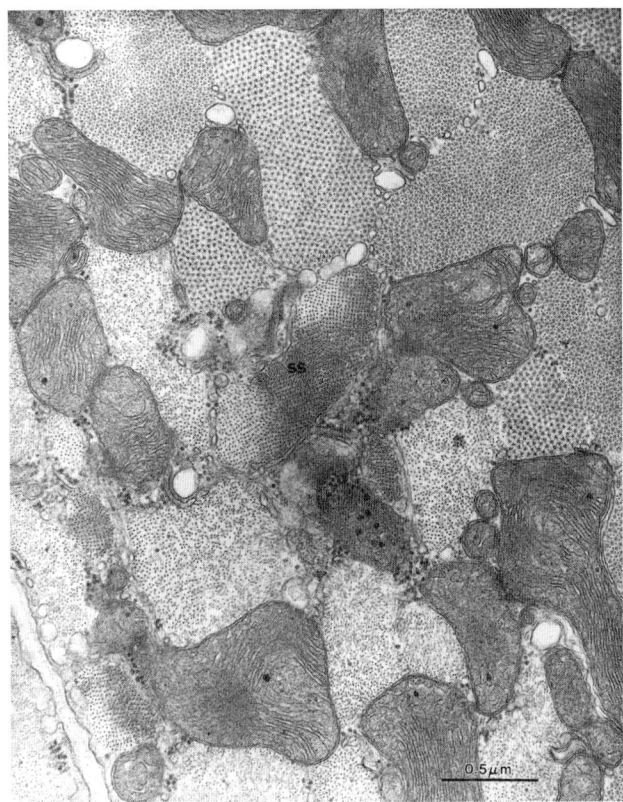

FIG. 1–68. Cross section of rat papillary muscle stretched in a bath containing 5 mM EGTA in 100 mM PIPES buffer, pH 7.2. Note the uniform small square (ss) appearance of the cardiac Z-band in relaxed muscle. Empty T-tubules and dark granules in mitochondria are both signs of altered calcium distribution in the cell due to chelation of calcium by EGTA.

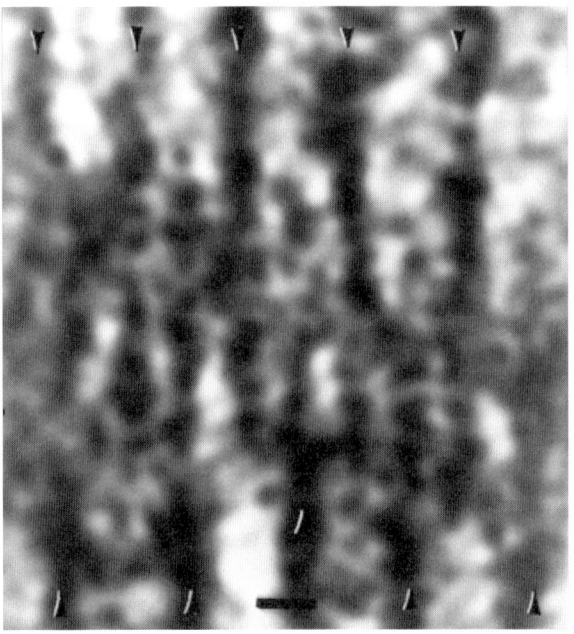

FIG. 1–70. A projection of a 25 nm-thick longitudinal section taken from a three-dimensional reconstruction of the Z-band from unstimulated skeletal muscle. Axial filaments enter the Z-band from top and bottom of the figure (*arrowheads*). Crossconnecting Z-filaments appear to connect the axial filaments in this "chevron" (1,0) orientation projection (scale bar = 10nm). (276) (Reprinted by permission of Rockefeller University Press.)

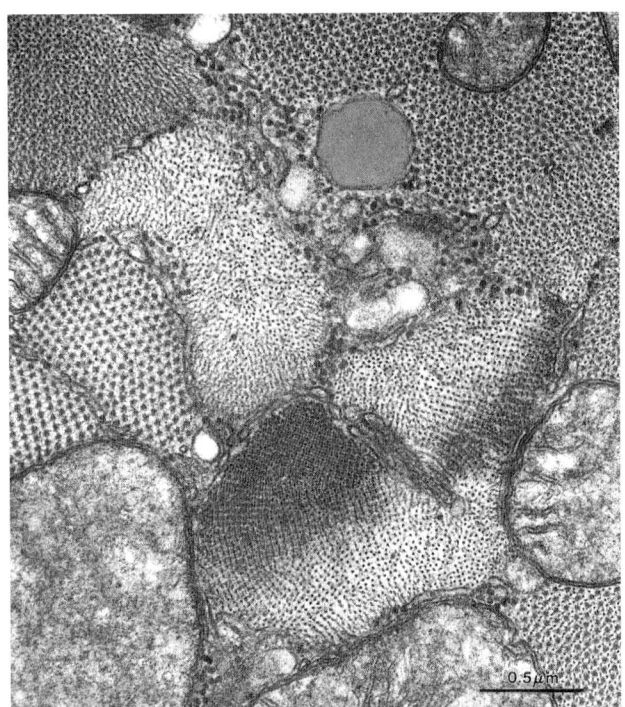

FIG. 1–69. Electron micrograph of EGTA treated cardiac muscle in cross section showing the Z-band in the ss form. (102) (Reprinted by permission of the American Physiological Society.)

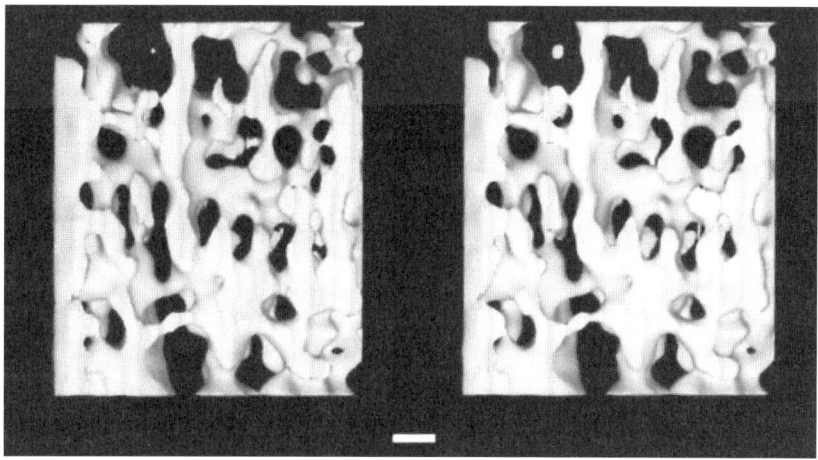

FIG. 1–71. A stereo-shaded solid rendering of the three-dimensional reconstruction of Plate 1. Compare to Figures 1–72 and 1–74; scale bar = 10 nm.

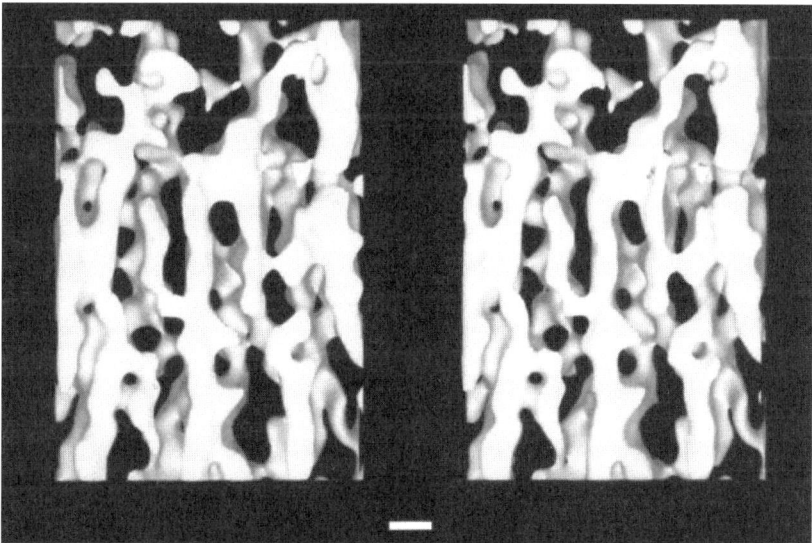

FIG. 1–72. Stereo-shaded solid rendering of a longitudinal section from a three-dimensional reconstruction of rigor skeletal muscle. Axial filaments enter from the top and bottom of the figure and are interconnected at the edges of the Z-band by an array of cross-connecting Z-filaments. There appear to be fewer crossconnections in this rigor Z-band than in the unstimulated muscle shown in Plate 1 and Figures 1–70 and 1–71. The vertical spacing between crossconnections is larger than in the unstimulated muscle; scale bar = 10 nm.

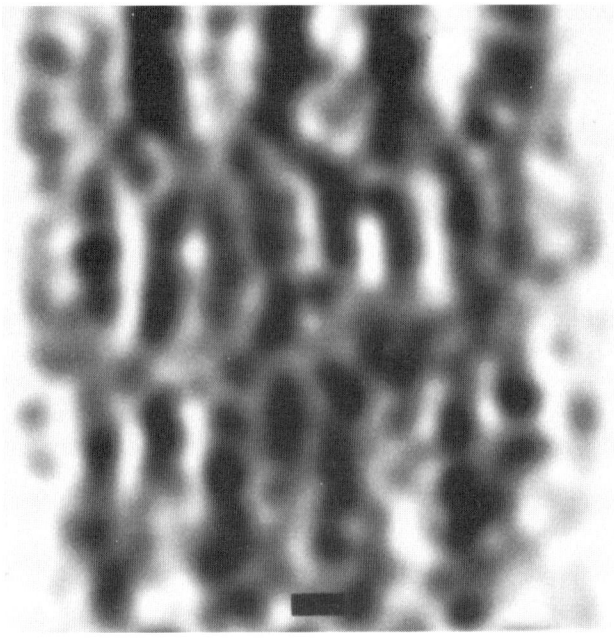

FIG. 1–73. Projection of a 20 nm longitudinal slice from a preliminary three-dimensional reconstruction of unstimulated cardiac Z-band. Compare similar projection view of longitudinal slice from three-dimensional reconstruction of unstimulated skeletal muscle sseen in Figure 1–70; scale bar = 10 nm.

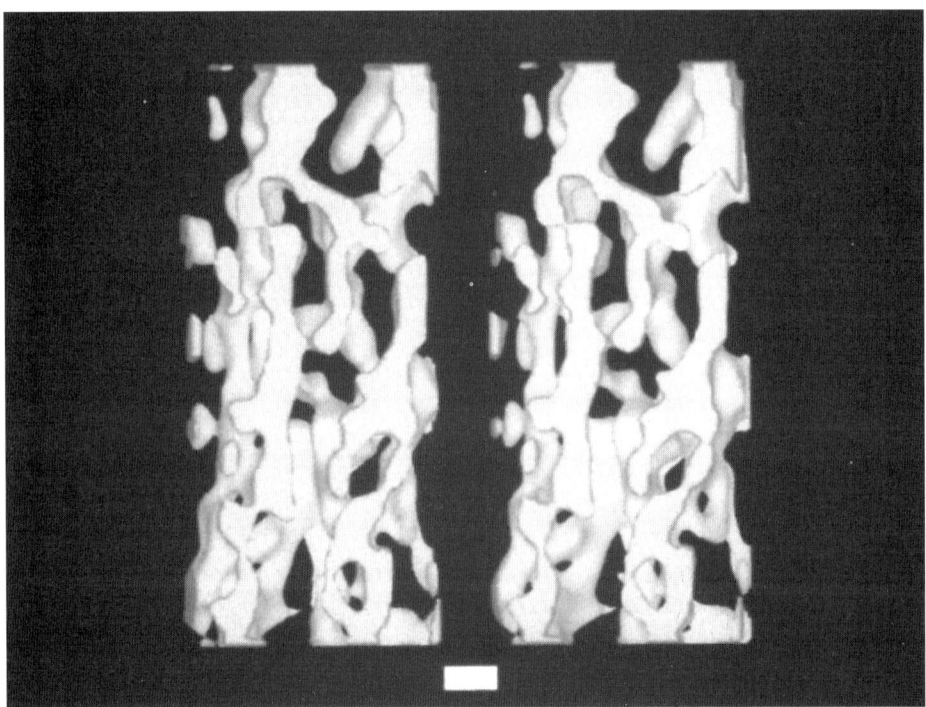

FIG. 1–74. Grey-scale shaded solid stereo pair of a portion of a three-dimensional reconstruction of the Z-band lattice in unstimulated rat cardiac muscle, shown in a longitudinal orientation. This muscle exhibits the basket weave form of the lattice in cross section. Thin axial filaments enter the Z-band from the top and bottom the figure, where they are interconnected by an array of Z-band cross-connecting filaments. In this view, the cross-connecting filaments attach at intervals of ~20 nm along the axial filament; scale bar = 10 nm.

coordinated through the Z-band and how mechanical forces are transmitted through various structural levels down to the Z-band. Recognition of the Z-band as an integral part of the contractile lattice is starting to occur, but the importance of the Z-band and its contribution to the contractile process is not yet appreciated.

We anticipate that much work will be done in the next five to ten years to understand the relationship between three-dimensional structure below the nanometer level and the transfer of energies and rearrangement of contractile components necessary to meet functional demands. The structure of thick and thin filaments is not a finished story. As our understanding of muscle physiology becomes more sophisticated and we assign precise functions to previously known "structural components," we may be forced to find new structures below the nanometer level to explain new physiological puzzles.

APPENDIX: IMAGING AND ANALYZING CARDIAC ULTRASTRUCTURE

Until the invention of the electron microscope (EM), optical microscopy was the tool of choice for examination of cardiac structure. Optical techniques were essential in delineating the structure of the myocardium by recognizing such basic elements as the sarcolemma (17), the intercalated disk (53, 148, 320), the myofibril and sarcomere (17, 149, 173), and other fundamental structures (5, 149). With the advent of the electron microscope, these structures could be studied at much higher resolution (1 nm for the EM vs 200 nm for the conventional optical microscope). Despite lower resolution, optical microscopes are still used in comparative studies, since fluorescent labeling of important structures is possible with optical microscopy, as is the ability to avoid heavy metal staining, some EM fixation artifacts, and the inevitable damage that the electron beam does to the specimen. In particular, optical confocal microscopes have been used in complementary studies to provide optical resolution three-dimensional information. Probe microscopies such as atomic force microscopy promise to provide even more choices for the ultrastructural examination of cardiac muscle.

Concurrent advances in electron microscopy have driven the resolution of the scanning electron microscope to the ~1 nm figure attainable in biological transmission electron microscopy (TEM), while the development of the environmental scanning electron microscope (SEM) has aided in the reduction of dehydration artifacts. The development of field emission electron guns and such devices as imaging energy filters has produced higher contrast images. As with optical microscopy, computerized acquisition and postacquisition image processing have aided in the enhancement and quantification of image properties, as well as the possibility of reconstruction of cardiac structures in three dimensions.

Transmission Electron Microscopy

Electrons are used in a variety of ways to image cardiac muscle. Most commonly, magnetic lenses direct electrons emitted by an electron source (gun) through a thin tissue specimen to a focal plane, in a manner analogous to light microscope imaging. However, imaging by TEM introduces several complications to the imaging process, all of which affect the quality and interpretability of the image. Spherical aberration of the magnetic lenses requires a very small aperture in the system. This limits the resolution of the microscope to something in the neighborhood of .1–.5 nm, and increases the depth of field to several microns (200). TEM images are therefore approximate two-dimensional projections of objects containing much three-dimensional information (123). This effect can make interpretation of a single micrograph difficult due to the superposition of many different structures. On the other hand, projected views acquired at many different angles may be combined to reconstruct the three-dimensional structure of the section (134). Thin sectioning of the material becomes necessary to decrease the confusion of many superposed structures as well as to increase the resolution of tomographically reconstructed images (245). Since the electron beam is coherent, additional interference effects modulate the microscope transfer function, affecting the resolving power of the instrument. The interference effects also result in opposite contrast for differing spatial frequencies (feature sizes) in the image. The situation is complicated further since the sample typically exhibits both phase and amplitude contrast, with relative strengths varying depending upon sample physical properties and preparation effects (60). These effects may be adjusted by modifying the point of focus and energy of the electrons. Chromatic aberration (energy spread) of the electrons emitted from the gun may also introduce artifacts reducing resolution in the final image. Chromatic aberration effects can be minimized by employing a field emission gun, which provides a much narrower energy spread than do thermal emission electron sources (52).

Unstained tissue is not an efficient electron scatterer at the 10–1000 kV energies used in standard and high-voltage TEM. Tissue postfixed in osmium tetroxide exhibits more electron scatter because of the osmium bound to proteins and phospholipids. Additional scattering can come from heavy metal stains such as uranyl acetate, lead citrate, and methylamine tungstate. These stains may be degraded or may migrate upon exposure to the electron beam (19, 131).

Despite the relative transparency of muscle tissue to electrons, a damaging amount of energy may be deposited into the specimen. Shrinkage of thin sections of 30%–50% upon exposure to conventional dose (> 100 electrons/angstrom squared) has been reported (12, 38, 181). Thus, many studies rely upon an initial exposure of the specimen so that it will become stable in the beam. It is possible to reduce shrinkage effects by employing a low-temperature cryo-holder for the thin section (92, 183). Many workers have introduced methods to reduce the total dose to the specimen (20, 22, 334), and doses as low as 10–20 electrons/square angstrom have been attained.

Scanning Electron Microscopies

Scanning microscopies depend upon scanning a small (<10 nm) electron beam spot across the specimen. Simultaneously, a detector picks up a signal induced by the scanned beam. The signal normally consists of secondary electrons emitted by the surface layers of the specimen. Since the secondary electron emission fraction depends on the angle between the surface and the scanned beam, EMS images typically provide a quite striking shaded rendering of the specimen surface. Additionally, since the effective aperture is on the order of the beam size, a very large depth of field (at low magnifications, much larger than that for optical microscopes) results (62, 150). Newer high-resolution scanning electron microscopes (HRSEM) with field emission electron guns can attain resolutions <1 nm, as good as that for TEM (94, 151). Images may be formed with accelerating voltages ranging from near zero to 40 kV, with the lower voltages more compatible with high resolution (19, 233). The conventional scanning microscopy technique is limited in that only the surface is imaged. As with TEM the specimen must be initially fixed by chemical or freezing methods. Dehydration then stabilizes the specimen for exposure to the microscope vacuum chamber. It is usually necessary to coat the surface with a conductor such as gold, chromium, or carbon to avoid charging effects (87). The scanning electron microscope may provide more easily interpretable images from freeze-fractured and freeze-etched specimens (see below), since specimen surface topography is more easily visualized than with TEM.

In addition to imaging with the secondary electrons, scanning electron microscopes may also make use of signals consisting of backscattered electrons (150, 260), Auger electrons (94, 187), cathodoluminescent emission of light (52, 133), transmitted electrons (172, 200), or even X-ray emission induced by the incident beam (68). The spectrum of the backscattered electrons may be used to detect the elemental composition of the sample surface, but at a much lower resolution (~1000 nm) than the secondary electron image (8, 259). The X-ray emission can provide a higher resolution compositional map through analysis of the spectrum of the emitted X-rays in a process known as energy dispersive spectroscopy (EDS) (68, 116, 147). The transmitted electrons may be used to form an image comparable to that from a standard transmission electron microscope (37, 58, 172, 200), as well as to detect specimen thickness effects and composition through electron energy loss spectroscopy (EELS) (59, 147).

A relatively recent innovation known as environmental scanning electron microscopy (ESEM) employs a small aperture to isolate a relatively high pressure (0.1–50 torr) sample chamber from the high vacuum (10^{-7} torr) column of the microscope. This provides an environment in which modestly hydrated samples may be observed with the enhanced depth of field of scanning EM. Unfortunately, in the higher pressure environmental SEM, the secondary electrons do not have enough energy to reach the detector, forcing reliance on the higher energy backscattered electrons to form a lower resolution image (46, 94).

Specimen Preparation

Specimen preparation can induce artifacts in a microscope image. Indeed, despite its lower resolution, optical microscopy provides the advantage that less specimen preparation is required than for nearly any type of electron microscopy. This is due to the EM requirement that samples be stabilized for exposure to high voltage electrons in a vacuum. Before a specimen is viewed in the electron microscope, it must generally be fixed, embedded for ease of sectioning, and stained so that it exhibits enough contrast to produce an interpretable image (200, 207). For electron microscopy, specimens may be prepared by the more standard room temperature techniques employing chemical fixation, or they may be prepared by rapid cooling employing cryogens.

(Near) Room Temperature Preparation. Fixation refers to the process of halting biological or chemical activity in the sample and stabilizing the tissue so that the sample structure will be preserved during the further preparative steps, as well as during imaging. Fixation may be performed by excising tissue and immersing it in fixative or by perfusion of the material. In either case, the chemical fixative diffuses into the tissue, stopping chemical reactions and crosslinking the material. Since diffusion times are on the order of minutes, the region fixed in a somewhat natural state

is considered to be within 1 mm of the surface (124, 135). Osmium tetroxide was initially employed as a primary fixative. It has the advantage that its heavy metal component also provides staining contrast. However, it is a slow diffuser, inactivates enzymes, and slowly denatures proteins. Additionally, OsO_4 aggregates DNA and causes some swelling of the material (52). Aldehyde fixation (formaldehyde, acrolein, glutaraldehyde) is superior to osmium alone, though OsO_4 is often employed as a secondary fixative after aldehyde fixation (19, 259). Glutaraldehyde is a rapid diffuser but reacts only with some phospholipids, hence the usual employment of a secondary fixative. Glutaraldehyde also inactivates some enzymes. It is known to cause shrinkage of the specimen (52, 91, 159).

After fixation, the sample is embedded (usually in a resinous plastic) to preserve the structure during sectioning, staining, and exposure to the electron beam (177). Originally done with wax, there are now a number of plastic embedding materials that allow sectioning on an ultramicrotome to produce slices as thin as 40 nm (177, 331). The specimen is initially dehydrated by immersion in an agent such as ethanol or acetone. Then the embedding medium is infiltrated into the specimen (282). Epoxide resins such as Araldite or LX112 are soluble in the dehydrating agent and are thus easily infused into the sample, where they are polymerized with heat or ultraviolet radiation (19, 177, 282). However, there are water-soluble resins, which can be infused into the tissue without solubulizing the lipids (145, 208, 282).

After fixation, the sample is ready for sectioning and staining. Staining with heavy metal electron scatterers increases contrast in the image. Positive staining, usually with uranyl acetate, may be performed before (en bloc) or after sectioning of the material. Counterstaining is most often done with lead citrate. Heavy metal stains of uranium, tungsten, and molybdenum can be used as negative stains for vesicles, filaments, and isolated proteins, where the stain surrounds the materials of interest and the final image approximates a negative of the projected material distribution in the sample (52). Uranyl stains are thought to interact with proteins by an ionic mechanism, and are also mordants for lead stains. In general the precise physical mechanism of stain interaction with the specimen is not well understood. Stains are subject to electron beam–induced damage or migration depending on the type of stain, the beam brightness, and beam energy.

Low-Temperature Preparation Methods. Fixation by conventional methods has the disadvantage that biological activity in the fixed material ceases only as the fixative diffusion front infuses the sample, i.e. in times of seconds to minutes. Rapid freezing of the sample (in times ranging from <1 msec to somewhat less than 1 sec for some SEM applications) can avoid artifacts resulting from the speed and nonuniformity of chemical fixation and embedding (225, 236, 261, 289). Rapid freezing may be accomplished by plunging the sample into a cryogen, such as liquid nitrogen–cooled propane, with a plunge-freezing device that ensures heat transfers in the range of 90,000°C/sec (52, 68). Even such rapid freezing induces ice crystal formation, but the surface layers (typically to a depth of 10–15 μm) are frozen rapidly enough that the ice remains amorphous, preserving the structure (6, 52). High-pressure freezing of the sample can extend the preservation depth to as much as .5 mm, comparable to the best attainable with chemical fixation (160). Other methods of rapid freezing for cardiac tissue are jet freezing, where the sample is sandwiched between two metal sheets that are cooled by jets of cryogen (68), and slam freezing, in which the sample is rapidly brought into contact with a cryogenically cooled polished metal mirror (52). Slam freezing allows the intriguing possibility of freezing an entire fiber, so that the surface layers, at least, are fixed under physiological conditions in 1–2 msec (45, 215, 285).

There are several methods of processing for microscopic examination after rapid freezing, some of which preserve structural detail, while others excel in localization of cytochemical reaction products. It is possible to transfer the cryo-fixed sample to a cryo-microtome, where it may be sectioned at low temperatures (280, 348). The sections may then be maintained at low temperature and transferred directly to a cryo-holder for examination in the microscope. Unfortunately, the contrast of such a specimen is quite low, so that additional heavy metal staining is usually required (19). Also, since light microscope examination is skipped in this procedure, it may be necessary to image a large number of samples to find one with proper preservation and correct orientation for the desired structures. Such problems can be avoided by the techniques of cryo-substitution (freeze substitution) in which the sample is raised to a temperature (typically −80°C) for dehydration in acetone or methanol, followed by infusion of chemical fixative. In this technique, the sample is maintained at too low a temperature for significant chemical activity to occur during fixative infusion. When the sample temperature is raised, the material is fixed simultaneously in all regions as the fixative reaches its active temperature (128, 261). Excellent preservation of muscle structures has been reported with this technique (40, 226). The sample is finally brought to room temperature for embedding, sectioning and staining. In a related but time-consuming method, the sample is freeze-dried by molecular distillation at low temperatures for 5–7 days. The temperature is then raised to −40°C, and the sample is infused with a low-temperature resin such as Lowicryl. The resin is polymerized with UV radiation before raising the temperature for sectioning and staining (176). Alternatively, fixative or stain may be infused into the freeze-dehydrated sample.

Related low-temperature techniques are freeze-fracture and freeze-etch, which avoid full fixation, as well as embedding, sectioning, and staining steps. For freeze-fracture, the sample is first lightly fixed to prevent shrinkage before infusion with a cryoprotectant such as 20%–25% glycerol. Rapid freezing is then followed by specimen fracture at low temperature in a vacuum chamber, after which the fractured surface is evaporatively coated with layers of metal and carbon. The specimen is then removed from the chamber and the replica metal-carbon layers are floated off for examination in the microscope (52, 83, 228). The replica is particularly useful in the imaging of membranes and intermembrane protein distributions (19, 321). Freeze-etching refers to an additional step in the process. After fracture of the specimen, water is extracted from the fractured surface by vacuum sublimation onto a metal surface. This process enhances protein relief (113).

While cryo-techniques avoid some of the artifacts resulting from conventional preparation, they have disadvantages. A primary difficulty is that only surface layers are well preserved in the most commonly used techniques. Also, the freezing front has been observed to be non-uniform, so that all structures are not preserved equally, even near the surface (52). Finally, slam freezing experiments must be carefully tailored to the particular specimen, so as to avoid crushing artifacts on the specimen surface(45). Nevertheless, these techniques have provided a wealth of information and are particularly useful in cytochemical and immunocytochemical studies (52, 261).

Cytochemistry and Immunocytochemistry

Cytochemistry and immunocytochemistry refer to methods used to locate and visualize reaction products, enzymes, and numerous other structures such as proteins. Since chemical fixation may disrupt reaction product spatial location or interfere with antigenicity, both techniques benefit from cryopreservation techniques (7, 52, 197).

Cytochemistry has been classically employed with chemical fixation to locate reaction products, enzymes, and calcium in the cell. Unfortunately, aldehyde fixation is known to deactivate enzymes to an extent depending upon the fixative. Formaldehyde, though a weak crosslinker, is preferred in this case because it inactivates a narrower range of enzymes (331). Cryofixation avoids these problems, but at the expense of a much smaller (~15 μm) depth of fixation. After fixation, the tissues are sectioned and exposed to stains that may label such cellular entities as enzymes, polysaccharides, or calcium. Unfortunately, it is often necessary to disrupt or permeabilize cellular membranes to infuse the labeling stains. These necessarily disrupt cellular structure to some extent. Typical stains used in electron microscopic visualization include peroxidase, lanthanum, lead, ferritin, and some silver stains (52). Colloidal gold may be conjugated to lectins or to enzymes such as phospholipase A2. Colloidal gold comes in a variety of diameters from 1 nm to 200 nm and thus will unambiguously label target sites (108, 125, 141, 264). Problems with the cytochemical approaches include nonspecific binding, diffusion of the target, and loss of reactivity during fixation.

A wide range of substances in the myocardium may be visualized using antibody labeling (294). This immunocytochemical procedure can correctly localize many complex substances, but it is not useful for simple reaction products such as calcium. Polyclonal or monoclonal antibodies are raised to a known target. The Fab region of the antibody is then infused into the tissue before fixation to bind to its target sites (126, 239). Alternatively, the surface may be labeled after fixation and staining, though this may result in artifacts caused by diffusion or loss of antigenicity during such processing (126, 263). Antibodies may be visualized by comparing images of similar structures with and without labeling, or by attaching labeling or staining compounds to them. Both ferritin and peroxidase may be conjugated with antibodies to provide staining density. Nonspecific binding can cause problems with ferritin, while peroxidase, which provides good visualization in the light microscope, may be compromised by the existence of endogenous peroxidase activity. However, these labeling materials have the advantage that they may diffuse through membranes and thus do not require structural disruption to function (52). Nonspecific labeling may be reduced by adding compounds such as bovine serum albumin to competitively bind to nonspecific "sticky" sites (141). Gold labeling of the antibody has the advantage that the bound gold particles are very electron dense, and do not occur naturally in biological material. Unfortunately, the gold labels are usually too large to penetrate cells and so demand some structural modification for binding. Gold labels can be colloidal gold (1–200 nm in diameter), or small gold clusters such as nanogold (20 gold atoms, 1.4 nm in diameter) or undecagold (11 gold atoms, diameter 0.8 nm) (9, 114, 115, 141, 323). The undecagold particles are small enough that they are hard to resolve in simple images of tissue, and so image processing may be required to discover their locations (114, 115).

Confocal Optical Microscopy

Confocal optical microscopy employs a highly focused, scanned beam from a laser or other light source to build up an image of the specimen. The scanned beam images structures in the focal plane. Coupled with computerized deconvolution techniques, this "optical sectioning" can image a region as thin as 0.7 μm, eliminating the image clutter resulting from depth-of-field effects in a conventional optical microscope. By varying the plane of focus between image scans, a stack of optical sections may be observed, from which a three-dimensional representation of the specimen can be generated (18, 39, 170). Additionally, the scanning of coherent light from a laser source results in an improvement of ~40% in lateral resolution over conventional light microscopy (39, 232).

Though the resolution of the confocal microscope is limited to that obtainable optically, it may be used for observation of dynamic events (at frame rates up to 30/sec) in living cells (146). Additionally, it may be used with fluorescent labeling to identify structures or reaction products of interest (202, 287). This microscopy is often used in conjunction with electron microscopy analysis to relate ultrastructure to dynamics.

Scanning Probe Microscopies

Scanning probe microscopies depend upon the measurement of an interaction property of a sample surface with a probe that is piezoelectrically scanned across it. The scanning tunneling microscope (STM) was the first such device. STM detects the tunneling current between a tiny probe tip and a conductive surface, and so requires coating of biological material with a conductor (1, 67, 117, 332). A related technique, atomic force microscopy (AFM) uses a cantilever arrangement to measure the force between the probe tip and the sample surface (67, 117, 167, 192). AFM has the advantage that images may be collected of nonconductive materials on solute-covered surfaces, so that the specimen may be fully hydrated. The height and in-plane resolution of these microscopies depend upon both the type of sample and the particular mode in which the microscope is operated. At best, the AFM can resolve surface contours of <1 nm with an in-plane resolution as good as that of electron microscopy (192). Of course, only surface information is collected; internal structure remains invisible. Additionally, the scanning rate must be limited to avoid perturbation of the sample surface, and so it is difficult to image dynamic structural changes. AFM has been used to characterize membrane channel architecture in cardiac membrane preparations (168), as well as the force-extension relation for titin (175a).

Image Processing and Analysis

Stereology and Morphometric Analysis. Ultrastructural analysis benefits from quantitation of morphological changes associated with differing muscle states. Quantitative measurements of numbers, surface areas, and volumes, among other features, can link structural changes to functional or disease states. These measurements may be made on digitized images using computer software to aid in the analysis or on micrograph prints. If the objects of interest are large enough that a single section may be regarded as a two-dimensional planar slice through the objects, the statistical methods of stereology can be applied to generate three-dimensional information from the initial measurements (21). These methods assume that the sections are randomly oriented and that the organelles of interest are randomly and isotropically distributed in the section volume (252). In the case of highly anisotropic structures such as the sarcomere, three-dimensional statistics can still be generated if the sections are collected isotropically or if the shape and orientation of the measured object is known (252).

Image Enhancement. Numerous computer methods now exist to enhance or make more visible objects of interest. Contrast manipulation by stretching, histogram equalization, or imposition of a upper or lower contour level can make dim or hard to differentiate components visible (206, 219). Image averaging (similar to Markham rotation or translation) may be used on presumed identical instances of the same structural component, once an appropriate translational and rotational alignment has been performed (78, 235). Similar to image averaging are the various forms of image enhancement that depend upon averaging or filtering of a regular lattice. These procedures are aimed primarily at increasing the signal-to-noise ratio in the image by discarding components judged to be noise (269, 275, 290). The impact of computerized image processing techniques has been primarily to aid in the visualization and characterization of hard to image or hard to quantitate structures. Image processing has been especially successful in providing interpretable images from the lower contrast techniques of cryo-electron microscopy (266).

Three-Dimensional Reconstruction. Imaging by TEM or STEM provides an image that approximates a projection of the three-dimensional structure of a thin section of tissue (123). Computer-aided mathematical techniques can be used to proceed from such projection data to the full three-dimensional structure of the objects (42, 49, 80). For larger structures for which the projection approximates a two-dimensional slice through the specimen, the techniques of serial section reconstruction can be used to characterize the three-dimensional structure (186, 190). For smaller objects, the three-dimensional structure can be derived from a set of tomographic projections taken at different angles (79, 80, 134, 245). A disadvantage of this latter technique is the requirement for a large enough number of projections so that beam damage to the specimen can become an important confounding factor. Methods for low-dose and automated tomographic data collection have somewhat alleviated this difficulty, but interaction of the specimen with the electron beam is still a significant problem (20, 50). If the specimen shows crystalline order, only a few projections may be necessary (49, 201, 246); otherwise a much larger data set (e.g. one degree tilt intervals) must be collected. In the later case the resulting structure will also be degraded in certain directions due to the difficulty of rotating the specimen through a full 180 degrees in the microscope (134, 245).

We gratefully acknowledge the technical assistance provided by the late David Murphy. We are grateful to Dr. Joy Frank for Figures 1–7 through 1–16. We thank Dr. Joy Frank and Mr. R. J. Edwards for helpful discussions. Support for this work was provided by grant HL17376 from the National Heart, Lung, and Blood Institute and by a NASA grant for the COSMOS program.

REFERENCES

1. Amrein, M. and H. Gross. Scanning tunneling microscopy of biological macromolecular structures coated with a conductive film. *Scanning Microsc.* 6:335–342, 1992.
2. Ashurst, D. E. The Z-line: its structure and evidence for the presence of connecting filaments. In Tregear, R. T., ed., *Insect Flight Muscle* Amsterdam: North-Holland 1977:57–73.
3. Ayoob, J. C., K. K., Turnacioglu, B., Mittal, J. M. Sanger, and J. W. Sanger. Targeting of cardiac muscle titin fragments to the Z-bands and dense bodies of living muscle and non-muscle cells. *Cell Motil. Cytoskel.* 45:67–82, 2000.
4. Bard, F. and C. Franzini-Armstrong. Extra actin filaments at the periphery of skeletal muscle myofibrils. *Tissue Cell* 23:191–197, 1991.
5. Barer, R. The structure of the striated muscle fibre, *Biol. Rev.* 23:159–200, 1948.
6. Barnard, T. Rapid freezing techniques and cryoprotection of biomedical specimens. *Scanning Microsc.* 1:1217–1224, 1987.
7. Baskin, T. I., D. D. Miller, J. W. Vos, J. E. Wilson and P. K. Hepler. Cryofixing single cells and multicellular specimens enhances structure and immunocytochemistry for light microscopy. *J. Microsc.* 182(Pt 2):149–161, 1996.
8. Becker, R. P. and J. S. Geoffroy, Backscattered electron imaging for the life sciences: Introduction and index to applications—1961 to 1980. *Scanning Electron Microsc.* 4:195–206, 1981.
9. Beesley, J. F. Bioapplication of colloidal gold in microbiological immunocytochemistry. *Scanning Microsc.* 2:1055–1068, 1988.
10. Behr, T., P. Fischer, W. Muller-Felber, M. Schmidt-Achert and D. Pongratz. Myofibrillogenesis in primary tissue cultures of adult human skeletal muscle: expression of desmin, titin, and nebulin. *Clin. Invest.* 72:150–5, 1994.
11. Belkin, A. M., N. I. Zhidkova and V. E. Koteliansky. Localization of talin in skeletal and cardiac muscles. *FEBS Lett* 200:32–36, 1986.
12. Bennett, P. M. Decrease in section thickness on exposure to the electron beam; the use of tilted sections in estimating the amount of shrinkage. *J. Cell Sci.* 15:693–701, 1974.
13. Berne, R. and M. Levy. Contraction of muscle cells. In *Physiology* 2nd ed. St. Louis: C. V. Mosby, 1988:315–334.
14. Bishop S. F. and C. R. Cole. Ultrastructure changes in canine myocardium with right ventricular hypertrophy and congestive heart failure. *Lab. Invest.* 20:219–229, 1969.
15. Blanchard, A., O. Vasken and D. Critchley. The structure and function of alpha-actinin. *J. Musc. Res. Cell Motil.* 10:280–289, 1989.
16. Borg, T. K., and J. B. Caulfield. Morphology of connective tissue in skeletal muscle. *Tissue Cell* 12:197–207, 1980.
17. Bowman, W., On the minute structure and movements of voluntary muscle. *Phil. Trans. R. Soc. Lond.* 130:457–501, 1840. Bowman coined the term "sarcolemma," and pointed out that skeletal muscle contraction is accompanied by a decrease in the distance between the transverse striations of the muscle fibril.
18. Boyde, A. Confocal optical microscopy. In Duke, P. J. and A. J. Michette, eds. *Modern Microscopies—Techniques and Applications*, New York: Plenum, 1990:185–204.
19. Bozzola, J. J. and L. D. Russell. In Jones, and Bartlett *Electron Microscopy—Principles and Techniques for Biologists*. Boston: 1992:108–120; 204; 44; 27–31; 110; 306–328.
20. Braunfeld, M. B., A. J. Koster, J. W. Sedat, and D. A. Agard. Cryo Automated electron tomography: towards high-resolution reconstructions of plastic-embedded structures, *J. Microsc.* 174: 75–84, 1994.
21. Briarty, L. G. Stereology: methods for quantitative light and electron microscopy. *Sci. Prog.* 62:1–32, 1975.
22. Bullough, P. and R. Henderson, Use of spot-scan procedure for recording low-dose micrographs of beam-sensitive specimens, *Ultramicroscopy* 21:223–230, 1987.
23. Burns, A. R., S. I. Simon, G. L. Kukielka, J. L. Rowen, H. Lu, L. H. Mendoza, E. S. Brown, M. L. Entman and C. W. Smith. Chemotactic factors stimulate CD18-dependent canine neutrophil adherence and motility on lung fibroblasts. *J. Immunol.* 156: 3389–3401, 1996.
24. Burridge, K. and P. Mangeat. An interaction between vinculin and talin. *Nature* 308:744–46, 1984.
25. Burridge, K. and L. Connell. A new protein of adhesion plaques and membrane ruffles. *J. Cell Biol.* 97:359–367, 1983.
26. Burridge, K. and L. Connell. Talin: a cytoskeletal component concentrated in adhesion plaques and other sites of actin–membrane interaction. *Cell Motil.* 3:405–417, 1983.
27. Caldwell, J. E., S. G. Heiss, V. Mermall and J. A. Cooper. Effects of CapZ, an actin capping protein of muscle, on the polymerization of actin. *Biochemistry* 28:8506–8514, 1989.
28. Campbell, S. E., A. M. Gerdes and T. D. Smith. Comparison of regional differences in cardiac myocyte dimensions in rats, hamsters, and guinea pigs. *Anat. Rec.* 219:53–59, 1987.
29. Carlsson, E., B. K. Grove, T. Wallimann, H. M. Eppenberger and L. E. Thornell. Myofibrillar M-based proteins in rat skeletal muscles during development. *Histochemistry* 95:27–35, 1990.
30. Cartwright, J., Jr. and M. A. Goldstein. Microtubules in the

heart muscle of the postnatal and adult rat. *J. Mol. Cell Cardiol.* 17:1–7, 1985.
31. Casella, J. F., J. Maack and S. Lin. Purification and initial characterization of a protein from skeletal muscle that caps the barbed ends of actin filaments. *J. Biol. Chem.* 261:10915–21, 1986.
32. Casella, J. F., S. W. Craig, D. L. Maack and A. E. Brown. CapZ$_{(36/32)}$, a barbed end actin-capping protein, is a component of the Z-line of skeletal muscle. *J. Cell Biol.* 105:371–379, 1987.
33. Caulfield, J. B. and T. K. Borg. The collagen network of the heart. *Lab. Invest.* 40:364–372, 1979.
34. Chen, F. B. Mottino, T. S. Klitzner, K. D. Philipson and J. S. Frank. Distribution of the Na$^+$/Ca^{2+} exchange protein in developing rabbit myocytes. *Am. J. Physiol.* 268 (*Cell Physiol.* 36): C1126–C1132, 1995.
35. Cheng, N. and J. F. Deatherage. Three-dimensional reconstruction of the Z disk of sectioned bee flight muscle. *J. Cell Biol.* 108:1761–1774, 1989.
36. Chowrashi, P. K. and F. A Pepe. The Z-band: 85000-dalton amorphin and alpha-actinin and their relation to structure. *J. Cell Biol.* 94:565–573, 1982.
37. Colliex, C., and C. Mory, Scanning transmission electron microscopy of biological structures, *Biol. Cell* 80:175–180, 1994.
38. Cosslett, V. E., Radiation damage in the high resolution electron microscopy of biological materials: a review. *J. Microsc.* 113: 113–129, 1978.
39. Cox, G. Trends in confocal microscopy. *Micron* 24:237–247, 1993.
40. Craig, R., L. Alamo and R. Padron. Structure of the myosin filaments of relaxed and rigor vertebrate striated muscle studied by rapid freezing electron microscopy. *J. Mol. Biol.* 228:474–487, 1992.
41. Craig, S. W and J. V. Pardo. Gamma actin, spectrin, and intermediate filament proteins colocalize with vinculin at costameres, myofibril-to-sarcolemma attachment sites. *Cell Motil.* 3:449–462, 1983.
42. Crowther, R. A., D. J. DeRosier and A. Klug. Three-dimensional reconstruction from projections and its application to electron microscopy. *Proc. R. Soc. Lond. A* 317:319–340, 1970.
43. Crowther, R. A. and P. K. Luther. Three-dimensional reconstruction from a single oblique section of fish muscle M-band. *Nature* 307:569–570, 1984.
44. Crowther, R. A., P. K. Luther and K. A. Taylor. Computation of a three dimensional image of a periodic specimen from a single view of an oblique section. *Electron Microsc. Rev.* 3:29–42, 1990.
45. Dalen, H., P. Scheie, R. Nassar, T. High, B. Scherer, I. Taylor, N. R. Wallace and J. R. Sommer. Cryopreservation evaluated with mitochondrial and Z line ultrastructure in striated muscle. *J. Microsc.* 165(Pt 2):239–254, 1992.
46. Danilatos, G. D. Introduction to the ESEM instrument, *Microsc. Res. Tech.* 25:354–361, 1993. This issue of *Microscopy Research and Technique* also contains several excellent articles detailing ESEM studies on different systems.
47. Davey, D. F. The relation between Z-disk lattice spacing and sarcomere length in sartorius muscle fibers from *Hyla cerula*. *Aust. J. Biol. Med. Sci.* 54:441–447, 1976.
48. Deatherage, J. F., N. Cheng and B. Bullard. Arrangement of filaments and cross-links in the bee flight muscle Z disk by image analysis of oblique sections. *J. Cell Biol.* 108:1775–1782, 1989.
49. DeRosier, D. J. The reconstruction of three-dimensional images from electron micrographs. *Contemp. Physics* 12:437–452, 1971.
50. Dierksen, K., D. Typke, R. Hegerl, A. J. Koster and W. Baumeister. Towards automatic electron tomography. *Ultramicroscopy* 40:71–87, 1992.
51. Dolber, P. C. and M. S. Spach. Conventional and confocal fluorescence microscopy of collagen fibers in the heart. *J. Histochem. Cytochem.* 41:465–469, 1993.
52. Dykstra, M. J. *Biological Electron Microscopy—Theory, Techniques, and Troubleshooting*, New York: Plenum, 1992:131–133; 237; 8–9; 17–18; 171–181; 251–258; 247; 264–267; 270; 249; 295–296; 297–308; 315–318.
53. Eberth, C. J. Die Elemente der quergestreiften Muskeln, *Arch. Pathol. Anat. Physiol.* 1866, as quoted by von Palczewska (1910) and by Jordan (1911).
54. Edwards, R. J., Goldstein, M. A., Schroeter, J. P. and Sass, R. L. The Z band lattice in skeletal muscle in rigor. *J. Ultrastruct. Mol. Struct. Res.* 102:59–65, 1989.
55. Eisenberg, B. R. and R. L. Milton. Muscle fiber termination at the tendon in the frog's sartorius: a stereological study. *Am. J. Anat.* 171:273–284, 1984.
56. Eisenberg, B. R. and Salmons, S. The reorganization of subcellular structure in muscle undergoing fast-to-slow type transformation. A stereological study. *Cell Tissue Res.* 220:449–471, 1981.
57. Elliott, G. F., J. Lowy and B. M. Millman. Low-angle X-ray diffraction studies of living striated muscle during contraction. *J. Mol. Biol.* 25:31–45, 1967.
58. Engel, A. and C. Colliex. Application of scanning transmission electron microscopy to the study of biological structure. *Current Opinion Biotech.* 4:403–411, 1993.
59. Egerton, R. F., *Electron Energy-Loss Spectroscopy in the Electron Microscope*. New York: Plenum, 1989.
60. Erickson, H. P. and A. Klug. Measurement and compensation of defocussing and aberrations by Fourier processing of electron micrographs, *Phil. Trans. R. Soc. Lond.* 261:105–118, 1971.
61. Ervasti, J. M. and K. P. Campbell. A role for the dystrophin–glycoprotein complex as a transmembrane linker between laminin and actin. *J. Cell Biol.* 122:809–823, 1993.
62. Everhart, T. E. and T. L. Hayes, The scanning electron microscope. *Sci. Am.* 226:54–68, 1972.
63. Fardeau, M. Ultrastructure de fibres musculaires squelettiqes (1). *Presse Med.* 77:1341–1344, 1969.
64. Faulkner, G., A. Pallavincini, E. Formentin, A. Comelli, C. Ievolella, S. Trevisan, G. Bortello, P. Scannapieco, M. Salamon, V. Mouly, G. Valle, and G. Lanfranchi. ZASP: a new Z-band alternatively spliced PDZ-motif protein. *J. Cell Biol.* 146:465–475, 1999.
65. Fawcett, D. W. and N. S. McNutt. The ultrastructure of the cat myocardium I. Ventricular papillary muscle. *J. Cell Biol.* 42:1–45, 1969.
66. Ferrans, V. J. and W. C. Roberts. Inter-myofibrillar and nuclear-myofibrillar connections in human and canine myocardium. An ultrastructural study. *J. Mol. Cell. Cardiol.* 5:247–257, 1973.
67. Firtel, M. and T. J. Bereridge. Scanning probe microscopy in microbiology. *Micron* 26:347–362, 1995.
68. Flegler, S. L., J. W. Heckman and K. L. Klomparens. *Scanning and Transmission Electron Microscopy, An Introduction*, New York: W. H. Freeman, 1993:173–196; 109; 108–113.
69. Flicker, P. F., R. A. Milligan and D. Applegate. Cryo-electron microscopy of S1-decorated actin filaments. *Adv. Biophys.* 27:185–196, 1991.
70. Flucher, B. E. and Franzini-Armstrong, C. Formation of junctions involved in excitation–contraction coupling in skeletal and cardiac muscle. *Proc. Natl. Acad. Sci. U.S.A.* 93:8101–8106, 1996.
71. Forbes, M. S. and N. Sperelakis. Ultrastructure of mammalian cardiac muscle. In Sperelakis, N., ed. *Physiology and Pathophysiology of the Heart.* Boston: Martinus Nijhoff, 1984:3–42.

72. Fowler, V. M. Regulation of actin filament length in erythrocytes and striated muscle. *Curr. Opin. Cell Biol.* 8:86–96, 1996.
73. Frank, J. S., and G. A. Langer. The myocardial interstitium: Its structure and its role in ionic exchange. *J. Cell Biol.* 60:586–601, 1974.
74. Frank, J. S. and S. Beydler. Intercellular connections in rabbit heart as revealed by quick-frozen, deep-etched, and rotary-replicated papillary muscle. *J. Ultrastruct. Res.* 90:183–193, 1985.
75. Frank, J. S. and R. Yung. The myocyte–connective tissue interface. In Robinson, T. F. and R. K. H. Kinne, eds. *Cardiac Myocyte–Connective Tissue Interactions in Health and Disease (Issues Biomed.* vol. 13). New York: Karger, 1990:79–98.
76. Frank, J. S., G. Mottino, D. Redi, R. S. Molday and K. D. Phillipson. Distribution of the Na^+-Ca^{2+} exchange protein in mammalian cardiac myocytes: an immunofluorescence and immunocolloidal gold-labeling study. *J. Cell Biol.* 117:337–345, 1992.
77. Frank, J. S., G. Mottino, F. Chen, V. Peri, P. Holland and B. S. Tuana. Subcellular distribution of dystrophin in isolated adult and neonatal cardiac myocytes. *Am. J. Physiol.* 267 (*Cell Physiol.* 36):C1707–1716, 1994.
78. Frank, J. The role of correlation techniques in computer image processing. In Hawkes, P. W., ed. *Computer Processing of Electron Microscope Images.* Berlin: Springer Verlag, 1980:187–222.
79. Frank, J., B. F. McEwen, M. Radermacher, J. N. Turner and C. L. Rieder. Three-dimensional tomographic reconstruction in high voltage electron microscopy. *JEM Tech.* 6:193–205, 1987.
80. Frank, J. Introduction: Principles of electron tomography. In Frank, J. ed. *Electron Tomography—three-dimensional imaging with the transmission electron microscope.* New York: Plenum, 1992:1–16.
81. Franzini-Armstrong, C. and D. A. Fischman. Morphogenesis of skeletal muscle fibers. In Engel, A. G. and Franzini-Armstrong, C. eds, *Myology.* New York: McGraw-Hill, 1994:74–96.
82. Franzini-Armstrong, C. and A. O. Jorgensen. Structure and development of E-C coupling units in skeletal muscle. *Annu. Rev. Physiol.* 56:509–534, 1994.
83. Fujikawa, S. Freeze-fracture techniques. In Harris, J. R. ed., *Electron Microscopy in Biology: A Practical Approach.* Oxford: Oxford University Press, 1991:173–202.
84. Funatsu, T., H. Higuchi and S. Ishiwata. Elastic filaments in skeletal muscle revealed by selective removal of thin filaments with plasma gelsolin. *J. Cell Biol.* 110:53–62, 1990.
85. Funatsu, T., E. Kono, H. Higuchi, S. Kimur, S. Ishiwata, T. Yoshioka, K. Maruyama and S. Tsukita. Elastic filaments *in situ* in cardiac muscle: deep-etch replica analysis in combination with selective removal of actin and myosin filaments. *J. Cell Biol.* 120: 711–24, 1993.
86. Furst, D. O., R. Nave, M. Osborn and K. Weber. Repetitive titin epitopes with a 42 nm spacing coincide in relative position with known A band striations also identified by major myosin-associated proteins. An immunoelectron-microscopical study on myofibrils. *J. Cell Sci.* 94:119–125, 1989.
87. Gabriel, B. L., *Biological Scanning Electron Microscopy.* New York: Van Nostrand Reinhold, 1982:43–50.
88. Gautel, M., E. Lehtonen and F. Pietruschka. Assembly of the cardiac I-band region of titin/connectin: expression of the cardiac-specific regions and their structural relation to the elastic segments. *J. Musc. Res. Cell Motil.* 17:449–61, 1996.
89. Geisler, J. G., R. J. Palmer, L. J. Stubbs, and M. L. Mucenski. Nspl1, a new Z-band–associated protein. *J. Musc. Res. Cell Motil.* 20:661–668, 1999.
90. Gerdes, A. M. and F. H. Kasten. Morphometric study of endomyocardium and epimyocardium of the left ventricle in adult dogs. *Am. J. Anat.* 159:389–394, 1980.
91. Gerdes, A. M., J. Kriseman and S. P. Bishop. Morphometric study of cardiac muscle: the problem of tissue shrinkage. *Lab. Invest.* 46:271–274, 1982.
92. Glaeser, R. M., and K. A. Taylor. Radiation damage relative to transmission electron microscopy of biological specimens and low temperature: a review, *J. Microsc.* 112:127–138, 1978.
93. Goldmann, W. H., V. Niggli, S. Kaufmann, and G. Isenberg. Probing actin and liposome interaction of talin and talin-vinculin complexes: A kinetic, thermodynamic, and lipid labeling study. *Biochemistry* 31:7665–7671, 1992.
94. Goldstein, J. I., D. E. Newbury, P. Echlin, D. C. Joy, A. D. Rornig Jr., C. E. Lyman, C. Fiori and E. Lifshin. *Scanning Electron Microscopy and X-Ray Microanalysis*, 2nd ed. New York: Plenum, 1992:219–230; 142; 255–259.
95. Goldstein, M. A., J. P. Schroeter and R. L. Sass. Optical diffraction of the Z lattice in canine cardiac muscle. *J. Cell. Biol.* 75:818–836, 1977.
96. Goldstein, M. A. Ultrastructure of the ischemic myocardium. *Cardiovasc. Res. Center Bull.* 18:1–33, 1979.
97. Goldstein, M. A., J. P. Schroeter and R. L. Sass. The Z lattice in canine cardiac muscle. *J. Cell Biol.* 83:187–204, 1979.
98. Goldstein, M. A. and M. L. Entman. Microtubules in mammalian heart muscle. *J. Cell. Biol.* 80:183–195, 1979.
99. Goldstein, M. A., M. H. Stromer, J. P. Schroeter and R. L. Sass. Optical reconstruction of nemaline rods. *Exp. Neurol.* 70:83–97, 1980.
100. Goldstein, M. A., D. L. Murphy, W. B. Van Winkle and M. L. Entman. Cytochemical studies of a glycogen–sarcoplasmic reticulum complex. *J. Musc. Res. Cell Motil.* 6:177–187, 1985.
101. Goldstein, M. A. Cardiac sarcomere. In Gotto, A. M. and R. Paoletti, eds. *Arteriosclerosis Reviews, 14.* New York: Raven, 1986:183–212.
102. Goldstein, M. A., L. H. Michael, J. P. Schroeter and R. L. Sass. Two structural states of Z bands in cardiac muscle. *Am. J. Physiol.* 256 (*Heart Physiol.* 25):H552–H559, 1989.
103. Goldstein, M. A., J. P. Schroeter and R. L. Sass. Two structural states of the vertebrate Z band. *Electron Microsc. Rev.* 3:227–248, 1990.
104. Goldstein, M. A., J. P. Schroeter and L. H. Michael. Role of the Z band in the mechanical properties of the heart. *FASEB J.* 5: 2167–2174, 1991.
105. Goldstein, M. A., R. J. Edwards and J. P. Schroeter. Cardiac morphology after conditions of microgravity during COSMOS 2044. *J. Appl. Physiol.* 73(Suppl.):94S–100S, 1992.
106. Goldstein, M. A., J. Cheng and J. P. Schroeter. The effects of increased gravity and microgravity on cardiac morphology. *Aviat. Space Environ. Med.* 69:(Suppl.):A12–16, 1998.
107. Goll, D. E., W. R. Dayton, I. Singh and R. M. Robson. Studies of the alpha-actinin/actin interaction in the Z-disk by using calpain. *J. Biol. Chem.* 266:8501–8510, 1991.
108. Goodman, S. L., G. M. Hodges, and D. C. Livingston. A review of the colloidal gold marker system. *Scan. Elec. Microsc.* (Pt 2):133–146, 1980.
109. Granzier, H. L. and T. C. Irving. Passive tension in cardiac muscle: contribution of collagen, titin, microtubules, and intermediate filaments. *Biophys. J.* 68:1027–1044, 1995.
110. Gregorio, C. C., K. Trombitas, T. Centner, B. Kolmerer, G. Stier, K. Kunke, K. Suzuki, F. Obermayr, B. Herrmann, H. Granzier, H. Sorimachi, and S. Labeit. The NH_2 terminus of titin spans the Z-disc: its interaction with a novel 19-kD ligand (T-cap) is required for sarcomeric integrity. *J. Cell Biol.* 143: 1013–1027, 1998.
111. Gruver, C. L., F. DeMayo, M. A. Goldstein and A. R. Means. Targeted developmental overexpression of calmodulin induces proliferative and hypertrophic growth of cardiomyocytes in transgenic mice. *Endocrinology* 133:376–388, 1993.

112. Guerrero, J. R. and R. Padron. The substructure of the backbone of the thick filament from tarantula muscle. *Acta Microsc.* 1:63–83, 1992.
113. Haggis, G. H. Sample preparation for electron microscopy of internal cell structure. *Microsc. Res. Tech.* 22:151–159, 1992.
114. Hainfeld, J. F. Site-specific cluster labels. *Ultramicroscopy* 46: 135–144, 1992.
115. Hainfeld, J. F. and F. R. Furuya. A 1.4 nm gold cluster covalently attached to antibodies improves immunolabeling. *J. Histochem. Cytochem.* 40:177–184, 1992.
116. Hall, T. A. Suggestions for the quantitative X-ray microanalysis of thin sections of frozen-dried and embedded biological tissues. *J. Microsc.* 164:67–79, 1991.
117. Hansma, P. K., V. B. Elings, O. Marti and C. E. Bracker. Scanning tunneling microscopy and atomic force microscopy: application to biology and technology. *Science* 242:209–216, 1988.
118. Harford, J., P. Luther and J. Squire. Equatorial A-band and I-band X-ray diffraction from relaxed and active fish muscle—further details of myosin crossbridge behavior. *J. Mol. Biol.* 239:500–512, 1994.
119. Harris, P. and P. A. Poole-Wilson, eds. *Advances in Myocardiology*, vol. 5, New York: Plenum, 1985.
120. Haselgrove, J. C. X-ray evidence for conformational changes in the myosin filaments of vertebrate striated muscle. *J. Mol. Biol.* 92:113–143, 1975.
121. Hasselink, M. K., H. Kuipers, P. Geurten, H. Van Straaten. Structural muscle damage and muscle strength after incremental numbers of isometric and forced lengthening contractions. *J. Musc. Res. Cell Motil.* 17:335–341, 1996.
122. Hausmanowa-Petrusewicz, I., A. Fidzianska and B. Badurska. Unusual course of nemaline myopathy. *Neuromusulc. Disord.* 2:413–418, 1992.
123. Hawkes, P. W. The electron microscope as a structure projector. In J. Frank, ed., *Electron Tomography—Three-Dimensional Imaging with the Transmission Electron Microscopy*. New York: Plenum, 1992:17–38.
124. Hayat, M. A. *Introduction to Scanning Electron Microscopy*. Baltimore: University Park Press, 1978, 96 p.
125. Hermann, R., P. Walther and M. Muller. Immunogold labeling in scanning electron microscopy. *Histochem. Cell Biol.* 106:31–39, 1996.
126. Herrara, G. A. Ultrastructural immunolabeling: a general overview of techniques and applications. *Ultrastruct. Pathol.* 16: 37–45, 1992.
127. Hesketh, J. Translation and the cytoskeleton: a mechanism for targeted protein synthesis. *Mol. Biol. Rep.* 19:233–243, 1994.
128. Hippe-Sanwald, S. Impact of freeze substitution on biological electron microscopy. *Microsc. Res. Tech.* 24:400–422, 1993.
129. Hirakow, R. and T. Gotoh. A quantitative ultrastructural study on developing rat heart. In M. Lieberman, and T. Sano, eds., *Developmental and Physiological Correlates of Cardiac Muscle*. New York: Raven, 1975:37–49.
130. Hirose, K. C. Franzini-Armstrong, Y. E. Goldman and J. M. Murray. Structural changes in muscle crossbridges accompanying force generation. *J. Cell Biol.* 127:763–778, 1994.
131. Hobbs, L. W. Murphy's law and the uncertainty of electron probes. *Scan. Microsc. Suppl.* 4:171–183, 1990.
132. Holmes, K. C., D. Popp, W. Gebhard and W. Kabsch. Atomic model of the actin filament. *Nature* 347:44–49, 1990.
133. Holt, D. B. New directions in scanning electron microscopy cathodoluminescence microcharacterization. *Scanning Microsc.* 6:1–21, 1992.
134. Hoppe, W. and R. Hegerl, Three-dimensional structure determination by electron microscopy (non-periodic specimens). In Hawkes, P. W., ed., *Computer Processing of Electron Microscope Images*. Berlin: Springer Verlag, 1980:127–186.
135. Hopwood, D. and G. Milne. Fixation. In Harris, J. R. ed., *Electron Microscopy in Biology: A Practical Approach*. Oxford: Oxford University Press, 1991:1–16.
136. Horowits, R. and R. J. Pololsky. The positional stability of thick filaments in activated skeletal muscle depends on sarcomere length: evidence for the role of titin filaments. *J. Cell Biol.* 105:2217–2223, 1987.
137. Horowitz, A. K., K. Duggan, C. Buck, M. C. Geckerle and K. Burridge. Interaction of plasma membrane fibronectin receptor with talin—A transmembrane linkage. *Nature* 320:531–33, 1986.
138. Houmeida, A., J Holt, L. Tskhovrebova and J. Trinick. Studies of the interaction between titin and myosin. *J. Cell Biol.* 131: 1471–1481, 1995.
139. Huxley, H. E. and W. Brown. The low-angle x-ray diagram of vertebrate striated muscle and its behavior during contraction and rigor. *J. Mol. Biol.* 30:383–434, 1967.
140. Huxley, H. E., A. Stewart, H. Sosa and T. Irving. X-ray diffraction measurements of the extensibility of actin and myosin filaments in contracting muscle. *Biophys. J.* 67:2411–2421, 1994.
141. Hyatt, A. D. Immunogold labeling techniques. In Harris, J. R. ed., *Electron Microscopy in Biology: A Practical Approach*. Oxford: Oxford University Press, 1991:59–82.
142. Irving, T. C., Q., Li, B. A., Williams, and B. M. Millman, Z/I and A-band lattice spacings in frog skeletal muscle: effects of contraction and osmolarity. *J. Musc. Res. Cell Motil.* 19:811–823, 1998.
143. Isaacs, W. B., L. S. Kin, A. Struve and A. B. Fulton. Association of titin and myosin heavy chain in developing skeletal muscle. *Proc. Natl. Acad. Sci. U.S.A.*, 89:7496–7500, 1992.
144. Jacobson, K., E. D. Sheets and R. Simson. Revisiting the fluid mosaic model of membranes. *Science* 268:1441–1442, 1995.
145. Jakubiec-Puka, A., D. Frosch and R. Rudel. Ultrastructure of the contractile apparatus of rat skeletal muscle embedded in an aqueous medium. *Gen. Physiol. Biophys.* 8:185–202, 1989.
145a. Jarosch, R. Muscle force arises by actin filament rotation and torque in the Z-filaments. *Biochem. Biophys. Res. Commun.* 270(3):677–682, 2000.
146. Jester, J. V., P. M. Andrews, W. M. Petroll, M. A. Lemp and H. D. Cavanagh. In vivo, real-time confocal imaging. *JEM Tech.* 18:50–60, 1991.
146a. Jin, J. P. Titin-thin filament interaction and potential role in muscle function. *Adv. Exp. Med. Biol.* 481:319–333, 2000.
147. Johnson, D., K. Izutsu, M. Cantino, and J. Wong. High spatial resolution spectroscopy in the elemental microanalysis and imaging of biological systems, *Ultramicroscopy* 24:221–235, 1988.
148. Jordan, H. E. The structure of the heart muscle of the hummingbird with special reference to the intercalated discs. *Anat. Rec.* 5:517–529, 1911.
149. Jordan, H. E. The structural changes in striped muscle during contraction, *Physiol. Rev.* 13:301–324, 1933.
150. Joy, D. C. Beam interactions, contrast and resolution in the SEM. *J. Microsc.* 136:241–258, 1984.
151. Joy, D. C. and J. B. Pawley. High-resolution scanning electron microscopy. *Ultramicroscopy* 47:80–100, 1992.
152. Karkoura, A., P. Tangkawattana, S. Yamano, K. Takehana, Y. Isumisawa, J. Masty and M. Yamaguchi. Hypertrophic Z-line observed in aged one-humped camel (*Camelus dromedarius*). *Acta Anat.* 153:220–225, 1995.
153. Katz, A. M. *Physiology of the Heart*. New York: Raven, 1992.
154. Kaufmann, S., T. Piekenbrock, W. H. Goldmann, M. Barmann

and G. Isenberg. Talin binds to actin and promotes filament nucleation. *FEBS Lett* 284:187–191, 1991.
155. Kawamura, Y., H. Kume, Y. Itoh, S. Ohtsuka, S. Kimura and K. Maruyuma. Localization of three fragments of connectin in chicken breast muscle sarcomeres. *J. Biochem.* 117:201–207, 1995.
156. Kelly, D. E. Models of muscle Z-band fine structure based on a looping filament configuration. *J. Cell Biol.* 37:507–520, 1967.
157. Kelly, D. E. and M. A. Cahill. Filamentous and matrix components of skeletal muscle Z disks. *Anat. Rec.* 172:623–642, 1972.
158. Khan, M. A. An ultrastructural study of the stretch-induced hypertrophy of skeletal muscle. *Cell Biol. Int.* 10:955–962, 1986.
159. King, M. V. Dimensional changes in cells and tissues during specimen preparation for the electron microscope. *Cell Biophys.* 18:31–55, 1991.
160. Kiss, J. Z. and L. A. Staehelin. High pressure freezing. In Severs, N. J. and D. M. Shotton, eds., *Rapid Freezing, Freeze Fracture, and Deep Etching*. New York: Wiley and Sons, 1995: 89–104.
161. Knappeis, G. G. and R. Carlsen. The ultrastructure of the Z disc in skeletal muscle. *J. Cell Biol.* 13:323–335, 1962.
162. Kreis, T. and R. Vale. *Guidebook to the Extracellular Matrix and Adhesion Proteins*. New York: Oxford University Press, 1993.
163. Kreis, T. and R. Vale. *Guidebook to the Cytoskeletal and Motor Proteins*. New York: Oxford University Press, 1993.
164. Kuisk, I. R., H. Li, D. Tran and Y. Capetanaki. A single MEF2 site governs desmin transcription in both heart and skeletal muscle during mouse embryogenesis. *Dev. Biol.* 174:1–13, 1996.
165. Kuroda, M., T. Tanaka and T. Masaki. Eu-actin, a new structural protein of the Z line of striated muscles. *J. Biochem.* 89:297–310, 1981.
166. Labeit, S., B. Kolmerer and W. A. Linke. The giant protein titin. Emerging roles in physiology and pathophysiology. *Circ. Res.* 80:290–294, 1997.
167. Lal, R. and S. A. John. Biological applications of atomic force microscopy. *Am. J. Physiol.* 266(*Cell Physiol.* 35):C1–C21, 1994.
168. Lal, R., S. A. John, D. W. Laird and M. F. Arnsdorf. Heart gap junctions preparations reveal hemiplaques by atomic force microscopy. *Am. J. Physiol.* 268 (*Cell Physiol* 37):C968–C977, 1995.
169. Landon, D. N. Change in Z-disc structure with muscular contraction. *J. Physiol.* (*Lond.*) 211:44–45, 1970.
170. Laurent, M., B. Johannin, N. Gilbert, L. Lucas, D. Cassio, P. X. Petit and A. Fleury. Power and limits of laser scanning confocal microscopy. *Biol. Cell* 80:229–240, 1994.
171. Lazarides, E. Intermediate filaments as mechanical integrators of cellular space. *Nature* 283:247–256, 1980.
172. Leapman, R. D. and S. B. Andrews. Analysis of directly frozen macromolecules and tissues in the field-emission STEM. *J. Microsc.* 161:3–19, 1991.
173. Leeuwenhoek mentioned the transverse striations of muscle in his letters, as quoted by Bowman, 1840.
174. Legato, M. J. Sarcomerogenesis in human myocardium. *J. Mol. Cell. Cardiol.* 1:425–437, 1970.
175. Linke, W. A., M. L. Bertoo and G. H. Pollack. Spontaneous sarcomeric oscillations at intermediate activation levels in single isolated cardiac myofibrils. *Circ. Res.* 73:724–734, 1993.
175a. Linke, W. A. Stretching molecular springs: elasticity of titin filaments in vertebrate striated muscle. *Histol. Histopathol.* 15:799–811, 2000.
176. Linner, J. G., S. A. Livesay, D. S. Harrison and A. L. Steiner. A new technique for removal of amorphous phase tissue water without ice crystal damage: a preparative method for ultrastructural analysis and immunoelectron microscopy. *J. Histochem. Cytochem.* 34:1123–1135, 1986.
176a. Liversage, A. D., D. Holmes, P. J. Knight, L. Tskhovrebova, J. Trinick. Titin and the Sarcomere Symmetry Paradox. *J. Mol. Biol.* 305:401–409, 2001.
177. Luft, J. H. Embedding media—old and new. In Koehler, J. H., ed., *Advanced Techniques in Biological Electron Microscopy*, New York: Springer-Verlag, 1973:1–34.
178. Luna, E. J. and A. L. Hitt. Cytoskeleton–plasma membrane interactions. *Science* 258:955–964, 1992.
179. Luther, P. K. and J. M. Squire. Three-dimensional structure of the vertebrate muscle A band. II. The myosin filament superlattice. *J. Mol. Biol.* 141:409–439, 1980.
180. Luther, P. K. and J. M. Squire. Three-dimensional structure of the vertebrate muscle M-region. *J. Mol. Biol.* 125:313–324, 1978.
181. Luther, P. K., M. C. Lawrence, and R. A. Crowther, A method for monitoring the collapse of plastic sections as a function of electron dose. *Ultramicroscopy* 24:7–18, 1988.
182. Luther, P. K. Three-dimensional reconstruction of a simple Z-band in fish muscle. *J. Cell Biol.* 113:1043–1055, 1991.
183. Luther, P. K., Sample shrinkage and radiation damage. In J. Frank, ed., *Electron Tomography—Three-Dimensional Imaging with the Transmission Electron Microscope*, New York: Plenum, 1992:39–60.
184. Luther, P. K. Symmetry of a vertebrate muscle basketweave Z-band. *J. Struct. Biol.* 115:275–282, 1995.
185. Luther, P. K. Three-dimensional structure of a vertebrate muscle Z-band: implications for titin and alpha-actinin binding. *J. Struct. Biol.* 129:1–16, 2000.
186. Macagno, E. R., C. Levinthal and I. Sobel. Three-dimensional computer reconstruction of neurons and neuronal assemblies. *Annu. Rev. Biophys. Bioeng.* 8:323–351, 1979.
187. MacDonald, N. C. Auger electron spectroscopy for scanning electron microscopy. *Scanning Electron Microsc.* 1971:88–96, 1971.
188. Maguruma, M., S. Matsumura and T. Fukazawa. Direct interaction between talin and actin. *Biochem. Biophys. Res. Commun.* 171:1217–1223, 1990.
189. Maher, P. A., G. F. Cox and S. J. Singer. Zeugmatin: a new high molecular weight protein associated with Z lines in adult and early embryonic striated muscle. *J. Cell Biol.* 101:1871–1883, 1985.
190. Marko, M., A. Leith and D. Parsons. Three-dimensional reconstruction of cells from serial section and whole cell mounts using multilevel contouring of stereo micrographs. *JEM Tech.* 9:395–412, 1988.
191. Maron, B. J., V. J. Ferrans and W. C. Roberts. Ultrastructural features of degenerated cardiac muscle cells in patients with cardiac hypertrophy. *Am. J. Pathol.* 79:387–434, 1975.
192. Marti, O. SXM: an introduction. In Marti, O. and M. Amrein, eds., *STM and SFM in Biology*. New York: Academic, 1993: 78–88.
193. Martin, W. D. Time course of change in soleus muscle fibers of rats subjected to chronic centrifugation. *Aviat. Space Environ. Med.* 49:792–297, 1978.
194. Maruyama, K., T. Endo, H. Kume, Y. Kawamura, N. Kanzawa, Y. Nakauchi, S. Kimura, S. Kawashima and K. Maruyama. A novel domain sequence of connectin localized at the I band of skeletal muscle sarcomeres: homology to neurofilament subunits. *Biochem. Biophys. Res. Commun.* 194:1288–1291, 1993.
195. Maruyama, K. Connectin, an elastic protein of striated muscle. *Biophys. Chem.* 50:73–85, 1994.

196. Matsubara, I. and B. M. Millman. X-ray diffraction studies on cardiac muscle. In *The Physiological Basis of Starling's Law of the Heart*. Amsterdam: North-Holland, 31–41, 1974.
197. McDonald, K. L. Electron microscopy and EM immunocytochemistry. *Meth. Cell Biol.* 44-411–44, 1994.
198. McDonald, K. A., M. Lakonishok and A. F. Horowitz. alpha-v and alpha-3 integrin subunits are associated with myofibrils during myofibrillogenesis. *J. Cell Sci.* 108:975–983, 1995.
199. McGough, A., M. Way and D. DeRosier. Determination of the alpha-actinin site on actin filaments by cryoelectron microscopy and image analysis. *J. Cell Biol.* 126:433–443, 1994.
200. Meek, G. A., *Practical Electron Microscopy for Biologists*, 2nd Edition. New York: John Wiley & Sons, 1976:81–83; 376–384; 414–415.
201. Mellema, J. E. Computer reconstruction of regular biological objects. In Hawkes, P. W. ed., *Computer Processing of Electron Microscope Images*, Berlin: Springer Verlag, 1980:89–126.
202. Messerli, J. M. and J. C. Perriard. Three-dimensional analysis and visualization of myofibrillogenesis in adult cardiomyocytes by confocal microscopy. *Microsc. Res. Tech.* 30:521–30, 1995.
203. Millevoi, S., K., Trombitas, B., Kolmerer, S., Kostin, J., Schaper, K., Pelin, H., Granzier, and S. Labeit. Characterization of nebulette and nebulin and emerging concepts of their roles for vertebrate Z-discs. *J. Mol. Biol.* 282:111–123, 1998.
204. Milligan, R. A., M. Whittaker and D. Safer. Molecular structure of F-actin and location of surface binding sites. *Nature* 348:217–221, 1990.
205. Milner, D. J., G. Weitzer, D. Tran, A. Bradley and Y. Capetanaki. Disruption of muscle architecture and myocardial degeneration in mice lacking desmin. *J. Cell Biol.* 134:1255–1270, 1996.
206. Misell, D. L. Image analysis, enhancement and interpretation. In A. M. Galauert, ed., *Practical Methods in Electron Microscopy, Vol. 7*. New York: North Holland, 1978:125–197.
207. Mohanty, S. B. *Electron Microscopy for Biologists*. Springfield, Il: Charles C. Thomas, 1982:183.
208. Mollenhauer, H. H. Artifacts caused by dehydration and epoxy embedding in transmission electron microscopy. *Microsc. Res. Tech.* 26:496–512, 1993.
209. Molony, L., D. McCaslin, J. Abernethy, B. Paschal and K. Burridge. Properties of talin from chicken gizzard smooth muscle. *J. Biol. Chem.* 262:7790–7795, 1987.
210. Moncman, C. L. and K. Wang. Nebulette: a 107 kD nebulin-like protein in cardiac muscle. *Cell Motil. Cytoskel.* 32:205–225, 1995.
211. Moncman, C. L. and K. Wang. Assembly of nebulin into the sarcomeres of avian skeletal muscle. *Cell Motil. Cytoskel.* 34:167–84, 1996.
212. Moncman, C. L. and K. Wang. Architecture of the thin filament-z-line junction lessons from nebulette and nebulin homologies. *J. Musc. Res. Cell Motil.* 21:153–169, 2000.
213. Mora, M., C. Di Blasi, R. Barresi, L. Morandi, B. Brambati, L. Jarre and F. Cornelio. Developmental expression of dystrophin, dystrophin-associated glycoproteins and other membrane cytoskeletal proteins in human skeletal and heart muscle. *Brain Res.*, 91:70–82, 1996.
214. Morris, E. P., G. Nneji and J. M. Squire. The three-dimensional structure of the nemaline rod Z-band. *J. Cell Biol.* 111:2961–2978, 1990.
215. Nassar, R., N. R. Wallace, I. Taylor and J. R. Sommer. The quick-freezing of single intact skeletal muscle fibers at known time intervals following electrical stimulation. *Scanning Electron Microsc.* I:309–328, 1986.
216. Nave, R., D. O. Furst and K. Weber. Visualization of the polarity of isolated titin molecules: a single globular head on a long thin rod as the M band anchoring domain? *J. Cell Biol.* 109:2177–2187, 1989.
217. Niggali, V., K. S. Kaufmann, W. H. Goldmann, T. Weber and G. Isenberg. Identification of functional domains in the cytoskeletal protein talin. *Eur. J. Biochem.* 227:951–57, 1994.
218. Noguchi, S., E. M. McNally, K. Ben Othmane, Y. Hagiwara, Y. Mizuno, M. Yoshida, H. Yamamoto, C. G. Bonnemann, E. Gussoni, P. H. Denton, et al. Mutations in the dystrophin-associated protein gamma-sarcoglycan in chromosome 13 muscular dystrophy. *Science* 270:819–822, 1995.
219. Oberholzer, M., M. Ostreicher, H. Christen and M. Bruhlmann. Methods in quantitative image analysis. *Histochem. Cell Biol.* 105:333–335, 1996.
220. Obermann, W. M., M. Gautel, F. Steiner, P. F. van der Ven, K. Weber and D. O. Furst. The structure of the sarcomeric M band: localization of defined domains of myomesin, M-protein, and the 250 kD corboxy-terminal region of titin by immunoelectron microscopy. *J. Cell Biol.* 134:1441–1453, 1996.
221. Obermann, W. M., M. Gautel, K. Wever and D. O. Furst. Molecular structure of the sarcomeric M band: mapping of titin and myosin binding domains in myomesin and the identification of a potential regulatory phosphorylation site in myomesin. *EMBO J.* 16:211–220, 1997.
222. Ohlendieck, I. Towards an understanding of the dystrophin-glycoprotein complex: linkage between the extracellular matrix and the membrane cytoskeleton in muscle fibers. *Eur. J. Cell Biol.* 69:1–10, 1996.
223. Ohtsuka, H., H. Yajima, K. Maryune and S. Kimura. Binding of the N-terminal 63 kDa portion of connectin/titin to alpha actinin as revealed by the yeast two-hybrid system. *FEBS Lett.* 401:65–67, 1997.
224. Otto, J. J. Vinculin. *Cell Motil. Cytoskel.* 16:1–6, 1990.
225. Padron, R., L. Alamo, R. Craig and C. Caputo. A method for quick-freezing live muscles at known instants during contraction with simultaneous recording of mechanical tension. *J. Microsc.* 151:81–102, 1988.
226. Padron, R., G. Maristela, L. Alamo, J. R. Guerrero and R. Craig. Visualization of myosin helices in sections of rapidly frozen relaxed tarantula muscle. *J. Struct. Biol.* 108:269–276, 1992.
227. Palmer, R. E. and K. P. Roos. Extent of radial sarcomere coupling revealed in passively stretched cardiac myocytes. *Cell Motil. Cytoskel.* 37:378–388, 1997.
228. Pameijer, C. H. Replica techniques for scanning electron microscopy—a review. In Becker, R. P. and O. Johari, eds., *Scanning Electron Microscopy/1978/II.*, Scanning Electron Microscopy, Inc., AMF O'Hare, Illinois, 1978:831–836.
229. Papa, I. C. Astier, O. Kwiatek, F. Raynaud, C. Bonnal, M.-C. Lebart, C. Roustan, and Y. Benyamin, Alpha actinin–CapZ, an anchoring complex for thin filaments in Z-line. *J. Musc. Res. Cell Motil.* 20:187–197, 1999.
230. Pardo, J. V., J. D. Siliciano and S. W. Craig. A vinculin-containing cortical lattice in skeletal muscle: transverse lattice elements ("costameres") mark sites of attachment between myofibrils and sarcolemma. *Proc. Natl. Acad. Sci. U.S.A.* 80:1008–1012, 1983.
231. Pask, H. T., K. L. Jones, P. K. Luther and J. M. Squire. M-band structure, M-bridge interactions and contraction speed in vertebrate cardiac muscles. *J. Musc. Res. Cell Motil.* 15:633–645, 1994.
232. Pawley, J. B. Fundamental limits on confocal microscopy. In Pawley, J. B., ed., *Handbook of Biological Confocal Microscopy, rev. ed.* New York: Plenum, 1990:15–26.
233. Pawley, J. B., and S. L. Erlandsen, The case for low voltage high resolution scanning microscopy of biological samples. *Scanning Microsc. Suppl.* 3:163–178, 1989.

234. Peachey, L. D., and C. Franzini-Armstrong. Structure and function of membrane systems of skeletal muscle cells. In Peachey, L. D., R. H. Adrian and S. R. Geiger, eds. *Handbook of Physiology: Skeletal Muscle*, Bethesda, MD: American Physiological Society, 1983:23–71.
235. Penczek, P., M. Radermacher and J. Frank. Three-dimensional reconstruction of single particles embedded in ice. *Ultramicroscopy* 40:33–53, 1992.
236. Penman, S. Rethinking cell structure. *Proc. Natl. Acad. Sci. U.S.A.* 92:5251–5257, 1995.
238. Phillips, G. N., J. P. Fillers and C. Cohen. Tropomyosin crystal structure and muscle regulation. *J. Mol. Biol.* 192:111–131, 1986.
239. Polack, J. M. Monoclonal antibodies at the electron microscopical level. *Int. J. Cancer Suppl.* 2:2–7, 1988.
240. Pollack, G. H. Muscle contraction mechanism: are alternative engines gathering steam. *Cardiovasc Res.* 29:737–746 (discussion 747–757), 1995.
241. Pollack, G. H. Phase transitions and the molecular mechanism of contraction. *Biophys. Chem.* 59:315–328, 1996.
242. Price, M. Striated muscle endosarcomeric and exosarcomeric lattices. In: Malhotic, S. K., ed. *Advances in Structural Biology Vol. 1.* Greenwich, CT: Jo's Press, 1990:175–207.
243. Price, M. G. and R. H. Gomer. Skelemin, a cytoskeletal M-disc periphery protein, contains motifs of adhesion/recognition and intermediate filament proteins. *J. Biol. Chem.* 268:21800–21810, 1993.
244. Price, M. G. and E. Lazarides. Expression of intermediate filament-associated proteins paranemin and synemin in chicken development. *J. Cell Biol.* 97:1860–1874, 1983.
245. Radermacher, M. Weighted back-projection methods. In Frank, J. ed., *Electron Tomography—three-dimensional imaging with the transmission electron microscope.* New York: Plenum, 1992:91–116.
246. Radermacher, M. Three-dimensional reconstruction of single particles from random and nonrandom tilt series. *JEM Tech.* 9:359–394, 1988.
247. Rappaport, L. and J. L. Samuel. Microtubules in cardiac myocytes. *Int. Rev. Cytol.* 113:101–143, 1988.
248. Rayment, I. R. R. Wojciech, K. Schmidt-Base, R. Smith, D. R. Tomchick, M. M. Benning, D. A. Winkelmann, G. Wesenberg, and H. M. Holden. Three-dimensional structure of myosin subfragment-1: a molecular motor. *Science* 261:50–57, 1993.
249. Rayment, I., H. M. Holden, M. Whittaker, C. B. Yohn, M. Lorenz, K. C. Holmes and R. A. Milligan. Structure of the actin–myosin complex and its implications for muscle contraction. *Science* 261:58–65, 1993.
250. Reddy, M. K., J. D. Etlinger, M. Rabinowitz, D. A. Fischman and R. Zak. Removal of Z lines and alpha-actinin from isolated myofibrils by a calcium activated neutral protease. *J. Biol. Chem.* 250:4278–4284, 1975.
251. Reedy, M. K. The structure of actin filaments and the origin of the axial periodicity in the I substance of vertebrate striated muscle. *Proc. R. Soc. Lond. B* 160:458–460, 1964.
252. Reith, A. and T. M. Mayhew. *Stereology and Morphology in Electron Microscopy—Problems and Solutions.* New York: Hemisphere Publishing, 1988.
253. Riley, D. A., S. Ellis, C. S. Giometti, J. F. Y. Hoh, E. I. Ilyina-Kakueva, V. A. Oganov, G. R. Slocum, J. L. W. Gain and F. R. Sedlak. Muscle sarcomere lesions and thrombosis after spaceflight and suspension loading. *J. Appl Physiol.* 73 (Suppl.):33S–43S, 1992.
254. Robinson, T. F. and S. Winegrad. The measurement and dynamic implications of thin filament lengths in heart muscle. *J. Physiol.* 286:607–619, 1979.
255. Robinson, T. F. Lateral connections between heart muscle cells as revealed by conventional and high voltage transmission electron microscopy. *Cell Tissue Res.* 211:353–359, 1980.
256. Robinson, T. F. and S. Winegrad. A variety of intercellular connections in heart muscle. *J. Mol. Cell Cardiol.* 13:185–195, 1981.
257. Robinson, T. F., L. Cohen-Gould and S. M. Factor. Skeletal framework of mammalian heart muscle: arrangement of inter- and pericellular connective tissue structures. *Lab. Invest.* 49:482–498, 1983.
258. Robinson, T. F., S. M. Factor, J. M. Capasso, B. A. Wittenberg, O. O. Blumefeld and S. Seifter. Morphology, composition, and function of struts between cardiac myocytes of rat and hamster. *Cell Tissue Res.* 249:247–255, 1987.
259. Robinson, D. G., U. Ehlers, R. Herken, B. Herrman, F. Mayer and F.-W. Shurmann. *Methods of Preparation for Electron Microscopy—An Introduction for the Biomedical Sciences.* Berlin: Springer-Verlag, 1987:24.
260. Robinson, V. N. E. Materials characterization using the backscattered electron signal in scanning electron microscopy. *Scanning Microsc.* 1:107–117, 1987.
261. Roos, N. Freeze-substitution and other low temperature embedding methods. In Harris, J. R. ed., *Electron Microscopy in Biology: A Practical Approach.* Oxford: Oxford University Press, 1991:39–58.
262. Rosenbloom, J., W. R. Abrams and R. Mechan. Extracellular matrix 4: the elastic fiber. *FASEB J.* 7:1208–1218, 1993.
263. Roth, J. Post-embedding cytochemistry with gold labelled reagents: a review. *J. Microsc.* 143(Pt 2):125–137, 1986.
264. Roth, J. The silver anniversary of gold: 25 years of the colloidal gold marker system for immunocytochemistry and histochemistry. *Histochem. Cell Biol.* 106:1–8, 1996.
265. Rowe, R. W. D. The ultrastructure of the Z discs from white, intermediate, and red fibres of mammalian striated muscles. *J. Cell Biol.* 57:261–277, 1973.
266. Ruiz, T., I. Erk and J. Lepault. Electron cryo-microscopy of vitrified biological specimens: towards high spatial and temporal resolution. *Biol. Cell* 80:203–210, 1994.
267. Saide, J. D. and W. C. Ullrick. Fine structure of the honeybee Z disk. *J. Mol. Biol.* 79:329–377, 1973.
268. Sanger, J. M., B. Mittal, M. B. Pochapin and J. W. Sanger. Myofibrillogenesis in living cells microinjected with fluorescently labeled alpha-actinin. *J. Cell Biol.* 102:2053–2066, 1986.
269. Saxton, W. D. and W. Baumeister. The correlation averaging of a regularly arranged bacterial cell envelope protein. *J. Microsc.* 127:127–138, 1982.
270. Schachat, F. H., A. C. Canine, M. M. Brigs, and M. C. Reedy. The presence of two skeletal muscle alpha-actinins correlates with troponin-tropomyosin expression and Z-line width. *J. Cell Biol.* 101:1001–1008, 1985.
271. Schafer, D. A., J. A. Waddle and J. A. Cooper. Localization of CapZ during myofibrillogenesis in cultured chicken muscle. *Cell Motil. Cytoskel.* 25:317–335, 1993.
272. Schafer, D. A., C. Hug and J. A. Cooper. Inhibition of CapZ during myofibrillogenesis alters assembly of actin filaments. *J. Cell Biol.* 128:61–70, 1995.
273. Schaper J. R. Froede, S. Hein, A. Buck, H. Hashizume, B. Speiser, A. Friedl and N. Bleese. Impairment of the myocardial ultrastructure and changes of the cytoskeleton in dilated cardiomyopathy. *Circulation* 83:504–514, 1991.
274. Schollmeyer, J. V., D. E. Goll, M. H. Stromer, W. Dayton, I. Singh and R. Robson. Studies on the composition of the Z-disk. *J. Cell Biol.* 63:303a, 1974.
275. Schroeter, J. P., J.-P. Bretaudiere and M. A. Goldstein. Similar features in Z bands of both skeletal and cardiac muscle revealed by image enhancement. *JEM Tech.* 18:296–304, 1991.
276. Schroeter, J. P., J.-P. Bretaudiere, R. L. Sass and M. A. Gold-

stein. Three-dimensional structure of the Z band in a normal mammalian skeletal muscle. *J. Cell Biol.* 133:571–583, 1996.
277. Schultheiss, T., J. Choi, Z. X. Lin, C. Dilullo, L. Cohen-Gould, D. Fischman and H. Holtzer. A sarcomeric alpha-actinin truncated at the carboxyl end induces the breakdown of stress fibers in PtK2 cells and the formation of nemaline-line bodies and breakdown of myofibrils in myotubes. *Proc. Natl. Acad. Sci. U.S.A.* 89:9282–9286, 1992.
278. Shear, C. R. and R. J. Bloch. Vinculin in subsarcolemmal densities. *J. Cell Biol.* 101:240–256, 1985.
279. Shy, G. M., W. K. Engel, J. E. Somers and T. Wanko. Nemaline myopathy. A new congenital myopathy. *Brain* 86:793–810, 1963.
280. Sjostrom, M., J. M. Squire, P. Luther, E. Morris and A. C. Edman. Cryoultramicrotomy of muscle: improved preservation and resolution of muscle ultrastructure using negatively stained ultrathin cryosections. *J. Microsc.* 163(Pt 1):29–42, 1991.
281. Small, J. V., D. O. Furst and L.-E. Thornell. The cytoskeletal lattice of muscle cells. *Eur. J. Biochem.* 208:559–572, 1992.
282. Smith, M. and S. Croft. Embedding and thin section preparation. In Harris, J. R. ed., *Electron Microscopy in Biology: A Practical Approach*. Oxford: Oxford University Press, 1991: 17–37.
283. Sommer, J. R. and R. B. Jennings. Ultrastructure of mammalian cardiac muscle. In Fozzard, H. A., ed., *The Heart and Cardiovascular System*. New York: Raven, 1986:61–100.
284. Sommer, J. R. and E. A. Johnson. Ultrastructure of cardiac muscle. In Berne, R. A. and N. Sperelakis, eds., *The Handbook of Physiology—The Cardiovascular System*, vol 2. Baltimore: American Physiological Society, 1980:113–186.
285. Sommer, J. R., E. A. Johnson, N. R. Wallace and R. Nassar. Cardiac muscle following quick-freezing: preservation of in vivo ultrastructure and geometry with special emphasis on intracellular clefts in the intact frog heart. *J. Mol. Cell Cardiol.* 20:285–302, 1988.
286. Sommer, J. R. and R. A. Waugh. The ultrastructure of the mammalian cardiac muscle cell, with special emphasis on the tubular membrane systems. A review. *Am. J. Pathol.* 82:192–232, 1976.
287. Stelzer, E. H. K. and R. W. Wijnaendts-van-Resand. Optical cell splicing with the confocal fluorescence microscope: Microtomoscopy. In Wilson, T., ed., *Confocal Microscopy*, New York: Academic Press, 1990:199–212.
288. Stevenson, S., S. Rothery, M. J. Cullen and N. J. Severs. Dystrophin is not a specific component of the cardiac costamere. *Circ. Res.* 80:269–280, 1997.
289. Stewart, M. Transmission electron microscopy of frozen hydrated biological material. *Elec. Microsc. Rev.* 2:117–121, 1989.
290. Stewart, M. Introduction to the computer image processing of electron micrographs of two dimensionally ordered biological structures. *JEM Tech.* 9:301–324, 1988.
291. Stoker, M. E., A. M. Gerdes and J. F. May. Regional differences in capillary density and myocyte size in the normal human heart. *Anat. Rec.* 202:187–191, 1982.
292. Stromer, M. H. and D. E. Goll. Studies on purified alpha-actinin. II. Electron microscopic studies on the competitive binding of alpha-actinin and tropomyosin to Z-line extracted myofibrils. *J. Mol. Biol.* 67:489–494, 1972.
293. Stromer, M. H. Immunocytochemical localization of proteins in striated muscle. *Int. Rev. Cytol.* 142:61–144, 1992.
294. Stromer, M. H. Immunocytochemistry of the muscle cell cytoskeleton. *Microsc. Res. Tech.* 31:95–105, 1995.
295. Takahashi, K., A. Hattori, R. Tatsumi and K. Takai. Calcium-induced splitting of connectin filaments into beta-connectin and a 1,200 kDa subfragment. *J. Biochem.* 111:778–782, 1992.
296. Tameyasu, T., N. Ishide and G. H. Pollack. Discrete sarcomere length distribution in skeletal muscle. *Biophys. J.* 37:489–492, 1982.
297. Tangkawattana, P., A. Karkoura, M. Muto, S. Yamano, H. Taniyama and M. Yamaguchi. Cardiac rod body: hypertrophic Z-line in an aged pony. *Acta Anat.* 155:266–273, 1996.
298. Taylor, K. A. and D. W. Taylor. Formation of two-dimensional complexes of F-actin and crosslinking proteins on lipid monolayers: demonstration of unipolar alpha-actinin–F-actin crosslinking. *Biophys. J.* 67:1976–1983, 1994.
299. Thomason, D. B., P. R. Morrison, V. Oganov, E. Ilyina-Kakueva, F. W. Booth and K. M. Baldwin. Altered actin and myosin expression in muscle during exposure to microgravity. *J. Appl. Physiol.* 73(Suppl.):90S–93S, 1992.
300. Thornell, L.-E. and M. G. Price. The cytoskeleton in muscle cells in relation to function. *Biochem. Soc. Trans.* 19:1116–1120, 1991.
301. Tidball, J. G., T. O'Halloran and K. Burridge. Talin at myotendinous junctions. *J. Cell Biol.* 103:1465–1472, 1986.
302. Tidball, J. G. and K. L. Andolina. Structure and protein composition of sites of papillary muscle attachment to chordae tendineae in avian hearts. *Cell Tissue Res.* 270:527–533, 1992.
303. Tirion, M. M., D. ben-Avraham, M. Lorenz and K. C. Holmes. Normal modes as refinement parameters for the F-actin model. *Biophys. J.* 68:5–12, 1995.
304. Tokuyasu, K. T., A. H. Dutton, B. Geiger and S. J. Singer. Ultrastructure of chicken cardiac muscle as studied by double immunolabeling in electron microscopy. *Proc. Natl. Acad. Sci. U.S.A.* 78:7619–7623, 1981.
305. Tokuyasu, K. T., A. H. Dutton and S. J. Singer. Immunoelectron microscopic studies of desmin (skeletin) localization and intermediate filament organization in chicken cardiac muscle. *J. Cell Biol.* 96:1736–1742, 1983.
306. Tokuyasu, K. T., P. A. Maher, and S. J. Singer. Distributions of vimentin and desmin in developing chick myotubes in vivo. II. Immunoelectron microscopic study. *J. Cell Biol.* 100:1157–1166, 1985.
307. Traeger, L. A. and M. A. Goldstein. Thin filaments are not of uniform length in rat skeletal muscle. *J. Cell Biol.* 96:100–103, 1983.
308. Trinick, J. Understanding the functions of titin and nebulin. *FEBS Lett.* 307:44–48, 1992.
309. Trombitas, K., G. H. Pollack, J. Wright and K. Wang. Elastic properties of titin filaments demonstrated using a "freeze-break" technique. *Cell Motil. Cytoskel.* 24:274–283, 1993.
310. Trombitas, K. and G. H. Pollack. Elastic properties of the titin filament in the Z-line region of vertebrate striated muscle. *J. Musc. Res. Cell Motil.* 14:416–422, 1993.
311. Trombitas, K. and G. H. Pollack. Elastic properties of connecting filaments along the sarcomere. *Adv. Exp. Med. Biol.* 332:71-79, 1993.
311. Trombitas, K. K., A. Redkar, T. Centner, Y. Wu, S. Labeit, and H. Granzier. Extensibility of isoforms of cardiac titin: variation in contour length of molecular subsegments provides a basis for cellular passive stiffness diversity. *Biophys. J.* 79:3226–3234, 2000.
312. Truex, R. C. Myocardial cell diameters in primate hearts. *Am. J. Anat.*, 135:269–280, 1972.
313. Turnacioglu, K. K., B. Mittal, J. M. Sanger and J. W. Sanger. Partial characterization of zeugmatin indicates that it is part of the Z-band region of titin. *Cell Motil. Cytoskel.* 34:108–121, 1996.
314. Turnacioglu, K. K., B. Mittal, G. A. Dabiri, J. M. Sanger, and J. W. Sanger. Zeugmatin is part of the Z-band targeting region of titin. *Cell Struct. Funct.* 22:73–82, 1997.
315. Ullrick, W. C., P. A. Toselli, J. D. Saide and W. P. C. Phear. Fine

structure of the vertebrate Z-disc. *J. Mol. Biol.* 115:61–74, 1977.
316. Van der Ven, P. F., Oberman, W. M., Lemke, B., Gautel, M., Weber, K. and Furst, D. O. Characterization of muscle filamin isoforms suggests a possible role of gamma-filamin/ABP-L in sarcomeric Z-disc formation. *Cell Motil. Cytoskel.* 45:149–162, 2000.
316a. Van der Ven, P. F., W. M., Obermann, K. Weber, and D. O. Furst. Myomesin, M-protein and the structure of the sarcomeric M-band. *Adv. Biophys.* 33:91–99, 1996.
317. Vanderloop, F., G. Schaart, W. Langmann, F. Ramaekers and C. Viebahn. Expression and organization of muscle specific proteins during the early developmental stages of the rabbit heart. *Anat. Embryol.* 185:439–450, 1992.
318. Vigoreaux, J. O. The muscle Z band: lessons in stress management. *J. Musc. Res. Cell Motil.* 15:237–255, 1994.
319. Vinkemeier, U., W. Obermann, K. Weber and D. O. Furst. The globular head domain of titin extends into the center of the sarcomeric M band. cDNA cloning, epitope mapping and immunoelectron microscopy of two titin-associated proteins. *J. Cell Sci.* 106:319–330, 1993.
320. von Palczewska, I., Uber die Struktur der menschlichen Herzmuskelfasern. *Arch. fur Mikros. Anat.* 41–100, 1910.
321. Wade, J. B., W. A. Kachadorian and V. A. DiScala. Freeze-fracture electron microscopy: relationship of membrane features to transport physiology. *Am. J. Physiol.* 232 (*Renal Fluid Electrolyte Physiol.* 1):F77–83, 1977.
322. Wakabayashi, K., Y. Sugimoto, H. Tanaka, Y. Ueno, Y. Takezawa and Y. Amemiya. X-ray diffraction evidence for the extensibility of actin and myosin filaments during muscle contraction. *Biophys. J.* 67:2422–435, 1994.
323. Wall, J. S., J. F. Hainfeld, P. A. Bartlett and S. J. Singer. Observation of an undecagold cluster compound in the scanning transmission electron microscope. *Ultramicroscopy* 8:397–402, 1982.
324. Wallgren-Pettersson, C., B. Jasani, G. R. Newman, G. E. Morris, S. Jones, S. Singhrao, A. Clarke, I. Virtanen, C. Holmberg and J. Rapola. Alpha-actinin in nemaline bodies in congenital nemaline myopathy: immunological confirmation by light and electron microscopy. *Neuromuscal. Disord.* 5:93–104, 1995.
325. Wallimann, T., T. C. Doetschman and H. M. Eppenberger. Novel staining pattern of skeletal muscle M-lines upon incubation with antibodies against creatine kinase. *J. Cell Biol.* 96: 1772–1779, 1983.
326. Wang, K. and R. Ramirez-Mitchell. A network of transverse and longitudinal intermediate filaments is associated with sarcomeres of adult vertebrate skeletal muscle. *J. Cell Biol.* 96: 562–570, 1983.
327. Wang, K., R. McCarter, J. Wright, J. Beverly and R. Ramirez-Mitchell. Viscoelasticity of the sarcomere matrix of skeletal muscles. The titin-myosin composite filament is a dual stage molecular spring. *Biophys. J.* 64:1161–1177, 1993.
328. Wang, K. Titin/connectin and nebulin: giant protein rulers of muscle structure and function. *Adv. Biophys.* 33:123–134, 1996.
329. Wang, L., M. M. Rahman, H. Iida, T. Inai, S. Kawabata, S. Iwanaga and Y. Shibata. Annexin V is localized in association with Z-line of rat cardiac myocytes. *Cardiovasc. Res.* 30:363–371, 1995.
330. Wang, S. M., C. J. Jeng and M. C. Sun. Studies on the interaction between titin and myosin. *Histol. Histopathol.* 7:333–337, 1992.
331. Weakley, B. S. *A Beginner's Handbook in Biological Transmission Electron Microscopy.* London: Churchill Livingstone, 1981:62–63; 142–144.
332. Welland, M. E. and M. E. Taylor. Scanning tunneling microscopy. In Duke, P. J. and A. J. Michette, eds., *Modern Microscopies—Techniques and Applications.* New York: Plenum, 1990:231–254.
333. Whiting, A., J. Wardale and J. Trinick. Does titin regulate the length of muscle thick filaments? *J. Mol. Biol.* 205:263–268, 1989.
334. Williams, R. C. and H. W. Fisher, Electron microscopy of tobacco mosaic virus under conditions of minimal beam exposure. *J. Mol. Biol.* 52:121–123, 1970.
335. Winkler, J., H. Lunsdorf and B. M. Jockusch. Energy filtered electron microscopy reveals that talin is a highly flexible protein composed of a series of globular domains. *Eur. J. Biochem.* 243:430–436, 1997.
336. Worton, R. Muscular dystrophies: diseases of the dystrophin-glycoprotein complex. *Science* 270:755–756, 1995.
337. Wright, J., Q. Q. Huang and K. Wang. Nebulin is a full-length template of actin filaments in the skeletal muscle sarcomere: an immunoelectron microscopic study of its orientation and span with site-specific monoclonal antibodies. *J. Musc. Res. Cell Motil.* 14:476 83, 1993.
338. Yamaguchi, M., R. M. Robson, M. H. Stromer, D. S. Dahl and T. Oda. Actin filaments form the backbone of nemaline myopathy rods. *Nature* 271:265–267, 1978.
339. Yamaguchi, M., R. M. Robson and M. H. Stromer. Evidence for actin involvement in cardiac Z-lines and Z-line analogs. *J. Cell Biol.* 96:435–442, 1983.
340. Yamaguchi, M., R. M. Robson, M. H. Stromer, N. R. Cholvin and M. Izumimoto. Properties of soleus muscle Z-lines and induced Z-line analogs revealed by dissection with Ca^{2+}-activated neutral protease. *Anat. Rec.* 206:345–362, 1983.
341. Yamaguchi, M., M. Izumimoto, R. M. Robson and M. H. Stromer. Fine structure of wide and narrow vertebrate muscle Z lines. *J. Mol. Biol.* 184:621–644, 1985.
342. Yamaguchi, M., G. A. Fuller, W., Klomkleaw, S., Yamano, T. Oba, Z-line structural diversity in frog single muscle fiber in the passive state. *J. Musc. Res. Cell Motil.* 20:371–381, 1999.
343. Yarom, R. and U. Meiri. N lines in striated muscle: a site of intracellular Ca^{2+}. *Nature* [*New Biol.*] 234:254–256, 1971.
344. Young, P. C., Ferguson, S., Banuelos, and M. Gautel. Molecular structure of the sarcomeric Z-disk: two types of titin interactions lead to a asymmetrical sorting of alpha-actinin. *EMBO J.* 17:1614–1624, 1998.
344a. Young, P. and M. Gautel. The interaction of titin and alpha-actinin is controlled by a phospholipid-regulated intramolecular pseudoligand mechanism. *EMBO J.* 19:6331–6340, 2000.
345. Yu, L. C., R. W. Lymn and R. J. Podolsky. Characterization of a non-indexible equatorial x-ray reflection from frog sartorius muscle. *J. Mol. Biol.* 115:455–464, 1977.
346. Yu, L. C. Analysis of equatorial x-ray diffraction patterns from skeletal muscle. *Biophys. J.* 55:433–440, 1989.
347. Yung, R. and J. S. Frank. Extracellular matrix-sarcolemmal surface interconnections: a quick-freeze deep-etch study. *J. Ultrastruct. Mol. Struct. Res.* 96:160–171, 1986.
348. Zierold, K. Preparation and transfer of ultrathin frozen-hydrated and freeze-dried cryosections for microanalysis in scanning transmission electron microscopy. *Scanning Elec. Microsc.* (Pt 3):1205–1214, 1982.
349. Zimmer, D. B. and M. A. Goldstein. Immunolocalization of alpha-actinin in adult chicken skeletal muscles. *JEM Tech.* 6: 357–366, 1987.

2. Cellular basis of physiological and pathological myocardial growth

PIERO ANVERSA
GIORGIO OLIVETTI

Department of Medicine, New York Medical College, Valhalla, New York

CHAPTER CONTENTS

Morphometric Analysis of Cell Size and Number in the Ventricular Myocardium
    Myocyte dimensional properties and number: methodological considerations
    Confocal microscopic measurements of myocyte cell volume
Morphometric Analysis of the Coronary Vasculature
Physiological Myocardial Growth: Maturation of the Heart
    Ventricular remodeling
    Myocyte adaptations
    Cytoplasmic adaptations in myocytes
    Capillary adaptations
    Conclusions
Aging of the Heart
    Aging and ventricular remodeling
    Aging and myocyte number
    Aging and myocyte reactive hypertrophy
    Aging and the coronary arterial and capillary tree
    Conclusions
Pressure and Volume Overload Hypertrophy
    Cardiac hypertrophy and ventricular remodeling
    Cardiac hypertrophy and myocyte size, shape, and number
    Cardiac hypertrophy and volume composition of myocytes
    Cardiac hypertrophy and the coronary arterial and capillary tree
    Conclusions
Ischemic Cardiomyopathy
    Ischemic cardiomyopathy and ventricular remodeling
    Ischemic cardiomyopathy, myocyte cell loss, and ventricular function
    Ischemic cardiomyopathy and myocyte cellular hypertrophy and hyperplasia
    Ischemic cardiomyopathy and volume composition of myocytes
    Ischemic cardiomyopathy and the coronary capillary tree
    Conclusions

THE PHENOMENON OF MYOCARDIAL GROWTH involves coordinated adaptations at three principal levels of structural organization: tissue, cellular and subcellular. The proportion and distribution of myocytes, endothelial cells, connective tissue cells, vascular components, collagen framework, and other extracellular constituents comprise the architecture of the tissue level; the quantities and configurational properties of the cytoplasmic organelles characterize the subcellular level. It is at the intermediate cellular level, however, that the fundamental mechanisms of growth, cell proliferation, and cellular hypertrophy are defined. Although endothelial and connective tissue cells can increase in number and volume, because these cell populations constitute only a small fraction of the myocardium, their changes have only modest effects on cardiac anatomy. Conversely, myocytes represent the major portion of the tissue, and modifications in their number, size, and shape have important consequences for ventricular dimension. These cellular responses characterize the various phases of postnatal myocardial growth as well as the different stages of induced cardiac hypertrophy in the adult. An additional variable relevant for understanding the structural adaptability of the maturing and overloaded heart is myocyte cell death, which may have a significant impact on ventricular remodeling. Myocyte cell death, programmed and necrotic in nature, may affect the myocardium, contributing to the restructuring of the heart during development, aging, and cardiac hypertrophy.

Changes in the dimensional properties of myocytes by cellular hypertrophy imply expansion of the subcellular components responsible for oxygen consumption and adenosine triphosphate (ATP) synthesis, i.e., the mitochondria, and those components responsible for ATP utilization, i.e., the myofibrils. Moreover, the pattern by which contractile proteins and sarcomeres are added in the cytoplasm determines increases in myocyte diameter and length that have significant effects on cardiac anatomy. The insertion of new cells to existing myocytes, in parallel or in series, can also alter wall thickness and chamber diameter. An equally important growth variable in the myocardium is the expansion of the capillary network, as new capillary units are necessary to maintain an adequate oxygen supply to the rapidly expanding ventricular mass. The proportionate or disproportionate growth of the coronary vasculature and microvasculature during enlargement of the myocyte compartment of the ventricle can be anticipated to preserve or decrease the oxygenation potential of the tissue, possibly limiting cell function and myocardial structural integrity.

This chapter reviews the quantitative morphologic characteristics of the ventricular myocardium in an attempt to document how measurements of cell size, number, shape, and cytoplasmic composition have contributed to the identification of critical parameters implicated in the maturation of the heart from birth to adult life. Moreover, the structural adaptation of the coronary microcirculation in this period of accelerated physiologic myocardial growth will be discussed to emphasize the intimate relationship between the muscle and vascular compartments of the myocardium in their ability to respond to the sudden increase in work demands imposed on the heart shortly after birth. In addition, the effects of aging on the ventricular myocardium, both at the myocyte and vascular levels, will be addressed to emphasize the implications of quantitative changes in these two major tissue constituents in the aging process of the heart. Finally, the quantitative structural properties of the myocardium in pressure and/or volume overload hypertrophy as well as in different forms of ischemic cardiomyopathy will be described to indicate how myocardial damage and tissue regeneration by cellular growth reserve mechanisms participate in ventricular wall remodeling and ultimate myocardial dysfunction. This information has been collected by the application of morphometric techniques to the quantitative assessment of the ventricular myocardium in normal and pathologic conditions. Therefore, the basis of this methodological approach will be described before introducing the actual results.

MORPHOMETRIC ANALYSIS OF CELL SIZE AND NUMBER IN THE VENTRICULAR MYOCARDIUM

The quantitative estimation of the ventricular myocardium requires application of morphometric methods that are noteworthy for their simplicity. Starting from a collection of representative two-dimensional samples, such as tissue sections, and a superimposed grid of test points and line segments, it is possible to determine the three-dimensional volume, surface area, number, and length of recognizable components simply by counting. Since the practical techniques and theoretical bases of morphometry have been described in complete detail in several texts and reviews (6, 307–309, 448, 510, 533–540), only some fundamental principles will be discussed.

The terms *morphometry* and *stereology* are frequently used interchangeably. However, stereology is the study of mathematical relationships between three-dimensional structures and their representation in two-dimensional samples, whereas morphometry refers to the measurement of structures using stereologic principles. Acquisition of morphometric data starts with the application of a test grid to magnified images of tissue sections of ventricular myocardium. The test grid contains a field of uniformly spaced sampling points, depicted by the intersections of lines in the grid, a set of sampling lines whose aggregate length is known, and a boundary that defines the area sampled by the grid (535). With highly oriented tissue like muscle, it is frequently advantageous to orient sectioning planes as precisely as possible in the directions that are transverse or longitudinal to the fiber axis. Some of the stereologic formulas can be simplified in these conditions (306). In general, transversely sectioned myocardium is frequently preferred to longitudinally oriented tissue because the identification of the different structures is facilitated in this preparation.

The population of cells of any given type distributed within a tissue may be considered in general terms to be a group of individual compartments existing in a spatial volume. Biologically meaningful characteristics of such a cell population are the number of cells per unit volume of tissue, N_V, the volume fraction of tissue occupied by the population, V_V, and the average compartment size or mean cell volume, V. These parameters are related by the expression:

$$V = \frac{V_V}{N_V} \qquad (1)$$

With the aid of a test grid, it is possible to estimate the area fraction, A_A, of the micrograph occupied by myocytes, endothelial cells, and connective tissue cells by counting the fraction of all of the points that lie over profiles of those components, P_P:

$$A_A = P_P \qquad (2)$$

Conversion of the morphometric area measurements, A_A, to their three-dimensional counterparts is accomplished by stereologic formulas. For any component its volume fraction, V_V, volume per unit volume, is directly equal to its area fraction:

$$V_V = A_A = P_P \qquad (3)$$

Since V_V is measured easily, evaluation of V depends on the determination of N_V. If the cells in a given population have only a single nucleus, their enumeration is greatly simplified by the counting of nuclear profiles, since nuclei are always clearly separated and can be stained for greater contrast and visibility. In cell populations containing multinucleate cells, such as liver cells or cardiac myocytes, the significant volume equivalent to cell volume is the cell volume per nucleus (305, 307).

For discrete convex objects, counts of their profiles per unit area, N_A, will be proportional to the number of such objects per unit volume, N_V, and their mean diameter, $\bar{D}$:

$$N_V = \frac{N_A}{\bar{D}} \quad (4)$$

The mean diameter, $\bar{D}$, can be determined rather easily for nearly spherical objects from the mean diameter, $\bar{d}$, of their circular profiles:

$$\bar{D} = \frac{4\bar{d}}{\pi} \quad (5)$$

However, cell nuclei often are irregularly shaped, and the measurement of their volume density by equation 4 is complicated by the fact that their mean diameter, $\bar{D}$, is neither known nor easily calculable. A solution to this problem was found by making additional measurements based on the observation that profile density in sections, N_A, is dependent not only on N_V and $\bar{D}$ but also on section thickness, t:

$$N_A = N_V (\bar{D} - 2p + t) \quad (6)$$

This more general relationship (152, 192, 306, 307, 535, 536) also includes a factor p equal to the minimal visible thickness of grazing nuclear slices. If this equation is rearranged in the form

$$N_A = N_V t + N_V (\bar{D} - 2p) \quad (7)$$

it is evident that N_A varies linearly with t and the proportionality factor is N_V. Thus, if values of N_A are measured in sections of different known thicknesses, a graph of N_A versus t yields a straight line whose slope is a direct determination of N_V independent of the unknown variables $\bar{D}$ and p. This relationship is illustrated in Figure 2–1. The mean cell volume then can be obtained from equation 1 and the quantity $(\bar{D} - 2p)$ can be deduced from the N_A intercept of the linear graph. The knowledge of N_V, in combination with the estimation of the absolute volume of ventricular myocardium, V_T, allows the calculation of the total number of cells in the ventricle, N_T. The quantity V_T is easily obtained by dividing ventricular weight by the tissue density of muscle, 1.06 gm/ml (335):

$$N_T = N_V \cdot V_T \quad (8)$$

Although the approach described above applies to the morphometric estimation of cell volume for all types of cells, measurements of myocyte cell volume per nucleus, V_m, and number of myocyte nuclei per unit volume, $N_{(m)V}$, can be obtained by rearranging and simplifying equation 7 (12, 307):

$$N_{(m)V} = \frac{N_{(m)A}}{(\bar{D}_m - 2p + t)} \quad (9)$$

It has been shown that under control conditions of tissue sectioning and orientation of plastic embedded myocardium, $-2p$ and $+t$ are essentially compensating each other (307). Therefore, the quotient of the number of myocyte nuclei per unit area of tissue, $N_{(m)A}$, measured in transversely sectioned cells, and the average nuclear length, $\bar{D}_m$, determined from mid-sections of nuclei in longitudinally oriented myocytes (Fig. 2–2), yields the number of myocyte nuclei per unit volume of myocardium, $N_{(m)V}$ (12):

$$N_{(m)V} = \frac{N_{(m)A}}{\bar{D}_m} \quad (10)$$

It should be emphasized that for the evaluation of $\bar{D}_m$, only nuclei in which the nuclear envelope is sharply defined at both ends, and in which clusters of mitochondria are clearly visible in the areas adjacent to the nuclear edges, can be utilized (12).

Although morphometric results concerning the volume fraction of myocytes, $V_{(m)V}$, number of myocyte nuclei per unit area of transverse myocardial sections, $N_{(m)A}$ and average length of myocyte nuclei in longitudinally oriented cells, $\bar{D}_m$, can be easily obtained at the light microscopic level of resolution (Fig. 2–2), the relative quantities of endothelial cells and connective tissue cells in the tissue can be measured only by electron microscopy (306, 309). Light microscopy does not provide sufficient resolution for accurate measurements because cell identification may be difficult and surface boundaries may be ill defined. The same limitations apply to the counting of muscle cell profiles, a parameter necessary for the computation of the numerical density of myocytes in the tissue and the average cross-sectional area or diameter of these cells. In addition, spacing between margins of adjacent myocytes is often too narrow to be visible by light microscopy. Myocytes have irregular outlines and spaces between them often measure only approximately 0.2 µm, the limit of resolution in light microscopy, and are unlikely to be visible even in semithin sections (306,

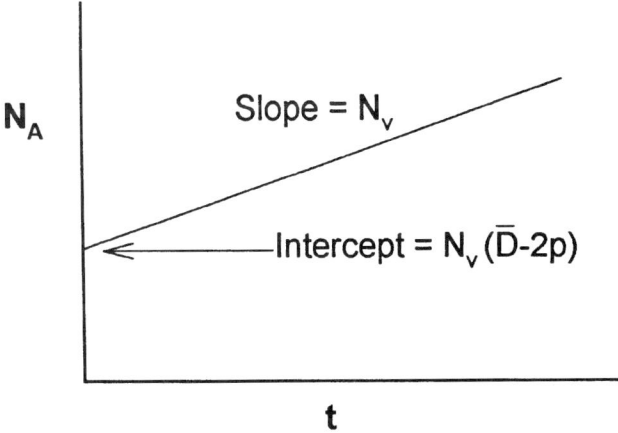

FIG. 2–1. Schematic graph of equation 7.

78 HANDBOOK OF PHYSIOLOGY ~ THE HEART

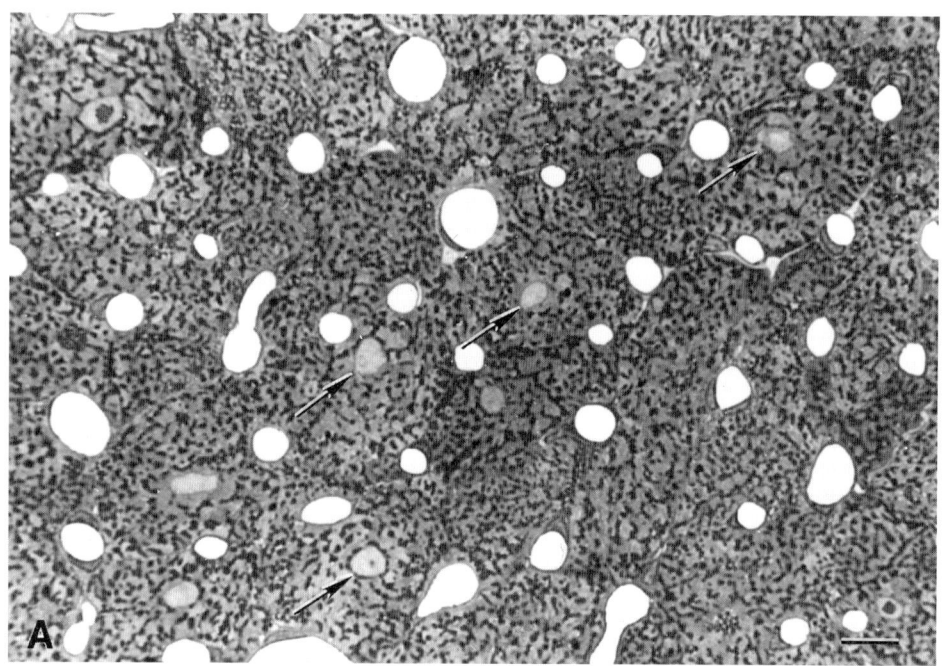

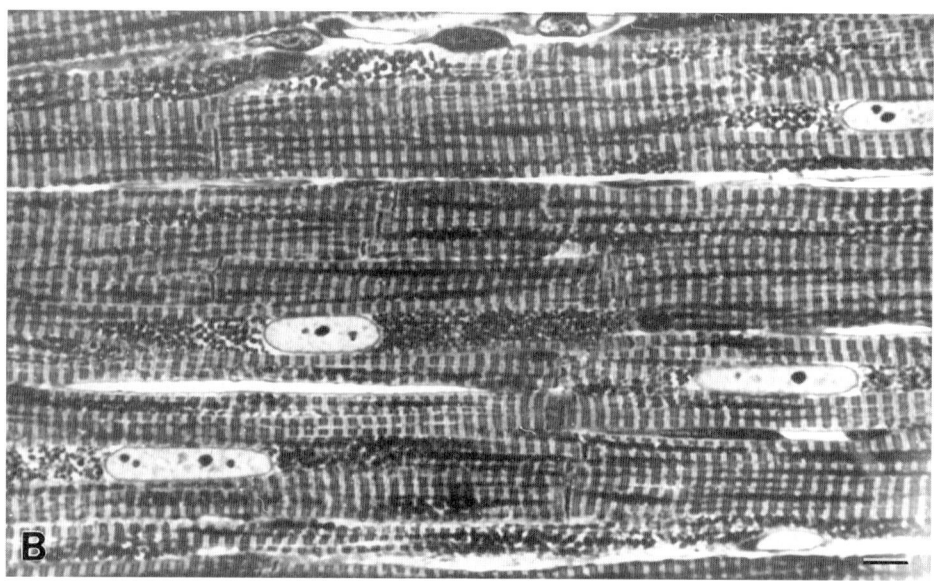

FIG. 2-2. Sections of plastic-embedded tissue of ventricular myocardium with myofibers oriented transversely (A) and longitudinally (B). A: several myocyte nuclear profiles (*arrows*) are seen in the center of transversely sectioned cells. B: Mid-sections of myocyte nuclei are shown. The nuclear envelope is defined at both ends, and clusters of mitochondria are visible at the nuclear poles. Methylene blue and safranin staining. A and B: bars = 10 μm.

309). The higher resolving power of electron microscopy also produces clearer endothelial cell boundaries enabling an accurate estimation of capillary volume and surface densities.

Since the area fraction of myocytes in transversely sectioned myocardium, $V_{(m)V}$, is the product of the number of myocytes per unit area of tissue, $N_{(m)A}$, and the average cross-sectional area of these cells, $\bar{A}_{(m)}$, this latter parameter can be obtained easily:

$$\bar{A}_{(m)} = \frac{V_{(m)V}}{N_{(m)A}} \qquad (11)$$

In view of the cylindrical configuration of myocytes, mean myocyte cell length, $\bar{L}_m$, can be determined from the quotient of their average cell volume, V_m, and their average transverse cross-sectional area, $\bar{A}_m$:

$$\bar{L}_m = \frac{V_m}{\bar{A}_m} \qquad (12)$$

The premise of equation 11 is the degree of accuracy by which myocytes are oriented in tissue section. With a highly oriented tissue, some of the stereologic formulas can be simplified (535, 536). For example, in transverse sections through longitudinally oriented muscle cells, it can be shown that their length per unit volume, $L_{(m)V}$, is equal to their number per unit area, $N_{(m)A}$, in the same dimensional unit.

$$L_{(m)V} = N_{(m)A} \quad (13)$$

However, even in the most careful control of myocyte orientation and examination of sections by electron microscopy, micrographs of transversely oriented myocardium clearly show some periodic Z-band structures, documenting that the sections are not oriented perfectly perpendicular to the long axis of every muscle cell. It is common experience that even under the best circumstances of orientation of tissue blocks, variation in the alignment of myocytes within the ventricular wall usually leads to the presence of several Z-band images in typical low power electron microscopic fields. The observed spacing, S, between Z-bands in approximately transverse muscle sections is an accurate and sensitive guide for calculating the obliquity of the sectioning plane; i.e., the angular deviation, θ, between the section and Z-band plane:

$$\sin \theta = \frac{L}{S} \quad (14)$$

where L is the true sarcomere length measured in longitudinal sections. Morphometric investigations of myocardium have to follow the practical rule, based on equation 14, that transverse sections include only those in which $S > 2L$, i.e., $\theta < 30°$. Oblique orientation of myocardial sections does not affect the evaluation of tissue volume fractions. Such misalignment, however, introduces some error into morphometric measurements by decreasing the numerical density and surface density of longitudinally oriented structures such as myocytes. The effect on these parameters is the same as that which would occur with a unidirectional stretching of a transverse tissue section, converting circular profiles into ellipses having an increased area, perimeter, and spacing. Since this effect is the reverse of the unidirectional shrinkage of sections caused by compression artifact during the sectioning process (42, 308), the appropriate correction factors are mathematically analogous. Sections cut at an oblique angle θ will show a numerical density, $N'_{(m)A}$, for longitudinal structures that is related to their true transverse numerical density, $N_{(m)A}$, by the expression:

$$N_{(m)A} = \frac{N'_{(m)A}}{\cos \theta} \quad (15)$$

The observed mean cross-sectional area, A'_m, of enclosed profiles is related to their real area, A_m, by:

$$A_m = A'_m \cos \theta \quad (16)$$

An additional relevant aspect of myocytes is the surface area of their sarcolemmal membrane. The surface area of myocyte membranes per unit volume of myocardium, $S_{(m)V}$, is related to the length of their profiles per unit area, $L_{(m)A}$, by the ratio $4/\pi$:

$$S_{(m)V} = \frac{4 L_{(m)A}}{\pi} = 2 I_{L(m)} \quad (17)$$

However, in perfectly oriented transverse sections,

$$S_{(m)V} = L_{(m)A} = I_{L(m)} \quad (18)$$

In oblique sections the measured surface density, S_v', of longitudinal membranes is altered from its true value, $S_{(m)V}$, by two effects: reduced because profiles are spread apart (equation 15) and increased because profiles are elongated by the amount that the perimeter of a circle of radius α is increased when it is distorted into an ellipse with semiaxes α and $\alpha/\cos \theta$. Thus,

$$S_{(m)V} = S'_{(m)V}\sqrt{(1 + \cos^2 \theta)/2} \quad (19)$$

Despite the variability in the alignment of tissue components and the visual error in orienting tissue blocks for transverse sectioning, it reasonably can be expected that resulting sections will be clustered near their true transverse orientation. If a worst case situation is assumed in which the obliquity of usable sections is uniformly distributed between 0° and 30°, the resulting maximal underestimation error of $N_{(m)A}$ would be 4.5%:

$$N'_{(m)A} = 6 N_{(m)A}/\pi \int_0^{\pi/6} \cos \theta \, d\theta = 0.955 N_{(m)A} \quad (20)$$

Similarly, the maximum overestimation of mean cross-sectional area would be 4.7%, and the underestimation of $S_{(m)V}$ would be 2.2%. Since, for these parameters the overall standard deviation among animals, including biologic variation, is in excess of 10%, it is clear that the limitation $S > 2L$ is sufficient to maintain a small error due to obliquity in section and/or myocyte orientation.

In summary, the higher resolution of electron microscopy is essential for counting individual myocyte profiles in transverse myocardial sections in order to determine their numerical density and mean cross-sectional area and the capillary-to-myocyte ratio. It has been demonstrated that as much as a twofold error can result when these measurements are attempted by light microscopy (28, 307). This is so because muscle cells in the myocardium are tightly packed, with the spacing between cells often measuring less than the limiting resolving power of the light microscope. Furthermore, the interdigitation of cardiac myocytes results in numerous small myocyte profiles with irregular boundaries that can only be reliably recognized in electron micrographs. The perceived advantage of light microscopic sampling in morphometry is the easier acquisition of a larger area for examination. A larger sample, however, cannot compensate for systematic errors introduced by inadequate resolution of structural details. Furthermore, sampling with the electron microscope seldom imposes a significant limitation on the area of tissue examined. This type of approach has to be employed for the analysis of the relationship between myocytes such as the mean center-to-center distance, d_{c-c}, between cells. This parameter can be calculated from the number of profiles counted per unit area of tissue, $N_{(m)A}$, in transverse myocardial sections by assuming the tendency for these roughly cylindrical cells to pack in a close hexagonal pattern:

$$d_{c-c} = \sqrt{\frac{2}{\sqrt{3} \cdot N_{(m)A}}} = \frac{1.0746}{\sqrt{N_{(m)A}}} \qquad (21)$$

The preference for a hexagonal pattern in the distribution of myocytes in the myocardium is based on the morphometric measurements of cell cross section and myocyte surface/volume ratio (28). The same concept can be used to estimate the average number of myocytes across the ventricular wall, that is, the number of myocytes that would be transversed by a thin transmural probe inserted perpendicular to the surface of the wall. In a hexagonal pattern, the spacing between planes of adjacent cells varies with the orientation of the hexagonal array from a maximum of d_{c-c} to a minimum of $d_{c-c}\sqrt{3}/2$ and has a mean value, $\bar{d}$, given by

$$\bar{d} = \frac{3d_{c-c}\sqrt{3}}{\pi} \int_0^{\pi/6} \frac{d\theta}{\cos\theta} = 0.9085\, d_{c-c} \qquad (22)$$

Thus, the transmural number, $\bar{N}_{(m)tm}$, of myocytes across a wall of thickness, W, can be found from

$$\bar{N}_{(m)tm} = W/\bar{d} = 1.0243\, W\, \sqrt{N_{(m)A}} \qquad (23)$$

The stereologic theoretical basis for morphometry requires that the sections from which data are drawn should be infinitely thin, free of distortion, and have a known orientation with respect to anisotropic structures. Deviations from the ideal have led to the derivation of various correction factors for section thickness, compression, and the effects of orientation (42, 306, 308, 539). Correction factors for systematic errors, such as thickness and compression, do improve the morphometric determination of absolute tissue measurements but often are unnecessary when only relative values are compared between groups subject to the same degrees of error.

Myocyte Dimensional Properties and Number: Methodological Considerations

The in situ morphometric procedure discussed above employs nuclear measurements to obtain cellular measurements. By this methodology, two fundamental parameters of the muscle compartment of the myocardium are estimated: (1) myocyte cell volume per nucleus and (2) total number of myocyte nuclei in the ventricle. However, myocyte cell volume per nucleus is identical to the mean cell volume strictly in mononucleated cell populations. The same premise applies also to the translation of the total number of myocyte nuclei to absolute number of cells in the entire ventricular myocardium. This limitation is particularly relevant to the morphometric analysis of the heart in different species, because large variations exist in the proportion of mononucleated and multinucleated myocytes in mammals (64, 73, 81, 169, 202, 217, 255, 262, 263, 344, 346, 456, 457, 472). In addition, the estimation of the percentage of multinucleated myocytes in tissue sections has been problematic. For example, in the rat, the most investigated animal model, histologic sections of the heart reveal mostly mononucleated muscle cells (307, 443). Conversely, cell suspensions from the dissociated ventricular wall show 80% or more binucleated cardiac myocytes (255, 345, 512). However, significantly lower values have been reported in rat atrial tissue (351).

Although the percentages of binucleated myocytes measured shortly after birth in the rat appear to agree in histologic preparations (38) and cell suspensions (119, 255), major discrepancies have been found in the adult rat heart (255, 307, 345, 443, 512). The controversy seems to revolve about the questions of whether isolated myocytes constitute a representative sampling of the whole myocyte population and whether binucleated pairs are recognizable microscopically in proportion to their true frequency in longitudinal tissue sections. It is obvious that lateral displacement of the nuclei in a binucleated cell or variation in the longitudinal orientations of either cells or sections leads to a sharp reduction in the apparent number of binucleated images (307). Such an effect should be less pronounced with increasing section thickness for myocytes with transverse diameter in the range of the thickness of the section examined. This may provide an explanation for the consistency in the results obtained in neonatal rats (38, 255). However, adult myocytes have large cell diameters, which present a greater possibility for error due to the displacement of nuclei within the cytoplasm and/or the non-optimal longitudinal alignment of muscle cells in the preparation (404). Therefore, the in situ evaluation of myocyte size and number by current morphometric methodologies can provide accurate information in terms of the relative and absolute numerical density of myocyte nuclei and the mean myocyte cell volume per nucleus, leaving still undefined the actual number of myocytes in the ventricle and the real volumes of mononucleated and multinucleated muscle cells. This pertains not only to the rat heart but also to the mammalian heart in general. In several other species, binucleated cardiac myocytes are usually absent at birth but accumulate during development (38, 73, 255, 344). The human heart also contains both mononucleated and multinucleated myocytes (5, 64, 217, 262, 356, 448).

In the last three decades, several methodologies have been described for the evaluation of myocyte size and number in the ventricular myocardium. Based on the cylindrical shape of cardiac myocytes, estimations of myocyte diameter and length have been obtained from tissue sections and mean cell volume calculated (59, 60, 103, 261, 292). However, the direct determination of myocyte diameter in routine histologic preparations is limited and measurements of cell length between two spaced intercalated disks is quite variable. Moreover, myocyte length has been determined by assessing the distance between two nuclei in an attempt to overcome the complexity of recognizing cell ends (59, 60, 292). The consequence of this approach is the computation of myocyte cell volume per nucleus, not average cell volume. Three-dimensional section reconstruction has also been employed in the analysis of average cell volume (262), but this technique permits only very small sampling and has the inherent problems of light microscopic detection of cell boundaries.

In recent years another technique has become available for the determination of myocyte volume and number, through preparation of enzymatically dissociated muscle cells (75, 88, 154, 162, 255). However, this procedure cannot be used for the measurement of these cellular parameters in the same heart because it has two limitations. First, cell size cannot be obtained in a reliable and accurate manner. As a result of flattening and spreading of the isolated cells when placed on the surface of a microscope slide, the mean myocyte cell volume is grossly overestimated. Second, the percentage of myocardium constituted by parenchymal cells cannot be determined with this approach. This information is essential for the computation of the aggregate volume of the myocyte compartment in the entire ventricle. Such a value can then be divided by the average cell volume to yield the total number of cells in the whole ventricular tissue. Furthermore, the volume composition of the myocardium cannot be assumed to be constant, because the quantities of muscle cells and other tissue constituents may vary significantly during pathologic processes characterized by cell loss and scar formation within the myocardium (27, 39). Problems also exist in the estimation of myocyte cell volume by the use of a Coulter counter (163). Such a methodology will yield an average myocyte volume without discriminating between mononucleated and binucleated cells, as well as between non-myocyte cells and cell fragments. Cell isolation may preferentially preserve one population of cells.

Although the possibility cannot be excluded that during the enzymatic dissociation of the myocardium smaller mononucleated or larger multinucleated cells may be more resistant to the methodology, altering the proportion of the various cell populations in the cell suspension, the frequency of myocytes with different numbers of nuclei per cell can be easily obtained with this technique (44, 75, 246, 255). This is the major advantage of cell isolation. Moreover, this procedure has been markedly improved in recent years so that large quantities of ventricular myocytes can be collected, minimizing the potential limitation of sampling error (106, 110, 245, 246, 284, 302). Systems also are available for the simultaneous isolation of cells from several hearts. At present, the average number of myocytes that can be obtained from the left and right ventricles of a rat heart varies from 6–8 $\times$ 10^6 and 2–3 $\times$ 10^6, respectively (106, 110, 284, 302). Nuclei can be stained by fluorescent dyes that bind specifically to DNA, making their recognition and distribution very apparent (Plate 2).

In conclusion, the morphometric analysis of tissue sections offers an in situ approach that yields reliable information on volume composition and number of myocyte nuclei in the tissue. In contrast, myocyte isolation provides accurate data on the frequency distribution of nuclei per cell. By employing both techniques, the number of mononucleated, binucleated, trinucleated, and tetranucleated myocytes in the ventricle can be calculated. This computation takes into account the total number of myocyte nuclei in the ventricle and the distribution of nuclei in the different cell populations (44). Such an approach has been employed using several animal models to document changes in myocyte number as a result of experimental conditions mimicking pathologic states in the human heart (44, 246, 364). An identical analysis has been performed in the human (357). In contrast, the evaluation of the average volume of mononucleated and multinucleated cells has been difficult and the methodology has been developed only recently for assessment of the size of these cells and the percentage of myocardium occupied by the various myocyte populations in the tissue (245, 356, 418).

Confocal Microscopic Measurements of Myocyte Cell Volume

The limitations mentioned above have been overcome by a technique that combines an in situ morphometric

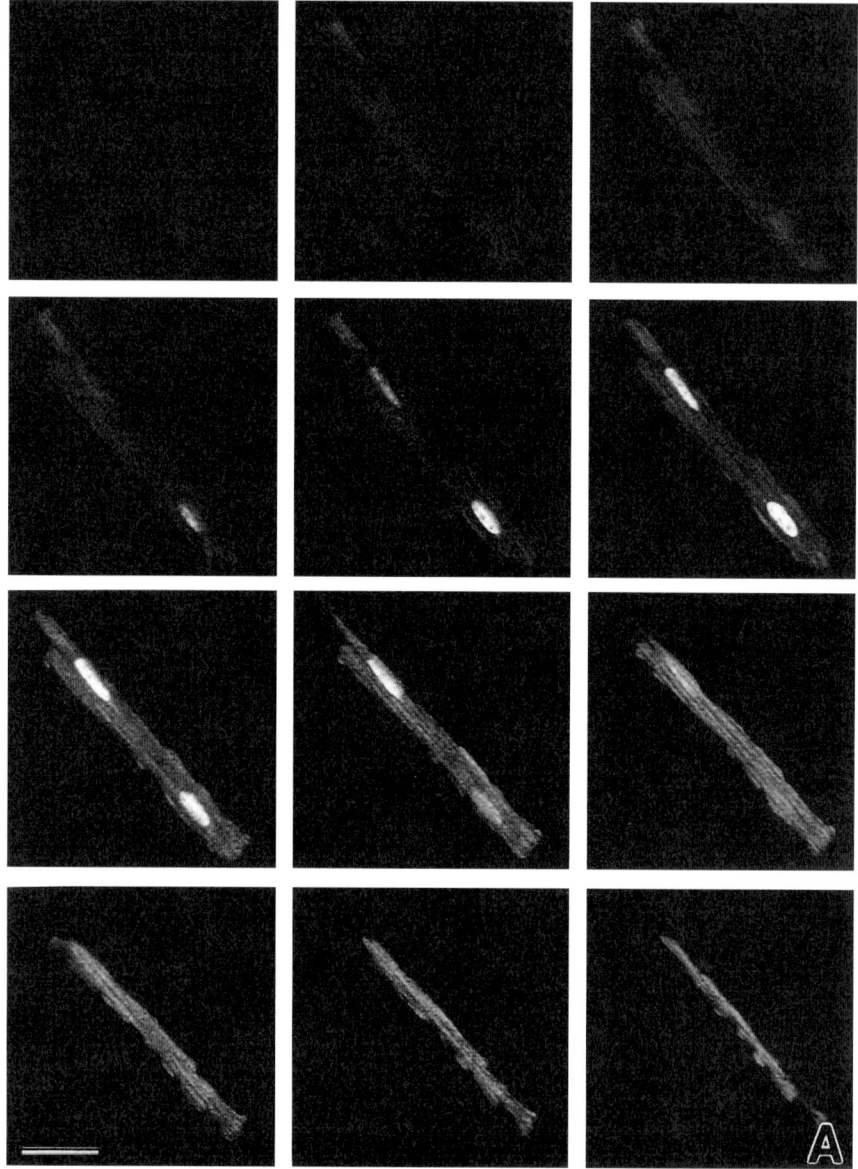

FIG. 2–3. Three-dimensional optical section reconstruction by confocal microscopy of a left ventricular myocyte from a dog heart (A) and a right ventricular myocyte from a rat heart (B). Fluorescein and propidium iodide staining. A and B: bars = 50 μm.

analysis with the determination of cell configuration and dimensions of isolated myocytes. By the use of confocal microscopy, three-dimensional optical reconstruction of single myocytes can be obtained (Fig. 2–3). With this technique, the contribution of each myocyte population to the overall muscle mass of the ventricular myocardium can be determined, as can the volumes of mononucleated and multinucleated cells and their changes in different physiologic and pathologic conditions. Isolated cells when placed in physiologic medium assume a cross-sectional area that resembles a flattened ellipse. The ratio of the minor axis (b) to the major axis (a) of the ellipse can be determined by confocal microscopy. Cell volume, V_C, is calculated assuming an elliptical cross-section with a major axis that is equivalent to cell width and a minor axis that is computed from the measured ratios. Cell length, L_C, is measured directly:

$$V_C = \left[\pi \cdot \left(\frac{a}{2}\right) \cdot \left(\frac{b}{2}\right) \right] L_C \quad (24)$$

Specifically, measurements of the average volume of mononucleated, $V(c)_n$ binucleated, $V(c)_{2n}$, trinucleated, $V(c)_{3n}$, and multinucleated, $V(c)_{mn}$, myocytes in the ven-

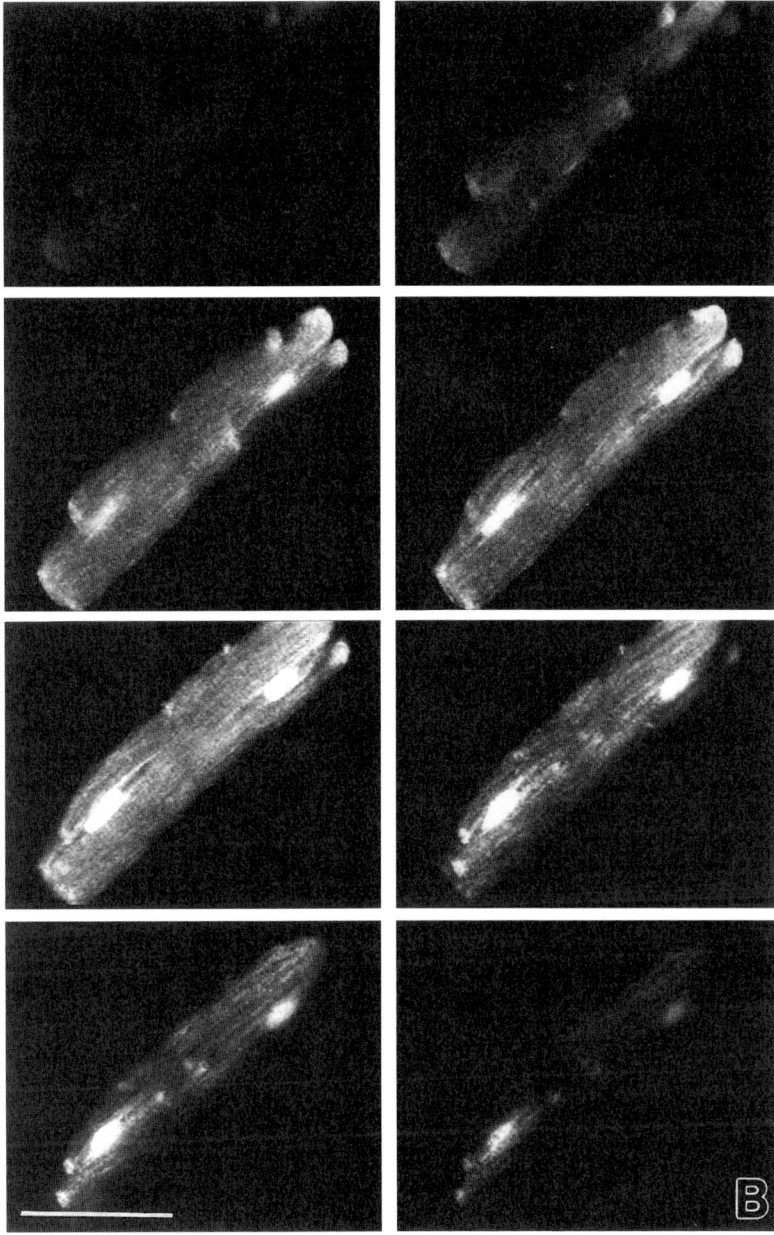

tricular myocardium can be obtained as follows: isolated myocytes are stained with fluorescein isothiocyanate to visualize the cell cytoplasm and with propidium iodide to label the nuclei. Subsequently, measurements of cell area for mononucleated, $\bar{A}(c)_n$, binucleated, $\bar{A}(c)_{2n}$, trinucleated, $\bar{A}(c)_{3n}$, and multinucleated, $\bar{A}(c)_{mn}$ myocytes can be collected by confocal microcopy. Importantly, with the same system, it is possible to measure the thickness, $\dot{t}(c)_n$, $\dot{t}(c)_{2n}$, $\dot{t}(c)_{3n}$, and $\dot{t}(c)_{mn}$, of these different cell populations by optical sectioning of each cell in the Z-plane (Fig. 2–4). Therefore, the average volume of each cell type, $V(c)_n$, $V(c)_{2n}$, $V(c)_{3n}$ and $V(c)_{mn}$ is computed from:

$$V(c)_n = \bar{A}(c)_n \cdot \dot{t}(c)_n \qquad (25)$$

Direct measurements of myocyte cell volumes by confocal microscopy are time consuming and can only be applied to a limited number of cells (245, 356, 418). However, myocyte geometric dimensions can be collected in a large number of enzymatically dissociated cells through the aid of computerized image analysis systems. Subsequently, the ratio between the minor and major axis can be derived from a restricted number of determinations by confocal microscopy and this relationship employed for the computation of the mean volume of each myocyte population (245, 356, 418).

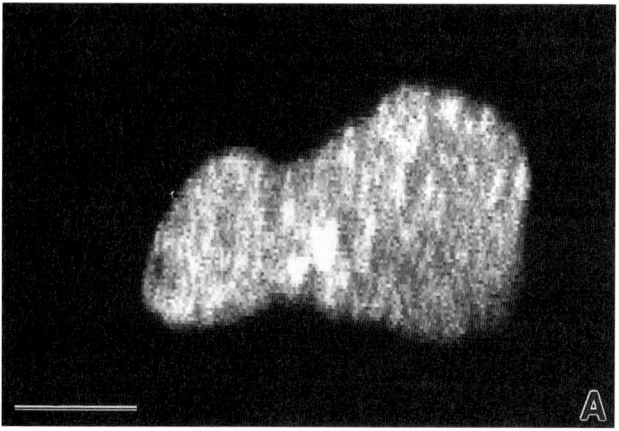

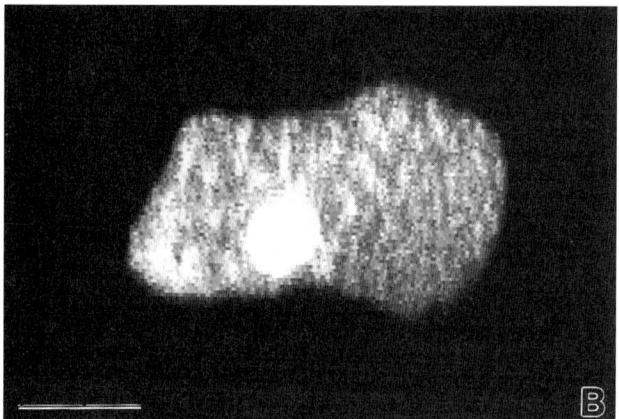

FIG. 2–4. Confocal microscopic images of cross-sectional areas of two rat ventricular myocytes on the surface of a microscopic slide. These images were obtained by three-dimensional optical reconstruction in the Z-plane of the cell. A and B: bars = 10 μm.

The evaluation of the aggregate number of myocytes in the ventricular myocardium requires the combination of measurements obtained by the in situ analysis of the tissue with the estimations of myocyte cell volume collected from enzymatically dissociated cells. The total volume of the ventricular myocardium, V_T, is first determined (335); the aggregate myocyte volume in the ventricle, $V(c)_T$, then is calculated from V_T and the volume fraction of myocytes in the tissue, $V(c)_V$:

$$V(c)_T = V_T \cdot V(c)_V \quad (26)$$

From the morphometric measurement of the volume fraction of myocytes in the myocardium, $V(c)_V$, and the proportion of mononucleated, $F(c)_n$, binucleated, $F(c)_{2n}$, trinucleated, $F(c)_{3n}$, and multinucleated, $F(c)_{mn}$, cells determined in enzymatically dissociated myocytes, the volume percent of mononucleated, $V(c)_{V_n}$, binucleated, $V(c)_{2n}$, trinucleated, $V(c)_{3n}$, and multinucleated cells, $V(c)_{mn}$, in the tissue is obtained:

$$V(c)_{V_n} = \frac{V(c)_n \cdot F(c)_n}{(V(c)_n \cdot F(c)_n) + (V(c)_{2n} \cdot F(c)_{2n}) + (V(c)_{3n} \cdot F(c)_{3n}) + (V(c)_{mn} \cdot F(c)_{mn})} \quad (27)$$

This information combined with the quantitative evaluation of the absolute volume of myocytes in the ventricle, $V(c)_T$, allows the estimation of the aggregate volume of mononucleated, $V(c)_{T_n}$, binucleated, $V(c)_{T2n}$, trinucleated, $V(c)_{T3n}$, and multinucleated, $V(c)_{T_{mn}}$, cells:

$$V(c)_{T_n} = V(c)_T \cdot V(c)_{V_n} \quad (28)$$

Finally, the number of mononucleated, $N(c)_n$, binucleated, $N(c)_{2n}$, trinucleated, $N(c)_{3n}$, and multinucleated, $N(c)_{mn}$, cells in the ventricle is computed:

$$N(c)_n = \frac{V(c)_{T_n}}{V(c)_n} \quad (29)$$

This methodology, which requires confocal microscopy, offers the most reliable approach for the quantitative analysis of the average volume of the different myocyte populations of the heart. In addition, it allows evaluations of structural parameters of the tissue and cells that were not previously available. Finally, the contribution of each cell population to the ventricular myocardium can be determined and the effects of physiological and pathological states of the heart on these cellular properties carefully measured (245, 356, 418). However, the acquisition of individual myocytes by enzymatic digestion does not permit the assessment of the multiple relationships between the myocyte compartment of the myocardium and the other tissue components, including the vascular framework. For example, the ratio of capillary profiles to myocyte profiles, which frequently is used as an index of the proportional and disproportional growth adaptations of these two tissue constituents (67, 204, 233, 398, 401, 485, 487, 490), cannot be obtained by this approach.

MORPHOMETRIC ANALYSIS OF THE CORONARY VASCULATURE

The principal elements of a tissue are its parenchymal cell population and its microvasculature. Quantitative estimation of the volume fraction of the cellular compartment relates to the amount of the tissue's functional capacity. The microvasculature, on the other hand, is appropriately characterized by three fundamental properties (216, 314, 534): (1) capillary luminal volume density, which is related to the volume of capillary blood available for gas exchange within the tissue; (2) capillary luminal surface density, which represents the capillary area available for oxygen transport from the blood to the tissue; and (3) the average maximum diffusion distance from the capillary wall to the mitochondria of the working cells, where oxygen is predominantly consumed in generating ATP through the process of oxidative phosphorylation. Measurement of these properties at a specific time can be used to characterize a tissue in some particular stage, whereas measurements at different times can reveal magnitudes of changes produced by normal growth or the quantitative effects of experimentally induced processes or pathological conditions (11, 203, 226, 395, 425, 459, 487, 502, 550).

Capillary luminal volume density, surface density, and length density can be obtained easily by applying the same principles described for the myocyte compartment in the preceding sections. The diffusion distance for oxygen, R, is calculated from the capillary profile density in transverse myocardial sections (306) according to the equation

$$R = \sqrt{\frac{1}{N_{Acap} \pi}} - \sqrt{\frac{A_{cap}}{\pi}} \quad (30)$$

where N_{Acap} corresponds to the number of capillaries per unit area of myocardium and A_{cap} is the average cross-sectional area of capillary lumen. This measurement, based on the Krogh's cylinder model for gas exchange in tissue (265), assumes that capillaries are uniformly distributed in the myocardium and that the mitochondria are dispersed evenly in the myocyte cytoplasm. It should be recognized, however, that questions have been raised concerning the functional significance of the Krogh's cylinder model because oxygen tension differs at the two extremes of the capillary unit (314, 400, 507, 509, 534). This may require more complex modeling (400, 507, 509) and better characterization of the distribution and interrelationships of capillary profiles within the tissue. To address this deficiency, the capillary domain model has been developed (507, 509), and by this approach the surface area surrounding each capillary can be measured. This analysis takes into account the variability in the distribution of capillary profiles in the myocardium and more closely reflects the characteristics of tissue oxygenation (314, 400, 507, 509). The heterogeneity in capillary spacing, which is an independent determinant of myocardial oxygenation (509), may be assessed by measuring capillary domain areas, defined as polygonal regions on a tissue cross-section that are closer to a given capillary than to any other (411). Moreover, the capillary domain method allows for local evaluation of capillary supply, which cannot be assessed by more general morphometric parameters. Additionally, relevant aspects of the capillary network can be obtained using a double-staining method, which distinguishes between the arteriolar and venular portions of capillaries. This approach yields values of capillary segment length (distance between two consecutive branch points), minimal capillary length (the shortest contiguous pathway from terminal arteriole to collecting venule), and capillary set length (sum of all capillary segments, originating from the same arteriole and ending in the same venule) (65). These structural properties are more easily determined in longitudinal sections of the myocardium. Combination of measurements on cross sections of myocardium (capillary domain) and longitudinal sections (capillary segment) yields the so-called capillary supply unit, which is the smallest tissue supply volume that can be modelled in three dimensions with some degree of accuracy (399). Capillary supply volume is significantly larger in capillary segments close to arterioles than in capillary segments close to venules (the venular portions of capillaries). Moreover, numerical values of these supply units are similar to the volumes of myocytes (204, 400).

The morphometric analysis of the arterial tree raises some methodological problems that have to be discussed. The conventional morphometric approach for measuring the length of arterial vessels in the myocardium would consist of counting the number, N, of artery profiles in a measured total area, A, of tissue sections. On the assumption that the sectioned vessels are randomly oriented, it is a well-established morphometric principle (535) that the length density equals twice the number of profiles per unit area, N_A:

$$L_V = 2N_A = \frac{2N}{A} \quad (31)$$

Multiplying L_V by the total myocardial volume gives the total arterial length. This technique is not used because it has important shortcomings for a useful analysis of the arterial tree. The quantitative analysis of the intramural branches of the coronary vasculature is complicated by three critical factors: (1) the orientation of the arterial tree within the ventricular myocardium does not conform to the criterion of random orientation, because intermediate and small-sized arteries and arterioles have a preferential radial distribution; (2) there are no established anatomic and/or functional parameters to be applied in the classification of arteries of varying size; and (3) the frequency of arterial and arteriolar profiles in tissue sections is rather small, requiring sampling of large amounts of tissue. These difficulties have been dealt with in a methodology that allows the estimation of the length density of vessels arranged in any variety of orientations (14, 26). This approach is based on the evaluation of each vascular profile individually as it is encountered. The theoretical basis and practical application of this technique are discussed below and are illustrated in Figure 2–5.

Figure 2–5A shows a cube of tissue with sides of unit length. The top surface may be considered to be a unit

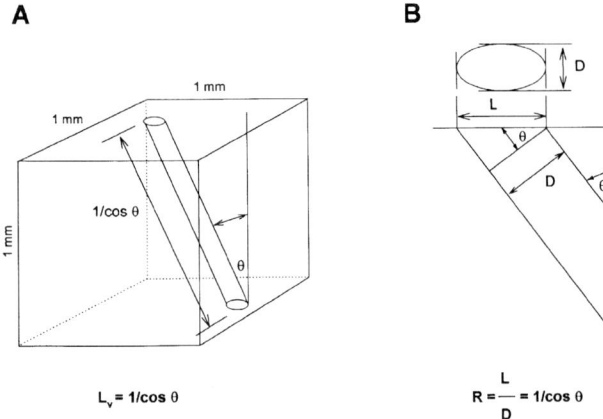

FIG. 2–5. Schematic representation of a vessel profile in the myocardium (A) and its projection on sectioning plane (B). L, major axis; D, minor axis. See text for details.

area in a thin tissue section. The cube of tissue has a unit volume. Inside the cube is shown a narrow cylinder oriented at an angle θ from a normal to the sectioning plane. The cylinder penetrates the top surface and will be counted as a single profile in the unit area. The length of the cylinder in the unit volume, L_V, is

$$L_V = \frac{1}{\cos \theta} \quad (32)$$

Thus, the length per unit volume represented by a profile per unit area is determined by the angular orientation of the elongate structure with respect to the plane of sectioning. Figure 2–5 B shows that the axial ratio, R = Length/Width, of the elliptical profile of an obliquely sectioned circular cylinder also has the same value:

$$R = \frac{1}{\cos \theta} \quad (33)$$

For a single profile per unit area, equation 32 becomes:

$$L_V = R \quad (34)$$

For N profiles counted in an area, A, the general result is:

$$L_V = 1/A \sum_{i=1}^{n} R_i = (R_1 + R_2 + R_3 + \ldots\ldots\ldots R_n)/A \quad (35)$$

This formula describes the morphometric determination of the length density of vessels having any orientation, simply from measurements of the axial ratios of their individual profiles. It should also be evident from Figure 2–5 B that the width or minor axis of the elliptical profile is identical to the cylinder diameter. Thus, measurement along the minor axis of an arterial profile gives the true dimensions of vessel diameter, luminal diameter, and wall thickness, from which one can calculate luminal, wall and vessel cross-sectional areas and the wall thickness-to-diameter ratio. Any of these characteristics may be used to classify the collected data.

Additional information about the vascular distribution in the myocardium can be derived from this morphometric analysis. For example, it can be determined whether any class of vessels, perhaps a size range of arterioles, are randomly oriented. In the case of random orientation, all values and rotations of the angle θ are equally likely and it can be shown (510) that the average value of $\cos \theta = 1/2$. Therefore, it is evident from equation 33 that for randomly oriented vessels the average value of R is 2 and equation 35 reduces to equation 31. Mean values of R substantially greater or less than 2 imply that the distribution of vessel orientations is more nearly parallel or perpendicular, respectively, to the section plane. When vessels are sectioned only transversely, as is the case when capillaries are counted in sections cut perpendicular to the fiber axis, $\cos \theta = 1$, all $Rs = 1$ and equation 35 becomes $L_V = N_A$. A more sensitive test for the random distribution of vessels can be made from the fact that 86.6% of all profiles of random cylinders will have axial ratios less than 2, 96.8% less than 4, 99.2% less than 8, and only 0.8% greater than 8 (141). The general formula for this result is $\% = 100 \cos (\sin^{-1} 1/R)$. Finally, in certain cases the angular orientation of the major axis of elliptical profiles may yield useful information. In the myocardium, vessel profiles can be examined in tissue sections cut transverse to the apex–base axis of the heart. In these sections, therefore, the radial direction, perpendicular to the ventricular wall, is easily identified. It can be expected, for example, that the size class of penetrating vessels will have elliptical profiles more often oriented radially than tangentially and, as noted above, a mean axial ratio greater than 2.

PHYSIOLOGICAL MYOCARDIAL GROWTH: MATURATION OF THE HEART

Ventricular Remodeling

Physiologic hypertrophy represents the response of the heart to the hemodynamic overloads that accompany the process of maturation and the evolution of life before aging effects become apparent. The fetal heart differs from the adult heart in structure and function. The work required by the two ventricles is approximately equal during intrauterine life, even though the left ventricle does less work and the right ventricle does more work than after birth (206, 435). This hemodynamic condition is characteristic of several animal species, including humans, and may account for the similarity in weight between the two ventricles at birth (38, 209, 276). With closure of the foramen ovale and ductus arteriosus after birth, blood flows in series through the right and left ventricles, resulting in a greater volume work load on each ventricle. In the same period, pulmonary resistance is lowered by expansion of the collapsed lungs (260), peripheral resistance increases with loss of the placental circulation (436), and the pressure load on the left ventricle becomes significantly greater than that on the right ventricle (58). The combination of these effects induces a faster growth of the left ventricle, leading to its relatively larger muscle mass typical of the adult heart (276). Thus, growth of the myocardium during the early postnatal period must accommodate not only the increasing demands of the rapidly growing body mass but also the relatively abrupt changes in the patterns of blood flow and circulatory resistance occurring shortly after birth. When these major adaptations have taken place, the process of maturation continues and the heart is influenced by the expansion in circulating blood volume, which increases the preload on both chambers (47).

A relative increase in the rate of growth of the right ventricle in comparison with the left ventricle has been observed during the last period of gestation in humans (209). Thus, the right ventricle becomes heavier than the left (142). At birth the walls of the two ventricles show approximately the same thickness (483), although the right ventricular weight is at least equal to but frequently heavier than the left (208, 414). Similar results have been shown in newborn pigs (77), rabbits (120), and dogs (274). In fetal lambs the right ventricle ejects about two-thirds of combined ventricular output while only one-third is sustained by the left ventricle (57, 129, 434, 437). The right ventricular preponderance has been attributed to the high resistance of the fetal pulmonary blood vessels probably related to pH, Po_2 and Pco_2 levels (206). Related observations have shown that newborns who died of pulmonary disease had a relatively hypertrophic right ventricle contrasting with a poorly developed left ventricle, functionally unable to supply the increased work demand required after birth (208). This unbalanced growth leads to a relative failure of the left ventricle with inadequate pulmonary circulation that may result in pulmonary disease (208).

The changes in the overall circulatory system lead to a reverse functional heterogeneity between the ventricles. Most of the information regarding the fetal circulation has been derived from the sheep, and it cannot be assumed that development in different species is the same at similar stages of the gestational period. Inherent species differences must always be kept in mind.

Within a few days of postnatal growth, the mean fetal pulmonary pressure of 55 mm Hg decreases abruptly, reaching values of 18 mm Hg (209). In contrast, only a slight variation occurs in the mean aortic pressure that rises from 55 mm Hg to 60 mm Hg. A pulmonary arterial pressure somewhat higher than that in the adult persists for several months. The sudden fall in pulmonary resistance is responsible for the lower growth rate of the right ventricle (209) that does not keep pace with the rapid postnatal hypertrophy of the left ventricle. Thus, the proportion of both ventricles reaches the adult type.

The dimension and weight of the right and left ventricle change disproportionately after birth (430). The left ventricle gets larger and the wall thickens rapidly. In contrast, although the right ventricle becomes larger, it has a thinner wall. Since calculated wall tension is inversely proportional to wall thickness (337), the faster thickening newborn left ventricle begins to approximate the adult in its stress–strain relations, while the right ventricular wall thickness and stress–strain relations are still similar to the fetus (156). The heart weight-to-body weight ratio is higher in newborns than in the fetus and adult, resulting from a greater left ventricular weight-to-body weight ratio (156). However, the fetus has a greater heart weight-to-body weight ratio than the adult because of a greater right ventricular mass. Measurements in rodents have shown that mean arterial blood pressure is approximately 14 mm Hg at birth (298), 35 mm Hg at 5 days (86), 52–56 mm Hg during the second postnatal week (269) and nearly 120 mm Hg in young adult animals (71, 363). The combination of these effects induces a faster growth in the left ventricular myocardium leading to its relatively larger muscle mass in the fully developed heart. In male rats, augmentation in weight of the left ventricle occurs at a rate of 7.1 mg/day, which is 3.7 times greater than that of the right ventricle, which increases by 1.9 mg/day (47). These differential growth rates result in a progressive elevation of the left-to-right ventricular weight ratio during the first month of postnatal life. Subsequently, this ratio remains nearly constant (396).

Little information is available concerning the mechanisms of ventricular remodeling in the late stages of fetal life, during which similar magnitudes of loading are present on both ventricles. However, two essential processes occur during the prenatal morphogenesis of the heart: (*1*) myocyte mitotic division; and (*2*) maturational events intracellularly, consisting of the synthesis and organized alignment of myofibrillar and other sarcoplasmic structures (50, 316, 318). The formation of these contractile and noncontractile elements late in gestation can be postulated to occupy the undifferentiated cytoplasmic region of these cells with little alterations of their size. Thus, myocyte hyperplasia may account for most of the increases in chamber volume and wall thickness in the fetal heart. On the other hand, quantitative data are lacking, and so this possibility can only be suggested on the basis of limited morphologic, morphometric, and autoradiographic findings from studies on the adaptation of the heart during the transition from the fetal to the adult circulatory pattern (38, 50, 353).

As a result of the increase in preload and afterload on the left ventricle, dictated by the transition from the fetal to the adult circulatory system, significant changes occur in the anatomical determinants of ventricular size and shape, i.e. wall thickness and chamber volume (38,406). These adaptations are the consequence of the changes in the number, volume, and dimensional characteristics of the myocyte population of the rapidly growing tissue. Importantly, these are all quantitative parameters that have been evaluated through application of the morphometric methodology summarized in the preceding section. In addition, these structural modifications characterize the ability of the myocardium to respond in an orderly manner to the variations in diastolic and systolic wall stress that occur with postnatal maturation. In this regard, an increasing pressure load on the left ventricle induces concentric ventricular hypertrophy, in which wall thickness increases without chamber enlargement (47, 175, 176). In contrast, an increasing volume load typically induces enlargement of the ventricular chamber volume without a relative increase in its wall thickness, i.e. eccentric hypertrophy (47, 175, 176). The hemodynamic condition of pressure overload on the left ventricle is counteracted by a striking increase in wall thickness achieved by the addition in parallel of newly formed myocytes (47, 353). The process of myocyte cellular hyperplasia occurs predominantly shortly after birth, and the magnitude of this growth mechanism reflects almost identical increases in the number of cells across the ventricular wall (47, 353, 397). Moreover, myocyte diameter progressively increases so that early wall thickening is caused by both these phenomena (47). When cellular enlargement rather than increased cell number becomes the main growth pattern (255, 402), lateral expansion of myocytes is responsible for subsequent increases in wall thickness with age. The increase in myocyte diameter with maturation is also accompanied by lengthening of myocytes, which is the cellular growth process involved in the dilation of the ventricular chamber and the normalization of the volume overload stress on the myocardium, dictated by the expansion in circulating blood volume with postnatal development. These phenomena are illustrated in Figure 2–6 that presents data obtained in the rat, a model extensively studied in the last two decades (47).

In contrast to the observations in the left ventricle, the contribution of myocyte proliferation to right ventricular growth occurs through the addition in series of new cells and chamber dilation; the number of cells across the right ventricular wall does not change significantly with postnatal development (353). Moreover, myocyte lengthening is the predominant mechanism of cellular hypertrophy, further expanding chamber volume on this side of the heart (38, 255). These structural adaptations at the cellular level tend to accommodate the increased preload and decreased afterload on the right ventricle shortly after birth (435). Thus, myocyte hypertrophy and hyperplasia participate in myocardial growth biventricularly, but their relative contribution, configurational changes, and architectural arrangement within the tissue vary in the two ventricles. As a result of these cellular adaptations, cardiac anatomy becomes markedly transformed and, while the left ventricle is characterized by thickening of the wall and chamber dilation, the right ventricle expands mainly by increasing cavitary volume with modest changes in right ventricular wall thickness. Later in adult life, the increases in cavitary diameter are paralleled by corresponding increases in wall thickness so that the adult shape of the heart is maintained up to senescence. Postnatal changes in the human heart (209, 276, 362) are consistent with these observations. The thickness of the left ventricle increases shortly after birth and with maturation (138), whereas right ventricular wall thickness remains constant in the heart of children from birth to 15 years of age (433). Although these results have been confirmed by echocardiographic analysis (350), a modest increase in the mural thickness of the right ventricle has been reported with postnatal myocardial growth in combination with a marked increase in the thickness of the left ventricular wall (131, 138). In particular, left ventricular wall thickness increases with age from the second to the eighth decade of life (164, 397, 462). Age-related changes in the dimensional characteristics of the heart also have been described in dogs (224), and several other mammalian species, including cat, sheep, and rabbit (276). Modest variations in the basic geometry of the heart have been noted in rats (99, 174, 460), but most parameters have been found to be comparable (397). *In summary, the circulatory changes occurring shortly after birth are important determinants of the nature, characteristics, and magnitudes of regional myocardial growth and the hypertrophic and hyperplastic response of myocytes. In essence, right ventricular growth is analogous to eccentric hypertrophy, whereas left ventricular growth represents a combination of eccentric and concentric hypertrophy.*

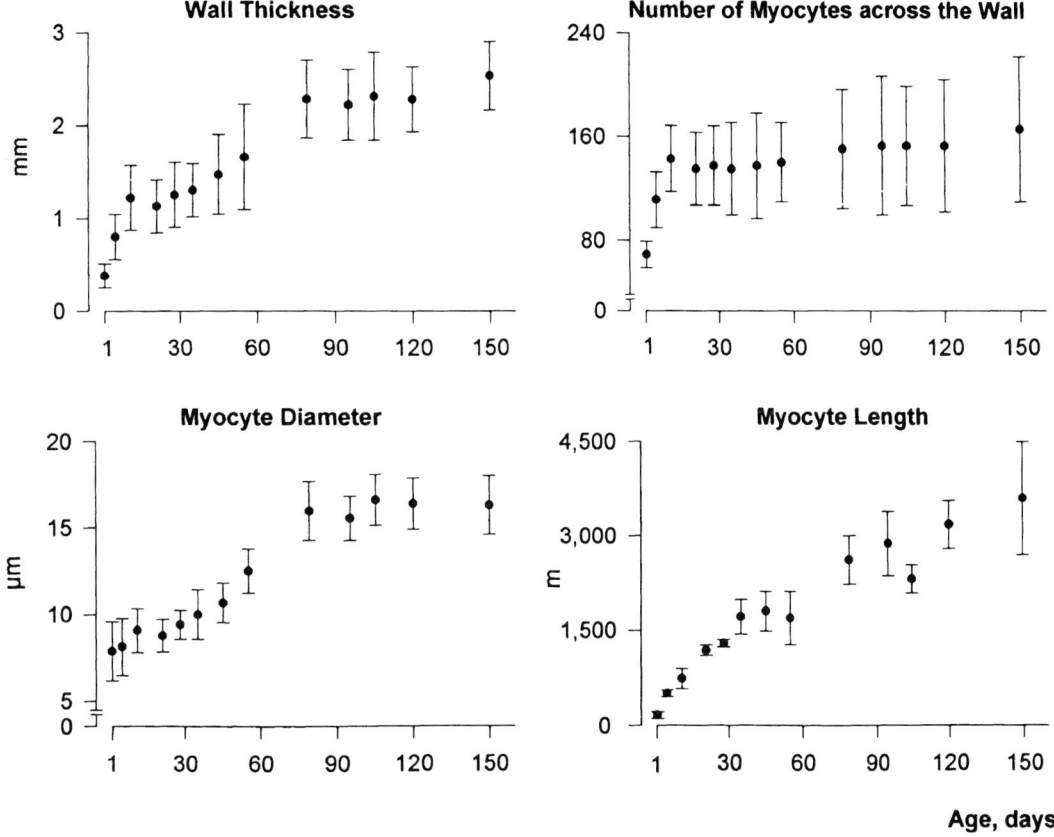

FIG. 2–6. Effects of postnatal development on wall thickness, mural number of myocytes, myocyte diameter, and aggregate length of myocytes in the left ventricle of the rat heart. Results are presented as mean ± SD.

Myocyte Adaptations

The expansion of cardiac mass during postnatal physiological growth is accomplished by increases in myocyte size and number (397). Moreover, the pattern by which new cells are added within the tissue—that is, myocyte cellular hyperplasia—and preexisting cells increase in diameter and length—that is, myocyte cellular hypertrophy—proceeds in a highly predictable manner, reflecting the nature and magnitude of the loading state on the myocardium. Numerous observations in the mammalian heart (47, 255, 261, 397, 405, 442, 457) indicate that postnatal myocardial growth is primarily the result of an increasing volume of contractile cells. However, limited information is available on the human heart. Shortly after birth, myocyte diameter is comparable in the two ventricles (56), but later in life left ventricular myocytes are larger than right ventricular myocytes (362). The total number of ventricular myocytes at birth is approximately 1×10^9 (2, 3), but this quantity is extremely variable (52, 439). In a recent report, the heart of young adults, from 17 to 30 years of age, has been shown to possess an average of 6.0×10^9 and 2.2×10^9 myocytes in the left and right ventricular myocardium, respectively (362). Similar results have also been obtained in other investigations (2, 439, 440). Although these findings suggest that a significant magnitude of myocyte proliferation may occur postnatally, claims have been made that myocardial growth may be completely dependent on an increase in volume of existing myocytes with little or no cell proliferation (397, 554). This calculation is based on the documentation that myocyte diameter increases from 5 μm in infants to 14 μm in the adult (53) and the assumption that the length-to-width ratio of myocytes remains constant with cardiac development (397). Myocyte cell number has been proposed to reach an adult value by 5 months after birth (52). However, the measurements of myocyte number varied from 4×10^9 to 10×10^9. Difficulties exist in the quantitative analysis of the human heart, and more studies with careful selection of patient populations and medical histories must be performed before a reasonable conclusion can be drawn about actual changes in number and size of ventricular myocytes from birth to adulthood.

In experimental animals, the rat model has been investigated extensively. Cardiac myocytes in the rat retain their capacity for proliferation up to the age of weaning, although significant hyperplasia may cease earlier (116–118, 554). Average size of myocytes also increases in parallel with postnatal body growth (255), and myocytes possess the capacity for additional hypertrophy in response to an added workload (39, 261). During embryonic and fetal development of the myocardium both undifferentiated cells and cells containing contractile proteins divide (50, 167, 316, 317, 322, 438, 541). The presence of myofilaments organized in well-aligned myofibrils does not act as an inhibitor of DNA synthesis, contrasting the growth of skeletal muscle cells where DNA synthesis and the synthesis of specific proteins are mutually exclusive (213, 478). DNA synthesis in rat ventricular myocytes has been reported to become undetectable between 2 and 6 weeks after birth (116–118, 133, 554). However, these observations have been challenged, and low levels of DNA synthesis in muscle cell nuclei have been shown to persist later in life in the heart (320). In the adult myocardium, 0.21% (109, 420) to 0.45% (320) of myocytes have been found to be labeled by bromodeoxyuridine (BrdU) and thymidine, respectively. Since BrdU labeling involves more than 10% of myocytes at birth (109), these observations document that the level of DNA synthesis is markedly diminished in adult rat ventricular myocytes. However, the number of cells and nuclei increases rapidly with maturation (38, 255), so that the decrease in the fraction of BrdU-labeled myocytes does not reflect a comparable reduction in the absolute number of cells synthesizing DNA in the entire ventricle. The left ventricle of the rat heart contains approximately 7.5×10^6, 13.1×10^6, 21.8×10^6, 30.2×10^6 and 40.3×10^6 myocyte nuclei at 1, 5, 11, 21, and 60 days after birth (29, 38, 47), and the corresponding percentages of BrdU-positive cells at these intervals are 13%, 7.7%, 5.5%, 0.52%, and 0.21% (109). This implies that nearly one million myocytes in the entire left ventricle undergo DNA synthesis at 1, 5, and 11 days postnatally. At 21 and 60 days, 157×10^3 and 85×10^3 myocytes are engaged in DNA replication. A value of 140×10^3 has also been reported for the adult myocardium (320). Nuclear and/or cell division in myocardial myocytes is greater and persists longer in the left ventricle than in the right ventricle during early postnatal development. The outcome of this difference is the conversion of the left-to-right ventricular ratios of weight and myocyte number from neonatal values approximating 1:1 to normal adult values near 2:1 (29, 47, 355).

Light microscopic autoradiographic detection of thymidine-labeled myocyte nuclei (320) or BrdU immunofluorescence localization in nuclei (109,420) does not determine whether the DNA synthetic activity is coupled with nuclear hyperplasia, ploidy formation, or DNA repair. This issue is particularly relevant during postnatal development because the proportion of mononucleated and binucleated myocytes changes with maturation. For this reason, nuclear mitotic division also cannot be equated with myocyte proliferation. In the mammalian heart, mononucleated myocytes constitute the major fraction of the muscle cell population at birth (38, 255, 397). However, the percentage of binucleated myocytes increases rapidly during early postnatal development in the rat (38, 255, 262), dog (73, 277, 278), mouse (82), and pig (169) heart. In the adult ventricle, 80%–90% of myocytes are binucleated; mononucleated cells constitute the second most frequent cell type. Trinucleated and tetranucleated myocytes also are present, but they constitute very small fractions of the entire myocyte population (44, 246, 397). In the human heart, the percentage of binucleated myocytes varies from 8% to 14% at birth (448), increases up to 33% in childhood, and subsequently decreases to 5%–10% in the adult (64, 217, 448). This reduction in the adult heart has been challenged (110). *In summary, postnatal myocardial growth is essentially the result of an increasing volume of myocytes, whereas the contribution of myocyte proliferation to expansion in ventricular mass is restricted primarily to the early postnatal period. The process of maturation involves changes in the number of nuclei per cell and a decrease in the DNA synthetic activity of myocytes, although low levels of DNA synthesis persist in the adult heart.*

Cytoplasmic Adaptations in Myocytes

The structural modifications of the subcellular components of myocytes with differentiation and growth have been determined mostly in different animal species (35, 122, 277, 278, 316, 457, 474, 499) because the need for electron microscopy in this type of analysis has limited the study of human tissue. However, the observations made have been very consistent and similar in all investigations. The process of differentiation of cardiac myocytes during normal development involves the continuing synthesis and organization of contractile proteins into characteristic cross-striated myofibrils. The myofibrils in embryonic myocardial cells first appear in a disordered array throughout the cytoplasm, without any specific cytoplasmic site of formation (50, 316). However, the ventricular myocardium of 19- to 21-day-old rat fetuses is composed of myocytes containing numerous myofibrils located predominantly near the sarcolemma and oriented parallel to each other and to the long axis of the cell (50). The corresponding distribution of newly synthesized proteins evaluated autoradiographically after the injection of ³H-leucine was found to be higher over the sarcolemma, smooth endoplasmic reticulum, and myofibrils; intermediate in the mitochondria; and below average at the level of the sarcoplasmic matrix. The high concentration of protein labeling near the sarcolemma may be related to the imminent development of the T-system and its associated channels of sarcoplasmic reticulum (327, 375). Furthermore, studies of myofibrillogenesis in embryonic chick heart suggest a continuity between the dense amorphous substance of the specialized intercellular junctions and the underlying Z lines that may be responsible for the initial positioning of the primitive myofibrils (185, 473). With further development, the myofibrils become more abundant and more oriented, and the muscle cells begin to resemble those in the adult heart (316, 318). Autoradiographic studies on both skeletal (341) and cardiac muscle cells (16, 184, 342) undergoing myofibrillogenesis demonstrate a selective localization of newly synthesized proteins at the periphery of the myofibrils, suggesting that the surface of these contractile units is the main region in which the process of deposition of contractile proteins occurs.

The volume composition of myocyte cytoplasm changes rapidly after birth. The volume fractions of myofibrils, mitochondria, and smooth endoplasmic reticulum increase and are accompanied by a commensurate loss of the cytoplasmic matrix compartment (353). The relative volumes of mitochondria and myofibrils at day one are greater than in fetal life (50, 353) and reach adult levels within two weeks in the rat (375, 376). The combined volume of mitochondria and myofibrils in fetal rat ventricular muscle cells is 47% of the sarcoplasmic volume (50), compared with values greater than 80% in the adult (28, 376). Even at one week of postnatal development (185), the combined mitochondrial and myofibrillar volume is 82% of the sarcoplasm, indicating a rapid change in the 7–10 day period following birth. In addition, the surface-to-volume ratio of sarcolemmal plus T-system area/unit cell volume is nearly constant postnatally as a result of the compensatory accumulation of T-tubular membranes. The ratio of sarcotubular membrane area to myofibrillar volume also remains constant (375). The increasing volume fraction of myofibrils is consistent with the observed increase in compliance of the myocardium with maturation (430, 474). Similarly, the contractile properties of the tissue appear to be related to the amounts of mitochondria and myofibrils in the cytoplasm (128, 215). In this regard, the volume ratio of mitochondria to myofibrils does not change from weaning to adult stages, implying a growth of these components proportional to each other and to the cell volume as a whole (375). Physiologically, isometric passive and active length tension curves of fetal cardiac muscle have been compared with those obtained in the adult heart. Fetal myocardium develops a considerably greater tension at rest when stretched than does adult myocardium (156), probably because of the lower volume fraction of contractile material in fetal myocytes (50). Thus, a reduced compliance of fetal muscle has been suggested. Also, when stimulated, fetal myocardium develops less tension at any resting length than does adult myocardium. However, when the cross-sectional area of myocytes and the relative concentration of myofibrils in fetal and adult myocardium are taken into account, it appears that myofilaments in the two situations are capable of similar force generation (156). The continuous synthesis and deposition of structural proteins in the myocyte cytoplasm lead to an increase in myocyte cell volume and a change in the proportion of the myocyte and nonmyocyte compartment of the myocardium. Results obtained from different morphometric studies indicate that the fetal ventricular myocardium (50) possesses a greater fraction of muscle cell tissue, 89.5%, than hearts of one-week-old rats, 74% (184), or the adult rat heart, 83% (32). However, the volume composition of adult myocardium varies significantly between the endocardial, 84.9%, and epicardial, 79.4%, regions of the left ventricle (28). The normally smaller epicardial fraction is composed of myocytes that are larger than those of the endocardium (28). The average configuration of all normal myocytes is that of an elongated cell that is, however, longer and smaller in diameter in the epicardium (307). The significance of this difference may be related to the lesser wall tension existing in the outer layer of the ventricle according to the law of Laplace (415).

In summary, cardiac maturation is characterized by the accumulation of structural proteins in the myocyte cytoplasm, resulting in changes in myocyte size and shape that may reflect differences in the stress distribution across the ventricular wall.

Capillary Adaptations

Although the growth process of cardiac myocytes has been described in some detail, considerably less information is available regarding the specific differentiation and composition of the interstitium at different stages of intrauterine life and postnatal development. Limited results indicate that the percentage of myocardium occupied by the extracellular space does not change with maturation in the canine heart (277). In contrast, a decrease of this tissue constituent has been shown in cat myocardium (457). The partial volume of the overall noncontractile portion of fetal rat ventricular myocardium, 10.5% (50), is more than double one week after birth, 26% (184), slightly decreasing in the adult heart, with differences between the endocardial, 15.1%, and epicardial, 20.5%, layers of the left ventricle (28). The most prominent fraction of the interstitium is represented by the capillary network, whereas larger vessels, connective tissue cells, and collagen matrix comprise minimal quantities of the myocardium (14, 26). The work potential of muscle tissue is clearly dependent on the blood supply to the muscle cells. The changes in ventricular loading shortly after birth and later, during the different phases of maturation, continuously alter the oxygen needs of the rapidly expanding ventricular mass, which adapts to the increasing work demands of the growing animal. A relevant issue is whether physiological hypertrophy of the ventricle is accompanied by a proportional or disproportional growth response of the capillary network, which may tend to preserve tissue oxygenation and normal hemodynamics (227). As discussed in the summary of morphometric methods, the principal structural variables of the microvasculature of the heart that are functionally relevant to tissue oxygenation are (216, 314, 534): (*1*) capillary luminal volume density, which is related to the volume of capillary blood available for gas exchange within the tissue; (*2*) capillary luminal surface density, which represents the capillary area available for oxygen transport from the blood to the tissue; and (*3*) the average diffusion distance from the capillary wall to the surrounding tissue, where oxygen is predominantly consumed in the mitochondria of myocytes by generating ATP through the process of oxidative phosphorylation. The alterations in capillary volume and surface densities, and in the diffusion distance for oxygen, are greatly influenced by the extent of capillary proliferation within the tissue. There are three principal morphometric parameters of the capillary network that have been employed frequently for the estimation of capillary proliferation during physiologic myocardial growth: (*1*) the numerical density of capillary profiles per unit area of myocardium (310, 353, 409, 410, 502); (*2*) the ratio of capillary profiles to myocyte profiles in the tissue (353, 397, 502); and (*3*) the aggregate length of capillaries in the whole ventricle (33, 353).

Measurements of capillary numerical density represent a meaningful estimation of capillary growth. An increase of this parameter with myocardial enlargement would unequivocally indicate capillary proliferation, because such a change can only be the result of the lateral addition of new capillary units. The insertion of new capillaries among myocytes will increase the ratio of capillary profiles to myocyte profiles (353, 396) and will effectively decrease or maintain the average diffusion distance for oxygen (146, 199, 402). In the human heart, there is nearly one capillary for every six myocytes in the newborn, whereas a value of approximately one in the capillary-to-myocyte ratio has been reported in the adult (425, 525, 526). Although the normal value for capillary numerical density has been found in early studies to vary from less than 2,000 per mm^2 of myocardium to more than 4,000 (218–220, 223), a recent analysis humans has documented that this parameter is 3,300 in infants, 2,400 in children, and 2,250 in the adult (401). Similar changes in the proportion of capillaries and myocytes have been described in the rabbit heart (459). Moreover, capillaries in the canine myocardium appear to have a much thicker wall shortly after birth than later, with maturation (277). A detailed quantitative analysis of the structural variables of the capillary bed in the rat (46, 47) has shown that the volume composition of the myocardium changes significantly after birth as a result of a decrease in the volume fraction of the myocyte population and an increase in the capillary vasculature inclusive of the capillary endothelium.

The volume percent of capillary lumen in the myocardium is 4.3% at 1 day and 15.9% at 28 days, demonstrating a 3.7-fold increase during this interval (Fig. 2–7). This tissue component progressively decreases, reaching a value of 8%–9% at approximately 2 months, and remains nearly constant up to 5 months. In addition to the greater concentration of capillary luminal volume percent in young myocardium, it has been shown that in the adult heart this capillary parameter is higher in the subepicardial layer of the ventricular wall than in the subendocardial layer (28), and that the papillary muscle possesses the largest volume fraction of capillary lumen (42). These observations, indicating the possibility of a greater capillary blood flow per unit volume of tissue in the young heart, adult epicardium, and papillary muscle are consistent with evidence of the lesser vulnerability of these tissues to ischemia (236, 319, 513). However, the transmural gradient in capillary volume has not been confirmed in other investigations (33, 369), raising the question of whether the well-known greater vulnerability of the endocardium in ischemic episodes has a structural basis.

During postnatal development significant changes occur in the luminal area of capillaries, the area available for oxygen transport (Fig. 2–7). Like the volume density of capillary lumen, the luminal surface area per unit volume of myocytes increases rapidly after birth, being 31 mm^2/mm^3 at 1 day and expanding up to 170 mm^2/mm^3 at 28 days. This parameter then begins to decline, and relatively constant values, 80–90 mm^2/mm^3, are found from 2 to 5 months of age. A corresponding analysis of the changes in the average distance from the capillary wall to the myocardial tissue (Fig. 2–8), the diffusion path length for oxygen molecular transport to the myocytes, indicates that this linear dimension progressively decreases from a value of 13.0

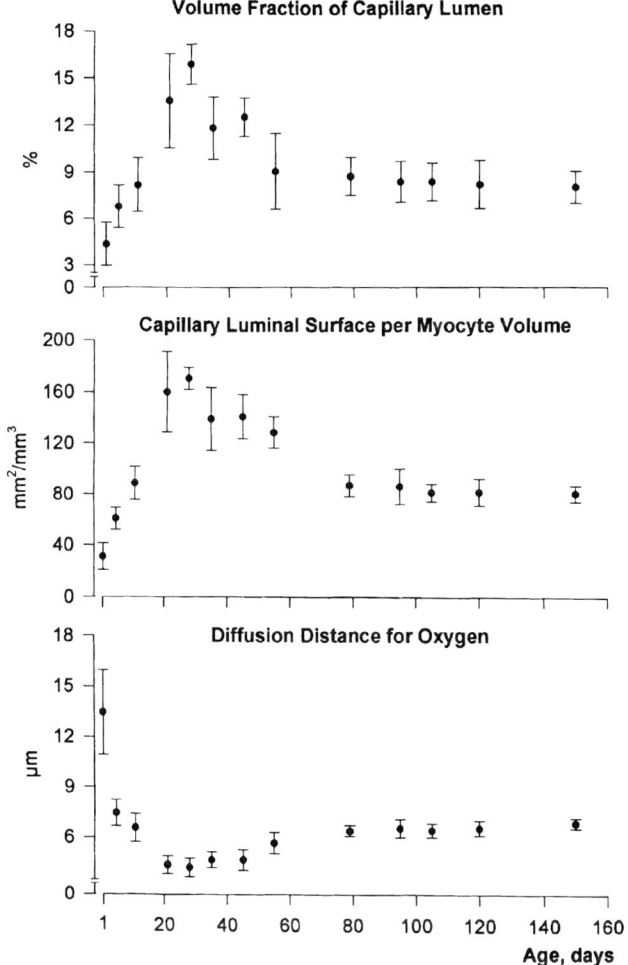

FIG. 2–7. Effects of postnatal development on the capillary properties implicated in tissue oxygenation in the rat left ventricle. Results are presented as mean ± SD.

μm at 1 day to values of 4.2 μm at 28 days and 5.7 μm at 2 months of age. Slightly greater values than 6 μm are seen during the later stages of postnatal development, reaching a mean value of 7.0 μm at 5 months of age. Similar age-related changes in intercapillary distance have been obtained by histometric methods (396, 409) and by direct in vivo estimations (146, 199). These adaptations of coronary capillaries with maturation are the consequence of capillary proliferation during the early postnatal period. Within the first 4 weeks of postnatal life, the ratio of capillary profiles to myocyte profiles in transverse myocardial sections increases severalfold in the ventricular myocardium (47, 57). One day after birth there is nearly one capillary for each 16 myocytes. This ratio decreases to one capillary for 5 myocytes at 5 days, 3 myocytes at 11 days, 1.7 myocytes at 21 days, 1.5 myocytes at 28 days, and subsequently achieves the adult ratio of 1 capillary for 1.1–1.3 myocytes. Increases in capillary numerical density and in the ratio of capillary-to-myocyte profiles can be considered to be only minimal indices of capillary proliferation. The estimation of the changes of total capillary length in the ventricle offers a direct measurement of capillary growth. There is an average capillary lengthening of 23 m per day, from birth to 5 months of age (47). The estimations of the changes in the aggregate luminal volume, luminal surface, and length of capillaries in the left ventricle during the first 5 months of postnatal life increase linearly with age, maintaining the proportion between capillaries and myocytes relatively constant in this period of development.

Conclusions

Hypertrophy of the ventricular myocardium with maturation shows a well-coordinated compensatory response of the heart to the increasing circulatory demands of the rapidly increasing body weight and the rather abrupt changes in the patterns of blood flow and circulatory resistance that occur shortly after birth. Parenchymal cells, subcellular components of myocytes, and capillary microvasculature all grow at a rate comparable to that of the increase in cardiac mass. Myocyte cellular hypertrophy and myocyte cellular hyperplasia both contribute to the expansion of the muscle compartment of the myocardium, and these growth adaptations are paralleled by intense capillary proliferation, which maintains capillary luminal volume, capillary luminal surface, and the diffusion distance for oxygen nearly constant in the adult heart. However, in the early postnatal period, capillary growth exceeds myocyte growth, and this phenomenon may provide an adequate oxygen supply to the muscle cells during the transition from the fetal to the adult circulatory system and the sudden increase in work load on the myocardium.

AGING OF THE HEART

One of the major difficulties encountered in the study of the effects of age on the cardiovascular system is the differentiation of the aging process itself from the presence of specific disease states. Atherosclerosis, diabetes, and ischemic heart disease are common events in humans, and the severity of these pathological conditions increases with age. Because the contribution of these variables to the alterations of the aged myocardium cannot easily be separated from the aging phenomenon alone, the changes of the heart throughout life are therefore the result of multifactorial events in which aging plays an important but indistinguishable role (542). There is no temporal reference point that can be used to distinguish between maturational changes beyond sexual maturity and the aging changes per se, since they both are controlled by time as a critical factor (272, 273, 542). Thus, the issue of whether aging of the heart has to be regarded as a successful adaptation or as a progressive disease state is a matter of controversy, with data being accumulated in support of both possibilities (17, 45, 154, 183, 229, 230). The aging phenotype remains to be characterized not only in the heart, but in other organs as well. Several theories of aging have been introduced; the applicability of one model versus another remains still debatable (89, 179, 237, 239, 465, 466). As discussed in the preceding section, in both humans and animals the growth of the heart is mediated by myocyte proliferation early after birth, whereas, during the later phases of postnatal life, myocyte division progressively declines and the expansion in cardiac mass is controlled by hypertrophy of myocytes and hyperplasia of capillary endothelial cells and interstitial fibroblasts (18, 109, 397, 555). Although DNA synthesis with ploidy formation in adult human cardiac myocytes has been described (2, 443, 482, 517), this phenomenon does not alter the number of muscle cells and/or muscle cell nuclei in the tissue, so that the total number of myocytes or myocyte nuclei in the ventricle can be used as an absolute reference parameter for the evaluation of the effects of aging on the myocardium. This approach forms the basis of the discussion below, which attempts to demonstrate how the application of morphometric methodologies has allowed identification of the basic cellular mechanisms implicated in cardiac aging. Moreover, the concept of myocyte cell loss has been introduced first in the analysis of the aging process of the heart (17) and has been raised as a potential etiologic factor underlying the occurrence of ventricular dysfunction and failure in the elderly (531). Before discussing the cellular changes accompanying the evolution of life in humans and animals, the alterations in the gross anatomical characteristics of the heart will be summarized.

Aging and Ventricular Remodeling

It is a general conviction that cardiac hypertrophy develops with age (272, 531). Studies in humans have suggested that heart weight increases by 1 g/year in men and 1.5 g/year in women (297). However, little attention has been given to the effects of pathological states of the heart and blood vessels on cardiac size (195, 297, 463). Normal aging was not distinguished from the superimposition of hypertension, valvular disorders, diabetes, and ischemic heart disease, all of which increase in the elderly. Moreover, these aging-associated events affect the absolute weight of the heart and its major subdivisions. An additional factor concerns the modality by which the anatomical properties of the heart are examined. Epicardial fat increases with age (297, 416, 463) and has to be carefully dissected before weight measurements are obtained. Early studies have been challenged recently by observations indicating that the aging process of the heart is characterized by a consistent loss in myocardial mass in the male heart (357, 362), while the female heart remains essentially constant (357). Whether these contrasting results are dependent on the criteria followed in the selection of the hearts to be examined and in the exclusion of epicardial fat from these determinations is difficult to ascertain. A recent analysis of data from the Framingham Study (126) tends to indicate that cardiac hypertrophy is not a necessary consequence of aging. Such a conclusion was derived from echocardiographic evaluation of left ventricular mass in healthy individuals (126), findings consistent with the physiological properties of the old heart. Although a reduced capacity of the aged heart to adapt to a mechanical stress has been shown repeatedly, cardiac pump performance at rest is preserved in the elderly (270, 272, 531). Thus, there is no functional basis for the possibility of a hemodynamic overload with age, which could sustain growth mechanisms in the myocardium and lead to organ hypertrophy. Similar observations have been made in different animal models, in which normal physiological responses of the aged heart have been found in terms of global cardiac function (17, 181), muscle mechanics (552, 553), and cell mechanics (154). These in vivo and in vitro studies tend to favor the concept that the modest alterations in the isotonic and isometric contraction characteristics of the aging myocardium represent adaptive phenomena that result in energy preservation (270, 272). However, the hypertrophic growth of myocytes is attenuated with age, limiting the reaction of the old heart to abnormal increases in wall stress associated with experimental conditions mimicking human diseases (110, 481).

An additional relevant aspect of the aging process of the heart in both men and women concerns the lack of changes in the thickness of the left and right ventricular free wall. In the male heart, wall thickness measures an average of 13.6 ± 1.4 mm in the left ventricle and 4.9 ± 0.5 mm in the right ventricle (357). Corresponding values in the female heart are 13.2 ± 1.3 mm and 5.04 ± 0.44 mm. Moreover, histologic analysis of the myocardium fails to reveal major qualitative structural changes. Occasionally, small foci of replacement fibrosis are observed in combination with areas of interstitial and perivascular fibrosis (Fig. 2–8). The tissue is, for the most part, well preserved and no specific forms of damage can be detected and linked to the aging phenomenon. Because of the difficulty in assessing of ventricular cavitary volume in postmortem studies,

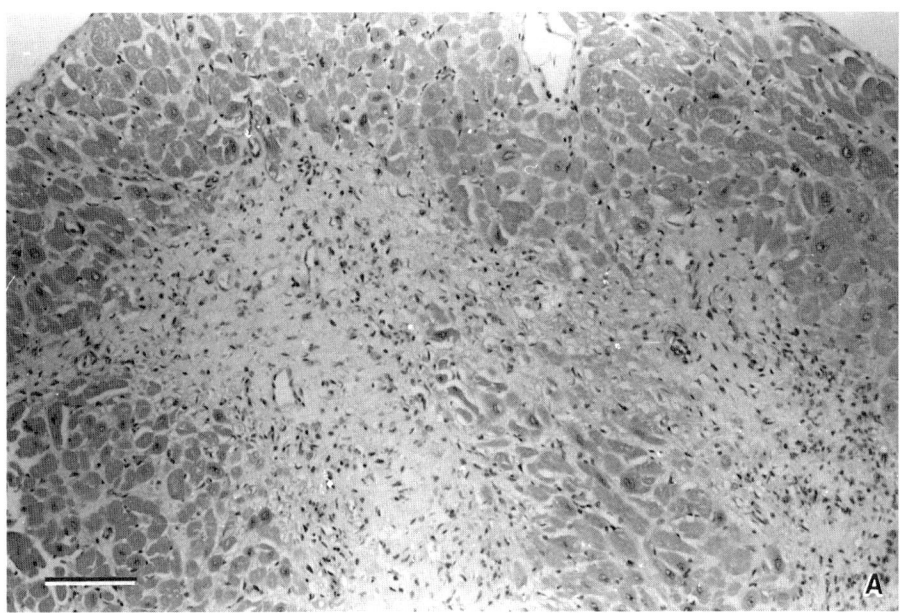

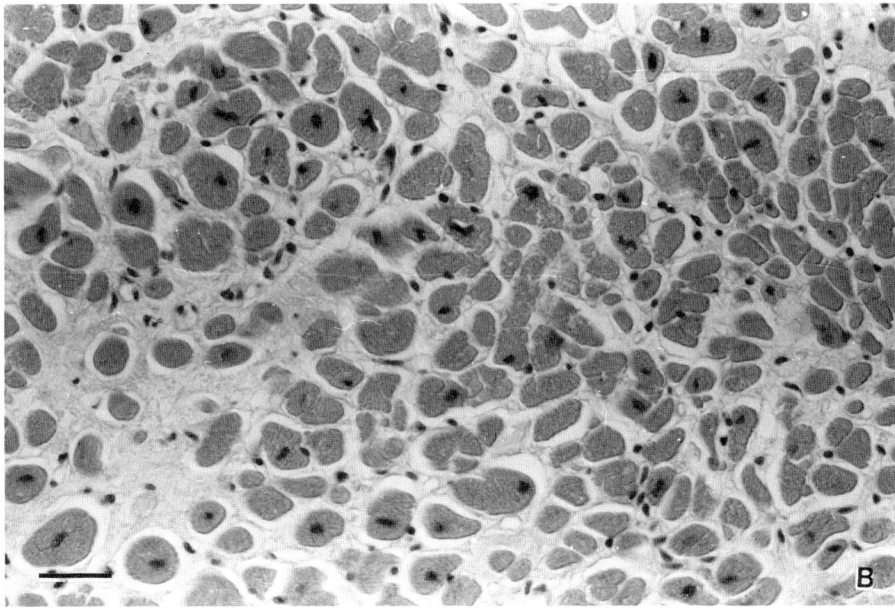

FIG. 2–8. Light microscopic tissue sections of methacrylate-embedded left ventricular myocardium collected from a 74-year-old woman. A: Two small foci of replacement fibrosis located in the subendocardial region of the wall. B: An area of interstitial fibrosis separating individual myocytes. Hematoxylin and eosin staining. A: bar = 50 μm. B: bar = 10 μm.

changes in ventricular wall area can be used as an index of chamber size. The calculation of ventricular wall area, which is obtained by dividing wall volume by wall thickness (47), assumes that the ventricular wall may be treated as a thin sheet. Thus, increases in wall area imply larger chamber volumes. However, this anatomical parameter does not change significantly with age, suggesting that ventricular dilation is not a relevant component of cardiac aging in humans (357, 362).

The effects of aging on the gross anatomical characteristics of the human heart differ from those detected in various strains of rats. In rodents, body weight continues to increase with age and heart weight tends to follow a similar pattern (17, 154, 552, 553). Small but significant increases in collagen content in the myocardium, coupled with the appearance of discrete sites of interstitial and reparative fibrosis, occur in old rats (17, 369, 543, 544). The Fischer 344 rat, developed by the National Institute of Aging, is considered the most appropriate small animal model of normal aging. This strain has been studied extensively in an attempt to identify the critical variables involved in the transition from normal compensated adult myocardium to abnormal, decompensated, aged ventricular tissue. Of relevance, body weight remains essentially constant in adult, aged, and senescent animals (232). Since cell loss, scar formation, and indirect evidence of subendocardial ischemia take place with the progression of life in this rat model (44, 45, 183, 229, 230), the consequences of these interrelated events on the anatomical properties of the heart have been examined. This is because ventricular remodeling with wall thinning and chamber dilation affects the loading state of the myocardium in spite of unaltered diastolic and systolic ventricular pressures (468). Although impairment of cardiac hemodynamics becomes apparent only late in the old and senescent rat (44, 99, 229, 230), the analysis of changes in wall stress has provided important information for the understanding of the progression of the detrimental effects of aging on the myocardium (99). An enlargement in chamber volume has been measured early in life in Fischer 344 rats, and this anatomical modification is the primary mechanism responsible for the abnormal systolic myocardial loading detected several months before pump failure is observed (99). Under any condition of overload, stress as a function of pressure, chamber radius, and wall thickness is believed to reach a new equilibrium, which is illustrated as a static event by the Laplace relation (337, 415). On such a basis, an increasing systolic loading on the left ventricle evokes an enlargement of myocardial cells until the load per unit volume of myocardium returns to normal (468). When this relationship is not maintained, stress remains elevated and ventricular hypertrophy is not adequate for the normalization of wall stress, as appears to be the case in the young Fischer 344 rat (99). With the progression of life, chamber size continues to expand without a corresponding increase in wall thickness and a secondary volume load becomes superimposed on the already overloaded and compromised ventricle, so that cardiac failure ensues at senescence (99, 284). Thus, the evolution of the aging process of the heart in this model can be subdivided into three phases: a first phase of normal cardiac hemodynamics and abnormal systolic stress, a second phase of preserved cardiac performance and altered diastolic and systolic stress, and a third phase of severe ventricular dysfunction and very high increases in diastolic and systolic stress on the myocardium. Importantly, the anatomical changes in cavitary volume and ventricular wall thickness precede the functional alterations in cardiac pump performance.

The possibility that the aging phenomenon alone may result in ventricular dysfunction and failure in the Fischer 344 rat model raises significant questions in terms of the relevance of these findings to the human condition. This is so because comparable studies are not available in the human heart in view of the difficulty in determining whether cardiac failure in the elderly is the consequence of aging alone or whether atherosclerosis, diabetes, hypertension, and ischemic heart disease play a major role in the initiation and evolution of the impairment in ventricular performance in the old population. Moreover, chronic progressive nephropathy, a spontaneous disease, is common in aging laboratory rats (167), making it difficult to distinguish between aging effects and age-related events in this model. Multiple neoplasms are detected with advancing age in rats (312), and, together with renal pathology, these may contribute to the development of the hemodynamic alterations of the heart. Cardiac failure is the leading cause of death in the elderly, but the impact of aging per se on ventricular pump function is unclear. Finally, myocardial hypertrophy occurs with age in rodents (273), whereas a loss in cardiac muscle mass characterizes the evolution of life in humans (357, 362). It should be emphasized, however, that changes in myocardial contractility have been found experimentally with age. The duration of isometric contraction and relaxation is increased and may result in impeded diastolic filling (97, 98, 271, 273). Resting tension increases, and this is usually associated with a decrease in diastolic and perhaps systolic compliance. The hypertrophied aged myocardium shortens considerably less during isotonic contraction, even though there is a measured increase in the duration of shortening. The isotonic velocity of muscle shortening and relengthening becomes depressed (97, 99, 197), and this decline in myocardial contractility is paralleled by a decrease in actomyosin enzymes from a faster isoenzyme, V_1, to a slower, V_3, enzymatic form (98). An increased electromechanical delay time (97, 98, 271, 273, 532) and a marked prolongation of transmembrane action potential duration (97, 98, 532) also have been found with aging, and these changes may have important implications in the regulation of mechanical timing parameters in the old heart. Moreover, it should be apparent that prolongation of contraction duration results in prolonged systolic and diastolic stresses on the ventricular wall and on individual myocytes during each cardiac cycle. These effects represent significant variables that have to be considered in the characterization of the magnitude and duration of the load on the wall and the myocytes with aging. The interaction between depressed muscle contractile performance and abnormal loading creates a conditioned state of the myocardium in which the growth reserve mechanisms are activated, leading to cardiac hypertrophy (17, 44, 273). Whether aging per se may have a similar influence on the human heart, resulting in defects in the contractile behavior of the myocardium, elevation in ventricular loading, cardiac hypertrophy, and the development of ventricular failure remains an important unanswered question. *In summary, the aging process of the heart in humans is characterized by a chronic loss of ventricular muscle mass, but whether this pathologic phenomenon is responsible for the initiation and progression of ventricular dysfunction and failure remains to be determined.*

Aging and Myocyte Number

Numerous studies have been conducted in both humans and animals in which the influence of variables extraneous to aging have been minimized to provide a means for elucidating of the pathophysiologic mechanisms implicated in the detrimental effects of aging on the heart (17, 44, 181, 198, 259, 271, 273, 280, 287, 357, 360–362, 369, 428, 4451, 463, 531, 532). In particular, the possibility has been raised that aging of the myocardium may be defined on the basis of the changes in number of ventricular myocytes with time (17, 44, 154, 362). This approach has established morphologic criteria for the recognition and quantification of the onset and progression of myocardial damage with aging in the mammalian heart. In addition, the loss of ventricular myocytes would suggest that aging of the heart has to be considered as a cardiac disease process and not as a successful adaptation of the myocardium. Myocyte cell death also potentiates other risk factors such as coronary artery disease and hypertension (69, 296, 361), which are common in the old population (531). Myocyte cell death is a consistent characteristic of the failing heart of different etiology (49). Therefore, the phenomenon of myocyte cell loss has been advanced as the potential underlying cause of ventricular dysfunction and failure in the elderly (531). These significant issues have been addressed by the quantitative analysis of the heart in animals and humans through the application of the methodology discussed at the beginning of this chapter under "Morphometric Analysis of Cell Size and Number in the Ventricular Myocardium." Specifically, by combining measurements of myocyte nuclei in situ and evaluations of the distribution of nuclei in the cells, the adaptations of the different myocyte populations with age have been characterized in the female and male human heart (357, 362) as well as in the rat myocardium (17, 44).

Average heart weight in men and women is considered to be 320 g and 280 g (139), respectively. An upper limit of 450 g and 400 g for men and women, respectively, has been established to compensate for a 10% higher body surface of the male population (461), and an approximately 45% variation in maximum heart weight due to the increase in epicardial fat with age in both genders (362). In the male heart (Fig. 2–9), the absolute number of mononucleated myocytes decreases by 50 million per year in the left ventricle and by 20 million per year in the right ventricle (357). In contrast, binucleated myocytes increase 5.0 million per year and 1.0 million per year in the left and right ventricles. These reductions result in a total loss of 45 million myocytes per year in the left ventricle and 19 million myocytes per year in the right ventricle, leading to a total loss of 64 million myocytes per year in the male heart. In contrast, the female heart contains an average $3.6 \pm 0.43 \times 10^9$ mononucleated myocytes and $0.67 \pm 0.08 \times 10^9$ binucleated myocytes in the left ventricle, and $1.05 \pm 0.14 \times 10^9$ mononucleated and $0.36 \pm 0.005 \times 10^9$ binucleated myocytes in the right ventricle. The total number of myocytes is calculated to be $4.31 \pm 0.52 \times 10^9$ and $1.42 \pm 0.18 \times 10^9$ in the left and right ventricles, respectively. Aging does not affect the aggregate number of myocytes in either ventricle (Fig. 2–9). The continuous loss of myocytes with aging in the male heart does not permit the calculation of an average number of left and right ventricular myocytes throughout the life span of the male population.

Observations of myocyte numbers indicate that in women from 20 to 95 years of age the total number of myocytes in the left and right ventricles remains essentially constant. In contrast, a loss of nearly 1% of myocytes per year takes place in both ventricles of the male population. A young man possesses approximately 5.8×10^9 (mononucleated: 5.4×10^9; binucleated: 0.4×10^9) and 2.0×10^9 (mononucleated: 1.8×10^9; binucleated: 0.2×10^9) myocytes in the left and right ventricles. The same individual, at 70 years of age, has 3.6×10^9 (mononucleated: 2.9×10^9; binucleated: 0.7×10^9) and 1.0×10^9 (mononucleated: 0.8×10^9; binucleated: 0.2×10^9) myocytes in the two ventricles. Such a change is the consequence of a 38% and 50% overall loss in the aggregate number of myocytes in the left and right sides of the heart during a 50 year interval (357, 362).

The basis for the differential effect of aging on ventricular myocytes in the two genders is unknown. Although the incidence of cardiovascular events in women increases after menopause, sex hormones do not appear to influence myocyte cell death in the myocardium with aging. The number of myocytes in the left and right ventricles shows no tendency to decrease in women from 55 to 95 years, whereas comparable losses of myocytes are observed in both ventricles of men from young to old age. This phenomenon suggests that a common mechanism may be involved in the activation of myocyte cell death in the left and right ventricular myocardium men. Capillary numerical density and the volume percent of capillary lumen in the tissue decrease as a function of age in the human heart, and this alteration is coupled with an increase in capillary spacing and diffusion distance for oxygen (401). How-

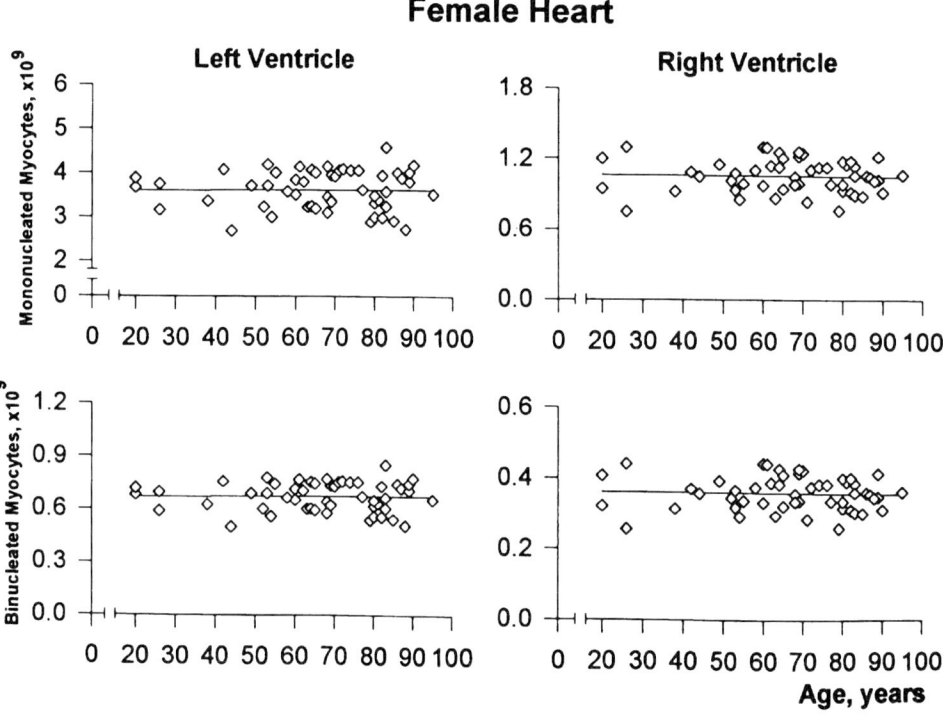

FIG. 2–9. Effects of aging on the number of mononucleated and binucleated myocytes in the left and right ventricles of the male and female heart. *Male heart*: left ventricle = mononucleated myocytes: $y = 6.4 - 0.05\times$; $r = 0.84$, $p = 0.0001$; binucleated myocytes: $y = 0.3 - 0.005 \times$; $r = 0.63$; $p = 0.0001$; right ventricle = mononucleated myocytes: $y = 2.2 - 0.02\times$; $r = 0.84$; $p = 0.0001$; binucleated myocytes: $y = 0.16 + 0.001 \times$; $r = 0.45$; $p = 0.0003$. Female heart: left ventricle = mononucleated myocytes: $y = 3.8 - 0.002\times$; $r = 0.09$; $p = 0.5$; binucleated myocytes: $y = 0.7 - 0.0004\times$; $r = 0.08$; $p = 0.5$; right ventricle: mononucleated myocytes: $y = 1.07 - 0.0002\times$; $r = 0.03$; $p = 0.82$; binucleated myocytes: $y = 0.36 - 0.00008\times$; $r = 0.03$; $p = 0.82$.

ever, this information is limited to the left ventricle in men and gender differences have not been investigated. Unfortunately, there are no reports on the quantitative structural characteristics of the coronary vasculature and microvascular of the human female heart. The phenomenon of myocyte loss in the male heart may be mediated by local ischemia and tissue injury, but whether the preservation of the number of myocytes in the female heart with aging is due to the integrity of the coronary circulation is an important unanswered question. The inability to obtain myocardial samples from human hearts fixed by coronary perfusion has complicated the quantitative analysis of the coronary vascular tree in both genders. Moreover, the loss of ventricular myocytes with aging has not been documented in all investigations of human hearts from birth to senescence (52, 480). The number of cells in these studies has been found to remain constant in both the left and right ventricles up to 90 years of age. However, hearts with concentric and eccentric hypertrophy associated with valvular defects, hypertension, chronic pulmonary diseases, and congenital abnormalities have been included in the quantitative analysis (52, 480). Although this difference is difficult to explain, the suggestion can be made that a cellular hyperplastic response in the hypertrophied ventricles (296, 361) may have masked the phenomenon of cell loss noted in more recent studies in humans (357, 362).

The possibility that the aging process may be associated with myocyte cell loss in the heart has also been examined experimentally in male Sprague-Dawley (17) and Fischer 344 (44) rats. In the first strain of rats, an 18% loss of cells takes place from 3 to 19 months of age in the left ventricle, whereas myocyte cell number remains essentially constant in the right ventricle during the same age interval. Myocyte cell loss is also a characteristic aspect of the aging heart in male Fischer 344 rats, but such a phenomenon becomes apparent at an earlier age than in Sprague-Dawley rats (17, 44). Moreover, the right ventricle is affected as well. In the period between 4 and 12 months, a reduction of nearly 19% in the total number of myocytes occurs in both ventricles. Myocyte cell death is restricted to binucleated myocytes, since the aggregate number of mononucleated myocytes does not change in either the left or right ventricle during this interval. This differential response of the myocardium of male Fischer 344 and Sprague-Dawley rats may be simply because Sprague-Dawley rats live longer and are characterized by a preservation of cardiac hemodynamics (17, 181) and muscle mechanical behavior (101, 369) up to almost 2 years of age. Although the proportions of mononucleated and binucleated myocytes has been reported to remain constant in the adult rat heart (255, 261, 397), the findings in Fischer 344 rats indicate that the phenomenon of cell loss affects binucleated cells exclusively, so that a change in the relative percentage of these two myocyte populations occurs with aging. Importantly, muscle cell loss in this model precedes the occurrence of ventricular dysfunction (17, 44, 99). Similarly, myocyte cell loss in the left ventricle of Sprague-Dawley rats occurs before indices of depressed cardiac performance become apparent (17, 181). These experimental findings, in combination with the results in the human heart, are consistent with the contention that myocyte cell loss is a feature of the detrimental effect of aging on the male mammalian heart.

The mechanisms responsible for the loss of myocytes in the myocardium remain unknown. However, myocyte cell death can occur by necrosis (27) or apoptosis (168, 244). It should be recognized that myocyte cell loss mediated by ischemic necrosis is characterized by activation of interstitial fibroblasts, which leads to the formation of foci of replacement fibrosis in the myocardium. Conversely, interstitial fibrosis may occur independently from necrotic myocyte cell death (113) and may be modulated by humoral factors (527, 528). However, the volume composition of the aging myocardium in men typically shows a progressive increase in the volume fraction of the myocyte compartment and the absence of multiple sites of reparative fibrosis across the ventricular wall. On a qualitative basis, the structural integrity of the tissue is well preserved throughout life. This observation challenges ischemia as the prevailing etiologic factor of myocyte cell loss in the male heart. In contrast, programmed cell death is characterized by the lack of an inflammatory reaction and collagen deposition (55, 127, 551). This process is insidious, difficult to detect by standard methodologies at any point in time, and has important cumulative effects (244). Apoptotic cell death involves the formation of DNA strand breaks at the level of the nucleus, leaving the sarcolemmal membrane and cytoplasmic structures intact (36, 127). In essence, the findings accumulated so far cannot exclude the possibility that programmed myocyte cell death may constitute a relevant component of the aging process of the human heart. This hypothesis is supported by results in rats during development (244) and aging (242).

Although the possibility may be advanced that the coronary microcirculation remains intact in the female heart, and that this condition prevents necrotic myocyte cell death, it seems unlikely that apoptosis does not affect cardiac muscle cells in this gender. Cell death by apoptosis occurs in a wide range of physiological events, including embryogenesis (207), organ involution (136), immunological reactions (458), and the end of the life span of differentiated cells (303). This phenomenon is common to various organs (55, 551) including the myocardium (21, 23, 36, 180, 193, 311,

352). The assumption that myocyte loss may characterize not only the male but also the female heart, implies that new cardiac muscle cells may be formed continuously to maintain constant the aggregate number of cells in the ventricle. Recent observations in humans (361, 393) and in animal models (246) have documented that ventricular myocytes are not terminally differentiated cells and that DNA replication, mitosis and cell proliferation are relevant aspects of the growth reserve mechanism of the mammalian heart (18, 90, 246, 420). Modest levels of DNA synthesis have also been detected in the adult heart under normal conditions (320), suggesting that a small degree of myocyte regeneration is present in the myocardium. Importantly, aging does not inhibit the ability of myocytes to undergo DNA synthesis, nuclear mitotic division, and myocyte cellular hyperplasia in animal models (15, 18, 44, 91, 419). The human heart seems to possess similar characteristics (361). *In summary, the aging process leads to myocyte cell loss in the male mammalian heart, whereas the existence of a similar phenomenon in the female heart remains to be determined.*

Aging and Myocyte Reactive Hypertrophy

It is a general belief that, as the heart reaches senescence, it undergoes a modest degree of hypertrophy (273, 531). However, myocyte cell volume increases only in the male heart (357, 362), whereas this cellular parameter is not altered by the aging process in the female heart (355). In men, myocyte size expands by 158 µm^3 per year in the left ventricle and 167 µm^3 per year in the right ventricle (Fig. 2–10). The mechanisms implicated in myocardial cellular hypertrophy in the aging male human heart are unknown. There are no functional alterations that can be linked to the increase in myocyte volume. Systemic and cardiac hemodynamic parameters as well as body mass are not found to be abnormal with aging. However, loss of myocytes in the ventricle can be expected to generate an increase in work load on the surviving cells proportional to the amount of myocyte loss (468). A similar phenomenon has been shown to be operative in experimental cardiomyopathies (143, 145) and after acute and chronic myocardial infarction (40, 264) in animal models. Thus, the diffuse focal loss of cardiac cells observed in the male human heart leaves a larger stress on the remaining myocytes, which undergo reactive hypertrophy in response to the increased load. Since this process occurs in the presence of normal arterial and ventricular pressures, the resulting condition can be defined as normotensive overload at the cellular level (468). The lack of changes in the aggregate number of myocytes in the female human heart may provide a basis for the absence of a cellular overload and myocyte hypertrophy in this gender as a function of age. The changes in number of myocytes discussed above and in myocyte cell volume described here in the male heart indicate that measurements of organ hypertrophy by weight changes are a crude, often misleading, oversimplification of the growth mechanisms of the ventricular myocardium. In this regard, ventricular weight decreases with age as does the aggregate volume of the myocyte mass in the heart, suggesting atrophy of this tissue compartment more than hypertrophy. Therefore, estimations of myocyte size and number (40–43, 49) are fundamental for an accurate analysis of the reactive hypertrophic response of myocytes with age.

Studies in animal models have been consistent in documenting that the aging process of the heart is characterized by a certain magnitude of myocyte cellular hypertrophy. Changes in myocyte cross-sectional area (491, 496, 552), mean myocyte cell volume (17, 44), and average volume of collagenase dissociated myocytes (92, 154) have been used to characterize aging-induced cardiac hypertrophy at the cellular level of organization. In a manner comparable to that indicated above in the human heart, the enlargement of myocytes exceeds the expansion in volume of the ventricular myocardium in the old Sprague-Dawley rat (17). This result points to the need to obtain information on the volume and aggregate number of cells to detect the actual degree of hypertrophic response of the muscle compartment of the heart with age. It should be emphasized, however, that it is impossible at present to distinguish the magnitude of growth dependent on the increase in body mass with age from that resulting from the loss of myocytes in the ventricle. The question arises because there is no adequate control for an aging animal. Physiologic hypertrophy does occur in the aging myocardium, but the contribution of pathologic hypertrophy remains to be determined.

An additional relevant variable that has been characterized in Fischer 344 rats consists of the participation of myocyte cellular hyperplasia in the growth reaction of the old myocardium (15, 44). On this basis, measurements of myocyte cell volume alone may result in a significant underestimation of the extent of myocyte growth occurring with age. Identical limitations have been observed experimentally in long-term pressure-overload hypertrophy (43) and in humans with markedly enlarged hearts (59, 60, 296, 361). Although the changes in the products of myocyte cell volume and number with time can be expected to provide a valid assessment of the hypertrophic growth adaptation of the myocyte compartment of the heart (17, 44, 361), the simultaneous presence of myocyte loss complicates the estimation of the real amount of newly generated tissue in the ventricle. For example, in the Fischer 344 rat, the volume fraction of collagen in the

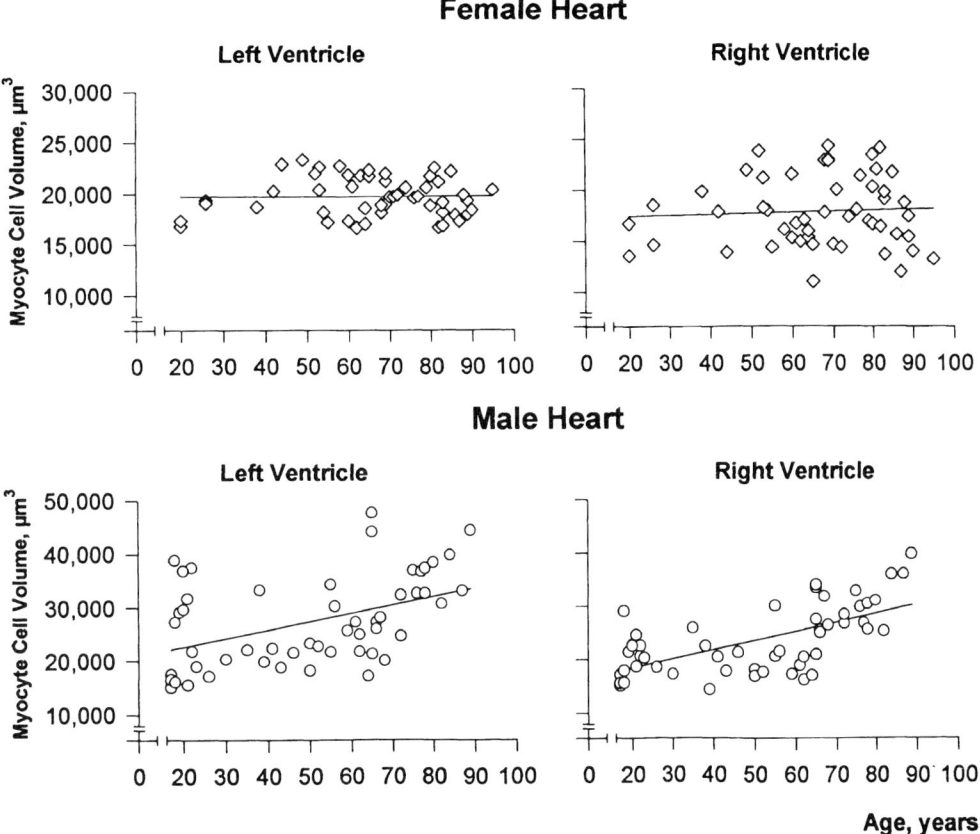

FIG. 2-10. Effects of aging on myocyte cell volume in the left and right ventricles of the female and male human heart. Female heart: left ventricle: $y = 19{,}718 + 0.5 \times$; $r = 0.0049$; $p = 0.97$; Right ventricle: $y = 17{,}204 + 10.6 \times$; $r = 0.057$; $p = 0.68$. Male heart; left ventricle: $y = 19{,}406 + 158 \times$; $r = 0.45$; $p = 0.001$; Right ventricle: $y = 15{,}106 + 167 \times$; $r = 0.63$; $p = 0.0001$.

myocardium continues to increase with age and this change is paralleled by an increase in the number of foci of replacement fibrosis across the wall (44, 99). Ongoing myocyte apoptosis and necrosis also increase as a function of age (242). These observations indicate that myocyte death accompanies the evolution of life in this model, in spite of an increased or constant number of myocytes in the senescent heart (44).

As discussed previously, the changes in shape of myocytes are important determinants of ventricular remodeling, because they represent the structural consequences of the variations in pressure and/or volume loads on the myocardium (13, 40, 47, 49). Myocyte diameter expands in the male human heart in both the left and right ventricles (357, 362), and this adaptation leads to a preservation of ventricular wall thickness with age. Although these findings are consistent with a prevailing increase in the lateral rather than longitudinal dimension of the cells in humans myocyte lengthening typically occurs in aging Wistar (154) and Fischer 344 (92) rats. The distribution of myocyte length is evenly balanced around the mean value in the young heart. Moreover, the majority of cells are close to the mean. With aging, there is a significant decrease in the number of cells in proximity of the average value, resulting in a decrease in the height of the Gaussian distribution curve (92). The curve is also moved to the right, since more cells have longer dimensions and a more uniform number of myocytes is now included in the various classes. Myocyte width does not follow a similar pattern. An increase in myocyte diameter, however, has been shown both age in Sprague-Dawley rats (369). Importantly, measurements of the volume composition of the myocyte cytoplasm have indicated that the fraction of myofibrils and mitochondria remains essentially constant with age with no apparent difference between left and right ventricular myocytes (369). On this basis, it is not clear whether cell loss with aging provokes a pressure and/or volume overload stress on the myocardium. The results in humans suggest an augmentation in the afterload on the myocyte population and concentric hypertrophy, whereas the findings in rodents indicate a prevailing increase in preload and an eccentric form of hypertrophic growth (47, 175, 176).

In summary, myocyte cellular hypertrophy typically occurs in the male human heart with aging, but such a response is not apparent in the female heart.

Aging and the Coronary Arterial and Capillary Tree

Morphometric methodologies have been applied extensively to the analysis of the quantitative structural characteristics of the coronary vasculature and microvasculature of the aging heart. However, these observations have been mainly made in experimental animals (26, 76, 132, 369, 396, 397, 402, 403, 408, 410, 487, 494, 519, 553), whereas results in humans are relatively rare (53, 140, 218, 220, 223, 397, 401, 525, 526). These studies have attempted to address the question of whether the aging process of the heart is characterized by a proportional or disproportional growth adaptation of the capillary microcirculation with respect to the myocyte compartment of the myocardium. This is so because the work potential of the myocardium is greatly influenced by the magnitude of blood supply to the muscle cells, and aging effects can be anticipated to preserve or alter the capillary parameters governing tissue oxygenation—namely, capillary luminal volume and surface densities—and the average distance from the capillary wall to the surrounding myocytes (216, 534). Maintenance of these structural properties of the capillary bed in the myocardium may reflect an adequate tissue oxygenation and functional capacity. Conversely, decreases of capillary luminal volume percent and luminal area in the myocardium, and an increase in the diffusion distance for oxygen, may be accompanied by the development of myocytolytic necrosis, with subsequent replacement and interstitial fibrosis and changes in the collagen content and composition in the tissue (26, 273, 328, 329, 369, 544) These quantitative parameters are easily measurable by the methodology discussed at the beginning of this chapter, which was developed in Weibel's laboratory (216, 534, 535). Such an approach emphasizes the possibility that structural abnormalities may form the bases for the reduced ventricular function potential of the old heart and for its progression into cardiac failure (98, 229, 230, 273, 481, 531, 542). Although several studies have analyzed the adaptive response of coronary capillaries during maturation and aging, the modifications of the intramural branches of the coronary circulation have been characterized only partially (26, 408). In spite of limited information, this work has attempted to establish whether maturational growth is accompanied by the addition of intermediate-sized arteries and arterioles or whether the coronary vasculature loses its ability to grow, resulting in an inadequate adaptation of the intramural branches of the coronary circulation in the myocardium. With the advancement of life, this abnormality may become progressively more severe and may limit coronary vascular reserve and impair coronary vascular resistance (183, 486). These functional defects may be the consequence of an inhibited capacity of the coronary bed to grow with age, or the result of an increase in the myocyte compartment which exceeds the vascular component of the tissue, or a combination of both. These phenomena would decrease the oxygenation potential of the old heart.

The observations made at the capillary level in experimental animals can be subdivided in relation to the presence of normal ventricular performance or ventricular dysfunction and failure. In the first case, most studies are in agreement that cardiac hypertrophy develops with age, but in contrast to parenchymal cells, which retain their capacity to grow (17, 255), the coronary vasculature loses this property much earlier in life, resulting in insufficient vascularization of the myocardium (369, 403, 410, 487, 552). This disproportionate growth between coronary capillaries and myocytes decreases capillary luminal volume percent and luminal area in the tissue, and increases the diffusion distance for oxygen (Fig. 2–11). These structural changes can be responsible for a reduction in the oxygenation potential of the ventricle and ischemic injury. Importantly, they have been found to accompany myocyte loss in the senescent heart (17, 369). In the rat, myocyte dropout and areas of interstitial and replacement fibrosis in the subendocardium develop at approximately 2 years (17), whereas reductions in capillary blood volume and endothelial surface, and a greater path length for oxygen molecular transport to the myocytes are first seen at 1 year of age (369). Further deterioration of these capillary parameters controlling oxygen distribution occurs with advancing age, and this change is accompanied by a significant loss in the number of left ventricular myocytes. The possibility that this type of injury is mediated by ischemia derives additional support from the fact that alterations in coronary blood flow appear early in life in the rat, becoming apparent from 4 to 12 months (183). Moreover, at 20 months, a marked decrease in the endocardial-to-epicardial flow ratio of the left ventricle has been detected following maximal vasodilation. These results are in agreement with findings showing that coronary blood flow decreases under stressful conditions in senescent rats (155, 522, 544) and guinea pigs (486). However, scattered myocyte death, apoptotic and necrotic in nature, occurs in the young heart and increases with age (242), complicating the recognition of the primary event responsible for the aging phenotype.

The potential influence of the structural variables of the capillary network on myocyte cell death can be understood further by the changes in these quantitative

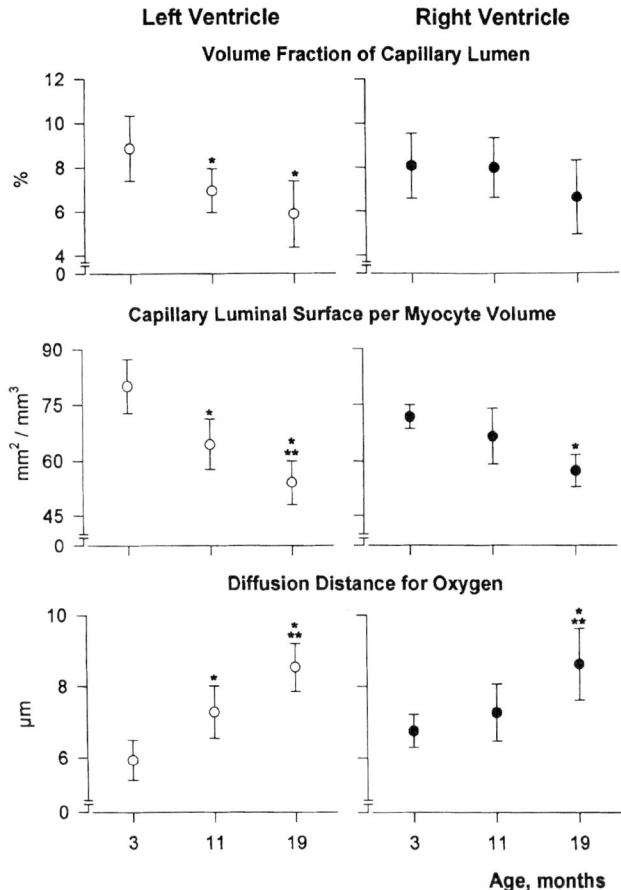

FIG. 2–11. Changes in the volume fraction of capillary lumen, capillary luminal surface per unit volume of myocytes, and diffusion distance for oxygen in the left and right ventricular myocardium of Sprague-Dawley rats at 3, 11, and 19 months of age. *Indicates a statistically significant difference from 3-month-old rats. **Indicates a statistically significant difference from 11-month-old rats. Results are presented as mean ± SD.

parameters in the right ventricular free wall with age (369). Myocyte cell loss does not take place in this side of the heart at the same age interval affecting the left ventricle (17) and the capillary microcirculation and myocyte number are both preserved up to 1 year of age in the right ventricle of Sprague-Dawley rats (17, 369). An insufficient growth of capillaries, however, has been measured at 2 years (369), indicating that aging effects are comparable in the two ventricles, being simply delayed in the right side. The mechanism of this temporal difference is unknown. The progressive increase in blood volume with body mass as a function of age results in an increased volume load on the heart, a condition in which an identical additional work load is applied to both ventricles. On the other hand, the left ventricle is subjected to a greater pressure load since systemic arterial pressure is significantly higher than pulmonary pressure. The combination of these effects on the left ventricle, associated with a deficit in the coronary microcirculation, may exceed its compensatory capacity, leading to loss of myocytes. Moreover, the smaller functional reserve of underperfused capillaries in the subendocardium (214) renders this region more susceptible to ischemic injury with the occurrence of tissue fibrosis (22, 271, 328, 329, 543) than the intermediate and outer layers of the wall. This phenomenon may not apply to the right ventricular free wall. Based upon an analysis of these quantitative indices of myocardial structure, aging of the heart can be proposed as a form of disproportionate growth of the coronary vasculature with respect to the myocyte compartment of the myocardium. A progressive increase in cardiac weight with aging (17, 183, 195, 228, 251, 297, 397, 416, 463, 488) that is not accompanied by corresponding expansion of the coronary tree, inclusive of the capillaries (26, 76, 132, 369, 396, 397, 402, 403, 410, 487, 494, 519, 552), may lead to an imbalance between oxygen supply and demand and local myocardial damage. The adaptations of the coronary vasculature in the human heart are consistent with this contention (401).

More complex is understanding the role of the intramural branches of the coronary circulation and capillary network in the Fischer 344 rat with aging, since in this animal model cardiac failure develops at 20–24 months (99, 229, 230) and the extensive myocardial damage (99, 230) is accompanied by myocyte proliferation (44, 45). Early with aging, the decrease in capillary luminal volume and capillary numerical density, together with the increase in the diffusion distance for oxygen (26), parallel the occurrence of myocyte cell loss in the ventricles (44). This phenomenon takes place from 4 to 12 months, but the alterations in the capillary properties are no longer apparent later in life (26), even though myocardial damage continues to occur. Importantly, capillary proliferation has been demonstrated in the senescent animal, with a complete normalization of the structural parameters involved in the oxygenation of the myocardium (26). In contrast, the length density of resistance vessels from 6 to 20 µm in diameter markedly decreases by 12 months of age, and this defect persists throughout life (Fig. 2–12). The inner, middle, and outer layers of the ventricular wall all are affected by this reduction in intramural branches of the coronary circulation. The length density of arteries 21–40 µm in diameter is low in the ventricular myocardium of the rat, making quantitative analysis of arteries complex. Wall thickness measurements of arterioles and arteries ranging from 6–40 µm in diameter have not been able to detect any aging effect on this parameter. Thus, aging leads to a significant decrease in the length density of arterioles 6–20 µm in diameter, whereas capillary numerical density is only temporarily

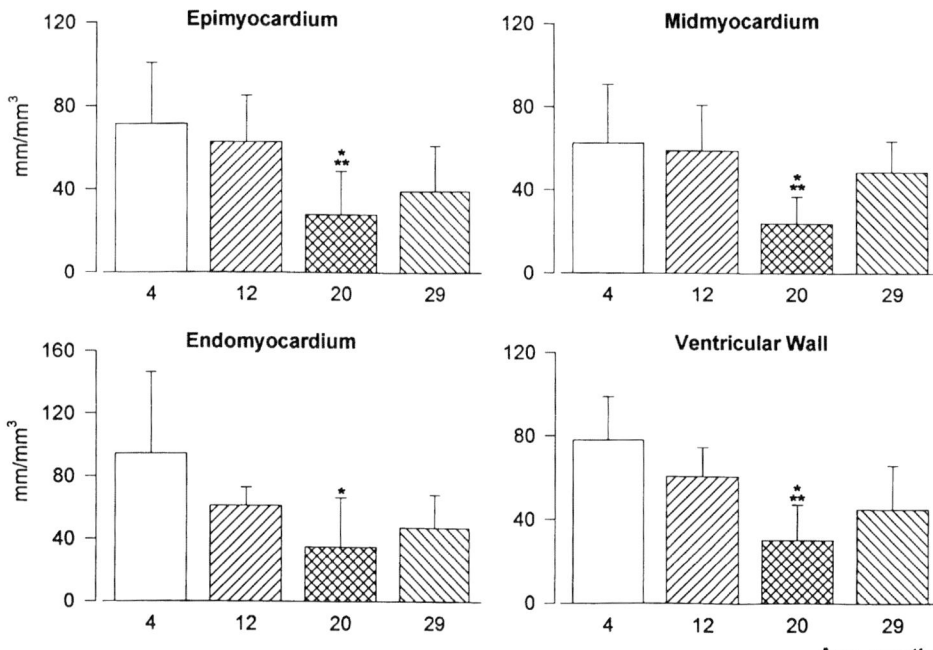

FIG. 2-12. Effects of age on length density of arterioles 6–20 µm in diameter in the principal layers of the left ventricular wall. *Indicates a statistically significant difference from 4-month-old rats. **Indicates a statistically significant difference from 12-month-old rats. Results are presented as mean ± SD.

reduced and returns to control values in the aged and senescent myocardium. The normalization of the capillary network later in life is accomplished by capillary proliferation, but such a growth adaptation is not apparent at the level of the supplying arteries and arterioles. These modifications of the coronary vasculature and microvasculature are accompanied by myocardial damage and collagen accumulation in the ventricular wall, which progressively increases with aging. However, the preservation of the capillary properties implicated in tissue oxygenation suggest that ischemia may not be the only factor responsible for tissue injury, myocyte cell loss, and the development of cardiac dysfunction and failure in the old heart.

Mechanisms responsible for the decrease in the length density of resistance vessels in the ventricle with aging have not yet been defined. Myocardial growth may involve a prevailing expansion in muscle mass, which may not be accompanied by a commensurate lengthening of coronary arterioles. This phenomenon leads to rarefaction of the coronary vasculature and microvasculature affecting coronary blood flow hemodynamics (80, 173, 183, 412, 498, 500). On the other hand, tissue injury may include the intramural branches of the coronary circulation, provoking a similar effect (14). Since the aggregate length of 6–20 µm arterioles is reduced in the aged heart (26) in combination with myocardial damage (17, 99, 229, 230), aging most likely results in a destruction of these resistance vessels. Therefore, tissue injury and dispropor-tionate myocyte growth may both contribute to the structural modifications of the coronary arterial tree of the old heart. Because the class of vessels 6–20 µm in diameter constitutes the major component of the coronary arterial tree, the increase in minimal coronary vascular resistance and decrease in coronary vascular reserve documented in this model as a function of age may have a structural basis. The reduction in the number of parallel pathways represented by arterioles 6–20 µm in diameter in the myocardium may have a major impact on the physiological abnormalities of the aging heart. Similar structural modifications have been observed in long-term renal hypertension (14, 413, 500), a condition also characterized by abnormalities in coronary vascular resistance and reserve (62). The possibility of vascular rarefaction as a mechanism of alteration in coronary vascular resistance and reserve has been implicated also in pressure-overload cardiac hypertrophy and failure, as well as after myocardial infarction (210, 250, 413, 498, 500). It should be emphasized that proliferation of coronary resistance vessels may occur in prolonged hypertension with normalization of coronary blood flow characteristics (501). Although capillary proliferation maintains a constant capillary luminal volume percentage and capillary numerical density in the aged heart, this protective effect is limited by the reduction in the length density of small-sized arterioles. This implies that a larger number of capillaries is supplied by a single arteriole, and this phenomenon may have reduced the potential beneficial impact of capillary neogenesis in the old heart. A similar variation in the magnitude of capillary and arteriolar growth occurs in long-term hypertension (14), although different results have been obtained as well (80, 413). Changes in the average length of individual capillary units and capillary domains (508) may also affect the oxygenation of the myocardium locally, creating discrete sites of myocardial ischemia. In either case, these alterations may play a prominent role in the occurrence of cardiac dysfunction and failure with age (531) and may represent the basis for the decreased ability of the heart to sustain an elevation in pressure (230) or volume (229) load late in life. *In summary, on the basis of these quantitative indices of myocardial structures, the decrease in the length densities of the intramural branches of the coronary circulation, capillary numerical density and surface density, as well as the increase in the average diffusion distance for oxygen, appear to differentiate the well-compensated adaptive phenomena of the maturing heart from those associated with the aging process. When cardiac decompensation occurs, capillary proliferation tends to minimize the potential detrimental effects of the rarefaction of coronary arterioles on the myocardium by preserving the oxygenation potential of the old and senescent failing heart.*

Conclusions

The aging process of the heart is characterized by multiple alterations of the structural properties of the myocardium, which are consistent with the inability of the coronary vasculature and microvasculature to grow in proportion to the muscle mass. However, it is not clear whether this inadequate growth response of the intramural branches of the coronary arterial tree and capillary network results in local ischemia, tissue damage, fibroblast activation, collagen deposition in the ventricular wall, and abnormalities in the loading state of the heart. Myocyte cell loss and myocyte cellular reactive hypertrophy are the critical events responsible for the transition from the mature compensated adult myocardium to the abnormal decompensated aged ventricular tissue. Although the general belief is that cell necrosis is the exclusive mechanism of muscle cell death in the myocardium, the possibility that the suicide program of myocytes may be activated in the heart has to be considered. Myocyte cell death, by necrosis, apoptosis, or both, is a major component of chamber and wall remodeling and may constitute a critical variable in the progression of aging toward end-stage cardiac failure. Myocyte cell loss of either etiology may initiate a sequence of integrated functional, morphological, and molecular responses that lead to additional cell death, scar formation, wall thinning, chamber dilation, and, over time, to the structural template of the congestive cardiomyopathic senescent heart. It should be emphasized, however, that myocyte cell death has been documented in animal models of normal aging and in the male human heart exclusively. Whether aging per se may produce a comparable detrimental impact in the female human population remains an important unanswered question. The basis for the differential effect of aging on ventricular myocytes in the two genders currently is unknown.

PRESSURE AND VOLUME OVERLOAD HYPERTROPHY

In the last three decades of the twentieth century, several morphometric investigations of pressure and volume overload hypertrophy were performed in an attempt to quantify alterations in critical structural parameters of the stressed myocardium (47, 373, 376, 379). The major objective of these studies was recognition of deficiencies in the reactive growth adaptation of tissue, and cellular and subcellular components that may play a role in the transition from compensated to decompensated cardiac hypertrophy. Congestive heart failure is a disease process that develops over time in the presence of pressure and/or volume overload hypertrophy. The clinical manifestations of these physiological abnormalities are mechanical and systemic hypertension, aortic insufficiency, and complex valvular defects. In addition, with acute myocardial infarction, massive infection, and intoxication, a large amount of ventricular tissue can be lost, in which case heart failure occurs as a result of the extensive destruction in muscle mass (40, 49). More obscure, however, is our understanding of the pathogenetic mechanisms responsible for the initial adaptation and subsequent deterioration of cardiac performance when a chronic excessive circulatory load is imposed on the heart. In particular, morphometric methodologies have been employed to determine whether structurally, hypertrophy, rather than being a compensatory process, constitutes the first step toward depressed myocardial function, and whether early ventricular deadaptation develops from an inadequate growth response of the myocyte compartment of the tissue, or the coronary vasculature, or both. Although early work emphasized the analysis of the subcellular constituents of ventricular myocytes (16, 325, 330, 379), more recent quantitative studies have described the cellular basis of ventricular remodeling (43, 88, 100, 123, 160, 188, 191, 300, 301, 321, 364, 366, 368, 464, 511) and the relationship between the vascular and nonvascular portions of the wall (14, 28, 33, 41, 42, 65, 279, 315, 358, 359, 407, 485, 500–502, 504, 520). Of relevance, the contribution of myocyte cell loss and proliferation to the progression of the cardiac myopathy also has been investigated (43, 59, 60, 204, 296, 360, 361, 516). Myocardial damage with cell loss and scar formation, leads to a profound change in the anatomical characteristics of the ventricle, consisting of relative wall thinning and chamber dilation. These gross anatomical modifications may have a significant impact on the magnitude of mural and myocyte stress, and they may become crucial variables in the development of intractable ventricular dysfunction and failure. Moreover, the changes in myocyte size, number, and shape have been determined morphometrically to define the cellular counterparts of the anatomical properties of the severely impaired overloaded heart.

Cardiac Hypertrophy and Ventricular Remodeling

Hypertrophy represents a response of the heart to a hemodynamic overload that tends to preserve normal cardiac function. Several studies in animals and humans have demonstrated that as a result of a severe increase in afterload, the affected ventricle grows relatively rapidly (47, 175, 397), so that the expanded ventricular mass compensates for the enhanced work demand, after which no further hypertrophy occurs (176). A similar response has been observed following volume overload (176), although the anatomical characteristics of the heart vary in these two hemodynamic conditions (172, 282, 288, 468). Increasing pressure load in the adult heart induces concentric ventricular hypertrophy, in which wall thickness increases without chamber enlargement (47, 175, 176, 288). This phenomenon is accomplished by lateral expansion of myocytes with no change in the number of cells across the wall, or in average myocyte length (47, 175, 176). According to the law of Laplace, the greater myocyte diameter would produce a proportional thickening of the wall that should offset the higher peak systolic wall stress resulting from the elevation in pressure (176). These morphologic modifications correspond to concentric hypertrophy in its compensated form, in which the selective increase in mural thickness leads to an increase in mass-to-chamber volume ratio. In contrast, an increasing volume load induces enlargement of the ventricular chamber without a relative increase in its wall thickness, that is, eccentric hypertrophy. Chamber enlargement appears to be brought about through lengthening of myocytes (10, 24), with only slight variations in myocyte cross-sectional area and no change in sarcomere length (10, 24). Lengthening of myocytes would have the effect of counteracting the greater end-diastolic wall stress (176) by contributing to the enlargement in chamber volume that would otherwise occur by spatial rearrangement or lateral slippage of myocardial fibers within the wall, or both. These factors characterize eccentric hypertrophy in the well-balanced stage, in which chamber dilation is accompanied by a proportional increase in wall thickness, so that the wall thickness-to-chamber radius ratio is not altered and the mass-to-chamber volume ratio remains constant. When these relations are not preserved, decompensated concentric and eccentric hypertrophy develop (59, 60, 70, 296, 361).

Although determination of the mechanism by which the initial mechanical message of increased stress is translated by the myocytes into increased synthesis of contractile proteins remains an unresolved problem, the myocardial cells are assumed to enlarge until the load per unit of myocardium returns to normal (175, 176, 337, 468). On the basis of the Laplace equation, the changes in the dimensional properties of myocytes lead to restoration of wall stress within normal values through integrated structural processes occurring at the cellular level of organization. Under any condition of overload, stress (σ) as a function of pressure (p), chamber radius (r), and wall thickness (h) will reach a new equilibrium, which is illustrated as a static event by the relationship (176): $\sigma = p \times r/2h$. However, observations made in humans and in animal models clearly indicate that not only the severity of the pathologic state but also the duration of the mechanical load play an important role in the outcome of ventricular hypertrophy and its progression into irreversible congestive heart failure (100, 159, 229, 230, 248). Thus, the evolution of the hypertrophied cardiomyopathic heart can be subdivided into two phases: a first phase of apparent compensatory hypertrophy and normal cardiac performance (338, 386, 387, 389, 390, 422) followed by a second phase in which long-standing work overload may result in further enlargement of the ventricular mass, with marked abnormalities in cardiac function (61, 137, 186, 286, 338, 386, 387, 447, 505). The implication is that, for a given elevation in preload or afterload, time becomes one of the most significant variables for the progression of hypertrophy and the occurrence of ventricular dysfunction. Should this be the case, the time factor (t) may have to be added to the Laplace relation to characterize wall stress in a more dynamic fashion: stress (σ) would then be a function of pressure (p), chamber radius (r), wall thickness (h), and time (t), i.e., $\sigma(p,r,h,t)$. It should be emphasized that time plays a role only if stress is not normalized and such an effect can be assumed to be proportional to the magnitude of the overload. On this basis, short- and long-term studies have been performed, and the duration of the overload has been shown to be an important phenomenon in the alterations in the proportions between wall thickness and chamber diameter in different animal models of pressure and volume overload hypertrophy (10, 12, 28, 42, 100, 368, 528). The preservation of the anatomical variables implicated in the loading state of the myocardium is paralleled by normal ventricular performance (338, 382). Conversely, a disproportionate increase in chamber size with relative thinning of the wall is associated with abnormalities in cardiac function, and excessive cavitary dilation typically occurs in the presence of intractable congestive heart failure (100, 286, 386, 387).

The anatomical aspects of ventricular remodeling briefly described above have been characterized carefully in the human heart by Linzbach (296), who also introduced the concept of physiologic hypertrophy to define the increase in myocardial mass associated with exercise (289). Adaptation to exercise is specific for a given model of physical activity (257), and events requiring dynamic exercise and endurance training are accompanied by an increased preload on the heart (134, 423), a functional condition that progresses into biventricular hypertrophy (10, 288). As demonstrated by Linzbach in humans (289, 296) and experimentally in rats (10, 24, 27), the increase in cavitary volume is associated with a corresponding thickening of the wall, i.e., compensated eccentric hypertrophy (47). The preservation of these dimensional parameters in volume hypertrophy has also been observed in vivo (27, 47, 115, 340, 446). With the exception of exercise, however, prolonged increases in preload associated with valvular insufficiency in humans are accompanied by a dilation of the ventricular chamber that exceeds mural thickness (296). Although this form of pathological hypertrophy is commonly detected in the long-term evolution of the cardiac myopathy (78, 158, 201, 296, 313, 431, 452, 471), it does correspond to decompensated eccentric hypertrophy. In a comparable manner, pressure overload is counteracted initially by an increase in wall thickness with no changes in chamber diameter (176). On the other hand, some left ventricular chamber enlargement has been observed following the sudden pressure increase produced experimentally by aortic stenosis in rats (41) and dogs (444, 513, 521). The more gradual increase in pressure load occurring in renal hypertension shows no evidence of chamber enlargement shortly after the imposition of the overload (28); however, with time, diastolic and systolic chamber diameters increase and these indices of ventricular decompensation are paralleled by impairment of cardiac pump performance (286). The terminal phase is characterized by extensive ventricular remodeling with an increase in the transverse and longitudinal chamber axes and a decrease in wall thickness (100). Thus, a sustained pathological elevation in afterload leads first to compensated concentric hypertrophy which evolves into the decompensated form (100, 286). Although anatomical studies analyzing the effects of pressure overload on the human heart are limited (360), available information suggests that the sequence of events identified in animal models applies to the human heart as well. However, systemic hypertension in the absence of cardiac failure in man is associated with right ventricular hypertrophy (360), a condition not commonly observed experimentally. The etiology of this phenomenon remains to be clarified. *In summary, increasing pressure and volume loading induces concentric and eccentric hypertrophy in which the duration of the overload is a critical determinant in the evolution of compensated myocardial hypertrophy into overt cardiac failure.*

Cardiac Hypertrophy and Myocyte Size, Shape, and Number

The gross morphological indices of ventricular dimensions, wall thickness and chamber radius, are the expression of a combination of parameters that include number of myocytes across the wall, average myocyte cross-sectional diameter and length, and proportion between viable myocardium and scarred tissue in the ventricle (13, 40). For example, chamber dilation and mural thinning may come about from side-to-side slippage of myocytes, which results in a reduction in the average number of muscle cells within this wall (70, 221, 288, 353–355, 547). Even if this phenomenon were to occur, however, the total number of myocytes in the whole ventricle might remain constant. Conversely, cell loss and scar formation could produce the same effect on ventricular size and shape: decreasing wall thickness and ratio of wall thickness-to-chamber radius (13). In contrast, myocyte proliferation may lead to mural thickening by the addition in parallel of newly formed cells (246, 353, 364, 368) and/or ventricular dilation through the insertion in series of dividing myocytes (246, 353, 361, 364). On a cellular basis, myocyte hypertrophy may be accomplished by an increase in myocyte diameter, length, or both. When cellular enlargement rather than increased cell length becomes the main growth mechanism, the lateral expansion of myocytes is responsible for subsequent increases in wall thickness with no changes in chamber volume. In contrast, myocyte lengthening alone can be expected to result in a larger cavitary volume without affecting wall thickness. A disproportionate increase in average cell length with respect to its diameter results in a decrease in the cell diameter-to-cell length ratio and, thus, in chamber enlargement with relative thinning of the wall. Therefore, the changes in number, size, and shape of myocytes in response to abnormal pressure and volume loads are the major determinants of concentric and eccentric ventricular hypertrophy in its compensated and decompensated forms. Moreover, as indicated in the preceding section, the duration of the overload is a critical variable in the modulation of the cellular growth response of the myocyte population in the ventricle. Before illustrating specific examples of the cellular basis of wall remodeling, the issue of myocyte proliferation in long-term cardiac hypertrophy will be discussed in an attempt to demonstrate the critical role played by this form of cell growth in pathological cardiac states.

The possibility that the human heart may not respond to an increase in pressure and volume loads by hypertrophy of preexisting myocytes alone but also by myocyte cellular hyperplasia has been a matter of controversy for several decades (111, 258, 397, 469, 554, 555). The critical heart weight theory introduced by Linzbach in the late 1940s and early 1950s (289–294) emphasizes the fact that, in the presence of a cardiac weight of 500 g or greater, hyperplasia of myofibers begins and this cellular process constitutes the prevailing growth mechanism of the heart. The initial findings were restricted to the left ventricle, but similar adaptations have been shown at the level of the right ventricle (60), indicating that the entire heart may respond to a sustained increase in workload by the generation of new myocytes through mitotic division of the existing muscle cells (59, 60, 296). This contention implies that myocyte cellular hypertrophy occurs first and, when this cellular response is exhausted, myocyte cellular hyperplasia is induced, further expanding ventricular weight. However, not only the existence of myocyte proliferation but also this postulated sequence of events have been challenged (43, 366, 554, 555). This challenge came about because experimental studies demonstrated that short-term cardiac hypertrophy in the adult heart results from an enlargement of preexisting myocytes with little DNA synthesis in myocyte nuclei, possibly representing polyploid cells (74, 177, 178, 343). Thus, it has become a general belief that no division of muscle nuclei occurs under normal conditions or following the imposition of an overload once cell division has ceased, shortly after birth, in the mammalian myocardium (258, 469).

These contrasting observations have raised a number of questions concerning, on one side, the validity of the conclusions drawn in humans, and, on the other, the difficulty of obtaining experimentally the degrees of hypertrophy found in the human. The critical heart weight theory, however, has neglected the role of time as a determinant of the cellular mechanisms implicated in long-standing cardiac hypertrophy. The possibility has been raised that this cellular process has to be regarded as a late event in response to a sustained mechanical stress more than as a compensatory mechanism that takes place in the presence of a defined degree of cardiac hypertrophy (43, 366, 368). Moreover, observations in humans (18, 23, 59, 60, 170, 243, 290–296, 360, 361, 393, 516) and animals (18, 22, 23, 43, 90, 91, 246, 366, 418–420, 530) suggest that the hemodynamic condition created by the overload may be the most important variable in the initiation of myocyte hypertrophy or hyperplasia. Following a gradual and moderate increase in workload on the heart, myocyte cellular hypertrophy predominates (28, 31, 41, 42, 75, 160, 177, 178, 261, 300, 301, 321, 464, 511), whereas a severe increase in ventricular loading, acute or chronic in nature, may engender DNA synthesis, nuclear mitotic division, and myocyte proliferation experimentally (18–20, 22, 23, 246, 299, 419, 420, 454) and in the human (18, 20, 23, 243, 296, 361, 393). Thus, in the absence of cardiac decompensation, myocardial growth may be accomplished exclusively by enlargement of myocytes, and myocyte cellular hyperplasia may take place only in the presence of ventricular dysfunction and overt failure, independent of a specific increase in cell size or myocardial mass. In addition, the negative results claimed experimentally have been based on a limited number of studies performed in animal models of cardiac hypertrophy in which little or no thymidine labeling has been found in the stressed myocardium (74, 178, 343, 441, 530). De novo DNA synthesis was restricted to the nonmyocyte populations of the ventricle, suggesting the absence of myocyte cellular hyperplasia during the development of cardiac hypertrophy. However, the functional state of the overloaded ventricle was ignored. Recent results have indicated that the number of myocyte nuclei incorporating labeled thymidine is 8.0×10^5 at birth and 1.4×10^5 in the adult rat heart (320). Similar levels of bromodeoxyuridine (BrdU) labeling have also been found in independent studies in the mammalian heart (246, 420), suggesting that myocytes may retain their capacity to replicate DNA throughout life. These observations support the contention that increases in load may activate DNA synthesis and myocyte mitotic division, as documented almost 30 years ago in pressure overload hypertrophy in the adult rat (530). Conversely, light microscopic autoradiographic detection of thymidine-labeled myocyte nuclei (320) or BrdU immunofluorescence localization in nuclei (246, 419, 420) does not determine whether the DNA synthetic activity is coupled with nuclear hyperplasia, ploidy formation, or DNA repair. Although changes in the distribution of ploidy in the overloaded myocardium have not been found consistently experimentally (177, 246), ploidy formation is a well-established event of the decompensated hypertrophied human heart (1, 4, 5, 516), where it correlates closely with the increases in myocardial mass (1). Aging does not affect this process (4).

A relevant aspect of the characterization of the terminal and nonterminal differentiation of ventricular myocytes in the adult heart concerns the documentation of mitotic figures in the cells. Nuclear mitotic divisions have been observed repeatedly, but quantifications of this process have been limited. Difficulty exists in establishing whether an individual image is associated with a myocyte nucleus, a fibroblast, or an endothelial cell. During mitosis, myocytes may not retain their characteristic morphological appearance. Colchicine administration increases the number of mitoses in both myocytes and noncontractile cells, but this alkaloid alters the configuration of metaphase chromosomes (476) and does not improve the distinction between myocytes and nonmyocytes. The complexity of establishing the cell of origin in the presence of mitosis was indicated more than two decades ago (177), and current histological observations confirm this contention (393). Only a few examples have been published of mitosis in myocyte nuclei in both the normal (371) and hypertrophied rat heart (246, 419, 420, 530). Such limitation in the recognition of mitosis may represent one of the most critical reasons for the controversy on the existence of myocyte cellular hyperplasia in the heart. However, in spite of these problems, DNA synthesis and nuclear mitotic figures have been shown in adult ventricular myocytes (246, 299, 393). Most importantly, the difficulty in identifying mitotic images in myocytes has been overcome by the use of confocal microscopy (18, 23). By this approach, a myocyte mitotic index has been measured in normal and failing human hearts (243). Therefore, the dogma that ventricular myocytes are terminally differentiated cells can be challenged, first, on the basis of nuclear events including cytokinesis, and second, in view of the findings of myocyte proliferation discussed below.

The significance of the alterations in ventricular function in the activation of the DNA synthetic machinery of myocytes and nuclear mitotic division has been shown in aging Fischer 344 rats in the absence of any intervention (15, 44, 91). Ventricular myocytes retain their capacity to undergo nuclear mitotic division in adulthood and senescence. Metaphase chromosomes have been detected at all stages of postnatal life in left and right ventricular myocytes, but the fraction of nuclei entering mitosis markedly increases in the overloaded failing old heart (15). Thus, low levels of myocyte replication may persist throughout the life span in this strain of rats. Similar observations have not been made in Sprague-Dawley rats of comparable ages (17), a discrepancy that is difficult to explain and that may reflect not only strain differences but also the precocious effects of aging on the Fischer heart, which lead to abnormalities in ventricular loading in young adult animals (99, 229, 230). The hemodynamic profile (15, 17, 44, 91, 99, 181), the mechanical characteristics (45, 101, 369), and the biochemical properties (98, 102) of the heart vary among strains of rats, and these factors may be responsible for their distinct life spans (104, 121) and the variability in the capacity of myocytes to proliferate. Decompensated cardiac hypertrophy in the senescent human heart is characterized by a 36% and 59% increase in the number of myocyte nuclei in the left and right ventricles, respectively (361). This proliferative response of the myocardium accounts for most of the increase in myocyte mass of both ventricles. However, these degrees of nuclear hyperplasia cannot be assumed to represent identical magnitudes of cellular hyperplasia. This phenomenon may reflect a change in the number of nuclei per cell without a real increase in myocyte number. This is so because the myocardium is composed of mononucleated and binucleated myocytes (5, 64, 81, 217, 262, 448), and the proportion between these two cell populations is not readily obtainable from quantitative analysis of tissue sections (306). Such a limitation complicates the computation of the changes in the absolute cell number in the ventricle because the relative contribution of mononucleated and binucleated cells to total cell number may change with cardiac hypertrophy.

Available information indicates that in the human heart, ~75%–85% of myocytes are mononucleated and only 15%–20% of myocytes are binucleated (5, 64, 217, 262). On the other hand, cardiac hypertrophy in humans has been claimed to be associated with increases in the percentage of binucleated cells in both the left and right ventricular myocardium (448). This phenomenon would lead to an overestimation of the actual magnitude of myocyte cellular hyperplasia when this process is evaluated on the basis of nuclear counts (43, 44, 366). Under extreme conditions, the fraction of binucleated cells was reported to increase from 13.5% to 25.5% in the left ventricle and from 7.1% to 11.1% in the right ventricle (448). If similar modifications in the percentage of binucleated cells occurred in hypertrophic senescent hearts, then the 36% and 59% increases in the aggregate number of myocyte nuclei would correspond to increases in myocyte cell number of 25% and 54% in the left and right ventricles (361). However, recent measurements in the distribution of nuclei in human myocytes, after enzymatic dissociation of cells, have demonstrated that mononucleated and binucleated myocytes constitute nearly 75% and 25% of the entire myocyte population (356). These values apply to both ventricles and are not affected by age, cardiac hypertrophy or ischemic cardiomyopathy. Together, these observations are consistent with the capacity of myocytes to reenter the cell cycle at all stages of postnatal life, providing strong supportive evidence for the contention that myocyte proliferation occurs in the old human heart.

Another issue that has been repeatedly raised against the ability of ventricular myocytes in humans to undergo nuclear mitotic division, and eventually cell proliferation, was the lack of demonstration of mitotic figures in cardiac muscle cells under normal and pathological states. However, recent observations have provided such documentation in patients affected by chronic intractable congestive heart failure (243, 393). For the first time, a quantitative estimate of this phenomenon was obtained in control and diseased hearts. Ventricular decompensation was characterized by a ten-fold increase in the number of dividing myocytes; cytokinesis was documented unequivocally (243). The frequency of mitosis in the nonmyocyte cell population also has been measured (393). Comparable data have been collected in dogs (299, 454), in which a myocyte mitotic index was evaluated separately in tissue sections and enzymatically dissociated myocytes (454). Some examples of mitotic figures in the failing heart in humans and in animal models of congestive heart failure are illustrated in Plate 3, whereas Figure 2–13 show the values of mitotic index collected in humans by confocal microscopy (243).

The ability of myocytes to proliferate and replace dying cells (180, 352) is markedly enhanced in the failing myocardium, in which 140 myocyte nuclei per 10^6 were found in mitosis, while only 14 nuclei per 10^6 were measured in control tissue (Fig. 2–13). The mitotic indices collected necessitate some comments to appreciate the magnitude of cell regeneration that can be achieved with these levels of mitosis (243). In a relatively young man, 5.8×10^9 myocyte nuclei, which represent only one-third of the entire number of cells (554), are present in the left ventricle (357, 362); a mitotic index of 14×10^6 implies that 81,200 myocyte nuclei are in mitosis. In most cell systems, mitosis is completed in less than one hour (243), indicating that nearly 0.71×10^9 myocyte nuclei are produced in one year in the unaffected left ventricle. Because in the left ventricular myocardium 74% of myocytes are mononucleated and 26% are binucleated (356), 0.61×10^9 new myocytes are formed. Conversely, in the same ventricle, in the presence of heart failure, 812×10^3 myocyte nuclei are in mitosis, resulting in an accumulation of 7.12×10^9 myocyte nuclei in one year. The fractions of mononucleated and binucleated myocytes is not altered by cardiac diseases (356), implying that this increase in nuclei may reflect the generation of 6.19×10^9 new myocytes in the decompensated ventricle (243). Moreover, mitotic figures have never been found positive for apoptosis, excluding myocyte death at this stage of the cell cycle (23, 454). Myocyte apoptosis exceeds the level of myocyte proliferation in the failing heart (180, 352), although at present a direct comparison between these two events is impossible. The time required for the completion of the apoptotic process in myocytes is unknown. The same problem exists for the duration of the cell cycle. No information is available concerning the length of any of the phases of the cell cycle in neonatal and adult myocytes in vitro and in vivo. The magnitude of myocyte proliferation suggested here is consistent with quantitative results in the severely hypertrophied human heart (59, 60, 296). It should be emphasized that in these calculations the assumption is made that myocyte nuclei divide only one time. Documentation of consistently high levels of myocyte regeneration have been obtained only in the presence of profound alterations in ventricular pump function and congestive heart failure (243, 361, 393). In contrast, cellular hypertrophy may be the dominant growth mechanism of the stressed myocardium in its compensated stage (360).

The demonstration of DNA replication, nuclear mitotic division, and nuclear proliferation in myocytes of human (243, 361, 393), rat (246, 419, 420), and dog (299, 454) hearts affected by cardiac failure does not necessarily imply myocyte cellular hyperplasia. This cellular process defines an increase in the total number of myocytes in the ventricular wall and can be documented exclusively by morphometric methodologies. No other technique allows this type of determination. However, an important complicating factor in the quantitative analysis of myocyte proliferation involves the concurrent presence of myocyte cell loss in the myocardium (17, 180, 246, 352). Myocyte cell death complicates the estimation of the real amount of newly formed cells in the ventricle. Myocyte loss results in

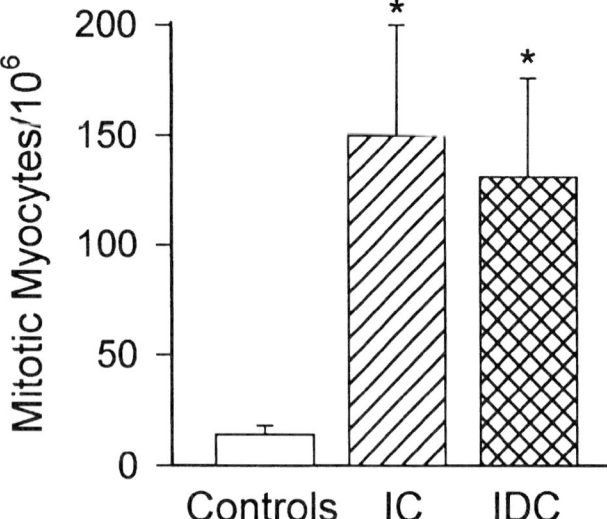

FIG. 2–13. Mitotic index in myocytes from control hearts (*Controls*), and hearts affected by ischemic cardiomyopathy (*IC*) and idiopathic dilated cardiomyopathy (*IDC*). Results are presented as means ± SD. *Indicates a statistically significant difference from controls. Reproduced from (243); copyright © 1998 National Academy of Sciences, USA.

underestimation of myocyte cellular hyperplasia in the tissue, whereas myocyte hyperplasia leads to underestimation of the magnitude of myocyte death in the myocardium. Thus, the event of myocyte proliferation may be obfuscated by the occurrence of myocyte loss, and the morphometric evaluation of the aggregate numbers of cells in the ventricle may not provide evidence of cell regeneration (17, 246). To overcome these limitations, the morphometric measurements of cell number have to be complemented with the detection of DNA synthesis and mitotic division in myocytes to obtain other indices of cell proliferation. The two examples of remodeling illustrated below demonstrate how increases in cell size and number in the absence of myocyte cell loss affect cardiac restructuring in short- and long-term pressure overload hypertrophy. In the first case, the papillary muscle, because of its easily dissectable elongated form and highly oriented histological structure, was employed as a simplified model for the quantitative estimation of the cellular mechanisms implicated in aortic banding–induced cardiac hypertrophy (42).

Constriction of the abdominal aorta in rats leads, in 8 days, to a 51% increase in the mass of the papillary muscle that results from a corresponding increase in mean cross-sectional area with no change in length (Fig. 2–14). This gross adaptation is accompanied by similar changes in the myocyte population, in which a 53% cellular enlargement is essentially identical to the 55% augmentation in average myocyte transverse area. This lateral expansion of myocytes is characterized by a significant increase in contractile material produced entirely by hyperplasia of myofibrillar units through the parallel addition of newly formed structures of approximately the same size. Thus, the number of myofibrillar profiles per cell cross section expands by 84%. It has been speculated that myofibrillar growth involves the accumulation of myofilaments at the surface of existing bundles (16, 375) that subsequently split to form new myofibrils. The maintenance of myofibrillar

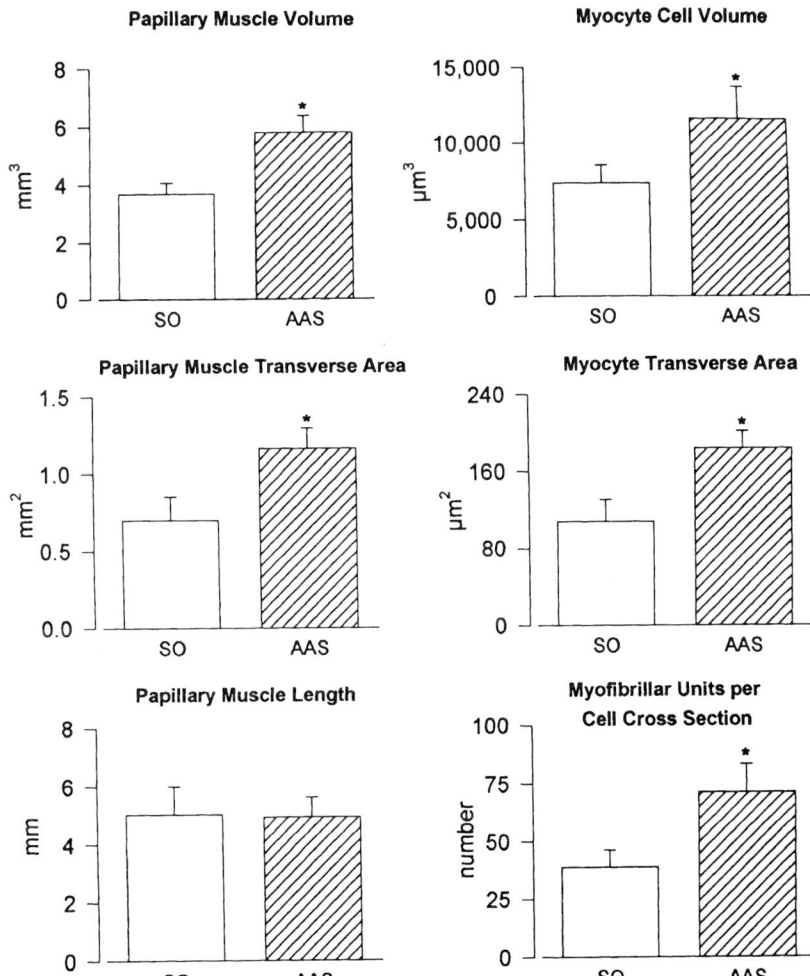

FIG. 2–14. Papillary muscle hypertrophy, eight days after abdominal aortic stenosis (*AAS*) in rats. Relationships between the anatomical characteristics of the papillary muscle and the structural properties of myocytes. *Indicates a statistically significant difference between sham-operated (*SO*) and aortic-banded rats. Results are presented as mean + SD.

size may be due to the existence of a critical perimitochondrial radius that is needed to supply ATP to the contractile proteins (373). A different type of cellular response characterizes the prolonged pressure load imposed by pulmonary artery banding on the right ventricle (Fig. 2–15). Under these conditions, right ventricular wall thickness increases 76%, and this phenomenon results from a 24% increase in myocyte diameter and a 44% parallel increase in the number of myocytes across the ventricular wall (368). These cellular alterations are accompanied by a 41% increase in the total number of myocyte nuclei in the ventricular myocardium (366), indicating that myocyte cellular hyperplasia can occur in response to a sustained mechanical stress on the ventricular wall. Functionally, increases in right ventricular end-diastolic pressure, systolic pressure, and central venous pressure are present in this model, but these indices of ventricular dysfunction are not associated with liver congestion, pleural effusion, or ascites, all of which indicate overt cardiac failure. The phenomenon of myocyte proliferation can be viewed as a compensatory reaction that tends to reduce the magnitude of systolic and diastolic cell stress in chronic pressure hypertrophy. These observations are consistent with findings in humans, in which the process of myocyte proliferation appears to characterize the transition from compensated physiological hypertrophy to cardiac dysfunction and failure (296, 360, 361). More complex is the remodeling of the ventricular wall when multiple foci of replacement fibrosis and diffuse myocyte loss are present in the myocardium in decompensated hypertensive hypertrophy (100, 286, 386, 528). Cardiac pump function is severely compromised and the phenomenon of cell proliferation (43) cannot preserve normal wall thickness (100). Ventricular dilation predominates, and this modification of heart anatomy suggests that newly formed myocytes are added in series, contributing to the expansion in cavitary volume and the reduction in mass-to-chamber volume ratio.

In contrast to pressure overload hypertrophy, the evolution of volume hypertrophy has been less characterized in both animals and humans. Only a few studies have analyzed the effects of volume overload hypertrophy on the changes in number and size of ventricular myocytes (160, 191, 300, 301, 321, 364, 511). Although the consequences for the myocardium of dynamic exercise (10, 24, 48, 309), arteriovenous fistula (160, 191, 300, 301), interatrial septal defect (321), mitral regurgitation (157, 511) and aortic regurgitation (157) have been examined in terms of chamber enlargement and myocyte lengthening, the potential contribution of myocyte hypertrophy and proliferation to ventricular growth has been measured only in iron- and copper-induced hypochromic anemia (364). Myocyte cell length consistently increases in the volume overloaded ventricle (88, 191, 300, 301, 511), but different results have been described in terms of the variations in myocyte diameter. Claims have been made that this cellular parameter remains unchanged (160, 300, 301), increases in proportion to cell length (10, 24, 27, 191), or constitutes the predominant aspect of myocyte cellular growth (157, 321). These contrasting observations leave undefined the cellular basis of ventricular remodeling in volume overload cardiac hypertrophy.

Before introducing the adaptation of myocytes in hypochromic anemia, its hemodynamic consequences will be described. In this experimental condition, peripheral vascular resistance typically diminishes, because blood viscosity is reduced and vasodilation of muscular arteries and arterioles takes place (475). These events are

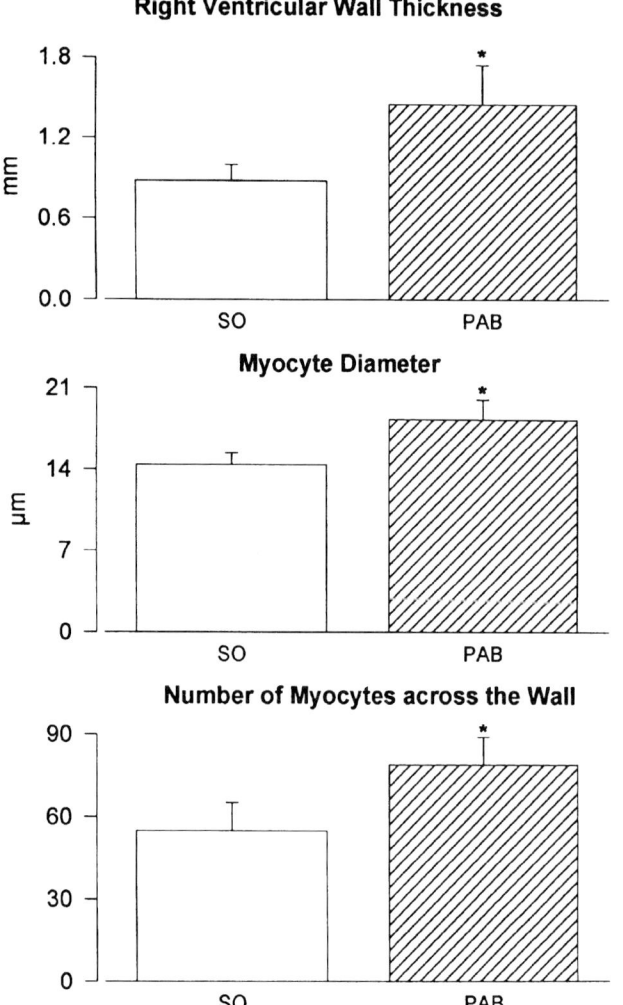

FIG. 2–15. Effects of chronic pulmonary artery banding (*PAB*) on wall thickness, myocyte diameter, and transmural number of myocytes in the right ventricular wall. *Indicates a statistically significant difference between sham operated (*SO*) and PAB rats. Results are presented as mean ± SD

mediated, respectively, by the decrease in number of circulating red blood cells and the impaired oxygen-carrying capacity of the blood (347, 479). Both systolic and diastolic arterial blood pressures decrease, but the latter is affected more than the former, leading to an increase in differential pressure. The combination of these circulatory adaptations results in a volume overload on the left and right ventricular myocardium and a reduction in afterload on the left side of the heart (72). In addition, cardiac output increases because stroke volume is elevated, and heart rate remains essentially constant (475). This hemodynamic state typically results in decompensated eccentric left ventricular hypertrophy, in which the marked increase in cavitary volume is the consequence of lengthening of myocytes and the in-series addition of newly formed cells in the myocardium (364). Thus, myocyte hypertrophy by replication of sarcomeres in series and cell proliferation through an identical pattern of insertion of dividing myocytes in the tissue both are responsible for the progressive decrease in ventricular mass-to-chamber volume ratio in this model (364). *In summary, the changes in myocyte size, shape, and number are the principal determinants of ventricular cavitary volume and wall thickness in pressure and volume overload cardiac hypertrophy. Disproportionate ventricular dilation with respect to mural thickness corresponds to the phase of decompensated eccentric hypertrophy in which myocyte cellular hyperplasia occurs and may constitute the ultimate response of the heart to a sustained mechanical stress before intractable congestive heart failure supervenes.*

Cardiac Hypertrophy and Volume Composition of Myocytes

Early in the hypertrophic response associated with pressure overload there is a relative enlargement of the mitochondrial compartment leading to an elevation of the mitochondrial-to-myofibrillar ratio (330). Corresponding measurements of the size and shape of individual mitochondria indicate that the growth in this compartment probably is due entirely to enlargement of preexisting mitochondrial units (32). Determinations of both mitochondrial respiratory enzymes and the incorporation of labeled amino acids into different myocardial subcellular fractions indicate that mitochondrial proteins are synthesized rapidly after cardiac overload (394, 455, 470, 556). Mitochondrial membranes are preferentially formed early after constriction of the ascending aorta in rats (7). Biochemical studies measuring differences in the temporal responses of muscle cell constituents during the initial stress of hypertrophy demonstrate that the enhanced protein synthesis is selectively directed toward energy producing structures, whereas the synthesis of contractile proteins occurs at later intervals (149). Observations at 20 hours after the production of subdiaphragmatic aortic stenosis in rats showed a significant increase in mitochondrial volume and little change in myofibrillar volume (32). However, reduction of the mitochondrial-to-myofibrillar volume ratio is a consistent subcellular alteration that occurs in myocytes after relatively short-term pressure overload hypertrophy (39, 373, 376). On the other hand, in prolonged pressure hypertrophy, the volume fractions of mitochondria and myofibrils return to control values (368, 498), possibly through proliferation of individual mitochondrial units (42). Because the generation of ATP in the mitochondrial cristae represents the primary source of energy for myofibrils, the restoration of an optimum concentration of mitochondria and myofibrils in myocytes may provide adequate energy supply and prevent the precocious impairment of heart muscle function. In contrast to the observations in pressure hypertrophy, the volume fractions of mitochondria and myofibrils remain nearly constant with volume hypertrophy (10, 24). The maintenance of a constant mitochondrial-to-myofibrillar volume ratio has been shown in several models of volume overload hypertrophy (10, 24, 514), although there is one report in which the volume percent of mitochondria was found to be decreased after aortocaval fistula in dogs (381). The changes in the dimensional properties of myocytes with a commensurate growth of the cytoplasmic structures responsible for energy production and utilization may constitute the morphologic counterpart for the normal or improved contractile (549) and relaxation (171) properties of the myocardium in volume overload hypertrophy.

The smooth endoplasmic reticulum (SER) in myocytes has been measured with respect to its volume and membrane surface area in the cytoplasm (28, 275, 375–377). The SER in hypertrophy due to pressure overload responds with a significant increase in volume relative to the volume of myofibrils (16, 28, 32). This increase appears not to be accompanied by any significant changes in the surface-to-volume ratio, implying that the tubules maintain their normal conformation and that the volume increases are also equivalent to a proportional elongation. The SER is a simple plexus of tubules of rather uniform caliber, freely anastomosing at all levels of the cross-banded pattern of the sarcomeres, surrounding the myofibrils. The SER in cardiac muscle, like that in skeletal muscle, functions in excitation–contraction coupling by the release and subsequent uptake of calcium (254). A reduced calcium-binding capacity of this system has been shown in hypertrophy (187). The increase in SER volume and surface demonstrated by means of morphometric techniques possibly indicates another of the complex compensatory mechanisms occurring in the myocytes in response to an increased work load. However, the adaptability of the SER cannot be appreciated fully if the changes in this component are not correlated with the changes in the strictly connected myofibrillar units. Variations in shape, size, volume and surface of the myofibrils may alter the structural as well as the functional relationship between SER and contractile material. Like the SER, an expansion of the T-system occurs in developing cardiac hypertrophy as a result of a proportional increase in both its volume and surface (28), indicating an elongation of the T-tubules without a change in size and shape. This result is consistent with the increased lateral dimension of the myocytes in hypertrophy (39). In contradistinction to the T-system, the surface area of the external sarcolemma of hypertrophying cardiac myocytes expands much less, since the cells assume a more nearly spherical configuration (28). The summation of T-system and external sarcolemma, however, varies nearly in proportion to the differences in myocyte volume in normal growth as well as in hypertrophy (28, 375, 376). *In summary, the quantitative structural adaptations of the subcellular components of myocytes in hypertrophy correspond to a well balanced form of physiologic accelerated growth. There may be components of incomplete compensations but it is not clear whether these modest alterations represent the interface between physiologic and pathologic cardiac hypertrophy.*

Cardiac Hypertrophy and the Coronary Arterial and Capillary Tree

The work potential of muscle myocardial tissue is clearly dependent on its blood supply. Thus, the hypertrophic response of the myocytes must be related in part to the capillary microvasculature, as higher metabolic requirements are needed to meet the needs of enhanced cell growth and increased function. The mechanisms controlling vascular growth in the mammalian heart are poorly understood (227, 411, 489). Capillary proliferation is very active in the early postnatal period (47, 353, 397) but becomes limited in the adult heart (397, 487). Moreover, as a result of a sudden and severe increase in afterload, the affected ventricle increases in size very rapidly. The expansion of the muscle compartment of the tissue, however, is not accompanied by a proportional growth response of the coronary capillary bed, so that myocyte enlargement provokes a corresponding decline in capillary density within the myocardium (42, 47, 413, 500). Yet, capillary endothelial cell hyperplasia does occur in cardiac hypertrophy (42, 74, 177, 178, 343), so that questions have been raised about the role of this cellular process in the presence of a reduced extent or absence of capillary proliferation. This paradox becomes even more apparent when the observations obtained in humans are taken into account. Capillary proliferation has been documented in humans under a variety of pathologic states that impose a large and prolonged stress on the myocardium, leading to a marked increase in ventricular mass (59, 60, 296). Because the human disease is an evolving condition that progresses over a number of years, and because animal models have mostly been examined shortly after the imposition of the overload, the time factor has to be considered as an important determinant of the tissue processes implicated in cardiac hypertrophy. This variable has to be taken into account in the characterization of the adaptive response of the coronary vasculature in models of pressure and volume overloads on the heart.

There are three principal morphometric parameters of the capillary network that have been used frequently for the estimation of capillary proliferation during induced myocardial growth: the ratio of capillary profiles to myocyte profiles in the tissue (353, 397, 402), the numerical density of capillary profiles per unit area of myocardium (310, 353, 409, 410, 502), and the total aggregate length of capillaries in the whole ventricular mass (33, 353, 358, 359). However, a change in the capillary-to-myocyte ratio cannot be considered an accurate measurement of the magnitude of capillary growth. Cardiac hypertrophy is associated with alterations in cell shape, characterized by an increased lateral diameter of the cell that induces a significant spreading of the capillary profiles and reduces the numerical density of muscle cells (33). Moreover, cell loss may also alter this ratio. How changes in myocyte size and number interact with changes in capillary density in the capillary-to-myocyte ratio cannot be determined easily. Thus, the capillary-to-myocyte ratio is only a qualitative indicator of capillary growth. Measurements of capillary numerical density, in the absence of myocyte loss, represent a more meaningful estimation of capillary adaptation to hypertrophy. An increase of this parameter with myocardial enlargement unequivocally indicates capillary proliferation because such a change can only be the result of the lateral addition of new capillary units. However, a decrease in capillary numerical density in hypertrophy does not imply loss of capillaries, because it is the result of the lateral separation of the vascular profiles associated with myocyte hypertrophy. The estimation of total capillary length in the ventricle offers a direct measurement of capillary growth. This morphometric quantity, although highly relevant for the evaluation of the overall response of the capillary bed, does not discriminate among the various mechanisms involved in the adaptation of the capillary network in hypertrophy. Lengthening of the whole capillary vasculature (33, 353, 358, 359) could be due either to an increase in length of individual capillary units or to capillary proliferation in series, or both (33, 353). These changes may affect tissue oxygenation differently. Thus, several structural characteristics of coronary capillaries can be measured and have been measured in an attempt to define the vascular reaction of the hypertrophied myocardium.

The importance of the quantitative tissue parameters of the capillary network mentioned above relates to their influence on the values of volume percent of capillary lumen in the myocardium, capillary luminal surface per unit volume of myocytes, and average distance from the capillary wall to the surrounding myocytes. These structural properties of the capillary bed are functionally related to the volume of capillary blood available for gas exchange, to the capillary area available for oxygen transport, and to the diffusion path length to the sites of oxygen consumption (216, 534). Morphometric results indicate that the initial phases of cardiac hypertrophy may be seen as a form of growth in which the inadequate expansion of the capillary bed (47) may generate conditions that leave the myocardium more susceptible to ischemia (412, 413, 498, 503). Short-term pressure overload hypertrophy of the left and right ventricles consistently shows a decrease in the capillary concentration within the tissue (413, 500) in association with a reduction in capillary luminal volume and surface densities and an increase in the path length for oxygen molecular transport to the myocytes (47, 412, 500, 503). In contrast, these parameters are not altered in volume overload hypertrophy (65, 105, 300, 321), although an inadequate growth adaptation of the capillary bed through changes in capillary numerical density also has been reported (407). Elevations in preload associated with dynamic exercise do not result, over a relatively short time period, in an amelioration of the capillarization of the myocardium in either normotensive (10) or hypertensive rats (413). Exercise also has no beneficial effect on hypertensive hypertrophy in terms of coronary blood flow amount and distribution and minimal coronary vascular resistance (413, 497). Brief durations of running exercise are not able to restore capillary numerical density in the hypertrophied myocardium (497). However, dynamic exercise stimulates capillary growth in young spontaneously hypertensive rats (114). In addition, thyroxine-induced hypertrophy has been found to elicit a similar response of coronary capillaries (79, 112, 124, 256, 315, 496, 519). The type and duration of the inciting stimulus as well as the age of the experimental animal, are important contributing elements modulating the magnitude and characteristics of the response of the heart (397, 492, 493).

Measurements of capillary luminal volume density, capillary luminal surface density, and diffusion distance from the capillary wall to the mitochondria of myocytes also have been undertaken to determine the impact of a prolonged and sustained pressure load on the principal structural variables of the microvasculature of the heart that are functionally relevant to tissue oxygenation. During this form of hypertrophic response, none of the capillary parameters implicated in myocardial oxygen distribution are affected. This preservation in the oxygenation potential of the myocardium occurs despite an increase in the lateral dimension of myocytes, which has the effect of producing a lateral spreading of the adjacent capillaries, decreasing their concentration within the tissue (33, 397). In this setting, the capillary-to-myocyte ratio, the aggregate length of capillaries in the ventricle, and the number of capillary profiles across the wall all increase (Fig. 2–16). These changes are consistent with the neogenesis of capillary units in long-standing pressure overload cardiac hypertrophy (358). Because the duration of the overload on the myocardium is the most apparent difference between short- and long-term cardiac hypertrophy, time seems to play an important primary role in the growth mechanisms of the capillary microcirculation in the enlarging myocardium. A similar time-dependent response has been shown to occur in spontaneously hypertensive rats, in which the long-term effects of genetically determined hypertension and hypertrophy lead to capillary neogenesis and to the restoration of a normal capillary luminal volume and surface densities in the left ventricular myocardium (502). These observations also suggest that capillary growth can occur in the presence of an increase in perfusion pressure in the coronary circulation (502) or in the absence of such a factor, as observed in the right ventricle following prolonged pulmonary artery banding (358). Capillary proliferation has been demonstrated in severe human myocardial hypertrophy (59, 60, 296). In this case, it is of particular interest that myocyte proliferation also takes place and the capillary-to-myocyte ratio remains essentially constant. Both in humans (59, 60, 296) and in animal models (358, 366, 368), long-term cardiac hypertrophy evokes a proliferative response of coronary capillaries, which parallels the hyperplastic reaction of the myocyte compartment of the ventricular mass. However, not all studies in the human heart are in agreement (401).

With the exception of the data obtained in the human heart (59, 60, 296), the observations summarized above in the different animal models of pressure and volume overload hypertrophy have been collected in phases of cardiac hypertrophy characterized by the preservation of ventricular function or, at most, modest alterations in myocardial performance. On this basis, the findings appear to contradict the contention that defects at the level of coronary capillaries play a pri-

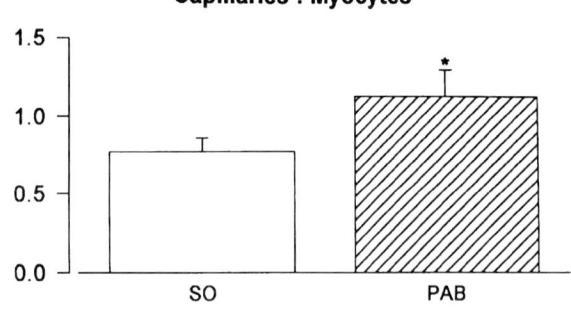
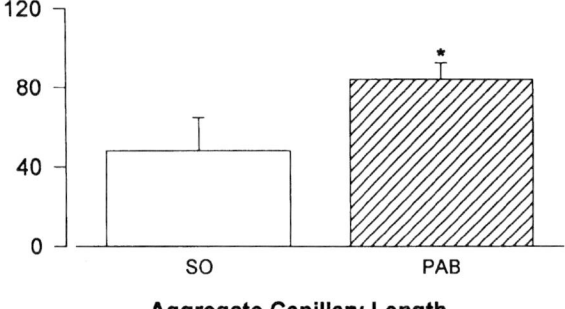
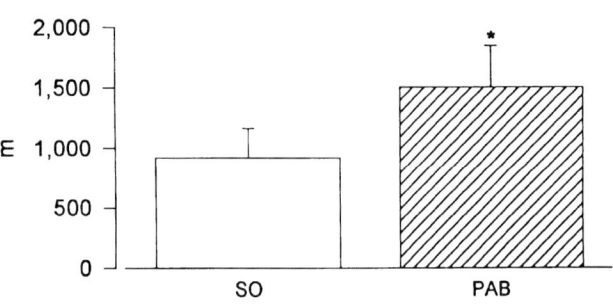

FIG. 2–16. Effects of chronic pulmonary artery banding (*PAB*) on the ratio of capillary profiles to myocyte profiles, number of capillaries across the wall, and aggregate length of capillaries in the right ventricle. *Indicates a statistically significant difference between sham-operated (*SO*) and PAB rats. Results are presented as mean ± SD

the capillary level. Diffusion distance for oxygen and capillary-to-myocyte ratio are not impaired in the hypertrophied decompensated human heart (296). Because the relationship between heart weight and the diameter of the coronary arteries is maintained in physiological (449, 518) but not in pathological (66, 289) hypertrophy, and because structural modifications are seen in the intramural branches of the coronary vascular tree even in the absence of myocardial hypertrophy (252, 295, 296, 529), alterations of the epicardial coronary arteries and coronary resistance vessels have been postulated to be the main cause of ischemic myocardial injury in the hypertrophied human heart (296).

In experimental cardiac hypertrophy, an impairment of coronary reserve and minimal coronary vascular resistance has been documented (62). However, the structural mechanisms responsible for these physiological alterations have not been clarified completely. Quantitative results have been inconsistent, because both thickening of the arterial wall (8) and no changes in wall thickness and luminal diameter of the different classes of the coronary artery branches (14, 500, 501) have been reported. However, the morphometric analysis of intermediate-sized coronary arteries and arterioles has shown that losses in these classes of vessels occur in long-term hypertension–induced ventricular failure (14). This phenomenon leads to rarefaction of coronary resistance vessels in the myocardium through the mechanism of destruction of arteries and arterioles 6–40 μm in diameter. These represent the major component of the arterial tree controlling the local distribution of blood flow in the myocardium. The inference has been made that rarefaction of the intramural branches of the coronary vasculature occurs as a result of an excessive enlargement of myocytes in the absence of a corresponding growth adaptation of the coronary arterial tree (501). This disproportionate growth reserve capacity of myocytes and vascular framework has been claimed to represent the structural template of the increase in minimal coronary vascular resistance found in pressure-overload cardiac hypertrophy (62, 413, 500) and failure (267), as well as in the pathological evolution of the aging process of the heart (26, 183) and after myocardial infarction (250). It should be pointed out, however, that proliferation of coronary resistance vessels may occur in prolonged pressure overload hypertrophy with normalization of coronary blood flow hemodynamics (501). This observation, in combination with findings characterizing the proliferative ability of capillaries (358) and myocytes (368), suggests that alterations in coronary blood flow properties may develop as a result of noncoordinated growth regulation of the vascular and myocyte compartments of the myocardium. Moreover, loss of intramural coronary vessels in association with myocardial

mary role in the genesis and evolution of myocardial hypertrophy toward cardiac dysfunction and failure (62, 397). Although decreases in capillary density within the tissue (47, 397, 498, 503) with reduction in the oxygenation potential of the myocardium have been demonstrated repeatedly and local sites of ischemia within the hypertrophy ventricle have been postulated to occur (214), these phenomena seem to be transient, returning to control conditions with time. The failing human heart also does not show clear indices of inadequate adaptation of the coronary microcirculation (59, 60, 296, 401). In particular, Linzbach in his classic review (296) challenged the concept that myocardial hypoxia develops in hypertrophy as a result of abnormalities dependent on tissue oxygenation at

damage and cell dropout (100) may impinge on the length density of the arterial tree in the left ventricle (14). Additionally, several reports have indicated that the intramural small-sized arteries and arterioles show practically no changes in wall thickness (14, 500). However, an increase in permeability to macromolecules of the myocardial microvasculature occurs during sustained pressure overload (267). The lack of an effect of hypertension on vessel wall dimension may occur because intramyocardial arteries are perfused primarily during the diastolic phase of the cardiac cycle. This portion of the coronary vasculature is protected from the elevated systolic pressure by the higher tissue pressure generated in the surrounding myocardium by the contracting cardiac muscle cells (268). In contrast, major epicardial arteries are exposed to both systolic and diastolic perfusion pressures, and hypertension leads to mural thickening and accumulation of fibrous protein in the vessel wall (34).

When overt cardiac failure is present, myocardial damage with areas of replacement fibrosis involves the different layers of the ventricular wall, and this phenomenon is associated with loss of capillary units. On the other hand, a proliferative response occurs in the remaining portion of the capillary network (14, 502). Thus, capillary proliferation takes place in combination with capillary loss, but the former process exceeds the latter so that the oxygenation potential of myocytes improves, possibly increasing their capacity to sustain the elevated load generated by the impairment in pump function. However, the lack of a similar growth response of the intramural branches of the coronary circulation in the failing ventricle may reduce the potential beneficial effects of capillary neogenesis. Such a possibility is consistent with the hypothesis introduced by Linzbach in the failing human heart (296), in which pathological structural changes of coronary resistance vessels (252, 289) were proposed to be associated with local reduction in myocardial perfusion, resulting in multiple foci of ischemic necrosis and replacement fibrosis in the ventricular wall. *In summary, alterations in the capillary properties implicated in tissue oxygenation characterize short-term cardiac hypertrophy in which ventricular pump function is essentially maintained, whereas defects of the intramural branches of the coronary circulation depict the long-term evolution of the hypertrophied heart in which myocardial structural damage occurs and cardiac dysfunction and failure are apparent.*

Conclusions

Hypertrophy represents a response of the heart to a hemodynamic overload that tends to preserve normal cardiac function. In short-term cardiac hypertrophy the myocardial adaptation consists of cellular enlargement with little or no DNA synthesis in the expanding myocytes. However, when the heart is subjected to a prolonged and sustained mechanical load, hyperplasia of myocytes occurs. The process of proliferation appears to characterize the phase of transition from compensated physiologic hypertrophy to cardiac deadaptation and ventricular failure. Myocyte loss is considered to be the initial triggering event responsible for the progression from nonpathological reversible hypertrophy to pathological irreversible hypertrophy. Cell loss and scar formation alter ventricular size and shape by decreasing wall thickness and the ratio of wall thickness-to-chamber radius. These anatomical modifications correspond to decompensated concentric and eccentric ventricular hypertrophy. Defects in the coronary vascular bed, mostly involving the intramural branches of the coronary circulation, develop and may result in local ischemia, myocyte necrosis, connective tissue cell activation, collagen deposition, and increased wall and chamber stiffness. These abnormalities, in combination with ventricular dilation, increase the magnitude of the overload on the remaining myocytes. The inability of the coronary vasculature continuously to meet the greater oxygen demands of the myocardium may generate a vicious cycle in which myocytolytic necrosis and reactive growth mechanisms in myocytes lead with time to the end-stage dilated cardiomyopathic heart.

ISCHEMIC CARDIOMYOPATHY

Ischemic heart disease is a complex and diverse clinical syndrome in which an imbalance between blood supply and demand is created by complete or partial occlusion of a major epicardial coronary artery, resulting in myocardial infarction and/or multiple isolated sites of tissue injury. In addition, alterations of the intramural arterial branches of the coronary vasculature or defects of the microcirculation may generate varying degrees of ischemia and scattered necrotic myocyte cell death (27, 49, 69, 85, 324, 380, 426, 453, 523). These types of myocardial damage frequently coexist in the patient population, leading to different forms of cardiac pathology which reflect the characteristics of myocyte loss in the myocardium (27, 69, 527, 528). On this basis, segmental fibrosis, replacement fibrosis, and interstitial fibrosis recently have been used as quantitative definitions of these aspects of myocyte cell death with collagen accumulation in the ventricular wall. In the human heart, segmental fibrosis has been considered to correspond to a healed myocardial infarct that comprises an area of myocardium >1 cm^2, whereas replacement fibrosis describes discrete areas of myocardial scarring developed as a result of focal myocyte cell loss (69). These smaller sites of myocardial injury are <1 cm² in size. Finally, interstitial fibrosis reflects widening of the extracellular space with collagen deposition between groups of myocytes, as a consequence of diffuse myocyte cell death in the wall. Interstitial fibrosis also may occur in the absence of myocytolytic necrosis through activation of fibroblasts via humoral and/or mechanical factors (527, 528). In all cases, the resulting clinical spectrum takes the form of a dilated ischemic myopathy in which myocyte loss, replacement scarring, and reactive growth mechanisms in the remaining viable cells are the major determinants of wall remodeling and chamber dilation. Thus, following coronary occlusion and infarction or coronary narrowing and focal damage, changes in myocyte size and number, in combination with restructuring of the nonmuscle compartment of the myocardium, become conditioning factors in the modification of cardiac anatomy and loading state of the heart (40, 49, 175, 326, 383, 468, 524). Morphometric methodologies have been applied in an attempt to characterize the consequences of a segmental—as opposed to diffuse—loss of myocytes in the onset and evolution of heart failure of ischemic origin. This approach has provided answers as to whether partial reductions in luminal diameter of a major coronary artery require the involvement of a quantity of myocardium similar to that necessary to impair cardiac pump function following coronary occlusion, and whether these anatomical conditions evoke comparable loading states and hypertrophic reactions on the remaining unaffected cells. In addition, the potential limitations in the regenerative capacity of the unaffected myocytes in the reconstitution of healthy viable myocardium have been identified.

Before discussing these issues in some detail, it is relevant to indicate that recent results have documented that cell death in the infarcted region of the wall is mediated by myocyte apoptosis and necrosis. However, programmed myocyte cell death is the principal form of myocardial damage produced by occlusion of a major epicardial coronary artery, whereas necrotic myocyte cell death follows apoptosis and contributes to the progressive loss of cells with time after infarction. Similar findings have been obtained in animal models and humans (63, 151, 231, 240). Conversely, in the surviving myocardium of the post-infarct heart, myocyte apoptosis predominates and this phenomenon persists chronically (63, 107, 231, 283, 365). This adaptation may be the consequence of the elevation in tension in the remaining viable myocardium (40); this process has been shown to be operative in vitro (108). Coronary artery narrowing leads to a different type of tissue injury acutely and chronically. In this setting, myocyte necrosis prevails and apoptosis constitutes a smaller fraction of dying myocytes (285).

Ischemic Cardiomyopathy and Ventricular Remodeling

Numerous studies have attempted to identify the functional (49, 354, 355, 382), biochemical (87), structural (49, 354, 355, 382), and molecular bases (106, 225, 331–334, 417, 419–421) for the evolution of ischemic cardiomyopathy toward terminal failure and death. Although these multiple observations have provided important information concerning the pathological changes in the myocardium, the alterations in contractile protein enzyme activity and the abnormalities in adrenergic and angiotensin II receptors and effector pathways associated with these receptors, the critical events responsible for the progressive deterioration of cardiac pump performance chronically after infarction or coronary artery narrowing remain unknown. Clinical and experimental results concur in the interpretation that ventricular dilation is an extremely accurate predictor of the unfavorable short- and long-term outcome of ischemic cardiomyopathy (40, 130, 165, 388). Dilation characterizes depressed ventricular function and correlates with poor survival in both patients and animal models (326, 382, 383, 524). Moreover, there is a major issue of whether ventricular dilation itself, resulting from the initial insult, may contribute to the continued deterioration in cardiac dynamics. The crucial question bears on the relation between ventricular size and diastolic loading in the onset, development, and progression of the dilated cardiomyopathy that follows coronary artery occlusion or coronary artery constriction.

A sudden occlusion of a coronary artery leads in one minute to loss of function in the supplied myocardium (253), affecting ventricular pump performance in proportion to the magnitude of tissue involved in the ischemic event (40, 49). This phenomenon results in a redistribution of cardiac loading as the remaining viable myocardium is called upon to maintain cardiac output and blood flow to the peripheral circulation. Diastolic wall stress markedly increases and the anatomical reaction consists of chamber dilation and thinning of the wall (211, 212, 355, 545). Similarly, shortly after coronary artery narrowing, transmural myocardial ischemia becomes apparent with depression in ventricular performance and elevation in systolic and diastolic wall stress (93, 94). The increase in diastolic stress induces dilation of the ventricular chamber, which would have the effect of decreasing ventricular diastolic pressure by generating a larger intracavitary volume. On the assumption that diastolic overload may be the initiating event and ventricular remodeling the inevitable consequence, the question concerns the process by which the chamber dilates and the wall adapts to the increase in cavitary volume. Acute mechanisms of adaptation may involve changes in sarcomere length or restructuring of muscle cell layers in the ventricular wall, or both. Observations regarding the relationship between cellular responses and acute (515), subacute (355), and chronic (354, 432) elevations in end-diastolic pressure consistently have shown that lengthening of sarcomeres in myocytes does not significantly contribute to increasing chamber volume. Conversely, architectural rearrangement of the wall, with side-to-side slippage of myocytes, accounts for the increase in cavitary volume and mural thinning (13, 355, 545, 546). This mechanism of restructuring of the wall is complex and requires some explanation.

Myocyte slippage implies that myocytes are capable of undergoing side-to-side translocation leading to wall thinning and increases in chamber diameter and longitudinal axis of the heart. Differences exist in the consequences of this architectural rearrangement depending upon whether it affects myocyte bundles oriented circumferentially to the transverse chamber diameter or to the longitudinal axis of the heart. In the first case, side-to-side slippage results in a reduction in the thickness of the wall and a corresponding increase in the transverse and longitudinal axis of the heart. On the other hand, slippage of cells within myocytes oriented circumferentially to the longitudinal axis of the heart is associated with wall thinning and increase of the transverse chamber diameter, with no change in the longitudinal axis of the ventricle. In both forms of slippage, the ring of cells that moves radially toward the epicardial region must enlarge to adapt to the new circumference associated with a greater chamber diameter. The immediate consequence is a sudden uniform increase in load on these cells. This elevation in stress may be transferred subsequently to a single cell of a hypothetical one-cell ring of myocytes generating a load that may become intolerable for that individual myocyte. The consequence of this extreme load may be activation of the suicide program, necking down of the cell body, and ultimately apoptotic cell death (93, 94, 107, 108). Side-to-side slippage of myocytes is the major determinant of the decrease in wall thickness-to-chamber radius ratio and ventricular dilation acutely after myocardial infarction both in animal models (355, 545) and humans (545). Anatomical changes and structural alterations in myocytes point to a similar form of ventricular remodeling shortly after coronary artery constriction (93, 94, 108). The possibility that rearrangements of myocytes within the wall constitute a mechanism of ventricular dilation in the failing heart was proposed originally by Linzbach in 1960 (296). The interdependence of chamber diameter wall thickness and mural number of myocytes in the characterization of the phenomenon of side-to-side slippage has been measured quantitatively in the acute phase of myocardial infarction in rats (355). The heterogeneity in distribution and magnitude of this process of wall restructuring also has been determined in the different regions of the surviving myocardium, bordering and remote from the infarct (Fig. 2–17). The participation of the capillary network in wall remodeling was documented as well. Lateral myocyte slippage has also

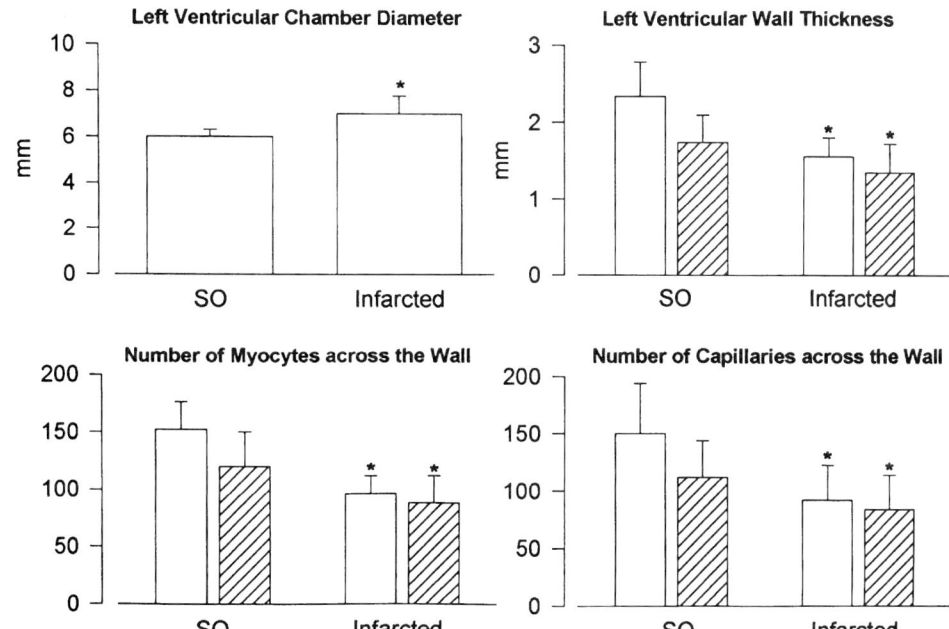

FIG. 2–17. Effects of occlusion of the left main coronary artery on left ventricular chamber diameter, ventricular wall (*open bars*), and septal (*hatched bars*) thickness, and number of myocytes and capillaries across the wall and septum. *Indicates a statistically significant difference between infarcted and sham operated (SO) rats. Results are presented as mean ± SD.

been inferred from wall thickness changes accompanying variations of ventricular volume in the intact heart in vitro (144) (1) following acute (515) and chronic (432) ventricular dysfunction, (2) as a result of transient but repeated episodes of myocardial ischemia (558), and (3) during the alterations in loading on the heart associated with the transition from the fetal to the adult circulatory system early after birth in the rat (353). The last case provides an experimental demonstration that side-to-side slippage of myocytes can occur in the ventricular wall with maturation, although the phenomenon is restricted to the muscle fibers without capillary involvement.

Some additional comments concerning the mechanisms of load dependent–induced myocyte death and translocation of cells may be relevant. Mechanical cell death implies that uniaxial circumferential cell stress (336, 337) is the determinant of myocyte cellular damage, triggering the endogenous cell death pathway (108). Whereas radial and compressive forces are relevant during systolic contraction, uniaxial stress prevails in diastole (336, 337) and is believed to be responsible for necking down of a finite region along the axis of the cell and ultimately myocyte cell death. Evidence for such a process that involves apoptosis has been obtained (94, 108). Unidirectional circumferential stress affects myocytes in a direction parallel to the length of the cells, regardless of their orientation in the wall. The possibility that mechanical stimuli may result in a nonischemic form of cell death and subsequently in an architectural rearrangement of myocytes in the myocardium has been demonstrated in vitro (108). Overstretching of papillary muscles is associated with the activation of programmed cell death and a reduction in the number of myocytes included in the transverse diameter of the muscle; physical forces, apoptotic cell death, and side-to-side slippage of cells are strictly related. On the basis of these observations, a potential sequence of events has been proposed: A segmental loss of myocardium or scattered tissue injury across the wall results in diastolic Laplace overloading, which may trigger apoptotic myocyte cell death, side-to-side slippage of cells, wall thinning, and chamber dilation (108). In this context, a spherical configuration corresponds to a condition of minimal and uniform stress distribution, while an ellipsoid pattern generates a greater and dissimilar distribution of stress along the myocardial surface, and a cylindrical shape is the least advantageous geometry (336, 337). As a consequence, the sliding of myocytes from the endocardial to the epicardial surface results in an increase in the longitudinal axis of the heart proportional to the extent of cell slippage (93, 354). The reduction of cells in the transverse direction leads to an increase in the number of cells in the longitudinal axis and ventricular dilation. The major axis of the ventricle increases by a factor that contains three variables: number of cells, average cell diameter, and the angle of orientation of muscle cells with respect to the longitudinal diameter of the heart (13). On the other hand, when the phenomenon of slippage affects myocytes included in the bundles of muscle cells oriented circumferentially to the longitudinal axis of the heart, wall thickness decreases through a reduction in the mural number of myocytes. This change generates an equivalent expansion in chamber diameter, leaving the major axis of the ventricle and its myocyte number nearly constant. The first mechanism of restructuring is associated with a more cylindrical aspect of the heart (354, 355), and the second form with a more spherical appearance (51). The recognition that side-to-side slippage of myocytes within the wall affects not only transverse chamber diameter but also the longitudinal axis of the ventricle has important implications for sudden increases in chamber volume and loading state of the myocardium (40). Moreover, the changes in the transverse direction may not be identical to those in the longitudinal direction, so that alterations in the shape of the heart occur (27). Physical alterations in the connective tissue compartment involving either breakage of the collagen structures that connect myocytes, or distortion of the collagen struts that tether muscle cells laterally (144) have to take place for this phenomenon to occur.

Although mural slippage of myocytes can be considered the major factor for acute expansions of cavitary volume in the ischemic cardiomyopathic heart, more complex are the mechanisms dictating changes in myocyte size and shape, which provide the structural template for chronic ventricular dilation (40, 49). On a cellular basis, myocyte hypertrophy may be accomplished by an increase in myocyte diameter, length, or both. When cellular enlargement rather than increased cell length becomes the main growth mechanism, lateral expansion of the myocytes is responsible for subsequent increases in wall thickness with no changes in chamber volume. In contrast, myocyte lengthening alone results in a larger cavity volume without affecting wall thickness. A disproportionate increase in average cell length with respect to its diameter generates a decrease in the cell diameter-to-cell length ratio and, thus, chamber enlargement with relative thinning of the wall. Importantly, the long-term consequences of cardiac restructuring are mandated by the acute events that establish the initial load on the viable tissue and the magnitude and characteristics of the growth reactions of the unaffected myocytes. Since changes in myocyte shape are strictly related to the nature of the prevailing load, the predominant increase in diastolic wall stress after coronary artery occlusion (354, 355) or constriction (51) is associated with a lengthening of the cells that exceeds the increase in their lateral dimension (9, 49, 354, 355, 419). Although the process of healing of both the infarcted region and the multiple foci of tissue injury associated with coronary artery narrowing results in thinning of the wall, contributing to the expansion in cavitary volume, myocyte lengthening in the radial and longitudinal directions is one of the major determinants of the changes in cardiac size and shape in ischemic cardiomyopathy. In contrast, the rigid collagen of the scar region may stretch very little over periods of months, participating minimally in chronic remodeling. The increase in myocyte length-to-diameter ratio with the long-term evolution of the ischemic myopathy produces an increase in the transverse and longitudinal axes of the heart, which together lead to a marked increase in cavitary volume (51, 354). The changes in volume of the ventricular chamber are greater than the increase in muscle mass, resulting in a decrease in ventricular mass-to-chamber volume ratio. Thus, decompensated eccentric hypertrophy characterizes the chronic phases of ischemic cardiomyopathy in which cavitary diameter increases and wall thickness decreases (Fig. 2–18).

Although the discussion above has emphasized the importance of the magnitude and characteristics of myocyte hypertrophy in ventricular remodeling after infarction and coronary artery constriction, recent observations indicate that myocyte cellular hyperplasia can occur in the ischemic cardiomyopathic heart (90, 243, 246, 393, 419–421), and such a mechanism of myocyte growth may play an important role in chronic changes of cardiac anatomy. This is so because the in-series addition of newly formed myocytes increases chamber volume more than ventricular mass, contributing to the development of decompensated eccentric hypertrophy. However, it is unknown whether the magnitude of myocyte regeneration is similar after coronary artery occlusion and constriction. Another potential difference between the impact of coronary artery narrowing and occlusion on myocardial pathology is that, in the former condition, myocyte cell death continues to occur chronically, and this phenomenon affects cavitary dilation. The possibility that ongoing isolated myocyte death plays a central role in the genesis of chamber enlargement is supported by the severe degrees of ventricular dilation observed with coronary artery narrowing in spite of limited amounts of myocyte cell loss (25, 51, 94, 96). In contrast, a single episode of extensive myocyte death in a segmental fashion does not provoke an expansion in cavitary volume unless regional damage involves more than 35% of the entire ventricular wall, early (95, 355) and late (354, 388) after the ischemic event. Similar observations have been made in humans (326, 382, 383, 524). However, long-term ischemic cardiomyopathy of any origin typically shows apoptotic and necrotic myocyte death, both of which participate in the evolution of the disease to terminal failure and death (180, 352). *In summary, ischemic cardiomyopathy is characterized acutely by ventricular dilation, mediated by an architectural rearrangement of myocytes within the wall, and chronically by decompensated eccentric hypertrophy in which myocyte lengthening, apoptotic and necrotic myocyte death, and the insertion in series of newly formed cells, all contribute to increased cavitary volume and severely depressed cardiac pump function.*

Ischemic Cardiomyopathy, Myocyte Cell Loss, and Ventricular Function

In a large number of patients affected by chronic coronary artery disease, the magnitude of constriction of the epicardial coronary arteries by atherosclerosis does not correspond to the severity of the clinical manifestations of myocardial dysfunction and failure (85, 190, 349, 427, 429, 523, 548). Similar degrees of coronary stenosis detected angiographically are associated with variable hemodynamic abnormalities, raising questions concerning the significance of these fixed obstructions of the coronary tree in the prediction of short- and long-term outcomes of ischemic heart disease clinically (85). This apparent inconsistency becomes even greater when anatomical findings are taken into account (84, 380, 424, 426, 453). Histologic examination of hearts of patients who died of congestive ischemic heart dis-

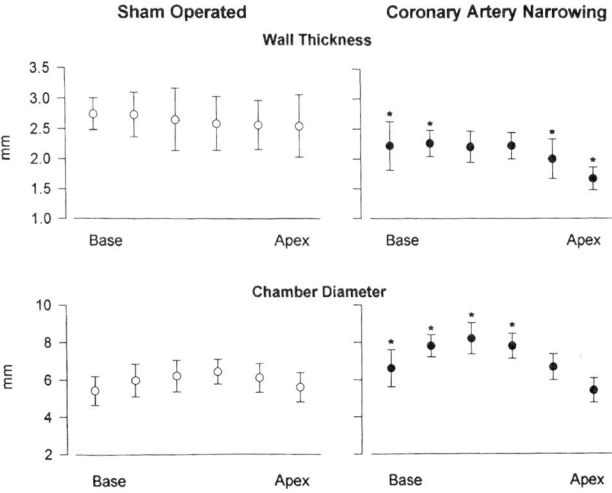

FIG. 2–18. Effects of chronic coronary artery narrowing on left ventricular wall thickness and chamber diameter, at six subsequent levels from the basal to the apical region of the heart. Sham-operated animals (*open circles*). Coronary artery narrowed animals with left ventricular failure (*solid circles*). *Indicates a value that is statistically significantly different from the corresponding value in sham-operated rats. Results are presented as mean ± SD.

ease reveals that only small quantities of viable myocardium have been replaced by scarred tissue (380, 453), suggesting that the overall extent of damage in the ventricular wall may not reflect a loss of myocytes that would be considered critical for the induction of irreversible cardiac failure and death.

Studies in humans (189, 374) and animals (29, 355) demonstrate that occlusion of a major coronary artery, resulting in acute transmural myocardial infarction, leads to overt cardiac failure when the destruction in muscle mass affects 40%–50% of the myocyte population of the ventricle. Moreover, ventricular decompensation persists during the healing process (150, 354, 384, 385) and long after (388, 391). Importantly, a direct relationship exists between healed infarct size and ventricular performance in animals (150) and humans (147, 484), further emphasizing potential differences in the genesis of cardiac failure produced by occlusive and nonocclusive coronary artery stenosis. This quantitative pathology issue was resolved by the determination of multiple structural variables, which allowed establishment of whether partial occlusion of a major epicardial coronary artery results in impairment of ventricular function when less than 40%–50% of myocytes are lost or whether this quantity is required to generate severe ventricular decompensation, mimicking the condition of myocardial infarction (51). The extent of damage produced by coronary occlusion may be determined easily shortly after the acute event when cell necrosis is present, but difficulties exist in the evaluation of the actual magnitude of tissue lost during the healing process and long after. This is so because there is a variable and unknown amount of swelling in the cells and interstitial spaces and a progressive lateral and radial shrinkage of the infarcted region (148, 238, 392). Scar formation, the contraction of necrotic tissue with time, and the growth of the unaffected cardiac mass, all represent dynamic processes that continuously change the proportions of viable and nonviable myocardium in the injured ventricle (12, 49). Similar concerns apply to the evolution of myocardial damage produced by coronary artery stenosis. These limitations have been resolved, at least in part, by morphometric methodologies that permit the estimation of the number of myocyte nuclei and/or cells lost as a result of coronary artery occlusion or coronary artery narrowing (49, 51, 246). This technique is based on the assumption that the number of myocyte nuclei or cells within the surviving ventricular tissue does not change with time, so that the fraction of myocytes or nuclei lost from the ventricle represents a valid measure of the number of lost myocytes. From the original volume of the ventricle, this fraction defines the volumes of damaged and spared myocardium from which several structural parameters can be obtained (12, 29, 30). In the absence of myocyte nuclear and cellular hyperplasia, the short- and long-term effects of coronary artery occlusion or constriction on the damaged and unaffected portions of the ventricle can be analyzed and interpreted with respect to original infarct size or extent of scattered tissue injury at any point in time after the initial event (12, 29, 30, 51, 246). However, in the presence of cell regeneration, this approach provides a quantitative estimate of the number of viable and nonviable myocytes in the ventricle, although the measured magnitude of myocytes lost corresponds to an underestimation of the actual number of dead cells (44). These two conditions are observed, respectively, with small infarcts and degrees of coronary artery narrowing not associated with ventricular failure, and large infarcts and coronary artery stenosis characterized by severe impairment of cardiac pump performance.

On the basis of quantitative morphological findings, the conclusion has been reached that a loss of myocytes, diffuse throughout the ventricle, has a much greater impact on cardiac performance than an identical loss of cells in a segmental fashion, acutely and chronically. In particular, coronary artery narrowing, associated with 5%–10% tissue damage, results in left-sided failure (94), whereas 45% damage of the wall is required for myocardial infarction to induce a comparable impairment in cardiac pump function (29, 355). However, a partial recovery in ventricular dynamics occurs chronically with coronary artery constriction, since myocyte losses involving 10% and 20% of the whole muscle cell population are accompanied by ventricular dysfunction and failure (51). In contrast, the hemodynamic characteristics of the heart are not altered by infarcts affecting less than 30%–35% of myocytes (150, 354, 384, 385). Moreover, in the presence of a 40%–50% infarct, ventricular performance does not improve during the evolution of the myopathy (12, 354, 355). An additional relevant difference between occlusive and nonocclusive coronary constriction is that, in the latter case, losses of discrete groups of cells are present chronically after the surgical intervention (25, 96, 286). Ongoing isolated myocyte death plays a central role in the genesis of chamber enlargement and ventricular performance. Cell loss, discrete in nature, can affect ventricular dimensions in two ways: acutely and chronically. The acute consequences reflect the early phase in which dying myocytes are overstretched in diastole and noncontracting in systole, leading to diastolic and systolic wall thinning. On the other hand, the chronic effects include the reparative processes associated with healing and scar formation. The simultaneous presence of these two aspects of myocardial damage contributes to the severe impairment in cardiac performance noted in this model of ischemic cardiomyopathy (22). A sudden change in coronary artery diameter may result in scattered loss of myocytes and profound impairment in ventricular performance, which may reverse if the abnormality in the vessel wall resolves (44). Conversely, a fixed lesion of the coronary artery, modest in nature, may provoke chronic and diffuse myocyte death, which may constitute a form of myocardial damage capable of continuously offsetting the reserve compensatory mechanisms of the injured ventricle, leading to irreversible myocardial dysfunction and overt congestive heart failure. Caution should be exercised in the translation of these experimental studies to the human population affected by atherosclerosis of the coronary arteries. Atherosclerosis is a disease state that progresses over a number of years, although acute hemorrhage within the atherosclerotic plaque may generate sudden constrictions in vessel luminal diameter.

Limited information is available on the quantitative structural characteristics of the human heart in ischemic cardiomyopathy. However, data have been obtained from patients undergoing cardiac transplantation as a result of chronic ischemic heart disease and refractory congestive heart failure (69). Hearts collected at autopsy from individuals who died from causes other than cardiovascular disease have been used as controls. Before emphasizing the similarities and differences between the animal model and the human disease, it should be recognized that ventricular dilation is not a common finding in humans (54, 83, 249), but most subjects requiring heart transplantation have dilated myopathy (194). Ventricular cavitary volume is increased severalfold, whereas the muscle mass-to-chamber volume ratio is markedly decreased. These individuals represent the fraction of patients with an unfavorable outcome due to severe diffuse coronary atherosclerosis of the three major vessels in all cases. At variance with the experimental conditions described above, coronary artery occlusion and coronary artery stenosis coexist with scattered foci of replacement fibrosis and diffuse interstitial fibrosis are found in conjunction with a healed infarct. As shown in Figure 2–19, interstitial and replacement fibrosis affect the noninfarcted myocardium of both ventricles. Collagen accumulation through these two processes exceeds the quantity associated with myocardial infarction and left ventricular scarring. Connective tissue comprises 28% of the left ventricle and 13% of the right ventricle. These percentages correspond to a 4.5-fold and 3.4-fold increase, indicating that the changes in the collagen compartment are major components of the remod-

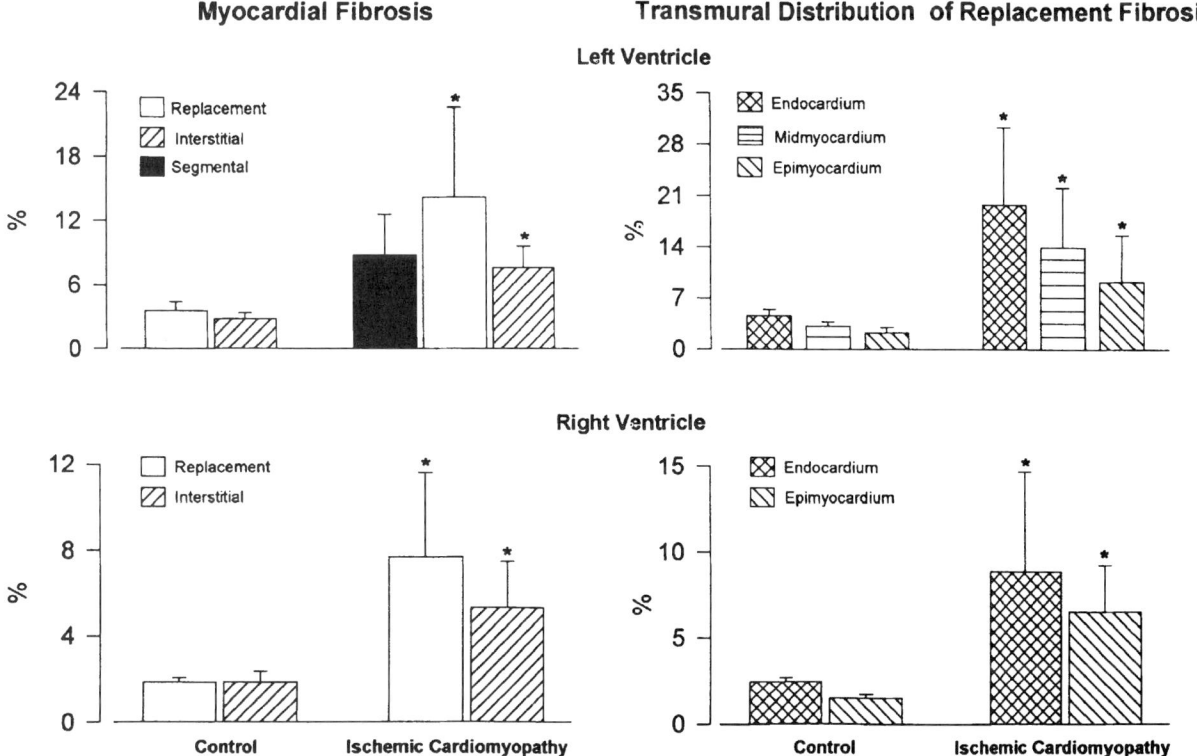

FIG. 2–19. Ischemic cardiomyopathy in humans: Relative amounts of segmental, replacement, and interstitial fibrosis in the myocardium. *Indicates a value that is statistically significantly different from the corresponding value in control hearts. Results are presented as mean ± SD.

eling of the ventricle with chronic ischemia. Myocyte cell loss, based on the number of ventricular myocyte nuclei (Fig. 2–20), involves only 35% of the myocyte population biventricularly (69). Therefore, in agreement with observations in the animal models, moderate losses of myocytes, diffuse in nature, have a greater impact on ventricular function than an equivalent loss of cells in a segmental fashion.

In recent years, several studies in humans and animals (445, 527, 528) have suggested that alterations of the collagen framework in the myocardium may play an important role in the genesis of ventricular dysfunction of ischemic and nonischemic origin. The possibility has been advanced that collagen deposition in the cardiac interstitium may constitute a primary event leading to a depression in myocardial and ventricular pump function (528). Although there is a general agreement that myocyte loss is the etiological factor of replacement fibrosis in the ventricular wall (527), less clear is the mechanism responsible for activation of the cardiac interstitium, resulting in the accumulation of fibrillar collagen between myocytes. Claims have been made that hormonal and/or hemodynamic overloads may trigger fibroblast proliferation and collagen neosynthesis in the myocardium, independent of myocytolytic necrosis and muscle cell loss. However, death of individual myocytes occurs with coronary artery constriction (94, 96, 285), and this phenomenon may stimulate healing, contributing to the expansion of the interstitium. However, the similarity in myocyte loss in the two ventricles (Fig. 2–22), despite differences in the fractional volumes of the collagen compartment, suggests that collagen neosynthesis has occurred in excess of the magnitude of myocyte loss. Alternatively, myocyte cellular hyperplasia might have been present in the left ventricle, resulting in an underestimation of the extent of myocyte cell loss. On the basis of quantitative findings in humans (69, 180), scattered myocyte loss leading to the formation of multiple foci of replacement fibrosis in the myocardium, in combination with interstitial fibrosis, appears to be the major cause of ventricular remodeling in the cardiomyopathic heart of ischemic origin. Myocardial infarction is a consistent determinant of this process and contributes to the alterations in size and shape of the heart, but it does not represent the principal etiologic factor of myocyte loss and the accumulation of collagen in the ventricle. This contention applies to conditions involving three-vessel disease in which segmental damage is only one aspect of the ischemic cardiomyopathic heart (54). *In summary, coronary artery constriction leads to scattered myocyte cell death, which has a more detrimental effect on ventricular pump function than an equivalent loss of cells in a segmental fashion as a result of coronary artery occlusion and myocardial infarction. However, both aspects of myocyte cell death contribute to the long-term evolution of ischemic cardiomyopathy toward end-stage cardiac failure.*

Ischemic Cardiomyopathy and Myocyte Cellular Hypertrophy and Hyperplasia

The phenomenon of myocyte cell loss in ischemic cardiomyopathy, in a segmental, focal, or diffuse pattern, complicates the analysis of the magnitude of reactive growth in the ventricular myocardium. Under these conditions, measurements of ventricular weight changes provide a significant underestimation of the actual magnitude of hypertrophy at the cellular level. Such a dissociation between the increase in organ weight and the increase in myocyte cell volume has been documented in humans (69, 70, 161, 357, 360–362) and animal models (51, 264, 354, 559). This problem applies not only to the ischemic cardiomyopathic heart but also to all cardiac disease states characterized by myocyte cell death in the ventricle. In particular, myocyte cell loss interferes with the determination of hypertrophic growth in aging (17, 44, 357, 362), hypertension (286, 360), and coronary artery constriction and hypertension combined (286). A direct relationship exists between the extent of cell death in the ventricle and the amount of reactive hypertrophy in the remaining viable muscle cells (40). However, this correlation persists only when ventricular performance is essentially maintained. In contrast, in the presence of acute, subacute, and chronic cardiac failure, an additional cellular response has been identified. Under the condition of severe impairment of ventricular function, DNA synthesis, myocyte nuclear mi-

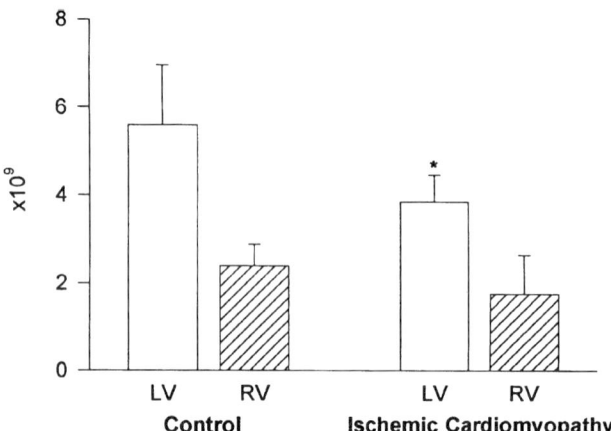

FIG. 2–20. Ischemic cardiomyopathy in humans: Total number of myocyte nuclei in the ventricle. *LV*: Left Ventricle; *RV*: Right Ventricle. *Indicates a value that is statistically significant different from the corresponding value in control hearts. Results are presented as mean ± SD.

totic division, and cellular hyperplasia occur, further complicating the analysis of the cellular mechanisms involved in the reactive growth adaptation of the injured ventricle (246, 393, 419, 420). Myocyte cellular hypertrophy is discussed first; myocyte proliferation, subsequently.

In the absence of myocyte proliferation, any loss of cardiac mass from ischemic necrosis results in a proportional loss of myocytes followed by the accumulation of a proportional amount of connective tissue scar in the ventricle (17, 37). However, the cellular reactions in the surviving myocardium differ with respect to their location to the damaged area. This phenomenon has been well documented after myocardial infarction (354, 355, 367), whereas more complex is the analysis of regional responses in the presence of diffuse myocardial injury following a constriction of a major epicardial coronary artery. The difficulty in discriminating viable from nonviable cells in the border zone of an infarct, using standard histological preparations of the myocardium, is well known and acknowledged by pathologists. This represents a particularly significant problem for defining the extent of an infarct and for estimating the potential additional loss of viable cells. An essential criterion for cell viability is the capacity of a cell to take up and incorporate free amino acids into its protein molecules (182) and, therefore, hypertrophy under conditions of stress (15). The prolonged and sustained effect of a segmental loss of tissue on discrete regions of the spared myocardium has been studied using methodologies capable of discriminating differences in cellular growth responses within the noninfarcted tissue (49). On this basis, the existence of a border zone has been extended to the entire evolution of the ischemic process (354, 355, 367). Once healing is completed, the surviving myocardium can be subdivided into two separate regions: the area bordering the infarct and that remote from the infarct. Myocyte cell volume in both zones increases in proportion to infarct size (Fig. 2–21). However, the hypertrophic growth of spared myocytes in the area adjacent to the scarred tissue is greater than that of cells in the portion remote from the infarct. The periinfarcted region participates in the myocardial adaptation to ischemic injury, creating a gradient in the hypertrophic response of the surviving myocardium. In addition, this gradient increases with infarct size, so that the impact of the border zone becomes progressively more significant in larger infarcts.

The mechanism by which myocardial infarction induces a greater hypertrophic growth in the myocytes adjacent to the scarred tissue is not clear. However, this region is stretched during ventricular contraction by the progressive thinning and bulging of the necrotic region (211, 212, 378), and passive stretch may be a

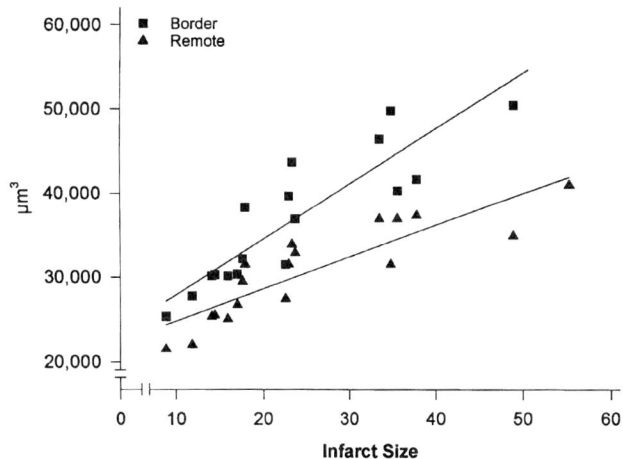

FIG. 2–21. Graphic comparison of myocyte cell volume measured in the border and remote regions of infarcted left ventricles. The upper linear regression line corresponds to the data collected in the border zone, whereas the lower regression line represents the values obtained in the remote region. Comparison of the two regression lines demonstrates a statistically significant difference between the two slopes ($p < 0.001$).

stimulus for muscle cell growth (125, 281, 467, 477). Because of the irregularity of the ventricular chamber produced by the aneurysmal extrusion of the scarred portion of the ventricle in systole, tension is greater in the border zone than in the remote portion of the wall. The interaction of the area of infarction with the viable myocardium also places obligatory constraints on the latter, resulting in altered series elasticity and an increased tension load, superimposed on the greater load associated with increased ventricular diameter and diastolic filling pressure (40). How the irregularity of chamber geometry and the fact that during systolic contraction only the viable myocardium shortens, further altering chamber architecture, interplay with the number of myocytes across the wall in the determination of stress at the cellular level is a central, unresolved issue. This information is crucial for the understanding of the multifactorial events implicated in global remodeling of the heart after ischemic myocardial injury.

Although regional differences in the myocyte cellular hypertrophic response have been measured in nonocclusive coronary artery constriction experimentally (51) and in the ischemic cardiomyopathic heart in humans (54, 69), the extent more than the pattern of myocyte cell death appears to influence the magnitude of hypertrophy in the unaffected muscle cells. Chronic coronary artery constriction associated with a 10% or 20% loss of ventricular myocytes is characterized by a corresponding 39% and 71% increase in myocyte size in the subendocardial region of the wall. An important aspect of the ischemic myopathy generated by coronary artery occlusion or constriction is the development of right ventricular hypertrophy (49, 51). The hypertrophic growth response of right ventricular myocytes is observed as early as 3 and 7 days after coronary artery occlusion (29, 331) and one week following coronary artery narrowing (106, 419, 557). Right ventricular myocyte hypertrophy also is present later during the evolution of the cardiac disease (246). However, experimentally, the magnitude of myocyte cellular hypertrophy in the ischemic left ventricle exceeds the extent of cellular growth in the right ventricle (106, 246, 419), whereas in the human heart comparable degrees of myocyte enlargement are present biventricularly (69). Three possibilities have been considered for the hypertrophic response of right ventricular myocytes after infarction: (1) an increase in right ventricular systolic pressure due to left-sided pump failure (385); (2) pulmonary hypertension as a primary stimulus, suggested by medial hypertrophy of the muscular branches of the pulmonary artery in infarcted subjects (506); and (3) the right ventricle may constitute a functional unit with the infarcted left ventricle, contributing to the emptying of the left ventricular chamber during systole (221, 222). These events, either independently or combined, lead to a greater pressure load on the right ventricle, resulting in concentric hypertrophy (12) before congestive heart failure develops (385, 388).

More complex is understanding the physiological mechanisms involved in the growth adaptation of the right ventricle with nonocclusive coronary artery constriction. The functional impairment of the left ventricle may affect the compliance properties of the right ventricle, and this phenomenon may account for diastolic overload and eccentric right ventricular myocyte hypertrophy (304, 323, 339). In addition, left ventricular dysfunction leads to an increase in left ventricular diastolic filling pressure, which, in turn, produces an increase in pulmonary arterial pressure. This provides a systolic load for the right ventricle that serves to stimulate concentric myocyte hypertrophy. Moreover, the intraventricular septum is shared by both ventricles, and its enlargement from left ventricular hypertrophy may transfer augmented filling pressures to the right ventricle. When left ventricular dilation and failure ensue, these loads for the right ventricle are enhanced further, and secondary right ventricular failure may develop. Although questions remain on the hemodynamic bases of myocyte reactive hypertrophy in ischemic cardiomyopathy, the quantitative evaluation of myocyte cell volume and its changes as a function of tissue injury has allowed characterization of the magnitude of cellular growth mechanisms in specific sites within the surviving myocardium of the left and right ventricles. Differences in the degree of cellular response exist; this heterogeneity seems to reflect variations in load on the myocardium that become more apparent with increasing quantities of myocyte cell loss in the ventricular wall.

The possibility that adult ventricular myocytes are not terminally differentiated cells and possess the capacity to proliferate in response to the hemodynamic overload generated by ischemic tissue injury is a matter of controversy. Although observations in humans (59, 60, 68, 243, 296, 361) and animals (15, 18–20, 23, 43, 44, 133, 246, 299, 364, 366, 3368, 371, 393, 418–420, 454) have indicated that myocyte hyperplasia may occur under a variety of pathological conditions, cardiac myocytes are commonly compared to neurons for their postulated inability to replace damaged myocardium. The bases for these opposing views are not clear, because only limited animal model data are available favoring the concept that myocytes cannot synthesize DNA and undergo mitotic division (177, 1178, 343, 469), whereas strong evidence has been obtained experimentally and in humans supporting the regenerative capacity of these cells. In addition, recent findings have indicated that cardiac failure, in combination with a marked elevation in diastolic wall stress, may be required for the initiation of the cellular hyperplastic response (90, 91). Unfortunately, very little emphasis has been given to the hemodynamic state as a major conditioning factor of the characteristics of myocyte growth in the heart. This limitation and the difficulty of establishing the cell of origin in the presence of mitosis (177, 246, 393), when confocal microscopy and histochemistry are not applied together (243), may represent the most important reasons for the controversy on the existence of myocyte cellular hyperplasia in the mammalian heart.

Myocardial damage is a consistent component of the failing, ischemic cardiomyopathic heart, and this phenomenon affects the analysis of the cellular processes involved in ventricular remodeling. In particular, the simultaneous presence of myocyte loss complicates the estimation of the number of newly formed cells in the myocardium by any methodological procedure currently available. The observation that segmental, replacement, and interstitial fibrosis are major factors in the restructuring of the ventricle demonstrates that a significant magnitude of myocyte loss occurs but does not provide a direct indication of its extent. Additionally, myocyte apoptosis occurs (180, 348, 352) and this form of cell death is not accompanied by an inflammatory reaction, fibroblast activation, and tissue fibrosis (21, 23, 36, 193, 235, 310). Cell loss complicates the analysis of myocyte proliferation because difficulties exist in the computation of the number of damaged cells from the relative and absolute amounts of fibrotic tissue in the myocardium. A graphical comparison between the aggregate volume of myocardial scarring and residual number of myocyte nuclei has been made chronically after infarction in an attempt to correlate collagen volume with loss of cells. This relationship shows that 1 mm³ of fibrotic tissue corresponds to the loss of approximately 60 times 10^3 myocytes (37). However, although such a value may be valid with a segmental loss of myocardium, it may not be applicable to small foci of replacement fibrosis and interstitial fibrosis. In this calculation, myocyte cell death is considered as the only source of collagen accumulation in the heart. The contribution of apoptosis to myocyte dropout is not taken into account, because of the impossibility of detecting this phenomenon after its completion.

In an effort to document that myocytes are not terminally differentiated cells and that cell proliferation occurs in ischemic cardiomyopathy, the presence of DNA synthesis, myocyte nuclear mitotic division, and an absolute increase in myocyte number in the left and right ventricular myocardium has been examined after coronary artery constriction in rats (246, 419). DNA replication and mitosis were present in the overloaded myocardium of the left and right ventricles, indicating that myocyte cellular hyperplasia contributed to biventricular remodeling in this setting (Plates 4 and 5). Similar findings have been observed after myocardial infarction (90, 420), in which the activation of the DNA synthetic machinery in the remaining viable myocytes and nuclear mitotic division (Fig. 2–25) occur initially in the region adjacent to the necrotic tissue and subsequently in the remote myocardium as well. This contention is supported by the observation that DNA synthesis does not result in ploidy formation or an increase in the number of nuclei per cell (246). A 40% increase in the aggregate number of cells in the right ventricle due to a 110% and 36% increase of mononucleated and binucleated myocytes (Fig. 2–22), has been measured chronically after coronary artery constriction. In contrast, myocyte proliferation in the left ventricle was not associated with an increase in the total number of myocytes. Myocardial damage and cell loss exceeded the hyperplastic response of muscle cells in this chamber, so that the left ventricle possessed 44% and 32% fewer mononucleated and binucleated muscle cells. These losses resulted in a 32% reduction in the number of myocytes in this ventricle. Importantly, the fraction of myocytes synthesizing DNA in the left ventricle was consistently higher than that in the right ventricle. However, the occurrence of myocyte cell death in the left ventricle made it impossible to establish with certainty the magnitude of cellular hyperplasia in this side of the heart. Conversely, based on the percentage of BrdU-labeled myocytes and the total number of muscle cell nuclei in the right ventricle (246), an aggregate number of

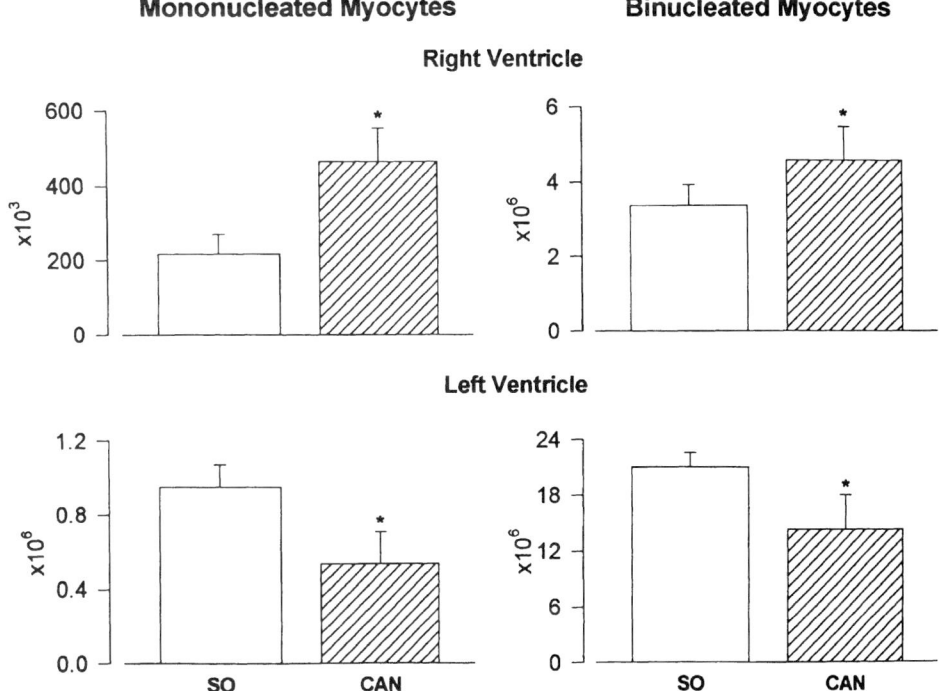

FIG. 2–22. Effects of coronary artery narrowing (CAN) on the total number of mononucleated and binucleated myocytes in the right and left ventricles. *Indicates a statistically significant difference between CAN and sham-operated (SO) rats. Results are presented as mean ± SD.

43,200 BrdU-positive nuclei was calculated for the right ventricle shortly after coronary stenosis. Such a magnitude of BrdU labeling resulted in the generation of 1.49 times 10^6 new myocytes in 3 months. If a similar relationship exists in the left ventricle, the corresponding 438,000 BrdU-labeled nuclei should result in the accumulation of 15.1 times 10^6 new myocytes at 3 months. This would imply that coronary artery constriction is accompanied by a 69% increase in the number of left ventricular myocytes during this period. Conversely, cell loss can be calculated to involve 60% of the myocyte population, or 13.3 times 10^6 myocytes. *In summary, adult ventricular myocytes can proliferate, and this process, in combination with myocyte cellular hypertrophy, leads to the restoration of large quantities of muscle mass lost as a result of ischemic myocardial injury.*

Ischemic Cardiomyopathy and Volume Composition of Myocytes

The volume fractions of mitochondria and myofibrils remain constant in left and right ventricular myocytes acutely after myocardial infarction (49). On the other hand, alterations in the mitochondria-to-myofibril volume ratio develop later in the evolution of the hypertrophic process when healing is complete. A reduction of the mitochondria-to-myofibril volume ratio has been measured in large infarcts 40 days after coronary occlusion in rats, indicating a disproportionate growth of these components relative to each other and to the cell volume as a whole (9). This phenomenon does not affect the post-infarcted hypertrophied right ventricle (12). Similarly, the composition of myocyte cytoplasm is not modified by small infarcts (9). The evolution of infarction-induced myocyte hypertrophy is characterized initially by an immediate, well-balanced compensatory response of the component structures involved in energy production and utilization that subsequently deteriorates with time. This becomes a potentially limiting factor in the functional capacity of the hypertrophied cardiac muscle cells following extensive ischemic injury of the myocardium. It should be emphasized, however, that no information is available concerning the effects of coronary artery constriction and diffuse myocyte loss on the subcellular structural properties of the unaffected myocytes. Moreover, it is unknown whether the long-term evolution of the post-infarction myopathy (388) is characterized by a restoration of the normal proportion of mitochondria and myofibrils, as documented in long-term pressure overload hypertrophy (368, 498). Although data on ischemic cardiomyopathy in humans are lacking, there is documentation that in cardiac failure, myocytes lose contractile material and that degenerative changes are present in the cytoplasm. Moreover, the nuclear cytoplasmic ratio is decreased, and myofilaments are irregularly arranged (196, 445, 450). These may represent common features of all cardiac disease states in their terminal phase. *In summary, ischemic cardiomyopathy results in multiple alterations of the mitochondrial and myofibrillar compartments of myocyte cytoplasm.*

Ischemic Cardiomyopathy and the Coronary Capillary Tree

An important issue concerning repair processes associated with myocardial damage is to establish whether hypertrophy of the spared tissue is accompanied by a proportionate or disproportionate growth of the capillary bed. Reconstitution of cardiac mass with a sufficient oxygen supply to the cells may improve the functional capacity of the ventricle, but an insufficient oxygen supply could contribute to its further deterioration. The volume fraction of capillary lumen in hypertrophying tissue of the left and right ventricles and the capillary luminal surface per unit volume of myocytes are both decreased shortly after coronary artery ligation (30, 355). The reduction in capillary luminal volume density indicates that an inadequate amount of capillary blood may be present per unit volume of tissue. On the other hand, studies in the dog heart have shown that occlusion of a major branch of the left coronary artery results in increased blood flow through the remaining arteries (135, 205). The mechanism by which increased blood flow through major coronary arteries can be achieved without proportional expansion of the capillary bed is difficult to explain. The morphometric measurements, however, cannot show the relative number of nonpatent capillaries that constitute the capillary reserve in the myocardium (200). Although it cannot be excluded that an increase in coronary blood flow may occur by the recruitment of capillaries after myocardial infarction, this process would reduce the normal reserve capacity of the capillary bed in the hypertrophied ventricle (200). A structural factor that further compromises tissue oxygenation in the hypertrophied left and right ventricles acutely after coronary artery occlusion is an increased average diffusion distance from the capillary wall to the mitochondria of myocytes (30, 355).

The lag in the growth response of the capillary microvasculature early after infarction raises a number of questions concerning the characteristics of the surviving myocardium later after the acute event. Moreover, regional differences in capillarity develop within the spared tissue with time, creating zones that may become particularly susceptible to ischemic injury. These issues have been addressed in a quantitative manner, and the results indicate that, after the healing process is complete, the concentration of capillary profiles per unit area of myocardium decreases progressively with infarct size (9, 354, 367, 506). Although the rate of change in capillary density is similar in the border zone and in the remote region, the capillarization of the former compartment is significantly lower than that of the latter in infarcts comprising more than 11% of the ventricular wall. Moreover, a similar gradient exists in the diffusion distance for oxygen, which is greater in the region bordering the infarct than in that remote from the scar. These alterations, combined with a decrease in capillary luminal volume and surface density, suggest that surviving myocytes, especially those located near the fibrotic area, are at high risk after healing. Comparable abnormalities of the capillary network have been found in the hypertrophied right ventricle chronically after coronary occlusion (12). Functional studies have documented a decrease in coronary vascular reserve and an increase in minimal coronary vascular resistance (250), suggesting that defects at the capillary level are accompanied by similar alterations in the transmural branches of the coronary vascular tree.

The presence of structural heterogeneity within the myocardium can have important clinical implications leading to local ischemic injury of the tissue and the occurrence of an arrhythmogenic response (370). In most patients who have coronary artery disease, ventricular tachyarrhythmias are the prevailing cause of sudden cardiac death and frequently are associated with myocardial ischemia (266) and cardiomegaly (234). Thus, the characteristics of the surviving tissue, in which there is marked heterogeneity in the hypertrophic response of the myocytes (Fig. 2–21) with an inadequate adaptation of the capillary microvasculature, may create a greater risk for the development of life-threatening arrhythmia. Arrhythmias may account for as much as 50% of sudden cardiac deaths in patients who have long-standing coronary artery disease and congestive heart failure (153, 372). In the presence of great destruction in myocardial mass, significant but insufficient tissue growth takes place in the surviving myocardium, and this is consistent with observations showing reduced cardiac output and lowered pressure-generating capacity (150, 385). Alterations in the structural integrity of the myocyte population (9) and in the capillary parameters controlling oxygen availability, diffusion, and transport (9, 62, 354, 367, 506) may also contribute to the deterioration of the physiological properties of the injured ventricle. Inadequate mass, reductions in the oxygenation potential of the hypertrophied myocardium, and decreases in the cytoplasmic component of myocytes responsible for energy production, all may be involved in the unfavorable long-term outcome of ischemic cardiomyopathy. *In summary, a deficit exists in the coronary vasculature in ischemic heart disease, and this inadequate adaptation may be one of the major factors involved in the development of the myopathy and its progression into irreversible congestive heart failure and death.*

Conclusions

Ischemic heart disease originates from an imbalance between oxygen supply and demand that, in turn, leads to myocyte loss, scarring, and ventricular failure. Cell loss occurs as a result of narrowing and/or occlusion of coronary arteries by atherosclerosis, spasm of the major or intramural arterial branches of the coronary vasculature, or alterations of the microcirculation, which, in an independent or combined fashion, create varying degrees of ischemia and tissue injury. The clinical spectrum ranges from acute myocardial infarction to chronic ischemic myopathy. The latter case may take the form of a dilated myopathy characterized by multiple focal sites of myocardial damage in the ventricular wall. In the most common manifestation, scattered foci of replacement fibrosis are found in conjunction with a healed myocardial infarct. Ventricular dilation is the predominant feature of the disease, and it exceeds the increase in ventricular muscle mass. The expansion in cavitary volume occurs acutely through an architectural rearrangement of myocytes within the wall consisting of side-to-side slippage of cells, whereas myocyte lengthening and reparative fibrosis are major determinants of chamber dilation chronically. Myocyte proliferation is a relevant component of wall remodeling and may contribute to the increase in cavitary size by the in-series addition of newly formed cells. This cellular process and the prevailing increase in myocyte length with hypertrophy result in a reduction in ventricular mass-to-chamber volume ratio and the development of decompensated eccentric hypertrophy. Moreover, a chronic, ongoing loss of myocytes throughout the wall appears to have a greater impact than a segmental loss of myocardium on cardiac anatomy and ventricular performance. Finally, defects in the coronary microcirculation may reduce the oxygenation potential of the hypertrophied spared tissue which, in combination with a reduction in the component structures of myocytes involved in energy production and utilization, may contribute to the progression of the myopathy to intractable congestive heart failure.

This work was supported by National Institutes of Health grants HL-38132, HL-39902, HL-43023, AG-15756, and AG-17042.

REFERENCES

1. Adler, C. P. Polyploidization and augmentation of heart muscle cells during normal cardiac growth and in cardiac hypertrophy. In: *The Development and Regenerative Potential of Cardiac Muscle*, edited by J. O. Oberpriller, J. O. Oberpriller, and A. Mauro. New York: Harwood Academic Publishers, 1991:227–252.
2. Adler, C. P. and U. Costabel. Cell number in human heart in atrophy, hypertrophy, and under the influence of cytostatics. *Recent Adv. Stud. Cardiol. Struct. Metab.* 6:343–355, 1975.
3. Adler, C. P. and U. Costabel. Myocardial DNA and cell number under the influence of cytostatics. I. Post-mortem investigations of human hearts. *Virchows. Arch. Cell Pathol.* 32:109–125, 1980.
4. Adler, C. P. and H. Friedburg. Myocardial DNA content, ploidy level and cell number in geriatric hearts: post mortem examination of human myocardium in old age. *J. Mol. Cell. Cardiol.* 18:39–53, 1986.
5. Adler, C. P. and W. Sandritter. Numerische Hyperplasie der Herzmuskelzellenbei Herzhypertrophie. *Deutsch. Med. Wochenschr.* 48:1895–1897, 1971.
6. Aherne, W. A. and M. S. Dunnill. *Morphometry*. London, Edward Arnold, 1982.
7. Albin, R., R. T. Dowell, R. Zak, and M. Rabinowitz. Synthesis and degradation of mitochondrial components in hypertrophied rat heart. *Biochem. J.* 136:629–637, 1973.
8. Anderson, P. G., S. P. Bishop, and S. B. Digerness. Vascular remodeling and improvement of coronary reserve after hydralazine treatment in spontaneously hypertensive rats. *Circ. Res.* 64:1127–1136, 1989.
9. Anversa, P., C. Beghi, Y. Kikkawa, and G. Olivetti. Myocardial infarction in rats: infarct size, myocyte hypertrophy and capillary growth. *Circ. Res.* 58:26–37, 1986.
10. Anversa, P., C. Beghi, V. Levicky, S. L. McDonald, and Y. Kikkawa. Morphometry of right ventricular hypertrophy induced by strenuous exercise in rat. *Am. J. Physiol.* 243 (Heart Circ. Physiol. 12):H856–H861, 1982.
11. Anversa, P., C. Beghi, V. Levicky, S. L. McDonald, Y. Kikkawa, and G. Olivetti. Effects of strenuous exercise on the quantitative morphology of left ventricular myocardium in the rat. *J. Mol. Cell. Cardiol.* 17:585–595, 1985.
12. Anversa, P., C. Beghi, S. L. McDonald, V. Levicky, Y. Kikkawa, and G. Olivetti. Morphometry of right ventricular hypertrophy induced by myocardial infarction in the rat. *Am. J. Pathol.* 116:504–513, 1984.
13. Anversa, P. and J. M. Capasso. Cardiac hypertrophy and ventricular remodeling. *Lab. Invest.* 64:441–445, 1991.
14. Anversa, P. and J. M. Capasso. Loss of intermediate-sized coronary arteries and capillary proliferation following left ventricular failure in rats. *Am. J. Physiol.* 260 (Heart Circ. Physiol. 29):H1552–H1560, 1991.
15. Anversa, P., D. Fitzpatrick, S. Argani, and J. M. Capasso. Myocyte mitotic division in the aging mammalian rat heart. *Circ. Res.* 69:1159–1164, 1991.
16. Anversa, P., M. Hagopian, and A. V. Loud. Quantitative radioautographic localization of protein synthesis in experimental cardiac hypertrophy. *Lab. Invest.* 29:282–292, 1973.
17. Anversa, P., B. Hiler, R. Ricci, G. Guideri, and G. Olivetti. Myocyte loss and myocyte hypertrophy in the aging rat heart. *J. Am. Coll. Cardiol.* 8:1441–1448, 1986.
18. Anversa, P. and J. Kajstura. Ventricular myocytes are not terminally differentiated in the adult mammalian heart. *Circ. Res.* 83:1–14, 1998.
19. Anversa, P., J. Kajstura, W. Cheng, K. Reiss, E. Cigola, and G. Olivetti. Insulin-like growth factor-1 and myocyte growth: the danger of a dogma. Part I. Postnatal myocardial development: normal growth. *Cardiovasc. Res.* 32:219–225, 1996.
20. Anversa, P., J. Kajstura, W. Cheng, K. Reiss, E. Cigola, and G. Olivetti. Insulin-like growth factor-1 and myocyte growth: the danger of a dogma. Part II. Induced myocardial growth: pathologic hypertrophy. *Cardiovasc. Res.* 32:484–495, 1996.
21. Anversa, P., J. Kajstura, and G. Olivetti. Myocyte death in heart failure. *Curr. Opin. Cardiol.* 11:245–251, 1996.
22. Anversa, P., J. Kajstura, K. Reiss, F. Quaini, A. Baldini, G. Olivetti, and E. H. Sonnenblick. Ischemic cardiomyopathy: myocyte cell loss, myocyte cellular hypertrophy, and myocyte cellular hyperplasia. In: *Annals of the New York Academy of Sciences*, edited by W. C. Claycomb and P. Di Nardo. New York: The New York Academy of Sciences, 1995:47–64.
23. Anversa, P., A. Leri, C. A. Beltrami, S. Guerra, and J. Kajstura. Myocyte death and growth in the failing heart. *Lab. Invest.* 78:767–786, 1998.
24. Anversa, P., V. Levicky, C. Beghi, S. L. McDonald, and Y. Kikkawa. Morphometry of exercise-induced right ventricular hypertrophy in the rat. *Circ. Res.* 52:57–64, 1983.
25. Anversa, P., P. Li, A. Malhotra, X. Zhang, M. V. Herman, and J. M. Capasso. Effects of hypertension and coronary constriction on cardiac function, morphology, and contractile proteins in rats. *Am. J. Physiol.* 265 (Heart Circ. Physiol. 34): H713–724, 1993.
26. Anversa, P., P. Li, E. H. Sonnenblick, and G. Olivetti. Effects of aging on quantitative structural properties of coronary vasculature and microvasculature in rats. *Am. J. Physiol.* 267 (Heart Circ. Physiol. 36):H1062–H1073, 1994.
27. Anversa, P., P. Li, X. Zhang, G. Olivetti, and J. M. Capasso. Ischemic myocardial injury and ventricular remodeling. *Cardiovasc. Res.* 27:145–157, 1993.
28. Anversa, P., A. V. Loud, F. Giacomelli, and J. Wiener. Absolute morphometric study of myocardial hypertrophy in experimental hypertension. II. Ultrastructure of myocytes and interstitium. *Lab. Invest.* 38:597–609, 1978.
29. Anversa, P., A. V. Loud, V. Levicky, and G. Guideri. Left ventricular failure induced by myocardial infarction. I. Myocyte hypertrophy. *Am. J. Physiol.* 248 (Heart Circ. Physiol. 17):H876–H882, 1985.
30. Anversa, P., A. V. Loud, V. Levicky, and G. Guideri. Left ventricular failure induced by myocardial infarction: II. Tissue morphometry. *Am. J. Physiol.* 248 (Heart Circ. Physiol. 17):H883–H889, 1985.
31. Anversa, P., A. V. Loud, and L. Vitali-Mazza. Morphometry and autoradiography of early hypertrophic changes in the ventricular myocardium of adult rat. A light microscopic study. *Lab. Invest.* 33:125–129, 1975.
32. Anversa, P., A. V. Loud, and L. Vitali-Mazza. Morphometry and autoradiography of early hypertrophic changes in the ventricular myocardium of adult rat. An electron microscopic study. *Lab. Invest.* 35:475–483, 1976.
33. Anversa, P., M. Melissari, C. Beghi, and G. Olivetti. Structural compensatory mechanisms in rat heart in early spontaneous hypertension. *Am. J. Physiol.* 246 (Heart Circ. Physiol. 15):H739–H746, 1984.
34. Anversa, P., M. Melissari, A. Tardini, and G. Olivetti. Connective tissue accumulation in the left coronary artery of young SHR. *Hypertension* 6:526–529, 1984.
35. Anversa, P., G. Olivetti, P. G. Bracchi, and A. V. Loud. Postnatal development of the M-band in rat cardiac myofibrils. *Circ. Res.* 48:561–568, 1981.
36. Anversa, P., G. Olivetti, A. Leri, Y. Liu, and J. Kajstura. Myocyte cell death and ventricular remodeling. *Curr. Opin. Nephrol. Hypertens.* 6:169–176, 1997.
37. Anversa, P., G. Olivetti, P. Li, M. V. Herman, and J. M. Capasso.

Myocardial infarction, cardiac anatomy and ventricular loading. *Cardioscience* 4:55–62, 1993.
38. Anversa, P., G. Olivetti, and A. V. Loud. Morphometric study of early postnatal development in the left and right ventricular myocardium of the rat. I. Hypertrophy, hyperplasia and binucleation of myocytes. *Circ. Res.* 46:495–502, 1980.
39. Anversa, P., G. Olivetti, and A. V. Loud. Morphometric studies of left ventricular hypertrophy. In: *Perspectives in Cardiovascular Research*, vol 8, edited by R. C. Tarazi and J. B. Dunbar. New York: Raven, 1983:27.
40. Anversa, P., G. Olivetti, L. G. Meggs, E. H. Sonnenblick, and J. M. Capasso. Cardiac anatomy and ventricular loading after myocardial infarction. *Circulation* [Suppl. VII] 87:22–27, 1983.
41. Anversa, P., G. Olivetti, M. Melissari, and A. V. Loud. Morphometric study of myocardial hypertrophy induced by abdominal aortic stenosis. *Lab. Invest.* 40:341–349, 1979.
42. Anversa, P., G. Olivetti, M. Melissari, and A. V. Loud. Stereological measurement of cellular and subcellular hypertrophy and hyperplasia in the papillary muscle of adult rat. *J. Mol. Cell. Cardiol.* 12:781–795, 1980.
43. Anversa, P., T. Palackal, G. Olivetti, and J. M. Capasso. Hypertensive cardiomyopathy: myocyte nuclei hyperplasia in the mammalian heart. *J. Clin. Invest.* 85:994–997, 1990.
44. Anversa, P., T. Palackal, E. H. Sonnenblick, G. Olivetti, L. G. Meggs, and J. M. Capasso. Myocyte cell loss and myocyte cellular hyperplasia in the hypertrophied aging rat heart. *Circ. Res.* 67:871–885, 1990.
45. Anversa, P., E. Puntillo, P. Nikitin, G. Olivetti, J. M. Capasso, and E. H. Sonnenblick. Effects of age on the mechanical and structural properties of myocardium of Fischer 344 rats. *Am. J. Physiol.* 256 (*Heart Circ. Physiol.* 25):H1440–H1449, 1989.
46. Anversa, P., R. Ricci, and G. Olivetti. Coronary capillaries during normal and pathological growth. *Can. J. Cardiol.* 2:104–113, 1986.
47. Anversa, P., R. Ricci, and G. Olivetti. Quantitative structural analysis of the myocardium during physiologic growth and induced cardiac hypertrophy: a review. *J. Am. Coll. Cardiol.* 7:1140–1149, 1986.
48. Anversa, P., R. Ricci, and G. Olivetti. Effects of exercise on the capillary vasculature of the rat heart. *Circulation* (Suppl I) 75:1–12, 1987.
49. Anversa, P. and E. H. Sonnenblick. Ischemic cardiomyopathy: pathophysiologic mechanisms. *Prog. Cardiovasc. Dis.* 33:49–70, 1990.
50. Anversa, P., L. Vitali-Mazza, and A. V. Loud. Morphometric and autoradiographic study of developing ventricular and atrial myocardium in fetal rats. *Lab. Invest.* 33:696–705, 1975.
51. Anversa, P., X. Zhang, P. Li, and J. M. Capasso. Chronic coronary artery constriction leads to moderate myocyte loss and left ventricular dysfunction and failure in rats. *J. Clin. Invest.* 89:618–629, 1992.
52. Arai, S. and A. Machida. Myocardial cell in left ventricular hypertrophy. *Tohoku J. Exp. Med.* 108:361–367, 1972.
53. Arai, S., A. Machida, and T. Nakamura. Myocardial structure and vascularization of hypertrophied hearts. *Tohoku J. Exp. Med.* 95:35–54, 1968.
54. Arbustini, E., R. Pozzi, M. Grasso, A. Gavazzi, M. Diegoli, M. Bramerio, G. Graziano, C. Campana, L. Angoli, S. De Servi, L. Martinelli, C. Goggi, M. Vigano, and G. Specchia. Pathologic substrates and clinical correlates of coronary artery disease and chronic congestive heart failure requiring cardiac transplantation. *Coronary Artery Dis.* 2:605–612, 1991.
55. Arends, M. J., R. G. Morris, and A. H. Wyllie. Apoptosis: the role of endonuclease. *Am. J. Pathol.* 136:593–608, 1990.
56. Ashley, L. M. A determination of the diameters of myocardial fibers in man and other mammals. *J. Anat.* 77:325–347, 1945.
57. Assali, N. S., T. M. Kirschbaum, and P. V. Diltis, Jr. Effects of hyperbaric oxygen on uteroplacental and fetal circulation. *Circ. Res.* 22:573–588, 1968.
58. Assali, N. S., J. A. Morris, and R. Beck. Cardiovascular hemodynamics in the fetal lamb before and after lung expansion. *Am. J. Physiol.* 208:122–129, 1965.
59. Astorri, E., R. Bolognesi, B. Colla, A. Chizzola, and O. Visioli. Left ventricular hypertrophy: a cytometric study on 42 human hearts. *J. Mol. Cell. Cardiol.* 9:763–775, 1977.
60. Astorri, E., A. Chizzola, O. Visioli, P. Anversa, G. Olivetti, and L. Vitali-Mazza. Right ventricular hypertrophy: a cytometric study on 55 human hearts. *J. Mol. Cell. Cardiol.* 2:99–110, 1971.
61. Averill, D. B., C. M. Ferrario, R. C. Tarazi, S. Sen, and R. Bajbus. Cardiac performance in rats with renal hypertension. *Circ. Res.* 38:280–288, 1976.
62. Bache, R. J. Effects of hypertrophy on the coronary circulation. *Prog. Cardiovasc. Dis.* 30:403–440, 1988.
63. Bardales, R. H., S. Hailey, S. S. Xie, R. F. Schaefer, and S. M. Hsu. In situ apoptosis assay for the detection of early acute myocardial infarction. *Am. J. Pathol.* 149:821–829.
64. Baroldi, G., G. Falzi, and P. Lampertico. The nuclear patterns of the cardiac muscle fiber. *Cardiologia* 51:109–123, 1967.
65. Batra, S., and K. Rakusan. Geometry of capillary networks in volume overloaded rat heart. *Microvasc. Res.* 42:39–95, 1991.
66. Bäurle, W. Die Coronarsklerose bei Hypertonie. *Beitr. Pathol. Anat.* 111:108–128, 1950.
67. Bell, R. D. and R. L. Rasmussen. Exercise and the myocardial capillary-fiber ratio during growth. *Growth* 38:237–244, 1974.
68. Beltrami, C. A., C. Di Loreto, N. Finato, M. Rocco, D. Artico, E. Cigola, S. R. Gambert, G. Olivetti, J. Kajstura, and P. Anversa. Proliferating cell nuclear antigen (PCNA), DNA synthesis and mitosis in myocytes following cardiac transplantation in man. *J. Mol. Cell. Cardiol.* 29:2789–2802, 1997.
69. Beltrami, C. A., N. Finato, M. Rocco, G. A. Feruglio, C. Puricelli, E. Cigola, E. H. Sonnenblick, G. Olivetti, and P. Anversa. Structural basis of end-stage failure in ischemic cardiomyopathy in humans. *Circulation* 89:151–163, 1994.
70. Beltrami, C. A., N. Finato, M. Rocco, G. A. Feruglio, C. Puricelli, E. Cigola, E. H. Sonnenblick, G. Olivetti, and P. Anversa. The cellular basis of dilated cardiomyopathy in humans. *J. Mol. Cell. Cardiol.* 27:291–305, 1995.
71. Beznak, M. The behavior of the weight of the heart and the blood pressure of albine rats under different conditions. *J. Physiol.* 124:44–63, 1954.
72. Bhatia, M. L. Circulatory adaptations in chronic severe anaemia. *Ind. Heart J.* 31:132–137, 1979.
73. Bishop, S. P. and P. Hine. Cardiac muscle cytoplasmic and nuclear development during canine neonatal growth. In *Recent Advances in Studies on Cardiac Structure and Metabolism*, edited by P. E. Roy, and P. Harris. Baltimore, University Park Press, 1975:77.
74. Bishop, S. P. and L. R. Melsen. Myocardial necrosis, fibrosis and DNA synthesis in experimental cardiac hypertrophy induced by sudden pressure overload. *Circ. Res.* 39:238–245, 1976.
75. Bishop, S. P., S. Oparil, R. H. Reynolds, and J. L. Drummond. Regional myocyte size in normotensive and spontaneously hypertensive rats. *Hypertension* 1:378–383, 1979.
76. Bloor, C. M. and A. S. Leon. Interaction of age and exercise on the heart and its blood supply. *Lab. Invest.* 22:160–165, 1970.
77. Booth, N. H., S. G. Hastings, M. L. Hopwood, and C. A. Maaske. Postnatal changes in the cardiac ventricles of the pig. *Proc. Soc. Exp. Biol. Med.* 122:186–188, 1966.
78. Borow, K. M., L. H. Green, T. Mann, L. J. Slon, E. Braunwald, J. J. Collins, L. Cohn, and W. Grossman. End systolic volume as a predictor of postoperative left ventricular performance in

volume-overload from valvular regurgitation. *Am. J. Med.* 68: 655–663, 1980.

79. Breisch, E. A., F. C. White, H. K. Hammond, S. Flynn, and C. M. Bloor. Myocardial characteristics of thyroxine stimulated hypertrophy. A structural and functional study. *Basic Res. Cardiol.* 84:345–358, 1989.

80. Breisch, E. A., F. C. White, L. E. Nimmo, and C. M. Bloor. Cardiac vasculature and flow during pressure-overload hypertrophy. *Am. J. Physiol.* 251 (*Heart Circ. Physiol.* 20):H1031–H1037, 1986.

81. Brodsky, V. Y. A. Cell ploidy in the mammalian heart. In: *The Development and Regenerative Potential of Cardiac Muscle*, edited by J. O. Oberpriller, J. C. Oberpriller, and A. Mauro. New York: Harwood Academic Publishers, 1991:253–292.

82. Brodsky, W. Y., A. M. Arefyeva, and I. V. Uryvaeva. Mitotic polyploidization of mouse heart myocytes during the first postnatal week. *Cell Tissue Res.* 210:133–144, 1980.

83. Bruschke, A. V. G., W. L. Pruodfit, and F. M. Sones. Progress study of 590 consecutive nonsurgical cases of coronary disease followed 5–9 years: II: ventriculographic and other correlations. *Circulation* 47:1154–1162, 1973.

84. Buja, L. M. and J. T. Willerson. Clinicopathologic correlates of acute ischemic heart disease syndromes. *Am. J. Cardiol.* 47:343–356, 1981.

85. Buja, L. M. and J. T. Willerson. The role of coronary artery lesions in ischemic heart disease:insight from recent clinicopathologic, coronary arteriographic, and experimental studies. *Hum. Pathol.* 18:451–461, 1987.

86. Burlingame, P., J. A. Long, and E. Ogden. The blood pressure of the fetal rat and its response to renin and angiotonin. *Am. J. Physiol.* 137:473–484, 1942.

87. Buttrick, P., C. Perla, A. Malhotra, D. Geenen, and J. Scheuer. Effects of chronic dobutamine on cardiac mechanics and biochemistry after myocardial infarction in rats. *Am. J. Physiol.* 260 (*Heart Circ. Physiol.* 29):H473–H479, 1991.

88. Campbell, S. E., A. M. Gerdes, and T. D. Smith. Comparison of regional differences in cardiac myocyte dimensions in rats, hamsters, and guinea pigs. *Anat. Rec.* 219:53–59, 1987.

89. Campisi, J. Replicative senescence:an old lives' tale? *Cell* 84: 497–500, 1996.

90. Capasso, J. M., S. Bruno, W. Cheng, P. Li, R. Rodgers, Z. Darzynkiewicz, and P. Anversa. Ventricular loading is coupled with DNA synthesis in adult cardiac myocytes after acute and chronic myocardial infarction in rats. *Circ. Res.* 71:1379–1389, 1992.

91. Capasso, J. M., S. Bruno, P. Li, X. Zhang, Z. Darzynkicwicz, and P. Anversa. Myocyte DNA synthesis with aging: correlation with ventricular loading in rats. *J. Cell Physiol.* 155:635–648, 1993.

92. Capasso, J. M., D. Fitzpatrick, and P. Anversa. Cellular mechanisms of ventricular failure: myocyte kinetics and geometry with age. *Am. J. Physiol.* 262 (*Heart Circ. Physiol.* 31):H1770–H1781, 1992.

93. Capasso, J. M., M. J. Jeanty, T. Palackal, G. Olivetti, and P. Anversa. Ventricular remodeling induced by acute nonocclusive constriction of coronary artery in rats. *Am. J. Physiol.* 257 (*Heart Circ. Physiol.* 26:H1983–H1993, 1989.

94. Capasso, J. M., P. Li, and P. Anversa. Nonischemic myocardial damage induced by nonocclusive constriction of coronary artery in rats. *Am. J. Physiol.* 260 (*Heart Circ. Physiol.* 29):H651–H661, 1991.

95. Capasso, J. M., P. Li, X. Zhang, and P. Anversa. Heterogeneity of ventricular remodeling after acute myocardial infarction in rats. *Am. J. Physiol.* 262 (*Heart Circ. Physiol.* 31):H486–H495, 1992.

96. Capasso, J. M., A. Malhotra, P. Li, X. Zhang, J. Scheuer, and P. Anversa. Chronic nonocclusive coronary artery constriction impairs ventricular function, myocardial structure, and cardiac contractile protein enzyme activity in rats. *Circ. Res.* 70:148–162, 1992.

97. Capasso, J. M., A. Malhotra, R. M. Remily, J. Scheuer, and E. H. Sonnenblick. Effects of age on mechanical and electrical performance or rat myocardium. *Am. J. Physiol.* 245 (*Heart Circ. Physiol.* 14):H72–H81, 1983.

98. Capasso, J. M., A. Malhotra, J. Scheuer, and E. H. Sonnenblick. Myocardial biochemical, contractile and electrical performance after imposition of hypertension in young and old rats. *Circ. Res.* 58:445–460, 1986.

99. Capasso, J. M., T. Palackal, G. Olivetti, and P. Anversa. Severe myocardial dysfunction induced by ventricular remodeling in aging rat hearts. *Am. J. Physiol.* 259 (*Heart Circ. Physiol.* 28): H1086–H1096, 1990.

100. Capasso, J. M., T. Palackal, G. Olivetti, and P. Anversa. Left ventricular failure induced by long-term hypertension in rats. *Circ. Res.* 66:1400–1412, 1990.

101. Capasso, J. M., E. Puntillo, G. Olivetti, and P. Anversa. Differences in load-dependence of relaxation between the left and right ventricular myocardium as a function of age in rats. *Circ. Res.* 65:1499–1507, 1989.

102. Capasso, J. M., J. E. Strobeck, A. Malhotra, J. Scheuer, and E. H. Sonnenblick. Contractile behavior of rat myocardium after reversal of hypertensive hypertrophy. *Am. J. Physiol.* 242 (*Heart Circ. Physiol.* 11):H882–H889, 1982.

103. Chalkley, D. T. The tetrakaidecahedron as the basis for the computation of cell volume and density. *Science* 118:599–600, 1953.

104. Charles River Technical Bulletin. Wilmington, Massachusetts: Charles River Laboratories, Inc., Vol 1, 1982:1–12.

105. Chen, Y., R. J. Torry, G. L. Baumbach, and R. J. Tomanek. Proportional arteriolar growth accompanies cardiac hypertrophy induced by volume overload. *Am. J. Physiol.* 267 (*Heart Circ. Physiol.* 36):H2132–H2137, 1994.

106. Cheng, W., J. Coupet, P. Li, K. Reiss, C. V. Hamby, J. M. Capasso, L. G. Meggs, and P. Anversa. Coronary artery constriction in rats affects the activation of α_1 adrenergic receptors in cardiac myocytes. *Cardiovasc. Res.* 28:1070–1082, 1994.

107. Cheng W., J. Kajstura, J. A. Nitahara, B. Li, K. Reiss, Y. Liu, W. A. Clark, S. Krajewski, J. C. Reed, G. Olivetti, and P. Anversa. Programmed myocyte cell death affects the viable myocardium after infarction in rats. *Exp. Cell. Res.* 226:316–327, 1996.

108. Cheng, W., B. Li, J. Kajstura, P. Li, M. S. Wolin, E. H. Sonnenblick, T. H. Hintze, G. Olivetti, and P. Anversa. Stretch-induced programmed myocyte cell death. *J. Clin. Invest.* 96:2247–2259, 1995.

109. Cheng, W., K. Reiss, J. Kajstura, K. Kowal, F. Quaini, and P. Anversa. Downregulation of the IGF-1 system parallels the attenuation in the proliferative capacity of rat ventricular myocytes during postnatal development. *Lab. Invest.* 72:646–655, 1995.

110. Cheng, W., K. Reiss, P. Li, J. M. J. Chun, J. Kajstura, G. Olivetti, and P. Anversa. Aging does not affect the activation of the myocyte insulin-like growth factor-1 autocrine system after infarction and ventricular failure in Fischer 344 rats. *Circ. Res.* 78:536–546, 1996.

111. Chien, K. R., K. U. Knowlton, H. Zhu, and S. Chien. Regulation of cardiac gene expression during myocardial growth and hypertrophy:molecular studies of an adaptive physiologic response. *FASEB J.* 5:3037–3046, 1991.

112. Chilian, W. M., R. D. Wangler, K. G. Peters, R. J. Tomanek, and M. L. Marcus. Thyroxine-induced left ventricular hypertrophy in the rat. Anatomical and physiological evidence for angiogenesis. *Circ. Res.* 57:591–598, 1985.

113. Chow, L. H., S. P. Yee, T. Pawson, and B. M. McManus. Progressive cardiac fibrosis and myocyte injury in v-fps transgenic mice:a model for primary disorders of connective tissue in the heart? *Lab. Invest.* 64:457–462, 1991.
114. Chrisman, R., P. B. Rittman, and R. J. Tomanek. Exercise induced myocardial capillary growth in the spontaneously hypertensive rat. *Microvasc. Res.* 30:185–194, 1985.
115. Clausen, J. P. Effect of physical training on cardiovascular adjustments to exercise in man. *Physiol. Rev.* 57:779–815, 1977.
116. Claycomb, W. C. DNA synthesis and DNA polymerase activity in differentiating cardiac muscle. *Biochem. Biophys. Res. Commun.* 54:715–720, 1973.
117. Claycomb, W. C. Biochemical aspects of cardiac muscle differentiation. Deoxyribonucleic acid synthesis and nuclear and cytoplasmic deoxyribonucleic acid polymerase activity. *J. Biol. Chem.* 250:3229–3235, 1975.
118. Claycomb, W. C. Cardiac-muscle hypertrophy. Differentiation and growth of the heart cell during development. *Biochem. J.* 168:599–601, 1977.
119. Clubb, F. J. and S. P. Bishop. Formation of binucleated myocardial cells in the neonatal rats. An index for growth hypertrophy. *Lab. Invest.* 50:571–577, 1984.
120. Cluck, L., N. S. Talner, T. H. Gardner, and M. V. Kulovich. RNA concentrations in the ventricles of full-term and premature rabbits following birth. *Nature* 202:770–771, 1964.
121. Coleman, G. L., S. W. Barthold, G. W. Osbaldiston, S. J. Foster, and A. M. Jonas. Pathological changes during aging in barrier-reared Fischer rats. *J. Gerontol.* 32:258–278, 1977.
122. Colgan, J. A., M. L. Lazarus, and H. G. Sachs. Post-natal development of the normal and cardiomyopathy Syrian hamster:a quantitative electron microscopic study. *J. Mol. Cell. Cardiol.* 10:43–54, 1978.
123. Cooper, G. IV, R. J. Tomanek, J. L. Ehrhardt, and M. L. Marcus. Chronic progressive pressure overload of the cat right ventricle. *Circ. Res.* 48:488–497, 1981.
124. Craft-Cormney, C. and J. T. Hansen. Early ultrastructural changes in the myocardium following thyroxine-induced hypertrophy. *Virchows. Arch. B Cell Pathol.* 33:267–273, 1980.
125. Csapo, A., T. Erdos, and C. R. Demattos. Stretch induced uterine growth, protein synthesis and function. *Nature* 207:1378–1379, 1965.
126. Dannenberg, A. L., D. Levy, and R. J. Garrison. Impact of age on echocardiographic left ventricular mass in a healthy population (*The Framingham Study*). *Am. J. Cardiol.* 64:1066–1068, 1989.
127. Darzynkiewicz, Z., S. Bruno, G. Del Bino, W. Gorczyca, M. A. Hotz, P. Lassota, and F. Traganos. Feature of apoptotic cells measured by flow cytometry. *Cytometry* 13:795–808, 1992.
128. Davies, P., J. Dewar, M. Tynan, and R. Ward. Post-natal development changes in the length–tension relationship of cat papillary muscles. *J. Physiol.* 253:95–102, 1975.
129. Dawes, G. S., J. C. Mott, and J. G. Widdicombe. The foetal circulation in the lamb. *J. Physiol.* 126:563–587, 1954.
130. DeFelice, A., R. Frering, and P. Horan. Time course of hemodynamic changes in rats with healed severe myocardial infarction. *Am. J. Physiol.* 257 (*Heart Circ. Physiol.* 26):H289–H296, 1989.
131. DeLa Cruz, M. V., G. Anselmi, A. Pomero, and G. Monroy. A qualitative and quantitative study of the ventricles and great vessels of normal children. *Am. Heart J.* 60:675–690, 1960.
132. Dobbs, S. L., D. M. Roth, C. M. Bloor, and F. C. White. Effects of age on coronary collateral development. *Coronary. Artery Dis.* 2:473–480, 1991.
133. Dowell, R. T., and R. E. McManus. Pressure-induced cardiac enlargement in neonatal and adult rats. Left ventricular functional characteristics and evidence of cardiac muscle cell proliferation in the neonate. *Circ. Res.* 42:303–310, 1978.
134. Dowell, R. T., C. M. Tipton, and R. J. Tomanek. Cardiac enlargement mechanisms with exercise training and pressure overload. *J. Mol. Cell. Cardiol.* 8:407–418, 1976.
135. Driscol, T. E. and R. W. Eckstein. Coronary inflow and outflow responses to coronary artery occlusion. *Circ. Res.* 20:485–495, 1967.
136. Duke, R. C., and J. J. Cohen. IL-2 addiction: withdrawal of growth factor activates a suicide program in dependent T cells. *Lymphokine Res.* 5:289–299, 1986.
137. Dunn, F. G., P. Chandraratna, J. G. R. de Carvallo, L. L. Basta, and E. D. Frohlich. Pathophysiologic assessment of hypertensive heart disease with echocardiography. *Am. J. Cardiol.* 39:789–795, 1977.
138. Eckner, F. A. O., B. W. Brown, D. L. Davidson, and S. Glagov. Dimensions of normal human hearts. *Arch. Pathol.* 88:497–507, 1969.
139. Edwards, W. D. Applied anatomy of the heart. In: *Cardiology: Fundamentals and Practice*, edited by R. O. Brandenburgh, V. Fuster, E. R. Giuliani, and D. C. McGoon. Chicago: Year Book, 1987, 47–112.
140. Ehrich, W., C. De La Chapelle, and A. E. Cohn. Anatomical ontogeny. B. Man (a study of the coronary arteries). *Am. J. Anat.* 49:241–282, 1931–32.
141. Elias, H., A. Sokol, and A. Lazarowitz. Contributions to the geometry of sectioning. II. Circular cylinders. *Z. Wiss Mikrosk* 62:20–31, 1954.
142. Emery, J. L., and M. D. MacDonald. The weight of ventricles in the later weeks of intra-uterine life. *Br. Heart J.* 22:563–570, 1960.
143. Factor, S. M., R. Bhan, T. Minase, H. Wolinsky, and E. H. Sonnenblick. Hypertensive-diabetic cardiomyopathy in the rat: an experimental model of human disease. *Am. J. Pathol.* 102:219–228, 1981.
144. Factor, S. M., M. Flomenbau, M. J. Zhao, C. Eng, and T. F. Robinson. The effects of acutely increased ventricular cavity pressure on intrinsic myocardial connective tissue. *J. Am. Coll. Cardiol.* 12:1582–1589, 1988.
145. Factor, S. M., T. Minase, S. Cho, R. Dominitz, and E. H. Sonnenblick. Microvascular spasm in the cardiomyopathic Syrian hamster: a preventable cause of focal myocardial necrosis. *Circulation* 66:342–354, 1982.
146. Feldstein, M. L., L. Henquell, and C. R. Honig. Frequency analysis of coronary intercapillary distances: site of capillary control. *Am. J. Physiol.* 235:(*Heart Circ. Physiol.* 4) H321–H325, 1978.
147. Field, B. J., R. O. Russell, J. T. Dowling, and C. E. Rackley. Regional left ventricular performance in the year following myocardial infarction. *Circulation* 46:679–689, 1972.
148. Fishbein, M. C., D. Maclean, and P. R. Maroko. Experimental myocardial infarction in the rat. Qualitative and quantitative changes during pathologic evolution. *Am. J. Pathol.* 90:57–70, 1978.
149. Fizelova, A. and A. Fizel. Cardiac hypertrophy and heart failure: dynamics of changes in proteins and nucleic acids. *J. Mol. Cell. Cardiol.* 1:389–402, 1970.
150. Fletcher, P. J., J. M. Pfeffer, M. A. Pfeffer, and E. Braunwald. Left ventricular diastolic pressure–volume relations in rats with healed myocardial infarction. *Circ. Res.* 49:618–626, 1981.
151. Fliss H. and D. Gattinger. Apoptosis in ischemic and reperfused rat myocardium. *Circ. Res.* 79:949–956, 1996.
152. Floderus, S. Untersuchungen über den Bau der menschlichen Hypophyse mit besonderer Berücksichtung der quantitativenmikromorphologischen Verhältnisse. *Acta. Pathol. Microbiol. Scand.* 53 [Suppl.]:1–276, 1944.

153. Franciosa, J. A., M. Wilen, and S. Ziesche. Survival in men with severe chronic left ventricular failure due to either coronary heart disease or idiopathic dilated cardiomyopathy. *Am. J. Cardiol.* 51:831–836, 1983.
154. Fraticelli, A., R. Josephson, R. Danziger, E. Lakatta, and H. A. Spurgeon. Morphological and contractile characteristics of rat cardiac myocytes from maturation to senescence. *Am. J. Physiol.* 257(*Heart Circ. Physiol.* 26): H259–H265, 1989.
155. Friberg, P., M. Nordlander, S. Lundin, and B. Folkow. Effects of aging on cardiac performance and coronary flow in spontaneously hypertensive and normotensive rats. *Acta. Physiol. Scand.* 125:1–11, 1985.
156. Friedman, W. F. The intrinsic physiologic properties of the developing heart. In: *Neonatal Heart Disease*, edited by W. F. Friedman, M. Lesch, and E. H. Sonnenblick. New York: Grune & Stratton, 1973:21–50.
157. Fukuda, J-I., J-I. Hayashi, T. Yoshimura, S-I. Ohtani, Y. Yamazaki, and S. Eguchi. Myocardial structure in volume-overloaded hearts before and after valve replacement. *Jpn. Circ. J.* 50:1033–1039, 1986.
158. Gault, J. H., J. W. Covell, E. Braunwald, and J. Ross Jr. Left ventricular performance following correction of free aortic regurgitation. *Circulation* 42:773–780, 1970.
159. Gavras, H. Hypertension and congestive heart failure: benefits of converting enzyme inhibition (Captopril). *J. Am. Coll. Cardiol.* 1:518–520, 1983.
160. Gerdes, A. M., S. E. Campbell, and D. R. Hilbelink. Structural remodeling of cardiac myocytes in rats with arteriovenous fistulas. *Lab. Invest.* 59:857–861, 1988.
161. Gerdes, A. M., S. E. Kellerman, J. A. Moore, L. C. Clark, P. Y. Reaves, K. B. Malec, K. E. Muffly, P. P. McKeown, and D. D. Schocken. Structural remodeling of cardiac myocytes from patient with chronic ischemic heart disease. *Circulation* 85:426–430, 1992.
162. Gerdes, A. M., J. Kriseman, and S. P. Bishop. Changes in myocardial cell size and number during the development and reversal of hyperthyroidism in neonatal rats. *Lab. Invest.* 48:598–602, 1983.
163. Gerdes, A. M., J. A. Moore, J. M. Hines, P. A. Kirkland, and S. P. Bishop. Regional differences in myocyte size in normal rat hearts. *Anat. Rec.* 215:420–426, 1986.
164. Gerstenblith, G., J. Frederiksen, F. C. Yin, N. J. Fortuin, E. G. Lakatta, and M. L. Weisfeldt. Echocardiographic assessment of a normal adult aging population. *Circulation* 56:273–278, 1977.
165. Ginzton, L. E., R. Conant, D. M. Rodriques, and M. M. Laks. Functional significance of hypertrophy of the noninfarcted myocardium after myocardial infarction in humans. *Circulation* 80:816–822, 1989.
166. Goldstein, M. A., W. C. Claycomb, and A. Schwartz. DNA synthesis and mitosis in well-differentiated mammalian cardiocytes. *Science* 183:212–213, 1974.
167. Goldstein, R. S., J. B. Tarloff, and J. B. Hook. Age-related nephropathy in laboratory rats. *FASEB J.* 2:2241–2251, 1988.
168. Gottlieb, R. A., K. O. Burleson, R. A. Kloner, B. M. Bablor, and R. L. Engler. Reperfusion injury induces apoptosis in rabbit cardiomyocytes. *J. Clin. Invest.* 94:1621–1628, 1994.
169. Grabner, W., and P. Pfitzer. Number of nuclei in isolated myocardial cells of pigs. *Virchows Arch. Cell Pathol.* 15:279–299, 1974.
170. Grajek, S., M. Lesiak, M. Pyda, M. Zajac. S. T. Pardowski, and E. Kaczmarek. Hypertrophy or hyperplasia in cardiac muscle, post-mortem human morphometric study. *Eur. Heart J.* 14:40–47, 1993.
171. Granger, C. B., M. K. Karimeddini, V. E. Smith, H. R. Shapiro, A. M. Katz, and A. L. Riba. Rapid ventricular filling in left ventricular hypertrophy. I. Physiologic hypertrophy. *J. Am. Coll. Cardiol.* 5:862–868, 1985.
172. Grant, C., D. G. Greene, and I. L. Bunnell. Left ventricular enlargement and hypertrophy. *Am. J. Med.* 39:895–904, 1965.
173. Greene, A. S., P. J. Tonellato, J. H. Lombard, and A. W. Cowley. Microvascular rarefaction and tissue vascular resistance in hypertension. *Am. J. Physiol.* 256 (*Heart Circ. Physiol.* 25): H126–H131, 1989.
174. Grimm, A. F., K. V. Katele, S. A. Klein, and H. L. Lin. Growth of the rat heart: left ventricular morphology and sarcomere lengths. *Growth* 37:189–201, 1973.
175. Grossman, W., B. A. Carabello, S. Gunther, and M. A. Fifer. Ventricular wall stress and the development of cardiac hypertrophy and failure. In: *Myocardial Hypertrophy and Failure*, edited by N. R. Alpert. New York: Raven, 1983:1–18.
176. Grossman W., D. Jones, L. P. McLaurin. Wall stress and patterns of hypertrophy in the human left ventricle. *J. Clin. Invest.* 56:56–64, 1975.
177. Grove, D., K. G. Nair, and R. Zak. Biochemical correlates of cardiac hypertrophy, III: changes in DNA content: the relative contributions of polyploidy and mitotic activity. *Circ. Res.* 25:463–471, 1969.
178. Grove, D., R. Zak, K. G. Nair, and V. Aschenbrenner. Biochemical correlates of cardiac hypertrophy, IV: observations on the cellular organization of growth during myocardial hypertrophy in the rats. *Circ. Res.* 25:473–485, 1969.
179. Guarente, L. Do changes in chromosomes cause aging? *Cell.* 86:9–12, 1996.
180. Guerra, S., A. Leri, X. Wang, N. Finato, C. Di Loreto, C. A. Beltrami, J. Kajstura, and P. Anversa. Myocyte death in the failing human heart is gender dependent. *Circ. Res.* 85:856–866, 1999.
181. Guideri, G., G. Olivetti, B. Hiler, R. Ricci, and P. Anversa. Increased incidence of isoproterenol-induced ventricular fibrillation in aging rats. *Can. J. Physiol. Pharmacol.* 65:504–508, 1987.
182. Guidotti, G. G., B. Luneburg, and A. F. Borghetti. Amino acid uptake in isolated chick embryo heart cells. Effect of insulin. *Biochem. J.* 114:97–105, 1969.
183. Hachamovitch, R., P. Wicker, J. M. Capasso, and P. Anversa. Alterations of coronary blood flow and reserve with aging in Fischer 344 rats. *Am. J. Physiol.* 256(*Heart Circ. Physiol.* 25): H66–H73, 1989.
184. Hagopian, M., P. Anversa, and A. V. Loud. Quantitative radioautographic localization of newly synthesized protein in the postnatal rat heart. *J. Mol. Cell. Cardiol.* 7:357–367, 1975.
185. Hagopian, M. and D. Spiro. Derivation of the Z line in the embryonic chick heart. *J. Cell Biol.* 44:683–687, 1970.
186. Hallback, M., O. Isaksson, and E. Noresson. Consequences of myocardial structural adaptation on left ventricular compliance and the Frank-Starling relationship in spontaneously hypertensive rats. *Acta. Physiol. Scand.* 94:259–270, 1975.
187. Hamrell, B. B., and N. R. Alpert. Cellular basis of the mechanical properties of hypertrophied myocardium. In: *The Heart and Cardiovascular System*, edited by H. A. Fozzard, R. B. Jennings, E. Haber, A. M. Katz, and H. E. Morgan. New York: Raven, 1986:1507–1524.
188. Hamrell, B. B., E. T. Roberts, J. L. Carkin, and C. L. Delaney. Myocyte morphology of free wall trabeculae in right ventricular pressure overload hypertrophy in rabbits. *J. Mol. Cell. Cardiol.* 18:127–138, 1986.
189. Harnarayan, C., M. A. Bennet, B. L. Pentecost, and D. B. Brewer. Quantitative study of infarcted myocardium in cardiogenic shock. *Br. Heart J.* 32:728–732, 1970.
190. Harrison, D. G., C. W. White, L. F. Hiratzka, D. B. Doty, D. H. Barnes, C. L. Eastham, and M. L. Marcus. The value of lesion

cross-sectional area determined by quantitative coronary angiography in assessing the physiologic significance of proximal left anterior descending coronary arterial stenosis. *Circulation* 69:1111–1119, 1984.
191. Hatt, P. Y., K. Rakusan, P. Gastineau, M. Laplace, and F. Cluzeaud. Aorto-caval fistula in the rat. An experimental model of heart volume overloading. *Basic Res. Cardiol.* 75:105–108, 1980.
192. Haug, H. Probleme und Methoden der Strukturzählung in Schnittpräparat. In: *Quantitative Methods in Morphology*, edited by E. R. Weibel, and H. Elias. New York: Springer-Verlag, 1967:58.
193. Haunstetter, A. and Izumo S. Apoptosis—Basic mechanisms and implications for cardiovascular disease. *Circ. Res.* 82:1111–1129, 1998.
194. Heck, C. F., S. J. Schumway, and M. Kape. The registry of the International Society for Heart Transplantation sixth official report 1989. *J. Heart Transplant.* 4:241–276, 1989.
195. Hegglin, R. Über Organvolumen und Organgewicht: Nebst Bemorkungen uber die Grobenbestimmungsmethoden. *Z. Konstitutionslehre* 18:110–134, 1934.
196. Hein, S., D. Scholz, N. Fujitani, T. Brand, A. Friedl, and J. Schaper. Altered expression of titin and contractile proteins in failing human myocardium. *J. Mol. Cell. Cardiol.* 26:1291–1306, 1994.
197. Heller, L. J., and W. V. Whitehorn. Age-associated alterations in myocardial contractile properties. *Am. J. Physiol.* 222:1613–1619, 1972.
198. Hellerstein, H. K., and D. Santiago-Stevenson. Atrophy of the heart: a correlative study of eighty-five proved cases. *Circulation* 1:93–126, 1950.
199. Henquell, L., C. L. Odoroff, and C. R. Honig. Coronary intercapillary distance during growth: relation to PO_2 and aerobic capacity. *Am. J. Physiol.* 231:1852–1859, 1976.
200. Henquell, L., C. L. Odoroff, and C. R. Honig. Intercapillary distance and capillary reserve in hypertrophied rat hearts beating in situ. *Circ. Res.* 41:400–408, 1977.
201. Henry, W. L., R. O. Bonow, J. S. Borer, J. H. Ware, K. M. Kent, D. R. Redwood, C. L. McIntosh, A. G. Morrow, and S. E. Epstein. Observations on the optimum time for operative intervention for aortic regurgitation. I. Evaluation of the results of aortic valve replacement in symptomatic patients. *Circulation* 61:471–483, 1980.
202. Henschel, E. Über Muskelfasermessungen und Kernveränderungen bei numerischer Hyperplasia des Myokards. *Virchows. Arch. Pathol. Anat.* 321:283–294, 1952.
203. Heron, M. I. and K. Rakusan. Geometry of coronary capillaries in hyperthyroid and hypothyroid rat heart. *Am. J. Physiol.* 267 (*Heart Circ. Physiol.* 36):H1024–H1031, 1994.
204. Heron, M. I., and K. Rakusan. Geometry of coronary capillaries in hyperthyroid and hypothyroid rat heart. *Am. J. Physiol.* 267 (*Heart Circ. Physiol.* 36):H1024–H1031, 1994.
205. Herzberg, R. M., R. Rubio, and R. M. Berne. Coronary occlusion and embolization: effect on blood flow in adjacent arteries. *Am. J. Physiol.* 210:169–175, 1966.
206. Heymann, M. A. and A. M. Rudolph. Effects of congenital heart disease on fetal and neonatal circulations. In: *Neonatal Heart Disease*, edited by W. F. Friedman, M. Lesch, and E. H. Sonnenblick. New York: Grune and Stratton, 1973:51–79.
207. Hinchliffe, J. R. Cell death in embryogenesis. In: *Cell Death in Biology and Pathology*, edited by I. D. Bowen and R. A. Lockshin. London: Chapman and Hall, 1981:35–78.
208. Hirokawa, K. A quantitative study on pre- and postnatal growth of human heart. *Acta. Pathol. Jpn.* 22:613–624, 1972.
209. Hislop, A. and L. Reid. Weight of the left and right ventricle of the heart during fetal life. *J. Clin. Pathol.* 25:534–536, 1972.
210. Hittinger, L. R., P. Shannon, S. P. Bishop, R. J. Gelpi, and S. F. Vatner. Subendomyocardial exhaustion of blood flow reserve and increased fibrosis in conscious dogs with heart failure. *Circ. Res.* 65:971–980, 1989.
211. Hochman, J. S. and B. H. Bulkley. Expansion of acute myocardial infarction. An experimental study. *Circulation* 65:1446–1450, 1982.
212. Hochman, J. S. and B. H. Bulkley. Pathogenesis of left ventricular aneurysms: an experimental study in the rat model. *Am. J. Cardiol.* 50:83–88, 1982.
213. Holtzer, H., T. M. Marshall, and H. Finck. Analysis of myogenesis by the use of fluorescent antimyosin. *J. Biophys. Biochem. Cytol.* 3:705–723, 1957.
214. Honing, C. R. and J. Bourdeau-Martini. Extravascular component of oxygen transport in normal and hypertrophied hearts with special reference to oxygen therapy. *Circ. Res.* 34/35: (Suppl 2) II-97–103, 1974.
215. Hopkins, S. F., E. P. McCutcheon, and D. R. Wekstein. Postnatal changes in rat ventricular function. *Circ. Res.* 32:685–691, 1973.
216. Hoppeler H, O. Mathieu, E. R. Weibel, R. Krauer, S. L. Lindstedt, and C. R. Taylor. Design of the mammalian respiratory system. VIII. Capillaries in skeletal muscles. *Respir. Physiol.* 44:129–150, 1981.
217. Hort, W. Quantitative histologische Untersuchungen an wachsenden Herzen. *Virchows. Arch. Pathol. Anat.* 323:223–242, 1953.
218. Hort, W. Quantitative Untersuchungen über die Kapillarisierung des Herzmuskels im Erwachsenen-und Greisenalter, bei Hypertrophie und Hyperplasia. *Virchows. Arch. Pathol. Anat.* 327:560–576, 1955
219. Hort, W. Morphologische Untersuchungen an Herzen vor, während und nach der postnatalen Kreislaufumschaltung. *Virchows. Arch. Pathol. Anat.* 326:458–484, 1955.
220. Hort, W. Mikrometrische Untersuchungen an verschieden weiten Meerschweinchenherzen. *Verhandl. Deutsch. Gesellsch. Kreislaufforsch.* 23:343–346, 1957.
221. Hort, W., S. da Canalis, and H. Just. Untersuchungen bei chronischem experimentellen Herzinfarkt der Ratte. *Arch. Kreisl-Forsch.* 44:288–299, 1964.
222. Hort, W. and H. Hort. Beiträge zur Histochemie der Blutgefäßendothelien und der Capillargrund häutchen. *Virchows Arch. Pathol. Anat.* 331:591–615, 1958.
223. Hort, W. and H. J. Severidt. Kapillarisierung und mikroskopische Veränderungen im Myokard bei angeborenen Herzfehlern. *Virchows. Arch. Pathol. Anat.* 341:192–203, 1966.
224. House, E. W. and H. E. Ederstrom. Anatomical changes with age in the heart and ductus arteriosus in the dog after birth. *Anat. Rec.* 160:289–296, 1968.
225. Huang, H., P. Li, C. V. Hamby, K. Reiss, L. G. Meggs, and P. Anversa. Alterations in angiotensin II receptor mediated signal transduction shortly after coronary artery constriction in the rat. *Cardiovasc. Res.* 28:1564–1573, 1994.
226. Hudlicka, O. Development of microcirculation: capillary growth and adaptation. In: *Handbook of Physiology Section 2. The Cardiovascular System. Vol IV, Microcirculation Part 1*, edited by E. M. Renkin, and C. C. Michel. Bethesda, MD: American Physiological Society, 1984:165–216.
227. Hudlická, O. Growth of capillaries in skeletal and cardiac muscle. *Circ. Res.* 50:451–561, 1982.
228. Hutchins, G. M. Structure of the aging heart. In: *The Aging Heart. Aging (Vol 12)*, edited by M. L. Weisfeld. New York: Raven, 1980:7–23.
229. Isoyama, S., W. Grossman, and J. Y. Wei. Effect of age on myocardial adaptation to volume overload in the rat. *J. Clin. Invest.* 81:1850–1857, 1988.

230. Isoyama, S., J. Y. Wei, S. Izumo, P. Fort, F. J. Schoen, and W. Grossman. Effect of age on the development of cardiac hypertrophy produced by aortic constriction in the rat. *Circ. Res.* 61: 337–345, 1987.
231. Itoh, G., J. Tamura, M. Suzuki, Y. Suzuki, H. Ikeda, M. Kioke, M. Nomura, T. Jie, and K. Ito. DNA fragmentation of human infarcted myocardial cells demonstrated by the nick end labeling and DNA agarose gel electrophoresis. *Am. J. Pathol.* 146: 1235–1331, 1995.
232. Iwasaki, K., C. A. Cleiser, E. J. Masoro, C. A. McMahan, E. J. Seo, and B. P. Yu. The influence of dietary protein source on longevity and age-related disease processes of Fischer rats. *J. Gerontol* 43:B5–B12, 1988.
233. Jacobs, T. B., R. D. Bell, and J. D. McClements. Exercise, age and the development of the myocardial vasculature. *Growth* 48:148–157, 1984.
234. James, T. N. Morphologic substrates of sudden death: Summary. *J. Am. Coll. Cardiol.* 5:81B–82B, 1985.
235. James, T. N. Apoptosis in cardiac disease. *Am. J. Med.* 107: 606–620, 1999.
236. Jarmakani, J. M., T. Nagatomo, M. Nakasawa, and G. A. Langer. Effect of hypoxia on myocardial high-energy phosphates in the neonatal mammalian heart. *Am. J. Physiol.* 235 (*Heart Circ. Physiol* 4):H475–H481, 1978.
237. Jazwinski, S. M. Longevity, genes, and aging. *Science* 273:54–59, 1996.
238. Jennings, R. B., H. M. Sommers, J. P. Kaltenbach, and J. J. West. Electrolyte alterations in acute myocardial ischemic injury. *Circ. Res.* 14:260–269, 1964.
239. Johnson, F. B., D. A. Sinclair, and L. Guarente. Molecular biology of aging. *Cell* 96:291–302, 1999.
240. Kajstura J, W. Cheng, K. Reiss, W. A. Clark, E. H. Sonnenblick, S. Krajewski, J. C. Reed, G. Olivetti, and P. Anversa. Apoptotic and necrotic myocyte cell death are independent contributing variables of infarct size of rats. *Lab. Invest.* 74:86–107, 1996.
241. Kajstura, J., W. Cheng, K. Reiss, and P. Anversa. The IGF-1–IGF-1 receptor system modulates myocyte proliferation but not myocyte cellular hypertrophy in vitro. *Exp. Cell Res.* 215:273–283, 1994.
242. Kajstura J., W. Cheng, R. Sarangarajan, P. Li, B. Li, J. A. Nitahara, S. Chapnick, K. Reiss, G. Olivetti, and P. Anversa. Necrotic and apoptotic myocyte cell death in the aging heart of Fischer 344 rats. *Am. J. Physiol.* 271 (*Heart, Circ. Physiol.* 40): H1215–H1228, 1996.
243. Kajstura J., A. Leri, N. Finato, C. Di Loreto, C. A. Beltrami, and P. Anversa. Myocyte proliferation in end-stage cardiac failure in humans. *Proc. Natl. Acad. Sci. U.S.A.* 95:8801–8805, 1998.
244. Kajstura, J., M. Mansukhani, W. Cheng, K. Reiss, S. Krajewski, J. C. Reed, F. Quaini, E. H. Sonnenblick, and P. Anversa. Programmed cell death and expression of the protooncogene bcl-2 in myocytes during postnatal maturation of the heart. *Exp. Cell Res.* 219:110–121, 1995.
245. Kajstura, J., X. Zhang, Y. Liu, E. Szoke, W. Cheng, G. Olivetti, T. H. Hintze, and P. Anversa. The cellular basis of pacing-induced dilated cardiomyopathy: myocyte cell loss and myocyte cellular reactive hypertrophy. *Circulation.* 92:2306–2317, 1995.
246. Kajstura, J., X. Zhang, K. Reiss, E. Szoke, P. Li, C. Lagrasta, W. Cheng, Z. Darzynkiewicz, G. Olivetti, and P. Anversa. Myocyte cellular hyperplasia and myocyte cellular hypertrophy contribute to chronic ventricular remodeling in coronary artery narrowing-induced cardiomyopathy in rats. *Circ. Res.* 74:383–400, 1994.
247. Kannel, W. B. Implications of Framingham Study data for treatment of hypertension: impact of other risk factors, In: *Frontiers in Hypertension Research*, edited by J. H. Laragh, R. F. Buhler, and D. W. Seldin. New York: Springer-Verlag, 1981:17–21.
248. Kannel, W. B. Role of blood pressure in cardiovascular morbidity and mortality. *Prog. Cardiovasc. Dis.* 17:5–24, 1974.
249. Kannel, W. B., P. Sorlie, and P. M. McNamara. Prognosis after initial myocardial infarction: the Framingham Study. *Am. J. Cardiol.* 44:53–59, 1979.
250. Karam, R., B. P. Healy, and P. Wicker. Coronary reserve is depressed in postmyocardial infarction reactive cardiac hypertrophy. *Circulation* 81:238–246, 1990.
251. Karsner, H. T., O. Saphir, and T. W. Todd. The state of the cardiac muscle in hypertrophy and atrophy. *Am. J. Pathol.* 1: 351–371, 1925.
252. Kathke, N. Die Veränderungen der Coronararterienzweige des Myocards bei Hypertonie. *Beitr. Path. Anat.* 115:405–422, 1955.
253. Katz, A. M. Effects of ischemia on the contractile processes of heart muscle. *Am. J. Cardiol.* 32:456–460, 1973.
254. Katz, A. M., H. Takenaka, and J. Watras. The sarcoplasmic reticulum. In: *The Heart and Cardiovascular System*, edited by H. A. Fozzard, R. B. Jennings, E. Haber, A. M. Katz, and H. E. Morgan. New York: Raven, 1986:731–746.
255. Katzberg, A. A., B. B. Farmer, and R. A. Harris. The predominance of binucleation in isolated rat heart myocytes. *Am. J. Anat.* 149:489–500, 1977.
256. Kerr, A., W. J. Bommer, and S. Pilota. Coronary-artery enlargement in experimental cardiac hypertrophy. *Am. Heart J.* 75: 144, 1968.
257. Keul, J., H. H. Dickhuth, G. Simon, and M. Lehman. Effect of static and dynamic exercise on heart volume, contractility and left ventricular dimensions. *Circ. Res.* 48 (Suppl I) I-163-I-170, 1981.
258. Kirsehbaum, L. A. and M. D. Schneider. The cardiac cell cycle, pocket proteins, and p300. *Trends. Cardiovasc. Med.* 5:230–235, 1995.
259. Kitzman, D. W., D. G. Scholz, P. T. Hagen, D. M. Ilstrup, and W. D. Edwards. Age-related changes in normal human hearts during the first 10 decades of life. Part II (Maturity): a quantitative anatomic study of 765 specimens from subjects 20 to 99 years old. *Mayo Clin. Proc.* 63:137–146, 1988.
260. Klopfenstein, H. S., and A. M. Rudolph. Postnatal changes in the circulation and responses to volume loading in sheep. *Circ. Res.* 42:839–845, 1978.
261. Korecky, B. and K. Rakusan. Normal and hypertrophic growth of the rat heart: changes in cell dimensions and number. *Am. J. Physiol.* 234 (*Heart Circ. Physiol.* 3):H123–H128, 1978.
262. Korecky, B., S. Sweet, and K. Rakusan. Number of nuclei in mammalian cardiac myocytes. *Can. J. Physiol. Pharmacol.* 57: 1122–1129, 1979.
263. Körner, F. Uber die direkte Teilung der Herzmuskelkerne. *Z. Mikrosk. Anat. Forsch.* 38:441–470,1935.
264. Kozlovskis, P. L., A. M. Gerdes, M. Smets, J. A. Moore, G. Koch, A. L. Bassett, and R. J. Myerburg. Regional increase in myocyte volume after healing of myocardial infarction in cats. *J. Mol. Cell. Cardiol.* 23:1459–1466, 1991.
265. Krogh, A. The number and distribution of capillaries in muscles with calculations of the oxygen pressure head necessary for supplying the tissue. *J. Physiol. (Lond.)* 52:409–415, 1919.
266. Kubler, W., A. Schomig, and J. Senges. The conduction and cardiac sympathetic system. Metabolic aspects. *J. Am. Coll. Cardiol.* 5:157B-161B, 1985.
267. Laine, G. A. Microvascular changes in the heart during chronic arterial hypertension. *Circ. Res.* 62:953–960, 1988.
268. Laine, G. A. and H. J. Granger. Microvascular, interstitial, and lymphatic interactions in normal heart. *Am. J. Physiol.* 249 (*Heart Circ. Physiol.* 18):H834–H842, 1985.

269. Lais, L. T., L. L. Rios, S. Boutelle, G. F. DiBona, and M. J. Brody. Arterial pressure development in neonatal and young spontaneously hypertensive rats. *Blood Vessels* 14:277–284, 1977.
270. Lakatta, E. G. Cardiovascular regulatory mechanisms in advanced age. *Physiol. Rev.* 73:413–467, 1993.
271. Lakatta, E. G., G. Gerstenblith, C. S. Angell, N. W. Shock, and M. L. Weisfeldt. Prolonged contraction duration in aged myocardium. *J. Clin. Invest.* 55:61–68, 1975.
272. Lakatta, E. G., J. H. Mitchell, A. Pomerance, and G. G. Rowe. Human aging: change in structure and function. *J. Am. Coll. Cardiol.* 10:42A–47A, 1987.
273. Lakatta, E. G. and F. C. P. Yin. Myocardial aging. Functional alterations and related cellular mechanisms. *Am. J. Physiol.* 244 (*Heart Circ. Physiol.* 13):H927-H941, 1982.
274. Latimer, H. B. The weight and thickness of the two ventricular walls in the newborn dog heart. *Anat. Rec.* 152:225–229, 1965.
275. Lazarus, M. L., J. A. Colgan, and H. G. Sachs. Quantitative light and electron microscopic comparison of the normal and cardiomyopathic Syrian hamster heart. *J. Mol. Cell. Cardiol.* 8: 431–441, 1976.
276. Lee, J. C., J. F. N. Taylor, and S. E. Downing. A comparison of ventricular weights and geometry in newborn, young, and adult mammals. *J. Appl. Physiol.* 38:147–150, 1975.
277. Legato, M. J. Cellular mechanisms of normal growth in the mammalian heart. I. Qualitative and quantitative features of ventricular architecture in the dog from birth to five months of age. *Circ. Res.* 44:250–262, 1979.
278. Legato, M. J. Cellular mechanisms of normal growth in the mammalian heart. II. A quantitative and qualitative comparison between the right and left ventricular myocytes in the dog from birth to five months of age. *Circ. Res.* 44:263–279, 1979.
279. Legault, F., J. L. Rovleau, C. Juneau, C. Rose, and K. Rakusan. Functional and morphological characteristics of compensated and decompensated cardiac hypertrophy in dogs with chronic infrarenal aorto-caval fistulas. *Circ. Res.* 66:846–459, 1990.
280. Lenkiewicz, J. E., M. J. Davies, and D. Rosen. Collagen in human myocardium as a function of age. *Cardiovasc. Res.* 6:549–555, 1972.
281. Lesch, M., R. Gorlin, and E. H. Sonnenblick. Myocardial amino acid transport in the isolated rabbit ventricular papillary muscle: general characteristics and effects of passive stretch. *Circ. Res.* 27:445–460, 1970.
282. Levine, N. D., S. D. Rockoff, and E. Braunwald. An angiocardiographic analysis of the thickness of the left ventricular wall and cavity in aortic stenosis and other valvular lesions. Hemodynamic-angiographic correlations in patients with obstruction to left ventricular outflow. *Circulation* 28:339–345, 1963.
283. Li, Q., B. Li, X. Wang, A. Leri, K. P. Jana, Y. Liu, J. Kajstura, R. Baserga, and P. Anversa. Overexpression of insulin-like growth factor-1 in mice protects from myocyte death after infarction, attenuating ventricular dilation, wall stress, and cardiac hypertrophy. *J. Clin. Invest.* 100:1991–1999, 1997.
284. Li, P., C. Park, R. Micheletti, B. Li, W. Cheng, E. H. Sonnenblick, P. Anversa, and G. Bianchi. Myocyte performance during evolution of myocardial infarction in rats: effects of propionyl-L-carnitine. *Am. J. Physiol.* 268 (*Heart Circ. Physiol.* 37): H1702–H1713, 1995.
285. Li, B., M. Setoguchi, X. Wang, A. M. Andreoli, A. Leri, A. Malhotra, J. Kajstura, and P. Anversa. Insulin-like growth factor-1 attenuates the detrimental impact of nonocclusive coronary artery constriction on the heart. *Circ. Res.* 84:1007–1019, 1999.
286. Li, P., X. Zhang, J. M. Capasso, L. G. Meggs, E. H. Sonnenblick, and P. Anversa. Myocyte loss and left ventricular failure characterise the long term effects of coronary artery narrowing or renal hypertension in rats. *Cardiovasc. Res.* 27:1066–1075, 1993.
287. Lie, J. T. and P. I. Hammond. Pathology of the senescent heart: anatomic observations on 237 autopsy studies of patients 90 to 105 years old. *Mayo Clin. Proc.* 63:552–564, 1988.
288. Lin, H-L., V. Kazimieras, and A. F. Grimm. Functional morphology of the pressure- and the volume-hypertrophied rat heart. *Circ. Res.* 41:830–836, 1977.
289. Linzbach, A. J. Mikrometrische und histologische Analyse hypertropher menschlicher Herzen. *Virchows Arch. Pathol. Anat.* 314:534–592, 1947.
290. Linzbach, A. J. Herzhypertrophie und kritisches Herzgewicht. *Klin. Wochenschr.* 26:459–463, 1948.
291. Linzbach, A. J. Die Muskelfaserkonstante und das Wachstumsgesetz der menschlichen Herzkammern. *Virchows Arch. Pathol. Anat.* 318:575–618, 1950.
292. Linzbach, A. J. Die Anzahl der Herzmuskelkerne in normalen, über-lasteten, atrophischen und mit Corhormon behandelten Herzkammern. *Z. Kreislaufforsch.* 41:641–658, 1952.
293. Linzbach, A. J. Quantitative Biologie und Morphologie des Wachstums. In: *Handbuch der Allgemeinen Pathologie, Vol 6*, edited by F. Büchner, E. Letterer, and F. Roulet. Berlin: Springer-Verlag, 1955, 181–306.
294. Linzbach, A. J. Über das Längenwachstum der Herzmuskelfasern und ihrer Kerne in Beziehung zur Herzdilatation. *Virchows Arch. Pathol. Anat.* 328:165–181, 1956.
295. Linzbach, A. J. Die Lebenswandlungen der Struktur des Herzens. *Verhandl. Deutsch. Gesellsch. Kreislaufforsch.* 24:3–15, 1958.
296. Linzbach, A. J. Heart failure from the point of view of quantitative anatomy. *Am. J. Cardiol.* 5:370–382, 1960.
297. Linzbach, A. J. and E. Akuomoa-Boateng. Alternsveranderungen des menschlinchen Herzens: I Das Herzgewicht im Alter. *Klin Wochenschr* 51:156–163, 1973.
298. Litchfield, J. B. Blood pressure in infant rats. *Physiol. Zool.* 31: 1–6, 1958.
299. Liu, Y, E. Cigola, W. Cheng, J. Kajstura, G. Olivetti, T. H. Hintze, and P. Anversa. Myocyte nuclear mitotic division and programmed myocyte cell death characterize the cardiac myopathy induced by rapid ventricular pacing in dogs. *Lab. Invest.* 73:771–787, 1995.
300. Liu, Z., D. R. Hilbelink, W. B. Crockett, and A. M. Gerdes. Regional changes in hemodynamics and cardiac myocyte size in rats with aortocaval fistulas. I. Developing and established hypertrophy. *Circ. Res.* 69:52–58, 1991.
301. Liu, Z, D. R. Hilbelink, and A. M. Gerdes. Regional changes in hemodynamics and cardiac myocyte size in rats with aortocaval fistulas. 2. Long-term effects. *Circ. Res.* 69:59–65, 1991.
302. Liu, Y., A. Leri, B. Li, X. Wang, W. Cheng, J. Kajstura, and P. Anversa. Angiotensin II stimulation in vitro induces hypertrophy of normal and postinfarcted ventricular myocytes. *Circ. Res.* 82:1145–1159, 1998.
303. Lockshin, R. A. and Z. Xakeri. Programmed cell death and apoptosis. In: *Apoptosis: The Molecular Basis of Cell Death, Current Communication Cell Mol. Biol., Vol 3*, edited by L. D. Tomei and F. O. Cope. Cold Spring Harbor, N.Y.: Laboratory Press, 1991, 47–60.
304. Lorell, B. H., I. Palacios, W. M. Daggett, M. L. Jacobs, B. N. Fowler, and J. B. Newell. Right ventricular distension and left ventricular compliance. *Am. J. Physiol.* 240 (*Heart Circ. Physiol.* 9):H87–H98, 1981.
305. Loud, A. V. A quantitative stereological description of the ul-

trastructure of normal rat liver parenchymal cells. *J. Cell Biol.* 37:27–46, 1968.

306. Loud, A. V., and P. Anversa. Morphometric analysis of biological processes. *Lab. Invest.* 50:250–261, 1984.

307. Loud, A. V., P. Anversa, F. Giacomelly, and J. Wiener. Absolute morphometric study of myocardial hypertrophy in experimental hypertension. I. Determination of myocyte size. *Lab. Invest.* 38:586–596, 1978.

308. Loud, A. V., W. C. Barany, and B. A. Pack. Quantitative evaluation of cytoplasmic structures in electron micrographs. *Lab. Invest.* 14:996–1008,1965.

309. Loud, A. V., C. Beghi, G. Olivetti, and P. Anversa. Morphometry of right and left ventricular myocardium after strenuous exercise in preconditioned rats. *Lab. Invest.* 51:104–111, 1984.

310. Lund, D. D. and R. J. Tomanek. Myocardial morphology in spontaneously hypertensive and aortic-constricted rats. *Am. J. Anat.* 152:141–152, 1978.

311. MacLellan, W. R. and M. D. Schneider. Death by design. Programmed cell death in cardiovascular biology and disease. *Circ. Res.* 81:137–144, 1997.

312. Maeda, H., C. A. Gleiser, E. J. Masoro, I. Murata, C. A. McMahan, and B. P. Yu. Nutritional influences on aging of Fischer 344 rats: II. Pathology. *J. Gerontol.* 40:671–688, 1985.

313. Magid, N. M., M. S. Young, D. C. Wallerson, R. S. Goldweit, J. N. Carter, R. B. Devereux, and J. S. Borer. Hypertrophic and functional response to experimental chronic aortic regurgitation. *J. Mol. Cell. Cardiol.* 20:239–246, 1988.

314. Mainwood, G. W. and K. Rakusan. A model for intracellular energy transport. *Can. J. Physiol. Pharmacol.* 60:98–102, 1982.

315. Mall, G., G. Zimmer, S. Baden, and T. Mattfeldt. Capillary neoformation in the rat heart—stereological studies on papillary muscles in hypertrophy and physiological growth. *Basic Res. Cardiol.* 85:531–540, 1990.

316. Manasek, F. J. Embryonic development of the heart. I. A light and electron microscopic study of myocardial development in the early chick embryo. *J. Morphol.* 125:329–365, 1968.

317. Manasek, F. J. Mitosis in developing cardiac muscle. *J. Cell Biol.* 37:191–196, 1968.

318. Manasek, F. J. Histogenesis of the embryonic myocardium. *Am. J. Cardiol.* 25:149–168, 1970.

319. Marcus, M. L. The coronary circulation in health and disease. New York: McGraw-Hill, 1983.

320. Marino, T. A., S. Haldar, E. C. Williamson, K. Beaverson, R. A. Walter, D. R. Marino, C. Beatty, and K. E. Lipson. Proliferating cell nuclear antigen in developing and adult rat cardiac muscle cells. *Circ. Res.* 69:1353–1360, 1991.

321. Marino, T. A., R. L. Kent, C. E. Uboh, E. Fernandez, E. W. Thompson, and G. Cooper. Structural analysis of pressure versus volume overload hypertrophy of cat right ventricle. *Am. J. Physiol.* 249 (*Heart Circ. Physiol.* 18):H371-H379, 1985.

322. Mark, G. E. and F. F. Strasser. Pacemaker activity and mitosis in cultures of newborn rat heart ventricle cells. *Exp. Cell Res.* 44:217–233, 1966.

323. Maruyama, Y., K. Ashikawa, S. Isoyama, H. Kanatsuka, E. Ino-Oka, and T. Takishima. Mechanical interactions between four heart chambers with and without pericardium in canine hearts. *Circ. Res.* 50:86–100, 1982.

324. Maseri, A. and S. Chierchia. Coronary artery spasm: demonstration, definition, diagnosis and consequences. *Prog. Cardiovasc. Dis.* 25:169–192, 1982.

325. McCallister, B. D. and A. L. Brown, Jr. A quantitative study of myocardial mitochondria in experimental cardiac hypertrophy. *Lab. Invest.* 14:692–700, 1965.

326. McKay, R. G., M. A. Pfeffer, R. C. Pasternak, J. E. Markis, G. C. Come, C. Nakao, N. D. Alderman, J. J. Ferguson, R. D. Safian, and W. Grossman. Left ventricular remodeling after myocardial infarction: A corollary to infarct expansion. *Circulation* 74:693–702, 1986.

327. McNutt, N. S., and D. W. Fawcett. The ultrastructure of the cat myocardium. II. Atrial muscle. *J. Cell Biol.* 42:46–67, 1969.

328. Medugorac, I. Collagen content in different areas of normal and hypertrophied rat myocardium. *Cardiovasc. Res.* 14:551–554, 1980.

329. Medugorac, I. and R. Jacob. Characterization of left ventricular collagen in the rat. *Cardiovasc. Res.* 17:15–21, 1983.

330. Meerson, F. Z., T. A. Zaletayeva, S. S. Lagutchev, and M. G. Pshennikova. Structure and mass of mitochondria in the process of compensatory hyperfunction and hypertrophy of the heart. *Exp. Cell. Res.* 36:568–578, 1964.

331. Meggs, L. G., J. Coupet, H. Huang, W. Cheng, P. Li, J. M. Capasso, C. J. Homcy, and P. Anversa. Regulation of angiotensin II receptors on ventricular myocytes after myocardial infarction in rats. *Circ. Res.* 72:1149–1162, 1993.

332. Meggs, L. G., H. Huang, P. Li, J. M. Capasso, and P. Anversa. Chronic nonocclusive coronary artery constriction in rats. β-adrenoreceptor signal transduction and ventricular failure. *J. Clin. Invest.* 88:1940–1946, 1991.

333. Meggs, L. G., H. Huang, P. Li, J. M. Capasso, and P. Anversa. Chronic coronary arterial stenosis impairs α_1-adrenoreceptor signaling and cardiac performance in rats. *Am. J. Physiol.* 263 (*Heart Circ. Physiol.* 31):H929–H938, 1992.

334. Meggs, L. G., J. Tillotson, H. Huang, E. H. Sonnenblick, J. M. Capasso, and P. Anversa. Noncoordinate regulation of alpha-1 adrenoreceptor coupling and reexpression of alpha skeletal actin in myocardial infarction–induced left ventricular failure in rats. *J. Clin. Invest.* 86:1451–1458, 1990.

335. Mendéz, J., and A. Keys. Density and composition of mammalian muscle. *Metabolism* 9:184–188, 1960.

336. Mirsky, I. Ventricular and arterial wall stresses based on large deformation analyses. *Biophys. J.* 13:1141–1159, 1973.

337. Mirsky, I. Elastic properties of the myocardium: a quantitative approach with physiological and clinical applications. In: *Handbook of Physiology, Vol 1: The Heart*, edited by R. M. Berne, N. Sperelakis, and S. R. Geiger. Bethesda, MD: American Physiological Society, 1979:497–531.

338. Mirsky, I., J. M. Pfeffer, M. A. Pfeffer, and E. Braunwald. The contractile state as the major determinant in the evolution of left ventricular dysfunction in the spontaneously hypertensive rat. *Circ. Res.* 53:767–778, 1983.

339. Momomura, S. I., A. B. Bradley, and W. Grossman. Left ventricular pressure–segment length relations and end-diastolic distensibility in dogs with coronary stenoses. An angina physiology model. *Circ. Res.* 55:203–214, 1984.

340. Monganroth, J., B. J. Maron, W. L. Henry, and S. E. Epstein. Comparative left ventricular dimensions in trained athletes. *Ann. Intern. Med.* 82:521–524, 1975.

341. Morkin, E. Postnatal muscle fiber assembly: localization of newly synthesized myofibrillar proteins. *Science* 167:1499–1501, 1970.

342. Morkin, E. Activation of synthetic processes in cardiac hypertrophy. *Circ. Res.* [Suppl. II] 35:37–48, 1974.

343. Morkin, E. and T. P. Ashford. Myocardial DNA synthesis in experimental cardiac hypertrophy. *Am. J. Physiol.* 215:1409–1413, 1968.

344. Muir, A. R. An electron microscope study of the embryology of the intercalated disc in the heart of the rabbit. *J. Biophys. Biochem. Cytol.* 3:193–202, 1957.

345. Muir, A. R. Further observations on the cellular structure of cardiac muscle. *J. Anat.* 99:27–46, 1965.

346. Munnell, J. F. and R. Getty. Nuclear lobulation and amitotic

division associated with increasing cell size in the aging canine myocardium. *J. Gerontol.* 23:363–369, 1968.
347. Murray, J. F., P. Gold, and B. L. Johnson. The circulatory effects of hematocrit variations in normovolemic and hypervolemic dogs. *J. Clin. Invest.* 42:1150–1159, 1963.
348. Narula, J., N. Haider, R. Virmani, T. G. DiSalvo, F. D. Kolodgie, R. J. Rajjar, U. Schmidt, M. F. Semigran, G. W. Dec, and B. A. Shaw. Apoptosis in myocytes in end-stage heart failure. *N. Engl. J. Med.* 335:1182–1189.
349. Oalmann, M. C., R. W. Palmer, M. A. Guzman, and R. A. Strong. Sudden death, coronary heart disease, atherosclerosis and myocardial lesions in young men. *Am. J. Epidemiol.* 112:639–649, 1980.
350. Oberhänsli, I., G. Brandon, G. Lacourt, and B. Friedli. Growth patterns of cardiac structures and changes in systolic time intervals in the newborn and infant. *Acta Paediatr. Scand.* 69:239–247, 1980.
351. Oberpriller, J. O., V. J. Ferrans, and R. J. Carroll. Changes in DNA content, number of nuclei and cellular dimensions of young rat atrial myocytes in response to left coronary artery ligation. *J. Mol. Cell. Cardiol.* 15:31–42, 1983.
352. Olivetti, G., R. Abbi, F. Quaini, J. Kajstura, W. Cheng, J. A. Nitahara, E. Quaini, C. Di Loreto, C. A. Beltrami, S. Krajewski, J. C. Reed, and P. Anversa. Apoptosis in the failing human heart. *N. Engl. J. Med.* 336:1131–1141, 1997.
353. Olivetti, G., P. Anversa, and A. Loud. Morphometric study of early postnatal development in the left and right ventricular myocardium of the rat. II. Tissue composition, capillary growth, and sarcoplasmic alterations. *Circ. Res.* 46:503–512, 1980.
354. Olivetti, G., J. M. Capasso, L. G. Meggs, E. H. Sonnenblick, and P. Anversa. Cellular basis of chronic ventricular remodeling after myocardial infarction in rats. *Circ. Res.* 68:856–869, 1991.
355. Olivetti, G., J. M. Capasso, E. H. Sonnenblick, and P. Anversa. Side-to-side slippage of myocytes participates in ventricular wall remodeling acutely after myocardial infarction in rats. *Circ. Res.* 67:23–34, 1990.
356. Olivetti, G., E. Cigola, R. Maestri, D. Corradi, C. Lagrasta, S. R. Gambert, and P. Anversa. Aging, cardiac hypertrophy and ischemic cardiomyopathy do not affect the proportion of mononucleated and multinucleated myocytes in the human heart. *J. Mol. Cell. Cardiol.* 28:1463–1477.
357. Olivetti, G., G. Giordano, D. Corradi, M. Melissari, C. Lagrasta, S. R. Gambert, and P. Anversa. Gender differences and aging: effects on the human heart. *J. Am. Coll. Cardiol.* 26:1068–1079, 1995.
358. Olivetti, G., C. Lagrasta, R. Ricci, E. H. Sonnenblick, J. M. Capasso, and P. Anversa. Long-term pressure-induced cardiac hypertrophy: capillary and mast cell proliferation. *Am. J. Physiol.* 257 (*Heart Circ. Physiol.* 26):H1766–H1772, 1989.
359. Olivetti, G., C. Lagrasta, F. Quaini, R. Ricci, G. Moccia, J. M. Capasso, and P. Anversa. Capillary growth in anemia-induced ventricular wall remodeling in the rat. *Circ. Res.* 65:1182–1192, 1989.
360. Olivetti, G., M. Melissari, T. Balbi, F. Quaini, E. Cigola, E. H. Sonnenblick, and P. Anversa. Myocyte cellular hypertrophy is responsible for ventricular remodeling in the hypertrophied heart of middle aged individuals in the absence of cardiac failure. *Cardiovasc. Res.* 28:1199–1208, 1994.
361. Olivetti, G., M. Melissari, T. Balbi, F. Quaini, E. H. Sonnenblick, and P. Anversa. Myocyte nuclear and possible cellular hyperplasia contribute to ventricular remodeling in the hypertrophic senescent heart in human. *J. Am. Coll. Cardiol.* 24:140–149, 1994.
362. Olivetti, G., M. Melissari, J. M. Capasso, and P. Anversa. Cardiomyopathy of the aging human heart. *Circ. Res.* 68:1560–1568, 1991.
363. Olivetti, G., M. Melissari, G. Marchetti, and P. Anversa. Quantitative structural changes of the rat thoracic aorta in early spontaneous hypertension. Tissue composition, and hypertrophy and hyperplasia of smooth muscle cells. *Circ. Res.* 51:19–26, 1982.
364. Olivetti, G., F. Quaini, C. Lagrasta, R. Ricci, G. Tiberti, J. M. Capasso, and P. Anversa. Myocyte cellular hypertrophy and hyperplasia contribute to ventricular wall remodeling in anemia-induced cardiac hypertrophy in rats. *Am. J. Pathol.* 141:227–239, 1992.
365. Olivetti, G., F. Quaini, R. Sala, C. Lagrasta, D. Corradi, E. Bonacina, S. R. Gambert, E. Cigola, and P. Anversa. Acute myocardial infarction in humans is associated with activation of programmed myocyte cell death in the surviving portion of the heart. *J. Mol. Cell. Cardiol.* 28:2005–2016, 1996.
366. Olivetti, G., R. Ricci, and P. Anversa. Hyperplasia of myocyte nuclei in long-term cardiac hypertrophy in rats. *J. Clin. Invest.* 80:1818–1822, 1987.
367. Olivetti, G., R. Ricci, C. Beghi, G. Guideri, and P. Anversa. Response of the border zone to myocardial infarction in rats. *Am. J. Pathol.* 125:476–483, 1986.
368. Olivetti, G., R. Ricci, C. Lagrasta, E. Maniga, E. H. Sonnenblick, and P. Anversa. Cellular basis of wall remodeling in long-term pressure overload-induced right ventricular hypertrophy in rats. *Circ. Res.* 63:648–657, 1988.
369. Olivetti, G., E. H. Sonnenblick, R. Ricci, E. Puntillo, and P. Anversa. Differences in the temporal effects of aging on the structure and function of rat myocardium. *Coronary Artery Dis.* 1:240–250, 1990.
370. Opie, L. H., D. Nathan, and W. F. Lubbe. Biochemical aspects of arrhythmogenesis and ventricular fibrillation. *Am. J. Cardiol.* 43:131–148, 1979.
371. Overy, H. R. and R. E. Priest. Mitotic cell division in postnatal cardiac growth. *Lab. Invest.* 15:1100–1103, 1966.
372. Packer, M. Sudden unexpected death in patients with congestive heart failure: A second frontier. *Circulation* 72:681–685, 1985.
373. Page, E. Quantitative ultrastructural analysis in cardiac membrane physiology. *Am. J. Physiol.* 235:C145–C158, 1978.
374. Page, D. L., J. B. Caulfield, J. A. Kastor, R. W. DeSanctis, and C. A. Sanders. Myocardial changes associated with cardiogenic shock. *N. Engl. J. Med.* 285:133–137, 1971.
375. Page, E., J. Early, and B. Power. Normal growth of ultrastructures in rat left ventricular myocardial cells. *Circ. Res.* [Suppl. II] 35:12–16, 1974.
376. Page, E. and L. P. McCallister. Quantitative electron microscopic description of heart muscle cells. Application to normal, hypertrophied and thyroxin-stimulated hearts. *Am. J. Cardiol.* 31:172–181, 1973.
377. Page, E., L. P. McCallister, and B. Power. Stereological measurements of cardiac ultrastructures implicated in excitation-contraction coupling. *Proc. Natl. Acad. Sci. U.S.A.* 68:1465–1466, 1971.
378. Page, E., and P. I. Polimeni. Ultrastructural changes in the ischemic zone bordering experimental infarcts in rat left ventricles. *Am. J. Pathol.* 87:81–104, 1977.
379. Page, E., P. I. Polimeni, R. Zak, J. Earley, and M. Johnson. Myofibrillar mass in rat and rabbit heart muscle: correlation of microchemical and stereological measurements in normal and hypertrophic hearts. *Circ. Res.* 30:430–439, 1972.
380. Pantely, G. A. and J. D. Bristow. Ischemic cardiomyopathy. *Prog. Cardiovasc. Dis.* 27:95–114, 1984.
381. Papadimitriou, J. M., B. E. Hopkins, and R. R. Taylor. Regres-

sion of left ventricular dilation and hypertrophy after removal of volume overload. *Circ. Res.* 34:127–135, 1974.
382. Pfeffer, M. A. and E. Braunwald. Ventricular remodeling after myocardial infarction. *Circulation* 81:1161–1172, 1990.
383. Pfeffer, M. A., G. A. Lamas, D. E. Vaughan, A. F. Parisi, and E. Braunwald. Effect of captopril on progressive ventricular dilation after anterior myocardial infarction. *N. Engl. J. Med.* 319:80–86, 1988.
384. Pfeffer, J. M., M. A. Pfeffer, and E. Braunwald. Influence of chronic captopril therapy on the infarcted left ventricle of the rat. *Circ. Res.* 57:84–95, 1985.
385. Pfeffer, M. A., J. M. Pfeffer, M. C. Fishbein, P. J. Fletcher, J. Spadaro, R. A. Kloner, and E. Braunwald. Myocardial infarct size and ventricular function in rats. *Circ. Res.* 44:503–512, 1979.
386. Pfeffer, J. M., M. A. Pfeffer, M. C. Fishbein, and E. D. Frohlich. Cardiac function and morphology with aging in the spontaneously hypertensive rat. *Am. J. Physiol.* 237 (*Heart Circ. Physiol.* 6):H461–H468, 1979.
387. Pfeffer, J. M., M. A. Pfeffer, P. J. Fletcher, and E. Braunwald. Alterations of cardiac performance in rats with established spontaneous hypertension. *Am. J. Cardiol.* 44:994–998, 1979.
388. Pfeffer, J. M., M. A. Pfeffer, P. J. Fletcher, and E. Braunwald. Progressive ventricular remodeling in rat myocardial infarction. *Am. J. Physiol.* 260 (*Heart Circ. Physiol.* 29):H1406-H1414, 1991.
389. Pfeffer, M. A., J. M. Pfeffer, and E. D. Frohlich. Pumping ability of the hypertrophying left ventricle of the spontaneously hypertensive rat. *Circ. Res.* 38:423–429, 1976.
390. Pfeffer, J. M., M. A. Pfeffer, I. Mirsky, and E. Braunwald. Regression of left ventricular hypertrophy and prevention of left ventricular dysfunction by captopril in the spontaneously hypertensive rat. *Proc. Natl. Acad. Sci. U.S.A.* 79:3310–3314, 1982
391. Pfeffer, M. A., J. M. Pfeffer, C. Steinberg, and P. Finn. Survival after an experimental myocardial infarction: beneficial effects of long-term therapy with captopril. *Circulation* 72:406–412, 1985.
392. Polimeni, P. I., and J. Al-Sadir. Expansion of extracellular space in the nonischemic zone of the infarcted heart and concomitant changes in tissue electrolyte contents in the rat. *Circ. Res.* 37: 725–732, 1975.
393. Quaini, F., E. Cigola, C. Lagrasta, G. Saccani, E. Quaini, C. Rossi, G. Olivetti, and P. Anversa. End-stage cardiac failure in humans is coupled with the induction of proliferating cell nuclear antigen and nuclear mitotic division in ventricular myocytes. *Circ. Res.* 75:1050–1063, 1994.
394. Rabinowitz, M., V. Aschenbrenner, R. Albin, N. J. Gross, R. Zak, and K. G. Nair. Synthesis and turnover of heart mitochondria in normal hypertrophied and hypoxic rat. In: *Cardiac Hypertrophy*, edited by N. Alpert. New York: Academic, 1971: 283–299.
395. Rakusan, K. Quantitative morphology of capillaries of the heart. *Methods Achiev. Exp. Pathol.* 5:272–286, 1971.
396. Rakusan, K. Postnatal development of the heart. In: *Heart and Heart-Like Organs*, Vol 1, edited by G. H. Bourne. New York: Academic, 1980:301–348.
397. Rakusan, K. Cardiac growth, maturation, and aging. In: *Growth of the Heart in Health and Disease*, edited by R. Zak. New York: Raven, 1984:131–164.
398. Rakusan, K. Microcirculation in the stressed heart. In: *The Stressed Heart*, edited by M. J. Legato. Boston: Martinus Nijhoff, 1987:107–123.
399. Rakusan, K., S. Batra, and M. I. Heron. A new approach for quantitative evaluation of coronary capillaries in longitudinal sections. In: *Oxygen Transport to Tissue XVI*, edited by M. C. Hogan, O. Mathieu-Costello, D. C. Poole, and P. D. Wager. New York: Plenum, 1994:407–415.
400. Rakusan, K., N. Cicutti, S. Kazda, and Z. Turek. Effect of Nifedipine on coronary capillary geometry in normotensive and hypertensive rats. *Hypertension* 24:205–211, 1994.
401. Rakusan, K., M. F. Flanagan, T. Geva, J. Southern, and R. Van Praagh. Morphometry of human coronary capillaries during normal growth and the effect of age in left ventricular pressure-overload hypertrophy. *Circulation* 86:38–46, 1992.
402. Rakusan, K., J. Jelinek, B. Korecky, M. Soukupova, and O. Poupa. Postnatal development of muscle fibers and capillaries in the rat heart. *Physiol. Bohemoslov.* 14:32–37, 1965.
403. Rakusan, K. and B. Korecky. The effect of growth and aging on functional capillary supply of the rat heart. *Growth* 46:275–281, 1982.
404. Rakusan, K. and B. Korecky. Cell size in experimental cardiomegaly. In: *Perspectives in Cardiovascular Research*, Vol 8, edited by R. C. Tarazi, and J. B. Dunbar. New York: Raven, 1983: 41–48.
405. Rakusan, K., B. Korecky, and V. Mezl. Cardiac hypertrophy and/or hyperplasia? In: *Biology of Myocardial Hypertrophy and Failure*, Vol. 7, edited by N. Alpert. New York: Raven, 1982:103–108.
406. Rakusan, K., B. Korecky, Z. Roth, and O. Poupa. Development of the ventricular weight of the rat heart with special reference to the early phases of postnatal ontogenesis. *Physiol. Bohemoslov.* 12:518–525, 1963.
407. Rakusan, K., J. Moravec, and P. Y. Hatt. Regional capillary supply in the normal and hypertrophied rat heart. *Microvasc. Res.* 20:319–326, 1980.
408. Rakusan, K. and J. Nagai. Morphometry of arterioles and capillaries in hearts of senescent mice. *Cardiovasc. Res.* 28:969–972, 1994.
409. Rakusan, K. and O. Poupa. Changes in the diffusion distance in the rat heart muscle during development. *Physiol. Bohemoslov.* 12:220–227, 1963.
410. Rakusan, K. and O. Poupa. Capillaries and muscle fibers in the heart of old rats. *Gerontologia* 9:107–112, 1964.
411. Rakusan, K. and Z. Turek. Protamine inhibits capillary formation in growing rat hearts. *Circ. Res.* 57:393–398, 1985.
412. Rakusan, K. and P. Wicker. Morphometry of the small arteries and arterioles in the rat heart: effects of chronic hypertension and exercise. *Cardiovasc. Res.* 24:278–284, 1990.
413. Rakusan, K., P. Wicker, M. Abdul-Samad, B. Healy, and Z. Turek. Failure of swimming exercise to improve capillarization in cardiac hypertrophy of renal hypertensive rats. *Circ. Res.* 61: 641–647, 1987.
414. Recavvaren, S. and J. Arias-Stella. Growth and development of the ventricular myocardium from birth to adult life. *Br. Heart J.* 26:187–192, 1964.
415. Regen, D. M., P. Anversa, and J. M. Capasso. Segmental calculation of left ventricular wall stresses. *Am. J. Physiol.* 264 (*Heart Circ. Physiol.* 33):H1411–H1421, 1993.
416. Reiner, L., A. Mazzoleni, F. L. Rodriguez, and R. R. Freudenthal. The weight of the human heart: I. Normal cases. *Arch. Pathol.* 68:58–73, 1959. 221
417. Reiss, K., J. M. Capasso, H. Huang, L. G. Meggs, P. Li, and P. Anversa. ANG II receptors, c-myc, and c-jun in myocytes after myocardial infarction and ventricular failure. *Am. J. Physiol.* 264 (*Heart Circ. Physiol.* 33):H760–H769, 1993.
418. Reiss, K., W. Cheng, A. Ferber, J. Kajstura, P. Li, B. Li, G. Olivetti, C. J. Homcy, R. Baserga, and P. Anversa. Overexpression of insulin-like growth factor-1 in the heart is coupled with myocyte proliferation in transgenic mice. *Proc. Natl. Acad. Sci. U.S.A.* 93:8630–8635, 1996.
419. Reiss, K., J. Kajstura, J. M. Capasso, T. A. Marino, and P. An-

versa. Impairment of myocyte contractility following coronary artery narrowing is associated with activation of the myocyte IGF-$_1$ autocrine system, enhanced expression of late growth related genes, DNA-synthesis and myocyte nuclear mitotic division in rats. *Exp. Cell Res.* 207:348–360, 1993.

420. Reiss, K., J. Kajstura, X. Zhang, P. Li, E. Szoke, G. Olivetti, and P. Anversa. Acute myocardial infarction leads to upregulation of the IGF-1 autocrine system, DNA replication, and nuclear mitotic division in the remaining viable cardiac myocytes. *Exp. Cell Res.* 213:463–472, 1994.

421. Reiss, K., L. G. Meggs, P. Li, G. Olivetti, J. M. Capasso, and P. Anversa. Upregulation of IGF$_1$, IGF-$_1$-receptor and late growth related genes in ventricular myocytes acutely after infarction in rats. *J. Cell. Physiol.* 158:160–168, 1993.

422. Remington, R. D. Interpretation of the hypertension detection and follow-up program. In: *Frontiers in Hypertension Research*, edited by J. H. Laragh, F. R. Buhler, and D. W. Seldin. New York: Springer-Verlag, 1981, 15–16.

423. Ritzer, T. F., A. A. Bove, and R. A. Carey. Left ventricular performance characteristics in trained and sedentary dogs. *J. Appl. Physiol.* 48:130–138, 1980.

424. Roberts, C. S. and W. C. Roberts. Cross-sectional area of the proximal portions of the three major epicardial coronary arteries in 98 necropsy patients with different coronary events. *Circulation* 62:953–959, 1980.

425. Roberts, J. T. and J. T. Wearn. Quantitative changes in the capillary–muscle relationship in human hearts during normal growth and hypertrophy. *Am. Heart J.* 21:617–633, 1941.

426. Roberts, W. C. The coronary arteries and left ventricle in clinically isolated angina pectoris: a necropsy analysis. *Circulation* 54:388–390, 1976.

427. Roberts, W. C. and A. A. Jones. Quantitation of coronary arterial narrowing at necropsy in sudden coronary death: analysis of 31 patients and comparison with 25 control subjects. *Am. J. Cardiol.* 44:39–45, 1979.

428. Roberts, W. C. Morphological features of the elderly heart. In: *Cardiovascular Disease in the Elderly Patient*, edited by D. D. Tresch and W. S. Aronow. New York: Marcel Dekker, 1994: 17–42.

429. Roeske, W. R., R. M. Savage, R. A. O'Rouke, and C. M. Bloor. Clinicopathologic correlations in patients after myocardial infarction. *Circulation* 63:36–45, 1981.

430. Romero, T., J. Covell, and W. F. Friedman. A comparison of pressure–volume relations of the fetal, newborn and adult heart. *Am. J. Physiol.* 222:1285–1290, 1972.

431. Ross, J., Jr., E. Braunwald, and A. G. Morrow. Clinical and hemodynamic observations in pure mitral insufficiency. *Am. J. Cardiol.* 2:11–23, 1958.

432. Ross, J., E. H. Sonnenblick, R. R. Taylor, H. M. Spotnitz, and J. W. Covell. Diastolic geometry and sarcomere lengths in the chronically dilated canine left ventricle. *Circ. Res.* 28:49–61, 1971.

433. Rowlatt, U. F., H. J. A. Rimoldi, and M. Lev. The quantitative morphology of the normal child's heart. *Pediatr. Clin. North Am.* 10:499–588, 1963.

434. Rudolph, A. M. and M. A. Heymann. Circulatory changes with growth in the fetal lamb. *Circ. Res.* 26:289–299, 1970.

435. Rudolph, A. M. *Congenital Disease of the Heart. Clinical Physiologic Considerations in Diagnosis and Management*. Chicago: Year Book 1974.

436. Rudolph, A. M. Fetal and neonatal pulmonary circulation. *Annu. Rev. Physiol.* 41:383–395, 1979.

437. Rudolph, A. M. and M. A. Heymann. The circulation of the fetus in utero: methods for studying distribution of blood flow, cardiac output and organ blood flow. *Circ. Res.* 21:163–184, 1967.

438. Rumyantsev, P. P. DNA synthesis and nuclear division in embryonical and postnatal histogenesis of myocardium. *Arch. Anat.* 47:59–65, 1964.

439. Sandritter, W. and C. P. Adler. Numerical hyperplasia in human heart hypertrophy. *Experientia* 27:1435–1437, 1971.

440. Sandritter, W. and C. P. Adler. Polyploidization of heart muscle nuclei as a prerequisite for heart growth and numerical hyperplasia in heart hypertrophy. *Recent Adv. Stud. Cardiol. Struct. Metab.* 12:115–127, 1978.

441. Sasaki, R., T. Morishita, S. Ichikawa, and S. Yamagata. Autoradiographic studies and mitosis of heart muscle cells in experimental cardiac hypertrophy. *Tohoku J. Exp. Med.* 102:159–167, 1970.

442. Sasaki, R., T. Morishita, and S. Yamagata. Mitosis of heart muscle cells in normal rats. *Tohoku J. Exp. Med.* 96:405–411, 1968.

443. Sasaki, R., Y. Watanabe, T. Morishita, and S. Yamagata. Estimation of the cell number of heart muscles in normal rats. *Tohoku J. Exp. Med.* 95:177–184, 1968.

444. Sasayama, S., J. Ross, Jr., D. Franklin, C. M. Bloor, S. Bishop, and R. B. Dilley. Adaptation of the left ventricle to chronic pressure overload. *Circ. Res.* 38:172–178, 1976.

445. Schaper, J., S. Hein, D. Scholz and H. Mollnau. Multifacetted morphological alterations are present in the failing human heart. *J. Mol. Cell. Cardiol.* 27:857–861, 1995.

446. Scheuer, J. and A. K. Bahn. Cardiac contractile proteins: ATPase activity and physiologic function. *Circ. Res.* 45:1–12, 1979.

447. Schlant, R. C., J. M. Felner, S. B. Heymsfield, C. A. Gilbert, N. B. Shulman, E. P. Tuttle, and B. A. Blumenstein. Echocardiographic studies of left ventricular anatomy and function in essential hypertension. *Cardiovasc. Med.* 2:477–499, 1977.

448. Schneider, R. and P. Pfitzer. Die Zahl der Kerne in isolierten Zellen des menschlichen Myokards. *Virchows Arch. B.* 12:238–258, 1973.

449. Schoenmackers, J. Die Herzkranzschlagadern bei der arteriokardialen Hypertrophie. *Kreislaufforsch.* 38:321–336, 1949.

450. Scholz, D., W. Diener, and J. Schaper. Altered nucleus/cytoplasm relationship and degenerative structural changes in human dilated cardiomyopathy. *Cardioscience* 5:127–138, 1994.

451. Scholz, D. G., D. W. Kitzman, P. T. Hagen, D. M. Ilstrup, and W. D. Edwards. Age-related changes in normal human hearts during the first 10 decades of life. Part I (Growth): a quantitative anatomic study of 200 specimens from subjects from birth to 19 years old. *Mayo Clin. Proc.* 63:126–136, 1988.

452. Schuler, G., K. L. Peterson, A. Johnson, G. Francis, G. Dennis, J. Utley, P. O. Daily, W. Ashburn, and J. Ross Jr. Temporal response of left ventricular performance to mitral valve surgery. *Circulation* 59:1218–1231, 1979.

453. Schuster, E. H. and B. H. Bulkley. Ischemic cardiomyopathy: a clinicopathologic study of fourteen patients. *Am. Heart J.* 100:506–512, 1980.

454. Setoguchi, M., A. Leri, S. Wang, Y. Liu, A. De Luca, A. Giordano, T. H. Hintze, J. Kajstura, and P. Anversa. Activation of cyclins and cyclin-dependent kinases, DNA synthesis, and myocyte mitotic division in pacing-induced heart failure in dogs. *Lab. Invest.* 79:1545–1558, 1999.

455. Shahab, L. and A. Wollenberger. Amino acid incorporation into mitochondria from hypertrophying hearts of rats with aortic constriction. *J. Mol. Cell. Cardiol.* 1:143–155, 1970.

456. Sheridan, D. J., M. J. Cullen, and M. J. Tynan. Postnatal ultrastructural changes in the cat myocardium: a morphometric study. *Cardiovasc. Res.* 11:536–540, 1977.

457. Sheridan, D. J., M. J. Cullen, and M. J. Tynan. Qualitative and quantitative observations on ultrastructural changes during postnatal development in the cat myocardium. *J. Mol. Cell. Cardiol.* 11:1173–1181, 1979.

458. Shi, Y. F., B. M. Sahai, and D. R. Green. Cyclosporin A inhibits activation-induced cell death in T-cell hybridomas and thymocytes. *Nature* 339:625–626, 1989.
459. Shipley, R. A., W. Shipley, and J. T. Wearn. The capillary supply in normal and hypertrophied hearts of rabbits. *J. Exp. Med.* 65:29–42, 1937.
460. Shreiner, T. P., M. L. Weisfeldt, and N. W. Shock. Effects of age, sex and breeding status on the rat heart. *Am. J. Physiol.* 217: 176–180, 1969.
461. Shub, C., A. L. Klein, P. K. Zachariah, K. R. Bailey, and J. Tajik. Determination of left ventricular mass by echocardiography in a normal population: effect of age and sex in addition to body size. *Mayo Clin. Proc.* 69:205–211, 1994.
462. Sjögren, A. L. Left ventricular wall thickness determined by ultrasound in 100 subjects without heart disease. *Chest* 60:341–346, 1971.
463. Smith, H. L. The relation of the weight of the heart to the weight of the body and the weight of the heart to age. *Am. Heart J.* 4:79–93, 1928.
464. Smith, S. H. and S. P. Bishop. Regional myocyte size in compensated right ventricular hypertrophy in the ferret. *J. Mol. Cell. Cardiol.* 17:1005–1011, 1985.
465. Smith, J. R. and O. M. Pereira-Smith. Replicative senescence: implications for in vivo aging and tumor suppression. *Science* 273:63–67, 1996.
466. Sohal, R. S. and R. Weindruch. Oxidative stress, caloric restriction, and aging. *Science* 273:59–63, 1996.
467. Sadoshima J, Y. Xu, H. S. Slayter, and S. Izumo. Autocrine release of angiotensin II mediates stretch-induced hypertrophy of cardiac myocytes in vitro. *Cell* 75:977–894, 1993.
468. Sonnenblick, E. H., J. E. Strobeck, J. M. Capasso, and S. M. Factor. Ventricular hypertrophy: models and methods. In: *Perspective in Cardiovascular Research, Vol 8, Cardiac Hypertrophy in Hypertension*, edited by R. C. Tarazi and J. B. Dunbar. New York: Raven, 1983:12–20.
469. Soonpaa, M. H. and L. J. Field. Survey of studies examining mammalian cardiomyocyte DNA synthesis. *Circ. Res.* 83:15–26, 1998.
470. Sordahl, L. A., W. B. McCollum, W. G. Wood, and A. Schwartz. Mitochondrial and sarcoplasmic reticulum function in cardiac hypertrophy and failure. *Am. J. Physiol.* 224:497–502, 1973.
471. Spagnuolo, M., H. Kloth, A. Taranta, E. Doyle, and B. Pasternack. Natural history of rheumatic aortic regurgitation. Criteria predictive of death, congestive heart failure, and angina in young patients. *Circulation* 44:368–389, 1971.
472. Spinale, F. G., J. L. Zellner, M. Tomita, F. A. Crawford, and M. R. Zile. Relation between ventricular and myocyte remodeling with the development and regression of supraventricular tachycardia-induced cardiomyopathy. *Circ. Res.* 69:1058–1067, 1991.
473. Spiro, D. and M. Hagopian. On the assemblage of myofibrils. In: *Formation and Fate of Cell Organelles*, edited by K. B. Warren. New York: Academic, 1967:71–98.
474. Spotnitz, W. D., H. M. Spotnitz, N. J. Truccone, T. S. Cottrell, W. Gersony, J. R. Malm, and E. H. Sonnenblick. Relations of ultrastructure and function: sarcomere dimensions, pressure–volume curves, and geometry of the intact left ventricle of the immature canine heart. *Circ. Res.* 44:679–691, 1979.
475. Sproule, R. S., J. H. Mitchell, and W. F. Miller. Cardiopulmonary physiological response to heavy exercise in patients with anemia. *J. Clin. Invest.* 39:378–388, 1960.
476. Stevens-Hooper, E. S. Use of colchicine for the measurement of mitotic rate in the intestinal epithelium. *Am. J. Anat.* 108:231–244, 1961.
477. Steward, D. M. and A. W. Martin. Hypertrophy of the denervated hemidiaphragm. *Am. J. Physiol.* 186:497–500, 1956.
478. Stockdale, F. E. and H. Holtzer. DNA synthesis and myogenesis. *Exp. Cell Res.* 24:508–520, 1962.
479. Stone, H. O., H. K. Thompson, Jr., and K. Schmidt-Nilsen. Influence of erythrocytes on blood viscosity. *Am. J. Physiol.* 214: 913–918, 1968.
480. Tadokoro, M. and S. Arai. Myocardial cell in right ventricular hypertrophy. *Tohoku. J. Exp. Med.* 106:5–16, 1972.
481. Takahashi, T., H. Schunkert, S. Isoyama, J. Y. Wei, B. Nadal-Ginard, W. Grossman, and S. Izumo. Age related differences in the expression of protooncogene and contractile protein genes in response to pressure overload in the rat myocardium. *J. Clin. Invest.* 89:939–946, 1992.
482. Takanatsu, T., K. Nayanishi, M. Fukuda, and S. Fujita. Cytofluorimetric nuclear DNA-determinations in infant, adolescence, adult and aging human hearts. *Histochemistry* 77:485–494, 1983.
483. Taussig, H. B. *Congenital Malformation of the Heart. Vol. I: General Considerations.* Cambridge: Harvard University Press, 1960.
484. Taylor, G. J., J. O. Humphries, E. D. Mellitis, B. Pitt, R. A. Schulze, L. S. C. Griffith, and S. C. Achoff. Predictors of clinical course, coronary anatomy and left ventricular function after recovery from acute myocardial infarction. *Circulation* 62:960–970, 1980.
485. Tharp, G. D. and C. T. Wagner. Chronic exercise and cardiac vascularization. *Eur. J. Appl. Physiol.* 48:97–104, 1982.
486. Toma, B. S., R. D. Wangler, D. F. Dewitt, and H. V. Sparks. Effect of development on coronary vasodilator reserve in the isolated guinea pig heart. *Circ. Res.* 57:538–544, 1985.
487. Tomanek, R. J. Effects of age and exercise on the extent of the myocardial capillary bed. *Anat. Rec.* 167:55–62, 1970.
488. Tomanek, R. J. Coronary vasculature of the aging heart. In: *The Aging Heart. Aging (Vol 12)*, edited by M. L. Weisfeld. New York: Raven, 1980:115–135.
489. Tomanek, R. J. Response of the coronary vasculature to myocardial hypertrophy. *J. Am. Coll. Cardiol.* 15:528–533, 1990.
490. Tomanek, R. J. Age as a modulator of coronary capillary angiogenesis. *Circulation* 86:320–321, 1992.
491. Tomanek, R. J. and M. R. Aydelott. Late onset renal hypertension in old rats alters left ventricular structure and function. *Am. J. Physiol.* 262 (*Heart Circ. Physiol.* 31):H531–H538, 1992.
492. Tomanek, R. J., M. R. Aydelotte, K. E. Anderson, and R. J. Torry. Coronary blood flow in senescent rats with late-onset hypertension. *Am. J. Physiol.* 264 (*Heart Circ. Physiol.* 33): H1854–H1860, 1993.
493. Tomanek, R. J., M. R. Aydelott, and C. A. Butters. Late-onset renal hypertension in old rats alters myocardial microvessels. *Am. J. Physiol.* 259 (*Heart Circ. Physiol.* 28):H1681–H1687, 1990.
494. Tomanek, R. J., M. R. Aydelotte, and R. J. Torry. Remodeling of coronary vessels during aging in purebred beagles. *Circ. Res.* 69:1068–1074, 1991.
495. Tomanek, R. J., P. A. Barlow, P. M. Connell, Y. Chen, and R. J. Torry. Effects of hypothyroidism and hypertension on myocardial perfusion and vascularity in rabbits. *Am. J. Physiol.* 265 (*Heart Circ. Physiol.* 34):H1638–H1644, 1993.
496. Tomanek, R. J., P. M. Connell, C. A. Butters, and R. J. Torry. Compensated coronary microvascular growth in senescent rats with thyroxine-induced cardiac hypertrophy. *Am. J. Physiol.* 268 (*Heart Circ. Physiol.* 37):H419–H425, 1995.
497. Tomanek, R. J., C. V. Gisolfi, C. A. Bauer, and P. J. Palmer. Coronary vasodilator reserve, capillarity and mitochondria in trained hypertensive rats. *J. Appl. Physiol.* 64:1179–1185, 1988.

498. Tomanek, R. J. and J. M. Hovanec. The effects of long-term pressure overload and aging on the myocardium. *J. Mol. Cell. Cardiol.* 13:471–488, 1981.
499. Tomanek, R. J. and U. L. Karlsson. Myocardial ultrastructure of young and senescent rats. *J. Ultrastruct. Res.* 42:201–220, 1973.
500. Tomanek, R. J., P. J. Palmer, G. L. Peiffer, K. L. Schreiber, C. L. Eastham, and M. L. Marcus. Morphometry of canine coronary arteries, arterioles and capillaries during hypertension and left ventricular hypertrophy. *Circ. Res.* 58:38–46, 1986.
501. Tomanek, R. J., K. A. Schalk, M. L. Marcus, and D. G. Harrison. Coronary angiogenesis during long-term hypertension and left ventricular hypertrophy in dogs. *Circ. Res.* 65:352–359, 1989.
502. Tomanek, R. J., J. C. Searls, and P. A. Lachenbruch. Quantitative changes in the capillary bed during developing, peak and stabilized cardiac hypertrophy in the spontaneously hypertensive rats. *Circ. Res.* 51:295–304, 1982.
503. Tomanek, R. J. and R. J. Torry. Growth of the coronary vasculature in hypertrophy: mechanisms and model dependence. *Cell. Mol. Biol. Res.* 40:129–136, 1994.
504. Tomanek, R. J., T. G. Wessel, and D. G. Harrison. Capillary growth and geometry during long-term hypertension and myocardial hypertrophy in dogs. *Am. J. Physiol.* 261 (*Heart Circ. Physiol.* 30):H1011–H1018, 1993.
505. Toshima, H., Y. Koga, H. Toshioka, T. Akijoshi, and N. Kimura. Echocardiographic classification of hypertensive heart disease. A correlative study with clinical features. *Jpn. Heart J.* 16:377–393, 1975.
506. Turek, Z., M. Grantner, K. Kubat, B. E. M. Ringnalda, and F. Kreuzer. Arterial blood gases, muscle fiber diameter and intercapillary distance in cardiac hypertrophy of rats with an old myocardial infarction. *Pflugers Arch.* 376:209–215, 1978.
507. Turek, Z., L. Hoofd, and K. Rakusan. Myocardial capillaries and tissue oxygenation. *Can. J. Cardiol.* 2:98–103, 1986.
508. Turek, Z. and K. Rakusan. Log normal distribution of intercapillary distance in normal and hypertrophic heart as estimated by the method of concentric circles: its effect on tissue oxygenation. *Pflugers Arch.* 391:17–21, 1981.
509. Turek, Z., K. Rakusan, J. Olders, L. Hoofd, and F. Kreuzer. Computed myocardial PO_2 histograms: effects of various geometrical and functional conditions. *J. Appl. Physiol.* 70:1845–1853, 1991.
510. Underwood, E. E. *Quantitative Stereology*. Reading, Massachusetts, Addison-Wesley, 1970.
511. Urabe, Y., D. L. Mann, R. L. Kent, K. Nakano, R. J. Tomanek, B. A. Carabello, and G. Cooper, IV. Cellular and ventricular contractile dysfunction in experimental canine mitral regurgitation. *Circ. Res.* 70:131–147, 1992.
512. Vahouny, G. V., R. Wei, R. Starkweather, and C. Davis. Preparation of beating heart cells from adult rats. *Science* 167:1616–1618, 1970.
513. Vinten-Johansen, J. and H. R. Weiss. Oxygen consumption in subepicardial and subendocardial regions of the canine left ventricle. The effector of experimental acute valvular aortic stenosis. *Circ. Res.* 46:139–145, 1980.
514. Vitali-Mazza, L. and P. Anversa. Myocardial hypertrophy by arterio-venous fistula in dogs. An ultrastructural quantitative study. In: *Colloque les Surcharges Cardiaques (Heart Overloading)*, edited by P. Y. Hatt. Paris, INSERM, 1972:55–57.
515. Vitali-Mazza, L., P. Anversa, F. Tedeschi, R. Mastandrea, V. Mavilla, and O. Visioli. Ultrastructural basis of acute left ventricular failure from severe acute aortic stenosis in the rabbit. *J. Mol. Cell. Cardiol.* 4:661–671, 1972.
516. Vliegen, H. W., A. Van Der Laarse, C. J. Cornelisse, and F. Eulderink. Myocardial changes in pressure overload–induced left ventricular hypertrophy: a study on tissue composition, polyploidization and multinucleation. *Eur. Heart J.* 12:488–494, 1991.
517. Vliegen, H. W., A. M. Vossepoel, A. Laarse, F. Eulderink, and C. J. Cornelisse. Methodological aspects of flow cytometric analysis of DNA polyploidy in human heart tissue. *Histochemistry* 84:348–354, 1986.
518. Vogelberg, K. Die Lichtungsweite der Coronarostien an normalen und hypertrophen Herzen. *Kreislaufforsch.* 46:101, 1957.
519. Wachtlova, M., B. Ostadal, and V. Mares. Thyroxine-induced cardiomegaly in rats of different age. *Physiol. Bohemoslov.* 34:385–395, 1985.
520. Wahlander, H., B. Haraldsson, and P. Friberg. Myocardial capillary diffusion capacity in rat hearts with cardiac hypertrophy due to pressure and volume overload. *Am. J. Physiol.* 265 (*Heart Circ. Physiol.* 34):H61–H68, 1993.
521. Walston, A., J. C. Rembert, J. M. Fedor, and J. C. Greenfield, Jr. Regional myocardial blood flow after sudden aortic constriction in awake dogs. *Circ. Res.* 42:419–425, 1978.
522. Wangler, R. D., K. G. Peters, M. L. Marcus, and R. J. Tomanek. Effects of duration and severity of arterial hypertension and cardiac hypertrophy on coronary vasodilator reserve. *Circ. Res.* 51:10–18, 1982.
523. Warnes, C. A. and W. C. Roberts. Sudden coronary death: relation of amount and distribution of coronary narrowing at necropsy to previous symptoms of myocardial ischemia, left ventricular scarring and heart weight. *Am. J. Cardiol.* 54:65–73, 1984.
524. Warren, S. E., H. D. Royal, J. E. Markis, W. Grossman, and R. J. McKay. Time course of left ventricular dilatation after myocardial infarction: influence of infarct-related artery and success of coronary thrombolysis. *J. Am. Coll. Cardiol.* 11:12–19, 1988.
525. Wearn, J. T. The extent of the capillary bed of the heart. *J. Exp. Med.* 47:273–291, 1928.
526. Wearn, J. T. Morphological and functional alterations of the coronary circulation. *Harvey Lect.* 35:243–270, 1939–40.
527. Weber, K. T. and C. G. Brilla. Pathological hypertrophy and cardiac interstitium. Fibrosis and renin-angiotensin-aldosterone system. *Circulation* 83:1849–1865, 1991.
528. Weber, K. T., J. S. Janicki, S. G. Shroff, R. Pick, R. M. Chen, and R. I. Bashey. Collagen remodeling of the pressure-overloaded, hypertrophied non-human primate myocardium. *Circ. Res.* 62:757–765, 1988.
529. Wegelin, C. Über Arteriolosklerose im Myocard. *Schweiz. Med. Wochenschr.* 74:57–60, 1944.
530. Wegner, G. and E. Mölbert. Das Verhalten des Myokards bei der experimentellen suupravalvulären Aortenstenose: autoradiographische und elektronenmikroskopische Untersuchungen an Rattenherzen. *Virchows Arch. A. Pathol. Anat.* 341:54–63, 1966.
531. Wei, J. Y. Age and the cardiovascular system. *N. Engl. J. Med.* 237:1735–1739, 1992.
532. Wei, J. Y., H. A. Spurgeon, and E. G. Lakatta. Excitation–contraction coupling in rat myocardium: alterations with adult aging. *Am. J. Physiol.* 246 (*Heart Circ. Physiol.* 15):H784–H791, 1984.
533. Weibel, E. R. Stereological principles for morphometry in electron microscopy cytology. *Int. Rev. Cytol.* 26:235–302, 1969.
534. Weibel, E. R. Oxygen demand and the size of respiratory structures in mammals. In: *Evolution of Respiratory Processes*, Vol 13 edited by S. C. Wood, and C. Lenfant. New York: Basel: Marcel Dekker, 1979:289–346.
535. Weibel, E. R. *Stereological Methods, Vol 1: Practical Methods for Biological Morphometry*. London, Academic, 1979.

536. Weibel, E. R. *Stereological Methods, Vol 2: Theoretical Foundations.* London, Academic, 1980.
537. Weibel, E. R. and R. P. Bolender. Sterological techniques for electron microscopic morphometry. In *Principles and Techniques of Electron Microscopy*, Vol 3, edited by M. A. Hayat. New York: Van Nostrand Reinhold, 1973:239.
538. Weibel, E. R. and D. Paumgartner. A principle for counting tissue structures on random sections. *J. Appl. Physiol.* 17:343–348, 1962.
539. Weibel, E. R. and D. Paumgartner. Integrated sterological and biochemical studies on hepatocytic membranes. II. Correction of section thickness effect on volume and surface density estimates. *J. Cell Biol.* 42:584–587, 1978.
540. Weibel, E. R., W. Stäubli, H. R. Gnägi, and F. A. Hess. Correlated morphometric and biochemical studies on the liver cell. I. Morphometric model, stereologic methods, and normal morphometric data for rat liver. *J. Cell Biol.* 42:68–91, 1969.
541. Weinstein, R. B. and E. D. Hay. DNA synthesis and mitosis in differentiated cardiac muscle cells of chick embryos. *J. Cell Biol.* 47:310–316, 1970.
542. Weisfeldt, M. L. Research on aging. In: *Aging, Volume 12: The Aging Heart: Its Function and Response to Stress*, edited by M. L. Weisfeldt. New York: Raven, 1980:1–6.
543. Weisfeld, M. L., W. A. Loeven, and N. W. Shock. Resting and active mechanical properties of trabeculae carneae from aged male rats. *Am. J. Physiol.* 220:1921–1927, 1971.
544. Weisfeldt, M. L., J. R. Wright, D. P. Shreiner, E. Lakatta, and N. W. Shock. Coronary flow and oxygen extraction in the perfused heart of senescent male rats. *J. Appl. Physiol.* 30:44–49, 1971.
545. Weisman, H. F., D. E. Bush, J. A. Mannisi, M. L. Weisfeldt, and B. Healy. Cellular mechanisms of myocardial infarct expansion. *Circulation* 78:186–201, 1988.
546. Weisman, H. F. and B. Healy. Myocardial infarct expansion, infarct extension and reinfarction: pathophysiologic concepts. *Prog. Cardiovasc. Dis.* 30:73–110, 1987.
547. Weitz, G. Über das unterschiedliche Verhalten der Lage der Herzmuskelfasern in kontrahiertem und dilatiertem Zustand. *Med. Klin.* 46:1031–1032, 1951.
548. White, C. W., C. B. Wright, D. B. Doty, L. F. Hiratza, C. L. Eastham, D. G. Harrison, and M. L. Marcus. Does the visual interpretation of the coronary arteriogram predict physiological significance of a coronary stenosis. *N. Engl. J. Med.* 310:819–824, 1984.
549. Wikman-Coffelt, J., W. W. Parmley, and D. T. Mason. The cardiac hypertrophy process. Analyses of factors determining pathological vs. physiological development. *Circ. Res.* 45:697–707, 1979.
550. Wright, A. J. A. and O. Hudlická. Capillary growth and changes in heart performance induced by chronic bradycardial pacing in the rabbit. *Circ. Res.* 49:469–478, 1981.
551. Wyllie, A. H. Apoptosis and the regulation of cell numbers in normal and neoplastic tissue: an overview. *Cancer Metast. Rev.* 11:95–103, 1992.
552. Yin, F. C. P., H. A. Spurgeon, K. Rakusan, M. L. Weisfeldt, and E. G. Lakatta. Use of tibial length to quantify cardiac hypertrophy: application in the aging rat. *Am. J. Physiol.* 243 (*Heart Circ. Physiol.* 12):H941–H947, 1982.
553. Yin, F. C. P., H. A. Spurgeon, M. L. Weisfeld, and E. G. Lakatta. Mechanical properties of myocardium from hypertrophied rat hearts: a comparison between hypertrophy induced by senescence and by aortic banding. *Circ. Res.* 46:292–300, 1980.
554. Zak, R. Development and proliferative capacity of cardiac muscle cells. *Circ. Res.* [Suppl. II] 35:17–26, 1974.
555. Zak, R. Overview of the growth process. In: *Growth of the Heart in Health and Disease*, edited by R. Zak. New York: Raven, 1984:1–24.
556. Zak, R., A. F. Martin, M. K. Reddy, and M. Rabinowitz. Control of protein balance in hypertrophied cardiac muscle. *Circ. Res.* 38: (Suppl I) 145–150, 1976.
557. Zhang, X., D. E. Dostal, K. Reiss, W. Cheng, J. Kajstura, P. Li, H. Huang, E. H. Sonnenblick, L. G. Meggs, K. M. Baker, and P. Anversa. Identification and activation of the autocrine renin–angiotensin system in adult ventricular myocytes in vivo. *Am. J. Physiol.* 269 (*Heart Circ. Physiol.* 38):H1791–H1802, 1995.
558. Zhao, M. J., H. Zhang, T. F. Robinson, S. M. Factor, E. H. Sonnenblick, and C. Eng. Profound structural alterations of the extracellular collagen matrix in postischemic dysfunctional ('stunned") but viable myocardium. *J. Am. Coll. Cardiol.* 10: 1322–1334, 1987.
559. Zimmer, H. G., A. M. Gerdes, S. Lortet, and G. Mall. Changes in heart function and cardiac cell size in rats with chronic myocardial infarction. *J. Mol. Cell. Cardiol.* 22:1231–1243, 1990.

3. Cell physiology and cell biology of myocardial cell caveolae

ERNEST PAGE | *Department of Medicine, University of Chicago, Chicago, Illinois*

HIROSHI IIDA | *Department of Agriculture, University of Kyushu, Japan*

DONALD D. DOYLE | *Department of Medicine, University of Chicago, Chicago, Illinois*

CHAPTER CONTENTS

Caveolae
Ultrastructure
Morphometric Studies
Accessibility of the Lumens of Caveolae to Extracellular Macromolecules
Opening and Closure of Cardiac Myocyte Caveolae
Reversible Changes in Myocardial Cell Caveolar Volume and Surface Density in Hypertonic Solutions
Hypertonic Solutions Increase Mean Caveolar Neck Surface Density and Diameter
Water-Channel Proteins in Mammalian Cardiac Myocytes
Temperature Dependence of the Co-localization of Aquaporin-1 with Caveolin3
Physiological Role of Aquaporin-1 in Human Cardiac Myocyte Caveolae
Relationship of Atrial Myocyte Caveolae to Atrial Granules
Localization of the Type B Atrial Natriuretic Peptide Receptor in Atrial Myocyte Cavaolae
Co-localization of Endothelium-Derived Nitric Oxide Synthase with Caveolin3 in Rat Cardiac Myocyte Caveolae
Endothelin and Protein Kinase C Isoforms in Cardiac Myocyte Caveolae
Immunoelectron Microscopic Localization of the Monocarboxylate Transporter, MCT-1 in In Situ Rat Left Ventricular Myocytes
Neuregulin Binding to its Receptor in Cardiac Myocyte Caveolae
Adenosine A1 Receptor in Adult Cardiac Ventricular Myocytes
Exploration of Possible Interactions of Cardiac Myocyte Caveolae with Extracellular Matrix and Cytoskeleton-Associated Proteins: Dystrophin and Dystroglycan
Dynamic Clustering of Sphingolipids and Cholesterol to Form Functional "Rafts" in Cellular Membranes
Development of More Efficient, Specific, and Sensitive Methods for Identifying the Intracaveolar and Caveolae-Bound Proteins of Cardiac Myocytes
Selected General Topics in Caveolar or Caveolae-Relevant Biology
    Physical considerations—caveolae as plasma membrane microdomains or plasma membrane-associated microdomains
    Caveolar Proteins
        Caveolin
        Caveolin isoforms
        Function of caveolin
    Other caveolar proteins: reality vs. artifact

PLASMA MEMBRANE–ASSOCIATED VESICLES CALLED CAVEOLAE are a conspicuous feature of mammalian heart muscle cells. As seen in transmission electron micrographs of ultrathin sections of hearts that have been fixed by conventional techniques and opacified with salts of uranium and lead (Fig. 3–1), these flask-shaped structures resemble vesicles first described in endothelial cells by Palade (92). Such vesicles were subsequently named "caveolae" (little caves) by Yamada (150). This name is now generally accepted, and is useful for distinguishing caveolae from other plasma membrane–associated vesicles present in cardiac myocytes: clathrin-coated vesicles, secretory granules, and coatomer-coated vesicles, which mediate both constitutive secretion via the default pathway and recycling of plasma membrane constituents. This chapter discusses the cell physiology and biology of myocardial cell caveolae, with emphasis on what is known about their structure and about the proteins within or closely associated with the caveolar membrane of in situ cardiac myocytes.

CAVEOLAE

It is becoming increasingly evident that caveolae from different mammalian tissues or from cell lines derived from such tissues differ between species in the number of proteins they contain or bind, but it is also worth noting that some properties of caveolae can be observed in a wide spectrum of tissues and cell lines. Among these properties of caveolae are their ultrastructure and their location in cells, and, at least to some extent, their lipid composition, some of the types of proteins associated with them, and their biophysical behavior. This introduction discusses briefly other putative caveolar properties whose features are still incompletely described and accepted: the roles of caveolae in signal transduction; caveolar internalization

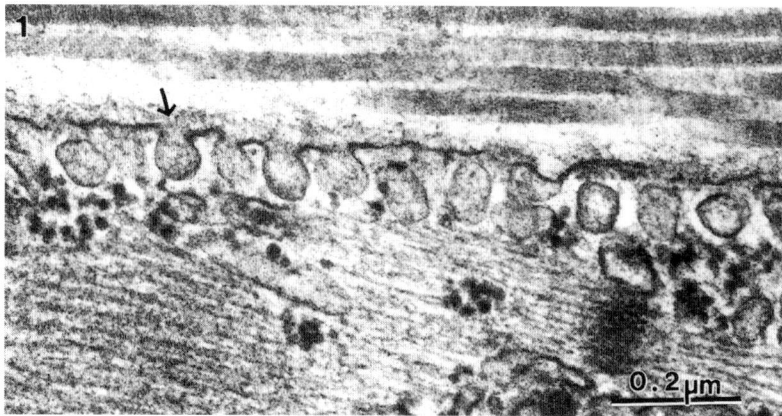

FIG. 3–1. Electron micrograph of a longitudinally oriented lead- and uranium-stained thin section through the cell surface of an unstretched, noncontracting isolated rat atrium incubated in physiological (isotonic) modified Krebs Henseleit (KH) solution at 37°C. Note multiple caveolar profiles beneath the sarcolemma, either open to the interstitial space (*arrow*) or apparently closed off from it. Figs. 3–1, 3–2, 3–5, 3–6, and 3–8 are from Kordylewski et al. (54).

of extracaveolar plasmalemmal receptor–ligand complexes by "potocytosis"; the putative localization of glycosyl-phosphatidylinositol (GPI)-anchored proteins exclusively or predominantly in caveolae; the interactions of caveolae with cytoskeletal proteins; the notion that caveolae may play a role in intercellular signaling; and the possibility that caveolae-associated transporters may control the intracaveolar Ca^{2+} concentration, the Ca^{2+} concentration in subplasmalemmal cytosolic microdomains immediately underlying the caveolae, or the concentrations in both of these loci. Particularly useful critical discussions of caveolar protein composition—the relevant methods, the assumptions and the limitations of method and interpretation—have been published by the laboratories of Anderson (128, 129), Lisanti (133), Page (20), Palade (136), Parton (59), Schnitzer (80), and Simons (123).

ULTRASTRUCTURE

The in situ sizes and shapes of caveolae in cells of different mammalian tissues are remarkably similar. To minimize duplication, in this chapter ultrastructural characteristics of caveolae are illustrated by electron micrographs of specimens of mammalian heart muscle cells, which have been extensively studied in several preparations. To date, ultrastructural studies on in situ plasmalemmal caveolae in heart muscle include morphometry of electron micrographs; studies of the accessibility of caveolar interiors (lumens) to extracellular electron-opaque tracers; studies of the relationship of caveolae to atrial granules; studies of the reversible swelling of caveolae in saline made hypertonic by the addition of sucrose, mannitol, or NaCl ("paradoxical" caveolar swelling); and immunoelectron microscopic localization of selected proteins present in caveolae or associated with caveolar membranes.

MORPHOMETRIC STUDIES

Following Palade's seminal discovery of caveolae in early transmission electron micrographs (93), structures resembling those described by Palade were found in multiple and diverse vertebrate cell types. Not surprisingly, such structures are clearly recognizable in early electron micrographs of thin-sectioned heart muscle and cardiac conduction system, (e.g., 28, 84, 99, 101, 131). The paper of Rayns et al. also for the first time showed the appearance of in situ myocardial cell caveolae in electron micrographs of the fracture faces, the artificial surfaces produced after freeze-fracture through the lipid bilayer of myocardial cell plasmalemma. Such qualitative studies, utilizing transmission electron micrographs of positively stained thin sections and freeze fractured, glutaraldehyde-fixed cardiac myocytes, were extended by other laboratories (38, 54, 64, 120) to include quantitative estimates of the surface density and size distributions of caveolae in the plasmalemmal fracture face.

Levin and Page (64) measured the diameter of caveolar profiles of cardiac myocytes in transmission electron micrographs from ultrathin sections of glutaraldehyde-fixed and osmium tetroxide post-fixed right ventricular papillary muscles from each of seven rabbits. The results, expressed as the mean diameter of the equivalent sphere, yielded a mean estimate (averaged over seven rabbits and excluding plasma membrane involved in complexes with sarcoplasmic reticulum) of 93 nm for the external sarcolemma and 89.7 nm for the T-tubules, with a standard error of 1 nm. Similar values for the mean diameters of rat atrial plasma membrane caveolae can be derived from data like those of Kordylewski et al. (54) (see Figure 7 of that paper). These authors also measured the diameters of caveolar necks in the plasma membrane fracture faces of three rat atria, and in this way obtained mean estimated values of 35.1, 35.7, and 39.7 nm, respectively. At a near-physiological diastolic mean sarcomere length of 2.1 μm, the mean percent increase in the sum of plasma membrane area and caveolar membrane area attributable to the contribution of area from caveolae was 10.7%, 21.4%, and 32.1%, assuming one, two, or three caveolae per caveolar neck, respectively. Diverse data discussed later in this chapter support the conclusion that mammalian cardiac myocyte caveolae are structures morphologically and functionally distinct from both the external plasmalemmal envelope and (in the rat ventricle), from the noncaveolar plasma membrane in the T-system. For the external plasmalemmal envelope, the magnitude of the caveolar component depends on how many caveolae there are on the average for each caveolar neck, a mean value that could not be measured precisely for technical reasons. While as many as four or five caveolae per neck were readily observed in selected samples (54), it remains unclear whether this number of caveolae per neck is rare or reasonably frequent, given the technical problems of sampling small, three-dimensional structures with the techniques available.

An issue of importance for the interpretation of electron micrographs of caveolae in heart muscle cells and for the validation of morphometric studies is whether conventional chemical fixation of this tissue for electron microscopy with glutaraldehyde or with glutaraldehyde followed by osmium tetroxide distorts the "native" structure of caveolae, or, in the worst case, creates membrane artifacts in the shape of caveolae (120). To address this issue, control experiments aimed at tissue preservation without chemical fixation have been done by rapidly freezing tissue to very low temperatures (about 16°K) using a liquid helium–cooled copper block that is rapidly slammed against the unfixed tissue (44, 45). Application of this method to skeletal muscle cells (97) yields the same number of caveolae as in skeletal muscle myocytes fixed conventionally with glutaraldehyde or with glutaraldehyde followed by osmium tetroxide. In meticulous experiments on cardiac muscle from frog, mouse, and bird hearts, Sommer et al. (132) confirmed that fixation by quick freezing to 10–20°K at freezing rates exceeding 40,000°C per second yields excellent structural preservation without detectable cryo-damage, including specifically preservation of cardiac myocyte caveolae. Preservation without chemical fixation as seen by electron microscopy was most unequivocally shown when rapid freezing was followed by freeze-fracture and freeze-etching, but was also evident in specimens subjected to freeze-substitution or to freeze-fracture and cryo-sectioning. These experiments, showing that caveolar structure and number in chemically fixed cardiac tissues are similar to those seen without chemical fixation, support the conclusion that the caveolae seen by classical electron microscopic techniques are not artifacts, and that caveolar shape, size, and surface density can be usefully approached by electron microscopy of tissues. This conclusion does not, however, vitiate the critique of Palade and coworkers (136), or the need for the development of additional techniques that permit observation of the dynamic behavior of cardiac myocyte caveolae in situ, including changes in their size, shape, number, and interactions in response to physiological, pharmacological, and developmental perturbations. Systematic and meticulous studies of the cytoplasmic surface of myocardial cell caveolae using the technique of quick freezing followed by deep-etching, as previously applied to various noncardiac tissues

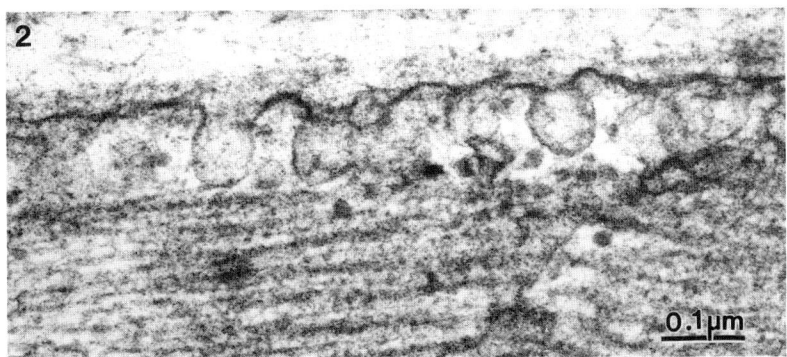

FIG. 3–2. Specimen similar to shown in Fig. 3–1, illustrates caveolar profiles open to the interstitial space or apparently closed off from it by a narrow diaphragm.

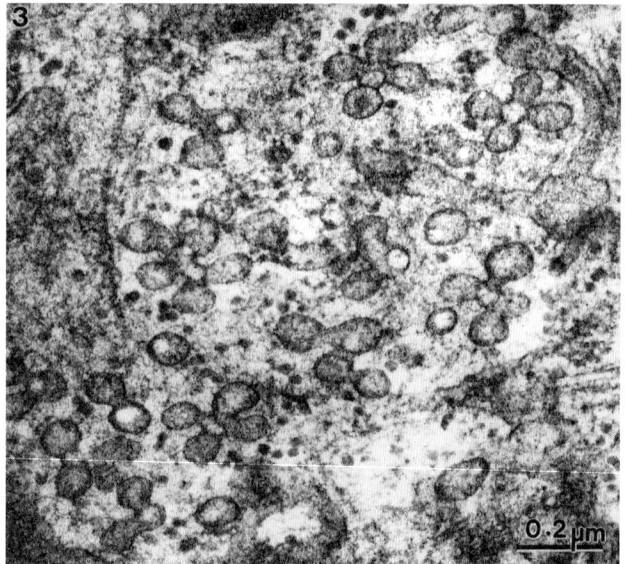

FIG. 3–3. Electron micrograph of rat atrium prepared as for Fig. 3–1, but thin-sectioned just below and parallel to the plasma membrane. Note multiple caveolar profiles (four or more) surrounding one caveolar neck in a "windmill" configuration, best seen just below the upper right corner of the micrograph.

(49), also seem worthwhile, but as yet remain to be done.

Figure 3–1 (54) is an electron micrograph of an in situ rat atrial myocyte that has been sectioned parallel to the long axis of the cell, after conventional fixation of the unstretched atrium with glutaraldehyde and osmium tetroxide, followed by opacification of the section with salts of lead and uranium. Two-dimensional "profiles" of caveolae are seen to be continuous with the linear profile of the plasma membrane. There they appear either as racemose sacs underlying and continuous with the linear profile of the plasma membrane, or as complete circular or elliptical profiles seemingly unconnected to the overlying plasma membrane. With this technique, the interior of some caveolar profiles appears continuous with the interstitial space, while that of other caveolar profiles seems separated from the interstitium by a narrow diaphragm (Figs. 3–1 and 3–2). If the atrial myocardial cell is sectioned tangentially to and just beneath the plasma membrane (Fig. 3–3), caveolar profiles can be shown to vary from single circles to complex pinwheel or cloverleaf configurations with as many as five caveolar profiles oriented around one central caveolar neck. Racemose or tree-like arrangements, in which subplasmalemmal caveolae appear as a continuous interconnected string of multiple caveolar profiles forming an apparently continuous compartment just under and parallel to the plasma membrane, are also seen in in situ rat atrial myocytes (Fig. 3–4).

ACCESSIBILITY OF THE LUMENS OF CAVEOLAE TO EXTRACELLULAR MACROMOLECULES

Accessibility of the caveolar interior or "lumen" to extracellular macromolecules was tested by equilibrating the endocardial surface of an intact rat atrium stretched with a physiological distending pressure by a 7 cm column of saline (equivalent to 5.1 mm Hg), and containing horseradish peroxidase (HRP, molecular weight about 40 kDa (89). In this way it could be shown by transmission electron microscopy (TEM) of thin-sectioned tissue that the interior of stretched myocardial cell caveolae is at least transiently capable of

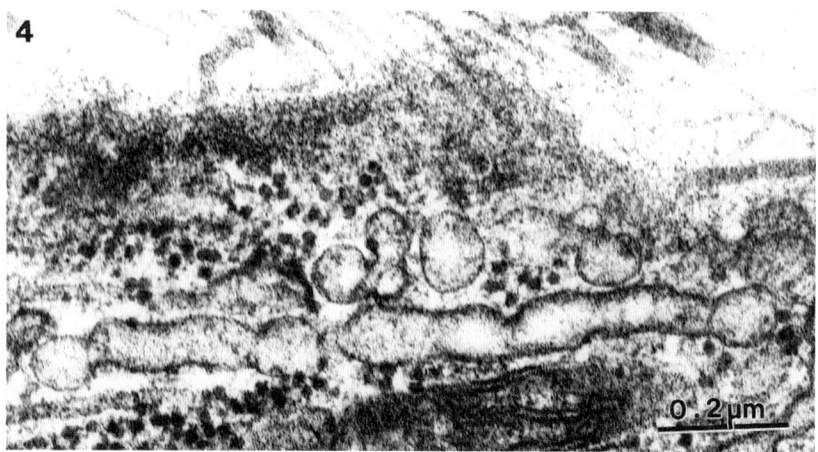

FIG. 3–4. Electron micrograph of rat atrium prepared and thin-sectioned as for Fig. 3–3 just below and parallel to the plasma membrane, showing multiple caveolar profiles in series forming a continuous elongated structure with a common lumen.

communicating with the extracellular space. This continuity between extracellular space and caveolar lumen is inferred from the observation that HRP readily penetrates into all myocardial cell caveolae (Fig. 3–5), and can be as readily and rapidly washed out of them by subsequent incubation in an HRP-free solution.

For in situ myocardial cells of the atrial and ventricular chambers, it is of particular interest to consider whether and how macromolecules in the blood plasma within the lumen of these chambers can traverse the endocardial barrier and enter the caveolae of the cardiac myocytes. In rat atria this barrier is made up predominantly of endothelium-like endocardial cells (89), which must be either crossed or bypassed in order for macromolecular probes to reach the myocardial cell caveolae. After crossing the endocardial barrier, and provided that (as is the case under normal conditions) the caveolar lumens are at least intermittently open to the interstitial space, macromolecular probes of appropriate size are taken up into the caveolar lumens. This uptake is of biological and medical interest, because multiple biologically active substances bound to plasma proteins (113, 122) could thus enter the caveolae of cardiac myocytes. Experiments on isolated in vitro preparations of rat hearts (54, 89) demonstrated that stretching the atria by the small, physiological distending pressure of 5.1 mm Hg renders the atrial endocardium permeable to the macromolecules HRP (40 kD; (Fig. 3–5), wheat germ agglutinin (WGH) labeled with HRP (70 kD), and ferritin (500 kD), whereas these macromolecules fail to traverse the endocardium of unstretched atria. The stretch-activated permeabilization of the endocardium was demonstrable within one minute and may well be functional much sooner. It was invariably rapidly reversed by releasing the distending hydrostatic pressure. Thus, when contracting at a physiological rate, myocardial cell caveolae may intermittently take up proteins from the cavities of the atria, an uptake perhaps synchronized with the intra-atrial pressure changes that accompany the cardiac contraction and relaxation cycle. Although it seems highly probable that a similar stretch-dependent and reversible macromolecule uptake mechanism exists for caveolae of ventricular myocytes, this possibility has not yet been experimentally tested.

OPENING AND CLOSURE OF CARDIAC MYOCYTE CAVEOLAE

The above-described experiments show that myocardial cell caveolae can rapidly take up macromolecules from the interstial space. The interior of these caveolae must therefore be in direct continuity with the interstitial space, either continually or by intermittent cycling (at an as yet undetermined range of frequencies) between open and closed states. Opening and closing could be achieved either by the opening and closing of a pore (e.g., the caveolar neck), or by intermittent cycles of neck insertion and withdrawal. In experiments on an epithelial cell line, Rothberg et al. (103) demonstrated that caveolae from this cell line are indeed intermittently open and closed, although the physiological relevance of this observation is controversial (72).

A similarly useful experimental design, both for studying whether myocardial cell caveolae are open or closed and for investigating the issues that affect this question, is to examine the *efflux* of HRP from isolated rat atria that have been preloaded with this physiologically inert macromolecular tracer by preequilibrating stretched atria with HRP on their endocardial surface. The atria can then be transferred in the stretched state to an HRP-free solution in which the ionic composition, temperature, and protein content can be varied, or to which inhibitors or stimulators of signal transduction pathways can be added. By performing conventional TEM on thin sections of such atria that have been fixed at various intervals after transfer to HRP-

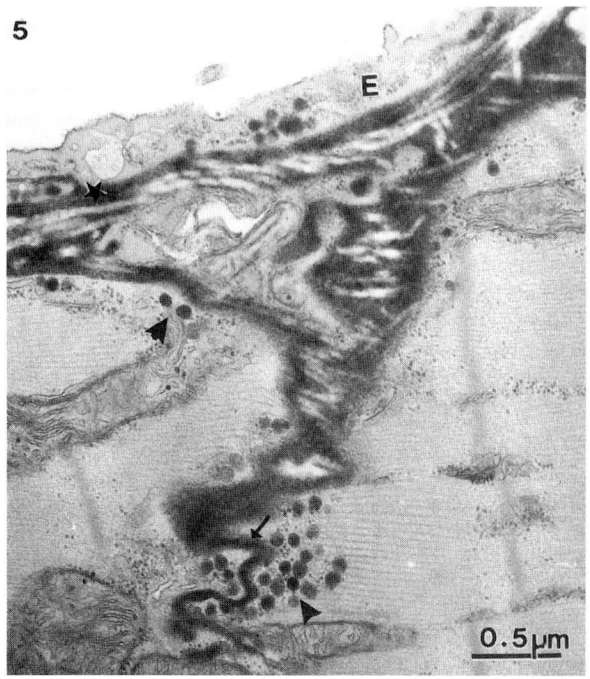

FIG. 3–5. Electron micrograph of stretched atrial preparation incubated at 18°C with horseradish peroxidase (HRP), stained histochemically for HRP, and counterstained with lead citrate. From the top downward note endocardial endothelial cell (E) with HRP-containing vesicular profiles, subendocardial space (star) heavily stained with HRP, interstitial space between atrial myocytes (*arrow*) that is opacified with HRP, and atrial myocyte caveolae (*arrowheads*) filled with HRP.

free solution, it is possible to determine whether a chosen inhibitor or perturbation prevents or significantly slows the efflux of HRP from myocardial cell caveolae (normally complete in 1–3 minutes at 37° or 20°C). This experiment is possible because HRP does not leak from the caveolae into the cytosol. To date, such experiments have been done on atria rendered noncontracting and relaxed by lowering the external Ca concentration ($[Ca^{2+}]_o$) to 0.2 mM, and inhibiting release of Ca from the sarcoplasmic reticulum into the cytosol with ryanodine (54). In this way it could be shown that intracaveolar HRP will diffuse out of caveolae of stretched atrial myocytes into an HRP-free medium over a temperature range from 4° to 37° C; i.e., even at very low temperature the caveolae appear to be open to the interstitial space for a significant fraction of time. A related experimental arrangement, designed to determine whether caveolae of in situ cardiac myocytes in stretched atria are open to or closed off from the interstitial space, tests whether selected perturbations prevent caveolar uptake of HRP from the interstitial space. This method was used for exploratory experiments showing that rat atrial myocyte caveolae are not prevented from taking up HRP by raising the cytosolic Ca^{2+} concentration with ionomycin, by α_1-adrenergic stimulation, by raising the cytosolic concentration of cyclic adenosine monophosphate (cAMP) with caffeine, and by sodium nitroprusside (54).

REVERSIBLE CHANGES IN MYOCARDIAL CELL CAVEOLAR VOLUME AND SURFACE DENSITY IN HYPERTONIC SOLUTIONS

The volumes of myocardial cell caveolae and the surface density (number per unit area of plasma membrane) of caveolar necks inserted into the lipid bilayer of the plasma membrane can be shown to undergo rapid and striking changes when intact isolated rat atria are incubated in otherwise physiological salt solution in which the osmolality has been raised by addition of 150 mM sucrose, 150 mM mannitol (54), or 75 mM NaCl (91). Figures 3–6A and B (53) are electron micrographs of caveolae thin-sectioned in the plane just under and parallel to the plasma membrane of an in situ rat atrial myocyte. The figures compare two halves of the same rat atrium, of which one half was exposed for 5 min at 37°C to the high-osmolality medium (Fig. 3–6A), while the control half, otherwise similarly treated (Fig. 3–6B), was incubated in a sucrose-free solution at physiological osmolality. Comparison of the two micrographs shows that the caveolar profiles of the atrium exposed to hypertonic sucrose are enlarged. At 37°C, the enlargement was already conspicuous after only one minute of exposure to the hypertonic medium. The caveolar enlargement could be readily reversed within 5 min or less by substituting isosmolar sucrose-free medium for the hypertonic, sucrose-containing medium. Raising the total solute concentration by addition of 150 mM mannitol instead of sucrose yielded similar enlargement of caveolar profiles, as did making the solution hypertonic with 75 mmol/L of NaCl, an observation suggesting

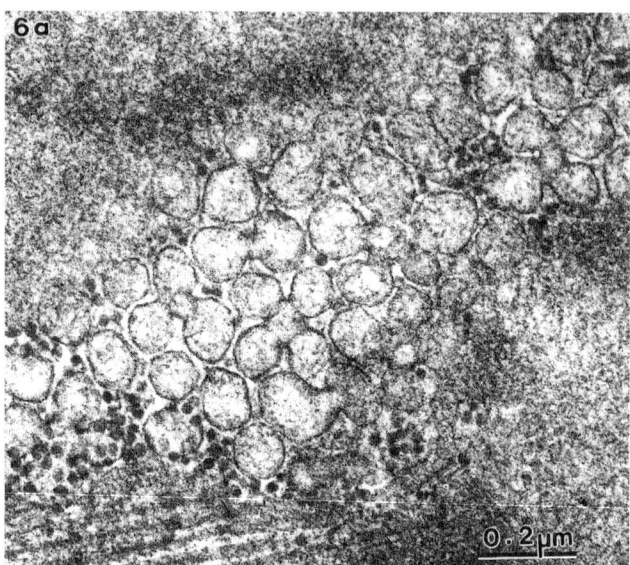

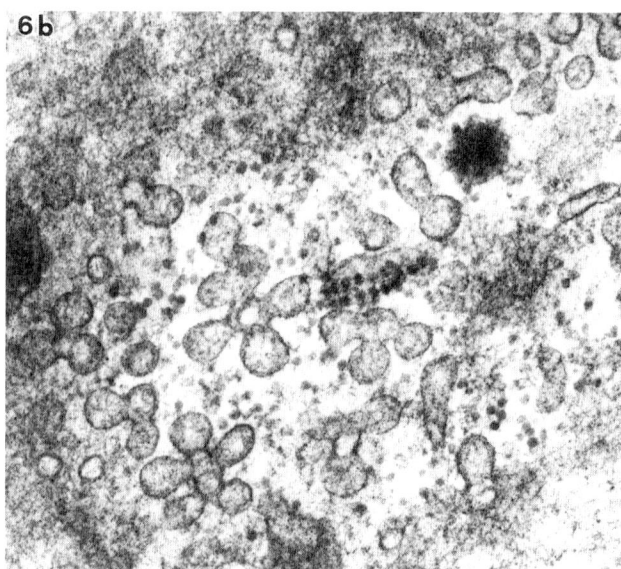

FIG. 3–6. Unstretched isolated half rat atria either incubated for 5 min at 37°C in control solution made hypertonic by adding 150 mM sucrose (A) or in otherwise identical sucrose-free isotonic control solution. Note swollen caveolae (A) and absence of swelling in isotonic control solution (B). Swelling in hypertonic sucrose was rapidly reversible by return to isotonic control solution (data not shown).

that the swelling mechanism was not sensitive to approximately doubling the ionic strength. Since caveolar swelling in hypertonic solutions is associated with closing off of the caveolar continuity with the interstitial space, and because swelling of vesicles in hypertonic solutions is unexpected, we have called this combination of phenomena *paradoxical caveolar closure and swelling* (PCCS).

Experiments on rat ventricular myocytes perfused in situ through the coronary circulation on the Langendorff cannula with solutions made hypertonic with 75 mM NaCl also resulted in swelling of ventricular myocyte caveolae (Fig. 3–7A and B), a change that was rapidly reversible by reperfusion with isotonic control solution [Fig. 3–7C; Page (91)]. (In this experiment on perfused rat ventricle, NaCl was used to raise the osmolality because the relatively high viscosity of hypertonic sucrose solutions interferes with perfusion of the coronary microcirculation.) By contrast to these in situ experiments, experiments in which freshly enzymatically dissociated and purified rat ventricular myocytes were suspended in control saline solution made hypertonic by adding 75 mM NaCl did not produce caveolar swelling.

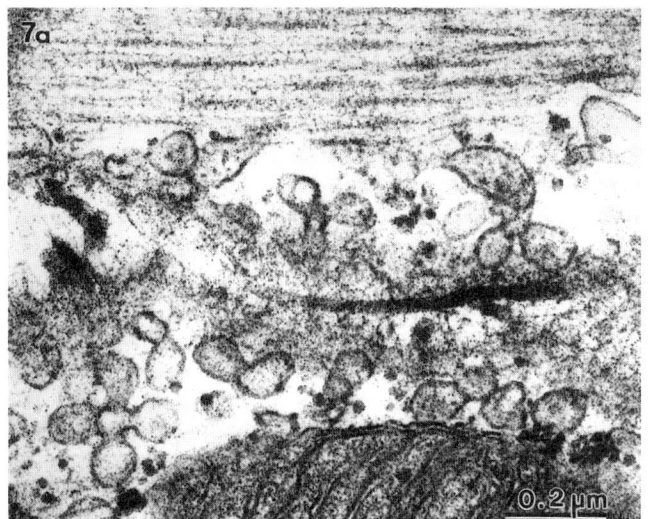
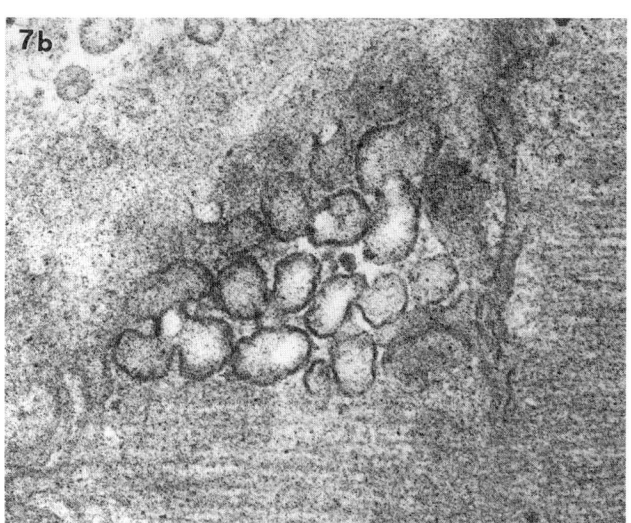
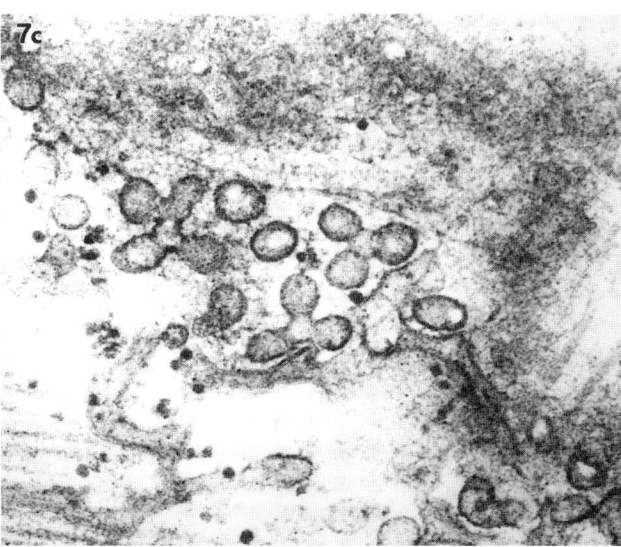

FIG. 3–7. Rat ventricular myocytes perfused in situ for 5 min. at 37°C through the coronary circulation on the Langendorff cannula with isotonic Krebs Henseleit solution (A), with an otherwise identical solution made hypertonic by adding 75 mM NaCl to isotonic control solution (B), or by reperfusing ventricles perfused with hypertonic solution with isotonic control solution (C). Note caveolar swelling in (B) and its regression in (C).

HYPERTONIC SOLUTIONS INCREASE MEAN CAVEOLAR NECK SURFACE DENSITY AND DIAMETER

In addition to causing caveolar swelling, exposure to hypertonic sucrose could be shown to increase the surface density of caveolar necks, i.e., the number of caveolar necks inserted into the lipid bilayer of the plasma membrane per unit of lipid bilayer area. This area was visualized in electron micrographs of platinum-shadowed replicas of the plasmalemmal fracture face observable after freeze-fracture and metal shadowing of the atria [Fig. 3–8A and B (54)]. In the same replicas, measurements of caveolar neck diameters confirmed that the mean diameter increases in hypertonic sucrose or mannitol solutions, and that this increase is rapidly reversible on returning the atria to sucrose-free

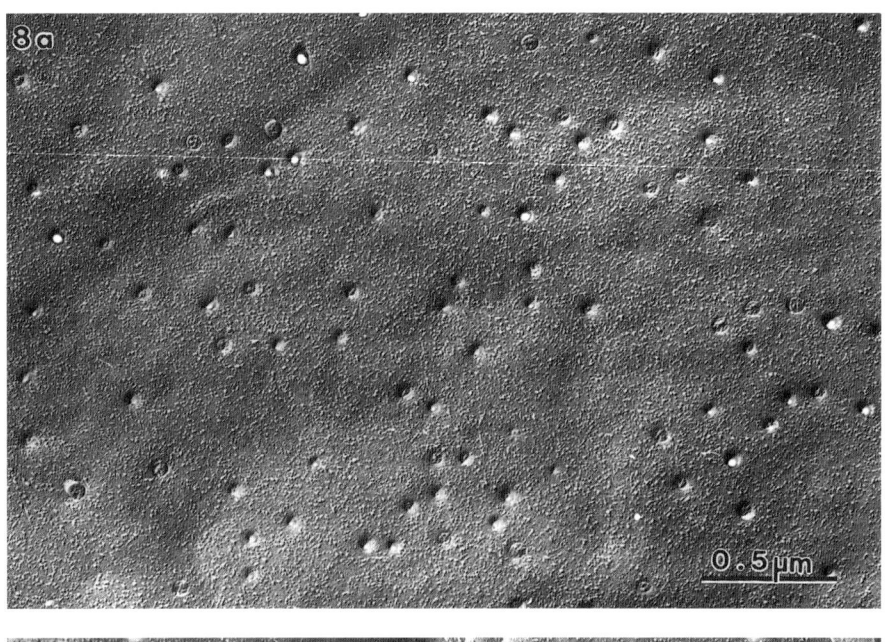

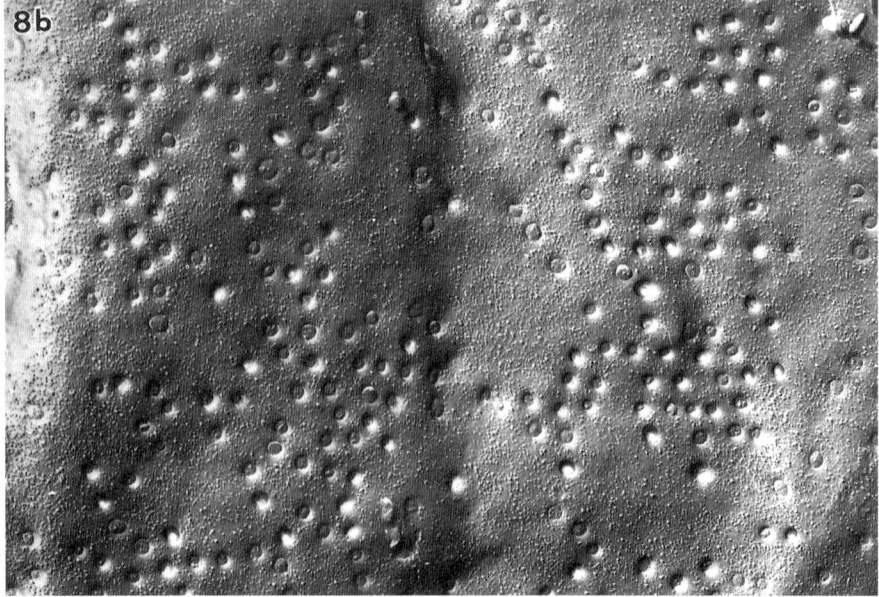

FIG. 3–8. Electron micrographs of replicas obtained by freeze-fracture of rat hemi-atria derived from the same atrium and incubated (before fixation, freeze-fracture, and platinum shadowing) for five min., either in isotonic physiological saline (A) or in an otherwise identical solution made hypertonic by raising the total osmolarity by addition of 150 mmoles/L of sucrose (B). Quantitative analysis of multiple such samples yields statistical confirmation that exposure to hypertonic solutions raises the mean surface density of caveolar necks and also increases their mean diameter.

or mannitol-free solutions. An attractive feature of these experiments is that, unlike many studies on myocardial cell caveolae, the results lend themselves to a statistical analysis. But attempts to extend these experiments to primary cultures of atrial myocytes (54) were unequivocally negative, as were, under the same conditions, attempts to induce caveolar swelling by exposure to hypertonic solutions in enzymatically dispersed (but not cultured) atrial or ventricular myocytes from adult rats (91). Failure to elicit either caveolar swelling or a change in the surface density of caveolar necks in dispersed myocyte preparations might be the result of phenotypic changes that atrial myocytes undergo in primary culture (46); but this mechanism clearly cannot explain the failure to elicit swelling of caveolae in freshly dissociated atrial or ventricular myocytes. Alternatively, the swelling observed in in situ myocytes could depend on a paracrine effect reflecting interaction of cardiac myocyte caveolae with nonmyocyte cell types—e.g., endothelial cells, fibroblasts, nerve cells, and/or any of the diverse other nonmyocyte cell types present in the intact atria or ventricles, but absent in preparations of purified dissociated myocytes. However this issue is resolved, it seems noteworthy that in situ cardiac myocyte caveolae in rat atria and ventricles appear to be sensors of extracellular osmolarity, and that they can change their volume and their continuity with the interstitial space in response to changes in the concentration (activity) of water to which the in situ myocyte is exposed. Before attempting to explain this sensitivity and the nature of PCCS, it is appropriate to discuss water channel proteins in cardiac myocytes.

WATER-CHANNEL PROTEINS IN MAMMALIAN CARDIAC MYOCYTES

As already noted, myocardial cell caveolae can be caused to swell and close off from the interstitial space by exposure of atria or ventricles to physiological saline made hypertonic by adding sucrose, mannitol, or NaCl. Under these conditions, the resultant caveolar swelling reflects a net caveolar uptake of water. In theory, such a net water uptake into the caveolae could be achieved in at least two ways: (1) by water-specific transport of water from the cytosol of the cardiac myocyte, through open aquaporin-1 (Ap-1) water channels inserted through the cytosolic faces of the caveolar membranes into the closed-off caveolar lumens or (2) by diffusion or osmotic flow of water from the cytosol, parallel to and bypassing the water channels, directly across the lipid bilayer of the caveolar membrane, into the closed-off caveolar lumens. Although we shall show that net inflow of water into caveolae through Ap-1 channels is absent in the *unphysiological* process of PCCS characteristically observed in hypertonic solutions, we will suggest that water flow through Ap-1 water channels inserted into the caveolar membranes of in situ cardiac myocytes could contribute significantly to the regulation of caveolar volume and water content under isotonic or near-isotonic conditions at 20° or 37°C.

The idea that it might be informative to look for a role of water channels in the maintenance of myocardial cell caveolar volume arises, as already discussed, because a family of water-selective plasma membrane channel proteins called aquaporins has recently been described [reviewed by Engel, Walz, and Agre (26), Zeidel et al., (151), and Van Os, Deen, and Dempster (143)]. Schnitzer et al. (114) have shown partial inhibition of aquaporin-1–mediated transendothelial tritiated water transport in lung endothelium by using the mercurial water channel inhibitors mercuric chloride at a concentration of 0.1 mM, or para-hydroxymercuribenzoic sulfonic acid (0.3 mM). Both of these mercurial inhibitors are known to target some aquaporin water channels. Water channels which are insensitive to mercurials have also been cloned (43b).

The above-described studies of PCCS from our laboratory (54, 91), showing that exposure to saline made hypertonic with sucrose, mannitol, or NaCl causes in situ rat atrial and ventricular myocyte caveolae to close off, take up water, and swell, raised an important issue: Which of the above two candidate mechanisms—water flow into and out of caveolae through Ap-1 water channels in the caveolar membrane, or diffusional and/or osmotic flow of water across the caveolar lipid bilayer—dominates during PCCS and its reversal in response to osmotic perturbations? Equally relevant for the normal cell physiology of water channels in cardiac myocytes is a related issue that arises under isotonic or near-isotonic conditions: Under these conditions, what is the relative magnitude of water flow through caveolar Ap-1 water channels inserted into and through the part of the caveolar membrane facing the cytosol, as compared to the magnitude of net water diffusion across the lipid bilayer of this membrane? These questions further suggested the desirability of identifying which, if any, of the known water channel isoforms are expressed in mammalian (rat) cardiac myocytes.

We have recently shown by confocal immunofluorescence microscopy that the water-channel protein isoform, aquaporin-1, forms a close association or "colocalizes" with the most nearly myocyte-selective caveolar marker protein isoform, caveolin3 (138, 147); at the external plasma membranes of rat atrial and ventricular myocytes (Page et al, 1998). The preparations in which the colocalization was observed included primary cultures of atrial myocytes (PCAM), freshly dissociated atrial myocytes (FDAM), and frozen sections of in situ cardiac myocytes from isolated rat atria and ventricles incubated in vitro in isotonic solutions at 20° or 37°C [shown in color in Figures 1, 2, 3 and 6, respectively, in Page et al., 1998 (91)]. These studies show clearly that aquaporin-1 water channels have a role in the "paradoxical swelling" response of in situ rat atrial and ventricular myocyte caveolae observable in hypertonic media. The evidence for this conclusion, shown for atria in Page et al., 1998 (91) includes the finding that the stimulus that elicits PCCS in intact atria at 20° or 37°C (raising the external osmolality by 150 mM with sucrose or NaCl), causes Ap-1 water channel protein to dissociate from its co-localization with caveolin3. Also shown is that the caveolin3 remains coating the caveolar membrane during PCCS, whereas the Ap-1 water channel protein is translocated away from its colocalization with the caveolin3 of the caveolar membrane, presumably by internalization to an as yet unidentified location. When the atrium is returned to sucrose-free isotonic solution, Ap-1 water channel protein recolocalizes with caveolin3 of the atrial myocyte caveolae. Thus PCCS is present in hypertonic solutions even when no discernible water channels are inserted into the caveolar membrane. The same observation of a reversible, hypertonic solution-evoked translocation of Ap-1 was made in in situ caveolae of rat ventricular myocytes (91).

The additional finding that PCCS can be readily elicited at 4°C, a temperature at which Ap-1 does not colocalize with caveolin3 by confocal microscopy, is further evidence that functional water channels inserted into the caveolar membrane are not a prerequisite for PCCS (91). Its persistent presence at low temperature also suggests that PCCS is not *directly* coupled to an input of metabolic energy, i.e., that it is a passive process. Since microtubules are depolymerized at 4°C, they also cannot be implicated directly in PCCS, which is readily demonstrable at that temperature (54).

TEMPERATURE DEPENDENCE OF THE CO-LOCALIZATION OF AQUAPORIN-1 WITH CAVEOLIN3

Page et al. (91) reported that the co-localization of Ap-1 with caveolin3 at the caveolar membrane interface separating the cytosol from the caveolar lumen, a phenomenon that is routinely observable by confocal microscopy at 20° and 37°C, is absent at 4°C, and becomes rapidly reestablished when the temperature is raised again from 4°C to 20° or 37°C. This finding suggests that the co-localization of Ap-1 with caveolin3 may entail one or more reversible energy-dependent steps or processes that are inhibited at 4°C.

PHYSIOLOGICAL ROLE OF AQUAPORIN-1 IN HUMAN CARDIAC MYOCYTE CAVEOLAE

One of the issues that emerges from the study of Page et al, (91) on rat hearts is, why it should be necessary for hearts to have water-specific channels in addition to the passive water flows down osmotic or diffusion gradients of water activity or water concentration. Schipke et al. (112b) approach this issue by pointing out that, in the mammalian heart, the magnitude of local myocardial blood flow to and from the in situ cardiac myocytes via the coronary circulation is highly correlated with the local rate of oxidative phosphorylation in mitochondria. They also emphasize that areas where flow and oxidative phosphorylation are elevated produce relatively large volumes of respiration-associated water, which cannot be allowed to accumulate, but must be efficiently removed by transport across the myocyte plasma membrane via water channel proteins.

RELATIONSHIP OF ATRIAL MYOCYTE CAVEOLAE TO ATRIAL GRANULES

Conclusions about functional relationships based entirely on structural associations and contiguities are problematical, given the limitations of inferring causality from the spatial or temporal association of two phenomena. Nevertheless, as visualized in electron micrographs of conventionally fixed and stained thin sections of mouse and rat atria (86, 88), the contiguities between profiles of atrial myocyte caveolae and profiles of the membranes surrounding atrial secretory granules (Fig. 3–9) are so compelling that it seems mandatory to determine whether a functional relationship exists between these two very different types of vesicles, both present in atrial myocytes.

Evidence for such a relationship has been obtained in mouse and rat atria by immunoelectron microscopy (88). With this method it was shown that plasma membrane caveolae contiguous with the limiting membranes of atrial granules in the underlying cytoplasm are specifically immunostained with colloidal gold-labeled antibody to atrial natriuretic peptide (ANP) (Fig. 3–10). Perturbations that markedly increase the rate of natriuretic peptide secretion by rat atria via the regulated pathway, including atrial stretch, atrial contractions, and increasing the external Ca^{2+} concentration (87, 90), did not detectably change immunostaining of caveolae with antibody against ANP. In addition

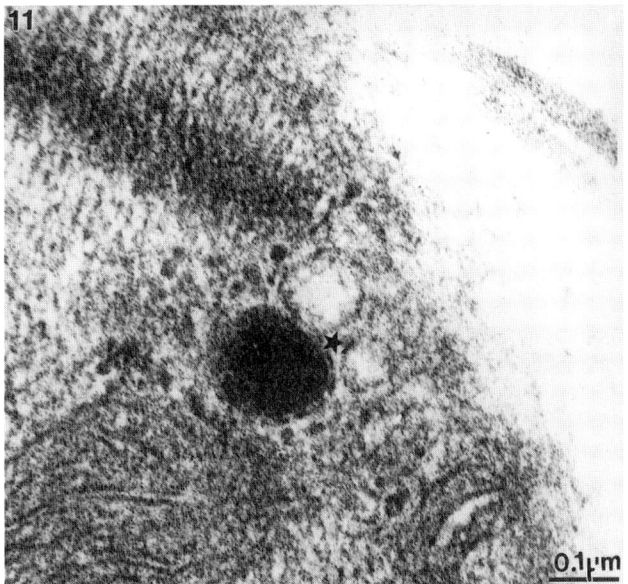

FIG. 3–9. Electron micrograph of a glutaraldehyde-fixed, osmium tetroxide post–fixed ultra-thin section of rat atrium stained with uranyl acetate and counter-stained with lead citrate. The section shows the profile of a plasma membrane–associated caveola apparently contiguous with an underlying atrial granule (*star*).

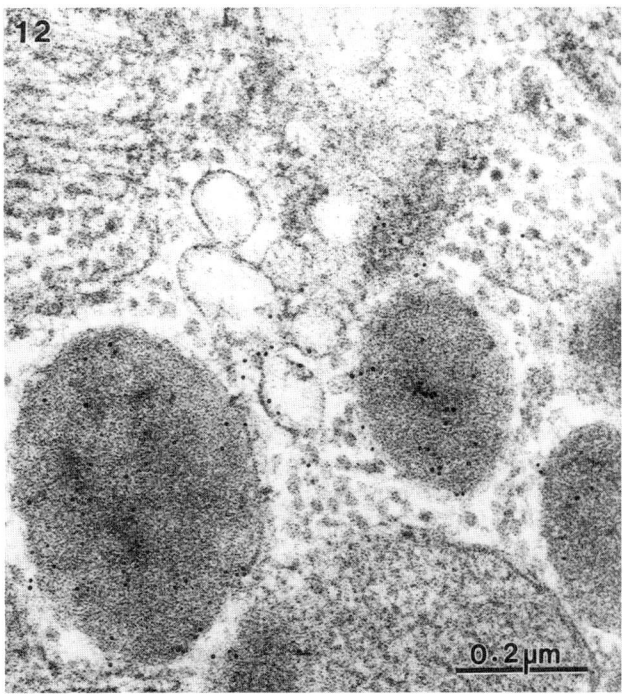

FIG. 3–10. Immunnoelectron micrograph showing a glutaraldehyde-fixed, osmium tetroxide post-fixed ultra-thin section of rat atrium that has been stained with uranyl acetate and lead citrate and immunostained with antibody against rat alpha atrial natriuretic peptide. A stereo-pair of this section (not shown) demonstrates colloidal gold decorating the inner edge of the caveolar membrane. From Page et al. (88), with permission.

to caveolae and atrial granules, this antibody also stained the Golgi cisternae and the trans-Golgi network (TGN) in the cytoplasm underlying the atrial granules.

The presence of ANP in caveolae of rat and mouse atrial myocytes raises several questions: If any fraction of intracaveolar ANP originates in underlying atrial granules, how does the ANP get from the granules to the interior of caveolae? Or, as seems a priori more probable, does most or all intracaveolar ANP originate from extracellular ANP that diffuses into the caveolar lumen through open caveolar necks? What fraction of intracaveolar ANP is bound to the ANP receptor? What fractions of the intracaveolar ANP of a given myocyte are derived, respectively, from the autocrine secretion of that myocyte, from the paracrine secretion of neighboring atrial myocytes, or, as an endocrine secretion, from the atrial blood supply? These questions remain to be answered by appropriately designed experiments.

LOCALIZATION OF THE TYPE B ATRIAL NATRIURETIC PEPTIDE RECEPTOR IN ATRIAL MYOCYTE CAVEOLAE

The finding of ANP in the caveolae of in situ atrial myocytes suggested that this peptide might be present in caveolae bound to an ANP receptor. By means of confocal immunofluorescence microscopy, and with the use of an antibody against the type B atrial natriuretic peptide receptor (ANP-RB) provided by Dr. Garbers (52), we were able to show that ANP-RB is indeed the isoform present in the caveolae of both primary cultures of atrial myocytes (PCAM) from adult rats and freshly enzymatically dissociated (but not cultured) rat atrial myocytes (21). There are three presently known natriuretic peptide (NP) hormones. The member of the family first discovered was ANP, which is synthesized in cardiac myocytes, where it is secreted constitutively in both the ventricle and atrium, as well as regulatively through granules in the atrium. Subsequently discovered in the brain, brain natriuretic peptide (BNP), and C-type natriuretic peptide (CNP) have both been localized in other tissues as well, including heart. There are presently three known NP receptors, NPR A, B, and C. All three, located in the plasmalemma of various cell types, traverse the membrane once. In an anomaly of nomenclature, NPR-A binds both ANP and BNP in the nmolar range, and CNP in the μmolar range, whereas NPR-B binds CNP in the pmolar range, and both ANP and BNP in the nmolar range (81b). Both these receptors have guanylyl cyclase (GC) activity in cytoplasmic tails which are associated with signal transduction and are also known as GC-A and GC-B (52). NPR-C, found most abundantly in the kidney, has a truncated cytoplasmic tail, lacks cyclase activity, and is believed to be involved in NP clearance. The full implications of the presence of the B-type NP receptor in atrial myocytes is not yet known. Effects of CNP on atrial contractility have been reported (4b, 45b, 63b).

CO-LOCALIZATION OF ENDOTHELIUM-DERIVED NITRIC OXIDE SYNTHASE WITH CAVEOLIN3 IN RAT CARDIAC MYOCYTE CAVEOLAE

Several recent publications (4, 29, 53) have demonstrated the generation of nitric oxide (NO) by rat ventricular myocyte preparations containing 90%–95% ventricular myocytes, and have reported the immunoprecipitation of the enzyme endothelial nitric oxide synthase (eNOS) with caveolin3. In parallel experiments with purified endothelial cells, only caveolin1 could be precipitated with the eNOS antibody. These and related immunochemical experiments led the authors to conclude that their experiments "establish expression of eNOS in cardiac myocyte caveolae and document tissue-specific and quantitative association of eNOS with caveolin." These investigators subsequently reported (30) the translocation of m2 muscarinic acetylcholine receptor to cardiac myocyte caveolae upon agonist stimulation. In a further study (31) these same investigators identified modulation of the eNOS-caveolin interaction by carbachol. They concluded that these "results suggest that acylated eNOS may couple muscarinic receptor activation to heart rate control." This is an important conclusion with potentially important implications for normal and pathological functions of cardiac myocytes.

ENDOTHELIN AND PROTEIN KINASE C ISOFORMS IN CARDIAC MYOCYTE CAVEOLAE

Rybin, Xu, and Steinberg (107) have published experiments on neonatal mouse hearts from which they concluded that three phorbol ester–sensitive isoforms of protein kinase C (PKC) are translocated to the caveolar compartment of the cardiac myocytes by phorbol 12-myristate 13-acetate (PMA), an activator of PKC. The authors also found that endothelin selectively induces translocation to caveolae of the alpha and epsilon isoforms of PKC. Rybin et al. concluded that their studies "identify cardiomyocyte caveolae as a meeting place for activated PKC isoforms and their downstream target substrates." They noted that the localization of PKC isoforms to caveolae could be clearly shown when fractionation was performed in the absence of detergents, but that localization was not detectable when fractionation included exposure to detergents. In addition, the authors also show the co-localization of mitogen-activated protein (MAP) kinases as well as of extracellular signal-related protein (ERK) kinase, MAP kinase kinase (MEK), and certain family proteins Raf—all components of the ERK cascade. Recently these same authors have published experiments on rat neonatal myocytes from which they concluded that β-adrenergic receptor types 1 and 2 and adenylyl cyclase are differentially targeted to myocyte caveolae (107b). Other authors have recently published experiments from which they conclude that proteins involved in signal transduction localize to cardiac myocyte caveolae upon β-adrenergic stimulation (19).

IMMUNOELECTRON MICROSCOPIC LOCALIZATION OF THE MONOCARBOXYLATE TRANSPORTER, MCT-1 IN IN SITU RAT LEFT VENTRICULAR MYOCYTES

Johannssen et al. (51) used a colloidal gold–labeled antibody to the C-terminus of the monocarboxylate transporter MCT-1 to investigate the distribution of this protein in in situ rat cardiac myocytes of the left ventricular free wall. They found that, although the most densely labeled parts of the cardiac myocytes were the non-gap junctional parts of the intercalated disks, there was also substantial labeling of the caveolae, whereas intracellular membrane-limited compartments remained unlabeled. They also pointed out that a high cellular content of MCT-1 need not reflect a high degree of MCT-1 activity. Thus both the relationship of this transporter to the functions of cardiomyocyte caveolae, and the role of caveolae in the functions of MCT-1 remain to be clarified.

NEUREGULIN BINDING TO ITS RECEPTOR IN CARDIAC MYOCYTE CAVEOLAE

Neuregulins (NRGs) and their receptors (the erbB family) induce growth and differentiation in a variety of cells. Zhao et al. determined that ErbB4 and its co-receptor erbB2 are instrumental in survival and growth of cardiac myocytes in neonates and adults through regulation by NRG1 (152). The same investigators (153) subsequently localized an erbB2/B4 heterocomplex to myocyte caveolae. Upon stimulation with NRG1, erbB4 is induced to translocate out of caveolae, while erbB2 remains. As the authors state, "[this event] supports the hypothesis that ligand-induced translocation of erbB4 terminates signaling by the erbB2/erbB4 heterodimer."

ADENOSINE A1 RECEPTOR IN ADULT CARDIAC VENTRICULAR MYOCYTES

Lasley and associates have shown that the adenosine A1 receptor, which has recently been localized to cardiac myocyte caveolae, also translocates out of the caveolar compartment upon stimulation by agonist (62). These authors also speculate that translocation of the receptor may be part of a desensitization process, possibly by inducing translocation of PKC delta from the caveolar compartment (81).

EXPLORATION OF POSSIBLE INTERACTIONS OF CARDIAC MYOCYTE CAVEOLAE WITH EXTRACELLULAR MATRIX AND CYTOSKELETON-ASSOCIATED PROTEINS: DYSTROPHIN AND DYSTROGLYCAN

Like the plasma membrane into which their necks are inserted, cardiac myocyte caveolae are strategically located at the interface between the extracellular and cytoplasmic compartments. How caveolae interact with proteins impinging on them from the two faces of the plasma membrane—proteins of the extracellular matrix and proteins of the predominantly subplasmalemmal cytoskeleton—is potentially of both scientific and medical interest. This notion is underscored by two recent reports in which a correlation between mutations in the caveolin3 gene and clinically observed muscular dystrophies is observed (77, 77). As in skeletal muscle, a portion of the dystrophin present in cardiac myocytes is bound to caveolae (22). Dystrophin bound to caveolae can be immunoprecipitated along with caveolin3 in the absence of dystroglycan, suggesting that dystroglycan and its associated complex of proteins do not reside in caveolae.

DYNAMIC CLUSTERING OF SPHINGOLIPIDS AND CHOLESTEROL TO FORM FUNCTIONAL "RAFTS" IN CELLULAR MEMBRANES

A paper by Simons and Ikonen (123), a subsequent paper from the laboratory of Simons (42), and a review by Kurzchalia and Parton (59) are seminal sources and yield a synthesis of ideas about caveolae and caveolae-related concepts. Emphasizing the clustering of sphingolipids and cholesterol to form detergent-insoluble glycolipid-rich (DIG) domains or "rafts" that move within the fluid lipid bilayer of the plasma membrane, the authors propose "that these rafts function as platforms for the attachment of proteins when membranes are moved around inside the cell during signal transduction." They point out that caveolae, which are known to (1) lack clathrin coats, (2) contain clusters of glycosphingolipids (141), and (3) require cholesterol to function (104), are a subset of DIG domains, but that "many proteins identified in DIGs were not localized to caveolae. DIGs even contained proteins from different cellular organelles." Exposure of myocardial cells to the cholesterol-binding agent filipin selectively perturbs the structure of caveolae as seen in electron micrographs of freeze-fractured rabbit hearts, suggesting that heart myocyte caveolar membrane is cholesterol-enriched (118, 119, 130). Analysis of a highly caveolin3-enriched membrane fraction prepared from adult rat ventricular myocytes reveals a high concentration of cholesterol in the fraction (62), suggesting that cardiac myocyte caveolae are DIG-type domains.

DEVELOPMENT OF MORE EFFICIENT, SPECIFIC, AND SENSITIVE METHODS FOR IDENTIFYING THE INTRACAVEOLAR AND CAVEOLAE-BOUND PROTEINS OF CARDIAC MYOCYTES

Although confocal immunofluorescence microscopy and immunoelectron microscopy are useful tools for screening myocardial cell caveolae for proteins thought to be present within the caveolae and/or interacting with the caveolar membrane, these methods are often either unhelpful or inefficient for identifying and then studying proteins whose presence is unsuspected. Similar criticisms hold for conventional biochemical techniques as applied to the proteins of cardiac myocyte caveolae. Clearly, more efficient, specific, and sensitive methods are desirable. Improvements in methodology seem attainable by combining much more sensitive and specific analysis of proteins with appropriate new techniques of presenting very small, caveolae-specific protein samples to the analytical apparatus. The technical advances that underlie this improvement depend on several recently developed techniques: a silica coating procedure for the separation of caveolae from associated noncaveolar membrane microdomains from lung tissue (114), as applied by Stan et al. (136) in the laboratory of Palade to plasma membrane-associated caveolae; rapid (one hour) density gradient centrifugation using iodixanol (trade name OptiPrpe) as an alternative to sucrose (128); the use of magnetic beads bound with caveolin-specific antibody for the immunopurification of caveolae (20, 136); protein microsequencing methods which are sensitive to and usable at femtomolar protein concentrations, and can be used for sequencing of proteins from one- or two-dimensional polyacrylamide gels by "nano-electrospray mass spectrometry"

(68); and tagging of relevant proteins with green fluorescent protein to assess dynamic properties of the protein relative to caveolae by fluorescence microscopy and biochemical analysis (39).

SELECTED GENERAL TOPICS IN CAVEOLAR OR CAVEOLAE-RELEVANT BIOLOGY

This section is designed to provide access to selected topics of caveolar or caveolae-relevant biology, most of which have not yet been directly addressed in studies of cardiac myocyte caveolae.

Physical considerations—caveolae as plasma membrane microdomains or plasma membrane-associated microdomains

It is useful to consider some of the physical properties of caveolae in more detail. For this purpose caveolae may be regarded as specialized microdomains in contact and interacting with the plasma membrane. What is known about this subject has so far been studied in noncardiac cells and tissues (for recent reviews see refs. 59, 83, 121, and 128), but the questions investigated and the methods used are sufficiently general to be relevant to and deserving of study in myocardial cells.

Lateral movements of membrane proteins in noncaveolar plasma membrane. Caveolae are membrane-limited organelles that are inserted into the noncaveolar plasma membrane. As a first step toward understanding how caveolae or caveolae-associated proteins may move in the plane of the plasma membrane (as well as the constraints on such movements), it seems useful to summarize recent concepts of how proteins move or are constrained from moving in *noncaveolar* plasma membrane (24, 25, 50, 60, 107). These concepts extend the classical fluid mosaic model of plasma membrane proposed by Singer and Nicolson (126), in which the membrane was considered to be "a two-dimensional oriented solution of integral proteins... in the viscous phospholipid bilayer." The extension is largely the result of applying three methods to the study of biological membranes: fluorescence recovery after photobleaching (FRAP); single particle tracking (SPT), in which antibody-coated membrane components labeled with submicrometer colloidal gold particles are tracked with nanometer level precision by digital imaging microscopy; and the determination of the barrier-free path (BFP) by dragging macromolecules labeled with submicrometer beads through the membrane with a laser beam acting as an experimental optical trapping device called "optical tweezers."

Although none of these methods has so far been applied to heart muscle or isolated cardiac myocytes, the results are potentially general enough so that they may be relevant to cardiac plasma membrane, and therefore to the environment in which myocardial cell caveolae exist and function. Kusumi, Sako, and Yamamoto (60) did indeed show by SPT in plasma membrane of a mouse keratinocyte cell line that both lipids and a fraction of the population of labeled proteins diffuse freely in the plane of the membrane. But, contrary to the predictions of the fluid mosaic model, SPT of these cells indicated that substantial fractions of labeled cadherins, neural cell adhesion molecules (NCAMs), and receptors for nutrients and growth factors were confined, at least transiently, to small plasma membrane domains. These observations led the investigators to propose the "membrane-skeleton fence" model, in which a spectrin-like meshwork that is closely apposed to the cytoplasmic face of the plasma membrane sterically confines membrane-spanning proteins to regions of a size given by the size of the cytoskeletal mesh. Edidin, Zuniga, and Sheetz (25) used both FRAP and BFP to compare lateral mobilities of wild-type class I major histocompatibility complex (MHC) plasma membrane glycoproteins, which have full-length, 31-residue cytoplasmic domains, with lateral mobilities of mutant class I MHC glycoproteins, which have truncated cytoplasmic domains of 7, 4, or zero residues. The experiment was designed to test whether the length of the cytoplasmic residues significantly affects lateral mobility of these glycoproteins in the plasma membrane. The results showed that mutants with only four residues or none were much more mobile in the lipid bilayer than mutants with seven or more residues, which resisted being dragged through the lipid bilayer. At room temperature, the corresponding BFPs for the critically truncated lipid-linked isoform and the membrane-spanning untruncated isoforms were, respectively, 1700 nm and 600 nm. A preliminary report (125) describes the results of SPT on a cell line derived from muscle. In these cells, about 28% of the population of a particular isoform of glycosylphosphatidylinositol (GPI)-linked NCAM showed a mixture of confined and random diffusion in the lipid bilayer. The temporary confinement zones were about 300 nm in diameter and lasted about 6 sec before the NCAM escaped from confinement. The authors suggested that a mosaic plasma membrane structure with regions of high and low obstacle concentrations could account for their findings.

Caveolar Proteins

Evidence is accumulating that caveolae have lipid and protein compositions that differ significantly from the lipid and protein compositions of noncaveolar plasma membrane. Caveolae are a subclass of detergent-insoluble domains (DIGs) enriched in cholesterol and sphingolipids, while non-DIG plasma membrane is enriched in phospholipids (59). DIG domains (also referred to as detergent resistant domains (DRMs) or "rafts") are lipids in a liquid ordered (l_0)-like phase which have a high degree of order and thus a high melting temperature (76). It is the high degree of order that confers on the domain its relative detergent insolubility (or imperviousness to sonication). Many proteins that target to such domains are acylated (usually dually), while few contain the bulkier branched prenyl side-chains. It is widely appreciated that the properties of caveolae and their specific functions in most tissues are unknown or only partially known, and myocardial cell caveolae are no exception. One approach to characterizing caveolae is to develop methods for identifying caveolar proteins or caveolae-associated proteins for a specific cell type like cardiac myocytes, on the premise that such identification will provide clues to caveolar functions in this cell type. While the logic of these assumptions is attractive, their experimental verification is complicated by the observation that the number and species of proteins within caveolae can vary depending on the method used to isolate the caveolae for biochemical analysis or to preserve the tissue or cell type for immunocytology (58, 71, 72, 93, 115, 116). Moreover, care must be taken to distinguish between caveolin-containing and non-caveolin-containig DIGs (e.g. see the later discussion of GPI-linked proteins). Because lipids seem to play important roles in caveolar biology, these poorly understood roles also need to be discussed. The following section, a condensed survey of selected data from the literature on caveolae of noncardiac tissues and cell lines, provides a background against which to judge the more limited information on caveolae of myocardial cells.

Caveolin: The biochemistry of caveolae did not advance rapidly until the discovery by Palade and associates that caveolae of capillary endothelial cells have a characteristic striped bipolar surface structure (95) which was recognized by the investigators to be clearly distinct from the coat of clathrin-coated pits. Since the publication of those findings, the interest in the protein composition of caveolae has intensified. A protein localized to the striped bipolar surface of plasma membrane–associated caveolae was isolated by Rothberg et al. (102). (For simplicity, the name *caveolin* will be used in this chapter.) This protein was found to be identical to a 22 kD tyrosine phosphoprotein expressed by chick embryo fibroblasts infected with the Rous sarcoma virus (40), one of the main substrates of *src* kinase in v-*src*-transformed cells. The chicken caveolin was nearly identical to a canine vesicular membrane protein of 21 kD named VIP21 by Glenney (41), which was found by Kurzchalia et al. (57) to be a constituent of trans-Golgi network (TGN). The presence of caveolin in both TGN and caveolae suggested that the protein might co-sort in the TGN with proteins and lipids destined for specific plasma membrane domains (23). Experimental expression of caveolin in a lymphocyte cell line which does not, in the control state, express either caveolin or electron microscopically identifiable caveolae, causes de novo formation of caveolae in the transfected cells (33). This finding suggests that caveolin is a key structural component required for caveolar biogenesis.

Caveolin Isoforms: Evidence for the existence of different isoforms of caveolin has emerged. Kurzchalia et al. (57) and Scherer et al. (112) described two isoforms of the protein component of the caveolar coat that are widely expressed in many nonmuscle cell lines and tissues, as well as in skeletal, cardiac, and smooth muscles. These proteins have been cloned and have masses of about 21 and 24 kDa, or 22 and 25 kDa. Way and Parton (147) subsequently identified and cloned an apparently muscle-specific isoform present in rat skeletal and heart muscle, and probably in smooth muscle as well. This isoform, which they named *M-caveolin* to distinguish it from the widely expressed V or (vesicular)-caveolin, targets muscle cells and is associated with muscle cell caveolae but is not found in noncaveolar plasma membrane, as judged by immunoelectron microscopy. M-caveolin is a protein of 151 amino acid residues with a predicted mass of 17.3 kDa. Way and Parton found that the expression of M-caveolin is tightly regulated, because it is expressed only after differentiation of myoblasts into myotubes. Since database searches with M- and V-caveolin suggested the existence of at least one additional caveolin homologue, Way and Parton concluded that M- and V-caveolin are members of an emerging family of caveolin-related proteins in mammalian cells (147). Experiments from the laboratory of Lisanti, which deal with 24 kDa and 21 kDa isoforms of caveolin-1 (denoted, respectively, alpha- and beta-caveolin ([137], showed by microsequencing that both isoforms contain identical internal residues 44–77. Scherer et al. also expressed caveolin in an Fischer rat thyroid (FRT) cell line which does not constitutively express caveolin. Since stable transfection with full-length caveolin cDNA resulted in expression of both the 21 kDa and the 24 kDa isoforms, the authors concluded that the two isoforms can be derived from a single gene through alternate initiation during translation. Additional experiments suggested that the isoforms differ in their N-terminal sequences: one isoform, alpha-caveolin, contains residues 1–178 and has a complete N-terminus;

the other isoform, beta-caveolin, contains residues 32–178 and lacks specific N-terminal sequences. Confocal immunofluorescence microscopy showed that the subcellular distributions of the two isoforms differ, although their distributions overlap. Only the beta isoform of caveolin-1 is phosphorylated in vivo, though both the alpha and beta forms can be phosphorylated in vitro. Further experiments from the laboratory of Tang et al. (137) led to cloning of "caveolin-3," a muscle-specific third caveolin isoform corresponding to Parton and Way's "M-caveolin" and discovered independently by the two laboratories. Although caveolin3 is undoubtedly the caveolin isoform expressed abundantly in muscle, a recent abstract (143) and paper (47) describing the abundant expression of caveolin3 in astrocytes from the brain, indicates that the specificity of caveolin3 for myocytes is less than perfect.

Function of caveolin: The notion that caveolae are the locus mediating diverse signaling events in many cell types has gradually gained favor over the past decade. The growing number of receptors found in caveolae, e.g. the muscarinic, endothelin, neuregulin, and adenosine receptors in cardiac myocytes addressed in the present review, as well as the presence of G proteins and kinases in cardiac myocytes and other cells, attests to the importance of this hypothesis. An overriding issue concerns how the many and diverse proteins associated with signaling events are targeted to caveolae. The hypothesis advanced by Lisanti (for a review see ref. 82) is that caveolins contain a peptide sequence that acts as a scaffolding domain for caveolin-binding proteins which contain the complimentary sequence motif $\Phi X \Phi XXXX \Phi XX \Phi$, where Φ denotes an aromatic residue. This scaffolding domain is found at residues 82–101 in caveolin1, 54–73 in caveolin2, and 55–74 in caveolin3. Moreover, the cholesterol-rich and spingolipid-rich nature of caveolae complements the specific protein associations of caveolin (59). As noted earlier, caveolin itself is a cholesterol-binding protein, and Kurzchalia and Parton noted that "caveolin regulation of cellular cholesterol may be equally as important as direct interactions of caveolin with signaling molecules in the regulation of signal transduction."

Effects of caveolin and caveolin-derived peptides on GTPase activity of G proteins: Residues 82–101 of the nonmuscle isoform caveolin1 are involved in functionally important interactions with G protein α-subunits and thereby in the suppression of the basal GTPase activity via inhibition of GDP/GTP exchange (64b). Tang et al. (137) reported that a corresponding highly conserved region of caveolin3 (residues 82–101) suppresses the GTPase activity of both trimeric G-0 and G-i2 in a dose-dependent fashion, with IC-50 values of 3 and 5μM, 80% inhibition for G-0, and total inhibition for G-i2, at inhibitor concentration of 10μM. In addition, and unlike the caveolin1-derived peptide, lower concentrations of caveolin3 were found to stimulate GTPase activity.

Caveolae of endothelial cells contain critical proteins known to mediate vesicle formation, vesicle docking, and vesicle fusion. These include vSNARE, VAMP-2, monomeric and trimeric GTPases, annexins II and VI, the NEM-sensitive fusion factor NSF (which may, alternatively be a molecular chaperone for the membrane docking and/or fusion mechanisms (78b), as well as the NSF attachment protein, SNAP (114). These proteins play important roles in membrane trafficking via the pathway entered through clathrin-coated vesicles. In addition, endocytosis of caveolin1-containing caveolae has been elegantly demonstrated to be regulated by dynamin (reviewed in 128). Internalization of cardiac myocyte caveolae has to date not been demonstrated. By contrast, it is unclear what role, if any, caveolin itself plays in membrane traffic involving caveolae.

In a cell culture derived from human skin, oxidation of caveolar cholesterol with the enzyme cholesterol oxidase rapidly displaces caveolin from the plasma membrane to intracellular vesicles that co-localize with the Golgi apparatus, a displacement reversed upon removal of the cholesterol oxidase (127). Murata et al. (79) studied lipid interactions of caveolin by reconstituting caveolin expressed in the bacterium *Escherichia coli* into liposomes. They observed that caveolin could be reconstituted into the lipid membrane of the liposomes only when more than 30mol% of cholesterol was present in the lipid mixture. They concluded that caveolin is a cholesterol-binding protein, and that its cholesterol-binding property serves a specific function in the formation of microdomains during membrane trafficking. Consistent with this conclusion, Li et al. (64c), who incorporated a full-length recombinant caveolin into synthetic lipid (1,2-dioleylphosphorylcholine) membranes, found that addition of cholesterol increased the incorporation of caveolin into the membranes 25- to 30-fold.

Evidence for microtubule-dependent cycling of caveolin between the plasma membrane and the Golgi complex (16) was obtained in cultures of human fibroblasts pretreated briefly with the microtubule depolymerizing agent nocodazole, and then with cholesterol oxidase and nocodazole. This treatment caused caveolin to relocate from the plasma membrane to the endoplasmic reticulum (ER), and thence to the ER/Golgi intermediate compartment (ERGIC), but not to the Golgi. Depolymerization of microtubules after removal of cholesterol oxidase did not slow translocation of caveolin to the plasma membrane from the Golgi. Conrad et al. (16) took advantage of the well-known observation that transport substrates that normally move to the Golgi from pre-Golgi compartments are inhibited from thus moving when the temperature is lowered to 15°C, and that transport substrates trapped at 15°C in pre-Golgi compartments can be abruptly caused to move to the Golgi and beyond by raising the temperature from 15° to 37°C. In this way it was possible to show that only ERGIC to Golgi transport of caveolin, (and not Golgi to plasma membrane transport) was microtubule-dependent. These experiments were interpreted by Conrad et al. (16) as suggesting the existence of "a constitutive transport cycle in which caveolin moves reversibly between plasma membrane caveolae and the Golgi complex in normal, unperturbed cells." That conclusion is valid only if the half-life of caveolin is much longer than the duration of the experiment, as was indeed shown to be the case by a measured half-life of about 10 hours. Conrad et al. (16) suggest a model for the constitutive cycling of caveolin from ERGIC to plasma membrane via the Golgi complex, and from plasma membrane via the ER to ERGIC, and they argue that the rate-limitng step in the cycle is the translocation from plasma membrane to ER. They further suggest that caveolin may function to carry exogenous fatty acids from uptake sites at the plasma mambrane to the ER, citing unpublished findings that caveolin binds long-chain fatty acids with high affinity.

It remains to be determined what fraction of the protein in the striped coat of caveolae observed by electron microscopy (and decorated by antibodies to caveolin by immunoelectron microscopy of caveolae [102]) can be accounted for by caveolin, as well as what other constituents may be present in the filaments of the coat. Caveolin is not solubilized by the non-ionic detergent Triton X-100 or by the non-denaturing zwitterionic detergent CHAPS. As already noted, caveolin is the product of a single gene (41) and can be derived from a single cDNA (112).

Monier et al. (78) have pointed out that caveolin, the only caveolar coat protein so far identified, is an integral membrane protein, whereas the two other major classes of coat proteins for noncaveolar vesicles in the clathrin-coated and coatomer-coated vesicular pathways consist almost entirely of soluble proteins. Treatment of trans golgic network (TGN)-derived vesicles, or of purified membrane fractions derived from lung or from cultures of Madlin-Darby cultured kidney (MDCK) cells with CHAPS or Triton X-114, yields caveolin in large, insoluble structures, referred to by Monier et al. as 200–400 kDa, and 600 kDa complexes, based on results of sodium dodecylsulfate polyacrylamide gel electrophoresis (SDS-PAGE). Monier et al. further found that these oligomers of the two isoforms of caveolin are formed early after their synthesis in the ER, that the hydrophobic domain of caveolin adopts an unusual loop or hairpin configuration, which exposes both the N- and C-flanking regions to the cytoplasm; and that formation of complexes is a very early post-translational process and does not require a vesicle fusion step. They consider the insolubility of the complexes in CHAPS and Triton as evidence for a structure rich in glycosphingolipids. The authors leave open the possibility that caveolin may not cross the entire membrane bilayer, i.e., that it could be a monotopic protein (6), as recently described for prostaglandin H2 synthase-1 (95). The existence of caveolin within caveolar membranes as a high molecular mass homo-oligomer has also been observed by Sargiacomo et al (109).

Other caveolar proteins: reality vs. artifact

An extensive literature documents that many and diverse proteins can be anchored to the external surface of the plasma membrane by covalently attached glycolipids containing inositol (see reviews in refs. 18, 27, and 69). These so called GPI anchors, covalently attached to the C-terminal carboxyl group of the protein, consist of a complex oligoglycan linked to a phosphatidylinositol molecule in the lipid bilayer of the membrane. Insofar as it involves a covalent interaction, a GPI-anchored protein differs from other integral membrane proteins that interact with the lipid bilayer only by non-covalent interactions. GPI linkages have also been found on the internal surfaces of secretory granule membranes (32, 63). As emphasized in a recent review (2), "Nearly every caveola has a cluster of GPI anchored proteins," and, within a cluster, the protein density can reach as high as 30,000 molecules per square micrometer. The latter figure was obtained by studies on the 5-methyltetrahydrofolate receptor, a GPI-anchored protein detected in caveolae by immunoelectron microscopy using antibodies against the protein (103). The clustering of the receptor in caveolae required the presence of cholesterol in the membrane (103). These experiments led to the conclusion that folate receptors (and perhaps other GPI-anchored plasma membrane proteins), cycle reversibly between noncaveolar plasma membrane and a transient intracaveolar location, a conclusion that has become controversial (71, 72; see below).

A second approach, most extensively represented by experiments from the laboratory of Lisanti (66, 67, 110), is based on the assumption that proteins co-isolating with caveolin (as a marker for caveolae), and resistant to solution by the detergent Triton X-100, are highly enriched in the proteins that are normally present in caveolae of the intact cell line or tissue *before treatment with detergent*. This approach presupposes that the presence of these proteins in the detergent-resistant fraction isolated by ultracentrifugation in a sucrose density gradient and identified by Western immunoblots was not an artifact of the detergent extraction. In response to criticisms of the use of detergent treatment, as discussed below, Lisanti (80, 128, 133, 136), and others replace detergent treatment by treatment with sonication in the isolation of caveolin-enriched membrane domains. These issues are important, since a diverse group of proteins have been classified as caveolar or caveolae-associated by these methods (e.g., numerous proteins, including albumin, osteopoetin, GPI-linked proteins, caveolin, the glycoprotein receptor CD 36, a receptor for advanced glycosylation end products, plasma membrane porin, Src-like kinases, PKC, gelsolin, actin, heterotrimeric G proteins, and the Ras-related GTPases rap 1, rab 5, and surfactant protein A—(a member of the family of C-type lectins that recognizes cell surface glycosphingolipids) have all been found in this fraction (66).

The assignment of a constitutive intracaveolar localization for GPI-anchored proteins, among and others, has been challenged on the basis of at least three arguments: (*1*) Immunoelectron micrographs made by reacting the tissue with primary antibodies to GPI-anchored plasma membrane proteins and then crosslinking the bound primary antibody with secondary antibody to the primary antibody (a very common experimental design) cannot be used to prove that, in the non-crosslinked state, these proteins are normally constitutively concentrated within caveolae. Instead, under these conditions, the concentration of GPI-anchored proteins in caveolae is or could be an artifact caused by crosslinking the protein–primary antibody complex with secondary antibody. (*2*) Insolubility in the nonionic detergent Triton X-100 (or imperviousness to sonication) and subsequent separation of ensuing insoluble fragments by density-gradient centrifugation are neither necessary nor sufficient for distinguishing intracaveolar or cavolae-bound proteins from plasmalemmal proteins not contained in or not bound to caveolae. This is so because the use of Triton X-100 creates an artifactual separation of proteins between caveolar and noncaveolar plasma membrane and because some non-caveolin-containing plasmalemma as well as membranes from other organelles are detergent- and sonication-resistant. (*3*) The properties of vesicular structures defined as caveolae in electron micrographs of conventionally prepared and heavy metal–stained ultrathin tissue sections, freeze-fracture replicas of the plasma membrane fracture face, or negatively stained preparations may not correlate well with biochemical data on caveolar proteins. It is also becoming evident that the properties and interactions of the lipid and glycolipid components of caveolae and of the membranes with which these components interact require extensive study.

Mayor, Rothberg, and Maxfield (72) have shown by both fluorescence microscopy and immunoelectron microscopy that folate receptors, previously reported by Anderson et al. (1) to be clustered in plasma membrane caveolae, are in fact not constitutively clustered in caveolae but become clustered there only as an artifact of crosslinking with polyclonal secondary antibodies. Resolution of this issue seems crucial for distinguishing the in situ distribution of GPI-anchored proteins from artifactual redistributions. In this regard, crosslinking of cell surface glycolipids and of GPI-anchored proteins has been shown to induce receptor-mediated cell activation in specific cell lines (55, 138, 139). In the absence of such nonphysiological crosslinking, the receptors remain distributed diffusely over the plasma membrane. While it is possible that the artifactual redistribution by crosslinking mimics a physiological process, such a process has not been identified. Colocalization of caveolin with endothelin A receptors under conditions said to preclude artifactual redistribution of these proteins has been reported for cultured COS cells by Chun et al. (13). In a separate study (Mayor and Maxfield 1995), the authors show that GPI-anchored proteins, which are diffusely distributed over the cell surface in the control state before exposure to detergent, are caused by detergent treatment to redistribute into a more clustered distribution. Mayor and Maxfield conclude that GPI-anchored proteins are intrinsically detergent-insoluble in the milieu of the plasma membrane, and that their co-purification with caveolin does not reflect their native distribution.

The insolubility of GPI-anchored proteins depends chiefly on the acyl or alkyl chain composition of the membrane lipids, the membrane cholesterol content, or the content of neutral glycolipid. The degree of saturation of the acyl or alkyl moiety of the GPI anchor is probably also important. Saturated alkyl or acyl chains are the predominant components of the lipid portions of the anchors (73).

In polarized cells like epithelial cells, the post-translational modification of protein carboxy terminals, which produces a GPI anchor, anchors the protein indiscriminately to caveolar and noncaveolar plasma membrane, showing no preference for an intracaveolar localization. The anchor is also thought to contain information targeting "glycolipid rafts" from the TGN to the plasma membrane (65, 124). Crosslinking of GPI-anchored proteins seems to be a prerequisite for the signaling functions of some GPI-anchored proteins (9, 100).

An original and potentially promising approach to defining the relationship of caveolae to associated microdomains of GPI-anchored proteins is to use cationic colloidal silica particles to separate caveolae from caveolin-free domains enriched in GPI-anchored proteins (116). By immobilizing membrane molecules, cationic silica particles can be induced to interact with negatively charged sites on the cell surface, thereby stabilizing the surface against vesiculation or lateral rearrangement (11). This method was applied to the surface of endothelial cells in rat lung. The silica-coated membrane pellets thus produced were enriched in markers for endothelial surface components and showed little contamination with other membrane components. Caveolae were then mechanically stripped away from the noncaveolar plasma membrane during homogenization at low temperature in the presence of Triton X-100. After sucrose density homogenization, vesicles that looked by electron microscopy like caveolae were recovered. This product was significantly enriched in caveolae-specific markers like caveolin and the caveolae-associated calcium ATPase (36) and inositol triphosphate receptor (37), whereas proteins normally restricted to noncaveolar plasma membrane were almost totally excluded. Significantly, the product was not enriched with respect to GPI-linked proteins; i.e., *when detergents were avoided during purification, the GPI-anchored plasma membrane proteins did not redistribute so as to cluster in caveolae,* as after exposure to Triton X-100. The authors found that, although insoluble in Triton X-100, the caveolae-enriched fraction was partially solubilized by the detergents beta-octyl glucoside, CHAPS, deoxycholate, and sodium dodecyl sulfate.

Schnitzer et al. (116) argue further that a substantial but variable fraction of GPI-anchored proteins is partitioned on the cell surface into detergent-resistant glycolipid microdomains. In this connection, it has been shown by immunoelectron microscopy (using colloidal gold–labeled cholera toxin, which binds to glycosphingolipids), that the ganglioside GM-1 is concentrated in plasma membrane caveolae and in non-clathrin-coated "endocytic" vesicles of the TGN, which also immunostain for caveolin (93). Whereas the profiles of caveolae purified from the silica-coated rat lung endothelial cell membranes were fairly uniform in size and were flask-shaped like caveolar profiles, the detergent-resistant membranes isolated without silica coating were a mixture of much larger vesicles with nonuniform shapes, interspersed with nonvesiculated linear sheets and with some caveolae-like profiles.

After taking precautions to minimize artifactual aggregation of GPI-anchored proteins, Schnitzer et al. (116) concluded nevertheless that "a substantial but variable fraction of GPI-anchored proteins exists on the cell surface dynamically partitioned into detergent-resistant glycolipid microdomains that are not likely to be simply a consequence of detergent extraction, and that the size of this fraction may depend on cell type, culture, and ligand or antibody exposure," and that some of these microdomains "may associate with caveolae as an annular region at the opening" (to the interstitium). In this model, crosslinking GPI-anchored proteins enhances their tendency to partition into the microdomains. Schnitzer et al. (116) also succeeded in isolating a detergent-insoluble plasma membrane fraction stripped of caveolae, and were able to show that this noncaveolar fraction was enriched in GPI-anchored proteins (carbonic anhydrase, 5'-nucleotidase, and urokinase plasminogen activator receptor), which were absent from the caveolar fraction. The authors briefly describe experiments in which caveolae, isolated without detergent, were found to be enriched in caveolin and ganglioside but to be nearly free of GPI-anchored proteins. They suggest that lipid anchors, like GPI, are involved in the selective partition of proteins into microdomains and they call attention to their published findings describing lipid-anchored nonreceptor tyrosine kinases, GTP-binding proteins, and small GTPases in their experimental systems (34, 43, 59, 114, 115). Similar notions of the nature of "raft" microdomains have been expressed by a consortium of European authors.

These issues have been addressed in cardiac myocytes by combined biochemical, confocal microscopic, and immunoelectron microscopic studies from our laboratory that focus on the truncated cadherin (T-cadherin) (20). The cadherins are a family of calcium ion-dependent adhesion proteins (97). T-cadherin is a major GPI-anchored protein, which, unlike other cadherins, expresses the extracellular, but not the intracellular, amino acid sequences characteristic of typical cadherins. Although T-cadherin is present in Triton X-100–insoluble domains of sheep heart sarcolemma, and although it is the major GPI-linked protein in the detergent-insoluble fraction from sheep heart, it does not co-purify with caveolin3 when caveolin3 and immunoelectron microscopically observed caveolae are immunoprecipitated (20). Further, immunocytochemical and immunocytological analyses of rat atrial myocytes in cell culture indicate that the immunostaining patterns of T-cadherin and caveolin3, although similar, are clearly not identical. These finding suggests that, in intact in situ cardiac myocytes, T-cadherin may occupy a membrane domain close to but distinct from that of caveolin3, and therefore distinct from that of cardiac myocyte caveolae.

That not all detergent- or sonication-resistant membrane domains are caveolar is empasized by similar observations on the isolation of non-caveolin-containing detergent- or sonication-resistant membrane domains, including domains that contain GM3, c-Src, Rho-A, cholesterol, and sphingomyelin from mouse melanoma cells (48), phosphoinositol 4-phosphate kinase in A431 cells (148), reggae and GPI-linked proteins in neuronal cells (61), and epidermal growth factor receptor in A431 cells (146).

This work was supported by USPHS National Heart, Lung, and Blood Institute grants HL-10503 and HL-20592.

REFERENCES

1. Anderson, R. G. W. Dissecting clathrin-coated pits. *Trends Cell Biol.* 2:177–199, 1992.
2. Anderson, R. G. W. Caveolae: where incoming and outgoing messengers meet. *Proc. Natl. Acad. Sci. U.S.A.* 90:10909–10913, 1993.
3. Anderson, R. G. W., B. A. Kamen, R. G. Rothberg, and S. W. Lacey. Potocytosis: sequestration and transport of small molecules by caveolae. *Science* 255:410–411, 1992.
4. Balligand, J.-L., R. A. Kelly, P. A. Marsden T. W. Smith, and T. Michel. Control of cardiac muscle cell function by an endogenous nitric oxide signalling system. *Proc Natl Acad. Sci. U.S.A.* 90:347–351, 1993.
4b. Beaulieu, P., R. Cardinal, P. Page, F. Francoeur, J. Tremblay, and C. Lambert. Positive chronotropic and ionotropic effects of C-type natriuretic peptide in dogs. *Am. J. Physiol.* 273:H1933–H1940, 1997.
5. Birkenkamp-Demtroeder, K., S. Bongartz, and J. D. Schipke. Expression of water channels in human heart. *Faseb J.* 89:1998.
6. Blobel, G. Intracellular protein topogenesis. *Proc. Natl. Acad. Sci. U.S.A.* 77:1496–1500, 1980.
7. Block, S. M. Leading the procession: new insights into kinesin motors. *J. Cell Biol.* 140:1281–1284, 1998.
8. Bloom, G. S. and L. S. B. Goldstein. Cruising along microtubule highways: how membranes move through the secretory pathway. *J. Cell Biol.* 140:1277–1280, 1998.
9. Brown, D. The tyrosine connection: how GPI-anchored proteins activate T-cells. *Curr. Opin. Immunol.* 5:349–354, 1993.
10. Carafoli, E. and D. Guerini. Molecular and cellular biology of plasma membrane calcium ATPase. *Trends Cardiovasc. Med.* 3:177–184, 1993.
11. Chaney, L. K. and B. S. Jacobson. Coating cells with colloidal silica for high yield isolation of plasma membrane sheets and identification of plasma membrane proteins. *J. Biol Chem.* 258:10062–10072, 1983.
12. Chang, M. P., W. G. Mallet, K. E. Mostov, and F. M. Brodsky. Adaptor self-aggregation, adaptor receptor recognition and binding of alpha-adaptin subunits to the plasma membrane contribute to recruitment of adaptor (AP2) components of clathrin-coated pits. *EMBO J.* 12:2169–2180, 1993.
13. Chun, M., U. K. Liyanage, M. P. Lisanti, and H. F. Lodish. Signal transduction of a G protein-coupled receptor in caveolae: colocalization of endothelin and its receptor with caveolin. *Proc. Natl. Acad. Sci. U.S.A.* 91:11728–11732, 1994.
14. Clemo, H. F., J. J. Feher, and C. N. Baumgarten. Modulation of rabbit ventricular cell volume and Na/K/2Cl cotransport by cGMP and atrial natriuretic factor. *J. Gen. Physiol.* 100:89–114, 1992.
15. Clemo, H. F., J. J. Feher, and C. M. Baumgarten. Modulation of rabbit ventricular cell volume and Na/K/2Cl cotransport by cGMP and atrial natriuretic factor. *J. Gen. Physiol.* 100:89–114, 1992.
16. Conrad, P. A., E. J. Smart, Y.-S. Ying, R. G. W. Anderson, and G. S. Bloom. Caveolin cycles between plasma membrane caveolae and the Golgi complex by microtubule-dependent and microtubule-independent steps. *J. Cell Biol.* 131:1421–1433, 1995.
17. Cook, R. F. and M. Sargiacomo. Characterization of caveolin-rich membrane domains isolated from an endothelial-rich source: implications for human disease. *J. Cell Biol.* 126:111–126, 1994.
18. Cross, G. A. M. Glycolipid anchoring of plasma membrane proteins. *Annu. Rev. Cell Biol.* 6:1–39, 1990.
19a. De Camilli, P., S. D. Emr, P. S. McPherson, and P. Novick. Phosphoinositides as regulators in membrane traffic. *Science* 271:1533–1539, 1996.
19b. De Luca, A., M. Sargiacomo, A. Puca, G. Sgaramella, P. De Paolis, G. Frati, C. Morisco, B. Trimarco, M. Volpe, and G. Condorelli. Characterization of caveolae from rat heart: localization of postreceptor signal transduction molecules and their rearrangement after norepinephrine stimulation. *J. Cell Biochem.* 77:529–539, 2000.
20. Doyle, D. D., G. E. Goings, J. Upshaw-Earley, E. Page, B. Ranscht, and H. C. Palfrey. T-cadherin is a major glycophosphoinositol-anchored protein associated with noncaveolar detergent-insoluble domains of the cardiac sarcolemma. *J. Biol. Chem.* 273:6937–6943, 1998.
21. Doyle, D. D., S. K. Ambler, J. Upshaw-Earley, A. Bastawropus, G. E. Goings and E. Page. Type B atrial natriuretic peptide receptor in cardiac myocyte caveolae. *Circ. Res.* 81:86–91, 1997.
22. Doyle, D. D., G. Goings, J. Upshaw-Earley, S. K. Ambler, A. Mondul, H. C. Palfrey, and E. Page. Dystrophin associates with caveolae of rat cardiac myocytes. *Circ. Res.* 87:480–488, 2000.
23. Dupree, P., R. G. Parton, G. Raposo, T. V. Kurzchalia, and K. Simons. Caveolae and sorting in the trans-Golgi network of epithelial cells. *EMBO J.* 12:1597–1604, 1993.
24. Edidin, M., S. C. Kuo, and M. P. Sheets. Lateral movements of membrane glycoproteins restricted by dynamic cytoplasmic barriers. *Science* 254:1379–1382, 1991.
25. Edidin, M., M. C. Zuniga, and M. P. Sheets. Truncation mutants define and locate cytoplasmic barriers to lateral mobility of membrane glycoproteins. *Proc. Natl. Acad Sci. U.S.A.* 91:3378–3382, 1994.
26. Engel, A., T. Walz, and P. Agre. The aquaporin family of membrane water channels. *Curr. Opin. Struct. Biol.* 4, 545–553, 1994.
27. Englund, P. T. The structure and biosynthesis of glycosyl phosphatidylinositol protein anchors. *Annu. Rev. Biochem.* 62:121–138, 1993.
28. Fawcett, D. W. The ultrastructure of the cat myocardium. I. Ventricular papillary muscle. *J. Cell Biol.* 42:1–45, 1969.
29. Feron, O., L. Belhassen, L. Kobzig, T. W. Smith, R. A. Kelly, and T. Michel. Endothelial nitric oxide synthase targeting to caveolae: specific interactions with caveolin isoforms in cardiac myocytes and endothelial cells. *J. Biol. Chem.* 271:22810–22814, 1996.
30. Feron, O., T. W. Smith, T. Michel, and R. A. Kelly. Dynamic targeting of the agonist-stimulated m2 muscarinic acetylcholine receptor to caveolae in cardiac myocytes. *J. Biol. Chem.* 272:17744–17748, 1997.
31. Feron, O., C. Dessy, D. J. Opel, M. A. Arstall, R. A. Kelly and T. Michel. Modulation of the endothelial nitric-oxide synthase–caveolin interaction in cardiac myocytes. Implications for the autonomic regulation of heart rate. *J. Biol. Chem.* 273:30249–30254, 1998.
32. Fouchier, F., P. Bastiani, T. Baltz, D. Aunis, and G. Rougon. Glycosylphosphatidylinositol is involved in the membrane attachment of proteins in granules of chromaffin cells. *Biochem J.* 256:103–108, 1988.
33. Fra, A. M., E. Williamson, K. Simons, and R. G. Parton. *De novo* formation of caveolae in lymphocytes by expression of

VIP21-caveolin. *Proc. Natl. Acad. Sci. U.S.A.* 92:8655–8659, 1995.
34. Friedrichson, T. and T. Kurzchalia. Microdomains of GPI-anchored proteins in living cells revealed by crosslinking. *Nature* 394:802–805, 1998.
35. Frigeri, A., M. A. Gropper, F. Umenishi, M. Kawashima, D. Brown, and A. S. Verkman. Localization of MIWC and GLIP water channel homologs in neuromuscular, epithelial and glandular tissues. *J. Cell. Sci.* 108:2993–3002, 1995.
36. Fujimoto, T. Calcium pump of the plasma membrane is localized in caveolae. *J. Cell Biol.* 120:1147–1149, 1993.
37. Fujimoto, T., S. Nakada, A. Miyawaki, A. Mikoshiba, and K. Ogawa. Localization of inositol 1,4,5-triphosphate receptor-like protein in plasmalemmal caveolae. *J. Cell Biol.* 119:1507–1513, 1992.
38. Gabella, G. Inpocketings of cell membrane (caveolae) in the rat myocardium. *J. Ultrastruct. Res.* 65:135–147, 1978.
39. Galbiati, F., D. Volonte, D. Meani, G. Milligan, D. M. Lublin, M. P. Lisanti, and M. Parenti. The dually acylated NH_2-terminal domain of G_{i1a} is sufficient to target a green fluorescent protein reporter to caveolin-enriched plasma membrane domains. Palmitoylation of caveolin-1 is required for the recognition of dually acylated G-protein a subunits in vivo. *J. Biol. Chem.* 274:5843–5850, 1999.
40. Glenney, J. R. and L. Zokas. Novel tyrosine kinase substrates from Rous sarcoma virus–transformed cells are present in the membrane cytoskeleton. *J. Cell Biol.* 108:2401–2408, 1989.
41. Glenney, J. R. The sequence of human caveolin reveals identity with VIP21, a component of transport vesiscles. *FEBS Lett.* 314:45–48, 1992.
42. Hansen, S. H., K. Sandvig, and B. van Deurs. Molecules internalized by clathrin-independent endocytosis are delivered to endosomes containing transferrin receptors. *J. Cell Biol.* 123:89–97, 1993.
43. Harder, T, P. Scheiffele, P. Verkade, and K. Simons. Lipid domain structure of the plasma membrane revealed by patching of membrane components. *J. Cell Biol.* 141:929–942, 1998.
43b. Hasegawa, H., T. Ma, W. Skach, and M. A. Matthay. Molecular cloning of a mercurial-insensitive water channel expressed in selected water-transporting tissues. *J. Biol. Chem.* 269:5497–5500, 1994.
44. Heuser, J. Three-dimensional visualization of coated vesicle formation in fibroblasts. *J. Cell Biol.* 84:560–563, 1980.
45. Heuser, J. E., T. S. Reese, M. J. Dennis, Y. Jan, L. Jan, and L. Evans. Synaptic vesicle exocytosis captured by quick freezing and correlated with quantal transmitter release. *J. Cell Biol.* 81:275–300, 1979.
45b. Hirose, M., Y. Furukawa, F. Kurogouchi, K. Nakajima, Y. Miyashita, and S. Chiba. C-type natriuretic peptide increases myocardial contractility and sinus rate mediated by guanylyl cyclase-linked natriuretic peptide receptors in isolated, blood-perfused dog heart preparations. *J. Pharm. Exp. Ther.* 286:70–76, 1998.
46. Iida, H., W. M. Barron, and E. Page. Monensin turns on microtubule-associated translocation of secretory granules in cultured atrial myocytes. *Circ. Res.* 62:1159–1170, 1988.
47. Ikezu, T., H. Ueda, B. D. Trapp, K. Nishiyama, J. F. Sha, D. Volonte, F. Galbiati, A. L. Byrd, G. Bassell, H. Serizawa, W. S. Lane, M. P. Lisanti, and T. Okamoto. Affinity-purification and characterization of caveolins from the brain: differential expression of caveolin-1,-2, and-3 in brain endothelial and astroglial cell types. *Brain Res.* 804:177–192, 1998.
48. Iwabuchi, K., K. Handa, and S. Hakomori. Separation of "glycolipid signaling domain" from caveolin-containing membrane fraction in mouse melanoma B16 cells and its role in cell adhesion coupled with signaling. *J. Biol. Chem.* 273:33766–33773, 1998.
49. Izumi, T., Y. Shibata, and T. Yamamoto. The cytoplasmic surface structures of uncoated vesicles in various tissues of rat as revealed by quick-freeze, deep-etching replicas. *J. Electron Microsc.* 38:47–53, 1989.
50. Jacobson, K., E. D. Sheets, and R. Simson. Revisiting the fluid mosaic model of membranes. *Science* 268:1441–1442, 1995.
51. Johannsson, E., E. Nagelhus, K. J. A. McCullagh, O. M. Sejersted, T. W. Blackstad, A. Bonen, and O. P. Ottersen. Cellular and subcellular expression of the monocarboxylate transporter MCT1 in rat heart: a high-resolution immunogold analysis. *Circ. Res.* 80:400–407, 1997.
52. Juen, P. S. T. and D. L. Garbers 1992. Guanylyl cyclase-linked receptors. *Annu. Rev. Neurosci.* 15:193–225, 1992.
53. Kelly, R., J.-L. Balligand, and T. W. Smith. Nitric oxide and cardiac function. *Circ. Res.* 79:363–380, 1996.
54. Kordylewski, L., G. E. Goings, and E. Page. Rat atrial myocyte plasmalemmal caveolae in situ. Reversible experimental increases in caveolar size and in surface density of caveolar necks. *Circ. Res.* 73:135–146, 1993.
55. Korty, P. E., C. Brando, and E. M. Shevach. *J. Immunol.* 146: 4092–4098, 1991: [Korty et al.] CD59 functions as a signal-transducing molecule for human T-cell activation.
56. Kreis, T. E. Regulation of vesicular and tubular membrane traffic of the Golgi complex by coat proteins. *Curr. Opin. Cell Biol.* 4:609–615, 1992.
57. Kurzchalia, T. V., P. Dupree, R. G. Parton, R. Kellner, H. Virta, M. Lehnert, and K. Simons. VIP21, a 21-KD membrane protein is an integral component of trans-Golgi network-derived transport vesicles. *J. Cell Biol.* 118:1003–1114, 1992.
58. Kurzchalia, T. V., E. Hartmann, and P. Dupree. Guilt by insolubility—does a protein's detergent insolubility reflect a caveolar location? *Trends Cell Biol.* 5:187–189, 1995.
59. Kurzchalia, T. V. and R. G. Parton. Membrane microdomains and caveolae. *Curr. Opin. Cell Biol.* 11:424–431, 1999.
60. Kusumi, A., Y. Sako, and M. Yamamoto. Confined membrane diffusion of membrane receptors as studied by single particle tracking (nanovid microscopy). Effects of calcium-induced differentiation in cultured epithelial cells. *Biophys. J.* 65:2021–2040, 1993.
61. Lang, D. M., S. Lommel, M. Jung, R. Ankerhold, B. Petraush, U. Laessing, M. F. Wiechers, H. Plattner, and C. A. Stuermer. Identification of reggie-t and reggie-2 as plasmamembrane-associated proteins which cocluster with activated GPI-linked cell adhesion molecules in non-caveolar micropatces in neurons. *J. Neurobiol.* 37:502–523, 1998.
62. Lasley, R. D., P. Narayan, A. Uittenbogaard, and E. J. Smart. Activated cardiac adenosine A_1 receptors translocate out of caveolae. *J. Biol. Chem.* 275:4417–4421, 2000.
63. LeBel, D. and M. Beattie. The major protein of pancreatic zymogen granule membranes (GP-2) is anchored via covalent bonds to phosphatidylinositol. *Biochem. Biophys. Res. Commun.* 154:818–823, 1988.
63b. Lee, S. J., S. Z. Kim, X. Cui, S. H. Kim, K. S. Lee, Y. J. Chung, and K. W. Cho. C-type natriuretic peptide inhibits ANP secretion and atria dynamics in perfused atria: NPR-B-cGMP signalling. *Am. J. Physiol. Heart Cir. Physiol.* 278: H208–H221, 2000.
64. Levin, K. R. and E. Page. Quantitative studies on plasmalemmal folds and caveolae of rabbit ventricular myocardial cells. *Circ. Res.* 46:244–255, 1980.
64b. Li, S., T. Okamoto, M. Chun, M. Sargiacomo, J. E. Casanova, S. H. Hansen, I. Nishimoto, and M. P. Lisanti. Evidence for a regulated interaction between heterotrimeric G proteins and caveolin. *J. Biol. Chem.* 270:15693-15701, 1995.

64c. Li, S., K. S. Song, and M. P. Lisanti. Expression and characterization of recombinant caveolin. Purification by polyhistidine tagging and cholesterol-dependent incorporation into defined lipid membranes. *J. Biol. Chem.* 271:568–573, 1996.

65. Lisanti, M. P. and E. Rodriguez-Boulan. Glycophospholipid membrane anchoring provides clues to the mechanism of protein sorting in polarized epithelial cells. *Trends Biochem. Sci.* 15:113–118, 1990.

66. Lisanti, M. P., P. E. Scherer, J. Vidugiriene, Z. L. Tang, A. Hermanowski-Vosatka, Y.-H. Tu, R. F. Cook, and M. Sargiacomo. Characterization of caveolin-rich membrane domains isolated from an endothlial-rich source: implications for human disease. *J. Cell Biol.* 126:111–1126, 1994.

67. Lisanti, M. P., Z. L. Tang, and M. Sargiacomo. Caveolin forms a hetero-oligomeric protein complex that interacts with an apical GPI-linked protein: implications for the biogenesis of caveolae. *J. Cell Biol.* 123:595–604, 1993.

68. Loo, J. A., and R. R. Ogorzalek Loo. Electrospray ionization mass spectroscopy of peptides and proteins. In *Electrospray Ionization Mass Spectrometry*, edited by R. B. Cole. New York: John Wiley & Sons, Inc., 1997:385–419.

69. Low, M. G. The glycosyl-phosphatidylinositol anchor of membrane proteins. *Biochim. Biophys. Acta* 988:427–454, 1989.

69b. Ma, T., B. Yang, and A. S. Verkman. Cloning of a novel and urea-permeable aquaporin from mouse expressed strongly in colon, placenta, liver, and heart. *Biochem. Biophys. Res. Commun.* 240:324–328, 1997.

70. Marsh, M. and D. Cutler. Membrane traffic: taking the Rabs off endocytosis. *Curr. Biol.* 3:30–33, 1993.

71. Mayor, S. and F. R. Maxfield. Insolubility and redistribution of GPI-anchored proteins at the cell surface after detergent treatment. *Mol. Biol. Cell* 6:929–944, 1995.

72. Mayor, S., K. G. Rothberg, and F. R. Maxfield. Sequestration of GPI-anchored proteins in caveolae triggered by cross-linking. *Science* 264:1948–1951, 1994.

73. McConville, M. J. and M. A. Ferguson. The structure, biosynthesis and function of glycosylated phosphatidylinositols in the parasitic protozoa and higher eukaryotes. *Biochem. J.* 294:305–324, 1993.

74. McNally, E. M., E. de Sa Moreira, D. J. Duggan, C. G. Bonnemann, M. P. Lisanti, H. G. W. Lidov, M. Vainzof, M. R. Passos-Bueno, E. P. Hoffman, M. Zatz, and L. M. Kinkel. Caveolin-3 in muscular dystrophy. *Hum. Mol. Genet.* 7:871–877, 1998.

75. Melancon, P. Vesicle traffic: "G Whizz." *Curr. Biol.* 3:230–233, 1993.

76. Melkonian, K. A., A. G. Ostermeyer, J. Z. Chen, M. G. Roth, and D. A. Brown. Role of lipid modifications in targeting proteins to detergent-resistant membrane rafts. Many raft proteins are acylated, while few are prenylated. *J. Biol. Chem.* 274:3910–3917, 1999.

77. Minetti, C., F. Sotgia, C. Bruno, P. Scartezzini, P. Broda, M. Bado, E. Masetti, M. Mazzocco, A. Egeo, M. A. Donati, D. Volonte, F. Galbiati, G. Cordone, F. D. Bricarelli, M. P. Lisanti, and F. Zara. Mutations in the caveolin-3 gene cause autosomal dominant limb-girdle muscular dystrophy. *Nature Genet.* 18:365–368, 1998.

78. Monier, S., R. G. Parton, F. Vogel, J. Behlke, A. Henske, and T. V. Kurzchalia. VIP21-caveolin, a membrane protein constituent of the caveolar coat, oligomerizes in vivo and in vitro. *Mol. Biol. Cell* 6:911–927, 1995.

78b. Morgan, A. and R. D. Burgoyne. A role for soluble NSF attachment proteins (SNAPS) in regulated exocytosis in adrenal chromaffin cells. *Embo. J.* 14:232–239, 1995.

79. Murata, M., J. Peranen, R. Schreiner, F. Wieland, T. Kurzchalia, and K. Simons. VIP21/caveolin is a cholesterol-binding protein. *Proc. Natl. Acad. Sci. U.S.A.* 92:10339–10343, 1995.

80. Oh, P. and J. E. Schnitzer. Immunoisolation of caveolae with high affinity antibody binding to the oligomeric caveolin cage. *J. Biol. Chem.* 274:23144–23154, 1999.

81. Narayan, P., H. H. Valdivia, R. M. Mentzer Jr., and R. D. Lasley. Adenosine A_1 receptor stimulation antagonizes the negative inotropic effects of PKC activator dioctanoylglycerol. *J. Mol. Cell Cardiol.* 30:913–921, 1998.

81b. Ohyama, Y., K. Miyamoto, Y. Morishita, Y. Matsuda, Y. Saito, N. Minamino, K. Kangawa, and H. Matsuo. Stable expression of natriuretic peptide receptors: effects of HS-142-1, a non-peptide ANP antagonist. *Biochem. Biophys. Res. Comm.* 189:336–342, 1992.

82. Okamoto, T., A. Schlegel, P. E. Scherer, and M. P. Lisanti. Caveolins, a family of scaffolding proteins for organizing "preassembled signaling complexes" at the plasma membrane. *J. Biol. Chem.* 273:5419–5422, 1998.

83. Ostrom, R. S. and P. A. Insel. Signal transduction pathways in caveolae. *Sci. Med.* Jan/Feb:44–53, 2000.

84. Page, E. Tubular systems in Purkinje cells of the cat heart. *J. Ultrastruct. Res.* 17:72–83, 1966.

85. Page, E., G. E. Goings, J. Upshaw-Earley, and D. A. Hanck. Endocytosis and uptake of lucifer yellow by cultured atrial myocytes and isolated intact atria from adult rats. Regulation and subcellular localization. *Circ. Res.* 75:335–346, 1994.

86. Page, E., G. E. Goings, B. Power, and J. Upshaw-Earley. Ultrastructural features of atrial peptide secretion. *Am. J. Physiol.* 251 (*Heart Circ. Physiol.* 20):H340–H348, 1986.

87. Page, E., G. E. Goings, B. Power, and J. Upshaw-Earley. Basal and stretch-augmented natriuretic peptide secretion by quiescent rat atria. *Am. J. Physiol.* 259 (*Cell Physiol.* 28):C801–C818, 1990.

88. Page, E., J. Upshaw-Earley, and G. E. Goings. Localization of atrial natriuretic peptide in caveolae of in situ atrial myocytes. *Circ. Res.* 75:949–954, 1994.

89. Page, E., J. Upshaw-Earley, and G. E. Goings. Permeability of rat atrial endocardium, epicardium, and myocardium to large molecules: stretch-dependent effects. *Circ. Res.* 71:159–173, 1992.

90. Page, E., J. Upshaw-Earley, G. E. Goings, and D. A. Hanck. Effect of external Ca^{2+} concentration on stretch-augmented natriuretic peptide secretion by rat atria. *Am. J. Physiol.* 260 (*Cell Physiol.* 29):C756–C762, 1991.

91. Page, E., J. Winterfield, G. E. Goings, A. Bastawrous, J. Upshaw-Earley, and D. D. Doyle. Water channel proteins in rat cardiac myocyte caveolae: osmolarity-dependent reversible internalization. *Am. J. Physiol.* 274 (*Heart Circ. Physiol.* 43):H1988–H2000, 1998.

92. Palade, G. E. Fine structure of blood capillaries. *J. Appl. Physics* 24, 1414, 1953 (Abstr).

93. Parton, R. G. Ultrastructural localization of gangliosides; GM-1 is concentrated in caveolae. *J. Histochem. Cytochem.* 42:155–166, 1994.

94. Parton, G. and K. Simons. Digging into caveolae. *Science* 269:1398–1399, 1995.

95. Peters, K.-R., W. W. Carley, and G. E. Palade. Endothelial plasmalemmal vesicles have a characteristic striped bipolar surface structure. *J. Cell Biol.* 101:2233–2238, 1985.

96. Picot, D., P. J. Loll, and R. M. Garavito. The X-ray crystal structure of the membrane protein prostaglandin H-2 synthase-1. *Nature* 367:243–249, 1994.

97. Poulos, A. C., J. E. Rash, and J. K. Elmund. Ultrarapid freezing reveals that skeletal muscle caveolae are semipermanent structures. *J. Ultrastruct. Res.* 96:114–124, 1986.

98. Ranscht, B., and M. T. Dours-Zimmermann. T-cadherin, a

novel cadherin cell adhesion molecule in the nervous system, lacks the conserved cytoplasmic region. *Neuron* 7:391–402, 1991.
99. Rayns, D. G., F. O. Simpson and W. S. Bertaud. Surface features of striated muscle. I. Guinea-pig cardiac muscle. *J. Cell Sci.* 3:467–474, 1968.
100. Robinson, P. J. Phosphatidylinositol membrane anchors and T-cell activation. *Immunol. Today* 12:35–41, 1991.
101. Rostgaard, J. and O. Behnke. Fine structural localization of adenine nucleoside. Phosphatase activity in the sarcoplasmic reticulum and the T system of rat myocardium. *J. Ultrastruct. Res.* 12:579–591, 1965.
102. Rothberg, K. G., J. E. Heuser, W. C. Donzell, Y.-S. Ying, J. R. Glenney, and R. G. W. Anderson. Caveolin, a protein component of caveolae membrane coats. *Cell* 68:673–682, 1992.
103. Rothberg, K. G., Y. Ying, J. F. Kolhouse, B. A. Kamen, and R. G. W. Anderson. The glycophospholipid-linked folate receptor internalizes folate without entering the clathrin-coated pit endocytic pathway. *J. Cell Biol.* 110:637–649, 1990.
104. Rothberg, K. G., Y.-S. Ying, B. A. Kamen, and R. G. W. Anderson. Cholesterol controls the clustering of the glycophospholipid-anchored membrane receptor for 5-methyltetrahydrofolate. *J. Cell Biol.* 111:2931–2938, 1990.
105. Rothman, J. E. and F. T. Wieland. Protein by transport vesicles. *Science* 272:227–234, 1996.
106a. Rybin, V. O., X. Xu, and S. F. Steinberg. Activated protein kinase C isoforms target to cardiomyocyte caveolae. Stimulation of local protein phosphorylation. *Circ. Res.* 84:980–988, 1999.
106b. Rybin, V. O., X. Xu, M. P. Lisanti, and S. F. Steinberg. Differential targeting of β-adrenergic receptor subtypes and adenylyl cyclase to cardiomyocyte caveolae. *J. Biol. Chem.* 275:41447–41457, 2000.
107. Sako, Y. and A. Kusumi. Compartmentalized structure of the plasma membrane for receptor movements as revealed by a nanometer-level motion analysis. *J. Cell Biol.* 125:1251–1264, 1994.
108. Sandvig, K., S. Olsnes, O. W. Petersen, and B. van Deurs. Acidification of the cytosol inhibits endocytosis from coated pits. *J. Cell Biol.* 105:679–689, 1987.
109. Sargiacomo, M., P. E. Scherer, Z.-L. Tang, E. Kubler, K. S. Song, M. C. Sanders, and M. C. Lisanti. *Proc. Natl. Acad. Sci. U.S.A.* 92:9407–9411, 1995. Oligomeric structure of caveolin: implications for caveolae membrane organization.
110. Sargiacomo, M., M. Sudol, Z. L. Tang, and M. P. Lisanti. Signal transducing molecules and glycosyl-phosphatidylinositol-linked prteins form a caveolin-rich insoluble complex in MDCK cells. *J. Cell Biol.* 122:789–807, 1993.
111. Schekman, R. and L. Orci. Coat proteins and vesicle budding. *Science* 271:1526–11533, 1996.
112. Scherer, P. E., Z. L. Tang, M. Chun, M. Sargiacomo, H. F. Lodish, and M. P. Lisanti. Caveolin isoforms differ in their N-terminal protein sequence and subcellular distribution. *J. Biol. Chem.* 270:16395–16401, 1995.
112b. Schipke, J. D., K. Birkenkamp-Demtroeder, and U. Schwanke. Myocardial hibernation: another view. *Z. Kardiol.* 89:259–263, 2000.
113. Schnitzer, J. E. Update on the cellular and molecular basis of capillary permeability. *Trends Cardiovasc. Med.* 3:124–130, 1993.
114. Schnitzer, J. E., J. Allard, and P. Oh. NEM inhibits transcytosis, endocytosis, and capillary permeability: implication of caveolae fusion in endothelia. *Am. J. Physiol.* 268 (*Heart Circ. Physiol.* 37):H48–H55, 1995.
115. Schnitzer, J. E., J. Liu, and P. Oh. Endothelial caveolae have the molecular transport machinery for vesicle budding, docking, and fusion including VAMP, NSF, SNAP, annexins, and GTPases. *J. Biol. Chem.* 270:14399–14404, 1995.
116. Schnitzer, J. E., D. P. McIntosh, A. M. Dvorak, J. Liu, and P. Oh. Separation of caveolae from associated microdomains of GPI-anchored proteins. *Science* 269:1435–1439, 1995.
117. Schnitzer, J. E., P. Oh, E. Pinney, and J. Allard. Filipin-sensitive caveolae-mediated transport in endothelium: reduced transcytosis, scavenger endocytosis, and capillary permeability of select macromolecules. *J. Cell Biol.* 127:1217–1132, 1994.
118. Severs, N. J. Localization of cholesterol in the Golgi apparatus of cardiac muscle cells. *Experientia* 37:1195–1197, 1981.
119. Severs, N. J. Comparison of the response of myocardial muscle and capillary endothelial nuclear membranes to the cholesterol probe filipin. *J. Submicrosc. Cytol.* 14:441–452, 1982.
120. Severs, N. J. Caveolae: static inpocketings of the plasma membrane, dynamic vesicles or plain artifact? *J. Cell Sci.* 90:341–348, 1988.
121. Shaul, P. W. and R. G. W. Anderson. Role of plasmalemmal caveolae in signal transduction. *Am. J. Physiol.* 275 (*Lung Cell Mol. Physiol.* 19):L843–L851, 1998.
122. Simionescu, N. and M. Simionescu. Receptor-mediated transcytosis of albumin: identification of albumin binding proteins in the plasma membrane of capillary endothelium. *Microcirculation*, vol. 1, edited by M. Tsuchiya et al. New York: Elsevier, 1987:67–82.
123. Simons, K. and E. Ikonen. Functional rafts in cell membranes. *Nature* 387:569–572, 1997.
124. Simons, K. and A. Wandinger-Ness. Polarized sorting in epithelia. *Cell* 62:207–210, 1990.
125. Simson, R., B. Yang, P. Doherty, S. Moore, F. Walsh, and K. Jacobson. The mosaic structure of cell membranes revealed by transient confinement of GPI-linked NCAM-125. *Biophys. J.* 68:436, 1995 (abstr).
126. Singer, S. J. and G. L. Nicolson. The fluid mosaic model of the structure of cell membranes. *Science* 175:720–731, 1972.
127. Smart, E. J., Y.-S. Ying, P. A. Conrad, and R. G. W. Anderson. Caveolin moves from caveolae to the Golgi apparatus in response to cholesterol oxidation. *J. Cell Biol.* 127:1185–1197, 1994.
128. Smart, E. J., Y.-S. Ying, C. Mineo, and R. G. W. Anderson. A detergent-free method for purifying caveolae membrane from tissue culture cells. *Proc. Natl. Acad. Sci. U.S.A.* 92:10104–10108, 1995.
129. Smart, E. J., G. A. Graf, M. A. McNiven, W. C. Sessa, J. A. Engelman, P. E. Scherer, T. Okamoto, and M. P. Lisanti. Caveolins, liquid-ordered domains, and signal transduction. *Mol. Cell. Biol.* 19:7289–7304, 1999.
130. Sommer, J. R., P. C. Dolber, and I. Taylor. Filipin-sterol complexes in the membranes of cardiac muscle. *J. Ultrastruct. Res.* 80:98–103, 1982.
131. Sommer, J. R. and E. A. Johnson. Comparative ultrastructure of cardiac membrane specializations. A review. *Am. J. Cardiol.* 25:184–194, 1970.
132. Sommer, J. R., E. A. Johnson, N. R. Wallace, and R. Nassar. Cardiac muscle following quick-freezing: preservation of in vivo ultrastructure and geometry with special emphasis on intercellular clefts in the intact frog heart. *J. Mol. Cell. Cardiol.* 20:285–302, 1988.
133. Song, K. S., S. Li, T. Okamoto, L. A. Quillam, M. Sargiacomo, and M. P. Lisanti. Copurification and direct interaction of Ras with caveolin, an integral membrane protein of caveolae microdomains: detergent-free purification of caveolae microdomains. *J. Biol. Chem.* 271:9690–9697, 1996.
134. Song, K. S., P. E. Scherer, Z. L. Tang, T. Okamoto, S. Li, M.

Chafel, C. Chu, D. S. Kohtz, and M. P. Lisanti. Expression of caveolin-3 in skeletal, cardiac, and smooth muscle cells. Caveolin-3 is a component of the sarcolemma and cofractionates with dystrophin and dystrophin-associated glycoproteins. *J. Biol. Chem.* 271:15160–15165, 1996.

135. Sperelakis, N., Tohse, N., Ohya, Y., and Masuda, H. Cyclic GMP regulation of calcium slow channels in cardiac muscle and vascular smooth muscle cells. *Adv. Pharmacol.* 26:217–151, 1994.

136. Stan, R.-V., W. G. Roberts, D. Predescu, K. Ihida, S. Saican, L. Ghitescu and G. E. Palade. Immunoisolation and partial characterization of endothelial plasmalemmal vesiscles (caveolae). *Mol. Biol. Cell* 8:595–605, 1997.

137. Tang, Z, P. E. Scherer, T. Okamoto, K. Song, C. Chu, D. S. Kohtz, I. Nishimoto, H. F. Lodish, and M. P. Lisanti. Molecular cloning of caveolin-3, a novel member of the caveolin gene family expressed predominantly in muscle. *J. Biol. Chem.* 271: 2255–2261, 1996.

138. Thompson, L. F., J. M. Ruedi, A. Glass, M. G. Low, and A. H. Lucas. Antibodies to 5'-nucleotidase (CD73), a glycophosphatidylinositol-anchored protein, cause human peripheral blood T-cells to proliferate. *J. Immunol* 143:1815–1821, 1989.

139. Thompson, T. E. and T. W. Tillack. Organization of glycosphingolipids in bilayers and plasma membranes of mammalian cells. *Annu. Rev. Biophys. Chem.* 14:361–386, 1985.

140. Tohse, N., H. Nakaya, Y. Takeda, and M. Kanno. Cyclic GMP–mediated inhibition of L-type Ca^{2+} channel activity by human natriuretic peptide in rabbit heart cells. *Br. J. Pharmacol.* 114:1076–1082, 1994.

141. Tran, D., J.-L. Carpentier, F. Sawamo, P. Goren, and L. Orci. Ligands internalized through coated or non-coated invaginations follow a common intracellular pathway. *Proc. Natl. Acad. Sci. U.S.A.* 84:7957–7961, 1987.

142. van Deurs, B., O. W. Petersen, S. Olsnes, and K. Sandvig. The ways of endocytosis. *Int. Rev. Cytol.* 117:131–177, 1989.

143. Van Os, C. H., P. M. T. Deen, and J. A. Dempster. Aquaporins: water selective channels in biological membranes. Molecular structure and tissue distribution. *Biochim. Biophys. Acta* 1197:291–309, 1994.

144. Vinten, J., J. Tranum-Jensen, and M. Foldstedlund. The caveolin-3 isoform of muscle is abundant in astrocytes. *Mol. Biol. Cell.* 8 [Suppl.] 208a, 1997.

145. Verkman, A. S., A. N. van Hoek, T. Ma. A. Frigeri, W. R. Skach, A. Mitra, B. K. Tamarappoo, and J. Farinas. Water transport across mammalian cell membranes. *Am. J. Physiol.* 270 (*Cell Physiol.* 39):C12–C30, 1996.

146. Watts, C. and M. Marsh. Endocytosis: what goes on and how? *J. Cell Sci.* 103:1–08, 1992.

147. Way, M., and R. G. Parton. M-caveolin, a muscle-specific caveolin-related protein. *FEBS Lett.* 376:108–112, 1995.

148. Waugh, M. G., D. Lawson, S. K. Tan, and J. J. Hsuan. Phosphatidylinositol 4-phosphate synthesis in immunoisolated caveolae-like vesicles and low density non-caveolar membranes. *J. Biol. Chem.* 273:17115–17121, 1998.

149. Waugh, M. G., D. Lawson, and J. J. Hsuan. Epidermal growth factor receptor activation is localized within low-buoyant density, non-caveolar membrane domains. *Biochem J.* 337:591–597, 1999.

150. Yamada, E. The fine structure of the gall bladder epithelium of the mouse. *J. Biophys. Biochem. Cytol.* 1:445–458, 1955.

151. Zeidel, M. L., S. Nielsen, B. L. Smith, S. V. Ambudkar, A. B. Maunsbach, and P. Agre. Ultrastructure, pharmacological inhibition, and transport selectivity of aquaporin channel-forming integral protein in proteoliposomes. *Biochem. J.* 33: 1606–1615, 1994.

152. Zhao, Y., D. R. Sawyer, R. R. Baglia, D. J. Opel, X. Han, M. A. Marchionni, and R. A. Kelly. Neuregulins promote survival and growth of cardiac myocytes. Persistence of erbB2 and erbB4 expression in neonatal and adult ventricular myocytes. *J. Biol. Chem.* 273:10261–10269, 1998.

153. Zhao, Y., O. Feron, C. Dessy, X. Han, M. A. Marchionni, R. A. Kelly. Neuregulin signaling in the heart: dynamic targeting of erbB4 to caveolar microdomains in cardiac myocytes. *Circ. Res.* 84:1380–1387, 1999.

4. Gap junctions in the cardiovascular system

DAVID C. SPRAY — *Departments of Neuroscience and Medicine, Albert Einstein College of Medicine, Bronx, New York*

SYLVIA O. SUADICANI — *Department of Neuroscience, Albert Einstein College of Medicine, Bronx, New York, and Universidade São Judas Tadeu, São Paulo, Brazil*

MIDUTURU SRINIVAS — *Department of Neuroscience. Albert Einstein College of Medicine, Bronx, New York*

DAVID E. GUTSTEIN — *Department of Medicine, Mount Sinai School of Medicine, New York, New York*

GLENN I. FISHMAN — *Departments of Medicine, Physiology and Biophysics, and Biochemistry and Molecular Biology, Mount Sinai School of Medicine, New York, New York*

CHAPTER CONTENTS

Cardiovascular Gap Junction Proteins
  Ultrastructural features
  Higher resolution through projection images
  The connexin multigene family
  Connexin and connexon topology
  Regional Connexin expression in the cardiovascular system
  Why are there multiple cardiovascular connexins?
Macroscopic Organization of the Heart (Cables, Bricks, and Textures)
  Gap junction organization within the tissue
  Modeling tissue connections
  Optical imaging of patterned cell cultures
  Microscopic and macroscopic discontinuities
Regulation of Gap Junction Expression, Formation, and Degradation
  Life and death of gap junctions
  Long-term changes in gap junction expression
  Transcriptional regulation of cardiac gap junction genes
Functional Properties of Cardiovascular Gap Junctions
  Cardiovascular gap junctions are K^+, Ca^{2+}, and second messenger channels
  Biophysical properties of junctional channels
  Gating of gap junctional channels by transjunctional voltage
  Properties of specific connexins expressed in exogenous systems
    Connexin43 expressed in exogenous systems
    Connexin40 expressed in exogenous systems
    Connexin45 expressed in SKHep1 cells and elsewhere
    Connexin37 expressed in exogenous systems
    Connexin50 expressed in exogenous systems
    Heterologous pairings of cells exogenously expressing different junctional proteins.
  Properties of gap junctions evaluated in cardiovascular cells
  Gating of gap junctions by other stimuli
    Sensitivity of gap junctions to protons and Ca^{2+}
    Sensitivity to lipophilic molecules
    Effects of phosphorylation on channel function
    Other agents that affect gap junction function and expression
Genetic and Somatic Disease States in Which Gap Junction Expression or Function Is Altered
  Somatic cardiac abnormalities
  Reversed physiology: Inferring gene function from its absence in knockout mice

---

GAP JUNCTIONS ARE IN A CLASS BY THEMSELVES. No other structure in vertebrate membranes forms enclosed channels crossing the extracellular space, and few other channels in the plasma membrane have pore diameters wide enough to allow both current-carrying ions and signaling molecules to pass by diffusion. Yet, like other membrane channels, those forming gap junctions possess mechanisms that regulate their opening and closing (a phenomenon termed "gating") and rapidly change their expression patterns in response to physiological and pathological stimuli. Such flexibility provides the opportunity for global, regional, or local alterations in conduction within the heart and signal transfer in vasculature and thus provides a substrate for disturbances of cardiac rhythm and vascular tone.

At a microscopic level, the higher resistance of gap junction channels than cytoplasm produces conduction discontinuities in the heart, so that action potentials regenerated in each cell are propagated from one cell to the next with tiny, but measureable, delays. Because gap junctions are not uniformly distributed on the myocyte surface, and because myocytes are longer than they are wide, the discontinuities at gap junctional contacts give rise to anisotropic conduction. Although this chapter is written from the standpoint of summarizing what is known regarding the physiology and cell biology of cardiac gap junction channels, which have largely been determined using cell pairs from dissociated cardiovascular tissues and transfected cell lines, we have attempted throughout to integrate such studies into current concepts regarding conduction in both normal and pathological heart (see 239). Truly integrative studies are only barely beginning, but by considering gap junctions in the context of both cellular and tissue environments, we have intentionally emphasized the importance of newly available strategies for understanding the roles of gap junctions in cardiovascular function (see also Chapter 12)

Research on cardiovascular gap junctions has a long history that has attracted the interest of many prominent physiologists. The earliest study of cardiac gap junctions generally cited is that of Engelmann (71), who described the physiological consequences of focal mechanical injury in frog heart. His simple experiments and insightful interpretation demonstrated that cells at or near the site of injury became refractory to further stimulation for a time thereafter, a phenomenon associated with the appearance of an injury potential that slowly disappeared during a period of "healing over." During this process of recovery, a boundary was believed to be formed between injured and uninjured regions. This behavior of injured cardiac muscle was paradoxical, in that the individually visible myocytes behaved syncytially. Contemporaneously in the field of neuroscience, a similar problem was being addressed by the conflict between the "reticular" and "neuronal" doctrines of neural connectivity. In both disciplines, the resolution of these paradoxes was achieved through the application of anatomical fine structural and intracellular electrophysiological methods introduced in the 1940s and 1950s.

Using cable equations developed a century ago to calculate the thickness required for transmission though transoceanic telephone lines, Sylvio Weidmann (293) determined the cable properties of sheep Purkinje fibers. Intracellular measurements revealed that longitudinal resistance of the fibers was low, even though many intercalated disks were interposed; the space constant corresponded to about 20 cell lengths. Woodbury and Crill (303) determined the length constant of cardiac tissue again, finding that it was much longer than the length of individual myocytes in both the longitudinal and the transverse directions. Despite physiological evidence of continuity between the cells, early thin section studies (229) clearly showed that intercalated disks in mouse hearts were boundaries between cells. Ultimately, when Barr et al. (8) provided anatomical evidence of the "nexus" or gap junction at the intercalated disk regions between cardiac myocytes, these anatomical substrates of cytoplasmic continuity were hypothesized to be conductive enough so that the cardiac strand behaved very much like a continuous cable.

CARDIOVASCULAR GAP JUNCTION PROTEINS

Ultrastructural Features

In the adult vertebrate heart, gap junctions are mainly concentrated at the ends of the myocytes, where they are located primarily in the adhesive "plicate" and "interplicate" regions of the intercalated disks (Fig. 4–1A; 150, 188). Lateral junctional contacts can frequently also be observed parallel to the long axes of ventricular cardiocytes, with intercalated disks and gap junctions appearing at any point along the cell body (109), so that a complex pattern of overlapping of cells characterizes the ventricular myocardium. This polarized distribution of cardiac gap junctions is progressively achieved during the time course of myocyte differentiation. Gap junctions appear at early stages during mouse heart ontogenesis, being rare at 10 days postcoitum (pc) and increasing in frequency and extent at 12 and 14 days pc (87). At these early stages, cardiac gap junctions form small aggregates of particles uniformly distributed in the myocyte membrane, but, as differentiation proceeds, the junctional plaques are gradually confined to the ends of the myocyte, finally becoming restricted to the intercalated disks (see Fig. 4–4; 81).

Investigation of the ultrastructural organization of the intercalated disks and associated structures gained great impetus with the advances that occured in electron microscopic technique in the 1950s and 1960s. The first anatomical observation of these regions of contact between cardiac myocytes was made by Sjostrand and colleagues in 1958, who described the junctional regions as fused osmophilic membranes between cardiac myocytes. Similar five-layered cell-to-cell junctions (see Fig. 4–1B) were observed by Dewey and Barr (60) between smooth muscle cells, where they were termed the "nexus" (*L.*, connection) and proposed as the sites of electrical coupling between smooth muscle cells. One year later, J. D. Robertson's (213) studies on Mauthner cells in goldfish brain contributed greatly to elucidating the structure of these junctions. The studies revealed that the electrical synapses in these cells were five-layered structures that contained polygonal sub-

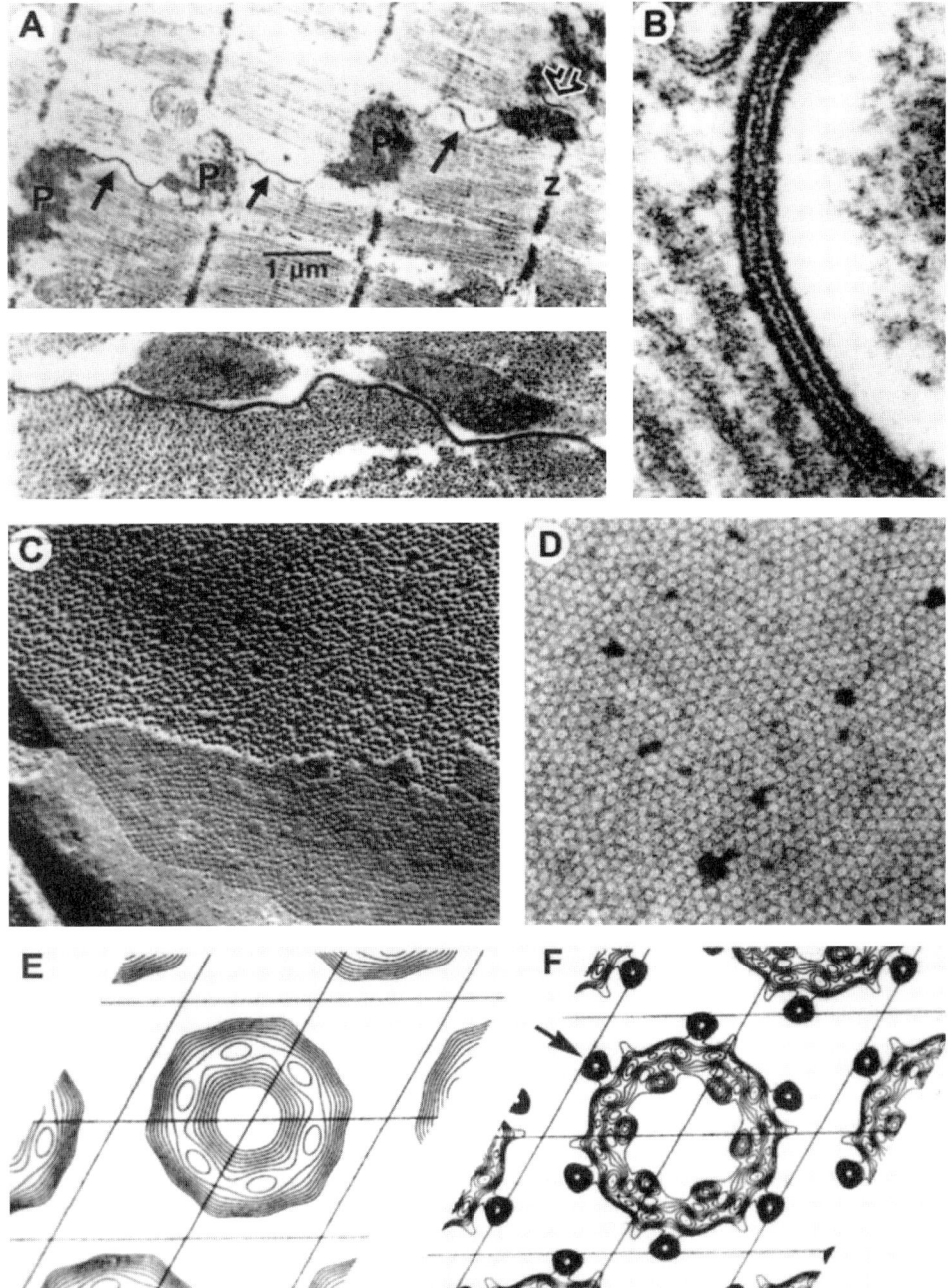

FIG. 4–1. Ultrastructural features of cardiac gap junctions: From thin section (A,B) and freeze-fracture (C) electron microscopy to negatively stained isolated junctional membranes (D) and projection density maps (E, F) of gap junctions. A: Transmission electron micrographs of canine myocardium showing the distribution of gap junctions at the intercalated disk. *Top panel:* The sarcomeric Z-line (Z) and the junctions within plicate (P, *open arrow*) and interplicate segments (*solid arrow*) are evident in this longitudinal section of the myocyte showing typical undulating geometry. *Bottom panel:* Undulations of apposed junctional membranes are also observed in a transverse section that emphasizes the long dimension of an interplicate gap junction. [From Luke and Saffitz, (150), with permission.] B: Higher power electron micrograph of gap junction between rat ventricular myocytes showing the characteristic seven-layered structure and the conspicuous fuzzy coating at both cytoplasmic surfaces. Fixed by vascular perfusion with osmium tetroxide and stained with uranyl acetate and lead citrate (magnification 156 × 10³). [From Manjunath et al. with permission (153).] C: Electron micrograph of replica of freeze-fractured gap junction between rat ventricular myocytes. Fixed by vascular perfusion with glutaraldehyde and unidirectionally shadowed with platinum-carbon. The particulate P-face and the pitted E-face of the junction are seen on the top and bottom sides of the picture, respectively (magnification 134 × 10³). [From Page and Manjunath with permission (188).] D: In an en face view of junctional membranes isolated from rat ventricle, the hexagonal structure of the connexons are outlined by phosphotungstate deposition around and within the core of the intercellular channels (magnification 241 × 10³). [From Page and Manjunath with permission 188).] E and F: Projection density maps of rat cardiac gap junction obtained at 1.5 nm resolution (E), showing individual hexameric connexons, and at 0.7 nm resolution (F), showing symmetrical circular densities that are interpreted as helices lining the channels, α helices that are most exposed to lipids (*arrow*) and two continuous dense bands that presumably represent the other two transmembrane α-helices. Spacing between grid bars is 4 nm [From Yeager and Nicholson (307) with permission.].

units, often packed in hexameric arrays, which were hypothesized to lie within the apposed outer leaflets of the two synaptic membranes. An almost identical pattern of hexagonally packed subunits was observed by Benedetti and Emmelot (15) in negatively stained isolated plasma membrane fractions (see Fig. 4–1D). In 1967, using uranium staining and lanthanum salts as a tracer of extracellular space, Revel and Karnovsky were able to distinguish two different types of junctions in the intercalated disks of mouse heart. One type (the tight junction) brought the membranes so closely into contact that the junctional region was not permeated by the lanthanum tracer; the other, outlined by lanthanum, was characterized by a 1.8 nm gap between apposing membranes, and in en face views showed the hexagonal subunits. Based on these differences, Revel (see 210) proposed the use of the term "gap junction" instead of nexus to avoid the confusion between tight junctions and those with the latter properties. The further use of freeze fracture techniques (258) to view the gap junctions in liver (124) and heart (158, 259) provided additional structural details of gap junction subunits and overall organization. These studies and those of Ernest Page and his group revealed that in freeze-fracture the gap junction is comprised of closely packed hexagonal arrays of pits on the E-face (the internal aspect of the lipid monolayer that is on the outside of the cell) and as particles or "contact cylinders" on the P (protoplasmic)-face (See Fig.4–1C; 188).

One initially puzzling aspect of cardiac gap junctions compared to similarly sized gap junctions in liver was that the images of cytoplasmic surfaces of cardiac gap junctions were reported to be less crisp, as if they were covered with a "fuzzy" layer (115, 153). Deep-etching of freeze-fractured cardiac samples revealed that the cytoplasmic aspect of the plaque was particulate, presumably accounting for the fuzzy coat seen in thin section micrographs (226). This fuzzy appearance of the cytoplasmic sides of cardiac gap junctions may reflect in part a difference in the connexon composition, which for liver consists of the β or group I connexins Cx26 and Cx32, and for heart the group II or α connexins Cx40, Cx43, and Cx45; as described in more detail below, the group II or α connexins have substantially longer cytoplasmic tail regions than do the β or group I connexins. An alternative explanation is that the particulate matter may represent one or more associated molecules (see next section).

Higher Resolution Through Projection Images

A prominent feature of gap junctions in freeze-fractured or negatively stained material is the high degree of order in the structure (see Fig. 4–1C, D). In some tissues, such as rodent liver and fish Mauthner neurons, the gap junction channels form a nearly two-dimensional crystalline array; in heart, isolated junctional membranes can be induced to form such ordered arrays through biochemical manipulations (153). The application of digital image processing techniques to electron microscope images initially resulted in two-dimensional projection maps of structure at about 2 nm resolution (Fig. 4–1F). The most notable differences between the two-dimensional membrane crystals obtained from liver and cardiac junctional membranes was the apparently larger diameter of the central region in junctions isolated from cardiac tissue, which was interpreted as representing a wider channel pore.

Technical improvements, mainly consisting of obtaining images while tilting the stage on which the specimens rested, led to three-dimensional intensity maps with resolutions at 1.8 nm, in which negatively stained and frozen hydrated liver gap junctions were shown to consist of units with six rod-like subunits about 2 nm long. These studies revealed that the hemichannels or connexons project about 2 nm into the extracellular space, accounting for the "gap" of 4 nm between the cells. Surprisingly, the cytoplasmic fuzzy projection that was predicted from thin-section and freeze-etch images to extend ~4–5 nm into the intracellular aspect of the channel was not discretely visualized, which has been attributed to the flexibility and noncrystalline structure of this domain.

These projection images supported the topological studies described below (connexin and connexon topology), wherein the gap junction proteins (connexins) are folded within the membrane and give rise to four transmembrane segments. Each of these transmembrane regions is long enough to form a membrane-spanning α helix, which Milks et al. (162) proposed would fold together within the area of each connexin domain, with an amphipathic domain contributed by each of the six connexins surrounding the central pore.

X-ray diffraction images from oriented gap junction membranes indicated sharp fringes at 0.47 nm on the meridian; this diffraction pattern was initially interpreted as indicative of β-sheet conformation, with strands oriented more parallel than perpendicular to the membrane (151). However, when this prediction was tested using models consisting of α-helical and β-sheet structures, the fringe was found more compatible with α-helical composition, and the difference from prediction was ascribed to a slight tilt of the subunits in the plane of the membrane (273). Subsequent circular dichroism studies on suspensions of isolated heart and liver junctions have estimated that the secondary structure of the connexins within gap junction structures is at least 40%–50% α-helical, presumably including the transmembrane domains M1, M2, M3, and M4.

The highest resolution projection images currently available have been obtained by Mark Yaeger and colleagues using recombinant Cx43 protein truncated at Lys 263 so as to remove most of the carboxyl terminus (276). Such truncated constructs form functional channels (78, 128), although pH sensitivity and interaction with other proteins would be expected to be altered. At 0.7 nm resolution, the projection intensity maps of negatively stained material reveal that each connexon has a diameter of 6.5 nm, with the connexin molecules forming each connexon arranged in a hexameric cluster around the channel pore (Fig. 4–1E). The 1.7 nm diameter central pore is immediately surrounded by circular densities interpreted as transmembrane domains roughly perpendicular to the membrane, a 3.3 nm ring that is farthest from the pore and closest to the lipid (interpreted as representing one of the other α-helical transmembrane domains), and a continuous band at 2.5 nm radius that presumably represents the other two transmembrane regions that are not individually resolved. Inner and outer rings of densities are displaced from one another by 30°, which is interpreted as providing rotational staggering of connexins, so as to increase interconnexin adhesion (199). In this latter model, connexons interlock tightly across a surface area that is maximized through corresponding convexities and concavities in each connexon subunit.

The Connexin Multigene Family

The first transcript encoding a gap junction protein was isolated using antibodies generated against an isolated liver gap junction protein, connexin32, which were used to screen a complementary liver DNA library (105, 127, 189). Subsequently, clones encoding Cx43 were identified by screening a rat heart cDNA library with the liver isoform at reduced stringency (19). These initial studies have led to an explosion in sequences determined in mammals, with numerous homologous connexins being found in nonmammalian vertebrates. Notably, however, connexin homologues have not been found in invertebrates, where intercellular communication has recently been attributed to an unrelated gene family termed the "innexins," which includes unc-7 in *Caenorhabditis elegans* and *passover* or *Shaking B* in *Drosophila* (47, 203).

At the time of this writing, fifteen distinct connexins have been detected in rodents (Cx26 Cx30, Cx30.3, Cx31, Cx31.1, Cx32, Cx33, Cx36, Cx37, Cx40, Cx43, Cx46, Cx47, Cx50, Cx57) and for most of these, human isologues are also recognized. The connexin genes have maintained highly conserved nucleic acid and amino acid sequence homology, and with only a single exception the genomic organization (Fig. 4–2C) is a hallmark of the family. This conservation implies critical constraints on the coding region of the gene to ensure functional protein as well as transcriptional control mechanisms. In all cases thus far examined (except for rat Cx36 and its skate homologue Cx35; 42, 185, 231), a small noncoding first exon is separated from a second exon by a long intervening intronic sequence; the second exon contains the coding region in a single uninterrupted stretch. (In rat Cx36 and skate Cx35, no upstream exon is identified, and the intron is contained within the reading frame.) The virtual uniformity in gene structure implies that a single precursor gene encoding an intercellular channel protein subunit underwent repeated duplications and subsequent mutations during vertebrate evolution, resulting in the formation of this large multigene family. In at least one case (human Cx43), a processed pseudogene has been incorporated into the genome (79).

Connexin and Connexon Topology

Each gap junction channel is made of two mirror-symmetric components contributed by each cell, called connexons or hemichannels (Fig. 4–2A; see refs. 16 and 125). Each connexon or hemichannel in turn is made up of six homologous subunits, the connexin molecules (Fig. 4–2B). Connexin proteins (18) share common membrane topology (deduced from protease digestion and antibody binding studies performed on isolated gap junction membranes, and also supported by Kyte-Doolittle hydropathy plots of sequences of cloned connexins).

As is illustrated in Figure 4–2B each connexin crosses the membrane four times (segments M1, M2, M3, and M4) and has both its amino-terminus (NT-domain) and carboxyl-terminus (CT-domain) on the cytoplasmic aspect of the channel. Extracellular loops (C1, C2) are structurally conserved, with three cysteines in each loop positioned identically in all of the known connexins (see color Plate 6). Presumably this feature accounts for the high-affinity interactions between many (but not all) different connexin molecules when cells expressing individual connexins are paired, thereby forming heterotypic channels from the end-to-end alignment of homomeric connexons. The part of the connexin molecule between M2 and M3 forms a loop or hinge region in the cytoplasm (CL) whose length (long or short) allows a useful separation of the different connexins into the group I (β) and group II

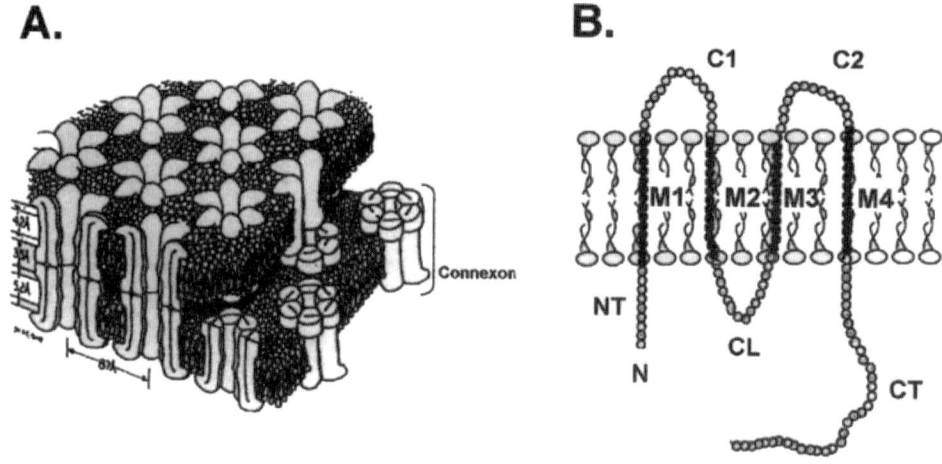

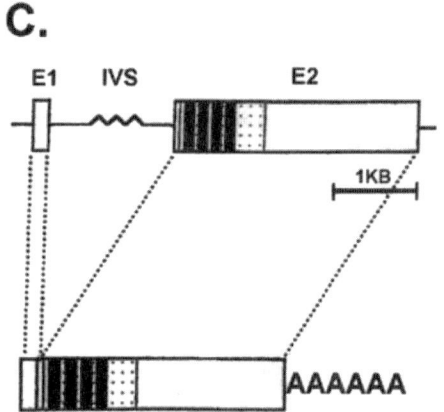

FIG. 4–2. Gap junction channels (*A*) are formed of hemichannels or connexons composed of connexin proteins (*B*) encoded by connexin genes (*C*). *A*: Schematic drawing of gap junction structure deduced from the classical study applying X-ray diffraction to gap junctions isolated from mouse liver (152). Two connexons dock across extracellular space to form the complete gap junction channel. *B*: The connexin protein and its membrane topology: the two extracellular loops (C1 and C2), the four transmembrane domains (M1, M2, M3, and M4), the intracellular loop (CL, short in group I or α subfamily and long in group II or β connexin subfamily), and the cytoplasmic amino- and carboxyl-terminal domains (NT and CT). *C, top*: Connexin gene (exons E1 and E2, intron IVS). *C, bottom*: Connexin transcript. Transmembrane domains of encoded protein indicated by *dark bars*.

(α) subfamilies (16, 125); the dissimilar gene structure of Cx36 indicates that it should probably be designated as the first member of a third subfamily (group III, or γ). The cardiovascular gap junction proteins Cx37, Cx40, Cx43, Cx45, Cx46, and Cx50 are all members of the group II (α) subfamily, perhaps implying that the cardiovascular connexins had common ancestry. The third transmembrane domain of the connexin molecules is the most amphipathic (with charged amino acid residues occuring at every third or fourth position in an otherwise predominantly hydrophobic sequence), and six of these M3 regions are believed to provide the hydrophilic face lining the lumen of the channel (16, 306; but see ref. 202 for evidence that other sequences may also participate in providing the pore-lining part of the molecular assembly).

The regions of greatest divergence among the connexins are the cytoplasmic loop (CL) region (connecting M2 and M3) and the carboxyl terminal tail extending beyond M4. These latter unique peptide sequences have proven quite useful in generating connexin-specific antibody probes; isoform sequences are nearly identical for most connexins in mammals, so that antibodies generated against peptides corresponding to rodent sequences have universally recognized the corresponding human connexin type.

Sequences corresponding to mouse and human isoforms of the cardiac connexins are presented in color Plate 6. Color codes above aligned sequences indicate whether the amino acid residues are highly conserved (red indicates 100% identity) or variant (shades of blue indicate most divergence). Arrows indicate regions of the connexins corresponding to M1, M2, M3, M4 in the topological drawing in Figure 4–2*B*. Note the longer length of the cytoplasmic loop region in Cx45 sequences, the especially high homology in the extracellular loops and M1 and M3 of these connexins, and the presence of abundant potentially phosphorylatable serine residues in the carboxyl terminal portion of the molecule. Note also the presence of a postulated PDZ-binding sequence at the most C-terminal portion of Cx43, with possibly homologous sequences in the other cardiovascular connexins, with the exception of Cx37.

Regional Connexin Expression in the Cardiovascular System

The individual cardiovascular connexins are expressed with overlapping temporal and spatial profiles. Although there is considerable interspecies variation in the types and abundance of different connexins in different regions of the cardiovascular system, general patterns of expression are outlined in the succeeding paragraphs and summarized in Table 4–1 and Figure 4–3.

Connexin43 is the most abundant gap junction channel gene expressed in the mammalian heart and blood vessel wall. This connexin is widely expressed in working atrial and ventricular myocytes, and in smooth muscle and endothelial cells of vessel walls. Although several reports have noted the absence of Cx43 in nodal tissues, immunocytochemistry on human atrioventricular node and dog sinus node have detected Cx43 expression in some individual cells (51, 129). In rodent hearts, Cx43 has been identified as early as 10 days pc in trabeculae and subendocardial regions of developing ventricles, the outflow tract, the interventricular septum, and the endocardial free wall (81, 89). Transcript levels increase substantially between midgestation and early neonatal stages (78, 81) and decline modestly in older animals (Fig. 4–4).

Connexin40 appears to be the second most abundant gap junction protein in the heart and cardiovascular system. In the heart, Cx40 is expressed in nodal tissue, in bundles within the conduction system, and in the atrium, whereas in ventricular muscle it is almost completely absent except in the coronary vasculature (86). In both muscular and elastic arteries, Cx40 expression is prominent in endothelial cells and may also be present in smooth muscle cells. In embryonic mouse

TABLE 4–1. *Distribution of Connexins in Cardiovascular Tissue*

	Cx37	Cx40	Cx43	Cx45	Cx46	Cx50
SA node	−	+	−/+	+	−	−
Atrium	−	+++	+++	++	−/+	−
AV node	−	+	−/+	+	−	−
Conduction system	−	+++	++/+++	++	−	−
Ventricle	−	−/+	+++	++	−/+	−
Vessel wall						
Smooth muscle	−	+	++	−	−	−
Endothelium	++	++	++	−	−	−

heart, Cx40 is widely expressed at atrial and ventricular primordia at 11 days PC; as embryonic development progresses, Cx40 expression is maintained in atrium, whereas its initial ventricular expression becomes confined to the differentiating conduction system (55, 280).

Connexin45 has been reported throughout the heart, in most cases co-localizing with, but at lower abundance than, Cx43. However, more recent studies with more specific Cx45 antibodies indicate that this gap junction protein may in large part be confined to the atrioventricular node and conduction system (44–46).

Three other connexins have been reported to be expressed in the cardiovascular system: Cx37, Cx46, and Cx50. Cx37 expression is quite high in endothelial cells throughout the vascular tree, including endocardial vessels, but it is absent in other regions of the heart. During embryogenesis, Cx37 is more widely distributed and can be detected in the developing murine ventricular myocardium, as well as in the area of the conotruncal ridges and atrioventricular cushions (94).

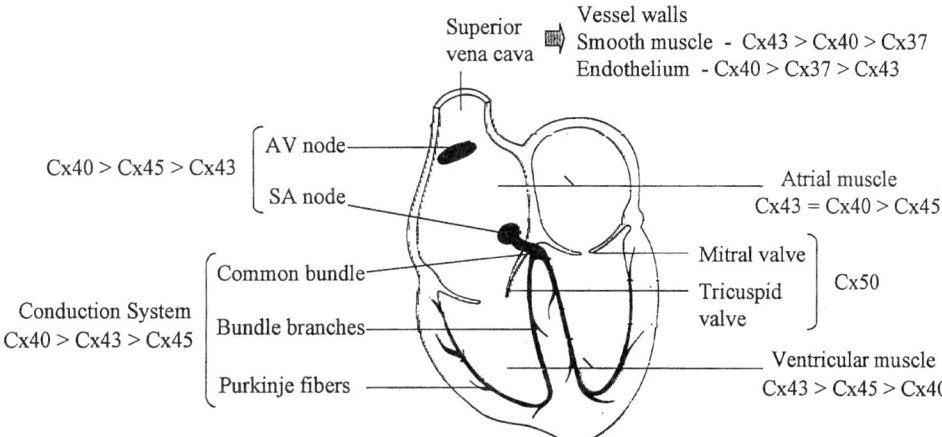

FIG. 4–3. Schematic diagram illustrating general pattern of distribution and relative abundance of connexin types expressed in different regions of the mammalian heart and vessel wall.

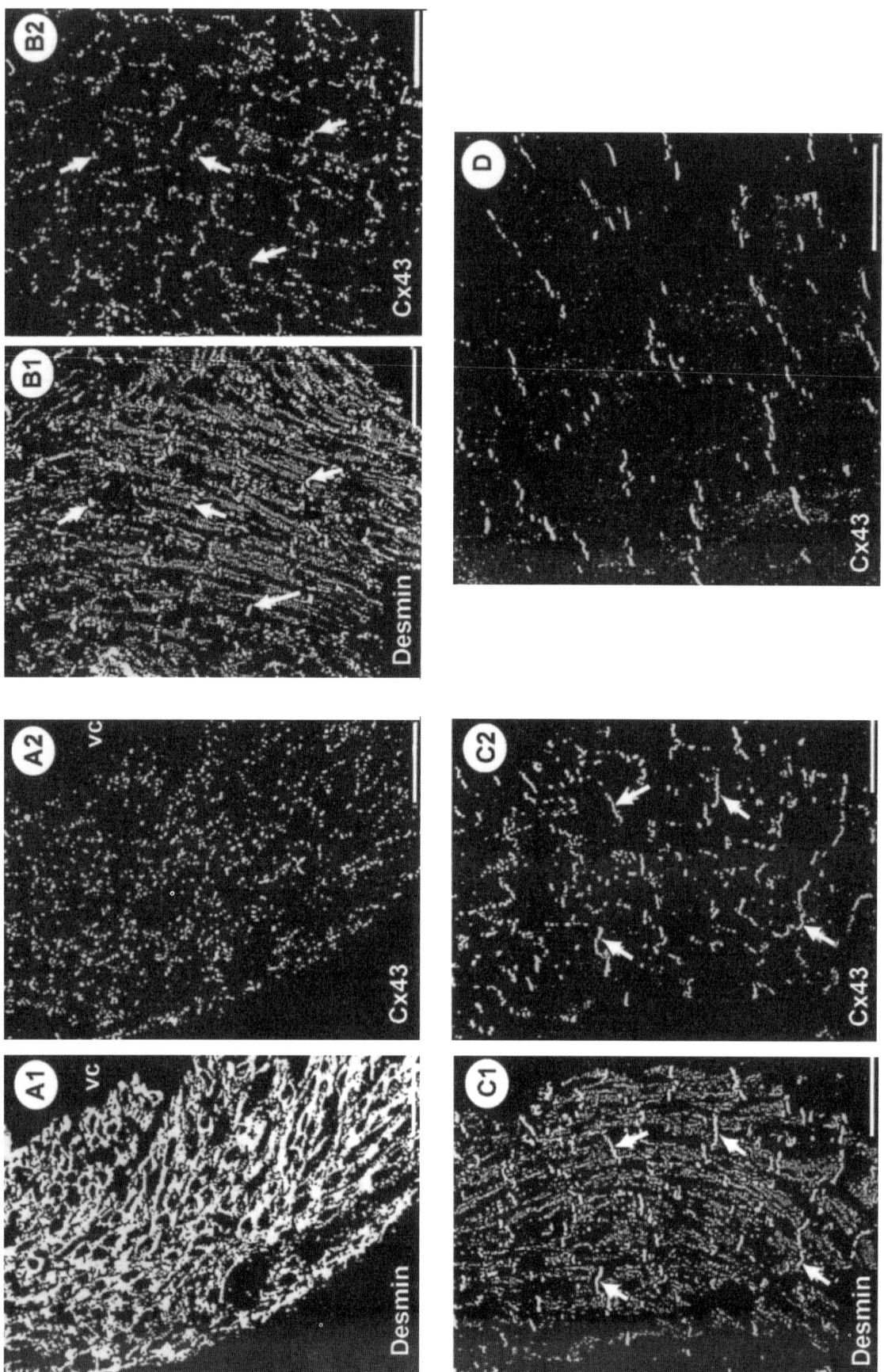

FIG. 4-4. Pattern of connexin 43 (Cx43) and desmin distribution during the developmental differentiation of mouse ventricle myocytes as viewed by double immunofluorescence. A: Cross-sections of newborn mouse ventricular wall showing desmin striations (identifying Z-lines of myofibrils) and the homogenous distribution of Cx43 between the myocytes. B: Longitudinal sections of two-week-old mouse ventricular wall showing the intercalated disks, which are strongly immunoreactive to anti-desmin antibodies (*white arrows*) and the initiation of polarized Cx43 expression that progressively becomes restricted to the opposite ends of the myocytes (intercalated disks, white arrows) and to the adjacent lateral regions. C: Longitudinal sections of three-week-old mouse ventricular wall showing the even more pronounced polarization of Cx43 expression at the intercalated disks (white arrows) that was first evident at two weeks postpartum. D: Longitudinal section of adult mouse ventricular wall showing that Cx43 expression is now confined to the intercalated disks. This pattern of expression is observed at the conclusion of myocyte differentiation and characterizes myocytes in adult ventricular tissue (bars = 50 µm). [From Fromaget et al. (81) with permission.]

Cx46 was initially detected in whole heart homogenates in a screen for expression of Cx46 mRNA in different tissues (190) and subsequently has been localized to infrequent contacts between human atrial and ventricular myocytes (51). Cx50 expression was detected in cardiac valves using antibodies prepared against isolated MP70 protein (89), which is a major component of gap junctions in the lens; significance of its expression in heart is unknown.

Why Are There Multiple Cardiovascular Connexins?

The expression of multiple types of gap junction proteins in the heart (and in other tissues) implies that either the common function provided by each of these channel types is so important that there is need for redundancy (the "safety in numbers" line of reasoning) or that each of the connexin types offers unique aspects of function, regulation, or binding that is useful under physiological or pathological conditions. If the latter argument is correct, there are several possibilities for why selective pressure for multiple connexin expression has been exerted during the process of evolution.

1. *Different connexons have different affinities for one another, either allowing communication between diverse cell populations or segregating these cells into isolated communication compartments.* Cell coupling is readily established between cells of different types in co-culture (72, 161). Although heterocellular communication might be due to channels formed of the same connexins (thereby forming "homotypic" channels), functional coupling between cells expressing different gap junction proteins ("heterotypic" channels) has been confirmed by exogenous expression studies using *Xenopus* oocytes injected with connexin cRNAs (see (182)) and with communication-deficient cells stably transfected with connexin cDNAs (70). Although such studies indicated that hemichannels formed of most connexins readily pair with those of other connexins, Cx43 and Cx40 were until very recently thought to be functionally incompatible (11, 26, 70, 98). In the cardiovascular system, regions where Cx40/Cx43 heterologous pairings might be expected to occur include the compartmental interface between endothelial and smooth muscle cells in the vessel wall. As David Paul's group has pointed out, such nonfunctional myoendothelial Cx40/Cx43 junctions in vasculature could serve to separate the endothelial and smooth muscle compartments (26). Perhaps more significantly, predominant expression of Cx40 by cells of the conduction system and of Cx43 by the ventricular mass would be expected to decrease electrical dispersion of the conducted impulse (11), further focussing excitation to the portals of contact between Purkinje cells and ventricular muscle (the P-V junctions; see ref. 206). The recent demonstration of functional Cx43/Cx40 channels (278) leaves open the possibility that such boundaries may still exist if the affinity of such pairing is less than each connexon has for an identical partner. For example, connexons formed of Cx45 appear to have higher affinity for Cx43 connexons than they have for themselves (170) and heterologous Cx43/Cx45 pairings might help to prevent retrograde conduction at the P-V junction or predispose ventricular areas to unidirectional block, due to the strong asymmetric voltage dependence that results from the heterotypic pairing of these connexons (170 see also 37 and below).

2. *Channels formed by different connexins have different functional properties and are differently gated,* thereby providing a functional advantage for the expression of certain connexins in specific tissues. Gap junction channels open and close in response to various stimuli, including transjunctional voltage, intracellular pH, phosphorylation of the connexin molecules and exposure to any of a wide variety of lipophilic molecules (see ref. 249; see also later, under Functional Properties of Cardiovascular Gap Junctions). From the standpoint of pathophysiology, each of these gating stimuli may play significant roles: during cardiac ischemia, appreciable transjunctional voltage gradients may develop, intracellular pH is radically lowered, phosphorylation substrates are reduced and phosphatases may be activated (157); moreover, lipophiles with uncoupling action are produced through lipid peroxidation and phospholipase action (304). Gap junction channels formed of different connexins are to at least some extent differentially sensitive to such stimuli (see below).

Moreover, the size of gap junction channels formed by different connexins differs, when evaluated either as conductance of individual channels (unitary conductance, γ_j) or assessed by the size limit or charge selectivity of the channels to permeant ions and molecules. Because unitary conductance of a channel determines its current-carrying capacity, a higher or lower single-channel conductance might be functionally facilitating or limiting for the processes of synchronous contraction and speed of conduction. Recordings from primary cardiovascular cells have detected unitary junctional currents corresponding to numerous channel sizes (249). While some of this diversity results from subconductance or alternate conductance states of the junctional channels (249), diversity also arises from the expression of multiple gap junction proteins in these cells. Finally, although it has been assumed that all gap junction channels were similarly permeable to molecules below a size limit (about 1 kDa), it is now clear that the gap junction channels formed of the cardiovascular connexins have markedly different permeabilities for anions than for cations. Thus, whereas Cx43 channels are freely permeant to lucifer yellow and other anions, Cx37 and Cx40 channels show much more restricted diffusion, and Cx45 channels are virtually anion impermeant (282, 283, 286). Implications of the findings for the cardiovascular system include the remarkable prediction that flow of anionic second messenger molecules (e.g., cAMP, cGMP, IP$_3$) will be impeded across certain types of gap junction channels, even though junctional current, which is carried predominantly by K$^+$ ions in situ, may be even higher in certain anion-impermeant junctional channels.

3. *Different connexins are differentially affected by transcriptional and post-transcriptional controls* such that hormonal and other stimuli may affect coupling in some tissues more than in others and that sequential transcript expression during development can be carefully timed. Numerous drugs, growth factors and hormones have been shown to affect connexin mRNA or protein levels and/or functional coupling over a time course of hours to days (1, 41, 56, 116, 159, 217, 257, 294). Both transcriptional and mRNA stabilizing signals differ among the few connexin proteins where gene regulatory sequences have been mapped or mRNA stability has been measured (5, 123, 141, 159, 165, 215, 313), presumably thereby allowing differential regulation of the same connexin in different cells and different connexins in the same cellular environment.

4. *Different connexins may bind differentially to other proteins, forming connexin-specific macromolecular complexes.* Although this possibility is yet to be fully explored, it is suggested by recent studies indicating high-affinity interactions between the carboxyl terminus of Cx43 and the PDZ domain of the tight junction–associated protein ZO-1 (85, 269) and of v-src to distinct regions (149), as well as an association between Cx43 and β-catenin (1). The extent to which other proteins are part of the nexus, and whether other connexins selectively bind other cytoplasmic components are questions of major current interest in the field.

MACROSCOPIC ORGANIZATION OF THE HEART (CABLES, BRICKS, AND TEXTURES)

Gap Junction Organization within the Tissue

The concept of anisotropic properties of cardiac tissue arose from demonstrations that both cable properties of cardiac tissue and conduction of impulse activity favored spread in the longitudinal direction over spread in the transverse direction (40, 222, 238, 303). Madison Spach and colleagues began investigating these directional differences in more detail in 1979, showing that the rate of rise of the action potential (V_{max}) was higher in the transverse direction than longitudinally (237). This anisotropy was ascribed to microscopic discontinuities in propagation at the interfaces between the myocytes, and in subsequent studies this group has maintained that changes in gap junction distribution can remodel the pathways of impulse propagation so as to create conditions susceptible to reentrant arrhythmias, including decremental and slow conduction and unidirectional block.

In a study that has had a long-lasting impact on subsequent modeling of results obtained from cardiac electrophysiological studies, Jeffrey Saffitz's group (218, 219) compared the cellular organization of canine left ventricle with that of crista terminalis (see Fig. 4–5). In the left ventricle, myocytes were typically found to be connected to an average of slightly more than eleven other myocytes, with gap junctions located both at the ends of the fibers and along their lateral borders. Whereas the length-to-width ratio of individual isolated cells was found to be 6:1, gap junction distribution in the overlapping cells within the tissue resulted in a much lower effective length-to-width ratio (3.4:1). This geometric organization thus accounts for the conduction velocity anisotropy observed when comparing propagation velocity in the longitudinal and transverse directions, because the propagated impulse encounters more cellular boundaries in transverse conduction than in longitudinal conduction.

In crista terminalis, the component cells were found to be smaller, although the same 6:1 length:width ratio was measured. However, gap junctions in this tissue were found to be localized almost exclusively at sites of end-to-end apposition (see Fig. 4–5); individual myocytes were only in contact with slightly more than six others and most of those contacts were at the fiber ends. As a consequence, the effective length-to-width ratio was 10:1, leading to pronounced anisotropy in propagation velocity with regard to transverse vs longitudinal conduction velocity. Not only was velocity severely attenuated in this tissue when measured in the transverse direction, but the wavefronts tended to become non-uniform as they passed in this direction.

Litchenberg et al. (145) provided important structure–function data supporting the importance of cellular gap junction distribution in determining cell-to-cell impulse conduction velocity. They showed that during postnatal growth in the rabbit, Cx43 distribution in the individual myocytes of the crista terminalis becomes increasingly polarized, correlating with changes in impulse propagation velocity.

In other cardiac compartments, the anatomical distribution of gap junctions between the component cells also appears to be a major determinant of conduction

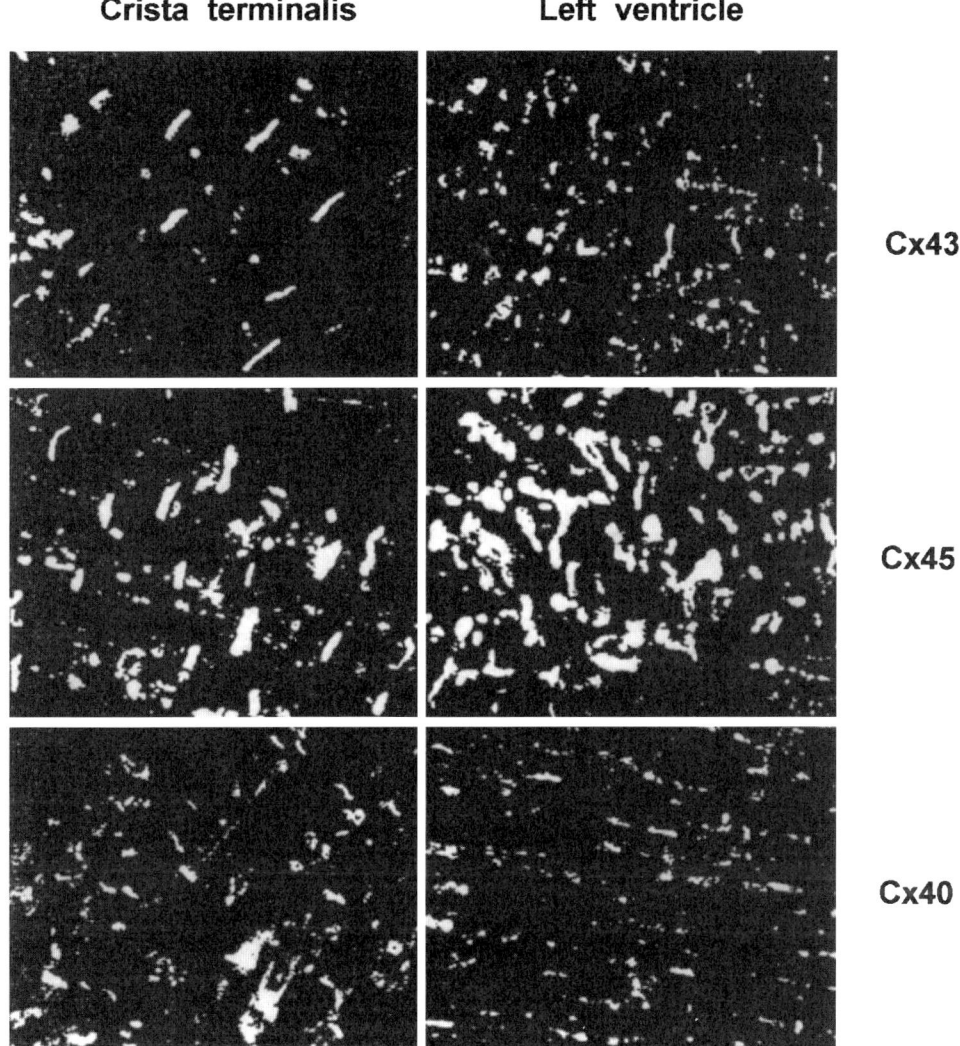

FIG. 4–5. Expression patterns of Cx43 (*top panels*), Cx45 (*middle panels*), and Cx40 (*bottom panels*) in the crista terminalis (*left panels*) and left ventricular muscle (*right panels*) viewed by immunofluorescence. In the crista terminalis, the distribution of immunoreactivity for the three connexins follows a regular and simple pattern, consistent with the localization of the intercalated disks at the true ends of the atrial myocytes. In the ventricle, the pattern is more complex with side-to-side as well as end-to-end staining, consistent with the more extensive intercellular junctions that occur between ventricular myocytes. [From Saffitz et al. (219).]

properties. For example, gap junctions are small and sparse in nodal tissue, presumably thereby favoring slow conduction and generation of pacemaking rhythms. In contrast, gap junctions in the conduction system are quite large and oriented at the fiber ends, thereby being positioned most effectively for longitudinal conduction.

As noted elsewhere in this chapter, gap junctions in mammalian heart are distributed all along the surface of myocytes until after birth, whereupon they assume their mature configuration in which they are primarily confined to intercalated disk regions of the cells. In the context of anisotropic conduction as a substrate of arrhythmias, it may be noteworthy that arrhythmia occurrence increases with age. In healed areas of infarct, gap junctions revert toward the neonatal pattern, with gap junctions near the infarcted region being smaller and less numerous than in regions far from the tissue insult (150). In the border zone, the number of cells connected to an individual myocyte decreases by half, primarily due to loss of side-to-side connections. As a result, wavefronts zig-zag, as is also seen in human papillary muscle, where local boundaries disrupt the wavefront (52). Such zig-zag propagation is found in both the setting of cardiac hypertrophy and in the atria and ventricles during aging, where microfibrosis creates connective tissue and collagenous septa, thereby separating the tissue into slowly conducting cell groups (232, 233).

Modeling Tissue Connections

Spach and colleagues have developed an elegant two-dimensional electrical model of cardiac conduction (234, 235), based closely on the anatomical detail presented by Saffitz and colleagues (109). In this model, cardiac cells are connected to one another by discrete resistances located at the ends and along the sides of the myocytes, as determined from electron micrographs. Conduction velocity in this model is 0.15 m/sec in the transverse direction and 0.45 m/sec longitudinally, for a threefold ratio of longitudinal to transverse conduction. The intra- and intercellular isochrones predicted for anisotropic conduction (1) show that different gap junctions support current flow in the two directions and (2) predict the observed difference in V_{max} for longitudinal and transverse current flow based on these anatomical discontinuities. Moreover, the model allows predicted voltage drops at the junctional barriers to be visualized, as shown in Figure 4–6.

Optical Imaging of Patterned Cell Cultures

Cardiac myocytes are readily dissociated in high yield from neonatal rodent hearts. When maintained in cell culture, such cells begin to beat spontaneously within 1–3 days, and by 3–5 days in high-density culture the monolayers display a high degree of synchronous beating (112). Presumably, these synchronized contractions are initiated by pacemaking cells in the population and are entrained within the population by gap junctions between the myocytes. Even though such cultures can be maintained for weeks, enabling studies of pharmacological and physiological responses, as well as analysis of the impact of assorted treatments on gene expression, a severe limitation to their more extensive use is that the neonatal myocytes in culture do not assume their in situ cardiac organization. Not only is the three-dimensionality of the heart lacking from such preparations, but also myocytes in culture do not normally exhibit the alignment that so uniquely characterizes their appearance in cardiac tissue.

Attempts to develop cell cultures with cellular morphologies that more closely resembled cardiac myocytes in situ were begun in a series of studies by Melvyn Lieberman and colleagues more than twenty-five years ago (108, 143, 144, 205). The approach of these studies was to impose longitudinal orientation onto the cardiac myocytes by growing them on nylon strands or in grooves scratched into the plastic culture dishes. Such "synthetic strands" of cardiac cells proved to be amenable to electrophysiological and pharmacological examination, mimicking the longitudinal conduction of impulse activity seen in cardiac tissue.

Major advances in the engineering of patterned cardiac myocyte cell growth in culture were achieved by Andre Kleber and Stefan Rohr and their colleagues. The first advance was to use "photoresist" technology originally developed for the computer chip industry to etch patterns of nonadherent substrate into the glass coverslips on which the neonatal myocytes are subsequently cultured. Because cells become packed into the confined spaces during plating, growth in such patterned substrates has proven to closely approximate the transverse/longitudinal anisotropy seen in cardiac tissue.

The second advance made by Kleber's group (121) in their studies of neonatal cardiocyte cultures was to use voltage-sensitive fluorescent dyes to simultaneously detect potential changes in large numbers of cells in the microscope field, thereby enabling optical mapping of wavefront propagation in these monolayer cultures. Because the dyes respond to membrane potential changes virtually instantaneously, such measurements can readily distinguish between cytoplasmic conduction time and the delay occurring at junctional membranes between the cells. When longitudinal conduction in wider strands was measured, it was found to be more rapid; such an averaging effect of lateral connections is attributable to the convergence and divergence of current flow at lateral and longitudinal boundaries and does not affect the overall conduction time.

Most recently, Kleber and colleagues (121) have used optical mapping of patterned cultures to investigate conduction discontinuities occurring at sites of mismatch between source and load impedances. (Chapter 12) For these studies, a narrow lane of cells rapidly expands into a large area, resulting in slowing of the impulse that can lead to block if the entrant level is sufficiently narrow compared to the expansion. A surprising result of these studies has been the finding that partial uncoupling of the cells with pharmacological agents can actually increase the safety factor for propagation at the region of expansion, because of a decrease in the load imposed by the extensive coupling in the expanded area. Thus, depending on geometric factors, decreasing junctional conductance between cardiac cells can actually reduce conduction discontinuities.

Optical mapping of intact hearts has recently been adapted to study genetically modified mice with cardiomyopathies, including those with arrhythmias such

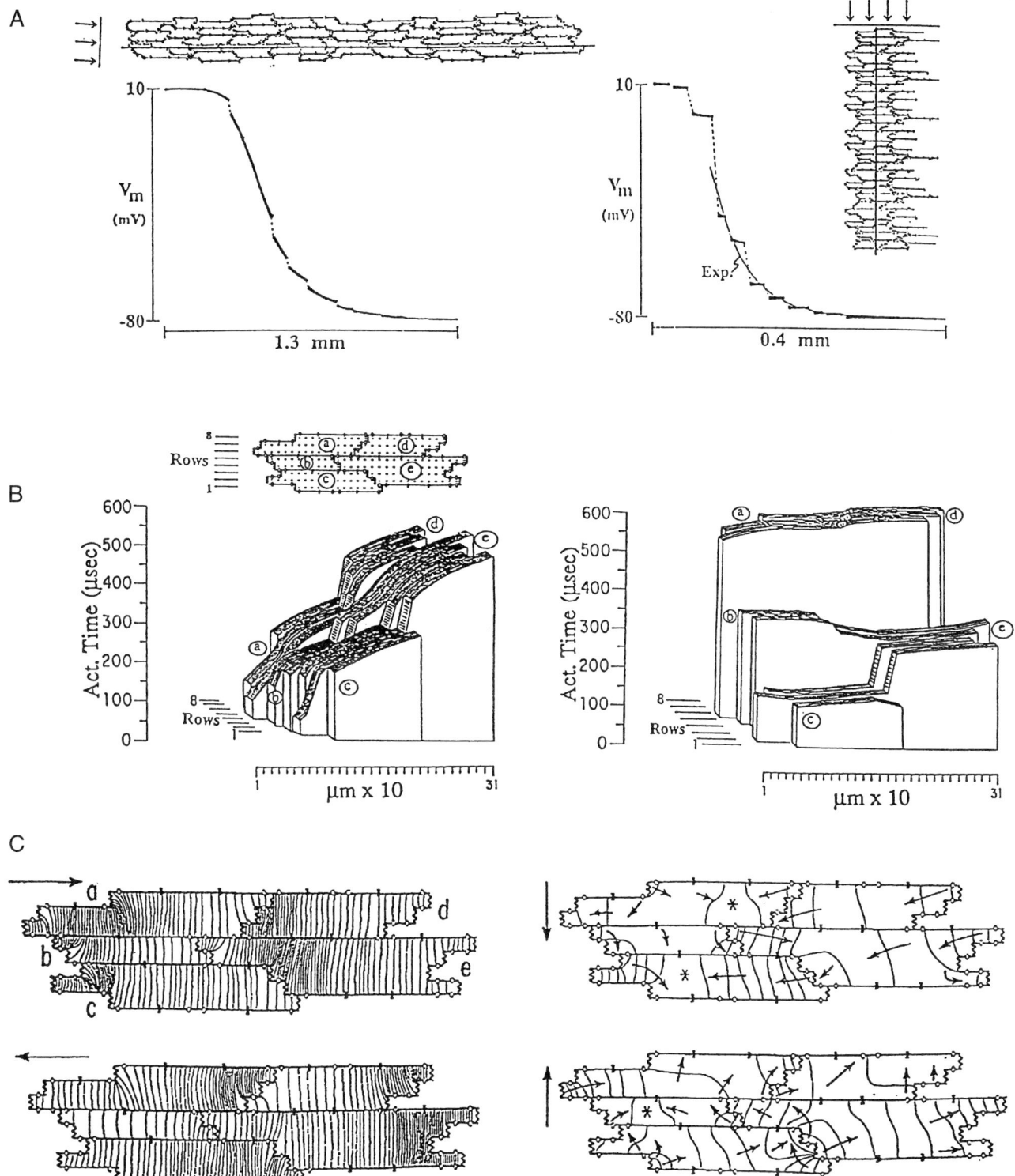

FIG. 4–6. Effect of gap junctions on longitudinal (*left panels*) and transverse propagation (*right panels*) in a 2D cellular network model. *A:* Spatial distribution of the depolarization (V_m) for longitudinal (*left*) and transverse (*right*) conduction. *Bold lines* represent changes of V_m within cells; *dashed lines* represent the step changes in V_m at the gap junctions. Note that *time scale on the right* is longer, so that signal is more rapidly attenuated (and discrete V_m drops at borders more profound) for transverse conduction. *B:* Time course of activation within a network of five myocytes (labeled a–e) in the 2D model, arranged longitudinally (*left*) or transversely (*right*). *C:* Excitation isochrones (separated by 4 μsec on the left and 3 μsec on the right) along the longitudinal (*left*) and transverse (*right*) axes of the myocytes. Direction of propagation is indicated by *arrows*. [From Spach and Heidlage, (235).]

181

as ventricular tachycardia. For example, targeted expression of diphtheria toxin A protein to the hearts of mice resulted in a dilated cardiomyopathy associated with spontaneous and inducible ventricular arrhythmias. A subset of the mice display markedly perturbed epicardial activation patterns associated with extensive remoding of Cx43-containing gap junction channels, providing some of the most direct evidence to date that connexin reorganization may contribute to the arrhythmogenic millieu (140). Studies of mice heterozygous for a connexin43 null allele have been somewhat contradictory. Optical mapping studies show no evidence of conduction slowing (174), in contrast to results obtained by direct epicardial electrode recordings (93). Using an isolated-heart preparation, this latter group found (142) no evidence of spontaneous arrhythmias in Cx43+/− mice, but an increased susceptibility to ischemia-induced arrhythmias.

Microscopic and Macroscopic Discontinuities

A major issue remaining to be resolved is the extent to which uniform microscopic conduction discontinuities provided by gap junctions between the cardiac cells are modified under pathological conditions, and whether the substrate for arrhythmic conduction necessarily involves the generation of abrupt conduction boundaries. Gating studies (considered below) have demonstrated that gap junction channels close in response to factors generated in ischemic myocardium (eg, intracellular acidosis and calcium loading, increased concentrations of lipophilic agents generated through lipid peroxidation and by phospholipases and by transjunctional voltage gradients). However, studies of intercellular coupling during an ischemic episode also indicate that the rise in junctional resistance is a slowly progressing event that may not make a significant impact on conduction until after arrhythmias appear (121).

On a macroscopic level, optical and electrophysiological mapping of wavefront propagation in cardiac tissues indicates that conduction is rather insensitive to the microscopic discontinuities imposed by gap junctions between individual myocytes. This is so because the large number of elements arranged both in parallel and in series have an averaging effect on one another. Modeling studies on macroscopic waves have indicated that wavefronts are not significantly distorted unless conduction barriers are encountered with lengths that are comparable to the wavefront curvature (33). Such anatomical discontinuities are modeled as "textures" in medium in which conduction occurs and may correspond to separation of myocardial bundles in regions of healed infarct or as occurs during the process of collagen deposition during aging. It should be noted, however, that normal myocardium is not a uniform conducting medium, but rather contains potential barriers for conduction that include blood vessels and interfaces between different cell types. A viewpoint that would unify the studies of macroscopic and microscopic discontinuities might be that the effective lengths of such anatomical barriers can be extended under conditions where gap junctional resistance is increased.

REGULATION OF GAP JUNCTION EXPRESSION, FORMATION, AND DEGRADATION

Life and Death of Gap Junctions

A major finding from studies first performed on rat liver in vivo (76, 310), then in cardiac myocytes, hepatocytes, and cell lines in culture (130, 132, 134, 302), and most recently in Langendorff-perfused rat hearts (12) is that connexin molecules are very short-lived. In the case of the heart, the measured decay of radioactivity in immunoprecipitated Cx43 was monoexponential, which was best fit by a half-life of only 1.3 hours! Thus, in cardiac tissue, there is a single pool of Cx43 protein that is completely turned over several times every day.

The rapid turnover of gap junction proteins reemphasizes the possibility that remodeling of communication compartments might occur over a short period of time and also stresses the importance of understanding the intracellular trafficking events that occur during this time frame (Figure 4–7A). Cx32 and Cx43 appear to be co-translationally inserted into the endoplasmic reticulum (ER) membrane, whereas there is evidence that Cx26 insertion may be either co- or post-translational (63, 74, 130, 302). Fatty acid acylation of Cx32 and Cx26 has been reported to be an early post-translational processing event that may occur as the protein folds into the membrane (63); whether Cx43 or the other cardiac connexins undergo similar modification remains to be determined and is an important missing data set from the standpoint of understanding the association of these connexins with membrane microdomains such as caveolae (207). Recent studies on Cx43 and Cx32 (74, 75) using in vitro translation in pancreatic microsomes indicate that the initial membrane folding event shows a tendency for proteolytic cleavage of the first membrane-spanning domain (TM1). Whether protein chaperones or co-translational protein modifications that nomally occur within cells stabilize the burial of TM1 within the plasma membrane remains to be determined. Newly synthesized connexins apparently remain as independent monomers as they begin their voyage along the secretory transport route from ER to Golgi apparatus. It remains to be determined exactly where it is that the

FIG. 4–7. Regulation of gap junction expression and degradation. *A:* Diagram of the life cycle of cardiac gap junctions. 1. MRNA is transcribed in the nucleus and translocated to the cytoplasm; 2. Protein is translated and inserted into the Endoplasmic reticulum. Mis-translated or mis-folded protein is proteolyzed by the Proteasome Ⓐ. Along the way from ER ② to Golgi ③, connexons are formed by connexin oligomerization. The connexons are then transported ④ to the cell surface where they meet and dock (⑤ and ⑥) with connexons of adjacent cells to form gap junction channels. Removal of gap junctions is through both proteasomal Ⓑ and lysosomal pathways Ⓒ. [Modified from Laing et al. (133).] *B:* Transcriptional activity of human connexin43-luciferase chimeric plasmids transfected into rat cardiac myocytes in vitro and adult rat ventricle myocytes in vivo. *On the right*, diagrams of the reporter gene constructs with nested deletions from the human Cx43 gene (−2400 to −50 base pairs, relative to transcription initiation). *On the left*, plot of relative luciferase activity generated by each construct, showing that the presence of at least 175 base pairs of 5′−flanking sequence is required for measurable transcription. Differences in transcription in in vitro and in vivo experiments was only seen with the 2400 base pair construct. In vivo this construct was 170-fold more active than the −50Cx43Lux plasmid, while in vitro it was only 30-fold more active. Each data point represents the mean ± S.E. from three to five different animals. Results in vivo are compared to myocytes in vitro by arbitrarily setting the −250Cx43Lux construct value to 1 for both systems. [Modified from De Leon et al. (153), with permission.]

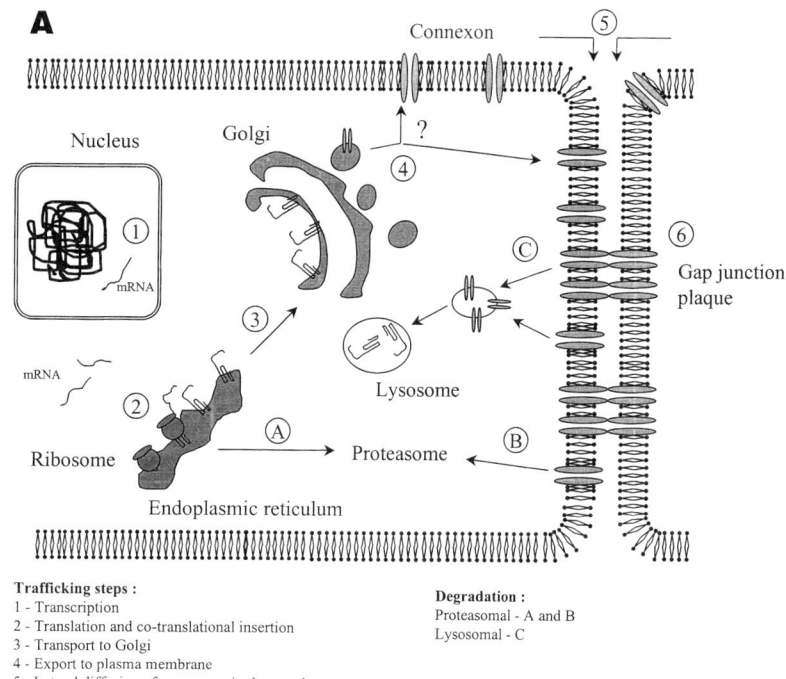

Trafficking steps:
1 - Transcription
2 - Translation and co-translational insertion
3 - Transport to Golgi
4 - Export to plasma membrane
5 - Lateral diffusion of connexons in the membrane
6 - Docking and formation of gap junction plaques

Degradation:
Proteasomal - A and B
Lysosomal - C

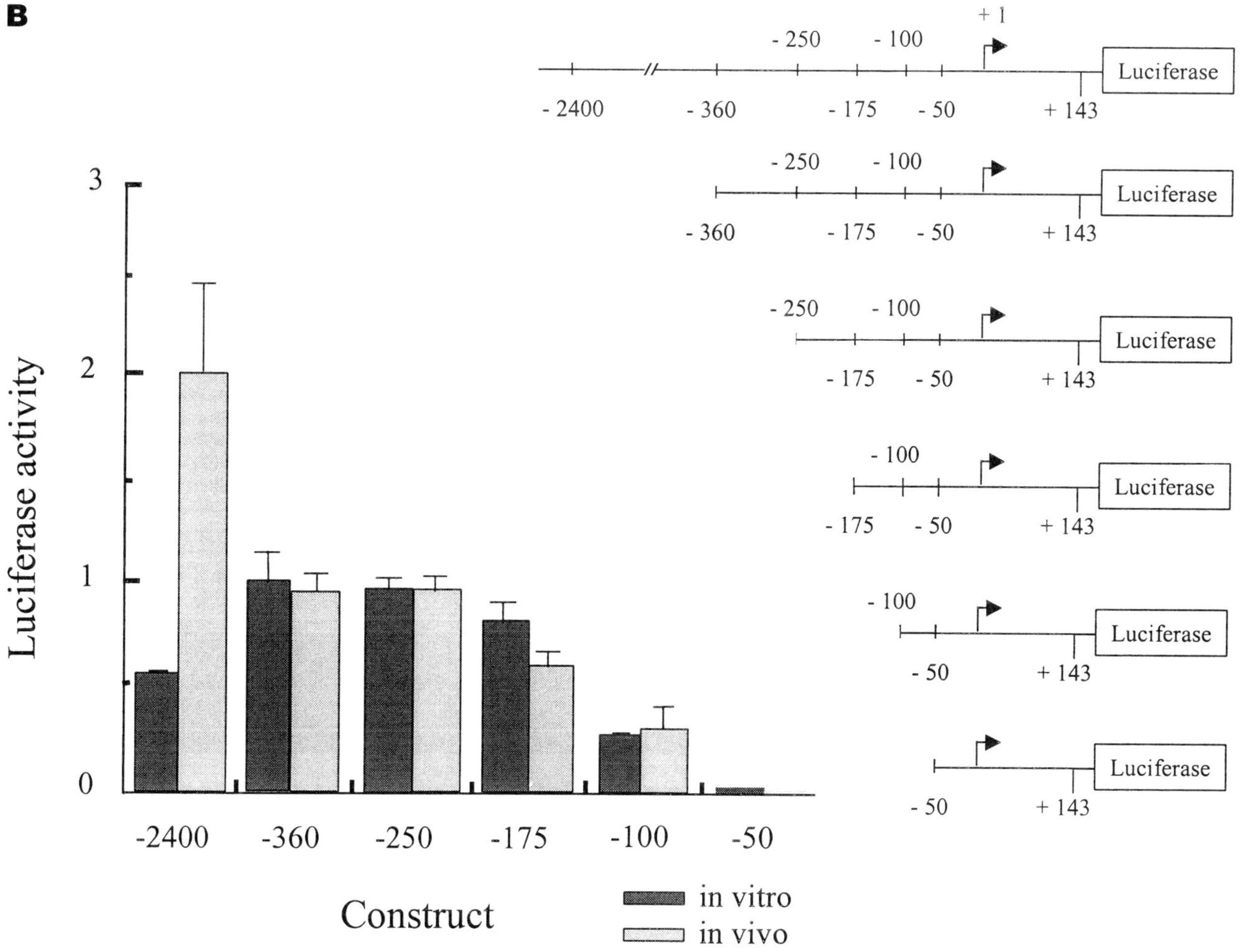

connexins coalesce into connexons, although recent evidence favors a more proximal site, near the ER–Golgi transition (63, 74), rather than in the distal *trans*-Golgi region as originally suggested (179). Where it is that connexins assemble may determine the probability of intermingling as heteromers. A curiosity is how the connexins can remain monomeric during their journey and why, once connexons form, they do not pair with contiguous connexons in apposed intracellular membranes. Indeed, in transfected cells overexpressing Cx43, such junctional structures are observed in intracellular membranes, and it is hypothesized that chaperone proteins, in low enough abundance as to be saturable by connexin overexpression, may perform this function in normal cells (126).

Movement of connexons from the distal Golgi to the junctional membrane remains mysterious. An unanswered question is whether delivery is random to anywhere on the cell surface, followed by diffusion until the connexon is trapped by high-affinity binding to an apposing hemichannel, or whether connexons are targeted to junctional plaques. The recent exciting finding that the second PDZ domain of the tight junction–associated protein ZO-1 binds the carboxyl terminus of Cx43 and links it to the cytoskeletal protein spectrin at intercalated disks of cardiac myocytes (85, 269) suggests that connexins may be centerpieces of a macromolecular complex or nexus. Next steps will involve testing whether scaffolds associated with gap junction proteins may generate the forces that aggregate junctional channels, direct their insertion or retrieval, or juxtapose modulatory molecules at the mouths of the junctional channels.

Connexins undergo other types of post-translational modification, including phosphorylation and ubiquitination (130). Where these modifications occur is not entirely clear, although Cx43 can be phosphorylated while in junctional plaques and phosphorylation has been suggested to facilitate channel formation (180). Whether such modifications as phosphorylation/dephosphorylation and ubiquitin incorporation into Cx43 provide binding sites for retrieval of connexin proteins from the membrane and ultimate degradation is unknown. Beardslee et al. (12) recently reported that selective pharmacological blockade of either lysosomal or proteasomal routes of degradation result in accumulation of junctional Cx43, indicating that both pathways normally contribute. An intriguing aspect of that study is that proteasomal inhibition caused accumulation of dephosphorylated Cx43, whereas treatment with lysosomal inhibitors increased the amount of phosphorylated Cx43 remaining in junctional membranes, suggesting that the phosphorylation state might provide one signal to direct the degradation pathway. It remains to be determined whether such differential breakdown might be responsible for foreshortened half-lives reported for Cx45 mutants lacking phosphorylatable serine residues (104).

Internalized annular gap junctions have been detected in dissociated cells (38, 155, 224) and more rarely in cells maintained in culture (e.g., 248), and it has been suggested that one cell may degrade both the connexins in its own connexons and those phagocytosed from the neighboring cell (135). A sequential contribution of proteasomal and lysosomal degradation pathways might allow such internalization and gap junction breakdown. Consistent with such a possibility, Laing et al. (132), using Chinese hamster ovary and transformed rat cardiocytes reported that Cx43 remained at the surface when the proteasome was inhibited but appeared in intracellular vesicles when the lysosome pathway was blocked.

Long-Term Changes in Gap Junction Expression

The rapid turnover dynamics of gap junction channels implies that gap junction–mediated circuitry in tissues might be a dynamic process that responds to local demands. The first example of a tissue in which gap junction expression was shown to undergo rapid changes was the pregnant myometrium (83), in which Cx43 expression is now known to be transcriptionally upregulated at the time of labor (38), presumably acting to coordinate and thereby intensify the contractions of the uterus.

The vessel wall is an organ that undergoes both physiological and pathological changes in response to mechanical stresses and upon exposure to hormonal stimuli. Vascular tissue consists of two communication compartments: smooth muscle, which predominantly expresses Cx43 (e.g., 39), and endothelial cells, which Gabriels and Paul (82) showed in undisturbed aorta express predominantly Cx40, somewhat less Cx37, and little or no Cx43. In culture, regulation of connexin expression by vascular smooth muscle and endothelial cells has been evaluated with regard to a variety of stimuli. For example, smooth muscle cells were recently shown to respond with upregulation of Cx43 and its mRNA within hours after application of 20% static stretch (46). Cultured endothelial cells have been shown to upregulate Cx43 in response to wounding (194, 195), application of shear stress (46), and after treatment with transforming growth factor-β (TGFβ; 138), and basic fibroblast growth factor (bFGF; 193), whereas expression of Cx43 has been reported to decrease in response to epidermal growth factor (EGF; 305) and tumor necrosis factor-α (TNFα; 279). It is interesting that in the few studies that have either measured transcription directly or evaluated mRNA stability through treatment with cycloheximide, the endothelial changes have been ascribed to altered mRNA stability (194, 195; see also ref. 122), whereas the changes in smooth muscle have been shown to be transcriptional (46).

Comparably fewer in vivo studies have been performed to evaluate effects of vascular manipulations on connexin expression, although the findings in arterial smooth muscle cells have been striking: Connexin43 is increased both in several hypertensive models (94, 292) and following balloon injury (312), whereas reduced Cx43 expression results from hypercholesterolemia-induced atherosclerosis (204).

It was recently reported that Cx43 is virtually absent in most regions of rodent aortic endothelium, except at sites where branching or flow division is expected to create high turbulence, and that Cx43 expression is reciprocally related to that of Cx37 (82). These observations may explain in part the anatomical finding that the shapes of the gap junction arrays connecting endothelial cells in regions of vascular turbulence are different from those in regions with laminar flow (110, 186), and the involvement of a shear stress–induced transduction mechanism might also relate to the reported high Cx43 expression in cardiac tissue below the mitral valve (312).

Gabriels and Paul (82) have also reported that Cx43 expression is dramatically induced in the coarcted region of the vasculature at 8 days after cuff ligation. This remarkable finding suggests a mechanism by which myoendothelial communication might be either established or intensified at regions of altered blood flow. Likely consequences of such changes in connexin expression might include altered vasomotor tone or vascular reactivity as either a compensation or maladaptation to such injury.

The rapid dynamics of gap junction turnover and the plasticity of gap junction expression in response to various stimuli offer the possibility for remodeling of the intercellular circuits both within and between communication compartments in the cardiovascular system. In the heart, such remodeling could exaggerate conduction discontinuities caused by tissue anisotropy and thus be arrhythmogenic (235). In the vessel wall, such altered expression may allow inter-compartmental signaling that is otherwise forbidden by the lack of heterotypic junction formation by the connexins normally expressed by smooth muscle and endothelial cells (26). The next step toward understanding the remodeling of gap junction–mediated circuits of intercellular signaling is the identification of *cis* and *trans*-activating elements responsible for the altered expression of the connexin genes in response to environmental stimuli. Although surprisingly few studies have thus far addressed these control mechanisms (e.g., 38), reports such as that of Gabriels and Paul (82) will likely stimulate such studies, leading not only to increased understanding of connexin gene regulation but also to strategies by which expression patterns might be therapeutically manipulated.

Transcriptional Regulation of Cardiac Gap Junction Genes

Studies of the transcriptional regulation of cardiac connexins have assumed increasing importance because of the growing numbers of reports indicating altered connexin expression in pathological situations (e.g., 11, 94). The first of these studies (53) examined transcriptional control of Cx43 in the heart by use of genomic clones encompassing putative 5' flanking regulation sequences of the human gene (Fig. 4–8B). Fusion of these sequences to that encoding firefly luciferase enzyme permitted assay of transcriptional activity both in cultured neonatal myocytes and after delivery into hearts in vivo using intracardiac DNA injection. In both culture and in vivo systems, substantial expression of the exogenous reporter gene was obtained by inclusion of as little as 175 bp of Cx43 5' flanking sequence. Inclusion of longer genomic sequence resulted in high levels of expression in vivo, but not in the culture system, suggesting that upstream regions between -175 and -2400 might be uniquely responsive to hemodynamic or neurohormonal effects.

The critical 100 bp sequence upstream of the transcription start sites are quite similar in Cx43 genes of human, rat, and mouse (53, 263, 313). The use of chloramphenicol acetyl transferase (CAT) constructs with deletions within this region have recently demonstrated both positive and negative *cis*-acting regulatory sequences in the mouse gene when expressed in myometrial cells (38). In addition, a site in this region has been demonstrated in the human promoter to be responsive to phorbol esters (84), and an estrogen response element has been found in the human sequence (313).

Recently, Wnt-1, a secreted ligand implicated in diverse development processes in a wide range of organisms, was shown to markedly induce Cx43 transcription in cultured neonatal cardiomyocytes. This effect appeared to work through the downstream effector beta-catenin, which heterodimerizes with T-cell factor family members to form a transcriptional transactivation complex (1). Interestingly, the expression of Wnt receptors (i.e. *frizzled*-like proteins) may be altered in diseased hearts, such as those with hypertrophy or following infarction, and this abnormality may play a role in the processes of gap junction remodeling and arrhythmogenesis (21, 22).

Analysis of Cx40 and Cx45 promoter regions might be expected to reveal regulatory elements that would explain their differential expression patterns compared to Cx43 in the cardiovascular system and could also lead to the generation of constructs that would be selectively targeted to endothelium or the cardiac conduction system. Although such studies are only just beginning, promoter analysis of the mouse Cx40 gene has revealed both positive and negative regulatory elements near the transcription start site (223).

FUNCTIONAL PROPERTIES OF CARDIOVASCULAR GAP JUNCTIONS

In excitable tissues including the heart, the preeminent role of gap junctions is in electrotonic spread of current, resulting in rapid and synchronized signal relay from one cell to the next. In some regions of the heart, such as the Purkinje fibers, it is the actual rapidity that is most important, and in other tissue areas, such as nodal structures, a paucity of junctional channels results in a delay that provides the timing necessary for rhythmic muscular contraction. Current spread from one cardiac myocyte to the next is mediated by the flow of ions. Because K^+ is the most abundant and most mobile intracellular ion, it is responsible for carrying most of the current between cells. In their role as electrotonic synapses, gap junction channels functionally operate as K^+ channels.

Cardiovascular Gap Junctions Are K^+, Ca^{2+}, and Second Messenger Channels

Besides the electrical coupling, gap junction channel permeability to larger ions and molecules (<1 kDa) allows them to couple the cells from the metabolic point of view, providing an intercellular pathway for communication of second messenger molecules such as cyclic adenosine or guanosine monophosphate, 1,4,5 inositol trisphosphate and adenosine disphosphate and triphosphate (cAMP, cGMP, IP_3, ATP, and ADP). Despite the abundant literature implicating Ca^{2+} ions in uncoupling cardiac cells, it is now generally recognized that Ca^{2+} sensitivity of gap junctions is low. Thus, instead of closing junctional channels, Ca^{2+} can actually diffuse through gap junction channels between cells, thereby acting as an intercellular messenger or signaling molecule.

The idea that Ca^{2+} ions could affect gap junction channel activity appeared with the studies on the mechanisms underlying the phenomenon of "healing over" which began with experiments in which the ionic solutions that bathed injured cardiac tissue were varied. Strikingly, removal of Ca^{2+} slowed or prevented recovery, from which it was concluded that Ca^{2+} ions entering the cardiac cell from the extracellular space could either directly occlude junctional channels or could close the channels by a conformational change in the channel protein or by altering binding or confomation of an intermediary molecule (such as calmodulin:see ref. 196). The hypothesis that sustained Ca^{2+} ions could act as an uncoupling agent reached its height of popularity about 25 years ago, when imaging experiments using aequorin introduced into transparent insect salivary gland cells revealed that injected Ca^{2+} caused gap junction closure only when the injected amounts were sufficient to reach the appositional membrane (214a). A major challenge to this Ca^{2+} hypothesis was raised at that time, with the demonstration by Turin and Warner (275) that intracellular acidification could close gap junctional channels, together with the subsequent demonstration that sensitivity to acidification was high in some systems and that sensitivity to Ca^{2+} was quite low. A unifying hypothesis that would allow control by both Ca^{2+} and H^+ involves action of both ions on a cytoplasmic intermediary molecule, either calmodulin itself or a calmodulin-like molecule.

One regrettable consequence of the belief that intracellular Ca^{2+} ions closed gap junction channels was that it prevented the appreciation that intercellular spread of Ca^{2+} ions might play a signaling role between coupled cells in the cardiovascular system. Although Ca^{2+} diffusion is normally limited to short intracellular distances due to high-affinity binding to cytoplasmic buffer molecules, the amplification mechanisms now known for Ca^{2+}-induced Ca^{2+} release have made the idea of such signaling a central aspect of intercellular coordination in many cell types.

The initial demonstration of intercellular signaling by Ca^{2+} was made by Dunlap, Takeda, and Brehm (64) on the hydrozoan *Obelia*, in which light-sensing cells are coupled to cells containing a Ca^{2+}-sensitive light-emitting protein related to aequorin. Subsequent studies involved direct injection of Ca^{2+} and IP_3 into hepatocytes or mechanical stimulation of airway epithelial cells (215, 220). Then, detecting local Ca^{2+} elevations with the EGTA-based ratiometric indicators developed by Roger Tsien clearly showed that Ca^{2+} rise evoked in one cell led to an elevation in adjacent cells and that this spread was blocked by substances that closed gap junction channels.

Spread of slow Ca^{2+} waves was soon demonstrated in a variety of other cell types, including astrocytes, endothelial cells, smooth muscle cells, osteoblasts, and chondrocytes, to name a few. In all these cell types, the spread has characteristic velocity, generally ranging from ~5–25 µm/sec. In many cell types, brief intracellular Ca^{2+} transients or oscillations can occur that are not transmitted to adjacent cells, indicating that a threshold concentration of messenger must diffuse to the second cell to elicit a propagated response. The current model for propagation of Ca^{2+} waves throughout a tissue (Fig. 4–8) involves the initial generation of IP$_3$ within the stimulated cell which diffuses to adjacent cells through gap junction channels, liberating Ca^{2+} from intracellular stores through activation of IP$_3$ receptors (IP3R). The spatial localization of IP3R quite close to the intercalated disk regions demonstrated in adult ventricular myocytes (117) provides an anatomical organization that might be ideal for such intercellular signaling. In some cell types, the spread is depressed by removal of extracellular Ca^{2+}, which is attributable to Ca^{2+}-induced opening of cation channels in the membrane. Whether ryanodine receptors (RYR) can sustain such Ca^{2+} waves is unknown.

Intercellular Ca^{2+} waves can also be propagated through release of ATP from a stimulated cell (see Fig. 4–8) and activation of purine and pyrimidine receptors (P$_2$-receptors) on its neighbors. Such an extracellular route of intercellular Ca^{2+} wavespread was first shown in rat mast cells by Osipchuk and Cahallan (187). This pathway apparently accounts for the observations that Ca^{2+} waves in cultured glial cells can leap small cell-free boundaries (97).

In the perfused whole rat heart, spontaneous intercellular Ca^{2+} waves can be seen propagating from one ventricular myocyte to others until they penetrate deep inside the myocardium (163). In neonatal mouse cardiac myocyte cultures, slow Ca^{2+} waves initiated by focal mechanical stimulation of a single cell propagate with velocity of 5–50 μm/sec (color plate 7). The transmission of Ca^{2+} signals relies mainly on gap junction channels and is modulated by P$_2$-receptor activation (260). Spread is inhibited by the gap junction channel blocker heptanol and is partially attenuated by duramin, a P$_2$-receptor blocker. In Cx43-null mouse cardiac myocytes the velocity of Ca^{2+} wave propagation as well as the efficacy of the Ca^{2+} signal spread are significantly reduced (260). The intercellular transmission of Ca^{2+} waves in cardiac myocytes seems to have a high safety factor, such that signal transmission in the absence of Cx43 can still be supported by the remaining connexins, as well as by ATP-mediated activation of P$_2$-receptors. The participation of this parallel panacrine pathway is also expected to be enhanced under abnormal conditions. Considering that ATP can be released by cardiac cells during ischemic injury, it is possible that ATP-mediated activation of P$_2$-receptors, in addition to direct Ca^{2+} entry into damaged cells, could initiate or sustain slow Ca^{2+} wave propagation. Application of ratiometric imaging techniques should allow more complete evaluation of this type of Ca^{2+} signaling in cardiac tissue, in much the same way that voltage-sensitive dyes are providing detailed maps of propagation of the much more rapid action potential wavefront. The nature of recruitment of the elemental Ca^{2+} release events ("Ca^{2+} sparks") into the propagated responses and the relative contribution of RYR and IP3R in the spread between cardiac myocytes are major issues that remain to be resolved.

Slow Ca^{2+} wave propagation mediated through both

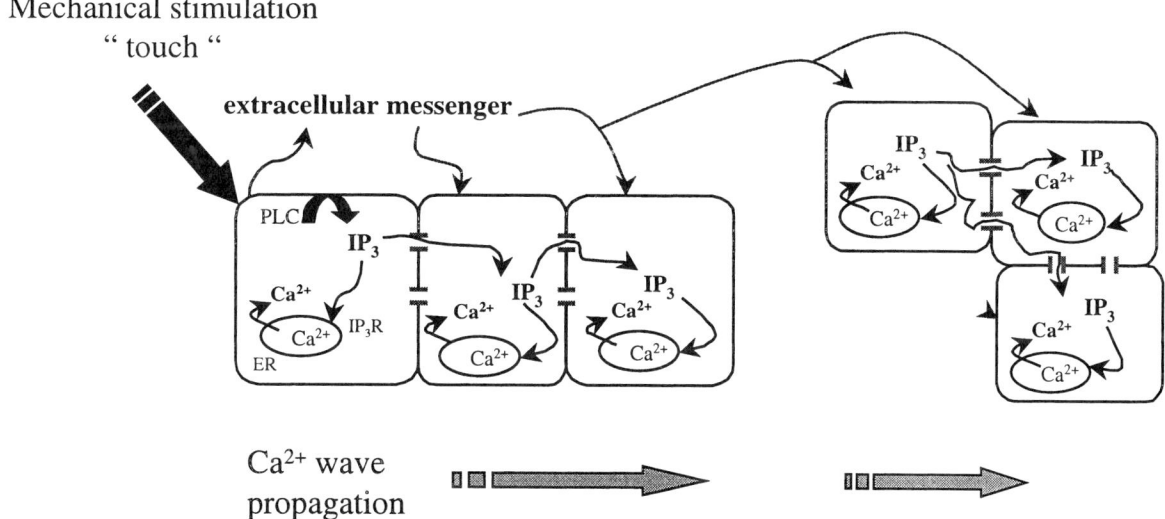

FIG. 4–8. Model for slow intercellular calcium wave propagation proposed by Sanderson and colleagues (221). Mechanical stimulation of a single cell in culture can induce the activation of phospholipase C (PLC) and synthesis of inositol trisphosphate (IP3), thereby activating IP3 receptors (IP3R) to release calcium from intracellular stores. The diffusion of IP3 to the neighboring cells, passing through gap junction channels, triggers the propagation of calcium waves from cell to cell. An extracellular pathway can also operate in parallel with the intercellular pathway. In this case, an extracellular messenger released from the stimulated cell diffuses from cell to cell and communicates the signal through activation of membrane receptors. In most cells that exhibit this mechanism, ATP has proven to be the extracellular messenger mediating the propagation of the calcium waves through activation of purinoceptors.

gap junction–dependent and gap junction–independent pathways may underlie "triggered propagated contractions" (TPC) in cardiac tissue and conducted vasomotor responses in vessel wall. Studies on both rat ventricular and human atrial trabeculae by ter Keurs and colleagues (48, 49, 175, 267, 300) have demonstrated that, following damage induced by local stretch, after-contractions caused by Ca^{2+} overload occur and can trigger arrhythmias as the after-contractions spread to neighboring myocardial regions (Fig.4–9). The velocity of these propagated contractions along undamaged parts of the trabeculae is constant with distance, at about 0.1–15 mm/sec, which is much slower than the propagation of electrical excitability in this tissue (nearly 1 m/sec), although the velocity of the intercellular Ca^{2+} wave that underlies the TPC (0.34–5.17 mm/sec, 164) appears to be somewhat faster than that of Ca^{2+} waves elicited in cultured cardiac myocytes by focal mechanical stimulation. Involvement of gap junctions in wave propagation is suggested by reduction of propagation velocity, triggering rate, and force of TPC in the presence of the gap junction channel blockers heptanol and octanol, without affecting the twitch force. The model proposed to account for the phenomenon of TPC includes local Ca^{2+} release from the sarcoplasmic reticulum in the damaged cell, leading to generation of slow Ca^{2+} waves that are communicated to the neighboring cells by Ca^{2+} diffusion through gap junction channels (267) with Ca^{2+}-induced Ca^{2+} release in the adjoining cell leading to the spreading contraction. Such Ca^{2+} entry and mobilization is also thought to result in depolarization (delayed with respect to the more rapidly conducted electrical activation), which may reach threshold and thereby trigger arrhythmias.

In vessel wall, Segal and Duling (225) showed that vasomotor responses could be spread over long distances even when innervation was blocked, and more recent evidence from a number of sources indicates that gap junctions between vascular smooth muscle can serve to maintain and modulate vessel tone (39). In addition, the provocative finding of myoendothelial junctional structures has prompted speculation that such contacts may be responsible for endothelial modulation of smooth muscle relaxation or contraction. Because of the geometry of the vessel, where a single endothelial cell may span multiple smooth muscle cells (147), endothelial gap junctional contacts may provide a rapid and extensive mechanism by which vasomotor tone can be regulated.

Biophysical Properties of Junctional Channels

The function of gap junction channels is to provide a pathway by which ions and small molecules (M_r <1000 Da) can diffuse from one cell to another. The ability of molecules to pass through gap junctions depends on the electrical conductance of the junctional membrane and its permeability to ions and molecules of different size and charge. The electrical conductance of the junctional membrane (g_j) depends on the number of junctional channels, the single-channel conductance, and the open probability of individual channels, whereas the junctional permeability to specific ions and molecules additionally depends on the extent to which passage is permitted by the connexins forming the gap junction channels.

Both macroscopic and single-channel conductances can be evaluated using electrophysiological techniques on pairs of cells. The dual voltage-clamp technique uses two microelectrodes in each cell of a pair to voltage clamp the cell and to measure the junctional current (247). This technique remains the method of choice for accurate measurement of macroscopic junctional conductance in oocytes and other large cells. The patch-clamp version of the technique, introduced more than ten years ago, uses one low-resistance patch electrode

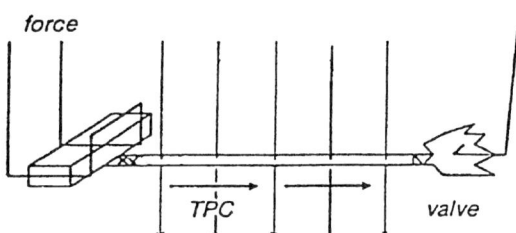

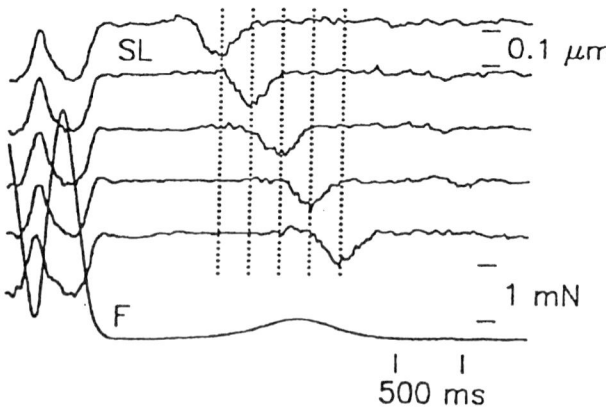

FIG. 4–9. Triggered propagated contraction (TPC) in rat trabeculae. The constant interval between the peak of sarcomere shortening (vertical dotted lines) recorded simultaneously at five different points (300 μm apart) along the trabeculae (length 2.9 mm) during a TPC indicates that the contraction propagates with a constant velocity (1.4 mm/sec) along the preparation. SL = sarcomere length; F = force of contraction. [From ter Keurs and Zhang, (267), with permission.]

per cell and makes it possible to record from mammalian cells (181, 299). Moreover, this technique has allowed the detection of single-channel currents under conditions where the input resistance of cells is high (≥ 1 GΩ) and when the number of channels between cells is low. With either version of the dual whole-cell method, both cells are initially clamped at a common holding potential and then one cell is either hyperpolarized or depolarized to impose a transjunctional voltage (V_j) gradient. The current measured in the stepped cell (I_1, delivered by the feedback amplifier to hold the voltage at the new level) corresponds to the sum of currents flowing through nonjunctional and junctional membranes; the current measured in the other cell's voltage-clamp circuit (I_2) is equal to the junctional current. This junctional current ($I_j = I_2$) is conventionally opposite in sign to the V_j command; the absolute value of the ratio of I_j to V_j is junctional conductance (g_j; normalized g_j values are usually indicated as G_j).

The open probability of gap junction channels is regulated by a wide range of stimuli including transjunctional voltage (i.e. the voltage difference across the junction), intracellular calcium and pH, and the phosphorylation state of the connexin molecules. It can be altered experimentally through the application of certain lipophilic molecules and other agents. The gating of junctional conductance by transjunctional voltage has been the most well-studied of these manipulations; therefore, in the following section, we discuss the regulation of macroscopic and single-channel conductance by V_j. It must be mentioned at the outset that a physiological role for the voltage dependence exhibited by gap junction channels has not yet been demonstrated. However, in some cases (e.g., homotypic Cx45 and heterotypic Cx43-Cx45), sensitivity to transjunctional voltage is high enough that it may play a role in some cardiac regions or at some compartmental interfaces. Moreover, determination of the properties of the different connexins has revealed that each connexin type has a different V_j sensitivity, thereby enabling gap junction physiologists to identify which types of connexins are functionally present in cardiac and other cell types, based in part on this property.

Gating of Gap Junctional Channels by Transjunctional Voltage

The dependence of junctional conductance on the transjunctional voltage was first demonstrated in amphibian embryonic cell pairs using the dual voltage-clamp technique (247). In these cells, application of large V_j steps of either polarity caused a strong decline of the junctional current to a non-zero steady-state level, whereas small V_j steps produced no appreciable change in junctional conductance. The sensitivity of junctional conductance to V_j of either polarity was found to be well described by the Boltzmann equation:

$$g_j = g_{ss} = \frac{g_{max} - g_{min}}{1 + \exp[A(V - V_0)]} + g_{min}$$

where g_{max} and g_{min} are the maximal and minimal conductances obtained at lowest and highest V_j; V_0 is the voltage at which the voltage-sensitive component of g_j ($g_{max} - g_{min}$) is reduced by 50%, and A is a slope factor from which the equivalent number of gating changes, n, can be calculated (245). Evaluation of voltage sensitivity after exogenous expression of connexins in mammalian cells or in weakly endogenously coupled cell pairs has indicated that for most connexins, the steady-state conductance is symmetrical around 0 mV and is well fit to Boltzmann relationships (Fig. 4–10). Moreover, Boltzmann parameters are now known to be distinct for gap junction channels formed of each connexin subtype, as described in more detail below.

For most of the gap junction channels that have been studied, the relaxation of junctional current from its initial level to the steady-state levels is well fit by a single exponential decay function for each voltage. This implies that a first-order process underlies channel closure by voltage. By determining the time constants for junctional current relaxation over the complete voltage range, together with curve fitting of the steady-state sensitivity to the Boltzmann relationship (G_{ss} at each V_j), the opening and closing rate constants (α and β, respectively) have been calculated as follows (96):

$$\alpha = \frac{G_{ss}}{\tau} \text{ and } \beta = \frac{1 - G_{ss}}{\tau}$$

Measurement of single gap junction channels from poorly expressing cells or from preformed cells provided additional insight into the gating of gap junction channels. At the microscopic level, junctional currents of most connexins exhibit direct, interconverting transitions between the fully open state (O) and the voltage-insensitive or residual conductance substate (O_s), as shown in Figures 4–11 and 4–12 (27, 171). The ratio of the unitary conductances of the main open state and the subconductance state has in all cases been found to be similar to the g_{min}/g_{max} ratio, thus indicating that the residual conductance g_{min} seen at high V_j arises from channel transitions occurring from the main state to the residual subconductance state (171). Single-channel open probability measurements further indicate that the voltage sensitivity of the macroscopic conductance is due to the ensemble activity of identical and independent channels (27, 256). Interestingly, single-channel studies reveal that most gap junction channels transit to the fully closed state at high V_j or when V_j

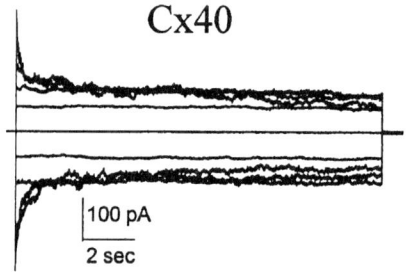
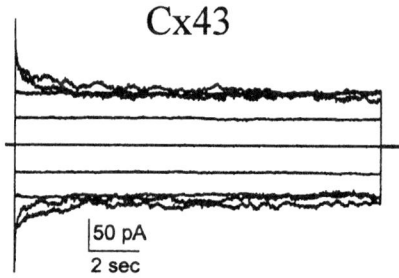
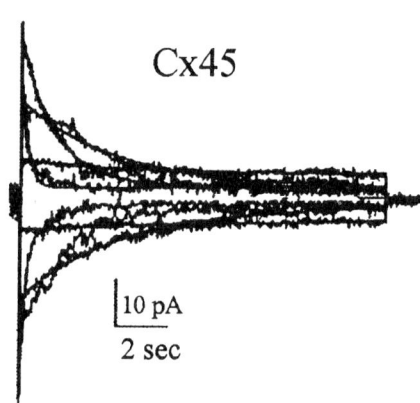
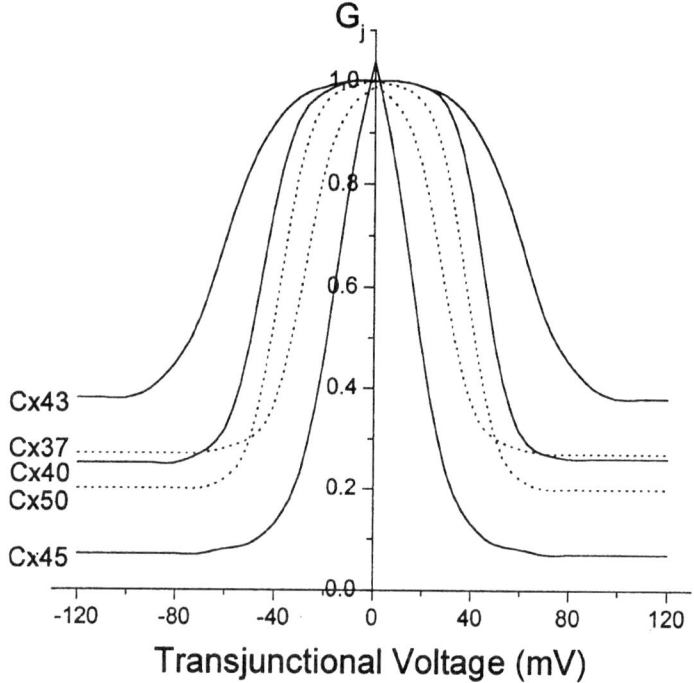

FIG. 4–10. Dependence of junctional conductance of Cx40, Cx43, and Cx45 gap junction channels on transjunctional voltage (V_j). *A:* Recordings of junctional current (I_j, lower traces) measured in one cell of a pair expressing each connexin individually in response to 8–15 sec long pulses from 0 to ± 80 mV (in 20 mV increments) that were applied to the other cell. Junctional currents were maximal at the beginning of the pulses and declined to steady-state values in a time- and voltage-dependent manner. *B:* Relationship between V_j and steady-state junctional conductance of Cx40, Cx43, and Cx45 gap junction channels (*solid lines*) and of Cx37 and Cx50 (*dotted lines*). The lines are a fit of the normalized steady-state junctional conductance (G_j, the ratio of the steady-state g_j to maximal g_j)-V_j relationship to a two state Boltzmann equation. The Boltzmann parameters for channels formed by each connexin type are listed in Table 4–2.

gradients are imposed for long durations (256). It remains to be determined whether this inactivation represents a "mode-shifting" behavior of the gap junction channel as proposed by Brink and colleagues (24) or is analogous to the inactivation of other voltage-gated channels. In either case, these transitions may underlie the slower decline in the macroscopic current that is observed at high V_j when sustained voltage pulses are applied. The state diagram for effects of V_j on gap junction channels is presented in Figure 4–12, consisting of a fully open state (O); a partially open or subconductance state (O_s) with single-order rate constants α and β, that is initially entered in response to V_j; and a fully closed state (C), representing the state entered during a sustained transjunctional potential.

The state diagram in Figure 4–12 has symmetrical but distinct states for depolarizing and hyperpolarizing responses. As mentioned, junctional conductance decreases symmetrically at about 0 mV, with identical kinetic properties for both polarities. Therefore, gap junction channels have been proposed to be comprised of two independent gates arranged in series (with each hemichannel providing one of the voltage-sensitive gates). This proposal is supported by potential reversal experiments (96, 167, 255). Changing the membrane potential from positive to negative values causes the junctional current to increase before the decline to steady-state levels. The fact that channels open first before closing in response to a transjunctional voltage of opposite polarity indicates that each hemichannel has a voltage-sensitive gate and that closure of one gate is contingent upon the other gate reopening (96).

Domains involved in voltage-dependent gating remain to be explicitly identified. Unlike other voltage-gated channels, connexins do not contain a highly charged helical motif upon which the voltage gradient

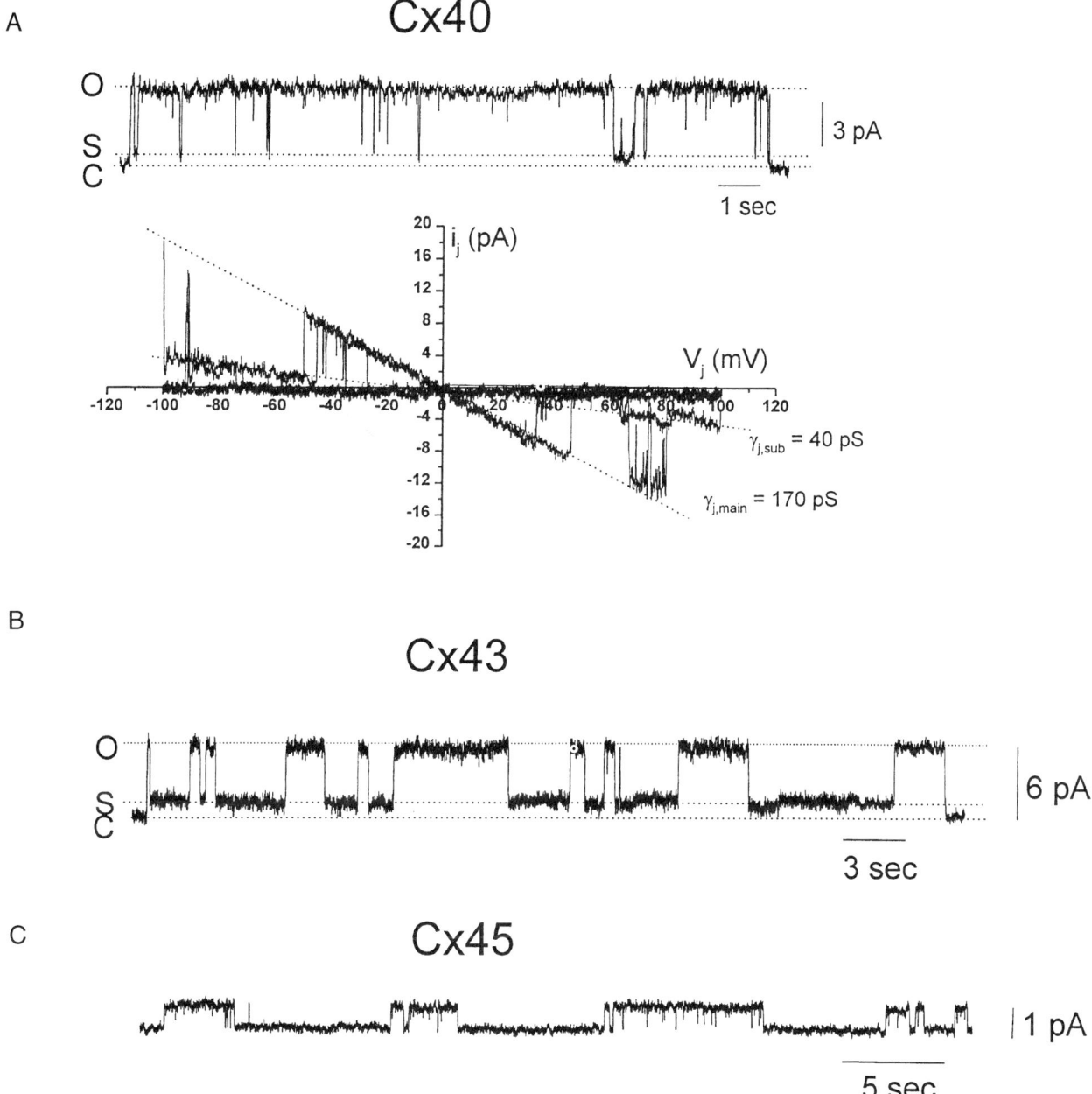

FIG. 4–11. Unitary conductances of gap junction channels formed by Cx40 (A), Cx43 (B), and Cx45 (C) measured with pipettes containing 130 mM CsCl. *A: Top.* Junctional currents measured in one cell of a Cx40-transfected N2A cell pair in response to 16 sec voltage step to 30 mV from a holding potential of 0 mV that was applied to the other cell. Single Cx40 channels were maximally open (O) from the baseline level (C) immediately upon application of a voltage pulse. The amplitude of the unitary current measured from all points amplitude histogram was 5.8 pA, corresponding to a single-channel conductance of 193 pS. *A: Bottom.* Single-channel current voltage (I_j-V_j) relationships of the junctional current constructed from responses of Cx40-transfected N2A cells to a series of ramps from −100 to +100 mV. The unitary conductance of the main state ($\gamma_{j, main}$) and the substate ($\gamma_{j, sub}$), measured as the slopes of the current–voltage relationships (solid lines), were 170 pS and 40 pS, respectively. The ratio of $\gamma_{j, sub}$ and $\gamma_{j, main}$ for Cx40 channels is similar to the g_{min}/g_{max} value obtained from macroscopic recordings. *B, C:* Single-channel currents from Cx43- and Cx45-transfected cell pairs at voltages close to the respective V_0 values obtained from macroscopic recordings. *B:* Single-channel current through Cx43 gap junction channels predominantly exhibits transitions between a subconductance state (S) and the open state (O) at a V_j of 75 mV. Transitions to the baseline level (C) were rare; only one such transition was observed during the 40-second pulse. Unitary conductances of the fully open state and the subconductance state were 80 pS and 26 pS, respectively. *C:* transitions of single-channel current from a Cx45-transfected cell pair at a V_j of 30 mV to the subconductance state is not clearly detected due to the small unitary conductance of these channels ($\gamma_{j, main}$ = 35 pS) and to the low g_{min}/g_{max} ratio for these channels. In addition, note that at these low voltages, open probability of Cx45 channels was low and comparable to that of Cx43 at a V_j of 75 mV.

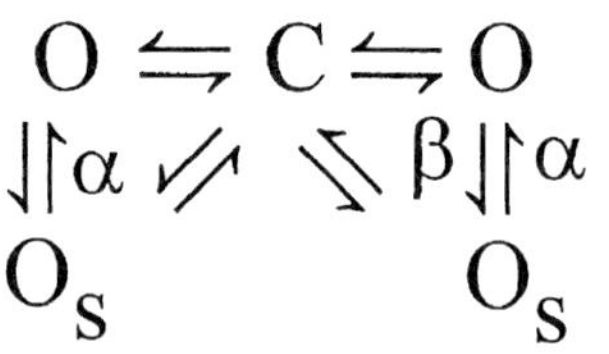

$$O \rightleftharpoons C \rightleftharpoons O$$
$$\beta \downarrow\uparrow \alpha \swarrow\nwarrow \searrow\nearrow \beta \downarrow\uparrow \alpha$$
$$O_s \qquad\qquad O_s$$

FIG. 4-12. State diagram of Cx50 gap junction channels. In this scheme, the channels are envisioned to possess two fully open states (O) and a single closed state (C). For each polarity of V_j, the equilibrium between fully open (O) and subconductance state (O_s) is determined by the opening and closing rate constants α and β. Transitions between O and C and O_s and C are not appreciably voltage sensitive and are presumably the targets of heptanol, halothane, and other uncoupling lipophiles.

is likely to act. Thus, it is conceivable that voltage dependence may arise out of interactions between several regions of the channel macromolecule. For example, mutation of Pro87 in M2 of Cx26 reverses the sign of voltage sensitivity when the mutant is paired with wild-type Cx26 in oocyte expression experiments (261). More detailed mutagenesis experiments on Cx32 and Cx26 have further implicated charged residues in the amino terminus and at the M1-E1 margin of these connexins (285). However, recent experiments from the laboratory of Luis Barrio (212) using carboxyl terminal truncation mutants of Cx43 clearly indicate that this domain is also important in channel closure in response to transjunctional voltage. A major conceptual deficit in the field is the lack of understanding of just which residues in connexins are the voltage sensors and how sensing of the voltage field is transduced into conformational change resulting in channel closure.

Properties of Specific Connexins Expressed in Exogenous Systems

Because multiple gap junction proteins are expressed in cells of most tissues, it has been desirable to evaluate the properties of channels formed of individual connexins in exogenous expression systems in which cRNA is injected into *Xenopus* oocytes (295) after prior inhibition of endogenous transcripts by antisense oligonucleotide injection (9), or DNA is introduced into communication-deficient mammalian cells using an expression vector (66, 79). Such exogenous expression in cells with minimal background has additionally allowed the functional evaluation of mutant connexin sequences, which, as noted, are expected to ultimately reveal which protein domains are involved in channel gating and in the assembly of the multimeric channel complex. The use of mammalian systems might be expected to lead to more faithful post-translational processing than in amphibian oocytes; moreover, the use of small, high-resistance cells allows assessment of channel properties through application of whole-cell recording methods to weakly coupled cell pairs.

Stable expression in mammalian cells requires genomic integration of the targeted construct, a very rare event. To select colonies of cells in which the gene is expressed, a selectable marker gene, conferring resistance to a specific antibiotic, is introduced either on the same plasmid or on a separate one. Treatment with antibiotic kills all cells that are not transfected with the marker, leaving some cells in which the target gene is also expressed. Communication-deficient cells that have been used thus far for transfection with gap junction cDNAs include SKHep1 (a highly metastatic human hepatoma cell line), PC12 (isolated from rat adrenomedullary tumor), HeLa (a human breast cancer line), and N2A (a rat spinal cord neuroblastoma cell line). It should be noted that none of these cells are truly devoid of endogenous gap junction channels (65, 172, 286, 287), although the high expression level obtained following transfection is generally believed to minimize this concern.

Activity of single gap junction channels is usually recorded in preparations in which the number of open channels is low enough to allow the detection of unitary events. However, in preparations where channel number is extremely high, as in the heart, single-channel events are usually recorded after exposure to uncoupling agents such as halothane, heptanol, or octanol. Because these agents reversibly reduce the number of open channels, presumably because of a decrease in P_o, they have been used to estimate the unitary conductance of gap junction channels. Alternately, unitary events have been resolved by an "induced" method, wherein two cells are pushed together and the sequential insertion of individual channels can be detected (28, 29, 214). All three preparations yield similar unitary conductance values, and data obtained with all methods are presented interchangeably in the discussion below.

Connexin43 Expressed in Exogenous Systems. Gap junction channels formed by Cx43 have been the best studied of all connexins known to date. Evaluation of Cx43 gap junction channel properties after expression in oocytes initially indicated little or no sensitivity of junctional conductance to transjunctional voltage (which was consistent with the earliest reports on heart cells using moderate transjunctional voltages; see below). Most recent studies in which space clamp conditions were improved by limiting analysis to lower conductance cell pairs indicated that these channels are weakly sensitive to V_j (298). Macroscopic conductance was shown to be reduced by V_j pulses of either polarity, although even at very high V_j values a large voltage-insensitive component (g_{min}) remains (Fig. 4–10; 171, 277). Parameters describing voltage sensitivity of Cx43 channels are given in Table 4–2. The proportion of junctional conductance that is voltage insensitive is quite high (40 % of total g_j), as is the voltage at which the voltage-sensitive component is reduced by 50 % ($V_0 = 60$ mV). In addition to the weak dependence of the junctional conductance on V_j, Cx43 channels expressed in oocytes appear to be modulated by the inside–outside potential (such that g_j is decreased by almost 50% upon depolarization from -100 to 0 mV). Such strong dependence of junctional conductance of Cx43 channels on the inside–outside potential has not been observed in mammalian cells (6).

Human connexin43 channels expressed in SKHep1 cells exhibit at least three discrete, non-zero conductance states, 30, 60–70 and 90–110 pS when recordings are done using internal solutions with highly mobile anions and cations. The 60–70 and 90–110 pS sizes appear to represent the phosphorylated and dephosphorylated unitary conductances of Cx43 channels, respectively (172), and the 30 pS events represent the residual subconductance state induced at high V_j values (172). The maximal unitary conductance of Cx43 channels is obtained under conditions in which phosphatase is introduced into the patch pipette or when protein kinases are inhibited by treatment with staurosporine. The intermediate conductance state is favored when phosphatases are inhibited (for example, by treatment with okadaic acid) or when cells are treated with membrane-permeant agents that promote protein phosphorylation (for example, tumor-promoting phorbol esters, 8Br-cAMP). These treatments alter Cx43 protein phosphorylation when applied under conditions similar to those used for electrophysiological studies. Regulation of unitary conductance of the Cx43 channel by phosphorylating agents appears to be species-specific. For example, recent studies have revealed that rodent Cx43 but not human Cx43 is phosphorylated by 8Br-cGMP and that g_j values of rodent but not human Cx43 channels are lower after such treatments (128). Whether this simply arises because there is a serine residue at position 257 in rat Cx43 but not human Cx43 remains to be resolved.

Parameters for steady-state voltage sensitivity do not appear to be appreciably affected by intracellular dialysis with phosphatase, implying that steady-state voltage sensitivity of open probability is not affected by phosphorylation. However, the decline in junctional current during a V_j step is accelerated after phosphatase treatment. Accelerated kinetics with similar steady-state voltage sensitivity could be explained by channel phosphorylation affecting both opening and closing rate constants to the same degree. However, this hypothesis needs to be validated by measurement of rate constants from single-channel recordings.

Cx43 channels do not discriminate to any great degree between anions and cations. They are highly permeant to the anionic dye lucifer yellow and appear to be similarly permeant to both anions and cations. This conclusion is based on ion-substitution experiments in which single-channel conductances were determined and compared to the aqueous diffusion coefficients of various ionic species (288). Interestingly, these studies measured a $P_{cation}:P_{anion}$ ratio of 8:1 for Cx43 channels, a value that is substantially higher than that predicted by ion-substitution experiments. One fundamental issue that remains is whether the permeability of the mainstate (O in the state diagram in Figure 4–10) is different from that of the residual conductance state (Os). For Cx43, a minor degree of reduced permeability has been claimed from experiments on neonatal cardiac myocytes (277). Studies on Cx37, which exhibits very high mainstate and substate conductances, indicate that conductances of all states are similarly affected by ionic substitutions; furthermore, the ratio

TABLE 4–2. *Properties of Cardiac Gap Junction Channels after Exogenous Expression in Mammalian Cells and Oocytes*

	Voltage Dependence			Unitary Conductance		
Connexin	V_0(mV)	n	g_{min}/g_{max}	Mainstate	Substate	References
mCx40	± 46	4.5	0.25	190	37	Bukauskas and Weingart, 1994; Traub et al, 1994
rCx40	± 48	3	0.28	180	30–40	Beblo et al., 1995; Hellman et al., 1996
hCx43	± 60	2.5	0.37	60–100	30	Moreno et al., 1994
rCx43	± 54	2.5	0.35	60–90	30	White et al., 1994; Veenstra et al., 1995
hCx45	± 13	2.7	0.06	32	ND	Moreno et al., 1995
hCx37	± 28	3	0.27	220	63	Reed et al., 1993
rCx37	± 29	2.5	0.10	260	80	Waltzmaan and Spray, 1994
mCx50	± 38	4	0.20	230	42	White et al., 1994; Srinivas et al., 1999

g_{min}/g_{max} in different solutions appears to be constant, implying that main state and substate permeabilities to small ions are not radically different (286).

Connexin40 Expressed in Exogenous Systems. The expression of rodent Cx40 in exogenous systems results in gap junction channels that are moderately sensitive to transjunctional voltage, with a half-inactivation voltage (V_0) of ±45 mV, a g_{min}/g_{max} ratio of about 0.25 (Fig.4–10; also see refs. pg. 101, 102, 271). These values are distinct from the Boltzmann parameters for Cx43 gap junction channels. Mouse and rat Cx40 channels expressed in communcation-deficient cells have a mainstate single channel conductance of 200 pS that is favored at low V_j values (Fig. 4–11; also see refs. 14, 27, 101). In addition, transitions to a subconductance state of 40 pS were detected at high transjunctional voltages. The ratio $\gamma_{j,sub}/\gamma_{j,main}$ (=0.2 for Cx40 channels) corresponds well with the ratio of g_{min}/g_{max} obtained from macroscopic g_j measurements, providing further support for the proposal that the residual conductance g_{min} seen at high V_j arises from channel transitions occurring from the mainstate to the residual subconductance state (171).

Cx40 is known to contain consensus sequence motifs for phosphorylation by protein kinases A, C, and G. Traub et al (271) have demonstrated that Cx40 can be phosphorylated by cAMP in transfected cells. Thus, it is conceivable that the channel properties of Cx40 can be modulated by phosphorylation, although such an effect remains to be demonstrated.

Gap junction channels formed by Cx40 and Cx45 (see below under Cx45 expressed in SKHep1 cells and elsewhere) are more selective for cations than for anions. This conclusion was initially based on the measurement of unitary conductances of Cx40 channels in equimolar KCl or K glutamate–containing pipette solutions (14). These studies indicated a KCl/ K glutamate single-channel conductance ratio of 1.4, a value that is higher than expected for a channel with a nonselective aqueous pore. This moderate selectivity of Cx40 channels to cations was also apparent when the relative permeabilities were directly estimated using assymmetric ionic gradients. For Cx40 channels expressed in N2A cells, Beblo et al. (14) have estimated a $P_{cation}:P_{anion}$ ratio of 5:1. However, the functional implications of this observation are unclear: because of the much higher unitary conductance of Cx40 channels, the total amount of current carried by anions through channels formed by these connexins should be similar.

Cx45 Expressed in SKHep1 Cells and Elsewhere. Cx45 forms gap junction channels that are more senstive to transjunctional voltage than those of any other mammalian connexin that has been characterized to date (Fig. 4–11). Junctional currents through endogenous Cx45 channels in SKHep1 cells is reduced even at low transjunctional voltages (Moreno et al., 1995a). Boltzmann parameters of hCx45 channels are listed in Table 4–2. Barrio and colleagues (8) have carried out a characterization of Cx45 channels from various species. Time constants for the decrease of the macroscopic junctional current were found to range between 4 and 8 seconds at low V_j and 100–200 msec at high V_j. In addition, the macroscopic current showed a small dependence on the membrane potential. These results suggest that in poorly coupled cells, significant change in junctional conductance could occur within the time course of a cardiac action potential.

Cx45 forms gap junction channels that have low unitary conductances. The single-channel conductance of Cx45 ranges between 20 and 30 pS depending on the species (hCx45: 170; chCx45: 282). Subconductance states of 10–15 pS were also reported. Cx45 channels do not allow the passage of lucifer yellow. Consistent with this finding, Cx45 channels have been shown to be only weakly permeable to anions (282). The lower anion permeability of Cx45 channels may have some functional relevance. Although there has been no direct demonstration of significance of the different selectivity profiles of cardiac gap junction channels, it may be speculated that such a low permeability would restrict the diffusion of second messenger molecules, many of which are negatively charged moieties under physiological conditions.

Connexin37 Expressed in Exogenous Systems. The cDNA encoding Cx37 protein has been cloned from mouse, rat, and human cells. Expression of human or rat Cx37 in N2A cells (283, 286, 287) results in channels that are moderately sensitive to the transjunctional voltage (V_0 = ± 28 mV). Both human and rat Cx37 exhibit a maximally open state corresponding to 300 pS at low transjunctional voltages and a subconductance state of 68 pS at high driving forces (209). Additional subconductance states were also observed for Cx37 channels. Cx37 channels have low anion permeability (relative anion/cation permeability ratio = 0.38; 283).

Connexin50 Expressed in Exogenous Systems. Cx50 gap junction channels were recently characterized after stable transfection of N2A cells with full-length DNA coding sequence for Cx50 (266). Macroscopic measurements using moderately long V_j pulses indicated that current flow through these gap junction channels responded with monoexponential declines to steady-state levels that appeared to be complete within the initial 10 sec of the pulse. Values for the Boltzmann parameters obtained from macroscopic measurements were $V_0 = \pm 38$ mV, n (equivalent gating charges) = 4 and $g_{min}/g_{max} = 0.21$; parameters obtained for positive and negative V_j were virtually identical, indicating that Cx50 channels are insensitive to inside–outside voltage ($V_{i\text{-}o}$) (see also ref. 298).

Unitary junctional conductances (g_j) measured from cell pairs exhibiting one or two open channels using both voltage ramp protocols and long voltage step protocols revealed a fully open state of about 220 pS (using 130 mM CsCl as internal solution) favored at low V_j values and a residual or substate g_j value of 45 pS whose occupancy was favored at V_j values beyond $\pm$ 40 mV. The results of this study also demonstrated that Cx50 gap junction channels have a large single-channel conductance and are more permissive to cation flux than to anions. Consistent with this selectivity profile, transfer of the negatively charged dye lucifer yellow was only rarely detected even in well-coupled Cx50 transfectants.

Heterologous Pairings of Cells Exogenously Expressing Different Junctional Proteins. Distribution of connexins in cardiac tissue is such that pairing of hemichannels formed of different connexins would be expected to occur throughout the heart and to be more prominent at compartmental boundaries. Other channel-forming proteins either require multiple subunits for function or permit functional participation of multiple subunits. For gap junction channels, multiple connexins have been detected at junctional interfaces, and immunoprecipitation with connexin-specific antibodies after treatment with crosslinking reagents has revealed that in certain tissues (lens, liver), distinct connexins are close enough to be crosslinked. Although close packing of connexons might allow such an opportunity, it is generally now assumed that these studies provide conclusive evidence for heteromeric composition of hemichannels (see 110a). As yet, crosslinking experiments have not been performed on cardiac tissue, and co-expression studies have not addressed whether such heteromers are functional. However, cells exogenously expressing individual connexins (as homomeric hemichannels) can be paired, and properties of these heterotypic homomers can be evaluated. Such expression studies were initially performed on *Xenopus* oocytes and indicated that certain heterotypic pairings are functional, whereas others are not (26). From the standpoint of cardiac function, the most important of these putatively nonfunctional heterotypic channels is probably Cx43/Cx40. Because Cx40 is a major component of the atrium and the conduction system, whereas Cx43 is the predominant connexin in ventricular muscle, nonfunctional Cx43/Cx40 channels could enhance the boundary between these compartments, limiting dispersion along the conduction pathway. It is thus of considerable interest that although initial studies on mammalian transfectants supported this incompatibility (70, 98), one study reported that such heterotypic junctions are indeed functional (278). Based on the expectation that Cx43/Cx40 pairings would be nonfunctional, several studies on cells expressing both connexins have interpreted multiple channel sizes as evidence for heteromeric assembly (69, 100, 146). Because of the recent report of functional Cx43/Cx40 heterotypic channels (278), such interpretation should be reevaluated. Lack of coupling between Cx43 and Cx50 hemichannels has also been found in *Xenopus* expression studies (298). The detection of Cx50 in heart valves raises the possibility that this functional compartment boundary arises in part due to heterologous connexin expression.

Heterologous pairings of Cx43 and Cx45 expressing mammalian transfectants indicates that these cardiac connexins form functional, high-affinity interactions. Both voltage sensitivity and single channel properties are as expected for the sum of properties contributed by hemichannels made of each connexin. Because of the great difference between voltage sensitivities of Cx43 and Cx45, the sum of the properties results in a strongly rectifying G_j–V_j relationship, such that steady-state G_j in response to depolarization of the Cx43 side is much lower than for depolarization of the Cx45 side (768). This biophysical asymmetry of Cx45 (Cx43 heterotypic channels) may be functionally important in reducing reentry from Purkinje cells to ventricular muscle or in impedance matching in nodal tissue.

Properties of Gap Junctions Evaluated in Cardiovascular Cells

Dual whole cell voltage clamping of pairs of freshly dissociated adult cardiac myocytes has revealed that junctional conductance values range from 30 to 1000 nS. Contrary to studies of connexins in expression systems, junctional conductance between cardiac myocytes exhibits only a slight sensitivity to the transjunctional voltage. Voltage sensitivity was at first regarded as absent in gap junctions from cardiac tissue. In part, this was because the range of V_j values tested in most studies was below ± 50 mV. Also, the underestimation of voltage sensitivity and the inadequacy of the space clamp on adult myocytes due to series resistance was not appreciated (167, 301). In most weakly coupled cell pairs or in preformed cell pairs where there is a sequential insertion of the gap junction protein, junctional conductance was shown to be sensitive to the transjunctional voltage (171, 172, 277). Junctional conductance between atrial myocytes in culture (for 18 h) ranges from 0.3 to 2 nS and is moderately sensitive to transjunctional voltage with V_0 of 43 mV, A = 0.2 and G_{min} = 0.22 (136). Similarly, Boltzmann parameters in preformed cell pairs of neonatal rat myocytes have been estimated (V_0 = ± 51, A = 0.11, and G_{min} = 0.28; 277).

Although we have limited our discussion to the properties of mammalian gap junction proteins and mammalian cardiac cells, the expression of different gap junction proteins in the heart was first observed in chick embryonic myocytes (281). Most recently, studies from DeHaan's laboratory (37) have described rectification similar to that found in studies on Cx43/Cx45 heterotypic pairings in mammalian cells (168).

The voltage sensitivity of connexins is unlikely to play a significant physiological role. The large V_0 values of various gap junction proteins (with the possible exception of Cx45 gap junction channels), as well as the slow kinetics of decrease of junctional current, would suggest that currents through gap junction channels formed by Cx40 and Cx43 are unlikely to be affected by existing voltage gradients between cells during the course of an action potential. In addition, theoretical calculations by Wilders and Jongsma (301) seem to indicate that the electric field density around a gap junction channel is dependent on the size of the plaque. These considerations would suggest that only a fraction of the true potential difference between adjacent cells is actually sensed by individual gap junction channels and further suggest that voltage sensitivity of Cx43 and Cx40 gap junctions is unlikely to play an important physiological role in the normal working myocardium. In contrast, the low V_0 and fast kinetics of closure of Cx45 channels lead us to speculate that these channels could play a role during the course of an action potential. The contribution of these channels to conduction in the heart, however, remains to be investigated.

Single-channel properties of cardiac gap junctions have now been evaluated from rat, guinea pig, and rabbit. Single-channel conductance of gap junctions between neonatal rat ventricular myocytes and SA nodal cells of various species range from 50 to 100 pS, a value that is in agreement with the expression of Cx43 in these cells (2, 32, 214). Listed in Table 4–3 are the unitary conductances that have been detected in the heart in various species. Although unitary conductance values from each study initially showed marked variation, these divergent results can now be attributed to differences in the cell type, species, and the composition of internal solution. Differences in unitary conductances between cell type and species arise predominantly as temporal expressions of connexins. For example, a single-channel conductance of 100 pS was determined in pairs of rabbit ventricular myocytes (284). In contrast, two different conductances corresponding to 185 pS and 100 pS were observed in atrial myocytes, in which both Cx40 and Cx43 were expressed (284). In comparison, rat atrial myocytes do not appreciably express Cx43, and therefore only one peak corresponding to Cx40 was observed in these species (136).

Gating of Gap Junctions by Other Stimuli

Sensitivity of Gap Junction Channels to Protons and Ca^{2+}. Gap junction channels are closed by intracellular acidification and by high levels of cytoplasmic Ca^{2+}. More than a century ago, Engelmann (71) discovered that when a small region of myocardium was cut in normal physiological salt solution, adjacent tissue was initially rendered quiescent but then recovered its responsiveness and contractility. Subsequent studies found that the recovery occurred less rapidly when Ca^{2+} was removed from the medium (54, 59), although it was accelerated in low Ca^{2+} solution if pH was lowered (58). These findings have been interpreted as indicating that both Ca^{2+} and H^+ ions can close gap junction channels, thereby allowing uninjured cells to repolarize when uncoupled from the damaged cells.

Cardiac myocytes and other cells types do uncouple

TABLE 4–3. *Unitary Conductance of Gap Junction Channels in the Heart*

Species	Cell Type	Unitary Conductance		References
		Mainstate	Substate	
Rat	Atrium	36		Lal and Ansdorf, 1992 (136)
	Ventricle			
Rabbit	SA node	60	30	Anumonwo et al., 1992 (2)
	Atrium	100 and 185		Verhuele et al., 1997 (284)
	Ventricle	100		Verhuele et al., 1997 (284)
Neonatal rat	Ventricle	40–70	12–30	Rook et al., 1988 (214); Valiunas et al. 1997 (277)
Chick	Ventricle	166 and 58		Veenstra and DeHaan, 1986 (281); Chen and DeHaan, 1996 (37)
Guinea pig	Ventricle	80		White et al., 1985 (299)

when Ca^{2+} is directly injected or when they are exposed to weak acids that cross the plasma membrane to acidify the cytoplasm (58, 250, 275). Major issues in the field are whether concentrations of either Ca or H ions required for closure of gap junction channels are obtained under physiological or pathological stiuations, whether the ions act independently or synergistically, whether all gap junction types respond similarly, and how the channel closure by these ions is transduced.

The answer to the first two sets of questions has depended on quantitative studies in which intracellular Ca^{2+} and pH are determined under pathophysiological conditions and in which intracellular Ca^{2+} and pH are independently varied while measuring junctional conductance. Simultaneous measurements of Ca^{2+}, pH_i, and g_j have proven to be somewhat difficult, although it is clear that under sufficiently long ischemic insults intracellular pH can fall to low levels, intracellular Ca^{2+} can be markedly elevated, and cardiac myocytes can become uncoupled. In one such careful study of the time course of these changes, Andre Kleber's group (121) determined junctional conductance changes occurring during the ischemic process, and noted that cellular uncoupling only occurred many minutes after tissue was deprived of oxygen. At that time, internal longitudinal resistance increased dramatically, and was associated with an increased tendency toward generation of arrhythmias.

Several studies have examined responses of junctional conductance to either changing pH or changing internal Ca^{2+} while concentration of the other ion was held constant. Such studies on internally perfused fish embryonic cells indicated that pH sensitivity was high (apparent pK_a about 7.3, Hill coefficient about 4), whereas Ca^{2+} sensitivity was low (apparent pK about 3.5, Hill coefficient about 1: 245, 252). Other workers, using different preparations and different methods, have obtained results that are at odds with each other and with the studies cited above. In an early study using cardiac myocyte pairs, in which one myocyte was broken open to allow direct manipulation of intracellular pH and Ca^{2+}, Noma and Tsuboi (184) measured an apparent pK for uncoupling by H ions (6.1) that was independent of Ca^{2+}, whereas the pK for uncoupling by Ca^{2+} was pH sensitive (6.6 to 5.6 at pH values of 7.4 and 6.5). Firek and Weingart (77) directly examined pH and Ca^{2+} sensitivity in neonatal cardiac myocytes in which ionic concentrations of each were well buffered. Their values for the apparent pK of Ca-induced channel closure were about 3.5, and those for H^+ ions were near 6; when concentrations of both Ca and H ions were increased, junctional conductance was reduced further, supporting an additive interaction of these cations in inhibition of junctional communication. White et al. (297), by contrast, reported the lack of appreciable uncoupling of cardiac myocytes with either low pH or high Ca^{2+} when the cytoplasmic concentration of the other ion was maintained at low levels.

If there is synergy between H^+ and Ca^{2+} ions in the closure of gap junction channels, this might arise from competition for the same sites on the connexin molecules, with different affinities for the two ions. Alternatively, an intermediary molecule with binding sites for both ions might be involved, such as calmodulin (198).

Gap junction channels composed of different connexins seem to have different pH sensitivities; whether Ca^{2+} sensitivity varies with connexin type is unexplored. Thus, Cx45 channels expressed in SKHep1 cells are mostly closed at an intracellular pH value of 6.7 (103), implying a pK value near pH 7 and a high Hill coefficient, whereas the apparent pK measured for Cx43 in SKHep1 cells, cardiac myocytes or paired oocytes is about 6.5, with a low Hill coefficient (103, 173, 242). The pH sensitivity of channels formed by the third major cardiac connexin, Cx40, has more recently been assessed and was found similar to that of Cx43 (91).

In early quantitation studies of gap junction sensitivity to pH, it was suggested that the Hill coefficient might reflect the cooperative titration of sites on the connexin molecules within the connexon (245). Based on the nearly neutral pK of the pH sensitivity, histidine residues initially seemed likely candidates for the pH sensor, and it was proposed that perhaps those residues located within the cytoplasmic loop of the connexin molecules might participate (243). Mutagenesis and expression of altered Cx43 and Cx32 sequences in Xenopus oocytes has revealed that this region does play a role in Cx43 but may not in Cx32. For Cx43, Mario Delmar, Steve Taffet and colleagues have shown that the most amino-terminal histidine residue within the cytoplasmic loop is a key player in the acidification-induced channel closure, but instead of being titrated by the acids, this residue appears to act as a binding site for a region within the carboxyl terminus (67, 68). Remarkably, pH sensitivity is low in Cx43 mutants lacking the carboxyl terminus or specific domains located therein, but it is restored by co-expression of a peptide corresponding to this region. In the view of these authors, pH gating involves a particle–receptor interaction of the carboxyl terminus with the cytoplasmic loop, comparable to mechanisms proposed for N-type inactivation of the potassium channel (Fig. 4–13).

For Cx32, whose pH sensitivity is lower than wild-type Cx43, and more like that of the truncated Cx43 constructs, mutagenesis studies by Camillo Peracchia's group have implicated postively charged residues at the

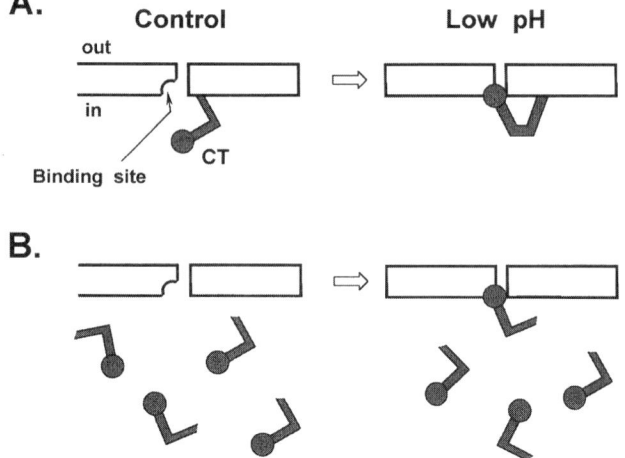

FIG. 4-13. pH sensitivity of Cx43 is mediated through a docking interaction between different domains of the connexin molecule. *A:* Under control conditions, the carboxyl terminus hangs freely in the cytoplasm; acidification causes a conformational change in which a domain in CT interacts with a binding site located in the cytoplasmic hinge region to close the channel. *B:* In experiments in which truncated Cx43, lacking CT, is co-expressed with a peptide corresponding to CT, acidification causes similar channel closure, which is envisioned to result from the same interaction between the blocking particle and the binding site. [Modified from Calero et al. (34).]

most N-proximal region of the carboxyl terminus as the pH responsive portions of the protein (290). Coexpression of low pH-sensitivity Cx32 mutant proteins, along with wild-type Cx32, has been reported to rescue wild-type pH sensitivity, implying that cooperativity between the titration of charges among the connexin subunits is not required for channel closure (289).

The mechanism of pH-induced gap junction channel closure differs from that caused by transjunctional voltage in several notable respects. First, there is no detectable substate associated with acidification-induced gating; closure of the channel by weak acids is thus complete. Second, the gating by pH and by V_j appear to be independently manipulatable. Certain pharmacological compounds (glutaraldehyde, EEDQ, retinoic acid) have been reported to effectively immobilize the pH gate without appreciably affecting voltage sensitivity (244). Moreover, although intracellular injection of strong acid can change the shape of the voltage sensitivity in amphibian blastomeres (17), substantial voltage sensitivity is retained at pH values sufficiently acidic to reduce open probability to very low levels (244). Further evidence that pH and voltage-sensitive gating involve distinct mechanisms is provided by single-channel studies on Cx43-transfected HeLa cells, in which acidification produced slow transitions between the open and closed states, in contrast to the rapid transitions between O and O_s caused by V_j (28).

Sensitivity to Lipophilic Molecules. Alcohols, specifically heptanol and octanol, were discovered by Fidel Ramon and his colleagues to uncouple crayfish axons (111). These compounds were shown to be effective in every mammalian tissue examined, and in cardiac myocytes the reduction in junctional conductance is rapid, complete, and reversible at concentrations in the range 0.1-3 mM (32). Halothane, a volatile anesthetic with arrhythmogenic properties, also totally and reversibly uncouples cardiac cell pairs from adult and neonatal rodents (32, 183). This action can occur at concentrations lower than those affecting excitability, implying relative specificity of their action on junctional channels. It has been proposed that these agents may act through membrane fluidity changes due either to increased bulk fluidity (266) or to decreased fluidity of cholesterol-rich domains (10), although an alternative mode of action involving domains at specific depths within the lipid bilayer is suggested by experiments performed on cardiac myocytes with doxyl stearic acid probes (31) and on astrocytes using oleamide derivatives (92). Like acidification-induced uncoupling, lipophile uncoupling does not induce substates in gap junction channels, but rather completely closes the channels to zero conductance.

It seems likely that the phenomenon of lipophile-induced uncoupling could play an important role in the ischemic heart. Arachidonic acid (4-20 μM) has been shown to uncouple neonatal rat cardiac myocytes (80, 154), and its mechanism of action is presumably similar to that of other lipophiles. Furthermore, Yamada et al. (308) showed that long-chain acyl carnitines increased rapidly after the onset of ischemia and uncoupled pairs of myocytes. Whether certain lipophiles may be more potent in reducing open times of some gap junction channels than others, as suggested by studies of oleic acid (106), is an important question with potential to provide the opportunity to selectively diminish electrical coupling within or between specific cardiac compartments. Interestingly, Burt's group has recently demonstrated that the sensitivity of heteromeric gap junction channels differs from those formed from single connexin types (99).

Effects of Phosphorylation on Channel Function. Cx43 is a phosphoprotein, and each of the other cardiac connexins contains consensus domains for phosphorylation by protein kinase. In heart cells and in most other Cx43-expressing cell types as well, two phosphorylated forms of Cx43 can be detected by autoradiographic analysis of ^{32}P-labeled Cx43 separated by sodium dodecyl sulfate-polyacrylamide gelelectropharesis (SDS-PAGE) (Fig. 4-14). These phosphorylated bands are recognizable in immunoblots due to their mobility shifts: unphosphorylated Cx43 runs at about 41 kDa,

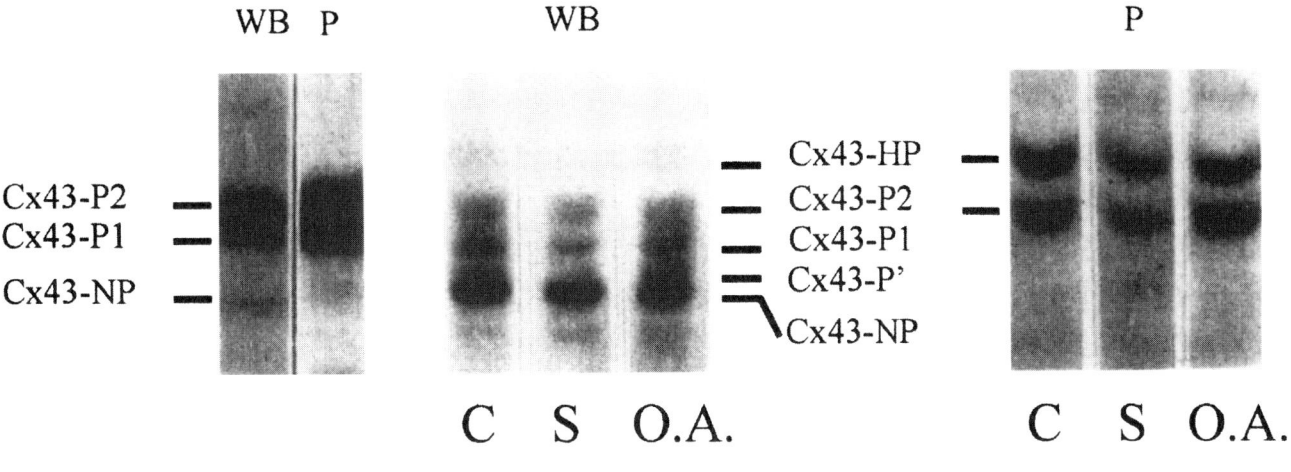

Cardiocytes

SKHep 1 cells

FIG. 4–14. Phosphorylation of Cx43 in rat cardiac myocytes and in hCx43 transfected SKHep1cells. Cx43 is a phosphoprotein; extent of phosphorylation depends on activity of protein kinases and phosphatases. Western blot (WB) shows that Cx43 appears in SDS-PAGE as a triplet of bands with distinct mobilities (labeled P2, P1 and NP in cardiocytes; in hCx43-transfectants a less mobile band appears that is labeled HP). In autoradiograms (P), only the upper forms are identified, indicating that NP is the dephosphorylated form. Treatment with the protein kinase inhibitor staurosporine (S) decreases phosphate incorporation, whereas treatment with the phosphatase inhibitor okadaic acid (O.A.) increases the intensity of the radiolabel compared to control (C) cultures. [From Spray et al, 1994, with permission.)

whereas the phosphorylated forms are retarded by about 2 and about 4 kDa in SDS-PAGE gels (Fig. 4–14). Why the incorporation of only one or two phosphate molecules induces such a profound retardation in mobility is unanswered. The nonphosphorylated forms of Cx43 may predominantly reside in the intracellular pools of this protein, and at least some phosphorylation occurs prior to plasma membrane insertion as indicated by the accumulation of intermediate phosphorylation states of Cx43 after treatment with brefeldin A and monensin agents that inhibit trafficking along the intracellular route (179, 180).

Numerous studies have shown that second messenger activation afftects junctional communication in adult and neonatal cardiac myocytes, including PKA, PKC and PKG (32, 128, 178). In addition, coupling in other cell types expressing endogenous or exogenous Cx43 is sensitive to mitogen-activated protein (MAP) kinase and tyrosine kinases (139, 264). The turnover rate of phosphate in Cx43 in cardiac myocytes has been reported to be similar to the half-life of the protein, suggesting that the protein stays phosphorylated for most of its lifetime (134). However, the results of other studies have shown rapid exchange of phosphate in at least a small portion of the Cx43 pool (217). In cardiac myocytes, treatment with the protein kinase inhibitor staurosporine was shown to reduce electrical and dye coupling between neonatal rat myocytes and to reduce steady-state incorporation of ^{32}P into Cx43 (217), whereas PKC has been found to increase coupling (243). Further acute treatment with 12-O-tetradecanoyl phorbol-13-acetate (TPA) reversed the uncoupling effect of staurosporine, presumably by overcoming the staurosporine inhibition. Protein kinase uncouples other cell types, and it has been shown in several instances to increase phosphate incorporation into Cx43 (217).

Identification of residues in Cx43 that are phosphorylated by PKC has not been completely straightforward. Although the PKC consensus sites Ser 368 and Ser 372 are phosphorylated by PKC in cardiac myocytes and in a recombinant Cx43 polypeptide (AA360–375), two-dimensional tryptic digests of a longer recombinant Cx43(AA243–382) showed additional phosphorylated residues, possibly due to activation of another kinase. Phosphorylation of serine residues 255, 279, 282 have been associated with cell uncoupling (113, 291), and candidate protein kinases mediating this effect include MAP kinase, which is activated by PKC.

Mutations in the consensus Cx43 phosphorylation sites that alter phosphate incorporation in cells transfected with these constructs have been reported to be associated with a subset of visceroatrial heterotaxia patients (25), although studies of more extensive populations with seemingly the same syndrome have not confirmed this finding (192).

In another cell type, Cx43 has been shown to be phosphorylated by a PKA pathway (90), and some studies on cardiac cells have shown increased coupling after treatment with cAMP (32, 57), whereas others have not found a change (265). Interestingly, rodent Cx43 contains a consensus phosphorylation site for PKG, and coupling is reduced and rCX43 is phosphorylated by membrane-permeant cGMP derivatives (128, 265). The human sequence, however, lacks this residue and coupling, and phosphorylation in SKHep1 cells transfected with hCx43 is not affected by elevated cGMP (128).

These studies imply that inotropic adrenoreceptors should exert changes in the phosphorylation status of Cx43 through elevation of cAMP (β-adrenergic receptors) or activation of PKC (α adrenoceptors) through release of diacylglycerol. The extent to which these biochemical changes in Cx43 modulate coupling and contribute to inotropic effects of adrenoreceptors on cardiac tissue remains to be completely understood.

Functional consequences of phosphorylation of consensus sites in the other cardiovascular connexins are virtually unexplored, despite the potential importance of such studies in revealing changes that might occur in selected cardiac compartments in response to neurotransmitters and hormones with their associated second messenger cascades.

Other Agents That Affect Gap Junction Function and Expression.

The search for a "silver bullet" that would block (or enhance) gap junctional communication without altering other ion channels or other cellular functions continues. Both environmental toxins such as dieldrin (155) and active ingredients in herbal remedies (such as glycyrrhetinic acid derivatives found in licorice: 50) appear to be potent inhibitors of at least some gap junction channel types in some systems. Although the mechanisms of action are presently unknown, the selective action reported for α and β glycyrretinic acids on gap junction channels have led to their use in studies evaluating the effects of cell uncoupling in various noncardiac tissues (e.g., ref. 177). Certainly, the nonvolatility of these agents simplifies their application in long-term studies. However, their effect has been to reduce junctional conductance, rather than to cause total blockade.

A totally different approach followed by several laboratories has been to apply connexin antibodies (23, 107) or polypeptides (36), corresponding to extracellular domains in the hope of occupying "binding sites" on the extracellular aspect of connexons, thereby inhibiting channel formation. The extent of blockade of functional coupling produced by these agents has been remarkable, similar to what has been achieved with oligonucleotides corresponding to antisense sequences of Cx43 and Cx40 sequences (86, 166, 228). The use of dominant-negative strategies, in which a connexin construct is expressed that inhibits functional channel formation by other connexins, has also been successfully used in studies of *Xenopus* and mouse development (191, 262). The refinement of these strategies is a goal of several laboratories and should prove useful in studies of transgenic animals and of cultured cells.

If coupling between cells of the heart is important for cardiac function, agents that increase coupling might be expected to improve cardiac performance and could be therapeutically useful. Stefan Dhein and his colleagues (61, 62), have recently pursued the mode of action and structure–activity relations of anti-arrhythmic peptides (AAPs). Synchronized beating of chick heart cell cultures by hexapeptides isolated from bovine atria was originally reported in 1980 by Kohana and colleagues (3, 4). These AAPs have subsequently been reported by Kohana and Dhein's groups to be anti-arrhythmic in certain mammalian cardiac preparations, including aconitine-induced arrhythmias in mice, ventricular fibrillation in dogs and rats, and ischemia–reperfusion associated arrhythmias (4, 61). Although the mechanism of action of AAPs has not been unambiguously identified, recent voltage-clamp studies of pairs of guinea pig ventricular myocytes using 10 nM concentrations of the synthetic AAP10 have revealed junctional conductance increase by as much as 25%–30%, and it was proposed that the increased coupling might be responsible for decreased susceptibility to arrhythmias (176).

GENETIC AND SOMATIC DISEASE STATES IN WHICH GAP JUNCTION EXPRESSION OR FUNCTION IS ALTERED

Somatic Cardiac Abnormalities

A number of naturally occuring human diseases or animal models have been examined to understand the potential relationship of altered gap junction expression or function and clinically relevant sequelae. Chagas' disease, a multisystem disorder caused by the parasite *Trypanosoma. cruzi*, often manifests as a cardiomyopathy with prominent rhythm disturbances. Interestingly, despite evidence for preserved connexin43 gap junctional abundance in chagasic hearts, marked disturbances in subcellular localization are observed, with prominent loss of appositional plaque formation (Fig. 4–15; 35). These data suggest that perturbations of connexin43 biotrafficking may contribute to the high incidence of arrhythmias in the chagasic heart. Substantial changes in gap junction expression are also reported following experimental myocardial infarction in rodents and larger mammalian species, such as the dog. Most reports describe a relative loss and/or reorganization of connexin43 within the epicardial border zones, a disturbance that may facilitate the development of re-entrant ventricular tachycardia (150, 201). Downregulation of connexin43 has also been observed at sites distant from the infarct, although in contrast to the epicardial border zones, the subcellular localization appears unchanged from normal myocardium. Similar quantitative and qualitative alterations in gap junction expression have been observed in tissue samples taken from humans with either ischemic or hypertrophic heart disease (114, 200, 224), supporting the utility of these animal models in the understanding of pathogenetic relationships between gap junction dysregulation and arrhythmogenesis. Accordingly, genetically modified mice have been employed to more fully characterize alterations in gap junction expression and/or function in the myopathic

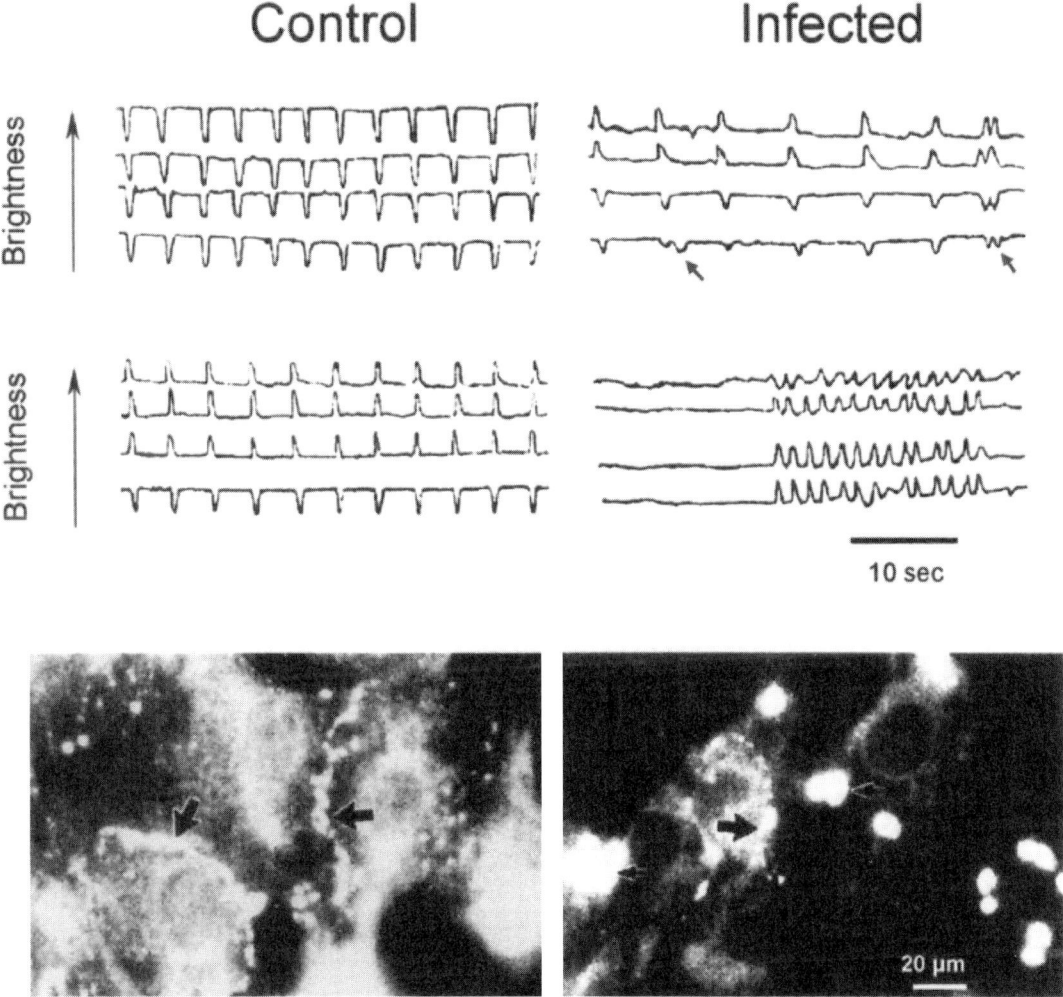

FIG. 4–15. Effects of infection of rat neonatal cardiac myocytes with *Trypanosoma cruzi* on synchronous beating and gap junction distribution. *Top:* Results of two experiments in which beat rates were recorded in matched cultures of uninfected (left) and *T. cruzi*-infected (right) cardiac myocytes. Beat rates were recorded in multiple areas of a microscope field using the brightness over time utility program in Image 1AT. Note constant interval between beats in control cultures and highly variable beat rates in infected cultures. *Bottom:* Redistribution of Cx43 immunoreactivity in *T. cruzi*-infected myocytes (right) compared to controls (left). In contrast to strong staining at appositional membranes in control cultures, infected cells exhibited little or no Cx43 immunoreactivity, whereas adjacent cells showed normal Cx43 expression levels. *Small arrows* indicate the parasites; *large arrows* point to junctional membranes. [From Campos de Carvalho et al. (35).]

heart. For example, conditional expression of diphtheria toxin A in the heart has been employed to achieve a novel cardiomyopathy with a high incidence of spontaneous cardiac arrhythmias (see color Plate 8), culminating in sudden death (140). Hearts from these mice show substantial downregulation of connexin43 gene expression, with reductions in both Cx43 mRNA and protein levels and loss of appositional Cx43 immunoreactivity. Mechanisms leading to this alteration in gap junction channel expression are uncertain, but may result in part from hemodynamic load-induced changes in myocardial gene expression as well as from post-translational effects, including alterations in the half-lives of connexin proteins. Ventricular arrhythmias are also more common after coronary occlusion in heterozygous Cx43 knockout mouse hearts than in wild-type control mouse hearts (142).

In addition to the increased arrhythmogenicity noted with decreased Cx43 expression, ventricular dysfunction in acquired heart disease has also been correlated with abnormal gap junction expression. Kaprielian et al. (114) demonstrated that immunostaining for Cx43 was decreased in ischemic heart disease, and Cx43 expression was most significantly downregulated in hibernating myocardium.

Reversed Physiology: Inferring Gene Function from Its Absence in Knockout Mice

Mice in which Cx43 was deleted by homologous recombination (Cx43-null or Cx43 −/− mice) were generated by a collaboration between the laboratories of Janet Roussant and Jerry Kidder in 1995 (208) and are now commercially available from the Jackson Laboratory (Bar Harbor, ME). These animals have right ventricular outflow tract obstruction and pulmonary oligemia, and they die at birth. Interestingly, the Cx43 knockout phenotype appears to be dependent on the loss of Cx43 in the cardiac neural crest, a loss partially restored by overexpression of Cx43 in the developing neural crest (73).

In cardiac myocytes obtained from Cx43-null mice and wild-type littermates, we have compared junctional conductance, single junctional channel properties, dye coupling, as well as synchrony of spontaneous contractions (78, 250). Junctional conductance in pairs of isolated myocytes primarily from ventricular tissue was lower in Cx43-null mice than in wild-type mice. However, transfer of intracellularly injected lucifer yellow dye was reduced to barely detectable in Cx43-null myocytes, as contrasted with strong dye coupling to contiguous and second-order myocytes from wild-type littermates. Consistent with the reduced junctional conductance and lucifer yellow transfer, propagation of Ca^{2+} waves between mechanically stimulated myocytes was markedly less extensive in Cx43-null than in wild-type myocyte primary cultures (260). When contraction synchrony was compared, interbeat intervals of Cx43-null myocytes were twice as long as for wild-type cells and showed much greater dispersion, reflected in a fivefold greater variability in inter-beat intervals (250).

Single-channel recordings reveal that the channels mediating coupling in Cx43-null myocytes are different from those in wild-type animals. Unitary conductances of wild-type myocytes were primarily of sizes associated with phosphorylated Cx43, whereas in Cx43-null myocytes, channels were of exclusively different sizes.

Cardiac myocytes of Cx43-null mice are thus deficient in intercellular coupling. Dye coupling is more profoundly reduced than electrical coupling, presumably reflecting the decreased anion permeability of the other cardiac gap junction proteins (Cx40 and Cx45) compared to Cx43. Conceivably, the reduced anion permeability of gap junctions in Cx43-null ventricular myocytes may contribute to the developmental abnormality by limiting diffusion of anionic morphogens.

In heterozygous Cx43 mice ($Cx43^{+/-}$), the deletion of a single copy of the Cx43 gene was reported to significantly affect the intraventricular but not the atrial conduction of the electrical impulse (93, 268). In the $Cx43^{(+/-)}$ hearts the electrocardiographic QRS complex was significantly longer than in the wild-type hearts (Fig. 4–16), with no differences in P wave parameters, heart rate, or propensity to arrhythmogenesis. The observed differences in atrial and ventricular conduction imposed by 50% reduction in Cx43 expression could be explained by the abundant expression of Cx40 in the atria, which would functionally compensate for the reduction in Cx43 expression (268). It should be noted, however, that more recent optical mapping studies have not confirmed these differences, showing that the conduction parameters of the $Cx43^{+/-}$ hearts are not significantly different from those of the wild-type (174). The lack of measurable differences in the cardiac impulse conduction is consistent with our findings that junctional conductance, lucifer yellow dye coupling, and the communication of the slow intercellular Ca^{2+} waves are not appreciably different between $Cx43^{+/-}$ and wildtype animals (250, 260).

In mice lacking Cx40 expression, the ECGs are abnormal (Fig. 4–16), with evidence of conduction slowing; in 6 of 31 Cx40-null mice, atrial rhythm disturbances were noted (118). Heart rates in wild-type and Cx40-null mice were similar, and sinus rhythms were

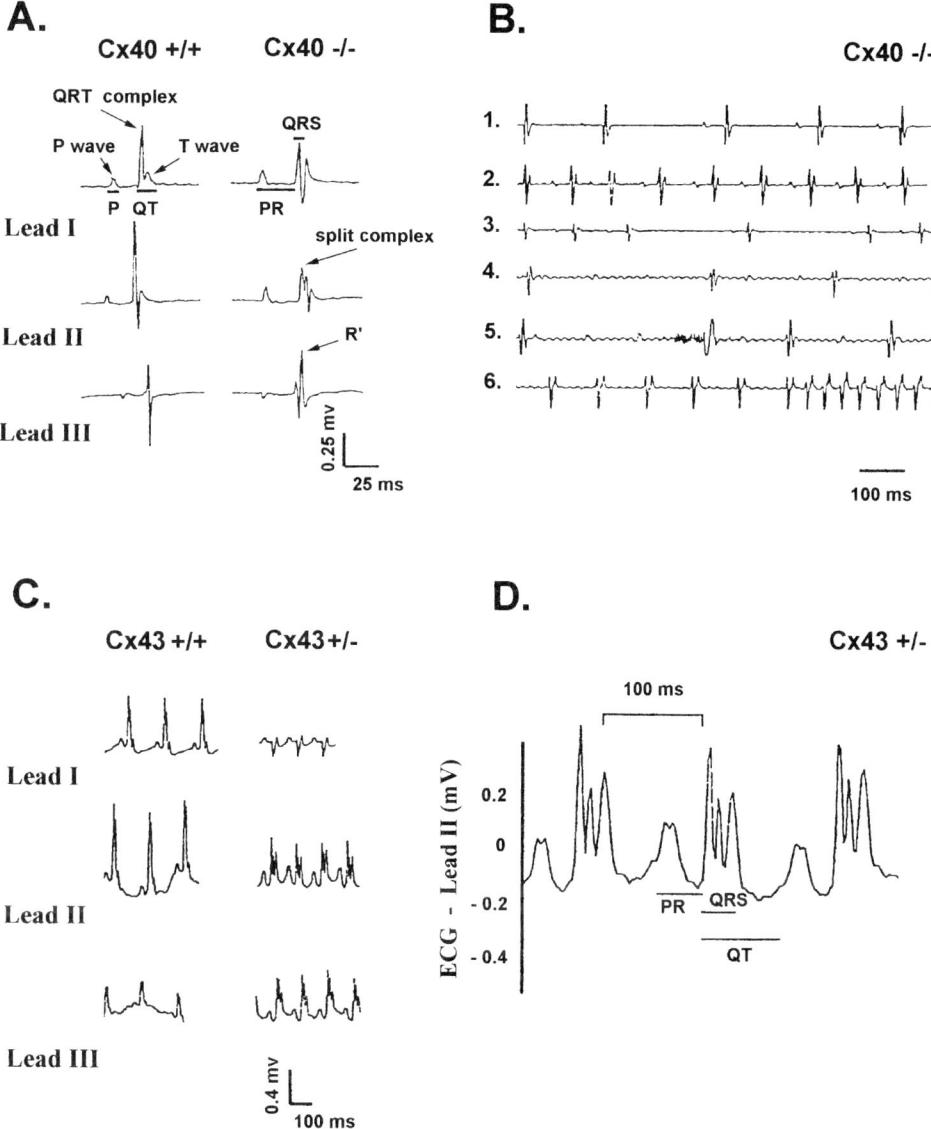

FIG. 4–16. Representative ECG recordings from wild-type, connexin40-null homozygous (Cx40$^{-/-}$) and connexin43 heterozygous (Cx43$^{+/-}$) mice. A: In Cx40-null hearts atrioventricular and intraventricular conductions are slower, with characteristic longer PR and QRS intervals; partial conduction blockage through His-Purkinje system leads to uncoordinated ventricular activation with a high incidence of split QRS complex and rSR= morpholog (227). B. Types of arrhythmias in hearts of Cx40$^{-/-}$ mice : (1) sinus arrhythmia; (2) atrial ectopia (third P wave of the tracing); (3) sinus arrhythmia or sino-atrial block; (4) total AV block; (5) total AV block with ventricular ectopic beat; (6) intra-atrial re-entrant tachycardia. (From Kirchhoff et al., 1998, with permission) C,D: Delayed intraventricular conduction and prolonged QRS interval are observed in Cx43$^{+/-}$ hearts, but other ECG parameters are similar to those recorded from wild-type mice. [From Thomas et al., with permission (268).]

normal but atrioventricular conduction was slower (PR interval 21% longer), as was intraventricular conduction (QRS complexes were 34% larger, presumably due to slowed conduction in portions of the specialized cardiac conduction system). In Cx40-null mice, 90% showed differences in ventricular activation as evidenced by split QRS complexes and atrial P waves 9% longer than in wild-types. These findings are generally consistent with the known expression pattern of Cx40 in the mouse (227).

In summary, genetically manipulated murine models in which the expression of specific connexin isoforms is altered are beginning to reveal the functional roles of connexins in normal impulse generation and propagation and precisely how perturbations of expression in myopathic hearts may be arrhythmogenic.

Research in the authors' laboratories is or has been supported by grants from FAPESP (SOS), The American Heart Association (National and Heritage Chapter and the Beatrice Parvin Grant-in-Aid and Participating Laboratory Awards), and the National Institutes of Health (DCS, GIF). Although this chapter is almost entirely rewritten and expanded, abbreviated versions of several sections have appeared elsewhere (241, 251).

REFERENCES

1. Ai, Z., A. Fischer, D. C. Spray, A. M. Brown and G. I. Fishman. Wnt-1 regulation of connexin43 in cardiac myocytes. *J. Clin. Invest.* 105:161–171, 2000.
2. Anumonwo, J. M., H. Z. Wang, E. Trabka-Janik, B. Dunham, R. D. Veenstra, M. Delmar and J. Jalife. Gap junctional channels in adult mammalian sinus nodal cells. Immunolocalization and electrophysiology. *Circ. Res.* 71:229–239, 1992.
3. Aonuma, S., Y. Kohama, K. Akai, et al. Studies on heart XIX: isolation of an atrial peptide that improves the rhythmicity of cultured myocardial cell clusters. *Chem. Pharm. Bull* 28:332–229, 1980.
4. Aonuma, S., Y. Kohana, T. Makino, et al. Studies on heart XXII: inhibitory effect of an atrial peptide on several drug induced arrhythmias in vivo. *Yakugaku Zasshi*, 103:662–666, 1983.
5. Bai, S., D. C. Spray and R. Burk. Characterization of rat connexin32 gene regulatory elements. In *Gap Junctions* (J. Hall, G. Zampighi and R. E. Davis, Eds), Elsevier. 1993; 291–297.
6. Banach, K., R. Weingart. Connexin43 gap junctions exhibit asymmetrical gating properties. *Pflugers Arch. Eur. J. Physiol.* 431:775–785, 1996.
7. Barr, L., M. M. Dewey and W. Berger. Propagation of action potentials and the structure of the nexus in cardiac muscle. *J. Gen. Physiol.* 48:797–823, 1965.
8. Barrio, L. C., J. Capel, J. A. Jarillo, C. Castro, and A. Revilla. Species-specific voltage-gating properties of connexin-45 junctions expressed in *Xenopus* oocytes. *Biophys. J.* 73:757–769, 1997.
9. Barrio, L. C., T. Suchyna, T. Bargiello, L. X. Xu, R. S. Roginski, M. V. Bennett and B. J. Nicholson Gap junctions formed by connexins 26 and 32 alone and in combination are differently affected by applied voltage. *Proc. Natl. Acad. Sci. U.S.A.* 88:8410–8414, 1991.
10. Bastiaanse, E. M., H. J. Jongsma, A. van dr Laarse, and B. R. Takens-Kwak. Heptanol-induced decrease in cardiac gap junctional conductance is mediated by a decrease in the fluidity of membranous cholesterol-rich domains.*J. Membr. Biol.* 136:135–145, 1993.
11. Bastide, B., L. Neyses, D. Ganten, M. Paul, K. Willecke and O. Traub. Gap junction protein connexin40 is preferentially expressed in vascular endothelium and conductive bundles of rat myocardium and is increased under hypertensive conditions. *Circ. Res.* 73:1138–1149, 1993.
12. Beardslee, M. A., J. G. Laing, E. C. Beyer and J. E., Saffitz. Rapid turnover of connexin43 in the adult rat heart. *Circ Res*, 83:629–635, 1998.
13. Beblo, D. A., H.-Z. Wang, E. C. Beyer, E. Westphale, and R. D. Veenstra. Unique conductance, gating and selective permeability properties of gap junction channels formed by connexin40. *Circ. Res.* 77:813–822, 1995.
14. Beblo, D. A. and R. D. Veenstra. Monovalent cation permeation through the connexin40 gap junction channel. Cs, Rb, K, Na, Li, TEA, TMA, TBA, and effects of anions Br, Cl, F, acetate, aspartate, glutamate, and NO3. *J. Gen. Physiol.* 109:509–522, 1997.
15. Benedetti, E. L., and P. Emmelot. Electron microscopic observations on negatively stained plasma membranes isolated from rat liver. *J. Cell. Biol.* 26:299–305, 1965.
16. Bennett, M. V. L., L. C. Barrio, T. A. Bargiello, D. C., Spray, E. Hertzberg and J. C. Saez. Gap junctions:new tools, new answers, new questions. *Neuron* 6:305–320, 1991.
17. Bennett, M. V., J. C. Saez, and D. C. Spray. Multiplicity of controls of gap junctional communication. *P.R. Health Sci J.* 7:126, 1988.
18. Bennett, M. V. L., X. Zheng and M. L. Sogin. The connexins and their family tree. In: *Molecular Evolution of Physiological Processes*, edited by D. Fambrough, 47th Annual Symposium of the Society of General Physiologists, vol. 49, 1994:223–233.
19. Beyer, E. C., D. L. Paul, and D. A. Goodenough. Connexin43: a protein from rat heart homologous to the gap junction protein from liver. *J. Cell. Biol.* 105:2621–2629, 1987.
20. Beyer, E. C., K. E. Reed, E. M. Westphale, H. L. Kanter, and D. M. Larson. Molecular cloning and expression of rat connexin40, a gap junction protein expressed in vascular smooth muscle. *J. Memb. Biol.* 127;69–76, 1992.
21. Blankesteijin, W. M., Y. P. Essers-Janssen, M. M. Ulrich and J. F. Smits. Increased expression of a homologue of *Drosophila* tissue polarity gene "frizzled" in left ventricular hypertrophy in the rat, as identified by subtractive hybridization. *J. Mol. Cell. Cardiol.* 29:1187–1191, 1996.
22. Blankesteijin, W. M., Y. P. Essers-Janssen, M. J. Verluyten, M. J. Daemen and J. F. Smits. A homologue of *Drosophila* tissue polarity gene frizzled is expressed in migrating myofibroblasts in the infarcted rat heart. *Nat. Med.* 3:541–544, 1997.
23. Boitano, S., E. R. Dirksen, and W. H. Evans. Sequence-specific antibodies to connexins block intercellular calcium signalig through gap junctions. *Cell Calcium* 23:1–9, 1998.
24. Brink, P. R., S. V. Ramanan, and G. J. Christ. Human conexin43 gap junction channel gating: evidence for mode shifts and/or heterogeneity. *Am. J. Physiol.* 271:C321–331, 1996.
25. Britz-Cunningham, S. H., M. M. Shah, C. W. Zuppan and W. H. Fletcher. Mutations of the connexin43 gap-junction gene in patients with heart malformations and defects of laterality. *N. Engl. J. Med.* 332:1323–1329, 1995.
26. Bruzzone, R., J.-A. Haefflinger, R. L. Gimlich, and D. L. Paul. Connexin40, a component of gap junctions in vascular endothelium, is restricted in its ability to interact with other connexins. *Mol. Cell. Biol.* 4:7–20, 1993.
27. Bukauskas, F. F., C. Elfgang, K. Willecke and R. Weingart. Biophysical properties of gap junction channels formed by mouse connexin40 in induced pairs of transfected human HeLa cells. *Biophys. J.* 68:2289–2298, 1995.
28. Bukauskas, F. F. and C. Peracchia. Two distinct gating mechanisms in gap junction channels: CO_2-sensitive and voltage-sensitive. *Biophys. J.* 72:2137–2142, 1997.
29. Bukauskas, F. F. and R. Weingart. Multiple conductance states of newly formed single gap junction channels between insect cells *Pflugers Arch.* 423:152–154, 1993.
30. Bukauskas, F. F. and R. Weingart. Voltage-dependent gating of single gap junction channels in an insect cell line. *Biophys. J.* 67: 613–625, 1994.
31. Burt, J. M. Uncoupling of cardiac cells by doxyl stearic acid specificity and mechanism of action. *Am. J. Physiol.* 256:C913-C924, 1989.

32. Burt, J. M. and D. C. Spray. Single channel events and gating behavior of the cardiac gap junction channel. *Proc. Natl. Acad. Sci, U.S.A.*, 85: 3431–3434, 1988.
33. Cabo, C., A. M. Pertsov, W. T. Baxter, J. M. Davidenko, R. A. Gray and J. Jalife. Wave-front curvature as a cause of slow conduction and block in isolated cardiac muscle. *Circ. Res.* 75: 1014–1028, 1994.
34. Calero, G., M. Kanemitsu, S. M. Taffet, A. F. Lau, and M. Delmar. A 17mer peptide interferes with acidification-induced uncoupling of connexin43. *Circ. Res.* 18:929–935, 1998.
35. Campos de Carvalho, A. C., H. B. Tanowitz, M. Wittner, R. Dermietzel, C. Roy, E. L. Hertzberg, and D. C. Spray. Gap junction distribution is altered between cardiac myocytes infected with *Trypanosoma cruzi*. *Circ. Res.* 70:733, 1992.
36. Chaytor, A. T., W. H. Evans, and T. M. Griffith. Peptides homologous to extracellular loop motifs of connexin43 reversibly abolish rhythmic contractile activity in rabbit arteries. *J. Physiol.* 15:99–110, 1997.
37. Chen, Y.-H. and R. L. DeHaan. Asymmetric voltage dependence of embryonic cardiac gap junction channels. *Am. J. Physiol.* 270: C276–C285, 1996.
38. Chen, Z. Q., D. Lefebvre, X. H. Bai, A. Reaume, J. Rossant, and S. J. Lye. Identification of two regulatory elements within the promoter region of the mouse connexin 43 gene. *J. Biol. Chem.* 270:3863–3868, 1995.
39. Christ, G. J., D. C. Spray, M. el-Sabban, L. K. Moore, and P. R. Brink. Gap junctions in vascular tissues. Evaluating the role of intercellular communication in the modulation of vasomotor tone. *Circ. Res.* 79:631–646, 1996.
40. Clerc, L. Directional differences of impulse spread in trabecular muscle from mammalian heart. *J. Phyisol. (Lond).* 125:221–224, 1954.
41. Cole, W. C. and R. E. Garfield. Evidence for physiological regulation of myometrial gap junction permeability. *Am. J. Physiol.* 251:C411–C420, 1986.
42. Condorelli, D. F., R. Parenti, F. Spinella, A. T. Salinaro, N. Belluardo, V. Cardile and F. Cicirata. Cloning of a new gap junction gene (Cx36) highly expressed in mammalian brain neurons. *Eur. J. Neurosci.* 10:1202–1208, 1998.
43. Coppen, S. R., E. Dupont, S. Rothery, and N. J. Severs. Connexin45 expression is preferentially associated with the ventricular conduction system in mouse and rat heart. *Circ. Res.* 82: 232–243, 1998.
44. Coppen, S. R., I. Kodama, M. R. Boyett, H. Dobrzynski, Y. Takagishi, H. Honjo, H. I. Yeh, and N. J. Severs. Connexin45, a major connexin of the rabbit sinoatrial node, is co-expressed with connexin43 in a restricted zone at the nodal-crista terminalis border. *J. Histochem. Cytochem.* 47:907–918, 1999.
45. Coppen, S. R., N. J. Severs and R. G. Gourdie. Connexin45(alpha 6) expression delineates an extended conduction system in the embryonic and mature rodent heart. *Dev. Genet.* 24:82–90, 1999.
46. Cowan, D. B., S. J. Lye and B. L. Langille. Regulation of vascular connexin43 gene expression by mechanical loads. *Circ. Res.* 82:786–793, 1998.
47. Curtin, K. D., Z. Zhang and R. J. Wyman. *Drosophila* has several genes for gap junction proteins. *Gene* 232:191–201, 1999.
48. Daniels, M. C., T. Kieser, and H. E. ter Keurs. Triggered propagated contractions in human atrial trabeculae. *Cardiovasc. Res.* 27:1831–1835, 1993.
49. Daniels, M. C. G. and H. E. D. ter Keurs. Spontaneous contractions in rat cardiac trabeculae: trigger mechanism and propagation velocity. *J. Gen. Physiol.* 95:1123–1137, 1990.
50. Davidson, J. S. and I. M. Baumgarten. Glycyrrhetinic acid derivatives: a novel class of inhibitors of gap-junctional intercellular communication. Structure-activity relationships. *J. Pharm Acol. Exp. Ther.* 246:1104–1107, 1988.
51. Davis, L. M., M. E. Rodefeld, K. Green, E. C. Beyer, and J. E. Saffitz. Gap junction protein phenotypes of the human heart and conduction system. *J. Cardiovasc. Electrophysiol.* 6:813–822, 1995.
52. De Bakker, J. M. T., F. J. L. van Capelle, M. J. Janse, et al. Slow conduction in the infarcted human heart Azig zag **course of activation.** *Circulation* 88:915–926, 1993.
53. De Leon, J. R., P. M. Buttrick, and G. I. Fishman. Functional analysis of the connexin43 gene promoter in vivo and in vitro. *J. Mol. Cell. Cardiol.* 26:379–389, 1994.
54. Deleze J. The recovery of resting potential and input resistance in sheep heart injured by knife or laser. *J. Physiol. (Lond.)* 208: 548–562, 1970.
55. Delorme, B., E. Dahl, T. Jarry-Guichard, I. Marics, J. P. Briand, K. Willcckc, D. Gros and M. Theveniau Ruissy. Developmental regulation of connexin40 gene expression in mouse heart correlates with the differentiation of the conduction system. *Dev. Dyn.* 204:358–371, 1995.
56. DeMaziere, A. M. G. L. and D. W. Scheuermann. Morphological analysis of gap-junctional area in parenchymal cells of the rat liver after administration of dibutyryl cAMP and aminophylline. *Cell Tissue Res.* 252:611–618, 1988.
57. De Mello, W. C. Effect of intracellular injection of cAMP on the electrical coupling of mammalian cardiac cells. *Biochem. Biphys. Res. Commun.* 119:1001–1107, 1984.
58. De Mello, W. C. The influence of pH on the healing-over of mammalian cardiac muscle. *J. Physiol.* 339:299–307, 1983.
59. De Mello, W. C., G. E. Motta, and M. Chapeau. A study on the healing-over of myocardial cells of toads. *Circ. Res.* 24:475–487, 1969.
60. Dewey, M. M. and L. Barr. Intercellular connection between smooth muscle cells: the nexus. *Science* 137:670, 1962.
61. Dhein, S. and T. Tudyka. Therapeutic potential of antiarrhythmic peptides: cellular coupling as a new antiarrhythmic target. *Drugs* 49:851–855, 1995.
62. Dhein, S., T. Tudyka, M. Schott, W. Gottwald, D. Piecha, A. Muller, and W. Klaus. Enhancement of cellular coupling as a possible new antiarrythmic mechanism. *Naunyn Schmiedeberg's Arch. Pharmacol.* 351, [Suppl]:R106. 1995.
63. Diez, J. A., S. Ahmad, and W. H. Evans: Biogenesis of liver gap junctions. In: *Gap Junctions*, edited by R. Werner. Amsterdam: IOS Press, 1998: 130–134.
64. Dunlap, K., K. Takeda and P. Brehm. Activation of calcium-dependent photoprotein by chemical signalling through gap junctions. *Nature* 325:60–62, 1987.
65. Eckert, R., A. Dunina-Barkovskaya and D. F. Hulser. Biophysical characterization of gap-junction channels in HeLa cells. *Pflugers Arch* 424:335–342, 1993.
66. Eghbali, B., J. A. Kessler and D. C. Spray. Expression of gap junction channels in a communication incompetent cell line after transfection with connexin32 cDNA. *Proc. Natl. Acad. Sci. U.S.A.* 87;1328–1331, 1990.
67. Ek, J. F., M. Delmar, R. Perzova, and S. M. Taffet. Role of histidine 95 on pH gating of the cardiac gap junction protein connexin43. *Circ. Res.* 74:1058–1064, 1994.
68. Ek-Vitorin, J. F., G. Calero, G. E. Morley, W. Coombs, S. M. Taffet, and M. Delmar. pH regulation of connexin43: molecular analysis of the gating particle. *Biophys. J.* 7:1273–1284, 1996.
69. Elenes, S., M. Rubart and A. P. Moreno. Junctional communication between isolated pairs of canine atrial cells is mediated by homogeneous and heterogeneous gap junction channels. *J. Cardiovasc. Electrophysiol.* 10:990–1004, 1999.
70. Elfgang, C., R. Eckert, H. Lichtembergy-Fiate, A. Butterweek, O. Traub, R. A. Klein, D. F. Huber and E. K. Willecke. Specific

permeability and selective formation of gap junction channels in connexin-transfected HeLa cells. *J. Cell. Biol.* 129:805–817, 1995.
71. Engelmann, T. W. Ueber die Leitung der Erregung im Herzmuskel. *Pflugers Arch. Physiol.* 11:465–480, 1877.
72. Epstein, M. L. and N. B. Gilula. A study of communication specificity between cells in culture. *J. Cell. Biol.* 75:769–787, 1977.
73. Ewart, J. L., M. F. Cohen, R. A. Meyer, G. Y. Huang, A. Wessels, R. G. Gourdie, A. J. Chin, S. M. Park, B. O. Lazatin, S. Villabon and C. W. Lo. Heart and neural tube defects in transgenic mice overexpressing the Cx43 gap junction gene. *Development* 124:1281–1292, 1997.
74. Falk, M. M., N. M. Kumar, and N. B. Gilula. Membrane insertion of gap junction connexins: polytopic channel forming membrane proteins. *J. Cell. Biol.* 127:343–355, 1994.
75. Falk, M. M., and N. B. Gilula. Connexin membrane protein biosynthesis is influenced by polypeptide positioning within the translocon and signal peptidase access. *J. Biol. Chem.* 273:7856–7864, 1998.
76. Fallon, R. F. and D. A. Goodenough. Five-hour half-life of mouse liver gap-junction protein. *J. Cell Biol.* 90:521–526, 1981.
77. Firek, L., and R. Weingart. Modification of gap junction conductance by divalent cations and protons in neonatal rat heart cells. *J. Mol. Cell. Cardiol.* 27:1633–1643, 1995.
78. Fishman G. I., A. P. Moreno, D. C. Spray, and L. A. Leinwand. Functional analysis of human cardiac gap junction channel mutants. *Proc. Natl. Acad. Sci U.S.A.* 88:3525–3529, 1991.
79. Fishman, G., D. C. Spray, and L. A. Leinwand. Molecular characterization and functional expression of the human cardiac gap junction channel. *J. Cell Biol.* 111:589–598, 1990.
80. Fluri, G. S., A. Rudisuli, M. Willi, S. Rohr and R. Weingart. Effects of arachidonic acid on the gap junctions of neonatal rat heart cells. *Pflugers Arch. Eur. J. Physiol.* 417:149–156, 1990.
81. Fromaget, C., A. El Aoumari, and D. Gros. Distribution pattern of connexin 43, a gap junction protein, during the differentiation of mouse heart myocytes. *Differentiation* 51:9–20, 1992.
82. Gabriels, J. E., and D. L. Paul: Connexin43 is highly localized to sites of disturbed flow in rat aortic endothelium while connexin37 and connexin40 are more uniformly distributed. *Circ. Res.* 83:636–643, 1998.
83. Garfield, R. E., S. M. Sims, M. S. Kannan, and E. E. Daniel. Possible role of gap junctions in activation of myometrium during parturition. *Am. J. Physiol.* 235:C168–C179, 1978.
84. Geimonen, E., O. Etchelsu, W. Jiang, et al. An AP-1 site in the human connexin43 promoter sequence mediates induction of transcription in uterine somooth muscle cells following treatment with phorbol ester. *Biol. Chem.* 271:23667–23674, 1996.
85. Giepmans, B. N. G., W. H. Moolenaar. The gap junction protein connexin43 interactions with the second PDZ domain of the zona occludens-1 protein. *Curr. Biol.* 8:931–934, 1998.
86. Goldberg G. S., K. D. Martyn, and A. F. Lau. A connexin 43 antisense vector reduces the ability of normal cells to inhibit the foci formation of transformed cells. *Mol. Carcinog.* 11:106–114, 1994.
87. Gros, D., and C. E. Challice. Early development of gap junctions between the mouse embryonic myocardial cells. A freeeze-etching study. *Experientia* 32:996–998, 1976.
88. Gros, D., T. Jarry-Guichard, L. Ten Velde, A. de Maziere, M. J. van Kempen, J. Davoust, J. P. Briand, A. F. Moorman, and H. J. Jongsma. Restricted distribution of connexin40, a gap junctional protein, in mammalian heart. *Circ. Res.* 74:839–851, 1994.
89. Gourdie, R., C. Green, N. Severs, and R. Thompson: Immunolabelling patterns of gap junction connexins in the developing and mature rat heart. *Anat. Embyryol.* 185:363–378, 1992.
90. Granot, I., and N. Dekel. Phosphorylation and expression of connexin-43 ovarian gap junction protein are regulatd by luteinizing hormone. *J. Biol. Chem.* 269:30502–30509, 1994.
91. Gu, H., J. F. Ek-Vitorin, S. M. Taffet, and M. Delmar. Coexpression of connexins 40 and 43 enhances the pH sensitivity of gap junctions: a model for synergistic interactions among connexins. *Circ. Res.* 86:E98-E103, 2000.
92. Guan, X., B. F. Cravatt, G. R. Ehring, J. E. Hall, D. L. Boger, R. A. Lerner, and N. B. Gilula. The sleep-inducing lipid oleamide deconvolutes gap junction communication and calcium wave transmission in glial cells. *J. Cell Biol.* 139:1785–1792, 1997.
93. Guerrero, P. A., R. B. Schuessler, L. M. Davis, E. C. Beyer, C. M. Johnson, K. A. Yamada, and J. E. Saffitz. Slow ventricular conduction in mice heterozygous for a connexin43 null mutation. *J. Clin. Invest.* 15:1991–1998, 1995.
94. Haefliger, J. A., E. Casatillo, G. Waeber, J. F. Aubert, P. Nicod, B. Waeber, and P. Meda. Hypertension differentially affects the expression of the gap junction protein connexin43 in cardiac myocytes and aortic smooth muscle cells. *Adv. Exp. Med. Biol.* 432:71–82, 1997.
95. Haefliger, J. A., R. Polikar, G. Schnyder, M. Burdet, E. Sutter, T. Pexieder, P. Nicod, and P. Meda. Connexin37 in normal and pathological development of mouse heart and great arteries. *Dev. Dyn.* 218:331–344, 2000.
96. Harris, A. L., D. C. Spray, and M. V. Bennett. Kinetic properties of a voltage-dependent junctional conductance. *J. Gen. Physiol.* 77:95–117, 1981.
97. Hassinger, T. D., P. B. Guthrie, P. B. Atkinson, M. V. L. Bennett, and S. B. Kater. An extracellular signaling component in propagation of astrocytic calcium waves. *Proc. Natl. Acad. Sci. U.S.A.* 93:13268–13273, 1996.
98. Haubrich, S., H. J., Schwarz, F. Bukauskas, H. Lichtenberg-Frate, O. Traub, R. Weingart and K. Willecke. Incompatibility of connexin 40 and 43 hemichannels in gap junctions between mammalian cells is determined by intracellular domains. *Mol. Biol. Cell* 7:1995–2006, 1996.
99. He, D. S., and J. M. Burt. Mechanism and selectivity of the effects of halothane on gap junction channel function. *Circ. Res.* 86:E104–109, 2000.
100. He, D. S., J. X. Jiang, S. M. Taffet, and J. M. Burt. Formation of heteromeric gap junction channels by connexins40 and 43 in vascular smooth muscle cells. *Proc. Natl. Acad. Sci. U.S.A.* 96:6495–6500, 1999.
101. Hellmann, P., E. Winterhager, and D. C. Spray. Properties of connexin40 gap junction channels endogenously expressed and exogenously overexpressed in human choriocarcinoma cell lines. *Eur. J. Physiol.* 432:501–509, 1996.
102. Hennemann, H., T. Suchyna, H. Lichtenberg-Frate, S. Jungbluth, E. Dahl, J. Schwartz, B. J., Nicholson, and K. Willecke. Molecular cloning and functional expression of mouse connexin40, a second gap junction gene preferentially expressed in lung. *J. Cell Biol.* 117:1299–310, 1992.
103. Hermans, M. M., P. Kortekaas, H. J. Jongsma, and M. B. Rook. pH sensitivity of the cardiac gap junction proteins, connexin 34 and 43. *Pflugers Arch* 431(1):138–140, 1995.
104. Hertlein, B., A. Butterweck, S. Haubrich, K. Willecke, and O. Traub: Phosphorylated carboxy terminal serine residues stabilize the mouse gap junction protein connexin45 against degradation. *J. Membr. Biol.* 162:247–257, 1998.
105. Heynkes, R, G. Kozjek, O. Traub, and K. Willecke. Identification of a rat liver cDNA and mRNA coding for the 28 kDa gap junction protein. *FEBS Lett.* 205:56–60, 1986.
106. Hirschi, K. K., B. N. Minnich, L. K. Moore, and J. M. Burt. Oleic acid differentially affects gap junction-mediated communication in heart and vascular smooth muscle cells. *Am. J. Physiol.* 265:C1517–1526, 1993.
107. Hofer, A., and R. Dermietzel. Visualization and functional

blocking of gap junction hemichannels (connexons) with antibodies against external loop domains in astrocytes. *Glia* 24: 141–154, 1998.
108. Horres, C., M. Lieberman, and J. Purdy. Growth orientation of heart cells on nylon monofilament. *J. Membr. Biol.* 34:313–329, 1977.
109. Hoyt, R. H., M. L. Cohen, and J. E. Saffitz. Distribution and three-dimensional structure of intercellular junctions in canine myocardium. *Circ. Res.* 64:563–574, 1989.
110. Huttner, I., P. M. Costabella, C. De Chastonay, and G. Gabbiani. Volume, surface, and junctions of rat aortic endothelium during experimental hypertension: a morphometric and freeze fracture study. *Lab. Invest.* 46:489–504, 1982.
110a. Jiang, J. X. and D. A. Goodenough. Heteromeric connexons in lens gap junction channels. *Proc. Natl. Acad. Sci. USA* 93: 1287–1291, 1996.
111. Johnston, M. F., S. A. Simon, and F. Ramon. Interaction of anaesthetics with electrical synapses. *Nature* 286:498–500, 1980.
112. Jongsma, H. J., M. Masson-Pevet, and L. Tsjernina. The development of beat-rate synchronization of rat myocyte pairs in cell culture. *Basic Res. Cardiol.* 82:454–464, 1987.
113. Kanemitsu, M. Y., L. W. Loo, S. Simon, A. F. Lau, and W. Eckhart. Tyrosine phosphorylation of connexin 43 by v-Src is mediated by SH2 and SH3 domain interactions. *J. Biol. Chem.* 272:22824–22831, 1997.
114. Kaprielian, R. R., M. Gunning, E. Dupont, M. N. Sheppard, S. M. Rothery, R, Underwood, D. J. Pennell, K. Fox, J. Pepper, P. A. Poole-Wilson, and N. J. Severs. Downregulation of immunodetectable connexin43 and decreased gap junction size in the pathogenesis of chronic hibernation in the human left ventricle. *Circulation* 97:651–660, 1998.
115. Kensler, R. W. and D. A. Goodenough. Isolation of mouse myocardial gap junctions. *J. Cell Biol.* 86:755–764, 1980.
116. Kessler J. A., D. C. Spray, J. C. Sáez, and M. V. L. Bennett. Determination of synaptic phenotype: insulin and cAMP independently initiate development of electrotonic coupling between cultured sympathetic neurons. *Proc. Natl. Acad. Sci. U.S.A.* 81: 6235–6239, 1984.
117. Kijima, Y., A. Saito, T. L. Jetton, M. A. Magnuson, and S. Fleischer. Different intracellular localization of inositol 1,4,5-triphosphate and ryanodine receptors in cardiomyocytes. *J. Biol. Chem.* 268:3499–3506, 1993.
118. Kirchhoff, S., E. Nelles, A. Hagendorff, O. Kruger, O. Truab, and K. Willecke. Reduced cardiac conduction velocity and predisposition to arrhythmias in connexin40-deficient mice. *Curr. Biol.* 299–302, 1998.
119. Kleber, A. G. Consequences of acute ischemia for the electrical and mechanical function of the ventricular myocardium. A brief review. *Experientia* 46:1162–1167, 1990.
120. Kleber, A. G., V. G. Faast, and S. Rohr. Microscopic conduction in cell cultures assessed by high-resolution optical mappin and computer simulation. In: *Discontinuous Conduction in the Heart*, edited by P. M. Spooner, R. W. Joyner, and J. Jalife. Armonk, NY: Futura 1997: 241–259.
121. Kleber, A. G., C. B. Riegger, and M. J. Janse. Electrical uncoupling and increase of extracellular resistance after induction of ischemia in isolated, arterially perfused rabbit papillary muscle. *Circ. Res.* 61:271–279, 1987.
122. Kosaki, K., J. Ando, R. Korenaga, T. Kurokawa, and A. Kamiya. Fluid shear stress increases the production of granulocyte–macrophage colony-stimulating factor by endothelial cells via mRNA stabilization. *Circ. Res.* 82:794–802, 1998.
123. Kren, B. T., N. M. Kumar, S. Q. Wang, N. B. Gilula, and C. J. Steer. Differential regulation of multiple gap junction transcripts and proteins during rat liver regeneration. *J. Cell. Biol.* 123:707–718, 1993.

124. Kreutziger, G. O. Freeze-etching of intercellular junctions of mouse liver. In: *Proceedings 26th Annual Meeting Electron Microscopy Society of America*, edited by C. J. Arceneaux. Baton Rouge, LA: Claitor's, 1968: 234–235.
125. Kumar, N. M. and N. B. Gilula. The gap junction communication channel. *Cell* 84:381–388, 1996.
126. Kumar, N. M., D. S. Friend, and N. B. Gilula. Synthesis and assembly of human beta 1 gap junctions in BHK cells by DNA transfection with the human beta 1 cDNA. *J. Cell. Sci.* 108: 3725–3734, 1995.
127. Kumar, N. M., and N. B. Gilula. Cloning and characterization of human and rat liver cDNAs coding for a gap junction protein. *J. Cell Biol.* 103:767–776, 1986.
128. Kwak, B. R., J. C., Sáez, R., Wilders, M. Chanson, G. I. Fishman, E. L., Hertzberg, D. C., Spray, and H. J. Jongsma. Effects of cGMP-dependent phosphorylation on rat and human connexin43 gap junction channels. *Eur. J. Physiol.* 430:770–778, 1995.
129. Kwong, K. F., R. B. Schuessler, K. G. Green, J. G. Laing, E. C. Beyer, J. P. Boineau, and J. E. Saffitz. Differential expression of gap junction proteins in the canine sinus node. *Circ. Res.* 23: 604–612, 1998.
130. Laing J. G., and E. C. Beyer. The gap junction protein connexin43 is degraded via the ubiquitin proteasome pathway. *J. Biol. Chem.* 270:26399–26403, 1995.
131. Laing, J. G., E. M. Westphale, G. L. Engelmann, and E. C. Beyer. Characterization of the gap junction protein, connexin45. *J. Membr. Biol.* 139:1–40, 1994.
132. Laing, J. G., P. N. Tadros, E. M. Westphale, and E. C. Beyer. Degradation of connexin43 gap junctions involves both the proteasome and the lysosome. *Exp. Cell. Res.* 236:482–492, 1997.
133. Laing, J. G., P. N. Tadros, and E. C. Beyer. Cx43 gap junction proteolysis involves both the lysosome and the proteasome. In: *Gap Junctions*, edited by R. Werner, The Amsterdam IOS Press 1998:112–116.
134. Laird, D. W. Turnover and phosphorylation of dynamics of connexin43 gap junction protein in cultured cardiac myocytes. *Biochem. J.* 273:67–72, 1991.
135. Laird, D. W. The life cycle of a connexin: gap junction formation, removal, and degradation. *J. Bioenerg. Biomembr.* 28: 311–318, 1996.
136. Lal, R. and M. F. Arnsdorf. Voltage-dependent gating and single-channel conductance of adult mammalian atrial gap junctions. *Circ. Res.* 71:737–743, 1992.
137. Larsen, W. J., H. N. Tung, S. A. Murray, C. A. Swenson, and W. Larsen. Evidence for the participation of actin microfilaments and bristle coats in the internalization of gap junction membrane. *J. Cell. Biol.* 83:576–587, 1979.
138. Larson, D. M., M. J. Wrobleski, G. D. Sagar, E. M. Westphale, and E. C. Beyer. Differential regulation of connexin43 and connexin37 in endothelial cells by cell density, growth, and TGF-beta1. *Am. J. Physiol.* 272:C405–C415, 1997.
139. Lau, A. F., W. E. Kurata, M. Y. Kanemmitsu, L. W. Loo, B. J. Warn-Cramer, W. Eckhart, and P. D. Lampe. Regulation of connexin43 function by activated tyrosine protein kinases. *J. Bioenerg. Biomembr.* 28:359–368, 1996.
140. Lee, P., G. Morley, Q. Huang, A. Fischer, S. Seiler, J. W. Horner, S. Factor, D. Vaidya, J. Jalife, and G. I. Fishman. Conditional lineage ablation to model human diseases. *Proc. Natl. Acad. Sci. U.S.A.* 95:11371–11376, 1998.
141. Lee, S. W., C. Tomasetto, D. Paul, K. Keyomarsi, and R. Sager. Transcriptional downregulation of gap-junction proteins blocks junctional communication in human mammary tumor cells. *J. Cell Biol.* 118:1213–1221, 1992.
142. Lerner, D. L., K. A. Yamada, R. B. Schuessler, and J. E. Saffitz. Accelerated onset and increased *incidence* of ventricular ar-

rhythmias induced by ischemia in Cx43-deficient mice. *Circulation* 101:547–552, 2000.
143. Lieberman, M., A. E. Roggeveen, J. E. Purdy, and E. A. Johnsson. Synthetic strands of cardiac muscle: growth and physiological implications. *Science* 175:909–911, 1972.
144. Lieberman, M., T., Sawanobori, J. M., Kootsey, E. A. Johnson. A synthetic strand of cardiac muscle. Its passive electrical properties. *J. Gen. Physiol.* 65:527–550, 1975.
145. Litchenberg, W. H., L. W., Norman, A. K., Holwell, K. L., Martin, K. W., Hewett, and R. G. Gourdie. The rate and anisotropy of impulse propagation in the postnatal terminal crest are correlated with remodeling of Cx43 gap junction pattern. *Cardiovasc. Res.* 45:379–387, 2000.
146. Li, X, and J. M. Simard. Multiple connexins form gap junction channels in rat basilar artery smooth muscle cells. *Circ Res* 84:1277–1284, 1999.
147. Little T. L. Connexin43 and connexin40 gap junctional proteins are present in arteriolar smooth muscle and endothelium in vivo. *Am. J. Physiol.* 268 (*Heart Circ. Physiol.*): H729–H739, 1995.
148. Liu, S., S. Taffet, L. Stoner, M. Delmar, M. L. Vallano and J. Jalife. A structural basis for the unequal sensitivity of the major cardiac and liver gap junctions to intracellular acidification: the carboxyl tail length. *Biophys. J.* 64:1422–1433, 1993.
149. Loo, L. W., M. Y. Kanemitsu and A. F. Lau. In vivo association of pp60v-src and the gap junction protein connexin43 in v-src-transformed fibroblasts. *Mol. Carcinog.* 25:187–195, 1999.
150. Luke, R. A., J. E. Saffitz. Remodeling of ventricular conduction pathways in healed canine infarct border zones. *J. Clin. Invest.* 87:1594–1602, 1991.
151. Makowski, L. X-ray diffraction studies of gap junction structure. *Adv. Cell. Biol.* 2:119–158, 1988.
152. Makowski L., D. L. D. Caspar, W. C. Phillips and D. A. Goodenough. Gap junction structures II. Analysis of the x-ray diffraction data. *J. Cell. Biol.* 74:629–645, 1977.
153. Manjunath, C. K., G. E. Goings and E. Page. Cytoplasmic surface and intramembrane components of rat heart gap junctional protein. *Am. J. Physiol.* 246 (*Heart Circ. Physiol.*): H865–H875, 1984.
154. Massey, K. D., B. N. Minnich, and J. M. Burt. Arachidonic acid and lipoxygenase metabolites uncouple neonatal rat cardiac myocyte cell pairs. *Am. J. Physiol.* 263:C494–C501, 1992.
155. Matesic, D. F., H. L. Rupp W. J. Bonney R. J. Ruch and J. E. Trosko. Changes in gap-junction permeability, phosphorylation, and number mediated by phorbol ester and non-phorbol-ester tumor promoters in rat liver epithelial cells. *Mol. Carc.* 10:226–236, 1994.
156. Mazet, F., B. A., Wittenberg and D. C. Spray. Fate of intercellular junctions in isolated adult rat cardiac cells. *Circ. Res.* 56:195–204, 1985.
157. McHowat, J., K. A. Yamada, J. Wu, G. X. Yan and P. B. Corr. Recent insights pertaining to sarcolemmal phospholipid alterations underlying arrhythmogenesis in the ischemic heart. *J. Cardiovasc. Electrophys.* 4:288–310, 1993.
158. McNutt, N. S., and R. S. Weinstein. The ultrastructure of the nexus: a correlated thin-section and freeze-cleave study. *J. Cell. Biol.* 47:666–688, 1970.
159. Mehta, P. P. and B. Rose. Expression of connexin43 and of functional cell-to-cell channels in a Morris hepatoma cell line is regulated by cAMP. *J. Cell Biol.* 111:154a, 1990.
160. Mehta P. P., M. Yamamoto and B. Rose. Transcription of the gene for the gap junctional protein connexin43 and expression of functional cell-to-cell channels are regulated by cAMP. *Mol. Biol. Cell.* 839–850, 1992.
161. Michalke, W. and W. R. Loewenstein. Communication between cells of different type. *Nature* 232:121–123, 1971.
162. Milks, J. C., N. M. Kumar, R. Houghton et al. Topology of the 32-kD liver gap junction protein determined by site-directed antibody localizations. *EMBO J* 7:2967–2975, 1988.
163. Minamikawa, T., S. H. Cody and D. A. Williams. In situ visualization of spontaneous calcium waves within perfused whole rat heart by confocal imaging. *Am. J. Physiol.* 272 (*Heart Circ. Physiol.*):H236–H243, 1997.
164. Miura, M., P. A. Boyden, and H. E. ter Keurs. Ca^{2+} waves during triggered propagated contractions in intact trabeculae. *Am. J. Physiol.* (*Heart Circ. Physiol.*):H266–H276, 1998.
165. Miller T., G. Dahl and R. Werner. Structure of a gap junction gene: connexin32. *Biosci. Rep.* 8:455–464, 1988.
166. Moore, L. K., and J. M. Burt. Antiarrythmic drugs have a minor effect on gap junction conductance. *Biophys. J.* 57:246a, 1990.
167. Moreno, A. P., B. Eghbali and D. C. Spray. Connexin32 gap junction channels in stably transfected cells. Equilibrium and kinetic properties. *Biophys. J.* 60:1267–1277, 1991.
168. Moreno, A. P., G. I. Fishman, E. C. Beyer and D. C. Spray. Voltage dependent gating and single channel analysis of heterotypic gap junction channels formed of Cx45 and Cx43. In *Gap Junctions* edited by Y. Kanno. *Progr. Cell. Biol.* 1995;405–408.
169. Moreno, A. P., G. I. Fishman and D. C. Spray. Phosphorylation shifts unitary conductance and modifies voltage dependent kinetics of human connexin43 gap junction channels. *Biophys. J.* 62:51–53, 1992.
170. Moreno, A. P., J. G. Laing, E. C. Beyer and D. C. Spray. Properties of gap junction channels formed of connexin45 endogenously expressed in human hepatoma (SKHep1) cells. *Am. J. Physiol.* 268:C356–C365, 1995.
171. Moreno, A. P., M. B. Rook, G. I. Fishman and D. C. Spray. Gap junction channels: Distinct voltage-sensitive and insensitive conductance states. *Biophys. J.* 67:113–119, 1994.
172. Moreno, A. P., J. C. Saez, G. I. Fishman and D. C. Spray. Human connexin43 gap junction channels: Regulation of unitary conductances by phosphorylation of the channel protein. *Circ. Res.* 74:1050–1057, 1994.
173. Morley, G. E., S. M. Taffet and M. Delmar. Intramolecular interactions mediate pH regulation of connexin43 channels. *Biophys J.* 70:1294–1302, 1996.
174. Morley, G. E., D. Vaidya, F. H. Samie, C. Lo, M. Delmar and J. Jalife. Characterization of conduction in the ventricles of normal and heterozygous Cx43 knockout mice using optical mapping. *J. Cardiovasc. Electrophysiol.* 10:1361–1375, 1999.
175. Mulder, B. J. M., P. P. de Tombe and H. E. D. J. ter Keurs. Spontaneous and propagated contractions in rat cardiac trabeculae. *J. Gen. Physiol.* 93:943–961, 1989.
176. Muller, A., T. Schaefer, W. Linke, T. Tudyka, M. Gottwald, W. Klaus and S. Dhein. Actions of the antiarrhythmic peptide AAP10 on intercellular coupling. *Naunyn Schmiedebergs Arch Pharmacol.* 356:76–82, 1997.
177. Munari-Silem, Y., M. C. Lebrethon, I. Morand, B. Rousset and J. M. Saez. Gap junction–mediated cell-to-cell communication in bovine and human adrenal cells. A process whereby cells increase their responsiveness to physiological corticotropin concentrations. *J. Clin. Invest.* 1429–1439, 1995.
178. Munster, P. N. and R. Weingart. Effects of phorbol ester on gap junctions of neonatal rat heart cells. *Pflugers. Arch. Eur. J. Physiol.* 423:181–188, 1993.
179. Musil, L. S. and D. A. Goodenough. Multisubunit assembly of an integral plasma membrane channel protein, gap junction connexin43, occurs after exit from the ER. *Cell* 74(6):1065–1077, 1993.
180. Musil, L. S. and D. A. Goodenough: Biochemical analysis of connexin43 intracellular transport, phosphorylation, and as-

sembly into gap junctional plaques. *J. Cell Biol.* 115:1357–1374, 1991.
181. Neyton, J. and A. Trautmann. Single-channel currents of an intercellular junction. *Nature* 317:331–335, 1985.
182. Nicholson, B. J., T. Suchyna, L. X. Xu, P. Hammernick, F. L. Cao, C. Fourtner, L. Barrio and M. V. L. Bennett. Divergent properties of different connexins expressed in *Xenopus* oocytes. *Progr. Cell Res.* 3L3014, 1993.
183. Niggli, E., A. Rudisuli, P. Maurer and R. Weingart. Effects of general anesthetics on current flow across membranes in guinea pig myocytes. *Am. J. Physiol.* 1989; 256:C273–281.
184. Noma, A. and N. Tsuboi. Dependence of junctional conductance on proton, calcium and magnesium ions in cardiac paired cells of guinea pig. *J. Physiol.* 382:193–211, 1987.
185. O'Brien, J., M. R. al-Ubaidi and H. Ripps. Connexin35: a gap-junctional protein expressed preferentially in the skate retina. *Mol. Biol. Cell* 7:233–243, 1996.
186. Okano, M. and Y. Yoshida. Junction complexes of endothelial cells in atherosclerosis-prone and atherosclerosis-resistant regions on flow dividers of brachiocephalic bifurcations in the rabbit aorta. *Biorheology* 31:155–161, 1994.
187. Osipchuk, Y. and M. Cahalan. Cell-to-cell spread of calcium signals mediated by ATP receptors in mast cells. *Nature* 359:241–244, 1992.
188. Page, E. and C. K. Manjunath. Communicating Junctions between cardiac cells. In: *The Heart and Cardiovascular System, Scientific Foundations,* Vol. 1, edited by Fozzard, E. Haber, R. B. Jennings, A. Katz, and H. Morgan, 1986:573–600. Raven Press, NY.
189. Paul, D. Molecular cloning of cDNA for rat liver gap junction protein. *J. Cell Biol.* 103:123–134, 1986.
190. Paul, D. L., L. Ebihara, L. J. Takemoto, K. I. Swenson and D. A. Goodenough. Connexin46, a novel lens gap junction protein, induces voltage-gated currents in nonjunctional plasma membrane of *Xenopus* oocytes. *J. Cell Biol.* 115:1077–1089, 1991.
191. Paul, D. L., K. Yu, R. Bruzzone, R. L. Gimlich and D. A. Goodenough. Expression of a dominant negative inhibitor of intercellular communication in the early *Xenopus* embryo causes delamination and extrusion of cells. *Development* 121:371–381, 1995.
192. Penman, Splitt M., M. Y. Tsai, J. Burn and J. A. Goodship. Absence of mutations in the regulatory domain of the gap junction protein connexin43 in patients with visceroatrial heterotaxy. *Heart* 77:369–370, 1997.
193. Pepper, M. S. and P. Meda. Basic fibroblast growth factor increases junctional communication and connexin 43 expression in microvascular endothelial cells. *J. Cell. Physiol* 153:196–205, 1992.
194. Pepper, M. S., D. C. Spray, M. Chanson, R. Montesano, L. Orci and P. Meda Junctional communication is induced in migrating capillary endothelial cells. *J. Cell Biol.* 109:3027–3038, 1989.
195. Pepper, M. S., R. Montesano, A. el Aoumari, D. Gros, L. Orci and P. Meda. Coupling and connexin 43 expression in microvascular and large vessel endothelial cells. *Am. J. Physiol.* C1246–C1257, 1992.
196. Peracchia, C. and S. J. Girsch. Functional modulation of cell coupling: evidence for a calmodulin-driven channel gate. *Am. J. Physiol.* 248 (*Heart Circ. Physiol.*):H765–H782, 1985.
197. Peracchia, C. and L. L. Peracchia. Gap junction dynamics: reversible effects of hydrogen ions. *J. Cell Biol.* 87719–727, 1980.
198. Peracchia, C., X. Wang, L. Li and L. L. Peracchia. Inhibition of calmodulin expression prevents low pH-induced gap junction uncoupling in *Xenopus* oocytes. *Pflugers Arch* 431:379–387, 1996.
199. Perkins, G. A., D. A. Goodenough and G. E. Sosinsky. Formation of the gap junction intercellular channel requires a 30 degree rotation for interdigitating two apposing connexons. *J. Mol. Biol.* 277:171–177, 1998.
200. Peters, N. S. New insights into myocardial arrhythmogenesis: distribution of gap-junctional coupling in normal, ischaemic and hypertrophied human hearts. *Clin. Sci.* 90:447–452, 1996.
201. Peters, N. S., J. Coromilas N. J. Severs and A. L. Wit. Disturbed connexin43 gap junction distribution correlates with the location of reentrant circuits in the epicardial border zone of healing canine infarcts that cause ventricular tachycardia. *Circulation* 18: 988–996, 1997.
202. Pfahnl, A., X.-W. Zhou, R. Werner and G. Dahl. Mapping of the pore of gap junction channels by cysteine scanning mutagenesis. *Biophys. J.* 70:A31, 1996.
203. Phelan, P., L. A. Stebbings, R. A. Baines, J. P. Bacon, J. A. Davies and C. Ford. Drosophila Shaking-B protein forms gap junctions in paired *Xenopus* oocytes. *Nature* 391:181–184, 1998.
204. Polacek, D., F. Bech, J. F. McKinsey, P. F. Davies. Connexin43 gene expression in the rabbit arterial wall: effects of hypercholesterolemia, balloon injury and their combination. *J. Vasc. Res.* 34(1):19–30, 1997.
205. Purdy J., M. Liebermann, A. E. Roggeveen and R. Kirk. Synthetic strands of cardiac muscle: growth and physiological implications. *J. Cell Biol.* 65:563–578, 1972.
206. Rawling, D. A. and R. W. Joyner. Characteristics of the junctional regions between Purkinje and ventricular muscle cells of the canine ventricular subendocardium. *Circ. Res.* 60:580–585, 1987.
207. Razani, B., A. Schlegel and M. P. Lisanti. Caveolin proteins in signaling, oncogenic transformation and muscular dystrophy. *J. Cell Sci.* 2103–2109, 2000.
208. Reaume, A. G., P. A. deSousa, S. Kulkarni, et al. Cardiac malformation in neonatal mice lacking connexin43. *Science* 267:1831–1834, 1995.
209. Reed, K. E., E. M. Westphale, D. M. Larson, H. Z. Wang, R. D, Veenstra and E. C. Beyer. Molecular cloning and functional expression of human connexin37, an endothelial cell gap junction protein. *J. Clin. Invest.* 91:997–1004, 1993.
210. Revel, J.-P. Contacts and junctions between cells. *Symp. Soc. Exp. Biol.* 28:447–461.
211. Revel, J.-P. and M. J. Karnovsky. Hexagonal array of subunits in intercellular junctions in the mouse heart and liver. *J. Cell. Biol.* 33:C7–C12, 1967.
212. Revilla, A., C. Castro and L. C. Barrio. Molecular dissection of transjunctional voltage dependence in the connexin-32 and connexin-43 junctions. *Biophys. J.* 77:1374–1383, 1999.
213. Robertson, J. D. The occurrence of a subunit pattern in the unit membranes of club endings in Mauthner cell synapses in goldfish brain. *J. Cell Biol.* 19:201–221, 1963.
214. Rook, M. B., H. J. Jongsma and A. C. G. van Ginneken. Properties of single gap junctional channels between isolated neonatal rat heart cells. *Am. J. Physiol.* 255 (*Heart Circ. Physiol.*): H770-H782, 1988.
214a. Rose, B. and W. R. Loewenstein. Permeability of cell junction depends on local cytoplasmic calcium activity. *Nature* 254:250–252, 1975.
215. Sáez, J. C., J. A. Connor, D. C. Spray and M. V. L. Bennett. Hepatocyte gap junctions are permeable to the second messenger, inositol 1,4,5-trisphosphate, and to calcium ions. *Proc. Natl. Acad. Sci. U.S.A.* 86:2708–2712, 1989.
216. Sáez, J. C., W. A. Gregory, T. Watanabe, R. Dermietzel, E. L. Hertzberg, L. Reid, M. V. L. Bennett and D. C. Spray. cAMP delays disappearance of gap junctions between pairs of rat he-

patocytes in primary culture. *Am. J. Physiol.* 257:C1–C11, 1989.
217. Sáez, J. C., A. C. Nairn, A. J. Czernik, G. I. Fishman, D. C. Spray and E. L. Hertzberg. Phosphorylation of connexin43 and the regulation of neonatal rat cardiac gap junctions. *J. Mol. Cell Cardiol.* 29:2131–2145, 1997.
218. Saffitz, J. E., L. M. Davis, B. J. Darrow, H. L. Kanter, J. G. Laing and E. C. Beyer. The molecular basis of anisotropy: role of gap junctions. *J. Cardiovasc. Electrophysiol.* 6:498–510, 1995.
219. Saffitz, J. E., H. L. Kanter, K. G. Green, T. K. Tolley and E. C. Beyer. Tissue-specific determinants of anisotropic conduction velocity in canine atrial and ventricular myocardium. *Circ. Res.* 74:1065–1070, 1994.
220. Sanderson, M. J., A. C. and Charles, E. R. Dirksen Mechanical stimulation and intercellular communication increases intracellular Ca^{2+} in epithelial cells. *Cell Regul.* 1:585–596, 1990.
221. Sanderson, M. J., K Paemeleire, A Strahonja and L. Leyvaert. Intercellular Ca^{2+} signaling between glial and endothelial cells. In: *Gap Junctions*, edited by R. Werner. Amsterdan IOS Press. Netherlands, 1998: 261–265.
222. Sano, T. N. Takayama and T. Shimamoto, Directional difference of conduction velocity in cardiac ventricular syncytium studied by microelectrodes. *Circ. Res.* 7:262–267 1959.
223. Seul, K. H., P. N. Tadros and E. C. Beyer. Mouse connexin40: gene structure and promoter analysis. *Genomics* 46:120–126, 1997.
224. Severs, N. J., K. S. Shovel, A. M. Slade, T. Powell, V. W. Twist, C. R. Green. Fate of gap junctions in isolated adult mammalian cardiomyocytes. *Circ. Res.* 65:22–42, 1989.
225. Segal, S. S. and B. R. Duling. Conduction of vasomotor responses in arterioles: a role for cell-to-cell coupling? *Am. J. Physiol.* 256 (*Heart Circ. Physiol.*):H838–H845, 1989.
226. Shibata, Y, C. K. Manjunath and E. Page Differences between cytoplasmic surfaces of deep-etched heart and liver gap junctions. *Am. J. Phsysiol.* 249: (*Heart Circ. Physiol.*) H690-H693, 1985.
227. Simon, A. M., D. A. Goodenough and D. L. Paul. Mice lacking connexin40 have cardiac conduction abnormalities characteristic of atrioventricular block and bundle branch block. *Curr. Biol.* 8:295–298, 1998.
228. Singh, M. V., R. Bhatnagar and S. K. Malhotra Inhibition of connexin43 synthesis by antisense RNA in rat glioma cells. *Cytobios* 91:103–123, 1997.
229. Sjostrand, F. S. and E. Anderson. Electron microscopy of the intercalated discs of cardiac muscle tissue. *Experientia* 9:369–371, 1954
230. Sjostrand, F. S., E. Andersson-Cedergren and M. M. Dewey. The ultrastructure of the intercalated discs of frog, mouse and guinea pig cardiac muscle. *Ultrast. Res.* 1:271–287, 1958.
231. Sohl, G., J. Degen, B. Teubner and K. Willecke. The murine gap junction gene connexin36 is highly expressed in mouse retina and regulated during brain development. *FEBS Lett.* 426: 27–31, 1998.
232. Spach, M. S. Changes in the topology of gap junctions as an adaptive structural response of the myocardium. *Circulation* 90:1103–1106, 1994.
233. Spach, M. S. and P. C. Dolber. Relating extracellular potentials and their derivatives to anisotropic propagation at a microscopic level in human cardiac muscle: evidence for electrical coupling of side-to-side iber connections with increasing age. *Circ. Res.* 58:356–371, 1986.
234. Spach, S. and J. F. Heidlage. A multidimensional model of cellular effects on the spread of electrotonic currents and on propagating action potentials. *Crit. Rev. Biomed. Eng.* 20:141–149, 1992.
235. Spach, S. and J. F. Heidlage. The stochastic nature of cardiac propagation at a microscopic level: an electrical description of myocardial architecture and its application to conduction. *Circ. Res.* 76:366–380, 1995.
236. Spach, M. S., W. T. Miller III and P. C. Dolber et al. The functional role of structural complexities in the propagation of depolarization in the atrium of the dog; cardiac conduction disturbances due to discontinuities of effective axial resistivity. *Circ. Res.* 50:175–191, 1982.
237. Spach, M. S., W. T. Miller 3d, E. Miller-Jones, R. B. Warren and R. C. Barr. Extracellular potentials related to intracellular action potentials during impulse conduction in anisotropic canine cardiac muscle. *Circ. Res.* 45:188–204, 1979.
238. Sperelakis, N and R. L. Macdonald. Ratio of transverse to longitudinal resistivities of isolated cardiac muscle fiber bundles. *J. Electrocardiol.* 7:301–314, 1974.
239. Spooner, P. M., R. W., Joyner and J. Jalife. *Discontinuous Conduction in the Heart.* Armonk, NY: Futura, 1997.
240. Spray, D. C. Gap junction channels: yes, there are substates, but what does that mean? *Biophys. J.* 67:491–492, 1994.
241. Spray, D. C. Gap junction proteins: where they live and how they die. *Circ. Res.* 83:679–681, 1998.
242. Spray, D. C. and M. V. Bennet. Physiology and pharmacology of gap junctions. *Annu. Rev. Physiol.* 47:281–303, 1985.
243. Spray, D. C. and J. M. Burt. Structure–activity relations of the cardiac gap junction channel. *Am J Physiol.* 258:LC195-C205, 1990.
244. Spray, D. C., A. C. Campos de Carvalho and M. V. Bennett. Sensitivity of gap junctional conductance to H ions in amphibian embryonic cells is independent of voltage sensitivity. *Proc. Natl. Acad Sci U.S.A.* 83:3533–3536, 1986.
245. Spray, D. C., A. L. Harris, M. V. Bennett. Gap junctional conductance is a simple and sensitive function of intracellular pH. *Science* 211:712–715, 1981.
246. Spray, D. C., A. L., Harris M. V. Bennett. Equilibrium properties of a voltage-dependent junctional conductance. *J. Gen. Physiol.* 77:77–93, 1981.
247. Spray, D. C., A. L. Harris and M. V. Bennett. Voltage dependence of junctional conductance in early amphibian embryos. *Science* 204:432–434, 1979.
248. Spray, D. C., A. P. Moreno, J. A. Kessler and R. Dermietzel Characterization of gap junctions between cultured leptomeningeal cells. *Brain Res* 568:1–14, 1991.
249. Spray, D. C., M. Rook, A. P. Moreno, J. C. Sá'ez, G. Christ, A. C. Campos de Carvalho and G. I. Fishman. Cardiovascular gap junctions: gating properties, function and dysfunction. In: *Ion Channels in the Cardiovascular System: Function and Dysfunction*, edited by P. M., Spooner, A. M. Brown, W. A. Catterall, G. J. Kaczorowski. H. C. Strauss, Mt. Kisco, NY: Futura 1994:185–217.
250. Spray, D. C. and E. Scemes. Effects of intracellular pH (and Ca^{2+}) on gap junction channels. In: *pH and Brain Function*, edited by K. Kaila and B. R. Ransom. New York: John Wiley & Sons, 1998: 477–489.
251. Spray, D. C., S. O. Suadicani, M. J. Vink and M. Srinivas. Gap junctions in the heart. In: *Physiology and Pathophysiology of the Heart*, edited by N. Sperelakis, Y. Kurachi, A. Terzic, M. J. Cohen 2000, San Diego, Academic Press. Pp 149–171.
252. Spray, D. C., J. H. Stern, A. L. Harris and M. V. Bennett. Gap junctional conductance: comparison of sensitivities to H and Ca ions. *Proc. Natl. Acad. Sci U.S.A.* 79:441–445, 1982.
253. Spray, D. C. and M. J. Vink. Cardiac gap junctions as K^+ (and Ca^{2+}) channels. In: *Potassium Channels in Normal and Pathological Conditions*, edited by J. Vereecke, F. Verdonck and P.-P. van Bogaert). Leuven, Belgium: Leuven University Press, 1995; 424–427.

254. Spray, D. C., M. J. Vink, E. Scemes, S. O. Suadicani, G. I. Fishman and R. Dermietzel. Characteristics of coupling in cardiac myocytes and CNS astrocytes cultured from wildtype and Cx43-null mice. In: *Gap Junctions*, edited by R. Werner. Amsterdam The Netherlands; IOS Press, 1998: 281–285.
255. Spray, D. C. R. L. White, A. C. de Carvalho, A. L. Harris, M. V. and Bennett. Gating of gap junction channels. *Biophys. J.* 45:219–230, 1984.
256. Srinivas, M., M. Costa, A. Fort, G. I. Fishman and D. C. Spray. Voltage dependence of macroscopic and unitary currents of gap junction channels formed by Cx50. *J. Physiol.* 517:673–689, 1999.
257. Stagg, R. B, A. M. Martinez, L. M. Green and W. H. Fletcher. cAMP regulation of connexin43 (Cx43) transcription in a variety of cell types: evidence for de novo transcription in a communication deficient mouse fibroblast cell line (CL-1D). *J. Cell Biol.* 111:155a; 1990.
258. Steere, R. L. Electron microscopy of structural detail in frozen biological spcimens. *J. Biophys. Biochem. Cytol.* 3:45–60, 1957.
259. Steere, R. L. and J. R. Sommer. Stereo ultrastructure of nexus faces exposed by freeze-fracturing. *J. Microsc. (Paris)* 15:205–218; 1972.
260. Suadicani, S. O., M. J. Vink and D. C. Spray Slow intercellular Ca^{2+} signaling in wild type and Cx43-null neonatal cardiac myocytes. *Am. J. Physiol.* (Heart Circ Physiol) 279:H3076–3088, 2000.
261. Suchyna, T. M., L. X. Xu, F. Gao, C. R. Fourtner, B. J. Nicholson. Identification of a proline residue as a transduction element involved in voltage gating of gap junctions. *Nature* 365: 847–849, 1993.
262. Sullivan, R. and C. W. Lo. Expression of connexin43/beta-galactosidase fusion protein inhibits gap junctional communication in NIH3T3 cells. *J. Cell. Biol.* 130:419–429, 1995.
263. Sullivan, R, C. Ruangvoravat, D. Joo, J. Morgan, B. L. Wang, X. K. Wang, and C. W. Lo. Structure, sequence and expression of the mouse Cx43 gene encoding connexin43. *Gene* 130:191–199, 1993.
264. Swenson, K. I, H. Piwnica-Worms, H. McNamee and D. L. Paul. Tyrosine phosphorylation of the gap junction protein connexin43 is required for the pp60v-src-induced inhibition of communication. *Cell Regul.* 1:989–1002, 1990.
265. Takens-Kwak, B. R. and H. J. Jongsma. Cardiac gap junctions: three distinct single channel conductances and their modulation by phosphorylating treatments. *Plugers Arch.* 422:198–200, 1992.
266. Takens-Kwak, B. R., H. J. Jongsma, M. B. Rook and A. C. Van Ginneken. Mechanism of heptanol-induced uncoupling of cardiac gap junctions: a perforated patch-clamp study. *Am J Physiol* 262:C1531-C1538, 1992.
267. ter Keurs, H. E. D. J. and Y. M. Zhang. Triggered propagated contractions and arrhythmias caused by acute damage to cardiac muscle. In: *Discontinuous Conduction in the Heart*. edited by P. M. Spooner, R. W. Joyner and J. Jalife, eds. Armonk, NY Futura 1997: 223–240.
268. Thomas, S. A., R. B. Schuessler, C. I. Berul, M. A. Beardslee E. C. Beyer, M. E. Mendelsohn and J. E. Saffitz. Disparate effects of deficient expression of connexin43 on atrial and ventricular conduction. *Circulation* 97:686–691, 1998.
269. Toyofuku, T., M. Yabuki, K. Otsu, T. Kuzuya, M. Hori and M. Tada. Direct association of the gap junction protein connexin-43 with ZO-1 in cardiac myocytes. *J. Biol Chem.* 273:12725–12731, 1998.
270. Tsien, R. H. W. and R. Weingart. Inotropic effect of cyclic AMP in calf ventricular muscle studied by a cut end method. *J Physiol. (Lond)* 260:117–141, 1976.
271. Traub, O., R. Eckert, H. Lichtenberg-Frate, C. Elfgang, B. Bastide, K. H. Scheidtmann and D. F. Hulser, K. Willecke. Immunochemical and electrophysiological characterization of murine connexin40 and-43 in mouse tissues and transfected human cells. *Eur. J Cell Biol.* 64:101–112, 1994.
272. ter Keurs, H. E., Y. M. Zhang, A. W. Davidoff, P. A. Boyden, V. Wakayama and M. Miura. Damage induced arrhymias: mechanisms and implications. *Canad. J. Physiol. Pharmacol.* 79:73–81, 2001.
273. Tibbits, T. T., D. L. D. Caspar, W. C. Phillips and D. A. Goodenough. Diffraction diagnosis of protein folding in gap junction connexons. *Biophys. J.* 57:1025–1036, 1990.
274. Tsien, R. W. and R. Weingart. Inotropic effect of cyclic AMP in calf ventricular muscle studied by a cut end method. *J. Physiol. (Lond.)* 260:117–141, 1976.
275. Turin, L. and A. E. Warner. Intracellular pH in early Xenopus embryos: its effect on current flow between blastomeres. *J. Physiol.* 300:489–504, 1980.
276. Unger, V. M., N. M. Kumar, N. B. Gilula and M. Yeager. Expression, two-dimensional crystallization and electron cryo-crystallography of recombinant gap junction membrane channels. *J. Struct. Biol.* 128:98–105, 1999.
277. Valiunas, V., F. F. Bukauskas and R. Weingart. Conductances and selective permeability of connexin43 gap junction channels examined in neonatal rat heart cells. *Circ. Res.* 80:708–719, 1997.
278. Valiunas, V., R. Weingart and P. R. Brink. Formation of heterotypic gap junction channels by connexins 40 and 43. *Circ. Res.* 86: E42-E49, 2000.
279. van Rijen, H. V, M. J. van Kempen, S. Postma and H. J. Jongsma. Tumour necrosis factor alpha alters the expression of connexin43, connexin40, and connexin37 in human umbilical vein endothelial cells. *Cytokine* 10:258–264, 1998.
280. Van Kempen, M. J., J. L. Vermeulen, A. F. Moorman, D. Gros, D. L. Paul and W. H. Lamers. Developmental changes of connexin40 and connexin43 mRNA distribution patterns in the rat heart. *Cardiovasc. Res.* 32:886–900, 1996.
281. Veenstra, R. D. and R. L. DeHaan. Measurement of single channel currents from cardiac gap junctions. *Science* 233:972–974, 1986.
282. Veenstra, R. D., H-Z, Wang, E. Beyer and P. R. Brink. Selective dye and ionic permeability of gap junction channels formed by connexin45. *Circ. Res.* 75:483–490, 1994.
283. Veenstra, R. D., H. Z. Wang, E. C. Beyer, S. V. Ramanan and P. R. Brink. Connexin37 forms high conductance gap junction channels with subconductance state activity and selective dye and ionic permeabilities. *Biophys. J.* 66:1915–1928, 1994.
284. Verheule, S, M. J. van Kempen, P. H. teWelscher, B. R. Kwak and H. J. Jongsma. Characterization of gap junction channels in adult rabbit atrial and ventricular myocardium. *Circ. Res.* 80:673–681, 1997.
285. Verselis, V. K., C. S. Ginter and T. A. Bargiello. Opposite voltage gating polarities of two closely related connexins. *Nature* 368:348–351, 1994.
286. Waltzman, M. and D. C. Spray. Anionic permeability of Cx37 channels is vanishingly low. *Biophys. J.* 68:A227, 1995.
287. Waltzman, M. N. and D. C. Spray. Exogenous expression of connexins for physiological characterization of channel properties: comparison of methods and results. In: *Intercellular Communication Through Gap Junctions*, edited by Y. Kanno, K. Kataoka, Y. Shiba, Y. Shibata and T. Shimazu. *Progr. Cell Res.*; 4:9–17, 1995.
288. Wang, H. H. Z. and R. D. Veenstra. Monovalent ion selectivity sequences of the rat connexin43 gap junction channel. *J. Gen. Physiol.* 109:491–507, 1997.
289. Wang, X. G. and C. Peracchia. Chemical gating of heteromeric

289. and heterotypic gap junction channels. *J Membr Biol* 162:169–176, 1998.
290. Wang, X. G. and C. Peracchia. Positive charges of the initial C-terminus domain of Cx32 inhibit gap junction gating sensitivity to CO_2. *Biophys. J.* 73:798–806, 1997.
291. Warn-Cramer, B. J. G. T. Cottrell, J. M. Burt, A. F. Lau. Regulation of connexin-43 gap junctional intercellular communication by mitogen-activated protein kinase. *J. Biol. Chem.* 273:9188–9196, 1998.
292. Watts, S. W. and R. C. Webb. Vascular gap junctional communication is increased in mineralocorticoid-salt hypertension. *Hypertension* 28:888–893, 1996.
293. Weidmann, S. The electrical constants of Purkinje fibres. *J. Physiol. (Lond).* 127:348–360, 1952.
294. Weiner, E. C. and W. R. Loewenstein. Correction of cell-cell communication defect by introduction of a protein kinase into mutant cells. *Nature* 305:433–435, 1983.
295. Werner, R., T. Miller, R. Azarnia and G. Dahl. Translation and functional expression of cell-cell channel mRNA in *Xenopus* oocytes. *J. Membr Biol* 87:253–268, 1985.
296. Wier, W. G., H. E. ter Keurs, E. Maban, W. D. Gao and C. W. Balke. Ca^{2+} 'sparks' and waves in intact ventricular muscle resolved by confocal imaging. *Circ. Res.* 81:462–469, 1997.
297. White, R. L., J. E. Doeller, V. K. Verselis and B. A. Wittenberg. Gap junctional conductance between pairs of ventricular myocytes is modulated synergistically by H^+ and Ca^{2+}. *J. Gen. Physiol.* 95:1061–1075, 1990.
298. White, T. W., R. Bruzzone, S. Wolfram, D. L. Paul and D. A. Goodenough. Selective interactions among the multiple connexin proteins expressed in the vertebrate lens: the second extracellular domain is a determinant of compatibility between connexins. *J. Cell Biol.* 125:879–892, 1994.
299. White, R. L., D. C. Spray, A. C. Campos de Carvalho, B. A. Wittenberg and M. V. Bennett. Some electrical and pharmacological properties of gap junctions between adult venticular myocytes. *Am. J. Physiol.* 249:C447–C455, 1985.
300. Wilders, R. and H. J. Jongsma. Limitations of the dual voltage clamp method in assaying conductance and kinetics of gap junction channels. *Biophys. J.* 63:942–953, 1992.
301. Willecke, K., O. Traub, J. Look, R. Stutenkemper and R. Dermietzel. Different protein components contribute to the structure and function of hepatic gap junctions. *Gap Junctions*, edited by E. L. Hertzberg, and R. G Johnson. New York: Alan R. Liss, 1988:41–52.
302. Woodbury, J. W. and W. E. Crill. On the problem of impulse conduction in the atrium. *Nervous Inhibition*, edited by E. Flovey. New York: Pergamon, 1961:124–135.
303. Wu, J., J. McHowat, J. E. Saffitz, K. A. Yamada and P. B. Corr. Inhibition of gap junctional conductance by long-chain acylcarnitines and their preferential accumulation in junctional sarcolemma during hypoxia. *Circ. Res.* 72:879–889, 1993.
304. Xie, H. Q. and V. W. Hu. Modulation of gap junctions in senescent endothelial cells. *Exp. Cell Res.* 214:172–176, 1994.
305. Yaeger, M. and N. B. Gilula. Membrane topology and quaternary structure of cardiac gap junction ion channels. *J. Mol. Biol.* 223:929–948, 1992.
307. Yaeger, M. and B. J. Nicholson Structure of gap junction intercellular channels. *Curr. Opin. Struct. Biol.* 6:183–192, 1996.
308. Yamada, K. A., J. McHowat, G. X. Yan, K. Donahue, J. Peirick, A. G. Kleber and P. B. Corr. Cellular uncoupling induced by accumulation of long-chain acylcarnitine during ischemia. *Cir. Res.* 74:83–95, 1994.
309. Yancey, S. B., S. A. John, R. Lal, B. J. Austin and J-P Revel. The 43-kD polypeptide of heart gap junctions: immunolocalization, topology and functional domains. *J. Cell. Biol.* 108:2241–2254, 1989.
310. Yancey, S. B., B. J. Nicholson and J. P. Revel. The dynamic state of liver gap junctions. *J. Supramol. Struct. Cell Biochem.* 221–232, 1981.
311. Yeh, H. I., F. Lupu, E. Dupont and N. J. Severs. Upregulation of connexin43 gap junctions between smooth muscle cells after balloon catheter injury in the rat carotid artery. *Arterioscler Thromb. Vasc. Biol.* 17:3174–3184, 1997.
312. Yeh, H. I., E. Dupont, S. Coppen, S. Rothery and N. J. Severs. Gap junction localization and connexin expression in cytochemically identified endothelial cells of arterial tissue. *J. Histochem. Cytochem.* 45:539–550, 1997.
313. Yu W, G. Dahl and R. Werner. The connexin43 gene is responsive to oestrogen. *Proc. R. Soc. Lond. B.* 255:125–132, 1994.

5. Vagal preganglionic neurons innervating the heart

K. MICHAEL SPYER | *Royal Free and University College Medical School, University College London, Royal Free Campus, Rowland Hill Street, London, United Kingdom.*

CHAPTER CONTENTS

Chronotropic Actions of Activating Vagal Efferent Fibers
B-Fibers and C-Fibers: Effect of Electrical Stimulation
The Location of the Somata of Preganglionic Vagal Neurons
Physiological Mapping
Biophysical Properties of Cardiac Vagal Neurons
Physiological Properties of Cardiac Vagal Motoneurons
Baroreceptor Input
Respiratory Influences on Cardiac Vagal Motoneuron Discharge
Mechanisms of Respiratory Patterning
Arterial Chemoreceptor Inputs
Pulmonary and Airway Inputs
   Slowly adapting pulmonary inputs
   Rapidly adapting pulmonary inputs
Pulmonary C-fibers
Upper Airway Receptors
Cardiac Receptors
CNS organization of reflex control
CNS pathways impinging on DVN and NA
Reflex Interactions: CNS Organization
Synaptic Effects Elicited by Baroreceptor Inputs in the Nucleus Tractus Solitarii
Synaptic Effects of Arterial Chemoreceptor Inputs
Central Modifications of Reflex Function
Role of Nucleus Tractus Solitarii in Reflex Adjustments
Respiratory influences of reflex transmission through the Nucleus Tractus Solitarius
Conclusions

HEART RATE is determined in a large part by the action of autonomic nervous innervation on the sino-atrial node and in consequence modulating the intrinsic pacemaker rhythm. From the now classical studies of Levy (137–139) it is clear that changes in vagal activity, at whatever the level of ongoing sympathetic efferent activity, exert the major effect on heart rate, and that this is adjusted on a beat-by-beat basis through reflex actions. Vagal efferent activity also affects both action potential conduction (dromotropic effects) and the force of cardiac contraction (inotropic state), but the role of vagal preganglionic motoneurons in the physiological control of these variables is much less well established than their role in control of cardiac chronotropy. From an extensive literature it is clear that the level of activity of cardiac vagal preganglionic motoneurons—neurons that control the activity of postganglionic neurons located in ganglia overlying the heart, is determined by interplay of excitatory and inhibitory synaptic inputs that impinge on these neurons. These inputs derive over complex neural pathways, both from peripheral receptors, many localized within the cardiovascular and respiratory systems, and from widely dispersed sensory receptors, and also from regions of the central nervous system (CNS) that are concerned with behavioral processes (229, 231, 232). These inputs act to maintain homeostasis by adjusting cardiac output, as a consequence of heart rate control, but also by modifying inotropic state and by ensuring a parallel change in respiratory minute volume. In some emergency responses this homeostatic role may be abrogated for a period, and the study of vagal control of the heart has been of some importance in developing an understanding of the CNS organization and integration of several aspects of the expression of behavioral activity. In this chapter the localization and morphology of cardiac vagal motoneurons (CVMs) is reviewed, concentrating on data from mammalian species and aspects of their physiological control. While a significant literature is now available concerning the physiological mechanisms controlling CVM activity, much less is known of the biophysical and pharmacological properties displayed by these neurons. However, this review focuses on actions that have been identified at the single-cell level rather than assessing actions from global pharmacological studies that have investigated the actions of centrally acting drugs in cardiac control.

CHRONOTROPIC ACTIONS OF ACTIVATING VAGAL EFFERENT FIBERS

It has been known since the nineteenth century that electrical stimulation of the vagus nerve will slow and ultimately stop the heart, depending on the intensity and pattern of stimulation (98). Two specific components to the response to vagal stimulation were recognized in, and subsequent to, the early experiments of Donders (53). This observation was most clearly defined by Brown and Eccles (18, 19), who noted the two components most clearly: the more rapid initial component (100–200 ms latency) was observed later by recording intracellularly from the sinoatrial (SA) node (106) and shown to be a consequence of hyperpolarization. The second, longer latency component merely reduced the slope of the pacemaker potential. The relatively long latency of the first component—between 100 and 200 ms was surprising, since it was believed to result from actions of small myelinated efferent fibers (B-fibers; Fig. 5–1) whose conduction velocity was such that only a few milliseconds would account for conduction from the cervical vagus to the cardiac ganglia. Accordingly the major component of the delay would be expected to result from ganglionic transmission, and subsequent neuro-effector delays resulting from acetylcholine (ACh) release from the postganglionic neurons. ACh increases a potassium conductance by the coupling of heterotrimeric G protein to the muscarinic M2 receptor. The potassium current so influenced leads to a hyperpolarization of the SA node. Opening of the ACh gated potassium channel has a lag of approximately 100 ms (83) and an appropriate time constant for activation (circa 100 ms with 10 mmol ACh) to account fully for the latency of vagal activation as demonstrated above.

B-FIBERS AND C-FIBERS: EFFECT OF ELECTRICAL STIMULATION

The cervical vagus and cardiac vagal branches are known to contain both small myelinated and unmyelinated C-fiber efferents in mammals. Electrical stimulation at low intensity can evoke responses solely attributed to B-fibers, but at higher intensity both B- and C-fibers will be activated (Fig. 5–1). The most sensitive means of assessing vagal actions is to measure R-R intervals, and B-fiber activation has been shown to lead to a rapid and maintained lengthening of that electrocardiographic feature (Fig. 5–1). In general it has been maintained in the cat that slowing is mediated entirely (128, 165) or largely (85) by B-fibers, and that this extends to actions on atrial contraction and atrioventricular (A-V) conduction (128). Increasing the intensity of vagal stimulation provokes an enhanced effect, but this has been explained most often as a consequence of the recruitment of additional B-fibers. However, in several species—turtle (84); rat (185); rabbit (69, 253)—a C-fiber component to the bradycardia has been demonstrated. This was recognized by using anodal block techniques (2, 253), which have been further exploited in a recent study that demonstrated in cat, rat, and rabbit a significant C-fiber–evoked bradycardia (Fig. 5–1). This bradycardia had characteristics unlike the effects elicited by B-fiber activation alone, in that it was both smaller in magnitude and slower in onset.

There is also evidence of clear differences in the pharmacology of ganglionic transmission underlying B- and C-fiber actions. While atropine will block the cardiac actions of both B- and C-fibers through its action at M_2 muscarinic atrial receptors, B-fiber actions are also fully blocked by the nicotinic ganglion blocker hexamethonium (69, 162, 221, 254). Actions attributed to C-fibers are, however, left unaffected by hexamethonium. They are however, blocked by the application of pirenzapine, a M_1 muscarinic receptor antagonist (110, 221). These findings are consistent with the demonstration that excitatory transmission through the cardiac ganglion is mediated by both fast and slow excitatory postsynaptic potentials (epsps), which are elicited by the activation of nicotinic and M_1 muscarinic receptors, respectively (4, 224, 254).

These observations suggest that the actions of B- and C-fibers may be different, and that they may mediate diverse physiological responses. Perhaps distinct populations of ganglionic neurons receive innervations from either B- or C-fibers. Indeed, preliminary studies (103) suggest that while B-fibers diverge and innervate several, perhaps many, postganglionic neurons, C-fibers have a restricted and largely nondivergent innervation of ganglion cells. These conclusions rest on observations drawn from studies in which fluorescent tracers were injected into specific brain stem nuclei known to contain vagal motoneurons (see later under the location of the Somata of Preganglionic Vagal Neurons). Whether the different ganglia overlying the heart (see refs. 197–199) have distinctive patterns of innervation from preganglionic B-and C-fibers remains to be resolved (see ref. 104 for discussion).

THE LOCATION OF THE SOMATA OF PREGANGLIONIC VAGAL NEURONS

There is compelling evidence that both B- and C-fibers in the cervical vagus and cardiac branches exert profound cardiac effects (see Fig. 5–1). In understanding the mechanisms that control the activity of these two classes of vagal efferent, it has been necessary to identify the localization of their cell bodies within the medulla oblongata. The extensive literature on this subject has been reviewed widely (23, 104, 121, 146, 229, 231). The earliest studies were undertaken using histological analyses that involved searching for neurons demonstrating retrograde degeneration after section of the vagus and its peripheral branches. These studies indicated the presence of CVMs in both the dorsal va-

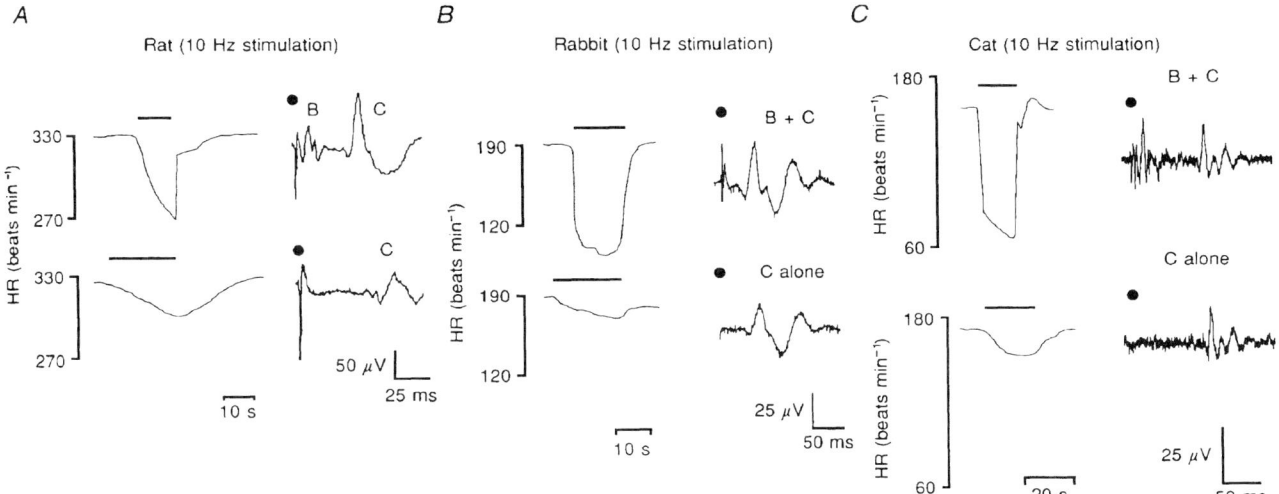

FIG. 5-1. Traces show the heart rate responses produced by electrical stimulation of the cervical vagus (1 msec, 10 V, 10 Hz). Responses to stimulating B + C fibers were evoked with the cathode facing the heart and no anodal block. Responses to stimulating C fibers alone were evoked with the anode facing the heart and the anodal block technique applied. [Reprinted with permission from Jones, Wang, and Jordan (111).]

gal nucleus (DVN); (78, 173, 180), among others) and the nucleus ambiguus (NA) (20, 134, 247). This latter distribution was confirmed when Szentagothai (239) demonstrated Wallerian degeneration in cardiac and pulmonary vagal branches following lesions placed in the NA. For reasons that still can not be explained, lesions in the DVN failed to produce equivalent degeneration in that study, but Calaresu and Cottle (21) showed convincingly such degenerative changes following DVN lesions.

This dual source of cardiac vagal neurons was further substantiated when more sensitive tracing techniques became available during the last twenty years of the twentieth century (Fig. 5-2). The retrograde transport of horseradish peroxidase (HRP) (134, 136) confirmed the presence of these neurons in both sites within the medulla (Fig. 5-2). There may, however, be species differences in their location: both cat and rat vagal preganglionic motoneurons relaying to the heart are localized within both the DVN and NA, and in the region between these two medullary nuclei (the intermediate zone) (10, 75, 102, 121, 172, 176, 184, 238). Notably, the neurons in the NA are found not in the compact region of the nucleus or in the columns of cells that give rise to the axons innervating the striated muscle of the larynx, pharynx, and esophagus, but are scattered in the ventral areas of the nucleus that is termed the *periambigual area* (see refs. 11, 104, 120, 247; and Fig. 5-2 and 5-3). The neurons of the DVN that give rise to the innervation of the heart are localized in the lateral regions of the nucleus approaching the nucleus tractus solitarii (NTS) (10, 102, 184) (see Fig. 5-2).

More recently, injections of pseudorabies virus into the myocardium have been used to determine retrograde labeling of CVMs. Distributions of CVMs seen in the rat (237) are equivalent to those demonstrated with conventional anatomical techniques. Although certain viral strains result in both DVN and NA labeling, others fail to label DVN neurons. Standish et al., (237) have also suggested that a specific subset of CVMs may innervate ganglion cells which have a solely ventricular projection.

Aside from their restricted localization in the medulla, CVMs in the DVN tend to have smaller perikarya than those localized within the NA (75, 76, 195, 238), but ultrastructural studies have failed to reveal any distinct morphological differences other than size between CVMs in these two principal locations (104, 241). All CVMs had smooth, unindented nuclei and cytoplasm rich in organelles, characteristics similar to those demonstrated by motoneurons in general.

These kinds of studies have provided important evidence regarding the localization of CVMs in general, but they are unable to distinguish directly the distribution of those containing B- and C-fibers or to identify the physiological role of the identified neuron, demonstrating only their pattern of axonal projection. The capricious nature of many of the tracing techniques, and the variation in detail between different studies, may reflect differences in transport characteristics of B- and C-fibers, but that remains a supposition. To distinguish between the distributions of B- and C-fiber neurons, there is the need to use neurophysiological techniques linked to a precise mapping of recording sites.

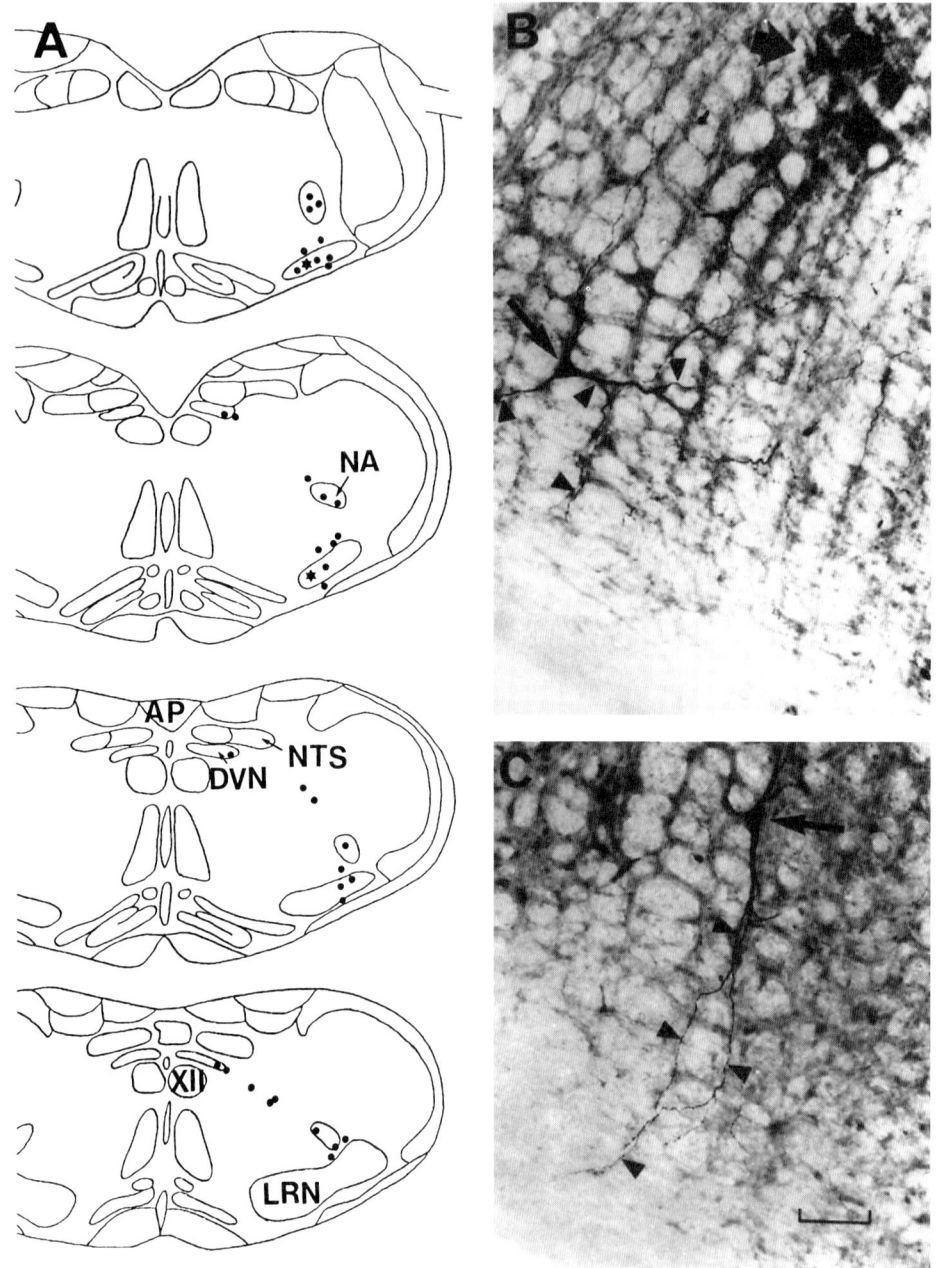

FIG. 5–2. *A*: Schematic representation of the position of retrogradely labeled neurons (l), at four levels of the medulla, after the application of cholera toxin conjugated to horseradish peroxidase (CT-HRP) into the myocardium. AP-area postrema; DVN-dorsal motor nucleus of the vagus nerve; LRN-lateral reticular nucleus; NA-nucleus ambiguus; XII-hypoglossal motonucleus; NTS-nucleus tractus solitarii. *B,C*: Light micrographs showing cardiac vagal preganglionic motoneurones (CVMs) in the ventral regions of the nucleus ambiguus retrogradely labeled after the application of CT-HRP into the myocardium (*long arrows*), the positions of which are represented in *A* by *asterisks*. Often the dendrites (*arrowheads*) of labeled neurons in this region extended as far as the ventral surface of the medulla (*C*). After some of the cardiac injections, a diffuse labeling of the compact group resulted (*broad arrow*), similar to that observed in control injections into the thoracic cavity (*B*). Scale bar: 50 mm. [Published with permission from Izzo and Spyer (104).]

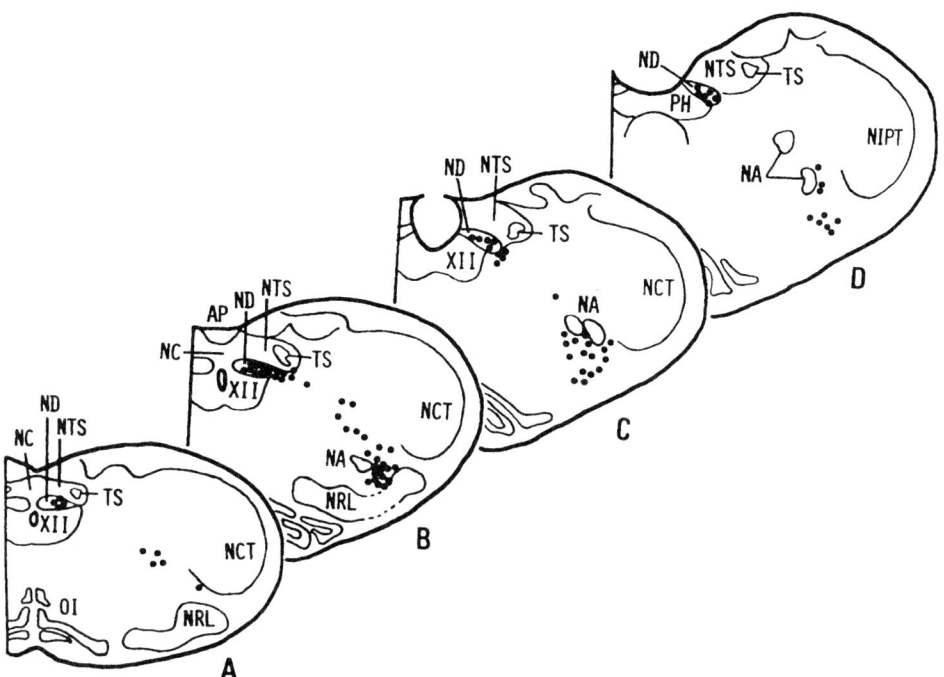

FIG. 5–3. Distribution of cell somata labeled with HRP following microiontophoretic application to the cardiac branch of the vagus nerve. All HRP-labeled cells in one animal were collectively plotted on the nearest of the four representative sections. A, B, C, and D: sections at the level of the obex, 420 m, 780 m, and 1,080 m rostral to it, respectively. [Published with permission from Nosaka et al. (186).]

PHYSIOLOGICAL MAPPING

While many of the anatomical studies predated physiological investigation, it is interesting to note that the more recent and detailed anatomical description of the localization of CVMs has merely confirmed what was established using electrophysiological approaches (see refs. 104, 229–231, for review). Indeed, the electrophysiological approach has many advantages since under certain circumstances the functional role of identified neurons has been established.

The first definitive physiological description of CVMs was provided in the cat (159–161), where they were identified using antidromic activation on stimulating the intrathoracic cardiac branches of the vagus (Fig. 5–4 A, B, C). While considerable care was taken to identify vagal branches that exerted major chronotropic effects on the heart, contamination with vagal fibers supplying other structures was only minimized, and not excluded. However, using an array of physiological stimuli it proved possible to distinguish between those vagal motoneurons with cardiac function and those with influences on airway smooth muscle (159). Subsequent studies in the rat (186) and the rabbit (115) have provided equivalent information, and some limited data are available also in the dog (75).

While the anatomical studies have indicated the broad distribution of vagal motoneurons through the medulla oblongata, they were unable to distinguish localization of those neurons with B- or C-fibers. In the cat, there was a clear separation—CVMs with small myelinated axons (B-fibers; conduction velocity 3–16 ms: bCVM) were restricted to the NA (Fig. 5–5), while those with C-fiber axons (conduction velocity >1 ms: cCVM) to the DVN (159). In the rabbit, bCVMs were seen in both DVN and NA (115) while in the rat, the DVN was shown to contain largely cCVM, but some neurons with B-fibers have also been described (186) (Fig. 5–2). Interestingly, in both cat and rabbit, ionophoretic application of DL-homocysteic acid, or glutamate, onto bCVMs elicited falls in heart rate (115, 160), the changes often appearing consistent with the evoked discharge of a single, or a few, neurons. Evidence was also obtained that indicated that injury discharges evoked small but measurable falls in heart rate (160). Many subsequent studies have shown that the microinjection of excitant amino acids or other ligands into DVN or NA can induce falls in heart rate, but the large volumes used (up to 100 μl or more) of relatively concentrated solutions indicate responses involving the activation of a significant population of neurons. The ob-

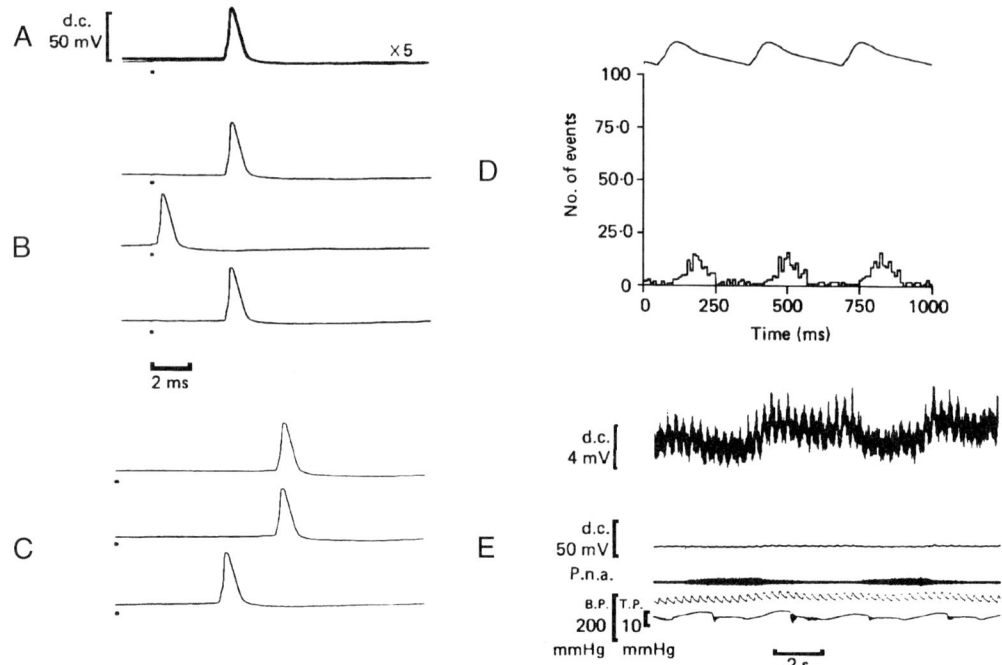

FIG. 5–4. Intracellular recording from CVM. *A*: Stimulating cervical vagus (0.1 ms, 6 V) at 1 Hz. Five superimposed sweeps. *B*: Three consecutive sweeps illustrating the collision of an othodromic spike, in the middle trace, with the antidromic spike. *D: Lower Trace*: electrocardiogram-(ECG) triggered histogram of ongoing discharge of the CVM identified in *A, B, C, D* (110 sweeps, 10 ms bins). *Upper trace*: femoral arterial waveform averaged over the same course and triggered from ECG (100 sweeps). *C*: stimulation of the cardiac branches of the right vagus (0.1 mecs, 3 V). Three consecutive sweeps, collision with orthodromic spike in tower trace. Stimulus marked by (l) in *A, B, C, E*: Intracellular recording from a CVM showing respiratory-related changed in membrane potential. The cell stopped firing action potentials 5 min after the cell was penetrated. In each panel traces from above; high and low gain d.c. recordings of membrane potential, phrenic nerve activity, arterial blood pressure, and tracheal pressure. [Modified and reproduced with permission from Gilbey et al. (79).]

servation that measurable changes in heart rate can be evoked by the activity of single (or few) CVM is consistent with a strongly divergent pattern of innervation of cardiac ganglia by B-fibers described earlier (104).

The maps of CVM distribution in the medulla that have been constructed using electrophysiological approaches and anatomical tracing, share some common features (compare Figures 5–2, 5–3, and 5–5 for the rat). It appears that CVMs in both DVN and NA are distributed in longitudinal columns (Figs. 5–4 and 5–5). Those in the DVN occupy lateral regions of the nucleus, while those in the NA are situated separately from the vagal motoneurons innervating the striated muscle of the larynx, pharynx, and esophagus (see above under The Location of the Somata of Preganglionic Vagal Neurons) and also the preganglionic neurons with bronchomotor function. There is some overlap, but CVMs tend to be localized ventrally to the compact region of the NA and may be further subdivided into functional groupings. Massari and his colleagues suggest on the basis of cardiac responses to restricted microinjections of glutamate in the dog, that distinct zones within the NA evoke chronotropic, inotropic, and dromotropic (71, 156) responses, implying that neurons with restricted function are localized in discrete regions of the NA (71, 156). There was not a total separation of zones and mixed responses were also observed. Some substantiation for this organization of vagal neurons has been obtained from equivalent studies in the in situ working heart–brain stem preparation (217).

Definitive electrophysiological confirmation of Massari's claim is awaited, as is support for an early study in the cat (75) that suggested that CVMs in the DVN might play a role in inotropic and not chronotropic responses. This has not as yet been confirmed by other laboratories. There does appear to be some functional correlation between preganglionic vagus neurons and the cardiac ganglia (155).

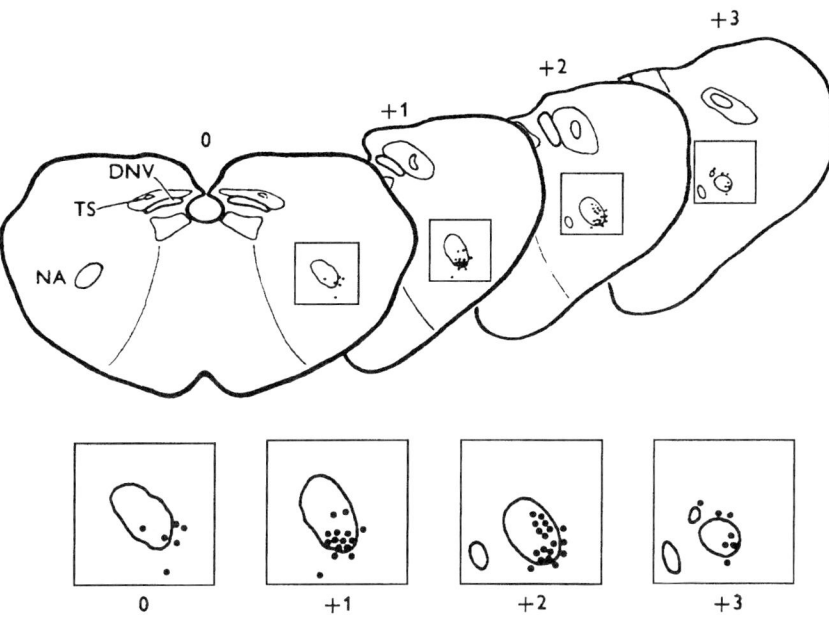

FIG. 5–5. Location. The positions of forty-six cardiac efferent neurons are shown on four standard sections of the medulla taken at obex level, and at 1 mm intervals rostrally. *Inserts*, 2 mm square, show details of their relation to the structure of the nucleus ambiguus. Abbreviations: *TS*, tractus solitarius; *DNV*, dorsal motor nucleus of the vagus; *NA*, nucleus ambiguus. [Published with permission from McAllen and Spyer (158).]

BIOPHYSICAL PROPERTIES OF CARDIAC VAGAL MOTONEURONS

The firing patterns of CVMs, as with other neurons, are determined by the interplay of their synaptic inputs and their basic membrane properties. While evidence has been accumulated concerning the range and magnitude of synaptic input, very little is yet known specifically about the basic membrane properties of either bCVMs or cCVMs (see ref. 233). What information is available has been extrapolated from the wide range of studies undertaken on vagal motoneurons of the DVN. The inferences may thus have direct relevance to c-CVMs and it is probable that the general properties are also shared by bCVMs.

From the extensive literature that exists with regard to DVN neurons, primarily from investigations in brain slices or cultured neurons taken from the rat and guinea pig (95, 183, 210, 211, 212, 255 among others), it is believed that in many respects vagal neurons are not very different from motoneurons in general (Fig. 5–6). They have somewhat distinctive features with regard to the falling phase of the action potential, where they have a more prominent after-depolarization than is seen in spinal motoneurons, and this is a consequence of a high threshold Ca current (Fig. 5–6). Calcium currents are indeed prominent in these neurons which display calcium-mediated action potentials in the presence of tetrodotoxin (TTX) (213). There may be two forms of action potential that are insensitive to TTX—a low and a high threshold form (213, 214, 245). There is also a prolonged and large afterhyperpolarization mediated in part by a calcium-dependent K current (I_{AHP}) which is supplemented by a transient and slowly inactivating K current (I_A) (213). These currents together are responsible for the effective hyperpolarization of vagal neurons (VN) that persists for as long as 2000 ms (see Fig. 5–6A). These currents will affect powerfully the excitability of VN and contribute to their low resting discharge. Furthermore, DVN neurons do not display low threshold and transient calcium currents that are so prominent in other brain stem neurons (109). They are also claimed to have an insignificant number of K_{ATP} channels, which are seen prominently in hypoglossal motoneurons (109). However, in some 20% of DVN neurons recorded in the whole-cell configuration (242), a tolbutamide-sensitive outward current has been described. The suggestion of the presence of K_{ATP} channels that were spontaneously active was further reinforced by the fact that the K_{ATP} channel agonist diazoxide activated a tolbutamide-sensitive current in up to 33% of DVN neurons. The conclusion must be that DVN neurons do in fact express K_{ATP} channels, but their activity must depend on the intracellular milieu, which may be modified significantly through dialysis in whole-cell recordings. The physiological role of these channels must therefore remain in question.

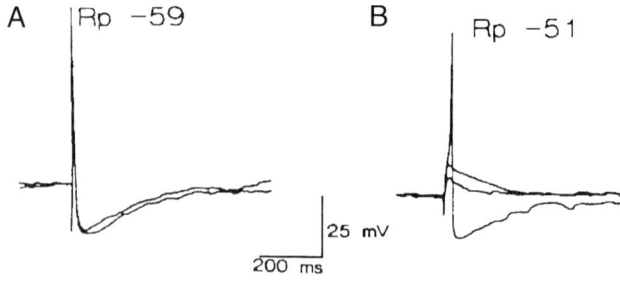

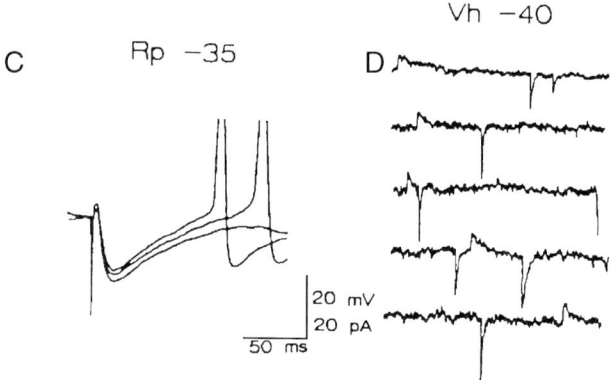

FIG. 5–6. *A*: Antidromically evoked action potential in the dorsal vagal nucleus (*DMV*) neuron upon vagal stimulation. *B*: Orthodromically evoked epsp and action potential in a DMV neuron upon perivagal stimulation. *C*: Orthodromic mixed epsp-ipsp in a DMV neuron during steady current injection to hold the cell resting membrane potential at a depolarized level of −35 mV. Action potentials were often triggered after the ipsps. *D*: At a holding potential of −40 mV, spontaneous miniature epsps and spontaneous miniature ipsps were observed as inward (downward) and outward (upward) currents, respectively, and were not abolished by the presence of 1 mM TTX. [Reproduced with permission from Travagli and Gillis (244).]

Recent studies on retrogradely labeled CVM localized in the NA of the rat have shown similar voltage-gated currents (171). A prominent K (I_A) current was revealed together with a long-lasting delayed rectified K current.

In view of the accumulated data, it is possible to infer that basic membrane properties exert a major influence on the excitability of VN and, presumably, also CVM. While these appear to act to minimize spike discharge frequency, in the slice, DVN neurons often show discharge (0.5–5 Hz) that is independent of synaptic input. This discharge has led to the suggestion that they may have some pacemaker-like properties. However, in this regard it may reflect nothing more than an example of the capability of all, or at least most, neurons under appropriate circumstances to exhibit beating or pacemaker-like activity. However the DVN neurons do have prominent Ca^{2+} and Ca^{2+} dependent K^+ channels that are known to be essential for both bursting and pacemaker type activity. In physiological situations the interplay of passive and ligand-gated channels will determine the effectiveness of synaptic input, and the pharmacology of the control of VN (and CVM) is of major interest.

Recent studies in rat have used retrograde fluorescent tracers to back-label NA neurons projecting to the heart. These neurons were then visualized in 250 μm transverse sections taken from the medulla, and whole-cell patch recordings were made (164, 171) These studies revealed voltage-gated Na^+ and K^+ currents and Ca^{2+}-activated K^+ currents that correspond closely to those described above for vagal neurons in general.

PHYSIOLOGICAL PROPERTIES OF CARDIAC VAGAL MOTONEURONS

There is an enormous body of information regarding the properties of vagal efferent fibers in the cervical

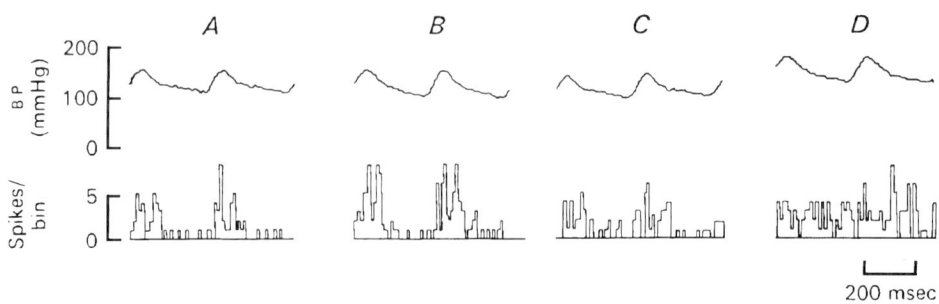

FIG. 5–7. The cardiac rhythm of a c.v.m. (aortic baroreceptors denervated). Pulse-triggered histogram of c.v.m. activity (*lower trace*) and pulse-triggered average of femoral pulse wave (*upper trace*). 128 superimposed cycles, 10 msec bin width. *A*: both common carotid arteries open; *B*: contralateral carotid occluded; *C*, ipsilateral carotid occluded; *D*, bilateral carotid occlusion. Unit firing in response to 8 nA DLH. [Reproduced with permission from McAllen and Spyer (161).]

vagus and cardiac vagal branches. These often meticulous studies (reviewed in refs. 219 and 229) have shown that across mammalian species the firing patterns of CVMs are very similar. Major studies have been conducted in dog and cat (100, 101, 107, 108, 135, among others), and all have indicated a powerful sensitivity of these fibers to baroreceptor input with discharge showing a marked cardiac rhythmicity (see also refs. 124, 125). Furthermore, when investigated, the discharge was seen to be modulated by respiratory activity, with discharge being most prevalent during expiration (see also ref. 123). All these studies had been undertaken in anesthetized preparations, and anesthesia is reported to have a particularly marked suppressive effect on vagal activity, especially in the cat, where vagal tone is notoriously low. Jewett (107, 108) discerned several different categories of vagal fiber in the cervical vagus (based in large part on action potential size) and was convinced that many neurons with small axons, presumably C-fibers, were usually silent but as with all CVMs, these neurons were excited powerfully by baroreceptor inputs. As a consequence of these and other studies, McAllen and Spyer (160, 161), recording from the perikarya in the medulla of the cat, concluded that the major excitatory input to the CVMs—at least those with B-fiber axons—originated from the arterial baroreceptors (see Figs. 5–4 A and 5–7) Subsequently the importance of central modulation of this input for cardiac control was revealed (see later under Mechanisms of Respiratory Patterning).

Recent studies on the cCVMs in a range of species (111–113a) have indicated that these neurons do not receive a significant baroreceptor input and their activity shows no relationship to central respiratory drive lung inflation or the cardiac cycle (113a). They are highly sensitive to inputs from pulmonary C-fiber afferents, and both powerful and prolonged excitatory responses can be elicited in them by injections of phenyl biguanide into the right atrium. These injections also excite bCVMs, but it is argued (110, 111, 113) that the C-fiber reflex pathway may represent an important defense mechanism preserved from gill-breathing ancestors (and present in fish and amphibia today) that seeks to minimize gill blood flow in the presence of potentially harmful chemicals in the water or the local environment. These effects may be mediated by a monosynaptic glutaminergic pathway from the NTS (252).

The conventional bCVMs are excited by many additional inputs, for example those arising from the arterial chemoreceptors, cardiac receptors, trigeminal inputs, and a particularly powerful input from the superior laryngeal nerve fibers. They are also subject to input from many sites in the central nervous system, and contribute to the adjustment in cardiac output that occurs in relation to behavioral activity. This role and the interplay between CNS evoked actions and reflex inputs will form an important additional component of the review.

BARORECEPTOR INPUT

As described above, cardiac vagal efferent fibers, and CVMs, receive a powerful excitatory input from the arterial baroreceptors (Figs. 5–4D and 5–7), although those CVMs with C-fiber axons may have distinctly different properties showing weak or absent baroreceptor inputs (see ref. 111). The apparently restricted localization of cCVMs within the DVN (see refs. 159, 160, 161, 184–186) has led to the belief that the two classes of vagal neurons might be regulated by different pathways or synaptic mechanisms, even though they share a relatively common morphology.

The marked influence of the baroreceptors on the activity of bCVMs can be seen from the post-R-wave correlation of discharge in studies undertaken in both cat and dog (reviewed in Spyer, 1981 (229; Figs. 5–4D and 5–7). Similarly, recordings made with extracellular microelectrodes (159, 160, 162) have shown that the discharges of bCVMs, either those with ongoing activity or those provoked to fire by the ionophoresis of excitant amino acids (160, 161) have a clear cardiac rhythm (Figs. 5–4D and 5–7). By making simultaneous recordings of sinus nerve (SN) activity, McAllen and Spyer were able to demonstrate that the latency of the influence from the carotid sinus baroreceptors to the onset of the cardiac-related burst of bCVM activity was some 20–110 ms (161). Further when the SN was stimulated electrically the onset of the stimulus-evoked response was somewhat shorter, presumably as a consequence of the synchronization of afferent input. Together, these data suggested that a disynaptic pathway could underlie the fast component of the stimulus-evoked response but that a more complex pathway might be responsible for a significant portion of that response (see refs. 229, 231 for discussion). The complexities of connection within the NTS (see later) and the fact that SN contains both myelinated and unmyelinated afferents with as yet unresolved physiological roles (see ref. 222), makes the interpretation of the effects of SN stimulation fraught with difficulties (note that the SN also contains chemoreceptor afferents). It should be noted that the actions of the baroreceptor input at the level of the NTS, the primary relay nucleus, is complex, the NTS functioning to process afferent inputs and limiting the frequency of the transmission (see ref. 220 and subsequent discussion). However, there is now clear evidence that monosynaptic glutaminergic pathways connect to DVN neurons (see above) and to

CVM in NA (182). NTS stimulation in rat medullary slices leads to glutaminergic currents mediated by both NMDA and non-N-methyl-D-aspartic acid (NMDA) receptors with a latency of 8–18 ms (182).

With regard to the importance of baroreceptor inputs in setting the level of excitability of bCVMs in anesthetized and paralyzed preparations, in which vagal "tone" is notoriously low, selective denervation of the aortic and sinus baroreceptors resulted in a progressive decrease of bCVM discharge so that the cardiac-related discharge was abolished by bilateral SN and aortic nerve section (161; Fig. 5–7).

Observations (186) in the rat imply that SN-evoked responses are mediated primarily by bCVMs located in the NA, while those in the DVN (cCVM) do not participate in reflex-evoked responses. Conversely vagal C-fiber activation resulted in a significant activation of DVN neurons. In the rabbit, bCVMs are localized within both DVN and NA and appear to show the same patterns of response to reflex inputs.

A predominant role of bCVMs in the NA in the mediation of baroreceptor inputs is further supported by both neuroanatomical (see 181) evidence for direct connections from the NTS to the NA and ultrastructural evidence that NA neurons and specifically CVMs, receive monosynaptic excitatory connections from the NTS (see refs. 51, 102, 104 for discussion). Whether these mediate baroreceptor actions remains to be resolved, as excitation of the arterial chemoreceptors (see ref. 38 for review) exerts powerful influences on bCVM discharge, and this reflex input, as well as others, is also processed within the NTS. Together with the in vitro electrophysiology data, this constitutes compelling evidence for a monosynaptic pathway from NTS mediating baroreceptor control of CVM activity.

RESPIRATORY INFLUENCES ON CARDIAC VAGAL MOTONEURON DISCHARGE

There is clear evidence that bCVMs (Fig. 5–3E) (79, 80, 159–161), vagal efferent fibers in the cervical vagus (100, 101, 107, 108 among others) and those in the cardiac branches (135) show fluctuations in firing coinciding with the pattern of central respiratory activity (Fig. 5–8A). It was concluded largely from fiber recordings that bCVMs fired in expiration, but a detailed neurophysiological analysis of their discharge has shown that they fire predominantly during postinspiration, the first phase of expiration, with a variable discharge during expiration, but that they are hyperpolarized during inspiration (79) (Figs. 5–4E and 8B). These studies, and earlier studies using extracellular recordings (160, 161; see Fig. 5–8A) were in preparations in which central respiration was dissociated from lung

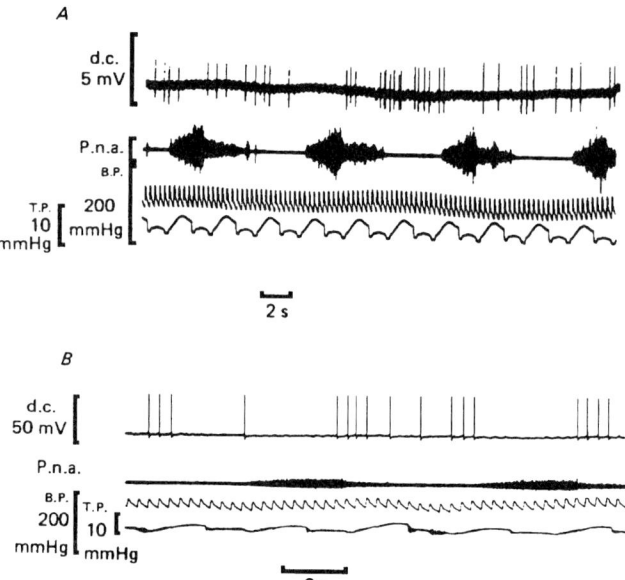

FIG. 5–8. *A*: extracellular recording from a c.v.m. (see ref. 189) *B*: intracellular recording from a c.v.m. (see ref. 73) Traces, from top to bottom: low gain recording of c.v.m. activity, phrenic nerve activity (p.n.a.), femoral arterial blood pressure (B.P.), and tracheal pressure (T. P.). [Reproduced with permission from Gilbey et al. (79).]

movements as the animals were artificially ventilated, open-chested and often paralyzed (Figs. 5–4E and 5–8). Lung inflation has long been known to evoke a tachycardia (see ref. 36 for detailed review) and was considered a major factor in respiratory arrythmias (6, 7), because lung inflation would be expected to inhibit bCVM discharge. Intracellular recordings from bCVMs (see ref. 79) have failed to reveal any major membrane potential fluctuations related to lung movements in animals prepared as above, where tidal volume was maintained at a relatively low level (Figs. 5–4E and 8B). Conversely, Daly (36, 37, 42, 43) has provided considerable data illustrating not only phasic effects of lung inflation on heart rate control exerted by vagal efferents but also effective modulation of other reflex effects on the heart by lung inflation. These effects have been beautifully illustrated in fiber recordings (48).

These apparent discrepancies might be reconciled if cCVMs, which are restricted in large part to the DVN (see above), were the target for lung inflation inputs. This does not appear to be the case (see refs. 110–113a); rather, cCVMs participate in C-fiber chemoreflexes (see above).

MECHANISMS OF RESPIRATORY PATTERNING

From intracellular recordings it is evident that bCVMs are hyperpolarized during inspiration by a Cl⁻ dependent process (79; Figs. 5–8B and 5–9)). Cl⁻ injection into CVMs, or the application of hyperpolarizing current, leads to a reversal of the inspiratory-related hyperpolarization to a depolarization as the equilibrium potential for Cl⁻ is passed (Fig. 5–9). Since the inhibition involves Cl⁻, it was reasoned to be mediated by the synaptic release of either GABA acting at $GABA_A$ receptors, or glycine. A detailed neuropharmacological study (79, 120) has, however, revealed the involvement of a cholinergic muscarinic synapse with neither bicuculline nor strychnine (antagonists at $GABA_A$ and glycine receptors, respectively) having an influence on inspiratory-related inhibitions of bCVM discharge. Atropine applied ionophoretically was effective (79), and bicuculline was shown to antagonize other inhibitory inputs such as those induced by stimulation within certain regions of the hypothalamus (see ref. 120, 235). GABA certainly acts centrally to modulate cardiac vagal tone in humans, although its site of action is unresolved (63) Immunocytochemical studies have shown that CVMs labeled retrogradely with HRP have symmetrical synapses on their perikarya and dendrites and that these often contain GABA (17, 149). Microionophoresis of GABA is certainly effective in inhibiting these neurons, yet other studies provided clear evidence that ACh is localized within terminals within the NA. However, in recent in vitro slice studies Mendelowitz (personal communication) has been unable to demonstrate an inhibitory action of ACh, rather observing a nicotine-sensitive excitatory action. Whether the atropine-sensitive action of ACh is acting at a presynaptic locus remains to be resolved. It is notable that no evidence of an M-current was revealed in NA neurons.

It thus remains an open question whether the respiratory modulated excitability of CVMs depends on a cholinergic synapse localized directly on the bCVM or a cholinergic (excitatory synapse) onto an inhibitory interneuron or a presynaptic action of ACh. The lack of action of bicuculline in antagonizing inspiratory inhibition makes the second suggestion largely untenable if GABA only acts via $GABA_A$ receptors. $GABA_B$ receptors, while predominately localized presynaptically, may also feature as postsynaptic receptors, but no study of their role in the process of respiratory modulation of CVM activity, nor of $GABA_C$ receptors, has yet been undertaken. In vitro studies on putative CVMs in NA have failed to identify an inhibitory or excitatory muscarinic action, but they have shown that nicotine exerts excitatory actions (182). It has a postsynaptic depolarizing action, and a presynaptic facilitation of glutamate release. A claim for a postsynaptic modulation of non-NMDA currents has been made, but this remains controversial.

The pattern of activity of bCVMs resembles closely that of postinspiratory (PI) neurons (see ref. 204 for discussion). It is conceivable that, rather than sharing common inputs, PI neurons (see Discussion) might function to control bCVM activity. Notably CVMs are at their most depolarized during postinspiration (see Figs. 5–4E, 5–8, and 5–9) and so might receive an excitatory input from these interneurons which are known to play a dominant role in the patterning of the respiratory rhythm (see ref. 201–203,). If this were the case, inspiratory inhibition of CVMs would be a consequence of disfacilitation, an effect that could not readily be accounted for by the increased Cl⁻ current observed during inspiration (79). The details of the synaptic mechanisms underlying this inhibitory action thus remain unresolved, although the phenomenon of inspiratory "inhibition" is now firmly established.

It is perhaps worth noting that sinus arrhythmia mediated by vagal activity is suppressed in cats and dogs by doses of atropine that are one-tenth/hundredth those required for vagal blockade at the heart (see ref. 124). This central effect of atropine is consistent with an action at the level of the NA given the data presented by Gilbey et al. (79). Respiratory sinus arrhythmia is prominent in humans, and it appears that the mechanisms underlying its appearance are the same or at least similar to those in other higher vertebrates (218).

A further factor that may exacerbate respiratory sinus arrhythmia mediated by vagal efferent activity is the phasic arrhythmia variations in arterial blood pressure that accompany normal ventilation. These variations may result in part from the changes in intrathoracic pressure that occur during the ventilatory cycle

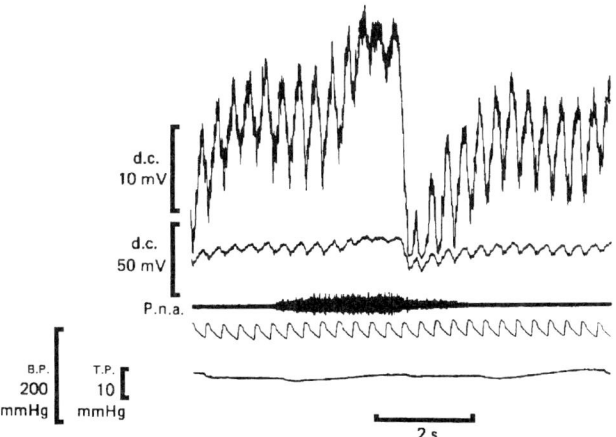

FIG. 5–9. Respiratory modulation of pulse-rhythmic epsps. Recording in a cell in which ipsps had been reversed previously by Cl⁻ injection (3 nA for 5 min). Further details in text. *Traces from top to bottom*: high and low gain d.c. recordings of membrane potential, phrenic nerve activity, femoral arterial blood pressure, and tracheal pressure. [Reproduced with permission from Gilbey et al. (79).]

and that influence venous return and hence cardiac output. Arterial blood pressure may, as a consequence, fluctuate with respiration (see 220), these fluctuations representing Traube-Hering waves (86, 220, 243). Since the major excitatory drive to CVMs arises from the arterial baroreceptors (see ref. 160), these changes may induce reflex cardiac effects by reducing bCVM activity during inspiration. However, the intracellular recording studies in cat (79) would seem to argue strongly that the major influence is that exerted centrally by inspiratory related inhibition of bCVM activity because baroreceptor-evoked epsps are shunted by the accompanying fall in membrane input resistance observed during inspiration (Fig. 5–9). These factors have been reviewed in detail by Daly (38). Alternatively, the alterations in the activity of cardiopulmonary receptors localized within the thorax that occur in parallel with intrathoracic pressure changes modify vagal (and sympathetic) outflow in a phasic manner.

The phenomenon of sinus arrhythmia has long been assumed to provide an indication of the level of vagal tone, but there is evidence of a sympathetic component to the phenomenon (49, 80). Either ganglionic blockade or combined vagosympathetic section results in an abolition of sinus arrhythmia, and cardiac transplanted dogs fail to demonstrate sinus arrhythmia until parasympathetic reinnervation is evident in most cases (241). However, there is evidence in human heart transplant recipients that sinus arrhythmia is reversed; i.e. tachycardia occurs during expiration and bradycardia occurs during inspiration (218). Conversely, in ganglionic blockade, normal subjects often show a small residual non-neural component of sinus arrhythmia, presumably resulting from atrial stretch (22).

ARTERIAL CHEMORECEPTOR INPUTS

There is a considerable literature describing the cardiac effects of exciting the arterial chemoreceptors (see ref. 38). To summarize, a brief chemoreceptor stimulus timed to occur during inspiration provokes an increased inspiratory effort together with cardio-acceleration that is largely, if not exclusively, due to vagal withdrawal (48, 70, 160, 161, 196; see Fig. 5–10). During expiration the equivalent stimulus elicits a bradycardia, together with a prolongation of expiration (see ref. 38 for references and discussion). Clearly, these brief, and intense, stimuli to the carotid body chemoreceptors are not physiological: but could respiratory related fluctuations in arterial Pco_2 and pH evoke significant influences of heart rate through actions on CVMs? Certainly more prolonged chemoreceptor afferent excitation elicits a marked effect on heart rate, the effect usually following closely the change in respiration (see above and Fig. 5–11).

The oscillations in Pco_2 and pH during the respiratory cycle that are observed usually result in the effective stimulus to the chemoreceptors being greater during expiration (13, 14, 58, 59), implying that chemoreceptor discharge may contribute under resting conditions to the respiration-related firing pattern of bCVMs. During expiration bCVMs are released from inspiration-related inhibition, and so are maximally excitable at that time. This excitability could be sustained, or enhanced, by any changes that occur in the level of chemoreceptor drive (see Fig. 5–11). Eldridge et al. (60) have described in some detail the long-term respiratory changes evoked by chemoreceptor (or sinus nerve) stimulation, indicating that the respiratory rate and depth may be changed for considerable periods after cessation of the initial stimulus. This is termed the *afterdischarge*. In much the same way, long-term changes in bCVM activity may be observed after intense activation of the arterial chemoreceptors, and in these situations sinus arrhythmia is also more marked (see ref. 204). Whether this is a consequence of enhanced respiration-related oscillations in arterial Pco_2 and pH remains to be resolved, but it is unlikely that these are in any way the trigger for sinus arrhythmia. Rather, they may be a manifestation of sinus arrhythmia acting to substantially reinforce its existence.

PULMONARY AND AIRWAY INPUTS

The importance of inputs from the airways and lungs in modifying CVM activity has already been discussed briefly. In this section the role of different classes of receptor responsible for these effects is reviewed as, in both physiological mechanisms and pathophysiological events, the interplay between reflex inputs and heart rate are of major significance. This subject has been reviewed extensively (26, 27, 36, 38, 151, 231).

Slowly Adapting Pulmonary Inputs

As indicated earlier, artificial lung inflation with pressures of <15 mm Hg invariably results in a tachycardia in the dog that is largely, if not exclusively, the consequence of vagal withdrawal (5, 6, 37, 39, 40, 44, 45, 108; see Fig. 5–10). This depends on the activity of vagal afferents with pulmonary endings that relay to the CNS with myelinated axons (250, 251). In the cat, cardiac effects are often smaller, but with raised vagal tone; as a consequence, for example, of superior laryngeal nerve stimulation, marked effects can be demonstrated (44). As indicated earlier, vagal tone is notori-

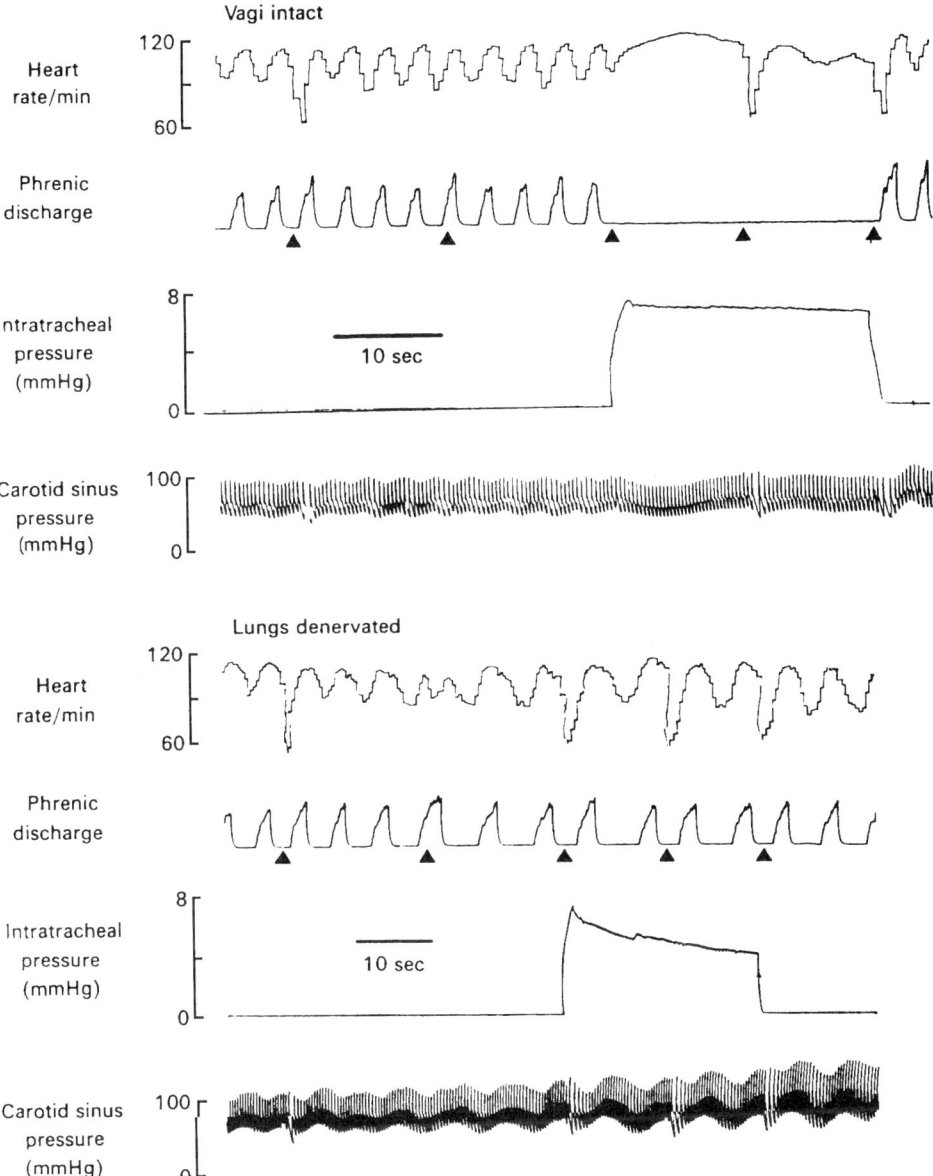

FIG. 5-10. Dog, anaesthetized with chloralose and paralyzed with D-tubocurarine. *Upper and lower panels* show heart rate, integrated phrenic activity, intratracheal pressure, and carotid sinus blood pressure, recorded during periods of temporary cessation of artificial ventilation. The effects of chemoreceptor stimuli (intracarotid injections of CO_2–saline at markers) on heart rate are seen. When the vagi are intact (*upper panel*), chemoreceptor stimuli evoke bradycardia, except when delivered during period of inspiration (second of the stimuli shown) or while the lungs are expanding in response to a rise in intratracheal pressure (third stimulus). After denervation of the lungs (*lower panel*), the stimuli remain ineffective during periods of central inspiratory activity (second stimulus), but now evoke a large bradycardia when delivered while the lungs are expanding in response to a rise in intratracheal pressure. [Published with permission from Gandevia, McCloskey, and Potter (70).]

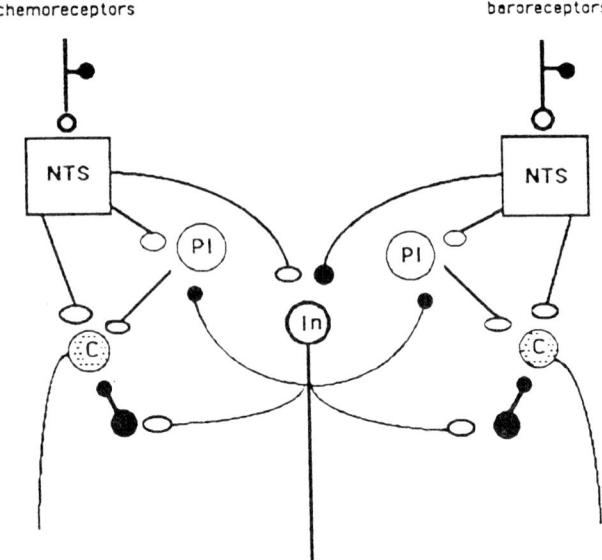

FIG. 5–11. Control of CVM activity: inspiratory and reflex inputs. Diagrammatic representation of the inputs to CVM (C) that determine their sensitivity to baroreceptor and chemoreceptor inputs. Inspiratory neurons (*In*) directly or via interneurons (e.g. *PI*, postinspiratory neurons) or inhibitory interneurons (shown in *black*) control of the excitability of CVM. Baroreceptor and chemoreceptor inputs are processed initially in the nucleus tractus solitarii (*NTS*) and send excitatory connections to CVM localized in the nucleus ambiguus, but these inputs act differentially on inspiratory neurons. *Open symbols:* excitatory: *filled symbols:* inhibitory.

ously low in the open-chest, artificially ventilated cat, and the need to elevate tone is thus not surprising. In contrast, in rats, lung inflation fails to produce cardiac effects while eliciting typical Breuer-Hering reflex changes in ventilation (152). Studies in primates, including humans, also indicate relatively weak influences of slowly adapting reflex receptors on heart rate (see ref. 151 for review).

Rapidly Adapting Pulmonary Inputs

It is widely accepted that activation of rapidly adapting pulmonary receptors, which often occurs during high-pressure lung inflation. For example, in dogs > 15 mm Hg can lead to bradycardia (5, 81). These receptors are again mediated by myelinated vagal afferents, but because of their sensitivity to a wide variety of modes of stimulation, Widdicombe (249) has termed them "irritant" receptors. They respond to mechanical stimulation (i.e. lung inflation, pneumothorax, atelectasis, pulmonary congestion, and also micro-emboli).

While their most notable reflex effects are bronchoconstriction and secretion, they exert considerable respiratory effects and usually provoke falls in heart rate involving vagal activation.

PULMONARY C-FIBERS

Work by Paintal (187–190) and the Coleridges (25, 26, 28, 29, 30) has shown conclusively that vagal C-fibers innervate receptors located in the pulmonary circulation. These receptors are powerfully excited by right atrial injections of phenyl biguanide, but they are affected naturally by either deflation or collapse of the lungs. From their position in the alveoli, they may also be sensitive to chemical irritants (for reviews, see refs. 27, 38). Evidence has been provided that these receptors are located in the juxtapulmonary capillaries, and they have been termed *J-receptors* (189, 190), suggesting that they play a role in terminating exercise. However, it is now clear that they are distributed widely through the lung (both pulmonary and bronchial distributions). Their activation invariably leads to a powerful and sustained bradycardia, usually with suppression of respiratory movements. The bradycardia is largely of vagal origin and appears to involve activation of CVMs with both B- and C-fiber axons. Notably in the rabbit, the cessation of ventilation provoked by their activation is in postinspiration, the phase when bCVMs are at their most excitable.

UPPER AIRWAY RECEPTORS

There is plentiful evidence that receptors in the upper airways—nasopharynx, larynx and trachea—act as defense mechanisms to prevent the aspiration of particulate matter or noxious chemicals into the lungs (249, 251). Activating these receptors produces a wide range of respiratory responses from apnea to cough, and accompanying these are marked cardiac effects. Influences that promote apnea invariably generate bradycardia, and stimulating the superior laryngeal nerve that innervates both mechano- and chemosensitive receptors in the larynx induces a powerful bradycardia. Essentially activating these receptors leads to parallel changes in ventilation and heart rate. The respiratory responses are often complex and long lasting, and phasic changes in heart rate are usually observed.

Several studies have used superior laryngeal nerve (SLN) stimulation as a means of enhancing cardiac vagal tone in order to assess the role of other inputs on cardiac control that would otherwise remain subliminal (see refs. 37, 41, 42, 147, 148, and others). Much of this can be attributed to the evoked inhibition of inspiratory activity or prolongation of post-inspiration (see above), but there may also be a major convergence of reflex inputs at an earlier stage in afferent processing, so that reflex facilitation may not merely reflect change in CVM excitability through respiration-related changes (see later).

CARDIAC RECEPTORS

There is literature showing that changes in heart rate accompany the activation of various receptors located within the chambers of the heart. While many of the effects are mediated by alteration in activity in vagal and sympathetic outflows (82, 140), there are also suggestions that some of the effects are mediated by short-loop reflexes that involve the modulation of ganglion cell activity (199, 200). This latter pathway would be expected to modulate the activity of conventional reflex pathways but may also imply more localized and distinctive patterns of control. Atrial receptors, located in the region of the venous drainage into the atria and diffusely distributed through the atrial wall, relay to the CNS through small myelinated fibers. There is a considerable literature indicating that their activation leads to a tachycardia, and that this is mediated by changes in sympathetic efferent activity alone (140). Stimulating myelinated afferent fibers in the vagal cardiac branches in the cat failed to evoke changes in bCVM activity (142). Conversely unmyelinated cardiac vagal afferents—with receptor endings widely dispersed through the ventricles but perhaps also in the atria—when stimulated, evoke a vagal bradycardia that may be intense, and this is elicited by a evoked excitation of bCVM (43, 142). Details of the role of different classes of cardiac receptor are available, but there is a general pattern of action conforming to this division between the effects of activating myelinated and unmyelinated afferents (see ref. 82 for review). Much less is known of the precise respiratory actions, if any, of these afferents.

CNS ORGANIZATION OF REFLEX CONTROL

The activity of CVMs depends on their intrinsic properties, which are as yet poorly described, and the interplay of excitatory and inhibitory synaptic control. Two major synaptic inputs have been defined that appear to provide the major extrinsic control of bCVM activity. These are the excitatory input from the arterial baroreceptors mediated via the NTS, and an inhibitory input that coincides with inspiration and involves synaptic processes restricted to the NA (Fig. 5–11). A second excitatory input may originate from post-inspiratory neurons, but this is not proven. In the case of cCVMs a single major excitatory input appears to maintain their discharge.

CNS PATHWAYS IMPINGING ON THE DORSAL VENTRAL NUCLEUS AND THE NUCLEUS AMBIGUUS

While there is an extensive literature describing the origin of afferent inputs to both the DVN and the NA, the specific inputs to cCVM and bCVM have not been resolved. As reviewed by Loewy and Spyer (146), numerous CNS regions send afferents to these two nuclei. Table 5–1 summarizes these data, but it is unlikely that this is in any way an exhaustive description. Electrical stimulation within all these sites elicits changes in heart rate—increases or decreases that are mediated in part through changes in vagal activity.

REFLEX INTERACTIONS: CNS ORGANIZATION

The full range of receptors outlined above, both cardiovascular and respiratory, relay to the NTS via the IXth and Xth cranial nerves. The specific pattern of projections of the branches of these two cranial nerves and of their individual afferents have been mapped extensively using both anatomical and physiological approaches (23, 24, 46, 119, 121, 218, 229, 232). The most detailed information has been derived by studying the individual projections of physiologically defined afferents using

TABLE 5–1. *Summary Description of CNS Regions Sending Afferents to the Dorsal Vagal Nucleus (DVN) and the Nucleus Ambiguus (NA)*

CNS Region	DVN	NA
Insular cortex	✓	✓
Central nucleus of amygdala	✓	✓
Bed nucleus of stria terminalis	✓	✓
Substantia innominata		✓
Lateral hypothalamic area		✓
Paraventricular nucleus	✓	✓
Dorsomedial hypothalamic area	✓	✓
Posterior hypothalamus	✓	✓
Mesenchephalic reticular form		✓
Parabrachial nucleus	✓	✓
A5 cell group		✓
Nucleus tractus solitarius	✓	✓
Medullary reticular formation	✓	✓
Raphe obscurus (and others)	✓	✓

For ref. see 146.

antidromic mapping techniques (reviewed in ref. 119). From these studies, it is clear that individual classes of afferent have distinctive patterns of innervation of the NTS, but that each subnucleus of the NTS receives convergent input from several different classes of afferent. Accordingly each NTS neuron may receive convergent inputs from several sources.

The details of projection of myelinated and unmyelinated baroreceptor afferents (in cat, rabbit), arterial chemoreceptors, pulmonary stretch, and rapidly adapting pulmonary afferents, have all been defined in this way (47, 54–56). However, these are not recapitulated in this review; rather, attempts are made to identify principles of organization that may have important implications for cardiac control. (For the details of the afferent innervation of the NTS, see refs. 46, 119, 230, 231.)

SYNAPTIC EFFECTS ELICITED BY BARORECEPTOR INPUTS IN THE NUCLEUS TRACTUS SOLITARII

Neurons in the NTS have been identified functionally on the basis of electrical stimulation of the SN together with some form of natural stimulation of the arterial baroreceptors (34, 96, 141, 177–179, 223, 236). In general low-intensity electrical stimulation of the SN (or the aortic nerve; AN) has been used to minimize problems associated with current spread, and a general consensus has been achieved that SN evoked monosynaptic actions are restricted to the NTS. In more recent studies (166–170, 225–228, 232) intracellular recordings were taken from NTS and the postsynaptic events were analyzed in some detail (Fig. 5–12). It is clear that the NTS has a complex intranuclear organisation, and neurons whose cell bodies are localized within many of its subnuclei, and even beyond in the neighboring reticular formation, receive either monosynaptic or polysynaptic inputs on SN stimulation, or both (232). There is a belief from limited intracellular labeling studies that the region overlying the tractus solitarius—the dorsal cap—has a particularly high density of monosynaptically activated neurons (223, 232), but the SN input is distributed more widely through the nucleus. Further, many "baroreceptor" sensitive neurons with excitatory inputs from the carotid sinus baroreceptors also receive convergent excitatory input from AN and from other afferent inputs (Fig. 5–12 B–E; see later).

The complex organization of the NTS is exemplified further by the fact that the NTS also contains neurons inhibited on baroreceptor stimulation, many of which are excited by arterial chemoreceptor inputs (see later under Synaptic Effects of Arterial Chemoreceptor Inputs). Sinus nerve evoked responses often consist of waves of epsps and ipsps. This is an indication of a clear integrative function of these particular neurons.

In addition to convergence between inhibitory baroreceptor and excitatory chemoreceptor effects, and the excitatory convergence of SN, AN, and baroreceptor inputs, further examples of convergence have recently emerged (Fig. 5–13).

As an example, the reflex effects of activating the SLN often mimic the arterial baroreceptor reflex in that hypotension, bradycardia and an arrest of ventilation in the post-inspiratory state are evoked (50). Stimulation of mechanoreceptor endings in the larynx (by balloon inflation or gentle touching) also evokes this triad of responses. Many NTS neurons shown to be affected by SN and baroreceptor inputs were also shown to receive convergent inputs from the SLN (Fig. 5–12 B, C), and to be affected by mechanical activation of laryngeal receptor endings (50, 168). This would suggest that NTS neurons may be coded not for a specific reflex input—although some show exclusive influences from one class of peripheral receptor—but rather for a pattern of cardiovascular (and respiratory) effect (226, 227, 232). For example baroreceptor-sensitive neurons, which have laryngeal mechanoreceptor inputs (and other inputs perhaps), appear to have properties that are compatible with their affecting sympathetic, vagal, and respiratory outflows in a stereotypic manner. This patterning becomes more relevant when other central inputs that affect these neurons are considered. The pattern of response to multiple inputs many provide a means of classifying the roles of individual NTS neurons (see Fig. 5–13). These observations have enhanced the significance of the baroreceptor input as the primary physiologically relevant excitatory input to b-CVMs (see Fig. 5–11), since its effectiveness is clearly modulated by other afferent inputs.

SYNAPTIC EFFECTS OF ARTERIAL CHEMORECEPTOR INPUTS

Arterial chemoreceptor afferents project to distinct regions of the NTS. Aside from influencing indirectly the activity of the respiratory neurons of the ventrolateral subnucleus (143) many neurons *without* a central respiratory firing pattern are excited by chemoreceptor stimulation (166, 167, 225, 227, 234).

A significant proportion of these neurons are concentrated in the commissural and medial NTS at the level of the obex and caudal to it in the cat. These do not appear to receive excitatory input from the arterial baroreceptors (166, 167, 223, 227, 234), although some are inhibited by baroreceptor stimulation (see above). In extracellular recording studies it has been reported that some neurons in the vicinity of the NTS may receive convergent excitatory input from the arterial chemoreceptors and baroreceptors (144). This

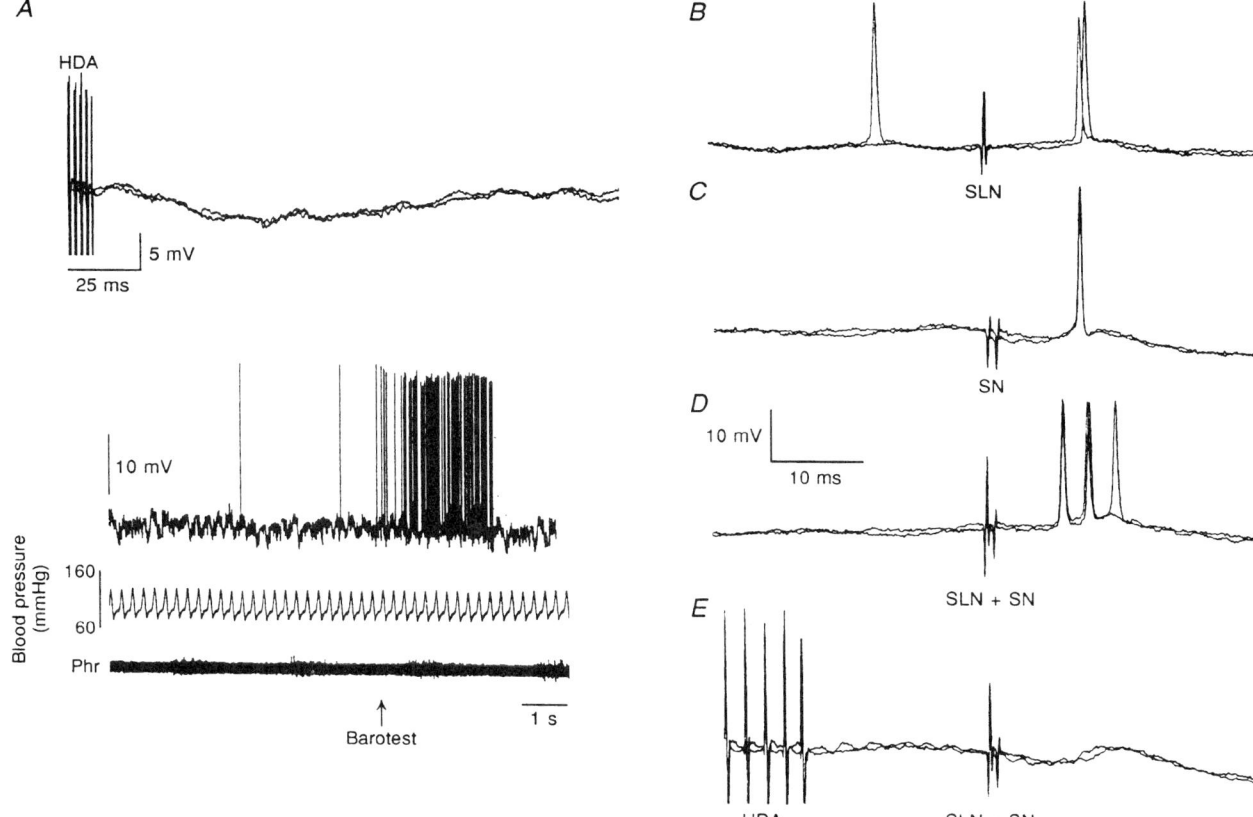

FIG. 5–12. Additional evidence for HDA inhibitory actions on SLN-evoked responses. Intracellular recording of a cell within the NTS (membrane potential, −62 mV). A: this neuron responded to stimulation of the HDA (5 pulses, 500 Hz, 0.1 mA, given at 1 Hz) with an ipsp (*upper traces*). The unit was baroreceptive, as shown in the *lower left panel,* since inflation of the ipsilateral carotid sinus (Barotest) evoked a burst of action potentials. B, SLN stimulation (1 pulse, 0.1 ms, 7 V at 1 Hz) evoked an excitatory response. C: epsp and action potentials evoked on stimulation of the SN (2 pulses, 0.1 ms, 1 kHz, 9V at 1 Hz). D: simultaneous stimulation of both nerves (Sn + SLN) evoked an enhanced response. The latency was shortened and a third spike was evoked in 80% of the stimulations. Stimulating parameters as in B and C. E: conditioning stimulus to the hypothalamus (HDA) suppressed the combined effects of SLN + SN stimulation (compare with D). Neuronal recordings in A (upper traces) B, C, D, and E are shown as 2 superimposed traces. [Reproduced with permission from Dawid-Milner et al. (50).]

has not been confirmed in recent intracellular recording studies on NTS neurons, making it likely that these are located in the vicinity of the NTS (66, 226). Several NTS neurons with excitatory inputs from the arterial chemoreceptors have been shown to receive convergent excitatory inputs on SLN stimulation, but indications have been obtained that the input results from the activation of chemosensitive laryngeal afferents (50). Recent studies in both the cat (in vivo, 228) and the mouse (in situ, 192) suggest a convergence onto NTS neurons of chemosensory inputs. It appears that pulmonary C-fiber inputs, ventricular chemosensory inputs relaying through the vagus, and arterial chemoreceptor inputs converge on NTS neurons. These appear to be largely unaffected by baroreceptor input.

The actions of the arterial chemoreceptors on heart rate mediated by bCVMs, appear to be the result of activating a relatively direct neural pathway originating in the NTS (see Fig. 5–11). This pathway would be expected to be accessed by other afferent inputs. Whether there is convergence of the "baroreceptor" and "chemoreceptor" pathways onto a single class of interneuron prior to a final synapse on the bCVM remains to be elucidated, but its location does not appear to be within the NTS.

CENTRAL MODIFICATIONS OF REFLEX FUNCTION

Interactions between reflex inputs in the control of heart rate have been illustrated over many years. At least a portion of these facilitatory or inhibitory interactions can be explained on the basis of interactions within the NTS (see above and refs. 169, 170, 226, 227, 232). The potential for the modification of reflex function as a consequence of activating regions of the

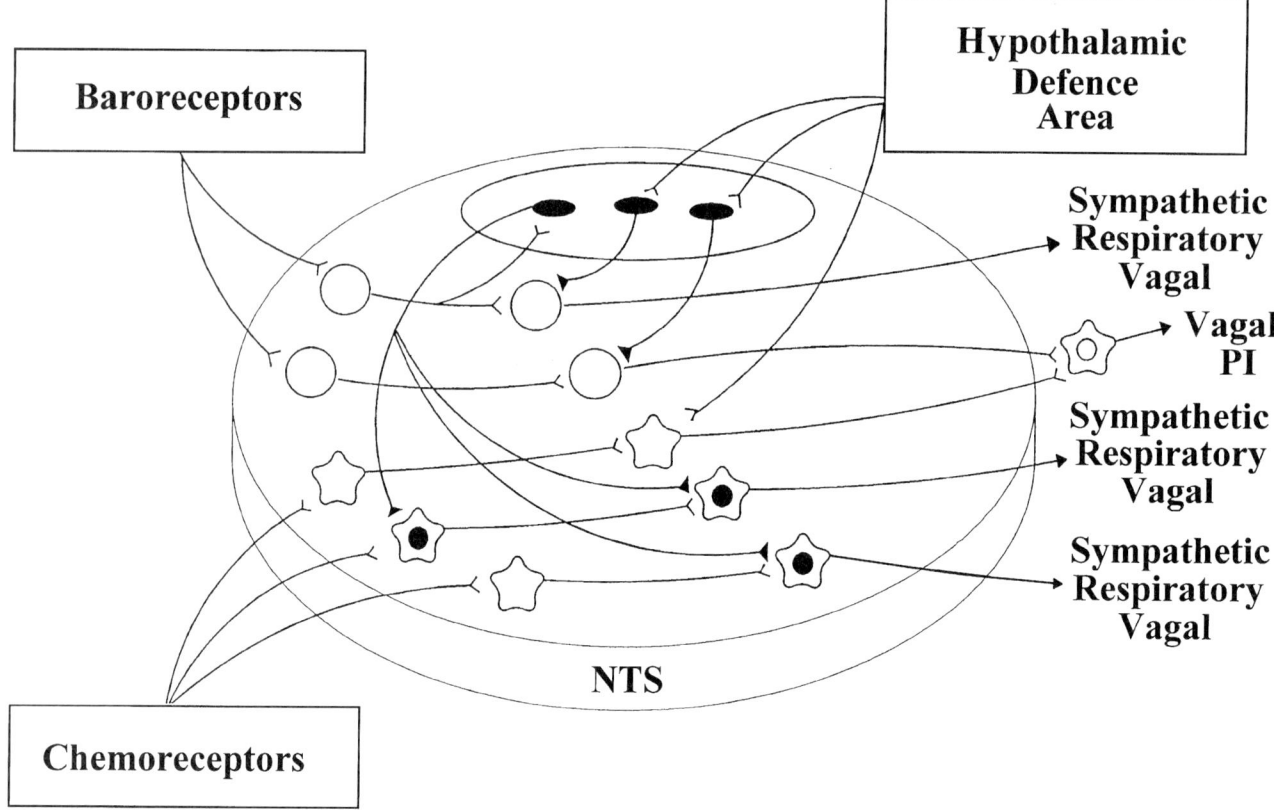

FIG. 5-13. Schematic diagram of the connections within the nucleus tractus solitarii (NTS) that mediate arterial chemoreceptor inputs and interaction with the arterial baroreceptors. Inputs to NTS from baroreceptors, chemoreceptors and HDA are shown. Exclusively baroreceptor-sensitive neurons are shown as ○; chemoreceptors are ☆. Excitatory inputs are shown as ∧ and inhibitory as ▲. Neurons receiving convergent baroreceptor and chemoreceptor inputs are shown as combined symbols: when baroreceptor influence is excitatory, when inhibitory. [Reproduced with permission from Silva-Carvalho et al. (227).]

CNS, or in naturally evoked behaviors has also been illustrated. With regard to CVM activity, this could be achieved merely by altering the level of excitability of CVMs as a consequence of changing the level of activity in the numerous pathways that impinge on NA and DVN (see Table 5-1). Indeed, the literature abounds with information on changes in heart rate in response to stimulation within the CNS, and also accompanying changes in behavioral state.

There is a consensus that reflex function is modulated during CNS stimulation, and certain experimental paradigms have been used to demonstrate this effectively. Perhaps the most significant example is the interaction between activating those areas of the brain stem concerned with affective behaviour and the baroreceptor reflex (Fig. 5-12 A, B). In the 1960s Hilton and colleagues (1, 88-90, 94) built on the work of Hess and Brugger (87) to identify regions of the hypothalamus and amygdala that were involved in the integration of the visceral and somatic components of the defense reaction. It was shown that activating the perifornical region of the hypothalamus, the central nucleus of the amygdala (CEN), and subsequently the periaqueductal gray, could effectively suppress the cardiovascular components of the baroreceptor reflex (32, 88, 93). There were conflicting attitudes regarding the magnitude and mechanisms underlying this interaction, with many studies indicating the particular susceptibility of the cardiac component of the reflex to central suppression (64, 67, 68, 73, 74, 97, amongst others), with the sympathetic arm remaining partially unaffected. Subsequently it was shown that stimulation in the hypothalamic defense area elicited a facilitation of the arterial chemoreceptor reflex (91, 92, 150, 225, 226).

The particular sensitivity of the cardiac component of reflexes appears to reflect the powerful respiratory modulation of bCVM activity (see above and Figs. 5-4E and 5-8, through 5-11), because stimulation at sites in the CNS that elicit cardiovascular changes invariably produce respiratory changes consistent with the observed changes in heart rate (see ref. 204 for discussion).

With regard to hypothalamically evoked cardiac effects, it has been shown that a GABA-mediated inhibitory control of bCVM activity can be evoked that is independent of respiratory control (73, 74). This appears to offer a powerful hypothalamic mode of control of bCVM activity. There are indications, however, that the NTS is a primary target of outputs from numerous CNS sites that are concerned with cardiovascular control, including the hypothalamus (see refs. 145, 146).

THE ROLE OF THE NUCLEUS TRACTUS SOLITARII IN REFLEX ADJUSTMENTS

McAllen (158) indicated that stimulation in the hypothalamus could provoke long-lasting inhibitory effects on those NTS neurons that received excitatory input from the arterial baroreceptors. The synaptic mechanism underlying the response was only resolved in the 1980s when in an intracellular recording study (170) it was demonstrated that NTS neurons receiving excitatory synaptic inputs from SN and the arterial baroreceptors were invariably inhibited on hypothalamic defense area (HDA) stimulation through a Cl^- mediated ipsp of long duration (170). This was subsequently shown to be mediated by GABA acting on $GABA_A$ receptors on those NTS neurons (116). Evidence has since been accumulated that the effect is the result of the activation of a pool of GABA-containing neurons localized within the NTS (50, 105, 226, 227). Furthermore many of the NTS neurons receiving baroreceptor input also were shown to receive SLN inputs (mechanosensitive) and the SLN evoked effects on heart rate, blood pressure, and respiration are also "blocked" by long trains of stimuli delivered to the HDA (50). Other studies have indicated that stimulation in the pontine parabrachial nucleus (65) and the uvula cortex of the posterior cerebellar vermis (193, 194) can exert similar influences on baroreceptor reflex function, mediated at least in part by the NTS, and presumably involving the same pool of intrinsic NTS GABA-containing neurons.

This synaptic process would lead to a reduced excitatory drive to the bCVM of the NA, but if this neural circuit is tonically active, a reduction in its level of activity would facilitate bCVM activity. Accordingly, bCVM activity will be highly sensitive to the interactions between reflex inputs and central drives. This would also provide an explanation for the state-dependent changes in heart rate that reflect the changing levels of arousal in the individual. This process is further enhanced by the demonstration that in other forms of affective behavior such as the "playing-dead" response, the NTS neurons receiving baroreceptor input are excited, perhaps as a consequence of disinhibition resulting from a reduced drive from the HDA, but perhaps also as a result of a direct excitatory input (see refs. 226, 227, 232; Fig. 13). In the rabbit stimulation in both hypothalamus and CEN evokes bradycardia and hypotension (8, 33, 62, 191), and here NTS "baroreceptor" sensitive neurons are activated. Equally in the cat, which under certain circumstances shows primarily a visceral alerting response to a threatening stimulus, the playing-dead response can be evoked (see 33, 114), and stimulation in the HDA can elicit an excitatory response in NTS neurons that were otherwise inhibited if $GABA_A$ receptors were pharmacologically blocked using bicuculline (116). In more recent studies, even in the absence of bicuculline, similar facilitatory interactions have been observed (227), suggesting that two distinct pathways emanating from the hypothalamus mediate the two extreme patterns of behavior, and that these are likely to be co-activated on electrical stimulation (232). This has major physiological importance, because it implies an essential integrative role of the NTS in cardiac control. Crude experimental paradigms may indicate reflex suppression or some degree of facilitation, but physiologically the output of the NTS will depend on the interplay of numerous inputs that will be highly state-dependent and hence nonlinear. Hilton's original observation of an abrogation of the baroreceptor reflex on HDA stimulation (90), and the more restricted observations of many laboratories that indicated merely a particular sensitivity of the cardiac arm of the reflex (see above) may be explained by both the complexity of integration within the NTS and the variability of the stimulus parameters between laboratories. This will be further complicated by the multiple sites of interaction in the reflex pathway. Any minor difference in experimental procedure will result in major differences in the degree of interaction. This is further illustrated by considering the cardiovascular changes that occur during exercise. These appear to be the result of interactions between central programing and reflex inputs.

The neural substrate underlying the central program for exercise is still a matter for conjecture, but subthalamic and hypothalamic structures have been implicated (61, 152, 174, 175, 248). The rise in heart rate, and cardiac output that is a characteristic of the exercise response includes a reduction in cardiac vagal activity. There have been both speculation and experimental studies in humans and other vertebrates indicating that modulation of baroreceptor reflex function might underlie these changes (9, 31, 163). While no consensus is available, evidence would seem to indicate a change in either gain or set-point of the reflex (57). Afferent inputs arising from exercising muscles and joints contribute significantly to the patterning of the cardiovascular, and respiratory, changes in exercise (126, 127, 129, 174). Stimulating muscle afferents (group III and IV) has been shown to modify baroreceptor reflex transmission in the NTS by an action involving a GABA synapse (163). It is thus plausible that, in exercise, use is made of the same general synaptic mechanism to adjust reflex performance as in affective behavior. This may have further implications, because emotional factors are known to influence the preparatory responses at the initiation of exercise, and this would provide a continuum of action through a single synaptic mechanism.

RESPIRATORY INFLUENCES OF REFLEX TRANSMISSION THROUGH THE NUCLEUS TRACTUS SOLITARIUS

In affective behavior and exercise, cardiovascular changes are paralleled by changes in respiration (27, 114, 232). The importance of reflex modulation as a basis for the patterning of cardiorespiratory activity in complex behaviors—such as in exercise and affective responses—has led to the awareness of a pivotal role of the NTS. Since the NTS is a site of interaction between reflex inputs and is implicated in both cardiovascular and respiratory control processes, it might be expected that much of the influence exerted by respiration on cardiovascular, and specifically CVM activity, might be the consequence of synaptic actions in the NTS. Even as long ago as the 1960s, Koepchen and colleagues (130, 131) postulated that the respiratory fluctuations in heart rate were an expression of a respiratory modulation of reflex inputs that affect CVM discharge. From our earlier discussions, it is clear that this would involve specifically the arterial baroreceptor and chemoreceptor reflexes (see above). The emphasis on these reflexes must, however, be revised in part in view of the complex reflex interactions within the NTS (50, 226, 227, 232). Current research would not, however, support a role for the NTS in the control of efficacy of either arterial baroreceptor and chemoreceptor reflexes in relation to respiratory state (166, 169, 234).

From intracellular recordings in anaesthetized, paralyzed, and artificially ventilated cats, NTS neurons with either baroreceptor (169) or chemoreceptor (166, 234) inputs have been identified, and the influence of lung inflation and central respiratory activity on the magnitude of synaptically evoked responses has been assessed. Neither respiratory input was effective in modifying synaptic events, although exhaustive investigations into lung inflation–mediated effects have not been conducted, as observations have been concentrated on inflation volumes below maximal levels. The literature abounds with evidence of presynaptic regulation of afferent inputs including actions on vagal afferents that terminate within the NTS (206–209, among others). There is, however, compelling evidence that this does not occur in the case of SN afferents (117, 118), and any significant influences of respiratory inputs acting presynaptically would be discerned as changes in evoked epsp or ipsp magnitude. These have not been observed.

Accordingly, these data imply that while the NTS is a site of major reflex modification—both up regulation and downregulation—through the pre- and postsynaptic actions of GABA, released by intrinsic GABA-containing neurons, respiratory influences on CVM control are not mediated through this synaptic process (see Fig. 5–13). Respiratory control is exerted specifically and directly by synaptic actions within the NA that involve mechanisms resulting in an inspiratory inhibition of CVM activity (see Fig. 5–11).

CONCLUSIONS

As yet little is known of the specific cellular properties of bCVM and cCVM, although both exert profound influences on the heart. Certain assumptions have been drawn from the extensive literature concerning DVN, and it is clear that the interplay of intrinsic membrane properties and synaptically evoked responses is of paramount importance in determining ongoing heart rate, and presumably other indices of cardiac function as well. The individual CVM is a site of integration—in the case of bCVM, a target for two principal inputs—an inhibitory input correlated with central inspiratory activity, and an excitatory input originating from the NTS whose magnitude is determined largely, but not exclusively, as a consequence of arterial baroreceptor discharge. Several other inputs, excitatory and inhibitory, have been identified, and at any moment the prevailing heart rate is a consequence of these synaptic interactions at the level of the bCVM and at the NTS whose output is a major determinant of synaptic drive to bCVM. CNS processes that involve alterations in cardiorespiratory activity exert their influences on heart rate in part through either direct synaptic influences on bCVM or by modulating respiratory activity or alternatively by modulating reflex transmission at the level of the NTS. These synaptic actions allow for an exquisite modulation of CVM discharge that can regulate heart rate on a beat-by-beat basis and correlate heart rate, and hence cardiac output, with respiratory minute volume.

The role of cCVMs remains as yet unresolved. They clearly can affect heart rate and may be of importance in emergency or protective mechanisms. Their physiological interactions with bCVM at the level of the cardiac ganglia remain to be identified. The appreciation of the pharmacology of CVM control is as yet rudimentary, and the relevance of this as a means of exerting or modifying cardiovascular control in humans has barely been examined. The prospect of modulating CVM activity as a therapy in cardiovascular disease other than by blocking its effects on the heart with atropine remains to be investigated.

REFERENCES

1. Abrahams, V. C., S. M., Hilton and A. Zbrozyna. Active muscle vasodilatation produced by stimulation of the brainstem: its significance in the defence reaction. *J. Physiol. (Lond.)* 154:491–513, 1960.
2. Accornero, N., G., Bini, G. L Lenzi and M. Manfredi. Selective activation of peripheral nerve fibre groups of different diameter by triangular shaped stimulus pulses. *J. Physiol. (Lond.)* 273: 539–560. 1977.
3. Al-Ali, M., A. S., Forkins, J. N., Townend and J. H. Cottoe. Respiratory sinus arrhythmia and central respiratory drive in humans. *Clin. Sci.* 90: 235–241, 1996.
4. Allen, T. G. J. and G. Burnstock. M_1 and M_2 muscarinic receptors mediate excitation and inhibition of guinea-pig intracardiac neurones in culture. *J. Physiol. (Lond.)* 422:463–480, 1990.
5. Angell-James, J. E. and M. de B. Daly. The effects of artificial lung inflation on reflexly induced bradycardia associated with apnoea in the dog. *J. Physiol. (Lond.)* 274:349–366, 1978.
6. Anrep, G. V., W. Pascual, and R. Rössler. Respiratory variations of heart rate. I. The reflex mechanism of the respiratory arrhythmia. *Proc. R. Soc. Lond. B* 119:191–217, 1936.
7. Anrep, G. V., W. Pascual, and R. Rössler. Respiratory variations of the hart rate. II. The central mechanism of respiratory arrhythmia and the inter-relationships between central and reflex mechanisms. *Proc. R. Soc. Lond. B* 119:218–230, 1936.
8. Applegate, C. D., B. S. Kapp, M. D. Underwood, and C. L. McNaoll. Autonomic and somomotor effects of amygdala central nucleus stimulation in awake rabbits. *Physiol. Behav.* 31: 353–360, 1983.
9. Barron, W. and J. H. Coote. The contribution of articular receptors to cardiovascular reflexes elicited by passive limb movement. *J. Physiol. (Lond.)* 235:423–436, 1973.
10. Bennett, J. A., C. Kidd, A. B. Latif, and P. M. McWilliam. A horseradish peroxidase study of vagal motoneurones with axons in cardiac and pulmonary branches of the cat and dog. *Q. J. Exp. Physiol.* 66:145–154, 1981.
11. Bieger, D., and D. A. Hopkins. Viscerotopic representation of the upper alimentary tract in the medulla oblongata in the rat: the nucleus ambiguus. *J. Comp. Neurol.* 252:546–562, 1987.
12. Billman, G. E., R. S. Hoskins, D. C. Randall, W. C. Randall, R. L. Hamlin, and Y. C. Lin. Selective vagal postganglionic innervation of the sinoatrial and atrioventricular nodes in the nonhuman primate. *J. Auton. Nerve. Syst.* 26:27–36, 1989.
13. Black, A. M. S. and R. W. Torrance. Chemoreceptor effects in the respiratory cycle. *J. Physiol. (Lond.)* 189:59–61, 1967.
14. Black, A. M. S. and R. W. Torrance. Respiratory oscillations in chemoreceptor discharge in the control of breathing. *Respir. Physiol.* 13:221–237, 1971.
15. Blinder, K. J., L. W. Dickerson, A. L., Gray, J. M. Lauenstein, J. T., Newgsome, M. Bingaman, P. J. Tti, R. A. Gillis, and V. J. Massari. Control of negative inotropic vagal preganglionic neurons in the dog: synaptic interactions with substance P afferent terminals in the nucleus ambiguus? *Brain Res.* 810: 251–256, 1998.
16. Blinder, K. J., P. J. Gatti, T. A. Johnson, J. M. Lauenstein, W. P. Coleman, A. L. Gray, and V. J. Massari. Untrastructural circuitry of cardiorespiratory reflexes; there is a monosynaptic path between the nucleus of the solitary tract and vagal preganglionic motoneurons controlling atrioventricular conduction in the cat. *Brain Res.* 785:143–57, 1998.
17. Brooks, P. A., P. M. Izzo, and K. M. Spyer. Brainstem GABA pathways and the regulation of baroreflex activity. In: *Central Neural Mechanisms in Cardiovascular Regulation*, Vol. 2, edited by G. Kunos, and J. Cirello, Boston: Birkhauser, 1992: 321–337.
18. Brown, G. L. and J. C. Eccles. The action of a single vagal volley on the rhythm of the heart beat. *J. Physiol. (Lond.)* 81:211–240, 1934.
19. Brown, G. L. and J. C. Eccles. Further experiments on vagal inhibition of the heart beat. *J. Physiol. (Lond.)* 81:241–257, 1934.
20. Bunzl-Federn, E. Der centrale ursprung des nervous vagus. *Psychiatr. Neurol.* 5:1–22, 1899.
21. Calaresu, F. R. and M. K. Cottle. Origin of cardiomotor fibres in the dorsal nucleus of the vagus in the cat: a histological study. *J. Physiol. (Lond.)* 176:252–260, 1965.
22. Casadei, B., J. Mood, and A. Caiazza. Respiratory sinus arrhythmia does not reflect cardiac vagal tone during exercise. *J. Physiol. (Lond.)* 473:66, 1993.
23. Ciriello, J. and F. R. Calaresu. Medullary origin of vagal preganglionic axons to the heart of the cat. *J. Auton. Nerv. Syst.* 5: 9–22, 1982.
24. Ciriello, J. and F. R. Calaresu. Distribution of vagal cardioinhibitory neurons in the medulla of the cat. *Am. J. Physiol.* 238 (*Renal Fluid Electrolyte Physiol.* 7): R57–R64. 1980.
25. Coleridge, H. M. and J. C. G. Coleridge. Impulse activity in afferent vagal C-fibres with endings in the intrapulmonary airways of dogs. *Respir. Physiol.* 29:125–142. 1977.
26. Coleridge, H. M. and J. C. G. Coleridge. Integration of ventilatory and cardiovascular control systems. In: *The Lung; Scientific Foundations*. 2nd Ed. edited by R. G. Crystal, J. B. West, et al., Philadelphia: Raven Press, pp. 1405–1418, 1996.
27. Coleridge, H. M., J. C. G. Coleridge, and D. Jordan. Integration of ventilatory and cardiovascular control systems. In: *The Lung: Scientific Foundations*, 2nd Ed., edited by R. G. Crystal, J. B. West, et al. Philadelphia: Lippincott-Raven, 1991:13601–13611.
28. Coleridge, H. M., J. C. G. Coleridge, and A. M. Roberts. Rapid shallow breathing evoked by selective stimulation of airway C-fibres in dogs. *J. Physiol. (Lond.)* 340:415–433, 1983.
29. Coleridge, J. C. G. and H. M. Coleridge. Chemoreflex regulation of the heart. In *Handbook of Physiology, Section 2, The Cardiovascular system, Vol 1: The Heart*, edited by R. M. Berne. Bethesda, MD: Am. Physiol. Soc. 1979: 653–676.
30. Coleridge, J. C. and H. M. Coleridge. Afferent vagal C Fibre innervation of the lungs and airways and its functional significance. *Rev. Physiol. Biochem. Pharmacol.* 99:1–110, 1984.
31. Coote, J. H. Cardiovascular responses to exercise: central and reflex contribution. In: *Cardiovascular Regulation*, edited by D. Jordan, and J. Marshall. London: Portland Press, 1995: 93–111.
32. Coote, J. H., S. M. Hilton, J. F. Perez-Gonzalez. Inhibition of the baroreceptor reflex on stimulation in the brainstem defence centre. *J. Physiol. (Lond.)* 288:549–560, 1979.
33. Cox, G. E., D. Jordan, P. Moruzzi, J. S. Schwaber, K. M. Spyer, and S. A. Turner. Amygdaloid influences on brainstem neurones in the rabbit. *J. Physiol. (Lond.)* 381:135–148., 1985.
34. Crill, W. E., and D. J. Reis. Distribution of carotid sinus and depressor nerves in the cat brain stem. *Am. J. Physiol.* 214:269–276, 1975.
35. Czachurski, J., K., Remborsky, H. Seller, R. Nobling, and R. Tangner. Morphology of electrophysiologically identified baroreceptor afferents and second order neurons in the brainstem of the cat. *Arch. Ital. Biol.* 126:129–144, 1988.
36. Daly, M. de B. Interactions between respiration and circulation. In *Handbook of Physiology*, Section 3, *The Respiratory System*,

Vol. II: *Control of Breathing*, part 2, edited by N. S. Cherniack, and J. G. Widdicombe. Bethesda MD: American Physiological Society, 1986: 529–594.

37. Daly, M. de B. Some reflex cardioinhibitory responses in the cat and their modulation by central inspiratory neuronal activity. *J. Physiol. (Lond.)* 439:559–577, 1991.

38. Daly, M. de B. Peripheral arterial chemoreceptors and respiratory-cardiovascular integration. *Monogr. Physiol. Soc.* (1997)

39. Daly, M. de B. and J. L. Hazzledine. The effects of artificially induced hyperventilation on the primary cardiac reflex response to stimulation of the carotid bodies in the dog. *J. Physiol.* 168: 872–889, 1963.

40. Daly, M. de B., J. L. Hazzledine, and A. Ungar. The reflex effects of alterations in lung volume on systemic vascular resistance in the dog. *J. Physiol.* 188:331–351, 1967.

41. Daly, M. de B. and E. Kirkman. Cardiovascular responses to stimulation of pulmonary C fibres in the cat: their modulation by changes in respiration. *J. Physiol. (Lond.)* 402:43–63, 1988.

42. Daly, M. de B. and E. Kirkman. Differential modulation by pulmonary stretch afferents of some reflex cardioinhibitory responses in the cat. *J. Physiol. (Lond.)* 417:323–341, 1989.

43. Daly, M. de B., E. Kirkman, and L. M. Wood. Cardiovascular responses to stimulation of cardiac receptors in the cat and their modification by changes in respiration. *J. Physiol. (Lond.)* 407: 349–362, 1988.

44. Daly, M. de B., A. S. Litherland, and L. M. Wood. The modification of the respiratory, cardiac and vascular responses to stimulation of the carotid body chemoreceptors by a laryngeal input in the cat. *IRCS Med. Sci.* 11:861–862, 1983.

45. Daly, M. de B. and M. J. Scott. The effect of stimulation of the carotid body chemoreceptors on the heart rate in the dog. *J. Physiol.* 141:32–33, 1958.

46. Dampney, R. A. L. Functional organization of central pathways regulating the cardiovascular system. *Physiol. Rev.* 74:323–364, 1994.

47. Davies, R. O. and L. Kubin. Projection of pulmonary rapidly adapting receptors to the medulla of the cat: an antidromic mapping study. *J. Physiol. (Lond.)* 373:63–86, 1986.

48. Davidson, N. S., S. Goldner, and D. I. McCloskey. Respiratory modulation of baroreceptor and chemoreceptor reflexes affecting heart-rate and cardiac vagal efferent nerve activity. *J. Physiol. (Lond.)* 259:523–530, 1976.

49. Davis, A. L., D. I. McCloskey, and E. K. Potter. Respiratory modulation of baroreceptor and chemoreceptor reflexes affecting heart rate through the sympathetic nervous system. *J. Physiol. (Lond.)* 272:691–703, 1977.

50. Dawid-Milner, M. S., L. Silva-Carvalho, G. E. Goldsmith, and K. M. Spyer. Hypothalamic modulation of laryngeal reflexes in the anaesthetized cat: role of the nucleus tractus solitarii. *J. Physiol. (Lond.)* 487:739–749, 1995.

51. Deuchars, J. and P. M. Izzo. Demonstration of a monosynaptic pathway from the nucleus tractus solitarius to regions of ventrolateral medulla with specific reference to vagal motoneurones in the nucleus ambiguus of the anaesthetized cat: a neurophysiological study. *J. Physiol. (Lond.)* 438:80, 1991.

52. Dickerson, L. W., D. J. Rodak, T. J. Fleming, P. J. Gatti, V. J. Massari, J. D. McKenzie, and R. A. Gillis. Parasympathetic neurons in the cranial medial ventricular fat pad on the dog heart selectively decrease ventricular contractility. *J Auton. Nerv. Syst.* 70 (1–2); 129–41, 1998,

53. Donders, F. C. Zur physiologie des nervus vagus. *Pflugers Arch.* 1:334–361, 1868.

54. Donoghue, S., R. B. Felder, D. Jordan, and K. M. Spyer. The central projections of carotid baroreceptors and chemoreceptors in the cat: a neurophysiological study. *J. Physiol. (Lond.)* 347: 397–410, 1984.

55. Donoghue S., M. Garcia, D., Jordan, and K. M. Spyer. Identification and brain-stem projections of aortic baroreceptor afferent neurons in nodose ganglia of cats and rabbits. *J. Physiol. (Lond.)* 322:337–352, 1982.

56. Donoghue S., M. Garcia, D. Jordan, and K. M. Spyer. The brainstem projections of pulmonary stretch afferent neurones in cats and rabbits. *J. Physiol. (Lond.)* 322:353–363, 1982.

57. Eckberg, D. L. and P. Sleight. *Human Baroreflex in Health and Disease*. *Monogr. Physiol Soc. Lond.*, 1992.

58. Eldridge, F. L. The importance of timing on the respiratory effects of intermittent carotid sinus nerve stimulation. *J. Physiol. (Lond.)* 222:297–318, 1972.

59. Eldridge, F. L. The importance of timing on the respiratory effects of intermittent carotid body chemoreceptor stimulation. *J. Physiol. (Lond.)* 222:319–333, 1972.

60. Eldridge, F. L., P Gill-Kumar, and D. E. Millhorn. Input-output relationship of central neural circuits involved in respiration in cats. *J. Physiol. (Lond.)* 311:82–95, 1981,

61. Eldridge, F. L., D. E. Millhorn, J. P. Kiley, and T. G. Waldrop. Stimulation by central command of locomotion, respiration and circulation during exercise. *Respir. Physiol.* 59:313–337, 1985.

62. Evans, M. H. Facilitation of reflex bradycardia by hypothalamic stimulation in the anaesthetized rabbit. *J. Physiol. (Lond.)* 265: 33–34, 1977.

63. Farmer, M. R., J. C. Vaile, F. Osman, H. F. Ross J. N. Townend, and J. H. Coote. A central gamma-aminobutyric acid mechanism in cardiac vagal control in man revealed by studies with intravenous midazolam. *Clin. Sci.* 95(3); 241–8, 1998.

64. Feigl, E., Johansson, B. & Löfving, B. Renal vasoconstriction and the 'defence reaction'. *Physiol. Scand.* 62:425–435, 1964.

65. Felder, R. B., and S. W. Mifflin. Modulation of carotid sinus afferent input to nucleus tractus solitarius by parabrachial nucleus stimulation. *Circ. Res.* 63:35–43, 1988.

66. Felder, R. B. and S. W. Mifflin. Baroreceptor and chemoreceptor afferent processing. In *The Solitary Tract Nucleus*, edited by I. R. A. Barracco. London: CRC Press, 1994: 169–186.

67. Folkow, B., B. Lisander, R. S. Tuttle, and S. C. Wang. Changes in cardiac output upon stimulation of the hypothalamic defence area and the medullary depressor area in the cat. *Acta Physiol. Scand.* 72:220–233, 1968.

68. Folkow, B., B. Öberg, and E. H. Rubinstein. A proposed differentiated neuro-effector organisation in muscle resistance vessels. *Angiologica* 1:197–208, 1964.

69. Ford, T. W. and P. N. McWilliam. The effects of electrical stimulation of myelinated and non-myelinated vagal fibres on heart rate in the rabbit. *J. Physiol. (Lond.)* 380:341–347. 1986.

70. Gandevia, S. C., D. I. McCloskey, and E. K. Potter. Inhibition of baroreceptor and chemoreceptor reflexes on heart rate by afferents from the lungs. *J. Physiol. (Lond.)* 276:369–381, 1978.

71. Gatti, P. J., T. A. Johnson, V. J. Massari. Can neurons in the nucleus ambiguus selectively regulate cardiac rate and atrioventricular conduction? *J. Auton. Nerv. Syst.* 57:123–127, 1996.

72. Gatti, P. J., T. A. Johnson, J. McKenzie, J. M. Lauenstein, A. Gray, and V. J. Massari. Vagal control of left ventricular contracility is selectively mediated by a cranioventricular intracardiac ganglion in the cat. *J Auton. Nerv. Syst.* 66:138–44; 1997.

73. Gebber, G. L. and L. R. Klevans. Central nervous system modulation of cardiovascular reflexes. *Federation Proc.* 31:1245–1252, 1972.

74. Gebber, G. L. and D. W. Snyder. Hypothalamic control of baroreceptor reflexes. *Am. J. Physiol.* 218:124–131, 1970.

75. Geis, G. S., J. W. Kozelka, and R. D. Wurster. Organisation and

reflex control of vagal cardiomotor neurons. *J. Auton. Nerv. Syst.* 3:437–450, 1981.
76. Geis, G. S. and R. D. Wurster. Horseradish peroxidase localization of cardiac vagal preganglionic somata. *Brain Res.* 182:19–30, 1980.
77. Geis, G. S. and R. D. Wurster. Cardiac responses during stimulation of the dorsal motonucleus and nucleus ambiguus in the cat. *Circ. Res.* 46:606–611, 1980.
78. Getz, B. and T. Sirnes. The localisation within the dorsal motor vagal nucleus. *J. Comp. Neurol.* 90:95–110, 1949.
79. Gilbey, M. P., D. Jordan, D. W. Richter, and K. M. Spyer. Synaptic mechanisms involved in the inspiratory modulation of vagal cardio-inhibitory neurones in the cat. *J. Physiol. (Lond.)* 356:65–78, 1984.
80. Gilbey, M. P. and K. M. Spyer. Cardiorespiratory regulation. In: *Neural Control of the Respiratory Muscles*, edited by A. D., Miller, A. L. Bianchi, and B. P. Bishop. Boca Ratan London: CRC Press, 1996: 261–271.
81. Hainsworth, R. Circulatory responses from lung inflation in anaesthetized dogs. *Am. J. Physiol.* 226:247–255, 1974.
82. Hainsworth, R. Reflexes from the heart. *Physiol. Rev.* 71:617–658, 1991.
83. Hartzell, H. J. C., P. F., Mery, R. Fischmeister, and G. Szabo. Sympathetic regulation of cardiac calcium current is due exclusively to cAMP-dependent phosphorylation. *Nature* 351:573–576, 1991.
84. Heinbecker, P. The effect of fibres of specific types in the vagus and sympathetic nerves on the sinus and atrium of the turtle and frog heart. *Am. J. Physiol.* 98:220–229, 1931.
85. Heinbecker, P. and G. J. Bishop. Studies on the extrinsic and intrinsic nerve mechanisms of the heart. *Am. J. Physiol.* 114:212–223, 1935.
86. Hering, E. Über den Einfluss der Athmung auf den Kreislauf. *Sitzungsberichte der Akademie der Wissenschaften in Wein* 64: Abt.2, 829–856, 1869.
87. Hess, W. R. and M. Brugger, Das subkorticale zentrum der affektiven-abwehrreaktion. *Acta Physiol. Helv.* 1:33–52, 1943.
88. Hilton, S. M. Inhibition of baroreceptor reflexes on hypothalamic stimulation. *J. Physiol. (Lond.)* 165:56–67, 1963.
89. Hilton, S. M. Hypothalamic control of the cardiovascular responses in fear and rage. *Sci. Basis Med.* XIII 217–233, 1965.
90. Hilton, S. M. Hypothalamic regulation of the cardiovascular system. *Br. Med. Bull.* 22:243–248, 1966.
91. Hilton, S. M. and N. Joels. Facilitation of chemoreceptor reflexes during the defence reaction. *J. Physiol. (Lond.)* 176:20–22, 1965.
92. Hilton, S. M. & J. M. Marshall. The pattern of cardiovascular response to carotid chemoreceptor stimulation in the cat. *J. Physiol.* 326:495–513, 1982.
93. Hilton, S. M. and W. S. Redfern. A search for brain stem cell groups integrating the defence reaction in the rat. *J. Physiol. (Lond.)* 165:160–173, 1963.
94. Hilton, S. M. and A. W. Zbrozyna. Amygdaloid region for defence reactions and its efferent pathway to the brain stem. *J. Physiol. (Lond.)* 165:160–173, 1963.
95. Hocherman, S. D., R. Werman, and Y. Yarom. An analysis of the long-lasting after-hyperpolarization of guinea-pig vagal motoneurones. *J. Physiol. (Lond.)* 456:325–349, 1992.
96. Humphrey, D. R. Neuronal activity in the medulla oblongata of the cat evoked by stimulation of the carotid sinus nerve. In: *Baroreceptors and Hypertension*, edited by P. Kezdi. Oxford: Pergamon, 1967: 131–168.
97. Humphreys, P. W., N. Joels, and R. M. McAllen. Modulation of the reflex response to stimulation of carotid sinus baroreceptors during and following stimulation of the hypothalamic defence area in the cat. *J. Physiol. (Lond.)* 216:461–482, 1971.
98. Hunt, R. Experiments on the relation of the inhibitory to the accelerator nerves of the heart. *J. Exp. Med.* 2:252–279, 1897.
99. Irisawa, H., J. F. Brown, and W. Giles. Cardiac pacemaking in the sinoatrial node. *Physiol. Rev.* 73:197–227, 1993.
100. Iriuchijima, J. and M. Kumada. Efferent cardiac vagal discharge of the dog in response to electrical stimulation of sensory nerves. *Jpn. J. Physiol.* 13:599–605, 1963.
101. Iriuchijima, J. and M. Kumada. Activity of single vagal fibers efferent to the heart. *Jpn. J. Physiol.* 14:479–487, 1964.
102. Izzo, P. N., J. Deuchars, and K. M. Spyer. Localization of cardiac vagal preganglionic motoneurones in the rat: immunocytochemical evidence of synaptic inputs containing 5-hydroxytraptamine. *J. Comp. Neurol.* 327:572–583, 1993.
103. Izzo, P. N. and J. F. X. Jones. Identification of vagal efferent fibres and their putative target neurones in cardiac ganglia of the anaesthetized rat. *J. Physiol. (Lond.)* 481:14, 1994.
104. Izzo, P. M. and K. M. Spyer. The parasympathetic innervation of the heart. In: *The Autonomic Nervous System*, Vol 11, edited by G. Burnstock. Harwood Academic Publishers. 1997.
105. Izzo, P. M., R. M. Sykes, and K. M. Spyer. γ-amino butyric acid immunoreactive structures in the nucleus tractus solitarius: a light and electron microscopic study. *Brain Res.* 591:69–79, 1992.
106. Jalife, J. and G. K. Moe. Phasic effects of vagal stimulation on pacemaker activity of the isolated sinus node of the young cat. *Circ. Res.* 45:595–607, 1979.
107. Jewett, D. L. Activity of single vagal efferent cardiac fibres in the dog. *J. Physiol. (Lond.)* 142:110–126, 1962.
108. Jewett, D. L. Activity of single efferent fibres in the cervical vagus nerve of the dog with special reference to possible cardioinhibitory fibres. *J. Physiol. (Lond.)* 175:321–357, 1964.
109. Jiang, C., T. R. Cummins, and G. G. Haddad. Membrane ionic currents and properties of freshly dissociated rat brainstem neurons. *Exp. Brain Res.* 100:407–420, 1994.
110. Jones, J. F. X. The central control of the pulmonary chemoreflex. Ph.D thesis, University of London, 1993.
111. Jones, J. F. X., Y. Wang, and D. Jordan. Activity of C fibre cardiac vagal efferents in anaesthetized cats and rats. *J. Physiol (Lond.).* 507:869–880, 1998.
112. Jones, J. F. X., Y. Wang, and D. Jordan. Activity of cardiac vagal preganglionic neurones during the pulmonary chemoreflex in the anaesthetized cat. In: *Arterial Chemoreceptors: Cell to System*, edited by R. O'Regan. et al., New York: Plenum Press, 1994: 301–303.
113. Jones, J. F. X., Y. Wang, and D. Jordan. Heart rate responses to selective stimulation of cardiac vagal C fibres in anaesthetized cats, rat and rabbits. *J. Physiol. (Lond.)* 489:203–214, 1995.
113a. Jones, J. F. X., Y. Wang, and D. Jordan. Activity of C fibre cardiac vagal efferents in anaesthetized cats and rats. *J. Physiol.* 507:869–80, 1998.
114. Jordan, D. Autonomic changes in affective behaviour. In *Central Regulation of Autonomic Functions*, edited by A. D. Loewy, and K. M. Spyer. New York: Oxford University Press, 1990: 349–367.
115. Jordan D., M. E. M. Khalid, N. Schneiderman, and K. M. Spyer. The location and properties of preganglionic vagal cardiomotor neurones in the rabbit. *Pflugers Arch.* 395:244–250, 1982.
116. Jordan, D., S. W. Mifflin, and K. M. Spyer. Hypothalamic inhibition of neurones in the nucleus tractus solitarius of the cat is GABA mediated. *J. Physiol. (Lond.)* 399:389–404, 1988.
117. Jordan, D. and K. M. Spyer. The distribution and excitability of myelinated aortic nerve afferent terminals. *Neurosci. Lett.* 8:113–117, 1978.
118. Jordan, D. and K. M. Spyer. Studies on the excitability of sinus

nerve afferent terminals. *J. Physiol. (Lond.)* 297:123–134, 1979.
119. Jordan, D. and K. M. Spyer. Brainstem integration of cardiovascular and pulmonary afferent activity. In *Prog. Brain Res.* Vol. 67, *Visceral Sensation,* edited by F. Cervero, and J. F. B. Morrison. Amsterdam: Elsevier 1986: 295–314.
120. Jordan, D. and K. M. Spyer. Central neural mechanisms mediating respiratory–cardiovascular interactions. In: *Neurobiology of the cardiorespiratory System,* edited by E. W. Taylor Manchester: Manchester University Press 1987: 322–341.
121. Kalia, M. and M. M. Mesulam. Brain stem projections of sensory and motor components of the vagus complex in the cat. II. Laryngeal, tracheobronchial, pulmonary, cardiac and gastrointestinal branches. *J. Comp. Neurol.* 193:467–508, 1980.
122. Kasparov, S. and J. F. Paton. Changes in baroreceptor vagal reflex performance in the developing rat. *Pflugers Arch. Eur. J. Physiol.* 434:438–44, 1997.
123. Katona, P. G. and F. Jih. Respiratory sinus arrhythmia. Noninvasive measure of parasympathetic cardiac control. *J. Appl. Physiol.* 39:801–805. 1975.
124. Katona, P., D. Lipson, and P. J. Dauchot. Opposing central and peripheral effects of atropine on parasympathetic cardiovascular control. *Am. J. Physiol.* 232:146–151, 1977.
125. Katona, P., J. Poitras, U. Barnett, and B. Terry. Cardiac vagal efferent activity and heart period in the carotid sinus reflex. *Am. J. Physiol.* 218:1030–1037, 1970.
126. Kaufman, M. P., J. C. Longhurst, K. J. Rybicki, J. H. Wallach, and J. H. Mitchell. Effects of static muscular contraction on impulse activity of groups III and IV afferent in cats. *J. Appl. Physiol.* 55:105–112, 1983.
127. Kaufman, M. P. and K. J. Rybicki. Discharge properties of group III and IV muscle afferents: their responses to mechanical and metabolic stimuli. *Circ. Res.* 61 (Suppl): I.60–I.65, 1987.
128. Kidd, C. and P. N. McWilliam. The action of myelinated and non-myelinated vagal efferent fibres on heart rate, atrioventricular conduction and atrial contraction in cat and rabbit. *J. Physiol. (Lond.)* 330:77–78, 1982.
129. Kniffki, D.-D., S. L. Mense, and R. F. Schmidt. Muscle receptors with fine afferent fibers which may evoke circulatory reflexes. *Circ. Res.* 48:25–31, 1987.
130. Koepchen, H. P., P. H. Wagner, and H. D. Lux. Untersuchungen über Zeitbedarf und zentrale Verarbeitung des pressoreceptischen Herzreflexes. *Pflugers Arch* 273:413–430, 1961.
131. Koepchen, H. P., P. H. Wagner, and H. D. Lux. Über die zusammenhänge zwischen zentraler erregbarkeit reflektorischen atemrhythmus bei der nervösen steuerung der herzfrequenz. *Pflugers Arch* 273:443–465, 1961.
132. Korner, P. I. Integrative neural cardiovascular control *Physiol. Rev.* 51:312–367, 1971.
133. Kosaka, K. Über die vaguskerne des hundes. *Neurol. Centralbl.* 28:406–410. 1909.
134. Kristenson, K. and Y. Olsson. Retrograde axonal transport of protein. *Brain Res.* 29:363–365, 1971.
135. Kunze, D. L. Reflex discharge patterns of cardiac vagal efferent fibres. *J. Physiol.,* 222:1–15, 1972.
136. LaVail, J. H. and M. M. LaVail. Retrograde axonal transport in the central nervous system. *Science* 176:1416–1417, 1972.
137. Levy, M. N. Parasympathetic control of the heart. In: *Neural Regulation of the Heart,* edited by W. C. Randal New York: Oxford University Press, 1977: 95–130.
138. Levy, M. N. and P. Martin. Parasympathetic control of the heart. In: *Nervous Control of Cardiovascular Function,* edited by W. C. Randall. New York: Oxford University Press, 1984: 68–94.
139. Levy, M. N. and H. Zieske. Autonomic control of cardiac pacemaker activity and atrioventricular transmission. *J. Appl. Physiol.* 27:465–470, 1969.
140. Linden, R. J. The function of atrial receptors. In: *Cardiogenic Reflexes,* edited by R. Hainsworth, P. N. McWilliam, and D. A. S. G. Mary. Oxford: Oxford Science Publications, 1985: 18–39.
141. Lipski, J., R. M. McAllen, and K. M. Spyer. The sinus nerve and baroreceptor input to the medulla of the cat. *J. Physiol. (Lond.)* 251:61–78, 1975.
142. Lipski, J., R. M. McAllen, and K. M. Spyer. Synaptic activation of cardiac vagal moto-neurones. *J. Physiol. (Lond.)* 256:68, 1976.
143. Lipski, J., R. M. McAllen, and K. M. Spyer. The carotid chemoreceptor input to the respiratory neurones of the nucleus of tractus solitarius. *J. Physiol. (Lond.)* 269:797–810, 1977.
144. Lipski, J., R. M. McAllen, and A. Trzebski. Carotid baroreceptor and chemoreceptor inputs onto single medullary neurones. *Brain Res.* 107:132–135, 1976.
145. Loewy, A. C. Central autonomic pathways. In *Central Regulation of Autonomic Functions,* edited by A. D. Loewy, and K. M. Spyer. New York: Oxford University Press, 1990: 88–103.
146. Loewy, A. C. and K. M. Spyer. Vagal preganglionic neurons. In *Central Regulation of Autonomic Functions,* edited by A. D. Loewy, and K. M. Spyer. New York: Oxford University Press, 1990: 68–87.
147. Lopes, O. U. and J. F. Palmer. Proposed respiratory 'gating' mechanism for cardiac slowing. *Nature* 264:454–456, 1976.
148. Lopes, O. U. and J. F. Palmer. Mechanism of hypothalamic control of cardiac component of sinus nerve reflex. *Q. J. Exp. Physiol.* 63:231–254, 1978.
149. Maqbool, A., T. F. C. Batten, and P. N. McWillian. Ultrastructural relationships between GABAergic terminals and cardiac vagal preganglionic motoneurones and vagal afferents in the cat: a combined HRP tracing and immunogold labelling study. *Eur. J. Neurosci.* 3:501–513, 1991.
150. Marshall, J. M. Contribution to overall cardiovascular control made by the chemoreceptor-induced alerting defence response. In *Neurobiology of the Cardiorespiratory System,* edited by E. W. Taylor, Manchester: Manchester University Press, 1987: 221–249.
151. Marshall, J. M. Peripheral chemoreceptors and cardiovascular regulation. *Physiol. Rev.* 74:543–594, 1994.
152. Marshall, J. M. and J. D. Metcalfe. Analysis of the cardiovascular changes induced in the rat by graded levels of systemic hypoxia. *J. Physiol (Lond.).* 407:385–403, 1988.
153. Marshall, J. M. and R. J. Timms. Experiments on the role of the subthalamus in the generation of the cardiovascular changes during locomotion in the cat. *J. Physiol. (Lond.)* 301: 92–93, 1980.
154. Massari, V. J., T. A., Johnson, R. A. Gillis, and P. J. Gatti. What are the roles of substance P and neurokinin-1 receptors in the control of negative chronotropic or negative dromotropic vagal mononeurones? A physiological and ultrastructural analysis. *Brain Res.* 715:197–207, 1996.
155. Massari, V. J., L. W. Dickerson, A. L. Gray, J. M. Lauenstein, K. J. Blinder, J. T. Newsome, D. J. Rodak, T. J. Fleming, P. J. Gatti, and R. A. Gillis. Neural control of left ventricular contractility in the dog heart; synaptic interactions of negative inotropic vagal preganglionic neurons in the nucleus ambiguus with tyrosine hydroxylase immunoreactive terminals. *Brain Res.* 802:205–20, 1998.
156. Masssari, V. J., T. A. Johnson, and P. J. Gatti. Cardiotopic organization of the nucleus ambiguus? An anatomical and physiological analysis of neurons regulating atrioventricular conduction. *Brain Res.* 679:227–240, 1995.

157. Massari, V. J., T. A. Johnson, I. J. Llewellyn-Smith, and P. J. Gatti. Cardiotopic organisation of the nucleus ambiguus? An anatomical and physiological analysis of neurons regulating atrio-ventricular conduction. *Brain Res.* 679:227–240 1995.
158. McAllen, R. M. The inhibition of the baroreceptor input to the medulla by stimulation of the hypothalamic defence area. *J. Physiol. (Lond.)* 257:45–46, 1976.
159. McAllen, R. M. and K. M. Spyer. The location of cardiac vagal preganglionic motoneurones in the medulla of the cat. *J. Physiol. (Lond.)* 258:187–204, 1976.
160. McAllen, R. M. and K. M. Spyer. Two types of vagal preganglionic motoneurones projecting to the heart and lungs. *J. Physiol. (Lond.)* 282:353–364, 1978.
161. McAllen, R. M. and K. M. Spyer. The baroreceptor input to cardiac vagal motoneurons. *J. Physiol. (Lond.)* 282:365–374, 1978.
162. McWilliam, P. N. and D. C. Woolley. The effect of supranodose vagotomy on the hexamethonium resistant bradycardia in the anaesthetized rabbit. *J. Auton. Nerve. Syst.* 29:227–230, 1990.
163. McWilliam, P. N., T. Yang, and L. X. Chen. Changes in the baroreceptor reflex at the start of muscle contraction in the decerebrate cat. *J. Physiol. (Lond.)* 436:549–558, 1991.
164. Mendelowitz, D. Firing properties of identified parasympathetic cardiac neurons in nucleus ambiguus. *Am. J. Physiol.*, 271: 40: H2609–H2614. (*Heart Circ. Physiol.* 40)
165. Middleton, S., H. H. Middleton, and H. Grundfest. Spike potentials and cardiac effects of mammalian vagus nerve. *Am. J. Physiol.* 162: 553–559, 1950.
166. Mifflin, S. W. Arterial chemoreceptor input to nucleus tractus solitarius. *Am. J. Physiol.* 263 (*Renal Fluid Electrolyte Physiol.* 32): R368–R375, 1992.
167. Mifflin, S. W. Inhibition of chemoreceptor inputs to nucleus of tractus solitarius neurons during baroreceptor stimulation. *Am. J. Physiol.* 265 (*Renal Fluid Electrolyte Physiol.* 34): R14–R20, 1993.
168. Mifflin, S. W. Laryngeal afferent inputs to the nucleus of the solitary tract. *Am. J. Physiol.* 265 (*Renal Fluid Electrolyte Physiol.* 34):R269–R276, 1993.
169. Mifflin, S. W., K. M. Spyer, and D. J. Withington-Wray. Baroreceptor input to the nucleus tractus solitarius in the cat: postsynaptic actions and the influence of respiration. *J. Physiol. (Lond.)* 399:349–367, 1988.
170. Mifflin, S. W., K. M. Spyer, and D. J. Withington-Wray. Baroreceptor inputs to the nucleus tractus solitarius in the cat: modulation by the hypothalamus. *J. Physiol. (Lond.)* 399:369–387, 1988.
171. Mihalevich, M., R. A. Neff, and D. Mendelowitz. Voltage-gated currents in identified parasympathetic cardiac neurons in the nucleus ambiguus. *Brain Res.* 739:258–262.
172. Miller, R. Identification of vagal efferent neurones: a horseradish peroxidase study. *J. Physiol. (Lond.)* 256:69–70, 1976.
173. Mitchell, G. A. G. and R. Warwick. The dorsal vagal nucleus. *Acta Anat.* 25:371–395, 1955.
174. Mitchell, J. H. Cardiovascular control during exercise: central and reflex neural mechanisms. *Am. J. Cardiol.* 55:34D–41D, 1985.
175. Mitchell, J. H., M. P. Kaufman, and G. A. Iwamoto. The exercise pressor reflex: cardiovascular effects, afferent mechanisms and central pathways. *Annu. Rev. Physiol.* 45:229–242, 1983.
176. Miura, M. and J. Okada. Cardiac and non-cardiac preganglionic neurones of the thoracic vagus nerve: an HRP study in the cat. *Jpn. J. Physiol.* 31:53–66, 1988.
177. Miura, M. and D. J. Reis. Electrophysiological evidence that the carotid sinus nerve fibers terminate in the bulbar reticular formation. *Brain Res.* 9:394–397, 1968.
178. Miura, M. & D. J. Reis. Termination and secondary projections of the carotid sinus nerve in the cat brainstem. *Am. J. Physiol.* 217:142–153, 1969.
179. Miura, M. and D. J. Reis. The role of the solitary and paramedian reticular nuclei in mediating cardiovascular reflex responses from carotid baro- and chemoreceptors. *J. Physiol. (Lond.)* 225:525–548, 1972.
180. Mohlant, M. Le nerv vagus: Les connxions anatomiques et la valeur functioneue en noyar en vagus. *Nevraxe* 11:131, 1910.
181. Morest, D. K. Experimental study of the projections of the tractus solitarius and the area postrema in the cat. *J. Comp. Neurol.* 130: 277–300, 1967.
182. Neff, R. A., J. Humphrey, M. Mihalevich, and D. Mendelowitz. Nicotine enhances presynaptic and postsynaptic glutamatergic neurotransmission to activate cardiac parasympathetic neurons. *Circ. Res.* 83: 1241–1247, 1998.
183. Nitzan, R., I. Segev, and Y. Yarom. Voltage behaviour along the irregular dendritic structure of morphologically and physiologically characterized vagal motoneurons in the guinea pig. *J. Neurophysiol.* 63:333–346, 1990.
184. Nosaka, S., Yamamoto, T. and Yasunaga, K. Localisation of vagal cardioinhibitory preganglionic neurones within the rat brain stem. *J. Comp. Neurol.* 186:79–92, 1979.
185. Nosaka, S., K. Yasunaga, and M. Kawano. Vagus cardioinhibitory fibers in rats. *Pflugers Arch.* 379: 281–285, 1979.
186. Nosaka, S., K. Yasunaga, and S. Tamai. Vagal cardiac preganglionic neurons: distribution, cell types and reflex discharges. *Am. J. Physiol.* 243 (*Renal Fluid Electrolyte Physiol.* 12):R92–R98, 1982.
187. Paintal, A. S. Impulses in vagal afferent fibres from specific pulmonary deflation receptors. The response of these receptors to phenyl diguanide, potato starch, 5-hydroxytryptamine and nicotine, and their role in respiratory and cardiovascular reflexes. *Q. J. Exp. Physiol.* 40:89–111. 1955.
188. Paintal, A. S. Block of conduction in mammalian myelinated nerve fibres by low temperatures. *J. Physiol. (Lond.)* 180:1–19, 1965.
189. Paintal, A. S. Mechanism of stimulation of type J-pulmonary receptors. *J. Physiol. (Lond.)* 203: 511–532, 1969.
190. Paintal, A. S. The mechanism of excitation of type J receptors and the J reflex. In: *Breathing: Bering-Breuer Centenary Symposium*, edited by R. Porter, London: Churchill, 1970: 59–71.
191. Pascoe, J., D. J. Bradley, and K. M. Spyer. Interactive responses to stimulation of the amygdaloid central nucleus and baroceptor afferents in the rabbit. *J. Auton. Nerv. Syst.* 26:157–167, 1989.
192. Paton, J. F. R. Pattern of cardiorespiratory afferent convergence to solitary tract neurons driven by pulmonary vagal C-fiber stimulation in the mouse. *J. Neurophysiol.* 79:2365–2373, 1998.
193. Paton, J. F. R., L. Silva-Carvalho, G. E. Goldsmith, and K. M. Spyer. Inhibition of barosensitive neurones evoked by lobule IXb of the posterior cerebellar cortex in the decerebrate rabbit. *J. Physiol. (Lond.)* 427:124–129, 1990.
194. Paton, J. F. R. and K. M. Spyer. Brainstem regions mediating the cardiovascular responses elicited from the posterior cerebellar cortex in the rabbit. *J. Physiol. (Lond.)* 427: 533–552, 1990.
195. Plecha, D. M., W. C. Randall, G. S. Geis, and R. D. Wurster. Localization of vagal preganglionic somata controlling the sinoatrial and atrioventricular nodes. *Am. J. Physiol.* 255 (*Renal Fluid Electrolyte Physiol.* 24):R703–R708, 1988.
196. Potter, E. K. Inspiratory inhibition of vagal responses to baro-

receptor and chemoreceptor stimuli in the dog. *J. Physiol. (Lond.)* 316:177–190, 1981.
197. Randall, W. C. and J. L. Ardell. Selective parasympathectomy of automatic and conductile tissues of the canine heart. *Am. J. Physiol.* 248 (*Heart Circ. Physiol.* 17):H61–H68, 1985.
198. Randall, W. C., J. L. Ardell, D. Calderwood, M. Milosavljevic, and S. C. Goyal. Parasympathetic ganglia innervating the canine atrioventricular nodal region. *J. Auton. Nerv. Syst.* 16: 311–323, 1986.
199. Randall, W. C., J. L. Ardell, R. D. Wurster, and M. Milosavljevic. Vagal postganglionic innervation of the canine sinoatrial node. *J. Auton. Nerv. Syst.* 20: 13–23, 1987.
200. Randall, W. C. and R. D. Wurster. Peripheral innervation of the heart. In: *Vagal Control of the Heart: Experimental Basis and Clinical Implications*, edited by M. N. Levy, and P. J. Schwartz. Armonk, NY: Futura 1994: 21–32.
201. Remmers, J. E., D. W. Richter, D. Ballantyne, C. R. Bainton, and J. P. Klein. Reflex prolongation of stage I of expiration. *Pflugers Arch.* 407:190–198, 1986.
202. Richter, D. Generation and maintenance of the respiratory rhythm. *J. Exp. Biol.* 100: 93–107, 1982.
203. Richter, D. W. and D. Ballantyne. A three phase theory about the basic respiratory pattern generation. In: *Central Neuron Environment*, edited by M. E., Schläfke, H. P. Koepchen, and W. R. See. Berlin: Springer-Verlag, 1983: 164–174.
204. Richter, D. W. and K. M. Spyer. Cardiorespiratory control. In *Central Regulation of Autonomic Functions*, edited by A. D. Loewy, and K. M. Spyer. New York: Oxford University Press, 1990: 189–207.
205. Rose, W. C. and J. S. Schwaber. Analysis of heart rate-based control of arterial blood pressure. *Am. J. Physiol.* 271 (*Heart Circ. Physiol.* 40):H812–22, 1996.
206. Rudomin, P. Pharmacological evidence for the existence of interneurones mediating primary afferent depolarisation in the solitary tract nucleus of the cat. *Brain Res.* 2:181–183, 1966.
207. Rudomin, P. Primary afferent depolarisation produced by vagal visceral afferents. *Experientia* 23:117–119, 1967.
208. Rudomin, P. Presynaptic inhibition induced by vagal afferent volleys. *J. Neurophysiol.* 30:964–981, 1967.
209. Rudomin, P. Excitability changes of superior laryngeal, vagal and depressor afferent terminals produced by stimulation of the solitary tract nucleus. *Exp. Brain Res.* 6:156–170, 1986.
210. Sah, P. Role of calcium influx and buffering in the kinetics of a Ca^{2+}-activated K^+ current in rat vagal motoneurons. *J. Neurophysiol.* 68:2237–2247, 1992.
211. Sah, P. Kinetic properties of a slow apamin-insensitive Ca^{2+}-activated K^+ current in guinea pig vagal neurons. *J. Neurophysiol.* 69: 361–366, 1993.
212. Sah, P. and E. M. McLachlan. Ca^{2+}-activated K^+ currents underlying the after hyperpolarization in guinea pig vagal neurons: a role for Ca^{2+}-activated CA^{2+} release. *Neuron* 7:257–264, 1991.
213. Sah, P. and E. M. McLachlan. A slow voltage-activated potassium current in rat vagal neurons. *Proc. R. Soc. Lond.* 249 (1324):71–76, 1992.
214. Sah, P. and E. M. McLachlan. Potassium currents contributing to action potential repolarization and the after hyperpolarization in rat vagal motoneurons. *J. Neurophysiol.* 68: 1834–1841, 1992.
215. Sah, P. and E. M. McLachlan. Differences in electrophysiological properties between neurones of the dorsal motor nucleus of the vagus in rat and guinea pig. *J. Auton. Nerv. Syst.* 42:89–98, 1993.
216. Sakmann, B. Acetylcholine activation of single muscarinic potassium channels in isolated pacemaker cells of the mammalian heart. *Nature* 303:250–253, 1983.
217. Sampaio, K. N., H. Mauad, T. W. Ford, and K. M. Spyer. Chronotropic and dromotropic effects of L-glutamate (L-Glu) injected into the rat nucleus ambiguus (NA). *Auton. Neurosci.* 82:62, 2000.
218. Saul, J. P. and R. J. Cohen. Respiratory sinus arrhythmia. In: *Vagal Control of the Heart: Experimental Basis and Clinical Implications*, edited by M. N. Levy, and P. J. Schwartz. Armonk, NY: Futura 1994: 511–536.
219. Schwartz, P. J. and D. Cerati. Cardiac vagal efferent nerve activity. In: *Vagal Control of the Heart: Experimental Basis and Clinical Implications*, edited by M. N. Levy, and P. J. Schwartz. Armonk, NY: Futura 1994: 77–87.
220. Schweitzer, A. Rhythmical fluctuations of the arterial blood pressure. *J. Physiol. (Lond.)* 104:25–26, 1945.
221. Seabrook, G. R., L. A. Fieber, & D. J. Adams. Neurotransmission in neonatal rat cardiac ganglia *in situ*. *Am. J. Physiol.* 259 (*Heart Circ. Physiol.* 28):H997–H1005, 1990.
222. Seagard, J. L., F. A. Hopp, H. A. Drummond, D. M. VanWynsberghe. Selective contributions of two types of carotid sinus baroreceptors to the control of blood pressure. *Circ. Res.* 72:1011–1022, 1993.
223. Seller, H. and M. Illert. The localization of the first synapse in the carotid sinus baroreceptor reflex pathway and its alteration of the afferent input. *Pflugers Archiv.* 306:1–19, 1969.
224. Selyanko, A. A. and V. I. Skok. Acetylcholine receptors in rat cardiac neurones. *J. Autonom. Nerv. Syst.* 40: 33–48. 1992.
225. Silva-Carvalho, L., M. S. Dawid-Milner, G. E. Goldsmith, and K. M. Spyer. Hypothalamic-evoked effects in cat nucleus tractus solitarius facilitating chemoreceptor reflexes. *Exp. Physiol.* 78:425–428, 1993.
226. Silva-Carvalho, L., M. S. Dawid-Milner, G. E. Goldsmith, and K. M. Spyer. Hypothalamic modulation of the arterial chemoreceptor reflex in the anaesthetized cat: role of the nucleus tractus solitarii. *J. Physiol. (Lond.)* 487:751–760, 1995.
227. Silva-Carvalho, L., M. S. Dawid-Milner, and K. M. Spyer. The pattern of excitatory inputs to the nucleus tractus solitarii evoked on stimulation in the hypothalamic defence area in the cat. *J. Physiol. (Lond.)* 487:727–737, 1995.
228. Silva-Carvalho, L., J. F. R. Paton, I. Rocha, G. E. Goldsmith, and K. M. Spyer. Convergence properties of solitary tract neurons responsive to cardiac receptor stimulation in the anesthetized cat. *J. Neurophysiol.* 79:2374–2382, 1998.
229. Spyer, K. M. Neural organization and control of the baroreceptor reflex. *Rev. Physiol., Biochem. and Pharmacol.* 88:23–124, 1981.
230. Spyer, K. M. Central control of the cardiovascular system. In *Recent Advances in Physiology*, edited by P. F. Porter. Edinburgh; Churchill Livingstone 1984: 163–200.
231. Spyer, K. M. The central nervous organization of reflex circulatory control. In *Central Regulation of Autonomic Functions*, edited by A. D. Loewy, and K. M. Spyer. New York: Oxford University Press, 1990: 168–188.
232. Spyer, K. M. Central nervous mechanisms contributing to cardiovascular control *J. Physiol. (Lond.)* 474:1–19, 1994.
233. Spyer, K. M., P. A. Brooks, and P. N. Izzo. Vagal preganglionic neurones supplying the heart, Chap. 4. In: *Vagal Control of the Heart*. edited by M. N. Levy, and P. J. Schwartz, Armonk, NY: Futura. 1994:45–63.
234. Spyer, K. M., P. N. Izzo., R. J. Liu, J. F. R. Paton, L. F. Silva-Carvalho, and D. W. Richter. The central nervous organization of the carotid body chemoreceptor reflex. In *Chemoreceptors and Chemoreceptor Reflexes,* edited by H. Acker, A. Trzebski, and R. O'Regan. New York: Plenum 1990. 317–321.
235. Spyer, K. M. and D. Jordan. Electrophysiology of the nucleus ambiguus. In: *Cardiogenic Reflexes*, edited by R. Hainsworth, P. N. McWilliam, and D. A. S. G. Mary, 1987. 237–249.

236. Spyer, K. M. and J. H. Wolstencroft. Problems of the afferent input to the paramedial reticular nucleus, and the central connections of the sinus nerve. *Brain Res.* 26:411–414, 1971.
237. Standish, A., L. W. Enquist, and J. S. Schwaber. Innervation of the heart and its central medullary origin defined by viral tracing. *Science* 263:232–234, 1994.
238. Stuesse, S. L. Origins of cardiac vagal preganglionic fibres: a retrograde transport study. *Brain Res.* 236: 15–25, 1982.
239. Szentagothai, J. The general visceral efferent column of the brain stem. *Acta Morphol. Acad. Sci. Hung.* 2:313–328, 1952.
240. Taylor, E. W., D. Jordan, and J. H. Coote. Central control of the cardiovascular and respiratory systems and their interactions in vertebrates. *Physiol. Rev.* 79:855–916, 1999.
241. Thames, M. D., H. A. Kontosm and R. R. Lower. Sinus arrhythmia in dogs after cardiac transplantation. *Am. J. Cardiol.* 24:54–58, 1969.
242. Trapp, S., K. Ballanyi, and D. W. Richter. Spontaneous activation of KATP current in rat dorsal vagal neurones. *NeuroReport* (5): 1285–1288, 1994.
243. Traube, L. Über periodische Thätigkeits-Äusserungen des vasomotorischen und Hemmungs-Hervencentrums. *Zentralbl. Med Wissen., Berlin* 56:881–885, 1865.
244. Travagli, R. A. and R. A. Gillis. Hyperpolarization activated currents, I_H and I_{KIR}, in rat dorsal motor nucleus of the vagus (DMV) neurones in vitro. *J. Neurophysiol.* 71:1308–1317, 1994.
245. Travagli, R. A., R. A. Gillis, C. D. Rossiter, and S. Vincini Fida. Glutamate and GABA-mediated synaptic currents in neurons of the rat dorsal motor nucleus of the vagus. *Am. J. Physiol.* 260 (*Gastrointest. Liver Physiol.* 23):G531–G536, 1991.
246. Ulman, L. G., E. K. Potter, D. I. McCloskey, and M. J. Morris. Post-exercise depression of baroreflex slowing of the heart in humans. *Clin. Physiol.* 17:299–309, 1997.
247. Van Gehuchten, A. *Les Centres Nerveus Cerebo-spinaux.* A. Louvain: Uystpruyst-Dieudonne, 1908.
248. Waldrop, T. G., R. M. Bauer, and G. A. Iwamoto. Microinjection of GABA antagonists into the posterior hypothalamus, locomotor activity and a cardiorespiratory activation. *Brain Res.* 444:84–94, 1988.
249. Widdicombe, J. G. Nervous receptors in the respiratory tract and lungs. In: *Regulation of Breathing*, Part I *Lung Biology in Health and Disease*, Vol 17, edited by T. F. Hornbein. New York: Marcel Dekker, 1981: 429–472.
250. Widdicombe, J. G. Pulmonary and respiratory tract receptors. *J. Exp. Biol.* 100:41–57, 1982.
251. Widdicombe, J. G. Reflexes from the upper respiratory tract. In *Handbook of Physiology*, section 3, *The Respiratory System*, Vol.II: *Control of Breathing*, part 1, edited by N. S. Cherniack, and J. G. Widdicombe. Bethesda, MD: American Physiological Society, 1986: 363–429.
252. Willis, A., M. Mihalevich, R. A. Neff, and D. Mendelowitz. Three types of postsynaptic glutamatergic receptors are activated in DMNX neurons upon stimulation of NTS. *Am. J. Physiol*, 271 (*Renal Fluid Electrolyte Physiol.* 34):R1614–R1619. 1996.
253. Woolley, D. C., P. M. McWillian, T. W. Ford, and R. W. Clarke. The effect of selective electrical stimulation of non-myelinated vagal fibres on heart rate in the rabbit. *J. Auton. Nerv. Syst.* 21:215–221, 1987.
254. Xi-Moy, S. X., W. C. Randall, and R. D. Wurster. Nicotinic and muscarinic synaptic transmission in canine intracardiac ganglion cells innervating the sinoatrial node. *J. Auton. Nerv. Syst.* 42:201–214, 1993.
255. Yarom, J., M. Sugimore, and R. Llinas. Ionic currents and firing patterns of mammalian vagal motoneurons in vitro. *Neuroscience* 16:719–737, 1985.

6. Kinetics of the actin–myosin interaction

JEFFERY W. WALKER | *Department of Physiology, University of Wisconsin, Madison, Wisconsin*

CHAPTER CONTENTS

Crossbridges and Sliding Filaments
Regulation
Myosin and Actomyosin ATPase
   Rates of specific steps
   Energetics of specific steps
   Cardiac versus skeletal actomyosin ATPase
The Crossbridge Cycle in Muscle
   Energy transduction and muscle mechanics
   Transient Kinetics in Fibers Using Caged Compounds
   Analysis of Specific Steps
      ATP binding and detachment
      ATP cleavage
      P_i dissociation and force generation
      ADP dissociation
   Cardiac Muscle
In Vitro Motility
Atomic Structures of Actin and Myosin
   Myosin S1
   Actomyosin
   Comparison of Structural Models to Other Models
Recent Progress
Regulation
   The steric blocking model
   Kinetic regulation
   Dual regulation of the crossbridge cycle
   Phosphorylation and protein isoform switching
Summary and Concluding Comments

THE KINETIC MECHANISM OF ADENOSINE TRIPHOSPHATE HYDROLYSIS (ATPase) by actomyosin has been established in large part by measurements of rate and equilibrium constants of isolated actin and myosin in solution. It is necessary, however, to modify and extend the actomyosin ATPase mechanism deduced in this manner if one is to account for the vectorial processes of force generation and motion in muscle fibers. The primary goal of this chapter is to summarize current understanding of the actin–myosin interaction cycle in striated muscle by integrating key findings in kinetics, thermodynamics, structure, and mechanics. Most investigations of contractile mechanisms have focused on fast skeletal muscle; therefore, much of the discussion emphasizes work with isolated proteins and tissue taken from fast skeletal muscle.

A secondary goal of the chapter is to summarize what is known about actin–myosin interactions in cardiac muscle. The proteins involved in cardiac muscle contraction and its regulation are likely to be uniquely tuned to support the physiological function of the heart. This review is not intended to be comprehensive in its coverage of the literature. For a more complete overview of the muscle literature, the reader is referred to a number of excellent reviews of kinetics (29, 34, 38, 95, 99), thermodynamics (18, 55, 75), mechanics (49, 88), and structure (30, 37, 69, 78, 84, 91) as well as general monographs on muscle contraction (4, 43, 112).

CROSSBRIDGES AND SLIDING FILAMENTS

In the sliding filament mechanism of muscle contraction (41, 44), partially overlapping filaments of actin and myosin slide past each other, causing the sarcomere to shorten (Fig. 6–1). Shortening of many sarcomeres in series along the length of the fiber results in muscle shortening. The driving force for filament sliding is ATP hydrolysis on the globular heads of myosin, often called crossbridges because they appear to form cross-links between myosin and actin filaments when viewed in the electron microscope (80). Crossbridges project away from the myosin filament and bind to the actin filament in such a way that each cycle of crossbridge attachment and detachment causes 5–20 nm or more of relative displacement of the filaments (9). The precise numerical value of filament displacement per attachment–detachment cycle, commonly called the myosin step size, is under debate. Many estimates of myosin step size are based on measurements of filament travel distance per ATP hydrolyzed, and such measurements assume that the attachment–detachment cycle for each crossbridge is tightly coupled to the hydrolysis of a single ATP molecule (9). Invariably, discussion of myosin step size is accompanied by discussion of the related issue of coupling, in particular, whether the chemical events of ATP hydrolysis are tightly or loosely coupled to mechanical transitions that produce force and displacement. Also under debate is whether the crossbridge generates force by a thermal rachet type of mechanism (40, 53) or by a tilting of some portion of the myosin head (30, 47, 48).

There are at least three compelling reasons to pursue a complete understanding of the cycle of myosin cross-

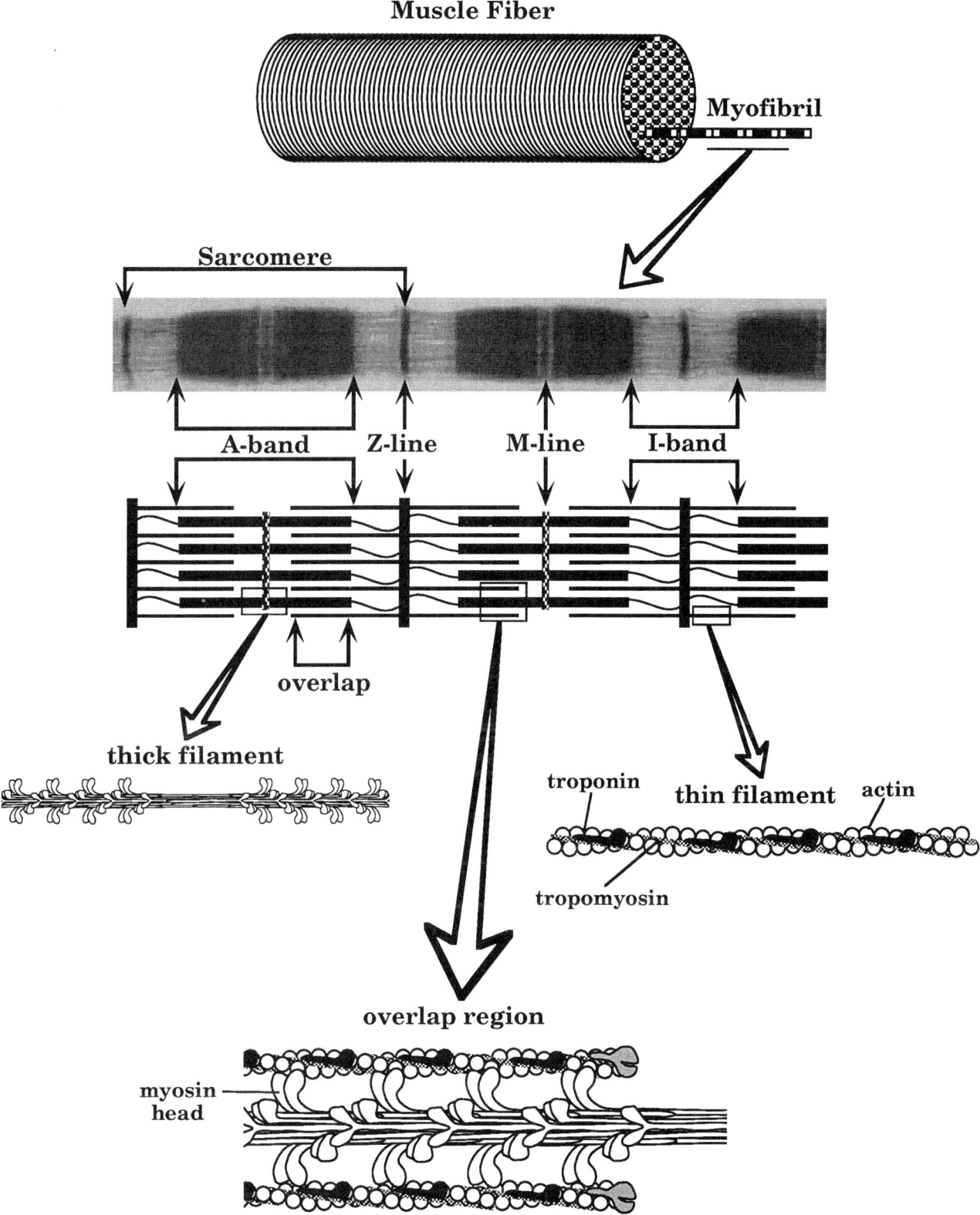

FIG. 6–1. Muscle fiber ultrastructure. Fibers are comprised of bundles of myofibrils, each containing alternating dark bands (A-bands) and light bands (I-bands) when viewed in the light microscope. Illustrated in diagrams below the micrograph is the arrangement of proteins that underlie this banding pattern. The dark band corresponds to the thick myosin filament which has a bare zone or light stripe at its center. The light band corresponds to thin actin filaments which are anchored at the Z-line in the center of the I-band. The outer segments of the dark band represent the region of overlap between actin and myosin filaments where crossbridges are located and where productive actin–myosin interactions occur. A sarcomere is the structure between two Z-lines, and when the sarcomere shortens the distance between Z-lines decreases.

bridge interactions with actin. First, it is a prime example of free energy transduction in biology, the details of which will provide insight into how chemical energy is converted to work at the molecular level. Second, it is an essential starting point in understanding how muscle contraction is regulated (for example, by Ca^{2+}, by protein phosphorylation, and by protein isoform switching). Third, it is becoming clear that point mutations or other molecular defects in skeletal or cardiac myosin that alter the energy transduction process are manifested clinically as myopathies. Development of effective therapeutic strategies for such muscle myopathies will depend on understanding these defects in detail.

In defining the actin–myosin interaction, kinetic measurements with isolated proteins establish the pathway of ATP hydrolysis by myosin, as well as the mechanism by which actin activates the myosin ATPase. Determining kinetic constants of elementary transitions also provides thermodynamic information, because ratios of rate constants are related to basic free energy changes (18, 29, 34). Of particular interest here is using thermodynamic principles to identify the precise step or steps in the ATP hydrolysis pathway where chemical free energy is made available for the system to perform work. As mentioned at the beginning of this chapter, understanding the processes of force generation and movement in muscle is more challenging than simply elucidating the enzymatic mechanism of ATP hydrolysis. Kinetic measurements must also be carried out in muscle fibers to establish exactly how mechanical processes like force generation and shortening are coupled to the chemical events of ATP hydrolysis. It is clear from such measurements that there is considerable complexity due to the ensemble behavior of myosin molecules in organized filaments. To address this state of affairs, remarkable progress has been made in recent years toward the goal of investigating force, displacement, and ATP hydrolysis by individual myosin molecules. These studies are beginning to reveal the nature of elementary mechanical and chemical events, at the single molecule level, that ultimately will facilitate understanding of crossbridge function in muscle.

REGULATION

Understanding regulation of the crossbridge cycle is another major challenge. In striated muscle, the primary mode of regulation is via Ca^{2+} binding to the thin filament protein troponin, which results in movement of tropomyosin on the actin filament. Recent evidence suggests that the thin filament regulatory proteins are much more than a Ca^{2+}-sensitive switch that controls myosin binding. In addition to regulation of myosin binding to actin, rates of specific chemical or mechanical transitions in the crossbridge cycle appear to be controlled by Ca^{2+} binding and by phosphorylation of myofilament proteins. Regulation of kinetic transitions is important, in part because it permits the rate, efficiency, and economy of muscle contraction to be altered to optimize muscle performance under different conditions. Changes in muscle protein isoform expression also influence muscle performance by affecting the kinetics of actin–myosin interactions.

MYOSIN AND ACTOMYOSIN ATPase

A central feature of the sliding filament model is that each crossbridge is considered to be an independent force generator (31, 42). Considerable information has been obtained by studying the proteolytic fragment of myosin, subfragment 1 (S1), which is in effect the isolated crossbridge. It was established early on that myosin S1 binds and hydrolyzes ATP to adenosine diphosphate (ADP) and inorganic phosphate (P_i). Moreover, in vitro motility assays showed that myosin S1 can support movement of actin filaments (98), and that the globular myosin S1 heads can generate forces of the magnitude expected for force generators in muscle (23, 71).

Rates of Specific Steps

The ATP hydrolysis reaction on myosin S1 takes place in discrete steps (labeled 1–4 in Scheme 1): ATP binding, ATP cleavage in the active site, P_i dissociation, and ADP dissociation. Each step may represent several processes such as formation of a collision complex between the protein and a ligand (ATP, ADP or P_i) followed by one or more conformational changes. For simplicity, only a single composite conformational change will be considered here for each step. The shorthand notation for Scheme 1 is M = myosin or S1, and

Scheme 1

$$M \xrightarrow[1]{ATP} M.ATP \xrightarrow[2]{} M.ADP.P_i \xrightarrow[3]{P_i} M.ADP \xrightarrow[4]{ADP} M$$

ATP, ADP and P_i are ligands that form noncovalent complexes with M. The true substrate for the ATPase is MgATP (99), so unless otherwise stated reference to ATP means MgATP. Analysis of rate constants for each step in the myosin ATPase showed that the slowest step in the reaction sequence was P_i dissociation occurring at $0.05\ s^{-1}$ ($t_{1/2} = 14\ s$) (62, 99). This slow rate accounts for the overall ATPase rate, and thus P_i dissociation is considered to be the rate-limiting step for ATP hydrolysis by myosin S1. Rapid mixing of myosin S1 with ATP reveals a rapid phase of ATP hydrolysis called the *phosphate burst* (62). This burst has been interpreted as the first turnover of ATP cleavage that occurs in the nucleotide binding pocket, and is detected as a burst of free P_i because the proteins are denatured with acid prior to the assay for P_i. As expected from this interpretation, the number of moles of P_i formed during the burst is close to the number of moles of active sites (Fig. 6–2). After the first turnover of ATP cleavage, further ATP hydrolysis requires dissociation of P_i and of ADP, which occurs more slowly and limits the rate of further ATP hydrolysis (Fig. 6–2). Estimates of equilibrium constants for each step revealed that two of the steps, ATP binding and P_i dissociation, occur with large equilibrium constants (99). A large equilibrium constant means that these are chemical or conformational transitions in the ligand–protein complex where a significant change (i.e. release) of free energy occurs.

Addition of actin to S1 accelerates the overall ATP hydrolysis rate but the same four steps are involved (Scheme 2; A.M=actomyosin) (95). Again a phosphate burst is detected when actomyosin S1 is rapidly mixed with ATP (Fig. 6–2), and the rate of ATP cleavage during the burst is similar with and without actin (i.e. similar for actomyosin S1 and for myosin S1) (95). Both

Scheme 2

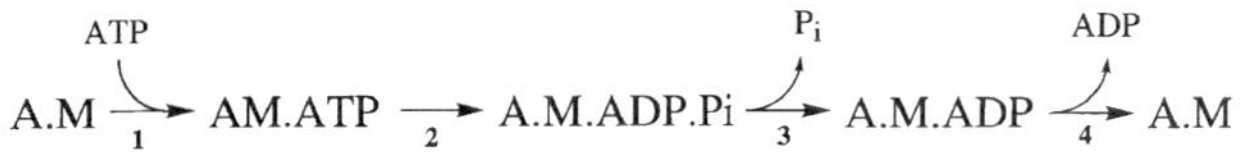

$$A.M \xrightarrow[1]{ATP} AM.ATP \xrightarrow{2} A.M.ADP.P_i \xrightarrow[3]{P_i} A.M.ADP \xrightarrow[4]{ADP} A.M$$

the steady-state ATPase rate and the size of the P_i burst are dependent on actin concentration. As the actin concentration increases, the degree of association of myosin with actin increases, and the rate-limiting product dissociation steps are accelerated. At very high actin concentrations, the product dissociation rate is at least 200-fold faster than for myosin S1 and approaches the rate of the ATP cleavage step. Thus, the P_i burst, which is due to slow P_i dissociation compared to ATP cleavage, becomes less readily detectable (Fig. 6–2). The precise step in the sequence that is rate limiting for actomyosin S1 continues to be controversial, as ATP cleavage (82), P_i dissociation (108), and isomerizations between them, have been proposed as limiting the steady-state rate. It is likely that these steps occur at similar rates and that all contribute to limit the overall ATP hydrolysis rate in the presence of high concentrations of actin.

Recent studies of myofibrillar ATPase, which approximates the filament organization of muscle fibers, showed that the phosphate burst amplitude is significant. Therefore, P_i release appears to be rate limiting at the effective actin concentrations in myofibrils (63). Further studies in myofibrils have confirmed that the phosphate burst is due to ADP + P_i which are tightly bound to myosin. In these experiments, a fluorescent phosphate binding protein was used to monitor *free* phosphate produced by ATP hydrolysis, and no change in free phosphate was detected during the burst (59). Thus, the P_i burst is a reflection of phosphate that is tightly but non-covalently bound to myosin. It is important to note that the P_i burst is not especially meaningful in a physiological context, but is an indication that ATP binding, dissociation of A.M to A + M.ATP, and ATP cleavage in the active site are much more rapid than release of hydrolysis products. These observations have helped to focus attention on the product release steps as being those that limit the actomyosin S1 ATPase rate at intermediate and low actin concentrations.

Identifying rate-limiting steps in a reaction pathway is important because kinetic intermediates that occur just prior to the rate-limiting step will be highly populated. For example, identification of ATP cleavage as

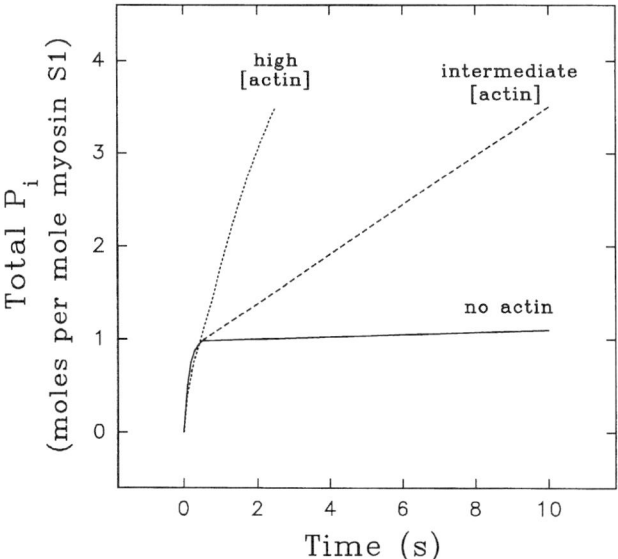

FIG. 6–2. Time course of ATP hydrolysis catalyzed by myosin S1 and actomyosin S1 measured by formation of total P_i. Rapid mixing of ATP with myosin produces a P_i burst in the first few tenths of a second, followed by a slower rate of P_i formation (*solid line*). The burst is approximately equal in moles to the number of moles of myosin S1 present, and represents the first cycle of ATP hydrolysis bound to myosin S1. Further ATP hydrolysis (and P_i formation) requires product dissociation, which is very slow ($t_{1/2}$=14 s) in the absence of actin. At intermediate actin concentrations, this second phase increases in rate but the overall time course remains distinctly biphasic. At very high actin concentration, the second phase approaches the rate of the initial (burst) phase making the burst less discernible.

a rapid step and P_i release as a rate-limiting step for myosin S1 alone suggests that $M.ADP.P_i$ is a major intermediate in relaxed muscle (the position of the equilibrium between M.ATP and $M.ADP.P_i$ also favors $M.ADP.P_i$). In addition, rates of conformational transitions in the actomyosin ATPase place limits on how fast mechanical processes can take place in muscle. For instance, the rate of tension development and the rate of relaxation may be dictated by transition rates into and out of force-generating states, which are likely to be controlled by specific chemical steps in the cycle. Similarly, filament sliding velocity is limited by the myosin step size and the rate of the slowest transition among attached states in the cycle (87). A goal is to establish the rate-limiting step for each mechanical process (force generation, shortening, relaxation) under physiological conditions. It will then be possible to better understand regulation (for example, by Ca^{2+} and by phosphorylation) of rate-limiting steps and their mechanical correlates, in addition to establishing the influence of experimental and pathological factors such as pH, ionic composition, temperature, and mechanical load.

Energetics of Specific Steps

Hydrolysis of ATP catalyzed by myosin and actomyosin does not alter the total free energy released from ATP, which under prevailing conditions within the cell is $\Delta G = \Delta G^\circ + RT \ln [ADP][P_i]/[ATP] = -11 + RT \ln [0.1 \text{ mM}][1 \text{ mM}]/[5 \text{ mM}] = -14$ kcal/mol. Instead, these enzymes partition the free energy change into discrete steps. Measurements of equilibrium constants for elementary steps in the pathway revealed that most of the free energy change for actomyosin S1 is associated with P_i dissociation (110). This differs from myosin S1 alone, where the largest proportion of the free energy change is associated with ATP binding. This occurs because myosin S1 has a high free energy content (it is energetically unstable), and much of this free energy is released when strong bonds form between ATP and myosin S1. A large free energy release also occurs when strong bonds form between myosin S1 and actin, giving rise to the very stable rigor complex (A.M in Scheme 2). When ATP binds to the actomyosin S1 rigor complex, considerably less free energy is released, because strong bonds between actin and myosin are replaced by strong bonds between ATP and myosin. In effect, the free energy available from binding of ATP to myosin S1 is thermodynamically coupled to dissociation of the energetically stable actomyosin rigor bonds.

The reversibility of several steps during ATP hydrolysis has been demonstrated by isotope-exchange experiments. Reversibility is an important property to establish because free energy changes associated with reversible steps are small. Actomyosin S1 in the presence of ATP incorporates labeled phosphate ($^{18}O\text{-}PO_4$ or $^{32}P\text{-}PO_4$) into ATP, suggesting that ATP binding, ATP cleavage, and P_i dissociation are readily reversible. However, acto-S1 without ATP but in the presence of ADP (or MgADP) and labeled phosphate does not give labeled ATP, showing that $A.M + ADP + P_i$ cannot be reversed to A. M.ATP. Taken together, these two exchange experiments show that a step after P_i dissociation is effectively irreversible for isolated actomyosin S1 (89). The results also indicate that the A. M.ADP state formed by mixing ADP (or MgADP) with A.M is different (unable to react with phosphate) than an A.M.ADP state formed during the hydrolysis cycle (which can react with phosphate). Thus, two A.M.ADP states are typically included in the actomyosin ATPase mechanism, A.M'.ADP and A.M.ADP. A.M'.ADP can be considered a high-energy conformation of A.M.ADP. Scheme 3 is obtained by combining the hydrolysis pathways for myosin S1 and actomyosin S1, and by inclusion of reversible steps where appropriate. These are the elementary states of the actomyosin ATPase. States that are not in bold are included for completeness, but these are not considered to be significantly populated during normal operation of the ATPase cycle. For instance, equilibria involving the M state substantially favor A.M (in the absence of ATP) and M.ATP (in the presence of ATP). Similarly, M.'ADP and M.ADP states are not populated because P_i dissociation from $M.ADP.P_i$ (lower row) is at least 100-fold slower than from $A. M.ADP.P_i$ (upper row), and A.M'.ADP and A.M.ADP are strongly attached states, so their detached counterparts M'.ADP and M.ADP become insignificant.

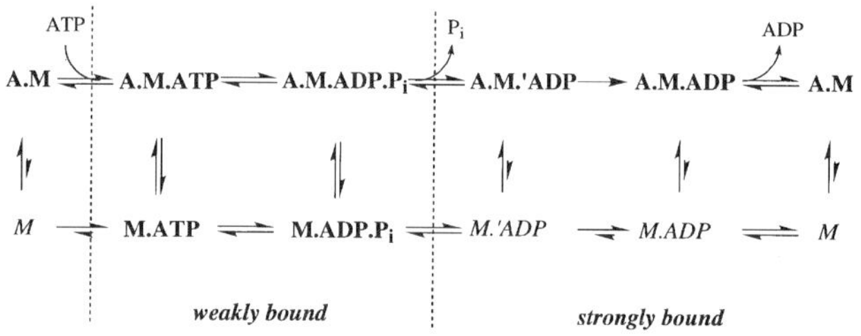

Scheme 3

$$A.M \rightleftharpoons A.M.ATP \rightleftharpoons A.M.ADP.P_i \rightleftharpoons A.M.'ADP \rightarrow A.M.ADP \rightleftharpoons A.M$$
$$\updownarrow \quad \updownarrow \quad \updownarrow \quad \updownarrow \quad \updownarrow \quad \updownarrow$$
$$M \rightleftharpoons M.ATP \rightleftharpoons M.ADP.P_i \rightleftharpoons M.'ADP \rightleftharpoons M.ADP \rightleftharpoons M$$

weakly bound | *strongly bound*

In many models the simplification is made that there are two general types of states, "weakly bound" and "strongly bound," as indicated in Scheme 3. Weak binding states are characterized by a rapid equilibrium between attached and detached states, while strong binding states are characterized by high-affinity interactions between actin and myosin. In such models, crossbridges generate force by cycling between weak and strong binding states (8). The transition from the strongly bound A.M state to the weakly bound A.M.ATP was described above as thermodynamic coupling of the energetically favorable binding of ATP to myosin with the unfavorable dissociation of A.M. The transition from weakly bound A.M.ADP.P_i state to the strongly bound A.M.ADP involves dissociation of P_i allowing for re-formation of stronger bonds between actin and myosin, eventually returning to the highly stable rigor complex on dissociation of ADP. Free energy minima for A.M.ADP.P_i and A.M.ADP are thought to differ along the filament axis in such a way that relative filament sliding in the direction appropriate for sarcomere shortening moves sequentially toward the free energy minima for A.M.ADP.P_i then A.M.ADP (18). In this way, the binding energy derived from formation of strong bonds between actin and myosin is transformed into vectorial filament motion. This concept is developed later, under CROSSBRIDGE CYCLING IN MUSCLE.

Efficient transduction of chemical energy into mechanical energy in muscle is due to the partitioning of free energy release into specific steps of the cycle, rather than permitting free energy loss at each step. Because the majority of the free energy change occurs during or immediately after the P_i dissociation step, this chemical transition is the one that is coupled in some way to a power-generating conformational change in the actin–myosin complex. The sequential release of P_i and ADP also contributes to efficient mechanochemical energy transduction, because P_i release initiates the formation of stronger bonds between actin and myosin, then slower ADP release ensures that the free energy made available from this interaction is converted into the appropriate conformational change, rather than lost as heat when ATP dissociates the complex. In effect, bound ADP prevents ATP from dissociating the complex before the conversion of binding energy into work is complete. Progress toward understanding the nature of the work performing conformational change, hypothesized to be a rotation of the crossbridge (45), is discussed later, under Atomic STRUCTURE OF ACTIN AND MYOSIN.

Cardiac versus Skeletal Actomyosin ATPase

The same pathway of ATP hydrolysis occurs with cardiac actomyosin. There are two main isotypes of myosin heavy chains in cardiac tissues, α and β, which form homodimers V_1 (αα) and V_3 (ββ) in cardiac thick filaments. α-Myosin S1 ATPase is 2–3 fold faster than β-myosin S1 ATPase (74), even though their sequence homology is 93% (27). Comparative studies have focused mostly on identifying differences between fast skeletal, β-cardiac and smooth muscle myosin S1. The rank order of actomyosin S1 ATPase rates is fast skeletal (10 sec^{-1}) > β-cardiac (2 sec^{-1}) > smooth (0.2 sec^{-1}) (82). Several steps in the actomyosin ATPase cycle differ quantitatively when β-cardiac and fast skeletal actomyosin S1 are compared. ATP-induced detachment has been shown to be slower by about 2–3 fold in β-cardiac than in fast skeletal (rabbit psoas muscle) actomyosin S1. The apparent rate of binding of myosin S1.ATP to actin is also slower with β-myosin (86). This has been interpreted as being due to slower P_i release, because P_i release is required for tight binding of myosin S1.ATP to actin. The association constant for ADP binding was found to be an order of magnitude greater in cardiac muscle than in fast skeletal muscle due in large part to an order of magnitude slower ADP dissociation rate constant (86). Other steps are similar between β-cardiac myosin and fast skeletal myosin, including the association constant for actin and unliganded myosin, and the ATP cleavage step. The implication of observed differences in terms of reaction speed is that the overall steady-state ATPase rate for β-cardiac actomyosin is slower by 5–10-fold, largely because of slower release of both P_i and ADP.

In terms of free energy partitioning, the A.M.ADP complex in cardiac actomyosin S1 is about four-fold more stable energetically than the same complex in fast skeletal actomyosin S1 (86). This means that in cardiac muscle there is less free energy available during ADP dissociation, but probably more free energy released in the overall A.M.ADP.P_i to A.M.ADP transition (A.M.ADP.P_i to A.M.′ADP to A.M.ADP). Thus, energetically the possibility exists that the transduction of chemical energy into work is more efficient (or into force is more economic) for cardiac muscle than for fast twitch skeletal muscle in part because ADP binds more tightly and dissociates more slowly.

THE CROSSBRIDGE CYCLE IN MUSCLE

In muscle fibers, actin and myosin are organized into arrays of filaments, an arrangement that alters the actin–myosin interaction in several ways. The effective actin concentration is fixed in fibers, the number of possible orientations between actin and myosin is restricted, and most importantly, some of the free energy released by ATP hydrolysis can be harnessed to do work by moving the filaments against a load. The latter process of coupling a chemical free energy change with mechanical events is expected to alter the energetics and kinetics of specific steps in the ATPase cycle (18,

34). Consider a reversible state transition that results in a force (F) applied to the filaments, as shown in Scheme 4, where A is a non-force state with basic free

Scheme 4

$$A \underset{k_-}{\overset{k_+}{\rightleftharpoons}} B$$

energy G_A^{chem}, and B is a force-generating state. If the force in B is approximated by a Hookean spring (F α displacement) then the basic free energy of B will depend upon force according to:

$$G_B = G_B^{chem} + \int F(x)dx \quad \text{with } F(x) = \kappa x$$

and

$$G_B = G_B^{chem} + \frac{\kappa x^2}{2}$$

where G_B^{chem} is the chemical component and $\kappa x^2/2$ is the mechanical component of the basic free energy content of B; x is the displacement of a spring-like element from its mechanical free energy minimum (Fig. 6–3 and 6–4), and κ is the spring constant or stiffness. The equilibrium constant, K_{AB}, and the rate constants, k_+/k_-, for the A to B transition will depend on the basic free energy change according to:

$$\frac{k_+}{k_-} = K_{AB} = \frac{\exp(\Delta G_{AB})}{RT} = \frac{\exp(G_B^{chem} + \kappa x^2/2 - G_A^{chem})}{RT}$$

The result is that the position of the equilibrium between states A and B will depend on the displacement (x) of B from its mechanical free energy minimum. The kinetics of the transition will also be altered as a result of this mechanical influence; either the reverse rate constant (k_-) will be faster, the forward rate constant (k_+) will be slower, or both. By contrast, in studies of actomyosin in solution, the proteins are always at their mechanical free energy minima so there are no mechanical influences on rates or equilibria (Figs. 6–3 and 6–4).

Energy Transduction and Muscle Mechanics

When muscles contract, the rate of shortening depends on the external load on the muscle in a predictable way defined by the load–velocity or force–velocity relationship (Fig. 6–5). Because free energy transduction involves converting chemical energy into work (work = force × distance) the rate of work output (or power where power = force × velocity = work/time) approaches zero at the extremes of the curve (force=0 or distance=0) and reaches a maximum at about ⅓ of maximum force and about ⅓ of maximum shortening

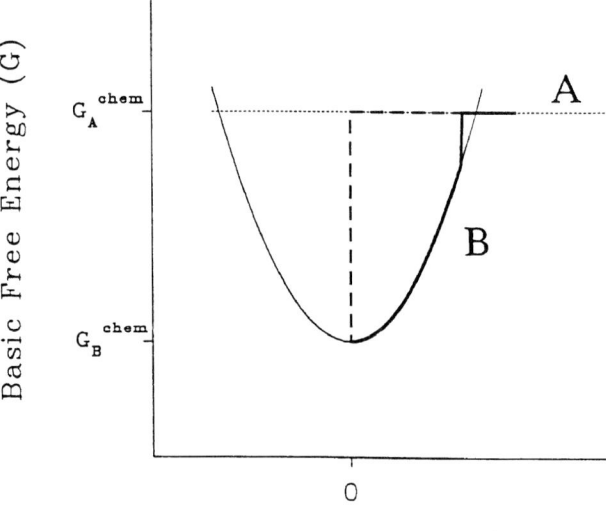

FIG. 6–3. Transduction of chemical free energy into a mechanical process for a simple one step reaction. State A is a non-force generating state so its basic free energy (G_A^{chem}) is independent of displacement. State B is a force generating state whose force is linearly related to displacement (F = κx) and whose mechanical free energy is parabolically related to displacement ($G_B^{mech} = \kappa x^2/2$). The *dashed line* indicates a pathway where all of the free energy is lost as heat and no work is done (as for isolated proteins in solution). The equilibrium constant for the A to B transition, K_{AB}, would be large for the dashed pathway and the reaction would not be readily reversible. The A to B transition can be used to drive a vectorial mechanical process if A is converted to B at some displacement away from the free energy minimum of B (G_B^{chem}; where $G_B^{mech} = 0$). The *heavy line* indicates the pathway for an A to B transition where free energy is efficiently transformed into external work. If after the A to B transition the displacement toward x = 0 were prevented, then the equilibrium constant, K_{AB}, would be small and the reaction would be readily reversible.

velocity (Fig. 6–5). Efficiency of energy transduction is defined as the rate of work output divided by the rate of ATP hydrolysis, and efficiency peaks at about 40%–50% efficiency at intermediate forces and velocities. Efficiency approaches zero at the extremes of force and velocity (49, 112). Efficiency is zero for an isometric contraction because velocity and work are zero, but ATP is still hydrolyzed at a measurable rate. The ratio of isometric force to ATPase rate is called *economy*, which is an index of how much isometric force is achieved at a given level of ATP consumption. The reciprocal of economy is called *tension cost*, which is how much ATP hydrolysis is required to sustain a certain level of isometric tension. The generalization has

shortening velocity (75). Smooth muscle is a highly economical muscle type, optimized for sustained contractile activity, whereas fast muscles optimized for sound production trade force for speed and are energetically costly to operate (81).

By employing heat measurements, Fenn (20) was the first to demonstrate that muscle possesses a fundamental property that enables it to adjust its energy cost to prevailing mechanical conditions. Thus, an important energetic distinction between shortening muscle and isometric muscle is that energy liberation is greater in shortening muscle whether measured as heat + work or as ATPase activity (55). The precise molecular mechanism of this property of muscle remains to be elucidated, but it indicates that rates of energy liberating reactions in the actomyosin interaction cycle are dependent on load. The force–velocity relationship illustrates how rates of mechanical transitions that govern shortening are dependent on load. Further evidence for load-dependent crossbridge cycling comes from mechanical stiffness measurements, which show that the number of strongly bound crossbridges is reduced by three-fold in muscle shortening against no load compared to an isometric contraction (25, 50). Thus, load appears to alter (increase) the fraction of cycle time each crossbridge spends in strongly bound states. In the

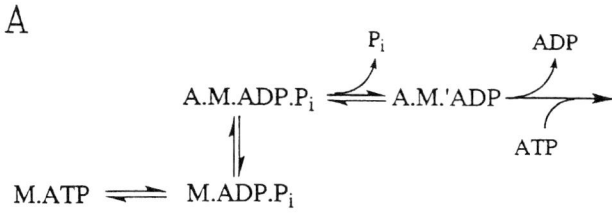

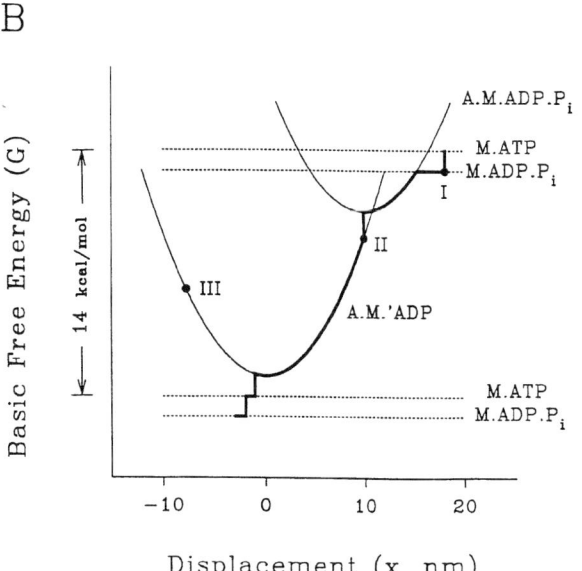

FIG. 6–4. *A*: A simplified chemical pathway for crossbridges undergoing attachment, force generation, and filament sliding in muscle. Two detached states, M.ATP and M.ADP.P$_i$, and two attached states, A.M.ADP.P$_i$ and A.M.'ADP, from Scheme 3 are shown. *B*: Free energy diagram for the two detached x-independent states, and the two attached x-dependent states. The *heavy line* represents the pathway for crossbridges performing work as they move through the crossbridge cycle. Vertical steps indicate heat loss; movement along x indicates external work. During isometric contraction, movement along x is prevented so crossbridges become mechanically trapped near position II. These crossbridges would be readily reversible back to A.M.ADP.P$_i$, M.ADP.P$_i$ and M.ATP (for instance in the presence of high P$_i$) because of the high free energy content of A.M.'ADP at position II. However, after A.M.'ADP reaches its free energy minimum due to filament sliding or because the proteins are not constrained within the filament (i.e. for ATPase in solution), the A.M.'ADP to A.M.ADP.P$_i$ transition is much less readily reversed. Vectorial force generation and filament sliding require attachment of crossbridges away from their free energy minima. For example, mechanical free energy minima for A.M.ADP.P$_i$ and A.M.'ADP must be displaced relative to one another in the direction appropriate for shortening.

been made that the maximum efficiency of muscle contraction that reflects the optimal conversion of chemical energy into work does not vary dramatically for different muscle types (75). By contrast, the economy of muscle contraction does vary widely among muscle types and is approximately inversely related to muscle

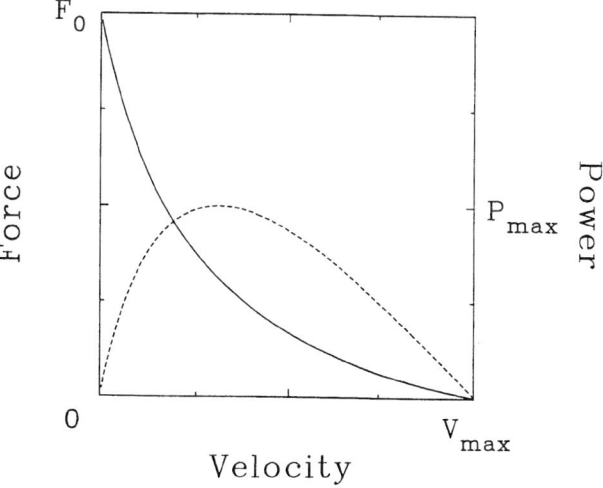

FIG. 6–5. An idealized force-velocity relationship (*solid line*) derived from the normalized Hill equation: $V/V_{max} = (1-F/F_o)/(1+(F/F_o)(F_o/\alpha))$. This equation describes the observed inverse relationship between force (or load) and velocity with a characteristic curvature (F_o/α) for each fiber type. The left extreme of the curve is dominated by the action of positively strained crossbridges, the right side by detachment of negatively strained crossbridges, and the middle by dynamic mixtures of positively and negatively strained cycling bridges. A power-load relationship (*dashed line*) derived from the idealized forced-velocity data shows maximum power at $0.3V_{max}$. The power-load curve and efficiency also depend upon the F_o/α factor for a given fiber type (49, 112).

terminology of molecular motors, this fraction is called the *duty ratio*, and so load appears to increase the duty ratio.

A classical explanation of the load dependence of crossbridge cycling comes from the 1957 model of A. F. Huxley (40). Huxley speculated that in an isometric muscle, crossbridges are displaced from their equilibrium in such a way as to have a strain favoring productive filament sliding (i.e. positively strained crossbridges) (Fig. 6–6). In isotonic contractions when the filaments are allowed to slide, some crossbridges would be dragged beyond their equilibrium positions (free energy minimum) into positions that would impede productive filament sliding (i.e. negatively strained crossbridges); (Fig. 6–6). He further postulated that the detachment rate of positively strained crossbridges was considerably slower than detachment of negatively strained crossbridges. In an unloaded muscle, a dynamic equilibrium would then arise between positively strained and negatively strained bridges, and the rate of sliding would be limited by the detachment rate of negatively strained bridges that oppose sliding. In this view, load-dependent changes in the number of strongly bound crossbridges (and possibly load-dependent changes in energy liberation) are due to strain-dependent differences in rates of crossbridge detachment.

How a crossbridge senses strain is an interesting and unresolved question. A popular view is that a spring-like elastic element is present near the neck of myosin S1 (Fig. 6–6), which becomes stretched as a consequence of head rotation if the filaments are held fixed (42). In this way crossbridges with varying amounts of displacement of their elastic elements will experience different amounts of strain. Also, because stretching the spring requires internal work, inclusion of an elastic element helps to visualize how free energy might be stored during isometric contraction, then be released when the filaments are permitted to slide.

It should be clear from the above discussion that a broad spectrum of crossbridges bearing different levels of positive and negative strain will exist in shortening muscle. Crossbridge strain may also be heterogeneous in isometric muscle, because in vertebrate skeletal and cardiac muscles the periodicity of myosin heads along the thick filament does not match that of actin monomers in the thin filament. [Specifically, the myosin filament has a spacing between neighboring monomers of 14.5 nm and a helical pitch of 42.9 nm, whereas actin monomers are separated by 5 nm and have a helical pitch of 37 nm (4)]. Thus, all crossbridges may not enter the crossbridge cycle in the same orientation relative to an actin partner. One consequence of this is that measurements of ensemble crossbridge properties in isometric fibers may be heterogeneous,

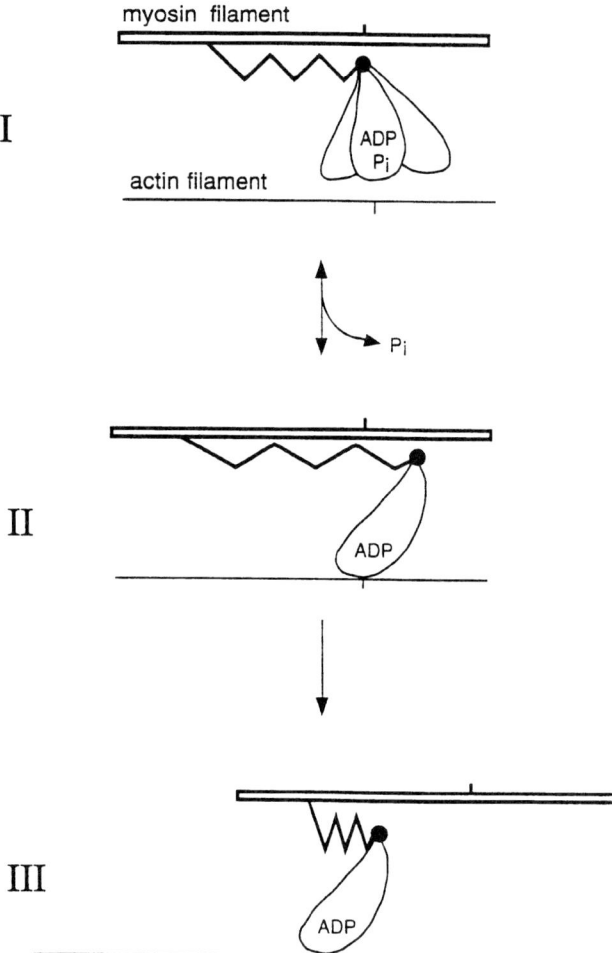

FIG. 6–6. Schematic representation of crossbridges in three states. I. Detached or weakly attached. In this state the crossbridge can assume many distinct orientations due to a flexible hinge where an elastic spring element attaches to the globular head. II. Strongly attached positively strained. This state would occur during isometric contraction after attachment, P_i release, and rotation of the crossbridge to stretch the spring. III. If the filaments are released the spring will recoil causing filament displacement. This state would occur if filaments were to slide beyond the mechanical equilibrium position to a position where the spring is compressed. This is a negatively strained crossbridge that impedes further sliding. Approximate locations of I–III on the free energy diagram are given in Figure 6–4B.

as observed with ^{18}O exchange (108). Similarly, differential effects of P_i on fiber ATPase and isometric force have been attributed to a non-uniform distribution of strain among attached crossbridges (11). There are other complications that confound analyses of crossbridge properties in muscle fibers. One is that individual crossbridges are not intrinsically synchronized in the cycle, but at any given moment there exists a broad distribution of states. Another complication is that each native myosin molecule is comprised of two crossbridge heads, and it is unclear whether each head of the pair acts independently to produce force or whether the mechanochemical status of one influences the other.

Transient Kinetics in Fibers Using Caged Compounds

In order to test the actomyosin S1 ATPase mechanism in muscle fibers, it has been useful to have caged nucleotides and caged phosphate compounds that afford rapid perturbation of different chemical steps in the cycle (38). Caged compounds are a class of synthetic molecules designed to be converted rapidly to specific biological molecules by brief flashes of near-ultraviolet light. Caged compounds permit rapid and uniform elevation of small molecules like ATP, Ca^{2+}, and phosphate within the fiber lattice, which effectively overcomes diffusional delays inherent in bath application of these agents. Caged Ca^{2+} and caged phosphate compounds have the general structure and photolysis reactions shown in Figure 6–7.

Analysis of Specific Steps

ATP Binding and Detachment. Caged ATP has been useful in studies of muscle contraction in skinned fibers, because it permits initiation of the crossbridge cycle starting from rigor (no ATP) with a time resolution dictated by the photochemical conversion of caged ATP to ATP. This conversion requires about 5 ms (107), or 0.1 ms for a newer version of caged ATP (96), and is therefore much faster than "waiting" for ATP to diffuse into the fiber interior from the bathing solution. Use of caged ATP to initiate crossbridge cycling from the rigor state also creates (at least initially) a population of synchronized crossbridges. It also permits crossbridge strain to be altered by either stretching or releasing the fiber prior to photogeneration of ATP (28). Photorelease of ATP within rigor fibers has shown that ATP binding and detachment of crossbridges from the A.M state is rapid, as predicted by the minimum actomyosin ATPase model. In fact, ATP binding and detachment occur by an apparent bimolecular process with a rate constant of 10^5–10^6 M^{-1} s^{-1} (28). This means that at a normal physiological ATP concentration of 5 mM, the detachment process would have a rate constant of 500–5000 s^{-1} (5×10^{-3} M times 10^5 M^{-1} s^{-1} = 500 $^{-1}$) which translates to a half-time of 0.1–1 ms (ln 2/500 s^{-1}) and would be too fast to limit the rate of ATP hydrolysis or many mechanical processes in muscle. It also indicates that the so-called ternary complex, A.M.ATP, has a very short lifetime (0.1–1 ms) and probably does not build up to a significant extent during isometric muscle contraction. These rate constants for ATP-induced detachment of rigor bridges are not highly sensitive to crossbridge strain introduced by stretching the fiber and are in fact similar to those measured with isolated actin and myosin (28). This suggests that the filament organization and load only modestly influence ATP binding and subsequent detachment steps, and that load must affect other steps in the cycle. This seems incompatible at first glance with A. F. Huxley's idea that crossbridge detachment is a major strain-dependent step in the cycle. However, what limits the rate of detachment of cycling crossbridges probably occurs before ATP binding (e.g. closer to ADP dissociation). It is the nature of these pre-ATP binding steps that remain to be defined and characterized in terms of their rates, their dependencies on crossbridge strain, and their potential role as sites of regulation.

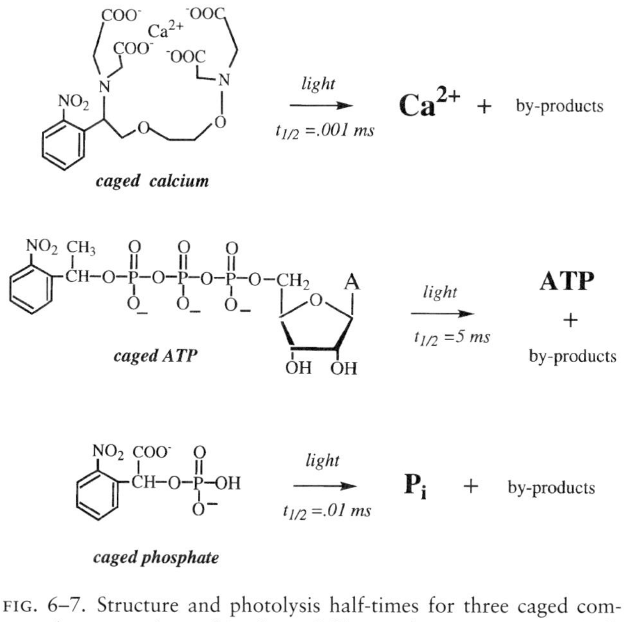

ATP Cleavage. According to the minimum actomyosin ATPase model in Scheme 3, before reattachment can occur for those crossbridges detached by ATP, the bound ATP must be hydrolyzed to bound ADP+P_i. Experiments with radiolabeled caged ATP have demonstrated that a rapid phase of ATP cleavage occurs in fibers that is analogous to the phosphate burst seen with myosin S1 and actomyosin S1 in solution (21, 22). The rate constant for this process has been estimated to be 60 s^{-1} both for relaxed fibers and fibers at full Ca^{2+} activation. This indicates that the cleavage step takes place on detached crossbridges and is fast ($t_{1/2}$ = 10 ms) for both actomyosin and myosin in fibers. After the burst phase, the steady state rate of ATP hydrolysis is 2 s^{-1} per myosin head (2 moles P_i or ADP formed/

FIG. 6–7. Structure and photolysis half-times for three caged compounds commonly used in skinned fiber studies. Approximate half-times are listed for the rate-limiting photochemical reactions under near physiological conditions, pH 7, 21°C. The version of caged Ca^{2+} illustrated is nitrophenyl EGTA (20).

mole myosin head/s) during Ca^{2+} activation and at least 10-fold slower in relaxed fibers. It should be re-emphasized that the P_i or ADP burst is not a physiological phenomenon because activation of fibers by a jump in ATP concentration does not mimic a physiological situation. The burst is simply an indication that ATP binding, crossbridge detachment, and ATP cleavage are all rapid compared to product release. Overall, the data are consistent with product release steps being responsible for limiting the steady-state rate of ATP hydrolysis in muscle fibers.

P_i Dissociation and Force Generation. When muscle fibers in rigor are activated by photorelease of ATP, rigor bridges initially detach. If physiological levels of Ca^{2+} are present to activate the regulatory system, crossbridges reattach in the A.M.ADP.P_i state, and active force develops. Active force development probably involves dissociation of P_i from the A.M.ADP.P_i complex. Evidence for this comes from inclusion of high P_i (10 mM) in the medium, which increases the rate and decreases the extent of force development (2, 14, 106). Similarly, if relaxed skinned fibers are stimulated to contract by photorelease of Ca^{2+} from caged Ca^{2+} (Fig. 6–8), the rate and extent of force development are altered by inclusion of 10 mM P_i in the solution bathing the fiber (Fig. 6–8A). Both of these observations are compatible with the model in Scheme 5, in which a reversible

Scheme 5

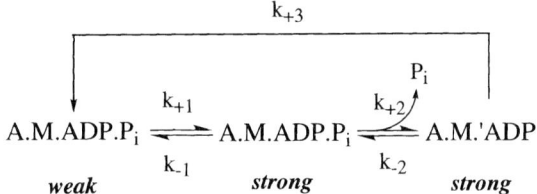

force-generating step is coupled to a reversible P_i dissociation step. This is where the ATPase cycle in muscle fibers begins to differ significantly from that measured with isolated soluble actomyosin. For example, in solution, P_i is a weak inhibitor of ATPase because it has a low affinity for isolated actomyosin (k_{-1} and/or k_{-2} values are very small). In contracting muscle, P_i binds with higher affinity to the nucleotide site (k_{-1} and/or k_{-2} are much larger). These differences in myosin P_i affinity in solution versus in muscle fibers have been clearly established by monitoring myosin catalyzed isotope exchange between labeled P_i and ATP (or water) (7, 108). A consequence of these differences in P_i affinity is that the P_i release step is much more reversible in muscle, consistent with the fact that high P_i concentrations can decrease active force development, presumably by shifting the force-generating equilib-

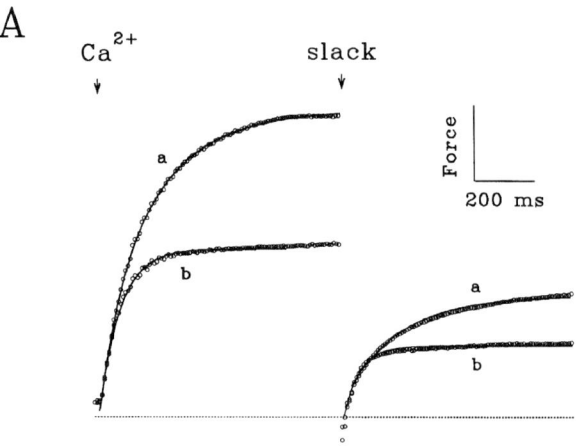

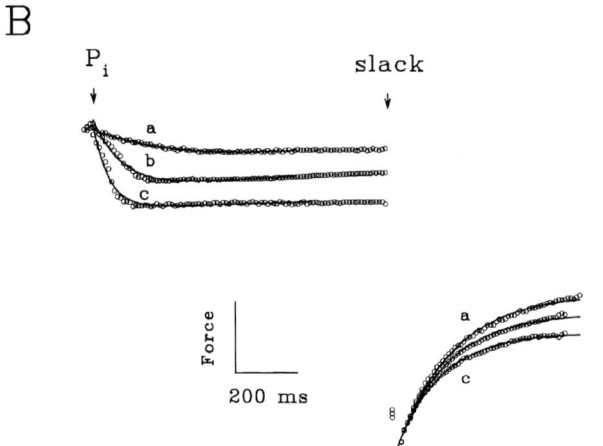

FIG. 6–8. Close coupling between force generation and P_i release in skinned cardiac myocytes. A: Isometric force development after photochemical elevation of free Ca^{2+} within the filament lattice. The time course prior to "slack" shows that both the rate and extent of force development were altered by the presence of 10 mM added P_i (b) compared to no added P_i (a). P_i depressed the amplitude of the force response and accelerated the rate of approach to the final amplitude, consistent with Scheme 4. B: A complimentary experiment in which P_i was produced rapidly within isometric Ca^{2+}-activated myocytes. Increasing concentrations of photoreleased P_i, (a) 0.5 mM P_i, (b) 1 mM P_i and (c) 2.7 mM P_i, caused both a greater and more rapid depression of isometric force, consistent with Scheme 4. For comparison, P_i at 0.5 to 10 mM has no effect on the ATPase of isolated actomyosin. Data from (2) with permission.

rium toward weak binding states. One possible explanation for these differences in reversibility is that in muscle some of the free energy change associated with P_i dissociation is stored mechanically in the A.M'.ADPstate (Fig. 6–3 and 6–4), possibly in an elastic element (Fig. 6–6). For myosin in solution, the lack of a filament organization does not allow released chemical free energy to be stored mechanically, so the A.M'.ADP states in solution do not have the same high energy conformation and P_i binding properties as those in muscle fibers.

Further evidence for a close association between force generation and P_i release comes from photorelease of P_i within actively contracting fibers (Figure 6–8B). A rapid photochemical jump in P_i produces a decrease in force with an observed rate constant and an amplitude that increase with P_i concentration (2, 14, 106). The dependence of these parameters on P_i concentration is most compatible with a reversible P_i release process, and the data permit rate constants to be derived for the model given in Scheme 5. The rate constants are similar to those obtained from caged ATP tension transients at full Ca^{2+} activation or caged Ca^{2+} tension transients in the presence of various concentrations of P_i. Moreover, these rate constants are considerably larger than the steady-state ATPase rate. If one assumes that most crossbridges are bound during isometric muscle contraction (i.e. the duty cycle is high, ≥50% of all crossbridges are bound and generating force), then rapid P_i release and slow ATPase rates suggest that the slowest steps in the cycle occur after P_i dissociation. This conclusion also implies that ADP-bound states, like A.M'.ADP and A.M.ADP, build up during isometric contraction, and probably represent crossbridge states that generate force on the filaments (68). A reliable number for the proportion of crossbridges participating in force generation during isometric contraction (the isometric duty ratio) remains to be established; values as low as 15% have been obtained from in vitro motility measurements (91) and as high as 70%–90% from stiffness and X-ray diffraction (25, 43, 112).

ADP Dissociation. Direct measurements of ADP dissociation from actively cycling crossbridges have yet to be accomplished. Most information about the ADP dissociation process has been obtained indirectly. For example, isotope exchange has been carried out in muscle fibers to examine the reversibility of different steps. As observed in actomyosin ATPase in solution, ^{32}P-labeled P_i becomes incorporated into ATP if the fibers are actively contracting in the presence of ATP and Ca^{2+} (7). This suggests the presence of an A.M.'ADP state that can bind labeled P_i at the active site and reform ATP by reversal of ATP cleavage. Interestingly, it was found that P_i bound tighter and isotope exchange was faster in isometrically contracting fibers than in actomyosin ATPase in solution. This was taken as evidence that more crossbridges were in the A.M.'ADP state and possibly in a different conformation in muscle fibers due to the effects of strain on P_i dissociation, ADP dissociation, or isomerizations near these steps (7). No incorporation of labeled P_i into ATP was observed in rigor fibers in the presence of ADP (A.M + ADP + P_i), consistent with the idea that a large free energy change occurs between A.M'.ADP and A.M.ADP, which makes this step effectively irreversible (7). Again, its likely that this large free energy change associated with product release is harnessed for the purpose of force generation.

Attempts to determine the ADP release rate by use of caged compounds have taken two approaches. Photorelease of ADP in isometrically contracting fibers to reverse ADP dissociation identified an *increase* in force, which is due to MgADP binding to nucleotide-free crossbridges (61). If the power stroke was linked to crossbridge flux through the ADP release step, one would expect a reversal of the power stroke and a *decrease* in force on binding ADP. The observed increase of force and the kinetics of the force rise are consistent with ADP binding and release occurring at the end of the power stroke. At this point most of the free energy of ATP hydrolysis would have been used or lost, which makes reversal into active force-generating states by ADP binding energetically improbable. Therefore, the force increase caused by ADP appears to be due to competition between ADP and ATP at the end of the cycle. Bound ADP prevents detachment by ATP, resulting in crossbridges being detained in the A.M.ADP state and net accumulation of states that contribute to force.

Given the competition between ADP and ATP for binding rigor crossbridges, the influence of ADP on caged ATP tension transients has been used to probe ADP dissociation kinetics (13). ADP slows relaxation from rigor following caged ATP photolysis because ADP must dissociate before ATP can bind and detach crossbridges. The rate constant for this process has been estimated to be 20 s^{-1} for positively strained crossbridges (those predominating in isometric muscle) and 6–8 times faster for negatively strained crossbridges (those that would be significantly populated in shortening muscle) (Fig. 6–6). Thus, some of the difference in ATPase rates in isometric versus shortening muscle may be due to strain dependence of ADP dissociation. However, the rate constants are not completely consistent with ADP dissociation being the limiting step in the cycle, as 20 s^{-1} is faster than the 2 s^{-1} per myosin head turnover rate for ATPase and 150 s^{-1} is somewhat too slow to permit maximal unloaded shortening of fibers, but the change in rate constants with changes in strain are substantial and in the appropriate direction (13).

An alternative kinetic method, referred to here as *sinusoidal analysis*, has been used to characterize specific steps in the crossbridge cycle (114). With sinusoidal analysis, the force response of muscle fibers subjected to small length oscillations applied over a range of frequencies provides information regarding mechanical crossbridge transitions. When used in conjunction with perturbation of specific chemical steps by variations in P_i, ADP, and ATP, sinusoidal analysis has led to a fairly complete mechanochemical model of the crossbridge cycle (114). An important conclusion from these studies is that an isomerization just prior to ADP dissociation is the slowest step in the cycle; unfortunately this method also does not measure this step directly. It will be necessary in the future to measure the isomerization that controls ADP dissociation directly (e.g. by use of fluorescent ADP analogues or ADP indicators) to determine its kinetic properties, temperature dependence, and sensitivity to strain to more rigorously test current crossbridge models. Important questions concerning ADP-bound states remain: Does ADP dissociation play a direct role in the power stroke? Is ADP dissociation (or isomerizations nearby) the slowest step(s) in the cycle? Are these steps faster during muscle shortening and do they account for the apparent strain dependencies of crossbridge cycling rate and ATP hydrolysis rate?

Cardiac Muscle

Transient kinetic measurements have not been carried out as extensively in cardiac fibers as in skeletal fibers. This is in part because of increased series elastic compliance in multicellular preparations such as papillary and trabecular muscles. Internal shortening and sarcomere non-uniformity can be significant, and can create problems in interpretation of tension transients. Recent technical advances, including the use of single cardiac myocytes which eliminates compliance between cells, and better attachment procedures, have improved the quality of mechanical measurements in cardiac tissues. Investigations with caged ATP show that the rate of detachment of rigor bridges by ATP is an order of magnitude slower in cardiac muscle than in fast skeletal muscle (6, 65). Also, ADP binds more tightly to cardiac crossbridges in rigor (66), which is consistent with the A.M.ADP state being more energetically stable in cardiac muscle than in fast twitch skeletal muscle.

Sinusoidal analysis of cardiac trabeculae has identified several differences in the crossbridge cycle in fast skeletal versus cardiac muscle (52). ATP binds more tightly and P_i binds more weakly in cardiac muscle. Moreover, two critical steps, the force-generating step and the step that limits the overall ATPase and cycling rates, are an order of magnitude slower in cardiac muscle. Thus, nucleotide (ATP or ADP) binding is more favorable in cardiac muscle and P_i binding is less favorable. Free energy partitioning in cardiac muscle is such that more free energy is available (released) when ATP binds and when P_i dissociates, but less is available when ADP dissociates. Experiments with caged phosphate also show a lower P_i binding affinity in cardiac muscle and a slower force-generating transition coupled to P_i dissociation (2). Overall, the mechanical transitions that are slower in cardiac muscle than in fast skeletal muscle are the rate of force development and the velocity of shortening. These are most likely the result of slower conformational changes in cardiac myosin that control rates of P_i dissociation and ADP dissociation, respectively.

IN VITRO MOTILITY

The in vitro motility assay, introduced by Spudich and colleagues in the 1980s, has revolutionized our understanding of the molecular basis of movement mediated by molecular motors (84, 91). This assay is based on measurements of the movement of fluorescent actin filaments over myosin molecules immobilized on a glass surface. Because it is an assessment of the mechanical function of isolated myosin it has been an ideal assay to exploit site-directed mutagenesis and protein domain analysis afforded by molecular biology. It also represents a simple way to compare actomyosin ATPase rates, shortening velocity, and force-generating capability for a variety of myosin isotypes under the same conditions. As found in muscle (5), the velocity of filament sliding correlates with the ATPase rate when smooth, β-cardiac, α-cardiac, and fast skeletal myosins are compared. However, experiments where domains of skeletal and cardiac myosins were interchanged reveal an uncoupling of the ATPase rate and the filament sliding rate (102), showing that this correlation is not absolute. Specifically, a loop domain near the actin site (loop 2) was found to be responsible for conferring skeletal-type or cardiac-type ATPase activity, but shortening velocity was determined by the catalytic domain of myosin S1 (102). Thus shortening velocity and ATPase rate are not required to be tightly coupled, and the observed correlation in muscle suggests that these rates are tuned in parallel to serve specific purposes such as rapid shortening velocity, high power output, or high economy.

Elementary mechanical transitions have recently been observed for single myosin molecules in vitro by use of optical traps (23, 32, 71, 88). Optical traps are devices that use forces available in focused laser light beams to manipulate molecular structures or measure molecular forces (Fig. 6–9). Application of optical traps to studies of isolated myosin revealed unitary events of force and motion produced by individual myosin subfragments (either myosin S1 or heavy meromyosin fragments containing two S1s connected at the neck). These unitary events generated 1–5 pN of force under near isometric conditions, and approximately 11 nm of displacement under unloaded conditions (Fig. 6–9).

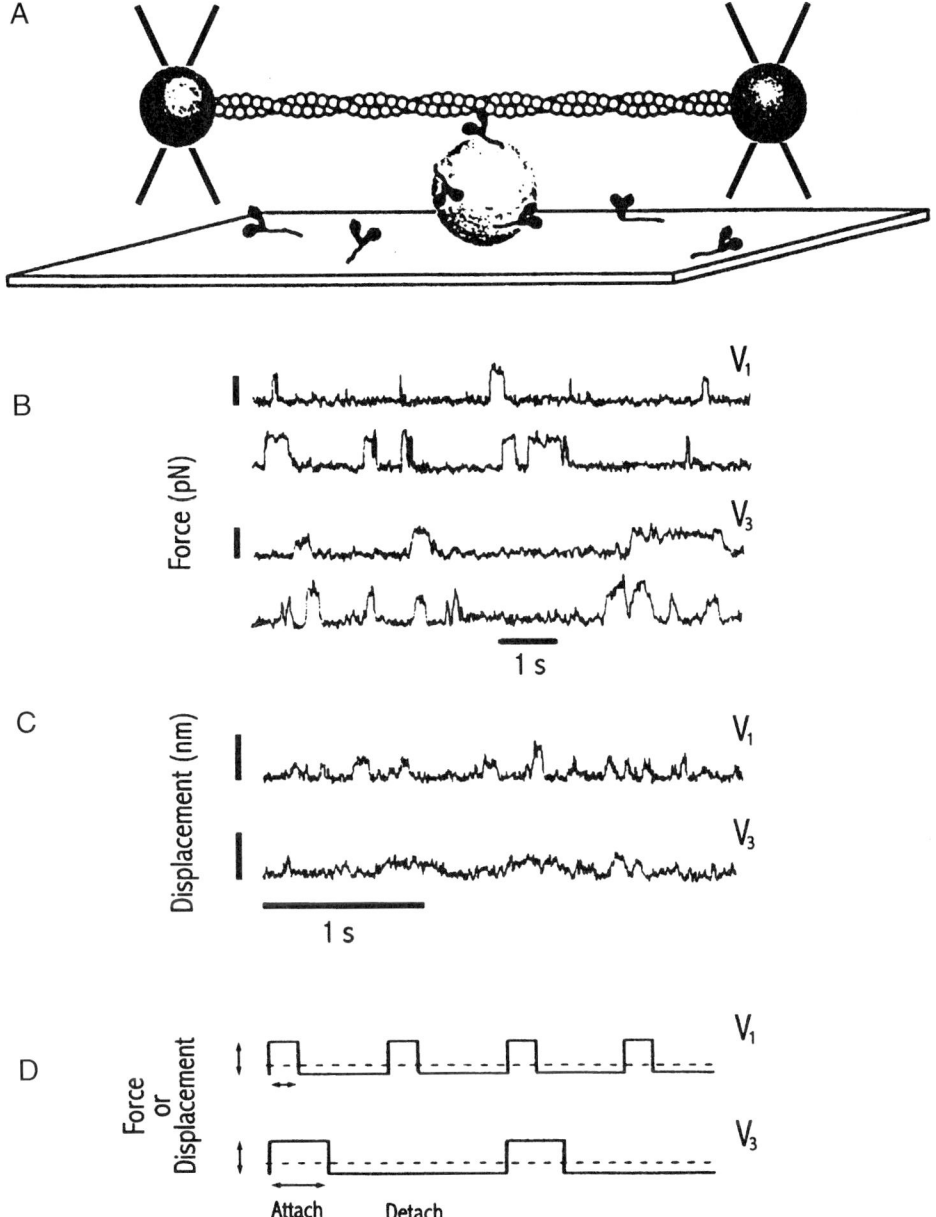

FIG. 6–9. Elementary transitions in single myosin molecules. *A:* Experimental arrangement for optical trap measurements of unitary force and displacement by actomyosin. The actin filament is attached at each end to a bead (dark spheres). Each bead is controlled by a laser trap. The actin filament is lowered onto another bead (white sphere) coated with a low density of myosin molecules. From (23) with permission. *B, C:* Records of force and displacement produced by individual V_1 and V_3 cardiac myosin isoforms. The unitary force and displacements are similar for V_1 and V_3, but V_3 events are prolonged. Verticle scale bars are 2 pN and 20 nm, respectively. [From (91) with permission.] *D:* Schematic of unitary events in cardiac myosin. In principle, myosins can differ by amplitude of unitary force or displacement on the y-axis, by mean duration of attached strong binding states, or by duration of detached or weak binding states. Dotted lines illustrate time-averaged force or displacement.

These values are similar to those derived from mechanical measurements of crossbridge populations in muscle fibers (42, 88). Moreover, the duration of unitary isometric events averaged 18 ms, whereas the duration of the elementary displacement events averaged 7 ms. Because the duration of the attached event is directly related to the probability of detachment, these studies reveal an apparent load dependence of crossbridge detachment at the single-molecule level (23).

The in vitro motility assay including single-molecule

force measurements also reveals interesting differences among myosin isoforms. For instance, smooth muscle myosin was shown to generate 3–4 times more time averaged force than fast skeletal myosin (32). By using a laser trap to measure forces produced by single molecules, the latter study showed that the higher force output of smooth muscle myosin is due to a greater duty ratio. That is, smooth muscle myosin spends a greater proportion of time in force generating conformations during each turnover of the cycle rather than in intrinsically generating more unitary force. The situation for cardiac myosin isoforms may be similar (Fig. 6–9). α-Cardiac myosin hydrolyzes ATP and supports actin filament sliding 2–3-fold faster than β-cardiac myosin. Comparison of elementary events with the laser trap technique showed identical unitary forces and displacements, but longer duration events for β-cardiac myosin (92, 104). Whether this observation can be generalized to all myosin isoforms remains to be determined, but the early indication is that myosin isoforms produce a similar unitary force by a similar molecular mechanism. Greater economy of contraction and a higher time-averaged force output can be achieved by a given isoform by populating force-generating conformations for a longer fraction of the duty cycle. The trade-off for the motor is that greater force output is typically accompanied by a slower turnover rate and a reduction in shortening velocity.

A variety of investigations including those using skinned fibers, in vitro motility assays on isolated proteins, and structural analysis of actomyosin are also shedding light on inherited defects associated with cardiac actin–myosin interactions. Identification of natural mutations in myosin has uncovered the underlying cause of some forms of familial hypertrophic cardiomyopathy in humans (56, 79). Correlating the location of these mutations in specific regions of the myosin molecule with defects in function has provided insight into the mechanism of muscle contraction in normal and diseased heart muscle (92).

ATOMIC STRUCTURES OF ACTIN AND MYOSIN

Myosin S1

The crystal structure of myosin S1 from chicken skeletal muscle was reported by Rayment and colleagues in 1993 (76). It revealed a highly asymmetric molecule with a number of recognizable "domains." Two light chains were identified wrapped around an α-helical neck region that extended approximately 10 nm from the globular portion where the nucleotide pocket and actin interaction site reside. The heavy chain was resolved into three segments, a 25K, a 50K and a 20K segment (Fig. 6–10). These segments are connected by disordered loops that are not resolved in the structure, presumably because of their flexibility. In addition to the extended α-helix containing the light chains, the molecule had two deep clefts. One cleft was lined with side chain residues labeled by nucleotide-directed probes, and the other cleft split the actin interaction site into two separate domains (Fig. 6–10). Early models proposed to explain coupling of ATP hydrolysis to crossbridge rotation featured opening and closing of the nucleotide cleft during various states of the crossbridge cycle. This cleft motion was thought to be translated to the light chain binding region, which could then act as a lever arm to displace the myosin filament relative to the actin filament (76).

This model had to be revised when the crystal structure of S1 complexed with nucleotide (ADP plus various phosphate analogues) was solved (24, 33). The nucleotide was located in the expected cleft with the γ-phosphate at the bottom of the pocket. The hydroxyls of ribose protruded out of the mouth of the cleft, free to interact with solvent. However, the dimensions of the cleft and the domains on either side did not appear to change dramatically with nucleotide bound, and this was inconsistent with the original nucleotide site cleft opening and closing model. Perhaps the most interesting observation was that the γ-phosphate was not only at the bottom of the nucleotide pocket, but it also appeared to be at the bottom of the actin interaction site cleft (Fig. 6–10). The γ-phosphate could be "seen" at the base of the actin interaction site and could presumably interact with solvent in that cleft. This observation led Yount and colleagues to suggest that the second cleft provides an escape route for P_i dissociation as well as a means for the nucleotide pocket to communicate with the actin interaction site (113). In this revised view, then, some other conformational change linked to P_i dissociation besides nucleotide cleft opening and closing must be transmitted to the rigid lever arm to accomplish filament sliding on the order of 5–20 nm per cycle.

The idea that the long helical portion of myosin S1 acts as a rigid lever arm stabilized by the binding of two light chains (Fig. 6–10) has been tested with in vitro motility measurements. Both the presence of tightly bound light chains (60, 84, 103), and a 10 nm extended arm (84) are required for rapid filament sliding and force generation in vitro. Remarkably, elongation of the lever and addition of extra light chains further enhances the speed of filament sliding (35, 37). Thus, the rigid lever arm concept proposed by Rayment and colleagues (76, 77) has received considerable experimental support.

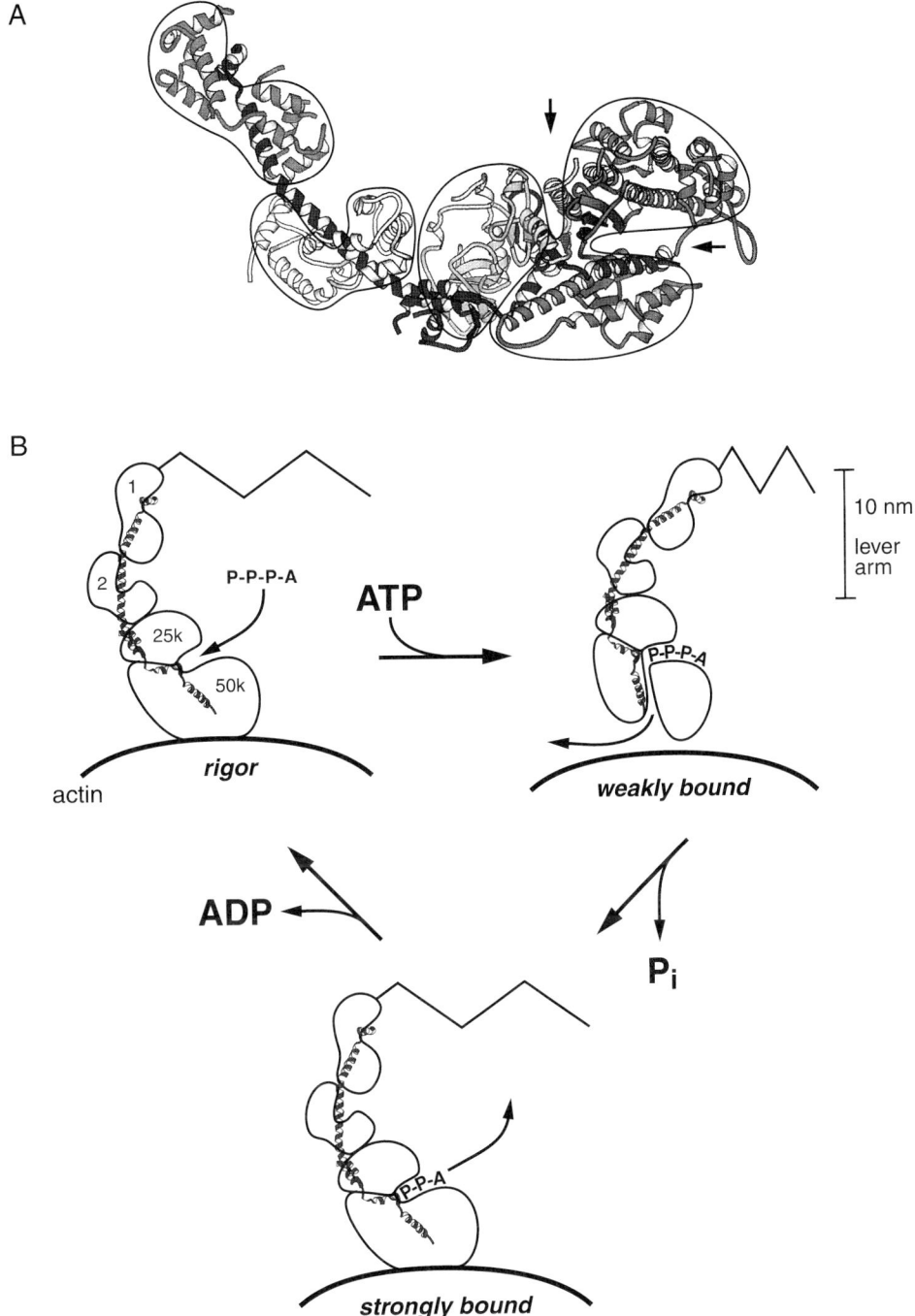

FIG. 6-10. Domains and clefts of myosin S1. *A:* Outlines of major domains are superimposed on a ribbon diagram taken from the crystal structure of chicken myosin S1 (76, 78). Also shown are the nucleotide cleft (*vertical arrow*) and actin site cleft (*horizontal arrow*). *B:* Schematic representation of myosin S1 including 20K (long helix), 25K, 50K, LC_1, LC_2, and an elastic element. In the nucleotide-free state (*left*), the nucleotide site at the 25K–50K interface is open, but the actin interaction site at the 20K–50K interface is closed and S1 is tightly bound to actin. ATP binding in the nucleotide pocket results in large changes in the actin interaction site causing a greatly weakened interaction between myosin S1 and actin (*right*). Dissociation of P_i out of the actin site cleft permits the 20K–50K interface to close and strong bonds between S1 and actin to reform (*bottom*). An appropriate change in the angle of the 10 nm extended arm of the 20K domain, stabilized by light chains, could stretch an elastic element or displace the actin and myosin filaments relative to one another.

Actomyosin

In 1992, Holmes and colleagues reported the structure of G-actin complexed with DNase I (to prevent actin polymerization) (36). They then used this information to obtain high-resolution structures for the actin filament by image reconstruction and low-angle X-ray diffraction. A high-resolution view of the actin–myosin interaction became available when Rayment and colleagues joined forces with Holmes, Milligan, and colleagues to see how myosin might dock onto the actin filament (70, 77, 85). By modeling, they succeeded in docking nucleotide-free myosin with the actin filament by, among other things, closing the cleft in the actin interaction site, allowing the two domains of this site to come together. It now appears that opening and closing of this cleft in the actin interaction site could occur in different states of the crossbridge cycle and could be translated to movement of the extended lever arm (Fig. 6–10). Yount and colleagues have suggested that one of the roles of the γ-phosphate on ATP is to open the actin interaction cleft and promote dissociation of actin and myosin when ATP binds. The γ-phosphate could keep the cleft open even after ATP cleavage, thereby preventing optimal interactions between myosin and actin. When phosphate dissociates out the "back door", this allows much more contact between actin and myosin, which, if thermodynamically favorable, will release free energy. This model provides a very attractive and testable hypothesis that it is the energy of these specific protein–protein interactions that is harnessed for work and force production. One goal then is to determine precisely which domains and which amino acid residues are most important in these free energy–releasing interactions. The precise pathway of phosphate dissociation out the back door also remains to be established.

Comparison of Structural Models to Other Models

In the two-state mechanical models, when ATP or ADP+P_i is bound to the complex myosin is "weakly bound" to actin. In the structural model, this is so because the actin site cleft is open. After P_i dissociation and cleft closure, myosin would be "strongly bound" to actin. For actomyosin ATPase in solution and in fibers, there is good evidence that P_i dissociates before ADP (12, 99). The structural model accommodates this observation particularly well, by revealing how ATP could enter the nucleotide cleft with the γ-phosphate leading, and then P_i could exit the nucleotide pocket through the actin site cleft without disturbing the binding of ADP. Without this escape route, it is not clear how P_i would dissociate before ADP. Thus, the structural model shows how P_i dissociation might gate the fundamental conformational change that leads to strong actin–myosin interactions and force generation.

A major thrust in muscle research has been to identify the nature of the conformational change associated with the working stroke of the crossbridge. Low-angle X-ray diffraction has been used with high time resolution to demonstrate that the crossbridge (14.5 reflection) moves along the filament axis relative to actin during the power stroke (47). This is consistent with but does not prove that the power stroke involves a change in angle of the crossbridge head relative to the actin filament. Orientation-sensitive probes such as fluorophores attached to myosin light chains reveal motions consistent with rotation of the extended arm of myosin relative to the filament axis (48), although the changes are considerably smaller than the expected 45° angle change. In reconstructed electron microscopic (EM) images of actin filaments decorated with myosin S1, a significant difference has been observed in the angle of the light chain region of bound myosin S1 compared to bound myosin S1.ADP (111). This is also generally supportive of the notion that crossbridge rotation occurs during the power stroke. However, in these studies differences in binding angles for myosin S1.ADP and myosin S1 suggest that rotation occurs *during or after* ADP release, although thermodynamic considerations indicate that A.M(S1).ADP represents a low-energy conformation thought to be like A.M(S1) near the end of the power stroke. The idea that ADP binding and/or disssociation plays a key role in the force-generating power stroke is gaining momentum, however (111, 109).

Other orientation-sensitive probes such as spin labels attached to a reactive sulfhydryl (SH1) on myosin heavy chain have likewise provided important information (97). In relaxed muscle fibers, two different, highly disordered conformations are observed, presumably representing M.ATP and M.ADP.P_i in rapid equilibrium with their attached counterparts. In isometrically contracting muscle, these two disordered conformations remain, but a new highly ordered population (20%–30% of the total signal) is observed. The disordered populations probably represent weakly attached crossbridges and the ordered population strongly attached crossbridges (Fig. 6–6). The data are consistent with a minimal interaction between actin and myosin that is non-stereospecific and therefore disordered when the γ-phosphate is present. When the γ-phosphate is allowed to dissociate, such as during steady state contraction, a much more extensive interaction occurs that is stereospecific and ordered. By attaching spin probes to light chains, the magnitude of the angle change associated with this transition has recently been estimated to be 36° (3).

The chemical nature of interactions between actin and myosin in the different states is not yet well defined. The weakly bound state is highly sensitive to ionic strength suggestive of ionic interactions, which can be non-stereospecific. The change that occurs on dissociation of P_i is stereospecific, not highly ionic strength dependent, and releases free energy. A good candidate for the strong binding interaction would be a series of complementary hydrophobic interactions between two surfaces of substantial area. Indeed, the actin site cleft is lined with potentially complementary hydrophobic residues, and the actin myosin interaction for nucleotide-free S1 has considerable hydrophobic character (69). The temperature dependence of different transitions in the crossbridge cycle suggests a large entropy change following P_i release, which is consistent with displacement of water from hydrophobic surfaces (114). The most complete structural model to date indicates that the actin–myosin interface in rigor contains a large hydrophobic surface surrounded on three sides by flexible surface loops on myosin, which form ionic and hydrogen bonds with actin (69).

RECENT PROGRESS

One area of significant progress has been to define functionally relevant conformational changes in subdomains of the myosin molecule. The ability to obtain crystal structures of myosin molecules with intact lever arms has been a major reason for this progress (16, 39). By growing such crystals in the presence or absence of various nucleotides, the influence of bound nucleotide on the angle of the lever arm has been demonstrated. Myosin with bound analogues that mimic ATP (so-called pre-hydrolysis states) give rise to an extended conformation of the lever arm, whereas analogues that mimic bound ADP+Pi (so-called posthydrolysis states) result in a more compact structure (16, 35, 39).

Progress has also been made toward defining the function of hypervariable loops on the surface of the globular myosin head. One loop near the mouth of the nucleotide pocket (loop 1) has been suggested to control nucleotide-exchange rates and therefore ADP dissociation (72). Another loop that links the 50 kD and 20 kD domains (loop 2) influences the actin-activated myosin ATPase rate, presumably because it is in the vicinity of the actin binding cleft (57, 101, 102). Yet another loop (the P loop) resides at the bottom of the nucleotide pocket, where it binds the γ-phosphate of ATP in a manner that is conserved among many diverse nucleotide binding proteins, including G proteins. The P loop appears to undergo shifts during P_i dissociation, suggesting a central role in the gating of P_i release and initiation of force generation. Considerable attention is being focused on the region of the myosin molecule where the nucleotide cleft, actin cleft, and lever arm all converge. Large conformational changes in this region, often referred to as the *converter* or *fulcrum* region, are thought to initiate lever arm motions. Detailed structure–function analyses by site-directed mutagenesis are just beginning to reveal the subdomain interactions important in specific transitions of the crossbridge cycle (93).

High-resolution measurements of force-generation by single myosin molecules are beginning to realize their potential to reveal details of force generating transitions. For example, a direct comparison of single-headed myosin and double-headed myosin from skeletal muscle showed differences in the elementary force-generating transition between the two. Specifically, two-headed myosin generated force steps and displacement steps that were twice the magnitude observed for single-headed myosin (100). According to this study, native two-headed myosin is designed in such a manner that the two heads cooperate to generate twice the force per event than can be generated by a single head. Measurements of force generation in single myosin molecules has recently been combined with single-molecule fluorescence to monitor nucleotide binding and force generation in parallel (26). As expected, a good correlation was found between nucleotide binding and force generation for most individual events. However, in a significant fraction of events myosin continued to generate force after the nucleotide dissociated (27), suggesting loose coupling or some form of protein memory.

Finally, recent studies of non-muscle myosins have produced some rather novel findings. First, myosin VI was shown by actin decoration experiments and by in vitro motility assays to carry out a power stroke that is the reverse of what other myosins undergo (109). In other words, myosin VI is the first minus-end-directed, actin-based motor protein. All other known myosins move toward the plus (barbed) end of actin. Also, studies of myosin I from intestinal brush border membranes by single-molecule force measurements have revealed a two-step force-generating process (105). Such a mechanism has not been found in striated muscle myosins, possibly because faster kinetic transitions make them difficult to resolve, or perhaps because of smaller duty ratios. It remains an open question whether the two-step nature is a common feature of all myosins or is unique to slow, high duty cycle motors. It is also unclear whether the two force steps correlate with specific steps of the ATPase cycle such as P_i release and ADP release.

REGULATION

The Steric Blocking Model

The modern era of studies on regulation of contraction by Ca^{2+} began with the identification of the thin filament proteins troponin and tropomyosin by Ebashi (17). Troponin, a heterotrimer (with C, I, and T-subunits), is a globular protein with Ca^{2+} binding sites on the C-subunit. Tropomyosin is an elongated molecule that binds in the major groove of the actin helix. The steric blocking model originated in part from low-angle X-ray diffraction studies, which showed that tropomyosin was in a position on actin to physically block the interaction between myosin and actin (46, 73). The steric blocking model also received support from time resolved low-angle X-ray studies that showed movement of tropomyosin occurring significantly before force development (54). In addition, stiffness measurements, which are sensitive to crossbridge binding, show that Ca^{2+} increases crossbridge attachment even in the presence of the nonhydrolyzable analog ATP(γS), which prevents the crossbridge cycle from proceeding through product release steps (15). There is also compelling evidence from high-resolution image reconstruction analysis of actin filaments that tropomyosin is positioned over clusters of amino acids required for myosin binding (58).

Kinetic Regulation

One of the first indications that a steric blocking mechanism might not be the whole story came from studies of the binding of myosin S1 to regulated actin (regulated actin is filamentous actin with tropomyosin and troponin in place) (10). Eisenberg and colleagues found that S1 bound to regulated actin even in the absence of Ca^{2+}, but the ATP hydrolysis rate was very low (0.1 s^{-1}). Addition of Ca^{2+} increased the hydrolysis rate to 10 s^{-1} as expected for solution ATPase. It was further shown that in the absence of Ca^{2+}, inhibition of myosin S1 ATPase by troponin-tropomyosin was due to a decrease in V_{max} with little change in K_m (10). These observations led to the proposal that the troponin-tropomyosin system controlled the kinetics of some early step in the ATPase mechanism, such as P_i dissociation, rather than the initial actin–myosin binding interaction (10, 83). Enthusiasm for this idea was tempered by the fact that these studies were carried out at nonphysiological ionic strengths (0.02 M) to promote actin–myosin binding, and it has been argued that these conditions could interfere with normal operation of the regulatory system.

Mechanical studies in fibers under more physiological conditions revealed rather large effects (e.g. tenfold) of variation in free Ca^{2+} levels on the kinetics of tension development (1, 8, 67). These effects of Ca^{2+} on crossbridge kinetics are not compatible with a simple steric blocking mechanism. As discussed above, the step(s) in the cycle that control tension development rate are believed to be early in the crossbridge cycle and close to the P_i dissociation step. Direct tests of the hypothesis that P_i dissociation is kinetically regulated by Ca^{2+}, however, have shown, at most, modest effects of variations in free Ca^{2+} on the rate of P_i dissociation in fibers (2, 68, 106). A model that accommodates the effects of Ca^{2+} both on ATPase rates and on tension development rates invokes dual (i.e. steric blocking and kinetic) regulation of the crossbridge cycle by the thin filament regulatory system.

Dual Regulation of the Crossbridge Cycle

Given that there is good evidence for both a steric blocking and a kinetic mode of regulation, it is worthwhile to try to reconcile these apparently opposing views. Several lines of evidence help to clarify this situation. First, high-resolution studies of the structure of the regulated actin filaments clearly show that actin residues involved in myosin binding are at least partly covered by tropomyosin (58). Thus, tropomyosin movement in response to Ca^{2+} binding would be expected to relieve this steric constraint and permit actin–myosin interactions. But, Ca^{2+} binding to troponin C alone does not uncover all sites on actin filaments required for tight binding (70). Second, results from equilibrium and kinetic myosin S1 binding experiments suggest that regulated thin filaments exist in at least three states (64). A blocked state occurs in the absence of Ca^{2+} in which actin–myosin interactions are prevented. This converts to a closed state in the presence of Ca^{2+}, where actin and myosin can interact weakly. Only in the presence of strongly bound crossbridges can the regulatory system be switched into the open state that permits further strong interactions between myosin and actin. Third, studies of actomyosin in solution and in fibers show that the regulatory system is not fully activated by Ca^{2+} alone but requires strongly bound crossbridges to reach full activation (94). One of the properties of a partially activated thin filament under conditions of an insufficient number of bound crossbridges is a reduced rate of tension development. Thus, the apparent kinetic regulation observed in a number of studies at submaximal levels of activation could be due to an insufficient number of strongly bound crossbridges to complete tropomyosin movement.

A dual regulation model that accounts for most of the data is that Ca^{2+} binding to troponin-tropomyosin regulates the recruitment of weak binding crossbridges into the cycle. The next phase of tropomyosin movement depends on the transition of those recruited crossbridges to strongly bound states. The apparent rate of this process depends on the number of strongly bound crossbridges and the amount of Ca^{2+} bound to troponin C in the vicinity. Therefore, Ca^{2+} binding to troponin influences both recruitment of crossbridges into the cycle and their rate of transition through the cycle. Whether a single step or many kinetic steps in the cycle are influenced by the regulatory system is not known. The observation that strongly bound crossbridges are required for complete activation of the troponin-tropomyosin system suggests that some of the free energy released from this strong interaction is used to move tropomyosin. As a result, the rate and energetics of specific steps in the crossbridge cycle and the rate and extent of activation of the regulatory system are likely to be interdependent.

Phosphorylation and Protein Isoform Switching

There is growing evidence that phosporylation of myofilament proteins plays a critical role in regulating the crossbridge cycle in cardiac muscle. The best characterized example of this is phosphorylation of troponin I by protein kinase A (cAMP-dependent protein kinase). This phosphorylation of troponin I appears to reduce myofilament Ca^{2+} sensitivity, accelerate Ca^{2+} dissociation from troponin C, and speed crossbridge kinetics (90). Other phosphorylations are less well characterized, particularly in terms of functional consequences. Examples include phosphorylation of myosin light chains by myosin light chain kinase or by protein kinase C, phosphorylation of troponin I and troponin T by protein kinase C (90), and phosphorylation of C protein by protein kinases A and C and by calmodulin kinase II. Another important mechanism of regulation is by changes in the isoform of a given myofilament protein that confers distinct kinetic or regulatory properties on cardiac muscle. Such protein isoform switches in the heart are particularly important during development or in various disease states. An important and widely studied example of this is the observation that failing hearts often revert to a fetal pattern of protein isoform expression for myofilament proteins such as troponin, tropomyosin, myosin heavy chains, and actin (90). This adaptation is thought to reflect a need to minimize the energy cost of contraction when the heart is failing.

SUMMARY AND CONCLUDING COMMENTS

A plausible description of the actin–myosin interaction cycle is as follows: ATP is a good source of chemical energy in biological systems because its free energy content in aqueous solution is much higher than the free energy content of its hydrolysis products, ADP and P_i. Some of this free energy of ATP is used on binding to myosin to dissociate the energetically stable actin–myosin bond. The precise mechanism of ATP-induced dissociation depends upon the location of the γ-phosphate deep within myosin, which may "push" open a cleft that physically separates two domains that make up the actin interaction site. Thus, ATP binding, largely through positioning of the γ-phosphate, disrupts optimal actin–myosin interactions. Bound ATP is then transformed into bound ADP+P_i which can dissociate back into solution in an energetically stable form. In addition, the subsequent ejection of P_i from the nucleotide pocket (via a different route than it entered) removes a major barrier to formation of the most stable bonds between myosin and actin. The binding energy derived from the ensuing protein–protein interactions is used to do work, i.e. rotate the crossbridge.

P_i dissociation may be slower than ATP binding and ATP cleavage, in part because during P_i dissociation the crossbridge must be ordered, oriented, and channeled into a specific pathway to begin a vectorial conformational change. P_i release is one step where the actomyosin ATPase in solution is significantly different than in fibers. Rotation of the crossbridge against a load requires a large part of the chemical energy to be converted to mechanical work, and this influences the energetics and kinetics of the conformational changes involved. In solution, the crossbridge would be expected to rotate unimpeded as ATP hydrolysis proceeds, and the free energy would be released as heat rather than stored and later released as work. In muscle fibers, ADP remains bound while crossbridge rotation occurs, preventing ATP from binding and short-circuiting the process. ADP release is also likely to be significantly different in fibers than in solution as its rate is somehow controlled by the orientation of or strain on the crossbridge. The probability of ADP dissociation is low (it occurs slowly) when crossbridges are bearing positive strain. This allows the crossbridge to finish its conformational change and has the beneficial effect of causing attached crossbridges to build up during isometric contraction to maximize force.

ADP release is faster for unstrained or negatively strained crossbridges, which permits ATP to bind and the cycle to begin anew. This also has the beneficial effects of allowing more rapid cycling and reducing the number of attached crossbridges during high-speed filament sliding.

This view of the actin–myosin interaction in which P_i and/or ADP release are strain dependent accommodates the load dependence of muscle contraction including the Fenn effect and the force–velocity relationship. However, the precise mechanisms of strain-dependent product release rates remain unknown. Other unresolved issues include the precise nature of conformational changes that produce force, the location of elastic elements, the characteristics of protein–protein interactions that underlie the large free energy release, and the nature of interactions between the two heads of myosin.

It is likely that the crossbridge cycle and its regulation are similar in fast skeletal and cardiac muscle, but cycling is slower by 5–10-fold in cardiac muscle. Two different myosin heavy chain isoforms, α- and β-, as well as a number of natural mutations in the β-isoform are known that probably underlie differences in contraction rates and economies for cardiac muscles in different species, developmental stages, and pathological conditions.

Several recent advances hold great promise for elucidation of molecular mechanisms of actomyosin-based force generation. One is the availability of high-resolution structures for the myosin head and for filamentous actin, which makes possible rational testing of existing models of the ATPase cycle against the molecular details of interactions among myosin, nucleotides, and actin. Resolution of structural detail in the regulated actin filament will also provide insight into mechanisms of regulation of the cycle by Ca^{2+}. Other emerging approaches that hold great promise include the ability to measure unitary force, unitary displacement, and ATP hydrolysis by single myosin molecules (26), which, combined with molecular biological techniques, provides an exciting new frontier for analysis of the molecular basis of muscle contraction.

The author thanks many colleagues who provided inspiration and insight during the preparation of this chapter, especially Drs. Robert Barsotti, Darl Swartz, and Richard Moss. I am indebted to Darl Swartz and Seth Robia for assitance with figures.

REFERENCES

1. Araujo, A. and J. W. Walker. Kinetics of tension development in skinned cardiac myocytes measured by photorelease of Ca^{2+}. *Am. J. Physiol.* 267 (*Heart Circ. Physiol.* 36):H1643–H1653, 1994.
2. Araujo, A. and J. W. Walker. Phosphate release and force generation in cardiac myocytes investigated with caged phosphate and caged Ca^{2+}. *Biophys. J.* 70:2316–2326, 1996.
3. Baker, J. E., I. Brust-Mascher, S. Ramachandran, L. E. LaConte, and D. D. Thomas. A large and distinct rotation of the myosin light chain domain occurs upon muslce contraction. *Proc. Nat. Acad. Sci. U.S.A.* 95:2720–2722, 1998.
4. Bagshaw, C. R. *Muscle Contraction*, London: Chapman Hall, 1993.
5. Barany, M. ATPase activity of myosin correlated with speed of muscle shortening. *J. Gen. Physiol.* 50:197–218, 1967.
6. Barsotti, R. J. and M. A. Ferenczi. Kinetics of ATP hydrolysis and tension production in skinned cardiac muscle of the guinea pig. *J. Biol. Chem.* 263:16750–16756, 1988.
7. Bowater, R. and J. Sleep. Demembranated muscle fibers catalyze a more rapid exchange between phosphate and adenosine triphosphate than actomyosin subfragment 1. *Biochemistry* 27:5314–5323, 1988.
8. Brenner, B. Effect of Ca^{2+} on cross-bridge turnover kinetics in skinned single rabbit psoas fibers: Implications for regulation of muscle contraction. *Proc. Natl. Aced. Sci. U.S.A.* 85:3265–3269, 1988.
9. Burton, K. Myosin step size: estimates from motility assays and shortening muscle. *J. Muscle Res. Cell Motil.* 13:590–607, 1992.
10. Chalovich, J. M. and E. Eisenberg. Inhibition of actomyosin ATPase activity by troponin–tropomyosin without blocking the binding of myosin to actin. *J. Biol. Chem.* 257:2432–2437, 1982.
11. Cooke, R. Actomyosin interaction in striated muscle. *Physiol. Rev.* 77:671–697, 1997.
12. Dantzig, J. A. and Y. E. Goldman. Suppression of muscle contraction by vanadate. *J. Gen. Physiol.* 86:305–327, 1985.
13. Dantzig, J. A., M. A. Hibberd, D. R. Trentham, and Y. E. Goldman. Crossbridge kinetics in the presence of MgADP investigated by photolysis of caged ATP in rabbit psoas muscle fibers. *J. Physiol. (Lond.)* 432:639–680, 1991.
14. Dantzig, J. A., Y. E. Goldman, N. C. Millar, J. Laktis, and E. Homsher. Reversal of the cross-bridge force-generating transition by photogeneration of phosphate in rabbit psoas muscle fibers. *J. Physiol. (Lond.)* 451:247–278, 1992.
15. Dantzig, J. A., J. W. Walker, D. R. Trentham, and Y. E. Goldman. Relaxation of muscle fibers with ATP(γS) and by laser photolysis of caged ATP(γS): Evidence for Ca^{2+} dependent affinity of rapidly detaching zero force cross-bridges. *Proc. Natl. Acad. Sci. U.S.A.* 85: 6716–6720, 1988.
16. Dominquez, R., Y. Freyzon, K. M. Trybus, and C. Cohen. Crystal structure of a vertebrate smooth muscle myosin motor domain and its complex with the essential light chain: visualization of the pre-power stroke state. *Cell* 94:559–571, 1998.
17. Ebashi, S. Calcium ions and muscle contraction. *Nature* 240: 217–218, 1972.
18. Eisenberg, E. and T. L. Hill. Muscle contraction and free energy transduction in biological systems. *Science* 227:999–1006, 1985.
19. Ellis-Davies, G. C. R. and J. A. Kaplan. Nitrophenyl EGTA, a photolabile chelator that selectively binds Ca^{2+} with high affinity and rapidly releases it upon photolysis. *Proc. Natl. Acad. Sci. U.S.A.* 91:187–191, 1994.
20. Fenn, W. O. A quantitative comparison between the energy liberated and the work performed by the isolated sartorius of the frog. *J. Physiol. (Lond.)* 58:175–203, 1923.
21. Ferenczi, M. A., E. Homsher, and D. R. Trentham. The kinetics of magnesium adenosine triphosphate cleavage in skinned muscle fibres of the rabbit. *J. Physiol. (Lond.)* 352:575–599, 1984.
22. Ferenczi, M. A. Phosphate burst in permeable muscle fibers of the rabbit. *Biophys. J.* 50:471–477, 1986.
23. Finer, J. T., R. A. Simmons, and J. A. Spudich. Single myosin

molecule mechanics: piconewton forces and nanometre steps. *Nature* 368:113–119, 1994.
24. Fisher, A. J., C. A. Smith, J. Thoden, R. Smith, K. Sutoh, H. Holden, and I. Rayment. Structural studies of myosin:nucleotide complexes: a revised model for the molecular basis of muscle contraction. *Biophys. J.* 68:19s–26s, 1995.
25. Ford, L. E., A. F. Huxley, and R. M. Simmons. Tension responses to sudden length changes in stimulate from muscle fibers near slack length. *J. Physiol. (Lond.)* 269:441–515, 1977.
26. Ishijima, A., H. Kojima, T. Funatsu, K. Tokunaga, H. Higuchi, H. Tanaka, and T. Yanagida. Simultaneous observation of individual ATPase and mechanical events by a singly myosin molecule during interation with actin. *Cell* 92:161–171, 1998.
27. Goodson, H. V. and J. A. Spudich. Molecular evolution of the myosin family: relationships derived from comparisons of amino acid sequences. *Proc. Natl. Acad. Sci. USA* 90:659–663, 1993.
28. Goldman, Y. E., M. G. Hibberd, and D. R. Trentham. Relaxation of rabbit psoas muscle fibers from rigor by photochemical generation of adenosine-5'-triphosphate. *J. Physiol.* 354:577–604, 1984.
29. Goldman, Y. E. Kinetics of the actomyosin ATPase in muscle fibers. *Annu. Rev. Physiol.* 49:637–654, 1987.
30. Goldman, Y. E. Wag the tail: structural dynamics of actomyosin. *Cell* 93:1–4, 1998.
31. Gordon, A. M., A. F. Huxley, and F. J. Julian. The variation in isometric tension with sarcomere length in vertebrate muscle fibers. *J. Physiol.* 184:170–192, 1966.
32. Guilford, W. H., D. E. Dupuis, G. Kennedy, J. Wu, J. B. Patlak, and D. M. Warshaw. Smooth muscle and skeletal muscle myosins produce similar unitary forces and displacements in the laser trap. *Biophys. J.* 72:1006–1021, 1997.
33. Gulick, A. M. and I. Rayment. Structural studies of myosin II: communication between distant protein domains. *Bioessays* 19:561–569.
34. Hibberd, M. G. and D. R. Trentham. Relationships between chemical and mechanical events during muscular contraction. *Annu. Rev. Biophys. Biophys. Chem.* 15:119–161, 1986.
35. Highsmith, S. Lever arm model of force generation by actin-myosin-ATP. *Biochemistry* 38:9791–9797, 1999.
36. Holmes, K. C., D. Popp, W. Gebhard, and W. Kabsch. Atomic model of the actin filament. *Nature* 347:44–49, 1990.
37. Holmes, K. C. The swinging lever-arm hypothesis of muscle contraction. *Curr. Biol.* 7:R112–R118, 1997.
38. Homsher, E. and N. C. Millar. Caged compounds and striated muscle contraction. *Annu. Rev. Physiol.* 52:875–896, 1990.
39. Houdusse, A., V. N. Kalbokis, D. Himmel, A. G. Szent-Gyorgyi, and C. Cohen. Atomic structure of scallop myosin subfragment S1 complexed with MgADP: a novel comformation of the myosin head. *Cell* 97:459–470, 1999.
40. Huxley, A. F. Muscle structure and theories of contraction. *Prog. Biophys. Biophys. Chem.* 7:255–318, 1957.
41. Huxley, A. F. and R. Niedergerke. Structural changes in muscle during contraction. *Nature* 173:971–973, 1954.
42. Huxley, A. F. and R. M. Simmons. Proposed mechanism of force generation in muscle fibers. *Nature* 233:533–538, 1971.
43. Huxley, A. F. *Reflections on Muscle*. Princeton, NJ: Princeton University Press, 1980.
44. Huxley, H. E. and J. Hanson. Changes in the cross-striations of muscle during contraction and stretch and their structural interpretation. *Nature* 173:973–976, 1954.
45. Huxley, H. E. The mechanism of muscular contraction. *Science* 164:1356–1366, 1969.
46. Huxley, H. E. Structural changes in actin- and myosin-containing filaments during contraction. *Cold Spring Harbor Symp. Quant. Biol.* 37:361–376, 1973.
47. Irving, M., V. Lombardi, G. Piazzesi, and M. A. Ferenczi. Myosin head movements are synchronous with the elementary force-generating process in muscle. *Nature* 357:156–158, 1992.
48. Irving, M., T. S. C. Allen, C. Sabido-David, J. S. Craik, B. Brandmeier, J. Kendrick-Jones, J. E. T. Corrie, D. R. Trentham, and Y. E. Goldman. Tilting of the light-chain region of myosin during step length changes and active force generation in skeletal muscle. *Nature* 375:688–691, 1995.
49. Josephson, R. K. Contraction dynamics and power output of skeletal muscle. *Annu. Rev. Physiol.* 55:527–54, 1993.
50. Julian, F. J. and M. R. Sollins. Variation of muscle stiffness with force at increasing speeds of shortening. *J. Gen. Physiol.* 66:287–302. 1975.
51. Kabsch, W., H. G. Mannherz, D. Suck, E. F. Pai, and K. C. Holmes. Atomic structure of the actin:DNaseI complex. *Nature* 347:21–22, 1990.
52. Kawai, M., Y. Saeki, and Y. Zhao. Cross-bridge scheme and the kinetic constants of elementary steps deduced from chemically skinned papillary and trabecular muscles of the ferret. *Circ. Res.* 73:35–50, 1993.
53. Kitamura, K., M. Tokunaga, A. H. Iwane, and T. Yanagida. A single myosin head moves along actin filaments with regular steps of 5.3 nanometers. *Nature* 397:129–134.
54. Kress, M., H. E. Huxley, A. R. Farqui, and J. Hendrix. Structural changes during activation of frog muscle studied by time-resolved x-ray diffraction. *J. Mol. Biol.* 188:325–342, 1985.
55. Kushmerick, M. J. and R. E. Davies. The chemical energetics of muscle contraction. II. The chemistry, efficiency and power of maximally working sartorius muscle. *Proc. R. Soc. London B* 174:315–353, 1969.
56. Lankford, E. B., N. D. Epstein, L. Fananpazir, and H. L. Sweeney. Abnormal contractile properties of muscle fibers expressing beta-myosin heavy chain gene mutations in patients with hypertrophic cardiomyopathy. *J. Clin. Invest.* 95:1409–1414, 1995.
57. Lauzon, A. M., M. J. Tyska, A. S. Rovner, Y. Freyon, D. M. Warshaw, and K. M. Trybus. A 7-amino acid insert in the heavy chain nucleotide binding loop alters the kinetics of smooth muscle myosin in the laser trap. *J. Muscle Cell Res. Cell Motil.* 19:825–837, 1998.
58. Lehman, W., P. Vibert, P. Uman, and R. Craig. Steric blocking by tropomyosin visualized in relaxed vertebrate muscle filaments. *J. Mol. Biol.* 251:191–196, 1995.
59. Lionne, C., M. Brune, M. R. Webb, F. Travers, and T. Barman. Time resolved measurements show that phosphate release is the rate limiting step on myofibrillar ATPase. *FEBS Lett.* 364:59–62, 1995.
60. Lowey, S., G. S. Waller, and K. M. Trybus. Skeletal muscle light chains are essential for physiological speeds of shortening. *Nature* 365:454–456, 1993.
61. Lu, Z., R. L. Moss, and J. W. Walker. Tension transients initiated by photogeneration of MgADP in skinned skeletal muscle fibers. *J. Gen. Physiol.* 101:867–888, 1993.
62. Lymn, R. W. and E. Taylor. Mechanism of adenosine triphosphate hydrolysis by actomyosin. *Biochemistry* 10:4617–4624, 1971.
63. Ma, Y. Z. and E. W. Taylor. Kinetic mechanism of myofibril ATPase. *Biophys. J.* 66:1542–1553, 1994.
64. McKillop, D. F and M. A. Geeves. Regulation of the acto.myosin subfragment 1 interaction by troponin/tropomyosin. *Biophys. J.* 65:693–701, 1993.
65. Martin, H. and R. J. Barsotti. Relaxation from rigor of skinned trabeculae of the guinea pig induced by laser photolysis of caged ATP. *Biophys. J.* 66:1115–1128, 1994.
66. Martin, H. and R. J. Barsotti. Activation of skinned trabeculae of the guinea pig induced by laser photolysis of caged ATP. *Biophys. J.* 67:1933–1941, 1994.
67. Metzger, J. M., M. L. Greaser, and R. L. Moss. Variations in

cross-bridge attachment rate and tension with phosphorylation of myosin in skinned skeletal muscle fibers. *J. Gen. Physiol.* 93: 855–883, 1989.
68. Millar, N. C. and E. Homsher. The effect of phosphate and calcium on force generation in glycerinated rabbit skeletal muscle fibers. *J. Biol. Chem.* 265:20234–20240, 1990.
69. Milligan, R. A. Protein-protein interactions in the rigor actomyosin complex. *Proc. Natl. Acad. Sci. U.S.A.* 93:21–26, 1996.
70. Milligan, R. A., M. Wittaker, and D. Safer. Molecular structure of F-actin and location of surface binding sites. *Nature* 348:217–221, 1990.
71. Molloy, J. E., J. E. Burns, J. Kendrick-Jones, R. T. Tregear and D. C. S. White. Force and movement produced by a single myosin head. *Nature* 378:209–212, 1995.
72. Murphy, C. T. and J. A. Spudich. The sequence of the myosin 50–20K loop affects myosins affinity for actin throughout the actin–myosin ATPase cycle and its maximum ATPAse activity. *Biochemistry* 38:3785–3792, 1999.
73. Parry, D. A. D. and J. M. Squire. Structural role of tropomyosin in muscle regulation: analysis of the X-ray diffraction patterns from relaxed and contracting muscle. *J. Mol. Biol.* 75:33–55, 1973.
74. Pope, B., J. F. Y. Hoh, and A. Weeds. The ATPase activities of rat cardiac myosin isoenzymes. *FEBS Lett.* 118:205–208, 1980.
75. Rall, J. A. Energetic aspects of skeletal muscle contraction: implications of fiber types. *Exerc. Sports Sci. Rev.* 13:33–74, 1985.
76. Rayment, I., W. R. Rypniewski, K. Schmidt-Base, R. Smith, D. R. Tomchick, M. M. Benning, D. A. Winkelman, G. Wesenberg, and H. M. Holden. Three dimensional structure of myosin subfragment 1: a molecular motor. *Science* 261:35–36, 1993.
77. Rayment, I., H. M. Holden, M. Wittaker, C. B. Yohn, M. Lorenz, K. C. Holmes, and R. A. Milligan. Structure of the actin-myosin complex and its implications for muscle contraction. *Science* 261:58–65, 1993.
78. Rayment, I. and H. Holden. The three dimensional structure of a molecular motor. *Trends Biochem. Sci.* 19:129–134, 1994.
79. Rayment, I., H. M. Holden, J. R. Sellers, L. Fananapazir, F. Epstein. Structural interpretation of the mutations in the β-cardiac myosin that have been implicated in familial hypertropic cardiomyopathy. *Proc. Natl. Acad. Sci. U.S.A.* 92:3864–3868, 1995.
80. Reedy, M., K. C. Holmes, and R. T. Tragear. Induced changes in orientation of the cross-bridges of glycerinated insect flight muscle. *Nature* 207:1276–1280, 1965.
81. Rome, L. C., C. Cook, D. A. Syme, M. A. Connaughton, M. Ashley-Ross, A. Klimov, B. Tikunov and Y. E. Goldman. Trading force for speed: why superfast crossbridge kinetics leads to superlow forces. *Proc. Nat. Acad. Sci. U.S.A.* 96:5826–5831, 1999.
82. Rosenfeld, S. S. and E. W. Taylor. The ATPase mechanism of skeletal and smooth muscle acto-subfragment 1. *J. Biol. Chem.* 259:11908–11918, 1984.
83. Rosenfeld, S. S. and E. W. Taylor. The mechanism of regulation of acto-subfragment 1 ATPase. *J. Biol. Chem.* 262:9984–9993, 1987.
84. Ruppel, K. M., M. Lorenz, and J. A. Spudich. Myosin structure/function: a combined mutagenesis-crystallographic approach. *Curr. Opin. in Struct. Biol.* 5:181–186, 1995.
85. Schroder, R. R., D. J. Manstein, W. Jahn, H. Holden, I. Rayment, K. C. Holmes, and J. A. Spudich. Three-dimensional atomic model of F-actin decorated with *Dictyostelium* myosin S1. *Nature* 364:171–174, 1993.
86. Siemankowski, R. F. and H. D. White. Kinetics of the interaction between actin, ADP and cardiac myosin S1. *J. Biol. Chem.* 259: 5045–5053. 1984.
87. Siemankowski, R. F., M. O. Wiseman, and H. D. White. ADP dissociation from actomyosin subfragment 1 is sufficiently slow to limit the unloaded shortening velocity in muscle. *Proc. Natl. Acad. Sci. U.S.A.* 82:658–666, 1985.
88. Simmons, R. Molecular motors: single-molecule mechanics. *Curr. Biology* 6:392–394.
89. Sleep, J. A. and R. L. Hutton. Exchange between inorganic phosphate and adenosine 5'-triphosphate in the medium by actomyosin subfragment 1. *Biochemistry* 19:1276–1283, 1980.
90. Solaro, R. J. and H. M. Rarick. Troponin and tropomyosin: proteins that switch on and tune in the activity of cardiac myofilaments. *Circ. Res.* 83:471–480, 1998.
91. Spudich, J. A. How molecular motors work. *Nature* 372:515–518, 1994.
92. Suguira, S. N. Kobayakawa, H. Fujita, H. Yamashita, S. Momomura, S. Chaen, M. Omata, and H. Sugi. Comparison of unitary displacements and forces between 2 cardiac myosin isoforms by the optical trap technique: molecular basis for cardiac adaptation. *Circ. Res.* 82:1029–1034, 1998.
93. Sweeney, H. L. and E. L. F. Holzbar. Mutational analysis of motor proteins. *Annu. Rev. Physiol.* 58:751–792, 1996.
94. Swartz, D. R. and R. L. Moss. Influence of a strong binding myosin analogue on calcium sensitive mechanical properties of skinned skeletal muscle fibers. *J. Biol. Chem.* 267:20497–20506, 1992.
95. Taylor, E. W. Mechanism of actomyosin ATPase and the problem of muscle contraction. *CRC Crit. Rev. Biochem.* 6:103–164, 1979.
96. Thirlwell, H., J. E. T. Corrie, G. P. Reid, D. R. Trentham, and M. A. Ferenczi. Kinetics of relaxation from rigor of permeabilized fast-twitch skeletal fibers from the rabbit using a novel caged ATP and apyrase. *Biophys. J.* 67:2346–2447, 1994.
97. Thomas, D. D., S. Ramachandran, O. Roopnarine, D. W. Hayden, and E. Ostap. The mechanism of force generation in muscle: a disorder-to-order transition coupled to internal structural change. *Biophys. J.* 68:135s–141s, 1995.
98. Toyoshima, Y. Y., S. J. Kron, E. M. McNally, K. R. Niebling, C. Toyoshima, and J. A. Spudich. Myosin subfragment 1 is sufficient to move actin filaments in vitro. *Nature* 328:536–539, 1987.
99. Trentham, D. R., J. F. Eccleston and C. R. Bagshaw. Kinetic analysis of ATPase mechanisms. *Q. Rev. Biophys.* 9:217–281, 1976.
100. Tyska, M. J., D. E. Dupuis, W. H. Guilford, J. B. Patlak, G. S. Waller, K. M. Trybus, D. M. Warshaw, and S. Lowey. Two heads of myosin are better than one for generating force and motion. *Proc. Nat. Acad. Sci. U.S.A.* 96:4402–4407, 1999.
101. Uyeda, T. Q. and J. A. Spudich. A functional recombinant myosin II lacking a regulatory light chain binding site. *Science* 262: 1867–1870, 1993.
102. Uyeda, T. Q., K. M. Ruppel, and J. A. Spudich. Enzymatic activities correlate with chimeric substitutions at the actin-binding face of myosin. *Nature* 368:567–569. 1994.
103. VanBuren, P., G. S. Waller, D. E. Harris, K. M. Trybus, D. M. Warshaw, and S. Lowey. The essential light chain is required for full force production by skeletal muscle myosin. *Proc. Natl. Acad. Sci. U.S.A.* 91:12403–12407, 1994.
104. VanBuren, P., D. E. Harris, N. R. Alpert and D. M. Warshaw. Cardiac V1 and V3 myosins differ in their hydrolytic and mechanical activities in vitro. *Circ. Res.* 77:439–444, 1995.
105. Veigel, C., L. M. Coluccio, J. D. Contes, J. C. Sparrow, R. A. Milligan, and J. E. Molloy. The motor protein myosin I produces its working stroke in two steps. *Nature* 398:530–533, 1999.
106. Walker, J. W., Z. Lu and R. L. Moss. Effects of Ca2+ on the

kinetics of phosphate release in skeletal muscle. *J. Biol. Chem.* 267:2459–2466, 1992.

107. Walker, J. W., G. Reid, J. A. McCray, and D. R. Trentham. Photolabile 1-(2-nitrophenyl)ethyl phosphate esters of adenine nucleotide analogues. Synthesis and mechanism of photolysis. *J. Am. Chem. Soc.* 110:7170–7177, 1988.

108. Webb, M. R., M. G. Hibberd, Y. E. Goldman, and D. R. Trentham. Oxygen exchange between Pi in the medium and water during ATP hydrolysis mediated by skinned fibers from rabbit skeletal muscle. *J. Biol. Chem.* 261:15557–15564, 1986.

109. Wells, A. L., A. W. Lin, L. Q. Chen, D. Safer, S. M. Cain, T. Hasson, B. O. Caragher, R. A. Milligan and H. L. Sweeney. Myosin VI is an actin-based motor that moves backwards. *Nature* 401:431–432, 1999.

110. White, H. D. and E. W. Taylor. Energetics and mechanism of actomyosin adenosine triphosphatase. *Biochemistry* 15:5818–5826, 1976.

111. Wittaker, M., E. M. Wilson-Kubalik, J. E. Smith, L. Faust, R. A. Milligan and H. L. Sweeney. A 35-A movement of smooth muscle myosin on ADP release. *Nature* 378:748–757, 1995.

112. Woledge, R. C., N. A. Curtin, and E. Homsher. *Energetic Aspects of Muscle Contraction* London: Academic Press, 1985.

113. Yount, R. G., D. Lawson, and I. Rayment. Is myosin a "back door" enzyme? *Biophys. J.* 68:44s–47s, 1995.

114. Zhao, Y. and M. Kawai. Kinetic and thermodynamic studies of the crossbridge cycle in rabbit psoas muscle fibers. *Biophys. J.* 67:1655–1658, 1994.

7. Modulation of cardiac myofilament activity by protein phosphorylation

R. JOHN SOLARO | Department of Physiology and Biophysics, and Program in Cardiovascular Sciences, College of Medicine, University of Illinois at Chicago, Chicago, Illinois

CHAPTER CONTENTS

Modulation of Cardiac Myofilament Activity as a Physiological Regulatory Device
Major Functional Sarcomeric Proteins and the Transition from Diastole to Systole
  Thin filament proteins in diastole and systole
  Thick filament proteins in diastole and systole
Crossbridge and thin filament states in diastole and in systole
cTnI Function and Phosphorylation
  Primary structure of cTnI and potential sites of phosphorylation
    The near NH_2-terminal region (residues 32–135)
    The inhibitory region of cTnI (residues 136–149)
    The C-terminal domain of TnI (residues 152–210)
  cTnI protein kinase A sites
  Functional effects of phosphorylation of cTnI by protein kinase A
  cTnI protein kinase C sites
  Functional effects of phosphorylation of cTnI by protein kinase C
  Integration of signals for cardiac myocyte hypertrophy/failure with cTnI protein phosphorylation
cTnT Function and Phosphorylation
  cTnT primary structure and functional domains
  cTnT sites of phosphorylation
Tropomyosin Function and Phosphorylation
  Tropomyosin isoforms and cardiac function
  Tropomyosin phosphorylation
MLC2 Function and Phosphorylation
  Primary structure of MLC2 and functional domains
  Metal binding to MLC2
  MLC2 and modulation of striated muscle contraction
  MLC2 phosphorylation and regulation of crossbridges
Phosphorylation and Function of Cardiac Myosin Binding Protein C
  Primary structure of MyBP-C and functional domains
  Phosphorylation sites of cardiac MyBP-C
Summary and Conclusions

THE CRITICAL COMPONENT OF THE REMARKABLE BIOLOGICAL MACHINE that gives heart muscle its ability to work is myosin, a molecular motor. The motor or crossbridge, which is formed by the globular head of myosin, protrudes from sarcomeric thick filaments (Fig. 7–1) and is powered by adenosine triphosphat (ATP) hydrolysis. The reaction of the crossbridge with actin induces ATP hydrolysis that is coupled to a series of mechanical events that translate the thin filaments toward the center of the sarcomere (Fig. 7–1). The chemomechanical coupling process is the fundamental mechanism by which the sarcomeres develop force and shorten and by which the cardiac chambers develop pressure and eject blood.

MODULATION OF CARDIAC MYOFILAMENT ACTIVITY AS A PHYSIOLOGICAL REGULATORY DEVICE

The intensity of cellular force (pressure) and the extent of shortening (ejection) against a particular load is determined by the number of crossbridges reacting with the thin filament actins and by the force generated by each motor. At rest or during diastole of the heart, the ATPase and mechanical activity of the myosin is essentially turned off by chemical and physical processes in the thin filament that impede the availability of sites on actin for reaction with the crossbridges. In systole, release from this inhibition is initiated by membrane-controlled fluxes of Ca^{2+} into the myofilament space. These Ca^{2+} ions bind to the thin filament and trigger activation, but activation of the myofilaments is sustained by a complex process involving long- and short-range cooperative interactions elicited by the actin–myosin reaction itself (58, 226, 252). In basal physiological states the sarcomeres appear to operate at about 25% of maximum activity. This leaves a reserve of crossbridge activation that is available to meet increasing hemodynamic demands. Short-term mechanisms for recruiting this reserve of crossbridges include the following: (1) variations in the amounts of Ca^{2+} released into the myofilament space as determined by neurohumoral signaling, the prevailing chemical environment, and sarcomere length; and (2) variations in the response of the myofilament to Ca^{2+}. The response of the myofilaments to Ca^{2+} is modulated in the short term by the sarcomere length (as determined by the prevailing preload and afterload, and associated feedback effects of crossbridge binding on activation), by the chemical environment, and by the state of myofilament protein phosphorylation as determined by the net activity of kinases and phosphatases. In the long term the response to Ca^{2+} may be modified by shifts in the isoform population of myofilament proteins.

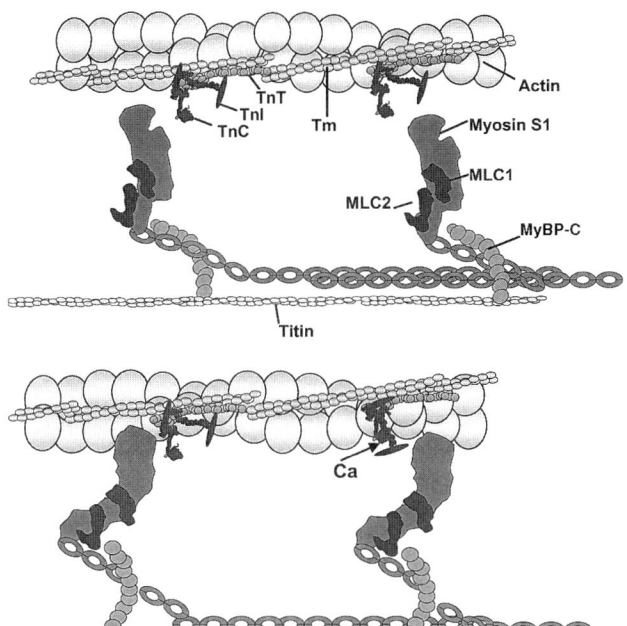

FIG. 7–1. Structural units of the myofilaments in the diastolic and systolic state. Both panels show an edge of the thick filament with myosin heads (S1) extending toward the thin filament. The crossbridge is shown as comprised of the S1 portion of the myosin heavy chain with a globular head and a lever arm formed by an α-helix that extends from the long tail making up the thick filament. Associated with the crossbridge are two light chains, MLC1 and MLC2. Associated with myosin is myosin binding protein C (MyBP-C), which connects to titin, a structural protein. One MyBP-C molecule is shown attached to the S2 region of myosin. Three such molecules may wrap around the thick filament. A. Diastole. In this state, Ca^{2+} is not bound to the regulatory site on troponin C (cTnC), cTnI is tethered to actin, and cTnT binds tightly to the actin-Tm. This disposition of the thin-filament proteins holds Tm and Tn in a position that physically blocks the actin-myosin interaction and may also allosterically affect actin reactivity with myosin. B. Systole in which crossbridges are generating force. Ca^{2+}-binding to cTnC has triggered a reversal of the inhibited state of the thin filament and caused Tn and Tm to move on thin filament. Note that the bound crossbridge has moved Tm further on the thin filament than could have occurred with Ca^{2+} binding alone. The result is that the near-neighbor crossbridge is shown reacting with actin in a force-generating complex without Ca^{2+} bound to TnC. See text for further details.

When heart muscle works well, these control devices ensure the ability of the heart pump to accommodate the venous return over manyfold increases. For example, during strong exercise the cardiac output is matched to venous return by reducing the end-systolic volume while maintaining end-diastolic pressures at optimal economy of contraction at low peripheral venous pressures. To maintain this homeostasis, there is an extensive array of control mechanisms with effectors—channels, exchangers, and pumps—at the surface and the intracellular membranes that regulate the flows of Ca^{2+} to and from the myofilament contractile machine of working heart cells (see Chapter 9, this volume). When hearts fail to work well and these control mechanisms are weak, the matching of cardiac output to venous return is maintained, but there is a compromise in which end-diastolic pressures increase, giving rise to a decreased economy of contraction, the threat of edema, and, with increasing myocardial strain, engagement of a pathological hypertrophic process. In this review, I present considerable evidence that the myofilaments are not passively controlled by membrane-determined Ca^{2+} homeostasis; there are extensive control mechanisms involving the myofilament response to Ca^{2+}. This is not surprising inasmuch as modulation of the myofilament response to Ca^{2+} offers the considerable advantage of reducing the energetic cost of transporting Ca^{2+} as well as reducing the threat of the pathology of Ca^{2+} overload.

Modulation of myofilament response to Ca^{2+} involves the two most prominent mechanisms for regulating cardiac output: extrinsic regulation by signaling through neurohumoral pathways, and intrinsic regulation reflected in Starling's law. Processes that modulate myofilament activation track signals arising from adrenergic and cholinergic signaling pathways by alterations in the state of phosphorylation of key myofilament regulatory proteins. Variations in myofilament protein phosphorylation constitute an important element in matching of cardiac output to venous return by providing a mechanism to vary the intensity and dynamics of cardiac contraction and relaxation independent of adjustments in membrane-regulated cellular Ca^{2+} flows (226). The myofilaments also sense and respond to the mechanical state of the heart imposed by changes in sarcomere length associated with variations in preload, afterload, and contractility. There is excellent evidence that this myofilament signaling pathway and length-dependence of activation are not mutually exclusive. For example, there is evidence that the length sensor is modified by protein phosphorylation (107, 108). This review presents strong evidence that phosphorylation of myofilaments is a vital mechanism in both intrinsic regulation of cardiac output according to the Frank-Starling mechanism as well as in extrinsic regulation of cardiac output by neurohumoral mechanisms.

MAJOR FUNCTIONAL SARCOMERIC PROTEINS AND THE TRANSITION FROM DIASTOLE TO SYSTOLE

Myofilament proteins react in complex allosteric, steric, and cooperative mechanisms that promote the transition from the diastolic to the systolic state. Here I view diastole as a state in which crossbridges do not react with actin in a force-generating reaction. According to concepts illustrated in Figures 7–1, 7–2, 7–3 as

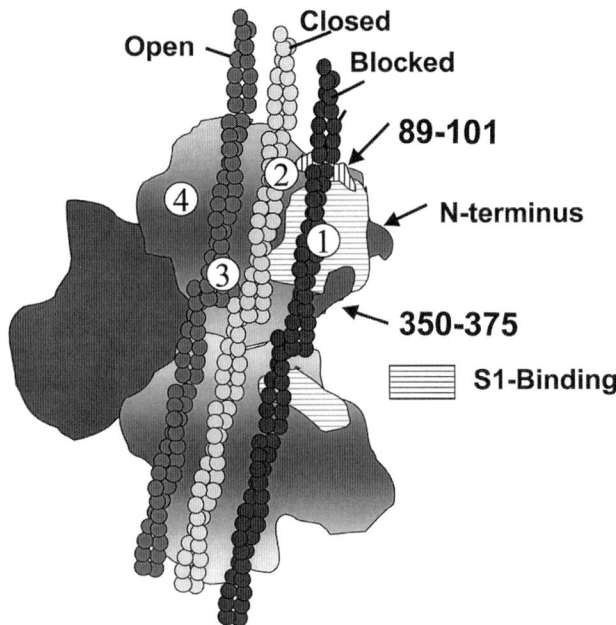

FIG. 7–2. Actin domains and the three states of the myofilaments. Three actins are shown with an illustration of positions of Tm in the various states of the myofilaments. Striped domains and amino acid numbers indicate myosin binding regions. Numbers 1–4 indicate subdomains of actin, which themselves may move upon transition from the blocked to the open state.

developed by Lehrer, Geeves, and colleagues (119, 135, 141), diastole may be perceived as a condition in which crossbridges are either in a "blocked" state, in which they are physically impeded from interacting with actin, or in a "closed" state, in which there are relatively weak, rapid on–off interactions between actin and myosin that do not generate force and do not hydrolyze Mg-ATP. I view systole as equivalent to the "open" state in which crossbridges react with actin in a strong state of binding and at a high rate of Mg-ATP hydrolysis. Figures 7–1 and 7–2 illustrate states of the array of thick and thin myofilament proteins in a fundamental structural unit of the sarcomere during diastole (closed or blocked state) and in systole (open state). The structural changes occurring in this transition reveal the complexity and extent of linked protein–protein interactions that are triggered by Ca^{2+} binding to the thin filament (see 44, 222, 223, 226, 252 for reviews). Figures 7–1 and 7–2 show a stretch of actins that forms the double helix of the thin filament. Associated with the actin helix are tropomyosin (Tm) and troponin (Tn), a hetero-trimer of distinct gene products: cardiac TnC (cTnC), the Ca^{2+} receptor; cTnI, an inhibitor of the actin–myosin reaction that toggles between binding to actin and to cTnC; and, TnT, a Tm-binding protein that transduces the Ca^{2+}-binding signal by interacting with cTnI and cTnC. Myofilament activation triggered by Ca^{2+} is likely to involve movements of Tm and Tn as well as sub-domains of actins (226, 230). There are seven actins for each Tn, but it is apparent that this structural unit is most likely not the functional unit (58, 135, 165). Figure 7–1 shows the edge of the thick filament with crossbridges extending from the core. The crossbridge is formed from the globular head of the heavy chain of myosin. Myosin is a hexameric protein complex composed of two heavy chains (MHC), each with two sets of light chains (MLC). Modulation of the activity, movement, and flexibility of the crossbridges is under the control of MLC2 and MLC1, and myosin-binding protein C (MyBP-C), another modulatory protein associated with the thick filament (Fig. 7–1). MyBP-C in turn interacts with titin, a third filament of the sarcomere.

Proteins undergoing reversible phosphorylation/dephosphorylation include Tm, cTnT, cTnI, MyBP-C, and MLC2. These proteins are substrates for multiple kinases and phosphatases. Here I focus on detailed descriptions of the myofilament regulatory proteins and how their function may be modulated by changes in protein phosphorylation. Although the kinases and phosphatases that determine the state of phosphorylation are considered in general, detailed description of regulation of these enzymes is beyond the scope of this chapter.

Thin Filament Proteins in Diastole and Systole

Consideration of current understanding of the protein–protein interactions that occur in the transition from the diastolic to systolic state reveals the wealth of potential sites for modulation of myofibrillar activity by protein phosphorylation. Triggering of the actin–myosin reaction involves both a movement and a rotation of Tm on the thin filament, and a change in actin structure (132, 229, 231). Although often depicted as a billiard ball, actin is a highly dynamic and flexible molecule. The crystal structure is known (87, 102), and models of the thin-filament–myosin head interaction have been built based on this information, together with analysis through cryoelectron microscopy. The molecule is a flattened structure approximately 5 nm across. A larger and smaller actin domain is shown in Figure 7–2; each of these domains is composed of two subdomains numbered 1–4. Figure 7–2 also depicts the positions of Tm on the actin surfaces in the blocked, open, and closed states illustrated in Figure 7–3. Subdomains 3 and 4 of actin are localized toward the core of the thin filament, and subdomains 1 and 2 extend into the outer regions of the helix and form the interface with myosin subfrequent 1 (S1). Subdomain 1 at the N-terminus of actin is highly acidic and is likely to interact with basic, lysine-rich loops on the myosin

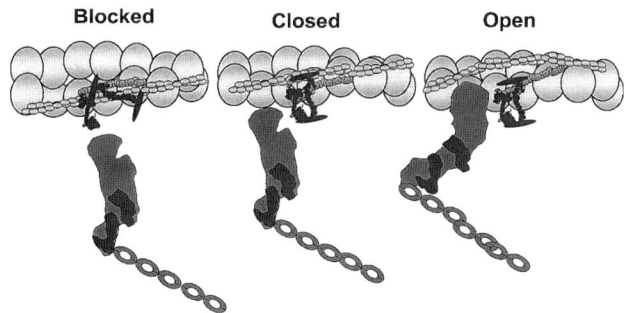

FIG. 7–3. Schematic illustration of a myofilaments in the blocked, closed, and open states. These states are determined by the position of Tm and Tn on the thin filament, which, in the absence of Ca^{2+}-binding to cTnC, holds the crossbridges either in weakly attached (closed) state or physically hindered (blocked state) from reacting with actin in a force-generating complex. Transition to the open, force-generating state is promoted by Ca^{2+} binding to cTnC and interaction of the crossbridge with the thin filament.

head. Subdomain 1 also contains binding sites for Tm and TnI. Interactions of Tn-Tm with subdomain 3 are also suggested from the data of Korman and Tobacman (108a), who showed that mutations in this region destabilize the binding of Tn-Tm to actin in the presence of Ca^{2+}. These findings are not surprising in that a general concept that is emerging is that Tn as well as Tm may be positioned on the thin filament at different sites on the actin monomer. By fitting X-ray diffraction data from a variety of sources, Squire et al. (229, 231) computed that the subdomains of actin move extensively in the transition from relaxed to active muscle. These movements are associated with movements of Tm. Direct evidence that Tm moves on the thin filament has come from changes in the X-ray diffraction pattern on the actin layer line that occur with muscle activation (92). The changes that occur are biggest on the second layer line, but other changes occur that are not clearly explained based on the atomic structure of actin. These changes are correlated with the extent of overlap with the thick filament, and therefore they could be associated with a change in actin structure associated with binding of the myosin head. Movement of proteins in the Tn complex may also be responsible for these changes in the X-ray diffraction pattern (230).

Tm is a double-stranded α-helical protein consisting of two chains that wind around each other to form a parallel coiled-coil (140, 145, 196) that extends to the ends of the molecule (61). As illustrated in Figure 7–1, the Tm coiled-coil intertwines as a polymer, overlapping a contiguous Tm by some 5–10 residues along the thin filament actins at a ratio of 1 Tm per 7 actin monomers. As with generic coiled-coils, Tm contains a heptad repeat of amino acids in which every fourth residue in the pseudo repeat is hydrophobic and interacts with a corresponding hydrophobic residue in the neighboring α-helix. McLachlan and Stewart (144) identified a seven-fold pseudo repeat of domains in the α-helix approximately 39–42 amino acids long. The repeats are regular, span an actin monomer, and provide sites that interact with the seven actins associated with Tm. The interaction with actin involves charged side chains of Tm that are mobile and accessible to the solution (132). Studies by Hitchcock-DeGregori and An (80) revealed that relatively high-affinity binding of Tn-Tm to actin is insensitive to the changes in sequence of the repeating motifs, but does require that the repeats be integral and that the coiled-coil exist along the entire length of Tm. The repeats were proposed by Hitchcock-DeGregori and An to serve as weakly interacting spacers that are important in aligning the ends of Tm on the thin filament. These nonspecific ionic mechanisms also appear important in permitting versatile and mobile interactions of Tm with different faces of the actin monomers as it winds around the helix. (132).

The mechanism by which contraction is turned on and modified by Tm was clarified by data elucidating the position of Tm on the thin filament in various states of the myofilaments. In the absence of crossbridges and Tn, the position of Tm was shown by Lorenz et al. (132) to make contact largely with C-terminal residues in the subdomain 4 regions of actin, as well as with residues in subdomain 3. This position of Tm on the actin helix resembles that occurring after the transition from the relaxed state to the Ca^{2+}-activated state (closed state illustrated in Fig. 7–3) in the native thin filaments (117). In this transition Tm moved radially and azimuthally closer to the cleft formed by the two actin strands and away from actin subdomain 1, the main site of myosin binding. This position of Tm, close to the cleft with a binding radius of about 38°A, is essentially the same as that determined from cryoelectron microscopy by Milligan and Flicker (150) and Milligan et al. (151). Similar binding of myosin S1 to Tm-actin and Ca^{2+}-Tn-Tm indicates a similar position of Tm in these two states (278). An atomic model (132) of the unregulated thin filament obtained by X-ray diffraction on oriented actin–tropomyosin gels also indicated that one position of Tm on the thin filament could represent either the Ca^{2+}-activated state or the Tn free state. However, these states were shown to be different from that occurring in the rigor state, in which the position of Tm was located toward the cleft formed by the actin array (open state in Fig. 7–3). A reasonable conclusion from these observations is that binding of rigor (strong) crossbridges is able to impel Tm further into the cleft than Ca^{2+} binding alone.

The interaction of Tm with the seven actins that it spans, the flexibility of Tm, and communication between the ends of contiguous Tm molecules are likely to provide a mechanism for promoting and spreading activation along the thin filament. One aspect of this spread of activation involves cooperative interactions between adjacent actins that may turn on as a unit in a concerted mechanism requiring Tm (160, 163). A second aspect of the spread of activation involves crossbridge-induced movements of Tm that may extend beyond the unit of seven actins by overlaps of the C- and N-terminal ends of contiguous Tm molecules along the thin filament (Fig. 7–1). Near-neighbor overlapping contacts between the ends of the Tm molecule (residues 1–9 and 275–284), which are highly conserved, thus appear to serve a special function. It has been known for some time that removal of C-terminal residues results in a reduction in the steepness of the relation between Ca^{2+} and myofilament activation (245). Cooperative binding of myosin S1 to actin-Tn-Tm is also reduced when the overlapping contacts are removed in Tm (184). In essence this means that the binding of one crossbridge promotes the binding of a near-neighbor crossbridge. Changes in apparent cooperativity could come about because of changes in the size of a cooperative unit—i.e. the number of actins affected by the binding of one crossbridge. On the basis of a variety of in vitro measurements of pre-steady state ATPase activity, Tm state, and S1 binding (226), it is apparent that the size of the cooperative unit is greater than the structural unit of seven actins and may be as big as 14–21 actins (164). It now seems likely that the loss of end–end interactions between contiguous Tm molecules in the complex with Tn-actin, would most likely reduce the size of the cooperative unit from this value. The ability of contiguous structural units to interact in a cooperative manner appears to involve flexibility in the Tm. Early models depicted Tm as a rigid rod; however, the Tm polymer on the thin filament is now perceived as a continuous flexible strand. Determination of the structural state of Tm indicates that the central region demonstrates flexibility, whereas the ends appear to be rather rigid (256). Flexibility in the Tm molecule is also suggested by the major shifts in position of Tm as it moves on the surface of the thin filament (116, 117). As illustrated in Figure 7–1, a flexible Tm provides a basis for the ability of strongly bound crossbridges to promote binding of near-neighbor crossbridges. The effect of strong crossbridges on binding of near-neighbor myosin heads has been directly demonstrated in skinned fibers by fluorescently labeled N-ethylmaleimide (NEM) modified S1 (239). Moreover, a flexible Tm molecule is an integral part of the mechanism for thin filament activation proposed by Maytum et al. (135), in which the size of the cooperative unit is regulated by the Ca–Tn complex. In this scheme, Maytum and associates introduced a modification of the three-state model that includes a term for variation in the size of the cooperative unit.

In the transition from diastole to systole, movements of Tm and possible actin sub-domains are triggered by a sequence of protein–protein interactions triggered by Ca^{2+} binding to cTnC. Interactions among the components of the Tn complex and Tm are illustrated in Figure 7–4. cTnC is a highly acidic protein comprising two globular domains joined by a central linker (52, 228). The NH_2-terminal globular domain contains a single helix-loop-helix motif that binds Ca^{2+} in the physiological range. This differs from the case in fast skeletal TnC, in which there are two competent sites in the NH_2-terminal domain. The single metal binding site in the NH_2-terminal domain of cTnC is relatively specific for Ca^{2+}, binds Mg^{2+} weakly, and is able to exchange Ca^{2+} fast enough to regulate the diastolic/systolic transition (210) The C-terminal domain of cTnC contains two helix-loop-helix motifs that bind both Mg^{2+} and Ca^{2+} with relatively high affinity. Exchange of metals at these C-terminal sites occurs too slowly to regulate activation of the myofilaments (187).

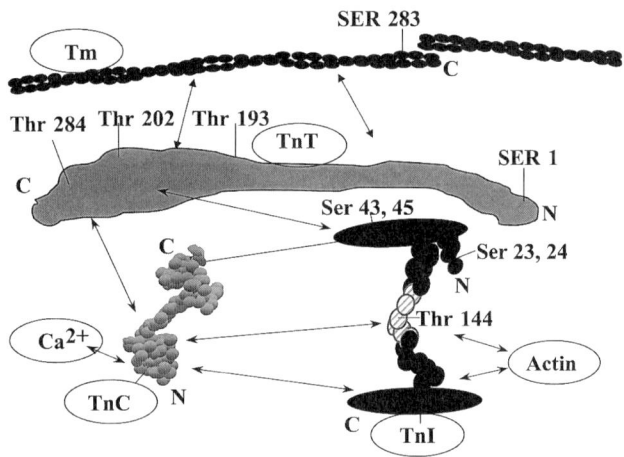

FIG. 7–4. Schematic representation of a functional unit of the thin filament illustrating regional locations of sites of protein phosphorylation. During diastole, Ca^{2+} or Mg^{2+} is bound exclusively to the high-affinity binding sites located in the C-terminus of TnC. The near N-terminus of cTnI is bound to the C-termini of cTnT and cTnC. The inhibitory region of TnI (*cross-hatched region in the middle of TnI*), is bound to actin-tropomyosin as is a second actin binding site (residues 156–168 in the C-terminus of cTnI). These interactions inhibit the actin–myosin force-generating reaction. During systole, Ca^{2+} is bound to a single site in the N-terminal domain of cTnC. This induces a conformational change in cTnC, which is transmitted through the thin filament proteins. There is a weakening in the interaction between TnI and actin-Tm and a strengthening in the interaction between cTnI and cTnC as well as between cTnC and cTnT. This occurs in part because of a switch in binding of the cTnI inhibitory region from actin-Tm to the C-terminal half of TnC. These changes in thin filament conformation release the thin filament from its inhibited state and promote the force-generating actin-myosin reaction.

A main role for these sites, which also exist in fsTnC, is to anchor cTnC tightly to the NH_2 terminus of cTnI (105). The solution structure of cTnI remains unclear. However, small-angle X-ray and neutron scattering data of Olah et al. (181), who analyzed the fsTnC (fast skeletal TnC)–TnI–$4Ca^{2+}$ complex, provide a reasonable picture of the shape for cTnI in its complex with TnC. Based on the model of Olah and Trewhella, Figures 7–1, 7–3 and 7–4 depict cTnI as an elongated structure with a central spiral connecting elliptical toroids at each end. The maximum linear dimension of the fsTnI (fast skeletal TnI) in the fsTnI–fsTnC complex is 11.8 nm. This molecular length in the cTnI–cTnC complex appears to be about the same, despite the larger mass of the cardiac variant, which contains an additional 32 amino acids (Trewella, Chandra, and Solaro, unpublished observations). cTnI makes multiple contacts with its neighbors on the thin filament. Its arrangement with cTnC is anti-parallel, making a strong apparently structural contact between the cTnI N-terminus and the C-terminus of cTnC (Fig. 7–4). C-terminal residues of cTnI and a stretch of highly basic amino acids (inhibitory peptide; Ip) make contact with actin in diastole. cTnI is thus tethered to actin when the regulatory binding site on cTnC is in its apo state. With binding of Ca^{2+} to cTnC, cTnI moves a substantial distance on the thin filament, shifting its binding from actin to cTnC (248). These changes in state of cTnC and of cTnI are sensed by cTnT in a signaling cascade that is ultimately responsible for movement of Tm and actin subdomains.

cTnT is a highly asymmetric protein (Figs. 7–1 and 7–4) with a globular C-terminal head and an N-terminal tail. As the biggest and longest component of the cTn complex, cTnT has the potential for extensive interactions with other thin myofilament proteins. The skeletal variant (fsTnT) is 19 nm long (150) cTnT, which has an NH_2-terminal extension, may be about 2 nm longer (252). Versatile interactions of cTnT are also possible, owing to multiple cardiac specific isoforms with variable NH_2-terminal regions generated by alternative splicing (5). The C-terminal half of cTnT interacts with cTnC, cTnI, and Tm, and thus forms a Ca^{2+}-sensitive domain (Fig. 7–4). The hypervariable N-terminal half of cTnT anchors the cTn complex to Tm independent of Ca^{2+} (217, 226, 252). This region of cTnT also binds to the region of overlap between contiguous Tm molecules. The role of the N-terminal region is not entirely clear. Its location at the region of end–end interactions of Tm suggests that the size of the cooperative unit should be influenced by this region of the TnT. Studies by Geeves and Lehrer (58) indicated that fsTnT may indeed modify the strength of the interactions between adjacent Tm' subdomains on the thin filament and thus increase the size of the cooperative unit. More direct evidence supporting this concept came from studies in which an N-terminal fragment of TnT (TnT_1) was demonstrated to induce an increase in the size of the cooperative unit (217). The size of the cooperative unit was also shown to be regulated by Ca binding to TnC (135) in the absence of crossbridge binding. Although the mechanism for this effect is not clear, a reasonable interpretation is that, in diastole, binding of TnT or TnI to actin-Tm may restrict the motions of Tm on the thin filaments that are critical to the flexible state involved in increasing the cooperative unit. A role for TnI binding to actin-Tm is indicated by recent findings reported by Zhou et al. (280) indicating that the binding of the TnI–TnC–Ca^{2+} complex is substantially weakened by the presence of strongly bound crossbridges. Zhou et al. interpret these data to mean that TnI binds to Tm in this vicinity of Tm-Cys 190 in the closed state and that it acts as an allosteric inhibitor of the actin–myosin interaction. These data thus provide strong evidence that TnI binding to Tm may restrict the movement of Tm, and that crossbridge binding to the thin filament not only must "push" Tm into the groove of the actin helix but also must overcome allosteric inhibition by TnI.

Thick Filament Proteins in Diastole and Systole

Figures 7–1 and 7–3 show the myosin crossbridges of the thick filament in various states of the myofilaments. The crossbridges contain actin and nucleotide binding sites and consist of the globular N-terminal region and long C-terminal α-helical tail of the myosin heavy chains (MHC). The backbone of the thick filament is formed by an assembly of a large portion of the myosin tail, with the head and a short segment of the tail, the crossbridges, projecting from the thick filament. Attached noncovalently to each head are two different light chains (Fig.7–1). One light chain (MLC1; 27 kD) is releasable in alkali and is also called the alkali light chain (ALC) or essential light chain (ELC). The second light chain (MLC2; 18 kD), which is phosphorylatable and binds Mg^{2+} and Ca^{2+}, is also called the P light chain (PLC) or regulatory light chain (RLC). The globular head region of the myosin molecule can be cleaved from the tail portion by proteolysis to yield a two-headed fragment called heavy meromyosin (HMM) or a single-headed fragment called subfragment 1 (S1). Both HMM and S1, which retain the actin-binding and ATPase sites, are often used in biochemical studies because they are soluble at physiological ionic strength. A major advance in our understanding of how myosin works came with X-ray analysis of crystals of myosin S1.(203, 204). These studies brought into focus earlier structural studies and revealed that the head of the myosin molecule is approximately 17 nm long, that the catalytic domain of the MHC consists of an actin-binding cleft and an ATP-binding cleft located on opposite sides of the molecule, and that an extended α-helical domain to which the light chains bind connects these domains to the thick filament proper. ATP binding, hydrolysis, and release of the products drive the chemomechanical process in which a cycle of reactions with actin move the myosin lever and translate the thin filament. Whether the heads function independently or in a cooperative manner remains an open question. There is also a poorly understood secondary site of interaction between the NH_2-terminal end of the ELC and actin (7). The positively charged NH_2-terminus ELC, which appears to be flexible, is likely to make electrostatic contacts with the negatively charged residues in the C-terminus of actin. While this interaction has been viewed as tethering the crossbridge to the thin filament and regulating the speed of contraction (160, 202), there is no clear evidence that this is the case. There is, however, evidence that MLC2 modulates the rate of crossbridge binding to the thin filament. This has been demonstrated from studies in which the light chain has been dissociated from the thick filament (82), and is inferred from studies on the effects of phosphorylation (148) and Ca^{2+} binding (189) to MLC2 on myofibrillar mechanics. These effects appear to arise from the ability of MLC2 to modulate the flexibility of the myosin head (126). Whereas the modulation of crossbridge activity by MLC2 seems certain, there is no evidence that Ca^{2+} binding to MLC2 can trigger contraction (186).

Attached to myosin at the head–neck region is MyBP-C (or C-protein), which was discovered in the 1970s as an abundant thick filament–associated component by Offer and colleagues (179, 180). Immunocytochemical analysis localized MyBP-C on the thick filament and demonstrated that it exists in 10 nm transverse stripes with 43 nm intervals along the thick filament in two 200 nm zones separated by 400 nm on either side of the M-line (179). The stoichiometry with myosin suggested that three MyBP-C molecules wrap transversely around the thick filament. In Figure 7–1 one of the monomers is shown wrapping around the thick filament. Although not clearly established, MyBP-C appears to function both as a regulator of crossbridge activity (70, 158) and as a factor stabilizing thick filament structure and assembly (49). MyBP-C has multiple sites for phosphorylation by multiple kinases (56, 69, 129, 219). Although early studies indicated that MyBP-C may alter its reaction with actin in the transition between a relaxed and an activated state, such a mechanism has not been demonstrated in a definitive experiment. It is most likely that effects of MyBP-C on the flexibility or mechanical activity of myosin serves a modulatory role in myofibrillar activation. This flexibility may be altered by the state of MyBP-C phosphorylation (269).

Crossbridge and Thin Filament States in Diastole and in Systole

Figure 7–3 illustrates another perception of the myofilament functional unit in the relaxed and active state. This model (141, 226, 230) includes three states that determine whether the crossbridges are sterically hindered from binding ("blocked state"), are bound weakly and stereospecifically ("closed" or "cocked" state), or bind in a force-generating complex ("strong" or "open" state). The blocked state of the thin filaments requires Tm–Tn interactions and a level of ambient Ca^{2+} below the threshold for binding to the regulatory site on cTnC. Classically, the blocked state was hypothesized to involve a particular position of Tm on the thin filament, as revealed by mass movements determined by X-ray diffraction of muscle fibers in the relaxing and contracting condition. However, as pointed out by Squire and Morris (230), potential mass movements of Tn were not generally considered in the analysis. Evidence indicates that cTnI and cTnT extend across several actins and that both may move on the thin filament during activation. Figures 7–1 and 7–3 thus show that Tn may physically block the crossbridges from binding and, along with Tm, contribute to the blocked state. However, although Tm alone is able to induce the closed and open states of the thin filament, Tn is required for the blocked state. There is evidence that during relaxation crossbridges are also bound weakly in the closed state, and the crossbridges go through the weak binding state as an essential step in force generation (109). Release from the blocked state moves crossbridges to a weak binding state in which it is apparent that control by Tm becomes prominent. The equilibrium between the three states was defined as K_{Tm} by Lehrer (118), McKillip and Geeves (141) and Lehrer and Geeves (119). The closed and open states demonstrate different affinities for myosin S1. Binding of S1 induces switching between these states such that myosin S1 binding curves show typical sigmoid characteristics of a cooperative process. The ability of the binding of one S1 to influence the subsequent binding of S1 is related to the size of the cooperative unit (n, number of actins turned on). In turn, the size of the cooperative unit appears to be determined by the physical and chemical state of the C-terminus of Tm. Thus, upon transition of a seven-actin unit to the open state, there is a "spread" of activation to a near-neighbor unit.

Our hypothesis relating to the model in Figure 7–4 to molecular signaling in the myofilaments is that Ca^{2+}

binding to cTnC releases the C-terminal domains and the inhibitory peptide of cTnI from actin and alters the reaction of an NH$_2$-terminal domain of cTnI with C-terminal regions of cTnT. The result is that steric effects of Tm, cTnI, or cTnT that maintain the blocked state may be removed. Moreover, as a result of the Ca^{2+}-activation process, actin subdomains move and Tm becomes free to move from its blocking position. As important aspect of the activation process is that strong crossbridge binding itself shifts the equilibrium of the thin filament to the open state and spreads activation along the thin filament, as strongly bound crossbridges promote movements of Tm and, most likely, actin S1, cTnT, and cTnI.

Diastolic and systolic states of the myofilaments are modified when key residues on thick and thin filament proteins change their state of phosphorylation. The following major questions drive research in this area:

- What are the potential sites of phosphorylation on the major cardiac myofilament regulatory proteins?
- Does the state of phosphorylation of these proteins change in various physiological and pathophysiological states?
- How and by what mechanism does the phosphorylation alter myofilament activity and its modulatiion by the prevailing chemical environment and mechanical state?
- How does modulation of myofilament activity by protein phosphorylation integrate with the other modes of short and long term regulation of cardiac function?

Although controversy and incomplete answers are evident, in some cases, research findings have brought us a long way toward answers to these questions. Perhaps the best example is our state of knowledge regarding the role of cTnI phosphorylation.

cTnI FUNCTION AND PHOSPHORYLATION

Primary Structure of cTnI and Potential Sites of Phosphorylation

Shown below are primary structures comparing human cTnI and human slow skeletal TnI (ssTnI), the embryonic isoform, and identifing the following regions of the molecule that have been defined functionally: (1) an N-terminal extension (residues 1–30) that is unique to the cardiac variant, (2) a near N-terminal region (residues 31–135) that interacts with both cTnC and cTnT, (3) a highly basic stretch of amino acids forming the inhibitory peptide (Ip; residues 136–147), and (4) a C-terminal regulatory domain (residues 148–210) that contains regions that, like the Ip, react in a Ca^{2+}-dependent manner with both actin and TnC.

The NH$_2$-Terminal Extension (Residues 1–31). An outstanding structural feature of the cardiac variant is an NH$_2$-terminal domain that consists of approximately

```
                                    ↕↕
CTNI (HUMAN)  1  MADGSSDAAR EPRPAPAPIR RRSSNYRAYAT 31
SSTNI (HUMAN)
                         ↕ ↕
             32  EPHAKKKSKISASRKLQLK TLLLQIAKQELEREAEERRG EKGRALSTRC 80
              1  MPEVERKPKITASRKLLLKSLMLAKAKECWEQEHEEREAEKVRYLAERI

             81  QPLELAGLGF AELQDLCRQL HARVDKVDEE RYDIEAKVTKNITEIADLTQ KIFD 135
                 PT LQTRGLSLSALDQDLCRELHAKVEVVDEERYDIEAKCLHNTREIKDLKLKVMD 103

                         ↕
            136  LRGKFK RPTLRRVRIS 151
            104  LRGKFK RPPLRRVRVS 119


            152  ADAMMQALLG ARAKESLDLR AHLKQVKKEDTEKENREVGD WRKNIDAL 198
            120  ADAMLRALLGSKHKVSMDLRANLKSVKKEDTEKERPV--VGD WRKNVEA  167


            199  SG MEGRKKKFES           210
            168  MSG MEGRKKMFDAANAPTSQ   187
```

30 amino acids that are not present in either the ssTnI or the fast skeletal (fsTnI) variant (272). Serines at positions 23 and 24 (Fig. 7–4) in this region of cTnI possess the sequence homology to be substrates for cAMP-dependent protein kinase (PKA) (27, 241); in some conditions these sites may also be phosphorylated by protein kinase C (171). When the sites are phosphorylated, pCa-force and pCa-ATPase activity relations are shifted to the right (42, 171, 224). The desensitization occurs through a phosphorylation dependent reduction in Ca^{2+} binding to cTnC(88, 210). It is also apparent that both sites need to be phosphorylated for this desensitization to be exhibited (37, 279).

The Near NH$_2$-Terminal Region (Residues 32–135).

The near NH$_2$-terminal region of cTnI is relatively highly conserved among the three isoforms of TnI and forms part of an interface with the C-terminus of cTnC and the C-terminus of cTnT (Fig. 7–4). The interaction appears not only to serve a structural role in anchoring cTn to the thin filament but also as a regulator of crossbridge activity. Binding to the C-terminus of cTnC requires the presence of occupied metal binding sites in the C-terminus of cTnC. Thus the arrangement of the TnI–TnC complex is anti-parallel (105, 114). In the case of fsTnI, there is a similar anti-parallel arrangement of the sTnI–sTnC interaction with the fragment sTnI$_{1-98}$ (corresponding to cTnI$_{31-128}$) binding to the C-terminus of sTnC (44, 45). A synthetic peptide of fsTnI residues 1–40 (corresponding to cTnI$_{31-71}$) is able to block the TnI–TnC interaction (169), as well the interaction of fsTnC with the fsTnI inhibitory peptide (residues 104–115). To address the role of the N-terminus of cTnI in heart muscle, we (200) generated wild-type mouse cardiac TnI (WT-cTnI; 211 residues) and three N-terminal deletion mutants of mouse cTnI: cTnI$_{31-211}$ (cTnI/NH$_2$ or N-cTnI; missing the N-terminal extension, cTnI$_{54-211}$ (missing 53 residues), and cTnI$_{80-211}$ (missing 79 residues). All of these mutants bound to F-actin. In fact, N-cTnI retained nearly the same ability to activate the ATPase activity of reconstituted myofibrils as the native full-length cTnI (65). Assays of protein–protein interactions demonstrated that cTnI$_{54-211}$ lost its ability to bind to cTnC, whereas, cTnI$_{80-211}$ bound weakly to cTnC. We determined the effects of these mutants on myofibrillar Mg-ATPase activity by reconstitution into Ca^{2+}-insensitive myofibrils lacking endogenous cTnI–cTnC. Ca^{2+} activation was lost in preparations reconstituted with cTnI$_{54-211}$. However, the cTnI$_{80-211}$/cTnC complex restored Ca^{2+} activation to nearly 50% of that obtained with WT-cTnI/cTnC. Thus, removal of the structural cTnC binding site on cTnI (mutant cTnI$_{54-211}$) eliminated Ca^{2+}-activation, whereas further truncation partially restored Ca^{2+}-activation.

Studies on the interaction of these N-terminal truncation mutants provided the first functional evidence for a cTnT-binding domain on cTnI and suggested that the differential Ca^{2+} activation of the myofilaments reconstituted with cTnI$_{54-211}$ and cTnI$_{80-211}$ was due to altered interactions of these mutants with cTnT. Earlier studies with fsTn complex had demonstrated that, in addition to binding to TnC, there are amino acid residues within the NH$_2$-terminus of fsTnI that bind to fsTnT. For example, deletion of residues 1–54 of fsTnI (corresponding to cTnI residues 31–85) eliminates binding to fsTnT (197). Residues within 40–100 of fsTnI (corresponding to cTnI residues 72–132) had also been shown to bind to fsTnT (23, 24, 80). In agreement with the data of Potter et al. (197) we found that cTnI$_{80-211}$ lost the ability to bind to cTnT. However, cTnI$_{54-211}$ retained the ability to bind to cTnT. Our interpretation of these results was that cTnT binding to the N-terminus of cTnI (most likely residues 53–79) is a negative regulator of activation. Modulation during physiological regulation of the interaction of the near NH$_2$ domain of cTnI with the rest of the thin filament may be accomplished through Protein Kinase C (PKC) dependent phosphorylation of serine residues Ser 42 and Ser 43 (178). Compared to dephosphorylated controls, phosphorylation of these sites has been shown to inhibit maximum acto-S1 ATPase rate in reconstituted preparations (178).

The Inhibitory Region of cTnI (Residues 136–149).

The cross-hatched region within cTnI in Figure 7–4 represents a key element in the molecular switch of myofilaments, the inhibitory peptide (Ip). This basic region of the TnI molecule binds either to actin or to Ca-TnC (242, 245, 257). Studies with fsTnI indicated that binding of Ca^{2+} to the regulatory sites on fsTnC induced binding of this region (fsTnI$_{104-116}$; cTnI$_{137-148}$), to the fsTnC E-helix in the C-terminal domain of sTnC (168). The Ip is highly conserved, except for a Thr residue at position 144 in human cTnI that substitutes for a Pro 113 in the human slow skeletal TnI sequence. Thr 144 is a substrate for PKC, and it would be expected that phosphorylation of this residue would affect myofilament activity. Whether this occurs or not remains controversial. Studies by Noland et al. (178) could not demonstrate any differences in maximum acto-S1 ATPase rate or Ca^{2+} sensitivity in preparations reconstituted with cTnI phosphorylated at Thr 144, whereas Malhotra et al. (137) have reported a decrease in maximum ATPase rate. Charge is not the only determinant of the interaction between the Ip and TnC. Reconstitution with a mutant TnI (K105G) containing a point mutation in the Ip induced an increase in the Ca sensitivity of cardiac skinned fiber bundles (236). The interaction of the Ip of fsTnI with fsTnC involves both hydrophobic and charge-dependent processes that may serve different steps in the switching process (32, 50, 258, 264). Evidence that the Ip is sufficient for causing relaxation through inhibition of the acto–myosin interaction and for release of the inhibition, came from studies in skinned fiber bundles of cardiac muscle. In these studies cTnI and cTnC were extracted by exposure to high concentrations of vanadate. The fiber bundles reconstituted with Ip and cTnC were able to undergo sequential contraction–relaxation cycles. Thus, an apparently functional regulatory complex could be reconstituted with the Ip alone in the Tn complex (212). This result has not been confirmed and is difficult to reconcile with data described in the next section, indicating that regions of cTnI C-terminal to the Ip are also required for full Ca^{2+}-dependent regulation.

The C-Terminal Domain TnI (Residues 152–210). The C-terminus of TnI extending from the inhibitory peptide is highly conserved among the various isoforms. This region appears critical for TnI to function in Ca-dependent control of thin filament activation. There is convincing evidence casting doubt on the idea that the inhibitory peptide (Ip) is necessary and sufficient for Ca^{2+} control of the myofilaments. To address the question of the significance of the C-terminus of cTnI in cardiac myofilament Ca^{2+} regulation, we (201) expressed and purified the following recombinant proteins, all of which retained the Ip: mouse WT-cTnI, $cTnI_{1-199}$ (missing 12 residues), $cTnI_{1-188}$ (missing 23 residues), and $cTnI_{1-151}$ (missing 60 residues). Each mutant bound to actin and to cTnC, as would be expected in preparations retaining the N-terminal TnC binding domain as well as the Ip. When the inhibitory activity of these mutants was compared to WT-cTnI, we found that addition of increasing amounts of exogenous WT-cTnI or $cTnI_{1-199}$ to cTnT-treated myofibrils (myofibrils missing cTnI–cTnC) at pCa 8 caused a similar concentration-dependent inhibition of the maximum ATPase activity. Yet, $cTnI_{1-188}$ was able to inhibit the ATPase activity only to about 75% of that of the WT-cTnI; $cTnI_{1-151}$ inhibited the activity only to 50% of that achieved with WT-cTnI. A complex of $cTnI_{1-188}$ with cTnC complex restored Ca^{2+} sensitivity to a fraction of that restored by WT-cTnI, whereas the $cTnI_{1-151}$-cTnC complex was unable to restore any Ca^{2+} sensitivity. Our results indicate that residues 152–199 (C-terminal to the inhibitory region) of cTnI are essential for full inhibitory activity and Ca^{2+} sensitivity of myofibrillar ATPase activity in the heart.

Studies with skeletal muscle preparations support the conclusion that regions C-terminal to the Ip of cTnI are critical for control of the myofilaments by Ca^{2+}. C-terminal residues extending from the fsIp $fsTnI_{116-133}$ (corresponding to residues $cTnI_{148-163}$) interact with the N-terminal domain of $sTnC_{46-78}$ (106, 125, 264). In the case of fsTnI residues 96–148 have been shown to bind more tightly to TnC than the inhibitory peptide, $fsTnI_{96-114}$ (193), suggesting that a more extensive interaction of TnI with TnC than that between the inhibitory peptide and TnC. Crosslinking studies (44, 106) demonstrated that $fsTnI_{132-141}$ interact with the NH_2-half of TnC, whereas residues in $fsTnI_{108-113}$ interact with the C-terminal half of TnC. Using mutants with the C-terminal domain of sTnI truncated, Farah et al. (44) reported that this region is important for Ca^{2+} sensitivity of the myofilaments. Therefore, TnI residues 136–179 and TnC may control Ca^{2+} sensitivity. Interestingly, within this C-terminal region is a second actin-binding site located in skeletal TnI residues 136–148 (cTnI residues 156–168), which also contributes to the blocked state by stabilization of the shorter TnI inhibitory region (255).

cTnI Protein Kinase A Sites

Phosphorylation of myofilament proteins by cAMP-dependent protein kinase (PKA) has been proposed to be an important mechanism for negative feedback in the transition from the basal state to the state of adrenergic stimulation, and explicitly in the increased rate of relaxation during β-adrenergic stimulation of the heart (222, 224, 227). This proposal arose from the surprising finding (41, 42, 224) that myofilaments containing cTnI phosphorylated at Ser residues in its unique N-terminal extension were desensitized with regard to Ca^{2+} activation. Thus at a time when the contractile state of the heart is stimulated to accommodate increased venous return during exercise, the myofilament response to Ca^{2+} is attenuated. Holroyde et al. (88) reported that Tn in the myofilament lattice bound Ca^{2+} with lower affinity following PKA-dependent phosphorylation. Later experiments demonstrated that the mechanism for the reduced myofilament sensitivity to Ca^{2+} was an increase in the "off rate" for Ca^{2+} exchange with TnC that occurred in the ternary complex with cTnT, and cTnI that had been phosphorylated with PKA (211). Bisphosphorylation of the cTnI at the PKA sites also has also been shown to modulate Ca^{2+}-sensitive binding of myosin S1 to regulated thin filaments (205). Studies using a mutant cTnI lacking the amino-terminal extension demonstrated that phosphorylation of TnI by PKA is both necessary and sufficient to induce the reduction in the Ca^{2+} sensitivity of myofilament activity (65, 267). This is an important finding inasmuch as MyBP-C is also a substrate for PKA phosphorylation and has also been demonstrated to be phosphorylated in hearts stimulated by β-adrenergic stimulation (55). Support for the idea that the increased off rate for TnC–Ca^{2+} exchange is functionally significant comes from pre-steady measurements in which Ca-activated force of skinned heart muscle preparations was quickly inhibited by photolytic release of Ca chelators (278). Myofilaments with dephosphorylated TnI relaxed about 1.5 times slower than myofilaments with TnI phosphorylated at the PKA sites when Ca^{2+} concentration was instantly lowered to relaxed levels. However, the experiments of Johns et al. (100) did not confirm this finding. There is also conflicting evidence on whether PKA-dependent phosphorylation of the myofilaments affects crossbridge cycling. Some laboratories (85, 213, 235) report an increase in crossbridge cycling with PKA-dependent phosphorylation, whereas others find no effect (81, 95). It is possible that these discrepancies are due to differences in age and strain of rat, in which variations in the basal level of myofilament phosphorylation may occur.

The molecular and structural mechanism by which phosphorylation of cTnI influences Ca^{2+} binding to cTnC appears to involve a depression in the affinity of cTnC for cTnI resulting from a global change in cTnI structure associated with the PKA-dependent phosphorylation. Recent evidence also points to the possibility that the N-terminal extension of cTnI has a direct effect on the conformation of the N-terminal regulatory domain of cTnC (1, 54). We proposed (65, 267) that phosphorylation induced a new conformation in cTnI on the basis of experiments that showed that Ca^{2+} sensitivity of reconstituted preparations was nearly the same whether the preparations contained dephosphorylated full-length cTnI or $cTnI/NH_2$, which is missing the N-terminal extension. We therefore determined conformational changes in the N-terminal segment induced by phosphorylation by using a monocysteine mutant—cTnI(S5C/C81I/C98S—of cTnI, in which a Cys residue was engineered at position 5 (40), as well as a monocysteine mutant missing the N-terminal extension (S9C/C50I/C67S). An 2-(4-(iodoacetamido) anilino) hapthalene-6-sulfonic acid probe attached to Cys 5 demonstrated a shift in emission spectrum upon PKA-dependent phosphorylation of Ser 23 and Ser 24. Changes in global rotational correlation time indicated a decrease in the axial ratio of the cTnI protein alone and in a binary complex with cTnC. These results, together with analysis of quenching of the fluorescence with acrylamide, were interpreted as indicative of a more compact hydrodynamic shape of the phosphorylated cTnI mutant. We concluded (41) that phosphorylation of the N-terminal segment induces a folded conformation in the protein. Results of studies using the same mutant of cTnI (S5C/C81I/C98S) confirmed earlier data showing that phosphorylation induced a substantial decrease in the affinity of cTnC for the full-length cTnC mutant. The binding of the truncated mutant was nearly the same as the full-length mutant containing unphosphorylated cTnI. Thus, as suggested from previous studies (65) on effects of the truncated mutant, $cTnI/NH_2$, in myofilament Ca^{2+}-activation, the N-terminal segment of cTnI itself may have little influence on the binding of cTnI to cTnC. Measurement of the molecular distance between Cys 5-IAANS and the native residue, Trp 192, were determined by analysis of the efficiency of fluorescence resonance energy transfer between these N-terminal and C-terminal sites. Phosphorylation of cTnI resulted in a 9–12 °A decrease in the mean distance, which was carried over in the cTnI–cTnC complex. Clear evidence that the N-domain of cTnI may directly affect the regulatory N-domain of cTnC has come from high-resolution nuclear magnetic resonance (NMR) studies (1, 54). These studies showed first evidence for conformational exchange in the regulatory domain of Ca^{2+}-saturated cTnC when bound to the isolated N-domain (1–80) of cTnI. This effect of the N-terminus of cTnI was reversed when serial Ser residues that are substrates for PKA were either phosphorylated or mutated to Asp residues (1). Abbott et al. (1) also reported that the cardiac-specific N-terminus comprised of residues 1–32 was capable of inducing conformational changes in the N-terminal regulatory domain of cTnC.

We think that these data provide a beginning to an understanding of the structural basis for the modulation of cTnI activity. We considered the question of how a change in phosphorylation that originates at the N-terminus of cTnI could be transmitted to the distant N-terminus of cTnC in the anti-parallel configuration of these proteins. One possibility is that the conformational changes induced in the N-terminus by PKA-dependent phosphorylation are transmitted through the C-terminus of cTnC via the linker region to the N-terminal regulatory sites. Another is that the signal is sensed by the C-terminus of cTnI and thus influences its interaction with the cTnC N-terminus. To probe these possibilities, we generated cTnC fragments (and $cTnC_{90-162}$), that corresponded to the N- and C-terminal halves of the molecule. Compared to the complex containing unphosphorylated cTnI, there was a significant reduction in Ca^{2+} affinity of $cTnC_{1-89}$ complexed with phosphorylated cTnI. Moreover, upon phosphorylation, the affinity of cTnI for $cTnC_{1-89}$ was reduces about fourfold. This finding indicates that the linker region of cTnC is not required for the reduction in cTnC Ca^{2+} affinity induced by cTnI PKA-dependent phosphorylation. Thus, we (20) favor a mechanism involving a global change in cTnI structure in which PKA phosphorylation at the N-terminus affects the Ip and C-terminal regulatory regions, altering their interaction with cTnC and reducing the affinity of the cTnC regulatory domain for Ca^{2+}. Induction of distinct structural states by mono- and bisphosphorylated cTnI has not been extensively investigated, but studies of Reiffert et al. (205) indicate that with graded increases in phosphorylation from mono- to bisphosphorylation states there is no change in dissociation rate constants but a graded decrease in the association rate constants of cTnI for cTnC and for cTnT, as studied using surface plasmon resonance (SPR) spectroscopy. However, when rate constants were determined in the ternary complex—that is, with cTnI/cTnC complex binding to cTnT—the dissociation rate constant was increased, and there was no change in the association rate constant. It is therefore apparent that the interaction of the N-terminal cTnT binding sites of cTnI with cTnT is also influenced by the state of phosphorylation. There are also data indicating that the phosphorylation of cTnI alters its interaction with actin-Tm. In studies comparing binding of fsTnI and cTnI to actin-Tm, Al-Hillawi et al. (3) reported that cooperative binding of cTnI to actin-Tm occurred only with the cardiac variant. This result suggests that the NH_2-terminal extension is able to alter actin or actin-Tm conformation and thus increase the probability of cTnI binding to actin. Interestingly, when phosphorylated in this domain, cooperative binding of cTnI to actin-Tm was abolished (3).

Vassylyev et al. (260) reported the first evidence on the partial structure of the fsTnI–fsTnC complex derived from crystallographic analysis. They formed a cocrystal of the C-terminal domain of fsTnC in a complex with 47 N-terminal residues of fsTnI. Polar and van der Waals interactions occurred between a 31 residue α-helical region of fsTnI with the C-terminal domain of fsTnC. Although the conformation of the C-terminal domain was the same whether or not the $fsTnI_{1-47}$ was bound, the D/E helix unwound into an extended linker in the complex. This structural change allowed the N- and C-terminals to come into closer proximity, forming a narrow interdomain cleft in the complex. The conclusion from this approach is different from that obtained from NMR investigations of the cTnC complex with cTnI. These results do not generally agree with the findings of Dong et al.(41), in which the interaction of the full-length cTnI with cTnC appeared to induce an extension of cTnC, at least in the binary complex. As already mentioned, an extended conformation of cTnI may be an important feature of its role in the "blocked" state of thin filaments (118). Interestingly, following phosphorylation of the Ser 22, Ser 23, the conformation of cTnI is extended, both alone and in the TnI–TnC complex. Changes in the extension of the cTnI molecule also occur in its reaction with cTnC. We (105) have used selective carbon-13 isotope enrichment of the ten methionines in a monocysteine derivative of cTnC(C35S) to determine the influence of TnI binding on the conformation of cTnC. Complex formation with cTnI decreased inter-domain flexibility and maintained cTnC in an extended conformation resembling the crystallographic structures of sTnC.

Functional Effects of Phosphorylation of cTnI by Protein Kinase A

Although there is substantial evidence that phosphorylation of cTnI at sites in its unique N-terminal domain alters the myofilament response to Ca^{2+}, the exact role of TnI phosphorylation in the modulation of cardiac function has remained elusive. The identification of how cTnI phosphorylation is integrated with other regulators of cardiac function is complicated by simultaneous phosphorylation of several key proteins. These include (1) phospholamban (PLB), (2) the regulatory protein of the sarcoplasmic reticulum (SR), (3) the Ca^{2+}-ATPase pump, (4) the sarcolemmal proteins-Ca^{2+} channels and phospholemman (110, 254) and (5) the ryanodine receptor (131). Thus, approaches that correlate the levels of phosphorylation with function are difficult to interpret because of multiple proteins that become phosphorylated and because of multi-site phosphorylation within a particular protein. An excellent example of the problem is study of the mechanism of enhanced relaxation associated with β-adrenergic stimulation of the heart. Associated with β-adrenergic stimulation is in situ phosphorylation of MyBP-C, cTnI, and PLB. Phospholamban inhibits the SR Ca^{2+} pump in its unphosphorylated state (130, 220), mainly by reducing its affinity for Ca^{2+} (28, 111). This inhibition is released with phosphorylation of PLB. There have also been reports that phosphorylation of MyBP-C desensitizes myofilaments to Ca^{2+} and alters the actin–myosin interaction (70). Experiments comparing the concentration dependence of isoproterenol (ISO) on relaxation, cAMP levels, and protein phosphorylation indicate that during increases in the relaxant rate at low concentrations of ISO and relatively low increases in cAMP, TnI was preferentially phosphorylated when compared to PLB (103). Although this suggests that cTnI phosphorylation may play a role in the relaxant effect, other studies comparing the time course of the relaxant effect of β-adrenergic stimulation with the time course of substrate phosphorylation concluded that phosphorylation of PLB is the main mechanism for the relaxant effect (55, 110, 227). In these studies the time course of enhanced relaxation following pulse perfusion with maximally activating concentrations of ISO correlated most closely with phosphorylation of PLB and not particularly well with cTnI phosphorylation, which outlasted the relaxant effect. A lack of correlation between levels of cTnI phosphorylation and enhanced relaxation could be related to the requirement that *both* PKA-sites (Ser 22, Ser 23) be phosphorylated for changes in cTnI function to occur (152, 279). As pointed out by Al-Hillawi and associates (3) there are four possible phosphorylation states that may be correlated with different functional states (unphosphorylated, either Ser 22 or Ser 23 phosphorylated alone, and both residues phosphorylated).

Our hypothesis is that enhanced relaxation with β-adrenergic stimulation is due to a concerted effect involving an increased rate of uptake of Ca^{2+} by the SR, promotion of Ca^{2+} release from cTnC, and enhanced crossbridge cycling. Mutant mice in which the PLB gene has been ablated have provided an important tool with which to approach the relative contribution of this and other phosphoproteins in the response to β-adrenergic agonists (133). Isolated work-performing hearts from these mice demonstrated interesting properties when compared to wild-type controls. Not only was basal contractility enhanced but also there was little or no response to β-adrenergic stimulation. However, measurements on isolated cells demonstrated that, as with the wild-type controls, ventricular myocytes from phospholamban (PLB)-ablated mice responded to ISO treatment (275), although with a reduced increase in activity. The results obtained in isolated cells fit well with echocardiographic data, which showed that some contractile parameters of PLB-deficient hearts were increased in situ after ISO administration (86). Li et al. (128), however, reported that PLB-ablated mouse heart cells stimulated with ISO demonstrated no alteration in the time constant (tau) of relaxation if muscle preparations were allowed to shorten. In PLB-ablated muscle preparations stimulated with ISO and developing increasing levels of isometric force, there was progressive acceleration of relaxation by about 17%. In wild-type myocytes, ISO stimulation reduced tau of cell relaxation by 30%–50%. These results indicate the interesting possibility that the mechanism by which cTnI phosphorylation induces a relaxant effect of β-adrenergic stimulation becomes manifest only when a substantial portion of crossbridges are in the strong binding state. This dependence on the presence of strong crossbridges indicates that enhanced crossbridge cycling rate or decreased crossbridge affinity for actin associated with PKA phosphorylation of cTnI may be the main physiological effect.

Transgenic (TG) models offer an exciting approach to understanding the relative role of TnI and PLB in the relaxant effect. Apart from the PLB-deficient mouse, two other transgenic models appear promising. The first is a transgenic mouse harboring a skeletal β-Tm transgene with expression restricted to the heart (167, 182). In this model, the native α-Tm had been largely replaced in the myofilament lattice by β-Tm. No other changes are apparent. These hearts demonstrate a slowing of relaxation in the basal condition and also significantly less of a relaxant effect of β-adrenergic stimulation, particularly at relatively low concentrations of ISO (167). Studies on skinned fiber preparations from these hearts show that the pCa-force relationship is left-shifted in the TG-βTm preparations, when compared to the nontransgenic controls (183). Moreover, although both myofilament preparations demonstrated phosphorylation of TnI by PKA, only in the wild-type preparations was there a desensitizing effect. The increased Ca^{2+} sensitivity of the myofilaments fits with the slowing of relaxation in the basal state of isolated work-performing heart preparations (167). Moreover, Muthuchamy et al. (167) reported a blunting of the relaxant effect of ISO stimulation of these hearts at the lower concentrations on the dose–response relationship. This blunting of the relaxant effect could be due to a blunting of the desensitizing effect of cTnI phosphorylation in the skinned fiber bundles. A second TG mouse that provides a useful experimental model is one in which ssTnI is overexpressed in the heart (46). Hearts from these mice also demonstrate a blunting of the relaxant effect of catecholamines (46). Myofilaments from these mice demonstrated complete replacement of cTnI with ssTnI. Studies with detergent-extracted single myocytes showed a lack of response of the pCa-force relation to PKA-dependent phosphorylation. In these cells, MyBP-C was phosphorylated, but there was no detectable phosphorylation of cTnI, confirming the disappearance of the cardiac isoform from the cells. This change in effect of phosphorylation was reflected in isolated intact myocytes and in isolated perfused hearts as impaired diastolic function associated with a diminished relaxant effect of ISO stimulation. Much work needs to be done to establish these transgenic mouse models as useful in approaching the question of the relative role of TnI phosphorylation in cardiac contractility. Yet, this is a compelling approach, especially with the possibility of varying the proportions of PLB in the heart by using heterozygotes that express about half the phospholamban and varying the proportions of β-Tm, and α-Tm, as well as ssTnI and cTnI, by using transgenic animals containing different copy numbers of the transgene.

cTnI Protein Kinase C Sites

Sites of phosphorylation of cTnI by PKC occur in regions of the molecule where one would expect a change in charge to affect function (Fig. 7–4). One site is at Thr 144, a cardiac-specific residue (Pro in skeletal ssTnI and fsTnI) located in the inhibitory peptide. Two other sites are at Ser 42 and Ser 44 of cTnI in the N-terminal domain that binds to cTnC and cTnT. Studies using a variety of approaches to investigate the role of cTnI phosphorylation by PKC in the regulation of cardiac muscle have not brought us to a clear consensus. A series of papers from the laboratory of J. F. Kuo (104, 172, 175) indicated that PKC-dependent phosphorylation inhibits the actin–crossbridge reaction but does not greatly affect Ca^{2+} sensitivity. These studies were done for the most part in reconstituted thin filament–myosin S1 preparations containing either unphosphorylated or fully phosphorylated cTnI. Phosphorylation of PKC sites on cTnI also caused a decrease in the apparent affinity of myosin S1 for the thin filament. Kuo's laboratory first showed clear evidence that cardiac and skeletal muscle TnI are excellent substrates for PKC (104). Noland et al. (175) went on to demonstrate that free cTnI was phosphorylated in a region of the molecule containing Ser 42 and Ser 44 and at Thr 144 in the Ip. Importantly, the same residues could be phosphorylated in vitro when cTnI was incorporated into the Tn complex or into the myofilament lattice of myofibrillar preparations (172). Myofibrils treated with PKC demonstrated the inhibition of Ca^{2+}-stimulated Mg-ATPase activity with little change in the Ca^{2+} sensitivity, despite the fact that a number of proteins appeared to be phosphorylated in these preparations. As discussed in other sections of this chapter, these proteins are likely to be TnT, MLC2, and MyBP-C. To test the relative ability of cTnI to act as substrate, Noland et al. (175) used peptide substrates to determine K_m/V_{max} values for the phosphoryl group transfer by PKC. These results predicted that cTnI was a better PKC substrate than cTnT. The mechanism of the inhibitory effects of the phosphorylation cTnI by PKC appears to involve an increased competition of cTnI with myosin S1 for binding to actin—in other words, a mechanism involving promotion of the blocked state as described in Figures 7–1 and 7–3. Noland and Kuo (172) reported that although phosphorylation of TnI always induced a decrease in the Ca^{2+}-dependent ATPase rate of reconstituted actomyosin, the inhibition was partially overcome as the concentration of myosin or S1 increased. This was not the observation in the case of phosphorylated TnT in which inhibition was the same at concentrations of myosin or S1.

To determine more clearly the relative role of the various PKC sites on cTnI in regulating the actin-crossbridge interaction, we (176, 178) generated the following mutant forms of heart cTnI: cTnI-T144A, cTnI-S42A/S44A, and cTnI-S42A/S44A/T144A in which Thr and Ser residues were replaced by Ala. Other mutant forms of cTnI studies were cTnI-S23A/S24A (substitution of the PKA phosphorylation sites Ser 23/Ser 24) and N32 (in which missing the N-terminal peptide extension). In one set of studies a pan PKC isolated from brain was used as the kinase. Subtle changes in the kinetics of phosphorylation by pan PKC occurred, but all mutants could be maximally phosphorylated to various extents depending on the number sites retained in the molecule. These studies showed that PKC could cross-phosphorylate PKA sites, but PKA could not phosphorylate the PKC sites in any of the mutants or native preparations. In these studies, the ATPase rate of preparations reconstituted with wild-type TnI and T144A had the same sensitivity to Ca^{2+}. However, compared to the these preparations, ATPase rate of regulated actomyosin-S1 containing either unphosphorylated S42A/S44A, S42A/S44A/T144, S23A/S24A, or N32 demonstrated a decreased Ca^{2+} sensitivity. Thus, Ser 42/Ser 44 and Ser 23/Ser 24 in cTnI appear important for normal myofibrillar Ca^{2+} sensitivity. Following PKC phosphorylation of wild-type and all mutants except S42A/S44A and S42A/S44A/T144A, there was a marked reduction in both the maximum Mg-ATPase activity and apparent affinity of myosin S1 for reconstituted (regulated) actin. Moreover, when both Ser 23/Ser 24 and Ser 42/Ser 44 were phosphorylated, there was an additive effect at submaximal Ca^{2+} concentration resulting in a severe depression in ATPase activity as a result of a combination of a decrease in Ca^{2+} sensitivity and V_{max}.

In a second series of experiments investigating the regulation of Ca^{2+}-stimulated Mg-ATPase activity of reconstituted actomyosin S1, we (176) phosphorylated wild-type and mutant forms of cTnI by the PKC isozymes alpha and delta and by PKA. PKC-alpha (which gave results similar to PKC-epsilon), was equal in its ability to phosphoryalate TnI wild-type and all mutants. Both free cTnI and cTnI in the Tn complex exhibited discrete specificities for phosphorylation by the two PKC isozymes. PKC-delta, but not PKC-alpha, had a propensity to phosphorylate the consensus PKA sites (Ser 23/Ser 24), resulting in a reduction of the Ca^{2+} sensitivity of the reconstituted actomyosin S1 Mg-ATPase. As predicted by this finding, N32 was a much poorer substrate for PKC-delta than for PKC-alpha. Thus, PKC-delta appears to function as a hybrid of PKC-alpha and PKA. On the other hand, PKC-alpha preferred to phosphorylate Ser 42/Ser 44, and thus reduced the maximal Ca^{2+}-stimulated activity of the Mg-ATPase. The site specificities and hence functional differences between PKC-alpha and PKC-delta were most evident at low phosphorylation (1 mol of phosphate/mol) of TnI wild-type and were magnified when S42A/S44A and N32 were used as substrates. These results provided the first evidence that site-selective preferences of PKC-alpha and PKC-delta for phosphorylating a single substrate (cTnI) in the myocardium may lead to distinct functional consequences. Jideama et al. (99) have shown further evidence that the PKC isozymes alpha, delta, epsilon, and zeta, which are expressed in adult rat cardiomyocytes, demonstrate specificity for the phosphorylation of cTnI and cTnT. Bovine cTnI was the preferred substrate for PKC-alpha,-delta, and-epsilon when compared to cTnT, whereas cTnI was the preferred substrata for PKC-zeta.

Whatever the path of phosphorylation, our results indicate that Ser 42, Ser 44 are the sites largely responsible for the inhibitory effect of TnI PKC-phosphorylation on actomyosin ATPase activity, and furthermore, that phosphorylation of Thr 144 by PKC is relatively unimportant in modulating the activity of the Ip. Although earlier work (177) had indicated that Thr 144 in cTnI is important for the observed decrease of Ca^{2+}-stimulated actomyosin Mg-ATPase activity, results of studies (176, 178) with site-directed mutants provide strong evidence that this may not be the case. A different conclusion was reached by Malhotra et al. (137) in a study of regulated actomyosin preparations containing S22A/23A and TI44A. Although they agree with the work of Noland et al. (176, 178) that PKA sites are exclusively phosphorylated by PKA with a resulting decrease in Ca^{2+} sensitivity, they indicate a more prominent role of Thr 144 phosphorylation than for Ser 42/Ser 44. In contrast to the data reported by Noland et al. (178), the curve relating Ca^{2+} to the ATPase activity was substantially shited to the right, when wild-type TnI, which was phosphorylated by PKC, was employed for regulation. Moreover, this shift was markedly attenuated when T144A was incorporated into the preparations. Although not analyzed, a residual reduction in maximum ATPase activity was still seen in the preparations containing the T144A mutant. It is apparent that this could be due to phosphorylation of Ser 42/Ser 44.

Functional Effects of Phosphorylation of cTnI by Protein Kinase C

There is compelling evidence for the significance of PKC-dependent phosphorylation of cTnI, yet there is no clear evidence for either a physiological or a pathophysiological role. Apart from determination of the functional role of site-specific phosphorylations on cTnI, understanding the general role of PKC-dependent protein phosphorylation in regulating myofilament activity remains a difficult challenge. There are multiple myofilament substrates for PKC, including cTnT, MyBP-C, and MLC2. There are also multiple PKC isoforms, whose specific functions remain uncertain; multiple phosphorylation sites on the substrates; and multiple pathways for activation of PKC (199). Moreover, some of these phosphorylations (MLC2 and MyBP-C) appear to increase Ca^{2+} sensitivity of the ATPase rate with no effect on V_{max}, whereas others (cTnT and cTnI) depress V_{max}, with no effect on sensitivity. Studies on the effects of activation of the PKC pathway have reported both negative (18, 67, 101), and positive inotropic effects (250). Few studies have directly compared levels of phosphorylation of sites on cTnI to the inotropic state. Venema and Kuo (265) measured cTnI sites phosphorylated in rat cardiac myocytes exposed to the phorbol ester, TPA, or the α-adrenergic agonist, phenylephrine. Their results showed relatively little change in the level of phosphorylation of TnT sites and MLC2, but they did show predominant phosphorylation of cTnI at Ser 42 and Ser 44. Compared to untreated controls, the maximum Ca^{2+}-stimulated MgATPase rate of myofibrils purified from these cells was depressed, as predicted from the in vitro studies with preparations reconstituted with PKC-phosphorylated cTnI. However, Talosi and Kranias (250) could find no change in the level of phosphorylation of cTnI in rabbit hearts perfused with phenylephrine. They used a 10 μM concentration of phenylephrine, which was sufficient to incease $+dp/dt$ 1.54-fold and induce a redistribution of PKC activity, but which was without effect on cTnI phosphorylation. α_1-Adrenergic stimulation of single cardiac myocytes, followed by rapid Triton X-100 skinning and force measurement, has been used to investigate the effect of the PKC pathway on pCa-force relations. Pucéat et al. (198), who used this technique, reported that such treatment increased the sensitivity to Ca^{2+}. They also reported that treatment of the cells with phorbol esters could mimic this effect. In a follow-up to these experiments, Clement et al. (26) reported that PKC enhances the effect of myosin light chain kinase to induce an increase in the Ca^{2+} sensitivity of skinned heart cells. Addition of PKC was shown to be associated with MLC2 phosphorylation, as well as with an increase in phosphorylation of cTnI and cTnT. Thus, these experiments indicate that the synergistic effect of PKC and myosin light chain kinase (MLCK) on MLC2 phosphorylation may override the inhibitory effects of Tn phosphorylation.

Similar studies by Strang and Moss (234) on mechanical activity of single myocytes skinned after pre-treatment with the α_1-adrenergic agonist phenylephrine in the presence of the β-receptor antagonist propranolol showed no shifts in the pCa–force relation, but a significant depression of unloaded shortening velocity. This finding generally supports an important role for PKC-dependent phosphorylation of cTnI sites, which depresses ATPase rate. The physiological relevance of this effect is not clear, but Strang and Moss (234) make the reasonable suggestion that α_1-receptors have two effects—one to increase intracellular Ca^{2+} and one to inhibit V_{max} of unloaded shortening velocity and actomyosin ATPase V_{max}. In conditions where intracellular

Ca^{2+} has been increased by mechanisms such as a prevailing β-adrenergic stimulation, then activation of the PKC pathway by α$_1$-receptor agonists might be expected to have a small effect on time-averaged intracellular Ca^{2+}. This would result in a predominant effect of the negative inotropic actions, which we hypothesize are due to phosphorylation of Ser 42, Ser 44. Lester et al. (120) reported that exposure of single heart cells to both R-PIA an adenosine receptor agonist and the phorbol ester, DOG, followed by rapid Triton X-100 skinning resulted in a 25% decrease in V$_{max}$, with no change in the pCa–force relation. However, there was no detectable change in myofilament protein phosphorylation (122).

It is difficult to know exactly why the literature contains so many different findings regarding the role of the myofilaments in the functional effects of PKC activation. Certainly the complexity of the PKC cascade may be an important reason. In most of the studies, the basal level of phosphorylation is not clear. Moreover, it is evident that the multiple sites of PKC phosphorylation give rise to different effects, so that the integrated effect of these multiple pathways appears certain to depend on prevailing inotropic state. There may also be important age- and species-dependent differences that have not been thoroughly evaluated.

Integration of Signals for Cardiac Myocyte Hypertrophy/Failure with cTnI Protein Phosphorylation

Changes in the level of phosphorylation of cTnI at both PKA and PKC sites may be an important mechanism in the long-term regulation of cardiac function in the hypertrophic/failure process. Bartel et al. (11) reported that isoproterenol induced inotropic effects, and phosphorylation of myosin-binding protein C, cTnI, and phospholamban in failed human hearts was reduced roughly to half that induced in control heart preparations. Addition of dibutryl cAMP was able to fully phosphorylate these proteins. These data suggested impaired mechanisms for phosphorylation of myofilament proteins in heart failure. In agreement with this conclusion, Bodor et al. (12) reported that levels of cTnI phosphorylation are chronically low in heart failure. Wolff et al. (274) reported that tension developed by permeabilized cells from hearts of patients in end-stage failure was more sensitive to Ca^{2+} than controls. However, following phosphorylation by PKA both preparations exhibited the same sensitivity to Ca^{2+}. Thus, when treated with PKA, the Ca^{2+} sensitivity of preparations from failed hearts was more greatly reduced than that of controls. This is what would be expected if the levels of phosphorylation of cTnI in the failed preparations was relatively low.

Evidence from animal studies also strongly supports the idea that PKC activation is a signal in the hypertrophic process and that PKC-dependent phosphorylation of cTnI may be a critical factor in hypertrophy/failure. Malhotra et al. (138) reported that diabetic cardiomyopathy is accompanied by an increase in cTnI phosphorylation and an associated redistrubution of PKC-epsilon. As proposed by Malhotra et al. (138), this result suggests that an angiotensin II receptor-mediated activation of PKC and a loss of myofibrillar sensitivity to Ca^{2+} may contribute to the contractile dysfunction seen in chronic diabetes. Pressure overload and stretch of adult myocardium has also been shown to stimulate angiotensin II–mediated hydrolysis of phosphatidylinositol and PKC translocation (64, 190). Using a transgenic mouse model overexpressing PKC-β-2, Takeishi et al. (244) demonstrated that in vivo phosphorylation of cTnI was elevated and associated with a decrease in twitch parameters of isolated cells, with no change in the Ca^{2+} transient. This effect could be reversed by superfusion of the cells with a selective inhibitor of PKC-β-2. Similar results were reported by Bowman et al. (14). In the Bowman et al. (14) experiments, PKC activation was induced by conditional expression of PKC-beta in hearts of transgenic mice. When the transgene was expressed in the adult, there was a mild and progressive hypertrophy and impaired relaxation of the heart. However, expression in newborns was associated with sudden death and abnormal Ca^{2+} transients in the isolated myocytes. The findings with PKC-β overexpression fit well with earlier findings with a transgenic mouse overexpressing Gαq and resulting in constitutive activation of the PKC signaling pathway. These hearts showed hypertrophy, decompensation to pressure overload hypertrophy, and increased phosphorylation of cTnI (31, 214). Our own studies (171, 176) predict that the phosphorylation of cTnI at Ser 42, Ser 44 could induce a depression in maximum myofilament activity. Bowling et al. (15) have provided substantial evidence that these studies with animal models may have application to human heart failure. They reported that, compared to non-failed controls, explanted hearts with dilated or ischemic myopathy demonstrated increased activity and membrane expression of PKC-α, PKC-β1, and PKC-β2. The increase in enzyme expression and activity was not uniform, as PKC-ε expression was not significantly changed.

How is it that altered myofilament response to Ca^{2+} could be an important aspect of the hypertrophy/failure process? An inescapable aspect of hypertrophy/failure is that alterations in Ca^{2+} homeostasis and myofilament activity occur in concert with the signals (peptides, growth factors, and neurotransmitters) that promote transcription, translation, and assembly of myocyte components. Myofilaments sense most, if not all, of the same intrinsic and extrinsic signals that regulate the hypertrophic process. Changes in preload and afterload that result in elaboration of growth signals are associated with changes in sarcomere length and interfilament spacing that alter not only maximum tension but also the ability of Ca^{2+} to activate the myofilaments (226). In fact, length dependence of myofilament activation is a well-accepted mechanism for intrinsic regulation by Starling's law (4, 226). Changes in pH_i associated with stretch of the myocardium (226) are well known to alter the myofilament response to Ca^{2+} and would also be expected to promote hypertrophy (238). Hypertrophic signaling involves transduction through G protein–coupled receptors (GPCR), activation of the MAPK, and phosphorylation of transcription factors. Myofilaments also respond to signal transduction through G protein–coupled receptors and activation of second messenger cascades through functionally significant protein phosphorylations by PKC and PKA (227). These phosphorylations, which appear to involve cTnI in important ways (225), modify myofilament response to Ca^{2+} (88) and sarcomere length (108) and thereby alter cellular Ca^{2+} dynamics. It is now apparent that such changes in Ca^{2+} dynamics are geared to hypertrophic signaling through Ca^{2+}–calmodulin dependent activation of the phosphatase calcineurin (155). Calcineurin activates transcription by dephosphorylation of a nuclear transcriptional factor (NF-AT), thereby permitting its translocation to the nucleus. A role for Ca^{2+} in the hypertrophic response is strongly indicated from studies showing that overexpression of calmodulin (CaM) (63) or calsequestrin (214) induces hypertrophy. Direct evidence that gene transcription is regulated by Ca^{2+} oscillations, amplitude, and duration involving NF-AT has been presented by Dolmetsch et al. (38). Yet despite the obvious connections, schemes depicting cascades thought to result in cardiac myocyte hypertrophy (238), in general, have not explicitly integrated cellular Ca^{2+} homeostasis and Ca^{2+} responsiveness of the myofilaments into the signaling pathways. There is no better example of the linkage between Ca^2 homeostasis, myofilament response to Ca^{2+}, and hypertrophy than the identification of sarcomeric mutations that are causal in familial hypertrophic myopathy (FHC). In this case the central question of causality in cardiac hypertrophy begins with a defect in the myofilaments (183).

cTnT FUNCTION AND PHOSPHORYLATION

cTnT Primary Structure and Functional Domains

Shown below is the primary structure of cTnT, which is the biggest and most likely the longest member of the Tn complex. cTnT thus has the potential for the most extensive and versatile interactions with adjacent proteins of the thin filament. Moreover, the expression of multiple cTnT isoforms, which are generated by alternative splicing, also gives rise to versatility in the actions of cTnT (5, 6, 17). The C-terminal half of the molecule comprises a highly conserved Ca^{2+}-sensitive region that interacts with cTnC, cTnI, and Tm (Fig. 7–4). The NH_2-terminal half of cTnT anchors the cTn complex to Tm independently of the Ca^{2+} concentration surrounding the myofilaments.

The interactions of TnT with its neighbors on the thin filament have been well defined in studies using large N- and C-terminal fragments of fsTnT (161, 247). Using tyrosine reactivity as a marker of accessibility of residues of Tm, Mak and Smillie (134) reported that the TnT fragment, $fsTnT_{1-151}$, interacts with Tm at its C-terminus. Moreover, removal of the Tm C-terminal domain by carboxy-peptidase treatment in-

```
                    ┌─ EEEEDWREDE
  1 MSDIEEVVEE YEEEEQ EEAAV┴EEQEEAAEE DA EAEAETEE TRAEEDEEEE EAKEAEDGPM

 61 EESKPKPRSF MPNLVPPKIP DGERVDFDDI HRKRMEKDLN ELQALIEAHF ENRKKEEEEL

121 VSLKDRIERR RAERAEQQRI RNEREKERQN RLAEERARRE EEENRRKAED EARKKKALSN

181 MMHFGGYIQK QAQTERKSGK RQTEREKKKK ILAERRKVLA IDHLNEDQLR EKAKELWQSI

241 YNLEAEKFDL QEKFKQQKYE INVLRNRIND NQKVSKTRGK AKVTGRWK
```

Splice Variants of TnT3

TnT1 EEEEDWREDE inserted after EEAAV (aa 17-21) as indicated
TnT2 missing EAAVE
TnT4 missing EAAVE EEEEDWREDE

hibits the binding of TnT (1–158) to Tm (77, 134, 191). Co-crystallization of TnT with Tm indicates that fsTnT$_{1-158}$ makes up about 70% of the length of TnT and spans the Tm–Tm overlap region at the most proximal portion of this peptide (271). Schaertl et al. (217) showed that fsTnT$_{1-159}$ did not affect the rate of S1 binding to actin in regulated thin filament preparations. However, fsTnT$_{1-159}$ was able to increase the size of the cooperative unit from 6 to 9 and to 12 actins. This finding fits with the location of the N-terminus of TnI at the region of overlap between contiguous Tm molecules. In the case of cTnT, N- and C-terminal regions of the molecule have similar functional specializations. For example, Fisher et al. (47) showed that the affinity of fsTnT$_{159-259}$ for Tm and actin-Tm was 2 orders of magnitude lower than that of full-length TnT. Moreover, an effect of Ca^{2+} on the energetics of thin filament assembly could not be attributed to the N-terminal region, indicating that the change in state of the thin filament upon binding of Ca^{2+} was due in large part to altered interactions of the globular C-terminal regions with the thin filament. Chandra et al. (23) have also found that preparations reconstituted with cTnT missing a large portion of the N-terminus retained the same sensitivity to Ca^{2+} as preparations containing full-length cTnT.

The N-terminal half of human cTnT contains splice sites giving rise to four isoforms in the adult human heart (5, 146, 147). TnT1 contains the full complement of amino acids. TnT4 is smallest variant in which 15 amino acids from positions 18 to 32 are spliced out. TnT2 is missing amino acids 18–22, and TnT3 is missing amino acids 23–32. The most abundant isoform present in the adult human heart is TnT3, but all four appear to be present to some extent (5). Splice variants involve removal of acidic amino acids, and thus isoform switching as occurs with development (53, 140), heart failure (5), and diabetes (2) would be expected to alter the charge–charge interactions so important in thin filament regulation. In fact, cTnT isoform switching has been demostrated to alter the sensitivity of skinned fiber preparations to Ca^{2+} (2, 140, 253). Tobacman and Lee (253) have reported that the two beef cTnT isoforms (124, 125), which differ by five amino acids (EAAEE) are similar in their ability to promote tropomyosin polymerization. Moreover, there was no difference in the potentiation of the thin filament–activated Mg-ATPase rate by a high concentration of myosin S1. However, reconsituted preparations containing the smaller isoform demonstrated a Ca^{2+}-activation curve that was shifted 0.1–0.15 pCa units to the left of preparations containing the larger isoform. To understand the role of the N-terminus of cTnT in activation of the myofilaments, we have studied (22) a deletion mutant of cTnT missing residues 1–79. When reconstituted into skinned fiber bundles, this deletion mutant was able to elicit Ca^{2+}-sensitive regulation of force with a half-maximal activation identical to that of full-length cTnT. However, the magnitude of tension was depressed. We interpret this to mean that cTnT$_{1-79}$ may regulate the number of actins under the control of Tn, as suggested by the results of Schaertl et al. (216).

Our results with the cTnT missing 79 N-terminal amino acids also agree with the findings in studies on fsTnT indicating that C-terminal regions of cTnT are likely to be the most important in transmitting the Ca^{2+} binding signal from cTnC to the rest of the thin filament. Studies by Fisher et al. (47), who investigated effects of an N-terminal truncation of cTnT on thin filament assembly, indicated that that the globular C-terminal region of cTnT was most important in switching the thin filament from the relaxed state to the active state. However, on the basis of findings in fast skeletal muscle preparations, Schaertl et al. (216) reported that, although fsTnT$_{159-259}$ was able to impart Ca^{2+} sensitivity to the rate of S1 binding to actin-Tm, this fragment of fsTnT had no effect on co-operativity. Interestingly, in the absence of Ca^{2+}, fsTnT$_{159-259}$ was able to inhibit the initial binding of S1 to actin–Tm–Tn to about the same extent as full-length TnT. A delay in the rate of binding provided evidence for a blocked state of cross-bridges. The C-terminal end of fsTnT represented by residues fsTnT$_{159-259}$ binds to the region containing Cys 190 in Tm, and this interaction is weakened when Ca^{2+} binds to fsTnC. C-terminal regions of fsTnT have also been shown to interact with fsTnI and fsTnC. Refinements in the sites of interaction show that there is overlap between regions of fsTnT interacting with fsTnC (fsTnT$_{176-230}$) and with fsTnI (fsTnT$_{201-253}$) (98), which is located at fsTnI$_{1-57}$ (197, 233). A highly conserved motif of fsTnT in the C-terminal region forms a heptad repeat that is likely to react with a heptad repeat in cTnI, forming a coiled-coil (233). The region of interaction fsTnC with fsTnT has not been defined, although crosslinking studies indicate that the binding region is close to fsTnC-Cys 98 in the central helix (264). In the case of fsTnT, Ca^{2+}-sensitive interactions between fsTnT and fsTnC appear to involve potentiation of ATPase activity (197), in contrast to the interactions between fsTnC and fsTnI, which appear to involve a release from inhibition.

To identify regions of interaction between cTnI and the C-terminus cTnT, we generated a series of N-terminal truncation mutants of cTnI (cTnI$_{33-211}$, cTnI$_{54-211}$, and cTnI$_{80-211}$). In its unphosphorylated state, it is apparent that the unique NH$_2$-terminal extension of cTnI either does not interact with cTnT or has only weak interactions. cTnI$_{33-211}$, which is missing this region, was able to essentially fully restore Ca^{2+}-

sensitivity of ATPase rate in reconstituted myofibrillar preparations (65). However, in fully reconstituted systems containing regulated actin and myosin S1, the relationship between pCa and actomyosin Mg-ATPase activity was shifted to the right upon removal of residues 1–32 of cTnI, with no effect on maximum rate. Chandra et al. (21) showed a similar result in a detergent-extracted preparation in which the Tn complex was exchanged with a Tn complex missing TnI_{1-32}. In this case there was no depression in maximum tension, but there was a small but significant right shift of the pCa tension relation compared to preparations reconstituted with full-length cTnI. However, our results from studies with mutants $cTnI_{80-211}$ and $cTnI_{54-211}$ clearly identified amino acids 54–79 of cTnI as forming a region of interaction with cTnT. The $cTnI_{54-211}$ mutant retained an ability to bind to a cTnT affinity column, whereas the $cTnI_{80-211}$ mutant did not. Functional studies indicated that the interaction between residues 54–79 of cTnI with cTnT *inhibit* Ca^{2+}-dependent activation of cardiac myofilaments. The function of this interaction is different from that of the corresponding region in fsTnI-fsTnT, which appears to activate skeletal myofilaments (197).

cTnT Sites of Phosphorylation

The C-terminal region of cTnT, which is important in Ca^{2+}-dependent control of the actin–myosin reaction, also contains most of the sites of phosphorylation by PKC and Ca^{2+}-calmodulin–dependent protein kinase (CaM-kinase). A site of phosphorylation in the N-terminus at Ser 1, (66, 263) was described in early studies, but the functional significance of this phosphorylation remains unknown. When freshly isolated from beef heart, troponin T contains 1–2 mol phosphate per mole of protein. (240). There are phosphorylation sites at Ser 1 and in the C-terminal region of the molecule. The site at Ser 1 is a substrate for troponin T kinase, which is a casein kinase type 2 (66, 207). A second phosphorylation site at Thr 190 in the bovine sequence is phosphorylated by CaM-kinase II (Ca^{2+}-calmodulin–dependent protein kinase II) (94, 96). This site is also a site for phosphorylation by PKC (170). An interesting point is that phosphorylation of this site by CaM-kinase II can be demonstrated in the holotroponin complex, but not in the troponin–tropomyosin complex (94). Thus the site may be inaccessible in the presence of Ca^{2+}, a necessary constituent in the assay. Early studies (208) demonstrated that fast skeletal TnT could be phosphorylated at Ser 1 and possibly in the region 147–161, by phosphorylase kinase. However, it was apparent that the kinase preparations may have been contaminated with troponin T kinase.

PKC-phosphorylation sites on beef cardiac TnT are in the C-terminal half of the molecule at Thr 190, Ser 194, Thr 199 and Thr 280 (175). These sites correspond to Thr 193, Thr 202, and Thr 284 in the human sequence (Fig. 7–4). C-terminal sites are also phosphorylated by PKC in the case of fsTnT (209), which indicates that this modification may be of general significance in regulation of striated muscle contraction. Swiderek et al. (240) used ^{31}P-NMR (nuclear magnetic resonance) to identify sites phosphorylated on bovine cardiac TnT isolated from the muscle in a highly phosphorylated form. Their data indicate that both Ser 1 and Thr 194 contain covalent phosphate. It appears, therefore, that these sites are exposed in the myofilament lattice containing the holo-Tn complex. Phosphorylation of the Ser 194 was not detected in the experiments of Noland et al. (170). Phosphorylation at the bovine cardiac cTnT sites by PKC results in an inhibition of the maximum ATPase rate of reconstituted thin filament preparations activating myosin S1 (170, 172, 173, 177). Therefore, phosphorylation of TnT provides an additional mechanism for the regulation of crossbridge kinetics. These sites are located in a region of the TnT molecule thought to be important in Ca^{2+}-sensitive interactions with TnC and Tm (44). In the case of skeletal muscle, these Ca^{2+}-sensitive interactions appear to involve activation (potentiation) of ATPase activity (197), in contrast to the interactions between TnC and TnI, which appear to involve a release from inhibition. The phosphorylation of TnT is associated with a significant decrease in its affinity for actin-Tm and an inhibition of Ca-stimulated binding of myosin-S1-ADP to reconstituted thin filaments. It is unlikely that Ca affinity is altered, inasmuch as there is no effect of TnT phosphorylation of the pCa-activity relation of these reconstituted preparations. Determination of thin filament sites phosphorylated in rat cardiac myocytes exposed to the phorbol ester TPA or to the α-adrenergic agonist phenylephrine, showed relatively little change in the level of phosphorylation of the TnT sites (261). As in the case of cTnI, there is some isozyme specificity in PKC-phosphorylation sites. Jideama et al. (99) reported that PKC-zeta phosphorylated free cTnT more effectively than PKC isozymes α, δ, and ε.

In the case of cTnT, data generated so far indicate that phosphorylation of C-terminal sites decreases the maximum acto-S1 ATPase rate, with no effect on Ca^{2+} sensitivity. This is surprising in view of the location of the phosphoryation sites in the region of interaction with cTnI and cTnT. No studies have been done explicitly comparing mechanical properties of skinned fibers containing specific changes in cTnT phosphorylation. The inhibition of Ca^{2+}-stimulated Mg-ATPase activity of actomyosin containing phosphorylated TnT was shown by Noland and Kuo (174) to be associated with a 3.5-fold decrease in its apparent affinity for Tm-F-actin. There was also a decrease in maximum binding of phosphorylated cTnT compared to unphosphorylated to Tm-F-actin. In view of the present picture that the N-terminus and not the C-terminus of cTnT would be important in scaling maximum activation, these results suggest that phosphorylation of the C-terminal resudues in cTnT may affect the affinity of N-terminal sites for Tm-actin. This would fit with the findings of Chandra et al. (22), who showed that removal of a large stretch of the N-terminus of cTnT is associated with a fall in maximum force and ATPase rate with no change in Ca^{2+} sensitivity.

TROPOMYOSIN FUNCTION AND PHOSPHORYLATION

Tropomyosin isoforms and cardiac function

Tropomyosin contains a single site of phosphorylation located at Ser 283 at the far C-terminus (75). The charge change associated with this phosphorylation in a critical region of Tm appears certain to alter the mechanisms by which transitions in state occur in the myofilaments. To support this statement I first discuss charge changes associated with isoform switching of α- and β-Tm and with expresson of mutant Tm linked to famital hypertrophic cardiomyopathy (FHC; 251, 266). Shown below are the primary sequences of the alpha- and beta-isoforms of Tm. Skeletal muscle expresses the β-isoform, whereas the α-isoform is the predominant from in the heart. General sites of interaction of Tm with TnT are illustrated in Figure 7–4 as is a single site of phosphorylation at Ser 283.

Tm alone is able induce the closed and open states of the thin filament. The blocked state of the thin filaments also requires Tm–Tn interactions and a level of ambient Ca^{2+} below the threshold for binding to the TnC regulatory site. The equilibrium between these three states was defined as K_{Tm} by Lehrer (118), McKillop and Geeves (141) and Lehrer and Geeves (119). The open and closed states demonstrate different affinities for myosin-S1. Binding of S1 induces switching between these states such that myosin S1 binding curves show typical sigmoid characteristics of a cooperative process. The ability of the binding of one S1 to influence the subsequent binding of S1 is related to the size of the cooperative unit (n, number of actins turned on). In turn, the size of the cooperative unit appears to be determined by the physical and chemical state of the C-terminus of Tm. Lehrer et al. (121) compared cooperative binding of S1 to thin filaments containing smooth muscle, striated muscle, and nonmuscle Tm, which differ in C-terminal residues. The steepness of the binding curves was correlated with the cooperative unit as determined in separate kinetic studies. Variations in the C-terminus of Tm that modulate the strength of end-to-end iteractions appear to be responsible for these differences, which are described in an appealing model of thin filament regulation involving a continuous flexible strand of Tm (121). As mentioned earlier, this flexibility is best achieved by nonspecific charge–charge interactions that permit multisite interactions between Tm as it moves on the thin filament. The charged state of side groups of Tm have been demonstrated explicitly to confer flexibility (120).

Earlier studies had pointed to the importance of the Tm C-domain. Removal of the last 11 C-terminal amino acids results in loss of cooperative activation of the myofilaments most likely through a loss of an ability of Tm to polymerize and a weakening of Tm binding to actin (184, 249). The C-domain of Tm is also involved in cooperative binding of TnI-TnT to Tm (191). Althouth removal of the Tm overlap greatly reduced the cooperative binding of myosin S1 to reconstituted thin filaments, studies of Pan et al. (184) showed that a substantial residual cooperativity remains. This residual cooperativity is not to be due to the N-terminus of cTnT, which one might expect

```
ALPHA  1   MDAIKKKMQM LKLDKENAID RAEQAEADKK QAEDRCKQLE  EEQQALQKKL KGTEDEVEKY
BETA   1   MDAIKKKMQM LKLDKENALD RAEQAEADKK AAEDRSKQLE  DELVSLQKKL KGTEDELDKY

       61  SESVKEAQEK  LEQAEKKATD AEADVASLNR RIQLVEEELD RAQERLATAL QKLEEAEKAA
       61  SEALKDAQEK  LELAEKKATD AEADVASLNR RIQLVEEELD RAQERLATAL QKLEEAEKAA

       121 DESERGMKVI ENRAMKDEEK MELQEMQLKE AKHIAEDSDR  KYEEVARKLV ILEG E LERS E
       121 DESERGMKVI ESRAQKDEEK MEIQEIQLKE AKHIAEDADR  KYEEVARKLV IIES D LERA E

       181 ERAEVAESKC  GDLEEELKIV TNNLKSLEAQ ADKYSTKEDK YEEEIKLL E EKLKEAETRAE
       181 ERAELSEGKC  AELEEELKTV TNNLKSLEAQ AEKYSQKEDR YEEEIKVL S DKLKEAETRAE

       241 FAERSVAKLE KTIDDLEDEV YAQKMKYKAI SEELD  N ALND IT  S L 284
       241 FAERSVTKLE KSIDDLEDEL YAQKLKYKAI SEELD  H ALND MT  S L 284
```

would link the truncated Tm units along the thin filament (185). These results thus indicate that actin–actin interactions may be important in the cooperative response, although it must be pointed out that the studies by Pan et al. (185) were done at low ratios of S1 to actin, a condition in which crossbridge-dependent activation would be minimized.

In any case, together with other work in this area, there is ample evidence to support the hypothesis that charge alterations in a broad region of the Tm C-domain lead to physiologically relevant changes in myofilament response to Ca^{2+}. Isoform switching to the β-Tm isoform involves 39 amino acid substitutions, 25 of which occur in the C-domain with two important charge modifications—Ser229Glu and His276Asn (136). These substitutions give β-Tm a more negative charge than α-TM. This change in charge appears responsible for a weaker binding of β-Tm of fast skeletal muscle to the N-domain of TnT than α-Tm (191). Although such a change in interaction between TnT and Tm would be predicted to make myofilaments more sensitive to Ca^{2+}, this has been difficult to assess in the intact myofilament lattice until relatively recently.

Transgenic (TG) approaches have made it possible to test hypotheses derived from studies on the in vitro properties of tropomyosin (Tm) in the heart functioning in situ The idea that alterations in charge on Tm should have important effects on cardiac myofibrils in the intact lattice and on cardiac function has been supported by TG approaches in which the isoform population of Tm in mouse heart muscle was switched from essentially all α-Tm to one containing a preponderance of the β-Tm isoform (167, 183). Skinned fiber bundles from hearts of TG mice overexpressing β-Tm (TG-β-Tm) were more senstivie to Ca^{2+} than wild-type myofibrils (183, 276); but showed no differences in length-dependent activation (276). An unexpected finding in these preparations was the demonstration that the effect of PKA-dependent phosphorylation to decrease the sensitvity of myofibrils to Ca^{2+} was blunted in the skinned fiber bundles containing more β-Tm than α-Tm. Measurements of the inotropic response to ISO in working heart preparations also indicated that the relaxant effect of submaximal β-adrenergic stimulation was significantly reduced in the TG hearts compared to WT controls. Moreover, relaxation, as determined by minimum dp/dt and half-relaxation times ($RT_{1/2}$) under basal conditions was prolonged in the TG versus WT hearts. The TG hearts showed no alterations in expression of Ca^{2+}-pumps that would account for the impaired relaxation. Changes in cardiac function associated with Tm isoform switching are also seen at the level of the single cell. We (276) compared the mechanical dynamics of single intact cells isolated from TG and non-TG (NTG) mouse hearts with the dynamics of whole-heart contraction. TG-β–Tm cells showed no change in the extent of shortening when compared with WT myocytes. There were, however, significantly reduced maximal rates of shortening and relaxation. We (183, 276) concluded from these findings that the enhanced myofibrillar sensitivity to Ca^{2+} was responsible for a delay in relaxation. Measurements of force/ATPase ratios in the WT and TG skinned fiber bundles showed no differences. This indicated that crossbridge detachment was most likely unaffecterd by Tm isoform switching, and that crossbridge attachment may be altered. The results also indicated that the impaired ability of ISO to induce a relaxant effect in the working heart preparations was also due to impaired ability of cTnI phosphoryation to desensitize the myofilaments to Ca^{2+}. Molecular mechanisms for this difference in transduction of the cTnI phosphorylation signal are not yet clear. The data do, however, suggest that transmission of the signal from the N-terminus of cTnI to the C-terminus of cTnT and on to the isoforms of Tm may be affected by differences in C-terminal amino acids of Tm.

Two missense mutations in α-Tm linked to FHC (Asp175Asn and Glu180Gly) involve charge changes in C-terminal residues that induce altered regulation of the myofibrillar response to Ca^{2+}. Binding affinity of the Asp175Asn Tm mutant to actin was shown by Golitsina et al. (60) to be greater than than two-fold weaker than for the Glu180Gly mutant, which was similar to WT Tm. This is of some interest inasmuch as the Asp175Asn is better correlated with hypertrophy than the Glu180Gly mutant (251). However, there were differences between the mutant and WT tropomyosins in their apparent affinity for Tn. The mutations decreased the local stability or increased the local flexibility of Tm, and demonstrated differences in their response to myosin S1 binding to the actin–tropomyosin filament. We (43) have found that skinned fiber bundles from hearts of transgenic mice harboring the Asp175Asn mutation are more sensitive to Ca^{2+} than WT controls. Moreover, isolated working mouse hearts demonstrate a prolongation in relaxation, as determined by minimum dp/dt and half-relaxation times under basal conditions. The hearts expressing Asp175Asn Tm also show a prolongation of time to peak pressure maximum +dp/dt.

Tropomyosin Phosphorylation

Phosphorylation at Ser 283 of the C-domain of Tm provides another potentially important charge modification of Tm. Studies by Heeley et al. (76) and Heeley (75) demonstrated that phosphorylation of Ser 283 altered the interaction of the N-terminal fragment of

TnT (1–158) with Tm. This TnT fragment promoted end-to-end interactions of Tm as determined by measurements of relative viscosities, but the change in viscosity was significantly lower for preparations containing phosphorylated α-Tm than for those containing nonphosphorylated α-Tm. In addition, affinity chromatography experiments demonstrated that the interaction between the C-terminal fragment TnT (159–259) and phosphorylated α-Tm was strengthened relative to the nonphosphorylated control. The net effect of these altered protein–protein interactions appears to be a modulation of the actin–myosin interaction. The ATPase rate of reconstituted preparations containing myosin S1 and regulated thin filaments with unphosphorylated Tm was double the rate of preparations containing phosphorylated α-Tm (75). There were no differences in Ca^{2+} sensitivity or steepness of the Ca^{2+}-ATPase activity relations.

Little is known regarding the physiological significance of Tm phosphorylation, although it has been speculated there may be importance in thin-filament assembly during development by alterations in the TnT–Tm interactions. This speculation is based on data showing that the kinase responsible for the phosphorylation is abundant in embryonic muscle (35, 156). That kinase has been designated "tropomyosin kinase" because of its unique properties including specificity for striated muscle Tm and an activity that is not affected by Ca^{2+}, calmodulin, or cAMP. α-Tm is a better substrate for Tm kinase than β-Tm. The Tm kinase phosphorylates casein, but its activity is not inhibited by heparin, a potent inhibitor of casein kinase II.

In summary, in vitro functional effects of changes in the phosphorylation state of the C-terminus of Tm provide further evidence that localized charge changes in Tm may be amplified to have generalized effects on thin-filament regulation of the actin–myosin interaction. Investigation of the functional significance of the Tm phosphorylation has been limited to reconstituted systems, but with the advent of transgenic approaches it has become possible to investigate this question directly in the myofilament lattice and in the heart. Such studies may provide clues to why this mechanism seems to be used by mammals essentially exclusively during development. It is also important to note that phosphorylation of Tm in various muscle diseases including heart failure has not to my knowledge been investigated thoroughly.

MLC2 FUNCTION AND PHOSPHORYLATION

Primary Structure of MLC2 and Functional Domains

The primary structure of MLC2 in human ventricle is shown below. MLC2 is homologous with other important regulatory proteins—calmodulin and troponin C (337). It consists of two domains. However, unlike calmodulin and TnC, the central linker is distorted and the protein demonstrates a compact configuration in models of myosin S1 (204). The N-terminal end of MLC2, which is highly homologous with calmodulin, contains a phosphorylatable Ser 19 located toward the C-terminus of the lever arm of myosin. Ser 19 in the human ventricular MLC2 is a site of phosphorylation by the Ca^{2+}-calmodulin–dependent kinase designated myosin light chain kinase (MLCK) and by PKC. The N-terminus also has metal binding EF hand regions. Clusters of hydrophobic residues in the N-terminal region form an interface with hydrophobic residues on myosin S1.

There is substantial evidence that MLC2 itself modifies crossbridge kinetics and force generation. Metal binding and protein phosphorylation would be expected to modify these functional properties of MLC2. Moreover, the special role of MLC2 metal binding in serving as a trigger for invertebrate muscle activation, as well as the special role of MLC2 phosphorylation in the activation of smooth muscle contraction, strongly suggests an important role for metal binding and covalent modification in modulation of cardiac muscle contraction.

Metal Binding to MLC2

There is little doubt that Ca^{2+}-binding to the regulatory site on cTnC is the trigger for contraction of heart muscle fibers, yet metal binding–dependent control of the interaction of the MLC2 (primary structure shown below) with myosin appears certain to play an important role in modulating contractile activity. The idea of a myosin-linked regulatory mechanism in vertebrate striated muscle was inspired both by observations showing a Ca^{2+} binding–induced conformation changes in isolated thick filaments (162), and by early X-ray diffraction studies of frog muscle stretched beyond overlap, showing activation-related changes in intensity of equatorial reflections and suggesting crossbridge move-

```
1   MAPKKAKKRA GGANSNVFSM FEQTQIQEFK EAFTIMDQNR DGFIDKNDLR DTFAALRVNV

61  KNEEIDEMIK EAPGPINFTV FLTMFGEKLK GADPEETILN AFKVFDPEGK GVLKADYVRE

121 MLTTQAERFS KEEVDQMFAA FPPDVTGNLD YKNLVHIITH GEEKD
```

ment independent of thin filaments (113). The divalent ion binding sites of myosin of vertebrate striated muscle have been studied extensively. Myosin contains a relatively high-affinity, nonspecific, divalent ion binding site on each of the two light chains. The sites bind Ca^{2+} and Mg^{2+} competitively, with the affinity for Ca^{2+} being higher than that for Mg^{2+}. The reported affinities for Ca^{2+} and Mg^{2+} of the site vary greatly, but it is likely that the affinities are significantly lower than Ca^{2+} binding to TnC (89, 186). There are four domains in MLC2 sequence that are analogous to the Ca^{2+}-binding domains of parvalbumin and calmodulin; however, only one domain is complete. Bagshaw and Reed (8) demonstrated that the nonspecific high-affinity site is indeed located in domain 1. Equilibrium binding studies (186) show that either purified myosin or myosin in the myofilament lattice is able to bind a small amount of Ca^{2+} at pCa 5 in the presence of physiological levels of Mg^{2+} (1 mM). However, since the rate constant for dissociation of Mg is slow (0.05–0.06 s^{-1}), the exchange of Ca^{2+} and Mg^{2+} at the site is expected to take tens of seconds to complete and is apparently too slow to contribute to rapid initiation of contraction of striated muscle. The data are, therefore, against a mechanism involving direct Ca^{2+} interaction with myosin as a switch for activation of cardiac myofilaments. Myofilaments lacking the regulatory site on cTnC cannot be switched on by Ca^{2+}, whereas myofilaments reconstituted with a mutant MLC2 defective in the metal binding site can be switched on (36). As will be discussed, though, crossbridge kinetics and maximum tension are altered when the MLC2 metal binding site is defective. It is important to note that metal binding sites such as those of MLC2 may be titrated differentially by alterations in the frequency of stimulation. In this way MLC2 metal binding sites may serve to integrate the prevailing frequency of stimulation of the heart. Inasmuch as metal binding to calmodulin, the activator of MLCK, may serve also to integrate the frequency of stimulation, it seems likely that protein phosphorylation is also modified with changes in the frequency with which pulses of Ca^{2+} come into the cells. Indeed levels of phosphorylation of both cardiac (237) and skeletal muscle light chains have been demonstrated to increase with increases in the frequency of contraction (221). Metal binding to the MLC2 sites appears to be unaffected by the state of light chain phosphorylation (89).

MLC2 and Modulation of Striated Muscle Contraction

As indicated by its strategic location on the myosin crossbridge, MLC2 is an important controller of myofilament activity. In crystallograhic studies muscle, MLC2 was shown to wrap around a 10 nm segment of the α-helix that forms the lever at the C-terminal region of the myosin head of fast skeletal muscle. Irving et al. (93), using fluorescence polarization as a reporter of myosin head orientation, reported that this light chain binding segment of the myosin head tilts both during an imposed filament sliding and during the force recovery that is thought to signal the elementary force-generating event. Later studies (91) indicated that MLC2 undergoes a 60° change in angle, suggesting a combination of tilting of MLC2 itself relative to the lever axis and a rotation of MLC2 about its own axis. It thus seems highly likely that MLC2 interaction with myosin affects the stability or stiffness of the lever or the kinetics of its motion. Although numerous studies (222) have been done in biochemical systems to investigate this potential role of MLC2 in regulation, approaches in which the light chain is removed, exchanged, or reconstituted offer the clearest insights (182, 148, 243). Unfortunately, different results have been obtained using different extraction conditions, and most studies have been done in fast-twitch skeletal muscle. Hofmann et al. (82) investigated the effect of partial removal of MLC2 on isometric tension, stiffness, and maximum velocity of shortening at pCa values between 6.6 and 4.5. Their results showed that removal of MLC2 induced an increase in submaximal tension and stiffness with no effect at the maximally activating pCa value, and that the crossbridge detachment (which is rate-limiting in measurements of unloaded shortening velocity) was slowed. Using a different MLC 2 extraction protocol from that of Hofmann et al., Szczesna et al. (243) also measured effects of removal of MLC 2 on the steady-state relations between pCa and force, as well as on the kinetics of Ca^{2+} activation of contraction following photolysis of caged Ca^{2+}. In contrast to results of Hofmann et al. (82), Szczesna et al. reported that upon removal of MLC 2, Ca^{2+} dependence of force generated by the fibers demonstrated a *decrease* in Ca^{2+} sensitivity compared to the unextracted controls. However, the fibers reconstituted with MLC2 did not achieve the same level of Ca^{2+}-sensitivity as the unextracted fibers. This was not the case in the study by Hofmann et al. (82) in which MLC2 readdition fully restored the pCa-force relation.

Effects of MLC2 removal on Ca^{2+}-sensitive transitions in crossbridge state have also been studied by determination of k_{tr}, a measure of crossbridge cycling rate (151). The measurement of k_{tr} involves activation of steady isometric tension with Ca^{2+}, followed by rapid release and re-extension (16). The time course of redevelopment of tension, which is generally exponential, provides a value of k_{tr}. The values of k_{tr}, which increase sigmoidally with increasing Ca^{2+} concentration, were shown to increase upon partial extraction of MLC2. Similar results were obtained when rate of tension development was measured following a sudden release of

Ca^{2+} by flash-photolysis of DM-nitrophen (188). In the native fibers, rate of tension development was relatively low at submaximally activating levels of free Ca^{2+} and high at levels of Ca^{2+} where tension was maximum. Removal of MLC2 resulted in an increase in the rate of tension development following Ca^{2+} release to that of the maximum rate achieved in the controls. Importantly, rate of force development retained Ca^{2+} sensitivity if TnC was removed instead of MLC2. Szczesna et al. (243) also concluded that MLC2 is important in determining the kinetics of crossbridge cycling on the basis of results of studies in which force transients were generated by photolysis of nitrophenyl-EGTA. However, these studies indicated that MLC2 removal *decreased* rate of force development two-fold. Again, this disagreement may be due to use of extraction conditions that, while resulting in nearly complete removal of MLC2, produce a preparation in which some activities cannot be restored on reconstitution with MLC2. Whatever the case, results using different techniques indicate that Ca^{2+}-binding sites on MLC2 determine, at least in part, the Ca^{2+} sensitivity of rate of force development in fast skeletal muscle.

Further evidence that the metal binding sites on MLC2 are important with regard to regulation of crossbridge cycling rate comes from studies (36) in which the endogenous MLC2 was partially exchanged with the mutant MLC2 (D47A). This point mutation, which is within the Ca^{2+}/Mg^{2+} binding motif of MLC2, greatly reduced its affinity for divalent cations. Fibers containing about 50% endogenous MLC2 and 50% of the D47A mutant, demonstrated a 40% drop in maximum tension and a 30% drop in k_{tr}. Thus, it is apparent that the MLC2 with incompetent metal binding decreases the rate of transition of crossbridges to the force-generating state. Studies employing photolytic release of a Ca^{2+}-chelator also demonstrated that the fibers containing the D47A MLC2 mutant relaxed faster than the controls. These data indicate that divalent metal binding sites on MLC2 modulate force-generation by myofilaments by regulating both the rate of crossbridge attachment and the rate of crossbridge detachment. With removal of light chains it appears that submaximal tension increases at a given pCa value as crossbridges enter the strong, force-generating state faster and detach more slowly than fibers with their full complement of MLC2.

A reasonable speculation on the mechanism of these effects is that removal of the light chain induces increased flexibility in myosin heads, resulting in a tendency for the crossbridges to move away from the thick filament, thereby increasing their probability of attachment to actin at submaximal levels of activation. Levine et al. (126) tested the idea that MLC2 helps maintain the order of the thick filament by isolating thick filaments and examining them using electron microscopy and optical diffraction of negatively stained samples. Removal of MLC2 from the thick filaments resulted in a loss of order interpreted to indicate increased myosin head mobility and increased accessibility to actin. Levine et al. (126) concluded that interactions between MLC2 and the thick filament backbone maintain a reversible order of myosin heads.

MLC2 Phosphorylation and Regulation of Crossbridges

Although for many years the role of MLC2 phosphorylation in the heart was controversial and poorly understood, a clearer understanding has emerged from careful comparisons of levels of MLC2 phosphorylation and myofibrillar function, which has also pronded a more complete understanding of the kinases and phosphatases that regulate phosphorylation. Early studies (see ref. 224 for review) indicated that there was no effect of MLC2 phosphorylation on myosin ATPase or actomyosin ATPase rate. However Cooke et al. (29) subsequently reported that thio-phosphorylation of MLC2 in skinned psoas fibers held at constant length, and in myofibrils crosslinked with glutaraldehyde to prevent shortening, decreased the ATPase activity by a factor of two. This result suggested that for effects of MLC2 phosphorylation on myofibrillar function to be demonstrated, the intact filament structure was required. Cooke et al. (29) also suggested that the reduction in ATPase rate would decrease energy use and shortening velocity. In agreement with this finding, experiments of Crow and Kushmerick (30) on fast skeletal fibers demonstrated a good correlation between the increased phosphorylation of MLC2 and a decrease in the rate of high-energy phosphate utilization and a parallel decrease in the maximum velocity of shortening. It was suggested that MLC2 phosphorylation may be capable of down-modulation of the rate of crossbridge turnover in tetanized muscle. However, Barsotti and Butler (10) reported that tetanized fast skeletal muscles demonstrated no consistent relationship between the degree of MLC2 phosphorylation and the rate of chemical energy utilization, a finding arguing against a role of phosphorylation of MCL2 as a modulator of the rate of crossbridge cycling. These controversies began to be sorted out with the reports by Persechini and Stull (194), who demonstrated that whereas phosphorylation of MLC2 in isolated thick filaments had no effect on myosin ATPase rate, there was a two-fold decrease in the K_m for actin activation of myosin ATPase with no effect on V_{max}. They further showed that the demonstration of this effect depended on the age of the myosin preparation and the ionic strength.

There is general agreement that increases in MLC2

phosphorylation correlate with an increase in the force level at submaximal Ca^{2+} and an associated leftward shift of the pCa-force relation in permeabilized skeletal and cardiac muscle fibers (159, 195). A plausible mechanism for this increase in Ca^{2+} sensitivity is that phosphorylation increases the rate of transition of crossbridges from weak to strong force-generating attachments (148). It is also evident that the sensitization to Ca^{2+} involves cooperative, crossbridge-dependent activation of the thin filament. When Metzger et al. (148) extracted TnC from skinned fibers, a maneuver that greatly reduces cooperative activation of the thin filament, the effect of MLC2 phosphorylation on the pCa–force relation was no longer evident although crossbridge attachment rate as reflected in k_{tr} remained. Experiments of Patel et al. (189) have extended these findings. In their experiments, Patel et al. (189) performed measurements reflecting the transition from strong to weak crossbridges by induction of relaxation by photolysis of diazo-2, which transforms it into a high Ca^{2+}-affinity chelator. Relaxation rate was slower in the fibers with phosphorylated MLC2 than in the controls. The slowed relaxation was associated with full elaboration of thin filament activation, inasmuch as changes in relaxation rates induced by Ca^{2+} and crossbridge-dependent activation were virtually eliminated (189). Thus, these results indicate that in addition to enhancing the transition from weak to strong crossbridge interactions with actin, MLC2 phosphorylation slows the transition from the strong to the weak state. There are, however, experiments that indicate that phosphorylation of MLC2 may not alter the kinetics of attached crossbridges in heart muscle. Rossmanith et al. (21) reported that the positive inotropic effect of endothelin in rat ventricular muscle was associated with an increase in MLC2 phosphorylation, but no change in myosin head turnover rate as determined from complex stiffness values in which the frequency at which stiffness assumes a minimum value (f_{min}) is a measure of the kinetics of attached, force-generating crossbridges. Rossmanith et al. (211) concluded that the positive inotropic effect of endothelin was related to a change in the sensitivity of the myofilaments to Ca^{2+} resulting from the MLC2 phosphorylation. However, although they showed no change in cTnI phosphorylation in these experiments, they did not determine the relative importance of potential changes in the Ca^{2+}-transient or in intracellular pH.

A reversible increase in myosin head mobility and/or changed conformation, induced by MLC2 phosphorylation, provides a structural basis for the increases in submaximal force developed by skinned fiber preparations in striated muscle. This change in mobility is likely to be due to charge changes at the N-terminus of MLC2. Levine et al.(127) reported that upon MLC2 phosphorylation, the near-helical array of surface myosin heads seen in relaxed preparations was lost. They proposed that this disorder places the heads close to thin filaments, thereby potentiating actin–myosin interaction at low calcium levels. Support for this hypothesis has come from experiments in which the time that crossbridges spend near the actin binding site was optimized by increasing the sarcomere length or by shrinking the fiber myofilament lattice with dextran. Both of these manipulations reduce interfilament spacing, thereby placing the crossbridge close to actin without changing the level of MLC2 phosphorylation. In this case, one might expect the potential of submaximal force enhanced by MLC2 phosphorylation to be blunted. This is exactly what was found by Yang et al. (277) in their report that changes in inter-filament spacing mimic the effects of MLC2 phosphorylation. Modulation of crossbridge interactions by MLC2 phosphorylation clearly offers an energetic advantage by potentiating the response of the myofilaments to Ca^{2+}. It is potentially significant that there are reports of a reduction in MLC2 phosphorylation of atrial MLC2 associated with heart failure (161). Threats to this mode of economy of energy use include missense mutations in MLC2 in patients with FHC.

Although MLC2 phosphorylation appears to be important in post-tetanic potentiation in skeletal muscle (157), it role in heart muscle contraction remains unclear. It is relatively difficult to demonstrate changes in MLC2 phosphorylation during common mechanisms of inotropic stimulation of the heart.(78, 90, 270). Levels of phosphorylation remain at about 0.3–0.4 mol/mol in hearts beating at basal physiological rates and following inotropic interventions such as β-adrenergic stimulation. Clues to the possible mechanism for changing MLC2 phosphorylation came from early work of Sayers and Bárány (216), who reported that turtle hearts beating with a heart rate of about 4/min could undergo MLC2 phosphorylation and dephosphorylation during a beat. This suggested that the phosphorylation may be rate dependent and a function of the kinase/phosphatase ratio. Clear evidence that long-term changes in heart rate can modulate the levels of light chain phosphorylation came from the work of Silver et al. (221). When the frequency of stimulation of the heart muscles (perfused rabbit septal preparations) was increased from 0 to 126 beats/min for 30 min, there was a frequency-dependent increase in MLC2 phosphorylation from 0.1 to 0.4 mol phosphate/mol light chain. They also reported that short-duration inotropic interventions such as adrenergic stimulation for 30 sec were not associated with an increase in MLC2 phosphorylation. Moreover, the rates of MLC2 phosphorylation and dephosphorylation in ventricular muscle were much slower than rates of phosphorylation in either fast-twitch skeletal or smooth muscles. These findings suggest a rationale for findings of some investigators that inotropic interventions such as β-adrenergic agonist increase MLC2 phosphorylation (9).

An additional mechanism by which MLC2 may become phosphorylated physiologically is through the PKC pathway, as stimulated by endothelin, angiotensin, and α-adrenergic stimulation. It is apparent from studies of phospho-peptide maps obtained of MLC2 phosphorylated by PKC and MLCK that the site of phosphorylation is the same in each case (262). Therefore it is not surprising that the effect of phosphorylation by PKC is to increase sensitivity to Ca^{2+} of skinned fibers (26) and myofibrils (173, 262). There is also PKC-dependent phosphorylation of cTnI, cTnT, and MyBP-C. One of the remaining challenges is to understand the integrated effects of these phosphorylations. There is no clear consensus in the literature. For example, Clement et al. (26) reported that ATPase activity of myofibrils is increased with PKC phosphorylation despite a simultaneous phosphorylation of cTnI and cTnT, where as Venema et al. (266) conclude that the phosphorylation of cTnI and cTnT override the sensitizing effect of PKC phosphorylation of MLC2. Damron et al. (266) have addressed this question. Effects of arachidonic acid (AA) and endothelin on cardiac excitation–contraction coupling are a good example of the complexity of the cellular responses that may involve MLC2 phosphorylation. Damron et al. (34) reported that these signaling molecules potentiate Ca^{2+} transients and contractility via a PKC-dependent pathway that involves K^+ channels. They also showed that AA or endothelin induces phosphorylation of cTnI or MLC2 by a mechanism that did not require extracellular Ca^{2+} or intact intracellular Ca^{2+} stores. These phosphorylations could be mimicked by treatment of isolated myocytes with 13-acetate phorbol ester myristate, and were blocked by the PKC inhibitor calphostin C. With identification of phosphorylation sites on MLC2 and other regulatory proteins, it appears possible to understand the relative importance of these phosphorylations using transgenic approaches in which myofilament proteins are replaced by mutants lacking the phosphorylation sites.

PHOSPHORYLATION AND FUNCTION OF CARDIAC MYOSIN BINDING PROTEIN C

Primary Structure of MyBP-C and Functional Domains

Shown on the following page is the primary structure of human myosin-bonding protein C (MyBP-C or C-protein). The probable location of MyBP-C in the myofilament lattice is illustrated in Figure 7–1. The primary structure reveals tandem domains made up of relatively small globular domains consisting of about 90–100 amino acids.

MyBP-C is situated on the thick filaments, attached to myosin at the head–neck region. It was discovered as an abundant myosin-associated protein by Offer and colleagues (179, 180), who demonstrated that it was localized to the thick filament by immunocytochemical analysis that demonstrated that it exists in 10 nm transverse stipes with 43 nm intervals along the thick filament in two 200 nm zones separated by 400 nm on either side of the M-line (179). The stoichiometry with myosin suggested that three MyBP-C molecules wrap transversely around the thick filament; the exact disposition of the proteins on the thick filament is not clear. The special importance of the cardiac MyBP-C is indicated by evidence that this isoform is expressed specifically and in abundance during both human and murine development of the heart (48, 57). MyBP-C appears to function both as a regulator of crossbridge activity (70, 71, 83, 84, 154, 176) and as a factor stabilizing thick-filament structure and assembly (49, 51). MyBP-C interacts with regions of myosin distal to S1, termed "myosin subfragment-2" and "light meromyosin" (62, 232). MyBP-C consists of 10 globular motifs (I–X) each about 90–100 amino acids long. Experiments of Gilbert et al. (59) suggested strongly that MyBP-C is associated with the thick filament through its C-terminus. Using truncation mutants, they showed that the C-terminal regions (approximately VII–X) are sufficient to target to myosin in the A-band. The area on myosin where MyBP-C binds has been localized to a region consisting of 126 residues at the N-terminus of myosin S2 (62). This region of the myosin heavy chain is the locus of several missense mutation (R870H and E924K) linked to FHC (19, 265). Gruen and Gautel (62) have shown that, compared to controls, the binding affinity of MyBP-C for myosin containing these mutations is greatly reduced. MyBP-C also forms a complex with titin, a giant sarcomeric protein that appears to provide a molecular ruler in thick-filament assembly (115). It is likely that this ternary complex of myosin, titin, and MyBP-C serves a role in thick-filament assembly and stabilization of that assembly. The C-terminal domain of MyBP-C, where titin and myosin bind, is deleted in individuals harboring a mutation linked to FHC (19). A hallmark of this mutation is disarray in the myofilament lattice.

Although early studies suggested that MyBP-C may alter its reaction with actin in the transition between a relaxed and an activated state, this mechanism has not been demonstrated. The idea remains, though, that cardiac MyBP-C, which is an asymmetric molecule about 22 nm long, could reach out across the distance between thick and thin filament, and perhaps compete with actin for myosin binding (68, 154, 158). It is more likely that MyBP-C has more a subtle modulatory in myofilament regulation. When added to actomyosin, MyBP-C was shown to modulate ATPase activity, depending on the stoichiometric ratio (70, 71, 158), but the significance of these effects remains unclear. More definitive evidence that MyBP-C may regulate force and shortening of muscle has come from studies in which MyBP-C was partially extracted from skinned myocytes from rat heart (83, 84). Extraction of 60%–70% of the MyBP-C was associated with an increase in force at submaximally activating Ca^{2+} concentrations (83). After the extraction of MyBP-C, the relation between pCa and force was also less steep than controls, but there was no effect on maximum tension. MyBP-C extraction was also associated with a reduction in the slope of the pCa-tension relation, which indicates that cooperative activation of the myofilaments was reduced. This effect was interpreted to reflect a radial movement of crossbridges away from the thick filaments missing MyBP-C. As a consequence, the

```
   1 MPEPGKKPVS AFSKKPRSVE VAAGSPAVFE AETERAGVKV RWQRGGSDIS ASNKYGLATE

  61 GTRHTLTVRE VGPADQGSYA VIAGSSKVKF DLKVIEAEKA EPMLAPAPAP AEATGAPGEA

 121 PAPAAELGES APSPKGSSSA ALNGPTPGAP DDPIGLFVMR PQDGEVTVGG SITFSARVAG

 181 ASLLKPPVVK WFKGKWVDLS SKVGQHLQLH DSYDRASKVY LFELHITDAQ PAFTGSYRCE

 241 VSTKDKFDCS NFNLTVHEAM GTGDLDLLSA FRRTS LAGGGRRIS DSHEDT GILDFSSLLK

 301 KRDSFRTPRD SKLEAPAEED VWEILRQAPP SEYERIAFQY GVTDLRGMLK RLKGMRRDEK

 361 KSTAFQKKLE PAYQVSKGHK IRLTVELADH DAEVKWLKNG QEIQMSGSKY IFESIGAKRT

 421 LTISQCSLAD DAAYQCVVGG EKCSTELFVK EPPVLITRPL EDQLVMVGQR VEFECEVSEE

 481 GAQVKWLKDG VELTREETFK YRFKKDGQRH HLIINEAMLE DAGHYALCTS GGQALAELIV

 541 QEKKLEVYQS IADLMVGAKD QAVFKCEVSD ENVRGVWLKN GKELVPDSRI KVSHIGRVHK

 601 LTIDDVTPAD EADYSFVPEG FACNLSAKLH FMEVKIDFVP RQEPPKIHLD CPGRIPDTIV

 661 VVAGNKLRLD VPISGDPAPT VIWQKAITQG NKAPARPAPD APEDTGDSDE WVFDKKLLCE

 721 TEGRVRVETT KDRSIFTVEG AEKEDEGVYT VTVKNPVGED QVNLTVKVID VPDAPAAPKI

 781 SNVGEDSCTV QWEPPAYDGG QPILGYILER KKKKSYRWMR LNFDLIQELS HEARRMIEGV

 841 VYEMRVYAVN AIGMSRPSPA SQPFMPIGPP SEPTHLAVED VSDTTVSLKW RPPERVGAGG

 901 LDGYSVEYCP EGCSEWVAAL QGLTEHTSIL VKDLPTGARL LFRVRAHNMA GPGAPVTTTE

 961 PVTVQEILQR PRLQLPRHLR QTIQKKVGEP VNLLIPFQGK PRPQVTWTKE GQPLAGEEVS

1021 IRNSPTDTIL FIRAARRVHS GTYQVTVRIE NMEDKATLVL QVVDKPSPPQ DLRVTDAWGL

1081 NVALEWKPPQ DVGNTELWGY TVQKADKKTM EWFTVLEHYR RTHCVVPELI IGNGYYFRVF

1141 SQNMVGFSDR AATTKEPVFI PRPGITYEPP NYKALDFSEA PSFTQPLVNR SVIAGYTAML

1201 CCAVRGSPKP KISWFKNGLD LGEDARFRMF SKQGVLTLEI RKPCPFDGGI YVCRATNLQG

1261 EARCECRLEV RVPQ
```

actin–crossbridge reaction would be expected to be promoted at submaximally activating free Ca^{2+} but not at full activation. Hofmann et al. (83) also reported that partial extraction of MyBP-C was able to significantly increase V_{max} in a low-velocity phase of unloaded shortening of skinned fibers but that it had no effect on a high-velocity phase. The interpretation of these experiments, which were carried out at relatively low levels of Ca^{2+} activation, was that MyBP-C may impose an internal load either by binding to actin and myosin or by influencing mechanical properties of myosin crossbridges. Direct evidence that the state of MyBP-C may restrict the movement of the myosin head and affect the actomyosin ATPase rate was reported by Weisberg and Winegrad (268, 269), who used electron microscopy and optical diffraction to examine the structure of thick filaments isolated from rat ventricles. With filaments containing the α-myosin heavy-chain isoform, they found that phosphorylation of MyBP-C by PKA induced an extension of the crossbridges away from the thick-filament backbone. This effect was apparently correlated with an increase in the ATPase rate measured using histochemical techniques (143).

Phosphorylation Sites of Cardiac MyBP-C

Since the first experiments of Jeacock and England (97), the phosphorylation of MyBP-C was well known to occur in situ. Myofilament proteins from hearts stimulated with β-adrenergic agonists consistently demonstrate phosphorylation of MyBP-C (55, 69, 72, 112). However, the relative role of MyBP-C phosphorylation in regulation of myofilament activity and/or structure remains unclear. Sites on cTnI, phospholamban, the ryanodine receptor, and L-type Ca^{2+} channels are simultaneously phosphorylated by various agonists—for example, β-adrenergic stimulation. Thus, a specific role for MyBP-C phosphorylation has been difficult to determine. In the case of TG mice expressing ssTnI, that lacks PKA-dependent phosphorylation sites, effects of PKA-dependent phosphorylation on myofilament Ca^{2+}-sensitivity and unloaded shortening velocity were absent. Clearly, with the advent of TG techniques, this issue may soon be directly addressed. Moreover, precise determination of crossbridge kinetics may reveal a role of MyBP-C phosphorylation on myofilament activity. A role is strongly suggested from the tissue-specific expression of the cardiac isoform, its multi-site phosphorylation, and from the strategic location of the phosphorylation domain to the region of interaction with myosin S2 and titin.

It has been known for some time that MyBP-C has multiple sites for phosphorylation by PKC, PKA, and Ca^{2+}-dependent kinases (69, 70, 129, 219). The sites of phosphorylations are localized in the N-terminal domain of the molecule and are unique to the cardiac isoform. There are also interactions among the phosphorylation sites, suggesting a sequential switching mechanism. Mohammed et al. (153) have identified PKA and PKC phosphorylation sites in chicken cardiac MyBP-C. Three PKA sites were found that have homologous regions in the N-terminus of human cardiac MyBP-C. These correspond to a Ser at position 265, a Ser at position 274 and a Ser at position 304 in human sequence. Ser 265 and Ser 304 are cross-phosphorylated by PKC. A specific PKC site in a C-terminal region of the molecule was found in the chicken protein, and is apparently not present in the rat or human. A significant finding in the study by Mohammed et al. (153) was that all of the identified sites of phosphorylation in the N-terminus of cardiac MyBP-C were not present in skeletal muscle. The chicken heart isoform of MyBP-C has been shown to be readily phosphorylated by CaM kinase II. Phosphopeptide maps indicate that some of the sites may overlap with PKA sites (219). Schlender et al. (219) have also reported that PKA sites of bovine MyBP-C are substrates for phosphorylase kinase. Importantly, in this study it was shown that Ca^{2+-} and cAMP-*independent* kinases were unable to phosphorylate MyBP-C. Using site-directed mutagenesis, Gautel et al. (56) identified a key regulatory motif specific for the cardiac isoform of MyBP-C. The isoform-specific motif consists of LAGGGRRIS—a loop in the N-terminal region of cardiac MyBP-C, which was identified as the key substrate site for phosphorylation by both PKA and a CaM-kinase. A novel finding in this study was that phosphorylation of two further sites by PKA was induced by phosphorylation of this isoform-specific site. This phosphorylation switch can be mimicked by aspartic acid instead of phosphoserine.

Hartzell (69) reported the first evidence that phosphorylation of MyBP-C was correlated with relaxation time in the heart. The studies were done in frog heart and showed that relaxation time, which decreased with isoproterenol stimulation and increased with carbamylcholine administration, was well correlated temporally with the levels of MyBP-C phosphorylation. Enhanced relaxation associated with increases in stimulation frequency did not correlate with MyBP-C phosphorylation. An effect of MyBP-C phosphorylation on crossbridge kinetics could explain the enhanced relaxation, but it does not seem likely that the explanation is a desensitization of the myofilaments to Ca^{2+} as appears to be the case with cTnI phosphorylation. Experiments (55, 267) in which cTnI phosphorylation is specifically changed indicate that PKA phosphorylation of cTnI is both necessary and sufficient to elicit a desensitization of cardiac myofilament activity to activation by Ca^{2+}. In contrast to the case with amphibian hearts, Kranias et al. (110) showed that the temporal relation between enhanced relaxation following pulse perfusion of rabbit hearts with ISO did not correlate well with MyBP-C phosphorylation. This was also the case with cTnI phosphorylation. However, this lack of correlation may be due to multi-site phosphorylations that were not taken into account in this study. In fact, it may be possible that the lack of correlation of MyBP-C phosphorylation and frequency-dependent enhanced relaxation noted by Hartzell (69) may also be related to a failure to know the exact sites that are undergoing changes in phosphorylation and a potential requirement for multiple sites to be phosphorylated to see a change in activity.

SUMMARY AND CONCLUSIONS

This summary of current knowledge of how phosphorylation may alter the function of key proteins in a functional unit of the myofilaments emphasizes the complexity of potential regulation by covalent modifications. In many cases, I have pointed out the unique aspects of the phosphorylation sites in the case of heart muscle. This provides strong circumstantial evidence that covalent modification has a special role in heart versus skeletal striated muscle. One imagines from the functional changes induced by changes in phosphorylation that this special role (for example in the case of PKA-dependent phosphorylation of cTnI) is related to regulating the dynamics of the contraction–relaxation cycle as heart rate changes. Other phosphorylations appear to keep the system poised for optimal use of energy supply. For example, phosphorylation of MLC2 and MyBP-C appear to alter the order of crossbridges thereby affecting Ca^{2+} sensitivity. In contrast, phosphorylation of cTnT and cTnI by PKC appears to modulate crossbridge cycling rate. Yet despite all the detailed information presented above, we still do not have a clear picture of integrative biology of cardiac myofilament protein phosphorylation. This is certain to be clarified by the application of powerful techniques manipulating genetic expression of mutant forms and isoforms of the myofilament proteins. Even so, with muliple sites of phosphorylation existing in most of the proteins, and with multiple kinases and phosphatases acting to determine the relative levels of phosphorylation, there is much work to be done.

This review is dedicated to the memory of Dr. Miroslav Stoyanovich (1965–1998), who contributed greatly to some of the experiments described from our laboratory. Work described in this paper could not have been done without the help and inspiration of my many fine colleagues and teachers. I especially wish to acknowledge Professor S. Victor Perry, who taught me much, and got me started thinking about protein phosphorylation. I am grateful for grant-in-aid support from the Heart, Lung, and Blood Institute of the National Institutes of Health, United States Public Health Service.

REFERENCES

1. Abbott, M. B., V. Gaponenko, E. Abusamhadneh, N. Finley, G. Li, A. Dvoretsky, M. Rance, R. J. Solaro, and P. R. Rosevear. Regulatory domain conformational exchange and linker region flexibility in cardiac troponin C bound to cardiac troponin I. *J. Biol. Chem.* 275:20610–206107, 2000.
2. Akella, A. B., X. L. Ding, R. Cheng, and J. Gulati. Diminished Ca^{2+} sensitivity of skinned cardiac muscle contractility coincident with troponin T-band shifts in the diabetic rat. *Circ. Res.* 76: 600–606, 1995.
3. Al-Hillawi, E. D. G. Bhandar, H. R. Trayer, and I. P. Trayer. The effects of phosphorylation of cardiac troponin-I on its interactions with actin and cardiac troponin-C. *Eur. J. Biochem.* 228: 962–970, 1995.
4. Allen, D. G. and J. C. Kentish. The cellular basis of the length-tension relation in cardiac muscle. *J. Mol. Cell Cardiol.* 2;17: 821–840, 1985.
5. Anderson, P. A. W., N. N. Malouf, A. Oakeley, E. D. Pagani, and P. D. Allen. Troponin T isoform expression in humans: a comparison among normal and failing adult heart, fetal heart, and adult and fetal skeletal muscle. *Circ. Res.* 60:1226–1233, 1991.
6. Anderson, P. A. A. Greig, T. M. Mark, N. N. Malouf, A. E. Oakeley, R. M. Ungerleider, P. D. Allen, and B. K. Kay. Molecular basis of human cardiac troponin T isoforms expressed in the developing, adult, and failing heart. *Circ. Res.* 76:681–686, 1995.
7. Andreev, O. A. and J. Borejdo. Interaction of the heavy and light chains of cardiac myosin subfragment-1 with F-actin. *Circ. Res.* 81:688–693, 1997.
8. Bagshaw, C. R., and G. H. Reed. The significance of the slow dissociation of divalent metal ions from myosin regulatory light chains. *FEBS Lett.* 81:386–390, 1977.
9. Bárány M. and K. Bárány. Protein phosphorylation in cardiac and vascular smooth muscle. *Am. J. Physiol.* 241 (*Heart Circ. Physiol.* 10):H117–H1128, 1981.
10. Barsotti, R. and T. Butler. Chemical energy usage and myosin light chain phosphorylation in mammalian skeletal muscle. *J. Muscle Res. Cell Motil.* 5:45–64, 1984.
11. Bartel, S., B. Stein, T. Eschenhagen, U. Mende, J. Neumann, W. Schmitz, E. G. Krause, P. Karczewski, and H. Sholz. Protein phosphorylation in isolated trabeculae from nonfailing and failing human hearts. *Mol. Cell. Biochem.* 157:171–179, 1996.
12. Bodor, G. S. A. E. Oakely, P. D. Allen, D. L. Crimmins, J. H. Ladenson, and P. A. Anderson. Troponin I phosphorylation in the normal and failing adult human heart. *Circulation* 96:1495–1500 1997.
13. Bowling, N. R. A. Walsh, G. Song, T. Estridge, G. E. Sandusky, R. L. Fouts, K. Mintze, T. Pickard, R. Roden, M. R. Bristow, H. N. Sabbah, J. L. Mizrahi, G. Gromo, G. L. King, and C. J. Vlahos. Increased protein kinase C activity and expression of Ca^{2+}-sensitive isoforms in the failing human heart. *Circulation* 99:384–91, 1999.
14. Bowman, J. C., S. J. Steinberg, T. Jiang, D. L. Geenen, G. I. Fishman, and P. M. Buttrick. Expresson of protein kinase C beta in the heart causes hypertrophy in adult mice and sudden death in neonates. *J. Clin Invest* 100:2189–2195, 1997.
15. Bremel, R. D., J. M. Murray, and A. Weber. Manifestations of cooperative behavior in the regulated actin filament during actin activated ATP hydrolysis in the presence of calcium. *Cold Spring Harbor Symp. Quant. Biol.* 37:267–275, 1972.

16. Brenner, B. Effect of Ca^{2+} on cross-bridge turnover kinetics in skinned single rabbit psoas fibers: implications for regulation of muscle contraction. *Proc. Natl. Acad. Sci. U.S.A.* 85:3265–3269, 1988.
17. Brietbart, R. E., and B. Nadal-Ginard. Complete nucleotide sequence of the fast skeletal troponin T gene. Alternatively spliced exons exhibit unusual interspecies divergence. *J. Mol. Biol.* 188: 313–324, 1986.
18. Capogrossi, M. C., T. Kaku, C. R. Filburn, D. J. Pelto, R. G. Hansford, H. A. Spurgeon, and E. G. Lakatta. Phorbol ester and dioctanoylglycerol stimulate membrane association of protein kinase C and have a negative inotropic effect mediated by changes in cytosolic Ca^{2+} in adult rat cardiac myocytes. *Circ. Res.* 66: 1143–1155, 1990.
19. Carrier, L., G. Bonne, E. Bährend, B. Yu, P. Richard, F. Niel, B. Hainque, C. Cruaud, F. Gary, S. Labeit, J.-B. Bouhour, O. Dubourg, M. Desnos, A. A. Hagège, R. J. Trent, M. Komajda, and K. Schwartz. Organization and sequence of human cardiac myosin binding protein C gene (MYBPC3) and identification of mutations predicted to produce truncated proteins in familial hypertrophic cardiomyopathy. *Circ. Res.* 80:427–434, 1997.
20. Chandra M., W.-J. Dong, B.-S., Pan, H. C. Cheung, and R. J. Solaro. Effects of protein kinase A phosphorylation on signaling between cardiac troponin I and the N-terminal domain of cardiac troponin C. *Biochemistry* 36:13305–13311, 1997.
21. Chandra, M., J. J. Kim, and R. J. Solaro. An improved method for exchanging troponin subunits in detergent skinned rat cardiac fiber bundles. *Biochem. Biophys. Res. Commun.* 263:219–223, 1999.
22. Chandra, M., D. E. Montgomery, J. J. Kim, and R. J. Solaro. The N-terminal region of troponin T is essential for the maximal activation of rat cardiac myofilaments. *J. Mol. Cell. Cardiol.* 31: 867–880, 1999.
23. Chong, P. C. S, and R. S. Hodges. Proximity of sulfhydryl groups to the sites of interaction between components of the troponin complex from rabbit skeletal muscle. *J. Biol. Chem.* 257:2549–2555, 1982.
24. Chong, P. C. S, and R. S. Hodges. Photochemical cross-linking between rabbit skeletal troponin subunits. Troponin I-troponin T interactions. *J. Biol. Chem.* 257:11667–11672, 1982.
25. Cingolani, H. E., B. V. Alvarez, I. L. Ennis, M. C. Camilion de Hurtado. Stretch-induced alkalinization of the feline papillary muscle. An autocrine-paracrine system. *Circ. Res.* 83:775–780, 1998.
26. Clement, O., M. Puceat, M. P. Walsh, and G. Vassort. Protein kinase C enhances myosin light-chain kinase effects on force development and ATPase activity in rat single skinned cardiac cells. *Biochem. J.* 285:311–317, 1992.
27. Cole, H. A. and S. V. Perry. The phosphorylation of troponin I from cardiac muscle. *Biochem. J.* 149:525–533, 1975.
28. Colyer, J. and J. H. Wang. Dependence of cardiac sarcoplasmic reticulum calcium pump activity on the phosphorylation status of phospholamban. *J. Biol. Chem.* 266:17486–17493, 1991.
29. Cooke, R, Franks K, and J. T. Stull. Myosin phosphorylation regulates the ATPase activity of permeable skeletal muscle fibers. *FEBS Lett.* 144:33–37, 1982.
30. Crow, M. T. and M. J. Kushmerick. Myosin Light chain phosphorylation is associated with a decrease in the energy cost for contraction in fast twitch mouse muscle. *J. Biol. Chem.* 257: 2121–2124, 1982.
31. D'Angelo, D. D., Y. Sakata, J. N. Lorenz, G. P. Boivin, R. A. Walsh, S. B. Liggett, and G. W. Dorn II. Transgenic Gαq overexpression induces cardiac contractile failure in mice. *Proc. Natl. Acad. Sci. U.S.A.;* 94:8121–8126, 1997.
32. Dalgarno, D. C., R. J. A., Grand, B. A. Levine, A. J. G. Moir, G. M. M. Scott, and S. V. Perry. Interaction between troponin I and troponin C. *FEBS Lett.* 149:54–58, 1982.
33. Dalla Libera, L., E., Hoffmann, M. Floroff, and G. Jackowski Isolation and nucleotide sequence of the cDNA encoding human ventricular myosin light chain 2. *Nucleic Acids Res.* 17:2360, 1989.
34. Damron, D. S., A. Darvish, L. Murphy, W. Sweet, C. S. Moravec, and M. Bond. Arachidonic acid-dependent phosphorylation of troponin I and myosin light chain 2 in cardiac myocytes. *Circ. Res.* 76:1011–1019, 1995.
35. deBelle, I. and A. S. Mak. Isolation and characterization of tropomyosin kinase from chicken embryo. *Biochim Biophys Acta* 925:17–26, 1987.
36. Diffee, G. M., J. R. Patel, F. C. Reinach, M. L. Greaser, and R. L. Moss. Altered kinetics of contraction in skeletal muscle fibers containing a mutant myosin regulatory light chain with reduced divalent cation binding. *Biophys. J.* 71:341–50, 1996.
37. Dohet, C., E. al-Hillawi, I. P. Trayer, J. C. Ruegg. Reconstitution of skinned cardiac fibres with human recombinant cardiac troponin-I mutants and troponin-C. *FEBS Lett.* 377:131–134, 1995.
38. Dolmetsch, R. E., R. S. Lewis, C. C. Goodnow, and J. I. Healy. Differential activation of transcription factors induced by Ca^{2+} response amplitude and duration. *Nature* 386:855–858, 1997.
39. Dong, W.-J., M. Chandra, J. Xing, M. She, R. J. Solaro, and H. C. Cheung. Phosphorylation-induced distance change in a cardiac muscle Troponin I mutant. *Biochemistry* 36:6754–6761, 1997.
40. Dong, W.-J., M. Chandra, J. Xing, R. J. Solaro, and H. C. Cheung. Conformation of the N-terminal segment of a monocysteine mutant of Troponin I from cardiac muscle. *Biochemistry* 36:6745–6753, 1997.
41. Endoh, M. and J. R. Blinks. Actions of sympathomimetic amines on the Ca^{2+} transients and contractions of rabbit myocardium: reciprocal changes in myofibrillar responsiveness to Ca^{2+} mediated through α- and β-adrenoceptors. *Circ. Res.* 62:247–265, 1988.
42. England, P. J. Cardiac function and phosphorylation of contractile proteins. *Phil. Trans. R. Soc. Lond. B* 302: 83–90, 1983.
43. Evans, C., J. R. Pena, M. Muthuchamy, D. F. Wieczorek, R. J. Solaro, and B. M. Wolska. Altered hemodynamics and response to β-adrenergic stimulation in transgenic mice harboring a mutant tropomyosin linked to hypertrophic cardiomyopathy. *Am.J. Physiol. (Heart Circ. Physiol.)* 279:H2414–24123, 2000.
44. Farah, C. S. and F. C. Reinach. The troponin complex and regulation of muscle contraction. *FASEB J.* 9:755–767, 1995.
45. Farah, C. S., C. A. Miyamoto, C. H. I, Ramos, A. R. da Silva, R. B. Quaggio, K. Fujimori, L. B. Smillie, and F. C. Reinach. Structural and regulatory functions of the NH_2- and COOH-terminal regions of skeletal muscle troponin I. *J. Biol. Chem.* 269:5230–5240, 1994.
46. Fentzke, R. C., S. H. Buck, J. R. Patel, H. Lin, B. M. Wolska, M. O. Stojanovic, A. M. Martin, R. J. Solaro, R. L. Moss, and J. M. Leiden. Impaired cardiomycyte relaxation and diastolic function in transgenic mice expressing slow skeletal troponin I in the heart. *J. Physiol. (Lond.)* 517: 143–157, 1999.
47. Fisher, D., G. Wang, and L. S. Tobacman NH_2-terminal truncation of skeletal muscle troponin T does not alter the Ca^{2+} sensitivity of thin filament assembly. *J. Biol. Chem.* 270:25455–25460, 1995.
48. Fougerousse, F., A. L. Delezoide, M. Y. Fiszman, K. Schwartz, J. S. Beckmann, and L. Carrier. Cardiac myosin binding protein C gene is specifically expressed in heart during murine and human development. *Circ. Res.* 82:130–133, 1998.
49. Freiburg, A. and M. Gautel. A molecular map of the interactions between titin and myosin-binding protein C. Implications for

sarcomeric assembly in familial hypertrophic cardiomyopathy. *Eur. J. Biochem.* 235:317–23, 1996.
50. Fuchs, F., Y.-M. Liou and Z. Grabarek. The reactivity of sulfhydryl groups of bovine cardiac troponin C. *J. Biol. Chem.* 264: 20344–20349, 1989.
51. Fürst, D. O., U. Vinkemeyer, and K. Weber. Mammalian skeletal muscle C-protein: purification from bovine muscle, binding to titin and the characterization of a full-length cDNA. *J. Cell Sci.* 102:769–778, 1992.
52. Gagne, S. M., S. Tsuca, M. X. Li, L. B. Smillie, and B. D. Sykes. Structure of the troponin C regulatory domains in the apo and calcium-saturated states. *Nature Struct Biol.* 2:784–789, 1995.
53. Gao, L., J. M. Kennedy, and R. J. Solaro. Differential expression of TnI and TnT isoforms in rabbit heart during the perinatal period and during cardiovascular stress. *J. Mol. Cell. Cardiol.* 27:541–550, 1995.
54. Gaponenko, V., E. Abusamhadneh, M. B. Abbot, N. Finleyh, G. Gasmi-Seabrook, R. J. Solaro, M. Rance, and P. R. Rosevear. Effects of troponin I phosphorylation on conformational exchange in the regulatory domain of cardiac troponin C. *J. Biol. Chem.* 274:16681–16684, 1999.
55. Garvey, J. E., E. G. Kranias, and R. J. Solaro. Phosphorylation of C-protein, troponin I and phospholamban in isolated rabbit hearts. *Biochem. J.* 249:709–714, 1988.
56. Gautel, M., O. Zuffardi, A. Freiburg, S. Labeit. Phosphorylation switches specific for the cardiac isoform of myosin binding protein-C: a modulator of cardiac contraction? *EMBO J.* 14: 1952–1960, 1995.
57. Gautel, M., D. O. Furst, A. Cocco and S. Schiaffino. Isoform transitions of the myosin binding protein C family in developing human and mouse muscles: lack of isoform transcomplementation in cardiac muscle. *Circ. Res.* 82:124–129, 1998.
58. Geeves, M. A., and S. S. Lehrer. Dynamics of the muscle thin filament regulatory switch: the size of the cooperative unit. *Biophys. J.* 67:273–282, 1994.
59. Gilbert, R., M. G. Kelly, T., Mikawa and D. A. Fischman. The carboxyl terminus of myosin binding protein C (MyBP-C, C-protein) specifies incorporation into the A-band of striated muscle. *J. Cell Sci.* 109:101–111, 1996.
60. Golitsina, N., Y. An, N. J. Greenfield, L. Thierfelder, K. Iizuka, J. G. Seidman, C. E. Seidman, S. S. Lehrer, and S. E. Hitchcock-DeGregori. Effects of two familial hypertrophic cardiomyopathy–causing mutations on alpha-tropomyosin structure and function. *Biochemistry* 36:4637–4642, 1997.
61. Greenfield, N. J., G. T. Montelione, R. S. Farid, and S. E. Hitchcock-DeGregorio. The structure of the N-terminus of striated muscle alpha-tropomyosin in a chimeric peptide: nuclear magnetic resonance structure and circular dichroism studies. *Biochemistry* 37:7834–7843, 1998.
62. Gruen, M. and M. Gautel. Cardiomyopathy (FHC) mutations in beta-myosin S2 that cause familial Hypertrophic cardiomyopathy abolish the interaction with the regulatory domain of myosin-binding protein-C. *J. Mol. Biol.* 286:933–949, 1999.
63. Gruver, C. I., F. DeMayo, M. A. Goldstein, and A. R. Means. Targeted developmental overexpresson of calmodulin induces proliferative and hypertrophic growth of t cardiomyocytes in transgenic mice. *Endocrinology* 133:376–388, 1993.
64. Gu, X. and S. P. Bishop. Increased proein kinase C and isozyme redistribution in pressure-overloaded cardiac hypertophy in the rat. *Circ. Res.* 75:926–931, 1994.
65. Guo, X., J. Wattanapermpool, K. A. Palmiter, A. M. Murphy, and R. J. Solaro. Mutagenesis of cardiac troponin I: role of the unique NH_2-terminal peptide in myofilament activation. *J. Biol. Chem.* 269:15210–15216, 1994.
66. Gusev, N. B., A. B. Dobrovolskii, and S. E. Severin. Isolation and some properties of troponin T kinase from rabbit skeletal muscle. *Biochem. J.* 189:219–226, 1980.
67. Gwathmey, J. K. and R. J. Hajar. Effect of protein kinase C activation on sarcoplasmic reticulum function and apparent myofibrillar Ca^{2+} sensitivity in intact and skinned muscles from normal and diseased human myocardium. *Circ. Res.* 67:744–652, 1990.
68. Hartzell, H. C. and W. S. Sale. Structure of C protein purified from cardiac muscle. *J. Cell Biol.* 100:208–215, 1985.
69. Hartzell, C. and D. Glass. Phosphorylation of purified cardiac muscle protein by purified cAMP-dependent and endogenous Ca-calmodulin-dependent protein kinases. *J. Biol. Chem.* 259: 15587–15596, 1984.
70. Hartzell, C. Phosphorylation of C protein in intact amphibian heart muscle. *J. Mol. Biol.* 186:185–195, 1985.
71. Hartzell, H. C. Effects of phosphorylation and unphosphorylated C-protein on cardiac actomyosin ATPase. *J. Mol. Biol.* 186: 185–195, 1985.
72. Hartzell, H. C. and L. Titus. Effects of cholinergic and adrenergic agonists on phosphorylation of a 165,000-dalton myofibrillar protein in intact cardiac muscle. *J. Biol. Chem.* 257:2111–2120, 1982.
73. Hartzell, H. C. Phosphorylation of C-protein in intact amphibian cardiac muscle. Correlation between ^{32}P incorporation and twitch relaxation. *J. Gen. Physiol.* 83:563–588, 1984.
74. Heeley, D. H., L. B. Smillie, E. M. Lohmeier-Vogel. Effects of deletion of tropomyosin overlap on regulated actomyosin subfragment 1 ATPase. *Biochem. J.* 258:831–836, 1989.
75. Heeley, D. H. Investigation of the effects of phosphorylation of rabbit striated muscle alpha alpha-tropomyosin and rabbit skeletal muscle troponin-T. *Eur. J. Biochem.* 221:129–37, 1994.
76. Heeley, D. H., M. H. Watson, A. S. Mak, P. Dubord, and L. B. Smillie. Effect of phosphorylation on the interaction and functional properties of rabbit striated muscle alpha alpha-tropomyosin. *J. Biol. Chem.* 264:2424–430, 1989.
77. Heely, D. H., K. Golosinska, L. B. Smillie. The effects of troponin T fragments T1 and T2 on the binding of non-polymerizable tropmyosin to F-actin in the presence and absence of troponin I and troponin C. *J. Biol. Chem.* 262:9971–9978, 1987.
78. High, C. W., and J. T. Stull. Phosphorylation of myosin in perfused rabbit and rat hearts. *Am. J. Physiol.* 239 (*Heart Circ. Physiol.* 8):H756–H764, 1980.
79. Hitchcock-De Gregori, S. E. Study of the structure of troponin-I by measuring the relative reactivities of lysines with acetic anhydride. *J. Biol. Chem.* 257:7372–7380, 1982.
80. Hitchcock-DeGregori, S. E. and Y. An. Integral repeats and a continuous coiled coil are required for binding of striated muscle tropomyosin to the regulated actin filament. *J. Biol. Chem.* 271: 3600–3603, 1996.
81. Hoffman, P. A. and J. H. Lange III. Effect of phosphorylation of troponin I and C protein on isometric tension and velocity of unloaded shortening in skinned single cardiac myocytes from rats. *Circ. Res.* 74:718–726, 1995.
82. Hofmann, P. A. J. M. Metzger, M. L. Greaser, and R. L. Moss. Effects of partial extraction of light chain 2 on the Ca^{2+} sensitivities of isometric tension, stiffness, and velocity of shortening in skinned skeletal muscle fibers. *J. Gen. Physiol.* 95:477–498, 1990.
83. Hofmann, P. A., M. L. Greaser, and R. L. Moss. C-protein limits shortening velocity of rabbit skeletal muscle fibres at low levels of Ca^{2+} activation. *J. Physiol. (Lond.)* 439:701–715, 1991.
84. Hofmann, P. A., H. C. Hartzell, and R. L. Moss. Alterations in Ca^{2+} sensitive tension due to partial extraction of C-protein from rat skinned cardiac myocytes and rabbit skeletal muscle fibers. *J. Gen. Physiol* 97:1141–1163, 1991.

85. Hoh, J. F., G. H. Rossmanith, L. J. Kwan, and A. M. Hamilton. Adrenaline increases the rate of cycling of crossbridges in rat cardiac muscle as measured by pseudo-random binary noise-modulated perturbation analysis. *Circ. Res.* 62:452–461, 1988.
86. Hoit, B. D., E. G. Khoury, E. G. Kranias, N. Ball, and R. A. Walsh. In vivo echocardiographic detection of enhanced left ventricular function in gene-targeted mice with phospholamban deficiency. *Circ. Res.* 77:632–637, 1995.
87. Holmes, K. C., D. Popp, W. Gebhard, and W. Kabsch. Atomic model of the actin filament. *Nature* 347:44–49, 1990.
88. Holroyde, M. J., E. Howe, R. J. Solaro. Modification of calcium requirements for activation of cardiac myofibrillar ATPase by cAMP dependent phosphorylation. *Biochim. Biophys. Acta.* 586:63–69, 1979.
89. Holroyde, M. J., J. D. Potter, and R. J. Solaro. The calcium binding properties of phosphorylated and unphosphorylated cardiac skeletal myosins. *J. Biol. Chem.* 254:6478–6482, 1979.
90. Holroyde, M. J., D. A. Small, E. Howe, and R. J. Solaro. Isolation of cardiac myofibrils and myosin light chains with in vivo levels of light chain phosphorylation. *Biochim. Biopys. Acta* 587:628–637, 1979.
91. Hopkins, S. C., C. Sabido-David, J. E. Corrie, M. Irving, and Y. E. Goldman. Fluorescence polarization transients from rhodamine isomers on the myosin regulatory light chain in skeletal muscle fibers. *Biophys. J.* 74:3093–110, 1998.
92. Huxley, H. E. Structural changes in the actin- and myosin-containing filaments during contraction. *Cold Spring Harbor Symp. Quant. Biol.* 37:361–376, 1972.
93. Irving, M., T. St Claire Allen, C. Sabido-David, J. S. Craik, B. Brandmeier, J. Kendrick-Jones, J. E. Corrie, D. R. Trentham, and Y. E. Goldman. Tilting of the light-chain region of myosin during step length changes and active force generation in skeletal muscle. *Nature* 375:688–691, 1995.
94. Iwasa, T., N. Inoue, K. Fukunaga, T. Isobe, T. Okuyama, and E. Miyamoto. Purification and characterization of a multifunctional calmodulin-dependent protein kinase from canine myocardial cytosol. *Arch. Biochem. Biophys.* 248:21–29, 1986.
95. Janssen, P. M. L., and P. P. deTombe. Protein kinase A does not alter unloaded velocity of sarcomere shortening in skinned rat cardaic trabeculae. *Am. J. Physiol.* 273 (*Heart Circ. Physiol.* 42):H2415–H2422, 1997.
96. Jaquet, K., K. Fukunaga, E. Miyamoto, and H. E. Meyer. A site phosphorylated in bovine cardiac troponin T by cardiac CaM kinase II. *Biochim. Biophys. Acta* 1248:193–195, 1995.
97. Jeacocke, S. A., and P. J. England. Phosphorylation of a myofibrillar protein of Mr 150 000 in perfused rat heart, and the tentative indentification of this as C-protein. *FEBS Lett.* 122: 129–132, 1980.
98. Jha, P. K., P. C. Leavis, and S. Sarkar. Interaction of deletion mutants of troponin I and T: COOH-terminal truncation of troponin T abolishes troponin I binding and reduces Ca^{2+}-sensitivity of reconstituted regulatory system. *Biochemistry* 35: 16573–16580, 1996.
99. Jideama, N. M., T. A. Noland Jr, R. L., Raynor, G. C., Blobe, D. Fabbro, M. G., Kazanietz, P. M., Blumberg, Y. A., Hannun, and J. F. Kuo. Phosphorylation specificities of protein kinase C isozymes for bovine cardiac troponin I and troponin T and sites within these proteins and regulation of myofilament properties. *J. Biol. Chem.* 271:23277–23283, 1996.
100. Johns, E. C., S. J., Simnett, I. P., Mulligan and C. C. Ashley. Troponin I phosphorylation does not increase the rate of relaxation following laser flash photolysis of dizo-2 in guinea-pig skinned trabeculae. *Pflugers Arch.* 433:842–844, 1997.
101. Johnson, J. A. and D. Mochly-Rosen. Inhibition of the spontaneous rate of contraction of neonatal cardiac myocytes by protein kinase C isozymes. A putative role for the ε isozyme. *Circ. Res.* 76:654–663, 1995.
102. Kabsch, W., H. G., Mannherz, D. Suck, E. F., Pai and K. C. Homes. Atomic structure of the actin:DNase I complex. *Nature* 347:37–44, 1990.
103. Karczewski, P., S. Bartel, and E.-G. Krause. Differential sensitivity to isoprenaline of troponin I and phospholamban phosphorylation in isolated rat hearts. *Biochem. J.* 266:115–122, 1990.
104. Katoh, N., B. C., Wise, and J. F. Kuo. Phosphorylation of cardiac troponin inhibitory subunit (troponin I) and tropomyosin-binding subunit (troponin T) by cardiac phospholipid-sensitive Ca^{2+}-dependent protein *Biochem. J.* 209:189–195, 1983.
105. Kleerekoper, Q, J. W. Howarth, X. Guo, R. J. Solaro, and P. R. Rosevear. Cardiac troponin I induced conformational changes in cardiac troponin C as monitored by NMR using site-directed spin and isotope labeling. *Biochemistry* 34:13343–13352, 1995.
106. Kobayahsi, T., T. Tao, J. Gergely, and J. H. Collins. Structure of the troponin complex. *J. Biol. Chem.* 269:5725–5729, 1994.
107. Konhilas, J., B. M. Wolska, A. F. Martin, R. J. Solaro, and P. P. deTombe. PKA modulates length dependent activation in murine myocardium. *Biophys. J.* 78:108A, 2000.
108. Komukai, K., and S. Kurihara. Length dependence of Ca^{2+}-tension relationship in aequorin-injected ferret papillary muscles. *Am. J. Physiol.* 273 (*Heart Circ. Physiol.* 42):H10068–H10074, 1997.
108a. Korman, V. L., and L. S. Tobacman, Mutations in action subdomain 3 that impair their filament regulation by troponin and tropomyosin. *J. Biol. Chem.* 274:22191–22196, 1999.
109. Kraft, T., J. M. Chalovich, L. C. Yu, and B. Brenner. Parallel inhibition of active force and relaxed fiber stiffness by caldesmon fragments at physiological ionic strength and temperature conditions: additional evidence that weak cross-bridge binding to actin is an essential intermediate for force generation. *Biophys. J.* 68:2404–2418, 1995.
110. Kranias, E. G., and R. J. Solaro. Phosphorylation of troponin I and phospholamban during catecholamine stimulation of rabbit heart. *Nature* 298:182–184, 1982.
111. Kranias, E. G. Regulation of calcium transport by protein phosphatase activity associated with cardiac sarcoplasmic reticulum. *J. Biol. Chem.* 260:11006–11010, 1985.
112. Kranias, E. G., J. L. Garvey, R. D. Srivastava, and R. J. Solaro. Phosphorylation and functional modifications of sarcoplasmic reticulum and myofibrils in isolated rabbit hearts stimulated with isoprenaline. *Biochem. J.* 226:113–121, 1985.
113. Kress, M., H. E. Huxley, A. R. Faruqi, and J. Hendrix. Structural changes during activation of frog muscle studied by time resolved X-ray diffraction. *J. Mol. Biol.* 188:325–342, 1986.
114. Krudy, Q. Kleerekoper, X. Guo, J. W. Howarth, R. J. Solaro, and P. R. Rosevear. NMR studies delineating spatial relationships within the cardiac troponin I–troponin C complex. *J. Biol. Chem.* 269:23731–23735, 1994.
115. Labeit, S., M. Gautel, A. Lakey, and J. Trinick. Towards a molecular understanding of titin. *EMBO J.* 11:1711–1716, 1992.
116. Lehman, W., P. Vibert, P. Uman, and R. Craig. Steric-blocking by tropomyosin visualized in relaxed vertebrate muscle thin filaments. *J. Mol. Biol.* 251:191–196, 1995.
117. Lehman, W., R. Craig, and P. Vibert. Ca^{2+}-induced tropomyosin movement Limulus thin filaments revealed by three-dimensional reconstruction. *Nature* 368:65–67, 1994.
118. Lehrer, S. The regulatory switch of the muscle thin filament: Ca^{2+} or myosin heads? *J. Muscle Res. Cell Motil.* 15:232–236, 1994.
119. Lehrer, S. S., and M. A. Geeves. The muscle thin filament as a

classical cooperative/allosteric regulatory system. *J. Mol. Biol.* 277:1081–1089, 1998.
120. Lehrer, S. S., and A. Yuan. The stability of tropomyosin at acid pH: effects of anion binding. *J. Struct. Biol.* 122:176–179, 1998.
121. Lehrer, S. S., N. L. Golitsina, and M. A. Geeves. Actin-tropomyosin activation of myosin subfragment 1 ATPase and thin filament cooperativity. The role of tropomyosin flexibility and end-to-end interactions. *Biochemistry* 36:13449–13454, 1997.
122. Lester, J. W., K. F. Gannaway, R. A. Reardon, L. D. Koon, and P. A. Hofmann. Effects of adenosine and protein kinase C stimulation on mechanical properties of rat cardiac myocytes. *Am. J. Physiol.* 271 *Heart Circ. Physiol.* 40):H1778–H1785, 1996.
123. Lesyzk, J., Z. Grabarek, J. Gergely, and J. H. Collins. Characterization of zero-length cross-links between rabbit skeletal muscle troponin C and troponin I: evidence for direct interaction between the inhibitory region of troponin I and the NH2-terminal, regulatory domain of troponin C. *Biochemistry* 29:299–304, 1990.
124. Leszyk, J., R. Dumaswala, J. D. Potter, N. B. Gusev, A. D. Verin, L. S. Tobacman, and J. H. Collins. Bovine cardiac troponin T: amino acid sequences of the two isoforms. *Biochemistry* 26:7035–42, 1987.
125. Leszyk, J., J. H. Collins, P. C. Leavis, and T. Tao. Cross-linking of rabbit skeletal muscle troponin subunits: labeling of cysteine-98 of troponin-C with 4-maleimidobenzophenone and analysis of products formed in the binary complex wth troponins I and T. *Biochemistry* 27:6983–6987, 1988.
126. Levine, R. J., Z. Yang, N. D. Epstein, L. Fananapazir, J. T. Stull, and H. L. Sweeney. Structural and functional responses of mammalian thick filaments to alterations in myosin regulatory light chains. *J. Struct. Biol.* 122:149–61, 1998.
127. Levine, R. J., R. W. Kensler, Z. Yang, J. T. Stull, and H. L. Sweeney. Myosin light chain phosphorylation affects the structure of rabbit skeletal muscle thick filaments. *Biophys. J.* 71:898–907, 1996.
128. Li, L., J. Desantiago, G. Chu, E. G. Kranias, and D. M. Bers. Phosphorylation of phospholamban and troponin I in beta-adrenergic-induced acceleration of cardiac relaxation. *Am. J. Physiol.* 278 (*Heart Circ.Physiol.* 47): H769–H779, 2000.
129. Lim, M., and M. Walsh. Phosphorylation of skeletal and cardiac muscle C-proteins by the catalytic subunit of cAMP-dependent protein kinase. *Biochem. Cell Biol.* 64:622–630, 1986.
130. Lindemann, J. P., L. R. Jones, D. R. Hathaway, B. G. Henry, and A. M. Watanabe. β-adrenergic stimulation of phospholamban phosphorylation and Ca^{2+}-ATPase activity in guinea pig ventricles. *J. Biol. Chem.* 258:464–471, 1983.
131. Lokuta, A. J., T. B. Rogers, W. J. Lederer, and H. H. Valdivia. Modulation of cardiac ryanodine receptors of swine and rabbit by a phosphorylation–dephosphorylation mechanism. *J. Physiol. (Lond.)* 487:609–622, 1995.
132. Lorenz, M., K. J. V. Poole, D. Popp, G. Rosenbaum, and K. C. Holmes. An atomic model of the unregulated thin filament obtained by X-ray fiber diffraction on oriented actin-tropomyosin gels. *J. Mol. Biol.* 246:108–119, 1995.
133. Luo, W., I. L. Grupp, J. Harrer, S. Ponniah, G. Grupp, J. J. Duffy, T. Doetschman, and E. G. Kranias. Targeted ablation of the phospholamban gene is associated with markedly enhanced myocardial contractility and loss of β-agonist stimulation. *Circ. Res.* 75:401–409, 1994.
134. Mak, A. S., and L. B. Smillie. Structural interpretation of the two-site binding of troponin on the muscle thin filament. *J. Mol. Biol.* 149:541–550, 1981.
135. Maytum, R., S. S. Lehrer, and M. A. Geeves. Cooperativity and switching within the three-state model of muscle regulation. *Biochemistry* 38:1102–1110, 1999.
136. Mak, A. S., L. B. Smillie, and G. R. Stewart. Comparison of the amino acid sequences of rabbit skeletal muscle α- and β-tropomyosin. *J. Biol. Chem.* 255:3649–3655, 1980.
137. Malhotra, A., A. Nakouzi, J. Bowman, and P. Buttrick. Expression and regulation of mutant forms of cardiac TnI in a reconstituted actomyosin system: role of kinase dependent phosphorylation. *Mol. Cell. Biochem.* 170:99–107, 1997.
138. Malhotra, A., D. Reich, A. Nakouzi, V. Sanghi, D. L. Geenen, and P. M. Buttrick. Experimental diabetes is associated with functional activation of protein kinase C epsilon and phosphorylation of troponin I in the heart, which are prevented by angiotensin II receptor blockade. *Circ. Res.* 81:1027–1033.40, 1997a.
139. Martin, A. M., K. Ball, L. Gao, P. K. Kumar, and R. J. Solaro. Identification and functional significance of troponin I isoforms in neonatal rat heart myofibrils. *Circ. Res.* 69:1244–1252, 1991.
140. McAuliffe, J. J., L. Gao, and R. J. Solaro. Changes in myofibrillar activation and troponin C Ca^{2+}-binding associated with troponin T isoform switching in developing rabbit heart. *Circ. Res.* 66:1204–1216, 1990.
141. McKillop, D. F., and M. A. Geeves. Regulation of the interaction between actin and myosin subfragment 1: evidence for three states of the thin filament. *Biophys. J.* 65:693–701, 1993.
142. McLachlan, A. D., and M. Stewart. The 14-fold periodicity in α-tropomyosin and the interaction with actin. *J. Mol. Biol.* 103:271–298, 1976.
143. McClellan, G., A. Weisberg, and S. Winegrad. cAMP can raise or lower cardiac actomyosin ATPase activity depending on alpha-adrenergic activity. *Am. J. Physiol.* 267 (*Heart Circ. Physiol.* 36):H431–H442, 1994.
144. McLachlan, A. D., and M. Stewart. The 14-fold periodicity in alpha-tropomyosin and the interaction with actin. *J. Mol. Biol.* 103:271–298, 1976.
145. McLachlan, A. D., and M. Stewart. Tropomyosin coiled–coil interactions: evidence for an unstaggered structure. *J. Mol. Biol.* 98:293–304, 1975.
146. Mesnard, L., D. Logeart, S. Taviaux, S. Diriong, J. J. Mercadier, and F. Samson. Human cardiac troponin T: cloning and expression of new isoforms in the normal and failing heart. *Circ. Res.* 76:687–692, 1995.
147. Mesnard-Rouiller, L., J. J. Mercadier, G. Butler-Browne, M. Heimburger, D. Logeart, P. D. Allen, and F. Samson. Troponin T mRNA and protein isoforms in the human left ventricle: pattern of expression in failing and control hearts. *J. Mol. Cell. Cardiol.* 29:3043–3055, 1997.
148. Metzger, J. M., M. L. Greaser, and R. L. Moss. Variations in cross-bridge attachment rate and tension with phosphorylation of myosin in mammalian skinned skeletal muscle fibers. Implications for twitch potentiation in intact muscle. *J. Gen. Physiol.* 93:855–883, 1989.
149. Metzger, J. M., and R. L. Moss. Myosin light chain 2 modulates calcium-sensitive cross-bridge transitions in vertebrate skeletal muscle. *Biophys. J.* 63:460–468, 1992.
150. Milligan, R. A., and P. F. Flicker. Structural relationships of actin, myosin, and tropomyosin revealed by cryo-electron microscopy. *J. Cell Biol.* 105:29–39, 1987.
151. Milligan, R. A., M. Whittaker, and D. Safer. Molelcular structure of F-actin and location of surface binding sites. *Nature* 348:217–221, 1990.
152. Mittmann, K., K. Jaquet, and L. M. G. Heilmeyer Jr. Ordered phosphorylation of a duplicated minimal recognition motif for cAMP-dependent protein kinase present in cardiac troponin I. *FEBS Lett.* 302:133–137, 1992.

153. Mohamed, A. S., J. D. Dignam, and K. K. Schlender. Cardiac myosin-binding protein C (MyBP-C): identification of protein kinase A and protein kinase C phosphorylation sites. *Arch. Biochem. Biophys.* 358:313–319, 1998.
154. Moos, C., C. M. Mason, J. M. Besterman, I. N. M. Feng, and J. H. Dubin. The binding of skeletal muscle C-protein to F-actin and its relation to the interaction of actin with myosin. *J. Mol. Biol.* 124:571–586, 1978.
155. Molkentin, J. D., J.-R. Lu, C. Antos, B. Markham, J. Richardson, J. Robbins, S. R. Grant, and E. N. Olson. A calcineurin-dependent transcriptional pathway for cardiac hypertrophy. *Cell* 93:215–228, 1998.
156. Montgomery, K., and A. S. Mak. In vitro phosphorylation of tropomyosin by a kinase from chicken embryo. *J. Biol. Chem.* 259:5555–5560, 1984.
157. Moore, R. T., and J. T. Stull. Myosin light chain phosphorylation in fast and slow skeletal muscles in situ. *Am. J. Physiol.* 247 (*Cell Physiol.* 16):C462–C471, 1984.
158. Moos, C. and I. N. M. Feng. Effect of C-protein on actomyosin ATPase. *Biochem. Biophys. Acta* 632:141–149, 1980.
159. Morano, I., F. Hofmann, M. Zimmer, and J. C. Ruegg. The influence of P-light chain phosphorylation by myosin light chain kinase on the calcium sensitivity of chemically skinned heart fibres. *FEBS Lett.* 189:221–224, 1985.
160. Morano, I., O. Ritter, A. Bonz, T. Timek, C. F. Vahl, and G. Michel. Myosin light chain-actin interaction regulates cardiac contractility. *Circ. Res.* 76:720–725, 1995.
161. Morano, I., M. Wankerl, M. Bohm, E. Erdmann, and J. C. Ruegg. Myosin P-light chain isoenzymes in the human heart: evidence for diphosphorylation of the atrial P-LC form. *Basic. Res. Cardiol.* 84:298–305, 1989.
162. Morimoto, K. and W. F. Harrington. Evidence for structural changes in vertebrate thick filament induced by calcium. *J. Mol. Biol.* 88:693–709, 1974.
163. Morris, E. P. and S. S. Lehrer. Troponin-tropomyosin interactions. Fluorescence studies of the binding of troponin, troponin T and chymotryptic troponin T fragments to specifically labeled tropomyosin. *Biochemistry* 23:2214–2320, 1984.
164. Moss, R. L., J. D. Allen, and M. L. Greaser. Effects of partial extraction of troponin complex upon the tension–pCa relation in rabbit skeletal muscle. Further evidence that tension development involves cooperative effects within the thin filament. *J. Gen. Physiol.* 87:761–774, 1986.
165. Moss, R. L. Ca^{2+} regulation of mechanical properties of striated muscle: mechanistic studies using extraction and replacement of regulatory proteins. *Circ. Res.* 70:865–884, 1992.
166. Moss, R. L., L. O. Nwoye, and M. L. Greaser. Substituion of cardiac troponin C into rabbit muscle does not alter the length dependence of Ca^{2+} sensitivity of tension. *J. Physiol.* 440:273–289, 1991.
167. Muthuchamy, M., I. Grupp, G. Grupp, B. O'Toole, A. Kier, G. Bolvin, J. Neumann, and D. Wieczorek. Molecular and physiological effects of overexpressing striated muscle beta-tropomyosin in the adult murine heart. *J. Biol. Chem.* 270:30593–30603, 1995.
168. Ngai, S.-M., and F. D. Sönnichsen, R. S. Hodges. Photochemical cross-linking between native rabbit skeletal troponin C and benzoyl-troponin I inhibitory peptide residues 104–115. *J. Biol. Chem.* 269:2798–2802, 1994.
169. Ngai, S.-M., and R. S. Hodges. Biologically important interactions between synthetic peptides of the N-terminal region of troponin I and troponin C. *J. Biol. Chem.* 267:15715–15720, 1992.
170. Noland, T. A. Jr., R. L. Raynor, and J. F. Kuo. Identification of sites phosphorylated in bovine cardiac troponin I and troponin T by protein kinase C and comparative substrate activity of synthetic peptides containing the phosphorylation sites. *J. Biol. Chem.* 264:20778–20785, 1989.
171. Noland, T. A., X. Guo, R. L. Raynor, V. Averyhart-Fullard, N. M. Jideama, R. J. Solaro, and J. F. Kuo. Cardiac troponin I mutants: phosphorylation by protein kinases C and A and regulation of Ca^{2+}-stimulated MgATPase of reconstituted actomyosin S-1. *J. Biol. Chem.* 43:25445–25454, 1995.
172. Noland, T. A. Jr. and J. F. Kuo. Protein kinase C phosphorylation of cardiac troponin I and troponin T inhibits Ca^{2+}-stimulated MgATPase activity in reconstituted actomyosin and isolated myofibrils, and decreases actin-myosin interactions. *J. Mol. Cell. Cardiol.* 25:53–65, 1993.
173. Noland, T. A. and J. F. Kuo. Phosphorylation of cardiac myosin light chain 2 by protein kinase C and myosin light chain kinase increases Ca^{2+}-stimulated actomyosin ATPase activity. *Biochem. Biophy. Res. Commun.* 193:254–260, 1993b.
174. Noland, T. A. Jr. and J. F. Kuo. Protein kinase C phosphorylation of cardiac troponin T decreases Ca^{2+}-dependent actomyosin MgATPase activity and troponin T binding to tropomyosin–F-actin complex. *Biochem. J.* 288:123–129, 1992.
175. Noland, T. A. Jr., R. L. Raynor, and J. F. Kuo. Identification of sites phosphorylated in bovine cardiac troponin I and troponin T by protein kinase C and comparative substrate activity of synthetic peptides containing the phosphorylation sites. *J. Biol. Chem.* 264:20778–20785, 1989.
176. Noland, T. A. Jr., R. L. Raynor, N. M. Jideama, X. Guo, M. G. Kazanietz, P. M. Blumberg, R. J. Solaro, and J. F. Kuo. Differential regulation of cardiac actomyosin S-1 MgATPase by protein kinase C isozyme-specific phosphorylation of specific sites in cardiac troponin I and its phosphorylation site mutants. *Biochemistry* 35:14923–14931, 1996.
177. Noland, T. A. Jr., and J. F. Kuo. Protein kinase C phosphorylation of cardiac troponin I or troponin T inhibits Ca^{2+}-stimulated actomyosin MgATPase activity. *J. Biol. Chem.* 266:4974–4978, 1991.
178. Noland, T. A., Jr., X. Guo, R. L. Raynor, N. M. Jedeama, V. Averyhart-Fullard, R. J. Solaro, and J. F. Kuo. Cardiac troponin I mutants. Phosphorylation by protein kinases C and A and regulation of Ca^{2+}-stimulated MgATPase of reconstituted actomyosin S-1. *J. Biol. Chem.* 43:25445–25454, 1995.
179. Offer, G. C-protein and peridicity in the thick filaments of vertebrate skeletal muscle. *Cold Spring Harbor Symp. Quant. Biol.* 37:87–93, 1972.
180. Offer, G., C. Moos, and R. Starr. A new protein of the thick filaments of vertebrate skeletal myofibrils: extraction, purification and characterization. *J. Mol. Biol.* 74:653–676, 1973.
181. Olah, G. A., S. E. Rokop, C-L. A. Wang, S. L. Blechner, and J. Trewhella. Troponin I encompasses an extended troponin C in the Ca^{2+}-bound complex: a small-angle X-ray and neutron scattering study. *Biochemistry* 33:8233–8239, 1994.
182. Palmiter, K. A., Y. Kitada, M. Muthuchamy, D. F. Wieczorek, and R. J. Solaro. Exchange of β-tropomyosin for α-tropomyosin in hearts of transgenic mice induces changes in thin filament response to Ca^{2+}, strong cross-bridge binding, and protein phosphorylation. *J. Biol. Chem.* 271:11611–11614, 1996.
183. Palmiter, K. A., and R. J. Solaro. Molecular mechanisms regulating the myofilament response to Ca^{2+}: implications of mutations causal for familial hypertrophic cardiomyopathy. *Basic Res. Cardiol.* 92 (Suppl 1):63–74, 1997.
184. Pan, B. S., A. M. Gordon, and Z. X. Luo. Removal of tropomyosin overlap modifies cooperative binding of myosin S-1 to reconstituted thin filaments of rabbit striated muscle. *J. Biol. Chem.* 264:8495–8498, 1989.
185. Pan, B. S., A. M. Gordon, and J. D. Potter. Deletion of the first 45 NH2-terminal residues of rabbit skeletal troponin T

strengthens binding of troponin to immobilized tropomyosin *J. Biol. Chem.* 266:12432–12438, 1991.
186. Pan, B. S., and R. J. Solaro. Calcium-binding properties of troponin C in detergent-skinned heart muscle fibers. *J. Biol. Chem.* 262:7839–7849, 1987.
187. Pan, B. S., K. A. Palmiter, M. Plonczynski, and R. J. Solaro. Slowly exchanging calcium binding sites unique to cardiac/slow muscle troponin C. *J. Mol. Cell. Cardiol.* 10:1117–1124, 1990.
188. Patel, J. R., G. M. Diffee, and R. L. Moss. Myosin regulatory light chain modulates the Ca^{2+} dependence of the kinetics of tension development in skeletal muscle fibers. *Biophys. J.* 70:2333–2340, 1996.
189. Patel, J. R., G. M. Diffee, X. P. Huang, and R. L. Moss. Phosphorylation of myosin regulatory light chain eliminates force-dependent changes in relaxation rates in skeletal muscle. *Biophys. J.* 74:360–368, 1998.
190. Paul, K., N. A. Ball, G. W. Dorn II, and R. A. Walsh. Left ventricular stretch stimulates angionensin II–mediated phosphatidylinositol hydrolysis and prtein kinase ε isoform translocation in adult guinea pig hearts. *Circ. Res.* 81:643–650, 1997.
191. Pearlstone, J. R., and L. B. Smillie. Binding of troponin T fragments to several types of tropomyosin. Sensitivity to Ca^{2+} in the presnece of troponin-C. *J. Biol. Chem.* 257:10587–10592, 1982.
192. Pearlstone, J. R., and L. B. Smillie. Effects of troponin-1 plus-C on the binding of troponin-T and its fragments to α-tropomyosin. *J. Biol. Chem.* 258:2534–2542, 1983.
193. Pearlstone, J. R., and L. B. Smillie. Evidence for two-site binding of troponin I inhibitory peptides to the N and C domains of troponin C. *Biochemistry* 34:6932–6940, 1995.
194. Persechini, A. and J. T. Stull. Phosphorylaton kinetics of skeletal muscle myosin and the effect of phosphorylation on actomyosin adenosinetriphosphatase activity. *Biochemistry* 23:4144–4150, 1984.
195. Persechini, A., J. T. Stull, and R. Cooke. The effect of myosin phosphorylation on the contractile properties of skinned rabbit skeletal muscle fibers. *J. Biol. Chem.* 260:7951–7954, 1985.
196. Phillips, G. N., Jr., J. P. Fillers, and C. Cohen. Tropomyosin crystal structure and muscled regulation. *J. Mol. Biol.* 192:111–131, 1986.
197. Potter, J. D., Z. Sheng, B.-S. Pan, and J. Zhao. A direct regulatory role for troponin T and a dual role for troponin C in the Ca^{2+} regulation of muscle contraction. *J. Biol. Chem.* 270:2557–2562, 1995.
198. Pucéat, M., O. Clement, P. Lechene, J. M. Pelosin, R. Ventura-Clapier, and G. Vassort. Neurohormonal control of calcium sensitivity of myofilaments in rat single heart cells. *Circ. Res.* 67:517–524, 1990.
199. Pucéat, M. and G. Vassort. Signaling by protein kinase C isoforms in the heart. *Mol. Cell. Biochem.* 157:65–72, 1996.
200. Rarick, H. M., H.-P. Tang, X.-D. Guo, A. F. Martin, and R. J. Solaro. Interactions at the NH_2-terminal interface of cardiac troponin I modulate myofilament activation. *J. Mol. Cell. Cardiol.* 31:363–375, 1999.
201. Rarick, H. M., X. Tu, R. J. Solaro, and A. M. Martin. The C-terminus of cardiac troponin I is essential for full inhibitory activity and Ca^{2+}-sensitivity of rat myofibrils. *J. Biol. Chem.* 272:26887–26892, 1997.
202. Rarick, H. M., T. J. Opgenorth, T. W. von Geldern, and R. J. Solaro. An essential myosin light chain peptide stimulates cardiac myofibrillar ATPase activity. *J. Biol. Chem.* 271:27039–27043, 1996.
203. Rayment, I., W. R. Rypniewski, K. Schmidt-Base, R. Smith, D. R. Tomchick, M. M. Benning, D. A. Winkelmann, G. Wesenberg, and H. M. Holden. Three-dimensional structure of myosin subfragment-1: a molecular motor. *Science* 261:50–58, 1993.
204. Rayment, I., H. M. Holden, M. Whittaker, C. B. Yohn, M. Lorenz, K. C. Holmes, and R. A. Milligan. Structure of the actin-myosin complex and its implications for muscle contraction. *Science* 261:58–65, 1993.
205. Reiffert, S. U., K. Jaquet, L. M. Fr. Heilmeyer, M. D. Ritchie, and M. A. Geeves. Bisphosphorylation of cardiac troponin I modulates the $Ca^{(2+)}$-dependent binding of myosin fragment S1 to reconstituted thin filaments. *FEBS Lett.* 384:43–47, 1996.
206. Reiffert, S. U., K. Jaquet, L. M. Heilmeyer Jr., and F. W. Herberg. Stepwise subunit interaction changes by mono- and bis-phosphorylation of cardiac troponin I. *Biochemistry* 37:13516–13525, 1998.
207. Risnik, V. V., and N. B. Gusev. Some properties of the nucleotide-binding site of troponin T kinase–casein kinase type II from skeletal muscle. *Biochim. Biophys. Acta.* 790:108–116, 1984.
208. Risnik, V. V., A. B. Dobrovolskii, N. B. Gusev, and S. E. Severin. Phosphorylase kinase phosphorylation of skeletal-muscle troponin T. *Biochem. J.* 191:851–854, 1980.
209. Risnik, V. V., A. V. Vorotnikov, and N. B. Gusev. Phosphorylation of troponin T by Ca-phospholipid-dependent protein kinase. *Biomed. Biochim. Acta* 46:S444–S447, 1987.
210. Robertson, S. P., J. D. Johnson, M. J. Holroyde, E. G. Kranias, J. D. Potter, R. J. Solaro. The effect of troponin I phosphorylation on the Ca^{2+}-binding properties of the Ca^{2+}-regulatory site of bovine cardiac troponin. *J. Biol. Chem.* 257:260–263, 1982.
211. Rossmanith, G. H., J. F. Hoh, L. Turnbull, R. I. Ludowyke. Mechanism of action of endothelin in rat cardiac muscle: cross-bridge kinetics and myosin light chain phosphorylation. *J. Physiol.(Lond.)* 505:217–227, 1997.
212. Rüegg, J. C., C. Zeugner, J. Van Eyk, C. M. Kay, and R. S. Hodges. Inhibition of TnI–TnC interaction and contraction of skinned muscle fibres by the synthetic peptide TnI [104–115]. *Pflugers Arch.* 414:430–436, 1989.
213. Saeki, Y., K. Shiozawa, K. Yanagisawa, and T. Shibata. Adrenaline increases the rate of cross-bridge cycling in rat cardiac muscle. *J. Mol. Cell. Cardiol.* 22:453–460, 1990.
214. Sakata, Y., B. D. Hoit, S. B. Liggett, R. A. Walsh, and G. W. Dorn II. Decompensation of pressure-overload hypertrophy in Gαq overexpressing mice. *Circulation* 97:1488–1495, 1998.
215. Sato, Y., D. G. Ferguson, H. Sako, G. W. Dorn II, V. J. Kadambi, A. Yatani, B. D. Hoit, R. A. Walsh, and E. G. Kranias. Cardiac-specific overexpression of mouse cardiac calsequestrin is associated with depressed cardiovascular function and hypertrophy in transgenic mice. *J. Biol. Chem.* 273:28470–28477, 1998.
216. Sayers, S. T., and K. Bárány. Myosin light chain phosphorylation during contraction of turtle heart. *FEBS Lett.* 154:305–310, 1983.
217. Schaertl, S., S. S. Lehrer, and M. A. Geeves. Separation and characterization of the two functional regions of troponin T involved in muscle thin filament regulation. *Biochemistry* 34:15890–15894, 1995.
218. Schlender, K. K., T. J. Thysseril, and M. G. Hegazy. Calcium-dependent phosphorylation of bovine cardiac C-protein by phosphorylase kinase. *Biochem. Biophys. Res. Commun.* 155:45–51, 1988.
219. Schlender, K., and L. Bean. Phosphorylation of chicken cardiac C protein by calcium calmodulin-dependent protein kinase II. *Biol. Chem.* 266: 2811–2817, 1991.
220. Sham, J. S. K., L. R. Jones, and M. Morad. Phospholamban mediates the β-adrenergic-enhanced Ca^{2+} uptake in mamma-

lian ventricular myocytes. *Am. J. Physiol.* 261 (*Heart Circ. Physiol.* 30):H1344–H1349, 1991.
221. Silver, P. J., L. M. Buja, and J. T. Stull. Frequency-dependent myosin light chain phosphorylation in isolated myocardium. *J. Mol. Cell. Cardiol.* 18:31–37, 1986.
222. Solaro, R. J. Protein phosphorylation and the cardiac myofilaments. In: *Protein Phosphorylation in Heart*, edited by R. J. Solaro, Boca Raton, FL: CRC Press, 1986:129–156.
223. Solaro, R. J., and J. Van Eyk. Altered interactions among thin filament proteins modulate cardiac function. *J. Mol. Cell. Cardiol.* 28:217–230, 1996.
224. Solaro, R. J., A. J. G. Moir, S. V. Perry. Phosphorylation of troponin I and the inotropic effect of adrenalin in the perfused rabbit heart. *Nature* 262:615–617, 1976.
225. Solaro R. J. Heart failure and the response of cardiac myofilaments to Ca^{2+}. *Heart Failure* 10:150–155, 1994.
226. Solaro, R. J., and H. M. Rarick. Troponin and tropomyosin: proteins that switch on and tune in the activity of cardiac myofilaments. *Circ. Res.* 83:471–480, 1998.
227. Solaro, R. J. Modulation of activation of cardiac myofilaments by beta-adrenergic agonists. In: *Modulation of Cardiac Calcium Sensitivity*, edited by D. A. G. Allen, and J. A. Lee, Oxford. Oxford University Press 160–177, 1993.
228. Spyracoupoulos, L., M. X. Li, S. K. Sia, S. M. Gagne, M. Chandra, R. J., Solaro, and B. D. Sykes. Calcium-induced structural transition in the regulatory domain of human cardiac troponin C. *Biochemistry* 36:12138–12146, 1997.
229. Squire, J. M., J. J. Harford, and H. A. Al-Khayat. Molecular movements in contracting muscle: towards "muscle—the movie." *Biophys. Chem.* 50:87–96, 1994.
230. Squire, J. M., and E. P. Morris. A new look at thin filament regulaton in vertebrate skeletal muscle. *FASEB J.* 12:761–771, 1998.
231. Squire, J. M., H. A. Al-Khayat, and N. Yagi. Muscle thin filament structure and regulation: actin subdomain movements and the tropomyosin shift modelled from low angle X-ray diffraction. *J. Chem. Soc. Faraday Trans.* 89:2717–2726, 1993.
232. Starr, R. and G. Offer. The interaction of C-protein with heavy meromyosin and subfragment-2. *Biochem. J.* 171:813–816, 1978.
233. Stefancik, R., P. K. Jha, and S. Sarkar. Identification and mutagenesis of a highly conserved domain in troponin T responsible for troponin I binding: potential role for coiled-coil interaction. *Proc. Natl. Acad. Sci. U.S.A.* 95:957–962, 1998.
234. Strang, K. T., and R. L. Moss. α_1-Adrenergic receptor stimulation decreases maximum shortening velocity of skinned single ventricular myocytes from rats. *Circ. Res.* 77:114–120, 1995.
235. Strang, K. T., N. K. Sweitzer, M. L. Greaser, and R. L. Moss. β-Adrenergic receptor stimulation increases unloaded shortening velocity of skinned single ventricular myocytes from rats. *Circ. Res.* 74:542–549, 1994.
236. Strauss, J. D., J. E. Van Eyk, Z. Barth, L. Kluwe, R. J. Wiesner, K. Maeda, J. C. Ruegg, Recombinant troponin I substitution and calcium responsiveness in skinned cardiac muscle. *Pflugers Arch.* 431:853–862, 1996.
237. Stull, J. T., C. J. Sanford, D. R., Manning D. K. Blumenthal, and C. W. High. Phosphorylation of myofibrillar proteins in striated muscle, *Cold Spring Harbor Conf. Cell Prolif.* 8:823–891, 1981.
238. Sugden, P. H., and A. Clerk. Cellular mechanisms of cardiac hypertrophy. *J. Mol. Med.* 76:725–746, 1998.
239. Swartz, D. R., and R. L. Moss. Influence of a strong binding myosin analog on calcium sensitive mechanical properties of skinned skeletal muslce fibers. *J. Biol. Chem.* 267:20497–20506, 1992.
240. Swiderek, K., K. Jaquet H. E. Meyer, C. Schachtele, F. Hofmann, and L. M. Heilmeyer Jr. Sites phosphorylated in bovine cardiac troponin T and I. Characterization by 31P-NMR spectroscopy and phosphorylation by protein kinases. *Eur. J. Biochem.* 190:575–582, 1990.
241. Swiderek, K., K. Jaquet, H. E. Meyer, and M. G. Heilmeyer Jr. Cardiac troponin I, isolated from bovine heart, contains two adjacent phosphoserines. A first example of phosphoserine determination by derivatization to S-ethylcysteine. *Eur. J. Biochem.* 176:335–342, 1988.
242. Syska, H., J. M. Wilkinson, R. J. A. Grand, and S. V. Perry. The relationship between biological activity and primary structure of troponin I from white skeletal muscle of the rabbit. *Biochem. J.* 153:375–387, 1976.
243. Szczesna, D., J. Zhao, and J. D. Potter. The regulatory light chains of myosin modulate cross-bridge cycling in skeletal muscle. *J. Biol. Chem.* 271:5246–5250, 1996.
244. Takeishi, Y., G. Chu, D. M. Kirkpatrick, Z. Li, H. Wakasaki, E. G Kranias, G. L. King, and R. A. Walsh. In vivo phosphorylation of cardiac troponin I by protein kinase C β2 decreases cardiomyocyte calcium responsiveness and contractility in transgenic mouse hearts. *J. Clin. Invest.* 102:72–78, 1998.
245. Talbot, J. A., and R. S. Hodges. Synthetic studies on the inhibitory region of rabbit skeletal troponin I. *J. Biol. Chem.* 256:2798–2802, 1981.
246. Talosi, L., and E. G. Kranias. Effect of alpha-adrenergic stimulation on activation of protein kinase C and phosphorylation of proteins in intact rabbit hearts. *Circ. Res.* 70:670–678, 1992.
247. Tanokura, M., Y. Tawada, A. Ono, and I. Ohtsuki. Chymotryptic subfragments on troponin T from rabbit skeletal muscle. Interactions with tropomyosin, troponin I and troponin C. *J. Biochem. (Tokyo)* 93:331–337, 1983.
248. Tao, T., B.-J. Gong, and P. C. Leavis. Calcium-induced movement of troponin-I relative to actin in skeletal muscle thin filaments. *Science* 247:1339–1341, 1990.
249. Tawada, Y., H. Ohara, T. Ooi, and K. Tawada. Nonpolymerizable tropomyosin and control of the superprecipitation of actomyosin. *J. Biochem.* 78: 65–72, 1975.
250. Terzic, A., M. Puceat, O. Clement, F. Scamps, and G. Vassort. α_1-Adrenergic effects on intracellular pH and calcium and on myofilaments in single rat cardiac cells. *J. Physiol. (Lond.)* 447: 275–292, 1992.
251. Thierfelder, L., H. Watkins, C. MacRae, R. Lamas, W. McKenna, H. P. Vosberg, J. G. Seidman, and C. E. Seidman. Alpha-tropomyosin and cardiac troponin T mutations cause familial hypertrophic cardiomyopathy: a disease of the sarcomere. *Cell* 77:701–712, 1994.
252. Tobacman, L. S., Thin filament–mediated regulation of cardiac contraction. *Annu. Rev. Physiol.* 58:447–481, 1996.
253. Tobacman L. S., and R. Lee. Isolation and functional comparison of bovine cardiac troponin T isoforms. *J. Biol. Chem.* 262: 4059–4064, 1987.
254. Trautwein, W., and J. Hescheler. Regulation of cardiac L-type calcium current by phosphorylation and G proteins. *Annu. Rev. Physiol.* 52:257–274, 1990.
255. Tripet, B., J. E. Van Eyk, and R. S. Hodges. Mapping of a second actin–tropomyosin and a second troponin C binding site within the C terminus of troponin I, and their importance in the Ca^{2+}-dependent regulation of muscle contraction. *J. Mol. Biol.* 271:728–750, 1997.
256. Ueno, H. Local structural changes in tropomyosin detected by a trypsin-probe method. *Biochemistry* 23:4791–4798, 1984.
257. Van Eyk, J. E., and R. S. Hodges. The use of synthetic peptides to unravel the mechanism of muscle regulation. *Methods: A Companion to Methods in Enzymology.* 5:264–280, 1993.

258. Van Eyk, J. E., and R. S. Hodges. The biological importance of each amino acid residue of the troponin I inhibitory sequence 104–115 in the interaction with troponin C and tropomyosin–actin. *J. Biol. Chem.* 263:1726–1732, 1988.

259. Van Eyk, J. E., C. M. Kay, and R. S. Hodges. A comparative study of the interactions of synthetic peptides of the skeletal and cardiac troponin I inhibitory region with skeletal and cardiac troponin C. *Biochemistry* 30:9974–9981, 1991.

260. Vassylyev, D. G., S. Takeda, S. Wakatsuki, K. Maeda, and Y. Maeda. The crystal structure of troponin C in complex with N-terminal fragment of troponin I. The mechanism of how the inhibitory action of troponin I is released by Ca$(^{2+})$-binding to troponin C. *Adv. Exp. Med. Biol.* 453:157–167, 1998.

261. Venema, R. C., and J. F. Kuo. Protein kinase C-mediated phosphorylation of troponin I and C-protein in isolated myocardial cells is associated with inhibition of myofibrillar actomyosin ATPase. *J. Biol. Chem.* 268:2705–2711, 1993.

262. Venema, R. C., R. L. Raynor, T. A. Noland, and J. F. Kuo. Role of protein kinase C in the phosphorylation of cardiac myosin light chain 2. *Biochem. J.* 294:401–406, 1993.

263. Villar-Palasi, C. and A. Kumon. Purification and properties of dog cardiac troponin T kinase. *J. Biol. Chem.* 256:7409–7415, 1981.

264. Wang, Z. Y., S. Sarkar, J. Gergely, and T. Tao. $Ca^{2(+)}$-dependent interactions between the C-helix of troponin-C and troponin-I. Photocross-linking and fluorescence studies using a recombinant troponin-C. *J. Biol. Chem.* 265:4953–4957, 1990.

265. Watkins, H., D. Conner, L. Thierfelder, J. A. Jarcho, C. MacRae, W. J. McKenna, B. J. Maron, J. G. Seidman, and C. E. Seidman. Mutations in the cardiac myosin binding protein-C gene on chromosome 11 cause familial hypertrophic cardiomyopathy. *Nat. Genet.* 11:434–437, 1995.

266. Watkins, H., W. J. McKenna, L. Thierfelder, H. J. Suk, R. Anan, A. O'Donoghue, P. Spirito, A. Matsumori, C. S. Moravec, J. G. Seidman, and C. E. Seidman. Mutations in the genes for cardiac troponin T and α-tropomyosin in hypertrophic cardiomyopathy. *N. Engl. J. Med.* 332:1058–1064, 1995.

267. Wattanapermpool, J., X. Guo, and R. J. Solaro. The unique amino-terminal peptide of cardiac troponin I regulates myofibrillar ATPase activity only when it is phosphorylated. *J. Mol. Cell. Cardiol.* 27:1383–1391, 1995.

268. Weisberg, A. and S. Winegrad. Alteration of myosin cross bridges by phosphorylation of myosin-binding protein C in cardiac muscle. *Proc. Natl. Acad. Sci. U.S.A.* 93:8999–9003, 1996.

269. Weisberg, A., and S. Winegrad. Relation between crossbridge structure and actomyosin ATPase activity in rat heart. *Circ. Res.* 83:60–72, 1998.

270. Westwood, S. A., and S. V. Perry. The effect of adrenaline on the phosphorylation of the P light chain of myosin and troponin-I in the perfused rabbit heart. *Biochem. J.* 197:185–193, 1981.

271. White, S. P., C. Cohen, and J. G. N. Phillips. Structure of co-crystals of tropomyosin and troponin. *Nature* 325:826–828, 1987.

272. Wilkinson, J. M., and R. J. A. Grand. Comparison of amino acid sequence of troponin I from different striated muscles. *Nature* 271:31–35, 1978.

273. Williams, D. L., Jr., L. E. Greene, and E. Eisenberg. Cooperative turning on of myosin subfragment 1 adenosinetriphosphatase activity by the troponin–tropomyosin–actin complex. *Biochemistry* 27:6987–6993, 1988.

274. Wolff, M. R., S. H. Buck, S. W. Stoker, M. L. Greaser, and R. M. Mentzer. Myofibrillar calcium sensitivity of isometric tension is increased in human dilated cardiomyopathies: role of altered beta-adrenergically mediated protein phosphorylation. *J. Clin. Invest.* 98:167–176, 1996.

275. Wolska, B. M., M. O. Stojanovic, W. Luo, E. G. Kranias, and R. J. Solaro. Effect of ablation of phospholamban on dynamics of cardiac myocyte contraction and intracellular Ca^{2+}. *Am. J. Physiol.* 271 (*Cell Physiol.* 40): C391, 1996.

276. Wolska, B. M., R. S. Keller, C. C. Evans, K. A. Palmiter, R. M. Phillips, M. Muthuchamy, J. Oehlenschlager, D. F. Wieczorek, P. P. de Tombe, and R. J. Solaro. Correlation between myofilament response to Ca^{2+} and altered dynamics of contraction and relaxation in transgenic cardiac cells expressing β-tropomyosin. *Circ. Res.* 84:745–751, 1999.

277. Yang, Z., J. T. Stull, R. J. Levine, and H. L. Sweeney. Changes in interfilament spacing mimic the effects of myosin regulatory light chain phosphorylation in rabbit psoas fibers. *J. Struct. Biol.* 122:139–148, 1998.

278. Zhang, R., J. Zhao, A. Mandveno, and J. D. Potter. Cardiac troponin I phosphorylation increases the rate of cardiac muscle relaxation. *Circ. Res.* 76:1028–1035, 1995.

279. Zhang R., J.-J. Zhao, and J. D. Potter. Phosphorylation of both serine residues in cardiac troponin I is required to decrease the Ca^{2+} affinity of cardiac troponin C. *J. Biol. Chem.* 270:30773–30780, 1995.

280. Zhou, X., E. P. Morris, S. S. Lehrer. Binding of troponin I and the troponin I-troponin C complex to actin-tropomyosin. Dissociation by myosin subfragment 1. *Biochemistry* 39: 1128–1132, 2000.

8. Cardiac sarcoplasmic reticulum Ca²⁺-ATPase

MICHIHIKO TADA
TOSHIHIKO TOYOFUKU

Department of Medicine and Pathophysiology, Osaka University School of Medicine, Osaka, Japan

CHAPTER CONTENTS

Structure of Ca^{2+}-ATPase
  Structure of Sarcoplasmic Reticulum
  Isolation and characterization of cardiac sarcoplasmic reticulum
    Components of cardiac sarcoplasmic reticulum
    Reconstitution of cardiac sarcoplasmic reticulum
Function of Ca^{2+}-ATPase
  Ca^{2+} pumping function
    Ca^{2+} uptake by isolated sarcoplasmic reticulum vesicles
    Stoichiometry of Ca^{2+} binding sites
    The coupling ratio
    Electrogenicity of Ca^{2+} transport
    Comparison of Ca^{2+}-ATPases from cardiac and skeletal muscle sarcoplasmic reticulum
  Mechanism of Ca^{2+}-ATPase activity
    The reaction cycle
    Conformational changes
  Regulation of Ca^{2+}-ATPase activity
Structure and Function of Ca^{2+}-ATPase
  Primary sequences and structural models for Ca^{2+} ATPases
    Secondary structural model of the Ca^{2+}-ATPase
    Three-dimensional structure of Ca^{2+}-ATPase
  Chemical modifications of the Ca^{2+}-ATPase
    Probes of catalytic and Ca^{2+} binding domains
    Measurement of fluorescence resonance energy transfer
    Measurement of rotational diffusion
    Measurement of secondary structure with spectroscopy
    Measurement of resonance x-ray diffraction
  Site-directed mutagenesis of Ca^{2+}-ATPase
    Ca^{2+} binding and Ca^{2+} affinity mutants
    ATP binding and phosphorylation mutants
    Conformational change mutants
    Uncoupling mutant
    A model for Ca^{2+} transport
  Ca^{2+}-ATPase Isoform Chimeras
Regulation of Ca^{2+}-ATPase by Phospholamban
  Structure of phospholamban
    Primary sequences and structural model of phospholamban
  Function of phospholamban
    Phosphorylation of phospholamban
    Effect of phospholamban on the reaction sequence of Ca^{2+}-ATPase
  Interaction between Ca^{2+}-ATPase and phospholamban
    Phospholamban-interaction site in Ca^{2+}-ATPase
    Ca^{2+}-ATPase-interacting sites in phospholamban
    Molecular mechanism of interaction
  Physiological relevance of the phospholamban–Ca^{2+}-ATPase system
    Phospholamban gene targeting mice

Regulation of Ca^{2+}-ATPase and Phospholamban Genes
  Structure of the Ca^{2+}-ATPase gene
  Transcriptional regulation of the Ca^{2+}-ATPase gene
  Structure of the phospholamban gene
  Transcriptional regulation of the phospholamban gene

FLUCTUATION OF INTRACELLULAR Ca^{2+} LEVELS, regulated through the accumulation or release of Ca^{2+} by intracellular organelles and by flux through the plasma membrane, mediates a variety of intracellular functions (151). The sarcoplasmic reticulum is a tubular, membranous network within muscle cells, which is the analogue of the endoplasmic reticulum in nonmuscle cells. This organelle has a variety of functions, of which release of Ca^{2+} to the cytosol and reuptake into the interior compartment (the lumen) of the sarcoplasmic reticulum are the most important. An understanding of the molecular events involved in Ca^{2+} regulation by the sarcoplasmic reticulum has come about through analysis at three different levels: (1) The sarco-tubular system has been resolved into its component membrane systems and retention of function has been analyzed. (2) Individual proteins have been isolated, characterized, and functionally reconstituted. (3) cDNAs encoding these proteins have been cloned, expressed, and mutagenized, providing new insights into structure–function relationships within and between these proteins.

Rapid release of Ca^{2+} through a Ca^{2+} release channel (the ryanodine receptor) in the sarcoplasmic reticulum of skeletal muscle cells is responsible for muscle contraction: Reuptake of Ca^{2+} by the action of a Ca^{2+}-ATPase is responsible for muscle relaxation. Thus, these proteins play an essential role in excitation–contraction coupling in skeletal muscle cells (71). In cardiac muscle cells, however, the intracellular Ca^{2+} concentration is controlled not only by the sarcoplasmic reticulum but also by other pumps, channels, and exchangers located in the sarcolemma. Nonetheless, the sarcoplasmic reticulum of mammalian cardiac cells is well developed and has a major role in excitation–contraction coupling. In cardiac muscle, phospholamban participates in the relaxation process by regulating the activity of the Ca^{2+}-ATPase. Ca^{2+} fluxes through the sarcoplasmic reticulum membrane are influenced by luminal Ca^{2+}-binding proteins, of which calsequestrin is the most important. A comparable system in nonmuscle cells involves release of Ca^{2+} from the endoplasmic reticulum through a Ca^{2+} release channel, the IP$_3$ receptor, and reuptake through organellar or plasma membrane Ca^{2+}-ATPases. The sarcoplasmic and endoplasmic reticulum Ca^{2+}-ATPases are referred to as the SERCA family of Ca^{2+}-ATPase, and the plasma membrane Ca^{2+}-ATPases are referred to as the PMCA family of Ca^{2+}-ATPases (87, 166). In this chapter we focus on the structure and function of two components of cardiac sarcoplasmic reticulum, the Ca^{2+}-ATPase and phospholamban.

STRUCTURE OF THE Ca^{2+}-ATPase

Structure of Cardiac Sarcoplasmic Reticulum

The sarcoplasmic reticulum is a specialized form of the endoplasmic reticulum, a system of intracellular membranes found in virtually every cell. The endoplasmic reticulum in most cells is composed of two morphologically distinct membranes: (1) the rough endoplasmic reticulum, in which the outer surface is studded with ribosomes, and which is involved primarily in protein synthesis, and (2) the smooth endoplasmic reticulum, which, in nonmuscle cells, participates in a range of metabolic functions from dephosphorylation of glucose to drug detoxification. Although the sarcoplasmic reticulum in muscle cells is smooth in appearance, it differs from smooth endoplasmic reticulum in that its function is highly specialized for Ca^{2+} regulation. The sarcoplasmic reticulum is an extensive intracellular muscle membrane system that surrounds each myofibril like a water jacket. Each myofibril is segmented longitudinally into sarcomeric structures, the functional units of the contractile apparatus. The sarcoplasmic reticulum surrounding the sarcomere is also segmented, more or less in register with the sarcomere (59, 237; Fig. 8–1).

In mammalian skeletal muscle, the sarcoplasmic reticulum segments extend between A-I junctions. Each segment of the sarcoplasmic reticulum consists of longitudinal reticulum with terminal cisternae at either end. The terminal cisternae abut transverse tubules (T-tubules), invaginations of the sarcolemma that penetrate into the sarcoplasm at points near the A-I junction of each mammalian sarcomere. Because the junction between the circular transverse tubule and the two dilated terminal cisternae has the appearance of three

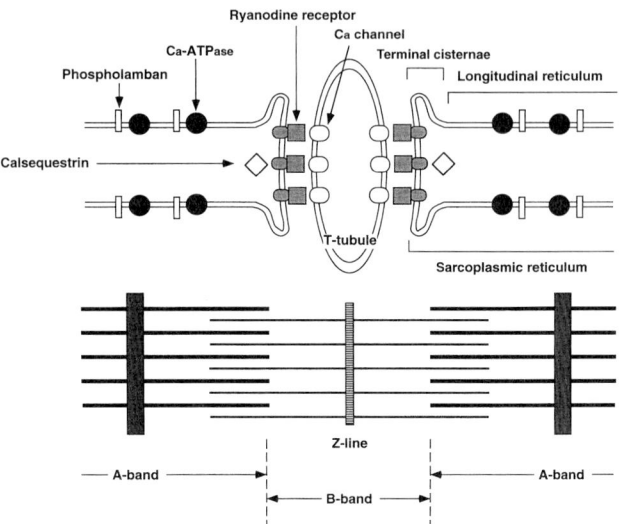

FIG. 8–1. Schematic model of the ultrastructure of the cardiac cell. Contractile proteins are arranged in a regular array of thick and thin filaments. The A-band represents the region of the sarcomere occupied by the thick filaments. Thin filaments extend variable distances into the A-band, from either side. The I-band represents the region of the sarcomere occupied excessively by thin filaments, which extend toward the center of the sarcomere from the Z-lines. The sarcomere, the functional unit of the contractile apparatus, is defined as the region between a pair of Z-lines, and contains two half I-bands and one A-band. The sarcoplasmic reticulum consists of the longitudinal reticulum and the terminal cisternae, which abut the transverse tubular system (T-tubule). The T-tubule is a sarcolemmal invagination, so that the lumen of the T-tubules is continuous with the extracellular space. Slow Ca^{2+} channels in the T-tubule are believed to be associated with the Ca^{2+} release channel in the junctional face of the terminal cisternae. In the lumen of the terminal cisternae, Ca^{2+}-binding proteins, calsequestrin, calreticulin, and histidine-rich Ca^{2+} binding protein also exist. In the longitudinal reticulum, Ca^{2+}-ATPase and phospholamban exist in the membrane, and glycoproteins of 53 kDa and 160 kDa are located in the lumen.

linked rings in longitudinal thin sections, the structure is referred to as a *triad*. The two junctional faces between the three membranes making up the triad are separated by a 150Å gap, which is partially filled with foot structures. The foot structures originate in the junctional face membrane of sarcoplasmic reticulum and bridge the gap to form an association with the T-tubule membrane (68, 73). It has recently become clear that the foot structure is a tetrameric complex of four 564,000 Da proteins making up both the Ca^{2+} release channel and the ryanodine receptor (36, 113, 116, 149) and that the most likely T-tubule protein with which the Ca^{2+} release channel associates is the slow Ca^{2+} channel protein, the dehydropyridine (DHP) receptor (259).

Cardiac and skeletal muscle sarcoplasmic reticulum have essentially the same structure. However, there are relatively fewer T-tubules in cardiac muscle and they have a larger diameter than those in skeletal muscle.

They often couple on only one side with the terminal cisternae of the sarcoplasmic reticulum, forming a *dyad* rather than a *triad* structure. *Dyads* also form with subsarcolemmal structures, and these couplings all contain a foot structure similar to that described in skeletal muscle. In avian cardiac cells, about 20% of terminal cisternae are associated with *dyads*, while the remainder are not associated with either transverse tubules or sarcolemma and exist as blind pouches referred to as *corbular structures* (126, 237).

Isolation and Characterization of Cardiac Sarcoplasmic Reticulum

In cardiac muscle, the sarcoplasmic reticulum network is less extensive than it is in skeletal muscle, and cell surface membranes, including sarcolemma and T-tubule, constitute much of the total membrane content of muscle cells. Consequently, it is more difficult to isolate highly purified sarcoplasmic reticulum vesicles from heart muscle than from skeletal muscle. To eliminate contaminating surface membrane vesicles, various procedures have been developed by many laboratories (41, 65, 91, 123, 156, 185, 212, 236).

Components of Cardiac Sarcoplasmic Reticulum. When muscle is homogenized, the sarcoplasmic reticulum membranes are fragmented, but they reseal spontaneously into small vesicles. These vesicles are a major component of the microsomal fraction. They are not sedimented by centrifugation of homogenized muscle at 10,000 × g for 10 min, but they are sedimented at 40,000 × g for 90 min (65, 91, 123, 212, 336). The resulting preparations are highly enriched in sarcoplasmic reticulum vesicles exhibiting high Ca^{2+} uptake and ATP hydrolytic activities. Both skeletal and cardiac sarcoplasmic reticulum membranes can be further fractionated into light and heavy fractions by sucrose density gradient centrifugation (41, 42, 91, 124, 185, 227). The light fraction corresponds predominantly to the longitudinal sarcoplasmic reticulum. The 110 kDa Ca^{2+}-ATPase is the major constituent, accounting for 35%–40% of the total protein associated with these vesicles (41, 42, 242). By contrast, the 110 kDa Ca^{2+}-ATPase accounts for about two-thirds of the protein in highly purified fractions of skeletal muscle sarcoplasmic reticulum (185). Luminal glycoproteins of 53 and 130 kDa (160 kDa in skeletal muscle) are also present in light fractions (44). Phospholamban (PLN), a homopentamer of 6 kDa subunits, is present in cardiac, but not in skeletal longitudinal reticulum. It fractionates with the Ca^{2+}-ATPase in cardiac muscle (125). In the heavy fraction, which corresponds to the terminal cisternae, the predominant proteins are the acidic Ca^{2+}-binding protein calsequestrin (175), calreticulin (72), a 170 kDa protein, the histidine-rich Ca^{2+}-binding protein (HCP; 100), and a high-molecular-weight protein, the Ca^{2+} release channel or ryanodine receptor (36, 115, 116). The Ca^{2+} release channel is the major protein in the junctional face membrane of the terminal cisternae, and the Ca^{2+}-storage protein, calsequestrin, is the major luminal protein (223, 224).

Reconstitution of Cardiac Sarcoplasmic Reticulum. Sarcoplasmic reticulum membrane vesicles with a high content of Ca^{2+}-ATPase have been used in reconstitution experiments to assess the function of the Ca^{2+}-ATPase. In the first such experiments, the active Ca^{2+}-ATPase was extracted from skeletal muscle sarcoplasmic reticulum using deoxycholate (184, 213). The reconstitution of active Ca^{2+}-ATPase into liposomes was carried out by the reversal of the process of dissociation. As detergents were removed by dialysis, the ATPase–phospholipid complexes were transferred into phospholipid vesicles. Highly purified and stable cardiac sarcoplasmic reticulum was also prepared using a combination of differential centrifugation and sucrose density gradient centrifugation (41, 42, 71, 124, 227), dissolved in Triton X-100, and reconstituted into phospholipid vesicles (113).

Vesicles reconstituted from whole sarcoplasmic reticulum had a protein composition similar to the original vesicles, but lacked a luminal Ca^{2+} binding protein such as calsequestrin. The reconstituted vesicles pumped Ca^{2+} at the expense of ATP hydrolysis (105, 113, 184, 213), but the Ca^{2+} loading rate of the reconstituted vesicles was only about 70% of that of the original cardiac sarcoplasmic reticulum, perhaps because of the bidirectional alignment of the Ca^{2+}-ATPase in reconstituted vesicles (105).

FUNCTION OF Ca^{2+}-ATPase

In most living cells, there is a remarkable cycle of events in which ATP, synthesized by oxidative or photosynthetic phosphorylation, is hydrolyzed to energize biological work and then rapidly and efficiently resynthesized to ATP. Cellular ATPases have been categorized as F-, V- and P-type ATPases (204). F-type ATPases are those of the F_0F_1 type, located in the mitochondrial inner membrane, and they are driven in the reverse direction to make ATP (ATP synthetases). V-type ATPases are located in vacuoles, the vacuolar H^+ ATPase being the archetype. P-type ATPases are those that form a phosphoprotein intermediate during their reaction cycle. They include a series of cation pumps, such as H^+/K^+-ATPases, Na^+/K^+-ATPases, Ca^{2+}-ATPases, Mg^{2+}-ATPases, and Cu^{2+}-ATPases. ATP formed by the mitochondrial ATP synthetase is available to other cellular ATPases for the performance of cellular work, in tightly coupled ATP hydrolytic reactions (84, 160, 204).

Ca²⁺ Pumping Function

Like all biological membranes, the sarcoplasmic reticulum is made up of an impermeable lipid bilayer in which various proteins are embedded to achieve selective movement of metabolites or regulatory molecules across the lipid barrier. The lipid bilayer serves as a barrier to the free diffusion of Ca^{2+}. Since the sarcoplasmic reticulum in situ consists of long tubes or sacs, disruption and resealing of the sarcoplasmic reticulum produces vesicles with a topology directly referable to the original membrane system: The cytoplasmic surface remains outside, and the luminal surface remains inside (42, 56, 91). The Ca^{2+}-ATPase accounts for 35%–40% of the total protein associated with isolated cardiac sarcoplasmic reticulum vesicles (42, 243). Isolated cardiac sarcoplasmic reticulum vesicles, therefore, provide an excellent system for the measurement of ATP hydrolysis coupled to Ca^{2+} transport.

Ca²⁺ Uptake by Isolated Sarcoplasmic Reticulum Vesicles. When cardiac sarcoplasmic reticulum vesicles are placed in a medium containing Ca^{2+}, Mg^{2+}, and sufficient ATP, they accumulate Ca^{2+} in luminal spaces (92, 93, 179, 293). Ca^{2+} uptake is usually measured as $^{45}Ca^{2+}$ retained after membrane filtration, a method that allows rapid separation of $^{45}Ca^{2+}$-loaded vesicles from the reaction medium. Transient and steady-state kinetics of Ca^{2+} uptake into vesicles have been analyzed under various conditions.

Ca^{2+} uptake by cardiac sarcoplasmic reticulum vesicles is nearly at steady state within 12 sec after initiation of the reaction (66, 74, 112, 255). The initial linear phase of Ca^{2+} uptake is quite fast, lasting only about 200 msec. Subsequently, the rate of Ca^{2+} uptake slows as internal Ca^{2+} binding sites are saturated and the increased luminal free Ca^{2+} inhibits further uptake by Ca^{2+}-ATPase (294). The initial phase of Ca^{2+} uptake can be measured on a time scale of milliseconds to seconds with stopped-flow or quench-flow methods. In the stopped-flow method, changes in the spectrum of Ca^{2+} indicator dyes such as murexide or arsenazo III, reflecting variation of the Ca^{2+} concentration in the medium, are measured spectrometrically. In the quench-flow method, $^{45}Ca^{2+}$ uptake by the vesicles is measured after rapid quenching of the uptake reaction with EGTA or La^{3+}. The initial rate of ATP-dependent Ca^{2+} uptake by cardiac sarcoplasmic reticulum vesicles, measured at 25°C with murexide by the stopped-flow technique, varied from 16 to 21 nmol Ca^{2+}/mg protein/ 150 msec (19), or, using a rapid-quenching apparatus, 33.4 nmol Ca^{2+}/mg protein/sec at 22°C (300).

Ca^{2+} accumulation by vesicles attains a plateau where both the rate of active Ca^{2+} influx by the Ca^{2+} ATPase and passive Ca^{2+} efflux are equal. This is a fairly slow process, occurring over several seconds to minutes. Steady-state Ca^{2+} accumulation levels depend on a number of factors such as pH, temperature, and the concentrations of Ca^{2+}, Mg^{2+}, ATP, and ADP. The maximal reported rates of Ca^{2+} uptake by cardiac sarcoplasmic reticulum vesicles, measured in the presence of oxalate, range from 0.2 µmol/mg protein/min at 25°C (243) to 1.5 µmol/mg protein/min at 37°C (236). Ca^{2+} uptake and Ca^{2+}-dependent ATP hydrolysis by cardiac sarcoplasmic reticulum vesicles are coactivated by Ca^{2+} in the reaction medium (179, 293). The rates of both activities rise with increasing Ca^{2+} concentrations, reaching a maximum at 3–10 µM Ca^{2+}. Half-maximal activation of both activities (K_{Ca}) occurs at 0.3–4.7 µM Ca^{2+} at pH 6.8–7.0 (91, 139, 212, 215, 230, 236, 255). Mg^{2+} is required for the rapid turnover of the Ca^{2+}-ATPase, and an equimolar complex of Mg^{2+} and ATP appears to serve as the physiological substrate for Ca^{2+} uptake and Ca^{2+}-dependent ATP hydrolysis. Divalent cation-binding studies showed that Mg^{2+}, derived from the complex of Mg^{2+} and ATP, remains bound to the Ca^{2+}-ATPase. Binding of this Mg^{2+} is responsible for the induction of a high rate of enzyme turnover (202, 231). ATPase activity is saturated at about 10 µM Mg-ATP (K_m = 1–2 µM), but a further increase in activity is observed at Mg-ATP concentrations of 180 µM (230, 279). The K_m value obtained at low ATP concentrations is similar to the K_m for formation of the phosphoenzyme intermediate of the ATPase, indicating that the low K_m site corresponds to the high-affinity catalytic site. The stimulatory effect of higher ATP concentrations is considered to arise from the regulatory action of the nucleotide on the turnover of the Ca^{2+}-ATPase. Besides ATP, the cardiac Ca^{2+}-ATPase utilizes other nucleotide triphosphates (93, 242, 258); the rates of utilization at 5 mM being in the order: ATP > CTP > ITP > GTP > UTP (65).

The pH dependence of the rates of Ca^{2+} uptake and Ca^{2+}-dependent ATP hydrolysis by cardiac sarcoplasmic reticulum vesicles exhibits a bell-shaped profile with an optimum at pH 6.2–6.5 for Ca^{2+} uptake and at pH 7.5–8.0 for ATP hydrolysis (230, 257, 290).

Thapsigargin, a tumor-promoting sesquiterpene lactone isolated from the plant *Thapsia garganica*, is a highly specific inhibitor of members of the sarco(endo)plasmic reticulum Ca^{2+}-ATPase (SERCA) family. It acts through suppression of Ca^{2+}-binding to the high-affinity transport sites (130, 222, 266). Thapsigargin interacts tightly with the Ca^{2+} ATPase in a 1:

1 stoichiometry in the absence of Ca^{2+}, forming a catalytically inactive dead-end complex (222).

Stoichiometry of Ca^{2+} Binding Sites. Ca^{2+} binding to the Ca^{2+}-ATPase produces a measurable enhancement of intrinsic protein fluorescence that can be used for measurement, by the stopped-flow method, of the kinetics of Ca^{2+} binding or dissociation (43, 61, 69, 86). The rates of Ca^{2+}-dependent fluorescence changes are rather slow, suggesting that they reflect conformational changes. Measurement of equilibrium Ca^{2+} binding to the Ca^{2+}-ATPase, using $^{45}Ca^{2+}$, shows that two high-affinity Ca^{2+} binding sites ($K_d = 10^{-6}$ M) are present for each ATPase phosphorylation site (44, 111, 184). Analysis of Ca^{2+} binding as a function of Ca^{2+} concentration demonstrates a cooperative mechanism in which binding to a first site is followed by development of higher affinity and binding to a second site. Measurement of the kinetics of exchange of $^{45}Ca^{2+}$ and $^{40}Ca^{2+}$ shows that the two Ca^{2+} binding sites are stacked and that dissociation of the two bound Ca^{2+} ions from the Ca^{2+} binding sites is ordered. Dissociation of the first Ca^{2+} ion from one of the sites triggers a conformational change, resulting in the dissociation of the second Ca^{2+} ion (109, 111). Thus, sequential Ca^{2+} binding accounts for the cooperativity of binding observed at equilibrium and for the cooperativity that is apparent in measurements of the Ca^{2+} dependence of Ca^{2+} uptake in the steady state. However, the cross-linking assay with cysteine mutations of Ca^{2+} binding helices 4 and 6 of SERCA1 indicated that two Ca^{2+} binding sites are positioned side-by-side in a Ca^{2+} binding "pocket" constructed by helices 4, 5, and 6 (174).

In contrast to this two-sites model, a four-sites model has been proposed by Jencks et al. (122) on the basis of measurement of phosphoenzyme formation at various concentrations of luminal Ca^{2+}. In this model, the free enzyme has two low-affinity, luminal Ca^{2+} binding sites and two high-affinity, cytoplasmic Ca^{2+} binding sites, which are independent of each other. Phosphorylation of the enzyme by ATP results in translocation of Ca^{2+} from the high-affinity to the low-affinity sites. Although the mechanisms of Ca^{2+} translocation appear to be different in the two models, the stoichiometry between Ca^{2+} ions translocated and ATP hydrolyzed remains at 2:1.

The Coupling Ratio. Ca^{2+} transport across the sarcoplasmic reticulum membrane is an energy-requiring process (92, 293). During Ca^{2+}-dependent hydrolysis of ATP by cardiac sarcoplasmic reticulum vesicles, the terminal phosphate of ATP is incorporated into the ATPase protein, forming the phosphoenzyme intermediate denoted by E~P (230, 242, 246, 255). The formation of E~P has been measured by the transfer of ^{32}P from [γ-^{32}P]ATP into a trichloroacetic acid (TCA) precipitate of the sarcoplasmic reticulum (306). The maximum amount of phosphoenzyme formed, which reflects the amount of ATPase protein in a typical preparation of cardiac sarcoplasmic reticulum, was up to 1.3 mmoles/mg protein (230, 243).

The coupling ratio between Ca^{2+}-dependent ATP hydrolysis and Ca^{2+} uptake is determined from simultaneous measurements of the rates of oxalate-supported Ca^{2+} uptake and ATP hydrolysis. These rates parallel each other under various conditions, indicating that they are tightly coupled. A number of experimental findings confirm that one mole of Ca^{2+}-ATPase transports two moles of Ca^{2+} ions from the cytoplasm to the luminal spaces at the expense of one mole of ATP hydrolysis (92, 110, 111, 293).

Electrogenicity of Ca^{2+} Transport. Several investigators, working with native sarcoplasmic reticulum vesicles and Ca^{2+}-ATPase incorporated into liposomes or planar lipid bilayers, have reported that ATP-dependent translocation of Ca^{2+} is electrogenic (288, 309, 313). In principle, electrogenicity would result if the charge stoichiometry of countertransport were uneven, as observed with the Na^+/K^+-ATPase (83). Countertransport of one H^+ per one Ca^{2+} and net positive charge displacement has been observed in studies of Ca^{2+} transport by the Ca^{2+}-ATPase reconstituted in planar lipid bilayers (309). A 1:1 Ca^{2+}/H^+ exchange at each binding site could explain the pH dependence of Ca^{2+} binding to the sarcoplasmic reticulum Ca^{2+}-ATPase in the absence of ATP (288). On the basis of these data, the overall catalytic and transport cycle may be written as:

$$2\ Ca^{2+}\ (out) + ATP + 2\ H^+\ (in) \rightarrow 2\ Ca^{2+}\ (in) + ADP + Pi + 2\ H^+\ (out)$$

Although electrogenicity is an intrinsic component of the mechanism of Ca^{2+} transport, its physiological role is probably not very important. Sarcoplasmic reticulum membranes are relatively permeable to cations and anions so that electrogenicity can only be measured in reconstituted proteoliposome systems. Moreover, a transmembrane potential of up to 40 mV had little effect on the kinetics of the Ca^{2+} pump (309).

Comparison of Ca^{2+}-ATPases from Cardiac and Skeletal Muscle Sarcoplasmic Reticulum. The basic features of the reaction cycle have been investigated extensively with the Ca^{2+}-ATPase from skeletal muscle sarcoplasmic reticulum (SERCA1a), and have been applied to the Ca^{2+}-ATPase from cardiac muscle sarcoplasmic reticulum (SERCA2a). Although the mechanism of Ca^{2+}

uptake and ATP hydrolysis by cardiac sarcoplasmic reticulum vesicles is generally similar to that by skeletal sarcoplasmic reticulum vesicles, significant differences are noted in the two preparations (37, 137, 231, 246, 254). Ca^{2+} uptake and ATP hydrolysis are considerably slower in cardiac preparations than in skeletal preparations and the difference is most pronounced with Ca^{2+} concentrations in the 100 nM to 1 μM range. In steady-state kinetic measurements, the maximum level of enzyme phosphorylation, which reflects the density of the ATPase protein, is about four-fold lower in cardiac preparations than in skeletal preparations. Studies of the ATP-dependence of ATP hydrolysis show that the K_m for ATP is similar in both preparations. However, the half-maximal activation of ATP hydrolysis or of Ca^{2+} transport by Ca^{2+} (K_{Ca}) from cardiac preparations is three- to fourfold higher for cardiac than for skeletal preparations. Therefore, the relatively slow rate of Ca^{2+} uptake by cardiac preparations reflects primarily the low content of the Ca^{2+}-ATPase and lower Ca^{2+} affinity of the enzyme, rather than a low enzyme turnover number. This conclusion is supported by studies of the activities of SERCA1a and SERCA2a expressed in homologous cell culture systems, where the intrinsic activities of these proteins can be compared in the absence of PLN. Under these conditions, the intrinsic activities of SERCA1a and SERCA2a were very similar (167, 272) and, in addition, the activities of both SERCA1a and SERCA2a could be regulated in identical fashion when they were coexpressed with PLN (275).

Mechanism of Ca^{2+}-ATPase Activity

The Ca^{2+}-ATPase of sarcoplasmic reticulum pumps Ca^{2+} from the cytoplasm of muscle to the lumen of the sarcoplasmic reticulum vesicle at the expense of ATP hydrolysis (55). The problem is to understand how this enzyme catalyzes the fully reversible coupled vectorial reaction:

$$2\ Ca^{2+}\ (out) + ATP + 2\ H^+\ (in) \rightarrow 2\ Ca^{2+}\ (in) + ADP + Pi + 2\ H^+\ (out)$$

Considerable effort has been directed toward characterization of pre–steady state events by rapid kinetic experiments (74, 112, 120, 148, 211, 282). The chemical reaction of ATP hydrolysis and the vectorial reaction of Ca^{2+} movement are coupled in such a way that neither ATP hydrolysis nor movement of Ca^{2+} will occur without the other. In the reaction pathway, coupling is brought about by changes in chemical and vectorial specificities. The chemical specificities are these: (1) the enzyme with bound Ca^{2+} in the transport sites can be phosphorylated reversibly with ATP, but not with P_i (inorganic phosphate), and (2) the enzyme with no bound Ca^{2+} can be phosphorylated reversibly with P_i, but not with ATP. The vectorial specificities are orthogonal to the chemical specificities: (1) Ca^{2+} is occluded, transported, and dissociated from its binding sites only when the enzyme has been phosphorylated from bound ATP, and (2) Ca^{2+} can bind to high-affinity sites in the Ca^{2+}-ATPase only when the enzyme is dephosphorylated.

The Reaction Cycle. To sustain active Ca^{2+} transport, the enzyme must alternate between at least two states with different affinity for Ca^{2+} and with opposite orientation of the Ca^{2+} binding sites with respect to the plane of the membrane. The reaction cycle has usually been described according to a model with two major states, E and E*, E and E', or E_1 and E_2 (55, 106, 108, 229), as shown in Figure 8–2. In the E_1-E_2 model, vectorial transport against a gradient can most readily be visualized as a transition between two conformations of the enzyme. The E_1 state of the enzyme has high-affinity Ca^{2+} binding sites, which face the cytoplasmic side of the membrane and are exposed to relatively lower concentrations of Ca^{2+}, and the E_2 state has low-affinity Ca^{2+} binding sites, which face the opposite side of the membrane and are, therefore, exposed to a higher concentration of Ca^{2+}. Micromolar Ca^{2+} stabilizes the E_1 conformation of the enzyme, whereas removal of Ca^{2+} from the medium at low pH and high temperature, or addition of vanadate, stabilizes the E_2 conformation of the enzyme (55, 207, 209). In the presence of saturating Mg^{2+}, neutral pH, and 25 °C, the K_{Ca} for the high-affinity Ca^{2+} binding sites of the enzyme (E_1) is estimated to be $10^{-6}\ M$, while the K_{Ca} for the low-affinity Ca^{2+} binding sites of the enzyme (E_2) is estimated to be less than $10^{-3}\ M$ (108).

In the initial step of the Ca^{2+} transport cycle, two

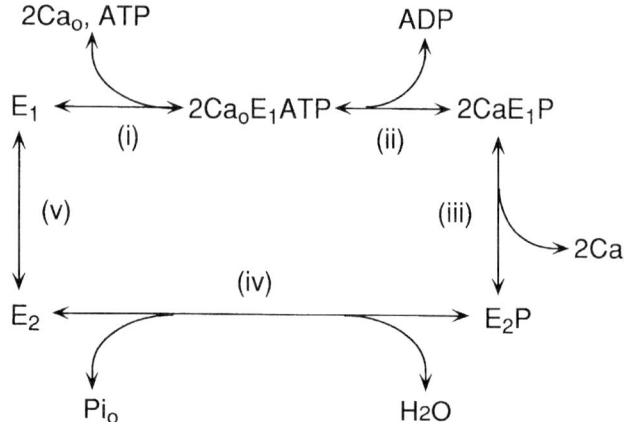

FIG. 8–2. The reaction cycle. Steps involved in the process of ATP hydrolysis and Ca^{2+} transport by the sarcoplasmic reticulum Ca^{2+}-ATPase. See text for details.

Ca^{2+} ions and one ATP bind to the enzyme (E$_1$) from the cytoplasmic side of the membrane (step i). When the γ-phosphate of ATP is covalently bound to Asp 351 of the enzyme, forming the phosphoenzyme (Ca^{2+})$_2$E$_1$~P, Ca^{2+} becomes occluded and can no longer dissociate to either side of the membrane (step ii). To this point, the reaction is reversible, since chemical energy is still conserved in the phosphoryl bond. The phosphoryl group can be transferred back to ADP to make ATP, accompanied by deocclusion of the bound Ca^{2+}. The next step (step iii) is the conformational transition between an ADP-sensitive phosphoenzyme intermediate, (Ca^{2+})$_2$E$_1$~P, and an ADP-insensitive phosphoenzyme intermediate (E$_2$~P). The conversion of the phosphoenzyme from a high-energy state to a low-energy state is coupled to the movement of Ca^{2+} from high-affinity binding sites facing the cytoplasmic surface to low-affinity binding sites facing the luminal surface of the membrane. Ca^{2+} now dissociates from the enzyme into the luminal side of the membrane. In step iv, the low-energy phosphoenzyme, E$_2$~P, is transformed to the (Ca^{2+})$_2$E$_1$ state as P$_i$ is lost to the cytoplasm, and the Ca^{2+} binding sites are reoriented from low-affinity to high-affinity states (step v).

Conformational Changes. When rapid kinetic measurements are initiated by adding 10 μM ATP to an enzyme preincubated with Ca^{2+}, the total amount of phosphoenzyme formed [(Ca^{2+})$_2$E$_1$~P form of the enzyme] increases with time to reach a maximum at 30 msec and then declines to a steady-state level (30, 246, 257). The liberation of P$_i$, however, shows a distinct lag phase and then increases linearly with time, indicating that P$_i$ is derived from the turnover of the phosphoenzyme. When enzyme phosphorylation is started by the addition of ATP without Ca^{2+} (E$_2$~P form of the enzyme), phosphoenzyme formation proceeds at a much slower rate and an overshoot of the steady-state level is not observed. These observations indicate that the E$_2$~P to (Ca^{2+})$_2$E$_1$ (step v), which is induced by Ca^{2+} addition, is slow and controls the rate of enzyme phosphorylation.

Two major conformations, of the enzyme, E$_1$ and E$_2$, have been observed in a number of different studies, including (*1*) proteolytic sensitivity at trypsin site T2 (*2*) measurement of changes in calculation of fluorescence from both intrinsic tryptophan residues (60) and extrinsic fluorophores such as iodoacetamide and N-substituted derivatives (16), (*3*) measurement of sensitivity to modifying reagents (106), (*4*) measurement of circular dichroism (81) and (*5*) time-resolved x-ray diffraction measurements (26, 27). However, all studies of Ca^{2+}-dependent phosphoenzyme formation from ATP have been difficult to interpret in terms of a simple E$_1$-E$_2$ model (121, 205, 206). Accordingly, Jencks et al. (120) have proposed that there are many conformational changes in the Ca^{2+} transport cycle and that none of them exist in the absence of either a phosphoryl or a Ca^{2+} ligand. A complete understanding of these conformational changes will require knowledge of the three-dimensional, high-resolution structure of the enzyme in its different chemical states.

Regulation of Ca^{2+}-ATPase Activity

When the kinetics of Ca^{2+} uptake and ATP hydrolysis are compared in sarcoplasmic reticulum vesicles from fast-twitch and cardiac muscles, the Ca^{2+}-ATPase from fast-twitch muscle has a higher activity than that from cardiac muscle (37, 137, 230, 254). This lower activity is due to lower amount of the protein and to its interaction with PLN (250). Phospholamban is an integral protein of the sarcoplasmic reticulum membrane in cardiac and slow-twitch muscle (251). Under β-adrenergic stimulation, it is phosphorylated by cyclic AMP–dependent protein kinase (PKA). The phosphorylation of phospholamban, either by PKA or by Ca^{2+}/calmodulin-dependent protein kinase, leads to an increase both in the maximal rate of Ca^{2+} uptake by the Ca^{2+} ATPase and in its affinity for Ca^{2+}.

Recently, Ca^{2+}/calmodulin-dependent protein kinase was found to phosphorylate SERCA2a at Ser 38. SERCA1a does not have a serine at position 38 and is not phosphorylated, even when an appropriate phosphorylation site is constructed (94, 270, 303). Although the Ca^{2+} uptake activity of phosphorylated SERCA2a was reported to be increased twofold by phosphorylation without any change in Ca^{2+} affinity, more recent studies have shown that the apparent increase in V$_{max}$ probably reflected a loss of control activity during preincubation (200).

There is evidence for long-term alterations of Ca^{2+}-ATPase activity under different physiological states. The content of sarcoplasmic reticulum and Ca^{2+}-ATPase and the amount of Ca^{2+} uptake and Ca^{2+}-dependent ATP hydrolysis are higher in adult cardiac muscle than in neonatal cardiac muscle (7, 10, 195). Cardiac hypertrophy is induced by thyroid hormone, pressure overload, and volume overload. In heart from hyperthyroid animals, the rate of Ca^{2+} uptake and Ca^{2+}-dependent ATP hydrolysis by sarcoplasmic reticulum were significantly increased, but the Ca^{2+} storage capacity and the steady-state level of Ca^{2+} uptake were unaltered (242). Hemodynamically loaded heart exhibited differential remodeling of sarcoplasmic reticulum in association with the degree of overload (1). In hearts with mild cardiac hypertrophy, an enhancement of Ca^{2+} uptake by Ca^{2+}-ATPase was reported. However, in more severely overloaded hearts, Ca^{2+} uptake and

Ca^{2+}-ATPase phosphoenzyme intermediate formation were significantly diminished (54, 150). Human heart samples from patients with hypertrophic cardiomyopathy after myomectomy have been used to measure intracellular Ca^{2+} transients (89). Isometric contraction and relaxation were prolonged, while end-diastolic intracellular Ca^{2+} concentrations were increased. Intracellular Ca^{2+} transients were also greatly prolonged (89).

The most widely used models of a failing heart are the BIO 14.6 and BIO 53.58 strains of hereditary cardiomyopathic Syrian hamster (17). Ca^{2+} uptake by cardiac sarcoplasmic reticulum vesicles from dilated cardiomyopathic hamsters between 3 and 11 months of age was significantly decreased, compared with vesicles from control hamsters (299).

In heart failure induced by chronic rapid ventricular pacing, Ca^{2+} uptake was diminished to half of that of control sarcoplasmic reticulum, and this decrease was positively correlated with left ventricular ejection fraction, an index of the degree of myocardial failure (199). Adriamycin (doxorubicin), an antineoplastic anthracycline antibiotic, provokes severe heart failure (Adriamycin cardiomyopathy; 308). A significant reduction in Ca^{2+}-ATPase activity was observed in chronically induced Adriamycin cardiomyopathy in dogs (269). Ca^{2+} uptake in human heart samples from dilated cardiomyopathy patients showed interesting discrepancies. A considerable decrease was measured in Ca^{2+} uptake by crude homogenates of the right ventricle (159), while Ca^{2+} uptake was normal in sarcoplasmic reticulum vesicles purified from the left ventricle (193).

STRUCTURE AND FUNCTION OF Ca^{2+}-ATPase

Primary Sequences and Structural Models for Ca^{2+}-ATPases

Although extensive efforts were made to sequence the Ca^{2+}-ATPase protein (3), molecular cloning of full-length cDNAs encoding SERCA2a (82), SERCA2b (166), SERCA1a (29), SERCA1b (28), and SERCA3 (32) eventually provided the primary sequences of each of these Ca^{2+}-ATPases. Three separate genes, ATP2A1, ATP2A2, and ATP2A3 encode SERCA1, SERCA2, and SERCA3 (144, 311). SERCA1 is expressed exclusively in fast-twitch skeletal muscle. It is alternatively spliced in the region encoding the carboxyl terminus, producing a short protein, SERCA1a, terminating in Gly, and a longer version, SERCA1b, terminating in Glu-Asp-Pro-Glu-Asp-Glu-Arg-Arg-Lys. SERCA1b is downregulated during neonatal development, while SERCA2a is upregulated, accounting for nearly 100% of the ATPase in adult muscle.

The SERCA2 transcript is also alternatively spliced in the region encoding the carboxyl terminus, producing SERCA2a and SERCA2b. SERCA2a, encoding a protein about 84% identical to the SERCA1 product and terminating in the sequence Ala-Ile-Leu-Glu, is the major spliced species of this gene expressed in striated muscle. SERCA1a is expressed in both neonatal and adult slow-twitch skeletal muscle and in cardiac muscle at all stages of development. The second transcript, SERCA2b, encodes a protein in which the last 4 amino acids in SERCA2a are replaced with an extended hydrophobic sequence of 49 amino acids containing a single transmembrane sequence (35, 87, 166). This transcript is the major Ca^{2+}-ATPase transcript found in most nonmuscle cells.

A third gene, SERCA3, encoding a protein about 75% identical to either the SERCA1 or SERCA2 products, has also been identified in a variety of muscle and nonmuscle tissues. The expression of SERCA3 is more restricted than that of SERCA2, but it is the major transcript in platelets (32).

Secondary Structural Model of the Ca^{2+}-ATPase.

Analysis of the primary sequences of SERCA1 and SERCA2 provided the first predicted topological and secondary structural model for P-type ATPases (29, 172, 264; Fig. 8–3). In this model, ten relatively hydrophobic sequences span the lipid bilayer in helical conformations with a small numbers of amino acids exposed to the lumen of the sarcoplasmic reticulum. Most of the remainder of the molecule forms cytoplasmic NH_2 and COOH terminal sequences and two domains that associate to form a cytoplasmic, globular headpiece structure that is connected to the transmembrane sequences through five α-helices, which are clustered to form a stalk-like structure. Mapping studies to localize immunologically reactive epitopes on potentially exposed luminal loops connecting transmembrane α-helices and ligand binding studies have, in general, supported the ten-helices model (48).

A comparison of the deduced amino acid sequences derived from cDNAs encoding P-type family members with different ion specificities reveals that several sequences within these proteins are highly conserved (85). These sequences are, presumably, involved in the common functions of ATP binding and hydrolysis, ion binding and dissociation, and the coupling of chemical energy to the alteration of ion binding sites.

Predictions of the secondary structure for the long cytoplasmic peptide loop between membrane-spanning segments M2 and M3 suggest that it folds into an antiparallel β-strand domain, containing several sequences that are highly conserved among P-type ATPases. The long hydrophilic segment between membrane-spanning segments M4 and M5 is predicted

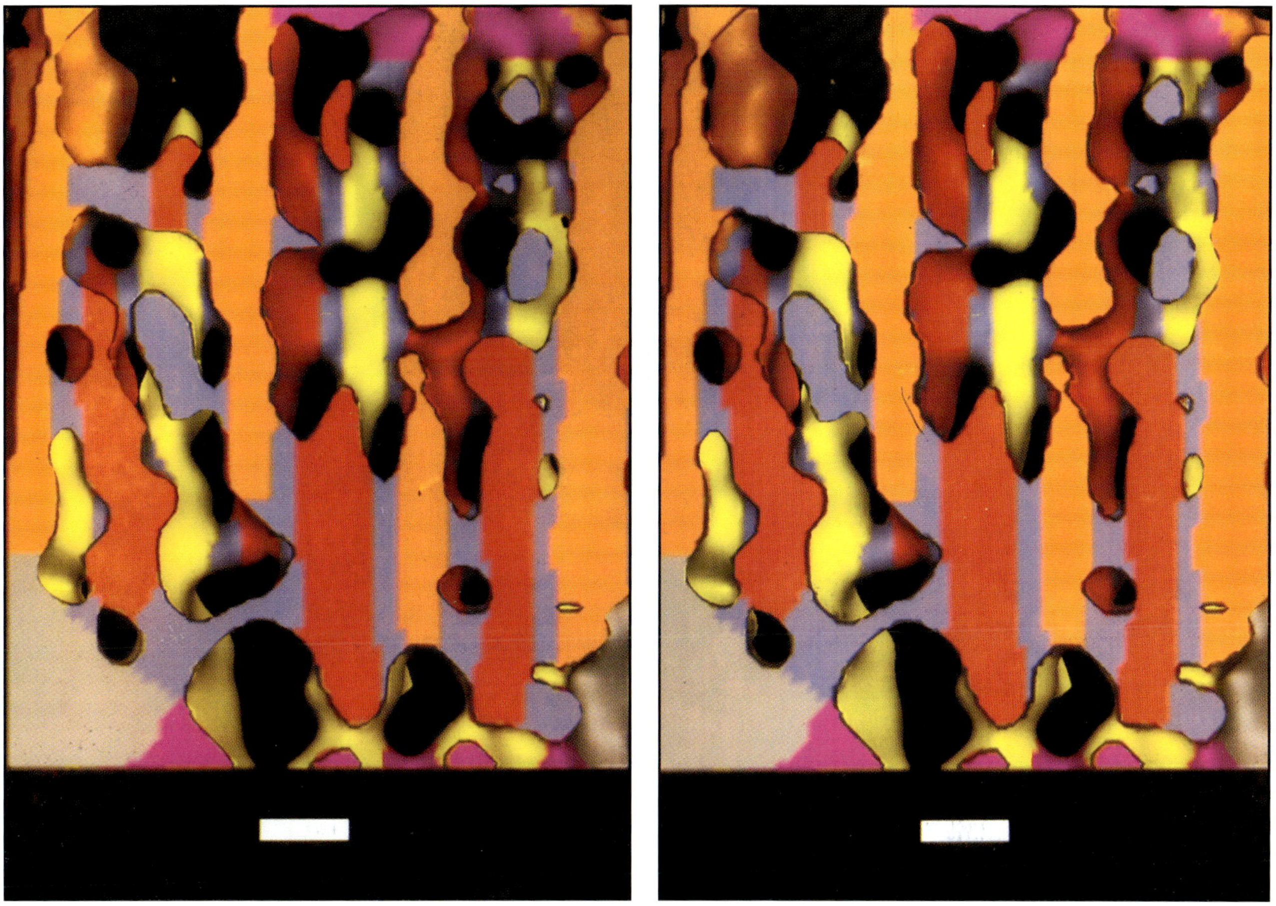

PLATE 1. False-color stereo shaded solid rendering of a section of a three-dimensional reconstruction of the Z-band from unstimulated rat soleus muscle. This 14 nm-thick longitudinal section shows the interdigitating axial filaments and the cross-connecting Z-filament array. Axial filaments enter the Z-band from the top (*yellow*) and bottom (*orange*) of the figure. The filaments are joined together by cross-connecting Z-filaments (*blue*), which also connect to the filamentous relaxed interconnecting body or Z-RIB (*red*). In the I-band near the top and bottom of the figure, some connections run directly between the axial filaments (*magenta*). Amorphous material (*gray*) obscures the filaments near the bottom corners of this section; scale bar = 10 nm). (276) [Reprinted by permission of Rockefeller University Press.]

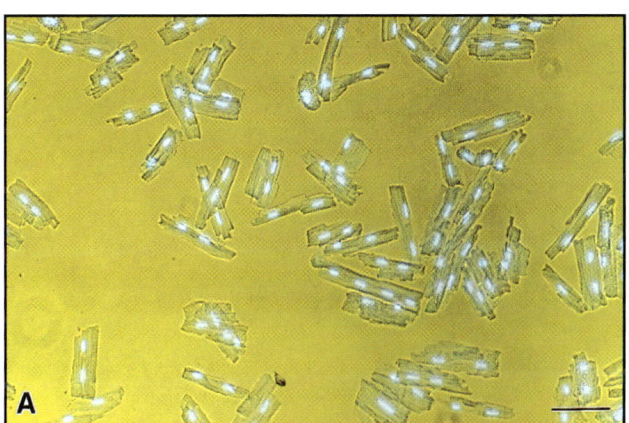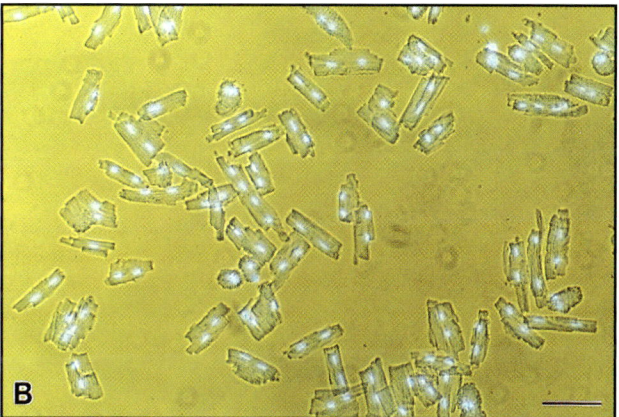

PLATE 2. Enzymatically dissociated left ventricular myocytes from adult dog *(A)* and rat *(B)*. Bisbenzimide staining. *A and B:* bars = 100 μm.

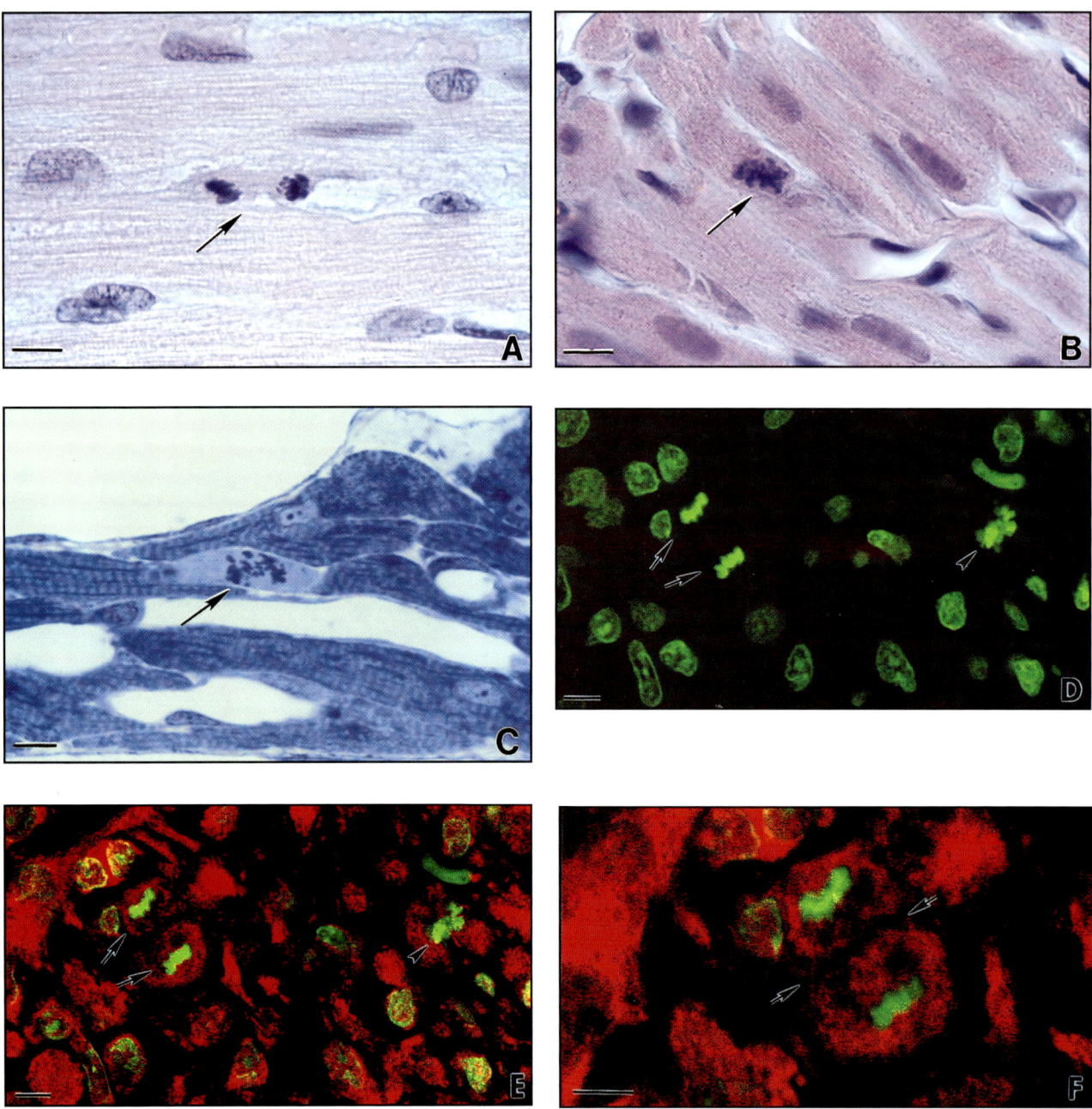

PLATE 3. Photomicrographs showing mitotic figures detected in the ventricular myocardium of the human (*A, B, D, E,* and *F*) and rat (*C*) heart. The light microscopic mitotic images in panels *A* and *B* were found in a patient who died as a result of an extensive acute myocardial infarction. *C* illustrates by light microscopy a mitotic figure in a severely anemic adult rat with ventricular dysfunction. The mitotic images shown by confocal microscopy in *D–F* were detected in a patient affected by end-stage dilated cardiomyopathy. Large field area, illustrating by propidium iodide labeling only (green fluorescence; *D*) and by a combination of propidium iodide and α-sarcomeric actin antibody staining of the myocyte cytoplasm (red fluorescence; *E*), a myocyte nucleus in metaphase (*arrowhead*) and a myocyte at completion of cytokinesis (*arrow*). Myocyte cytokinesis is shown at higher magnification in *F*. *A, B,* and *D–F*: Paraffin-embedded sections stained by hematoxylin and eosin (*A* and *B*) and propidium iodide (*D–F*) and α-sarcomeric actin (*E* and *F*). *C*: Semithin section of plastic-embedded tissue stained by toluidine blue. *A–F*: bars correspond to 10 μm. [*D–F*: reproduced from (243); copyright © 1998 National Academy of Sciences, USA.]

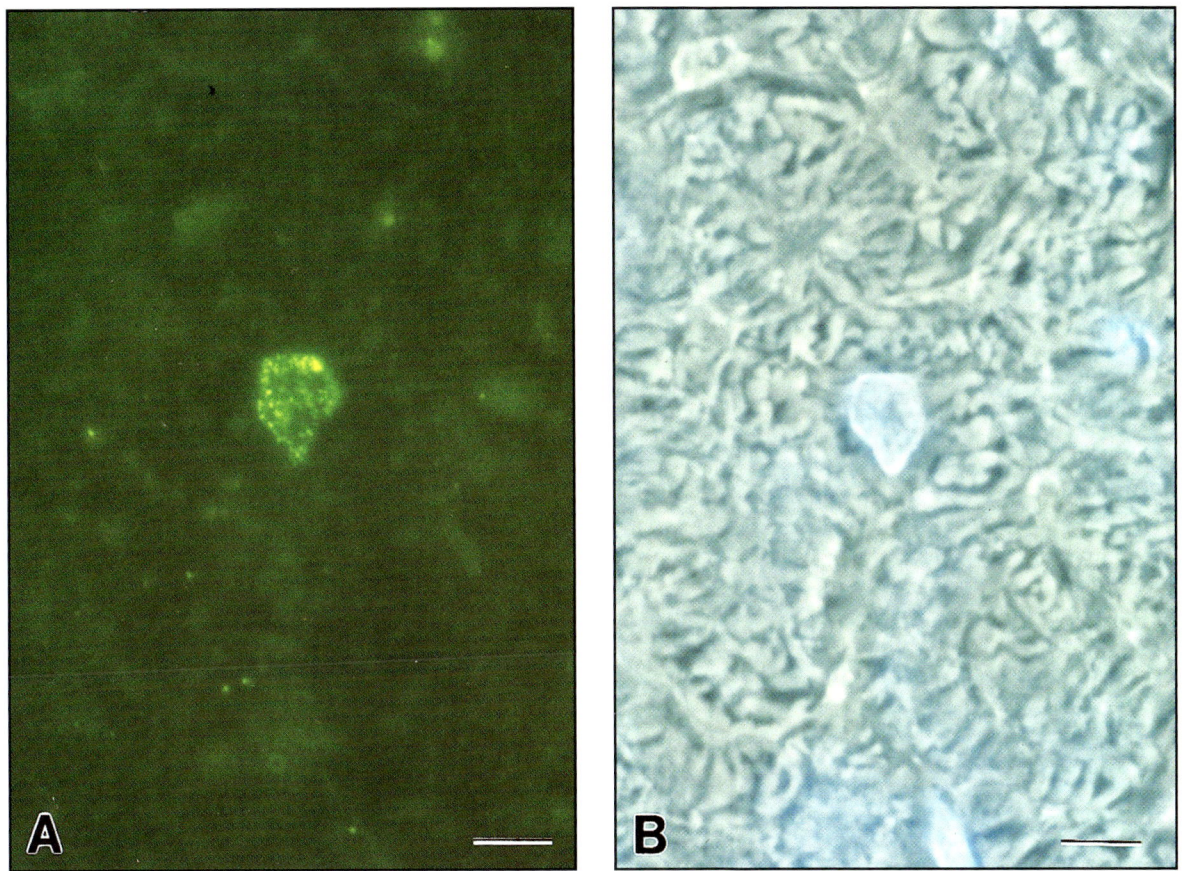

PLATE 4. Frozen sections of ventricular myocardium showing bromodeoxyuridine (BrdU) labeling of a myocyte nucleus after coronary artery narrowing. (A) BrdU labeling by immunofluorescence; (B): the same field shown by phase-contrast microscopy and bisbenzimide H33258 fluorescence. A and B: bars = 10 µm.

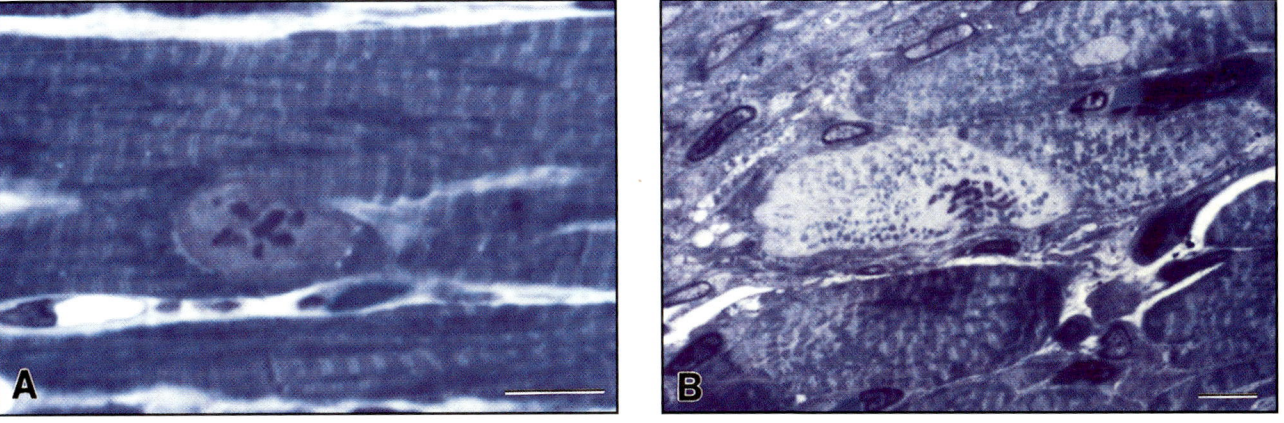

PLATE 5. Semithin sections of plastic-embedded rat ventricular myocardium after coronary artery narrowing (A) and coronary artery occlusion (B) showing mitotic figures. A: Methylene blue and safranin staining; B: Toluidine blue staining. A and B: bars = 10 µm.

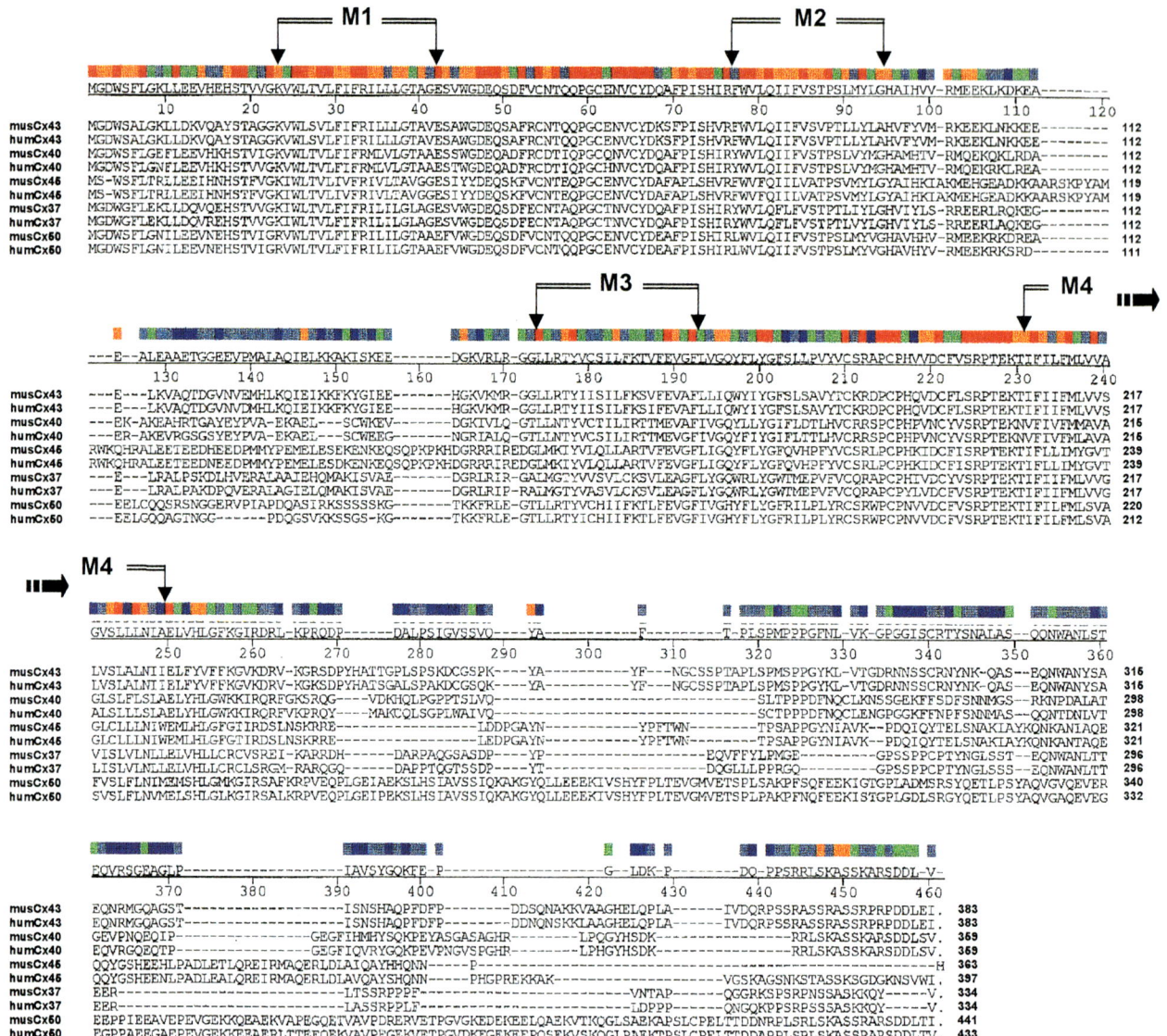

PLATE 6. Peptide sequence alignment of mouse and human cardiac connexins. The color bar code at the top of the alignment indicates the degree of homology among all cardiac connexins, where red indicates identity, dark blue very low homology, and intermediate colors moderate similarity. (Alignment provided by Ms. M. Urban, using Clustal method with PAM 100 residue weight table, Lasergene program, DNASTAR Inc.) Regions corresponding to membrane-spanning domains M1, M2, M3, M4 in Figure 4–2B are indicated.

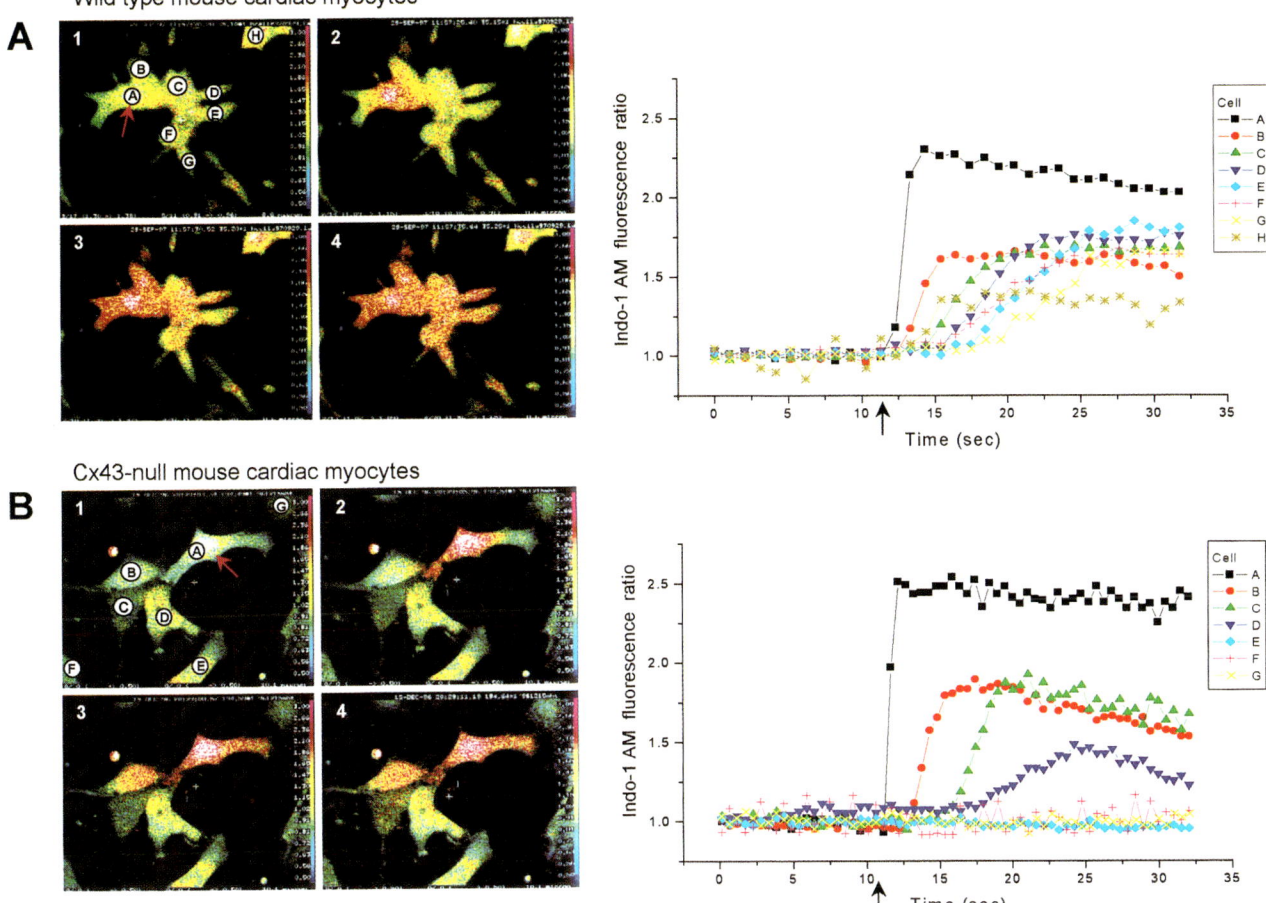

PLATE 7. Propagation of slow intercellular calcium waves between wild-type *(A)* and Cx43-null *(B)* neonatal mouse cardiac myocytes loaded with an intracellular calcium indicator (Indo-1AM) and imaged with real-time confocal microscopy (Nikon RCM 8000). The mechanical stimulation of a single myocyte in culture (cell A, red arrow, uper left frames) initiates the propagation of the calcium wave captured in the pseudocolored display at 5 sec intervals (green: low Ca^{2+}; red: high Ca^{2+}). Graphical representations of the phenomenon as a function of time are shown to the right of the photographs; arrows indicate the moment of the stimulation. Note that the absence of Cx43 expression does not prevent the communication of the calcium signal, but reduces the efficacy of calcium wave spread, which extends to fewer cells per field than in wild-type myocytes.

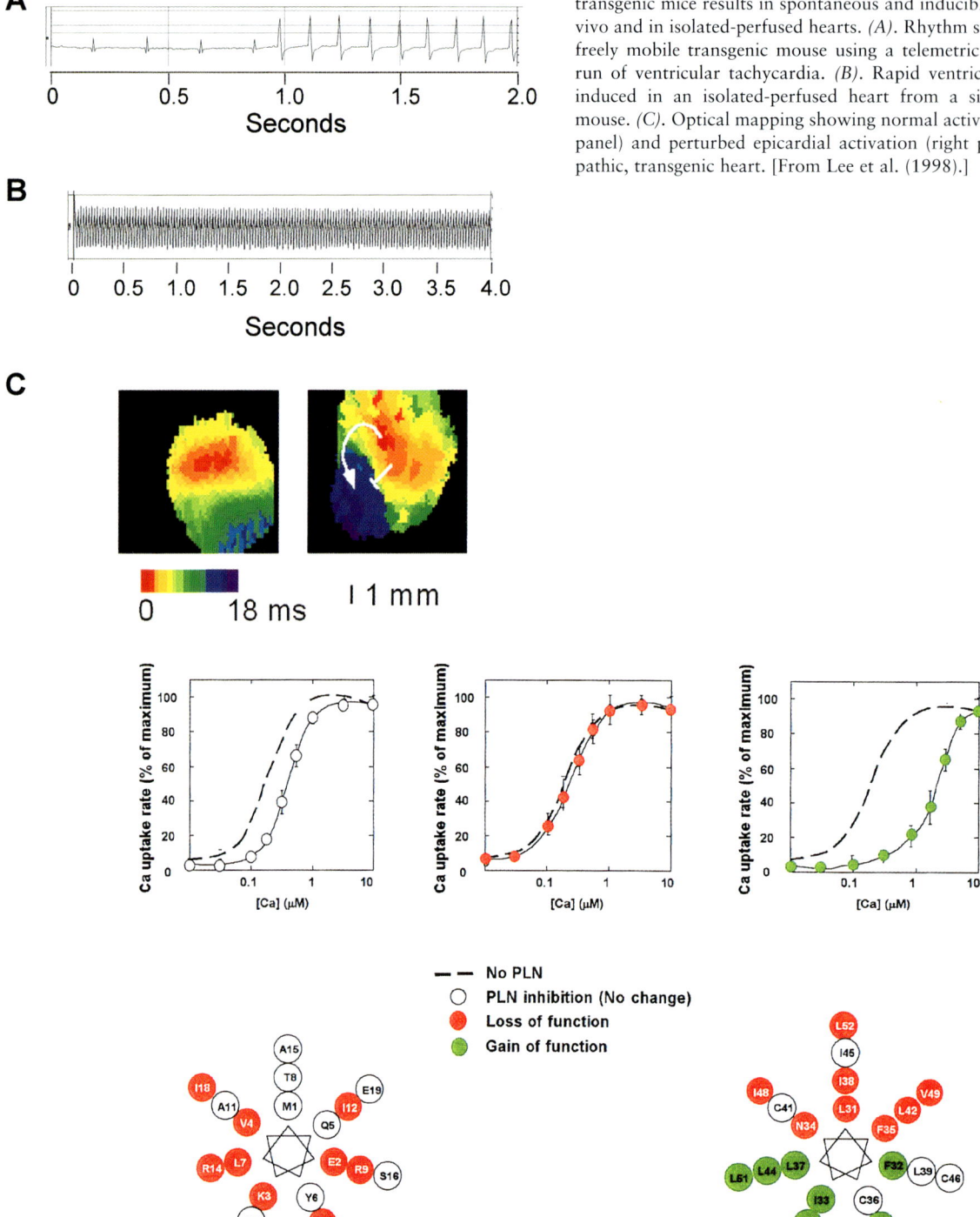

PLATE 8. Regulated expression of diphtheria toxin A in the hearts of transgenic mice results in spontaneous and inducible arrhythmias in vivo and in isolated-perfused hearts. *(A)*. Rhythm strip from awake, freely mobile transgenic mouse using a telemetric system shows a run of ventricular tachycardia. *(B)*. Rapid ventricular tachycardia induced in an isolated-perfused heart from a similar transgenic mouse. *(C)*. Optical mapping showing normal activation profile (left panel) and perturbed epicardial activation (right panel) in a myopathic, transgenic heart. [From Lee et al. (1998).]

Mutations of Cytoplasmic Domain Ia

Mutations of Transmembrane Domain II

PLATE 9. Effects of phospholamban mutations on apparent Ca^{2+} affinity of SERCA2 and location of residues in phospholamban that affect interaction with SERCA2 in cytoplasmic and transmembrane domains. Top: Ca^{2+}-dependence of Ca^{2+} uptake rates for SERCA2 were measured in the presence of coexpressed phospholamban (PLN) *(solid line)*, and in the absence of phospholamban *(dashed line)*. Ca^{2+}-dependence of Ca^{2+} uptake for SERCA2 coexpressed with wild-type and mutant PLN is classified into three types in accordance with the extent of inhibitory actions on Ca^{2+} uptake rate. Wild-type and no change phospholamban mutants lower the Ca^{2+} affinity for SERCA2 by about 0.34 pCa units *(open circles)*, loss of function mutants do not alter the Ca^{2+} affinity for SERCA2 *(red circles)*, and gain of function mutants diminish apparent Ca^{2+} affinity by up to 1 pCa unit, enhancing the inhibitory effect on Ca^{2+} uptake at low Ca^{2+} concentrations *(green circles)*. Bottom: Location of phospholamban mutations that affect apparent Ca^{2+} affinity for SERCA2, presented in an α-helical wheel configuration for both domain Ia and domain II. Each amino acid is classified into three types in accordance with the loss *(red circles)*, gain *(green circles)*, or no change *(open circles)* on inhibitory function. Phospholamban is abbreviated as PLN.

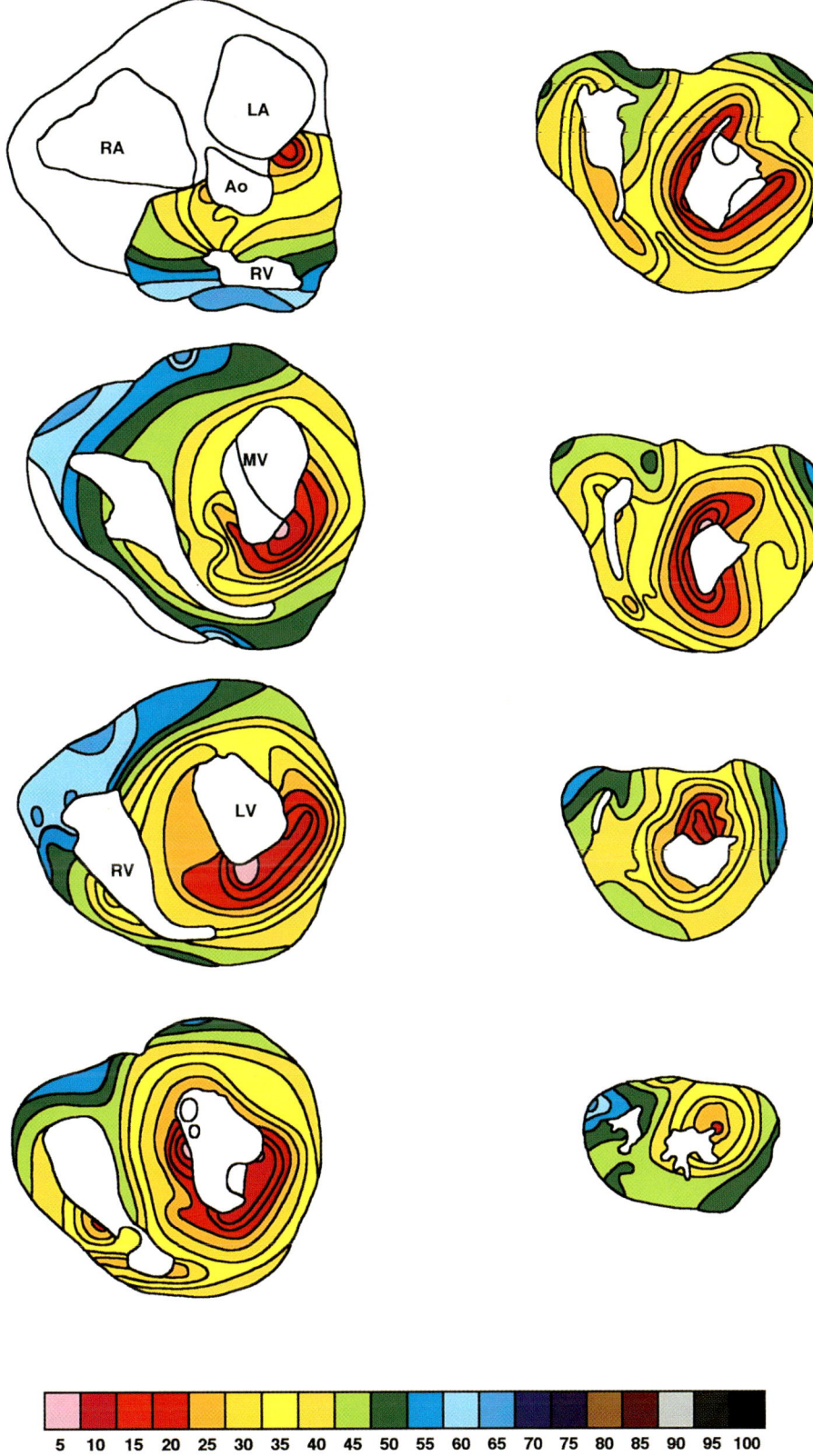

PLATE 10. Excitation of the isolated human heart. Isochrone map of the ventricular activation of an isolated human heart, based on measurements at 870 intramural electrode terminals. The horizontal planes into which the multi-electrodes were inserted, and into which the heart was sectioned, are depicted. Each color represents a 5-msec interval. Zero time is the beginning of the left ventricular cavity potential. White areas indicate either fatty tissue or parts of the myocardium for which no data are available. *RA* = right atrial cavity; *LA* = left atrial cavity; *Ao* = aorta; *LV* = left ventricular cavity; *RV* = right ventricular cavity; *MV* = mitral valve. [Reproduced with permission from reference 173.]

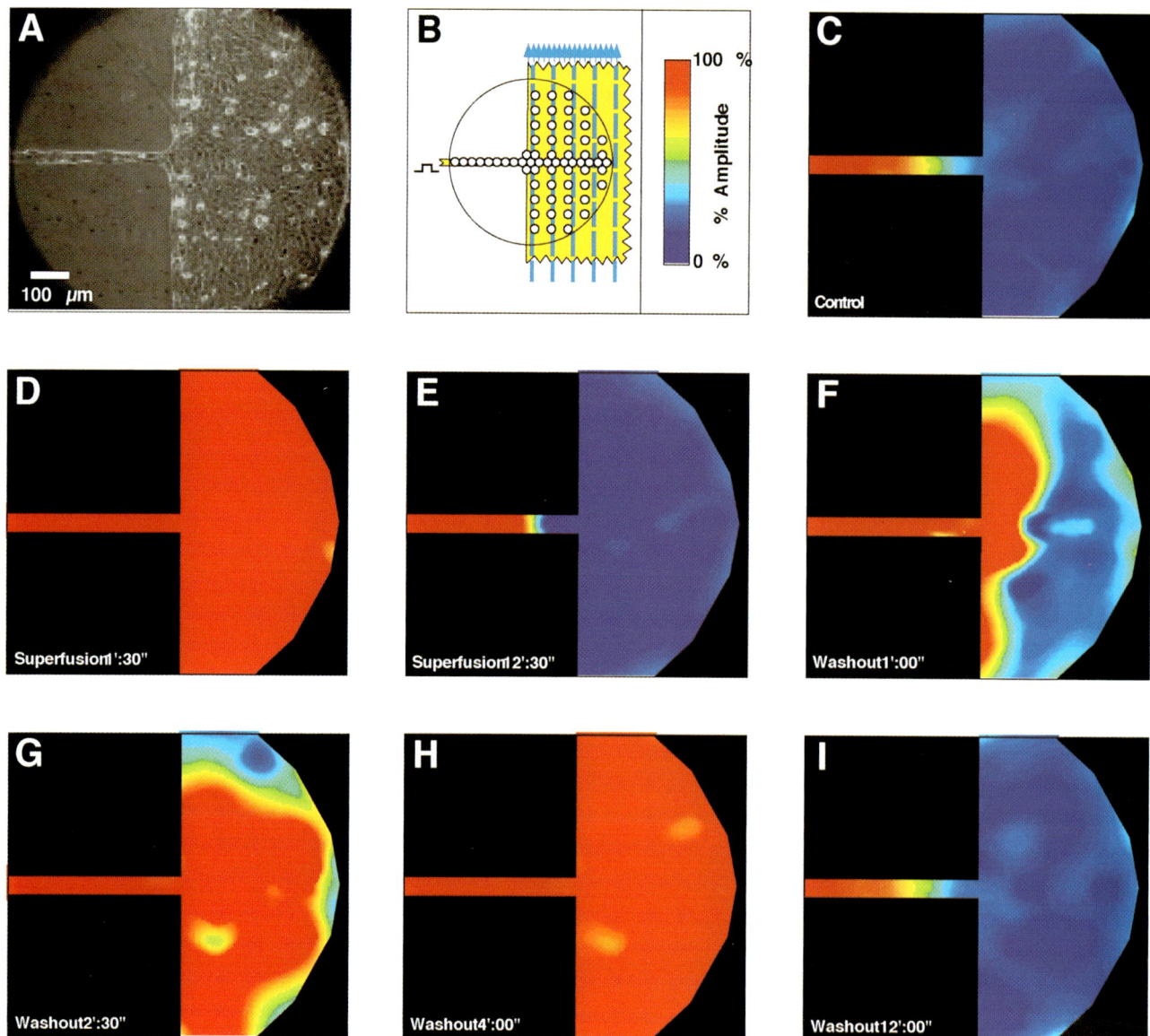

PLATE 11. Reversal of unidirectional block to bidirectional conduction by partial cell-to-cell uncoupling. Unidirectional block in patterned cell cultures (A) is produced by current-to-load mismatch at a geometrical expansion—i.e., an insertion of a small cell strand into a large tissue mass. The degree of electrical cell-to-cell coupling in the large area can be changed by application of a blocking agent (palmitoleic acid, 10 μmol/liter) through local superfusion (yellow area in B). During control (C) excitation (red) after stimulation of the strand is observed only in the small strand, while the unidirectional block leaves the large area at rest (blue), because of current-to-load mismatch at the expansion. Application of the uncoupling agent reverses block to bidirectional conduction during partial cell-to-cell uncoupling (D), and block is obviously observed again after total uncoupling (E). Washout of the uncoupling agent establishes conduction again transiently (F–H), while unidirectional block is observed after completion of washout. [Reproduced with permission from reference 327.]

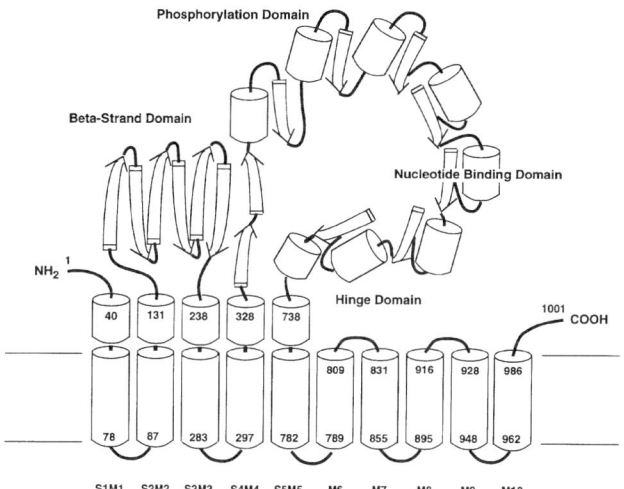

FIG. 8–3. Secondary structural model of the Ca^{2+}-ATPase molecule. This structural diagram is based on predictions of domain structure and a hydropathy plot (85). The bulk of the protein consists of a cytoplasmic globular headpiece structure and ten membrane-spanning segments (M1–M10), which are connected via a stalk-like cluster of α-helices. The large globular cytoplasmic part is composed of three domains: the β-strand domain, between segments M2 and M3; the phosphorylation domain, attached to segment M4 at one end and to the nucleotide-binding domain at the other. The nucleotide binding domain runs into a hinge domain, which is attached to segment M5. The folding of the cytoplasmic structure is indicated schematically in accordance with the general principles established for antiparallel or parallel β-sheet domains (218). The α-helical sequence and the β-sheet sequences are shown by *cylinders* and *arrows*, respectively. The *numbers at the top and bottom* of each transmembrane helix indicate the amino acid positions at each end of these helices.

Three-Dimensional Structure of the Ca^{2+}-ATPase.

The overall shape and distribution of SERCA1 with respect to the bilayer has been studied using electron microscopy and electron diffraction/image reconstitution techniques, applied to two-dimensional crystalline arrays of Ca^{2+}-ATPase (261, 262) and to three-dimensional microcrystals of detergent-solubilized Ca^{2+}-ATPase (260–262). In the lipid bilayer, two strands of Ca^{2+}-ATPase molecules were seen to be pointing in opposite directions to form a "dimeric ribbon." The size of the molecule fitted into a box 120 Å high × 50 Å perpendicular to the dimeric ribbon × 85 Å along the dimeric ribbon.

The three-dimensional structure of SERCA1 at 14 Å resolution has also been determined from two-dimensional crystals in a tubular array, using cryoelectron microscopy and helical image analysis (277; Fig. 8–4). The Ca^{2+}-ATPase appears to be a tall molecule consisting of cytoplasmic, transmembrane, and luminal parts, with much of the mass distributed on the cytoplasmic surface of the lipid bilayer. The cytoplasmic part resembles the head and neck of a bird. The "head," probably forming ATP binding and phosphorylation domains, is connected to the transmembrane domain through the "neck." The ATP binding site was proposed to lie in a groove formed by three cyto-

to consist of alternating α-helices and β-strands, which would form into parallel-stranded β-sheet structures analogous to those in other nucleotide-binding domains (64). This cytoplasmic sequence contains both Asp 351, the site of catalytic phosphorylation by ATP, and those residues predicted to comprise the nucleotide binding site. These sites are separated in the linear sequence by a very exposed tryptic cleavage site, T1. This exposed site is predicted to divide the cytoplasmic region into phosphorylation and nucleotide binding domains.

There is no direct sequence homology between the Ca^{2+}-ATPase and soluble kinases such as hexokinase, phosphoglycerate kinase, phosphofructokinase, or the adenylate kinases. In particular, there are no Gly-X-Gly-X-X-Gly or Gly-X-X-Gly-X-Gly-Lys motifs in the Ca^{2+}-ATPase that are characteristic of the nucleotide binding domain of many dehydrogenases and kinases. Nonetheless, pattern-matching techniques, based on comparisons between the known sequences of P-type Ca^{2+}-ATPases and those of various kinases, have been used to develop a model for the folding of the nucleotide binding domain of the Ca^{2+}-ATPase (264).

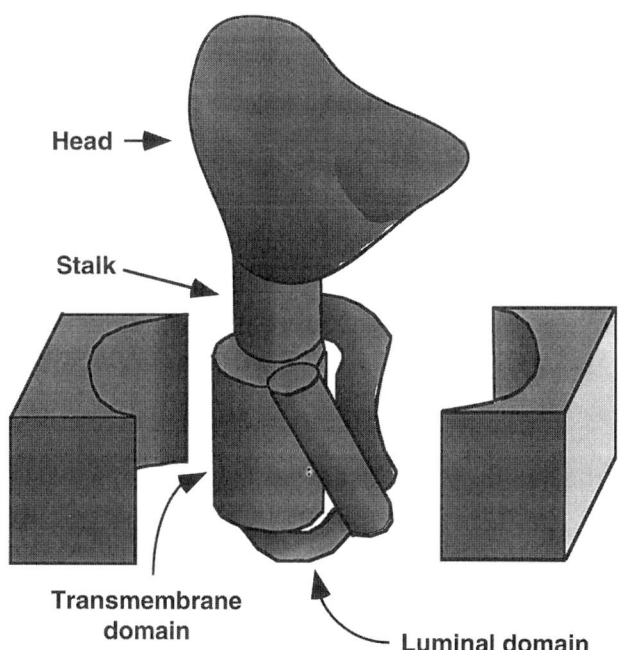

FIG. 8–4. Overall structure of Ca^{2+}-ATPase in the native sarcoplasmic reticulum membrane at 14 Å resolution. Three-dimensional structure of Ca^{2+}-ATPase in the native sarcoplasmic reticulum membrane was determined by cryoelectron microscopy and helical image analysis (277). The cytoplasmic part has a complex structure resembling the head and neck of a bird. The transmembrane domain has three segments and a luminal domain.

plasmic densities surrounding the "beak" in the bird-like model of the headpiece. The transmembrane part has three densities, one of which is highly inclined. Gross features of the structure appeared to be consistent with the ten-helices model proposed by MacLennan et al. (172), and, on the basis of unique features of the ten-helices model, each of the proposed transmembrane helices could be assigned to one of the three transmembrane densities. The three-dimensional structure of SERCA1 at 8 Å resolution, obtained by improved processing images, revealed clusters of rod-like densities in the transmembrane domain that presumably correspond to α-helices (312). Together with the results of site-directed mutagenesis, which localized the Ca^{2+} binding sites between M4, M5, and M6 (47, 216), and from disulfide links between pairs of cysteine introduced into M4 and M6 (217), the most favored assignments of these transmembrane helices M4, M5, and M6 were proposed to form a right-handed coiled-coil structure surrounding the distinctive cavity (312). The Ca^{2+}-bound structure documented by crystallographic analysis at 2.6 Å resolution by Toyoshima et al. (277a) offers many more insights into the mechanism of action of Ca^{2+}-ATPase. They identified new ligands, particularly mutation-sensitive backbone carbonyl groups on transmembrane helix M4, and a single water molecule, in the Ca^{2+} binding site, together with possible entry and exit pathways for Ca^{2+} that are lined by oxygen atoms. A distinctive feature of this region is the disruption of the M4 and M6 helices to form a Ca^{2+}-binding cavity. This was anticipated from earlier NMR studies of helix M6 (237a), and means that structural changes in the carbonyl termini of M4 and M6 may be the key to creating and closing off access to the Ca^{2+}-binding cavity. It is of utmost significance to examine how PLN could fit into the M4-M6 structures when co-crystallographic analysis of PLN/SERCA2a will be available.

The overall mechanism of ATP utilization by the Ca^{2+}-ATPase consists of the sum of the partial reactions, together with their equilibrium constants. The most important feature of the reversible cycle of ATP utilization coupled to Ca^{2+} transport is the sequential destabilization of phosphorylation and Ca^{2+} binding functions (98, 121, 295). Since these functions occur in widely separated domains in the molecule, intramolecular linkage between the phosphorylation domain and the Ca^{2+} binding domain must be considered to be a basic mechanistic device that couples catalytic and transport activities. This has been structurally resolved by analysis of two-dimensional structures of SERCA1 at 9 Å resolution showing that Ca binding to transmembrane domains induces large conformational changes in the cytoplasmic domain (201). Chemical derivatization, spectroscopic labeling, and site-directed mutagenesis have contributed to our present understanding of the localization of functional domains within the Ca^{2+}-ATPase molecule.

Chemical Modifications of the Ca^{2+}-ATPase

Since the Ca^{2+}-ATPase functions within a lipid bilayer, deductions concerning its structure should be referable to conditions in which the enzyme is capable of catalysis. This requirement often can be met by binding appropriate probes to specific points of reference within the Ca^{2+}-ATPase molecule and carrying out spectroscopic measurement of the probes under different experimental conditions. Chemical modification of certain residues through binding of specific exogenous probes has produced a wider range of reference points (21), and some of these fluorophores actually modify different steps in the Ca^{2+} transport cycle. The locations of binding of various fluorophores that either alter function or record conformational changes, leading to spectroscopic changes, have been determined by reference to the primary sequence. Controlled trypsin digestion of the labeled protein has released small peptides that, when purified and sequenced, have permitted the localization of the specific photolabeled amino acid residue.

Probes of Catalytic and Ca^{2+} Binding Domains. Adenosine triphosphate phosphorylates Asp 351 in the SERCA1 sequence (3, 18, 57). A few amino acid residues involved in nucleotide binding have been identified through their covalent binding of reagents that compete with ATP binding (Fig. 8–5). The lysine-reactive fluorophore, fluorescein isothiocyanate (FITC), has an intense fluorescence that has facilitated its use as a probe of nucleotide binding sites of several active transport proteins. FITC binds covalently to Lys 515 of SERCA1 (189), interfering with ATP utilization, but not inhibiting phosphorylation by P_i. High-affinity Ca^{2+} binding is retained, together with spectroscopic changes associated with Ca^{2+} occupancy of these sites (208, 238). Thus, FITC may occupy only a portion of the nucleotide binding site, without disrupting other aspects of the structure and function of the Ca^{2+}-ATPase.

Other useful fluorescent probes of the Ca^{2+}-ATPase nucleotide site include the trinitrophenylated derivatives of ATP, ADP, and AMP (TNP-ATP, TNP-ADP, and TNP-AMP). These nucleotide analogues exhibit a dramatic enhancement of fluorescence upon binding to the phosphorylated Ca^{2+}-ATPase in the presence of Ca^{2+}. By contrast, their fluorescence intensity is relatively low when bound to the nonphosphorylated enzyme (60, 289). The azido derivative of AMP, TNP-

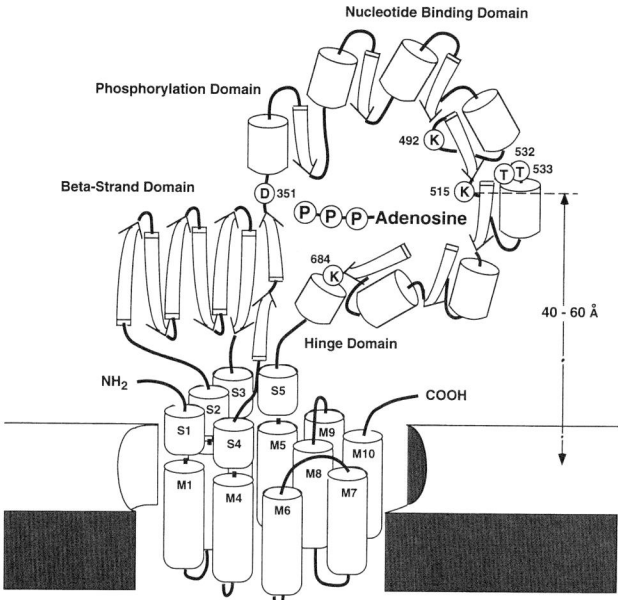

FIG. 8–5. Chemical modification of Ca^{2+}-ATPase. In this structural model, based on the predictions of Green and MacLennan (85), the helices of the stalk and membrane are clustered to show a channel for translocation of Ca^{2+}. Specific points of reference are shown in the extramembranous region, including Asp 351 (the phosphorylation site), Lys 492 (derivatized by TNP-8N$_3$-AMP), Lys 515 (derivatized by FITC), Thr 532 and Thr 533 (derivatized by 8N$_3$-[^{3}H]-ADP), and Lys 684 (derivatized by ATP-PLP).

8N$_3$-AMP, has also been found to photolabel Lys 492 of SERCA1 (182). The azido derivative of ADP, 8N$_3$-[^{3}H]-ADP, photolabels Thr 532 and Thr 533, resulting in irreversible inhibition of ATPase activity. The ATP binding site of SERCA1 has also been modified at Lys 684 with both pyridoxal phosphate and the affinity probe adenosine triphosphopyridoxal (PLP-ATP; 194, 305).

Crystal structures of Ca^{2+} binding proteins reveal that there is considerable diversity in the manner in which polypeptide chains fold to produce a Ca^{2+} binding site. "E-F hand" type Ca^{2+} binding sites can be deduced from primary sequences (146), as can Ca^{2+} binding sites in Ca^{2+}-dependent membrane-binding proteins (80). However, no such sequences are present in the sarcoplasmic reticulum Ca^{2+}-ATPase. Specific modification of the Ca^{2+}-ATPase with the fluorophore N-cyclohexyl-N'-(4-dimethylaminonaphthyl)-carbodiimide (NCD-4) inhibited high-affinity Ca^{2+} binding to the Ca^{2+}-ATPase without affecting any of the Ca^{2+}-independent partial reactions (39, 40, 210, 244). The location and nature of the Ca^{2+} binding sites has also been investigated through spectroscopic studies of the binding of lanthanide ions (102, 235). These paramagnetic ions, lanthanum (La^{3+}), gadolinium (Gd^{3+}), and terbium (Tb^{3+}), have similar ionic radii and ligand specificity to Ca^{2+}, allowing their use as probes of Ca^{2+} binding sites in a variety of proteins.

Measurement of Fluorescence Resonance Energy Transfer.

The nature of the protein environment around bound fluorophores has been investigated in energy-transfer experiments. The capacity of a fluorescent molecule for nonradiative energy transfer to a nearby absorbing species has been used as a convenient spectroscopic ruler for the measurement of molecular dimensions of biological macromolecules. The scale of this ruler covers the range between 10 Å and 80 Å (241). FITC has been employed as a resonance energy transfer donor in conjunction with lipid analogue acceptors in which headgroups are labeled with a fluorophore (88, 265). These studies indicate that bound FITC is located 40–60 Å away from the bilayer surface (Fig. 8–5). When compared to the dimensions of the Ca^{2+}-ATPase derived from image reconstruction techniques (260), this distance corresponds to a location that is near to the maximum height of the Ca^{2+}-ATPase. Thus, fluorescent energy transfer experiments are consistent with the model that the ATP binding site is located in the headpiece of the Ca^{2+}-ATPase.

The Ca^{2+} transport site has also been investigated by fluorescence energy transfer measurements. Studies of both Gd^{3+} and Tb^{3+} probes, which might act as analogues for the Ca^{2+} binding and transport sites, indicate that the protein-bound ion is substantially stripped of water, suggesting that the helices contributing to the Ca^{2+} binding site form a narrow channel (22, 95, 238, 239). A combination of sequencing and fluorescence energy transfer measurements using NCD-4 demonstrates that this fluorescent carbodiimide derivative introduces a perturbation within or near helices 3 or 4 of the membrane-spanning region of the Ca^{2+}-ATPase (245).

Measurement of Rotational Diffusion.

The anisotropic rotational diffusion of an intrinsic membrane protein is sensitive to both the fluidity of the surrounding bilayer and the radius of the rotating protein (267). Therefore, measurements of rotational diffusion can provide insight into the distribution of oligomeric structures and of protein–protein and lipid–protein interactions in the membrane. Several techniques have been employed for the measurement of microsecond rotational motions of the Ca^{2+}-ATPase, including saturation-transfer electron paramagnetic resonance (ST-EPR) of nitroxide spin labels (22, 240, 268), and time-resolved phosphorescence anisotropy (TPA) of long-lived triplet probes such as erythrosin and eosin (23, 99). A series of ST-EPR and TPA measurements of skeletal sarcoplasmic reticulum show that perturbations of the sarcoplasmic reticulum by changing temperature, selective crosslinking of the enzyme, delipidation, or two-dimensional crystallization of the ATPase using vanadate, induces aggregation of the Ca^{2+}-ATPase within the membrane and results in significant inhibition of enzymatic activity (22, 23, 240). The rotational mobility of the Ca^{2+}-ATPase in cardiac sarcoplasmic reticulum is lower than that in skeletal sarcoplasmic reticulum, apparently because of large-scale aggregation of the enzyme in the plane of the membrane (24). Recent development of frequency-domain phosphorescence specroscopy using the skeletal sarcoplasmic reticulum Ca^{2+}-ATPases covalently bound to erythrosin isothiocyanate revealed that Ca^{2+} binding, but not nucleotide binding or phosphoenzyme formation, induces global rotational dynamics involving the phosphorylation domain (103).

Measurement of Secondary Structure with Spectroscopy. Spectroscopic studies using circular dichroism (81, 196), infrared spectroscopy (12), and raman spectroscopy (161, 301) have been used to probe the asymmetry of the peptide bond or vibrational modes of both backbone and sidechain groups of the polypeptide chain without any introduction of an exogenous reporter group. Distinct peaks corresponding to α-helix, β-sheet, and random coil structures yield estimates for the secondary structural content of the Ca^{2+}-ATPase. These studies indicate that the Ca^{2+}-ATPase is highly α-helical (161, 301).

During Ca^{2+} transport, structural transitions in the Ca^{2+}-ATPase (E_1 and E_2 states) have been proposed to occur. Circular dichroism instrumentation (81) and infrared spectroscopy (12) have been used to detect Ca^{2+} binding or enzyme phosphorylation-induced increases in ellipticity of the native Ca^{2+}-ATPase. Thus, structural transitions from E_1 to E_2 and enzyme phosphorylation are associated with reorganization of the secondary structure of the Ca^{2+}-ATPase.

Measurement of Resonance X-Ray Diffraction. X-ray and neutron diffraction studies provide a cylindrically averaged profile structure, to approximately 15 Å resolution, of the Ca^{2+}-ATPase within the fully functional, isolated sarcoplasmic reticulum membrane (27, 96). This profile structure for the Ca^{2+}-ATPase is in general agreement with the three-dimensional structure derived from image reconstruction from electron micrographs of two-dimensional crystals (260–262, 277). Time-resolved x-ray diffraction studies employed synchrotron radiation sources and flash-photolysis of caged ATP to synchronize the phosphorylation of an ensemble of Ca^{2+}-ATPase molecules. Time-resolved x-ray diffraction measurements of the oriented membranes, carried out before and immediately after flash photolysis of caged ATP, revealed that large-scale changes occur in the relative electron dense profiles for the sarcoplasmic reticulum membrane and that these changes correspond to transitions between the (Ca^{2+})$_2$E$_1$ and (Ca^{2+})$_2$E$_1$~P forms of the Ca^{2+}-ATPase (27).

Resonance x-ray diffraction studies have also been used to determine the location of the La^{3+} and Tb^{3+} binding sites within the profile structure of the sarcoplasmic reticulum membrane (14, 58). These studies showed that the predominant lanthanide binding site was located in the stalk portion of the enzyme molecule, in agreement with the result of fluorescence energy transfer measurements (238).

Site-Directed Mutagenesis of Ca^{2+}-ATPase

The investigation of the functional consequences of specific amino acid substitutions in the Ca^{2+}-ATPase has provided novel insights into the domains of the protein responsible for Ca^{2+} binding, ATP binding, and conformational changes. Full-length cDNA clones encoding SERCA1 were first expressed in COS cells in amounts that permitted the analysis of overall Ca^{2+} transport or of the partial reactions of ATP-dependent Ca^{2+} transport (181). Mutagenesis using synthetic oligonucleotides was developed by Kunkel and colleagues (147). A synthetic oligonucleotide containing a mutated base is hybridized to a fragment of cDNA inserted into a single-stranded template. Synthesis of the second strand results in formation of a mutated strand and a wild-type strand. Isolation of the mutated strand provides the essential fragment for expression of a mutant protein. The mutated fragment is ligated back into its original position in the full-length cDNA, in a vector that will ensure a high level of expression in the mammalian cell line that will serve as the host for expression. Functional analyses are performed with microsomal vesicles prepared from the transfected cells 2–3 days after transfection. On the basis of the functional consequences of amino acid substitutions, Ca^{2+}-ATPase mutants can be classified into a number of categories, including Ca^{2+} binding mutants, Ca^{2+} affinity mutants, ATP binding mutants, phosphorylation mutants, conformational change (E$_1$~P to E$_2$~P) mutants, E$_2$P dephosphorylation mutants, and uncoupled mutants (171, 173; Fig. 8–6).

Ca^{2+} Binding and Ca^{2+} Affinity Mutants. An early prediction, derived from primary sequence analysis, was that the amphipathic, negatively charged stalk sector might contain high-affinity Ca^{2+} binding sites (28). When all of the negatively charged or amidated amino acids (Glu, Asp, Gln, and Asn) in stalk sequences 1, 2, and 3 were altered, either individually or in groups, the

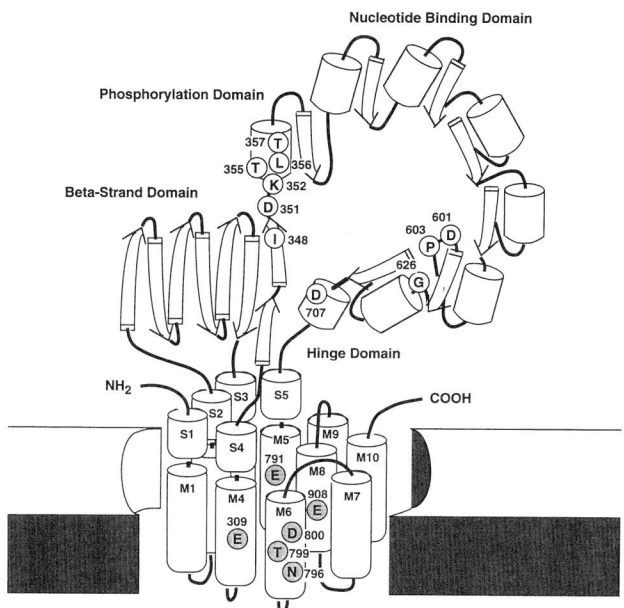

FIG. 8–6. Site-directed mutagenesis of the Ca^{2+}-ATPase molecule. In this structural model, based on the predictions of Green and MacLennan (85), the arrangements of the helices of the stalk and membrane are clustered to create a channel for translocation of Ca^{2+}. The locations of mutated residues are *circled* and the wild-type residues are identified by a *single letter code*. The six residues, in the transmembrane region, are related to Ca^{2+} binding. The ten residues, in the cytoplasmic globular region, are related to the ATP binding and phosphoenzyme formation.

high-affinity Ca^{2+} binding sites in the mutant proteins remained intact (180). Therefore, it is unlikely that the high level of lanthanide binding to the stalk sectors observed in x-ray diffraction studies (26) reflects an essential physiological role for this domain. Ca^{2+} binding in this domain might, however, facilitate Ca^{2+} concentration prior to Ca^{2+} transport.

In the next series of experiments, charged and polar residues in transmembrane sequences in the membrane were analyzed for their potential role as Ca^{2+} binding sites. Mutation of Glu 309 to Gln or Asp, Glu 771 to Gln or Asp, Asn 796 to Asp or Ala, Thr 799 to Ala, Asp 800 to Asn or Glu and Glu 908 to Asp or Ala, but not to Gln, abolished overall Ca^{2+} transport and also abolished the formation of the phosphoenzyme intermediate from ATP (step i in Figure 8–2). In addition, phosphorylation of these mutant Ca^{2+}-ATPases from inorganic phosphate (P_i) was not prevented in the presence of Ca^{2+}. Since phosphorylation of the enzyme from P_i occurs in the E_2 conformation and, since this phosphorylation is normally prevented by alteration of the equilibrium toward the E_1 conformation through Ca^{2+} binding to transiently formed high-affinity sites (step iv in Fig. 8–2), the inability of the enzyme to be phosphorylated from ATP and the inability of high levels of Ca^{2+} to prevent phosphorylation from P_i indicated that these mutant Ca^{2+}-ATPases lacked at least one of the two high-affinity Ca^{2+} binding sites. All of these residues lie within transmembrane helices 4, 5, 6, and 8, suggesting that these four helices form the pore through which Ca^{2+} is translocated (Fig. 8–6).

While the six Ca^{2+} binding mutants had unique properties that supported their roles in Ca^{2+} binding, it is clear that other residues in transmembrane helices 4, 5, and 6 also contribute in important ways to the structure of the two Ca^{2+} binding sites. Analysis of mutations in all of the polar (50) and nonpolar residues predicted to lie within the transmembrane segments of the molecule (51, 216, 283) indicated that other types of mutants exist in these sequences. Mutations of Ser 766, Ser 767, and Asn 768, although not abolishing Ca^{2+} transport function, decreased apparent Ca^{2+} affinity. Mutations of Pro 308 and Pro 803, located in transmembrane sequences 4 and 6, near the residues involved in Ca^{2+} binding, also lowered apparent Ca^{2+} affinity, with little effect on Ca^{2+} transport (283). These residues may be involved in the correct conformation of the Ca^{2+} binding sites.

Analysis of mutations in all of the residues in transmembrane sequence 4 revealed that a "patch" of mutation-sensitive residues could be delineated around Glu 308 and on the same face of the helix (51). Similar patches can be delineated on transmembrane sequences 5 and 6, but not on transmembrane sequence 8 (216). These patches are best delineated when V_{max} alterations, down to about 20% of wild-type, are ignored but K_m mutants are included. These studies provide a clear picture of the faces of transmembrane sequences 4, 5, and 6, which interact to form the Ca^{2+} binding sites, but cast doubt on the role of transmembrane sequence 8 in the formation of the Ca^{2+} binding sites. The packing of these transmembrane sequences was studied by the introduction of pairs of cysteine into selected positions and assay of the expressed products for crosslinking (217). Observed crosslinks at different positions of transmembrane sequences 4 and 6 favor the packing of these sequences as a right-handed supercoil at an angle of about 40°. Thus, correct orientation of transmembrane sequences 4, 5, and 6 must be crucial for the formation of high-affinity Ca^{2+} binding sites, and their reorientation coupled to movement of the cytoplasmic domains could cause occlusion and changes in Ca^{2+} affinity during the Ca^{2+} transport cycle. Insight from crosslinking assay also provides a model for the configuration of Ca^{2+} binding sites in which two Ca^{2+} binding sites are positioned side-by-side, so that all Ca^{2+} binding residues (Glu 309, Glu

771, Asn 796, Thr 799, Asp 800, and Glu 908) are exposed to the "pocket" constructed by sequences 4, 5, and 6 (174).

ATP Binding and Phosphorylation Mutants. Asp 351 has been identified as the site of phosphorylation within the protein (3). All mutations of Asp 351 and Lys 352 abolished both the formation of the phosphoenzyme intermediate and Ca^{2+} transport (181). Mutations of other residues surrounding Asp 351 indicated that highly conservative substitutions of amino acid residues at positions 348, 355, 356, and 357 permit formation of phosphoenzyme intermediate, while nonconservative substitutions of these residues abolish phosphoenzyme formation. Thus, their role may be to provide the correct enviroment to allow phosphorylation of Asp 351 from ATP (180). On the other hand, mutation of Ser 350 or Thr 353 abolished or drastically reduced Ca^{2+} transport without affecting phosphorylation, indicating that these residues may play a role in the conformational changes that occur after phosphorylation and are related to the transport of Ca^{2+} across the membrane.

The structural model of the nucleotide-binding domain of P-type ATPases predicted that certain residues would be involved in ATP binding (228, 264). Mutations of any of highly conserved residues Lys-Gly-Ala-Pro-Glu 519, Arg 615, Gly 618, Arg 620, and Lys-Lys 713 had no influence on either Ca^{2+} transport or phosphorylation of the enzyme (180). On the other hand, mutations of Asp 601, Pro 603, Thr 625, Gly 626, Asp 627, Asp 703, and Asp 707 abolished Ca^{2+} transport and, mutations of Asp 601, Pro 603, Thr 625, Gly 626, Asp 627, and Asp 707, abolished phosphorylation from either ATP or P_i (Fig. 8–6). The ability of the enzyme to bind ATP was tested by the method of Ross and McIntosh (221), which is based on the observation that ATP protects the enzyme against glutaraldehyde-induced intramolecular crosslinking. Thus, if the ATP binding site were altered, the protective effect of ATP would also be altered. Complete or partial loss of protection from crosslinking by ATP was observed for Asp 601, Pro 603, Gly 626, and Asp 707, indicating that these residues may be located in loops critical for ATP binding. Further, ATP binding affinity was directly measured through competitive inhibition of $[\gamma\text{-}^{32}P]$8-azido-TNP-ATP photolabeling (183). Phe 487, Arg 489, and Lys 492 were found to have altered ATP dependence of ATPase activity in wide ATP concentration ranges, indicating that they are involved in both catalytic and regulating ATP binding.

Mutation of Lys 515, the site of FITC modification of the enzyme, had only a moderate influence on Ca^{2+} transport and no effect on phosphoenzyme intermediate formation, indicating that these residues are unlikely to be involved directly either in conformational changes necessary for energy transduction or in ATP binding. Thus, the inhibition of ATPase activity by FITC is not likely to be a consequence of its interaction with Lys 515, but rather of its ability to bring about steric hindrance of ATP binding.

Conformational Change Mutants. There are many residues that, when mutated, abolish Ca^{2+} transport, but have no effect on Ca^{2+}-dependent phosphoenzyme formation. In these mutants, neither the Ca^{2+} binding sites nor the nucleotide binding sites have been destroyed. Results of these mutants are consistent with the idea that they interfere with the major rate-limiting conformational change of the protein. Some of these mutants appear to be blocked in a high-energy–phosphorylated conformation ($E_1\sim P$), which can support transfer of the high-energy phosphoryl group back to ADP, but which can go forward to the low-energy phosphorylated conformation ($E_2\sim P$) only slowly, if at all (5, 49, 50, 284). Examples of this class of mutants are found in different parts of the molecule, including the β-strand, stalk, phosphorylation domain, nucleotide binding domain, and transmembrane domain.

Another class of mutants permits those conformational changes that drive the enzyme from the $E_1\sim P$ to the $E_2\sim P$ conformation, but block the enzyme in an $E_2\sim P$ conformation, which cannot be dephosphorylated (6, 51). These mutations are found in only a small cluster of residues, including Ala 304, Ala 305 and Gly 310, near the center of transmembrane sequence M4, and surrounding Glu 309, one of the essential Ca^{2+} binding residues. This region of the Ca^{2+}-ATPase molecule, therefore, contains many residues essential for Ca^{2+} translocation.

Uncoupling Mutant. Mutation of Thr 317 to Gly led to a mutant protein that had no Ca^{2+}-transport activity, that was not blocked at any partial reaction step, and that had a high level of Ca^{2+}-ATPase activity (6). Since this residue is located near the cytoplasmic surface of transmembrane sequence 4, probably at the mouth of the Ca^{2+} translocation pore, it is conceivable that it is peripherally involved in formation of the Ca^{2+} binding site. Although two Ca^{2+} ions must initially be bound tightly enough to activate phosphoenzyme formation from ATP, the bound Ca^{2+} must be ejected to the cytoplasmic surface rather than to the luminal surface as the conformational changes that accompany Ca^{2+} transport proceed through the cycle.

A Model for Ca^{2+} Transport. These results of site-directed mutagenesis have permitted the development of a model for ATP-dependent Ca^{2+} transport (171,

173). In this model, long-range interactions occur between the ATP hydrolytic site in the cytoplasmic domain and the Ca^{2+} binding and transport site in the transmembrane domain. In E_1 conformations, the Ca^{2+} binding sites, made up from acidic and polar groups in several transmembrane sequences, have very high Ca^{2+} affinity. They are accessible to Ca^{2+} from the cytoplasm, but they do not have access to the lumen. When the protein is phosphorylated from ATP, a series of long-range conformational changes begin in the catalytic site in the cytoplasmic domain and are transmitted to the transmembrane Ca^{2+} binding and transport site. These conformational changes first result in the occlusion of Ca^{2+} in the transmembrane helices so that it becomes inaccessible to either the cytoplasm or the lumen. As the conformational changes progress, energy in the high-energy phosphoryl bond, which is initially able to phosphorylate ADP, is used up in conformational movement and the enzyme moves into a series of lower energy conformations. In these E_2 conformations, the Ca^{2+} binding sites are altered. They gain access to the lumen, they lose access to the cytoplasm, and their affinity for Ca^{2+} drops by at least three orders of magnitude. In this model, the structural basis for the transport of Ca^{2+} lies in a change in orientation of peptide strands constituting the Ca^{2+} binding sites, resulting in disruption of the high-affinity Ca^{2+} binding sites so that their affinity for Ca^{2+} is lost as they are exposed to the lumen.

Ca²⁺-ATPase Isoform Chimeras

Many of those functionally important residues that have been defined by site-directed mutagenesis of SERCA1 are conserved among the other SERCA isoforms, SERCA2 and SERCA3 (32). Since they also share a highly conserved primary structure, all of the SERCA isoforms are predicted to have essentially identical transmembrane topologies and tertiary structures. When the characteristics of the three SERCA isoforms, plus the two splice variants, were compared following their expression in COS-1 cells, all isoforms transported Ca^{2+} in an ATP-dependent fashion and in a cooperative manner with a Hill coefficient of 2. Both quantitative and qualitative properties of SERCA1a and SERCA2a were identical in all aspects. SERCA2b, however, exhibited a lower turnover rate for both Ca^{2+} transport and ATP hydrolysis. SERCA3 displayed a reduced apparent Ca^{2+} affinity, an increased apparent vanadate affinity, and an altered pH dependence (167, 275). Thus, functional differences among the SERCA isoforms, combined with tissue- or cell-specific expression, may impart unique properties of calcium homeostasis to certain cells.

Chimera formation and expression of the chimeric Ca^{2+}-ATPases in COS-1 cells have been used to identify those regions in the different molecules that determine the unique properties of the different proteins (117, 275). One of the most surprising results using chimeric proteins was the extent to which long linear sequences could be exchanged between members of P-type ATPases without destroying either expression or enzymatic properties.

Functional analysis of chimeric Ca^{2+}-ATPases formed between SERCA2a and SERCA3 revealed that the nucleotide binding/hinge domain of SERCA2, when swapped with the nucleotide binding/hinge domain of SERCA3, conferred high apparent Ca^{2+} affinity to the chimera. This domain plays a crucial role in determining the isoform-specific Ca^{2+} dependence of Ca^{2+} transport (275). Chimeras have also been used to show that the phosphorylation and nucleotide binding domains of SERCA2 contain sequences essential for the demonstration of functional interaction between SERCA molecules and PLN (275).

Chimeric recombinants between the Ca^{2+}-ATPase and the Na^+/K^+-ATPase have been used successfully to confirm that the Ca^{2+} binding region lies in the transmembrane region of SERCA1 (245). Other chimeras have been used to show that the binding site for thapsigargin, a highly specific inhibitor of SERCA type enzymes, lies in transmembrane sequences 3 and 4 (117, 198).

Coexpression of all three SERCA isoforms with PLN revealed that SERCA1 can be inhibited by PLN. This result suggests that the only reason that fast-twitch skeletal muscle function is not regulated by PLN is that PLN is not expressed in fast-twitch muscle. By contrast, SERCA3, when coexpressed with PLN, was regulated to only a minor degree.

REGULATION OF Ca²⁺-ATPase BY PHOSPHOLAMBAN

The β-adrenergic action of catecholamines represents a key control mechanism that regulates the metabolic, electrical, and mechanical performance of cardiac muscle. Cyclic AMP (cAMP), which is synthesized by the β-adrenergic activation of adenyl cyclase, is the major intracellular messenger that mediates the stimulatory effects of the sympathetic nervous system. Besides catalyzing phosphorylation of phosphorylase kinase and glycogen synthetase, resulting in a marked increase in glycogenolysis and glycolysis (31), intracellular cAMP alters several aspects of the excitation–contraction process in cardiac muscle through the stimulation of PKA (129, 278). When PKA acts on cardiac sarcoplasmic reticulum membranes, a 22 kDa protein is phosphorylated, and the phosphoprotein exhibits the stability characteristics of a phosphoester (252, 255). This phosphorylatable protein, phospholamban, is a key protein linking the two important intracellular messengers, Ca^{2+} and cAMP as modulators of the Ca^{2+}-ATPase.

Structure of Phospholamban

Phospholamban was first identified as a substrate for PKA in cardiac sarcoplasmic reticulum membranes, and it was postulated to function as a regulator of the Ca^{2+}-ATPase (138, 251, 254). The molecular weight of PLN was originally reported to be 22 kDa on the basis of its mobility in sodium dodecylsulfate–polyacrylamide gels (SDS-PAGE; 252). When cardiac sarcoplasmic reticulum was boiled in SDS prior to electrophoresis, the mobility of PLN was increased, consistent with a reduction in its mass to about 6 kDa (153, 296). Thus, PLN appears to exist as an oligomer in cardiac sarcoplasmic reticulum. Temperature-dependent, stepwise conversion between oligomer and monomer has also been demonstrated (152). On phosphorylation by PKA, the mobility of PLN is altered in a stepwise fashion, showing at least four intermediary components on SDS-PAGE (167, 296). The patterns of temperature-dependent and phosphorylation-dependent mobility shifts indicate that PLN is a homopentamer.

Primary Sequences and Structural Model of Phospholamban. Phospholamban has been purified by differential centrifugation and column chromatography in the presence of non-ionic detergents (114, 125). cDNA encoding PLN has been isolated from dog heart (78), rabbit slow-twitch muscle (75), pig stomach (280), and chicken heart (276). The amino acid sequence of PLN deduced from the nucleotide sequence is 52 amino acids, with a molecular weight of 6080. A model of PLN structure was formulated from its hydropathy profile and from secondary structural prediction of its deduced amino acid sequence (78; Fig. 8–7). In this model, domain I, from Met 1 to Gln 30, forms a hydrophilic, cytoplasmic domain. Domain IA, from Met 1 to Met 20 was predicted to be α-helical, while domain IB, from Pro 21 to Gln 30, was predicted to be less structured. Secondary structure analysis using circular dichroism supported this prediction (234). Domain II, comprised of Asn 31 to Leu 52 was predicted to form an uncharged, hydrophobic, transmembrane helix. Fourier transform infrared spectroscopy with site-directed isotope labeling as a probe of local secondary structure revealed domain II as an α-helix with an axial orientation of approximately 30° relative to the membrane (164).

Domain I contains the cAMP-dependent protein kinase phosphorylation site at Ser 16 and the Ca^{2+}/calmodulin-dependent protein kinase phosphorylation

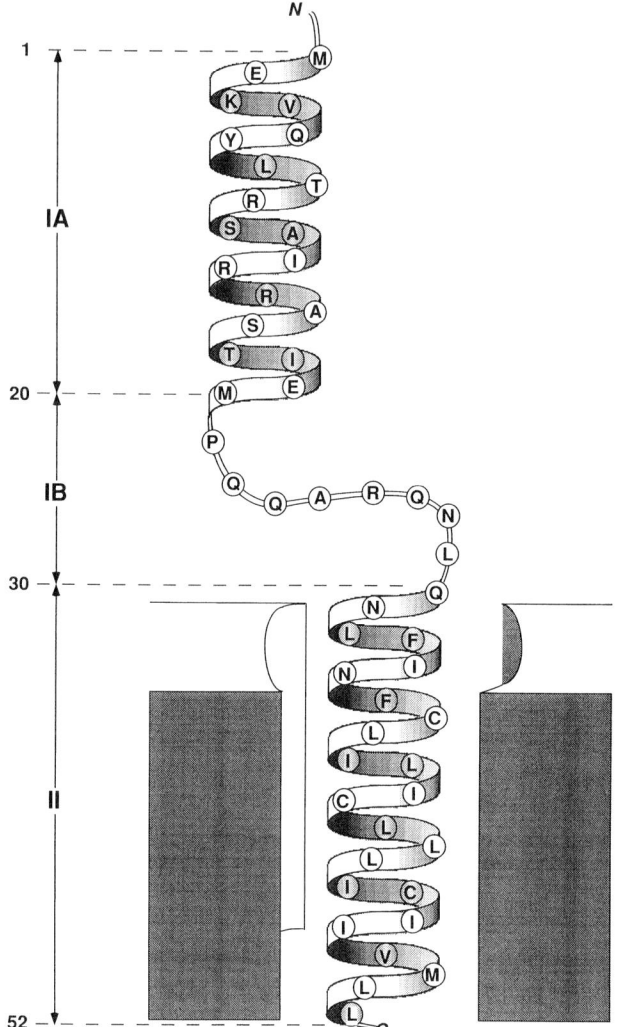

FIG. 8–7. Secondary structural model of phospholamban monomer. In this structural diagram, based on predictions of domain structure and hydropathy plots (78), the two α-helices with a 3.6 residues/turn, domain IA and domain II, are connected by domain IB, which is unstructural. Domain I is exposed at the cytoplasmic surface, whereas domain II is anchored in the sarcoplasmic reticulum membrane. The residues are identified by a single letter code. Ser 16 and Thr 17 are phosphorylated by cAMP-dependent protein kinase and Ca^{2+}/calmodulin-dependent protein kinase, respectively.

sites at Thr 17 (77, 232). Arg 13 and Arg 14, which form part of the consensus sequence, Arg-Arg-X-Ser-Thr, for the two protein kinases, have been shown to be essential by site-directed mutagenesis (77). It is, perhaps, relevant to an understanding of the dynamics of the PLN structure that the structure of a high-affinity (Ki = 2–3 nM) inhibitory peptide of PKA consists of a 9-residue α-helix, a four-residue turn, and a four-residue (Arg-Arg-X-Ser) phosphorylation site in an extended conformation (140, 263). Since this inhibitory peptide must bind to the same site in PKA as domain

I of PLN, then it is probable that phospholamban and the inhibitory peptide have similar structures. It is likely that the amphipathic α-helix at the N-terminus of PLN must unwind, at least partially, during phosphorylation by PKA. Studies using circular dichroism and fluorescence energy transfer analyses also showed the conformational changes following phosphorylation (61, 157).

Domain II contains the essential residues for oligomeric organization, because trypsinized PLN, which is devoid of most of domain I, remained pentameric (296). Three Cys residues (Cys 36, Cys 41, and Cys 46), which lie at every 5 residues in an α-helix, exist as free SH groups rather than forming disulfide bonds during pentamer formation (77, 233). Arkin et al. (11) predicted that the hydrophobic residues form a 3.5 residue/turn helix. This allows the construction of a model of the interacting surfaces in which the helices are associated in a left-handed pentameric coiled-coil configuration. Mutation of the hydrophobic residues Ile 40, Leu 43, and Ile 47 destabilizes the pentamer, consistent with the view that these residues are critical to homopentameric formation (11). Further mutational study of domain II indicated that a predicted coiled-coil structure is stabilized by a leucine zipper motif formed by close packing of Leu 37, Ile 40, Leu 44, Ile 47, and Leu 51 (233). Consistent with this notion are the data obtained by the structural analysis using electron paramagnetic resonance spectra, in which oligomeric proteins show decreased spin-labeled mobility compared with monomers. Compared with wild-type PLN, phospholamban with Leu 37 mutated to Ala increases its mobility (128), in accord with the previous data that this PLN mutant is predominantly monomeric.

Function of Phospholamban

When the kinetics of Ca^{2+} uptake are compared in sarcoplasmic reticulum vesicles from fast-twitch and cardiac muscles, the Ca^{2+}-ATPase from fast-twitch muscle has a higher activity than that from cardiac muscle (37, 137, 230, 254). A series of experiments indicates that this lower activity is due both to a lower amount of Ca^{2+}-ATPase protein in the cardiac vesicles and to its interaction with PLN (250, 251).

Phosphorylation of Phospholamban.
Binding of a β-adrenergic agonist to its receptor in muscle activates a sarcolemmal adenyl cyclase to produce cAMP through stimulatory G protein complexes (Gs; 129). Cytosolic levels of cAMP are also controlled by phosphodiesterases, which degrade cAMP by hydrolyzing one of the two ester bonds linking phosphate to ribose in the cyclic nucleotide. The synthesis and breakdown of cAMP occurs as follows:

$$\text{ATP} \xrightarrow{\text{Adenyl Cyclase}} \text{Cyclic AMP} \xrightarrow{\text{Phosphodiesterase}} \text{AMP}$$

Cyclic AMP, as an intracellular second messenger for regulatory processes, activates cAMP-dependent protein kinase (247). Protein kinases are enzymes that catalyze the transfer of the terminal phosphate of ATP to serine and threonine hydroxyl groups in target proteins. The signal generated by the formation of these phosphorylated proteins is turned off when the phosphoproteins are dephosphorylated by phosphoprotein phosphatases:

$$\text{Protein} + \text{ATP} \xrightarrow{\text{Protein Kinase}} \text{Phosphoprotein} \xrightarrow{\text{Phosphoprotein Phosphatase}} \text{Protein} + P_i$$

Phosphorylation of phospholamban by cAMP-dependent protein kinase increases Ca^{2+} affinity for the Ca^{2+}-ATPase about threefold at concentrations of Ca^{2+} that are half-maximal for activation of Ca^{2+} uptake. It also increases V_{max} of Ca^{2+} uptake. The phosphorylated cardiac sarcoplasmic reticulum appears to have about the same turnover number as SERCA1 in skeletal muscle sarcoplasmic reticulum (97, 230).

Phospholamban is also phosphorylated by Ca^{2+}/calmodulin-dependent protein kinase (145, 152, 249). The maximal amount of PLN phosphorylation by Ca^{2+}/calmodulin-dependent protein kinase occurs with 5–10 μM Ca^{2+} (249). The phosphorylation of PLN by the two protein kinases occurs independently and to about the same extent. The amount of phosphorylation by the two protein kinases is additive (249). Ca^{2+}/calmodulin-dependent phosphorylation has been shown to occur in the intact heart (297). Although the physiological significance of this stimulation on Ca^{2+} transport is not clear, a cooperative interaction with cAMP may accelerate the removal of Ca^{2+} from the cytosol.

Phospholamban can also be phosphorylated in vitro by a phospholipid-dependent protein kinase, protein kinase C (192). This enzyme is activated when Ca^{2+} is present together with diacylglycerol, one of the products of phosphatidylinositol hydrolysis. A role for protein kinase C phosphorylation in cardiac function has not yet been defined.

To regulate the phosphorylation state of PLN, phosphoprotein phosphatases are needed to turn off the signal initiated by phosphorylation. When phosphorylated sarcoplasmic reticulum vesicles are incubated with phosphoprotein phosphatase obtained from bovine heart, most of the phosphorylated PLN is dephosphorylated (136, 252, 253) and dephosphorylation leads to a complete reversal of the stimulation produced by protein kinase. A number of phosphoprotein phosphatases can dephosphorylate PLN. One such enzyme, a PLN phosphatase purified from cardiac cytosol, is a protein phosphatase-1, having a molecular weight of 160 kDa (169).

Effect of Phospholamban on the Reaction Sequence of Ca^{2+}-ATPase. Ca^{2+} uptake by sarcoplasmic reticulum vesicles is tightly coupled to Ca^{2+}-dependent ATP hydrolysis. When PLN is phosphorylated by cAMP-dependent protein kinase, Ca^{2+} uptake and ATP hydrolysis are accelerated and the coupling ratio is maintained at about 2 (254). Since there is no alteration of EP levels in the presence of saturating concentrations of Ca^{2+} and ATP, enhancement of Ca^{2+} ATPase activity must be due to the acceleration of the turnover of the enzyme (163, 255).

Studies of partial reactions of Ca^{2+} uptake, using pre-steady-state kinetic measurements, have been extensively performed (250, 257). The rate of $E_1 \sim P$ formation is enhanced by PLN phosphorylation when the ATPase reaction is initiated by adding ATP and Ca^{2+} to a reaction medium containing EGTA. The rate of $E_1 \sim P$ formation, is not altered significantly when ATP is added to a reaction medium already containing Ca^{2+} (250, 257). Thus, the effect of PLN phosphorylation is manifested in the formation of $(Ca^{2+})_2 E_1$ (step v in Fig 8–2), the rate-limiting step in $E_1 \sim P$ formation and not in the formation of $(Ca^{2+})_2 E_1 \sim P$ (step v in Fig. 8–2). The rate of $E \sim P$ decomposition was also markedly accelerated by PLN phosphorylation (145, 251, 255), indicating that the transition from $(Ca^{2+})_2 E_1 \sim P$ to $(Ca^{2+})_2 E_2$-P (step iii in Fig. 8–2), the rate-limiting step during phosphoenzyme decomposition, is accelerated. Thus, the two rate-limiting steps, the transition from E_2 to E_1 states and the transition from E_1 to E_2 states in the E_1-E_2 model are greatly enhanced when PLN is phosphorylated by cAMP-dependent protein kinase. It is interesting to note that PLN phosphorylation enhances the two rate-limiting steps in ATP hydrolysis in which significant conformational changes occur in the Ca^{2+}-ATPase, bringing about alterations in Ca^{2+} affinity.

Interaction Between Ca^{2+}-ATPase and Phospholamban

Advances in our understanding of the mechanism by which PLN interacts with the Ca^{2+}-ATPase have come from the use of biochemical and molecular biological techniques. Protein–protein interactions appear to occur between the Ca^{2+}-ATPase and PLN, and these are dependent on the phosphorylation state of the PLN. Evidence for a direct interaction between the Ca^{2+}-ATPase and PLN is as follows: the two proteins remain associated with each other after solubilization of microsomes (20, 152); a monoclonal antibody against PLN disrupts the inhibitory effects of PLN on Ca^{2+}-ATPase activity (192, 248); when the Ca^{2+}-ATPase and PLN are reconstituted into liposomes, the inhibitory effect of PLN can be observed (15, 113, 131, 225); and when Ca^{2+}-ATPase and PLN are coexpressed in heterologous cell culture, PLN inhibition of Ca^{2+}-ATPase activity is observed (76, 133, 134, 273–275, 280).

Phospholamban-Interaction Site in the Ca^{2+}-ATPase. James et al. (119) used the Denny-Jaffe crosslinking agent to conjugate purified PLN with the Ca^{2+}-ATPase from cardiac sarcoplasmic reticulum. The complex was formed only when PLN was in the dephosphorylated state and the Ca^{2+}-ATPase was in the Ca^{2+}-free state. Isolation and amino acid sequencing of the photoaffinity-labeled peptide from the Ca^{2+}-ATPase showed that Lys 397 and Lys 400, which are located just after the phosphorylation site (Asp 351) in the Ca^{2+}-ATPase were photolabeled. The functional significance of this sequence for PLN interaction was confirmed by measuring the effects of synthetic peptides covering this sequence on cardiac Ca^{2+}-ATPase activity (285). In the presence of the synthetic peptide, the Ca^{2+} transport activity of cardiac sarcoplasmic reticulum, but not that of skeletal sarcoplasmic reticulum, was accelerated. Since the major difference between the two types of sarcoplasmic reticulum is the presence of PLN, it was suggested that this peptide competes with cardiac Ca^{2+}-ATPase for PLN, resulting in the de-inhibition of Ca^{2+}-ATPase activity (285).

Analysis of the amino acid sequence in the phosphorylation domain of SERCA1, SERCA2, and SERCA3 showed that the amino acid sequence of the putative PLN binding region was nearly identical in SERCA1 and SERCA2, but not in SERCA3 (Fig. 8–8). When Ca^{2+} uptake rates for the three SERCA isoforms, coexpressed with or without PLN, were measured, the inhibitory effect of PLN on Ca^{2+} affinity was observed with SERCA2 and SERCA1, but not with SERCA3 (275; Fig. 8–9A).

An interesting observation in these studies was that SERCA3 has an intrinsically lower apparent affinity for Ca^{2+} than either SERCA1 or SERCA2. Measurement of the effect of PLN on Ca^{2+} dependence of Ca^{2+} transport for chimeric proteins constructed from different regions of SERCA2 and SERCA3 permitted the identification of the region in the SERCA molecules that interacts functionally with PLN. The nucleotide binding/hinge domain of SERCA3 was found to be responsible for the low apparent Ca^{2+} affinity of SERCA3, and the nucleotide binding/hinge domain of SERCA2 was found to be responsible for the high apparent Ca^{2+}

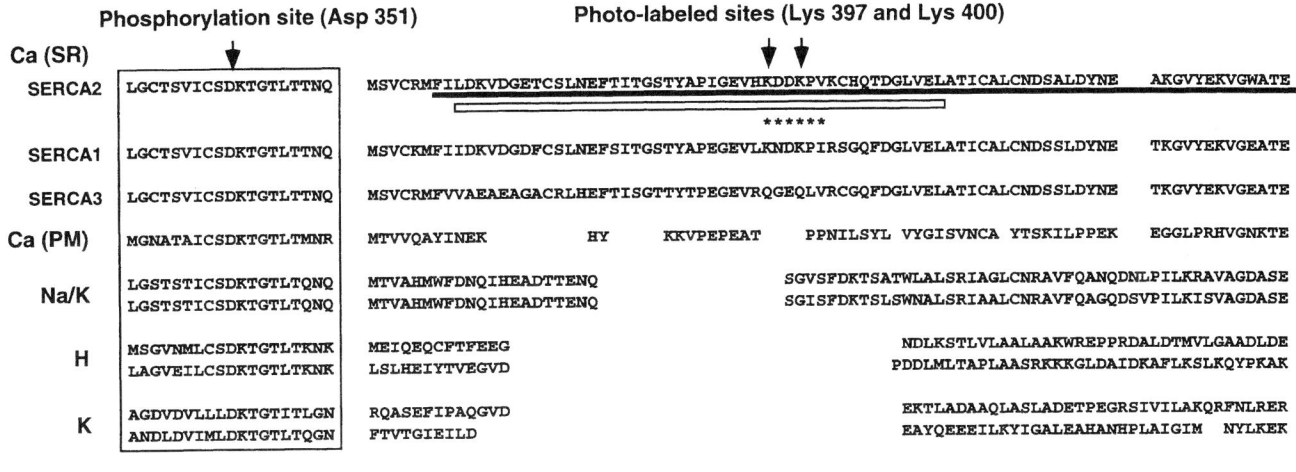

FIG. 8–8. Comparison of amino acid sequences among P-type ATPases in the cytoplasmic phospholamban-interacting site of the Ca²⁺-ATPase. The amino acid sequence around the phospholamban (PLN)-interacting site of SERCA2, presented in the single letter code, is aligned with homologous regions in other P-type ATPases. Each line represents a different ATPase sequence, which are, *from top to bottom:* rabbit slow-twitch/cardiac muscle sarcoplasmic reticulum Ca²⁺-ATPase (SERCA2), rabbit fast-twitch muscle sarcoplasmic reticulum Ca²⁺-ATPase (SERCA1), rat nonmuscle sarcoplasmic reticulum Ca²⁺-ATPase (SERCA3), human plasma membrane Ca²⁺-ATPase PMCA, sheep plasma membrane Na⁺/K⁺-ATPase, torpedo plasma membrane Na⁺/K⁺ ATPase, *Saccharomyces cerevisiae* H⁺-ATPase, *Neurospora crassa* H⁺-ATPase, *Escherichia coli* K⁺-ATPase, and *Streptococcus faecalis* K⁺-ATPase. *Filled arrow* indicates the aspartic acid 351 which is phosphorylated by ATP. *Two closed arrows* indicate Lys 397 and Lys 400, which can be crosslinked to PLN (119). The *thick bar* indicates a region corresponding to the ¹²⁵I-labeled peptides that appear to interact with PLN (49). The *open bar* indicates a synthetic peptide that was used to prevent the interaction between PLN and Ca²⁺-ATPase (285). The *asterisk* indicates the SERCA2 amino acid residues that were shown to interact functionally with PLN in studies using site-directed mutagenesis (273).

affinity of SERCA2. The nucleotide binding/hinge domain of SERCA2, which provided the high apparent Ca²⁺ affinity of SERCA2, was found to be essential for the demonstration of a functional interaction between PLN and a series of chimeric Ca²⁺-ATPases coexpressed with or without PLN. It is not clear that any essential PLN/Ca²⁺-ATPase interaction site is present in this domain. The phosphorylation domain, however, was found to be essential for interaction with PLN (Fig. 8–9B) (275).

Further dissection of the PLN-binding region of SERCA2, was accomplished using site-directed mutagenesis (274). A series of substitutions in the phosphorylation domain of SERCA2 had no functional effect, but substitution of any amino acids in the sequence Lys-Asp-Asp-Lys-Pro-Val 402 diminished the functional interaction between SERCA2 and PLN. When the SERCA2 sequence Lys-Asp-Asp-Lys-Pro-Val 402 replaced the SERCA3 sequence Gn-Gly-Glu-Gln-Leu-Val 402, functional interaction of SERCA3 with PLN was gained, proving the essentiality of this sequence for PLN/Ca²⁺-ATPase interaction (Fig. 8–9C).

In the mutational studies of PLN, mutation of amino acids both in the cytoplasmic domain and in the transmembrane helix led to the loss of PLN inhibition of SERCA2 (134, 274); the former was shown to associate with sequences Lys-Asp-Asp-Lys-Pro-Val 402 of SERCA2. Search for the transmembrane interacting sites has been achieved using PLN and SERCA1 mutants instead of SERCA2, because SERCA1 and SERCA2 are equally inhibited by the wild-type and mutant PLN (275), and because the sequences of transmembrane helices M4, M5, M6 and M8 are highly conserved among all three SERCA isoforms (32). Of these four helices, which was shown to form a Ca²⁺-transporting pocket or pouch (174), the studies on the effects of specific mutations on functional interactions, together with co-immunoprecipitation of wild-type and mutant PLN and SERCA1, implicate that transmembrane M6 and, in particular, Val795 and Leu802 directly serve to interact functionally with transmembrane helix of PLN (13). This study clearly demonstrated that PLN should associate with M6, one of four helices involved in Ca²⁺ binding and one of the tree helices that have been proposed to form a right-handed, coiled-coil Ca²⁺-binding structure in the SERCA transmembrane domain (174). By binding to one key helix, PLN would be in a favorable position to influence the Ca²⁺ binding properties of the four helix structure. Structure determination of the co-

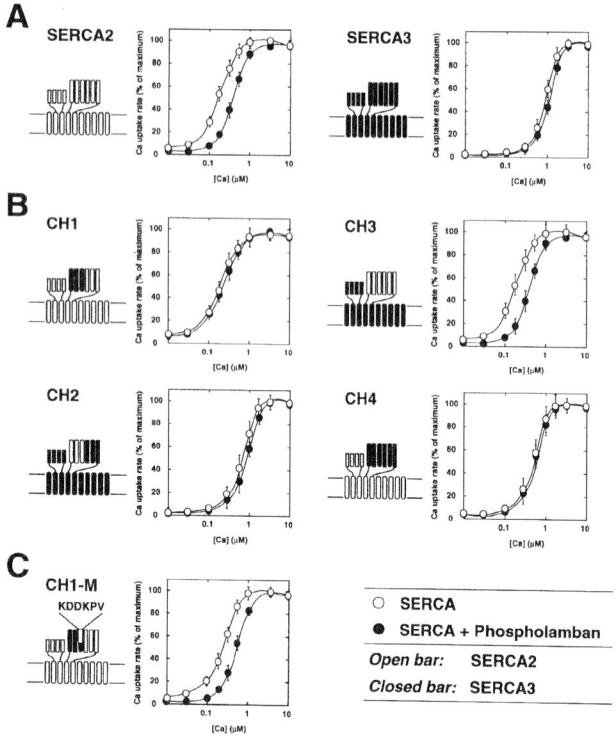

FIG. 8–9. Phospholamban-interacting site in the cytoplasmic domains of SERCA2. Ca^{2+}-dependence of Ca^{2+} uptake rates for SERCA 2 and SERCA3 (A) and chimeras between them (B and C) were measured with (●) or without (○) coexpressed phospholamban (PLN). The domain structure of the SERCA chimera shown in the left side of each graph is based on the structural predictions defined in Figure 8–3. The *open bars* indicate SERCA2 sequence and the *closed bars* indicate SERCA3 sequence. B: Chimeric Ca^{2+}-ATPases between SERCA2 and SERCA3 were constructed as follows: CH1: the phosphorylation domain is from SERCA3 and the remainder is from SERCA2; CH2: the phosphorylation domain is from SERCA2 and the remainder is from SERCA3; CH3: the phosphorylation and the nucleotide-binding/hinge domains are from SERCA2 and the remainder is from SERCA3; and CH4: the phosphorylation and the nucleotide-binding/hinge domains are from SERCA3 and the remainder is from SERCA2. CH3 showed functional interaction with PLN. C: Individual amino acid residues in the SERCA3 sequence in CH1 were replaced by the corresponding residues in SERCA2. Mutant CH1-M, in which 6 sequential amino acid residues Lys-Asp-Asp-Lys-Pro-Val 402 from SERCA2 were introduced into the corresponding SERCA3 sequence, restored functional interaction with PLN. Note that nomenclature of chimera and mutant constructs are modified from those originally described by Toyofuku et al. (274).

crystals of Ca-ATPase and PLN will eventually reveal the interaction between the two proteins (307).

Ca^{2+}-ATPase-Interacting Sites in Phospholamban.

Monoclonal antibodies against PLN are usually formed against epitopes in the cytoplasmic domain of PLN, lying between Gln 5 and Ser 16 (274). These antibodies frequently disrupt the inhibitory effects of PLN on Ca^{2+}-ATPase activity, suggesting that functional interactions occur between the cytoplasmic regions of PLN and the Ca^{2+}-ATPase (132, 192, 248). Individual amino acid residues in the cytoplasmic region of PLN have been systematically mutated to alter the net charge in the cytoplasmic domain of PLN, or to reduce hydrophobicity (273; Plate 9). When the net charge in the cytoplasmic domain of PLN was +2 or +1, function was retained. When the net charge was increased to +3 or reduced to 0 or less, for example by phosphorylation, function was lost.

Loss of hydrophobicity in domain IA of PLN also affected functional interactions. On the basis of the predicted structure of domain IA, an α-helical wheel with 3.6 residues per turn, charged amino acid residues of domain IA would be clustered on one side of the α-helical wheel, while hydrophobic residues would be on the other side. As hydrophobic interactions have been proposed to be a major factor in protein–protein interactions in general (46), this hydrophobic surface could possibly interact with a reciprocal hydrophobic surface on SERCA2. The hydrophilic surface of the helix would add to the stability of the complex by providing appropriate electrostatic interactions. High ionic strength (45) and polycations (304) can disrupt the inhibitory effects of PLN on the Ca^{2+}-ATPase activity in cardiac sarcoplasmic reticulum. Thus, if cytoplasmic domain IA forms an amphiphatic α-helix, it could fit compactly into a complementary pocket in SERCA2, utilizing both hydrophobic and electrostatic interaction between the two proteins.

Synthetic peptides representing the cytoplasmic and transmembrane sequences of PLN have been added to preparations of purified SERCA2 in an attempt to reconstitute the inhibitory interaction between PLN and SERCA2. Peptides corresponding to domain I were found to reduce the V$_{max}$ of SERCA2, while peptides corresponding to domain II affected Ca^{2+} affinity (225). Very high concentrations of peptides were required to achieve functional alteration, however, and there is a possibility that Ca^{2+} uptake and ATP hydrolysis may have been uncoupled in reconstitution experiments (214). These studies suggest that interactions may take place in the transmembrane helices of PLN and the Ca^{2+}-ATPase, as well as in the cytoplasmic domains of the two proteins. When domain II of PLN was fused with a variety of cytoplasmic eitopes, and then coexpressed with SERCA2, these chimeric PLN retained the inhibitory function on SERCA2 activity (134). A series of amino acid substitutions of domain II revealed three types of effect on SERCA2 activity; no change of function, showing wild-type PLN inhibitory effect; loss of function, showing no inhibitory effect; and gain of function, showing augmentation of inhibitory effect (134). As indicated in the helical wheel configuration of domain II, loss of function is associated with mutations on one face of transmembrane helix, and gain of function is associated with mutations on the opposite face (Plate 9). From these studies, it is clear that the cytoplasmic and transmembrane domains of PLN play an important role in the functional interaction between PLN and SERCA2.

Molecular Mechanism of Interaction. The interaction between PLN and SERCA2 can be regulated by the phosphorylation state of PLN. Phospholamban is an active inhibitor only if the net charge in domain IA is +1 or +2 (273). The charge in the corresponding KDDKPV 402 sequence of SERCA2 is also important in the interaction (274). Thus the reduction of net charge to −2 or less by phosphorylation of Ser 16 and/or Thr 17 has a deleterious effect on PLN function. Phosphorylation of Ser 16 has been shown to alter the accessibility of PLN to proteinases (104), implying that conformational changes must occur in the cytoplasmic part of PLN. Studies using circular dichroism analysis have also supported the view that conformational changes occur following phosphorylation (61). These conformational changes may also affect the functional interaction between PLN and SERCA2. Unphosphorylated PLN suppresses the Ca^{2+}-ATPase activity by binding to discrete sequences in the Ca^{2+}-ATPase. Suppression is reduced by phosphorylation of PLN, which induces changes in both its net charge and its conformation. These changes result in its dissociation from and activation of the Ca^{2+}-ATPase (Fig. 8–10).

Bee venom melittin, a basic, amphipathic, α-helical, 26 amino acid peptide structurally related to PLN, has been shown to induce immobilization of proteins in a lipid bilayer (292). The melittin–sarcoplasmic reticulum membrane interaction has been used as a model for investigation of the state of association between Ca^{2+}-ATPase molecules in the membrane and between Ca^{2+}-ATPase and PLN. Time-resolved phosphorescence anisotropy (TPA) and saturation-transfer electron paramagnetic resonance (ST-EPR) showed that mellitin strongly restricts the rotational mobility of Ca^{2+}-ATPase in the membrane, mainly through electrostatic interactions (176, 286). Phosphorylation of PLN increased the rotational mobility of the Ca^{2+}-ATPase in the cardiac sarcoplasmic reticulum membrane by a decrease in large-scale protein association, resulting in the acceleration of Ca^{2+}-ATPase activity (197, 287). Thus phospholamban may be involved in the self-association of Ca^{2+}-ATPase through electrostatic interactions.

Most PLN exists as a pentamer (291). It is of utmost importance to define how the monomer–pentamer conversion is related to the PLN-SERCA2 interaction. Measurement of the maximal incorporation of phosphoryl groups into the Ca^{2+}-ATPase and PLN resulted in the calculation of a stoichiometry of one PLN monomer per Ca^{2+}-ATPase monomer (249). By contrast, Colyer and Wang (52) calculated a ratio of two moles of PLN per one mole of Ca^{2+}-ATPase. Mutations of domain II of PLN provide insight into the stoichiometry of these proteins in the functional PLN-SERCA2 unit (15, 133, 273). The formation of a pentamer is considered to occur through domain II of PLN. Residues in this domain exhibit functionally polarized localization on a helical wheel diagram. When the stability of the pentamer was estimated by its mobility in SDS-PAGE, wild-type PLN was about 75% pentameric and 25% monomeric. A study using fluorescence energy transfer revealed that 7%–23% of the PLN subunits are monomeric in the lipid membrane (158). Gain of function mutants with a 2.5-fold increase in inhibitory function accompanied the 3- to 4-fold enhancement of monomer formation, suggesting that gain of function may be a direct consequence of enhanced monomer formation. In loss of function mutants, the pentamer stability remained unchanged compared with wild-type PLN, suggesting that the interacting surface for SERCA2 lies on one face of the helix—i.e. the exterior face of each helix in a PLN pentamer (133). Thus, PLN monomers are considered to represent the functional form, while PLN pentamers function as a reservoir for the active monomer, leading to the proposal that the key determinant of inhibitory function is the concentration of inhibited PLN monomer–SERCA2 complexes. This physical interaction between SECA2 and PLN revealed to be regulated during Ca^{2+}-transporting cycle. Recent study demonstrated

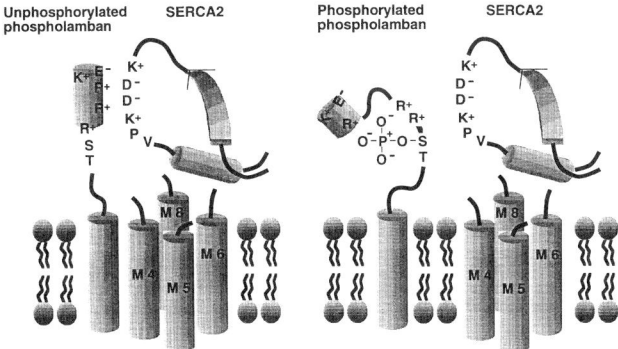

FIG. 8–10. A model for the PKA-regulation of the phospholamban-SERCA2 system. The interaction between phospholamban (PLN) and the Ca^{2+}-ATPase is proposed to take place in the cytoplasmic and transmembrane parts of the two proteins. Unphosphorylated PLN suppresses Ca^{2+}-ATPase activity by associating charged residues in domain IA with the six serial amino acid residues Lys-Asp-Asp-Lys-Pro-Val 402 in the cytoplasmic region of the Ca^{2+}-ATPase, and by forming an association between transmembrane sequences in both molecules. Phosphorylation of Ser16 in domain IA of PLN induces a conformational change resulting in dissociation of PLN from the Ca^{2+}-ATPase in both the cytoplasmic sequence and the transmembrane sequence.

that higher Ca^{2+} concentration disrupt the physical interaction between SERCA2 and PLN, but the phosphorylation of PLN did not. These data provided evidences that this physical interaction between two proteins is stabilized in the Ca^{2+}-free E_2 conformation (13a).

Physiological Relevance of Phospholamban–Ca^{2+}-ATPase System

During β-adrenergic stimulation, cathecholamines have two major effects on the myocardium, increased contractility and abbreviation of systole (251). When intracellular Ca^{2+} concentrations are measured with aequorin, a Ca^{2+}-sensitive bioluminescent protein, isoprotenenol (ISO) augments the initial rate of Ca^{2+} release from sarcoplasmic reticulum during the early phase of contraction. In addition, there is an enhancement of the rate of Ca^{2+} removal from the cytoplasm at the onset of relaxation (2). When skinned cardiac cells, which exhibit cycles of phasic contraction upon addition of Ca^{2+}, are preincubated with cAMP, these cells show an increased amplitude of contraction and faster rates of tension development and relaxation (152). These effects of catecholamines on contraction are believed to result from their effects on Ca^{2+} fluxes across the sarcoplasmic reticulum and sarcolemmal membranes of myocardial cells (251). Ca^{2+} influx through Ca^{2+} channels in the sarcolemmal membrane is activated by PKA (53). This "trigger" Ca^{2+} accelerates Ca^{2+}-induced Ca^{2+} release from sarcoplasmic reticulum. Cardiac sarcoplasmic reticulum Ca^{2+} release channels are also activated through phosphorylation by Ca^{2+}/calmodulin-dependent protein kinase (302). Thus, increased Ca^{2+} release through Ca^{2+} release channels in the sarcoplasmic reticulum could increase the rate and extent of myofibrillar contraction. Ca^{2+} uptake through the Ca^{2+}-ATPase is accelerated by phosphorylation of PLN by PKA, reversing its inhibitory effect on Ca^{2+}-ATPase activity. The addition of ISO to isolated hearts or heart slices perfused with [^{32}P]P_i resulted in increased ^{32}P incorporation into PLN in situ, with a simultaneous increase in the rates of contraction and relaxation (136, 152, 153). Thus, the increased rate of Ca^{2+} uptake by the sarcoplasmic reticulum results in the acceleration of relaxation of myocardium.

Phospholamban Gene Targeting Mice Mice lacking phospholamban as a result of gene targeting appear to be very healthy and to have equal, if not longer life spans than wild-type animals (165). Studies of these animals have enhanced our understanding of the role of PLN in mediating the contractile response of the heart to β-adrenergic agonists (101, 165). Isolated work-performing heart preparations from PLN-deficient mice show significant increases in contractile and relaxation parameters. These are similar to the maximal values produced in wild-type mouse hearts by Ca^{2+} loading, force-frequency response, and pressure and/or volume loading (165). Isolated microsomes from these mice show that the sarcoplasmic reticulum Ca^{2+}-ATPase has an increased affinity for Ca^{2+}. The left ventricular function of murine hearts can be assessed in vivo, by echocardiographic techniques (178). Phospholamban-deficient mice show different left ventricular functional parameters from wild-type mice in their response to β-adrenergic agonists (101). These parameters resemble those of a normal heart infused with ISO. Cardiac-specific overexpression of PLN shows the decrease in contractile parameters, which is abolished when PKA-catalyzed phosphorylation of PLN is induced by ISO stimulation. These studies have confirmed all of the predictions that were made concerning the physiological function of PLN.

The physiological hallmark of all forms of end-stage heart failure is the severe loss of cardiac contractile function. In this regard, decreases in peak calcium transients have recently been shown to be a feature of end-stage human dilated cardiomyopathy. Therefore, the potential role of calcium regulatory proteins such as SR Ca-ATPase and PLN has been of particular interest. Overexpression of a peptide inhibitor of the β-adrenergic receptor kinase (141) can rescue the heart failure phenotype of muscle-specific LIM domain protein (MLP)-deficient mice with dilated cardiomyopathy (219), suggesting the possibility that augmented Ca-ATPase activity by PLN phosphorylation should be important for the improvement of cardiac contractility. This has been proved by the evidence that ablation of PLN rescued the heart failure phenotype of MLP-deficient mice (187). Accordingly, the analysis of genetically engineered animals has revealed a significant role for PLN as a therapeutic target for heart failure.

REGULATION OF Ca^{2+}-ATPase AND PHOSPHOLAMBAN GENES

Skeletal and cardiac muscle share a similar spectrum of proteins involved in muscle contraction and excitation–contraction coupling, but the isoforms expressed in heart are frequently different from those expressed in skeletal muscle. It is of interest that there are cardiac-specific and fast-twitch skeletal muscle-specific isoforms of the Ca^{2+}-ATPase, the Ca^{2+} release channel, and calsequestrin. Slow-twitch skeletal muscle expresses the cardiac isoforms of the Ca^{2+}-ATPase and calsequestrin, but not the fast-twitch isoform of the Ca^{2+} release channel (166).

For skeletal muscle development, members of the MyoD family of transcription factors, which are characterized by a helix-loop-helix (HLH) structure, are unique in their abilities to activate skeletal muscle-specific genes and to transform a wide range of cell types into skeletal muscle (63, 298). By contrast, none of this family of helix-loop-helix transcription factors has been found in cardiac muscle cells. In fact, proliferation and differentiation are temporily distinct events during skeletal muscle development, while differentiation and proliferation occur simultaneously in cardiac muscle cells in fetal and early neonatal life (310). Despite an enormous amount of effort, little is yet known about the factors involved in production and maintenance of the differentiated cardiac phenotype.

Structure of the Ca^{2+}-ATPase Gene

From the time that a full-length cDNA clone encoding the rabbit cardiac sarcoplasmic reticulum Ca^{2+}-ATPase was first isolated (172), a family of sarcoplasmic and endoplasmic reticulum Ca^{2+}-ATPase (SERCA) cDNAs has been cloned and classified as SERCA1, SERCA2, and SERCA3 on the basis of primary sequence homology (28, 29, 32, 87, 166, 168, 172). Genes encoding SERCA1 and SERCA2 have been fully or partially characterized (144, 166, 311, 313), but the gene encoding SERCA3 has not been isolated (Table 8–1).

The SERCA1 genes from rabbit (144) are composed of 23 exons. SERCA1 is alternatively spliced in the region encoding the carboxyl terminus, producing two proteins, SERCA1a and SERCA1b. In the adult transcript (SERCA1a), splicing occurs between the splice site in the antepenultimate exon (exon 21) and the penultimate exon (exon 22), producing a Gly residue followed by a stop codon. The remaining sequence, including the sequence of the ultimate exon (exon 23), is untranslated. In the neonatal transcript (SERCA1b), the penultimate exon (exon 22) is excised, and the splicing of the antepenultimate exon (exon 21) to the ultimate exon (exon 23) encodes the highly charged sequence Asp-Pro-Glu-Asp-Glu-Arg-Arg-Lys that is found in the neonatal cDNA sequence (172).

Analysis of the nucleotide sequence in the 5' exon indicates that SERCA1a and SERCA1b are transcribed from the same transcription initiation site. "TATA" box (CATAAA) and "CAAT" box (CCAAT) are present within 100 base pairs relative to the transcription initiation site. In addition, Sp1-binding sequences (GGGCGC) (226), which are commonly found in the promoter sequences of housekeeping genes (62), are found in the 3' end instead of the 5' end of the gene.

The partial structure of the 5' end of the rabbit SERCA2 gene has been characterized (311). Analysis of the nucleotide sequence in the 5' exon indicates that SERCA2a and SERCA2b transcripts are transcribed from the same promoter and the same transcription initiation site in heart, slow-twitch, smooth muscle, and nonmuscle tissues. "TATA" box (GATAAA) and "CAAT" box (CCAAT) are present in the promoter, and the Sp1 binding sequence (GGCGGG) (226) is present four times in the 5' region. A common muscle regulatory element, the "CArG" box (188), is also

TABLE 8–1. *RNA Processing, Tissue Distribution, and Chromosomal Localization of SERCA Type*

SERCA Isoforms	Alternative Splicing of Carboxy Terminal Regions	Tissue Distribution	Chromosomal Localization in Human Genes
A SERCA1 gene			16
SERCA1a mRNA (994 aa.)		Fast-twitch skeletal muscle (adult)	
SERCA1b mRNA (1011 aa.)		Fast-twitch skeletal muscle (neonate)	
B SERCA2 gene			12
SERCA2a mRNA (997 aa.)		Slow-twitch skeletal muscle Cardiac muscle	
SERCA2b mRNA (1043 aa.)		Smooth muscle Nonmuscle tissues	

Diagrams: *A*: The upper line depicts the 3' end of the SERCA1 gene. Boxes represent exons, in which black boxes indicate translated regions and white boxes indicate nontranslated regions. The introns and the downstream flanking region are represented by a thinner line. The exons are numbered. Exons 1–21 are constitutive exons present in the two SERCA1 mRNAs. Exons 22 and 23 are alternatively included or excluded. Two classes of mRNA translate into two different proteins, SERCA1a or SERCA1b. The Letter A represents the poly A tail of mRNA. Amino acid numbers (*aa*) in the protein isoforms indicated in the parentheses. *B*: The upper line depicts the 3' end of the SERCA2 gene. Two classes of mRNA are made from constitutive exons 1–21, and exon 22 or 23 are alternatively included or excluded. Two classes of mRNA translate into two different proteins, SERCA2a or SERCA2b. The SERCA3 gene has not been isolated and is omitted in this table.

present in the 5' end of the gene. Interestingly, the SERCA2 gene contains a thyroid hormone receptor responsive element (CG(T/A/C)C(A/G), which is found in the rat growth hormone gene (44, 142) and the rat α-myosin heavy chain gene (108, 177). In fact, SERCA2 gene expression in cardiac muscle is positively regulated by thyroid hormone (135, 195, 220, 311). Induction of SERCA2 transcription results from the direct binding of the thyroid hormone receptor to the 5'-flanking sequences of the SERCA2 gene (311).

The 3' end of the SERCA2 gene, like the SERCA1 gene, is alternatively spliced, encoding two proteins, SERCA2a and SERCA2b (166). In the SERCA2a (cardiac and slow-twitch muscle) transcripts, alternative splicing occurs between the antepenultimate exon (exon 21) and the ultimate exon (exon 23) to encode the sequence Ala-Ile-Leu-Glu that is found in cardiac and slow-twitch muscle (172). In the SERCA2b (smooth muscle and nonmuscle) transcripts, the penultimate exon (exon 22) is not excised and it encodes 49 amino acids, which replace the 4 carboxyl terminal amino acids in SERCA2a. The remaining sequences, including the sequence in the ultimate exon (exon 23), are untranslated.

Chromosomal mapping of human Ca^{2+}-ATPase genes has shown that the SERCA1 gene is localized on chromosome 16p12.1 (34), while the SERCA2 gene is located on chromosome 12q23-q24.1 (203). The chromosomal locations of other human cardiac sarcoplasmic reticulum protein genes are: phospholamban, 6q22.1; calsequestrin, 1p11-p13.3; Ca^{2+} release channel, 1q42.1-q43. The chromosomal locations of other skeletal muscle sarcoplasmic reticulum protein genes are: calsequestrin, 1q21; Ca^{2+} release channel, 19q13.1 (170).

Transcriptional Regulation of the Ca^{2+}-ATPase Gene

The transcriptional activity of the SERCA2 gene was measured in transient transfection assays of deletion construct fused with reporter plasmids (70). The region from −284 base pairs to the transcriptional start site was revealed to be essential for high-level transcription of the SERCA2 gene in differentiating muscle cells and in fetal cardiac myocytes. During cardiac muscle development, the SERCA2a mRNA is the primary transcript in atrial and ventricular muscle, and its concentration increases gradually with time. Trace amounts of SERCA2b mRNA are also transcribed, but they do not increase significantly with time (10, 168, 195). SERCA2 mRNA is already present in the cardiogenic plate before the occurrence of the first contractions (191), and its concentration is reduced gradually as the hearts age. There is a 55% reduction in SERCA2 mRNA in 24-month-old adult rats, when compared with 1- to 2-month-old adult rats (162). SERCA1 is not expressed in cardiac muscle at any stage of development or in any pathological condition. There is considerable evidence that Ca^{2+}-ATPase mRNA levels change under different physiological conditions, in parallel with changes in Ca^{2+}-ATPase protein levels. The SERCA2a mRNA levels increase in hyperthyroid hearts but decrease in hypothyroid hearts (8, 135). Pressure-overload induces cardiac hypertrophy and decreases the level of SERCA2 mRNA. Thus mRNA levels are negatively correlated with left ventricular weight/body weight ratios, an index of cardiac hypertrophy (54, 143, 155, 195).

The relative levels of mRNAs encoding several sarcoplasmic reticulum proteins, including SERCA, phospholamban, calsequestrin, and Ca^{2+} release channel proteins, have been examined in human heart samples exhibiting various degrees of failure (7, 67, 186). The level of SERCA2a mRNA, the only SERCA isoform transcript in failing hearts, was greatly reduced with different etiologies. The levels of SERCA2 mRNA are positively correlated with cardiac function indices (186) and negatively correlated with the elevated expression level of atrial natriuretic factor (ANF) mRNA and of brain natriuretic factor (BNF) mRNA in failing human heart (7). Thus, the transcription of mRNAs encoding sarcoplasmic reticulum proteins is altered in a gene-specific manner in heart muscle under different physiological and pathological conditions. The data appear to be consistent with the view that altered expression of sarcoplasmic reticulum genes is the major cause of altered Ca^{2+} handling seen in heart failure and cardiac hypertrophy.

Structure of the Phospholamban Gene

cDNAs encoding PLN from different sources have been isolated and characterized (78, 276, 280). Different sized PLN transcripts have been observed, and these represent polyadenylated mRNAs with 3'-untranslated sequences of different lengths. The PLN genes from both rabbit and chicken have been characterized (79, 276). In both cases, the gene is composed of two exons. Analysis of the nucleotide sequence in the 5' exon has shown that "TATA" and "CAAT" boxes are both present within 100 base pairs of the transcription initiation site. Regulatory elements identified in other muscle-specific genes, for example, the "CArG" box (188) and the MEF-2 binding sequence (33), are present in the 5' end of the gene. Phospholamban gene expression in cardiac muscle is negatively regulated by thyroid hormone (195, 220). A partial thyroid hormone receptor responsive element motif, which is associated with negative regulation of thyroid hormone (38), is found in the gene. The full motif, GG(T/A/C)C(A/G), has not been found in the gene (25).

Transcriptional Regulation of the Phospholamban Gene

The transcriptional activity of the PLN gene was measured in transient transfection assays and transgenic mice using a deletion construct fused with reporter plasmids (90). The 7 kilo base pairs 5' flanking region including exon 1, the entire intron, and part of exon 2 was revealed to be essential for cardiac-specific expression of the phospholamban gene. Transcription of the PLN gene does not change significantly during development in rabbits (10) or chickens (271). The heart at the very early cardiac tube stage expresses phospholamban mRNA concomitant with mRNAs encoding other muscle contractile proteins, suggesting that excitation–contraction coupling is established in the early stages of heart development (191, 271).

Phospholamban mRNA levels are reduced in the heart in experimental animals with hyperthyroidism (8, 135), in hemodynamic overload (143, 155, 195), and in human heart failure (7, 67, 186). Ca^{2+}-ATPase mRNA levels were also reduced under conditions of hemodynamic overload and human heart failure, but they were not reduced in hyperthyroidism. Thus in two of the three cases, the stoichiometry between these proteins would not change significantly. It is not clear whether the changes in mRNAs levels are adaptive responses to a specific physiological condition or whether there is discordance in gene regulation.

REFERENCES

1. Afzal, N. and N. S. Dhalla. Differential changes in left and right ventricular SR calcium transport in congestive heart failure. *Am. J. Physiol.* 262 (*Heart Circ. Physiol.* 31):H868–H874, 1992.
2. Allen, D. G. and J. R. Blinks. Calcium transients in aequorin-injected frog cardiac muscle. *Nature* 273:509–513, 1978.
3. Allen, G. and N. M. Green. A 31-residue tryptic peptide from the active site of the [Ca^{2+}]-transporting adenosine triphosphatase of rabbit sarcoplasmic reticulum. *FEBS Lett.* 63:188–192, 1976.
4. Andersen, J. P. and P. L. Jorgensen. Conformational states of sarcoplasmic reticulum Ca^{2+}-ATPase as studied by proteolytic cleavage. *J. Membr. Biol.* 88:187–98, 1985.
5. Andersen, J. P., B., Vilsen, E. Leberer, and D. H. MacLennan. Functional consequences of mutations in the beta-strand sector of the Ca^{2+}-ATPase of sarcoplasmic reticulum. *J. Biol. Chem.* 264:21018–21023, 1989.
6. Andersen, J. P., B. Vilsen, and D. H. MacLennan. Functional consequences of alterations to Gly310, Gly770, and Gly801 located in the transmembrane domain of the Ca^{2+}-ATPase of sarcoplasmic reticulum. *J. Biol. Chem.* 267:2767–2774, 1992.
7. Arai, M., N. R. Alpert, D. H. MacLennan, P. Barton, and M. Periasamy. Alterations in sarcoplasmic reticulum gene expression in human heart failure. A possible mechanism for alterations in systolic and diastolic properties of the failing myocardium. *Circ. Res.* 72:463–469, 1993.
8. Arai, M., N. R. Alpert, and M. Periasamy. Cloning and characterization of the gene encoding rabbit cardiac calsequestrin. *Gene* 109:275–279, 1991.
9. Arai, M., K. Otsu, D. H. MacLennan, N. R. Alpert, and M. Periasamy. Effect of thyroid hormone on the expression of mRNA encoding sarcoplasmic reticulum proteins. *Circ. Res.* 69:266–276, 1991.
10. Arai, M., K. Otsu, D. H. MacLennan, and M. Periasamy. Regulation of sarcoplasmic reticulum gene expression during cardiac and skeletal muscle development. *Am. J. Physiol.* 262 (*Cell Physiol.* 31):C614–C620, 1992.
11. Arkin, I. T., P. D. Adams, K. R. MacKenzie, M. A. Lemmon, A. T. Brunger, and D. M. Engelman. Structural organization of the pentameric transmembrane alpha-helices of phospholamban, a cardiac ion channel. *Embo J.* 13:4757–4764, 1994.
12. Arrondo, J. L., H. H. Mantsch, N. Mullner, S. Pikula, and A. Martonosi. Infrared spectroscopic characterization of the structural changes connected with the E1–E2 transition in the Ca^{2+}-ATPase of sarcoplasmic reticulum. *J. Biol. Chem.* 262:9037–9043, 1987.
13. Asahi, M., Y. Kimura, K. Kurzydlowski, M. Tada, and D. H. MacLennan. Transmembrane helix M6 in sarco(endo)plasmic reticulum Ca^{2+}-ATPase forms a functional interaction site with phospholamban. *J. Biol. Chem.* 274:32855–32862, 1999.
13a. Asahi, M. E. McKenna, K. Kurzydlowski, M. Tada, and D. H. MacLennan Physical interactions between phospholamban and sarco(endo)plasmic reticulum Ca^{2+}-ATPases are dissociated by elevated Ca^{2+}, but not by phospholamban phosphorylation, vanadate, or thapsigargin, and are enhanced by ATP. *J. Biol. Chem.* 275:15034–15038, 2000.
14. Asturias, F. J. and J. K. Blasie. Location of high-affinity metal binding sites in the profile structure of the Ca^{2+}-ATPase in the sarcoplasmic reticulum by resonance x-ray diffraction. *Biophys. J.* 59:488–502, 1991.
15. Autry, J. M. and L. R. Jones. Functional co-expression of the canine cardiac Ca^{2+} pump and phospholamban in *Spodoptera frugiperda* (Sf21) cells reveals new insights on ATPase regulation. *J. Biol. Chem.* 272:15872–15880, 1997.
16. Baba, A., T. Nakamura, and M. Kawakita. Chemical modification and fluorescence labeling study of Ca^{2+}, Mg^{2+}-adenosine triphosphatase of sarcoplasmic reticulum using iodoacetamide and its N-substituted derivatives. *J. Biochem. Tokyo* 100:1137–1147, 1986.
17. Bajusz, E., J. R. Baker, C. W. Nixon, and F. Homburger. Spontaneous, herditary myocardial degeneration and congestive heart failure in a strain of Syrian hamsters. *Ann. N.Y. Acad. Sci.* 156:105–129, 1996.
18. Bastide, F., G. Meissner, S. Fleischer, and R. L. Post. Similarity of the active site of phosphorylation of the adenosine triphosphatase from transport of sodium and potassium ions in kidney to that for transport of calcium ions in the sarcoplasmic reticulum of muscle. *J. Biol. Chem.* 248:8385–8391, 1973.
19. Besch, H. R., Jr. and A. Schwartz. Initial calcium binding rates of canine cardiac relaxing system (sarcoplasmic reticulum fragments) determined by stopped-flow spectrophotometry. *Biochem. Biophys. Res. Commun.* 45:286–292, 1971.
20. Bidlack, J. M. and A. E. Shamoo. Adenosine 3',5'-monophosphate-dependent phosphorylation of a 6000 and a 22,000 dalton protein from cardiac sarcoplasmic reticulum. *Biochim. Biophys. Acta* 632:310–325, 1980.
21. Bigelow, D. J. and G. Inesi. Contributions of chemical derivatization and spectroscopic studies to the characterization of the

Ca^{2+} transport ATPase of sarcoplasmic reticulum. *Biochim. Biophys. Acta* 1113:323–338, 1992.
22. Bigelow, D. J. and D. D. Thomas. Rotational dynamics of lipid and the Ca^{2+}-ATPase in sarcoplasmic reticulum. The molecular basis of activation by diethyl ether. *J. Biol. Chem.* 262:13449–13456, 1987.
23. Birmachu, W. and D. D. Thomas. Rotational dynamics of the Ca^{2+}-ATPase in sarcoplasmic reticulum studied by time-resolved phosphorescence anisotropy. *Biochemistry* 29:3904–3914, 1990.
24. Birmachu, W., J. C. Voss, C. F. Louis, and D. D. Thomas. Protein and lipid rotational dynamics in cardiac and skeletal sarcoplasmic reticulum detected by EPR and phosphorescence anisotropy. *Biochemistry* 32:9445–9453, 1993.
25. Blanchard, E. M., L. A. Mulieri, and N. R. Alpert. The effects of acute and chronic inotropic interventions on tension independent heat of rabbit papillary muscle. *Basic. Res. Cardiol.* 82(Suppl 2):127–135, 1987.
26. Blasie, J. K., L. G. Herbette, D. Pascolini, V. Skita, D. H. Pierce, and A. Scarpa. Time-resolved x-ray diffraction studies of the sarcoplasmic reticulum membrane during active transport. *Biophys J.* 48:9–18, 1985.
27. Blasie, J. K., D. Pascolini, F. Asturias, L. G. Herbette, D. Pierce, and A. Scarpa. Large-scale structural changes in the sarcoplasmic reticulum ATPase appear essential for calcium transport. *Biophys. J.* 58:687–693, 1990.
28. Brandl, C. J., S. deLeon, D. R. Martin, and D. H. MacLennan. Adult forms of the Ca^{2+}-ATPase of sarcoplasmic reticulum. Expression in developing skeletal muscle. *J. Biol. Chem.* 262:3768–3774, 1987.
29. Brandl, C. J., N. M. Green, B. Korczak, and D. H. MacLennan. Two Ca^{2+}-ATPase genes: homologies and mechanistic implications of deduced amino acid sequences. *Cell* 44:597–607, 1986.
30. Briggs, F. N., R. M. Wise, and J. A. Hearn. The effect of lithium and potassium on the transient state kinetics of the (Ca^{2+} + Mg^{2+})-ATPase of cardiac sarcoplasmic reticulum. *J. Biol. Chem.* 253:5884–5885, 1978.
31. Brostrom, M. A., E. M. Reimann, D. A. Walsh, and E. G. Krebs. A cyclic 3',5'-AMP-stimulated protein kinase from cardiac muscle. *Adv. Enzyme Regul.* 8:191–203, 1970.
32. Burk, S. E., J. Lytton, D. H. MacLennan, and G. E. Shull. cDNA cloning, functional expression, and mRNA tissue distribution of a third organellar Ca^{2+} pump. *J. Biol. Chem.* 264:18561–18568, 1989.
33. Buskin, J. N. and S. D. Hauschka. Identification of a myocyte nuclear factor that binds to the muscle-specific enhancer of the mouse muscle creatine kinase gene. *Mol. Cell. Biol.* 9:2627–2640, 1989.
34. Callen, D. F., E. Baker, S. Lane, J. Nancarrow, A. Thompson, S. A. Whitmore, D. H. MacLennan, R. Berger, D. Cherif, I. Jarvela, et al. Regional mapping of the Batten disease locus (CLN3) to human chromosome 16p12. *Am. J. Hum. Genet.* 49:1372–1377, 1991.
35. Campbell, A. M., P. D. Kessler, and D. M. Fambrough. The alternative carboxyl termini of avian cardiac and brain sarcoplasmic reticulum/endoplasmic reticulum Ca^{2+}-ATPases are on opposite sides of the membrane. *J. Biol. Chem.* 267:9321–9325, 1992.
36. Campbell, K. P., C. M. Knudson, T. Imagawa, A. T. Leung, J. L. Sutko, S. D. Kahl, C. R. Raab, and L. Madson. Identification and characterization of the high affinity [³H]ryanodine receptor of the junctional sarcoplasmic reticulum Ca^{2+} release channel. *J. Biol. Chem.* 262:6460–6463, 1987.
37. Cantilina, T., Y. Sagara, G. Inesi, and L. R. Jones. Comparative studies of cardiac and skeletal sarcoplasmic reticulum ATPases. Effect of a phospholamban antibody on enzyme activation by Ca^{2+}. *J. Biol. Chem.* 268:17018–17025, 1993.
38. Carr, F. E. and N. C. Wong. Characteristics of a negative thyroid hormone response element. *J. Biol. Chem.* 269:4175–4179, 1994.
39. Chadwick, C. C. and E. W. Thomas. Inactivation of sarcoplasmic reticulum (Ca^{2+} + Mg^{2+})-ATPase by N-cyclohexyl-N'-(4-dimethylamino-alpha-naphthyl) carbodiimide. *Biochim. Biophys. Acta* 730:201–206, 1983.
40. Chadwick, C. C. and E. W. Thomas. Ligand binding properties of the sarcoplasmic reticulum (Ca^{2+} + Mg^{2+})-ATPase labelled with N-cyclohexyl-N'-(4-dimethylamino-alpha-naphthyl)-carbodiimide. *Biochim. Biophys. Acta* 769:291–296, 1984.
41. Chamberlain, B. K. and S. Fleischer. Isolation of canine cardiac sarcoplasmic reticulum. *Methods Enzymol.* 157:91–99, 1988.
42. Chamberlain, B. K., D. O. Levitsky, and S. Fleischer. Isolation and characterization of canine cardiac sarcoplasmic reticulum with improved Ca^{2+} transport properties. *J. Biol. Chem.* 258:6602–6609, 1983.
43. Champeil, P., M. P. Gingold, F. Guillain, and G. Inesi. Effect of magnesium on the calcium-dependent transient kinetics of sarcoplasmic reticulum ATPase, studied by stopped flow fluorescence and phosphorylation. *J. Biol. Chem.* 258:4453–4458, 1583.
44. Chevallier, J. and R. A. Butow. Calcium binding to the sarcoplasmic reticulum of rabbit skeletal muscle. *Biochemistry* 10:2733–2737, 1971.
45. Chiesi, M. and R. Schwaller. Involvement of electrostatic phenomena in phospholamban-induced stimulation of Ca^{2+} uptake into cardiac sarcoplasmic reticulum. *FEBS Lett.* 244:241–244, 1989.
46. Chothia, C. and J. Janin. Principles of protein-protein recognition. *Nature* 256:705–708, 1975.
47. Clarke, D. M., T. W. Loo, G. Inesi, and D. H. MacLennan. Location of high affinity Ca^{2+}-binding sites within the predicted transmembrane domain of the sarcoplasmic reticulum Ca^{2+}-ATPase. *Nature* 339:476–478, 1989.
48. Clarke, D. M., T. W. Loo, and D. H. MacLennan. The epitope for monoclonal antibody A20 (amino acids 870–890) is located on the luminal surface of the Ca^{2+}-ATPase of sarcoplasmic reticulum. *J. Biol. Chem.* 265:17405–17408, 1990.
49. Clarke, D. M., T. W. Loo, and D. H. MacLennan. Functional consequences of alterations to amino acids located in the nucleotide binding domain of the Ca^{2+}-ATPase of sarcoplasmic reticulum. *J. Biol. Chem.* 265:22223–22227, 1990.
50. Clarke, D. M., T. W. Loo, and D. H. MacLennan. Functional consequences of alterations to polar amino acids located in the transmembrane domain of the Ca^{2+}-ATPase of sarcoplasmic reticulum. *J. Biol. Chem.* 265:6262–6267, 1990.
51. Clarke, D. M., T. W. Loo, W. J. Rice, J. P. Andersen, B. Vilsen, and D. H. MacLennan. Functional consequences of alterations to hydrophobic amino acids located in the M4 transmembrane sector of the Ca^{2+}-ATPase of sarcoplasmic reticulum. *J. Biol. Chem.* 268:18359–18364, 1993.
52. Colyer, J. and J. H. Wang. Dependence of cardiac sarcoplasmic reticulum calcium pump activity on the phosphorylation status of phospholamban. *J. Biol. Chem.* 266:17486–17493, 1991.
53. Curtis, B. M. and W. A. Catterall. Phosphorylation of the calcium antagonist receptor of the voltage-sensitive calcium channel by cAMP-dependent protein kinase. *Proc. Natl. Acad. Sci. U.S.A.* 82:2528–2532, 1985.
54. de la Bastie, D., D. Levitsky, L. Rappaport, J. J. Mercadier, F. Marotte, C. Wisnewsky, V. Brovkovich, K. Schwartz, and A. M. Lompre. Function of the sarcoplasmic reticulum and expression of its Ca^{2+}-ATPase gene in pressure overload-induced cardiac hypertrophy in the rat. *Circ. Res.* 66:554–564, 1990.
55. de Meis, L. and A. L. Vianna. Energy interconversion by the

Ca^{2+}-dependent ATPase of the sarcoplasmic reticulum. *Annu. Rev. Biochem.* 48:275–292, 1979.
56. DeFoor, P. H., D. Levitsky, T. Biryukova, and S. Fleischer. Immunological dissimilarity of the calcium pump protein of skeletal and cardiac muscle sarcoplasmic reticulum. *Arch. Biochem. Biophys.* 200:196–205, 1980.
57. Degani, C. and P. D. Boyer. A borohydride reduction method for characterization of the acyl phosphate linkage in proteins and its application to sarcoplasmic reticulum adenosine triphosphatase. *J. Biol. Chem.* 248:8222–8226, 1973.
58. DeLong, L. J. and J. K. Blasie. Effect of Ca^{2+} binding on the profile structure of the sarcoplasmic reticulum membrane using time-resolved x-ray diffraction. *Biophys. J.* 64:1750–1759, 1993.
59. Dolber, P. C. and J. R. Sommer. Corbular sarcoplasmic reticulum of rabbit cardiac muscle. *J. Ultrastruct. Res.* 87:190–196, 1984.
60. Dupont, Y., Y., Chapron, and R. Pougeois. Titration of the nucleotide binding sites of sarcoplasmic reticulum Ca^{2+}-ATPase with 2',3'-O-(2,4,6-trinitrophenyl) adenosine 5'-triphosphate and 5'-diphosphate. *Biochem. Biophys. Res. Commun.* 106:1272–1279, 1982.
61. Dupont, Y. and J. B. Leigh, Transient kinetics of sarcoplasmic reticulum Ca^{2+} + Mg^{2+} ATPase studied by fluorescence. *Nature* 273:396–398, 1978.
62. Dynan, W. S. and R. Tjian. Control of eukaryotic messenger RNA synthesis by sequence-specific DNA-binding proteins. *Nature* 316:774–778, 1985.
63. Edmondson, D. G. and E. N. Olson. Helix-loop-helix proteins as regulators of muscle-specific transcription. *J. Biol. Chem.* 268:755–758, 1993.
64. Eklund, H., J. P. Samma, L. Wallen, C. I. Branden, A. Akeson, and T. A. Jones. Structure of a triclinic ternary complex of horse liver alcohol dehydrogenase at 2.9 Å resolution. *J. Mol. Biol.* 146:561–587, 1981.
65. Fanburg, B. and J. Gergely. Studies on adenosine triphosphate-supported calcium accumulation by cardiac subcellular particles. *J. Biol. Chem.* 240:2721–2728, 1965.
66. Feher, J. J. and F. N. Briggs. The effect of calcium load on the calcium permeability of sarcoplasmic reticulum. *J. Biol. Chem.* 257:10191–10191, 1982.
67. Feldman, A. M., P. E. Ray, C. M. Silan, J. A. Mercer, W. Minobe, and M. R. Bristow. Selective gene expression in failing human heart. Quantification of steady-state levels of messenger RNA in endomyocardial biopsies using the polymerase chain reaction. *Circulation* 83:1866–1872, 1991.
68. Ferguson, D. G., H. W. Schwartz, and C. Franzini Armstrong. Subunit structure of junctional feet in triads of skeletal muscle: a freeze-drying, rotary-shadowing study. *J. Cell Biol.* 99:1735–1742, 1984.
69. Fernandez Belda, F., M. Kurzmack, and G. Inesi. A comparative study of calcium transients by isotopic tracer, metallochromic indicator, and intrinsic fluorescence in sarcoplasmic reticulum ATPase. *J. Biol. Chem.* 259:9687–9698, 1984.
70. Fisher, S. A., P. M. Buttrick, D. Sukovich, and M. Periasamy. Characterization of promoter elements of the rabbit cardiac sarcoplasmic reticulum Ca^{2+}-ATPase gene required for expression in cardiac muscle cells. *Circ. Res.* 73:622–628, 1993.
71. Fleischer, S. and M. Inui. Biochemistry and biophysics of excitation-contraction coupling. *Annu. Rev. Biophys. Biophys. Chem.* 18:333–364, 1989.
72. Fliegel, L., K. Burns, M. Opas, and M. Michalak. The high-affinity calcium binding protein of sarcoplasmic reticulum. Tissue distribution, and homology with calregulin. *Biochim. Biophys. Acta.* 982:1–8, 1989.
73. Franzini-Armstrong, C. Studies of the triad. I. Structure of the junction in frog twitch fibers. *J. Cell. Biol.* 47:488–499, 1970.
74. Froehlich, J. P. and E. W. Taylor. Transient state kinetic studies of sarcoplasmic reticulum adenosine triphosphatase. *J. Biol. Chem.* 250:2013–2021, 1975.
75. Fujii, J., J. Lytton, M. Tada, and D. H. MacLennan. Rabbit cardiac and slow-twitch muscle express the same phospholamban gene. *FEBS Lett.* 227:51–55, 1988.
76. Fujii, J., K. Maruyama, M. Tada, and D. H. MacLennan. Co-expression of slow-twitch/cardiac muscle Ca^{2+}-ATPase (SERCA2) and phospholamban. *FEBS Lett.* 273:232–234, 1990.
77. Fujii, J., K. Maruyama, M. Tada, and D. H. MacLennan. Expression and site-specific mutagenesis of phospholamban. Studies of residues involved in phosphorylation and pentamer formation. *J. Biol. Chem.* 264:12950–12955, 1989.
78. Fujii, J., A. Ueno, K. Kitano, S. Tanaka, M. Kadoma, and M. Tada. Complete complementary DNA-derived amino acid sequence of canine cardiac phospholamban. *J. Clin. Invest.* 79:301–304, 1987.
79. Fujii, J., A. Zarain Herzberg, H. F. Willard, M. Tada, and D. H. MacLennan. Structure of the rabbit phospholamban gene, cloning of the human cDNA, and assignment of the gene to human chromosome 6. *J. Biol. Chem.* 266:11669–11675, 1991.
80. Geisow, M. J., U. Fritsche, J. M. Hexham, B. Dash, and T. Johnson. A consensus amino-acid sequence repeat in Torpedo and mammalian Ca2+-dependent membrane-binding proteins. *Nature* 320:636–638, 1986.
81. Girardet, J. L. and Y. Dupont. Ellipticity changes of the sarcoplasmic reticulum Ca^{2+}-ATPase induced by cation binding and phosphorylation. *FEBS Lett.* 296:103–106, 1992.
82. Glass, C. K., R. Franco, C. Weinberger, V. R. Albert, R. M. Evans, and M. G. Rosenfeld. A c-erb-A binding site in rat growth hormone gene mediates trans-activation by thyroid hormone. *Nature* 329:738–41, 1987.
83. Goldshleger, R., Y. Shahak, and S. J. Karlish. Electrogenic and electroneutral transport modes of renal Na$^+$/K$^+$ ATPase reconstituted into proteoliposomes. *J. Membr. Biol.* 113:139–154, 1990.
84. Gottesman, M. M. and I. Pastan. The multidrug transporter, a double-edged sword. *J. Biol. Chem.* 263:12163–12166, 1988.
85. Green, N. M. and D. H. MacLennan. ATP driven ion pumps: an evolutionary mosaic. *Biochem. Soc. Trans.* 17:819–822, 1989.
86. Guillain, F., P. Champeil, J. J. Lacapere, and M. P. Gingold. Stopped flow and rapid quenching measurement of the transient steps induced by calcium binding to sarcoplasmic reticulum adenosine triphosphatase. Competition with Ca^{2+}-independent phosphorylation. *J. Biol. Chem.* 256:6140–6147, 1981.
87. Gunteski Hamblin, A. M., J. Greeb, and G. E. Shull. A novel Ca^{2+} pump expressed in brain, kidney, and stomach is encoded by an alternative transcript of the slow-twitch muscle sarcoplasmic reticulum Ca^{2+}-ATPase gene. Identification of cDNAs encoding Ca^{2+} and other cation-transporting ATPases using an oligonucleotide probe derived from the ATP-binding site. *J. Biol. Chem.* 263:15032–15040, 1988.
88. Gutierrez Merino, C., F. Munkonge, A. M. Mata, J. M. East, B. L. Levinson, R. M. Napier, and A. G. Lee. The position of the ATP binding site on the (Ca^{2+} + Mg^{2+})-ATPase. *Biochim. Biophys. Acta.* 897:207–216, 1987.
89. Gwathmey, J. K., S. E. Warren, G. M. Briggs, L. Copelas, M. D. Feldman, P. J. Phillips, M. Callahan, Jr., F. J. Schoen, W. Grossman, and J. P. Morgan. Diastolic dysfunction in hypertrophic cardiomyopathy. Effect on active force generation during systole. *J. Clin. Invest.* 87:1023–1031, 1991.
90. Haghighi, K., V. J. Kadambi, K. L. Koss, W. Luo, J. M. Harrer, S. Ponniah, Z. Zhou, and E. G. Kranias. In vitro and in vivo promoter analyses of the mouse phospholamban gene. *Gene* 203:199–207, 1997.

91. Harigaya, S. and A. Schwartz. Rate of calcium binding and uptake in normal animal and failing human cardiac muscle. Membrane vesicles (relaxing system) and mitochondria. *Circ. Res.* 25:781–794, 1969.
92. Hasselbach, W. Regulatory mechanisms of the calcium transport system of fragmented rabbit sarcoplasmic reticulum. I. The effect of accumulated calcium on transport and adenosine triphosphate hydrolysis. *J. Gen. Physiol.* 57:50–70, 1971.
93. Hasselbach, W. The reversibility of the sarcoplasmic calcium pump. *Biochim. Biophys. Acta* 515:23–53, 1978.
94. Hawkins, C., A. Xu, and N. Narayanan. Sarcoplasmic reticulum calcium pump in cardiac and slow twitch skeletal muscle but not fast twitch skeletal muscle undergoes phosphorylation by endogenous and exogenous Ca^{2+}/calmodulin-dependent protein kinase. Characterization of optimal conditions for calcium pump phosphorylation. *J. Biol. Chem.* 269:31198–31206, 1994.
95. Henao, F., S. Orlowski, Z. Merah, and P. Champeil. The metal sites on sarcoplasmic reticulum membranes that bind lanthanide ions with the highest affinity are not the ATPase Ca^{2+} transport sites. *J. Biol. Chem.* 267:10302–10312, 1992.
96. Herbette, L., P. DeFoor, S. Fleischer, D. Pascolini, A. Scarpa, and J. K. Blasie. The separate profile structures of the functional calcium pump protein and the phospholipid bilayer within isolated sarcoplasmic reticulum membranes determined by X-ray and neutron diffraction. *Biochim. Biophys. Acta* 817:103–122, 1985.
97. Hicks, M. J., M. Shigekawa, and A. M. Katz. Mechanism by which cyclic adenosine 3':5'-monophosphate-dependent protein kinase stimulates calcium transport in cardiac sarcoplasmic reticulum. *Circ. Res.* 44:384–391, 1979.
98. Hill, T. L. *Free Energy Transduction in Biology*. New York: Academic Press, 1977.
99. Hoffmann, W., M. G. Sarzala, and D. Chapman. Rotational motion and evidence for oligomeric structures of sarcoplasmic reticulum Ca^{2+}-activated ATPase. *Proc. Natl. Acad. Sci. U.S.A.* 76:3860–3864, 1979.
100. Hofmann, S. L., M. S. Brown, E. Lee, R. K. Pathak, R. G. Anderson, and J. L. Goldstein. Purification of a sarcoplasmic reticulum protein that binds Ca^{2+} and plasma lipoproteins. *J. Biol. Chem.* 264:8260–8270, 1989.
101. Hoit, B. D., S. F. Khoury, E. G. Kranias, N. Ball, and R. A. Walsh. In vivo echocardiographic detection of enhanced left ventricular function in gene-targeted mice with phospholamban deficiency. *Circ. Res.* 77:632–637, 1995.
102. Horrocks, W. D., Jr. and D. R. Sudnick. Time-resolved europium(III) excitation spectroscopy: a luminescence probe of metal ion binding sites. *Science* 206:1194–1196, 1979.
103. Huang, S. and T. C. Squier. Enhanced rotational dynamics of the phosphorylation domain of the Ca^{2+}-ATPase upon calcium activation. *Biochemistry* 37:18064–18073, 1998.
104. Huggins, J. P. and P. J. England. Evidence for a phosphorylation-induced conformational change in phospholamban from the effects of three proteases. *FEBS Lett.* 217:32–36, 1987.
105. Hymel, L., and S. Fleischer. Reconstitution of skeletal muscle sarcoplasmic reticulum membranes: strategies for varying the lipid/protein ratio. *Methods Enzymol.* 157:302–314, 1988.
106. Ikemoto, N., J. F. Morgan, and S. Yamada. Ca^{2+}-controlled conformational states of the Ca^{2+} transport enzyme of sarcoplasmic reticulum. *J. Biol. Chem.* 253:8027–8033, 1978.
107. Imagawa, T., T. Watanabe, and T. Nakamura. Subunit structure and multiple phosphorylation sites of phospholamban. *J. Biochem. Tokyo* 99:41–53, 1986.
108. Inesi, G. Mechanism of calcium transport. *Annu. Rev. Physiol.* 47:573–601, 1985.
109. Inesi, G. Sequential mechanism of calcium binding and translocation in sarcoplasmic reticulum adenosine triphosphatase. *J. Biol. Chem.* 262:16338–16342, 1987.
110. Inesi, G. Mechanism of calcium transport. *Annu. Rev. Physiol.* 47:573–601, 1985.
111. Inesi, G., M. Kurzmack, C. Coan, and D. E. Lewis. Cooperative calcium binding and ATPase activation in sarcoplasmic reticulum vesicles. *J. Biol. Chem.* 255:3025–3031, 1980.
112. Inesi, G. and A. Scarpa. Fast kinetics of adenosine triphosphate dependent Ca^{2+} uptake by fragmented sarcoplasmic reticulum. *Biochemistry* 11:356–359, 1972.
113. Inui, M., B. K. Chamberlain, A. Saito, and S. Fleischer. The nature of the modulation of Ca^{2+} transport as studied by reconstitution of cardiac sarcoplasmic reticulum. *J. Biol. Chem.* 261:1794–1800, 1986.
114. Inui, M., M. Kadoma, and M. Tada. Purification and characterization of phospholamban from canine cardiac sarcoplasmic reticulum. *J. Biol. Chem.* 260:3708–3715, 1985.
115. Inui, M., A. Saito, and S. Fleischer. Isolation of the ryanodine receptor from cardiac sarcoplasmic reticulum and identity with the feet structures. *J. Biol. Chem.* 262:15637–15642, 1987.
116. Inui, M., A. Saito, and S. Fleischer. Purification of the ryanodine receptor and identity with feet structures of junctional terminal cisternae of sarcoplasmic reticulum from fast skeletal muscle. *J. Biol. Chem.* 262:1740–1747, 1987.
117. Ishii, T., M. V. Lemas, and K. Takeyasu. Na(+)-, ouabain-, Ca^{2+}-, and thapsigargin-sensitive ATPase activity expressed in chimeras between the calcium and the sodium pump alpha subunits. *Proc. Natl. Acad. Sci. U.S.A.* 91:6103–6107, 1994.
118. Izumo, S. and V. Mahdavi. Thyroid hormone receptor alpha isoforms generated by alternative splicing differentially activate myosin HC gene transcription [published erratum appears in *Nature* 1988 Oct 20;335(6192):744]. *Nature* 334:539–542, 1988.
119. James, P., M. Inui, M. Tada, M. Chiesi and E. Carafoli. Nature and site of phospholamban regulation of the Ca^{2+} pump of sarcoplasmic reticulum. *Nature* 342:90–92, 1989.
120. Jencks, W. P. How does a calcium pump pump calcium? *J. Biol. Chem.* 264:18855–18858, 1989.
121. Jencks, W. P. Utilization of binding energy and coupling rules for active transport and other coupled vectorial processes. *Methods Enzymol.* 171:145–164, 1989.
122. Jencks, W. P., T. Yang, D. Peisach, and J. Myung. Calcium ATPase of sarcoplasmic reticulum has four binding sites for calcium. *Biochemistry* 32:7030–7034, 1993.
123. Jones, L. R., H. R. Besch, Jr., J. W. Fleming, M. M. McConnaughey, and A. M. Watanabe. Separation of vesicles of cardiac sarcolemma from vesicles of cardiac sarcoplasmic reticulum. Comparative biochemical analysis of component activities. *J. Biol. Chem.* 254:530–539, 1979.
124. Jones, L. R. and S. E. Cala. Biochemical evidence for functional heterogeneity of cardiac sarcoplasmic reticulum vesicles. *J. Biol. Chem.* 256:11809–11818, 1981.
125. Jones, L. R., H. K. Simmerman, W. W. Wilson, F. R. Gurd, and A. D. Wegener. Purification and characterization of phospholamban from canine cardiac sarcoplasmic reticulum. *J. Biol. Chem.* 260:7721–7730, 1985.
126. Jorgensen, A. O. and K. P. Campbell. Evidence for the presence of calsequestrin in two structurally different regions of myocardial sarcoplasmic reticulum. *J. Cell. Biol.* 98:1597–1602, 1984.
127. Kadambi, V. J., S. Ponniah, J. M. Harrer, B. D. Hoit, G. W. Dorn, 2nd, R. A. Walsh, and E. G. Kranias. Cardiac-specific overexpression of phospholamban alters calcium kinetics and resultant cardiomyocyte mechanics in transgenic mice. *J. Clin. Invest.* 97:533–639, 1996.
128. Karim, C. B., J. D. Stamm, J. Karim, L. R. Jones, and D. D.

128. (continued) Thomas. Cysteine reactivity and oligomeric structures of phospholamban and its mutants. *Biochemistry* 37:12074–12081, 1998.

129. Katz, A. M. *Physiology of the Heart,* Volume 2. New York: Raven Press, Ltd., 1992.

130. Kijima, Y., E. Ogunbunmi, and S. Fleischer. Drug action of thapsigargin on the Ca^{2+} pump protein of sarcoplasmic reticulum. *J. Biol. Chem.* 266:22912–22918, 1991.

131. Kim, H. W., N. A. Steenaart, D. G. Ferguson, and E. G. Kranias. Functional reconstitution of the cardiac sarcoplasmic reticulum Ca^{2+}-ATPase with phospholamban in phospholipid vesicles. *J. Biol. Chem.* 265:1702–1709, 1990.

132. Kimura, Y., M. Inui, M. Kadoma, Y. Kijima, T. Sasaki, and M. Tada. Effects of monoclonal antibody against phospholamban on calcium pump ATPase of cardiac sarcoplasmic reticulum. *J. Mol. Cell. Cardiol.* 23:1223–1230, 1991.

133. Kimura, Y., K. Kurzydlowski, M. Tada, and D. H. MacLennan. Phospholamban inhibitory function is activated by depolymerization. *J. Biol. Chem.* 272:15061–15064, 1997.

134. Kimura, Y., K. Kurzydlowski, M. Tada, and D. H. MacLennan. Phospholamban regulates the Ca^{2+}-ATPase through intramembrane interactions. *J. Biol. Chem.* 271:21726–21731, 1996.

135. Kimura, Y., K. Otsu, K. Nishida, T. Kuzuya, and M. Tada. Thyroid hormone enhances Ca^{2+} pumping activity of the cardiac sarcoplasmic reticulum by increasing Ca^{2+}-ATPase and decreasing phospholamban expression. *J. Mol. Cell. Cardiol.* 26:1145–1154, 1994.

136. Kirchberger, M. A. and A. Raffo. Decrease in calcium transport associated with phosphoprotein phosphatase-catalyzed dephosphorylation of cardiac sarcoplasmic reticulum. *J. Cyclic Nucleotide Res.* 3:45–53, 1977.

137. Kirchberger, M. A. and M. Tada. Effects of adenosine 3':5'-monophosphate-dependent protein kinase on sarcoplasmic reticulum isolated from cardiac and slow and fast contracting skeletal muscles. *J. Biol. Chem.* 251:725–729, 1976.

138. Kirchberger, M. A., M. Tada, and A. M. Katz. Adenosine 3':5'-monophosphate-dependent protein kinase-catalyzed phosphorylation reaction and its relationship to calcium transport in cardiac sarcoplasmic reticulum. *J. Biol. Chem.* 249:6166–6173, 1974.

139. Kitazawa, T. Physiological significance of Ca^{2+} uptake by mitochondria in the heart in comparison with that by cardiac sarcoplasmic reticulum. *J. Biochem. Tokyo* 80:1129–1147, 1976.

140. Knighton, D. R., J. H. Zheng, L. F. Ten Eyck, N. H. Xuong, S. S. Taylor, and J. M. Sowadski. Structure of a peptide inhibitor bound to the catalytic subunit of cyclic adenosine monophosphate-dependent protein kinase. *Science* 253:414–420, 1991.

141. Koch, W. J., H. A. Rockman, P. Samama, R. A. Hamilton, R. A. Bond, C. A. Milano, and R. J. Lefkowitz. Cardiac function in mice overexpressing the beta-adrenergic receptor kinase or a beta ARK inhibitor. *Science* 268:1350–1353, 1995.

142. Koenig, R. J., G. A. Brent, R. L. Warne, P. R. Larsen, and D. D. Moore. Thyroid hormone receptor binds to a site in the rat growth hormone promoter required for induction by thyroid hormone. *Proc. Natl. Acad. Sci. U.S.A.* 84:5670–5674, 1987.

143. Komuro, I., M. Kurabayashi, Y. Shibazaki, F. Takaku, and Y. Yazaki. Molecular cloning and characterization of a Ca^{2+} + Mg^{2+}-dependent adenosine triphosphatase from rat cardiac sarcoplasmic reticulum. Regulation of its expression by pressure overload and developmental stage. *J. Clin. Invest.* 83:1102–1108, 1989.

144. Korczak, B., A. Zarain Herzberg, C. J. Brandl, C. J. Ingles, N. M. Green, and D. H. MacLennan. Structure of the rabbit fast-twitch skeletal muscle Ca^{2+}-ATPase gene. *J. Biol. Chem.* 263:4813–4819, 1988.

145. Kranias, E. G., F. Mandel, T. Wang, and A. Schwartz. Mechanism of the stimulation of calcium ion dependent adenosine triphosphatase of cardiac sarcoplasmic reticulum by adenosine 3',5'-monophosphate dependent protein kinase. *Biochemistry* 19:5434–5439, 1980.

146. Kretsinger, R. H. Calcium-binding proteins. *Annu. Rev. Biochem.* 45:239–266, 1976.

147. Kunkel, T. A. Rapid and efficient site-specific mutagenesis without phenotypic selection. *Proc. Natl. Acad. Sci. U.S.A.* 82:488–92, 1985.

148. Kurzmack, M., S. Verjovski Almeida, and G. Inesi. Detection of an initial burst of Ca^{2+} translocation in sarcoplasmic reticulum. *Biochem. Biophys. Res. Commun.* 78:772–776, 1977.

149. Lai, F. A., H. P. Erickson, E. Rousseau, Q. Y. Liu, and G. Meissner. Purification and reconstitution of the calcium release channel from skeletal muscle. *Nature* 331:315–319, 1988.

150. Lamers, J. M. and J. T. Stinis. Defective calcium pump in the sarcoplasmic reticulum of the hypertrophied rabbit heart. *Life. Sci.* 24:2313–2319, 1979.

151. Langer, G. A. *Calcium and the Heart.* New York: Raven Press, 1990.

152. Le Peuch, C. J., J. C. Guilleux, and J. G. Demaille. Phospholamban phosphorylation in the perfused rat heart is not solely dependent on beta-adrenergic stimulation. *FEBS Lett.* 114:165–168, 1980.

153. Le Peuch, C. J., J. Haiech, and J. G. Demaille. Concerted regulation of cardiac sarcoplasmic reticulum calcium transport by cyclic adenosine monophosphate-dependent and calcium-calmodulin-dependent phosphorylations. *Biochemistry* 18:5150–5157, 1979.

154. Le Peuch, C. J., D. A. Le Peuch, and J. G. Demaille. Phospholamban, activator of the cardiac sarcoplasmic reticulum calcium pump. Physicochemical properties and diagonal purification. *Biochemistry* 19:3368–3373, 1980.

155. Levitsky, D., D. de la Bastie, K. Schwartz, and A. M. Lompre. Ca^{2+}-ATPase and function of sarcoplasmic reticulum during cardiac hypertrophy. *Am. J. Physiol.* 261:23–26, 1991.

156. Levitsky, D. O., M. K. Aliev, A. V. Kuzmin, T. S. Levchenko, V. N. Smirnov, and E. I. Chazov. Isolation of calcium pump system and purification of calcium ion-dependent ATPase from heart muscle. *Biochim. Biophys. Acta.* 443:468–484, 1976.

157. Li, M., R. L. Cornea, J. M. Autry, L. R. Jones, and D. D. Thomas. Phosphorylation-induced structural change in phospholamban and its mutants, detected by intrinsic fluorescence. *Biochemistry* 37:7869–7877, 1998.

158. Li, M., L. G. Reddy, R. Bennett, N. D. Silva, Jr., L. R. Jones, and D. D. Thomas (1999). A fluorescence energy transfer method for analyzing protein oligomeric structure: application to phospholamban. *Biophys. J.* 76:2587–2599.

159. Limas, C. J., M. T. Olivari, I. F. Goldenberg, T. B. Levine, D. G. Benditt, and A. Simon. Calcium uptake by cardiac sarcoplasmic reticulum in human dilated cardiomyopathy. *Cardiovasc. Res.* 21:601–605.

160. Lin, S. H. and G. Guidotti. Cloning and expression of a cDNA coding for a rat liver plasma membrane ecto-ATPase. The primary structure of the ecto-ATPase is similar to that of the human biliary glycoprotein I. *J. Biol. Chem.* 264:14408–14414.

161. Lippert, J. L., R. M. Lindsay, and R. Schultz. Laser Raman characterization of conformational changes in sarcoplasmic reticulum induced by temperature, Ca^{2+}, and Mg^{2+}. *J. Biol. Chem.* 256:12411–12416.

162. Lompre, A. M., F. Lambert, E. G. Lakatta, and K. Schwartz. Expression of sarcoplasmic reticulum Ca^{2+}-ATPase and calsequestrin genes in rat heart during ontogenic development and aging. *Circ. Res.* 69:1380–1388, 1991.

163. Lu, Y. Z., Z. C. Xu, and M. A. Kirchberger. Evidence for an

effect of phospholamban on the regulatory role of ATP in calcium uptake by the calcium pump of the cardiac sarcoplasmic reticulum. *Biochemistry* 32:3105–3111, 1993.
164. Ludlam, C. F., I. T. Arkin, X. M. Liu, M. S. Rothman, P. Rath, S. Aimoto, S. O. Smith, D. M. Engelman, and K. J. Rothschild. Fourier transform infrared spectroscopy and site-directed isotope labeling as a probe of local secondary structure in the transmembrane domain of phospholamban. *Biophys. J.* 70: 1728–1736, 1996.
165. Luo, W., I. L. Grupp, J. Harrer, S. Ponniah, G. Grupp, J. J. Duffy, T. Doetschman, and E. G. Kranias. Targeted ablation of the phospholamban gene is associated with markedly enhanced myocardial contractility and loss of beta-agonist stimulation. *Circ. Res.* 75:401–409, 1994.
166. Lytton, J. and D. H. MacLennan. Molecular cloning of cDNAs from human kidney coding for two alternatively spliced products of the cardiac Ca^{2+}-ATPase gene. *J. Biol. Chem.* 263: 15024–15031, 1988.
167. Lytton, J., M. Westlin, S. E. Burk, G. E. Shull, and D. H. MacLennan. Functional comparisons between isoforms of the sarcoplasmic or endoplasmic reticulum family of calcium pumps. *J. Biol. Chem.* 267:14483–14489, 1992.
168. Lytton, J., A. Zarain Herzberg, M. Periasamy, and D. H. MacLennan. Molecular cloning of the mammalian smooth muscle sarco(endo)plasmic reticulum Ca^{2+}-ATPase. *J. Biol. Chem.* 264:7059–7065, 1989.
169. MacDougall, L. K., L. R. Jones, and P. Cohen. Identification of the major protein phosphatases in mammalian cardiac muscle which dephosphorylate phospholamban. *Eur. J. Biochem.* 196: 725–734, 1991.
170. MacKenzie, A. E., R. G. Korneluk, F. Zorzato, J. Fujii, M. Phillips, D. Iles, B. Wieringa, S. Leblond, J. Bailly, H. F. Willard, et al. The human ryanodine receptor gene: its mapping to 19q13.1, placement in a chromosome 19 linkage group, and exclusion as the gene causing myotonic dystrophy. *Am. J. Hum. Genet.* 46:1082–1089, 1990.
171. MacLennan, D. H. Molecular tools to elucidate problems in excitation–contraction coupling. *Biophys. J.* 58:1355–1365, 1990.
172. MacLennan, D. H., C. J. Brandl, B. Korczak, and N. M. Green. Amino-acid sequence of a Ca^{2+} + Mg^{2+}-dependent ATPase from rabbit muscle sarcoplasmic reticulum, deduced from its complementary DNA sequence. *Nature* 316:696–700, 1985.
173. MacLennan, D. H., D. M. Clarke, T. W. Loo, and I. S. Skerjanc. Site-directed mutagenesis of the Ca^{2+}-ATPase of sarcoplasmic reticulum. *Acta. Physiol. Scand. Suppl.* 607:141–150, 1992.
174. MacLennan, D. H., W. J. Rice, and N. M. Green. The mechanism of Ca^{2+} transport by sarco(endo)plasmic reticulum Ca^{2+}-ATPases. *J. Biol. Chem.* 272:28815–28818, 1997.
175. MacLennan, D. H. and P. T. Wong. Isolation of a calcium-sequestering protein from sarcoplasmic reticulum. *Proc. Natl. Acad. Sci. U.S.A.* 68:1231–1235, 1971.
176. Mahaney, J. E. and D. D. Thomas. Effects of melittin on molecular dynamics and Ca^{2+}-ATPase activity in sarcoplasmic reticulum membranes: electron paramagnetic resonance. *Biochemistry* 30:7171–7180, 1991.
177. Mahdavi, V., A. P., Chambers, and B. Nadal Ginard. Cardiac alpha- and beta-myosin heavy chain genes are organized in tandem. *Proc. Natl. Acad. Sci. U.S.A.* 81:2626–2630, 1984.
178. Manning, W. J., J. Y. Wei, S. E. Katz, S. E. Litwin, and P. S. Douglas. In vivo assessment of LV mass in mice using high-frequency cardiac ultrasound: necropsy validation. *Am. J. Physiol.* 266 (*Heart Circ. Physiol.*):H1672–H1675, 1994.
179. Martonosi, A. Biochemical and clinical aspects of sarcoplasmic reticulum function. *Curr. Top. Membr. Transp.* 3:83–197, 1972.
180. Maruyama, K., D. M. Clarke, J. Fujii, G. Inesi, T. W. Loo, and D. H. MacLennan. Functional consequences of alterations to amino acids located in the catalytic center (isoleucine 348 to threonine 357) and nucleotide-binding domain of the Ca^{2+}-ATPase of sarcoplasmic reticulum. *J. Biol. Chem.* 264:13038–13042, 1989.
181. Maruyama, K. and D. H. MacLennan. Mutation of aspartic acid-351, lysine-352, and lysine-515 alters the Ca^{2+} transport activity of the Ca^{2+}-ATPase expressed in COS-1 cells. *Proc. Natl. Acad. Sci. U.S.A.* 85:3314–3318, 1988.
182. McIntosh, D. B., D. G. Woolley, and M. C. Berman. 2',3'-O-(2,4,6-trinitrophenyl)-8-azido-AMP and ATP photolabel Lys-492 at the active site of sarcoplasmic reticulum Ca^{2+}-ATPase. *J. Biol. Chem.* 267:5301–5309, 1992.
183. McIntosh, D. B., D. G. Woolley, B. Vilsen, and J. P. Andersen. Mutagenesis of segment 487Phe-Ser-Arg-Asp-Arg-Lys492 of sarcoplasmic reticulum Ca^{2+}-ATPase produces pumps defective in ATP binding. *J. Biol. Chem.* 271:25778–89, 1996.
184. Meissner, G. ATP and Ca^{2+} binding by the Ca^{2+} pump protein of sarcoplasmic reticulum. *Biochim. Biophys. Acta.* 298:906–26, 1973.
185. Meissner, G. Isolation and characterization of two types of sarcoplasmic reticulum vesicles. *Biochim. Biophys. Acta.* 389:51–68, 1975.
186. Mercadier, J. J., A. M. Lompre, P. Duc, K. R. Boheler, J. B. Fraysse, C. Wisnewsky, P. D. Allen, M. Komajda, and K. Schwartz. Altered sarcoplasmic reticulum Ca^{2+}-ATPase gene expression in the human ventricle during end-stage heart failure. *J. Clin. Invest.* 85:305–309, 1990.
187. Minamisawa, S., M. Hoshijima, G. Chu, C. A. Ward, K. Frank, Y. Gu, M. E. Martone, Y. Wang, J. Ross, Jr., E. G. Kranias, W. R. Giles, and K. R. Chien. Chronic phospholamban-sarcoplasmic reticulum calcium ATPase interaction is the critical calcium cycling defect in dilated cardiomyopathy. *Cell* 99: 313–322, 1999.
188. Minty, A. and L. Kedes. Upstream regions of the human cardiac actin gene that modulate its transcription in muscle cells: presence of an evolutionarily conserved repeated motif. *Mol. Cell. Biol.* 6:2125–2136, 1986.
189. Mitchinson, C., A. F. Wilderspin, B. J. Trinnaman, and N. M. Green. Identification of a labelled peptide after stoichiometric reaction of fluorescein isothiocyanate with the Ca^{2+}-dependent adenosine triphosphatase of sarcoplasmic reticulum. *FEBS Lett.* 146:87–92, 1982.
190. Mohraz, M., E. Arystarkhova, and K. J. Sweadner. Immunoelectron microscopy of epitopes on Na^+,K^+-ATPase catalytic subunit. Implications for the transmembrane organization of the C-terminal domain. *J. Biol. Chem.* 269:2929–2936, 1994.
191. Moorman, A. F., J. L. Vermeulen, M. U. Koban, K. Schwartz, W. H. Lamers, and K. R. Boheler. Patterns of expression of sarcoplasmic reticulum Ca^{2+}-ATPase and phospholamban mRNAs during rat heart development. *Circ. Res.* 76:616–625 1995.
192. Morris, G. L., H. C. Cheng, J. Colyer, and J. H. Wang. Phospholamban regulation of cardiac sarcoplasmic reticulum (Ca^{2+}-Mg^{2+}-ATPase. Mechanism of regulation and site of monoclonal antibody interaction. *J. Biol. Chem.* 266:11270–11275, 1991.
193. Movsesian, M. A., M. R. Bristow, and J. Krall. Ca^{2+} uptake by cardiac sarcoplasmic reticulum from patients with idiopathic dilated cardiomyopathy. *Circ. Res.* 65:1141–1144, 1989.
194. Murphy, A. J. Sarcoplasmic reticulum adenosine triphosphatase: labeling of an essential lysyl residue with pyridoxal-5'-phosphate. *Arch. Biochem. Biophys.* 180:114–120, 1977.
195. Nagai, R., A. Zarain Herzberg, C. J. Brandl, J. Fujii, M. Tada, D. H. MacLennan, N. R. Alpert, and M. Periasamy. Regulation

of myocardial Ca^{2+}-ATPase and phospholamban mRNA expression in response to pressure overload and thyroid hormone. *Proc. Natl. Acad. Sci. U.S.A.* 86:2966–2970, 1989.
196. Nakamoto, R. K. and G. Inesi. Retention of ellipticity between enzymatic states of the Ca^{2+}-ATPase of sarcoplasmic reticulum. *FEBS Lett.* 194:258–262, 1986.
197. Negash, S., L. T. Chen, D. J. Bigelow, and T. C. Squier. Phosphorylation of phospholamban by cAMP-dependent protein kinase enhances interactions between Ca^{2+}-ATPase polypeptide chains in cardiac sarcoplasmic reticulum membranes. *Biochemistry* 35:11247–11259, 1996.
198. Norregaard, A., B. Vilsen, and J. P. Andersen. Chimeric Ca$^+$-ATPase/Na$^+$,K$^+$-ATPase molecules. Their phosphoenzyme intermediates and sensitivity to Ca^{2+} and thapsigargin. *FEBS Lett.* 336:248–254, 1993.
199. O. Brien, P. J., C. D. Ianuzzo, G. W. Moe, T. P. Stopps, and P. W. Armstrong. Rapid ventricular pacing of dogs to heart failure: biochemical and physiological studies. *Can. J. Physiol. Pharmacol.* 68:34–39, 1990.
200. Odermatt, A., K., Kurzydlowski, and D. H. MacLennan, The v_{max} of the Ca^{2+}-ATPase of cardiac sarcoplasmic reticulum (SERCA2a) is not altered by Ca^{2+}/calmodulin-dependent phosphorylation or by interaction with phospholamban. *J. Biol. Chem.* 271:14206–14213, 1996.
201. Ogawa, H., D. L. Stokes, H. Sasabe, and C. Toyoshima. Structure of the Ca^{2+} pump of sarcoplasmic reticulum: a view along the lipid bilayer at 9-A resolution. *Biophys. J.* 75:41–52, 1998.
202. Ogurusu, T., S. Wakabayashi, and M. Shigekawa. Activation of sarcoplasmic reticulum Ca^{2+}-ATPase by Mn^{2+}: a Mn^{2+} binding study. *J. Biochem. Tokyo* 109:472–476, 1991.
203. Otsu, K., J. Fujii, M. Periasamy, M. Difilippantonio, M. Uppender, D. C. Ward, and D. H. MacLennan. Chromosome mapping of five human cardiac and skeletal muscle sarcoplasmic reticulum protein genes. *Genomics* 17:507–509, 1993.
204. Pedersen, P. L. and E. Carafoli. Ion motive ATPases. I. Ubiquity, properties, and significance to cell function. *Trends. Biochem. Sci.* 12:146–150, 1987.
205. Petithory, J. R. and W. P. Jencks. Binding of Ca^{2+} to the calcium adenosinetriphosphatase of sarcoplasmic reticulum. *Biochemistry* 27:8626–8635, 1988.
206. Petithory, J. R. and W. P. Jencks. Phosphorylation of the calcium adenosinetriphosphatase of sarcoplasmic reticulum: rate-limiting conformational change followed by rapid phosphoryl transfer. *Biochemistry* 25:4493–4497, 1986.
207. Pick, U. The interaction of vanadate ions with the Ca^{2+}-ATPase from sarcoplasmic reticulum. *J. Biol. Chem.* 257:6111–9, 1982.
208. Pick, U. and S. Bassilian. Modification of the ATP binding site of the Ca^{2+}-ATPase from sarcoplasmic reticulum by fluorescein isothiocyanate. *FEBS Lett.* 123:127–130, 1981.
209. Pick, U. and S. J. Karlish. Regulation of the conformation transition in the Ca^{2+}-ATPase from sarcoplasmic reticulum by pH, temperature, and calcium ions. *J. Biol. Chem.* 257:6120–6126, 1982.
210. Pick, U. and M. Weiss. Spectral and catalytical properties of the sarcoplasmic reticulum Ca^{2+}-ATPase labeled with N-cyclohexyl-N'-(4-dimethylamino-1-naphthyl)-carbodiimide. *Eur. J. Biochem.* 152:83–89, 1985.
211. Pickart, C. M. and W. P. Jencks. Energetics of the calcium-transporting ATPase. *J. Biol. Chem.* 259:1629–1643, 1984.
212. Pretorius, P. J. W. G. Pohl, C. S. Smithen, and G. Inesi. Structural and functional characterization of dog heart microsomes. *Circ. Res.* 25:487–499, 1969.
213. Racker, E. Reconstitution of a calcium pump with phospholipids and a purified Ca^{2+}-adenosine triphosphatase from sarcoplasmic reticulum. *J. Biol. Chem.* 247:8198–8200, 1972.
214. Reddy, L. G., L. R. Jones, S. E. Cala, O. B. JJ, S. A. Tatulian and D. L. Stokes. Functional reconstitution of recombinant phospholamban with rabbit skeletal Ca^{2+}-ATPase. *J. Biol. Chem.* 270:9390–9397, 1995.
215. Repke, D. I. and A. M. Katz. Calcium-binding and calcium-uptake by cardiac microsomes: a kinetic analysis. *J. Mol. Cell. Cardiol.* 4:401–416, 1972.
216. Rice, W. J. and D. H. MacLennan. Scanning mutagenesis reveals a similar pattern of mutation sensitivity in transmembrane sequences M4, M5, and M6, but not in M8, of the Ca^{2+}-ATPase of sarcoplasmic reticulum (SERCA1a). *J. Biol. Chem.* 271:31412–31419, 1996.
217. Rice, W. J., N. M. Green, and D. H. MacLennan. Site-directed disulfide mapping of helices M4 and M6 in the Ca^{2+} binding domain of SERCA1a, the Ca^{2+} ATPase of fast twitch skeletal muscle sarcoplasmic reticulum. *J. Biol. Chem.* 272:31412–31419, 1997.
218. Richardson, J. S. The anatomy and taxonomy of protein structure. *Adv. Protein Chem.* 34:167–339, 1981.
219. Rockman, H. A., K. R. Chien, D. J. Choi, G. Iaccarino, J. J. Hunter, J. Ross, Jr., R. J. Lefkowitz, and W. J. Koch. Expression of a beta-adrenergic receptor kinase 1 inhibitor prevents the development of myocardial failure in gene-targeted mice. *Proc. Natl. Acad. Sci. U.S.A.* 95:7000–70005, 1998.
220. Rohrer, D. and W. H. Dillmann. Thyroid hormone markedly increases the mRNA coding for sarcoplasmic reticulum Ca^{2+}-ATPase in the rat heart. *J. Biol. Chem.* 263:6941–6944, 1988.
221. Ross, D. C. and D. B. McIntosh. Intramolecular cross-linking at the active site of the Ca^{2+}-ATPase of sarcoplasmic reticulum. High and low affinity nucleotide binding and evidence of active site closure in E2-P. *J. Biol. Chem.* 262:12977–12983, 1987.
222. Sagara, Y., F. Fernandez Belda, L. de Meis, and G. Inesi. Characterization of the inhibition of intracellular Ca^{2+} transport ATPases by thapsigargin. *J. Biol. Chem.* 267:12606–12613, 1992.
223. Saito, A., M. Inui, M. Radermacher, J. Frank, and S. Fleischer. Ultrastructure of the calcium release channel of sarcoplasmic reticulum. *J. Cell. Biol.* 107:211–219, 1988.
224. Saito, A., S. Seiler, and S. Fleischer. Alterations in the morphology of rabbit skeletal muscle plasma membrane during membrane isolation. *J. Ultrastruct. Res.* 86:277–293, 1984.
225. Sasaki, T., M. Inui, Y. Kimura, T. Kuzuya, and M. Tada. Molecular mechanism of regulation of Ca^{2+} pump ATPase by phospholamban in cardiac sarcoplasmic reticulum. Effects of synthetic phospholamban peptides on Ca^{2+} pump ATPase. *J. Biol. Chem.* 267:1674–1679, 1992.
226. Seed, B. Purification of genomic sequences from bacteriophage libraries by recombination and selection in vivo. *Nucleic Acids Res.* 11:2427–2445, 1983.
227. Seiler, S., A. D. Wegener, D. D. Whang, D. R. Hathaway, and L. R. Jones. High molecular weight proteins in cardiac and skeletal muscle junctional sarcoplasmic reticulum vesicles bind calmodulin, are phosphorylated, and are degraded by Ca^{2+}-activated protease. *J. Biol. Chem.* 259:8550–8557, 1984.
228. Serrano, R. Structure and function of proton translocating ATPase in plasma membranes of plants and fungi. *Biochim. Biophys. Acta* 947:1–28, 1988.
229. Shigekawa, M. and J. P. Dougherty. Reaction mechanism of Ca^{2+}-dependent ATP hydrolysis by skeletal muscle sarcoplasmic reticulum in the absence of added alkali metal salts. III. Sequential occurrence of ADP-sensitive and ADP-insensitive phosphoenzymes. *J. Biol. Chem.* 253:1458–1464, 1978.
230. Shigekawa, M., J. A. Finegan, and A. M. Katz. Calcium transport ATPase of canine cardiac sarcoplasmic reticulum. A comparison with that of rabbit fast skeletal muscle sarcoplasmic reticulum. *J. Biol. Chem.* 251:6894–6900, 1976.
231. Shigekawa, M., S. Wakabayashi, and H. Nakamura. Effect of

divalent cation bound to the ATPase of sarcoplasmic reticulum. Activation of phosphoenzyme hydrolysis by Mg^{2+}. *J. Biol. Chem.* 258:14157–14161, 1983.
232. Simmerman, H. K., J. H. Collins, J. L. Theibert, A. D. Wegener, and L. R. Jones. Sequence analysis of phospholamban. Identification of phosphorylation sites and two major structural domains. *J. Biol. Chem.* 261:13333–13341, 1986.
233. Simmerman, H. K., Y. M. Kobayashi, J. M. Autry, and L. R. Jones. A leucine zipper stabilizes the pentameric membrane domain of phospholamban and forms a coiled-coil pore structure. *J. Biol. Chem.* 271:5941–5946, 1996.
234. Simmerman, H. K., D. E. Lovelace, and L. R. Jones. Secondary structure of detergent-solubilized phospholamban, a phosphorylatable, oligomeric protein of cardiac sarcoplasmic reticulum. *Biochim. Biophys. Acta* 997:322–329, 1989.
235. Snyder, A. P., D. R. Sudnick, V. K. Arkle, and W. D. Horrocks, Jr. Lanthanide ion luminescence probes. Characterization of metal ion binding sites and intermetal energy transfer distance measurements in calcium-binding proteins. 2. Thermolysin. *Biochemistry* 20:3334–3339, 1981.
236. Solaro, R. J. and F. N. Briggs. Estimating the functional capabilities of sarcoplasmic reticulum in cardiac muscle. Calcium binding. *Circ. Res.* 34:531–540, 1974.
237. Sommer, J. R. and R. B. Jennings. Ultrastructure of cardiac muscle. In H. Fozzard, R. Jenny, B. Hader, A. Katz and H. Morgan, eds. *The Heart and Cardiovascular System.* New York: Raven, 1986:61–100.
237a. Soulié, S., J.-M. Neuman, C. Berthomieu, J. Møller, M. le Maire, and V. Forge. NMR conformational study of the sixth transmembrane segment of sarcoplasmic reticulum Ca^{2+}-ATPase. *Biochemistry* 38:5813–5821, 1999.
238. Squier, T. C., D. J. Bigelow, F. J. Fernandez Belda, L. deMeis, and G. Inesi. Calcium and lanthanide binding in the sarcoplasmic reticulum ATPase. *J. Biol. Chem.* 265:13713–13720, 1990.
239. Squier, T. C., D. J. Bigelow, J. Garcia de Ancos, and G. Inesi. Localization of site-specific probes on the Ca^{2+}-ATPase of sarcoplasmic reticulum using fluorescence energy transfer. *J. Biol. Chem.* 262:4748–4754, 1987.
240. Squier, T. C. and D. D. Thomas. Relationship between protein rotational dynamics and phosphoenzyme decomposition in the sarcoplasmic reticulum Ca^{2+}-ATPase. *J. Biol. Chem.* 263:9171–9177, 1988.
241. Stryer, L. Fluorescence energy transfer as a spectroscopic ruler. *Annu. Rev. Biochem.* 47:819–846, 1978.
242. Suko, J. The calcium pump of cardiac sarcoplasmic reticulum. Functional alterations at different levels of thyroid state in rabbits. *J. Physiol. Lond.* 228:563–582, 1973.
243. Suko, J. and W. Hasselbach. Characterization of cardiac sarcoplasmic reticulum ATP-ADP phosphate exchange and phosphorylation of the calcium transport adenosine triphosphatase. *Eur. J. Biochem.* 64:123–130, 1976.
244. Sumbilla, C., T. Cantilina, J. H. Collins, H. Malak, J. R. Lakowicz, and G. Inesi. Structural perturbation of the transmembrane region interferes with calcium binding by the Ca^{2+} transport ATPase. *J. Biol. Chem.* 266:12682–12689, 1991.
245. Sumbilla, C., L. Lu, D. E. Lewis, G. Inesi, T. Ishii, K. Takeyasu, Y. Feng, and D. M. Fambrough. Ca^{2+}-dependent and thapsigargin-inhibited phosphorylation of $Na^+,K(+)$-ATPase catalytic domain following chimeric recombination with Ca^{2+}-ATPase. *J. Biol. Chem.* 268:21185–21192, 1993.
246. Sumida, M., T. Wang, F. Mandel, J. P. Froehlich, and A. Schwartz. Transient kinetics of Ca^{2+} transport of sarcoplasmic reticulum. A comparison of cardiac and skeletal muscle. *J. Biol. Chem.* 253:8772–8777, 1978.
247. Sutherland, E. W. and T. W. Rall. The relation of adenosine-3',5'-phosphate and phosphorylase to the actions of catecholamines and other hormones. *Pharmacol. Rev.* 12:265–299, 1960.
248. Suzuki, T. and J. H. Wang. Stimulation of bovine cardiac sarcoplasmic reticulum Ca^{2+} pump and blocking of phospholamban phosphorylation and dephosphorylation by a phospholamban monoclonal antibody. *J. Biol. Chem.* 261:7018–7023, 1986.
249. Tada, M., M. Inui, M. Yamada, M. Kadoma, T. Kuzuya, H. Abe, and S. Kakiuchi. Effects of phospholamban phosphorylation catalyzed by adenosine 3':5'-monophosphate- and calmodulin-dependent protein kinases on calcium transport ATPase of cardiac sarcoplasmic reticulum. *J. Mol. Cell. Cardiol.* 15:335–46, 1983.
250. Tada, M., M. Kadoma, M. Inui, and J. Fujii. Regulation of Ca^{2+}-pump from cardiac sarcoplasmic reticulum. *Methods Enzymol.* 157:107–154, 1988.
251. Tada, M. and A. M. Katz. Phosphorylation of the sarcoplasmic reticulum and sarcolemma. *Annu. Rev. Physiol.* 44:401–423, 1982.
252. Tada, M., M. A. Kirchberger, and A. M. Katz. Phosphorylation of a 22,000-dalton component of the cardiac sarcoplasmic reticulum by adenosine 3':5'-monophosphate-dependent protein kinase. *J. Biol. Chem.* 250:2640–2647, 1975.
253. Tada, M., M. A. Kirchberger, and H. C. Li. Phosphoprotein phosphatase-catalyzed dephosphorylation of the 22,000 dalton phosphoprotein of cardiac sarcoplasmic reticulum. *J. Cyclic Nucleotide Res.* 1:329–338, 1975.
254. Tada, M., M. A. Kirchberger, D. I. Repke, and A. M. Katz. The stimulation of calcium transport in cardiac sarcoplasmic reticulum by adenosine 3':5'-monophosphate-dependent protein kinase. *J. Biol. Chem.* 249:6174–6180, 1974.
255. Tada, M., F. Ohmori, M. Yamada, and H. Abe. Mechanism of the stimulation of Ca^{2+}-dependent ATPase of cardiac sarcoplasmic reticulum by adenosine 3':5'-monophosphate-dependent protein kinase. Role of the 22,000-dalton protein. *J. Biol. Chem.* 254:319–326, 1979.
256. Tada, M., M. Yamada, M. Kadoma, M. Inui, and F. Ohmori. Calcium transport by cardiac sarcoplasmic reticulum and phosphorylation of phospholamban. *Mol. Cell. Biochem.* 46:73–95, 1982.
257. Tada, M., M. Yamada, F. Ohmori, T. Kuzuya, M. Inui, and H. Abe. Transient state kinetic studies of Ca^{2+}-dependent ATPase and calcium transport by cardiac sarcoplasmic reticulum. Effect of cyclic AMP-dependent protein kinase-catalyzed phosphorylation of phospholamban. *J. Biol. Chem.* 255:1985–1992, 1980.
258. Tada, M., T. Yamamoto, and Y. Tonomura. Molecular mechanism of active calcium transport by sarcoplasmic reticulum. *Physiol. Rev.* 58:1–79, 1978.
259. Tanabe, T., K. G. Beam, B. A. Adams, T. Niidome, and S. Numa. Regions of the skeletal muscle dihydropyridine receptor critical for excitation-contraction coupling. *Nature* 346:567–569, 1990.
260. Taylor, K. A., L. Dux, and A. Martonosi. Three-dimensional reconstruction of negatively stained crystals of the Ca^{2+}-ATPase from muscle sarcoplasmic reticulum. *J. Mol. Biol.* 187:417–427, 1986.
261. Taylor, K. A., L. Dux, S. Varga, H. P. Ting Beall, and A. Martonosi. Analysis of two-dimensional crystals of Ca^{2+}-ATPase in sarcoplasmic reticulum. *Methods Enzymol.* 157:271–289, 1988.
262. Taylor, K. A., N. Mullner, S. Pikula, L. Dux, C. Peracchia, S. Varga, and A. Martonosi. Electron microscope observations on Ca^{2+}-ATPase microcrystals in detergent-solubilized sarcoplasmic reticulum. *J. Biol. Chem.* 263:5287–5294, 1988.
263. Taylor, S. S., D. R. Knighton, J. Zheng, L. F. Ten Eyck, and

J. M. Sowadski. Structural framework for the protein kinase family. *Annu. Rev. Cell. Biol.* 8:429–462, 1992.
264. Taylor, W. R. and N. M. Green. The predicted secondary structures of the nucleotide-binding sites of six cation-transporting ATPases lead to a probable tertiary fold. *Eur. J. Biochem.* 179:241–248, 1989.
265. Teruel, J. A. and J. C. Gomez Fernandez. Distances between the functional sites of sarcoplasmic reticulum (Ca^{2+} + Mg^{2+})-ATPase and the lipid/water interface. *Biochim. Biophys. Acta* 863:178–84, 1986.
266. Thastrup, O., P. J. Cullen, B. K. Drobak, M. R. Hanley, and A. P. Dawson. Thapsigargin, a tumor promoter, discharges intracellular Ca^{2+} stores by specific inhibition of the endoplasmic reticulum Ca^{2+}-ATPase. *Proc. Natl. Acad. Sci. U.S.A.* 87:2466–2470, 1990.
267. Thomas, D. D. Rotational diffusion of membrane proteins. In: R. Cherry and I. Ragan, eds. *Techniques for Analysis of Membrane Proteins.* London: Chapman and Hall. 1986:377–431.
268. Thomas, D. D. and C. Hidalgo. Rotational motion of the sarcoplasmic reticulum Ca^{2+}-ATPase. *Proc. Natl. Acad. Sci. U.S.A.* 75:5488–5492, 1978.
269. Tomlinson, C. W., D. V. Godin, and S. W. Rabkin. Adriamycin cardiomyopathy: implications of cellular changes in a canine model with mild impairment of left ventricular function. *Biochem. Pharmacol.* 34:4033–4041, 1985.
270. Toyofuku, T., K. Curotto Kurzydlowski, N. Narayanan, and D. H. MacLennan. Identification of Ser38 as the site in cardiac sarcoplasmic reticulum Ca^{2+}-ATPase that is phosphorylated by Ca^{2+}/calmodulin-dependent protein kinase. *J. Biol. Chem.* 269:26492–26496, 1994.
271. Toyofuku, T., D. D. Doyle, R. Zak, and L. Kordylewski. Expression of phospholamban mRNA during early avian muscle morphogenesis is distinct from that of alpha-actin. *Dev. Dyn.* 196:103–113, 1993.
272. Toyofuku, T., K. Kurzydlowski, J. Lytton, and D. H. MacLennan. The nucleotide binding/hinge domain plays a crucial role in determining isoform-specific Ca^{2+} dependence of organellar Ca^{2+}-ATPases. *J. Biol. Chem.* 267:14490–14496, 1992.
273. Toyofuku, T., K. Kurzydlowski, M. Tada, and D. H. MacLennan. Amino acids Glu2 to Ile18 in the cytoplasmic domain of phospholamban are essential for functional association with the Ca^{2+}-ATPase of sarcoplasmic reticulum. *J. Biol. Chem.* 269:3088–3094, 1994.
274. Toyofuku, T., K. Kurzydlowski, M. Tada, and D. H. MacLennan. Amino acids Lys-Asp-Asp-Lys-Pro-Val402 in the Ca^{2+}-ATPase of cardiac sarcoplasmic reticulum are critical for functional association with phospholamban. *J. Biol. Chem.* 269:22929–22932, 1994.
275. Toyofuku, T., K. Kurzydlowski, M. Tada, and D. H. MacLennan. Identification of regions in the Ca^{2+}-ATPase of sarcoplasmic reticulum that affect functional association with phospholamban. *J. Biol. Chem.* 268:2809–2815, 1993.
276. Toyofuku, T., and R. Zak. Characterization of cDNA and genomic sequences encoding a chicken phospholamban. *J. Biol. Chem.* 266:5375–5383, 1991.
277. Toyoshima, C., H. Sasabe, and D. L. Stokes. Three-dimensional cryo-electron microscopy of the calcium ion pump in the sarcoplasmic reticulum membrane [published erratum appears in *Nature* 1993 May 20;363(6426):286]. *Nature* 362:467–471, 1993.
277a. Toyoshima, C., M. Nakasato, H. Nomura, and H. Ogawa. Crystal structure of the calcium pump of sarcoplasmic reticulum at 2.6 Å resolution. *Nature* 405:647–655, 2000.
278. Tsien, R. W. Cyclic AMP and contractile activity in heart. *Adv. Cyclic Nucleotide Res.* 8:363–420, 1977.
279. Van Winkle, W. B., C. A. Tate, R. J. Bick, and M. L. Entman. Nucleotide triphosphate utilization by cardiac and skeletal muscle sarcoplasmic reticulum. Evidence for a hydrolysis cycle not coupled to intermediate acyl phosphate formation and calcium translocation. *J. Biol. Chem.* 256:2268–2274, 1981.
280. Verboomen, H., F. Wuytack, H. De Smedt, B. Himpens, and R. Casteels. Functional difference between SERCA2a and SERCA2b Ca^{2+} pumps and their modulation by phospholamban. *Biochem. J.* 286:591–559 1992.
281. Verboomen, H., F. Wuytack, J. A. Eggermont, S. De Jaegere, L. Missiaen, L. Raeymaekers, and R. Casteels. cDNA cloning and sequencing of phospholamban from pig stomach smooth muscle. *Biochem. J.* 262:353–356, 1989.
282. Verjovski Almeida, S., M. Kurzmack, and G. Inesi. Partial reactions in the catalytic and transport cycle of sarcoplasmic reticulum ATPase. *Biochemistry* 17:5006–5013, 1978.
283. Vilsen, B., J. P. Andersen, D. M. Clarke, and D. H. MacLennan. Functional consequences of proline mutations in the cytoplasmic and transmembrane sectors of the Ca^{2+}-ATPase of sarcoplasmic reticulum. *J. Biol. Chem.* 264:21024–21030, 1989.
284. Vilsen, B., J. P. Andersen, and D. H. MacLennan. Functional consequences of alterations to amino acids located in the hinge domain of the Ca^{2+}-ATPase of sarcoplasmic reticulum. *J. Biol. Chem.* 266:16157–16164, 1991.
285. Vorherr, T., M. Chiesi, R. Schwaller, and E. Carafoli. Regulation of the calcium ion pump of sarcoplasmic reticulum: reversible inhibition by phospholamban and by the calmodulin binding domain of the plasma membrane calcium ion pump. *Biochemistry* 31:371–376, 1992.
286. Voss, J., W. Birmachu, D. M. Hussey, and D. D. Thomas. Effects of melittin on molecular dynamics and Ca^{2+}-ATPase activity in sarcoplasmic reticulum membranes: time-resolved optical anisotropy. *Biochemistry* 30:7498–7506, 1991.
287. Voss, J., L. R. Jones, and D. D. Thomas. The physical mechanism of calcium pump regulation in the heart [see comments]. *Biophys. J.* 67:190–196, 1994.
288. Wakabayashi, S., T. Ogurusu, and M. Shigekawa. Factors influencing calcium release from the ADP-sensitive phosphoenzyme intermediate of the sarcoplasmic reticulum ATPase. *J. Biol. Chem.* 261:9762–9769, 1986.
289. Watanabe, T. and G. Inesi. The use of 2′,3′-O-(2,4,6-trinitrophenyl) adenosine 5′-triphosphate for studies of nucleotide interaction with sarcoplasmic reticulum vesicles. *J. Biol. Chem.* 257:11510–11516, 1982.
290. Watanabe, T., D. Lewis, R. Nakamoto, M. Kurzmack, C. Fronticelli, and G. Inesi. Modulation of calcium binding in sarcoplasmic reticulum adenosinetriphosphatase. *Biochemistry* 20:6617–6625, 1981.
291. Watanabe, Y., Y. Kijima, M. Kadoma, M. Tada, and T. Takagi. Molecular weight determination of phospholamban oligomer in the presence of sodium dodecyl sulfate: application of low-angle laser light scattering photometry. *J. Biochem. Tokyo* 110:40–45, 1991.
292. Weaver, A. J., M. D. Kemple, and F. G. Prendergast. Fluorescence and ^{13}C NMR determination of side-chain and backbone dynamics of synthetic melittin and melittin analogues in isotropic solvents. *Biochemistry* 28:8624–8639, 1989.
293. Weber, A. Energized calcium transport and relaxaing factors. *Curr. Top. Bioenerg.* 1:203–254, 1966.
294. Weber, A. Regulatory mechanisms of the calcium transport system of fragmented rabbit sarcoplasmic rticulum. I. The effect of accumulated calcium on transport and adenosine triphosphate hydrolysis. *J. Gen. Physiol.* 57:50–63, 1971.
295. Weber, G. Energetics of ligand binding to proteins. *Adv. Protein Chem.* 29:1–83, 1975.
296. Wegener, A. D., H. K. Simmerman, J. Liepnieks, and L. R.

Jones. Proteolytic cleavage of phospholamban purified from canine cardiac sarcoplasmic reticulum vesicles. Generation of a low resolution model of phospholamban structure. *J. Biol. Chem.* 261:5154–5159, 1986.

297. Wegener, A. D., H. K. Simmerman, J. P. Lindemann, and L. R. Jones. Phospholamban phosphorylation in intact ventricles. Phosphorylation of serine 16 and threonine 17 in response to beta-adrenergic stimulation [published erratum appears in *J. Biol. Chem.* 1989 Sep 15;264(26):15738]. *J. Biol. Chem.* 264:11468–11474, 1989.

298. Weintraub, H., R. Davis, S. Tapscott, M. Thayer, M. Krause, R. Benezra, T. K. Blackwell, D. Turner, R. Rupp, S. Hollenberg, et al. The myoD gene family: nodal point during specification of the muscle cell lineage. *Science* 251:761–766, 1991.

299. Whitmer, J. T., P. Kumar, and R. J. Solaro. Calcium transport properties of cardiac sarcoplasmic reticulum from cardiomyopathic Syrian hamsters (BIO 53.58 and 14.6): evidence for a quantitative defect in dilated myopathic hearts not evident in hypertrophic hearts. *Circ. Res.* 62:81–85, 1988.

300. Will, H., J. Blanck, G. Smettan, and A. Wollenberger. A quench-flow kinetic investigation of calcium ion accumulation by isolated cardiac sarcoplasmic reticulum. Dependence of initial velocity on free calcium ion concentration and influence of preincubation with a protein kinase, Mg^{2+}ATP, and cyclic AMP. *Biochim. Biophys. Acta* 449:295–303, 1976.

301. Williams, R. W., J. O. McIntyre, B. P. Gaber, and S. Fleischer. The secondary structure of calcium pump protein in light sarcoplasmic reticulum and reconstituted in a single lipid component as determined by Raman spectroscopy. *J. Biol. Chem.* 261:14520–14524, 1986.

302. Witcher, D. R., R. J. Kovacs, H. Schulman, D. C. Cefali, and L. R. Jones. Unique phosphorylation site on the cardiac ryanodine receptor regulates calcium channel activity. *J. Biol. Chem.* 266:11144–11152, 1991.

303. Xu, A., C. Hawkins, and N. Narayanan. Phosphorylation and activation of the Ca^{2+}-pumping ATPase of cardiac sarcoplasmic reticulum by Ca^{2+}/calmodulin-dependent protein kinase. *J. Biol. Chem.* 268:8394–8397, 1993.

304. Xu, Z. C. and M. A. Kirchberger. Modulation by polyelectrolytes of canine cardiac microsomal calcium uptake and the possible relationship to phospholamban. *J. Biol. Chem.* 264:16644–16651, 1989.

305. Yamamoto, H., M. Tagaya, T. Fukui, and M. Kawakita. Affinity labeling of the ATP-binding site of Ca^{2+}-transporting ATPase of sarcoplasmic reticulum by adenosine triphosphopyridoxal: identification of the reactive lysyl residue. *J. Biochem. Tokyo* 103:452–457, 1988.

306. Yamamoto, T. and Y. Tonomura. Reaction mechanism of the Ca^{2+}-dependent ATPase of sarcoplasmic reticulum from skeletal muscle. I. Kinetic studies. *J. Biochem. Tokyo* 62:558–575, 1967.

307. Young, H. S., L. G. Reddy, L. R. Jones, and D. L. Stokes. Co-reconstitution and co-crystallization of phospholamban and Ca^{2+}-ATPase. In: R. G. Johnson, and E. G. Kranias, eds. *Cardiac Sarcoplasmic Reticulum Function and Regulation of Contractility. Ann. N.Y. Acad. Sci.* vol. 853:103–115, 1998.

308. Young, R. C., R. F. Ozols, and C. E. Myers. The anthracycline antineoplastic drugs. *N. Engl. J. Med.* 305:139–153, 1981.

309. Yu, X., S. Carroll, J. L. Rigaud, and G. Inesi. H^+ countertransport and electrogenicity of the sarcoplasmic reticulum Ca^{2+} pump in reconstituted proteoliposomes. *Biophys. J.* 64:1232–1242, 1993.

310. Zak, R. Factors controlling cardiac growth. In: R. Zak, ed. *Growth of the Heart in Health and Disease.* New York: Raven Press. 1984:165–185.

311. Zarain Herzberg, A., D. H. MacLennan, and M. Periasamy. Characterization of rabbit cardiac sarco(endo)plasmic reticulum Ca^{2+}-ATPase gene. *J. Biol. Chem.* 265:4670–4677, 1990.

312. Zhang, P., C. Toyoshima, K. Yonekura, N. M. Green, and D. L. Stokes. Structure of the calcium pump from sarcoplasmic reticulum at 8−°A resolution. *Nature* 392:835–839, 1998.

313. Zimniak, P. and E. Racker. Electrogenicity of Ca^{2+} transport catalyzed by the Ca^{2+}-ATPase from sarcoplasmic reticulum. *J. Biol. Chem.* 253:4631–4637, 1978.

9. Regulation of cellular calcium in cardiac myocytes

DONALD M. BERS | *Department of Physiology, Loyola University Chicago, Maywood, Illinois*

CHAPTER CONTENTS

General Aspects of Cellular Calcium Regulation
   Ca transport systems
   Cytosolic volume conventions
   Ca binding sites and buffering in cardiac myocytes
   Ca requirements for contractile activation
   Simplified kinetic considerations during a Ca transient
Sarcolemmal Ca Transport Systems
   Ca channels
      Types of Ca channels
      Ca current inactivation
      Amount of Ca entry during the ventricular action potential
      Ca channel regulation
   Na/Ca exchange
      Fundamental characterizations
      Cloning and structure/function
      Thermodynamics and Ca flux during action potentials
   Sarcolemmal Ca-ATPase
Intracellular Ca Transporters
   Sarcoplasmic reticulum Ca-ATPase and Sarcoplasmic reticulum Ca content
   Regulation of the SR Ca-ATPase
   Measurement of SR Ca transport in cells
   SR Ca content under physiological conditions
   Sarcoplasmic reticulum Ca release channels
      Amount of Ca released during E-C coupling
   Mitochondrial Ca transport
Ca Removal from the Cytoplasm During Relaxation
   Relative contributions of Ca transporters
      Quantitative analysis of cellular Ca fluxes during relaxation
   Species, developmental, and temperature dependence
   Ca recycling from mitochondria back to the SR
The Ca Supply that Activates Contraction
   Ca influx *vs* SR Ca release
      Quantitative analysis of cellular Ca fluxes
      Pharmacological interference with SR Ca release
   Fraction of SR Ca released during a twitch
Perturbations of Cellular Ca Balance
   Rest-dependent changes in cellular and SR Ca content
   Refilling depleted internal Ca stores
   Rest-decay and rest-potentiation of twitches
   Force-frequency relationships

CALCIUM (Ca) is a ubiquitous intracellular second messenger, important in the regulation of numerous cellular processes in virtually all living cells. Other chapters deal in more specific detail with certain key individual Ca-dependent processes in the heart. These include calcium channels and Na/Ca exchange in the sarcolemma, the Ca-ATPase pump and Ca release channels of the sarcoplasmic reticulum (SR), the process of excitation–contraction coupling (E-C coupling), and the activation of the contractile proteins by Ca. The aim of this chapter is to integrate some aspects of the calcium transport systems and their key regulatory sites into a comprehensive and somewhat quantitative picture of overall a calcium regulation in cardiac myocytes.

GENERAL ASPECTS OF CELLULAR CALCIUM REGULATION

Ca Transport Systems

Figure 9–1 summarizes the known basic calcium transport pathways in cardiac myocytes. Calcium can enter the cardiac myocyte during the action potential by sarcolemmal Ca channels or by the electrogenic Na/Ca exchange process. Calcium that enters the cell also triggers release of additional Ca from the SR, and this amplification of the Ca influx signal is what is often referred to as *excitation–contraction coupling*, although that term really applies to the whole process from electrical excitation to the resulting contractile force generated by the myofilaments. The combination of Ca influx and SR Ca release provide the Ca that activates contraction by binding to the Ca regulatory site on troponin C, in the thin filament. The degree of contractile activation depends on the amount of Ca bound to troponin C, and contraction can continue as either shortening or force production as long as Ca remains bound. The normal driving function for relaxation is transport of Ca out of the cytosol. As free cytosolic [Ca] ([Ca]$_i$) declines, Ca dissociates from troponin C and relaxation occurs. There are physical and Ca-independent kinetic factors that also contribute to mechanical relaxation, but these are better dealt with in Chapters 6 and 11 and will not be discussed here.

There are four main Ca transport systems responsible for removal of Ca from the cytoplasm in cardiac muscle. These are (*1*) the SR Ca-ATPase, (*2*) the sarcolemmal Na/Ca exchange, (*3*) the sarcolemmal Ca-ATPase, and (*4*) the mitochondrial Ca uniport system

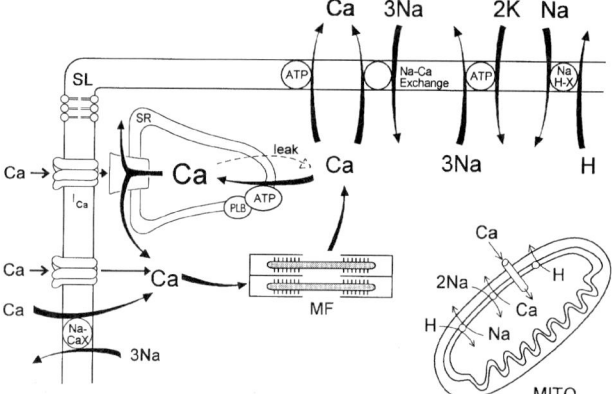

FIG. 9-1. Simplified cardiac myocyte Ca fluxes. Ca enters during the action potential via I_{Ca} and Na/Ca exchange (Na/CaX). Ca entry triggers Ca release from the SR and the combination activates the myofilaments (MF). Elevated $[Ca]_i$ stimulates Ca removal from the cytosol by the SR Ca-ATPase (modulated by phospholamban, PLB), the Na/Ca exchange, the sarcolemmal Ca-ATPase, and the mitochondrial uniporter. As $[Ca]_i$ declines Ca dissociates from the myofilaments allowing relaxation. The sarcolemmal (Na + K)ATPase and Na/H exchange are also indicated, along with other key mitochondrial ion transporters. [Modified from Bers (34).]

(17, 20, 34). The relative contributions of these Ca removal systems will be discussed more quantitatively below, but the SR Ca-ATPase (Chapter 8) and the sarcolemmal Na/Ca exchange (Chapter 10) are the dominant processes.

Cytosolic Volume Conventions

Before discussion of the amounts of Ca transport required to activate contraction and which are transported in and out of the cytosol during the normal cardiac cycle, it is useful to consider the volume that this transport occurs in. Measurements of Ca transport are made using numerous different preparations and techniques that have different advantages and disadvantages. Somehow, all of this information must be brought back to a common framework for overall quantitative consideration.

We usually talk about free concentrations of ions in moles per liter of volume. Inside the cell it makes sense then to consider $[Ca]_i$ in nM or μM and total cytosolic Ca in similar units, i.e. $\mu mol/liter$ cytosolic volume. Fabiato (104) suggested excluding mitochondrial volume as not readily accessible. Since mitochondria occupy 30%–35% of total cell volume in ventricular myocytes (summarized in Table 2 of Bers [34] and see ref. 14), this constitutes a substantial decrease from total cell volume. Nuclear volume is about 2% of cell volume in rat ventricular myocytes (249), but Ca probably passes through nuclear pores such that this volume should not be excluded. The SR also occupies 1%–3.5% of cell volume (see ref. 34, Table 2). While the SR is clearly a separate compartment, its absolute volume is less accurately known, and since it is small, it makes less difference whether it is included or not. Thus for cytosolic volume we typically use the non-mitochondrial cell volume. The myofilament space, which occupies almost 50% of the cell volume, is considered to be part of the cytosol.

When considering Ca fluxes into and out of the cytosolic compartment of ventricular myocytes, several different units have been used, depending on the type of preparation and experimental measurements. For example, Ca transport by SR vesicles may be reported in nmol Ca/mg SR protein, while integrated Ca current may be reported in pCoul/pF (or fmol/pF). Table 9-1 shows convenient conversion factors for some of the most commonly used units and preparations. These values are somewhat mixed with respect to species but are generally based on measurements from either rabbit or rat ventricle. The choice I have made here for the common units for Ca fluxes in Table 9-1 is somewhat arbitrary as described above, but reflects the cellular focus for this chapter. Another value that falls out of these calculations is the concentration of protein in a ventricular myocyte (109 mg cell protein/ml total cell volume; and either 9.2 µl cell volume or 5.95 µl cytosol per mg cell protein). It is my hope that putting these conversion factors in this format will be generally useful.

Ca Binding Sites and Buffering in Cardiac Myocytes

As in all cells Ca is very highly buffered in the cardiac myocyte. Indeed, while the free [Ca] transient in cardiac myocytes may go from a diastolic value of 100 nM to a peak near 1 µM, it takes 50–100 µM added to the cytosol to produce this change (see Fig. 9-9; Table 9-2). Having established some convention about cytosolic volume units, we can consider the cytosolic Ca binding sites in terms of their concentrations (in µmol/liter cytosol or simply µM) and using affinities in terms of their equilibrium dissociation constants (K_d, in µM).

While one of the main motivating factors is to assess the Ca requirements for activation of contraction, we must recognize that Ca that enters the cytosol may bind to any of numerous Ca binding ligands in addition to the Ca regulatory site on cardiac troponin C. Two general strategies have been used to evaluate intracellular Ca buffering: (1) calculations using the Ca binding properties of known cellular constituents based on measurements in isolated systems (104) and (2) attempts to directly measure the total Ca buffering properties in ventricular muscle or myocytes approaching in situ conditions (29, 145, 266). These

TABLE 9–1. *Conversion of Ca Fluxes from Different Units to a Common One*

Preparation	Measurement Units	Multiply by This Factor for Units μmol/Liter Cytosol
Ventricular muscle	μmol/kg wet weight	2.43[a]
Ventricular muscle	μmol/kg dry weight	0.49[b]
Ventricular homogenate	nmol/mg homog pn	292[c]
Ventricular myocytes	nmol/mg cell pn	168[d]
Subcellular fractions (e.g. SR or SL)	nmol/mg SR pn	29.2[e]
Ventricular myocytes	fmol/pF	7046[f]

[a] Using ventricular density, extracellular space measurements (109, 186) and 35% of cell volume occupied by mitochondria (249, 251). [1.06 kg wet wt/liter vent][1 liter vent/0.67 liter cell][1 liter cell/0.65 liter non-mito volume] = 2.434 or 2.509 kg wet wt/liter cytosol as in Fabiato (104) via a more complicated calculation. Without exclusion of mitochondrial volume the value is 1.58 kg wet wt/liter total cell volume.

[b] Similar to above, but including wet weight: dry weight = 5 (ref 183)

[c] Using [120 mg homog pn/g wet wt][2.4 kg wet wt/liter cytosol] = 292 g homog pn/liter cytosol.

[d] Using the 1.83-fold and 1.66-fold purification of dihydropyridine and ryanodine receptors in isolated myocytes (44, 145) [0.574 mg cell pn/mg vent homog pn][120 mg homog pn/g wet wt][2.43 kg wet wt/liter cytosol] = 168 g cell pn/ liter cytosol.

[e] Assuming a 10-fold purification factor for e.g. SR or sarcolemma (SL). [1 mg SR pn/10 mg homog protein][120 mg homog pn/g wet wt][2.43 g wet wt/ml cytosol] = 29.2 mg SR protein/ml cytosol]. More generically the conversion factor is 292/x, where x is the purification factor for a given organelle.

[f] Using 4.58 pF/pl for rabbit ventricular myocytes (294) [4.58 pF/pl][1 liter cell/0.65 liter cytosol] = 7.046 pF/pl cytosol [×1000 (pl/liter)(μmol/fmol)]. Satoh et al. (294) found higher values for ferret (5.39 pF/pl), young rats (6.76 pF/pl), and older rats (8.88 pF/pl), and these values are slightly different from the stereological measurements of Page (239) in rabbit and rat (0.6 and 0.46 μm²/μm³, respectively) which correspond to 6 and 4.6 pF/pl assuming 1 μF/cm² for cell membrane capacitance).

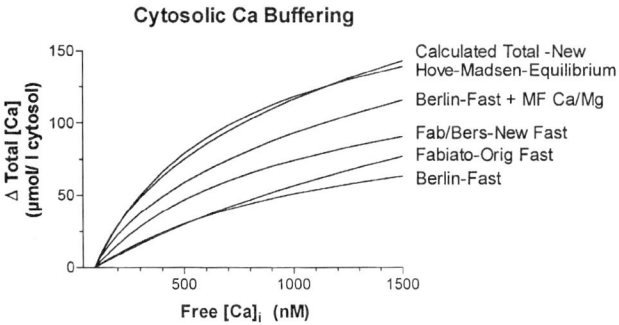

FIG. 9–2. Passive Ca buffering in cardiac myocytes. The six curves represent different estimates of how passive Ca buffering changes as [Ca]$_i$ increases from 100 to 1500 nM. These values are indicated as increments above the amount of Ca bound at 100 nM [Ca]$_i$ (see also Table 9–2 and discussion in text). Fabiato-Orig Fast, Berlin-Fast and Hove-Madsen-Equilibrium are taken directly from values in the relevant papers (29, 104, 145). Fab/Bers-New Fast updates some binding constants from the original estimates of Fabiato (104), as described in the text. Berlin-Fast+MF Ca/Mg adds known myofilament sites at which Ca and Mg compete. Calculated Total-New refers to values resulting from constants in Table 9–2.

approaches are described in the paragraphs that follow, and I will try to synthesize them into a current "best guess" composite that combines the two approaches.

Fabiato (104) made the first concerted effort to estimate the Ca requirements for contractile activation by collecting data concerning known concentrations and Ca binding characteristics of the following cardiac myocyte constituents: cardiac troponin C, the SR Ca-ATPase, calmodulin, ATP, creatine phosphate, and sarcolemmal sites (see lower Fabiato curve in Fig 9–2). This was an extremely useful first approximation and indicated that a total of ~57 μM total Ca would be required to raise free [Ca]$_i$ from 100 nM to 1 μM (or for activation of 70% of maximal contraction). However, it seems likely that this estimated Ca buffering is somewhat low, because there must be additional Ca binding sites in the cell not on the above list, which Fabiato did not account for, and because the K$_d$ values for Ca binding to troponin C and the SR Ca-ATPase used by Fabiato (2 μM and 1 μM, respectively) were probably too high (see below and Table 9–2). The curve labeled "Fab/Bers-New Fast" in Figure 9–2, is an update of the Fabiato compilation. It includes lower K$_d$ values for both the SR Ca-ATPase and the regulatory site on troponin C (0.6 μM), based on generally lower K$_d$ values in SR Ca transport studies (e.g. 146, 212) and in situ estimates of myofilament Ca sensitivity (116, 362). I have also updated the sarcolemmal Ca binding to include a slightly lower total, based on recent measurements of inner sarcolemmal sites from Post and Langer (269; B$_{max}$ = 42 μM, K$_d$ = 13 μM) and our own measured at low [Ca] (35 and Bers, unpublished; B$_{max}$ = 15 μM, K$_d$ = 0.3 μM). I also refer to this calculated total estimate as "fast buffering" since the major contributors are expected to bind rapidly (see below concerning slow binding).

Pierce et al. (266) were the first to try a direct Ca titration of whole ventricular homogenate (as well as particulate and soluble fractions). Their study might be expected to overestimate intracellular Ca buffering, because they include titration of sites on the external cell surface and additional non-myocyte sites as well. However, they would also include (appropriately) intracellular sites not included by Fabiato (104). This approach was refined somewhat by Hove-Madsen and Bers (145), where they performed similar Ca titrations on isolated ventricular myocytes that were permeabilized by digitonin and where SR and mitochondrial Ca transport were blocked by thapsigargin and ruthenium red, respectively. These equilibrium binding results of

Hove-Madsen and Bers (145; see the top curves in Figure 9-2) were a bit lower than reported by Pierce et al. (266), but might still include some external sarcolemmal sites. On the other hand, such external sarcolemmal sites may be small since passive Ca binding to the sarcolemma is asymmetric, with the Ca binding phospholipids situated almost exclusively on the inner sarcolemmal surface (268). As Hove-Madsen and Bers (145) pointed out, the SR Ca binding might be underestimated in the presence of thapsigargin, since this agent appears to lock the SR Ca-ATPase in a Ca-free E_1 state (168, 290). One of the upper curves in Figure 9-2 is labeled "Equilibrium," because these measurements were made on a very slow time scale and would thus be expected to include both rapidly and slowly equilibrating sites.

Berlin et al. (29) used a single cell intracellular titration strategy to assess intracellular Ca buffering using the fluorescent Ca indicator indo-1 and voltage clamp. They blocked the transport of Ca by the SR Ca-pump, Na/Ca exchange, sarcolemmal Ca-ATPase, and mitochondria respectively using thapsigargin, Na-free solutions, high $[Ca]_o$, and a mitochondrial uncoupler. Then they measured total Ca injected into the cytoplasm via I_{Ca} (using voltage clamp) and the change in free $[Ca]_i$ produced (Fig. 9-3A). Stepwise increases in $[Ca]_i$ accompany the I_{Ca} traces. Closer inspection of these $[Ca]_i$ steps (e.g. Fig 9-3B) reveals a rapid phase of $[Ca]_i$ increase followed by a slow decline. They argued that the rapid increase, which was in phase with the integral of Ca influx via I_{Ca}, was associated with very rapid Ca buffering. Note that entry of 9 µM total Ca only raises free $[Ca]_i$ by 0.1 µM, corresponding to 90:1 Ca buffering. Focusing on this rapid phase, Berlin et al. (29) used only the initial rapid $\Delta[Ca]_{bound}/\Delta[Ca]_i$ component to identify a mean lumped cytosolic buffering with a B_{max} = 123 µM and K_d = 960 nM (see bottom curve in Figure 9-2). Their results agree well with the fast buffering calculated by Fabiato (104).

The sag in $[Ca]_i$ in Figure 9-3B could be due to either a slower phase of Ca buffering or incomplete inhibition of Ca transport out of the cytosol. Berlin et al. (29) set up and tested conditions to ensure block of such transport, so residual transport is expected to be extremely small. It is reasonable to expect slow Ca buffering by sites initially occupied by Mg or protons. This is because Mg or H must dissociate before Ca can bind. This is why EGTA is a slower Ca buffer than BAPTA (i.e. it exists mainly as H_2EGTA at neutral pH). Troponin C and myosin both have divalent cation binding sites at which Ca and Mg compete (often referred to as "Ca/Mg" or "cal-mag" sites; 141, 142, 256). The Ca/Mg sites on troponin C and myosin are expected to bind Ca slowly because they are nearly saturated with

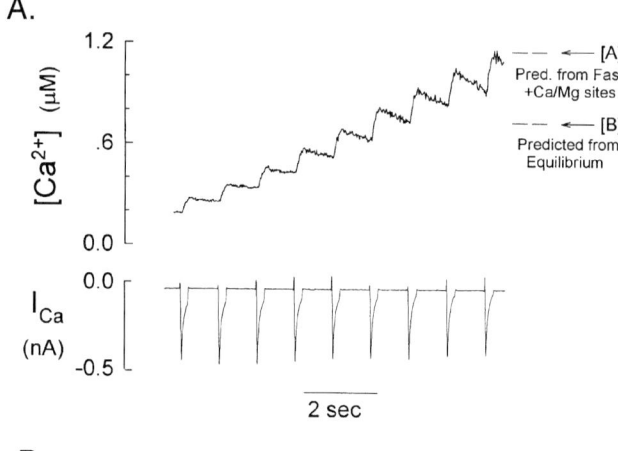

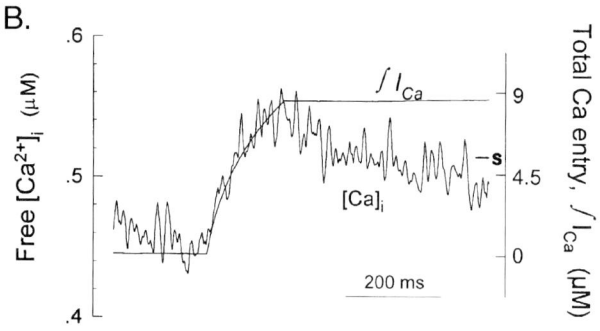

FIG. 9-3. Measurement of fast Ca buffering in a voltage clamped rat ventricular myocyte. Cells were exposed to 10 µM thapsigargin to prevent SR Ca uptake and were in Na-free conditions (inside and out) to prevent Na/Ca exchange. A. Voltage clamp pulses (200 ms from -40 to 0 mV) activated I_{Ca} and produced nearly step-like increases in $[Ca]_i$. B: The integral of the I_{Ca} from the fourth pulse in A ($\int I_{Ca}$) follows the kinetics of the rise in $[Ca]_i$. The sag in the $[Ca]_i$ trace may represent slow buffering that is not in phase with Ca entry via I_{Ca}. The "S" indicates where $[Ca]_i$ would be predicted to fall to eventually if the slow buffering by myofilament Ca/Mg sites are included with the fast buffering measured (see text). The points marked [A] and [B] in panel A are the predicted final settling points for $[Ca]_i$ if the slow buffering is included for the total $\int I_{Ca}$ throughout the train (as for S) and when the equilibrium buffering from Fig 9-2 and Table 9-2 is assumed, respectively [Modified from Berlin et al. (29).]

either Ca or Mg at resting levels of $[Ca]_i$ (285; and see Table 9-2). Simple inclusion of these sites along with the measured fast buffering sites in the cell in Figure 9-3B would cause $[Ca]_i$ to fall to the small horizontal line indicated with an "S" in the figure. Inclusion of these myofilament Ca/Mg sites would also move the overall buffering curve up, as indicated by the "Berlin-Fast + MF Ca/Mg" trace in Figure 9-2. This still doesn't explain all of the equilibrium buffering measured by Hove-Madsen and Bers (145) or all of the apparent slow buffering in Figure 9-3. For example, in Figure 9-3A the overall increase in $[Ca]_i$ expected from the total integrated Ca influx from the 9 pulses by the end of the trace would be to 1.75 µM for just the measured fast sites (off the scale of the graph). Inclusion of the calculated myofilament Ca/Mg sites would predict a final $[Ca]_i$ of 1.15 µM, indicated by [A] in Figure 9–3A. Clearly, free $[Ca]_i$ is falling below the [A] level, but perhaps not all the way down to the level predicted by the equilibrium buffering, [B]. There may well be additional slow Ca/Mg buffers such as the Mg-sensitive Ca binding sites on the inner sarcolemmal surface (35, 110) or other sites that contribute to equilibrium Ca binding (145).

Of course these calculations depend on accurate knowledge of the Ca, H and Mg affinities of the various binding sites, as well as on what the conditions are in the cell. For example, if the Mg affinity of the Ca/Mg sites is underestimated, then the "Berlin-Fast+ Ca/Mg" curve in Figure 9–2 could move up to the "Equilibrium" curve (29). Also, when Robertson et al. (285) did detailed calculations of the time course of Ca binding to cardiac myofilaments, they assumed that diastolic $[Ca]_i$ was 10 nM and free $[Mg]_i$ was 2 mM. This led them to predict that the Ca/Mg sites on troponin C were 91% saturated with Mg with little bound Ca at rest. Based on more recent data, diastolic $[Ca]_i$ is probably between 100 and 150 nM, and free $[Mg]_i$ is probably about 0.5 mM (49, 116, 226, 227). This means that at diastole, the Ca/Mg sites on troponin C would be 84% saturated with Ca and only 5% with Mg (see Table 9–2). Obviously the kinetics of binding will also be important to clarify further.

There is also a subtle additional consideration as to what really constitutes the accessible cytosolic volume. Our standard cytosolic volume defined above only excludes the cellular space occupied by mitochondria (~35%). If we also exclude the volume occupied by the SR (3.5%, ref 249) and physically occupied by the concentrated protein in the cytosol (~10%–15%), the

TABLE 9–2. *Passive Intracellular Ca Buffering*[a]

	K_d (µM)	B_{max}	Ca Bound at 100 nM $[Ca]_i$	at 1 µM $[Ca]_i$	Difference
			µmol Ca/Liter cytosol[b]		
FAST					
Troponin C	0.6	70	10	43.9	33.9
SR Ca-pump	0.6	47	6.8	29.6	22.8
Calmodulin total[c]	0.1–1	24	0.45	3.57	3.1
ATP	200	5,000	0.35	3.46	3.1
Creatine phosphate	71,073	12,000	0.02	0.17	0.2
Sarcolemma[d]	13	42	0.32	3.0	2.7
Membrane/High[e]	0.3	15	3.7	11.5	7.8
Free $[Ca]_i$	—		0.1	1.0	0.9
Fast total			21.7	96.2	74.5
SLOW: Ca/Mg					
Troponin C: Ca[f]	0.013	140	117	137	20
Mg (Mg bound)	1111		Mg 7.1	Mg – 0.8	
Myosin: Ca[g]	0.033	140	3	25	22
Mg (Mg bound)	3.64		Mg – 136	Mg – 114	
Slow total			120	162.2	42
Total Ca					117

[a] These constants describe the "Calculated Total-New" curve in Fig. 9–2. The values are mostly taken from references 34 and 104 and other sources noted in the text. Binding was calculated assuming [K] = 140 mM and [Mg] = 0.5 mM, where relevant (e.g. ATP, creatine phosphate, calmodulin, Ca/Mg sites).

[b] See Table 9–1 for unit conversion factors.

[c] Calmodulin results are from four classes of binding sites, which also exhibit specific affinities for Mg and K, and these characteristics were accounted for using the constants compiled by Fabiato (104) and Haiech et al. (126).

[d] Inner sarcolemmal binding measured by Post and Langer (269).

[e] This is based initially on our estimates of sarcolemmal Ca binding at low [Ca] with K_d ~0.3 µM. The B_{max} was reduced from our earlier estimates (34) because the moderate affinity sarcolemmal sites from Post and Langer (269) are now included. This modest B_{max} value was also adjusted some to make the calculated total buffering match the equilibrium measurements (top two traces in Fig. 9–2). These sites could also include some unaccounted for high-affinity sites from other sources.

[f] K_d values are from Pan and Solaro (256).

[g] Values are from Holroyde et al. (141) and Robertson et al. (285).

values for the curves in Figure 9-2 would have to be shifted up by another 15%–20%. The protein volume is based on cytosolic [protein] of 120 mg/ml cytosol and density of 1.2 g protein/ml. This would bring the "Berlin-Fast + MF Ca/Mg" up to the top "Calculated" curve and values in Table 9-2. Thus, it should be clear that these estimates of cellular Ca buffering have certain caveats and the quantitative considerations here are meant only to be a current "best guess" guide, subject to further clarification.

So how much total Ca is required to raise $[Ca]_i$ from 100 nM to 1 µM and produce a contraction (and to what does Ca bind)? It should be noted that the "slow" buffering discussed here is still occurring over only a few hundred msec and may thus be relevant to overall Ca fluxes during contraction. Thus, the bottom three curves in Figure 9-2 really serve as lower limits. Probably the real overall buffering relationship falls somewhere in the range of the upper three curves. For simple projections over the physiological range of $[Ca]_i$ it is satisfactory to use a single lumped Michaelis equation (Ca bound = $B_{max}/(1 + K_d/[Ca])$) with B_{max} = 232 µM and K_d = 455 nM (which fits the Hove-Madsen-Equilibrium data and which we routinely use) or one with two terms B_{max1} = 145 µM and K_{d1} = 22.3 nM and B_{max2} = 218 µM and K_{d2} = 1625 nM (for a curve more like Berlin-Fast + MF Ca/Mg). These will calculate total binding at a given [Ca] and produce the ΔCa total values in Figure 9-2 when the Ca bound at 100 nM is subtracted. These simple equations do not specify what Ca is binding to, but they predict that 94–117 µM Ca must be added to the cytosol to raise $[Ca]_i$ from 100 nM to 1 µM (> 100:1 Ca buffering). The Ca-buffering is also non-linear over the physiological range so 65–85 µM is still needed to produce half of that rise in $[Ca]_i$ (i.e. from 100 to 550 nM).

To be more specific about the binding sites and what might happen as $[Ca]_i$ rises from 100 nM to 1 µM, I have compiled some values in Table 9-2. While the specific assignment of binding sites is still provisional and subject to further refinement, this table provides a practical working model for the present. Not surprisingly, the proteins that show the largest change in bound Ca between 100 nM and 1 µM are the regulatory Ca binding sites on troponin C and the SR Ca-pump (which are present at 70 and 47 µM in the cytosol). However, these sites only account for about 50% of the total overall change in bound Ca (and 75% of the fast buffering). It can also be seen that even at the resting $[Ca]_i$ (100 nM) there is a substantial amount of Ca already bound (142 µM), with much of that at the Ca/Mg sites of troponin C. Furthermore, there are several constituents that don't make a large impact by themselves (e.g. calmodulin, ATP, and sarcolemma), but collectively make a buffering contribution that should not be considered negligible. These calculations are based on 0.5 mM $[Mg]_i$ at pH of 7–7.2 and mostly at room temperature. Obviously, changing conditions may also be expected to change the cytosolic Ca buffering.

Ca Requirements for Contractile Activation

It may also be noted that with the binding constants used in Table 9-2 10 µM Ca is already bound to troponin C at 100 nM $[Ca]_i$. In principle this might be expected to change resting activation of the myofilaments. However, Figure 9-4A shows that with the steep cooperativity reported for the myofilament Ca sensitivity in intact ventricular muscle (116, 362), there would still be less than 0.1% of maximal force at 100 nM $[Ca]_i$.

Figure 9-4A illustrates the impact of the Hill coefficient on the [Ca] dependence of cardiac myofilaments. Typically, measurements made in chemically skinned cardiac muscle fibers are fit with a Hill equation (Force = $F_{max}/\{1 + (K_m/[Ca])^n\}$) with a Hill coefficient (n) of ~2–3 and half-maximal force at K_m ~1–2 µM (e.g. 103, 129). Measurements of the myofilament Ca sensitivity in intact ventricular muscle have given both a higher affinity (K_m~0.6 µM) and Hill coefficient (n = 4–6), indicating greater cooperativity (8, 116, 362). The result is a very steep dependence of force on [Ca] between 300 an 800 nM (see Fig., 9-4A). The issue of cooperativity in tension development is further addressed in Chapter 7 and 11. Here I focus on the amount of Ca required for activation.

Figure 9-4B shows force as a function of the amount of Ca added to the cytosol from an initial free [Ca] of 150 nM using the Ca buffering from Table 9-2 and Figure 9-2 (Calculated-Total-New). It can be seen that very little force is developed with the first 30 µM Ca supplied. As the amount of Ca increases the relationship is fairly steep, such that most of the force development occurs between 40 and 80 µM of added Ca. The steady-state twitch in mammalian ventricular muscle is typically sufficient to reach ~40% of maximal force at 25°–30°C (129). This would require a free $[Ca]_i$ of 540 nM and about 62 µM of added total Ca. To reach 600 nM $[Ca]_i$ (the K_m for force in Figure 9-4) would require between 31 and 74 µM for the six curves in Figure 9-2 (from 150 nM resting $[Ca]_i$). Thus, while there are several quantitative points that could be known more precisely, a reasonable current estimate of the Ca that must be added to the cytosol to activate a normal ventricular twitch is 60 µM.

It should also be recognized that many factors can

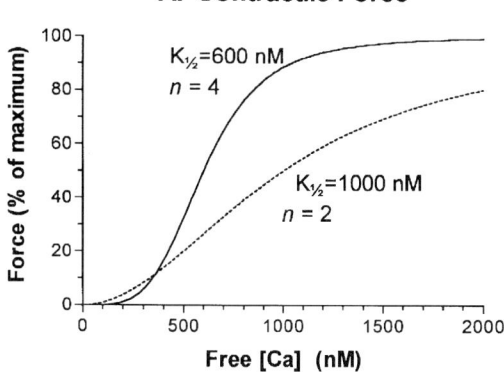

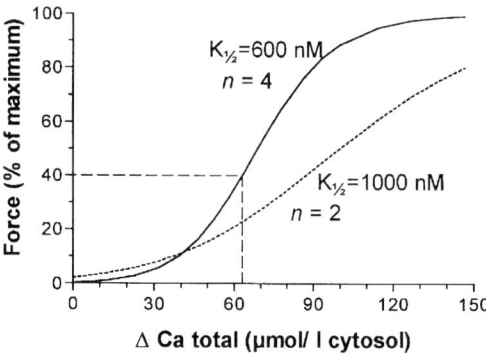

FIG. 9–4. Free and total Ca requirements for myofilament activation in cardiac myocytes. *A*: Two different sets of parameters are used for the Hill equation ($100/(1 + (K_m/[Ca])^n)$) describing the steady-state relationship between force and [Ca]. The *solid* curve ($K_m = 600$ nM and $n = 4$) is more consistent with recent estimates in intact ventricular muscle, whereas the lower *dotted* curve ($K_m = 1000$ nM and $n = 2$) is closer to traditional data from skinned muscle fibers (see text). *B*. The same relationships as in *A*, but the free [Ca] axis has been altered to account for the cytosolic Ca buffering relationship (Calculated-Total-New in Figure 9–2 and Table 9–2). Thus, this predicts the force as a function of the total amount of Ca added to the cytosol from a resting level of 150 nM free [Ca]. Coincidentally, almost the same curves are obtained if resting [Ca]$_i$ is assumed to be 100 nM and the intermediate buffering curve from Figure 9–2 is used (Berlin-Fast+MF Ca/Mg).

alter the cytosolic Ca buffering and Ca requirements for myofilament activation, such as pH and Mg. Under normal conditions intracellular pH is 7.1–7.2 and intracellular free [Mg] is probably ~0.5 mM (49, 116, 226, 227). Both acidosis and increased [Mg]$_i$ can occur in pathophysiological situations and would be expected to reduce cytosolic Ca buffering by competition. Elevated [Mg]$_i$ can occur as a consequence of decline in [ATP], most of which is bound to Mg under normal conditions (227). Of course there may be temperature- and species-dependent differences in cytosolic buffering, but these have not been addressed in a systematic manner.

Simplified Kinetic Considerations During a Ca Transient

So far I have dealt with cytosolic Ca buffering in a steady-state manner in Figures 9–2 and 9–4, without explicit consideration of kinetic aspects. Figure 9–5 shows a simplified kinetic model of a myocyte Ca transient. The starting point is a generic free [Ca]$_i$ signal, which starts at 100 nM, rises to a peak of 744 nM at 70 ms, and falls exponentially with a time constant $\tau = 300$ ms. This free [Ca]$_i$ transient is used as the driving function to determine Ca binding to the various cytosolic sites listed in Table 9–2 (e.g. using the expression $d[Ca\text{-}TnC]/dt = k_{on} \times [Ca]_i \times [TnC] - k_{off} \times [Ca\text{-}TnC]$). Not all of the kinetic parameters have been directly measured, so some approximations are used. Figure 9–5A shows the timecourse of free [Ca]$_i$ as well as the change in total cytoplasmic [Ca] (ΔTotal Ca$_{cyt}$) after considering on- and off-rates for Ca (and Mg) binding to the cellular ligands (see Table 9–3). Figure 9–5B shows how Ca bound to different ligands varies dynamically during the Ca transient. From these figures it can be appreciated that free [Ca]$_i$ peaks earlier than total cytosolic Ca and also comes back to near initial value faster due to these kinetic considerations. Relatively slow buffering can also create a "ratcheting" up of total cytosolic Ca (e.g. see Ca/Mg sites). This would be expected to be influenced by stimulation frequency. In this case the total cytosolic Ca is 6.5 μM higher at the end of 2 sec than it was before the pulse, and 5.3 μM of this is still bound to TnC Ca/Mg sites, with 1.1 μM still bound to myosin Ca/Mg sites.

Figure 9–5C adds a simplified consideration of Ca fluxes that may underlie the Ca transient in Figure 9–5A. This also serves as an introduction to the following sections where these fluxes will be addressed more directly. The fluxes in Figure 9–5C were calculated in the following manner (see Table 9–3): Ca current (I$_{Ca}$) was assumed to reach a peak of 6.8 pA/pF with a rising and falling time constants of 3 and 40 ms, respectively (bringing in a total of 16 μM Ca; ref 360). The Ca transported by the SR Ca-ATPase was calculated using a classic Michaelis-Menten relationship with a V$_{max}$ of 210 μM/sec, a K$_m$ of 300 nM, and a Hill coefficient of 2 (11, 17). The SR Ca leak was set to counterbalance the resting SR Ca-ATPase rate (21 μM/sec) and was allowed to vary in direct proportion to the calculated intra-SR free [Ca] ([Ca]$_{SR}$). The initial SR Ca content was set at 100 μmol/liter cytosol (24) with passive intra-SR Ca buffering (B$_{max}$ = 180 μmol/liter cytosol and K$_d$ = 600 μM; ref 305). The SR Ca release flux in this particular model ends up being predicted simply as the amount of change in total cytosolic [Ca] required for the initial free [Ca]$_i$ waveform and not accounted for by either I$_{Ca}$, SR Ca-ATPase, or SR Ca leak.

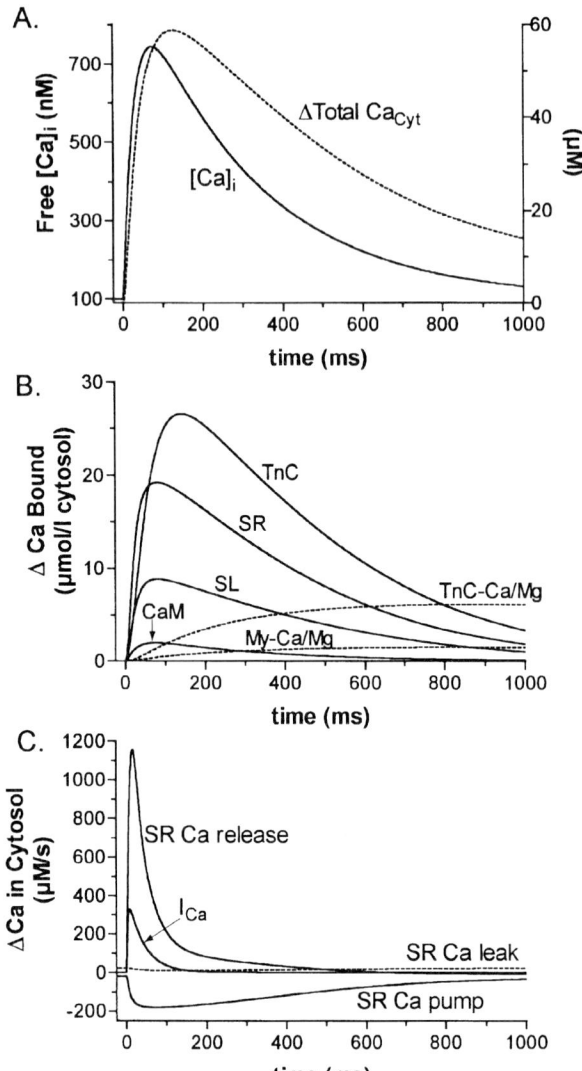

FIG. 9–5. Cytosolic Ca buffering and transport during a Ca transient. A. A Ca transient is calculated from the product of a rising and declining exponential which rises from 100 to 744 nM and back with time constants (τ) of 30 ms (rising) and 300 ms (falling). This was used as a driving function to calculate the time-dependent changes in binding to various cytosolic buffers (B) using the rate constants and concentrations in Table 9–3 (TnC is troponin C, SL is total sarcolemmal site in Table 9–3, CaM is calmodulin, TnC-Ca/Mg and My-Ca/Mg are Ca binding to Ca/Mg sites on TnC and myosin). The change in total cytosolic [Ca] (ΔTotal Ca_{Cyt} in A) is the sum of the curves in B and the free $[Ca]_i$ curve. C: Ca fluxes associated with the Ca transient. I_{Ca} activation was calculated by a rising (τ = 3 ms) and falling exponential (τ = 40 ms), peaking at 6.8 pA/pF and bringing in 16 μmol/l cytosol. The SR Ca-pump rate was $210/(1+(300\ nM/[Ca]_i)^2)$ in mol/l cytosol. The SR Ca leak was initiated to counterbalance the SR Ca-pump rate at rest, and changed linearly as a function of free [Ca] in the SR (based on intra-SR Ca buffering with a K_d = 600 μM and B_{max} equivalent to 180 μmol/l cytosol in an SR volume occupying 3.5% of cell volume). The SR Ca release flux was taken as the residual Ca flux required to produce the driving Ca transient.

TABLE 9–3. *Kinetic Parameters Used for Figure 9–5*[a]

	B_{max} (μM)	K_d (μM)	k_{off} (sec^{-1})	k_{on} (μM^{-1}sec^{-1})	Reference
Troponin C	70	0.6	19.6	32.7	116,285
Troponin C Ca/Mg	140	0.0135	0.032	2.37	256,285
(Mg sites)		1111	3.33	0.003	256,285
Myosin Ca/Mg	140	0.0333	0.46	13.8	285
(Mg sites)		3.64	0.057	0.0157	285
SR Ca-pump	47	0.6	60	100	Diffusion
Calmodulin total[b]	24	7	238	34	126
Sarcolemma	42	13	1300	100	269
Membrane/High	15	0.3	30	100	34,35

FLUX CALCULATIONS

SR Ca-ATPase	V = (210 μM/s)/(1 + {0.3 μM /[Ca]}^{2})
Ca current	I_{Ca} = (9 pA/pF) exp(−t/40 ms)(1−exp[−t/3 ms])
SR Ca leak	at t = 0 set at SR Ca-ATPase rate, changes proportional to $[Ca]_{SR}$
SR Ca content	initially 100 μM/liter cytosol; $[Ca]_{SR\text{-}bound}$ = 180 μM/(1 + 0.6 mM/$[Ca]_{SR}$) SR volume taken as 3.5% of cell volume
SR Ca release	Δtotal cytosolic Ca (accounting for I_{Ca}, SR Ca-ATPase and leak)

[a] B_{max} and K_d values are generally the same as in Table 9–2. In most cases values are only available for k_{on} or k_{off} such that the other was calculated using $K_d = k_{off}/k_{on}$. If neither k_{on} or k_{off} were available, diffusion limited k_{on} (100 μM^{-1}sec^{-1}) and K_d were used.
[b] The four Ca-calmodulin binding sites were lumped as a single site. The K_d was artificially increased so that the steady-state Ca-calmodulin binding was well predicted over the relevant range of $[Ca]_i$ (0.1 to 3 μM) without requiring separate kinetic calculations of Mg and K competition at each of the four sites (although these equilibrium interactions were included in Table 9–2 and Figures 9–2 and 9–4).

Thus, the SR Ca release flux is the residual of the calculations, but is similar to experimental estimates (e.g. 352).

In this section I have tried to summarize some quantitative information about Ca balance in the range of physiological $[Ca]_i$. This includes conventions for quantitative units with respect to cell volume, passive Ca buffering, and Ca requirements for activation of the myofilaments. The kinetic and Ca flux considerations in Figure 9–5 also lead into the discussion of flux of Ca across the various cellular membranes, which is the focus of the remainder of this chapter.

SARCOLEMMAL Ca TRANSPORT SYSTEMS

There are three main sarcolemmal Ca transport systems: (1) Sarcolemmal Ca channels provide a pathway for Ca influx down the electrochemical gradient. (2) Sarcolemmal Na/Ca exchange can move Ca either into or out of the cell, depending on the membrane potential (E_m) and the [Na] and [Ca] gradients. (3) The sarcolemmal Ca-ATPase can pump Ca out of the myocyte up an electrochemical gradient using the energy stored in ATP. While other cellular systems can affect the net Ca transport by these systems, these three systems are the final pathways that directly mediate the Ca fluxes across the cell membrane.

Ca Channels

Types of Ca Channels. There are two principal types of voltage-dependent Ca channels in cardiac myocytes. These are known as the L-type and the T-type (27, 28, 239), and many characteristics of these channels are described in chapters 14 and 18. Here I will only introduce the properties in a general way and focus more on the contribution of these channels to cellular Ca balance. There may also be some other channels that can permit Ca influx to occur, such as background or leak channels, stretch-activated channels and channels activated by extracellular ATP (e.g. 111). However, since the quantitative contribution of these channels to cellular Ca balance is not well characterized yet, I will not discuss them further.

T-type Ca channels are characterized by their transient timecourse, a threshold E_m for activation that is relatively negative, and a tiny single-channel conductance (240). In contrast L-type Ca channels generally have a longer lasting current, less negative E_m for activation, larger single-channel conductance, and are also sensitive to dihydropyridines such as nifedipine and Bay K 8644 (28, 343). L-type I_{Ca} appears to be prominent in all cardiac myocytes, whereas T-type I_{Ca} is present to variable extents and in only some cardiac myocytes.

Figure 9–6 A and B shows experimental separation of T-type and L-type I_{Ca} in dog atrial myocytes and also in dog Purkinje fiber cells, where T-type I_{Ca} is particularly prominent (about half of the L-type I_{Ca}). Two different holding E_m are used in each case. The I_{Ca} available from the more positive holding E_m (−30 or −50 mV) is taken to be L-type I_{Ca}, whereas that from E_m of −80 or −90 is a combination of L- and T-type I_{Ca}. Subtraction of the two traces then gives the T-type I_{Ca}, and the current-voltage relationships for both are shown on the right in Figure 9–6A and B. It should also be noted that since L-type I_{Ca} inactivation is Ca-dependent (see under Ca current Inactivation and Chapter 14), it also shows a relatively transient nature in cardiac myocytes. For this reason, it is most useful in separating these currents to use barium as the charge-carrying ion (as in Figure 9–6A), so that differences in both the voltage-dependence and the much slower inactivation of L-type I_{Ba} can be more easily discerned (28).

A. Dog Atrium (115 mM Ba; Bean, 1985)

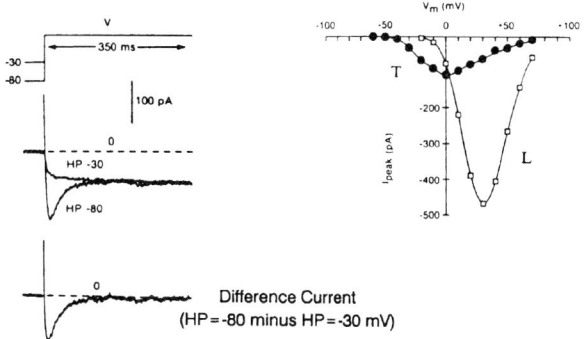

B. Dog Purkinje Fiber (2 mM Ca; Hirano et al., 1989)

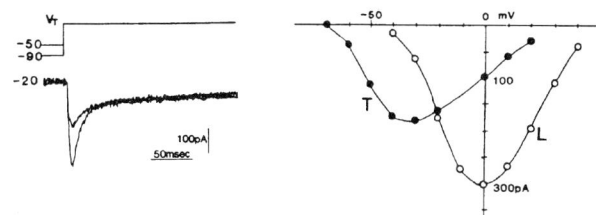

C. Several Species (Total I_{Ca})

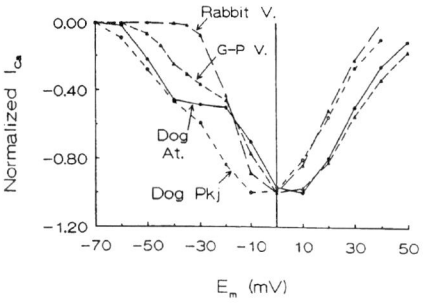

FIG. 9–6. Currents via T-and L-type Ca channels. *A*. Barium currents (with 115 mM Ba) induced by depolarizations to various test potentials from holding potentials of 80 or 30 mV. The E_m protocol is shown in the *top trace*, the currents in the *middle trace*, and the difference between these currents in the *bottom panel*. Peak I_{Ba} from 30 mV is attributed to L-type Ca channels and the additional transient difference current activated from 80 mV is attributed to T-type Ca channels. [From Bean (27), with permission.] *B*: I_{Ca} in dog Purkinje fiber cell with 2 mM Ca as charge carrier. [From Hirano et al. (139), with permission.] The more positive E_m required in I_{Ba} is due to the higher surface potential in 2 mM Ca vs 115 mM Ba. C: I_{Ca} from several species (from 80 to 100 mV), where the hump at ~−40 mV is due to T-type current and differs among the tissues studied. Dog Purkinje (ref. 139) and rabbit ventricle (G. M. Briggs and D. M. Bers, unpublished) are in 2 mM Ca. Dog atrium (ref. 27) and guinea-pig ventricle (from Mitra & Morad, 218) are with 5 mM Ca, but are shifted by 10 mV to compensate for surface potential differences. [From Bers (34) with permission).]

The function of the T-type I_{Ca} is not known. However, since it seems to be most prominent in either conductive or pacemaker cell types in the heart, it has often been speculated that it may serve those functions (125). Figure 9–6C illustrates that in addition to Purkinje fibers T-type I_{Ca} can be measured in atrial myocytes from some species (e.g. dog and guinea pig) and even a small amount in ventricular myocytes from the guinea pig (27, 28, 218). However, T-type I_{Ca} seems to be absent in ventricular myocytes from most species (e.g. bullfrog, calf, cat, rabbit, rat, and ferret) and also in atrial cells from calf and rabbit (28, 241, 358, 360). Thus T-type current is not a factor in most ventricular myocytes. Furthermore, quantitative Ca flux via T-type I_{Ca} in ventricular myocytes may be negligible anyway, since these channels would inactivate very rapidly during the peak of the action potential, and in conjunction with the low electrochemical driving force the net Ca influx would be extremely small. Thus, I will not consider it further in terms of cellular Ca balance.

Under normal conditions most of the Ca influx occurring during the ventricular muscle action potential is due to L-type I_{Ca}. This can be appreciated by considering the typical observation of many investigators that blocking Ca influx with nifedipine can virtually abolish contraction (but see later, under Na/Ca Exchange, and 34a). This is true even when participation of the SR Ca stores (which would complicate the assessment of Ca influx) is inhibited and there is a substantial SR independent contraction before I_{Ca} blockade (41).

Ca Current Inactivation. Inactivation of cardiac I_{Ca} is both voltage-dependent and Ca-dependent (123, 165, 187). It is increasingly clear that Ca-dependent inactivation is the dominant component under physiological conditions. This can be appreciated in a simplistic manner from Figure 9–7, which shows normalized currents through Ca channels with different charge carriers and conditions.

Figure 9–7 shows that I_{Ca} inactivates much faster than I_{Ba} at $E_m = 0$ mV. This can be attributed to Ca-dependent inactivation of the cardiac L-type Ca channels. Even in the ruptured patch with $[Ca]_i$ heavily buffered by 10 mM EGTA in the pipette, I_{Ca} inactivates faster than I_{Ba}. In the perforated patch, where the cell contracts and there are normal Ca transients, I_{Ca} inactivates much faster still. This is probably a consequence of even stronger Ca-dependent inactivation in the absence of exogenous Ca buffer and with both Ca entry and SR Ca release functioning. The mean halftimes of current decline were 17, 37, and 161 ms for I_{Ca} (perforated patch), I_{Ca} (ruptured patch + EGTA) and I_{Ba}, respectively (359). The fact that Ca-dependent inactivation is still so strong even when cytosolic Ca transients are strongly buffered by 10 mM EGTA in-

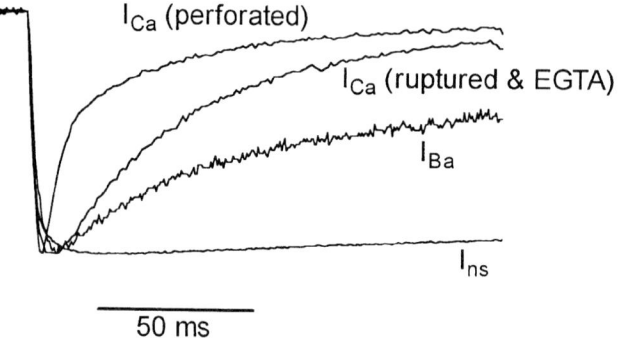

FIG. 9–7. Ca channel inactivation with different charge carriers. Normalized current amplitudes measured at 0 mV (except I_{ns} at −30 mV to match activation state). I_{Ca} was recorded under both perforated patch (allowing normal SR Ca release and Ca transients) and ruptured patch with cells dialyzed with 10 mM EGTA (to prevent global Ca transients). I_{Ba} was also recorded with ruptured patch (with 10 mM EGTA in the pipette). Extracellular [Ca] and [Ba] were both 2 mM and I_{ns} was measured in divalent-free conditions (10 mM EDTA inside and out) with $[Na]_o$ at 20 mM and $[Na]_i$ at 10 mM. Peak currents were 1370, 808, 780, and 5200 pA and were attained at 5, 7, 10, and 14 ms for I_{Ca} (perforated), I_{Ca} (ruptured), I_{Ba} and I_{ns} respectively. Halftimes of current decline were 17, 37, 161, and >500 ms, respectively. [Recordings made by Dr. W. Yuan.]

dicates that the site must be very close to the inner mouth of the Ca channel. Indeed, a key site that seems to be responsible for Ca-dependent I_{Ca} inactivation has been identified to be a region in the carboxy tail of the α_1-subunit of the cardiac L-type Ca channel (91). Recent work has also directly implicated calmodulin bound to the L-type Ca channel as the mediator of Ca-dependent inactivation (261, 274, 366).

Ca-dependent inactivation can be prevented when Ca channel currents are carried by Na or Cs, in the absence of divalent cations (3, 131). Under these conditions the channel shows relatively little selectivity among monovalent cations, so this current is commonly called I_{ns} or nonspecific current (209). Figure 9–7 shows that I_{ns} inactivation is very slow in comparison to I_{Ca} and I_{Ba}. This is somewhat exaggerated because the I_{ns} trace was recorded at a more negative E_m (−30 mV) than I_{Ca} and I_{Ba} (0 mV). However, the lack of surface charge screening in the absence of divalent cations (for I_{ns}) makes a −20 mV shift in the voltage that the channel senses (based on shifts in activation). Therefore, the relevant voltage difference is only about −10 mV. Although it is not as easy to compare I_{ns} and I_{Ba} directly, the slower decline in I_{ns} could reveal that Ba can very weakly substitute for Ca in Ca-dependent I_{Ca} inactivation.

The time to peak current was also increased as Ca-dependent inactivation was minimized in Figure 9–7. For I_{Ca} in perforated patch the peak I_{Ca} occurred in 4 msec, whereas it occurred at 6 msec in I_{Ca} (ruptured patch), 9 msec in I_{Ba}, and 15 msec for I_{ns}. This could be an indication that the peak I_{Ca} may even be curtailed by the rapid Ca-dependent inactivation of I_{Ca}.

Sipido et al. (311) demonstrated during very long voltage clamp depolarizations that I_{Ca} could be strongly suppressed during the cytosolic Ca transient, but then recover as $[Ca]_i$ declined (Figure 9–8). They compared I_{Ca} during pulses when the SR Ca content and Ca_i transient were small (a) with those after the SR was Ca loaded and the Ca_i transient was large (b). Indeed, even the kinetics of the Ca_i transient differences seemed to match those of the I_{Ca} depression (Fig. 9–8, bottom panel). Their results emphasize that even if peak I_{Ca} is the same, $[Ca]_i$ can feed back to alter the kinetics of Ca entry via I_{Ca}.

Amount of Ca Entry During the Ventricular Action Potential.

Most measurements of I_{Ca} have used traditional square voltage clamp pulses. Figure 9–9 shows the difference in I_{Ca} waveform when rabbit or rat ventricular myocytes are subjected to the usual square pulses vs a voltage waveform based on a recorded action potential from each species. It can be seen that the peak current during the action potential clamp is lower and occurs later in both species. This is so because the peak of the action potential activates Ca channels, but the driving force for Ca is initially low because E_m is close to the reversal potential for I_{Ca}. As E_m falls, the driving force apparently increases faster than the channels inactivate, producing a larger current at later times during the action potential. The current is more sustained during the action potential than during a square pulse.

In a study by Yuan et al. (360) several differences in

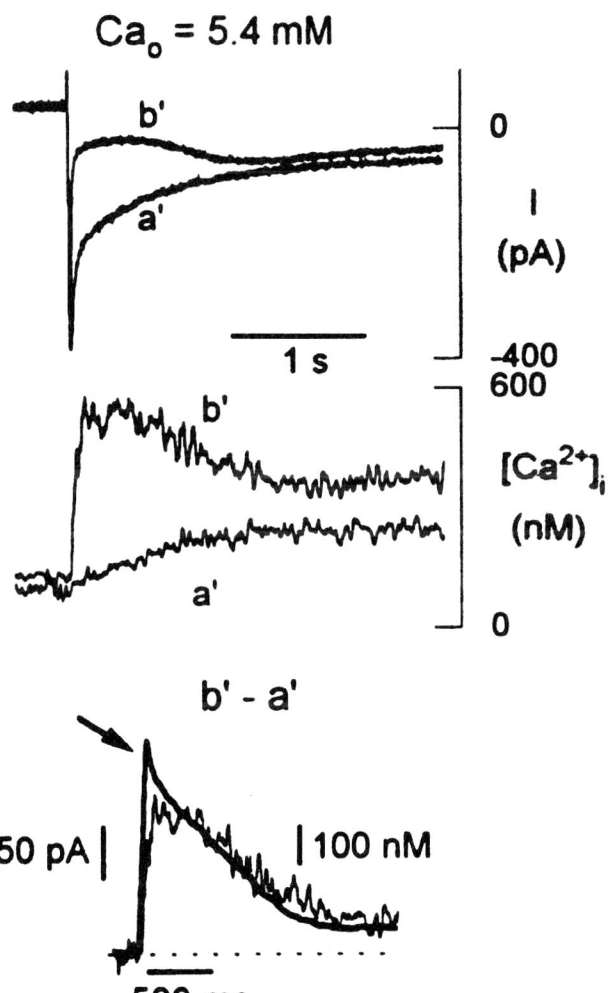

FIG. 9–8. Ca-dependent inactivation by SR Ca release and recovery of I_{Ca}. Long (4 sec.) voltage clamp pulses activated I_{Ca} and SR Ca release and Ca transient in Na-free conditions and 5.4 mM $[Ca]_o$. The pulse labeled *a* was the first pulse after depletion of the SR and *b* was after 5–10 pulses when the SR was loaded. The smaller Ca transient produces less I_{Ca} inactivation. The larger Ca transient produces marked inactivation, but the current partially recovers as $[Ca]_i$ declines. The lower difference traces show the similarity between the I_{Ca} inactivation and Ca_i transient [Modified from Sipido et al. (311), with permission.]

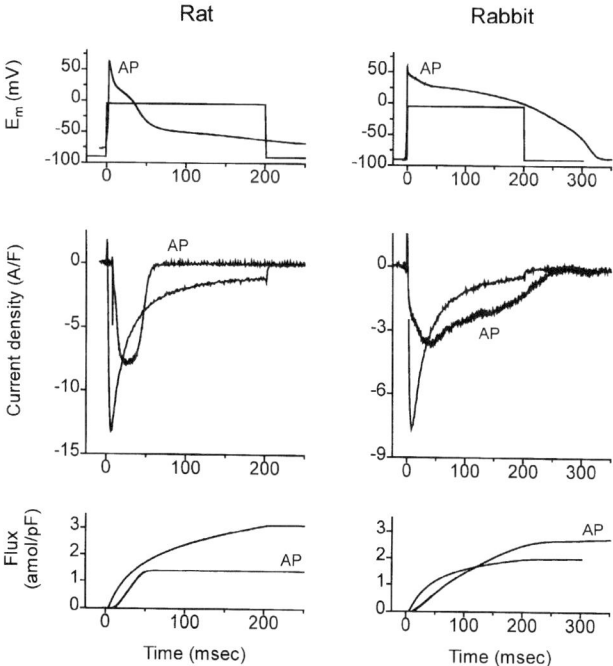

FIG. 9–9. Ca currents measured during square pulse and action potential clamp in rat and rabbit ventricular myocytes. Command E_m waveforms were either the traditional 200 ms square depolarization to 0 mV or an action potential (AP), which was recorded from normal rat and rabbit ventricular myocytes under more physiological conditions (i.e. normal Ca Na and K concentrations, ref 358). I_{Ca} was then recorded under conditions where all other currents were blocked (e.g. Na-free and Cs-rich inside and out). With the action potential waveform, the peak I_{Ca} is smaller in both species and occurs later (*middle panel*). The I_{Ca} integral (*lower panels*) for the AP clamp vs the square, pulses are smaller for the rat but larger for the rabbit (see ref. 358 for additional information).

fundamental properties of I_{Ca} were observed in rat vs rabbit ventricular myocytes. That is, the rat Ca channel showed slower Ca-dependent and E_m-dependent inactivation, a more negative activation E_m, and more positive steady-state inactivation E_m (creating a larger steady-state window I_{Ca}), and more rapid recovery from inactivation. These properties cause the amount of integrated Ca influx to be greater in rat (vs rabbit) for any given waveform (360). However, during the shorter rat ventricular action potential, the integrated Ca influx was less. After integration of I_{Ca} during the action potential and correction for myocyte surface-to-volume ratio (see Table 9–1, last entry) and 35% mitochondrial volume, mean Ca influx via I_{Ca} during the action potential can bring in 21–25 μM in rabbit and 9–14 μM in rat ventricular myocyte (depending on which surface-to-volume ratios are used). Grantham and Cannell (119) obtained integrated Ca influx of 4.5 amol/pF during action potential clamp in guinea pig ventricular myocyte, which corresponds to 34 μM Ca influx (assuming 5 pF/pl and 35% mitochondrial volume).

This brings the Ca influx via I_{Ca} into the range where it could contribute significantly to contractile activation, at least in the guinea pig and rabbit, but only marginally so in the rat. This is consistent with observations that blockade of the SR with ryanodine or thapsigargin can nearly abolish contractions and Ca transients in the rat, but only moderately depresses contractions and Ca transients in rabbit or guinea pig ventricular myocytes (31, 34, 159, 160, 323, 324).

The data in Figure 9–9 were obtained under conditions where Ca transients were suppressed by dialysis with intracellular EGTA. This minimizes complications due to other $[Ca]_i$-dependent currents (e.g. Na/Ca exchange) or to subsarcolemmal Ca accumulation and makes accurate measurements of I_{Ca} more practical. However, it surely overestimates the physiological Ca influx, because SR Ca release causes more rapid I_{Ca} inactivation (as discussed above). Unfortunately, it is rather difficult to assess the Ca entry via I_{Ca} during an action potential in a normally contracting cell because Ca-activated currents can complicate the interpretation. A prominent one is Na/Ca exchange (50, 134) but there is also evidence for Ca-activated Cl and nonselective currents. Although it is possible to measure the dihydropyridine sensitive current during an action potential clamp (5, 119), the block of I_{Ca} also prevents the Ca_i transient and alters the other currents. Thus the dihydropyridine-sensitive current may include more than the I_{Ca}.

Puglisi et al. (272) measured I_{Ca} during action potential clamp in rabbit ventricular myocyte at 25° and 35°C where SR Ca release occurred, but Na/Ca exchange was prevented by Na-free solutions inside and out. They found that the integral of Ca entry via I_{Ca} was ~12 μmol/liter cytosol at both temperatures when there was no SR Ca to be released, but this amount decreased by about 50% in the steady state when there was normal SR Ca release. This result implies that the SR Ca release inhibits about 50% of the Ca influx via I_{Ca} which would otherwise occur.

Despite having only imperfect measurements of Ca flux via I_{Ca} during an action potential, the knowledge of I_{Ca} biophysical properties has allowed the estimation of I_{Ca} flux during models of ventricular myocyte action potentials. Figure 9–10 shows calculations of a guinea pig ventricular action potential using the Oxsoft Heart program (Oxsoft Ltd, Oxford, UK) which has been developed over many years by Denis Noble's lab. The calculated I_{Ca} is not too different from the measurements in Figure 9–9, but the current inactivates more rapidly and produces a somewhat smaller integrated Ca flux via I_{Ca} of 18 μM (both as expected due to stronger Ca dependent inactivation). Figure 9–10 also shows a calculated Na/Ca exchange current, which will be discussed below. Another notable model integrating ionic currents and Ca transients during guinea pig ventricular action potential is that by Luo and Rudy (202) (See chapter 13). Integrating total I_{Ca} from their model produced about 15 μM Ca influx. J. L. Puglisi and I have also developed a user-friendly model called LabHeart.

Ca Channel Regulation. The sarcolemmal Ca channel is also a target for physiological and pharmacological modulation of Ca fluxes (see chapter 14). Catecholamines secreted by sympathetic nerve endings in the heart and by chromaffin cells in the adrenal medulla into the circulation activate cardiac β-adrenergic receptors. This G-protein–coupled receptor activates adenylate cyclase to form cyclic AMP (from ATP) and activates protein kinase A. Protein kinase A can phosphorylate the L-type Ca channel or an associated protein, increasing basal I_{Ca} in ventricular myocyte by a factor of 2–4 and shifting the voltage where activation occurs to more negative E_m. Acetylcholine and some other effectors can counteract this stimulatory effect of catecholamines, either by activation of G proteins, which inhibit adenylate cyclase, and probably also through other cellular cascades as well (see chapter 14; ref. 258). I_{Ca} can also be dramatically stimulated by dihydropyridine Ca channel agonists such as Bay K 8644, which increases the duration of individual channel openings (130). Bay K 8644 can also increase basal I_{Ca} about 3–4-fold. Several classes of Ca channel antagonists that block I_{Ca} have also been discovered and used (see Chapter 14 for further information).

In conclusion, the amount of Ca entry via I_{Ca} during the cardiac action potential is likely to vary somewhat

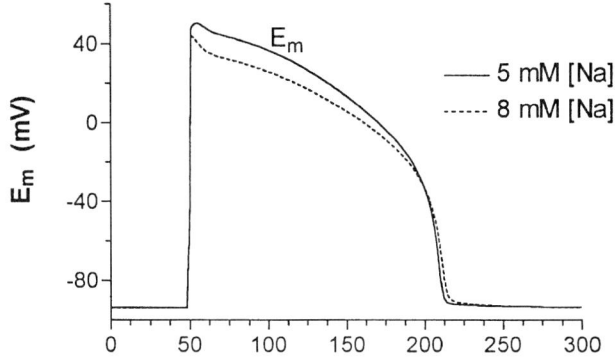
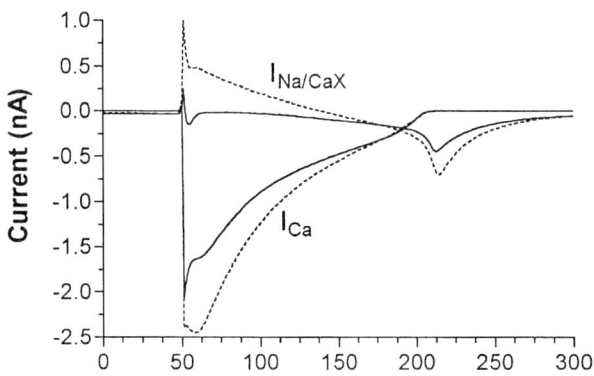
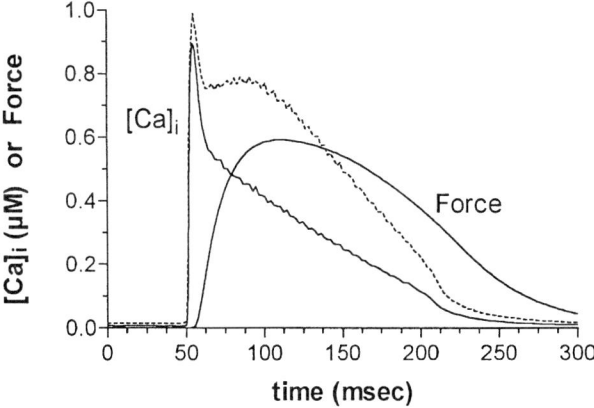

FIG. 9–10. Simulations of guinea-pig ventricular action potential using Oxsoft Heart (v 4.5). This comprehensive simulation created by Professor Denis Noble and colleagues (at Oxford, UK) calculates the E_m and many of the ionic currents that are known to flow during the action potential. Shown here are the E_m (top), I_{Ca}, $I_{Na/Ca}$ (*middle panel*), $[Ca]_i$, and force (*lower panel*) for two different initial $[Na]_i$ values (5 and 8 mM).

among species and depend on action potential configuration and the timecourse and amplitude of the intracellular Ca transient. Indeed, SR Ca release appears to produce large effects on I_{Ca} inactivation, even under conditions where the global cytosolic Ca transient is blocked by high concentrations of Ca buffer in the cytosol (1). This result is indicative of the close physical relationship between the L-type Ca channel and the SR Ca release channel or ryanodine receptor in cardiac muscle, such that crosstalk appears to work in both directions. That is, Ca influx via I_{Ca} acts locally to cause SR Ca release (even when cytosolic Ca is well buffered), and the released Ca from the SR can cause more rapid inactivation of I_{Ca} (for further discussion, see 34a). Thus Ca entry via I_{Ca} during the cardiac action potential is likely to bring in 10–20 μM Ca into the cytosol, mostly, but not exclusively during the early part of the action potential.

Na/Ca Exchange

Na/Ca exchange or countertransport was first demonstrated in heart (284) and in squid giant axon (9). Much work ensued during the next 25 years to characterize this system and understand its importance in the function of cardiac muscle and other tissues (see Chapter 10; and 34a, 50, 138, 263–265). It is now clear that the Na/Ca exchanger is the major pathway for Ca efflux from cardiac myocytes. The Na/Ca exchanger is also reversible so that Ca can also enter the myocyte via Na/Ca exchange. The factors determining the direction of net Ca flux will be discussed below.

Fundamental Characterizations. Much of the early characterization of the cardiac Na/Ca exchanger came from studies in isolated sarcolemmal vesicles, where the environment can be well controlled (e.g. 43, 73, 267, 277, 278). These studies showed transport of both Na and Ca, reversibility, voltage dependence, and electrogenicity of the exchanger. The electrogenicity, E_m-dependence, and early coupling ratios were all consistent with a transport stoichiometry of greater than 2 Na ions transported per Ca ion. Reeves and Hale (279) most clearly demonstrated the stoichiometry of 3Na:1Ca using a thermodynamic approach in sarcolemmal vesicles. They measured the [Na] gradient required to prevent net Ca transport at various membrane potentials. This stoichiometry is completely consistent with a wide array of other studies and is now generally accepted as the fixed stoichiometry of Na/Ca exchange in cardiac muscle (e.g. 263, 281, and Chapter 9), but there also have been recent challenges to this (101, 114). Since the stoichiometry appears to be fixed, for each Ca ion transported a single positive charge moves the other way (i.e. three monovalent Na ions are exchanged for each divalent Ca ion). This also allows Ca flux via Na/Ca exchange to be measured electrophysiologically as a Na/Ca exchange current ($I_{Na/Ca}$).

Horackova and Vassort (143) reported ionic currents that were probably attributable to Na/Ca exchange, but the results were somewhat equivocal because of limitations in multicellular voltage clamp techniques and lack of knowledge about expectations of the measured current. The parallel development of whole-cell patch voltage clamp, techniques for isolation of mammalian ventricular myocytes and progress from characterization of Na/Ca exchange in sarcolemmal vesicles allowed Kimura et al. (169, 170, 219) to provide a compelling electrophysiological characterization of Na/Ca exchange in intact ventricular myocytes. They blocked all other known ionic conductances [as well as the (Na + K)ATPase] and dialyzed the cell with known Na and Ca containing solutions. Figure 9–11 shows that without internal Ca, there was no current activated by 140 mM Na$_o$. However, after [Ca]$_i$ was raised from zero to 430 nM, application of 140 mM Na$_o$ activated an E_m-dependent current (Fig. 9–11 B–D) which was inward at E_m = -90 mV. Thus this inward current was dependent on [Na]$_o$, [Ca]$_i$, and E_m. They also demonstrated an E_m-dependent outward current that depended on [Na]$_i$ and [Ca]$_o$. The outward $I_{Na/Ca}$ (Na efflux and Ca influx) also appeared to require a certain amount of [Ca]$_i$ acting as an allosteric regulator ($K_{1/2}$ ~22 nM [Ca]$_i$; ref 219 or 125nM, ref 349a), qualitatively consistent with observations in sarcolemmal vesicles (280).

Hilgemann (133) developed the giant excised patch technique to study cardiac Na/Ca exchange under more controlled conditions in patches detached from the cell. By dialyzing patch pipettes and rapidly changing bath solution around the intracellular surface of the Na/Ca exchanger Hilgemann and colleagues produced a comprehensive characterization of cardiac Na/Ca exchange under conditions of experimental isolation, but in a relatively native membrane environment (81, 133–137, 210, 211). Figure 9–12 shows the E_m- and [Na]$_i$-dependence of $I_{Na/Ca}$ at two [Ca]$_i$ which may reflect resting and peak systolic [Ca]$_i$. These experiments were carried out at physiological [Na]$_o$ (140 mM) and [Ca]$_o$ (2 mM). The complex dependence of the $I_{Na/Ca}$ on Na, Ca, and E_m can be seen and is further addressed below (see Thermodynamics and Ca Flux During Action Potentials). These studies also uncovered a Na$_i$-dependent inactivation of Na/Ca exchange. That is, when [Na]$_i$ is high the Na/Ca exchange seems to inactivate in a time- and [Na]-dependent manner (136). The dynamics of the Ca$_i$-dependent activation and Na$_i$-dependent inactivation with respect to physiological function of the Na/Ca exchanger in intact cells are still not clear. However, the Ca$_i$-dependent activation could stimulate Ca extrusion by the exchanger when [Ca]$_i$ is relatively high and turn the exchanger off as [Ca]$_i$ falls to diastolic levels. This Ca$_i$-dependent activation could also stimulate greater Ca influx via Na/Ca exchange when conditions favor this direction of Ca flux. The Na$_i$-dependent inactivation could prevent excess Ca influx and cellular Ca overload under conditions of high

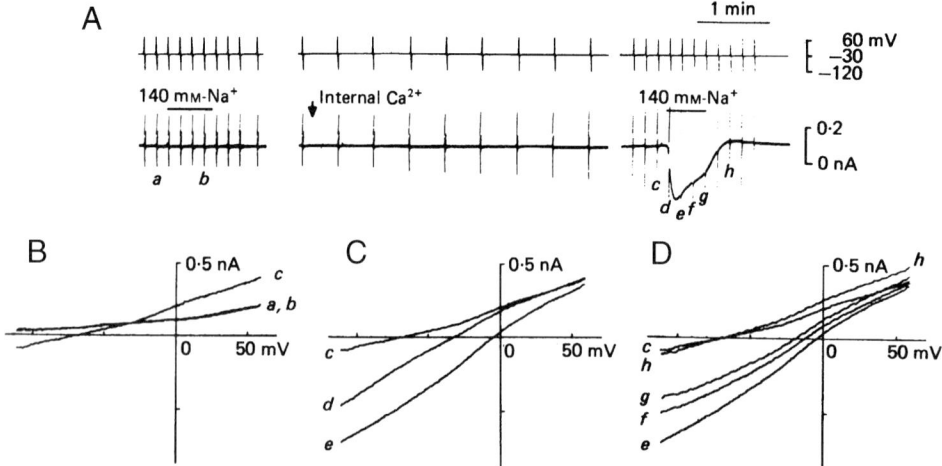

FIG. 9–11. Na/Ca exchange current in intact ventricular myocytes recorded under controlled conditions. A. Very slow speed recording of E_m (top) and $I_{Na/Ca}$ where the spikes are from ramp depolarizations that were used to generate the current voltage relationships in B, C, and D at the times indicated (a–h). The bars in A are when [Na]$_o$ was applied (replacing Li) to activate $I_{Na/Ca}$ ([Ca]$_o$ was 1 mM throughout). At the *arrow* [Ca]$_i$ was increased from nominally Ca free to 430 nM with 42 mM EGTA and 140 CsCl in the dialyzing pipette throughout. Ouabain, Ba, Cs, D600 and tetraethylammonium were used to inhibit other ionic currents. Application of [Na]$_o$ stimulated $I_{Na/Ca}$ only after [Ca]$_i$ was raised. The gradual decline in $I_{Na/Ca}$ (d–g) was supposed to be due to depletion of [Ca]$_i$. [From Kimura et al. (170), with permission.]

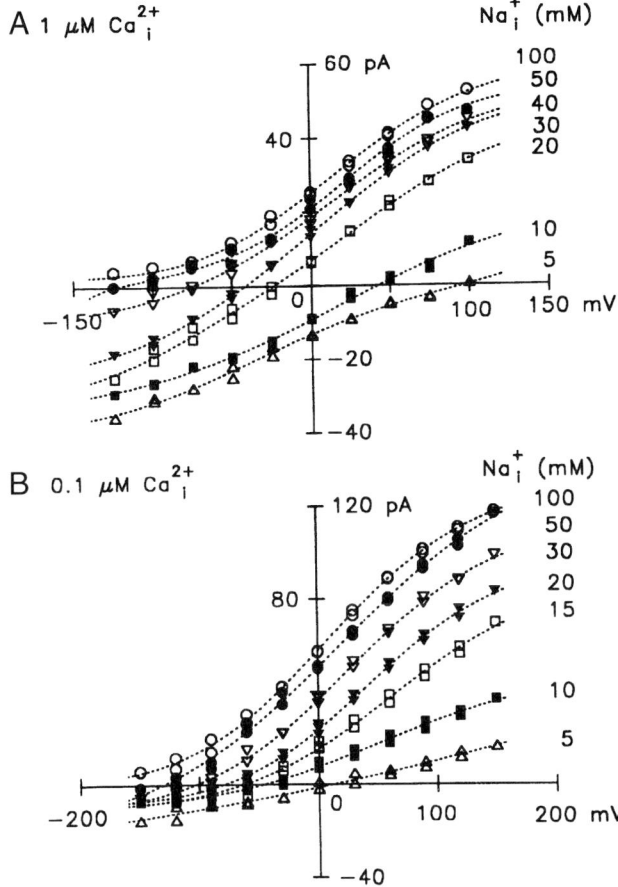

FIG. 9–12. Current–voltage relationships for $I_{Na/Ca}$ recorded in excised giant patches from guinea pig ventricular myocytes. The patches were treated with chymotrypsin to remove $I_{Na/Ca}$ inactivation and all other known currents were blocked (210). *A:* With constant $[Ca]_o$ (2 mM), $[Na]_o$ (150 mM) and $[Ca]_i$ (1 μM), the $[Na]_i$ was varied from 5 to 100 mM. The lower 3–4 curves probably reflect the $I_{Na/Ca}$ expected in intact cells when $[Ca]_i$ is high (e.g. peak systole). *B:* The same conditions as *A*, except $[Ca]_i$ is reduced to 100 nM, comparable to diastolic $[Ca]_i$. [From Matsuoka and Hilgemann (210), with permission.]

$[Na]_i$, where net Ca influx might be strongly favored. The very high $[Na]_i$ required to observe Na-dependent inactivation of $I_{Na/Ca}$ makes this regulation unlikely to be very important in the physiological modulation of the Na/Ca exchanger.

There is little evidence that phosphorylation by known kinases exerts any major regulatory role on cardiac Na/Ca exchange (252). However, MgATP reactivates Na/Ca exchange in the giant excised patch with a K_m of ~3 mM and may do so by activating a phospholipid translocase reorienting phosphatidylserine to the inner surface (81, 135). More likely, ATP activates a lipid kinase causing phosphorylation of phosphatidylinositol (PI) to form PIP_2 which increases Na/Ca exchange (134). This would be consistent with observations that acidic phospholipids also stimulate Na/Ca exchange (262).

Attempts to measure a transport $K_m(Ca_i)$ for the Na/Ca exchanger have provided a wide range of estimates in sarcolemmal vesicles and intact cells (mostly between 1 and 30 μM; refs 133, 219, 281). Part of the difficulty may be that it is difficult to distinguish the affinities for Ca binding to the transport site vs the allosteric regulatory site. Clearly the regulatory site has a lower apparent $K_m(Ca)$ (<1 μM), whereas the transport site has a much higher $K_m(Ca)$. Hilgemann et al. (137) reported a half-maximal inward $I_{Na/Ca}$ at ~3 μM $[Ca]_i$ in the giant excised patch. Another complication is that the experimentally measured $K_m(Ca)$ may be affected by other conditions such as [Na].

Data from intact cells may also provide practically useful information about the $[Ca]_i$-dependence of Ca extrusion via the Na/Ca exchanger. Figure 9–13 shows simultaneous measurement of $I_{Na/Ca}$ and Ca transients in a guinea pig ventricular myocyte where other channels and transporters including SR were blocked (13). During long depolarizing voltage clamp steps the Na/Ca exchanger can bring in enough Ca to produce a very high $[Ca]_i$ (>1 μM). Then on repolarization, $I_{Na/Ca}$ is also responsible for the inward tail currents in the lower traces in figure 9–13*A*, as well as $[Ca]_i$ decline. The plot of $I_{Na/Ca}$ as a function of $[Ca]_i$ is fairly linear, suggesting that Ca extrusion via Na/Ca exchange is not saturated even at relatively high physiological $[Ca]_i$. This result suggests that the functional $K_m(Ca_i)$ for the Na/Ca exchange is higher than 1 μM.

There is general agreement that the $K_m(Na_o)$ is on the order of 30 mM $[Na]_o$ and perhaps a bit lower at the intracellular surface (~15–20 mM, see Fig. 9–12). The apparent $K_m(Ca_o)$ is generally found to be in the range of 0.15 to 1 mM (210, 219), much higher than the $K_m(Ca_i)$. It should also be noted that these K_m values are only apparent and rough approximations, because Na, Ca, and protons can compete for the same sites on both sides, and the E_m can also alter the apparent K_m values (e.g. see Fig 9–12 and ref 210). Thus the specific experimental conditions are important in these apparent K_m values.

Cloning and Structure/Function. Philipson's group first cloned the heart Na/Ca exchange (234), and a current working model is shown in Figure 9–14. The translated protein consists of 970 amino acids (MW = 110 kDa) minus a leader peptide (32 amino acids) including a putative first transmembrane domain, which is removed posttranslationally and is not part of the mature functional protein (98, 234). There were originally thought to be eleven transmembrane domains and a very large cytoplasmic hydrophilic domain (264). However, new topological data suggest that there are

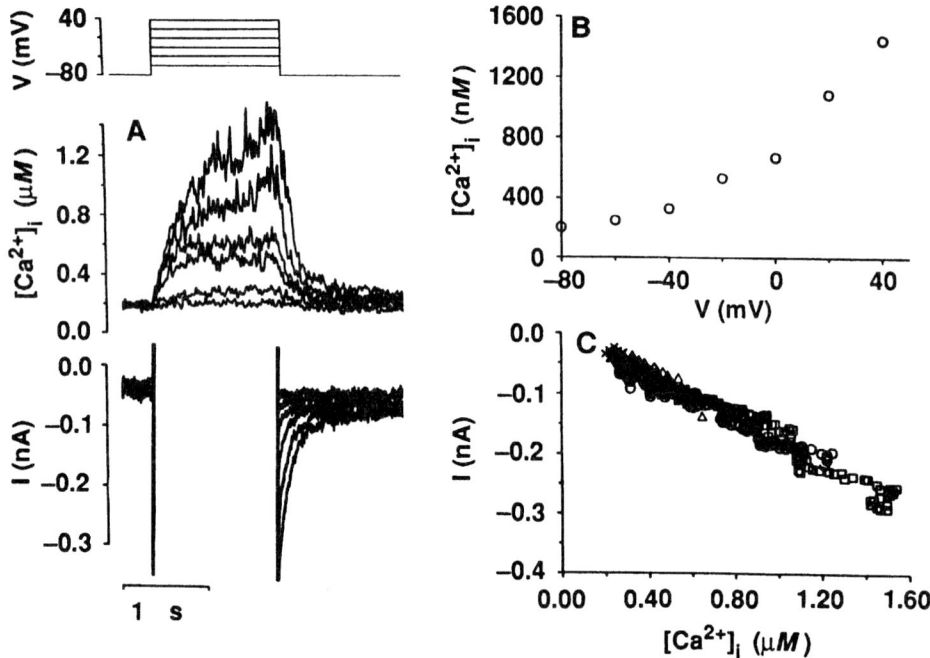

FIG. 9–13. Na/Ca exchange currents and [Ca]$_i$ in a guinea pig ventricular myocyte. The Ca transient (using fura-2) show that Ca influx via Na/Ca exchange can bring in large quantities of Ca during large sustained depolarizations (A and B). The [Na] in the dialyzing pipette was 7.5 mM. Outward currents during the depolarization were off-scale. C: The [Ca]$_i$-dependence of the "tail" current was observed upon repolarization to −80 mV. Other ionic currents are blocked by Cs, tetraethylammonium, verapamil, and ryanodine. [From Barcenas-Ruiz et al., (13), with permission.]

only nine transmembrane spans (Fig. 9–14) based on access of epitope-specific antibodies and of sulfhydryl reagents to substituted cysteine residues (157, 236). The structure has three potential glycosylation sites on the extracellular side, and one near the amino terminus appears to be glycosylated. The protein is highly acidic and bears some similarity to the (Na + K) ATPase having a 23 amino acid stretch with 48% identity (α repeats in Fig. 9–14). This region is also homologous to a region of the SR Ca-ATPase thought to be involved in Ca transport (79, 235). Indeed, the transmembrane domains must also be involved in the ion translocation steps, although this remains to be clarified.

On the large cytoplasmic domain (520 amino acids) near the amino end, there is a domain resembling the calmodulin binding regions of other proteins, which serve auto-inhibitory functions. Indeed, a peptide with this sequence, termed "exchange inhibitory peptide" (XIP), can strongly inhibit cardiac Na/Ca exchange activity (196). However, it should be noted that to date there is no clear evidence of regulation of the cardiac Na/Ca exchanger by either calmodulin or protein kinases (263). Recent results have suggested that the XIP region of the Na/Ca exchange molecule is also the region responsible for Na$_i$-dependent inactivation. The site for Ca$_i$-dependent activation has also been identified near the middle of the large cytoplasmic loop of the exchanger by studies combining mutagenesis, biochemical, and electrophysiological methods (211). Deletion of nearly the entire cytosolic loop or treatment with chymotrypsin results in a protein that still transports Na and Ca and carries I$_{Na/Ca}$ but loses secondary regulation (252). Thus the ion translocation steps do not require the large intracellular loop, but that loop seems to be essential for regulation. These types of combined molecular structure–function studies continue to provide valuable information about how the Na/Ca exchange works.

Thermodynamics and Ca Flux During Action Potentials. As indicated above, the direction and amount of net Ca movement by Na/Ca exchange depend on the concentrations of both Na and Ca on both sides of the membrane, as well as the E$_m$. If there is more energy in the inward [Na] gradient (for three Na ions) than in the inward [Ca] gradient (for one ion), Ca extrusion via this coupled transporter is thermodynamically favored (225). That is

$$n(E_{Na} - E_m) > 2(E_{Ca} - E_m) \qquad (1)$$

where n is the coupling ratio and E$_{Ca}$ and E$_{Na}$ are the thermodynamic equilibrium potentials for Ca and Na

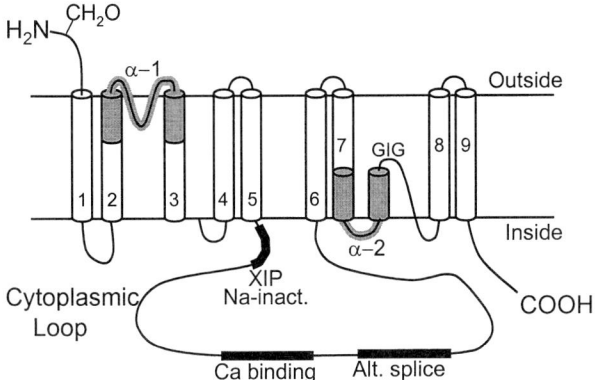

FIG. 9–14. Model of the Na/Ca exchanger based on recent work by Nicoll et al. (236) and Iwamoto et al.(157). The structure is consistent with 9 membrane spanning segments and a glycosylation site (CH_2O). The large cytoplasmic loop contains the Na/Ca exchange inhibitory peptide (XIP) domain (also associated closely with the region responsible for Na-dependent inactivation) and also contains the site for allosteric regulation by $[Ca]_i$. The two homologous α repeats (α-1 and α-2) are also indicated.

(e.g. $E_{Na} = (RT/zF) \log([Na]_o/[Na]_i)$). Then, for $n = 3$, the E_m value at which the gradients are exactly equal ($E_{Na/Ca}$) is the reversal potential of the $I_{Na/Ca}$. Hence,

$$E_{Na/Ca} = 3E_{Na} - 2E_{Ca} \quad (2)$$

When E_m is more positive than $E_{Na/Ca}$, outward $I_{Na/Ca}$ is favored. In other words, Ca entry via the exchanger is favored for $E_m > E_{Na/Ca}$ and Ca extrusion is favored (inward $I_{Na/Ca}$) when $E_m < E_{Na/Ca}$.

For typical diastolic values of $[Na]_o$ and $[Na]_i$ (140 and 8.9 mM respectively; $E_{Na} = +73$ mV) and $[Ca]_o$ and $[Ca]_i$ (2 mM and 150 nM, respectively; $E_{Ca} = +125.8$ mV) $E_{Na/Ca}$ would be -32.6 mV. Thus at a resting E_m of -80 mV Ca extrusion and inward $I_{Na/Ca}$ would be thermodynamically favored. This initial point corresponds to the time in Figure 9–15 before the action potential where $E_{Na/Ca}$ is more positive than E_m. During the action potential both E_m and $[Ca]_i$ change dynamically and this can be expected to change the thermodynamic driving force on the Na/Ca exchanger (for simplicity I will assume that $[Na]_i$ does not change). The changing $[Ca]_i$ during the Ca transient of course changes E_{Ca} and consequently $E_{Na/Ca}$ (see Eq. 2). Thus both E_m and $E_{Na/Ca}$ change during the action potential, as indicated in Figure 9–15. During the rapid upstroke of the action potential in Figure 9–15A E_m exceeds $E_{Na/Ca}$ such that Ca influx via Na/Ca exchange is favored for a brief period (indicated by cross-hatched area between the curves). However, in this case as $[Ca]_i$ rises to its peak (changing E_{Ca} to $+95$ mV), $E_{Na/Ca}$ is rising while E_m is declining and Ca influx via exchange must stop at the point where the E_m and $E_{Na/Ca}$ curves cross. This is exactly analogous to the reversal potential of an ion channel where there is no net driving force for ion movement. In Figure 9–15A $E_{Na/Ca}$ stays positive to E_m for the rest of the action potential such that the Na/Ca exchange works mainly in the Ca extrusion mode throughout the action potential, gradually returning to the diastolic condition that existed at the start of the trace. Since the difference between $E_{Na/Ca}$ and E_m is greater as E_m becomes more negative, it may be expected that Na/Ca exchange is better at extruding Ca at more negative E_m. This is also intuitively obvious from the stoichiometry and is apparent in Figures 9–1, 9–11, and 9–12.

Figure 9–15B shows another example where $[Na]_i$ has been increased to 12.7 mM (a$Na_i = 10$ mM) and the amplitude of the Ca transient is increased by 33%. In this case the $E_{Na/Ca}$ begins at -60 mV and during the action potential E_m exceeds $E_{Na/Ca}$ most of the time, such that Ca influx is favored almost throughout the action potential (cross-hatched region). Thus relatively modest changes in cellular conditions can strongly affect Ca movements by the Na/Ca exchange. Furthermore, if $[Na]_i$ were to rise to 16 mM, diastolic $E_{Na/Ca}$ would be -80 mV and Na/Ca exchange could no longer extrude Ca when $[Ca]_i$ is 150 nM at $E_m = -80$ mV. Since Na/Ca exchange is the main mechanism of Ca removal from cardiac myocytes, this suggests that situations that cause $[Na]_i$ to rise, such as repetitive Na channel activity, administration of cardioactive steroids (which inhibit the (Na + K) ATPase), and hypoxia, could put the cell at major jeopardy with respect to maintenance of normal Ca balance.

From Figure 9–15 it can be appreciated that the duration of Ca influx via Na/Ca exchange during the action potential is rather sensitive to changes in peak $[Ca]_i$, the time course of the Ca transient, the $[Na]_i$, and the shape of the action potential. This simple thermodynamic consideration is adequate to predict the direction of net Ca transport by Na/Ca exchange and the thermodynamic driving force ($E_{Na/Ca} - E_m$), but the amount of Ca moved and the amplitude of $I_{Na/Ca}$ also depend on kinetic factors. For example, during diastole in Figure 9–15A the driving force for Ca extrusion via Na/Ca exchange is large, but net Ca extrusion will be limited by the low diastolic $[Ca]_i$. Thus, more complete quantitative models of $I_{Na/Ca}$ must include both the thermodynamic driving force as well as the impact of ion concentrations on the amount of flux in either direction (e.g. 48, 96, 132, 210). These models vary in complexity and numbers of reaction steps considered. Some of the simpler forms are useful because they can be readily incorporated into models of the cardiac action potential and Ca fluxes (96, 202, 349a).

Figure 9–10 shows calculated $I_{Na/Ca}$ expected during the guinea pig ventricular action potential, based on the Oxsoft Heart program developed by Dr. Denis

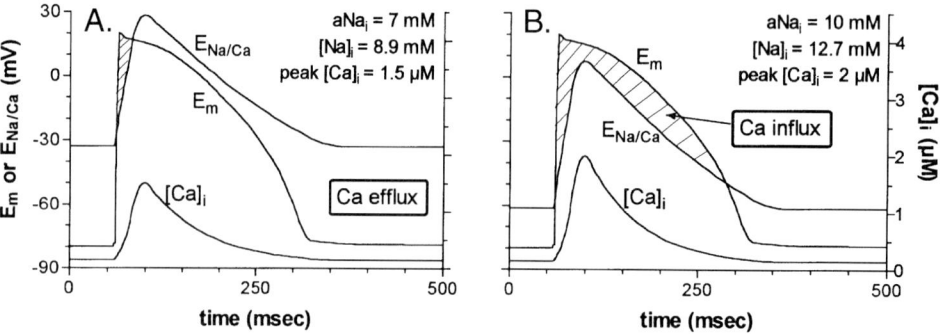

FIG. 9–15. Na/Ca exchange reversal potential ($E_{Na/Ca}$) during the rabbit ventricular action potential. This schematic diagram shows how $E_{Na/Ca}$ is expected to change during the action potential for two different levels of intracellular Na activity (aNa_i =5 and 8 mM), where aNa_i is roughly 0.78 · $[Na]_i$. When E_m is positive to $E_{Na/Ca}$, Ca influx via the Na/Ca exchange is thermodynamically favored (*shaded areas*). When E_m is negative to $E_{Na/Ca}$, Ca extrusion is favored. Resting $[Ca]_i$ =150 nM, $[Ca]_o$ =2 mM and aNa_o = 110 mM for both traces and aNa_i and peak $[Ca]_i$ are as indicated. The $[Ca]_i$ trace reaches a peak 40 msec after the action potential begins. [After Bers (32, 34).]

Noble and colleagues. The model of Luo and Rudy (202) produces similar results. For the 5 mM $[Na]_i$ trace it can be seen that there is an initial outward $I_{Na/Ca}$ during the very early part of the action potential which brings in a tiny amount of Ca (0.06 μM). This $I_{Na/Ca}$ quickly reverses to an inward $I_{Na/Ca}$ with two humps. The first hump is due to the large and rapid rise in $[Ca]_i$ early in the Ca transient and the second hump is during rapid repolarization and is attributable to the large increase in driving force ($E_{Na/Ca} - E_m$) at that time (see also Fig. 9–15). The integrated Ca extrusion via Na/Ca exchange during the trace shown is ~11 μM (compared to a calculated Ca influx of 18.5 μM via I_{ca}). The remaining 7.5 μM would have to be extruded between beats if this cell were in steady-state Ca balance.

The example in Figure 9–10 for $[Na]_i$ of 5 mM is probably rather low for $[Na]_i$ in intact myocytes. An additional trace for 8 mM $[Na]_i$ is also shown in Figure 9–10. Luo and Rudy (202) used 10 mM $[Na]_i$, and integration of Ca fluxes during their guinea pig ventricular action potential model yields an early Ca influx via outward $I_{Na/Ca}$ of 1.4 μM reversing somewhat later than in Figure 9–10, and ~11 μM Ca is extruded by Na/Ca exchange over the remainder of a comparable 300 ms trace. In this case I extrapolated an additional 4.4 μM to be extruded over the next 150 ms of diastole. Thus, the total Ca extrusion via Na/Ca exchange was ~15.5 μM whereas the total Ca influx was ~16 μM (1.4 via Na/Ca exchange and 14.7 via I_{ca}). It is clear that additional experimental verification of these fluxes via Na/Ca exchange would be quite valuable (although difficult). Nevertheless, these numbers provide a good working model and are reasonably consistent with the data so far available (but see complicating factors below).

Based on the foregoing, one might expect that there would be condition- and species-dependent differences in how or when most of the Ca flux occurs. This indeed seems likely, and Figure 9–16 shows an experimental manifestation of this difference in measurements of local $[Ca]_o$ in rat and rabbit ventricular muscle during the cardiac cycle (309). During the contraction in rabbit ventricle there was a net depletion of $[Ca]_o$, which recovered slowly later in the contraction and during diastole (consistent with Figures 9–10 and 9–15). However, in rat ventricle there was net Ca efflux and increased $[Ca]_o$ early in the contraction, indicating net Ca efflux (presumably via Na/Ca exchange). The early Ca extrusion may result from the very short rat ventricular action potential, such that repolarization

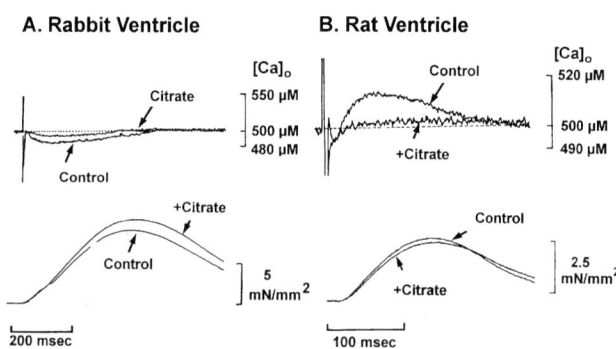

FIG. 9–16. Extracellular [Ca] depletion in rat-rabbit ventricular muscle. Changes in $[Ca]_o$ were measured with double-barreled Ca-selective microelectrodes during individual contractions in rabbit (*A*) and rat (*B*) ventricular muscle (0.5 Hz, 30°C). The traces show $[Ca]_o$ (*top*) and tension (*bottom*) in the absence and presence of 10 mM citrate (which limits $[Ca]_o$ depletion by buffering [Ca]. The bath $[Ca]_o$ was 0.5 mM and is indicated by the *dotted line*. [*A* is modified from Shattock and Bers (309) and composite from Bers (34), with permission.]

causes Ca extrusion to be favored more strongly very early in the contraction. Indeed, Figure 9–17 is like Figure 9–15 for these cases and supports this interpretation. The lower panels in Figure 9–17 show the thermodynamic driving force ($E_{Na/Ca} - E_m$) for Ca flux via Na/Ca exchange. Shattock and Bers (309) also measured intracellular Na activity (aNa_i) in rabbit and rat ventricle, so the measured values (7.2 and 12.7 mM) were used. It can be seen that in the rabbit, Ca influx is weakly favored during much of the action potential (and a small $[Ca]_o$ depletion is seen in Fig. 9–16A). By the time Ca efflux is strongly favored (by +40 mV) $[Ca]_i$ has declined, thereby limiting the amount of Ca extrusion (so $[Ca]_o$ does not change very fast in Fig. 9–16A). In the rat there is a large driving force for Ca extrusion as the brief action potential returns to -80 mV. In the rat this large driving force occurs only 50–100 ms after the upstroke when $[Ca]_i$ is high and would provide plenty of substrate for Ca efflux via Na/Ca exchange. Note that the rapid efflux of Ca, raising local $[Ca]_o$ in Figure 9–16B, is very similar to the shape of the driving force curve in Figure 9–17B. Shattock and Bers (309) also found that aNa_i was rather high in rat ventricle, suggesting that diastolic $E_{Na/Ca}$ is very close to E_m. If the Na/Ca exchange is really close to equilibrium in the rat heart at diastole, very small changes in $[Na]_i$ could have a large impact on cellular Ca balance. Thus if $E_{Na/Ca}$ is really below E_m, the cells cannot extrude Ca at rest and, in fact, could gain Ca during diastole. These shifts in transmembrane Ca via Na/Ca exchange can also be important in determining the SR Ca content during rest (see later under, Rest-Dependent Changes in Cellular and SR Ca Content).

A complicating factor in the estimation of the Na/Ca exchange flux during the twitch is that there are likely to be spatial gradients of [Ca] near the membrane and sites of SR Ca release (182). This point was raised by the results of Egan et al. (100). They interrupted the action potential by repolarization and measured the activation of a tail current attributed to $I_{Na/Ca}$. They inferred that this $I_{Na/Ca}$ could serve as a bioassay for the local $[Ca]_i$ sensed by the Na/Ca exchanger. Figure 9–18 shows another manifestation of this same effect. Application of 10 mM caffeine increases global $[Ca]_i$ (sensed by indo-1) and activates an inward $I_{Na/Ca}$. However, the kinetics of the global Ca transient and $I_{Na/Ca}$

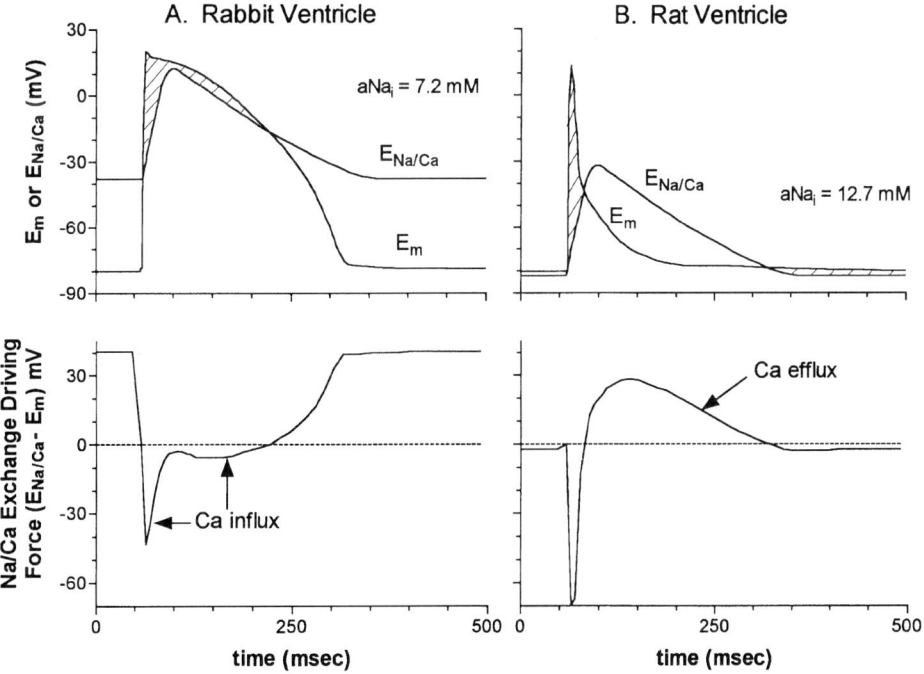

FIG. 9-17. Changes in Na/Ca exchange driving force during action potential in rat and rabbit ventricle. $E_{Na/Ca}$ is expected to change during the action potential and Ca transient in rabbit and rat ventricle (top). The estimated changes in the net electrochemical driving force for Na/Ca exchange ($E_{Na/Ca} - E_m$) are shown in the *bottom panel*. Na/Ca exchange stoichiometry of 3Na:1Ca was assumed, the aNa_i values were measured (309) and, for simplicity, the Ca transient accompanying the contraction, has been assumed to be the same for both species. Resting $[Ca]_i$ was assumed to be 150 nM, rising to a peak of 1 μM, 40 msec after the upstroke of the action potential. Note the similarity between the lower panels and the $[Ca]_o$ traces in Figure. 16. [Modified from Shattock and Bers (309) and Bers (34), with permission.]

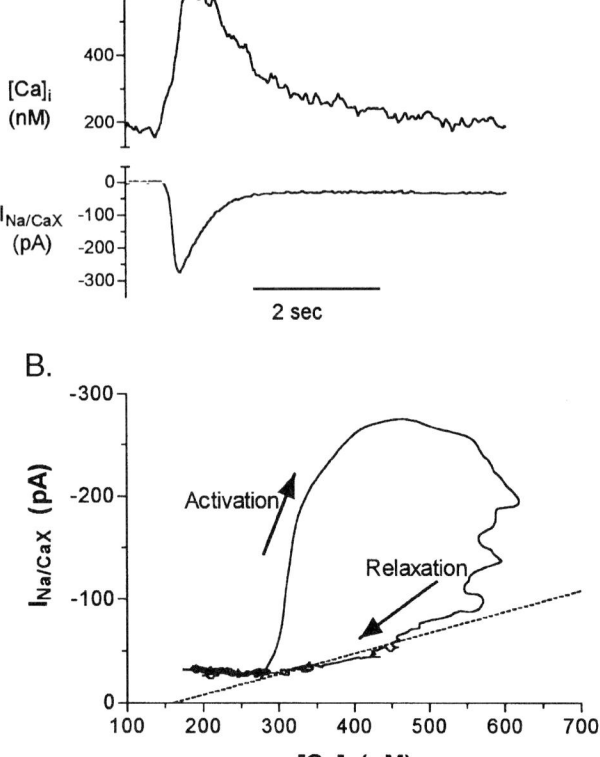

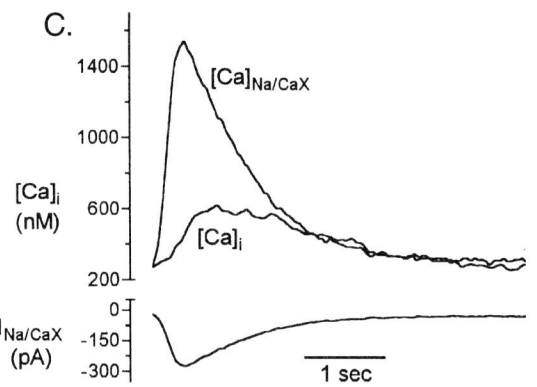

FIG. 9–18. Caffeine-induced Ca transient and Na/Ca exchange current in a ferret ventricular myocyte. A: After a steady-state series of voltage clamp pulses, 10 mM caffeine was rapidly and continuously applied to release SR Ca. Experimental conditions blocked most other ionic currents (e.g. Cs inside and out) and indo-1 was used as the Ca indicator. The inward $I_{Na/Ca}$ rises to a peak before the Ca transient. B: Instantaneous $I_{Na/Ca}$ from *panel A* is plotted as a function of the global $[Ca]_i$ reported by indo-1. The hysteresis shows that during the rising phase of the Ca transient, more inward $I_{Na/Ca}$ is observed for a given $[Ca]_i$ than during relaxation. The relationship between $I_{Na/Ca}$ and $[Ca]_i$ during relaxation was fit to a linear regression (for $[Ca]_i$ between 300 and 450 nM (*dashed line*; see also Fig. 9–13 C). C. $I_{Na/Ca}$ and $[Ca]_i$ data are reproduced from *panel A* and the subsarcolemmal $[Ca]_i$ sensed by the Na/Ca exchanger ($[Ca]_{Na/CaX}$) based on the linear regression in *panel B* is also shown. [Experiment performed by Dr. Li Li.].

are not the same, as emphasized by the hysteretical loop in Figure 9–18B which shows $I_{Na/Ca}$ as a function of global $[Ca]_i$ at each point in time. If we assume that spatial gradients are minimal as $[Ca]_i$ declines from 400 to 300 nM, we can use the extrapolated dotted line in Figure 9–18B to estimate the local $[Ca]_i$ that the Na/Ca exchanger senses at earlier time points. Thus the earlier rise of $I_{Na/Ca}$ (vs $[Ca]_i$) probably reflects the faster rise of subsarcolemmal $[Ca]_i$ than global $[Ca]_i$. Figure 9–18C shows that the predicted subsarcolemmal $[Ca]_i$ sensed by the Na/Ca exchange ($[Ca]_{Na/CaX}$) is much higher early in the Ca transient and then merges with the global Ca transient during $[Ca]_i$ decline. Figure 9–18 is meant solely for illustration of the principle. The exact relationship between global and subsarcolemmal $[Ca]_i$ will depend on where we assume the spatial gradients dissipate and on the real linearity of the $[Ca]_i$ vs $I_{Na/Ca}$ relationship (see Fig. 9–13).

Sarcolemmal Ca-ATPase

The plasma membrane Ca-pump first reported in erythrocytes (295) has since been demonstrated in many other cells (69, 71, 296, 297). The red cell plasma membrane Ca-pump has been most extensively characterized and appears closely related to that in other tissues. The purified protein is 138 kDa and is not particularly homologous with the SR Ca-pump protein, vs the (Na + K)-ATPase or proton pump (238, 346). A central stretch of ~80 kDa is all that is required for Ca transport, and a 30 kDa stretch at the carboxy terminal contains a 10 kDa regulatory calmodulin binding domain (158). The stoichiometry of the plasma membrane Ca-ATPase appears to be 1 Ca ion per ATP hydrolyzed (282), and Ca extrusion by this pump appears coupled to proton influx (177). The turnover rate of plasma membrane Ca-pumps may approach ~1000/min with $K_m(Ca)$ ~1 μM (297).

Caroni and Carafoli (72) first described activity of this pump in cardiac sarcolemmal vesicles. They also described stimulation by cAMP-dependent phosphorylation (~3-fold) and calmodulin on the pump (74, 75). They reported $K_m(ATP) \sim 30$ μM, $K_m(Ca) = 0.3$ μM and $V_{max} = 31$ nmol/mg protein/min in the presence of endogenous calmodulin *vs.* $K_m(Ca) = 11$ μM and $V_{max} = 10$ nmol/mg protein/min in calmodulin-depleted preparations. Table 9–4 compares cardiac sarcolemmal Ca-pump activation by calmodulin, cAMP-dependent protein kinase, or both (97). Dixon and Haynes (97) found that calmodulin had a profound effect on the $K_m(Ca)$ and V_{max}, while smaller affects were observed with cAMP-dependent protein kinase.

We can estimate the maximum cellular Ca transport rates from the values in Table 9–4 with the help of the conversion factors in Table 9–1 (assuming a sarcolem-

TABLE 9–4. *Kinetic Properties of the Cardiac Sarcolemmal Ca-Pump*

	V_{max} (nmol/mg pn/min)	$K_m(Ca)$ (nM)	n(Hill)
Basal	1.7 ± 0.3	1800 ± 100	1.6 ± 0.1
+cAMP-dependent protein kinase	3.1 ± 0.5	1100 ± 100	1.7 ± 0.1
+Calmodulin	15.0 ± 2.5	64 ± 1.4	3.7 ± 0.2
+Both	36.0 ± 6.5	63 ± 1.7	3.7 ± 0.1

Values are taken from Dixon and Haynes (97).

mal purification factor of 30). Thus the highest transport rate reported, 36 nmol/mg sarcolemmal protein/min (× 9.7 mg sarcolemmal protein/ml cytosol) corresponds to 5.8 μM/sec. This maximum transport rate is small compared to either the SR Ca-ATPase (~200 μM/sec), the Na/Ca exchange (e.g. ~75 μM/sec in Figure 9–11), or Ca current (7 pA/pF~200 μM/sec). Thus, while the sarcolemmal Ca-pump can have a high affinity for $[Ca]_i$, the transport rate is probably too slow for it to be of major importance to Ca fluxes during the cardiac cycle (see under Relative Contributions of Ca Transporters).

INTRACELLULAR Ca TRANSPORTERS

Sarcoplasmic Reticulum Ca-ATPase and Sarcoplasmic Reticulum Ca Content

Regulation of the SR Ca-ATPase. The SR Ca-ATPase is discussed in detail in Chapter 8. The focus here will be on quantitative aspects of Ca transport and functional regulation in the cell. The main physiological regulator of the SR Ca-ATPase is phospholamban (PLB), a 52 amino acid transmembrane protein that serves as an endogenous inhibitor of the Ca-pump (174, 328). Phospholamban is present at high concentration in ventricular myocytes, probably comparable to the concentration of the SR Ca-ATPase, although the absolute stoichiometry is not known. However, when PLB protein expression is doubled with respect to the SR Ca-ATPase in transgenic mice, there is a proportional shift to lower Ca affinity, suggesting that the Ca-pumps are not nearly saturated with PLB (163). There is much less PLB in atrial muscle, and it is also present in smooth muscle and slow skeletal muscle, but not in fast skeletal muscle (57). The main effect of PLB appears to be to reduce Ca affinity of the pump.

Figure 9–19 shows the [Ca] dependence of forward Ca-pumping by the SR Ca-ATPase. With endogenous PLB in ventricular SR, the K_m for Ca is typically around 600 nM. The maximal Ca-pump rate is shown in the cellular units used throughout this chapter and typical of that in rat ventricular myocytes (11, 17). Recent values for K_m in the literature vary considerably (e.g. from 234 to 1,200 nM; 146, 173, 200, 203, 212, 242, 276, 292, 337). Part of this variation might be the difficulty in making precisely calibrated Ca-EGTA buffers. Thus a K_m value of 600 nM is an educated guess, near the mean of a large number of reports in different preparations.

Phospholamban can be phosphorylated by cAMP-dependent protein kinase (PKA) at serine 16 and this largely reverses the Ca affinity shift, thus increasing the Ca affinity of the SR Ca-pump by 2–3-fold (consistent with a decrease in K_m to 250 nM in Figure 9–19). Thus for most relevant $[Ca]_i$ values (0.1–1 μM) there is a substantial increase in Ca-pump rate. Application of a PLB antibody, which interferes with the interaction between PLB and the SR Ca-ATPase, produces similar effects (303, 326). Furthermore when either the cardiac or skeletal muscle SR Ca-pump (SERCA2A or SERCA1) is expressed without PLB the Ca pumping and ATPase activity properties are like the endogenous PKA phosphorylated Ca-pump (e.g. 276, 337).

Phospholamban can also be phosphorylated by Ca-calmodulin dependent protein kinase II (CaMKII) at threonine 17 (310). Phosphorylation at this site can also increase SR Ca-ATPase, but it has somewhat smaller effect on reduction of K_m (vs PKA) and might also increase V_{max} (175, 212, 242, 292). Indeed, Bassani et al. (25) showed that CaMKII phosphorylation could contribute to frequency-dependent acceleration of SR Ca uptake and relaxation in intact cells. Phospholamban can also be phosphorylated by protein kinase C at serine 10, but substantial functional effects on Ca transport have not been described.

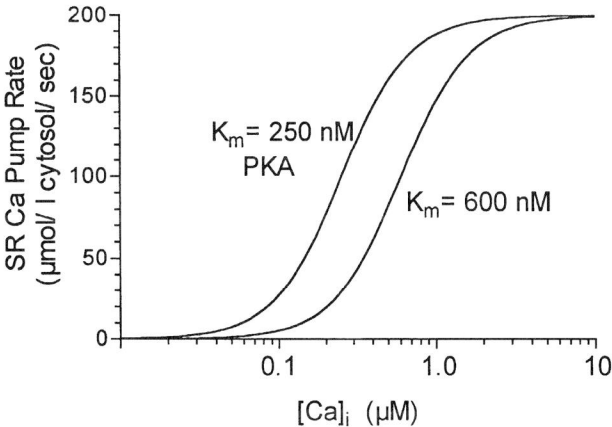

FIG. 9–19. Ca transport by the SR Ca-ATPase based on literature values (see text). Ca pump rates were calculated based on Eq. 3 using V_{max} = 200 μmol/liter cytosol, K_m = 600 nM and n= 2. Activation of protein kinase A (PKA) decreases the K_m to 250 nM, but does not affect V_{max}.

There were recent reports that CaMKII could directly phosphorylate the cardiac SR Ca-ATPase, increasing the V_{max} for Ca transport (338, 356). However, this result is still controversial and two major studies have directly contradicted this conclusion (242, 276). Thus, PLB and the phosphorylation state of this protein seems to be the main endogenous regulator of SR Ca-pump function. Of course, the Ca-ATPase is also sensitive to the concentrations of substrates (Ca and ATP) as well as pH and other small molecules (See chapter 8).

Measurement of SR Ca Transport in Cells. Numerous measurements of SR Ca uptake have been made in isolated SR vesicles and these have allowed extensive characterization of the SR Ca-ATPase. However, it is also important to attempt to assess the functional ability of the SR Ca-pump in its normal cellular environment. Figure 9-20 shows a procedure developed by Hove-Madsen and Bers (146) to measure SR Ca uptake in isolated ventricular myocytes. After cells were washed in Ca-free medium the sarcolemma was selectively permeabilized by digitonin and then 25 µM ruthenium red was added to inhibit both mitochondrial Ca uptake and SR Ca release; 12.5 mM creatine phosphate was added to provide an energy source and 10 mM oxalate was added to precipitate Ca transported into the SR and thus prevent intra-SR [Ca] from increasing and thereby opposing the forward Ca-pump flux.

Figure 9-20A shows recording of free [Ca] in the cuvette measured simultaneously with indo-1 and a Ca minielectrode during a Ca addition. The [Ca] rises to a peak and then declines as Ca is transported from the cuvette and cytosolic space into the SR. The decline in [Ca] is completely blocked by the selective SR Ca-

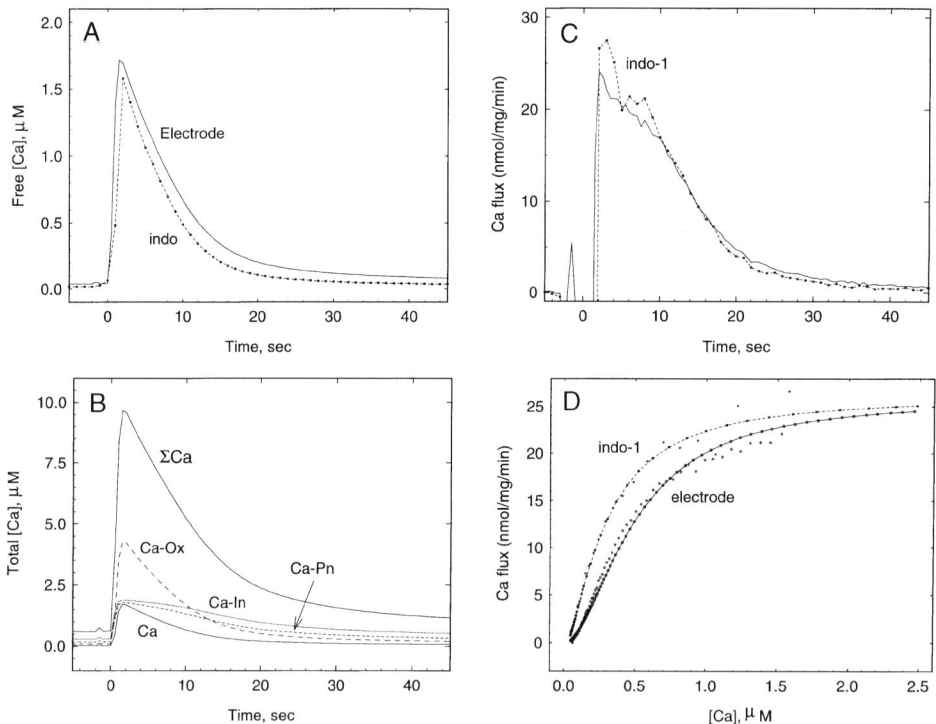

FIG. 9-20. Measurement of SR Ca uptake rate in digitonin permeabilized myocytes. A. Free [Ca] was measured simultaneously with indo-1 and Ca electrode. Ca was added at time 0 to a suspension of rabbit ventricular myocytes permeabilized with digitonin and incubated with 25 µM ruthenium red, 12.5 mM creatine phosphate, and 10 mM oxalate. B: The change in free [Ca] (Ca, *solid line*, from A), protein bound Ca (Ca-Pn), Ca-oxalate (Ca-Ox), Ca-indo (Ca-In), and the sum of free and bound Ca (ΣCa) after addition of 14 µM total Ca. After an initial increase in free [Ca], Ca uptake by the SR lowered the free [Ca] back to the level before the Ca addition. The Ca bound to protein, oxalate, and indo-1 was calculated from the passive Ca binding to permeabilized myocytes and indo-1 (144, 145). C. The Ca uptake rate was calculated as the rate of change in the total non-SR Ca with time (i.e. dΣCa/dt). D: [Ca] dependence of Ca uptake by the SR. The Ca uptake rate determined in C was plotted versus the corresponding free [Ca] measured in A. Data were fit with Eq. 3 to determine the maximal Ca uptake rate, K_m, and Hill coefficient. Data are shown for addition of two different amounts of Ca to the myocyte suspension (14 µM total Ca = *diamonds* and 43 µM total Ca = *circles*. [From Hove-Madsen and Bers (145), with permission.]

ATPase inhibitor, thapsigargin, verifying the SR Ca-ATPase as mediating [Ca] decline. However, we want to know the amount of total Ca transported by the SR per unit time, not just how free [Ca] changes. In Figure 9–20B the free [Ca] is translated to total non-SR cuvette [Ca] (ΣCa) from the free [Ca] and by calculating the amount of Ca bound to oxalate, indo-1 and cellular protein (note that the passive Ca buffering properties were measured separately with the SR Ca-pump blocked; 145, 146). Thus the rate of decline of the total non-SR Ca (dΣCa/dt) represents the rate of Ca flux into the SR and this derivative is shown in Figure 9–20 C. From panels A and C we know both the free [Ca] and flux rate at each point in time and can hence plot Ca flux rate as a function of free [Ca] in Figure 9–20D and obtain the entire Ca pump flux curve, allowing direct estimation of a V_{max}, K_m, and Hill coefficient (n) using the Hill equation:

$$\text{Ca flux} = V_{max}/(1 + \{K_m/[Ca]\}^n) \quad (3)$$

Indo-1 tracks the free [Ca] change more accurately and predicts a lower value of K_m, but the V_{max} values are similar. The values using indo-1 in rat myocytes in this study were V_{max} = 37 nmol/mg protein/min (104 μmol/liter cytosol/s), K_m = 250 nM and n = 2.1. In rabbit ventricular myocytes the values for V_{max}, K_m, and n were 15 (42), 260 and 2, respectively (in the same units). Thus, in rat ventricular myocytes the SR Ca-ATPase appears to have a 2–3 times higher V_{max} than in rabbit, and based on titration with thapsigargin, this seems likely to be due to a higher number of Ca-ATPase pump sites (146).

While the digitonin-permeabilized myocytes contain the Ca-pump in its native environment, the permeabilization could alter local concentrations of soluble proteins or other factors. We have also measured the SR Ca-pump rate in intact rat and rabbit ventricular myocytes using a similar strategy, where all of the other processes that remove Ca from the cytosol are blocked or accounted for (17; see later, under Quantitative Analysis of Ca Fluxes During Relaxation). The V_{max} values obtained there for rat and rabbit, respectively, were 207 and 82 μmol/liter cytosol/sec (with comparable K_m values). Again the rat V_{max} was 2–3 times higher, but the values in the intact cell are about twice as large as those in digitonin-permeabilized cells. Balke et al. (11) obtained very similar values in voltage clamped rat ventricular myocytes (V_{max} = 210 μmol/liter cytosol/sec, K_m = 280 nM).

Like most measurements in SR vesicles, these studies really only considered the forward mode of the SR Ca-pump. That is, they did not consider how the net Ca flux by the SR Ca-pump slows down as intra SR free [Ca] rises. While this is reasonable for the specific experimental conditions (where intra SR Ca is precipitated by oxalate), the situation in intact cells is likely to be more complex. As the Ca-pump loads up the SR with Ca, reverse Ca flux though the pump is expected (153). Shannon et al. (306) considered this in determining Ca fluxes during dynamic Ca transients. The simple Hill equation for the forward pump rate (Eq.3) can be made a step more general to allow both forward and reverse flux:

$$V_{net} = \frac{V_{mf}([Ca]_i/K_{mf})^2 - V_{mr}([Ca]_{SR}/K_{mr})^2}{1 + ([Ca]_i/K_{mf})^2 + ([Ca]_{SR}/K_{mr})^2} \quad (4)$$

where V_{mf} and V_{mr} are the forward and reverse maximum velocities, and K_{mf} and K_{mr} are the forward and reverse dissociation constants, respectively and $[Ca]_i$ and $[Ca]_{SR}$ are the free Ca in cytosol and SR, respectively. I have also made the simplifying assumption that n is 2 for flux in both directions. Of course with $[Ca]_{SR}$ = 0, this reduces to Eq. 3, but as $[Ca]_{SR}$ rises the reverse flux becomes more important and limits the net flux by the Ca-pump. Indeed, at steady state, where V_{net} = 0, then the numerator of Eq. 4 is also 0. If we assume that the maximal velocity of the pump can approach the same forward and reverse limit, then $V_{mf} = V_{mr} = V_{max}$ (329), and it follows that

$$K_{mr}/K_{mf} = [Ca]_{SR}/[Ca]_i \quad (5)$$

In this case the ratio of dissociation constants would equal the [Ca] gradient that can be established across the SR membrane. Shannon and Bers (305) measured $[Ca]_{SR}$ under conditions where leak fluxes were blocked and found this limiting gradient to be 7000 (implying that K_{mr} = 7000K_{mf}. This $[Ca]_{SR}/[Ca]_i$ gradient would require a free energy of 44 kJ/mol for ΔG = 2RT·ln($[Ca]_{SR}/[Ca]_i$), which is about 74% of the energy available from ATP in ventricular muscle (ΔG$_{ATP}$ = 59 kJ/mol; ref 2). In the limit of thermodynamic reversibility, this would constitute a relatively efficient transport. A very important consequence of this thermodynamic consideration is that any decline in ΔG$_{ATP}$ due to decline of [ATP] or increase in either [ADP] or [PO$_4$] (as in hypoxia or ischemia) would decrease the limiting thermodynamic [Ca] gradient. For example, if ΔG$_{ATP}$ drops from 59 to 47 kJ/mol during hypoxia (2) the $[Ca]_{SR}/[Ca]_i$ gradient would drop from 7000 to 1100 (using the same 74% apparent efficiency). This would reduce $[Ca]_{SR}$ from 700 μM to only 110 μM (for 100 nM $[Ca]_i$) and decrease the maximum SR Ca content by a factor of 5 (305).

Shannon and Bers (305) measured the $[Ca]_{SR}$ to be; ~1 mM for an ambient [Ca] of 150 nM with SR Ca leak blocked. This agrees with measurements of $[Ca]_{SR}$ by Chen et al. (77) in the intact beating heart using ^{19}F NMR and a low-affinity fluorine-containing Ca probe ($[Ca]_{SR}$=1 mM). It also raises the question of how much the diastolic leak of SR Ca is expected to displace the $[Ca]_{SR}$ from the thermodynamic equilibrium. This leak may well be due to the occasional opening of SR Ca release channels during Ca sparks (77), but some finite leak must occur no matter what the route. Bassani and Bers (24) measured the rate of unidirectional Ca leak from the SR in intact rat and rabbit ventricular myocytes when the SR Ca-pump was completely blocked by thapsigargin (0.3 µmol/liter cytosol/sec), and this is consistent with calculations based on Ca spark frequency and estimated Ca flux during these Ca sparks.

The importance of considering the backwards flux through the SR Ca-pump is emphasized by the following consideration (see Fig 9–21). At the steady state, SR Ca influx and efflux are equal, so the forward pump rate (V_f) is balanced by the reverse pump rate (V_r) plus the leak (V_L),

$$V_f = V_r + V_L \qquad (6)$$

Using Eq. 3 with cellular estimates above of V_{max}, K_m, and n (see values in Fig. 9–21) gives a V_f of 27 µmol/liter cytosol/sec. This is almost 100 times higher than the measured V_L with the unidirectional SR Ca leak (0.3) and suggests that V_r at steady state must be about 26.7 µmol/liter cytosol/sec. This sort of value for backwards Ca-pump flux would indeed be expected from the foregoing as $[Ca]_{SR}$ approaches millimolar levels (see also 106, 329). Including the backwards flux through the SR Ca-ATPase is certainly a more complete way to consider SR Ca balance than simply forward Ca pumping and a constant Ca leak. The magnitude of this backflux also explains why simpler Ca-pump-leak models (Fig. 9–5C; 11, 312, 352) have predicted a leak rate at diastolic $[Ca]_i$ that is much higher (~20 µmol/liter cytosol/sec) than the 0.3 µmol/liter cytosol/sec measured in the cell (24).

The impact of SR Ca leak on the maximum steady-state SR Ca load was addressed by Ginsburg et al. (117) in a study measuring maximal SR Ca load in intact voltage-clamped ventricular myocytes. The issue is whether the resting SR Ca leak significantly limits the SR Ca content. If the leak does limit SR Ca load, then accelerating the SR Ca-pump (with isoproterenol) or slowing the pump (with submaximal thapsigargin exposure) should alter SR Ca load accordingly. On the other hand, if the leak is inconsequential, then the Ca-pump should approach the thermodynamically limiting gradient even when the pump is significantly slowed. Ginsburg et al. (117) found that essentially the same SR Ca load could be attained when the SR Ca-pump was activated by isoproterenol, partially blocked by thapsigargin, or untreated. Thus the implication is that the normal resting SR Ca leak does not greatly limit the SR Ca load.

This can also be appreciated on quantitative theoretical grounds. Consider that V_{net} in Eq. 4 is equal to $V_f - V_r$ in Eq. 6 and that in the steady state V_{net} is balanced by V_L. Then Eq. 4–6 can be combined and rearranged to

$$[Ca]_{SR} = 7000 \left(\frac{[Ca]_i^2 (V_{max}/V_L - 1) - K_{mf}^2}{(V_{max}/V_L + 1)} \right)^{1/2} \qquad (7)$$

Thus $[Ca]_{SR}$ can be predicted as a function of $[Ca]_i$, V_{max}, V_L, and K_{mf}. Since the total SR Ca ($[Ca]_{SRT}$) is the sum of $[Ca]_{SR}$ and the Ca bound to intra-SR Ca buffers such as calsequestrin, $[Ca]_{SR}$ can be plugged into the following to calculate $[Ca]_{SRT}$.

$$[Ca]_{SRT} = [Ca]_{SR} + \left(\frac{B_{maxSR}}{1 + (K_{dSR}/[Ca]_{SR})} \right) \qquad (8)$$

where B_{maxSR} is the maximal binding capacity of the intra-SR Ca buffers and K_{dSR} is the dissociation constant. Figure 9–22 shows that the SR Ca load is not expected to be greatly decreased by the Ca leak until V_L approaches the forward rate of the pump. Further-

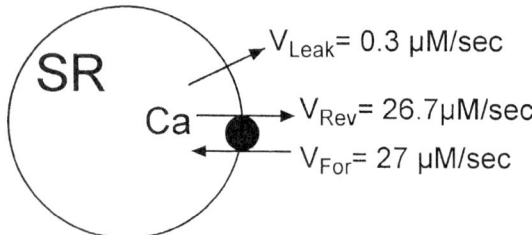

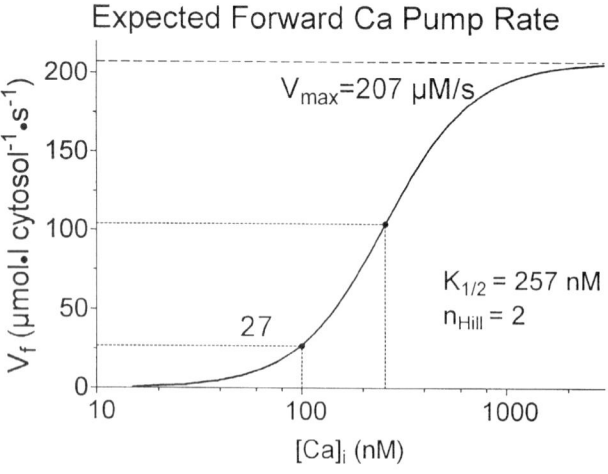

FIG. 9–21. Unidirectional SR Ca fluxes at rest. At rest when $[Ca]_{SR}$ is changing only very slowly, net SR Ca flux must be close to zero, implying the forward rate (V_{For}) is equal to the sum of reverse flux and leak from the SR ($V_{Rev} + V_{Leak}$). The forward rate predicted from the Hill curve is 27 µmol/liter cytosol/sec. For a V_{Leak} of 0.3 µmol/l cytosol/sec (24) the reverse flux must be 26.7 µmol/liter cytosol/sec.

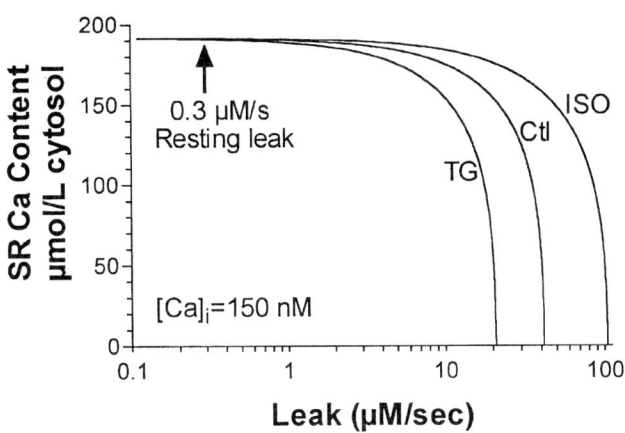

FIG. 9–22. The influence of SR Ca leak on SR Ca content. The effect of different leak values on steady-state SR Ca content with $[Ca]_i$ = 150 nM was calculated using Eq. 7 and 8 with V_{max} = 207 μmol/liter cytosol/sec, K_{mf} = 300 nM, B_{maxSR} = 3.95 mM and K_{dSR} = 600 μM. For pump inhibition by thapsigargin (TG) V_{max} was decreased by 50%. For Ca-pump stimulation by isoproterenol, K_m was reduced by 50%. The SR Ca leak rate (0.3 μmol/liter cytosol/sec) measured by Bassani and Bers (24) is indicated. (See text and ref 117 for further discussion.)

more, near the physiological leak rate (0.3 μmol/liter cytosol/sec), slowing or accelerating the Ca-pump does not affect the steady-state SR Ca load, although the time required to attain that load is altered accordingly. The control values used for Figure 9–22 are V_{max} = 207 μmol/liter cytosol/sec, K_{mf} = 300 nM, B_{maxSR} = 3.95 mM, and K_{dSR} = 600 μM. For pump inhibition by thapsigargin (TG) V_{max} was decreased by 50% and for Ca-pump stimulation by isoproterenol, K_m was reduced by 50%. Figure 9–22 also shows that if the 20 μmol/liter cytosol/sec leak required in the absence of backward SR Ca-pump flux (Fig. 9–5;352) is used, then thapsigargin and isoproterenol would be expected to produce major effects. This is not consistent with observed results and re-emphasizes the importance of considering this backflux in realistic models of SR Ca regulation in intact cells. Not all results agree with this interpretation. Indeed, blocking the ryanodine receptor with tetracaine can dramatically increase SR Ca content (122, 248), an effect that would not be expected if the leak were very small.

SR Ca Content under Physiological Conditions. A number of different experimental approaches have been used to measure the SR Ca content in ventricular muscle. These have included ^{45}Ca fluxes in intact cells and tissue as well as in homogenates and SR vesicles. Some of the more recent measurements in intact cells have come from the amplitude of caffeine-induced Ca transients, as well as integration of $I_{Na/Ca}$ during caffeine-induced contractures. Table 9–5 shows a compilation of some of the measurements where all are converted to the units μmol/liter cytosol. The top group are relatively high and are generally with an ambient [Ca] or $[Ca]_i$ higher than the diastolic level of 100–150 nM. Most of the values in the lower section are at physiological [Ca], and many are from intact cells. These values range from 32–58 μmol/liter cytosol in guinea pig ventricular myocytes to 210–260 μmol/liter cytosol in rat or ferret ventricle. I think this provides a realistic range and given the variety of experimental approaches, conditions and laboratories, it seems that a consensus is developing. For now, 80–130 μmol/liter cytosol is probably a reasonable estimate of steady-state SR Ca content in intact ventricular myocytes at typical frequencies of stimulation. For an SR volume of 3.5% of the cell, this would correspond to 1.5–3 mM total SR Ca.

Sarcoplasmic Reticulum Ca Release Channels

The SR Ca release channel has been clearly identified as the ryanodine receptor. Indeed, ryanodine has been used as a specific ligand allowing the purification of the ryanodine receptor from skeletal muscle (62, 152, 154, 178, 179) and cardiac muscle (155, 180) with estimated molecular weights ~320–450 kDa for a monomer. The purified ryanodine receptor was also incorporated into bilayers and retained the Ca channel characteristics from the native SR (151, 152, 179, 315). The ryanodine receptor appears to be a homo-tetramer, based on its quatrefoil appearance (179, 289, 348), gel permeation chromatography (149), and stoichiometry of high-affinity ryanodine binding (179, 181). Image processing allowed Wagenknecht et al. (348) to reconstruct a detailed three-dimensional architecture of the ryanodine receptor/Ca release channel. The complex is ~27 nm along each side and ~14 nm tall, measurements that correspond reasonably well with the width and length of the junctional "feet" observed in intact muscle (52). The skeletal and cardiac ryanodine receptors have been cloned and have monomeric MW of 565 kDa (208, 229, 247, 330, 365). The tetrameric nature of the ryanodine receptor in vivo implies a 2,260,000 Da structure. The overall evidence now seems compelling that this molecular entity is the ryanodine receptor, the SR Ca-release channel, and the "foot" process observed in electron micrographs

Electrophysiological studies of the cardiac ryanodine receptor incorporated into lipid bilayers and Ca flux studies in isolated SR vesicles have been extremely valuable (e.g. see ref. 215 and reviews 34, 82). Indeed, the ability to incorporate the cardiac ryanodine receptor into lipid bilayers and to record current carried by

TABLE 9-5. *SR Ca Content Measurements*

Reference	Species	Preparation	SR Ca Content (µmoll cytosol^{-1})	Conditions
Solaro and Briggs (318)	Dog	V homog	427	1 µM [Ca], ^{45}Ca
Dani et al. (87)	Rabbit	Perm V myo	171–512	< 1 µM [Ca], ^{45}Ca
Levitsky et al. (191)	Guinea pig	V homog	376	24 µM [Ca], ^{45}Ca
Bridge (56)	Rabbit	Papillary	645	0.5 Hz, 2.7 mM [Ca]$_o$, aa, rest-dep Ca loss
Hove-Madsen and Bers (145)	Rabbit	Perm V myo	884	> 7.5 µM [Ca]
Shannon and Bers (305)	Rat	Perm V myoc	880	~V1 µM [Ca]$_i$ ^{45}Ca
Kawai and Konishi (167)	Ferret	Perm papilary	372	1 µM [Ca], fl
Solaro and Briggs (318)	Dog	V homog	68	100 nM [Ca], ^{45}Ca
Hunter et al. (149)	Rat	Perfused heart	119	2.5 mM [Ca]$_o$, rest-dep ^{45}Ca loss
Fabiato (104)	Rat	Skinned fiber	142	~100 nM [Ca]
Callewaert et al. (61)	Rat	Isol V myo	90	66 nM [Ca]$_c$, caff, I$_{Na/Ca}$
	Guinea pig		32	~70 nM [Ca]$_c$, caff, I$_{Na/Ca}$
Hove-Madsen and Bers (145)	Rabbit	Perm V myo	~100	~100 nM [Ca]$_c$
Shannon and Bers (305)	Rat	Perm V myo	415	100 nM [Ca]$_i$ ^{45}Ca
Varro et al. (345)	Rat	Isol V myo	185	1 mM [Ca]$_o$, caff, I$_{Na/Ca}$
Pytkowski (273)	Rabbit	Papillary	408*	1 Hz, 1.8 mM [Ca]$_o$, ^{45}Ca
Langer and Rich (184)	Rat	Isol V myo	210*	1 mM [Ca]$_o$, ^{45}Ca flux, caff
Kawai and Konishi (167)	Ferret	Perm papilary	260	100 nM [Ca]$_c$, fl
Bassani et al. (22)	Ferret	Isol V myo	141	0.5 Hz, 2 mM [Ca]$_o$, caff, fl
Bassani and Bers (24)	Rat	Isol V myo	114	0.5 Hz, 1 mM [Ca]$_o$, caff, fl
	Rabbit	Isol V myo	106	0.5 Hz, 2 mM [Ca]$_o$, caff, fl
Terracciano et al. (334)	Guinea pig	Isol V myo	58	0.5 Hz, 2 mM [Ca]$_o$, caff, I$_{Na/Ca}$
Terracciano and MacLeod (332)	Guinea-pig	Isol V myo	38	0.5 Hz, 1 mM [Ca]$_o$, caff, I$_{Na/Ca}$
	Rat	Isol V myo	73	0.5 Hz, 1 mM [Ca]$_o$, caff, I$_{Na/Ca}$
Delbridge et al. (89)	Rabbit	Isol V myo	87	0.5 Hz, 2 mM [Ca]$_o$, caff, fl & I$_{Na/Ca}$
Ginsburg et al. (117)	Ferret	Isol V myo	149–190	0.5 Hz, 2 mM [Ca]$_o$, caff, fl & I$_{Na/Ca}$

SR Ca Content Measurements. The line separates measurements of maximum attainable SR Ca content (above) from those at normal cellular conditions.

*Represents caffeine and ryanodine sensitive component of kinetically defined ^{45}Ca washout curve (only ~20% of total component).

aa = atomic absorption spectroscopy, caff = caffeine-induced release, fl = Ca-sensitive fluorescence, Isol V myo. = isolated ventricular myocytes, I$_{Na/Ca}$ = Ca efflux measured via Na-Ca exchange current, Perm = sarcolemma permeabilized by digitonin or saponin, rest-dep = rest dependent loss of Ca.

Table prepared with help from Dr. T. R. Shannon.

single ryanodine receptor channels has provided unique insights into the properties of these channels, including their conductance, open time, open probability, and factors that alter channel-gating properties (e.g. 34, 121, 214, 286–288, 299, 336, 344). Table 9–6 lists some of the known modulators of the SR Ca release channel. These types of studies in the well-controlled bilayer chamber environment (or vesicles) have provided detailed evaluations of the regulation of ryanodine receptor channel gating by Ca, ATP, Mg, caffeine, ryanodine, phosphorylation, and other factors. These types of studies have been essential in the continuing development of our comprehensive understanding of cardiac excitation–contraction (E-C) coupling (34, 34a, 121). Clearly it is also important to consider more explicitly how the SR Ca release channel is regulated in situ in the intact ventricular myocyte, but this is dealt with in a new monograph by Bers (34a) and in recent reviews (45, 351).

Amount of Ca Released During E-C Coupling.

Without discussing the details of how E-C coupling and Ca-induced Ca-release work (34a, 45), it is in keeping with the theme of this chapter to consider quantitative aspects of SR Ca release flux. Bassani et al. (16, 19) measured that about 35%–43% of SR Ca content was released during a normal twitch, but that this fraction was sensitive to both the I$_{Ca}$ trigger and SR Ca load (and could vary from 4%–60%). For an SR Ca content of 120 µmol/liter cytosol this means that 42–52 µmol SR Ca/liter cytosol would be released at a twitch together with 5–15 µmol/liter cytosol of Ca entering as I$_{Ca}$ (see earlier, under Ca Channels). This combination

TABLE 9-6. *Factors That Alter SR Ca Release*

	Effective Concentration	Muscle Type	Reference
ENHANCERS OF Ca RELEASE			
Ca	0.3–10 µM	hrt	215, 288
Caffeine	~1–10 mM	hrt	104, 243, 288
ATP (or AMP-PCP)	1–5 mM	hrt	215, 286
Ryanodine	0.01–30 µM	hrt/sk	214, 287
Sulmazole (AR-L 115BS)	1 mM	hrt	353
Halothane	~0.5 mM	hrt/sk	244, 253, 321
Doxorubicin	7–25 µM	sk	228, 364
Quercetin	10–300 µM	sk	172, 253
Bromo-eudistomin D	~5 µM	sk	230
Sulfhydryl reagents			
$\quad$ AgNO$_3$	0.1–15 µM	sk	291
$\quad$ Ag$^+$ or Hg^{2+}	10–25 µM	hrt	270
$\quad$ Cu^{2+}/Cysteine	2–10 µM	sk	340
INHIBITORS OF Ca RELEASE			
Mg	1–3 mM	hrt	104, 215
Ruthenium red	10 µM	hrt	215
Ryanodine	>100 µM	hrt/sk	161, 181, 214
Dantrolene	2 µM	sk	88
Calmodulin	1 µM	hrt	215, 316
Tetracaine, procaine	0.1, 1 mM	sk	4, 252
Neomycin, gentamycin	60–200 nM	sk	254
Spermine, spermidine	20–200 µM	sk	254
FK binding protein	Endogenous	hrt/sk	59, 164

hrt = heart, sk = skeletal muscle, sm = smooth muscle. This table is based in part on tables compiled by Fleischer and Inui (107) and more extensive tables by Palade (253, 255) which were focused on skeletal muscle SR vesicles. This table is intended to focus on cardiac SR Ca release where data are available.

would provide the Ca (60 µmol/liter cytosol) needed for activation of the myofilaments (see Fig 9–4).

SR Ca release appears to occur via relatively stereotypical events referred to as "Ca sparks" (78) both during rest as well as during E-C coupling. Cheng et al. (78) estimated the Ca flux associated with a single Ca spark as $\sim 2 \times 10^{-19}$ mol, consistent with a single ryanodine receptor current of 4 pA for 10 ms (40 fC). To explain a resting SR Ca leak rate of 0.3 µmol/liter cytosol (24) would require about 50 Ca sparks/sec in the cell (or $\sim 2 \cdot$ pL$^{-1} \cdot$ s^{-1}). The 40 fC Ca spark flux used by Cheng et al. (78) is probably larger than the flux via a single ryanodine receptor channel current under physiological conditions (216), where a single ryanodine receptor channel flux of 2 fC (0.4 pA × 4 ms) may be more realistic (336). This would be consistent with ~20 ryanodine receptor release channels contributing to the Ca flux at a single Ca spark. This is also consistent with recent attempts to measure the number of RyR per Ca Spark (49a, 56a, 201a).

The normal Ca transient during the twitch in ventricular myocytes is composed of a temporal and spatial summation of many Ca sparks which are synchronized by the action potential and activation of Ca influx via Ca channels (64, 65, 198, 199). To attain the peak SR Ca release flux of 3 mM/sec estimated by Wier et al. (352) would require simultaneous activation of about 5,000 Ca sparks per 30 pL cell (within a few ms). If a Ca spark were due to a single ryanodine receptor, this would require only 0.3% of the ~1.7 million ryanodine receptors in a 30 pL rat ventricular myocyte (44). Even if 20 ryanodine receptors are required to produce the 40 fC of Ca flux above, this would still only require 5%–6% of the total number of cellular ryanodine receptors. Furthermore, a total SR Ca release flux of 50 µmol/liter cytosol would also require only ~5,000 Ca sparks (based on 40 fC/spark) or 5%–6% of the cellular ryanodine receptors (based on 2 fC/ryanodine receptor). Thus normal twitch activation only requires a small percentage of available release channels to function at any given twitch.

It is of interest to note here that opening of a similarly modest fraction of L-type Ca channels (2%–3%) is required to produce the measured whole-cell I_{Ca} (192). For example, there may be ~230,000 dihydropyridine receptors in a 30 pL rat ventricular myocyte and only ~5,000 Ca channels need to open (with a single channel current of 0.2 pA to produce a whole-cell current of 1 nA).

Mitochondrial Ca Transport

It is widely appreciated that mitochondria can accumulate massive amounts of Ca, especially when there is sufficient inorganic phosphate, which can precipitate insoluble Ca-phosphate in mitochondria, a process known as matrix loading (68, 70, 189). Indeed isolated mitochondria can take up 100 nmol Ca/mg mitochondrial protein (corresponding to 10,000 µmol/liter cytosol, assuming 40 mg mitochondrial protein/g wet weight) and can store several times more (67). While this is a potentially enormous capacity, it appears that under physiological conditions anticipated in vivo, mitochondria are likely to contain very much less (e.g. 1 nmol/mg; ref. 68). In conditions closer to in vivo conditions, Fry et al. (112) showed that mitochondrial Ca uptake was not appreciable in digitonin-permeabilized isolated cardiac myocytes until cytoplasmic [Ca] exceeded 1 µM (where Ca uptake rate of 2–5 µmol/liter cytosol/sec can be inferred).

Figure 9–23 illustrates the Ca cycle of mitochondria. Ca enters via a uniport system down a large electro-

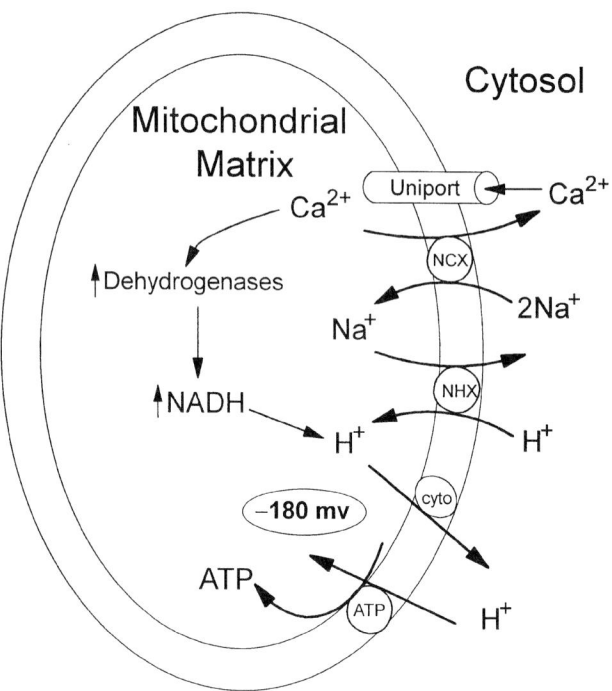

FIG. 9–23. Ionic fluxes across the mitochondrial membrane. Ca enters via a uniport, down an electrical gradient established by the proton pump at bottom. Ca can be extruded by a Na/Ca antiport and Na is extruded by Na/H exchange thereby completing the cycle. Elevated cytoplasmic [Ca] can lead to elevated mitochondrial [Ca] and increased activity of mitochondrial dehydrogenases and NADH production.

chemical gradient (about −180 mV) set up by proton extrusion linked to the passage of electrons down the cytochrome system in the respiratory chain. This Ca uniporter is blocked competitively by physiological $[Mg]_i$ (237) and also potently by ruthenium red (221), Ru 360 (357, 363), and lanthanides (213, 275). Ca entry via the uniport pathway exhibits a sigmoid dependence on [Ca] and under physiologic ionic conditions has a K_m above 30 μM for Ca. Thus, at the $[Ca]_i$ associated with the cardiac cycle (0.1–1 μM) the influx rate is expected to be quite low. In particular, Crompton (85, 86) developed a model to describe Ca uptake by isolated mitochondria. At 0.1 and 1 μM [Ca] mitochondrial Ca uptake is 0.1 and 3.1 μmol/liter cytosol/sec, respectively (assuming 40 mg mitochondrial protein/ml cell and 0.65 L cytosol/L cell). The ability of mitochondria to accumulate Ca led Lehninger (190) and Carafoli (67) to speculate that mitochondria may be involved in removing Ca from the cytoplasm during cardiac relaxation, but it turns out that the quantitative contribution is almost negligible. This issue is addressed more explicitly later (see Relative Contributions of Ca Transporters).

The main route of Ca extrusion from the mitochondria is via a Na/Ca antiporter, which may be electroneutral (2:1), but might also be > 2:1 (84–86, 162). The [Na] dependence of this Na/Ca antiporter is sigmoidal with half-maximal Ca extrusion at ~5–8 mM Na, making this system quite sensitive to changes of $[Na]_i$ in the physiological range (84, 113). While variations in bulk cytoplasmic [Na] during the cardiac cycle are probably insufficient to cause rapid release of mitochondrial Ca, large changes in [Na] can induce substantial mitochondrial Ca release in vitro (84). There is also a Na-independent extrusion of Ca from mitochondria which is less prominent in heart, but more so in tissues lacking the Na/Ca antiport activity (e.g. liver and kidney; 85). The inner mitochondrial membrane also has an active Na/H exchange system (217), which may be the means by which Na is extruded from the matrix, and which also completes the cycle. In this way the energy for Ca extrusion via Na/Ca exchange depends also on the proton movement during respiration and the consequently negative intramitochondrial potential.

Under relatively physiological conditions there is probably only a small [Ca] gradient across the inner mitochondrial membrane, with internal [Ca] being slightly lower than cytoplasmic [Ca] (223, 205). Based on the trans-mitochondrial potential (−180 mV), Ca would be at equilibrium when mitochondrial [Ca] is 100 mM–1 M. Ca is thus far from equilibrium, and considerable energy is required to extrude Ca from mitochondria up this electrochemical gradient. While the [Na] gradient may be the immediate source of energy, the Na gradient is created by the proton gradient. Thus the true energy source is respiration and the protonmotive force it generates. In intact cells, it appears that resting intra-mitochondrial free [Ca] ($[Ca]_M$) is lower than $[Ca]_i$ (220, 363). Figure 9–24 shows $[Ca]_M$ in intact cells (220) where $[Ca]_i$ was elevated by reduction in $[Na]_o$ (thereby promoting Ca entry via Na/Ca exchange). These results indicate that as resting $[Ca]_i$ rises to 650 nM the value of $[Ca]_M$ stays below $[Ca]_i$. However, as resting $[Ca]_i$ becomes very high, mitochondrial Ca uptake appears to be activated and $[Ca]_M$ exceeds $[Ca]_i$.

At present it seems clear that there is no detectable fluctuation in $[Ca]_M$ during an individual twitch in ventricular myocytes (120, 220, 363). Phasic Ca transients reported in heart mitochondria by Chacon et al. (76), which were kinetically identical to the cytosolic signal, may be due to artifactual contamination of the $[Ca]_M$ signal by $[Ca]_i$ (and the authors did not use any blockers of mitochondrial Ca uptake or quench of cytosolic indicator to confirm their interpretation). Crompton (85) also modeled the response of isolated cardiac mitochondria to the phasic changes in $[Ca]_i$ expected during the cardiac cycle. For a cytoplasmic [Ca] change

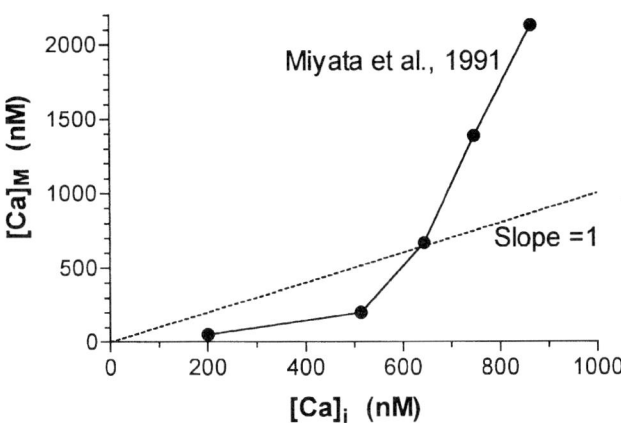

FIG. 9-24. Mitochondria free [Ca] ([Ca]$_m$) as a function of cytosolic [Ca] ([Ca]$_c$). Increases of [Ca]$_c$ in rat ventricular myocytes were induced by reduction of extracellular [Na] (i.e. via Na/Ca exchange). Mean [Ca]$_c$ was measured using indo-1 (loaded as the salt form) and [Ca]$_m$ was measured using indo-1 (loaded as the AM form) with Mn quench of cytosolic indo-1. Data are taken from Miyata et al., (220) and have been redrawn (without error bars) and including a broken line corresponding to [Ca]$_m$ = [Ca]$_c$ (slope = 1).

from ~200 nM to ~2 μM and back, [Ca]$_M$ increased by only ~2%. On the other hand, experiments have shown that very high frequency stimulation (4 Hz) or strong cellular Ca loading via the Na/Ca exchange cause a slow rise in [Ca]$_M$ over tens of seconds (220, 363). Indeed, Zhou et al. (363) demonstrated that under these conditions phasic increases of [Ca]$_M$ could be detected, but only when diastolic [Ca]$_i$ exceeded 400 nM. This is entirely consistent with the sigmoid dependence of mitochondrial Ca uptake (84, 112, 113) and the intact cell data in Figure 9-24.

Mitochondrial Ca fluxes might not be important quantitatively in E-C coupling, but the small gradual changes in mitochondrial [Ca] with frequency changes or cellular Ca load may help to regulate mitochondrial energy production. Three key mitochondrial matrix enzymes are activated by low μM [Ca] (pyruvate dehydrogenase, α-ketoglutarate dehydrogenase, and the NAD-dependent isocitrate dehydrogenase; 92–94, 127, 128). Thus, increases in mitochondrial Ca via the above mechanisms could occur when cytosolic [Ca] is relatively high and the energy demands are also high (i.e. when contractile activation and Ca pumping are consuming ATP at high rates). In this way, the rise in cytoplasmic (and mitochondrial) [Ca] can increase oxidative metabolism and thereby increase ATP production to meet increased demands. A potentially interesting twist on this is that cellular Ca loading is often secondary to cellular Na loading, via sarcolemmal Na/Ca exchange (e.g. when the Na-pump is inhibited by digitalis). In this case the increase of mitochondrial Ca, which *could* stimulate oxidative metabolism, may be minimized by the elevation of [Na]$_i$, which would deplete the mitochondria of Ca. Thus, energy supply may not go up to meet demands and the cytoplasmic Ca load will be more severe. This might favor more force production, but it could also elevate diastolic [Ca]$_i$ and compromise cardiac relaxation.

Brandes and Bers (55) have recently demonstrated a [Ca]$_i$-dependent stimulation of mitochondrial NADH production by measuring [NADH] in intact contracting ventricular muscle. With a sudden increase in stimulation frequency or [Ca]$_o$ there was a transient decrease in [NADH], consistent with NADH production not keeping up with the increased ATP and NADH consumption. However, this [NADH] decline was followed by recovery toward the initial value that was entirely dependent on increased average [Ca]$_i$. That is, a comparable increase in work by increasing sarcomere length was associated with the same initial NADH decline, but no recovery. They suggested that the increased average [Ca]$_i$ caused an increase in [Ca]$_M$ and stimulation of dehydrogenases and NADH production. Indeed, when the elevated [Ca]$_i$ was terminated, there was an overshoot of [NADH], which could be due to a slow loss of the Ca-dependent stimulation of mitochondrial dehydrogenases. The time course of this overshoot is also consistent with that of Ca efflux from mitochondria (20–40 sec; ref. 15).

It should be noted that mitochondria use the same pool of energy to phosphorylate ADP to ATP as to drive Ca uptake (i.e. the protonmotive force). Energized, isolated mitochondria have been shown to take up Ca at the expense of making ATP (347). This would obviously be a dangerous situation in vivo, but it appears that at physiological [Mg]$_i$ the uniport is inhibited strongly enough that mitochondrial energy is preferentially used to make ATP (319). This may not be the case when the cell is exposed to chronic elevated [Ca]$_i$, where mitochondrial Ca uptake gets much more active.

The ability of heart mitochondria to accumulate massive amounts of Ca under pathological conditions such as ischemia (283) may serve as an important safety device for heart cells. Cellular Ca overload is a common early component of cell injury in many cell types (304) and could quickly become disastrous in heart cells, because high cytosolic [Ca] would keep energy consumption by the myofilaments and Ca-ATPases high while mitochondrial Ca uptake could limit ATP synthesis. Sustained contracture could also worsen the situation by decreasing local blood flow by vascular compression. If the mitochondria can temporarily compensate for the cellular Ca load by taking up large amounts of Ca, permanent cell damage might be avoided. Unfortunately it is a double-edged sword, since Ca accumulation by the mitochondria diminishes ATP production and eventually compromises the mitochondria. Thus the survival of the cell might depend on whether the mitochondria can survive a given degree of Ca loading.

In conclusion, it seems that mitochondria play a very minor role in Ca movements during contraction and relaxation. However, with slower increases in "mean" $[Ca]_i$ mitochondrial Ca transport may play a more important role in increasing metabolism to meet increased metabolic demands. In more severe cellular Ca overload, mitochondria may also store massive amounts of Ca to protect the cytoplasm from very high Ca levels.

Ca REMOVAL FROM THE CYTOPLASM DURING RELAXATION

Relative Contributions of Ca Transporters

As pointed out earlier, four Ca transport systems can compete for cytoplasmic Ca during relaxation in cardiac muscle: (1) the SR Ca-ATPase, (2) the sarcolemmal Na/Ca exchange, (3) the sarcolemmal Ca-ATPase, and (4) the mitochondrial Ca uniport system. Obviously, Ca entering the cytosol from the extracellular space or SR is mostly bound to the various Ca buffers that were discussed with respect to Figs. 9–2 through 9–5 and Table 9–2. The focus here is the final fate of that Ca which entered the cytosol to activate contraction when the $[Ca]_i$ and bound Ca return toward their initial resting condition. That is, which of the four Ca transport processes described above are responsible for the removal of cytosolic Ca which allows relaxation to proceed? In particular how do these Ca transporters compete dynamically during relaxation?

Bassani et al. (20) evaluated this competition initially by using inhibition of each Ca transport system and observing the impact on the rate of $[Ca]_i$ decline and relaxation in rabbit ventricular myocytes. Figure 9–25 shows a summary of their results for relaxation, which were in close agreement with data from $[Ca]_i$ decline. The normal twitch relaxes with a half-time ($t_{1/2}$) of 170 ± 30 ms where all Ca removal systems are functional. Rapid and sustained application of 10 mM caffeine causes abrupt SR Ca release via ryanodine receptors, and with appropriate flow characteristics the rate of rise of $[Ca]_i$ can be comparable to that during the twitch. However, the sustained exposure to caffeine prevents net Ca reaccumulation by the SR, while the other Ca removal systems can still function. When SR Ca reaccumulation was inhibited in this way relaxation was slowed by a factor of 3 ($t_{1/2}$ = 540 ± 70 ms). This

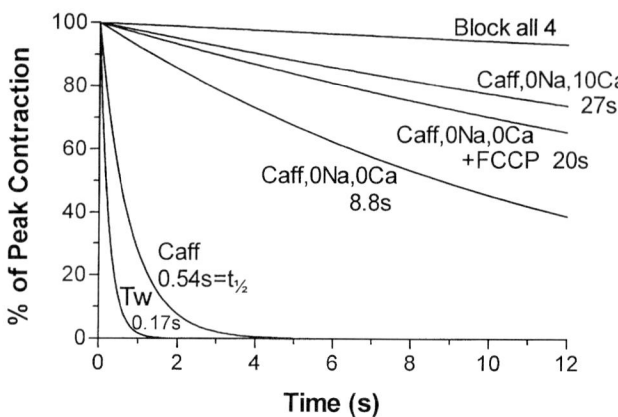

FIG. 9–25. Relaxation in rabbit ventricular myocyte with selective inhibition of Ca transporters. Normalized cell relaxations are shown and conditions were either (1) with all Ca transporters functional during relaxation of a steady-state twitch (Tw), (2) preventing net SR Ca uptake during a caffeine-induced contracture in NT (Caff), (3) additionally inhibiting Na/Ca exchange in 0Na, 0Ca solution (Caff,0Na,0Ca). To further analyze relaxation during Caff, 0Na, 0Ca, this was coupled with either (4) inhibition of mitochondrial Ca uptake with 1 μM FCCP + 1 μM oligomycin so only sarcolemmal Ca-ATPase was functional (Caff,0Na,0Ca + FCCP) or (5) inhibition of the sarcolemmal Ca-pump by elevating $[Ca]_o$ to 10 mM after pre-depletion of $[Na]_i$, so that only mitochondrial Ca uptake was functional (Caff,0Na,10Ca). All four Ca removal systems were also blocked by combining the caffeine application with 0Na, 10Ca and FCCP (after pre-depletion of $[Na]_i$). The traces are based on mean $t_{1/2}$ values (shown along the traces without standard error values) for relaxation measured in experiments described by Bassani et al. (20).

result makes it clear that SR Ca uptake is important in relaxation, but also that a reasonable rate of relaxation can be obtained by the other three systems. Next, the Na/Ca exchange was blocked at the same time as SR Ca reuptake by applying 10 mM caffeine in a Na-free, Ca-free solution containing EGTA (Caff, 0Na, 0Ca). It should be noted that this blocks Ca movement by Na/Ca exchange in both directions. This maneuver slowed relaxation and $[Ca]_i$ decline by almost 20-fold ($t_{1/2}$ 8.8 ± 1.0 s) compared to caffeine alone, which indicates that Na/Ca exchange is responsible for most of the relaxation and $[Ca]_i$ decline during a caffeine-induced contracture.

Even when both the SR Ca-ATPase and Na/Ca exchange are prevented, relaxation and $[Ca]_i$ decline still proceed, although very slowly. This slow relaxation and $[Ca]_i$ decline requiring tens of seconds could be due to Ca transport by the mitochondrial Ca uniporter or the sarcolemmal Ca-ATPase. To inhibit mitochondrial Ca uptake in the intact myocyte, Bassani et al. (20) used application of FCCP and oligomycin a few seconds before exposure to caffeine, 0Na, 0Ca solution. FCCP is a protonophore that dissipates the mitochondrial proton and membrane potential gradient, thereby eliminating the driving force responsible for Ca influx into mitochondria (oligomycin was included to minimize mitochondrial ATP consumption during the brief exposure to FCCP). Inhibition of mitochondrial Ca uptake in this way slowed the mean relaxation time by about twofold compared to caffeine, 0Na, 0Ca (20 sec vs 8.8 sec). Two different strategies were used to inhibit the sarcolemmal Ca-ATPase (thermodynamic and pharmacological). The thermodynamic approach used elevation of $[Ca]_o$ to 10–100 mM to limit the ability of the sarcolemmal Ca-pump by steepening the concentration gradient. However, to do this experiment in Na-free solution required that the cells first be depleted of intracellular Na by incubation in 0Na, 0Ca. Otherwise extracellular Ca would enter in exchange for intracellular Na, greatly complicating the interpretation. As seen in Figure 9–25, this slowed relaxation about threefold with respect to caffeine, 0Na, 0Ca ($t_{1/2}$ went from 8.8 sec to 27 sec). The second method employed carboxyeosin, a potent inhibitor of the sarcolemmal Ca-pump (115) and produced very similar results (22). That is, carboxyeosin slowed the $t_{1/2}$ of $[Ca]_i$ decline in rabbit ventricular myocytes during caffeine, 0Na, 0Ca from 7.5 ± 0.5 sec to 26.3 ± 2.1 sec. When all four Ca transport systems were blocked, relaxation and $[Ca]_i$ decline were nearly abolished (20, 22). This indicates that these are the only four Ca removal systems that need to be considered from any practical standpoint.

Based on this series of studies, it is possible to make a crude prediction of the relative rates of Ca extrusion by these four systems in rabbit ventricular myocytes (using ratios of $t_{1/2}$ values). Compared to the Na/Ca exchanger (assumed to be the main mechanism functioning during caffeine exposure) the SR Ca-ATPase was 2–3 times faster and the sarcolemmal Ca-ATPase and mitochondrial Ca transport were 37 and 50 times slower, respectively (20). Even at this basic level of analysis this might suggest that roughly 67%–75% of the Ca during relaxation in rabbit ventricle goes to the SR, with most of the rest extruded via Na/Ca exchange.

Bassani et al. (17) extended this work by comparing rat and rabbit ventricular myocytes and also developed a quantitative analysis scheme that allowed a more direct evaluation of how the Ca transport systems interact dynamically during $[Ca]_i$ decline. In both rat and rabbit ventricular myocytes $[Ca]_i$ decline during a caffeine-induced contracture in 0Na, 0Ca had a time constant (τ) of ~12 sec, indicating that the combined action of the mitochondrial Ca uptake and sarcolemmal Ca-pump were comparable between species. However, when caffeine was applied in normal Na-containing buffer, the rabbit myocytes relaxed much faster ($t_{1/2}$ = 0.6 vs 2.0 sec), indicating that the Na/Ca exchange is more powerful in rabbit than rat myocytes.

When the SR Ca-pump was also functional (during the twitch), rat myocytes relaxed much faster than rabbit myocytes ($t_{1/2}$ = 80 vs 180 ms). Thus it appears that the SR Ca-pump is much stronger in rat than rabbit ventricle and this more than compensates for the slower Ca removal by Na/Ca exchange. These results are consistent with anecdotal observations of $I_{Na/Ca}$ in ventricular myocytes (larger in rabbit) and stronger SR Ca-ATPase activity reported in rat, which was attributed to a higher density of SR Ca-pump sites (146).

One limitation with the type of experiments in Figure 9–25 is that twitches are being compared with caffeine-induced contractures. Thus, experimental protocols were developed to selectively block either the SR Ca-ATPase or the sarcolemmal Na/Ca exchange during an otherwise normal twitch contraction activated by an action potential (17). Figure 9–26 shows Ca transients during twitches in rabbit and rat myocytes before and after selective inhibition of the SR Ca-ATPase by thapsigargin. A key feature of this experiment was that the SR Ca-pump must be completely blocked, but the SR Ca load at the time of the twitch had to be the same. To achieve this state, after steady-state stimulation the cells were incubated for 2 min in 0Na, 0Ca solution, with 2.5 μM thapsigargin, just before switching back to NT and stimulation of a twitch. This specific protocol allowed the SR Ca load to remain at the normal level, but it also produced complete block of SR Ca uptake (as was tested directly by attempts to reload the SR after Ca depletion). Of course only one test twitch

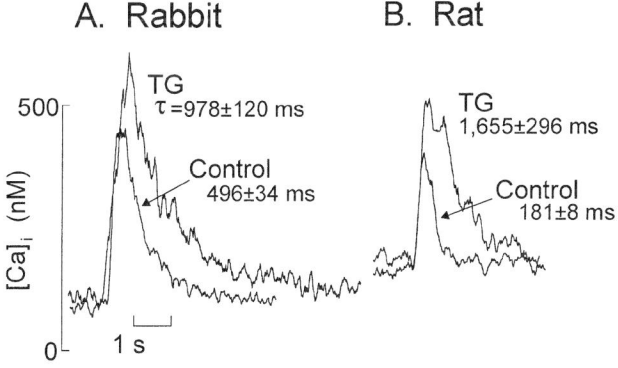

FIG. 9–26. Twitch Ca transients in rabbit and rat ventricular myocytes with SR Ca-ATPase blocked by thapsigargin. Ca transient were measured using indo-1 fluorescence during electrically stimulated twitches in rabbit (A) and rat (B) ventricular myocytes before (Control) and after treatment with 2.5 μM thapsigargin (TG). Twitches were evoked 10 sec after switching to control solution (after 5–7 min pre-perfusion with 0Na,0Ca solution). For the TG twitch the cells were exposed to TG for 2 min during the last part of the pre-perfusion period. SR Ca load was maintained despite complete block of the SR Ca-pump. Time constants (τ) of $[Ca]_i$ decline are shown [Modified from Bassani et al., (17).]

can be given (because SR Ca released is not reaccumulated). Also after much longer rest times in thapsigargin solution, the SR Ca content does gradually decline, even in 0Na, 0Ca solution.

Two key features are of note in Figure 9–26. First, the peaks of the Ca transients are larger after the SR Ca-pump is blocked. This is consistent with the idea that rapid Ca transport by the SR Ca-pump normally limits the peak of $[Ca]_i$, and this seems to be true for both rabbit and rat myocytes. Second, the time constant (τ) of $[Ca]_i$ decline is prolonged in the presence of thapsigargin. In rabbit $[Ca]_i$ decline is only slowed by a factor of 2 (τ increases from 496 ms to 978 ms). However, in rat myocytes thapsigargin slows $[Ca]_i$ decline by a factor of 9 (τ increases from 181 ms to 1.66 sec). This is certainly consistent with the foregoing results suggesting that SR Ca uptake is stronger in rat.

Bassani et al. (17) did analogous experiments with selective inhibition of the Na/Ca exchange. In this case cells were first depleted of $[Na]_i$ by superfusion for 5–7 min in 0Na, 0Ca solution. This allows the Na-pump to extrude Na and thereby prevents Ca influx via Na/Ca exchange when $[Ca]_o$ is subsequently elevated (even to 100 mM) in the continued absence of $[Na]_o$. Twitches in this case were activated in Na-free solution with Li in place of Na so that the measured action potentials were essentially normal and Na/Ca exchange in either direction was completely prevented. For rabbit cells, blocking Na/Ca exchange slightly increased the peak $[Ca]_i$ and slowed the τ of $[Ca]_i$ decline by 45% (from 406 ms to 588 ms). For rat, the effects of Na/Ca exchange inhibition were very modest: There was no significant increase in the amplitude of the Cai transient and there was only a 20% slowing of $[Ca]_i$ decline (consistent with voltage clamp results in rat ventricular myocyte [42]). These results indicate that the Na/Ca exchanger is considerably more important in rabbit than rat myocytes, as inferred above.

Blocking both the SR Ca-ATPase and Na/Ca exchange simultaneously greatly slowed the rate of $[Ca]_i$ decline in both rabbit and rat myocytes to a similar rate ($\tau \sim 12$ sec). This is also the same τ measured for the $[Ca]_i$ decline during caffeine, 0Na, 0Ca in these same cells. However, the amplitude of the twitch Ca transients (thapsigargin, 0Na, 0Ca) was only about half of that observed during caffeine, 0Na, 0Ca. This is probably because only about half of the SR Ca content is released during a normal twitch vs all during caffeine exposure (16, 19).

Quantitative Analysis of Cellular Ca Fluxes During Relaxation.
A second limitation of the experiments in Figure 9–25 and foregoing discussion of rates of relaxation and $[Ca]_i$ decline is that it does not deal directly with total Ca flux rates. The requisite information is, however, available to take this analysis to the next important quantitative level (17, 21). First the free $[Ca]_i$ can be converted to total cytoplasmic [Ca] ($[Ca]_t$), using the passive myoplasmic buffering characteristics measured by Hove-Madsen and Bers (146; see also Figure 9–2 and Table 9–2). This assumes that the Ca buffering is in rapid equilibrium, which may be a reasonable estimate during $[Ca]_i$ decline (though not during $[Ca]_i$ rise). Then differentiation of $[Ca]_t$ with respect to time ($d[Ca]_t/dt$) provides the rate of Ca transport from the myoplasm during relaxation. This transport rate must be the sum of the individual transport rates given by

$$d[Ca]_t/dt = J_{SR} + J_{Na/CaX} + J_{Slow} - \text{Leak} \quad (9)$$

where the three J terms refer to flux through the SR Ca-ATPase, Na/Ca exchange and the combined slow Ca transport by mitochondria and sarcolemmal Ca-ATPase. The Leak term is a constant Ca leak into the cytoplasm and was assumed to be small compared to other fluxes during $[Ca]_i$ decline. For simplicity J_{SR}, $J_{Na/CaX}$ and J_{Slow} can be empirically described as simple [Ca] dependent fluxes of the form

$$J_x = \frac{V_{max}}{1 + (K_m/[Ca]_i)^n} \quad (10)$$

J_{Slow} was first fit by using the decline of $[Ca]_i$ during a twitch in 0Na, 0Ca and thapsigargin, where J_{SR} and J_{NaCaX} are zero (and comparable results were found for caffeine, 0Na, 0Ca). In other words, we plot $d[Ca]_t/dt$ as a function of $[Ca]_i$ and fit it to Eq. 10. Then the determined V_{max}, K_m, and n for J_{Slow} are held constant for the additional analyses for a given cell type. Similarly, parameters for J_{NaCaX} can be measured during a twitch in thapsigargin where $d[Ca]_t/dt = J_{Na/CaX} + J_{Slow}$ (again the normal caffeine response gave similar values). Obviously, the same strategy can be used to obtain parameters for J_{SR} (using the twitch where Na/Ca exchange is prevented by Na-free intracellular and extracellular conditions). A good check for this analysis is to see if $d[Ca]_t/dt$ during the normal twitch Ca transient can be reasonably described by the sum in Eq. 9 (and this was the case). Figure 9–27 shows the resulting J_x functions estimated in this way. The V_{max} for the SR Ca-ATPase in rat is larger than in rabbit, but the situation is reversed for the Na/Ca exchange. The J_{Slow} is quite slow compared even to the J_{NaCaX}. It should also be noted that the Hill function (Eq. 10) used to describe J_x does not necessarily have to be a good mechanistic descriptor of the flux (e.g. not the case for Na/Ca exchange), as long as it provides a reasonably good

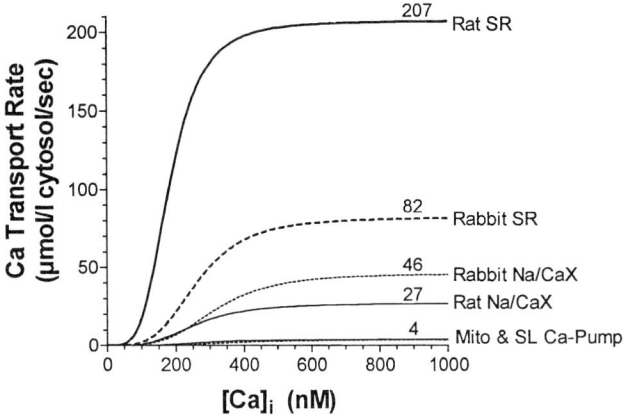

FIG. 9–27. Ca transport functions derived from Ca transients in intact rabbit and rat ventricular myocytes. Ca transport rates as functions of [Ca]$_i$ for the SR Ca-ATPase, Na/Ca exchange and combined slow systems (mitochondrial and sarcolemmal Ca-ATPase) were determined as described in the text and with respect to Eq. 9 and 10. Independent values obtained for J$_{SR}$, J$_{Na/CaX}$ and J$_{Slow}$ respectively were: V$_{max}$ (in μmol/liter cytosol/sec) = 82, 46 and 3.9 for rabbit and 207, 27 and 4 for rat; K$_m$ (in nM) = 264, 316, and 362 in rabbit and 184, 257 and 268 in rat; n = 3.7, 3.7, 3.2 in rabbit and 3.9, 3.4 an 3.5 in rat. [Based on data from Bassani et al. (17).]

empirical fit to the dependence of d[Ca]$_t$/dt on [Ca]$_i$ over the range of interest.

Figure 9–28 shows how we can then simulate the action of all systems working simultaneously during a normal twitch. Here we use the free [Ca]$_i$ during that twitch to calculate the instantaneous individual fluxes through each system. In this way we are directly estimating the dynamic competition of the individual transporters for free [Ca]$_i$. A point that could improve this analysis would be to calculate the back-fluxes for each of these transporters as described for the SR Ca-pump in Eq. 4. This would allow net flux via these systems to more closely approach zero as free [Ca]$_i$ returns to the resting level. Consideration of local spatial distributions of both Ca transporters and buffering sites could also make this sort of analysis more comprehensive (182; see also Fig. 9–18).

Figure 9–28 shows that during a normal twitch the fractions of Ca transported by the SR, Na/Ca exchange, and slow systems are 70%, 28% and 2%, respectively in rabbit myocytes and 92%, 7%, and 1% in rat myocytes. This 28% estimate of Ca flux by Na/Ca exchange in rabbit agrees with the 25%–33% estimated above, which was based only on the ratio of time constants during [Ca]$_i$ decline. The 7% value for rat also agrees with very similar experimental results in rat by Negretti et al. (233), but it is somewhat smaller than previous indirect estimates based on time constants of relaxation or [Ca]$_i$ decline (42, 83). Thus there seems to be a clear species difference in this competi-

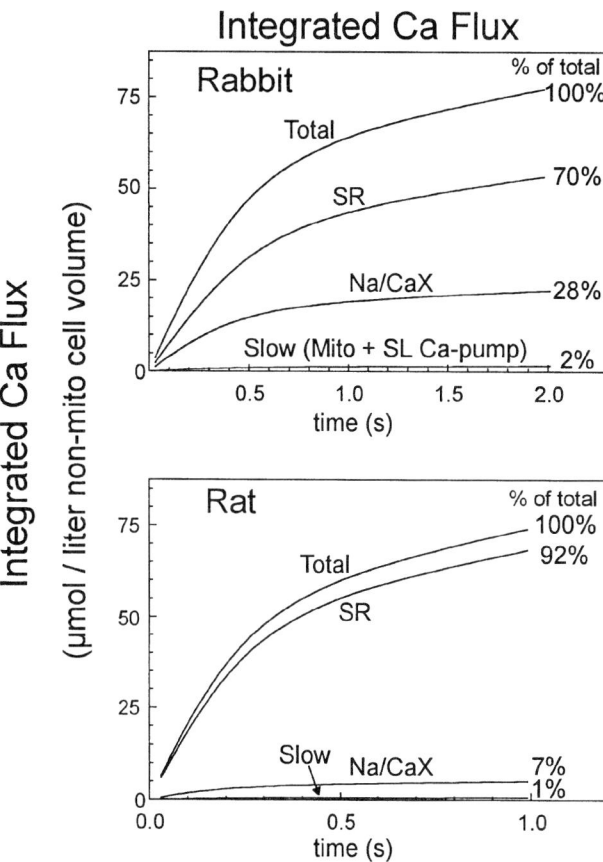

FIG. 9–28. Integrated Ca fluxes during twitch relaxation in rabbit and rat ventricular myocytes. Free [Ca]$_i$ during relaxation of a normal twitch was used as a driving function so that Ca flux via each system could be integrated over time using the [Ca]$_i$ dependence as described in Figure 9–27 and Eq. 9 and 10. [Modified from Bassani et al. (17).]

tion between the SR Ca-ATPase and the Na/Ca exchange.

This same sort of analysis can also be applied to caffeine-induced contractures (17, 21). This allows estimation of what fraction of the Ca removal flux is via Na/Ca exchange during a caffeine-induced contracture where net SR Ca uptake is prevented. As we will see below, this value is particularly useful in allowing the use of caffeine-activated Na/Ca exchange current to estimate total SR Ca contents (see also Table 9–5). For rabbit ventricular myocytes this value was 93% and for rat it was 87%. Negretti et al. (233) estimated this value at 67% in ventricular myocytes from a different strain of rats using a similar experimental strategy and ratios of time constants. Their work suggested a somewhat larger contribution of both sarcolemmal Ca-ATPase and mitochondrial Ca uptake vs Na/Ca exchange in rat (4% vs 1% during the twitch and 33% vs 13% during caffeine exposure).

Species, Developmental, and Temperature Dependence

The experiments and analyses in Figures 9–25 through 9–28 were done at room temperature. Since all of the membrane-transport systems are expected to be faster at more physiological temperature, it is reasonable to ask how this relative competition among Ca transport systems is altered at different temperatures. Puglisi et al. (271) performed such experiments and analysis for rabbit, ferret, and cat ventricular myocytes at 25° and 35°C. All the Ca transport systems are indeed faster at 35°C than at 25°C (with apparent Q_{10} in these experiments in the range of 1.7–2.5). For example, the V_{max} of the rabbit SR Ca-ATPase was increased from 73 to 189 μmol/liter cytosol/sec as temperature increased from 25° to 35°C. However, the relative contribution of the Na/Ca exchange or the SR Ca-ATPase to $[Ca]_i$ decline or relaxation was essentially the same. That is, for rabbit ventricular myocytes, analysis like that shown in Figure 9–28 at 25°C were 70: 27: 3% and at 35°C were 74: 23: 3% for SR: Na/Ca exchange: lumped slow systems respectively. Moreover, there was not a very great difference between rabbit, ferret, and cat (except that the sarcolemmal Ca-ATPase was notably stronger in the ferret). Some of the values derived from different studies on this issue are listed in Table 9–7.

Table 9–7 also shows results from studies in different mammalian species, using either the experimental and analytical strategy just described or paired rapid cooling contractures (RCCs) induced by sudden reduction in temperature to 0°–1°C (33, 34, 39, 40, 56, 313). The idea behind the paired RCCs is the following. The first RCC causes release of all of the SR Ca content while inhibiting Ca transport at 0°–1°C. Upon rewarming, the Ca transport systems are all re-activated and compete for cytosolic Ca. Thus a second RCC immediately after relaxation of the first will allow indirect assessment of the fraction of Ca resequestered by the SR, vs the fraction extruded from the cell. For example, Hryshko et al. (147) found that in rabbit ventricle the second RCC was ~75% of the first. In important control experiments they also found that this value was ~100% when Ca extrusion during the first RCC and rewarming was done with the Na/Ca exchange prevented in 0Na, 0Ca solution. These results indicated that the Ca responsible for 75% of contraction was taken back up by the SR with 25% extruded by Na/Ca exchange (consistent with the results in Fig. 9–28).

Developmental differences in this balance of Ca fluxes during relaxation are also apparent. For example, neonatal rabbit ventricular myocytes have a much higher level of functional expression of the Na/Ca exchanger and a lower level of the SR Ca-ATPase (6, 7,

TABLE 9–7. *Ca Transport During Ventricular Myocyte and Muscle Relaxation*

Species	Reference	Temp (°C)	Contribution to Relaxation (%)		
			Na/Ca X	SR	Slow
Rabbit $[Ca]_i$	Puglisi et al. (271)	35	27	70	3
	Puglisi et al. (271)	25	23	74	3
	Bassani et al. (17)	22	28	70	2
Rat $[Ca]_i$	Bassani et al. (17)	22	7	92	1
	Negretti et al. (233)	27	9	87	4
Mouse $[Ca]_i$	Li et al. (194)	23	9	90	1
Rat neonate $[Ca]_i$	Bassani et al. (18)	22	46	50	4
Ferret $[Ca]_i$	Bassani et al. (21)	22	29	64	4
Rabbit relax	Puglisi et al. (271)	25	28	70	2
	Puglisi et al. (271)	35	21	76	3
Ferret relax	Puglisi et al. (271)	25	30	63	7
	Puglisi et al. (271)	35	28	67	5
Cat relax	Puglisi et al. (271)	25	47	51	2
	Puglisi et al. (271)	35	32	66	2
PAIRED RCCS					
Rabbit relax	Hryshko et al. (147)	29	23	76	1
Rabbit relax	Hryshko et al. (147)	29	27	73	—
Guinea pig $[Ca]_i$	Bers et al. (40)	30	36	64	—
Guinea pig $[Ca]_i$	Terracciano and MacLeod (331)	22	30	67	3

53). Indeed, there are extensive data documenting the low SR Ca-ATPase levels during neonatal development in rat, rabbit, and sheep ventricle (206, 231, 232, 257). There are also ultrastructural data indicating that the T-tubule/SR system is gradually developing from the prenatal period through the first few weeks of life, although at different rates in different species (118, 140, 188, 245, 250, 260, 298).

The higher Na/Ca exchange and lower SR Ca-ATPase in the newborn can be expected to shift the balance of Ca fluxes during relaxation more in favor of the Na/Ca exchanger. In addition, the SR is able to attain a relatively normal Ca load in neonatal rabbit ventricular myocytes, but very little appears to be released during the twitch (10). The consequently high intra-SR [Ca] at the start of relaxation may further limit the ability of the SR to compete with the Na/Ca exchanger. The detailed quantitative analysis shown in Figure 9–28 has not been done in newborn ventricular myocytes. However, caffeine-induced contractures in neonatal rabbit ventricular myocytes relax as fast or faster than twitches, where the SR Ca-ATPase can function (10). This suggests that the Na/Ca exchange may be greatly dominant over the SR Ca-ATPase during the early postnatal period. The failure of substantial SR Ca release in the neonatal rabbit may also slow the SR Ca-ATPase (due to high [Ca]$_{SR}$, Eq. 4), allowing the stronger Na/Ca exchange to be even more dominant. That is, in the newborn rabbit ventricle the balance of fluxes between SR Ca-ATPase and Na/Ca exchange may be reversed from the adult so that most of the [Ca]$_i$ decline is due to Na/Ca exchange.

This same shift is likely to occur in neonatal rat ventricular myocytes. Indeed, quantitative analysis has suggested that the balance between the SR Ca-pump and Na/Ca exchange in the newborn rat myocyte is similar to that in the adult rabbit ventricular myocyte (18). Using t$_{1/2}$ values as discussed above with respect to Figure 9–25, the data of Bassani et al. (18) indicate 50% of [Ca]$_i$ decline is due to the SR Ca-ATPase, 46% due Na/Ca exchange and 4% due to slow systems. Thus there are both species and developmental differences in the balance between Na/Ca exchange and SR Ca-pump in contribution to [Ca]$_i$ decline during relaxation of the twitch.

Ca Recycling from Mitochondria Back to the SR

When Ca has been extruded from the cell by either Na/Ca exchange or the sarcolemmal Ca-ATPase, it is gone from the cell and must enter again via either Ca channels, Na/Ca exchange or Ca leak. The fate of Ca that is accumulated by the mitochondria is different. As described above, this amount is probably small on a normal beat to beat basis (<1 μmol/liter cytosol), but can change progressively because Ca extrusion from mitochondria is also slow. How fast does this Ca come back out of the mitochondria? This issue has been studied to a certain extent in isolated mitochondria and digitonin-permeabilized cells (see earlier, under Mitochondrial Ca Transport and ref. 85, 86, 112, 113) and also in intact rabbit ventricular myocytes (15).

In intact cells during relaxation of a caffeine-induced contracture in 0Na, 0Ca solution about 50% of the SR Ca is extruded by the sarcolemmal Ca-ATPase and ~50% goes into the mitochondria. This artificially large Ca shift into the mitochondria allowed Bassani et al. (15) to better track the redistribution of this Ca in the cell. They found that after removal of caffeine (in sustained 0Na, 0Ca solution with EGTA) this mitochondrial Ca was transported back to the SR with a time constant of 40 sec. It was inferred that this represented mainly the time constant of mitochondrial Ca efflux (with relatively rapid reuptake into the SR). Furthermore, the rate of Ca redistribution from mitochondria to SR was slowed when intracellular Na was removed (consistent with the Na-dependence of mitochondrial Ca efflux in cardiac myocytes). Thus, it seems clear that moderate transient increases in mitochondrial Ca may be expected to accumulate gradually over a large number of beats (e.g. during increased or more frequent cytosolic Ca transients) and also very gradually dissipate over 1–3 min when the initial steady state is resumed.

THE Ca SUPPLY THAT ACTIVATES CONTRACTION

Ca Influx vs SR Ca Release

The foregoing quantitative discussions have given a good general picture of cellular Ca fluxes associated with contraction and relaxation. Clearly, the two main sources of Ca involved in the normal activation of cardiac muscle contraction are Ca influx and SR Ca release. Two general strategies have been employed to evaluate how much of the activation of contraction depends on Ca influx vs SR Ca release: (1) quantitative analysis of cellular Ca fluxes and (2) pharmacological interference with SR Ca release.

Quantitative Analysis of Cellular Ca Fluxes. In the steady state the amount of Ca entry during the cardiac cycle must be the same as the amount of Ca efflux. Otherwise the cell will gain or lose Ca and not be in a steady state with respect to cellular Ca balance. The same is true for the SR. Thus the quantitative analysis of the contributions of the SR Ca-ATPase and Na/Ca exchange to relaxation should roughly reflect the fraction of activation by SR Ca release or Ca influx, respectively. Thus, based on Figure 9–28 we might expect Ca influx and SR Ca release to supply roughly 28% and 70% of the activating Ca respectively in rabbit (and 7% and 92% in rat).

Delbridge et al. (89, 90) used a more direct quantitative approach to assess this. They measured Ca influx via I$_{Ca}$, the SR Ca content by caffeine-induced I$_{Na/Ca}$ and used estimates of the fraction of this SR Ca content released during a twitch (16, 90). Figure 9–29 shows steady-state conditioning voltage clamp pulses, Ca transients, and I$_{Ca}$ in the left panels. In the right panels, 10 mM caffeine is applied, which causes a large and rapid Ca transient and an inward current that decreases as [Ca]$_i$ declines. This current was identified as Na/Ca exchange (I$_{Na/Ca}$) current because it was completely absent during caffeine-induced Ca transients when external Na was replaced by Li (89). This current also depended on [Ca]$_i$ (i.e. a second caffeine application did not activate this current when there was no Ca transient (right panel). Furthermore, one sustained caffeine application was sufficient to empty the SR, since the second caffeine did not cause any further release. The integral of the I$_{Ca}$ allows direct evaluation of Ca influx and the SR Ca content can be calculated from the integral of I$_{Na/Ca}$. Since Na/Ca exchange only re-

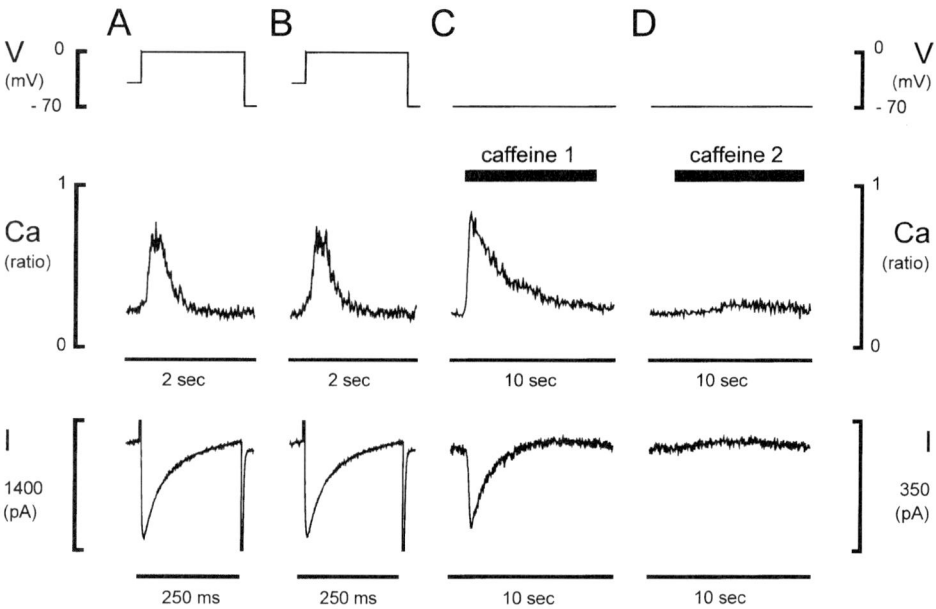

FIG. 9–29. Ca transients I_{Ca} during a twitch and $I_{Na/Ca}$ used to measure SR Ca content. Ca transients and inward currents (I_{Ca} and $I_{Na/Ca}$) in a rat ventricular cardiomyocyte (dialyzed with 50 μM indo-1) were recorded during the last two (of 8) conditioning voltage clamp pulses to 0 mV and during two rapid applications of 10 mM caffeine (bars, holding potential −70 mV). Amplitude and time scales for I_{Ca} (left) and $I_{Na/Ca}$ (right) are different. [From Delbridge et al. (90), with permission.]

moves 93% and 87% of the Ca during a caffeine-induced Ca transient in rabbit and rat, respectively (17), the SR Ca content is calculated by dividing the $I_{Na/Ca}$ integral by 0.93 or 0.87.

Table 9–8 summarizes quantitative analysis of data from this type of experiment in both rabbit and rat ventricular myocytes. After making corrections for surface to volume ratios in rabbit ventricular myocytes the integrated I_{Ca} is sufficient to increase total cytosolic Ca by 9.7 μM and the SR Ca content is 87 μmol/liter cytosol. Bassani et al. (16) measured the fractional SR Ca release in rabbit ventricular myocytes to be 43% (see below, under Fraction of SR Ca released during the Twitch). Thus during the twitch we have 9.7 plus 43% of the SR Ca content (43 × 87) giving 47 μmol/liter cytosol activating the twitch, with 23% coming from I_{Ca} and 77% from SR Ca release. These numbers are in rather good agreement with the experiments in Figure 9–28, where 28% of Ca extrusion was due to Na/Ca exchange and 70% due to SR Ca uptake. In Table 9–8, similar analysis for the rat agrees with the idea of about 7%–8% of activating Ca exchanging across the sarcolemma with 92% across the SR during the twitch (90).

Terracciano and MacLeod (332) used a slightly different approach to measure Ca entry during action po-

TABLE 9–8. *Fraction of Activator Ca from I_{Ca} and SR Ca Release*

	Rabbit		Rat	
	I_{Ca}	$I_{Na/CaX}$ (SR)	I_{Ca}	$I_{Na/CaX}$ (SR)
∫I dt (fC/pF)	221 ± 14	860 ± 118	185 ± 12	851 ± 70
Δ[Ca]$_i$ (μM)	9.7 ± 0.5	77 ± 11	6.5 ± 0.3	120 ± 8
SR Ca (μM)		87 ± 13		138 ± 9
Twitch Δ[Ca]$_i$ (μM)	9.7	+ 0.43·87	6.5	+ 0.55·138
Total		= 47		= 82
Activator Ca	23% ± 2%	77% ± 2%	7.9%	92%

Data for this table were taken from Delbridge et al. (89) for rabbit and from Delbridge et al. (90) and Yuan et al. (360) for rat ventricular myocytes. The columns labeled $I_{Na/CaX}$ (SR) reflect the use of integrated $I_{Na/Ca}$ to derive SR Ca content and in the last three lines refer to the amount of SR Ca release contributing to the twitch (vs Ca influx via I_{Ca}).

tential clamp and found that in rat ventricular myocytes the Ca entry via I_{Ca} was 3.5% of the SR Ca content. This would be equivalent to the results discussed above in rat regarding the fraction of activating Ca from Ca influx (i.e. 7%) if the fractional SR Ca release was ~50% (as measured in ref 90). They also carried out these studies in guinea pig ventricular myocytes at both 0.5 and 0.2 Hz and found that the Ca influx via I_{Ca} was a much larger fraction of the SR Ca content (~30 and 50% respectively). This is consistent with the higher transsarcolemmal Ca flux dependence in guinea pig in Table 9-7 (comparable to rabbit or even a bit more dependent on sarcolemmal Ca flux). At the lower frequency, the SR Ca content was lower, while I_{Ca} was slightly higher (secondary to less Ca-dependent inactivation). Consequently the ratio of I_{Ca} to SR Ca load was higher at lower frequency. Given the different methodologies and limitations ([Ca]$_i$ decline vs. current integration), this agreement seems remarkably good.

What about Ca entry via Na/Ca exchange during the cardiac action potential? This discussion has focused on Ca entry via Ca current, but during the early phase of the action potential some Ca entry via Na/Ca exchange may be expected (Fig. 9-10 and see earlier, under Thermodynamics and Ca Flux During Action Potential). As discussed earlier, the amount of Ca entry during a normal Ca transient is likely to be ≤1 μmol/liter cytosol and less than 10% of that entering via I_{Ca}. This quantity has also never been directly measured under physiological conditions, because this small transient outward current would be complicated by both the larger I_{Ca} and other Ca-activated currents when the normal Ca transient occurs. Thus, under normal physiological conditions it is expected that most of Ca influx is via I_{Ca} and only a very small fraction (<10%) is via Na/Ca exchange (119). On the other hand, when [Na]$_i$ is elevated, as in the case of digitalis-induced inhibition of the (Na + K)ATPase, this situation can change and substantial Ca can enter during the action potential (see Figs. 9-10 and 9-15; 32, 41), enough to activate substantial contractions directly.

In the newborn rabbit heart the situation may also be quantitatively very different where there are very few T-tubules. The expression of Na/Ca exchange and $I_{Na/Ca}$ in newborn rabbits is much higher than in the adult and the expression of L-type Ca channels, I_{Ca} density and number of ryanodine receptors is about four times smaller in the newborn (6, 7, 53, 58, 150, 246). Thus, although the SR in newborn ventricle can accumulate virtually normal amounts of Ca, there appears to be less released during normal E-C coupling (10). Furthermore, with the combination of lower I_{Ca}, lower SR Ca release, and higher Na/Ca exchange activity, enough Ca can enter the cell in newborn rabbit via Na/Ca exchange to support a nearly normal contraction amplitude (124). Thus there are also likely to be substantial developmental and species-dependent differences in this balance of Ca fluxes during the normal contraction.

Pharmacological Interference with SR Ca Release

A less complex analytical procedure to approach this issue has been to use agents that interfere with SR Ca transport (e.g. caffeine, ryanodine, thapsigargin, and cyclopiazonic acid) and assess the impact on the amplitude of twitch contractions or Ca transients. Figure 9-30 shows the effects of pre-equilibration with 10 mM caffeine or 100 nM ryanodine on steady-state twitch contractions in several cardiac muscle preparations. It can be seen that these agents depress twitch tension development to varying extents in different cardiac muscle preparations. This variation is apparent among different species (frog vs rabbit vs rat), at different stages of development (neonatal vs adult rat) and regionally in the heart (rabbit ventricle vs atrium). The concentration of ryanodine and caffeine required to produce a maximal effect does not appear to vary in different tissues, despite the difference in the extent of maximal effect on twitch amplitude (308, 323). While caffeine is well known to inhibit net SR Ca uptake by making the SR extremely leaky to Ca (and thereby preventing net Ca uptake [349]), it has many side effects. For example, it increases myofilament Ca sensitivity (e.g. 350) and increases Ca influx (30, 51, 342). Additionally, caffeine inhibits phosphodiesterases at the millimolar concentrations required for the effects on SR (60) and can thus elevate cyclic AMP. Ryanodine is much more specific in its interaction with the SR (K_d = nM), but its mechanism of action is somewhat more complex (39, 325).

High concentrations of caffeine (≥ 10 mM) cause a very rapid release of SR Ca and dramatically increase

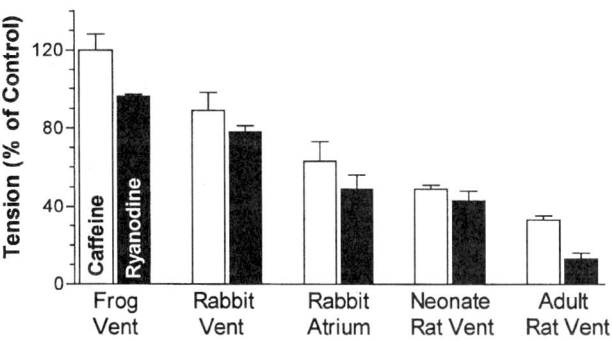

FIG. 9-30. Relative reliance on Ca influx in different cardiac muscle preparations. The effect of caffeine (10 mM) or ryanodine (100 nM) on steady-state twitch contraction amplitude (0.5 Hz at 30°C or 23°C for frog) in various cardiac muscle preparations. [Data are from refs 33, 34; modified from Bers (34).]

the open probability of the SR Ca release channel (288). This results in a short-circuiting of net SR Ca uptake, such that Ca leaks back into the cytoplasm as fast as it is pumped into the SR. Ryanodine (at concentrations of 10 nM to 10 μM) increases SR Ca release channel flux by locking the channel into a subconductance state (287), but the effect is extremely slow to equilibrate with all of the ryanodine receptors (probably many hours at normal ionic strength). Thus the experimentally induced leak in intact cells by moderate concentrations of ryanodine is not nearly as great as for 10 mM caffeine. This creates a situation in ryanodine where net SR Ca uptake can still occur during the twitch when [Ca]$_i$ is relatively high, but Ca then leaks out of the SR fairly rapidly during diastole (39). This explains why 0.1–1 μM ryanodine only slows the very terminal part of relaxation (38) whereas 10 mM caffeine slows the entire timecourse (20). After very long (>2 hr) exposures to 10–50 μM ryanodine, the effects of ryanodine can become more like caffeine, presumably because a sufficient number of SR Ca release channels are locked in the subconducting state to make a very large resting leak (i.e. sufficient to overcome the V_{max} of the SR Ca-pump). At very high ryanodine concentration (0.5–1 mM) individual SR Ca release channels are blocked by ryanodine (214), but in the intact cell it may be very difficult to drive enough release channels into the blocked state such that one really prevents leak of Ca from the SR. This is because in the cell (vs SR vesicles) all of the release channels are arranged in parallel, and just a few channels locked open could overcome the effect of blocking the others. In SR vesicles, the release channels are distributed to different vesicles so the effects on flux are less subject to this caveat.

Thapsigargin and cyclopiazonic acid are direct and rather specific inhibitors of the SR Ca-ATPase (171, 204, 290, 302, 335, 355). Because of the side effects of caffeine and the ability of the SR to still function as a transient Ca buffer in the presence of ryanodine, these agents are very useful tools to block SR function entirely. After ryanodine treatment or when the SR Ca content is rather low, thapsigargin can actually increase the amplitude of twitch Ca transients (16, 159). This is undoubtedly due to thapsigargin blockade of the Ca buffering action of the SR Ca-ATPase (even in the presence of ryanodine). While thapsigargin and cyclopiazonic acid work very well to completely block the SR Ca-ATPase in intact single cells (e.g. 16), they do not seem to completely block SR Ca accumulation in multicellular preparations (26). The reason for this is not known, but this places some practical limitations on the use of thapsigargin or cyclopiazonic acid in these preparations.

In summary, the sensitivity of tension to depression by interference with SR Ca transport has provided data which is indicative of the relative requirement for SR Ca release in the activation of the myofilaments. From greatest reliance on SR Ca to least, I would say the sequence is (V, ventricle; A, atrium): calf Purkinje fiber > adult rat V ~ mouse V > dog V ~ ferret V > rabbit A > neonate rat V > cat V ~ human V > rabbit V > guinea-pig V > neonate rabbit V > fetal V (human, cat & rabbit) > trout V > frog V ~ toad V (31, 34, 46, 102, 194, 207, 259, 301, 323, 324). Obviously this is an approximate sequence and can be expected to change under different conditions.

Fraction of SR Ca Released During a Twitch

The topic of E-C coupling is discussed in detail elsewhere (34a). I will limit the discussion here to global issues related to the fraction of SR Ca released and the quantity of Ca involved. It has been clear for some time that the amount of SR Ca released can be graded by the amount of Ca influx that triggers the release (47, 63, 104, 105, 197), However, the actual amount of SR Ca content and the fraction of the SR Ca content released at the twitch has not been widely studied.

Bassani et al. (16, 19) devised a protocol to measure the fraction and amount of SR Ca released at a twitch in ventricular myocytes and also used this to assess the effect of both trigger and SR Ca content on the fractional release (19, 307). In rabbit ventricular myocytes they found that during the normal twitch the SR released 43% of its Ca content and this value was 35% in ferret ventricular myocytes, where the SR Ca load was about 90 μmol/liter cytosol (16, 19). Figure 9–31A shows how the fractional release of SR Ca varies as a function of I_{Ca} trigger at constant SR Ca load. Not surprisingly, fractional SR Ca release increases with increasing trigger Ca influx. This is a basic tenet of Ca-induced Ca-release, but the data also show that the dynamic range of fractional SR Ca release is 10%–60% (9–56 μmol/liter cytosol).

Figure 9–31B shows how fractional SR Ca release is altered when the load is varied but the trigger is kept constant. The Normal SR Ca load at 0.5 Hz stimulation was 91 μmol/liter cytosol, and 35% was released at the normal twitch. When [Ca]$_o$ was elevated (to 8 mM) and myocytes were paced at 0.8 Hz the SR Ca load reached a maximum of 95 μmol/liter cytosol. This maximal point was when the cells were on the verge of Ca overload (i.e. just below the frequency where large spontaneous SR Ca release and waves occurred). It was somewhat surprising that the twitch Ca transients were so much larger with only a 4% increase in SR Ca load. Indeed the amount of SR Ca released was almost doubled (from 32 to 56 μmol/liter cytosol), but most of this increase was due to an increase in frac-

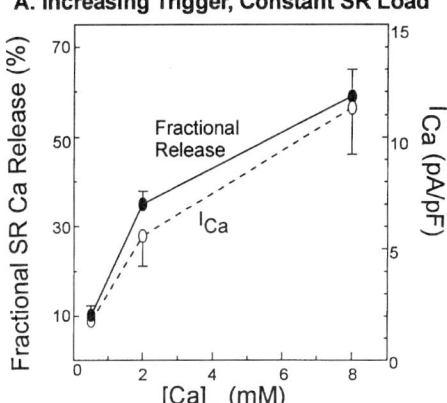 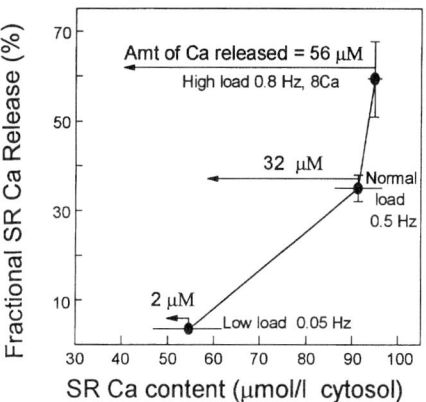

FIG. 9–31. Fractional SR Ca release during the twitch depends on both I_{Ca} trigger and SR Ca load in ferret ventricular myocytes. A. Cells were loaded to a constant level (by stimulation at 0.5 Hz). Extracellular [Ca] was changed just prior to the test contraction where the fraction of SR Ca release was measured. Thus increasing trigger (at constant SR Ca load) increases fractional release. Parallel voltage clamp experiments were done to evaluate how I_{Ca} changes over this range of $[Ca]_o$. B. Using a constant trigger (with 2 mM $[Ca]_o$) the SR of cells were Ca loaded to different levels by varying frequency (as indicated) and also increasing $[Ca]_o$ at the highest load. SR Ca content was determined by translating the peak and resting $[Ca]_i$ during caffeine-induced contractures to total cytosolic [Ca], using values determined by Hove-Madsen and Bers (145) for cytosolic Ca buffering. [Modified from Bassani et al. (19), with permission.]

tional SR Ca release (from 35% to 59%) rather than the amount available for release. This result suggests that intra-SR Ca can importantly regulate the E-C coupling process. It is possible that under the control conditions used, the intra-SR Ca buffers such as calsequestrin are nearly saturated so that with more aggressive stimulation free intra-SR [Ca] ($[Ca]_{SR}$) rises without much increase in SR Ca content. This possible rise in $[Ca]_{SR}$ may in turn exert some effect to increase ryanodine receptor gating and thereby fractional release. Luminal Ca has been reported to increase ryanodine receptor open probability in single channels (201, 314). In the skeletal muscle ryanodine receptor the effect of luminal Ca to increase open probability has been attributed to Ca coming out through the channel and acting at a cytoplasmic site (341), but this may not be the case in the cardiac SR Ca release channel (201).

Thus $[Ca]_{SR}$ may be important in and integral to the control of SR Ca release. Furthermore, what is usually referred to as spontaneous SR Ca release associated with cellular Ca overload, may really be Ca release triggered by intra-SR Ca. Moreover, increased fractional SR Ca release works synergistically with increases in Ca available for release and may even be the more important factor at relatively high SR Ca loads.

When SR Ca content is lowered, the fractional SR Ca release is dramatically reduced. In Figure 9–31B reduction of SR load by only 40% almost abolished SR Ca release. That is, only 4% of the SR Ca load was released (2 µmol/liter cytosol) and this amount is much less than even the amount of Ca that enters the cell via I_{Ca} (5–15 µmol/liter cytosol; see earlier, under Ca Channels). Thus at low levels of SR Ca load, the SR nearly stops participating in E-C coupling even though there is still a large pool of Ca available for release (55 µmol/liter cytosol).

PERTURBATIONS OF CELLULAR Ca BALANCE

Rest-Dependent Changes in Cellular and SR Ca Content

The delicate balance of Ca flux via Na/Ca exchange in the resting cell discussed earlier with respect to Figure 9–17 may be essential in understanding whether cells lose Ca during rest. In resting rabbit ventricular myocytes there is a strong thermodynamic driving force for Ca extrusion via Na/Ca exchange (Fig. 9–17A). Thus, when Ca leaks from the SR to the cytosol during rest it is subject to competition between the Na/Ca exchange and re-uptake by the SR Ca-ATPase. When some of this Ca is extruded by the Na/Ca exchange, the result is a net loss of SR Ca. Evidence for this interpretation is shown by the amplitude of post-rest caffeine-induced contractures (Caff) in Figure 9–32A (23). The rest-dependent decline of SR Ca content in rabbit ventricular myocytes (assessed by caffeine-induced contraction) was completely prevented when

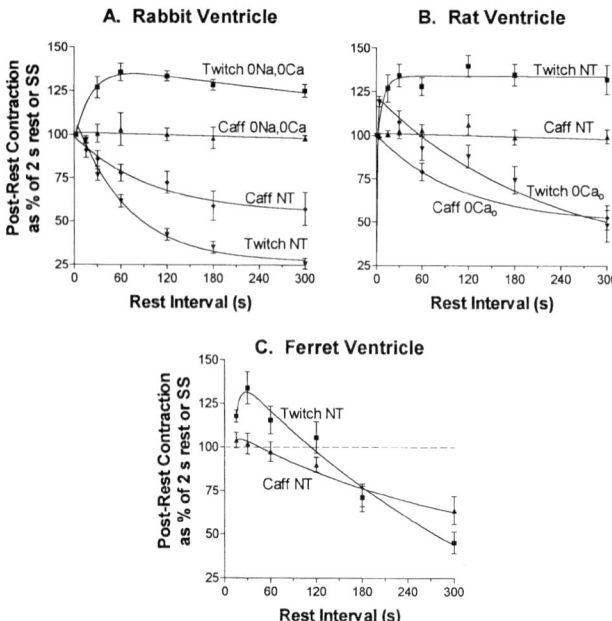

FIG. 9–32. Rest decay and rest potentiation of twitches and SR Ca content in rabbit, rat and ferret myocytes. Both post-rest twitches and caffeine-induced contractures (Caff) were measured either in a modified normal Tyrode's solution (NT), when Na/Ca exchange was blocked during the rest (0Na,0Ca) or after pre-depletion of $[Na]_i$ and rest in Ca-free, 140 mM Na solution ($0Ca_o$) to stimulate Ca efflux via Na/Ca exchange. Caff data are indicative of SR Ca load. SR Ca content data (Caff) was fit with $[Ca]_{SRC} = A \cdot \exp(-t/\tau_{RD})(1 - \exp\{-t/\tau_{RF}\}) + B$, where t is time, τ_{RD} is time constant, of rest decay of SR Ca content and τ_{RF} is a rest-dependent filling time constant used to explain the delay in rest decay of SR Ca content. A and B are constants for scaling and baseline respectively. Twitch data were fit with the expression $C[Ca]_{SRC}(1-\exp\{-t/\tau_{ECC}\}) + D$, where τ_{ECC} is the time constant for recovery of E-C coupling and C and D are scaling and baseline constants. A small second exponential factor was also included to explain the slow decline in twitch amplitude in rabbit ventricle after long rests in 0Na, 0Ca. [Data are from Bers et al. (36) and Bassani and Bers (23) and have been combined and reanalyzed.]

Na/Ca exchange was blocked by Na-free, Ca-free solution (0Na, 0Ca) during the rest. With Na/Ca exchange prevented, there is no serious competitor for the SR Ca-ATPase, allowing the SR to reaccumulate virtually all of the Ca that leaks to the cytosol (and thus maintain a constant load).

In rat ventricular myocytes, according to results of Shattock and Bers (309) and Figure 9–17B, the $E_{Na/Ca}$ is very close to the resting membrane potential. Thus there is little or no driving force for Ca efflux via Na/Ca exchange. In addition, the Na/Ca exchanger is weaker in rat ventricular myocytes. The result is that when Ca leaks from the SR in resting rat ventricular myocytes there is virtually no Ca extrusion via Na/Ca exchange and all of the Ca is taken back up by the SR. This explains why there is typically no resting loss in SR Ca in rat ventricular myocytes in normal solution (Caff-NT in Fig. 9–32B; ref 23). However, when extracellular [Ca] is removed during rest while normal 140 mM $[Na]_o$ is retained, the driving force for Ca extrusion via Na/Ca exchange is enhanced. In this case, the SR Ca content declines during rest, much as in control rabbit ventricular myocytes (Caff-$0Ca_o$ in Figure 9–32B; ref 23).

Furthermore if $[Na]_i$ is elevated in rabbit ventricular muscle by partial blockade of the (Na + K)ATPase by digitalis-related steroids, the rest-dependent decline in SR Ca content can be strongly depressed (37). In rat ventricular muscle there is also evidence that the cells and SR can actually gain Ca during rest (12, 33, 193, 309). Whether this situation actually occurs in a given experiment (as opposed to no change in SR Ca content with rest), may depend on the actual $[Na]_i$ in the cell and whether there is net efflux of Ca via Na/Ca exchange during the action potential (see Figs. 9–16B and 9–17B). It has also been shown that rest decay in rabbit and guinea pig ventricle is slowed by slowing Ca extrusion via Na/Ca exchange ($[Na]_o$ reduction, 0Na, 0Ca solution, or Na-pump blockade) or accelerating the SR Ca-pump with isoproterenol. Conversely rest decay is accelerated by increasing the rate of SR Ca leak or increasing the driving force for Ca extrusion via Na/Ca exchange (36, 39–41, 323). These effects are all consistent with the sort of competition between the SR Ca-pump and sarcolemmal Na/Ca exchange discussed above.

The rat (and perhaps mouse) ventricle seems to be an exception to the general rule that rest allows slow gradual depletion of the SR Ca content (which is clearly the case for rabbit, ferret, guinea pig, and canine ventricle). Interestingly, the rate of resting leak of Ca from the SR does not seem to differ between rabbit and rat ventricle (24). Thus the main determinant of whether rest decay of SR Ca content occurs (and its rate) appears to be how well the sarcolemmal Na/Ca exchange competes with the SR Ca-pump for the Ca that leaks from the SR. If the Na/Ca exchange is relatively potent in this regard (due to the number of exchangers and thermodynamic considerations), then rest decay will occur relatively rapidly (as in rabbit and guinea pig ventricle). If the Na/Ca exchanger protein is relatively poorly expressed and/or $E_{Na/Ca}$ is near the resting E_m then the SR Ca content will be well maintained. A complicating factor with ferret ventricle is that the sarcolemmal Ca-pump appears to be relatively strong and can produce gradual rest decay even when the Na/Ca exchanger is completely blocked (21). The fundamental mechanism in this case, however, is probably exactly the same as described above. That is, in ferret, the sarcolemmal Ca-ATPase is a weak but significantly stronger competitor with the SR Ca-ATPase.

A final point here is that rest decay does not have to proceed to completion, emptying the SR (e.g. see Fig 9–32). Indeed, Terraciano and MacLeod (333) have shown that in guinea pig ventricular myocytes the depleted SR can even partially refill during rest. This emphasizes the delicate and dynamic balance of resting Ca fluxes in the cell. It may also have something to do with the ability of the SR Ca-ATPase to establish a finite and substantial [Ca] gradient between the SR and the cytoplasm, even when resting $[Ca]_i$ is very low.

Refilling Depleted Internal Ca Stores

The SR Ca content can been depleted by either long rest periods or sustained exposure to caffeine (which causes SR Ca to be extruded from the cell via Na/Ca exchange; Fig. 9–29). Figure 9–33 shows that once the SR has been depleted of Ca, it takes only 5–10 beats to refill the SR again (16, 33). During the first beat after SR Ca depletion Ca influx is greater (due to less Ca-dependent inactivation of I_{Ca} and less inward $I_{Na/Ca}$). Also a large fraction of the Ca influx during the action potential can be taken up by the SR (32, 339). This is partly because the smaller Ca transient does not strongly activate Ca efflux via the Na/Ca exchanger, and the SR Ca-ATPase can also pump Ca more rapidly at low $[Ca]_{SR}$ because backflux through the pump is low (Eq. 4). As the next several pulses proceed, the Ca efflux during the twitch increases until at the steady state, the Ca influx and efflux are exactly equal and opposite (32, 339). Clearly the SR Ca load where this balance occurs will depend on a large number of factors (e.g. frequency, temperature, $[Ca]_o$, $[Na]_i$, action potential configuration, transport strength of the SR Ca-ATPase, and sarcolemmal Na/Ca exchange). The 5–10 beats required to refill the SR also makes reasonable sense with the foregoing quantitative discussions about Ca influx and SR Ca content. That is, if Ca influx during the action potential is 12–20 μmol/liter cytosol and the SR Ca content is ~100 μmol/liter cytosol, the measured refilling in 5–10 beats is consistent with these values.

Rest-Decay and Rest-Potentiation of Twitches

As the SR Ca content declines during rest (e.g. in rabbit, Fig. 9–32A) it is logical that the first post-rest twitch or Ca transient is smaller after longer rest intervals. That is almost surely the main explanation for the rest decay of twitch contraction that is routinely observed in rabbit and guinea pig ventricular myocytes. Another relevant factor is that as the SR Ca content goes down with rest, the fraction of SR Ca released during a twitch also decreases (Figure 9–31B; ref 19). Thus decreased SR Ca content, together with the consequent decreased fractional release, is likely to be responsible in large part for the rest decay of twitches and Ca transients.

The resting loss of SR Ca content during rest can be completely prevented in rabbit ventricular myocytes by incubation in 0Na, 0Ca solution during the rest period (Fig. 9–32A; ref 23). When this is done and normal solution is returned just prior to the post-rest twitch, rabbit ventricular myocytes demonstrate striking rest potentiation of twitch contractions (and Ca transients, Fig. 9–32A; ref 23). Indeed, the rest potentiation observed in this case in rabbit ventricle is almost the same as the rest potentiation normally observed in rat ventricle, when the SR Ca content does not change with rest (NT in Fig. 9–32B). Similar rest potentiation is also seen in ferret, dog, and cat ventricular myocytes at relatively short rest intervals (e.g. Fig. 9–32C; ref 36). This potentiation of twitches and Ca transients occurs despite data showing that there is no increase in SR Ca content, I_{Ca} trigger, or action potential duration or plateau (36). It was concluded that this increase in apparent fractional SR Ca release with rest is attributable to a very slow phase of recovery of the E-C coupling process after a previous excitation. This recovery may be due to a recovery of the SR Ca release channel from inactivation or adaptation (105, 121, 299). Interestingly, the same intrinsic recovery time appears to be apparent in the probability of resting Ca sparks at the

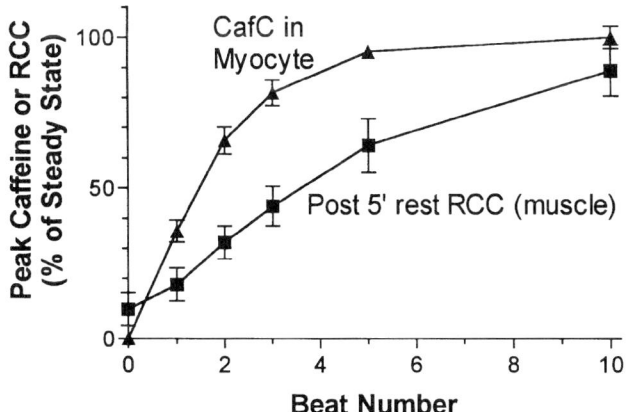

FIG. 9–33. Refilling of SR Ca stores after depletion in rabbit ventricle. SR Ca content was measured by either caffeine-induced contracture amplitude (in isolated myocytes at 23°C) or rapid cooling contractures (RCC) in trabeculae from rabbit ventricle (at 30°C). SR Ca was depleted by either a long rest (5 min) in normal solution (muscle) or a 10 sec application of 10 mM caffeine (myocyte). After SR Ca depletion, stimulation was started at 0.5 Hz and the SR Ca content was assessed after the beat number indicated. [Data are from Bers (33) and Bassani et al. (16).]

subcellular level (293). Thus this recovery process may indeed reflect an intrinsic stochastic behavior of individual ryanodine receptors (or clusters thereof).

From the ferret data in Figure 9–32C, it can be seen that the rest potentiation of twitches seen at short rest intervals gradually gives way to rest decay at longer rest intervals (>2 min). SR Ca content (Caff NT) declines throughout the 5 min period shown, although there seems to be some initial period where the rest decay of SR Ca content is delayed. Thus, at short rest intervals, the ferret ventricle may exhibit rest potentiation due mainly to the same sort of recovery of E-C coupling discussed above for rabbit and rat. At longer rests the strong negative effect of decreased SR Ca content (both on the amount and fractional release) may outweigh the positive effect of full recovery of the E-C coupling mechanism.

Moreover, all the curves shown in Figure 9–32 were fit to the data with a rather simple functional model. The SR Ca content (Caff curves) were assumed to change as a function of rest in a manner described by the product of a decreasing and increasing exponential. The declining exponential was the dominant feature, while the increasing factor allowed the delay in rest decay seen most notably in ferret. The twitch curves are then derived directly from the SR Ca content curves. Specifically, the SR Ca content function was multiplied by a scaling constant and a simple increasing exponential (to reflect the recovery of E-C coupling with rest). Thus the twitch was basically calculated as the product of the SR Ca content available for release times the fraction of SR Ca that is released. Obviously, this is an oversimplification of the dynamic interplay of many factors, but it may help focus on the two major factors responsible for changes in post-rest contraction amplitude (SR Ca content and recovery of E-C coupling).

Force-Frequency Relationships

The frequency dependence of contraction and Ca transients is obviously related to the post-rest behavior, but may be more complicated to fully understand. To make this simple, I will focus on just a few main factors that are probably critical in understanding force-frequency relationships. Increasing frequency of stimulation will tend to increase contractions for several reasons. First, an increased [Na]$_i$ occurs due to more Na influx per unit time (80). Second, there is higher Ca influx per unit time due to the higher frequency, a CaMKII dependent increase of I$_{Ca}$ (358) and possibly more Ca influx by Na/Ca exchange. These two factors tend to increase diastolic [Ca]$_i$ (due to less time for removal from the cytosol), limit the ability of the Na/Ca exchanger to extrude Ca, and also contribute to increased SR Ca content. There may also be an increase in fractional SR Ca release mediated by progressive activation of CaMKII (195). Thus these interacting factors would tend to increase diastolic [Ca]$_i$, SR Ca content and fractional SR Ca release.

With increasing frequency there are also factors that would tend to decrease the amplitude of the twitch and the Ca transient. One factor is a shortening of the action potential duration, which would tend to encourage Ca extrusion via Na/Ca exchange and gradually decrease cell Ca, SR Ca, and Ca transient amplitude (see Fig. 9–17; refs 156, 309, 320). Second, there may be accumulating encroachment on the time required for complete recovery of E-C coupling after the last stimulation. This is the logical extension of the foregoing discussion about rest potentiation. The L-type Ca channel also requires some time to recover from inactivation. This recovery depends on voltage and temperature and typically has a time constant of 50–100 ms at -80 mV and room temperature (e.g. 342, 358). Thus, incomplete recovery of I$_{Ca}$ from inactivation is only likely to depress function at relatively high heart rates. Historically, a delay for movement of SR Ca from an "uptake compartment" to a "release compartment" has been incorporated into some models of the force-frequency relationship to explain the slow phase of restitution of E-C coupling after Ca uptake by the SR (e.g. 99, 222, 354, 361). A possible source of this delay was considered to be diffusion of Ca from the longitudinal SR (where Ca uptake occurs) to the terminal cisternae (specialized for Ca release). However, there are no apparent membrane boundaries within the SR, and simple diffusion of Ca from longitudinal SR to junctional SR (<1 μm) should only take ~1 msec. Furthermore, SR Ca is fully available for release by either rapid cooling or caffeine long before it can be optimally released by E-C coupling (39). It seems that the slow phase of recovery of E-C coupling after a twitch, which requires several seconds, may be more appropriately explained by a recovery of the ryanodine receptor from previous adaptation or inactivation. Thus, the major negative influences on twitches with increasing frequency are probably refractoriness of E-C coupling and, at faster rates, some refractoriness of I$_{Ca}$. The overall effect of increasing frequency will depend on the balance of the various positive and negative factors described here.

Figure 9–34 shows abrupt changes in frequency in a rabbit ventricular muscle. The first twitch at higher frequency is smaller in amplitude, probably reflecting insufficient time for the Ca release channel to recover from inactivation or adaptation. The interpulse interval in this case is probably sufficient for recovery of I$_{Ca}$ from inactivation and for SR Ca to be available for release (34). Continued pacing at this higher frequency

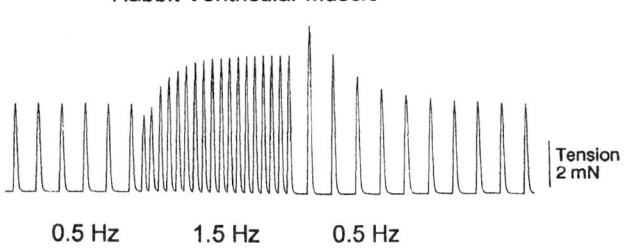

FIG. 9–34. Changes in contraction force with abrupt changes in frequency. Frequency of stimulation of a rabbit ventricular trabecula (at 30°C) was increased from 0.5 to 1.5 Hz and then returned to 0.5 Hz.

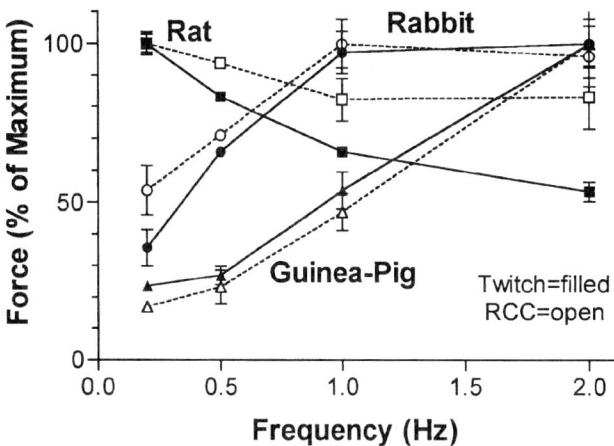

FIG. 9–35. Steady-state force-frequency relationships. The effect of frequency (from 0.5 to 2 Hz) on twitch force in rabbit (*circles*), rat (*squares*) and guinea pig (*triangles*) ventricular muscle. Data for rabbit and rat are at 30°C. [From Bers (33 and unpublished.] Data for guinea pig are at 36.5°C and were taken from Kurihara and Sakai (176). RCCs were initiated within 5 sec of the last steady-state stimulated contraction. [Redrawn from Bers (34).]

leads to a progressive positive "staircase" (which more than compensates for the infringement on restitution). This probably reflects the gradual increase in SR Ca content and fractional release (above) that take several pulses to accumulate. When the frequency is suddenly reduced, the first contraction is very large. This is probably due to the combination of the higher steady state SR Ca load (resulting from the higher frequency) and the increased time for recovery of E-C coupling. It may be noted that this large SR Ca release will tend to drive more Ca out of the cell via Na/Ca exchange and that starts the process of gradually unloading the cell and SR Ca content back toward the steady-state level at the lower frequency.

Figure 9–35 shows the effect of frequency on steady-state twitch amplitude and SR Ca content (assessed by RCC) in rabbit, guinea pig, and rat ventricle. In rabbit and guinea pig over this range there is a progressive increase in both SR Ca content as well as twitch force. This is consistent with the factors that increase force being dominant, and even being sufficient to overcome some degree of encroachment into the recovery process at higher frequency. In rat ventricle a negative force-frequency relationship is often observed, and this has been reported with either a slight decrease in SR Ca content (as in the RCC data in Fig. 9–35) or with unchanged SR Ca content (54). With unchanged SR Ca content, the negative force-frequency relationship in rat can be explained by the refractoriness of E-C coupling being a major limitation, since SR Ca content did not increase to compensate for this effect. It is possible that the rat SR Ca load is already very high at very low frequency. This, in turn might be a consequence of the higher resting $[Na]_i$ reported in rat vs rabbit ventricle (309). Thus, if SR Ca content fails to increase with increasing frequency, the negative effect of frequency on recovery of E-C coupling may become more apparent. The slight decline in SR Ca load in rat in Figure 9–35 may be due to the relatively large net Ca efflux during the twitch (Figs. 9–16B and 9–17B), such that

increasing frequency produces a slight decrease in cellular Ca (309). This is analogous to the way that spontaneous SR Ca release stimulates net Ca efflux of 15% of the SR Ca content via Na/Ca exchange when the SR is loaded to a nearly maximal or threshold level (95).

It should be noted that in rat ventricular myocytes and muscles both positive and negative force-frequency relationships have been reported (34, 66, 108, 300). I do not really consider this to be contradictory, especially given the dynamic interplay of factors. It is possible that rat myocytes where positive force-frequency relationships are observed begin with lower SR Ca load (and perhaps lower $[Na]_i$) than cells that exhibit negative force-frequency relationships (108). This discussion of force-frequency relationships is an appropriate place to finish, because this topic emphasizes the importance of integrating the many concepts and factors described in this chapter to develop a comprehensive understanding of the dynamic regulation of cellular Ca in cardiac myocytes.

The talented contributions of many collaborators during the past several years is most gratefully acknowledged, especially Drs. Rosana A. Bassani, José W. M. Bassani, Joshua R. Berlin, Lothar A. Blatter, John H. B. Bridge, Leanne M. D. Delbridge, Kenneth S. Ginsburg, Leif Hove-Madsen, Larry V. Hryshko, W. J. Lederer, Li Li, Eileen McCall, Ming Qi, Allen Samarel, Hiroshi Satoh Thomas R. Shannon, and Weilong Yuan. The influence of many other friends and colleagues has also shaped the view of cardiac Ca regulation that I have summarized here. This work was supported by grants from the United States Public Health Service (HL-30077, HL-44583, and HL-52478).

REFERENCES

1. Adachi-Akahane, S., L. Cleemann, and M. Morad. Cross-signaling between L-type Ca^{2+} channels and ryanodine receptors in rat ventricular myocytes. *J. Gen. Physiol.* 108:435–454, 1996.
2. Allen, D. G., P. G. Morris, C. H. Orchard and J. S. Pirolo. A nuclear magnetic resonance study of metabolism in the ferret heart during hypoxia and inhibition of glycolysis. *J. Physiol.* 361:185–204, 1985.
3. Almers, W. and E. W. McCleskey. Non-selective conductance in calcium channels of frog muscle: calcium selectivity in a single-file pore. *J. Physiol. Lond.* 353:585–608, 1984.
4. Antoniu, B., D. H. Kim, M. Morii, and N. Ikemoto. Inhibitors of Ca^{2+} release from the isolated sarcoplasmic reticulum. I. Ca^{2+} channel blockers. *Biochim. Biophys. Acta* 816:9–17, 1985.
5. Arreola, J., R. T. Driksen, R-C. Shieh, D. J. Willford, and S-S. Sheu. Ca^{2+} current and Ca^{2+} transients under action potential clamp in guinea pig ventricular myocytes. *Am. J. Physiol.* 261 (*Cell Physiol.* 30):C393–C397, 1991.
6. Artman, M. Sarcolemmal Na^+-Ca^{2+} exchange activity and exchanger immunoreactivity in developing rabbit hearts. *Am. J. Physiol.* 263 (*Heart Circ. Physiol.* 32):H1506–H1513, 1992.
7. Artman, M. Developmental Changes in Myocardial Inotropic Responsiveness. Austin, Texas-R. G. Landes Company, 1994.
8. Backx, P. H., W-D. Gao, M. D. Azan-Backx, and E. Marban. The relationship between contractile force and intracellular $[Ca^{2+}]$ in intact rat cardiac trabeculae. *J. Gen. Physiol.* 105:1–19, 1995.
9. Baker, P. F., M. P. Blaustein, A. L. Hodgkin, and R. A. Steinhardt. The influence of calcium on sodium efflux in squid axons. *J. Physiol. (Lond).* 200:431–458, 1969.
10. Balaguru, D., P. S. Haddock, J. L. Puglisi, D. M. Bers, W. A. Coetzee, and M. Artman. Role of the sarcoplasmic reticulum in contraction and relaxation of immature rabbit ventricular myocytes. *J. Mol. Cell. Cardiol.* 29:2747–2757, 1997.
11. Balke C. W., T. M. Egan, and W. G. Wier. Processes that remove calcium from the cytoplasm during excitation-contraction coupling in intact rat heart cells. *J. Physiol. (Lond).* 474:447–462, 1994.
12. Banijamali, H. S., W. D. Gao, and H. E. D. J. Ter Keurs. Induction of calcium leak from the sarcoplasmic reticulum of rat cardiac trebeculae by ryanodine. *Circulation* 82: Supl III abstract–215, 1990.
13. Barcenas-Ruiz L., D. J. Beuckelmann, and W. G. Wier. Sodium-calcium exchange in heart: membrane currents and changes in $[Ca^{2+}]_i$. *Science* 238:1720–1722, 1987.
14. Barth, E., G. Stammler, B. Speiser, and J. Schaper. Ultrastructural quantitation of mitochondria and myofilaments in cardiac muscle from 10 different animal species including man. *J. Mol. Cell. Cardiol.* 24:669–681, 1992.
15. Bassani, J. W. M., R. A. Bassani, and D. M. Bers. Ca^{2+} cycling between sarcoplasmic reticulum and mitochondria in rabbit cardiac myocytes. *J. Physiol. Lond.* 460:603–621, 1993.
16. Bassani, J. W. M., R. A. Bassani and D. M. Bers. Twitch-dependent SR Ca accumulation and release in rabbit ventricular myocytes. *Am. J. Physiol.* 265 (*Cell Physiol.* 34):C533–C540, 1993.
17. Bassani, J. W. M., R. A. Bassani, and D. M. Bers. Relaxation in rabbit and rat cardiac cells: species-dependent differences in cellular mechanisms. *J. Physiol. (Lond).* 476:279–293, 1994.
18. Bassani, J. W. M., M. Qi, A. M. Samarel, and D. M. Bers Contractile arrest increases SR Ca uptake and SERCa2 gene expression in cultured neonatal rat heart cells. *Circ. Res.* 74:991–997, 1994.
19. Bassani, J. W. M., W. Yuan, and D. M. Bers. Fractional SR Ca release is altered by trigger Ca and SR Ca content in cardiac myocytes. *Am. J. Physiol.* 268:C1313–C1319, 1995.
20. Bassani, R. A., J. W. M. Bassani, and D. M. Bers. Mitochondrial and sarcolemmal Ca transport can reduce $[Ca]_i$ during caffeine contractures in rabbit cardiac myocytes. *J. Physiol. (Lond).* 453: 591–608, 1992
21. Bassani, R. A., J. W. M. Bassani, and D. M. Bers. Relaxation in ferret ventricular myocytes: unusual interplay among calcium transport systems. *J. Physiol.* 476:295–308, 1994.
22. Bassani, R. A., J. W. M. Bassani, and D. M. Bers. Relaxation in ferret ventricular myocytes: role of the sarcolemmal Ca ATPase. *Pflugers Arch.* 430:573–579, 1995.
23. Bassani, R. A. and D. M. Bers. Na-Ca exchange is required for rest-decay but not for rest-potentiation of twitches in rabbit and rat ventricular myocytes. *J. Mol. Cell. Cardiol.* 26:1335–1347, 1994.
24. Bassani, R. A. and D. M. Bers. Rate of diastolic Ca release from the sarcoplasmic reticulum of intact rabbit and rat ventricular myocytes. *Biophys. J.* 68:2015–2022, 1995.
25. Bassani, R. A., A. Mattiazzi, and D. M. Bers. CaMK-II is responsible for activity-dependent acceleration of relaxation in rat ventricular myocytes. *Am. J. Physiol.* 268 (*Heart Circ. Physiol.* 77):H703–H712, 1995.
26. Baudet, S., R. Shaoulian, and D. M. Bers. Effects of thapsigargin and cyclopiazonic acid on twitch force and SR Ca content of rabbit ventricular muscle. *Circ. Res.* 73:813–819, 1993.
27. Bean, B. P. Two kinds of calcium channels in canine atrial cells. differences in kinetics, selectivity, and pharmacology. *J. Gen Physiol.* 86:1–30, 1985.
28. Bean, B. P. Classes of calcium channels in vertebrate cells. *Annu. Rev. Physiol.* 51:367–384, 1989.
29. Berlin, J. R., J. W. M. Bassani, and D. M. Bers. Intrinsic cytosolic calcium buffering properties of single rat cardiac myocytes. *Biophys. J.* 67:1775–1787, 1994.
30. Bers, D. M. Early transient depletion of extracellular [Ca] during individual cardiac muscle contractions. *Am. J. Physiol.* 244 (*Heart Circ. Physiol.* 13):H462–H468, 1983.
31. Bers, D. M. Ca influx and SR Ca release in cardiac muscle activation during postrest recovery. *Am. J. Physiol.* 248 (*Heart Circ. Physiol.* 17):H366–H381, 1985.
32. Bers, D. M. Mechanisms contributing to the cardiac inotropic effect of Na-pump inhibition and reduction of extracellular Na. *J. Gen. Physiol.* 90:479–504, 1987.
33. Bers, D. M. SR Ca loading in cardiac muscle preparations based on rapid cooling contractures. *Am. J. Physiol.* 256 (*Cell Physiol.* 25):C109–C120, 1989.
34. Bers, D. M. *Excitation-contraction coupling and cardiac contractile force*. Dordrecht: Netherlands: Kluwer Academic Press, 1991.
34a. Bers D. M. *Excitation-Contraction Coupling and Cardiac Contractile Force*., 2nd edition. Dordrecht: Netherlands, Kluwer Academic Press, (in press), 2001.
35. Bers, D. M., L. A. Allen, and Y. Kim. Calcium binding to cardiac sarcolemma isolated from rabbit ventricular muscle: it's possible role in modifying contractile force. *Am. J. Physiol.* 251: C861–C871, 1986.
36. Bers, D. M., R. A. Bassani J. W. M. Bassani, S. Baudet, and L. V. Hryshko. Paradoxical twitch potentiation after rest in cardiac muscle: increased fractional release of SR calcium. *J. Mol. Cell. Cardiol.* 25:1047–1057, 1993.
37. Bers, D. M. and J. H. B. Bridge. The effect of acetylstrophanthi-

din on twitches, microscopic tension fluctuations and cooling contractures in rabbit ventricular muscle. *J. Physiol. (Lond)*. 404:53–69, 1988.
38. Bers, D. M. and J. H. B. Bridge. Relaxation of rabbit ventricular muscle by Na-Ca exchange and sarcoplasmic reticulum Ca-pump: ryanodine and voltage sensitivity. *Circ. Res.* 65:334–342, 1989.
39. Bers, D. M., J. H. B. Bridge, and K. T. MacLeod. The mechanism of ryanodine action in cardiac muscle assessed with Ca selective microelectrodes and rapid cooling contractures. *Can. J. Physiol. Pharmacol.* 65:610–618, 1987.
40. Bers, D. M., J. H. B. Bridge, and K. W. Sptizer. Intracellular Ca transients during rapid cooling contractures in guinea-pig ventricular myocytes. *J. Physiol. (Lond)*. 417:537–553, 1989.
41. Bers, D. M., D. M. Christensen, and T. X. Nguyen. Can Ca entry via Na-Ca exchange directly activate cardiac muscle contraction? *J. Mol. Cell Cardiol.* 20:405–414, 1988.
42. Bers, D. M., W. J. Lederer and J. R. Berlin. Intracellular Ca transients in rat cardiac myocytes: role of Na/Ca exchange in excitation-contraction coupling. *Am. J. Physiol.* 258 (*Cell Physiol.* 27):C944–C954, 1990.
43. Bers, D. M., K. D. Philipson, and A. Y. Nishimoto. Sodium-calcium exchange and sidedness of isolated cardiac sarcolemmal vesicles. *Biochim. Biophys. Acta.* 601:358–371, 1980.
44. Bers, D. M. and V. M. Stiffel. The ratio of ryanodine:dihydropyridine receptors in cardiac and skeletal muscle and implications for E-C coupling. *Am. J. Physiol.* 264 (*Cell Physiol.* 33):C1587–C1593, 1993.
45. Bers, D. M., L. Li, H. Satoh, and E. McCall. Factors which control SR Ca release in intact ventricular myocytes. *Ann. N. Y. Acad. Sci.* 853:157–177, 1998.
46. Beuckelmann, D. J. Contributions of Ca^{2+} influx via L-type Ca^{2+} current and Ca^{2+} release from the sarcoplasmic reticulum to [Ca]$_i$ transients in human myocytes. *Basic Res. Cardiol.* 92 (Suppl 1):105–110, 1997.
47. Beuckelmann, D. J. and W. G. Wier. Mechanism of release of calcium from sarcoplasmic reticulum of guinea pig cardiac cells. *J. Physiol.* 405:233–255, 1988.
48. Beuckelmann, D. J., and W. G. Wier. Sodium-calcium exchange in guinea-pig cardiac cells: exchange current and changes in intracellular Ca^{2+}. *J. Physiol. (Lond)*. 414:499–520, 1989.
49. Blater, L. A., and J. A. S. McGuigan. Free intracellular magnesium concentration in ferret ventricular muscle measured with ion selective micro-electrodes. *Q. J. Exp. Physiol.* 71:467–473, 1986.
49a. Blater L. A, J. Hüser, E. Ríos. Sarcoplasmic reticulum Ca^{2+} release flux underlying Ca^{2+} sparks in cardiac muscle. *Proc Natl Acad Sci U S A*. 94:4176–4181, 1997.
50. Blaustein, M. P. and W. J. Lederer. Sodium/calcium exchange: its physiological implications. *Physiol. Rev.* 79:763–854, 1999.
51. Blinks, J. R., C. B. Olson, B. R. Jewell, and P. Braveny. Influence of caffeine and other methylxanthines on mechanical properties of isolated mammalian heart muscle: evidence for a dual mechanism of action. *Circ. Res.* 30:367–392, 1972.
52. Block, B. A., T. Imagawa, K. P. Campbell, and C. Franzini-Armstrong. Structural evidence for direct interaction between the molecular components of the transverse tubule/sarcoplasmic reticulum junction in skeletal muscle. *J. Cell Biol.* 107:2587–2600, 1988.
53. Boerth, S. R., D. B. Zimmer, and M. Artman. Steady-state mRNA levels of the sarcolemmal Na^+-Ca^{2+} exchanger peak near birth in developing rabit and rat hearts. *Circ. Res.* 74:354–359, 1994.
54. Bouchard, R. A. and D. Bose. Analysis of the interval-force relationship in rat and canine ventricular myocardium. *Am. J. Physiol.* 257 (*Heart Circ. Physiol.* 26):H2036–H2047, 1989.

55. Brandes, R. and D. M. Bers. Intracellular Ca^{2+} increases NADH production and redox potential during elevated work in intact cardiac muscle. *Circ. Res.* 80:82–87, 1997.
56. Bridge, J. H. B. Relationships between the sarcoplasmic reticulum and transarcolemmal Ca transport revealed by rapidly cooling rabbit ventricular muscle. *J. Gen. Physiol.* 88:437–473, 1986.
56a. Bridge J. H, P. R. Ershler, M. B. Cannell. Properties of Ca^{2+} sparks evoked by action potentials in mouse ventricular myocytes. *J. Physiol. (Lond)*. 518:469–478, 1999.
57. Briggs, F. N., K. F. Lee, A. W. Wechsler, and L. R. Jones. Phospholamban expressed in slow-twitch and chronically stimulated fast-twitch muscles minimally affects calcium affinity of sarcoplasmic reticulum Ca^{2+}-ATPase. *J. Biol. Chem.* 267:26056–26061, 1992.
58. Brillantes, A. B., S. Bezprozvannaya, and A. R. Marks. Developmental and tissue-specific regulation of rabbit skeletal and cardiac muscle calcium channels involved in excitation-contraction coupling. *Circ. Res.* 75:503–510, 1994.
59. Brillantes A. B., K. Ondrias, A. Scott, E. Kobrinsky, E. Ondriasova, M. C. Moschella, T. Jayaraman, M. Landers, B. E. Ehrlich, and A. R. Marks. Stabilization of calcium release channel (ryanodine receptor) function by FK-506 binding protein. *Cell* 77:513–523, 1994.
60. Butcher, R. W. and E. W. Sutherland. Adenosine 3',5'-phosphate in biological materials. I. Purification and properties of cyclic 3',5'-nucleotide phosphodiesterase and the use of this enzyme to characterize adenosine 3',5'-phosphate in human urine. *J. Biol. Chem.* 237:1244–1250, 1962.
61. Callewaert, G., L. Cleemann, and M. Morad. Caffeine-induced Ca^{2+} release activates Ca^{2+} extrusion via Na^+-Ca^{2+} exchanger in cardiac myocytes. *Am. J. Physiol.* 257 (*Cell Physiol.* 26):C147–C152, 1989.
62. Campbell, K. P., T. Imagawa, J. S. Smith, and R. Coronado. Purified ryanodine receptor from skeletal muscle sarcoplasmic reticulum is the Ca^{2+}-permeable pore of the calcium release channel. *J. Biol. Chem.* 262:16636–16643, 1987.
63. Cannell, M. B., J. R. Berlin, and W. J. Lederer. Effect of membrane potential changes on the calcium transient in single rat cardiac muscle cells. *Science* 238:1419–1423, 1987.
64. Cannell M. B., H. Cheng, and W. J. Lederer. Spatial non-uniformities in [Ca^{2+}]i during excitation-contraction coupling in cardiac myocytes. *Biophys. J.* 67:1942–1956, 1994.
65. Cannell, M. B., H. Cheng, and W. J. Lederer. The control of calcium release in heart muscle. *Science* 268:1045–1049, 1995.
66. Capogrossi, M. C., A. A. Kort, H. A. Spurgeon, and E. G. Lakatta. Single adult rabbit and rat cardiac myocytes retain the Ca^{2+} and species-dependent systolic and diastolic contractile properties of intact muscle. *J. Gen. Physiol.* 88:589–613, 1986.
67. Carafoli, E. Mitochondria, Ca^{2+} transport and the regulation of heart contraction and metabolism. *J. Mol. Cell. Cardiol.* 7:83–89, 1975.
68. Carafoli, E. Intracellular calcium homeostasis. *Annu. Rev. Biochem.* 56:395–433, 1987.
69. Carafoli, E. Biogenesis: plasma membrane calcium ATPase: 15 years of work on the purified enzyme. *FASEB J.* 8:993–1002, 1994.
70. Carafoli, E. and A. L. Lehninger. A survey of the interaction of calcium ions with mitochondria from different tissues and species. *Biochem. J.* 122:618–690, 1971.
71. Carafoli, E. and T. Stauffer. The plasma membrane calcium pump: functional domains, regulation of the activity, and tissue specificity of isoform expression. *J. Neurobiol.* 25:312–324, 1994.
72. Caroni, P. and E. Carafoli. An ATP-dependent Ca^{2+}-pumping system in dog heart sarcolemma. *Nature* 283:765–767, 1980.

73. Caroni, P., L. Reinlib, and E. Carafoli. Charge movements during the Na$^+$-Ca^{2+} exchange in heart sarcolemmal vesicles. *Proc. Natl. Acad. Sci. U.S.A.* 77:6354–6358, 1980.
74. Caroni, P., and E. Carafoli. The Ca^{2+}-pumping ATPase of heart sarcolemma. *J. Biol. Chem.* 256:3263–3270, 1981.
75. Caroni, P. and E. Carafoli. Regulation of Ca^{2+}-pumping ATPase of heart sarcolemma by a phosphorylation-dephosphorylation process. *J. Biol. Chem.* 256:9371–9373, 1981.
76. Chacon, E, H. Ohata, I. S. Harper, D. R. Trollinger, B. Herman, and J. J. Lemasters. Mitochondrial free calcium transients during excitation-contraction coupling in rabbit cardiac myocytes. *FEBS Lett.*, 382:32–36, 1996.
77. Chen, W., C. Steenbergen, L. A. Levy, J. Vance, R. E. London, and E. Murphy. Measurement of free Ca^{2+} in sarcoplasmic reticulum in perfused rabbit heart loaded with 1,2-bis(2-amino-5,6-difluorophenoxy) ethane-N,N,N'N'-tetraacetic acid by ^{19}F NMR. *J. Biol. Chem.* 271:7398–7403, 1996.
78. Cheng H., W. J. Lederer., M. B. Cannell. Calcium sparks: elementary events underlying excitation-contraction coupling in heart muscle. *Science* 262:740–744, 1993.
79. Clarke, D. M., T. W. Loo, G. Inesi, and D. H. MacLennan. Location of high affinity Ca^{2+}-binding sites within the predicted transmembrane domain of the sarcoplasmic reticulum Ca^{2+}-ATPase. *Nature* 339:476–478, 1989.
80. Cohen, C. J., H. A. Fozzard, and S.-S. Sheu. Increase in intracellular sodium ion activity during stimulation in mammalian cardiac muscle. *Circ. Res.* 50:651–662, 1982.
81. Collins, A., A. V. Somlyo, and D. W. Hilgemann. The giant cardiac membrane patch method: stimulation of outward Na$^+$-Ca^{2+} exchange current by MgATP. *J. Physiol.* 454:27–57, 1992.
82. Coronado, R., J. Morisette, M. Sukhareva, and M. Vaughan. Structure and function of the ryanodine receptors. *Am. J. Physiol.* 266 (*Cell Physiol.* 35):C1485–C1504, 1994.
83. Crespo, L. M., C. J. Grantham, and M. B. Cannell. Kinetics, stoichiometry and role of the Na-Ca exchange mechanism in isolated cardiac myocytes. *Nature* 345:618–621, 1990.
84. Crompton, M., M. Capana and E. Carafoli. The sodium-induced efflux of calcium from heart mitochondria: a possible mechanism for the regulation of mitochondrial calcium. *Eur. J. Biochem.* 69:453–462, 1976.
85. Crompton, M. The regulation of mitochondrial calcium transport in heart. *Curr. Top. Memb. Transp.* 25:231–276, 1985.
86. Crompton, M. The role of Ca^{2+} in the function and dysfunction of heart mitochondria. In: *Calcium and the Heart*, edited by G. A. Langer. New York: Raven Press, 1990:167–198.
87. Dani, A. M., A. Cittadini, and G. Inesi. Calcium transport and contractile activity in dissociated mammalian heart cells. *Am. J. Physiol.* 237 (*Cell Physiol.* 6):C147–C155, 1979.
88. Danko, S., D. H. Kim, F. A. Sreter and N. Ikemoto. Inhibitors of Ca^{2+} release from the isolated sarcoplasmic reticulum. II. The effects of dantrolene on Ca^{2+} release induced by caffeine, Ca^{2+} and depolarization. *Biochim. Biophys. Acta* 816:18–24, 1985.
89. Delbridge, L. M., J. W. M. Bassani, and D. M. Bers. Steady-state twitch Ca fluxes and cytosolic Ca buffering in rabbit ventricular myocytes. *Am. J. Physiol.* 270 (*Cell Physiol.* 39):C192–C199, 1996.
90. Delbridge, L. M. D., H. Satoh, W. Yuan, J. W. M. Bassani, M. QI, K. S. Ginsburg, A. M. Samarel, and D. M. Bers. Cardiac myocyte volume, Ca^{2+} fluxes and sarcoplasmic reticulum loading in pressure overload hypertrophy. *Am. J. Physiol.* 272 (*Heart Circ. Physiol.* 41):H2425–H2435, 1997.
91. Deleon, M., Y. Wang, L. Jones, E. Perez-Reyes, X. Wei, T. W. Soong, T. P. Snutch, and D. T. Yue. Essential Ca^{2+}-binding motif for Ca^{2+}-sensitive inactivation of L-type Ca^{2+} channels. *Science* 270:1502–1506, 1995.
92. Denton, R. M. and J. G. McCormack. On the role of the calcium transport cycle in heart and other mammalian mitochondria. *FEBS Lett.* 119:1–8, 1980.
93. Denton, R. M. and J. G. McCormack. Ca^{2+} transport by mammalian mitochondria and its role in hormone action. *Am. J. Physiol.* 249 (*Endocrinol. Metab.* 12):E543–E554. 1985.
94. Denton, R. M. and J. G. McCormack. Ca^{2+} as a second messenger within mitochondria of the heart and other tissues. *Annu. Rev. Physiol.* 52:451–466, 1990.
95. Díaz, M. E., A. W. Trafford, S. C. O'Neill, and D. A. Eisner. Measurement of sarcoplasmic reticulum Ca^{2+} content and sarcolemmal Ca^{2+} fluxes in isolated rat ventricular myocytes during spontaneous Ca^{2+} release. *J. Physiol.* 501:3–16, 1997.
96. Difrancesco, D., and D. Noble. A model of cardiac electrical activity incorporating ionic pumps and concentration changes. *Phil. Trans. R. Soc. Lond. B* 307:353–309, 1985.
97. Dixon, D. A. and D. H. Haynes. Kinetic characterization of the Ca^{2+}-pumping ATPase of cardiac sarcolemma in four states of activation. *J. Biol. Chem.* 264:13612–13622, 1989.
98. Durkin, J. T., D. C. Ahrens, Y.-C. E. Pan, and J. P. Reeves. Purification and amino-terminal sequence of the bovine cardiac sodium-calcium exchanger: evidence for the presence of a signal sequence. *Arch. Biochem. Biophys.* 290:369–375, 1991.
99. Edman, K. A. P. and M. Jóhannsson. The contractile state of rabbit papillary muscle in relation to stimulation frequency. *J. Physiol.* 254:565–581, 1976.
100. Egan, T. M., D. Noble, S. J. Noble, T. Powell, A. J. Spindler, and V. W. Twist. Sodium-calcium exchange during the action potential in guinea-pig ventricular cells. *J. Physiol.* 411:639–661, 1989.
101. Egger, M. and E. Niggli. Paradoxical block of the Na$^+$-Ca^{2+} exchanger by extracellular protons in guinea-pig ventricular rmyocytes. *J. Physiol.* 523:353–366, 2000
102. El-Sayed, M. F. and H. Gesser. Sarcoplasmic reticulum, potassium, and cardiac force in rainbow trout and plaice. *Am. J. Physiol.* 257 (*Renal Fluid Electrolyte Physiol.* 26):R599–R604, 1989.
103. Fabiato, A. Calcium release in skinned cardiac cells: variations with species, tissues, and development. *Federation Proc.* 41:2238–2244, 1982.
104. Fabiato, A. Calcium-induced release of calcium from the cardiac sarcoplasmic reticulum. *Am. J. Physiol.* 245 (*Cell Physiol.* 14):C1–C14, 1983.
105. Fabiato, A. Simulated calcium current can both cause calcium loading in and trigger calcium release from the sarcoplasmic reticulum of a skinned canine cardiac Purkinje cell. *J. Gen. Physiol.* 85:291–320, 1985.
106. Feher, J. J. Unidirectional calcium and nucleotide fluxes in sarcoplasmic reticulum. *Biophys. J.* 45:1125–1133, 1984.
107. Fleischer, S. and M. Inui. Biochemistry and biophysics of excitation-contraction coupling. *Annu. Rev. Biophys. Chem.* 18:333–364, 1989.
108. Frampton, J. E., S. M. Harrison, M. R. Boyett, and C. H. Orchard. Ca^{2+} and Na$^+$ in rat ventricular myocytes showing different force frequency relationships. *Am. J. Physiol.* 261 (*Cell Physiol.* 30):C739–C750, 1991.
109. Frank, J. S. and G. A. Langer. The myocardial interstitium: its structure and its role in ionic exchange. *J. Cell Biol.* 60:586–601, 1974.
110. Frankis, M. B. and G. E. Lindenmayer. Sodium-sensitive calcium binding to sarcolemma-enriched preparations from canine ventricles. *Circ. Res.* 55:676–688, 1984.
111. Friel, D. D. and B. P. Bean. Two ATP-activated conductances in bullfrog atrial cells. *J. Gen. Physiol.* 91:1–27, 1988.
112. Fry, C. H., T. Powell, V. W. Twist, and J. P. T. Ward. Net calcium exchange in adult rat ventricular myocytes: an assessment

of mitochondrial calcium accumulating capacity. *Proc. R. Soc. Lond.* 223:223–238, 1984.
113. Fry, C. H., T. Powell, V. W. Twist, and J. P. T. Ward. The effects of sodium, hydrogen and magnesium ions on mitochondrial calcium sequestration in adult rat ventricular myocytes. *Proc. R. Soc. Lond.* 223:239–254, 1984.
114. Fujioka Y, M. Komeda, and S. Matsuoka. Stoichiometry of Na^+-Ca^{2+} exchange in inside-out patches excised from guinea-pig ventricular myocytes. *J. Physiol.* 523:339–351, 2000.
115. Gatto, C. and M. A. Milanick. Inhibition of the red blood cell calcium pump by eosin and other fluorescein analogues. *Am. J. Physiol.* 264 (*Cell Physiol.* 33):C1577–C1586, 1993.
116. Gao, W., P. H. Backx, M. Azan-Backx, and E. Marban. Myofilament Ca^{2+} sensitivity in intact versus skinned rat ventricular muscle. *Circ. Res.* 74:408–415, 1994.
117. Ginsburg, K. S., C. R. Weber, and D. M. Bers. Control of maximum sarcoplasmic reticulum Ca load in intact ferret ventricular myocytes: effects of thapsigargin and isoproterenol. *J. Gen. Physiol.* 111:491–504, 1998.
118. Goldstein, M. A. and L. Traeger. Ultrastructural changes in postnatal development of the cardiac myocytes. In: *The Developing Heart*, edited by M. J. Legato. Boston: Martinus Nijhoff Publishing, 1985:1–20.
119. Grantham, C. J. and M. B. Cannell. Ca^{2+} influx during the cardiac action potential in guinea pig ventricular myocytes. *Circ. Res.* 79:194–200, 1996.
120. Griffiths, E. J., M. D. Stern, and H. S. Silverman. Measurement of mitochondrial calcium in single living cardiac myocytes by selective removal of cytosolic indo-1. *Am. J. Physiol.* 273 (*Cell Physiol.* 42):C37–C44, 1997.
121. Györke, S. and M. Fill. Ryanodine receptor adaptation:control mechanism of Ca^{2+}-induced Ca^{2+} release in heart. *Science* 260:807–809, 1993.
122. Györke S, V. Lukyanenko, and I. Györke. Dual effects of tetracaine on spontaneous calcium release in rat ventricular myocytes. *J. Physiol. (Lond.)* 500:297–309, 1997.
123. Hadley, R. W. and J. R. Hume. An intrinsic potential-dependent inactivation mechanism associated with calcium channels in guinea-pig myocytes. *J. Physiol.* 389:205–222, 1987.
124. Haddock, P. S., W. A. Coetzee, and M. Artman. Na^+/Ca^{2+} exchange current and contractions measured under Cl^--free conditions in developing rabbit hearts. *Am. J. Physiol.* 273 (*Heart Circ. Physiol.* 42):H837–H846, 1997.
125. Hagiwara, N., H. Irisawa, and M. Kameyama. Contribution of two types of calcium currents to the pacemaker potentials of rabbit sino-atrial node cells. *J. Physiol., (Lond.)* 359:233–253, 1988.
126. Haiech, J., B. Klee, and J. G. Demaille. Effects of cations on affinity of calmodulin for calcium:ordered binding of calcium ions allows the specific activation of calmodulin-stimulated enzymes. *Biochemistry* 20:3890–3897, 1981.
127. Hansford, R. G. Relation between mitochondrial calcium transport and control of energy metabolism. *Rev. Physiol. Biochem. Pharmacol.* 102:1–72, 1985.
128. Hansford, R. G. Relation between cytosolic free Ca^{2+} concentration and the control of pyruvate dehydrogenase in isolated cardiac myocytes. *Biochem. J.* 241:145–151, 1987.
129. Harrison, S. M., and D. M. Bers. The influence of temperature on the calcium sensitivity of the myofilaments of skinned ventricular muscle from the rabbit. *J. Gen. Physiol.* 93:411–427, 1989.
130. Hess, P., J. B. Lansman and R. W. Tsien. Different modes of Ca channel gating behavior favored by dihydropyridine Ca agonists and antagonists. *Nature* 311:538–544, 1984.
131. Hess, P., J. B. Lansman, and R. W. Tsien. Calcium channel selectivity for divalent and monovalent cations. Voltage and concentration dependence of single channel current in ventricular heart cells. *J. Gen. Physiol.* 88:293–319, 1986.
132. Hilgemann, D. W. Numerical probes of sodium-calcium exchange. In:*Sodium-Calcium Exchange*, edited by T. J. A. Allen, D. Noble, and H. Reuter. Oxford: Oxford University Press, 1989:126–152.
133. Hilgemann, D. W. Regulation and deregulation of cardiac Na^+-Ca^{2+} exchange in giant excised sarcolemmal membrane patches. *Nature* 344:242–245, 1990.
134. Hilgemann, D. W. and R. Ball. Regulation of cardiac Na^+,Ca^{2+} exchange and KATP potassium channels by PIP2. *Science* 273:956–959, 1996.
135. Hilgemann, D. W. and A. Collins. Mechanism of cardiac Na^+-Ca^{2+} exchange current stimulation by MgATP:possible involvement of aminophospholipid translocase. *J. Physiol. (Lond.)* 454:59–82, 1992.
136. Hilgemann, D. W., A. Collins, and S. Matsuoka. Steady-state and dynamic properties of cardiac sodium-calcium exchange. Secondary modulation by cytoplasmic calcium and ATP. *J. Gen. Physiol.* 100:933–961, 1992.
137. Hilgemann, D. W., S. Matsuoka, G. A. Nagel, and A. Collins. Steady-state and dynamic properties of cardiac sodium-calcium exchange. Sodium-dependent inactivation. *J. Gen. Physiol.* 100:905–932, 1992.
138. Hilgemann, D. W., K. D. Philipson, and G. Vassort. Sodium-Calcium Exchange:Proceedings of the Third International Conference. *Ann. N.Y. Acad. Sci.* 1996, vol. 779.
139. Hirano, Y., H. A. Fozzard, and C. T. January. Characteristics of L- and T-type Ca^{2+} currents in canine cardiac Purkinje cells. *Am. J. Physiol.* 256 (*Heart Circ. Physiol.* 25):H1478–H1492, 1989.
140. Hoerter, J., F. Mazet, and G. Vassort. Perinatal growth of the rabbit cardiac cell:possible implications for the mechanism of relaxation. *J. Mol. Cell. Cardiol.* 13:725–740, 1981.
141. Holroyde, M. J., E. Howe, and R. J. Solaro. Modification of calcium requirements for activation of cardiac myofibrillar ATPase by cyclic AMP dependent phosphorylation. *Biochim. Biophys. Acta* 586:63–69, 1979.
142. Holroyde, M. J., S. P. Robertson, J. D. Johnson, R. J. Solaro, and J. D. Potter. The calcium and magnesium binding sites on cardiac troponin and their role in the regulation of myofibrillar adenosine triphosphatase. *J. Biol. Chem.* 255:11688–11693, 1980.
143. Horackova, M. and G. Vassort. Sodium-calcium exchange in regulation of cardiac contractility. Evidence for an electrogenic, voltage-dependent mechanism. *J. Gen. Physiol.* 73:403–424, 1979.
144. Hove-Madsen, L. and D. M. Bers. Indo-1 binding in permeabilized myocytes alters its spectral and Ca binding properties. *Biophys. J.* 63:89–97, 1992.
145. Hove-Madsen, L. and D. M. Bers. Passive Ca buffering and SR Ca uptake in permeabilized rabbit ventricular myocytes. *Am. J. Physiol.* 264 (*Cell Physiol.* 33):C677–C686, 1993.
146. Hove-Madsen, L. and D. M. Bers. SR Ca uptake and thapsigargin sensitivity in permeabilized rabbit and rat ventricular myocytes. *Circ. Res.* 73:820–828, 1993.
147. Hryshko, L. V., V. M. Stiffel, and D. M. Bers. Rapid cooling contractures as an index of SR Ca content in rabbit ventricular myocyte. *Am. J. Physiol.* 257 (*Heart Circ. Physiol.* 26):H1369–1377, 1989.
148. Deleted
149. Hunter, D. R., R. A. Haworth, and H. A. Berkoff. Measurement of rapidly exchangeable cellular calcium in the perfused beating rat heart. *Proc. Natl. Acad. Sci. U.S.A.* 78:5665–5668, 1981.

150. Huynh, T. V., F. H. Chen, G. T. Wetzel, W. F. Friedman, and T. S. Klitzner. Developmental changes in membrane Ca^{2+} and K^+ currents in fetal, neonatal, and adult rabbit ventricular myocytes. *Circ. Res.* 70:508–515, 1992.

151. Hymel, L., M. Inui, S. Fleischer, and H. Schindler. Purified ryanodine receptor of skeletal muscle sarcoplasmic reticulum forms Ca^{2+}-activated oligomeric Ca^{2+} channels in planar bilayers. *Proc. Natl. Acad. Sci. U.S.A.* 85:441–445, 1988.

152. Imagawa, T., J. S. Smith, R. Coronado, and K. P. Campbell. Purified ryanodine receptor from skeletal muscle sarcoplasmic reticulum is the Ca^{2+}-permeable pore of the calcium release channel. *J. Biol. Chem.* 262:16636–16643, 1987.

153. Inesi G. and L. De Meis. Regulation of steady state filling in sarcoplasmic reticulum. *J. Biol. Chem.* 264:5929–5936, 1988.

154. Inui, M., A. Saito, and S. Fleischer. Purification of the ryanodine receptor and identity with feet structures of junctional terminal cisternae of sarcoplasmic reticulum from fast skeletal muscle. *J. Biol. Chem.* 262:1740–1747, 1987.

155. Inui, M., A. Saito, and S. Fleischer. Isolation of the ryanodine receptor from cardiac sarcoplasmic reticulum and identity with the feet structures. *J. Biol. Chem.* 262:15637–15642, 1987.

156. Isenberg, G. and M. F. Wendt-Gallitelli. Cellular mechanisms of excitation contraction coupling. In: *Isolated Adult Cardiomyocytes*, Volume II, edited by H. M. Piper and G. Isenberg. Boca Raton, Florida: CRC Press, 1989:213–248.

157. Iwamoto, T, T. Y. Nakamura, Y. Pan, A. Uehara, I. Imagawa, and M. Shigekawa. Unique topology of the internal repeats in the cardiac Na^+/Ca^{2+} exchanger. *FEBS Lett.* 446:264–268, 1999.

158. James, P., M. Maeda, R. Fischer, A. K. Verma, J. Krebs, J. T. Penniston, and E. Carafoli. Identification and primary structure of a calmodulin binding domain of the Ca^{2+} pump of human erythrocytes. *J. Biol. Chem.* 263:2905–2910, 1988.

159. Janczewski, A. M. and E. G. Lakatta. Buffering of calcium influx by sarcoplasmic reticulum during the action potential in guinea-pig ventricular myocytes. *J. Physiol.* 471:343–363, 1993.

160. Janczewski, A. M. and E. G. Lakatta. Thapsigargin inhibits Ca^{2+} uptake, and Ca^{2+} depletes sarcoplasmic reticulum in intact cardiac myocytes. *Am. J. Physiol.* 265 (*Heart Circ. Physiol.* 34):H517–H522, 1993.

161. Jones, L. R., H. R. Besch, J. L. Sutko and J. T. Willerson. Ryanodine-induced stimulation of net Ca++ uptake by cardiac sarcoplasmic reticulum vesicles. *J. Pharmacol. Exp. Ther.* 209:48–55, 1979.

162. Jung, D. W., K. Baysal, and G. P. Brierley. The sodium-calcium antiport of heart mitochondria is not electroneutral. *J. Biol. Chem.* 270:672–678, 1995.

163. Kadambi, V. J., S. Ponniah, J. M. Harrer, B. D. Hoit, G. W. Dorn II, R. A. Walsh, and E. G. Kranias. Cardiac-specific overexpression of phospholamban alters calcium kinetics and resultant cardiomyocyte mechanics in transgenic mice. *J. Clin. Invest.* 97:533–539, 1996.

164. Kaftan E, A. R. Marks, and B. E. Ehrlich. Effects of rapamycin on ryanodine receptor/calcium release. *Circ. Res.* 78:990–997, 1996.

165. Kass, R. S. and M. C. Sanguinetti. Inactivation of calcium channel current in the calf cardiac Purkinje fiber. Evidence for voltage- and calcium-mediated mechanisms. *J. Gen. Physiol.* 84:705–726, 1984.

166. Deleted

167. Kawai, M. and M. Konishi. Measurement of sarcoplasmic reticulum calcium content in skinned mammalian cardiac muscle. *Cell Calcium* 16:123–136, 1994.

168. Kijima, Y., E. Ogunbunmi, and S. Fleischer. Drug action of thapsigargin on the Ca^{2+} pump protein of sarcoplasmic reticulum. *J. Biol. Chem.* 266:22912–22918, 1991.

169. Kimura, J., A. Noma, and H. Irisawa. Na-Ca exchange current in mammalian heart cells. *Nature* 319:596–597, 1986.

170. Kimura, J., S. Miyamae, and A. Noma. Identification of sodium-calcium exchange current in single ventricular cells in guinea pig. *J. Physiol.* 384:199–222, 1987.

171. Kirby, M. S., Y. Sagara, S. Gaa, G. Inesi, W. J. Lederer, and T. B. Rogers. Thapsigargin inhibits contraction and Ca transient in cardiac cells by specific inhibition of the sarcoplasmic reticulum Ca pump. *J. Biol. Chem.* 267:12545–12551, 1992.

172. Kirino, Y. and H. Shimizu. Ca^{2+}-induced Ca^{2+} release from fragmented sarcoplasmic reticulum: a comparison with skinned muscle fiber studies. *J. Biochem.* 92:1287–1296, 1982.

173. Kiss, E., G. Jakab, E. G. Kranias, and I. Edes. Thyroid hormone-induced alterations in phospholamban protein expression. *Circ. Res.* 75:245–251, 1994.

174. Koss, K. L. and E. G. Kranias. Phospholamban: a prominent regulator of myocardial contractility. *Circ. Res.* 79:1059–1063, 1996.

175. Kranias, E. G. Regulation of calcium transport by protein phosphatase activity associated with cardiac sarcoplasmic reticulum. *J. Biol. Chem.* 260:11006–11010, 1985.

176. Kurihara, S. and T. Sakai. Effects of rapid cooling on mechanical and electrical responses in ventricular muscle of guinea pig. *J. Physiol.* 361:361–378, 1985.

177. Kuyayama, H. The membrane potential modulates the ATP-dependent Ca^{2+} pump of cardiac sarcolemma. *Biochim. Biophys. Acta* 940:295–299, 1988.

178. Lai, F. A., H. Erickson, B. A. Block, and G. Meissner. Evidence for a junctional feet-ryanodine receptor complex from sarcoplasmic reticulum. *Biochem. Biophys. Res. Commun.* 143:704–709, 1987.

179. Lai, F. A., H. F. Erickson, E. Rousseau, Q.-Y. Liu, and G. Meissner. Purification and reconstitution of the calcium release channel from skeletal muscle. *Nature* 331:315–319, 1988.

180. Lai, F. A., K. Anderson, E. Rousseau, Q.-Y. Liu, and G. Meissner Evidence for a Ca^{2+} channel within the ryanodine receptor complex from cardiac sarcoplasmic reticulum. *Biochem. Biophys. Res. Commun.* 151:441–449, 1988.

181. Lai, F. A., M. Misra, L. Xu, H. A. Smith, and G. Meissner. The ryanodine receptor-Ca^{2+} release channel complex of skeletal muscle sarcoplasmic reticulum. *J. Biol. Chem.* 264:16776–16785, 1989.

182. Langer, G. A. and A. Peskoff. Calcium concentration and movement in the diadic cleft space of the cardiac ventricular cell. *Biophys. J.* 70:1169–1182, 1996.

183. Langer, G. A., T. L. Rich, and F. B. Orner. Ca exchange under non-perfusion-limited conditions in rat ventricular cells:identification of subcellular compartments. *Am. J. Physiol.* 259 (*Heart Circ. Physiol.* 28):H592–H602, 1990.

184. Langer, G. A. and T. L. Rich. Further characterization of the Na-Ca exchange-dependent Ca compartment in rat ventricular cells. *Am. J. Physiol.* 265 (*Cell Physiol.* 34):C556–C561, 1993.

185. Deleted

186. Lee, C. O. and H. A. Fozzard. Activities of potassium and sodium ions in rabbit heart muscle. *J. Gen. Physiol.* 65:695–708, 1975.

187. Lee, K. S., E. Marban, and R. W. Tsien. Inactivation of calcium channels in mammalian heart cells:joint dependence on membrane potential and intracellular calcium. *J. Physiol. (Lond.)* 364:395–411, 1985.

188. Legato, M. Cellular mechanisms of normal growth in the mammalian heart. II. A quantitative and qualitative comparison between the right and left ventricular myocytes in the dog from birth to five months of age. *Circ. Res.* 44:263–279, 1979.

189. Lehninger, A. L., E. Carafoli, and C. S. Rossi. Energy linked ion movements in mitochondrial systems. *Adv. Enzymol.* 29:259–320, 1967.
190. Lehninger, A. L. Ca^{2+} transport by mitochondria and its possible role in the cardiac excitation-contraction-relaxation cycle. *Circ. Res.* 34/35(Suppl. III):83–89, 1974.
191. Levitsky, D. O., D. S. Benevolensky, T. S. Levchenko, V. N. Smirnov, and E. I. Chazov. Calcium-binding rate and capacity of cardiac sarcoplasmic reticulum. *J. Mol. Cell Cardiol.* 13:785–796, 1981.
192. Lew, W. Y. W., L. V. Hryshko, and D. M. Bers. Dihydropyridine receptors are primarily functional L-type Ca channels in rabbit ventricular myocytes. *Circ. Res.* 69:1139–1145, 1991.
193. Lewartowski, B. and K. Zdanowski. Net Ca^{2+} influx and sarcoplasmic reticulum Ca^{2+} uptake in resting single myocytes of the rat heart:comparison with guinea-pig. *J. Mol. Cell Cardiol.* 22:1221–1229, 1990.
194. Li, L., G. Chu, E. G. Kranias, and D. M. Bers. Cardiac myocyte calcium transport in phospholamban knockout mouse: Relaxation and endogenous CaMKII effects. *Am. J. Physiol.* 274 (*Heart Circ. Physiol.* 43):H1335–H1347, 1998.
195. Li, L., H. Satoh, K. S. Ginsburg, and D. M. Bers. The effects of CaMKII on cardiac excitation-contraction coupling in ferret ventricular myocytes. *J. Physiol.* 501:17–32, 1997.
196. Li, Z., D. A. Nicoll, A. Collins, D. W. Hilgemann, A. G. Filoteo, J. T. Penniston, J. N. Weiss J. M. Tomich, and K. D. Philipson. Identification of a peptide inhibitor of the cardiac sarcolemmal Na^+-Ca^{2+} exchanger. *J. Biol. Chem.* 266:1014–1020, 1991.
197. London, B. and J. W. Krueger. Contraction in voltage-clamped, internally perfused single heart cells. *J. Gen. Physiol.* 88:475–505, 1986.
198. López-López, J. R., P. S. Shacklock, C. W. Balke, and W. G. Wier. Local, stochastic release of Ca^{2+} in voltage-clamped rat heart cells: visualization with confocal microscopy. *J. Physiol. (Lond.).* 480:21–29, 1994.
199. López-López JR., P. S. Shacklock, C. W. Balke, and W. G. Wier. Local calcium transients triggered by single L-type calcium channel currents in cardiac cells. *Science.* 268:1042–1045, 1995.
200. Lu, Y.-Z. and M. A. Kirchberger. Effects of a nonionic detergent on calcium uptake by cardiac microsomes. *Biochemistry* 33:5056–5062, 1994.
201. Lukyanenko, I. Györke, and S. Györke. Regulation of calcium release by calcium inside the sarcoplasmic reticulum in ventricular myocytes. *Pflugers Arch.* 432:1047–1054, 1996.
201a. Lukyanenko V., I. Györke, S. Subramanian, A. Smirnov, T. F. Wiesner, S. Györke. Inhibition of Ca^{2+} sparks by ruthenium red in permeabilized rat ventricular myocytes. *Biophys J.* 79:1273–1284, 2000.
202. Luo, C.-H. and Y. Rudy. A dynamic model of the cardiac ventricular action potential. I. Simulations of ionic currents and concentration changes. *Circ. Res.* 74:1071–1096, 1994.
203. Luo, W., B. W. Wolska, I. L. Grupp, J. M. Harrer, K. Haghighi, D. G. Ferguson, J. P. Slack, G. Grupp, T. Doetschman, R. J. Solaro, E. G. Kranias. Phospholamban gene dosage effects in the mammalian heart. *Circ. Res.* 78:839–847, 1996.
204. Lytton, J., M. Westlin, and R. Hanley. Thapsigargin inhibits the sarcoplasmic and endoplasmic reticulum Ca-ATPase family of calcium pumps. *J. Biol. Chem.* 266:17067–17071, 1991.
205. McCormack, J. G., H. M. Browne, and N. J. Dawes. Studies on mitochondrial Ca^{2+}-transport and matrix Ca^{2+} using fura-2-loaded rat heart mitochondria. *Biochim. Biophys. Acta* 973:420–427, 1989.
206. Mahony, L. and L. R. Jones. Developmental changes in cardiac sarcoplasmic reticulum in sheep. *J. Biol. Chem.* 261:15257–15265, 1986.
207. Malécot, C. O., D. M. Bers, and B. G. Katzung. Biphasic contractions induced by milrinone at low temperature in ferret ventricular muscle: role of the sarcoplasmic reticulum and transmembrane Ca influx. *Circ. Res.* 59:151–162, 1986.
208. Marks, A. P., P. Tempst, K. S. Hwang, M. B. Taubman, M. Inui, C. Chadwick, S. Fleischer and B. Nadal-Ginard. Molecular cloning and characterization of the ryanodine receptor/junctional channel complex cDNA from skeletal muscle sarcoplasmic reticulum. *Proc. Natl. Acad. Sci. U.S.A.* 86:8683–8687, 1989.
209. Matsuda, H. Sodium conductance in calcium channels of guinea pig ventricular cells induced by removal of external calcium ions. *Pflugers Arch.* 407:465–475, 1986.
210. Matsuoka, S. and D. W. Hilgemann. Steady-state and dynamic properties of cardiac sdium-calcium exchange. Ion and voltage dependencies of the transport cycle. *J. Gen. Physiol.* 100:963–1001, 1992.
211. Matsuoka, S., D. A. Nicoll, L. V. Hryshko, D. O. Levitsky, J. N. Weiss, and K. D. Philipson. Regulation of the cardiac Na^+-Ca^{2+} exchanger by Ca^{2+}. *J. Gen. Physiol.* 105:403–420, 1995.
212. Mattiazzi, A., L. Hove-Madsen, and D. M. Bers. Protein kinase inhibitors reduce SR Ca transport in permeabilized cardiac myocytes. *Am. J. Physiol.* 267 (*Heart Circ. Physiol.* 36):H812–H820, 1994.
213. Mela, L. Inhibition and activation of calcium transport in mitochondria. Effect of lanthanides and local anaesthetic drugs. *Biochemistry* 8:2481–2486, 1969.
214. Meissner, G. Ryanodine activation and inhibition of the Ca^{2+} release channel of sarcoplasmic reticulum. *J. Biol. Chem.* 261:6300–6306, 1986.
215. Meissner, G. and J. S. Henderson. Rapid calcium release from cardiac sarcoplasmic reticulum vesicles is dependent on Ca^{2+} and is modulated by Mg^{2+}, adenine nucleotide, and calmodulin. *J. Biol. Chem.* 262:3065–3073, 1987.
216. Mejia-Alvarez, R., C. Kettlun, E. Rros, M. Stern, M. Fill. Unitary Ca^{2+} current through cardiac ryanodine receptors in physiological ionic conditions. *J. Gen. Physiol.* 113:177–186, 1999.
217. Mitchell, P. and J. Moyle. Respiration-driven proton translocation in rat liver mitochondria. *Biochem. J.* 105:1147–1162, 1967.
218. Mitra, R. and M. Morad. Two types of calcium channels in guinea pig ventricular myocytes. *Proc. Natl. Acad. Sci. U.S.A.* 83:5340–5344, 1986.
219. Miura, Y. and J. Kimuara. Sodium-calcium exchange current. *J. Gen. Physiol.* 93:1129–1145, 1989.
220. Miyata, H, H. S. Silerman, S. J. Sollott, E. G. Lakatta, M. D. Stern, and R. G. Hansford. Measurement of mitochondrial free Ca concentration in living single rat cardiac myocytes. *Am. J. Physiol.* 261 (*Heart Circ. Physiol.* 30):H1123–H1134, 1991.
221. Moore, C. L. Specific inhibition of mitochondrial Ca^{2+} transport by ruthenium red. *Biochem. Biophys. Res. Commun.* 42:298–305, 1971.
222. Morad, M. and Y. Goldman. Excitation-contraction coupling in heart muscle: membrane control of development of tension. *Prog. Biophys. Mol. Biol.* 27:257–313, 1973.
223. Moreno-Sanchez, R. and R. G. Hansford. Dependence of cardiac mitochondrial pyruvate dehydrogenase activity on intramitochondrial free Ca^{2+} concentration. *Biochem. J.* 256:403–412, 1988.
224. Deleted
225. Mullins, L. J. The generation of electric currents in cardiac fibers by Na/Ca exchange. *Am. J. Physiol.* 236 (*Cell. Physiol.* 5):C103–C110, 1979.

226. Murphy, E., C. C. Freudenrich, L. A. Levy, R. E. London, and M. Lieberman. Monitoring cytosolic free magnesium in cultured chicken heart cells by use of the fluorescent indicator furaptra. *Proc. Natl. Acad. Sci. U.S.A.* 86:2981–2984, 1989.
227. Murphy, E., C. Steenbergen, L. A. Levy, B. Raju, and R. E. London. Cytosolic free magnesium levels in ischemic rat heart. *J. Biol. Chem.* 264:5622–5627, 1989.
228. Nagasaki, K. and S. Fleischer. Modulation of the calcium release channel of sarcoplasmic reticulum by Adriamycin and other drugs. *Cell Calcium* 10:63–70, 1989.
229. Nakai, J., T. Imagawa, Y. Hakamata, M. Shigekawa, H. Takeshima and S. Numa. Primary structure and functional expression from cDNA of cardiac muscle ryanodine receptor/calcium release channel. *FEBS Lett.* 271:169–177, 1990.
230. Nakamura, Y., J. Kobayashi, J. Gilmore, M. Mascal, K. L. Rinehart, Jr., H. Nakamura, and Y. Ohizumi. Bromoeudistomin D, a novel inducer of calcium release from fragmented sarcoplasmic reticulum that causes contractions of skinned muscle fibers. *J. Biol. Chem.* 261:4139–4142, 1986.
231. Nakanishi, T. and J. M. Jarmakani. Developmental changes in myocardial mechanical function and subcellular organelles. *Am. J. Physiol.* 246 (*Heart Circ. Physiol.* 15):H615–H625, 1984.
232. Nayler, W. G. and E. Fassold. Calcium accumulation and ATPase activity of cardiac sarcoplasmic reticulum before and after birth. *Cardiovasc. Res.* 11:231–237, 1977.
233. Negretti N, S. C. O'Neill, and D. A. Eisner. The relative contributions of different intracellular and sarcolemmal systems to relaxation in rat ventricular myocytes. *Cardiovasc. Res.* 1993: 27:1826–1830.
234. Nicoll, D. A., S. Longoni, and K. D. Philipson. Molecular cloning and functional expression of the cardiac sarcolemmal Na^+-Ca^{2+} exchanger. *Science* 250:562–565, 1990.
235. Nicoll, D. A., L. V. Hryshko, S. Matsuoka, J. S. Frank, and K. D. Philipson. Mutation of amino acid residues in the putative transmembrane segments of the cardiac sarcolemmal Na^+-Ca^{2+} exchanger. *J. Biol. Chem.* 271:13385–13391, 1996.
236. Nicoll, D. A., M. Ottolia, L. Lu, Y. Lu, and K. D. Philipson. A new topological model of the cardiac sarcolemmal Na^+-Ca^{2+} exchanger. *J. Biol. Chem.* 274:910–917, 1999.
237. Nicholls, D. G. and K. E. O. Akerman. Mitochondrial calcium transport. *Biochim. Biophys. Acta* 683:57–88, 1982.
238. Niggli, V., E. S. Adunyah, J. T. Penniston and E. Carafoli. Purified (Ca^{2+}-Mg^{2+})-ATPase of the erythrocyte membrane. *J. Biol. Chem.* 256:395–401, 1981.
239. Nilius, B., P. Hess, J. B. Lansman, and R. W. Tsien. A novel type of cardiac calcium channel in ventricular cells. *Nature* 316:443–446, 1985.
240. Nowycky, M. C., A. P. Fox, and R. W. Tsien. Three types of neuronal calcium channel with different calcium agonist sensitivity. *Nature* 316:440–443, 1985.
241. Nuss, H. B., and S. R. Houser. T-type Ca^{2+} current is expressed in hypertrophied adult feline left ventricular myocytes. *Circ. Res.* 73:777–782, 1993.
242. Odermatt A, K. Kurzydlowski, and D. H. MacLennan. The Vmax of the Ca^{2+}-ATPase of cardiac sarcoplasmic reticulum (SERCA2a) is not altered by Ca^{2+}/calmodulin-dependent phosphorylation or by interaction with phospholamban. *J. Biol. Chem.* 271:14206–14213, 1996.
243. O'Neill, S. C., J. G. Mill, and D. A. Eisner. Local activation of contraction in isolated rat ventricular myocytes. *Am. J. Physiol.* 258 (*Cell Physiol.* 27):C1165–C1168, 1990.
244. Ohnishi, S. T. A method for studying the depolarization-induced calcium release from fragmented sarcoplasmic reticulum. *J. Biochem.* 86:1147–1150, 1979.
245. Olivetti, G., P. Anversa, and A. Loud. Morphometric study of early postnatal development in the left and right ventricular myocardium of the rat. II. Tissue composition, capillary growth, and sarcoplasmic alterations. *Circ. Res.* 46:503–512, 1980.
246. Osaka, T. and R. W. Joyner. Developmental changes in calcium currents of rabbit ventricular cells. *Circ. Res.* 68:788–796, 1991.
247. Otsu, K., H. F. Willard, V. J. Khana, F. Zorzato, N. M. Green and D. H. MacLennan. Molecular cloning of cDNA encoding the Ca^{2+} release channel (ryanodine receptor) of rabbit cardiac muscle sarcoplasmic reticulum. *J. Biol. Chem.* 265:13713–13720, 1990.
248. Overend, C. L., C. S. O'Niell and D. A. Eisner. The effect of tetracaine on stimulated contractions, sarcoplasmic reticulum Ca^{2+} content and membrane current in isolated rat ventricular myocytes. *J. Physiol.* 507:759–769, 1998.
249. Page, E. Quantitative ultrastructural analysis in cardiac membrane physiology. *Am. J. Physiol.* 235 (*Cell Physiol.* 4): C147–C158, 1978.
250. Page, E. and J. L. Buecker. Development of dyadic junctional complexes between sarcoplasmic reticulum and plasmalemma in rabbit left ventricular myocardial cells. *Circ. Res.* 48:519–522, 1981.
251. Page, E., L. P. McCallister and B. Power. Stereological measurements of cardiac ultrastructures implicated in excitation-contraction coupling. *Proc. Natl. Acad. Sci. U.S.A.* 68:1465–1466, 1971.
252. Palade, P. Drug-induced Ca^{2+} release from isolated sarcoplasmic reticulum. I. Use of pyrophosphate to study caffeine-induced Ca^{2+} release. *J. Biol. Chem.* 262:6135–6141, 1987.
253. Palade, P. Drug-induced Ca^{2+} release from isolated sarcoplasmic reticulum. II. Releases involving a Ca^{2+}-induced Ca^{2+} release channel. *J. Biol. Chem.* 262:6142–6148, 1987.
254. Palade, P. Drug-induced Ca^{2+} release from isolated sarcoplasmic reticulum. III. Block of Ca^{2+}-induced Ca^{2+} release by inorganic polyamines. *J. Biol. Chem.* 262:6149–6154, 1987.
255. Palade, P., C. Dettbarn, D. Brunder, P. Stein, and G. Hals. Pharmacology of calcium release from sarcoplasmic reticulum. *J. Bioenerg. Biomemb.* 21:295–320, 1989.
256. Pan, B. S. and R. J. Solaro. Calcium-binding properties of troponin C in detergent-skinned heart muscle fibers. *J. Biol. Chem.* 262:7839–7849, 1987.
257. Pegg, W. and M. Michalak. Differentiation of sarcoplasmic reticulum during cardiac myogenesis. *Am. J. Physiol.* 252 (*Heart Circ. Physiol.* 21):H22–H31, 1987.
258. Pelzer, D., S. Pelzer and T. F. McDonald. Properties and regulation of Ca channels in muscle cells. *Rev. Physiol. Biochem. Pharmacol.* 114:107–207, 1990.
259. Penefsky, Z. J. Studies on the mechanism of inhibition of cardiac muscle contractile tension by ryanodine. *Pflugers Arch.* 347:173–184, 1974.
260. Penefsky, Z. J. Perinatal development of cardiac mechanisms. In: *Perinatal Cardiovascular Function*, edited by N. Gootman and P. M. Gootman, NY, NY, 1983:109–200.
261. Peterson, B. Z., C. D. Demaria, and D. T. Yue. Calmodulin is the Ca^{2+} sensor for Ca^{2+}-dependent inactivation of l-type calcium channels. *Neuron* 22:549–558, 1999.
262. Philipson, K. D. Interaction of charged amphiphiles with Na^+-Ca^{2+} exchange in cardiac sarcolemmal vesicles. *J. Biol. Chem.* 259:13999–14002, 1984.
263. Philipson, K. D and D. A. Nicoll. Sodium-calcium exchange. A molecular perspective. *Annu. Rev. Physiol.* 62:111–133, 2000.
264. Philipson, K. D., and D. A. Nicoll. Molecular and kinetic aspects of sodium-calcium exchange. *Int. Rev. Cytol.* 137C:199–227, 1993.
265. Philipson, K. D. Myocardial ion transporters. In: *The Myocar-*

dium, 2nd Ed., edited by G. A. Langer. San Diego: Academic Press, 1997:143–179.
266. Pierce, G. N., K. D. Philipson, and G. A. Langer. Passive calcium-buffering capacity of a rabbit ventricular homogenate preparation. *Am. J. Physiol.* 249 (*Cell Physiol.* 18):C248–C255, 1985.
267. Pitts, B. J. R. Stoichiometry of sodium-calcium exchange in cardiac sarcolemmal vesicles. *J. Biol. Chem.* 254:6232–6235, 1979.
268. Post, J. A., G. A. Langer, J. A. F. Op Den Kamp, and A. J. Verkleij. Phospholipid asymmetry in cardiac sarcolemma. Analysis of intact cells and "gas-dissected" membranes. *Biochim. Biophys. Acta* 943:256–266, 1988.
269. Post, J. A. and G. A. Langer. Sarcolemmal calcium binding sites in heart: I. Molecular origin in "gas-dissected" sarcolemma. *J. Membr. Biol.* 129:49–57, 1992.
270. Prabhu, S. D. and G. Salama. The heavy metal ions Ag^+ and Hg^{2+} trigger calcium release from cardiac sarcoplasmic reticulum. *Arch. Biochem. Biophys.* 277:47–55, 1990.
271. Puglisi, J. L., R. A. Bassani, J. W. M. Bassani, J. N. Amin and D. M. Bers. Temperature and the relative contributions of Ca transport systems in cardiac myocyte relaxation. *Am. J. Physiol.* 270 (*Heart Circ. Physiol.* 39):H1772–H1778, 1996.
272. Puglisi, J. L., W. Yuan, J. W. M. Bassani, and D. M. Bers. Ca^{2+} influx through Ca^{2+} channels in rabbit ventricular myocytes during action potential clamp: influence of temperature. *Circ. Res.* 85:e7–e16, 1999.
273. Pytkowski, B. Rest- and stimulation-dependent changes in exchangeable calcium content in rabbit ventricular myocardium. *Basic Res. Cardiol.* 84:22–29, 1989.
274. Qin N, R. Olcese, M. Bransby, T. Lin, and L. Birnbaumer: Ca^{2+}-induced inhibition of the cardiac Ca^{2+} channel depends on calmodulin. *Proc. Natl. Acad. Sci. U.S.A.* 96:2435–2438, 1999.
275. Reed, K. C. and F. L. Bygrave. A kinetic study of mitochondrial calcium transport. *Eur. J. Biochem.* 55:497–503, 1975.
276. Reddy, L. G., L. R. Jones R. C. Pace, and D. L. Stokes. Purified, reconstituted cardiac Ca^{2+}-ATPase is regulated by phospholamban, but not by direct phosphorylation with by Ca^{2+}/calmodulin-dependent protein kinase. *J. Biol. Chem.* 271:14964–14970, 1996.
277. Reeves, J. P., and J. L. Sutko. Sodium-calcium exchange in cardiac membrane vesicles. *Proc. Natl. Acad. Sci. U.S.A.* 76:590–594, 1979.
278. Reeves, J. P., and J. L. Sutko. Sodium-calcium exchange activity generates a current in cardiac membrane vesicles. *Science* 208:1461–1464, 1980.
279. Reeves, J. P., and C. C. Hale. The stoichiometry of the cardiac sodium-calcium exchange system. *J. Biol. Chem.* 259:7733–7739, 1984.
280. Reeves, J. P., and P. Poronnik. Modulation of Na^+-Ca^{2+} exchange in sarcolemmal vesicles by intravesicular Ca^{2+}. *Am. J. Physiol.* 252 (*Cell Physiol.* 21):C17–C23, 1987.
281. Reeves, J. P. Na^+/Ca^{2+} exchange and cellular calcium homeostasis. *J. Bioeng. Biomembr.* 30:151–160, 1998.
282. Rega, A. F. and P. J. Garrahan. The Ca^{2+}-pump of plasma membranes. Boca Raton, FL: CRC Press, 1986:173.
283. Reimer, K. A. and R. B. Jennings. Myocardial ischemia, hypoxia, and infarction. In: *The Heart and Cardiovascular System*, edited by H. A. Fozzard et al. New York: Raven Press, 1986:1133–1201.
284. Reuter, H. and N. Seitz. The dependence of calcium efflux from cardiac muscle on temperature and external ion composition. *J. Physiol. Lond.)* 195:45–70, 1968.
285. Robertson, S. P., J. D. Johnson, and J. D. Potter. The time-course of Ca^{2+} exchange with calmodulin, troponin, parvalbumin, and myosin in response to transient increases in Ca^{2+}. *Biophys. J.* 34:559–569, 1981.
286. Rousseau, E., J. S. Smith, J. S. Henderson, and G. Meissner. Single channel and $^{45}Ca^{2+}$ flux measurements of the cardiac sarcoplasmic reticulum calcium channel. *Biophys. J.* 50:1009–1014, 1986.
287. Rousseau, E., J. S. Smith, and G. Meissner. Ryanodine modifies conductance and gating behavior of single Ca^{2+} release channel. *Am. J. Physiol.* 253 (*Heart Circ. Physiol.* 22):C364–C368, 1987.
288. Rousseau, E. and G. Meissner. Single cardiac sarcoplasmic reticulum Ca^{2+}-release channel: activation by caffeine. *Am. J. Physiol.* 256 (*Heart Circ. Physiol.* 25):H328–H333, 1989.
289. Saito, A., M. Inui, M. Radermacher, J. Frank, and S. Fleischer. Ultrastructure of the calcium release channel of sarcoplasmic reticulum. *J. Cell Biol.* 107:211–219, 1988.
290. Sagara, Y. and G. Inesi. Inhibition of the sarcoplasmic reticulum Ca^{2+} transport ATPase by thapsigargin at subnanomolar concentrations. *J. Biol. Chem.* 266:13503–13506, 1991.
291. Salama, G. and J. Abramson. Silver ions trigger Ca^{2+} release by acting at the apparent physiological release site in sarcoplasmic reticulum. *J. Biol. Chem.* 259:13363–13360, 1984.
292. Sasaki, T., M. Inui, Y. Kimura, T. Kuzuya, and M. Tada. Molecular mechanism of regulation of Ca^{2+} pump ATPase by phospholamban in cardiac sarcoplasmic reticulum. *J. Biol. Chem.* 267:1674–1679, 1992.
293. Satoh H., L. A. Blatter, and D. M. Bers. Effects of $[Ca]_i$, Ca^{2+} load and rest on Ca^{2+} spark frequency in ventricular myocytes. *Am. J. Physiol.* 272 (*Heart Circ. Physiol.* 41):H657–668, 1997.
294. Satoh, H., L. M. Delbridge, L. A. Blatter, and D. M. Bers. Surface:volume relationship in cardiac myocytes studied with confocal microscopy and membrane capacitance measurements: species-dependence and developmental effects. *Biophys. J.* 70:1494–1504, 1996.
295. Schatzmann, H. J. ATP dependent Ca^{2+} extrusion from human red cells. *Experientia* 22:364–368, 1966.
296. Schatzmann, H. J. The plasma membrane calcium pump of erythrocytes and other animal cells. In: *Membrane Transport of Calcium*, edited by E. Carafoli. London: Academic Press, 1982:41–108.
297. Schatzmann, H. J. The calcium pump of the surface membrane and of the sarcoplasmic reticulum. *Annu. Rev. Physiol.* 51:473–485, 1989.
298. Schiebler, T. and H. H. Wolff. Electronenmikroskopische Untersuchungen am Herzmuskel der Ratte wahrend der Entwicklung. *Z. Zellforsch. Mikrosk. Anat.* 69:22–40, 1962.
299. Schiefer A., G. Meissner, and Isenberg. Ca^{2+} activation and Ca^{2+} inactivation of cardiac sarcoplasmic reticulum Ca^{2+}-release channels. *J. Physiol.* 489:337–348, 1995.
300. Schouten, V. J. A. and H. E. D. J. ter Keurs. The force-frequency relationship in rat myocardium. *Pflugers Arch.* 407:14–17, 1986.
301. Seguchi, M., J. A. Harding, and J. M. Jarmakani. Developmental change in the function of sarcoplasmic reticulum. *J. Mol. Cell. Cardiol.* 18:189–195, 1986.
302. Seidler, N. W., I. Jona, M. Vegh, and A. Martonosi. Cyclopiazonic acid is a specific inhibitor of the Ca^{2+}-ATPase of sarcoplasmic reticulum. *J. Biol. Chem.* 264:17816–17823, 1989.
303. Sham, J. S. K., L. R. Jones, and M. Morad. Phospholamban mediates the β-adrenergic-enhanced Ca uptake in mammalian ventricular myocytes. *Am. J. Physiol.* 261 (*Heart Circ, Physiol.* 30):H1344–H1349, 1991.
304. Shanne, F. A. X., A. B. Kane, E. E. Young, and J. L. Farber. Calcium dependence of toxic cell death: a final common pathway. *Science* 206:700–702, 1979.
305. Shannon, T. R. and D. M. Bers. Assessment of intra-SR free

[Ca] and buffering in rat heart. *Biophys. J.* 73:1524–1531, 1997.

306. Shannon, T. R., K. S. Ginsburg, and D. M. Bers. Reverse mode of the SR Ca-pump and load-dependent Ca decline in voltage clamped cardiac ventricular myocytes. *Biophys. J.* 78:322–333, 2000.
307. Shannon, T. R., K. S. Ginsburg, and D. M. Bers. Potentiation of fractional SR Ca release by total and free intra-SR Ca concentration. *Biophys. J.* 78:334–343, 2000.
308. Shattock, M. J. and D. M. Bers. The inotropic response to hypothermia and the temperature-dependence of ryanodine action in isolated rabbit and rat ventricular muscle: implications for E-C coupling. *Circ. Res.* 61:761–771, 1987.
309. Shattock, M. J. and D. M. Bers. Rat vs. rabbit ventricle: Ca flux and intracellular Na assessed by ion-selective microelectrodes. *Am. J. Physiol.* 256 (*Cell Physiol.* 25):C813–C822, 1989.
310. Simmerman, H. K. B., J. H. Collins, J. L. Theiber, A. D. Wegener, and L. R. Jones. Sequence analysis of phospholamban. *J. Biol. Chem.* 261:13333–13341, 1986.
311. Sipido, K. R., G. Callewaert, and E. Carmeliet. Inhibition and rapid recovery of Ca^{2+} current during Ca^{2+} release from sarcoplasmic reticulum in guinea pig ventricular myocytes. *Circ. Res.* 76:102–109, 1995.
312. Sipido K. R. and W. G. Weir. Flux of Ca^{2+} across the sarcoplasmic reticulum of guinea pig cardiac cells during excitation-contraction coupling. *J. Physiol. (Lond.)* 435:605–630, 1991.
313. Sitsapesan, R., R. A. P. Montgomery, K. T. MacLeod, and A. J. Williams. Sheep cardiac sarcoplasmic reticulum calcium-release channels: modification of conductance and gating by temperature. *J. Physiol. (Lond.)* 434:469–488, 1991.
314. Sitsapesan R. and A. J. Williams. Regulation of the gating of the sheep cardiac sarcoplasmic reticulum Ca^{2+}-release channel by luminal Ca^{2+}. *J. Membr. Biol.* 137:215–226, 1994.
315. Smith, J. S., T. Imagawa, J. MA, M. Foll, K. P. Campbell, and R. Coronado. Purified ryanodine receptor from rabbit skeletal muscle is the calcium-release channel of sarcoplasmic reticulum. *J. Gen. Physiol.* 92:1–26, 1988.
316. Smith, J. S., E. Rousseau, and G. Meissner. Calmodulin modulation of single sarcoplasmic reticulum Ca release channels from cardiac and skeletal muscle. *Circ. Res.* 64:352–359, 1989.
317. Deleted.
318. Solaro, R. J. and F. N. Briggs. Estimating the functional capabilities of sarcoplasmic reticulum in cardiac muscle. *Circ. Res.* 34:531–540, 1974.
319. Sordahl, L. A. Effects of magnesium, ruthenium red and the antibiotic ionophore A-23187 on initial rates of calcium uptake and release by heart mitochondria. *Arch. Biochem. Biophys.* 167:104–115, 1975.
320. Spurgeon, H. A., M. D. Stern, G. Baartz, S. Raffaeli, R. G. Hansford, A Talo, E. G. Lakatta, and M. C. Capogrossi. Simultaneous measurement of Ca^{2+}, contraction and potential in cardiac myocytes. *Am. J. Physiol.* 258 (*Heart Circ. Physiol.* 27):H574–H586, 1990.
321. Su, J. H. and W. G. L. Kerrick. Effects of halothane on caffeine-induced tension transients in functionally skinned myocardial fibers. *Pflugers Arch.* 380:29–34, 1979.
322. Sutko, J. L., D. M. Bers, and J. P. Reeves. Postrest inotropy in rabbit ventricle: Na^+-Ca^{2+} exchange determines sarcoplasmic reticulum Ca^{2+} content. *Am. J. Physiol.* 250 (*Heart Circ. Physiol.* 19):H654–H661, 1986.
323. Sutko, J. L. and J. T. Willerson. Ryanodine alteration of the contractile state of rat ventricular myocardium. Comparison with dog, cat and rabbit ventricular tissues. *Circ. Res.* 46:332–343, 1980.
324. Sutko, J. L. and J. L. Kenyon. Ryanodine modification of cardiac muscle responses to potassium free solutions. Evidence for inhibition of sarcoplasmic reticulum calcium release. *J. Gen. Physiol.* 82:385–404, 1983.
325. Sutko, J. L., K. Ito, and J. L. Kenyon. Ryanodine: a modifier of sarcoplasmic reticulum calcium release. Biochemical and functional consequences of its actions on striated muscle. *Federation Proc.* 44:2984–2988, 1985.
326. Suzuki, T. and J. H. Wang. Stimulation of bovine cardiac sarcoplasmic reticulum Ca^{2+} pump and blocking of phospholamban phosphorylation and dephosphorylation by a phospholamban monoclonal antibody. *J. Biol. Chem.* 261:7018–7023, 1986.
327. Deleted.
328. Tada, M., M. A. Kirchberger, D. I. Repke, and A. M. Katz. The stimulation of calcium transport in cardiac sarcoplasmic reticulum by adenosine 3':5'-monophosphate-dependent protein kinase. *J. Biol. Chem.* 249:6174–6180, 1974.
329. Takenaka, H., P. N. Adler, and A. M. Katz. Calcium fluxes across the membrane of sarcoplasmic reticulum vesicles. *J. Biol. Chem.* 257:12649–12656, 1982.
330. Takeshima, H., S. Hishimura, T. Matsumoto, H. Ishida, K. Kangawa, N. Minamino, H. Matsuo, M. Ueda, M. Hanaoka, T. Hirose, and S. Numa. Primary structure and expression from complementary DNA of skeletal muscle ryanodine receptor. *Nature* 339:439–445, 1989.
331. Terracciano, C. M. N. and K. T. MacLeod. Effects of acidosis on Na^+/Ca^{2+} exchange and consequences for relaxation in guinea pig cardiac myocytes. *Am. J. Physiol.* 267 (*Heart Circ. Physiol.* 36):H477–H487, 1994.
332. Terracciano, C. M. N. and K. T. MacLeod. Measurements of Ca^{2+} entry and sarcoplasmic reticulum Ca^{2+} content during the cardiac cycle in guinea pig and rat ventricular myocytes. *Biophys. J.* 72:1319–1326, 1997.
333. Terracciano, C. M. N. and K. T. MacLeod. Reloading of Ca^{2+}-depleted sarcoplasmic reticulum during rest in guinea pig ventricular myocytes. *Am. J. Physiol.* 271 (*Heart Circ. Physiol.* 40):H1814–H1822, 1996.
334. Terracciano, C. M. N., R. U., Naqvi, and K. T. MacLeod. Effects of rest interval on the release of calcium from the sarcoplasmic reticulum in isolated guinea pig ventricular myocytes. *Circ. Res.* 77:354–360, 1995.
335. Thastrup, O, P. J. Cullen, B. K. Drobak, M. R. Hanley, A. P. Dawson. Thapsigargin, a tumor promoter, discharges intracellular Ca stores by specific inhibition of the endoplasmic reticulum Ca-ATPase. *Proc. Natl. Acad. Sci. U.S.A.*, 87:2466–2470, 1990.
336. Tinker A., A. R. G. Lindsay, and A. J. Williams. Cation conductance in the calcium release channel of the cardiac sarcoplasmic reticulum under physiological and pathophysiological conditions. *Cardiovasc. Res.* 27:1820–1825, 1993.
337. Toyofuku, T., K. Kurzydlowski, M. Tada, and D. H. MacLennan. Identification of regions in the Ca^{2+}-ATPase of sarcoplasmic reticulum that affect functional association with phospholamban. *J. Biol. Chem.* 268:2809–2815, 1993.
338. Toyofuku T., K. Kurzydlowski., N. Narayanan, and D. H. MacLennan. Identification of Ser38 as the site in cardiac sarcoplasmic reticulum Ca^{2+}-ATPase that is phosphorylated by Ca^{2+}/calmodulin dependent protein kinase. *J. Biol. Chem.* 269:26492–26496, 1994.
339. Trafford, A. W., M. E. Díaz, N. Negretti, and D. A. Eisner. Enhanced Ca^{2+} current and decreased Ca^{2+} efflux restore sarcoplasmic reticulum Ca^{2+} content after depletion. *Circ. Res.* 81:477–484, 1997.
340. Trimm, J. L., G. Salama, and J. Abramson. Sulfhydryl oxidation induces rapid calcium release from sarcoplasmic reticulum vesicles. *J. Biol. Chem.* 261:16092–16098, 1986.

341. Tripathy A. and G. Meissner. Sarcoplasmic reticulum lumenal Ca^{2+} has access to cytosolic activation and inactivation sites of skeletal muscle Ca^{2+} release channel. *Biophys. J.* 70:2600–2615, 1996.
342. Tseng, G. Calcium current restitution in mammalian ventricular myocytes is modulated by intracellular calcium. *Circ. Res.* 63:468–482, 1988.
343. Tsien, R. W., P. Hess, E. W. McCleskey, and R. L. Rosenberg. Calcium channels:mechanisms of selectivity, permeation and block. *Annu. Rev. Biophys. Chem.* 16:265–290, 1987.
344. Valdivia, H. H., J. H. Kaplan, G. C. R. Ellis-Davies, and W. J. Lederer. Rapid adaptation of cardiac ryanodine receptors:modulation by Mg^{2+} and phosphorylation. *Science* 267:1997–1999, 1995.
345. Varro, A., N. Negretti, S. B. Hester, and D. A. Eisner. An estimate of the calcium content of the sarcoplasmic reticulum in rat ventricular myocytes. *Pflugers. Arch.* 423:158–160, 1993.
346. Verma, A. K., A. Filoteo, D. R. Stanford, E. D. Wieben, J. T. Penniston, E. E. Strehler, R. Fischer, R. Heim, G. Vogel, S. Mathews, M.-A. Strehler-Page, P. James, T. Vorherr, J. Krebbs, and E. Carafoli. Complete primary structure of a human plasma membrane Ca^{2+} pump. *J. Biol. Chem.* 263:14152–14159, 1988.
347. Vercesi, A., B. Reynafarje, and A. L. Lehninger. Stoichiometry of H+ ejection and Ca^{2+} uptake coupled to electron transfer in rat heart mitochondria. *J. Biol. Chem.* 253:6379–6385, 1978.
348. Wagenknecht, T., R. Grassucci, J. Frank, A. Saito, M. Inui, and S. Fleischer. Three-dimensional architecture of the calcium channel/foot structure of sarcoplasmic reticulum. *Nature* 338:167–170, 1989.
349. Weber, A. and R. Herz. The relationship between caffeine contracture of intact muscle and the effect of caffeine on reticulum. *J. Gen. Physiol.* 52:750–759, 1968.
349a. Weber, C. R. K. S. Ginsburg, K. D. Philipson, T. R. Shannon and D. M. Bers. Allosteric regulation of Na/Ca exchange current by cytosolic Ca in intact cardiac myocytes. *J. Gen. Physiol.* 117:119–131, 2001.
350. Wendt, I. R. and D. G. Stephenson. Effects of caffeine on Ca-activated force production in skinned cardiac and skeletal muscle fibres of the rat. *Pflugers. Arch.* 398:210–216, 1983.
351. Wier W. G. and C. W. Balke. Ca^{2+} release mechanisms, Ca^{2+} sparks, and local control of excitation-contraction coupling in normal heart muscle. *Circ. Res.* 85:770–776, 1999.
352. Wier, W. G., T. M. Egan, J. R. López-López, and C. W. Balke. Local control of excitation-contraction coupling in rat heart cells. *J. Physiol. (Lond.)* 474:463–471, 1994.
353. Williams, A. J. and S. R. M. Holmberg. Sulmazole (AR-L 115BS) activates the sheep cardiac muscle sarcoplasmic reticulum calcium-release channel in the presence and absence of calcium. *J. Membr. Biol.* 115:167–178, 1990.
354. Wohlfart, B. Relationship between peak force, action potential duration and stimulus interval in rabbit myocardium. *Acta Physiol. Scand.* 106:395–409, 1979.
355. Wrzosek, A, H. Schneider, S. Grueninger, and M. Chiesi: Effect of thapsigargin on cardiac muscle cells. *Cell. Calcium* 13:281–292, 1992.
356. Xu A., C. Hawkins, N. Narayanan. Phosphorylation and activation of the Ca-pumping ATPase of cardiac sarcoplasmic reticulum by Ca/calmodulin-dependent protein kinase. *J. Biol. Chem.* 268:8394–8397, 1993.
357. Ying, W. L., J. Emerson, M. J. Clarke, and D. R. Sanadi. Inhibition of mitochondrial calcium ion transport by oxo-bridged dinuclear ruthenium amine complex. *Biochemistry* 30:4949–4952, 1991.
358. Yuan, W. and D. M. Bers. Ca-dependent facilitation of cardiac Ca current is due to Ca-calmodulin dependent protein kinase. *Am. J. Physiol.* 267 (*Heart Circ. Physiol.* 36):H982–H993, 1994.
359. Yuan, W. and D. M. Bers. Protein kinase inhibitor H-89 reverses forskolin stimulation of cardiac L-type calcium current. *Am. J. Physiol.* 267 (*Cell Physiol.* 36):C651–C659, 1995.
360. Yuan, W., K. S. Ginsburg, and D. M. Bers. Comparison of sarcolemmal Ca channel current in rabbit and rat ventricular myocytes. *J. Physiol. (Lond.)* 493:733–746, 1996.
361. Yue, D. T., D. Burkhoff, M. R. Franz, W. C. Hunter, and K. Sagawa. Postextrasystolic potentiation of the isolated canine left ventricle. *Circ. Res.* 56:340–350, 1985.
362. Yue, D. T., E. Marban, and W. G. Wier. Relationship between force and intracellular[Ca^{2+}] in tetanized mammalian heart muscle. *J. Gen. Physiol.* 87:223–242, 1986.
363. Zhou, Z., M. A. Matlib, and D. M. Bers. Cytosolic and mitochondrial Ca^{2+} signals in patch clamped ventricular myocytes. *J. Physiol.* 507:379–403, 1998.
364. Zorzato, F., G. Salviati, T. Facchinetti, and P. Volpe. Doxorubicin induces calcium release from terminal cisternae of skeletal muscle. *J. Biol. Chem.* 260:7349–7355, 1985.
365. Zorzato, F., J. Fujii, K. Otsu, M. Phillips, N. M. Green, F. A. Lai, G. Meissner, and D. H. Maclennan. Molecular cloning of cDNA encoding human and rabbit forms of the Ca^{2+} release channel (ryanodine receptor) of skeletal muscle sarcoplasmic reticulum. *J. Biol. Chem.* 265:2244–2256, 1990.
366. Zühlke, R. D., G. S. Pitt, K. Deisseroth, R. W. Tsien, and H. Reuter: Calmodulin supports both inactivation and facilitation of L-type calcium channels. *Nature.* 399:159–162, 1999.

10. The cardiac Na$^+$-Ca^{2+} exchanger

LARRY V. HRYSHKO | Institute of Cardiovascular Sciences, St. Boniface General Hospital Research Centre, University of Manitoba, Winnipeg, Manitoba, Canada

CHAPTER CONTENTS

A Brief Historical Perspective and Prelude to the Review
Physiological Role of the Cardiac Na$^+$–Ca^{2+} Exchanger
Reverse Na$^+$–Ca^{2+} Exchange as a Trigger for SR Ca^{2+} Release
Digitalis Effects
Immunolocalization
Transport Properties
   Stoichiometry
   Transport mechanism
   Turnover rates and exchanger density
   Ion selectivity
   Temperature dependence
Molecular Biology of the Na$^+$–Ca^{2+} Exchanger
   The prototypical canine cardiac Na$^+$–Ca^{2+} exchanger
   The exchanger superfamily
   Topology of the Na$^+$–Ca^{2+} exchanger
   The *Calx*-α and *Calx*-β repeats
   Alternative splicing of Na$^+$–Ca^{2+} exchangers
Regulation of Na$^+$–Ca^{2+} Exchange
   Ionic regulation
      Na$_i^+$-dependent inactivation
      Ca$_i^{2+}$-dependent regulation
   Structure–function relationships of ionic regulation
      The XIP region
      The regulatory Ca^{2+} binding site
   Regulation by phosphorylation
   Regulation by PIP$_2$
   Regulation by pH
   Cytoskeletal interactions
Pharmacology of Na$^+$–Ca^{2+} Exchange
   The exchanger inhibitory peptide, XIP
   Other peptide inhibitors
   KB-R7943
   Other inhibitors
Studies in Transgenic Mice
Adenoviral Transfection of Na$^+$–Ca^{2+} Exchange Proteins
Antisense Oligonucleotides
Fequency-dependent Behaviour of Na$^+$–Ca^{2+} Exchange
Developmental Changes
Species Differences
Pathophysiological Alterations in Na$^+$–Ca^{2+} Exchange
   Contribution of Na$^+$–Ca^{2+} exchange to cardiac injury
   Alterations in Na$^+$–Ca^{2+} exchange levels

THE LAST DECADE OF THE TWENTIETH CENTURY produced major progress in our understanding of the Na$^+$–Ca^{2+} exchange transport system. This plasmalemmal ion counter-transporter plays a prominent role in the maintenance of Ca^{2+} homeostasis in a variety of tissues. The role of Na$^+$–Ca^{2+} exchange is especially prominent in cardiac muscle, where this transport mechanism must remove nearly all of the Ca^{2+} entering on a beat-to-beat basis. This review focuses primarily on advances in our understanding of the cardiac Na$^+$–Ca^{2+} exchanger, NCX1.1. Accomplishing this goal requires digression to information concerning the diverse family of Na$^+$–Ca^{2+} exchangers and the technical accomplishments underlying those advances. Most important, an effort is made to highlight major deficiencies in our knowledge and to forecast impending developments.

The appearance of several comprehensive reviews of Na$^+$–Ca^{2+} exchange in the past few years (34, 74, 84, 163, 260, 270) obviates the need for simple reiteration of this vast body of literature. The interested reader should certainly consult these earlier comprehensive works, which provide exemplary historical accounts of this field that are not repeated here. There have been, however, a number of significant new developments. This chapter is intended as a companion to these extensive undertakings, and it expands upon and emphasizes specific aspects of the field that were dealt with in less detail in the previous publications. I have attempted to provide updates, where available, up to and including the 2000 Biophysical Society Meeting. In addition, Chapter 9 provides a detailed and quantitative description of Na$^+$–Ca^{2+} thermodynamics and fluxes in cardiac cells. I have tried to minimize unnecessary duplication in this subject matter. In this chapter, the personal bias of the author and the personal injury due to missing citations are both unavoidable.

A BRIEF HISTORICAL PERSPECTIVE AND PRELUDE TO THE REVIEW

The rich history of Na$^+$–Ca^{2+} exchange research has been described in several recent reviews (34, 84, 163, 260), and is not reiterated here. Rather, I focus on the last decade of the century, during which there has been an explosion of knowledge regarding the Na$^+$–Ca^{2+} exchange transport system. The trigger for this boom was the cloning of the cardiac Na$^+$–Ca^{2+} exchanger in 1990 (241). Consequently, investigations of Na$^+$–Ca^{2+}

exchange are now proceeding using the full arsenal of molecular biological approaches. To highlight briefly, the cloning of the cardiac Na$^+$–Ca^{2+} exchanger has led directly to the identification of a superfamily of Na$^+$–Ca^{2+} exchange proteins, including unique genes, alternatively spliced variants, and related transport proteins. The coincident availability of antibodies permits assessment of Na$^+$–Ca^{2+} exchange levels using either protein or transcript levels. Mutagenesis, in conjunction with heterologous expression systems, is increasingly employed to investigate Na$^+$–Ca^{2+} exchange structure–function relationships. Promoter analyses and gene mapping studies have been conducted and variations in exchanger levels under pathophysiological conditions have been identified. Recombinant Na$^+$–Ca^{2+} exchange protein is widely used for a variety of biochemical analyses including circular dichroism, Fourier transform infrared spectroscopy, ligand binding, and crystallization efforts. Finally, the applications of transgenic animal technology, antisense oligonucleotides, and adenoviral gene transfer have all been employed to investigate Na$^+$–Ca^{2+} exchange physiology and pathophysiology.

The development of the giant excised patch technique has been another major advance toward the investigation of Na$^+$–Ca^{2+} exchange function (126). The primary advantage of this approach is the superior temporal resolution provided for assessing Na$^+$–Ca^{2+} exchange activity compared to radiotracer-based analyses (133). Furthermore, this approach provides rapid access to the cytoplasmic face of the molecule. This is a significant benefit compared to cell-based assays (e.g. whole cell voltage clamping, Ca^{2+}$_i$ fluorescence measurements), as all regulatory mechanisms identified to date appear to involve this surface of the molecule. Rich kinetic details of Na$^+$–Ca^{2+} exchange activity have been revealed using giant excised patch clamping. Finally, the application of this approach, in combination with heterologous expression systems, has provided considerable information on structure–function relationships of Na$^+$–Ca^{2+} exchange proteins. Unfortunately, this technique has not become employed widely, despite its demonstrated utility.

Whole-cell electrophysiology, fluorescence-based techniques, and radiotracer flux measurements are all firmly established methodologies for investigation of Na$^+$–Ca^{2+} exchange. These approaches have been routinely and confidently employed in the past decade. Nevertheless, information on exchange function lags considerably behind the equivalent information for most ion channels. The major missing ingredients are the ability to study the properties of single Na$^+$–Ca^{2+} exchange molecules (equivalent to elementary current measurements) and the dearth of pharmacological tools to assess, label, and modify Na$^+$–Ca^{2+} exchange activity. Furthermore, insight into the molecular underpinnings of Na$^+$–Ca^{2+} exchange transport and regulation are poorly integrated into our understanding of physiological Na$^+$–Ca^{2+} exchange function. Overall, however, the next decade promises to be particularly informative with respect to understanding the role of Na$^+$–Ca^{2+} exchange under physiological and pathophysiological conditions.

PHYSIOLOGICAL ROLE OF THE CARDIAC Na$^+$–Ca^{2+} EXCHANGER

Rhythmic cardiac contractions occur in response to repetitive elevations and reductions in cellular Ca^{2+} levels. To enable cardiac relaxation, cellular Ca^{2+} must be lowered to sub-micromolar levels, typically ranging from 100 to 150 nM. The sarcolemmal Na$^+$–Ca^{2+} exchange system is generally viewed as the primary mechanism for the transsarcolemmal removal of Ca^{2+}. In general, the Na$^+$–Ca^{2+} exchanger is thought to remove the same quantity of Ca^{2+} that enters through L-type Ca^{2+} channels on a beat-to-beat basis. An elegant demonstration of this coupling was provided by Bridge et al. (40), where the total charge associated with Ca^{2+} entry via L-type Ca^{2+} channels was twice that mediated during Ca^{2+} efflux via the exchanger. Assuming a 3:1 stoichiometry for Na$^+$–Ca^{2+} exchange, this result indicated that all the Ca^{2+} entering the myocyte was subsequently removed by the exchanger (40). Several different approaches have provided similar conclusions. For example, O'Neill et al. (249) demonstrated that caffeine-evoked Ca^{2+} efflux from Langendorff-perfused hearts was indistinguishable from background Ca^{2+} efflux in the absence of extracellular Na$^+$. However, other experimental approaches by the same investigators suggested that additional pathways could be involved (249). Pharmacological and ion-substitution experiments employing rapid cooling contractures (23, 25, 39, 145) or caffeine-evoked contractions (13, 23, 24) have demonstrated a prominent role for Na$^+$–Ca^{2+} exchange in mediating contractile relaxation, post-rest decay, and the decline of the Ca^{2+} transient. In contrast, studies of this nature have not established a major role for the parallel transsarcolemmal Ca^{2+} efflux pathway, the plasmalemmal Ca^{2+}-ATPase. Furthermore, overexpression of the sarcolemmal Ca^{2+}-ATPase in transgenic rat hearts failed to produce any effects on the systolic Ca^{2+} transient or general cardiac performance despite an approximately twofold increase in expression levels (110). Here, the authors concluded that the sarcolemmal Ca^{2+}-ATPase played little role in the beat-to-beat regulation of cardiac contraction/relaxation. Thus, the concept has evolved that Na$^+$–Ca^{2+} exchange is the primary, if not singular, physiologically relevant pathway for the transsarcolemmal efflux of Ca^{2+} to mediate cardiac relaxation. This topic is reviewed extensively in Chapter 9.

While the notion that Na^+–Ca^{2+} exchange is the predominant mechanism for transsarcolemmal Ca^{2+} removal pervades most recent literature, this issue has become far more contentious in recent years. Several studies have demonstrated a significant role for the sarcolemmal Ca^{2+}-ATPase, primarily based on results obtained using carboxyeosin as a sarcolemmal Ca^{2+} ATPase inhibitor. In these studies, the role of the sarcolemmal Ca^{2+}-ATPase was found to represent 24%–45% of the total transsarcolemmal Ca^{2+} efflux (50, 51, 249, 319), far in excess of that previously suggested. Species differences have also been identified in the relative importance of the sarcolemmal Ca^{2+}-ATPase. For example, this pathway appears to be particularly prominent in ferret ventricular muscle, where it may contribute to the same degree as Na^+–Ca^{2+} exchange (14, 15). Furthermore, as the stoichiometry of Na^+–Ca^{2+} exchange has once again become the subject of contentious debate (98), electrophysiological assessments of Na^+–Ca^{2+} exchange currents (compared to Ca^{2+} entry via Ca^{2+} channels) may require reevaluation. As discussed below, over-expression of the wild-type Na^+–Ca^{2+} exchanger has also proven to be relatively benign, analogous to the results obtained with sarcolemmal Ca^{2+}-ATPase expression (110). Finally, the Na^+–Ca^{2+} exchange system has been postulated to serve as a Ca^{2+} entry mechanism during cardiac excitation (182). If Ca^{2+} does, in fact, enter myocytes through this mechanism, the amount of Ca^{2+} efflux required would be increased accordingly to maintain Ca^{2+} homeostasis. Thus, equality of Ca^{2+} fluxes associated with L-type Ca^{2+} channels and inward Na^+–Ca^{2+} exchange currents may overstate the role of the exchanger, as this would fail to account for Ca^{2+} entry via outward exchange currents. Despite these numerous caveats, however, it seems reasonable to conclude that Na^+–Ca^{2+} exchange is a primary, although not necessarily singular, mechanism for transsarcolemmal Ca^{2+} removal. Further work is clearly required to establish a more quantitative description of this role.

The quantitative coupling of Ca^{2+} entry and Ca^{2+} efflux is absolutely critical for viable cardiac function. While intuitively obvious, this point warrants emphasis as it is occasionally misunderstood and highlights one of the major limitations in our understanding of Na^+–Ca^{2+} exchange function. To begin, cardiac myocytes have very little tolerance for imbalance between Ca^{2+} entry and Ca^{2+} efflux. While minor imbalance in this coupling can occur over a brief period (e.g. several beats), it is essential that Ca^{2+} influx and Ca^{2+} efflux become matched over any extended period. Irrespective of the magnitude or direction of changes in Ca^{2+} entry, Ca^{2+} efflux must adjust to match these input levels. Moreover, if Na^+–Ca^{2+} exchange is a primary mediator of Ca^{2+} efflux, then this transport system must have the ability to respond to changes in Ca^{2+} influx levels. The sarcoplasmic reticulum and mitochondria do not contribute to this relationship other than by providing some temporal buffering for any imbalances in Ca^{2+} fluxes. Since both of these intracellular stores have finite capacities for Ca^{2+} sequestration and storage, they would quickly become depleted or overloaded if net transsarcolemmal Ca^{2+} fluxes did not achieve equality. This necessity for Ca^{2+} influx and efflux being equal remains true whether Na^+–Ca^{2+} exchange contributes 1% or 100% to normal cardiac relaxation. Obviously, any contribution of the parallel sarcolemmal Ca^{2+}-ATPase would offset or reduce the Ca^{2+} burden presented to the Na^+–Ca^{2+} exchanger. Similarly, any Ca^{2+} entry mediated by reverse Na^+–Ca^{2+} exchange would increase the amount of required Ca^{2+} efflux.

Ca^{2+} entry into cardiac myocytes varies over a wide range both physiologically and in response to pharmacological interventions (21, 28, 223, 256, 257). For example, Ca^{2+} entry via L-type Ca^{2+} channels varies physiologically in response to frequency changes, intracellular Ca^{2+} levels, and adrenergic stimulation. Pharmacologically, Ca^{2+} entry can be modulated both positively and negatively by several compounds such as dihydropyridines and adrenergic agents (124, 125, 285, 314). A great deal is known about how these various interventions influence cardiac contractility. In all cases where Ca^{2+} entry is modified, the Na^+–Ca^{2+} exchanger must adjust to match the different levels of Ca^{2+} influx. However, while we know that this must occur, we do not know how it occurs. Furthermore, many of the same interventions that influence Ca^{2+} channel function also appear to influence Na^+–Ca^{2+} exchange activity (e.g. intracellular Ca^{2+}, frequency, etc.). However, these modulating effects are not integrated in any cohesive way toward clarifying the relationship between Ca^{2+} entry and efflux. This aspect of Na^+–Ca^{2+} exchange function remains one of the most intriguing questions to be answered.

There are several possible ways in which Na^+–Ca^{2+} exchange activity could adapt to changes in Ca^{2+} influx. For example, simply having a large excess of Na^+–Ca^{2+} exchangers could provide the requisite capacity for handling increases in Ca^{2+} entry levels. This notion appears to have some support, as both the Na^+–Ca^{2+} exchanger and the sarcoplasmic reticulum have the ability to mediate cardiac relaxation independently, albeit at slightly slower rates (22). With reduced Ca^{2+} entry, Ca^{2+} efflux may simply turn off because of the relatively low Ca^{2+} affinity of the exchanger at the intracellular transport site. While estimates vary, the exchanger is generally considered to be a high-capacity, low-affinity Ca^{2+} efflux mechanism (34, 260). With higher Ca^{2+} levels, an excess of Na^+–Ca^{2+} exchangers could provide the necessary reserve capacity to accommodate an increase in Ca^{2+} influx. Thus, a simple excess of tonically active Na^+–Ca^{2+} exchangers could provide an appropriate safety margin to enable a range of Ca^{2+} entry levels. Alternatively, the activity and/or availability of the Na^+–Ca^{2+} exchanger population might be actively regulated to provide appropriate Ca^{2+} efflux levels over a wide range of inotropic states. At present there are only speculative reasons to suggest this latter possibility. That is, in addition to the thermodynamic consequences of changing Na^+ and Ca^{2+} gradients, there is some indirect evidence to suggest that the exchanger population is regulated. First, highly conserved ionic regulatory mechanisms have been identified for all Na^+–Ca^{2+} exchangers characterized to date (82, 123, 127, 198, 202, 251). As described below, these ionic regulatory mechanisms can substantially alter the population of active exchangers, independent of thermodynamic considerations. Second, ionic regulatory mechanisms have been demonstrated to operate in a variety of intact cellular preparations (54, 94, 316, 320), including cardiac myocytes (212, 217). Third, over-expression of wild-type Na^+–Ca^{2+} exchangers in transgenic mice has proven to be relatively benign with respect to physiological relaxation of the Ca^{2+} transient (3). It is somewhat difficult to reconcile this latter experimental result with the notion of an unregulated exchanger population. However, it should be emphasized that, at present, there is no cohesive understanding for the role of Na^+–Ca^{2+} exchanger regulation, if any, in the context of cardiac excitation-contraction coupling. Simply stated, we do not know:

1. how many exchangers there are in a cardiac myocyte,
2. how fast exchangers turn over (i.e. their transport rates) physiologically,
3. whether the active exchanger population is regulated, and ultimately
4. how Ca^{2+} influx and Ca^{2+} efflux are coupled over such a wide range of inotropic conditions.

The pharmacological modification of Ca^{2+} entry has proven to be of substantial therapeutic utility for a variety of cardiovascular ailments. Intuitively, modifying Ca^{2+} efflux could provide the same host of therapeutic opportunities. However, no clinically employed agents exist that specifically target the Na^+–Ca^{2+} exchanger. As discussed below, the utility of digitalis may reside in its ability to indirectly modify Na^+–Ca^{2+} exchange activity. While newer experimental agents targeting the Na^+–Ca^{2+} exchanger have become available (151, 327), these have yet to be used clinically. Nevertheless, there appears to be considerable optimism in the field with respect to the promise of deriving clinical benefit from modifying Na^+–Ca^{2+} exchange activity. However, until the tools become available to accomplish this goal, this therapeutic frontier remains largely unexplored.

REVERSE Na^+-Ca^{2+} EXCHANGE AS A TRIGGER FOR SR Ca^{2+} RELEASE

During the past decade, there has been major interest in the possibility that reverse Na^+–Ca^{2+} exchange plays an important physiological role in triggering Ca^{2+} release from the sarcoplasmic reticulum. That is, in addition to the conventional view that L-type Ca^{2+} channels trigger Ca^{2+}-induced Ca^{2+} release from the sarcoplasmic reticulum (21, 92), the Na^+–Ca^{2+} exchanger may also be involved in this process. The concept that Ca^{2+} entry through reverse Na^+–Ca^{2+} exchange can induce cardiac contractions is well established (26, 139). In particular, at high levels of membrane depolarization, and/or reduced Na^+ electrochemical gradients, Ca^{2+} entry via reverse exchange had been demonstrated to produce a slowly developing tonic contraction. However, in 1990, reverse Na^+–Ca^{2+} exchange was proposed to be involved in physiological Ca^{2+}-induced Ca^{2+}-release (182). The general premise for this notion is that subsarcolemmal Na^+ is sufficiently elevated during an action potential to induce a large reverse Na^+–Ca^{2+} exchange current. Ca^{2+} entry through this pathway then triggers Ca^{2+}-induced Ca^{2+} release from the sarcoplasmic reticulum. A great deal of effort has been expended in the past decade to verify or refute this possibility.

There is general agreement that reverse Na^+–Ca^{2+} exchange can trigger sarcoplasmic reticulum Ca^{2+} release, a phenomenon that has been demonstrated by many investigators (174, 188, 189, 190, 191, 193, 203, 206, 208, 322, 324). However, there is considerable disagreement as to the physiological relevance of this mechanism (for example, see references (37, 91, 235, 290, 291, 296, 297). Several major issues underlie this disparity of opinions. First, the levels of intracellular Na^+ required to observe this effect were initially above those thought to occur physiologically. The two problems associated with abnormally elevated Na^+ are that (1) this does not occur physiologically and (2) this creates an overloaded or "trigger happy" sarcoplasmic reticulum through reverse Na^+–Ca^{2+} exchange. Under these conditions, a small Ca^{2+} entry through incompletely blocked Ca^{2+} channels could presumably trigger a phasic Ca^{2+} release. In addition, to be physiologically relevant, this effect should be observable at membrane voltages normally visited during a cardiac action potential. Results obtained at extreme voltage levels (e.g., + 80 mV) do not provide a compelling case for physiological relevance. It is unclear whether there is a genuine species difference in the prominence of this mechanism. "Physiological" reverse Na^+–Ca^{2+} exchange mediated Ca^{2+} induced Ca^{2+} release has been reported in cardiac myocytes from a variety of species, almost equivalent to those for which it has been demonstrated to be absent. Finally, Ca^{2+} entry by reverse exchange must be appropriately localized to activate the Ca^{2+} release channels in the sarcoplasmic reticulum. While some studies have demonstrated a preferential localization of Na^+-Ca^{2+} exchangers to the t-tubules of cardiac myocytes (e.g. see ref. 96), others have suggested a more diffuse sarcolemmal localization (e.g. see ref. 167). Several groups have also shown that L-type Ca^{2+} channels have preferential access to the Ca^{2+} release channels of the sarcoplasmic reticulum (99, 290, 291, 295, 296, 297), whereas Na^+–Ca^{2+} exchange does not.

While the importance of reverse Na^+–Ca^{2+} exchange as a trigger for sarcoplasmic reticulum Ca^{2+} release must be considered unresolved, there appears to be some consensus developing around an alternative possibility. Specifically, reverse Na^+–Ca^{2+} exchange may modulate the gain of calcium-induced Ca^{2+} release from the sarcoplasmic reticulum. It is well documented that the Ca^{2+} load of the sarcoplasmic reticulum plays a major role in determining the amount of Ca^{2+} release (88, 225, 275). Furthermore, the activity of the Na^+-Ca^{2+} exchanger clearly plays a role in determining this Ca^{2+} content, as it competes directly with the sarcoplasmic reticulum Ca^{2+}-ATPase for cytoplasmic Ca^{2+} removal (see Chapter 9). As details of the Ca^{2+} release mechanism evolve (225, 321, 338), there is evidence to suggest that the Na^+–Ca^{2+} exchanger may play a role in determining local Ca^{2+} concentrations near the sarcoplasmic reticulum Ca^{2+} release channels (34, 60, 105, 106, 118, 179, 180) and therefore could affect the gain of Ca^{2+}-induced Ca^{2+} release. In smooth muscle cells, for example, a functional unit called a "plasmERosome" has been described (33). This region consists of the plasma membrane containing the high ouabain affinity Na^+,K^+-ATPase isoforms and Na^+-Ca^{2+} exchangers physically near the underlying junctional sarcoplasmic or endoplasmic reticulum. A "restricted" space separating these two membrane systems creates the possibility of unique ionic compositions within the plasmerosome compared to those of bulk cytosol. Similar structural entities may exist in cardiac and skeletal muscle and nerve. This possibility has been extensively described in a recent review by Blaustein and Lederer (34).

If reverse Na^+–Ca^{2+} exchange plays a prominent role in cardiac excitation–contraction coupling, then the amount of Ca^{2+} entering via this mechanism (plus that provided by L-type Ca^{2+} channels) must be removed by forward Na^+–Ca^{2+} exchange (and possibly the sarcolemmal Ca^{2+}-ATPase) on a beat-to-beat basis. This, again, would place Na^+–Ca^{2+} exchange function at a critical checkpoint in cardiac excitation–contraction coupling. Virtually all investigations in support of this possibility have employed thermodynamic arguments to complement experimental results. The anticipated changes in the reversal potential of Na^+–Ca^{2+} exchange (E_{NaCa}) corresponding to the dynamics of the Ca^{2+} transient have been modeled and compared to membrane potential changes (E_m) during the action potential (20) (see Chapter 9). While elegant studies of this nature provide insight into the thermodynamically favored modes of Na^+–Ca^{2+} exchange transport, it seems that incorporation of regulatory aspects of Na^+–Ca^{2+} exchange activity will be required in the near future. Specifically, thermodynamic considerations may not be the sole determinant of Na^+–Ca^{2+} exchange activity in either the forward or reverse mode of transport. In the extreme case, this is analogous to considering ion channel function without consideration of channel gating. However, much greater insight into the role of Na^+–Ca^{2+} exchange regulation is required before such treatments will become practical.

DIGITALIS EFFECTS

Despite their inherent toxicity and marginal therapeutic window, digitalis-like compounds remain an important component of chronic cardiac inotropic therapy for the treatment of congestive heart failure. Mechanistically, these compounds are likely to exert their positive inotropic actions through indirect effects on the Na^+–Ca^{2+} exchanger. Specifically, digitalis-like compounds inhibit the plasmalemmal Na^+,K^+–ATPase, leading to a small elevation of cytosolic Na^+ (2, 12, 185, 186, 192). From thermodynamic considerations, this results in a reduced capacity for Ca^{2+} efflux via the Na^+–Ca^{2+} exchanger, as well as increasing the ability of reverse exchange to promote Ca^{2+} entry. Competition between intracellular Na^+ and Ca^{2+} at the intracellular transport site may also contribute slightly to reduced Na^+–Ca^{2+} exchange efficiency. Overall, these alterations lead to an increase in intracellular Ca^{2+} levels and therefore positive cardiac inotropy. Toxicity, at least under experimental conditions, occurs when these alterations in exchange function promote Ca^{2+} overload. Clinically, the use of digitalis-like compounds requires careful titration, as the toxic effects are simply overzealous accomplishments of the desired effects.

Virtually all aspects of digitalis utilization and its mechanism of action can be considered controversial.

Despite its long history of clinical use in the treatment of congestive heart failure, most recent studies highlight the uncertainties of continuing this practice. For example, a recent large clinical trial by the Digitalis Investigation Group (DIG) revealed that digoxin did not alter mortality, although the rate of hospitalization was reduced as was the worsening of heart failure (1). Mechanistically, it appears that the sympatholytic effects of digitalis may be a primary mechanism of clinical utility and as such, its continued use with various multidrug therapies (e.g. ACE inhibitors, β-adrenergic antagonists, among others) remains questionable (4, 116, 117, 274, 302). Overall, the use of digitalis as a positive inotropic agent is likely to decline as more contemporary pharmacological approaches improve (116).

Mechanistically, alternative explanations have appeared to explain the inotropic basis of digitalis-like compounds. Recently, digitalis has been reported to modify the selectivity of cardiac Na^+ channels such that Ca^{2+} entry could contribute significantly to this conductance. This property, termed *slip-mode conductance*, could provide an additional mechanism for increasing intracellular Ca^{2+} levels in response to digitalis-like compounds (279). Digitalis has also been proposed to directly affect Ca^{2+} release from the sarcoplasmic reticulum, another potential means for improving cardiac inotropy (323). Considering the multiplicity of digitalis receptors (i.e. Na^+,K^+-ATPase isoforms), each with unique sensitivities to digitalis, the pharmacological consequences of digitalis treatment are complex (224). Furthermore, most mechanistic studies of digitalis have focused on the thermodynamic consequences of altering the Na^+ gradient. These ionic changes may also influence regulatory properties of the Na^+–Ca^{2+} exchanger, a possibility that has been largely ignored. Thus, even though the use of digitalis is in decline, there is still a great deal to be learned regarding the specific details of its mechanism of action.

It is unclear whether specific pharmacological agents targeting the Na^+–Ca^{2+} exchanger directly would provide an inotropy strategy preferable to that accomplished with digitalis. This is certainly a tantalizing possibility. For example, a graded reduction in Na^+–Ca^{2+} exchange activity might produce the same beneficial consequences as digitalis. Furthermore, the actions of digitalis lead to alterations in both Na^+ and K^+ gradients, whereas the undesired alterations in K^+ gradients might be circumvented by directly targeting the exchanger. Finally, the opportunity to modulate a specific transport mode of Na^+–Ca^{2+} exchange might create even greater therapeutic opportunities. Hypothetically, graded reduction in Ca^{2+} efflux (or augmentation of Ca^{2+} influx) via the exchanger might prove useful as a means of achieving positive inotropy. Alternatively, increasing net Ca^{2+} efflux by this pathway could prove useful toward alleviating pathologies induced by Ca^{2+} overload (e.g. ischemic or hypoxic injury). The absence of specific pharmacological tools with which to address these possibilities is a major problem in Na^+–Ca^{2+} exchange research. However, as discussed below, newer agents (e.g. KB-R7943) are becoming available to test these possibilities, and initial results show great promise. Mode-specific inhibition of Na^+–Ca^{2+} exchange has also been observed in response to treatment with protein phosphatase blockers (56), suggesting that transport mode–specific approaches may become increasingly fruitful.

IMMUNOLOCALIZATION

The cellular localization of cardiac Na^+–Ca^{2+} exchange proteins has been studied by a number of investigators. Frank et al. (97, 278) observed strong immunofluorescent labeling within the t-tubular system, whereas more diffuse staining was observed in the peripheral sarcolemma. This study, in guinea pig myocytes, also employed immunoelectron microscopy and similar results were obtained. In contrast, studies by Kieval et al. (167) identified a more homogeneous distribution of Na^+–Ca^{2+} exchangers in both peripheral and t-tubular sarcolemma. The reason for these differences remains unknown, but the issue is of considerable importance. Prominent localization of the Na^+–Ca^{2+} exchanger within the t-tubules (and therefore near the Ca^{2+} release channels of the sarcoplasmic reticulum) would seem to be necessary for reverse Na^+–Ca^{2+} exchange to contribute significantly to Ca^{2+}-induced Ca^{2+} release. The results of Kieval et al. (167) do not exclude this possibility but render it somewhat more unlikely. However, as both the roles of reverse Na^+–Ca^{2+} exchange in triggering sarcoplasmic reticulum Ca^{2+} release and the exact details of immunolocalization remain a subject for debate it may be specious reasoning to compare these findings in this context.

Subsequent studies have examined the developmental changes in Na^+–Ca^{2+} exchanger localization in rabbit myocytes (44, 45). It was found that the Na^+–Ca^{2+} exchanger exhibited a peripheral distribution at early developmental stages, but prominent labeling within the t-tubules was observed as soon as invaginations were formed (44). Previous studies by Philipson and co-workers (200) had demonstrated that the Na^+–Ca^{2+} exchanger binds ankyrin. The relationship between the subcellular distribution of ankyrin and the Na^+–Ca^{2+} exchanger was then evaluated in developing rabbit heart (45). Coincident localization of ankyrin and Na^+–Ca^{2+} exchange was observed within the t-tubules of adult myocytes. In contrast, neonatal cells exhibited peripheral Na$^+$–Ca^{2+} exchange, whereas ankyrin labeling was largely confined to the Z disks. A recent study by Haddock et al. (107) has also demonstrated prominent co-localization of the Na$^+$–Ca^{2+} exchanger and ryanodine receptors within the t-tubules of adult rabbit myocytes. In contrast, NCX1 exhibited a peripheral sarcolemmal distribution in both newborn and juvenile myocytes.

TRANSPORT PROPERTIES

Stoichiometry

The Na$^+$–Ca^{2+} exchanger is an electrogenic ion countertransporter with a generally accepted stoichiometry of 3 Na$^+$:1 Ca^{2+} (11, 61, 169, 181, 215, 216). Speculation concerning this stoichiometry is evident in the literature as early as 1969 during the discovery of Na$^+$–Ca^{2+} exchange in the squid axon (10). Several studies then provided evidence consistent with an electrogenic transport mechanism, although the exact stoichiometry remained a controversial matter (35, 87, 139, 184, 232, 233, 234). For example, Horackova and Vassort provided evidence for an electrogenic Na$^+$–Ca^{2+} exchange mechanism from voltage-clamp experiments in frog atrial muscle (140), consistent with a 3:1 stoichiometry. Reeves and Hale (271) used a convincing thermodynamic approach to demonstrate a 3 Na$^+$:1 Ca^{2+} stoichiometry in bovine sarcolemmal vesicles. In this study, ^{45}Ca^{2+} uptake and efflux were evaluated during manipulation of the membrane potential and Na$^+$ gradients. Conditions were identified where manipulation of the Na$^+$ gradient exactly offset the Ca^{2+} flux driven by the electrical gradient, with the results strongly supporting a 3:1 stoichiometry. Similar conclusions, albeit less compelling, had been reached earlier by Pitts (263). However, a review of this subject as late as 1985 concluded that there was no unambiguous evidence to support a 3 Na$^+$:1 Ca^{2+} stoichiometry or unequivocally attribute a particular membrane current to Na$^+$–Ca^{2+} exchange (87). From that time, a large body of evidence has developed to support the notion that Na$^+$–Ca^{2+} exchange transport is electrogenic with a consensus stoichiometry of 3 Na$^+$:1 Ca^{2+} (11, 40, 41, 61, 104, 154, 169, 170). Importantly, this stoichiometry forms the basis for much of our understanding of Na$^+$–Ca^{2+} exchange transport and physiology. That is, most electrophysiological analyses employ the assumption of a 3:1 stoichiometry to assess coupling ratios between Ca^{2+} entry and Ca^{2+} efflux via the Na$^+$–Ca^{2+} exchanger (e.g. references 61, 63, 319). Assessment of Na$^+$–Ca^{2+} exchange transport rates based on exchanger partial reactions also assumes this stoichiometry (128, 134, 157, 245).

A recent report has raised the possibility that the stoichiometry of Na$^+$–Ca^{2+} exchange may in fact be 4 Na$^+$:1 Ca^{2+} or variable depending upon ionic conditions (98). This study employed "macro" patches from intact guinea-pig ventricular myocytes, and the reversal potentials of Na$^+$–Ca^{2+} exchange currents were measured over a wide range of ionic conditions. Overall, the data were consistent with a 4:1 stoichiometry over most ionic conditions, although variable stoichiometry ranging from 3.3 to 8.7 was demonstrated. The implications from this study are far-reaching. In particular, if additional studies are able to validate this 4:1 or variable stoichiometry, that would affect interpretation of several aspects of Na$^+$–Ca^{2+} exchange function. In particular, with a 4:1 stoichiometry, several current estimates of Na$^+$–Ca^{2+} exchange transport rates based on partial transport reactions would be halved. The notion that the Na$^+$–Ca^{2+} exchanger operates in the reverse mode would seem far less likely over a much broader range of physiological potentials and ionic conditions. Furthermore, the additional energy imparted by this coupling ratio would provide the exchanger with the ability to lower intracellular Ca^{2+} far below the current estimates of diastolic Ca^{2+} levels. This would imply that active regulatory mechanisms exist to limit Ca^{2+} efflux via this mechanism. Based on these new results (98), it seems necessary to reexamine the issue of Na$^+$–Ca^{2+} exchange stoichiometry.

Interestingly, photoreceptor cells and neural tissue express a functionally related, though structurally distinct, family of Na$^+$–Ca^{2+} exchange proteins, termed NCKXs. The prototypical protein was first cloned from bovine rod photoreceptors (272), although since similar proteins, including alternatively spliced variants, have subsequently been identified in brain (264, 315). These proteins have a putative stoichiometry of 4 Na$^+$:1 Ca^{2+}, 1 K$^+$. This requirement for K$^+$ cotransport appears to exist for all members of the NCKX family (59, 268, 282, 283) (although see reference 238) and distinguishes them from the NCX exchangers. Members of the NCKX protein family are involved in Ca^{2+} efflux and their role has been best defined in visual transduction. Presumably, a similar function for these transporters occurs in neuronal tissue. Overall, there is very little structural similarity between NCKX and NCX proteins, although both serve as plasmalemmal Ca^{2+} transporters. Given the stoichiometry of the NCKX family, these transporters have the ability to lower intracellular Ca^{2+} to subnanomolar concentrations based on thermodynamic considerations (281, 284). However, regulatory mechanisms have been identified (described as time-dependent or Ca$^{2+}_i$-dependent) that lead to NCKX inactivation prior to attaining theoretical limits of Ca$^{2+}_i$

reduction (281, 284). The molecular details of these inactivation mechanisms remain largely unknown.

Transport Mechanism

Most recent studies support a consecutive mechanism for Na^+–Ca^{2+} exchange transport (134, 157, 158, 162, 196, 245, 253, 265). That is, the ion binding sites alternate between intracellularly and extracellularly facing configurations, with occluded states occurring during ion transport. In a simultaneous transport mechanism, ion-binding sites exist on both membrane surfaces and transport occurs only when both sites become occupied. A composite or hybrid model of these two extremes has also been postulated (226) based on results obtained from ferret red blood cells. This topic has been covered in detail in the recent review by Blaustein and Lederer (34), and is only briefly recounted here. At present, there are several lines of evidence providing direct support for a consecutive or "ping-pong" transport model. First, electrophysiological approaches have identified partial transport reactions associated with either Na^+ or Ca^{2+} translocation. Hilgemann et al. (134) used the giant excised patch technique to demonstrate charge movement associated with Na^+ translocation. Pipettes contained low concentrations of either Na^+ (5 mM) or Ca^{2+} (10 μM), initially in the absence of cytoplasmic Ca^{2+} and Na^+. Under these conditions, the only allowable transitions would orient all ion-binding sites to the cytoplasmic surface. Positive charge movement was observed upon application of cytoplasmic Na^+ but not with cytoplasmic Ca^{2+} application. Thus, the electrogenic step was proposed to occur during Na^+ translocation and/or Na^+ unbinding from the transport site (134). Somewhat different results were obtained by Niggli and Lederer (245), although both studies directly support a consecutive transport mechanism. These investigators identified charge movements, termed *conformation currents*, upon photorelease of caged Ca^{2+}_i in voltage-clamped myocytes, and these could be distinguished from net Na^+–Ca^{2+} exchange transport (245). Similarly, Kappl and Hartung identified partial exchanger reactions in giant excised membrane patches from guinea pig and rat myocytes (157). Here, photorelease of caged Ca^{2+} was used to activate transient and/or stationary currents depending upon the counter ions in the pipette, and net negative charge movement was identified during Ca^{2+} translocation. Interestingly, the latter two studies (157, 245) observed opposite effects for dichlorobenzamil (DCB) application, a nonselective Na^+–Ca^{2+} exchange inhibitor. Both the transient and stationary Na^+–Ca^{2+} exchange currents associated with photorelease of Ca^{2+} were blocked by 200 μM DCB applied to the cytoplasmic side in one study (157), whereas 1 mM intracellularly applied DCB (in the pipette) led to a sixfold increase in conformation currents and very little effect on stationary currents (245). The origin of this disparity remains unknown. More recently, Hilgemann and others (123, 128) have identified charge movements associated with partial reactions using either transport substrate and thus a consensus is developing that both limbs of the transport cycle are electrogenic. Furthermore, the Na^+–Ca^{2+} exchanger from squid, NCX-SQ1, exhibits major differences in charge movement of partial reactions, with Ca^{2+} movements being notably more electrogenic than that observed for NCX1 (123). Thus, species and/or isoform differences may ultimately be found to possess different electrophysiological profiles. Numerous studies have examined the electrophysiological profile and regulatory mechanisms for the squid giant axon Na^+–Ca^{2+} exchanger (e.g., references 67, 68, 70, 71, 72, 73, 75) and the recent availability of the cloned squid exchanger (123) should greatly facilitate this work. This topic has recently been reviewed by DiPolo and Beauge (74).

Additional evidence favoring a consecutive reaction scheme has been derived from studies examining the influence of the counter ion concentration on the apparent affinity of the other transported ion. As described by Lauger (181), reducing the concentration of one ion should increase the apparent affinity of the other in a consecutive reaction mechanism. Giant excised patch clamp experiments have demonstrated that the apparent ion affinities of steady state Na^+–Ca^{2+} exchange currents increase in response to decreases of the counter ion concentration (134). Voltage-clamp studies of intact myocytes have yielded similar results (196), and earlier work by Khananshvili (162) arrived at this conclusion using $^{45}Ca^{2+}$ uptake measurements in reconstituted proteoliposomes. Overall, the majority of recent evidence provides robust support for a consecutive reaction mechanism.

Turnover Rates and Exchanger Density

Several investigators have made elegant attempts to establish turnover rates for the cardiac Na^+–Ca^{2+} exchanger using a variety of different approaches. While some consensus on turnover rates has developed, in recent literature the estimates still vary considerably. For example, recent reports have indicated values of 5000 s^{-1} (128, 134), ~ 2000 s^{-1} (157), < 75 s^{-1} (265), 1000 s^{-1} (46), and 2500 s^{-1} (245). Perhaps this range of results (almost 2 orders of magnitude) is not surprising considering that all estimates are assumption based or model based and that distinct experimental techniques have been employed. Furthermore, these estimates of transport rates have been obtained from measurements of partial exchange reactions (i.e. half cycles) as well as from complete transport cycles. The specific stoichiometry of Na^+–Ca^{2+} exchange has recently been called into question, and if verified, this new data demonstrating 4:1 stoichiometry would immediately alter all estimates (98). Finally, there is simply no unequivocal means of establishing the number of exchangers contributing to a given signal. The inability to assess elementary current events directly and the absence of tools (e.g., radioligands) to count exchangers greatly confound studies of transport rates. The recent study by Hilgemann applying analysis of current noise associated with exchanger inactivation reactions is the closest approximation to obtaining elementary current measurements (128). Overall, our understanding of physiological turnover rates for Na^+–Ca^{2+} exchange transport (which would vary throughout the action potential and Ca^{2+}_i transient) is poor.

It should be noted that an accurate determination of the Na^+–Ca^{2+} exchange transport rates would have a major impact on our understanding of Na^+–Ca^{2+} exchange physiology. Immediately, this would place lower limits on the number of exchangers required to accomplish Ca^{2+} efflux from cardiac myocytes. Accurate knowledge of the exchanger density, combined with information on physiological transport rates, would contribute greatly to our understanding of Na^+–Ca^{2+} exchanger recruitment and regulation, if this exists. At present, we are left with describing global Na^+–Ca^{2+} exchange activity as increasing or decreasing with very limited knowledge of how this is accomplished. Some recent estimates of Na^+–Ca^{2+} exchanger density had provided values of 250 (245), 300–400 (128, 134), and > 1235 (265) exchangers per μm^2. It seems necessary to validate these estimates through independent experimental means, although few, if any, tools are available to accomplish this goal. Furthermore, it is unclear how changes in the site density of Na^+–Ca^{2+} exchangers would influence cardiac excitation–contraction coupling, even though this has become a widely used measure toward understanding cardiac pathophysiology. The results from transgenic animals studies (described below) highlight our limited knowledge of physiological Na^+–Ca^{2+} exchange function.

Ion Selectivity

Ion selectivity (or specificity) of Na^+–Ca^{2+} exchange has been studied extensively for both the cardiac and squid giant axon exchangers (reviewed in reference 34). This review focuses on more recent developments on this topic. The cardiac Na^+–Ca^{2+} exchanger has a strict specificity for Na^+ as the transported monovalent cation. However, this specificity can be reduced by mutagenesis to induce a significant Li^+ transport capacity (79). Less stringency is observed for the transported divalent cation with Sr^{2+} and Ba^{2+} being transported to various degrees (310, 312, 313). It appears that Sr^{2+} is nearly equivalent to Ca^{2+} as a transport substrate, whereas Ba^{2+} transport is considerably less, based on results obtained from sarcolemmal vesicles (310, 313). Na^+–Sr^{2+} exchange currents have also been characterized using electrophysiological approaches (104, 244, 312), although the ability to detect Na^+–Ba^{2+} exchange currents has been variable or absent in cardiac cells (98, 104, 169). Robust outward Na^+–Ba^{2+} exchange currents have been identified using the giant excised patch technique, whereas inward Na^+–Ba^{2+} exchange currents were barely detectable (312). In this study, Ba^{2+} was also able to substitute for Ca^{2+} at the high affinity regulatory Ca^{2+} binding site, although stimulation of the exchanger was reduced with respect to both affinity and efficiency (i.e. I_{max} was less) (312). Reeves and coworkers have also identified Na^+–Ba^{2+} exchange activity in Chinese hamster ovary cells expressing the cloned NCX1.1 exchanger and have found this activity to be regulated by both intracellular Ca^{2+} and ATP (54, 94, 320). Furthermore, regulatory Ca^{2+}-dependent stimulation of Na^+–Ba^{2+} exchange was absent when examined for a mutant exchanger devoid of the regulatory Ca^{2+} response (94). There is also evidence that Ni^{2+} and La^{3+}, commonly used inhibitors of Na^+–Ca^{2+} exchange, can substitute for Ca^{2+} as a transport substrate (85, 86, 266). Chimeric analyses of different exchangers have begun to identify specific residues involved in differential sensitivities to extracellular Ni^{2+} and Li^+ (148).

Temperature Dependence

Hypothermic cardioplegic approaches are widely employed to preserve myocardial function during cardiac surgery. This dictates that some consideration must be given to the consequences of lowering temperature for various ion transport systems. Mammalian Na^+–Ca^{2+} exchange activity is highly dependent on temperature, with reported Q_{10}s ranging from 2 to 4 depending on the temperature range examined (127, 157, 169, 311). Consequently, Na^+–Ca^{2+} exchange activity would be seriously compromised under hypothermic conditions. As an extreme example, rapid cooling contractures of cardiac muscle are a direct manifestation of inhibiting Ca^{2+} efflux via Na^+–Ca^{2+} exchange (25, 39, 145). In contrast, several studies have demonstrated that Na^+–Ca^{2+} exchange activity in poikilothermic species exhibit substantial exchange activity at low temperatures (309, 311). For example, the Na^+–Ca^{2+} exchanger from trout heart exhibits a Q_{10} of ~1.2 and shows substantial activity at 7° C, whereas mammalian exchangers are largely inactive at this temperature (311). This distinction in temperature dependence between homeotherms and poikilotherms is retained following reconstitution of the different exchangers in a common lipid environment (29, 259, 309, 311). Therefore, these studies concluded that differences in the temperature sensitivity reside within the Na^+–Ca^{2+} exchanger per se, as opposed to the native lipid environment.

The trout Na^+–Ca^{2+} exchanger was recently cloned and functionally expressed in *Xenopus laevis* oocytes (334). A chimeric analysis of trout and canine NCX1 exchangers was subsequently conducted using the giant excised patch technique to determine if the distinct temperature profiles were attributable to specific portions of the exchanger molecule (333). All chimeric molecules bearing canine sequence in the first third of the molecule exhibited a mammalian exchanger temperature dependence. In contrast, chimeras with trout sequence in the first third of the molecule exhibited a poikilothermic temperature profile. The remaining two-thirds of the exchanger did not contribute strongly to this temperature dependence (333).

MOLECULAR BIOLOGY OF THE Na^+–Ca^{2+} EXCHANGER

The Prototypical Canine Cardiac Na^+–Ca^{2+} Exchanger

The prototypical Na^+–Ca^{2+} exchanger, now referred to as NCX1.1, was cloned from a canine cardiac cDNA library (241). The identified clone encoded a protein of 970 amino acids with a calculated molecular weight of ~110 kD. Injection of cRNA transcribed from this clone into *Xenopus* oocytes produced robust Na^+–Ca^{2+} exchange activity. This fundamental advance has led to a tremendous increase in our understanding of the role of Na^+–Ca^{2+} exchange in cardiac and other tissues.

The Exchanger Superfamily

The cloning of the canine cardiac Na^+–Ca^{2+} exchanger has led directly to the identification of a superfamily of Na^+–Ca^{2+} exchangers and related proteins. At present, three mammalian Na^+–Ca^{2+} exchangers have been cloned and are referred to as NCX1 (241), NCX2 (198), and NCX3 (239). All three NCX members have been demonstrated to operate as Na^+–Ca^{2+} exchangers with similar functional attributes (202). Related proteins from the fruit fly (*Drosophila melanogaster*) and squid (*Loligo opalescens*) have been identified and observed to function as Na^+–Ca^{2+} exchangers (123, 143, 277, 288). Related proteins from *Caenorhabditis elegans* and *Arabidopsis thaliana* have been identified from large-scale sequencing projects but Na^+–Ca^{2+} exchange function has not been established (260). Both NCX1 and NCX3 undergo alternative splicing, as described below. A complete discussion of the exchanger superfamily appears in a recent review by Philipson and Nicoll (260).

Topology of the Na^+–Ca^{2+} Exchanger

The original topological model of the Na^+–Ca^{2+} exchanger was proposed in 1990 based on hydropathy analysis (241). This analysis identified twelve potential transmembrane segments, a large cytoplasmic domain (termed loop f), 6 potential N-linked glycosylation sites, and a potential phosphorylation site. Furthermore, the authors speculated that the protein might contain a cleavable NH_2-terminal signal sequence and identified a potential calmodulin-binding domain (now known as the XIP sequence [199]). Since this original description, newer experimental studies have provided evidence validating several of the original predictions but also necessitating a revision of the model. This review deals exclusively with the most recent topological model of the cardiac Na^+–Ca^{2+} exchanger.

The current topological model is based largely upon mutagenesis, cysteine susceptibility analysis, and epitope tagging studies (58, 149, 242). From the two most recent studies, the Na^+–Ca^{2+} exchanger is predicted to have 9 transmembrane spanning segments (149, 242). The large cytoplasmic domain, loop f, which separates the two sets of transmembrane segments (TMS 1–5 and TMS 6–9), comprises the majority of the exchange molecule, as originally modeled. Other major revisions include the placement of TM 6 within cytoplasmic loop f and the *Calx*-α motifs (also called α-1 and α-2 repeats (149, 242)) appearing on opposite membrane surfaces. These motifs may constitute portions of re-entrant membrane loops, analogous to the pore regions of ion channels. Earlier work established that the exchanger does possess a cleaved signal sequence and is glycosylated at a single site, Asn-9 (80, 144, 243). Functionally, glycosylation does not appear to modify the properties of the exchanger (144). Furthermore, elimination of the cleavage site of the signal sequence, or deleting this sequence entirely, does not prevent correct membrane insertion (101, 211, 278).

At present, the exchanger is thought to function as a monomer, although there is very little evidence supporting or refuting this possibility. Functionally important accessory proteins have not been identified. Furthermore, the cloned Na^+–Ca^{2+} exchanger has been studied in a variety of heterologous expression systems (e.g., *Xenopus*, insect, and mammalian cell lines) without major evidence for functional differences. Thus, these distinct expression systems either possess common accessory proteins or such proteins are not required for exchange function. An early study (109) employing irradiation inactivation-target sizing analyses provided evidence for an high molecular weight exchanger of ~225 kDa (roughly 2× the size of a monomer). This study, conducted prior to the cloning of NCX1, has not been verified by other experimental means. Overall, the notion that the exchanger functions as a monomer without accessory proteins is widespread, but poorly substantiated.

Two studies have shown Na^+–Ca^{2+} exchange activity following expression of highly truncated exchangers (essentially the amino terminus TM 1–5 and portions of the large cytoplasmic loop) (102, 197). This has led to the suggestion that the truncated exchanger could dimerize to form an active transporter (102). A much smaller truncation of NCX1 has also been identified and cloned from the BALB/c mouse heart, lacking 30 amino acids at the C-terminus because of the presence of a premature termination site (293). More recently, split Na^+–Ca^{2+} exchangers have been demonstrated to possess activity provided that both halves of the molecule were co-expressed (255). However, in contrast to the above two reports, exchange activity was not observed unless both halves were present. The reason for this discrepancy remains unknown. While this could reflect the different constructs examined, current topological models have placed the highly conserved and functionally important *Calx-α* repeats on opposite membrane surfaces (see below). The truncated exchangers would lack one such *Calx-α* domain. Clearly, more studies are required to resolve this issue.

The Calx-α and Calx-β Repeats

A Na^+-Ca^{2+} exchanger from *Drosophila* was cloned independently by two groups of investigators in 1997 (277, 288). The gene product, called *Calx* (288) or DroNCX (277), encodes a protein with ~55% identity with NCX1–NCX3 and shows similar transport functions (81, 143, 251, 277, 288). Two intragenic repeats were identified in CALX by Schwarz and Benzer and were originally referred to as the *Calx-α* and *Calx-β* motifs (288). These motifs are referred to as the α-and β-repeats in most literature. To retain information on the origin of these intragenic repeats, the original description of these domains used by Schwarz and Benzer (287, 288) is used in this review. Both of these motifs are highly conserved throughout the NCX1–NCX3 family of exchangers. In addition, the *Calx-α* motifs are conserved for mammalian and *Drosophila* Na^+,Ca^{2+},K^+-exchangers (NCKX family) (115, 315). Furthermore, specific residues within the *Calx-α* motifs of NCX1 have been shown to play an important role in ion transport (240). Several site-specific mutations within these regions have been shown to eliminate or alter ion transport properties (240). As currently modeled (149, 242), the *Calx-α* motifs are positioned on opposite sides of the membrane (in contrast to the original topological models (241)) and may form portions of re-entrant membrane loops. The role of the *Calx-β* motifs remains unknown although they overlap portions of the cytoplasmic loop involved in regulatory Ca^{2+} binding. Furthermore, these *Calx-β* motifs have been identified in integrin β4 and related proteins (287).

Alternative Splicing of Na^+–Ca^{2+} Exchangers

The demonstration of alternative splicing for the NCX1 exchanger was first shown in 1994 (173, 187). Prior to this discovery, a Na^+–Ca^{2+} exchanger was cloned from kidney and was found to be 29 amino acids shorter than the prototypical cardiac Na^+–Ca^{2+} exchanger (273). Alternative splicing occurs through the variable assembly of six cassette exons (exons A–F) toward the C-terminus of the large intracellular loop. The first two exons, A and B, are mutually exclusive, whereas the remaining 4 exons are found in various combinations for all splice variants. Of the 32 possible combinations permissible from this arrangement for NCX1, twelve splice variants have been identified, many of which are expressed in a tissue-specific manner (173, 187, 269). In general, splice variants containing the A exon are found in excitable tissue (such as brain, heart, and skeletal muscle), whereas B exon–containing variants are found in most other tissues (for example, kidney and smooth muscle).

Functionally, very little is known concerning the physiological consequences of alternative splicing. Alternatively spliced Na^+–Ca^{2+} exchangers with prominent expression in kidney (NCX1.3, BD exons), heart (NCX1.1, ACDEF exons), and brain (NCX1.4, AD exons) have all been shown to exhibit distinct patterns of ionic regulation (82, 252). Two splice variants have also been identified for the *Drosophila* Na^+–Ca^{2+} exchanger in the analogous region of the alternative splicing site of mammalian NCX1 (251, 277). These splice variants also exhibit unique ionic regulatory profiles (251). Furthermore, isoform-specific regulation by protein kinase A (PKA) was observed for NCX1.4 (AD exons), whereas NCX1.3 (BD exons) was unaffected (120). Overall, while differences between alternatively spliced Na^+–Ca^+ exchangers have been identified, these findings have not been integrated into our understanding of physiological Na^+–Ca^{2+} exchange function. Furthermore, there has been no functional characterization for any of the remaining NCX1 splice variants or for those of NCX3. Much remains to be learned regarding the role(s) of alternative splicing for Na$^+$–Ca^{2+} exchangers.

REGULATION OF Na$^+$–Ca^{2+} EXCHANGE

Ionic Regulation

Both of the transported ions, Na$^+$ and Ca^{2+}, exert regulatory effects on Na$^+$–Ca^{2+} exchange activity. These effects have been extensively characterized for NCX1.1, although the effects are also apparent in other members of the Na$^+$–Ca^{2+} exchanger family. Most characterization efforts have employed the giant excised patch technique, although the regulatory behaviors have also been identified using whole-cell patch clamping, fluorometric, and ^{45}Ca^{2+} flux experiments. Furthermore, the regulatory responses have been identified in preparations expressing the native exchanger (i.e. sarcolemmal membrane "blebs" or intact myocytes) and in a variety of heterologous expression systems [e.g. *Xenopus* oocytes, Chinese hamster ovary (CHO) cells]. Finally, the majority of evidence favors the notion that these ionic regulatory properties are intrinsic to the exchanger per se rather than through accessory proteins or reactions. However, this latter possibility has not been thoroughly investigated.

Na$_i^+$-Dependent Inactivation Na$_i^+$-dependent inactivation was originally identified in sarcolemmal membrane blebs using the giant patch technique (127). This process, subsequently called I$_1$ inactivation, describes the ability of cytoplasmic Na$^+$ to promote entry into an inactive state of the exchanger (128, 129, 131). Na$_i^+$-dependent inactivation is apparent in outward Na$^+$–Ca^{2+} exchange current measurements as the progressive decay in currents associated with increases in Na$_i^+$. The similarity between Na$_i^+$ affinities for current production and current decay underlies the postulate that the Na$_i^+$-dependent (I$_1$) inactive state arises from the 3-Na$^+$-loaded conformation of the exchanger. That is, upon Na$_i^+$ binding, the exchanger partitions between active and inactive conformations. If current–voltage relationships were obtained at various time points during the decaying current transients, all resulting traces had identical slopes upon scaling (131). This indicates that Na$_i^+$-dependent inactivation simply alters the population of available exchangers, rather than altering global transport behavior (128, 131). Thus, the availability of exchangers can be controlled by this mechanism.

The physiological significance of Na$_i^+$-dependent inactivation is unknown. While the operation of this mechanism has been identified in intact cardiac myocytes (217), the conditions required to demonstrate this process are unlikely to represent those occurring physiologically. Specifically, Na$_i^+$-dependent inactivation is most prominent at elevated Na$_i^+$ levels (e.g., 25–100 mM), far in excess of those thought to occur physiologically. While species-dependent variations are known to exist, most estimates of intracellular Na$^+$ in mammalian myocytes range from 8 to 12 mM, a concentration at which Na$_i^+$-dependent inactivation would not occur. Furthermore, physiological concentrations of ATP appear to alleviate Na$_i^+$-dependent inactivation almost completely (132). These observations make it difficult to envision a role for the Na$_i^+$-dependent inactivation process. While the idea of a restricted sub-sarcolemmal space (183), where local Na$_i^+$ does rise to levels sufficient to activate this mechanism, could be invoked, this possibility remains to be established. Certainly, increased stimulation frequency and digitalis-like compounds would elevate the concentration of intracellular Na$_i^+$, although it is unclear that this elevation would promote I$_1$ inactivation. Thus, at present, there is no compelling evidence supporting a physiological role for Na$_i^+$-dependent inactivation. More likely, we have not yet asked the correct questions.

Ca$_i^{2+}$-Dependent Regulation Ca^{2+}-dependent, or I$_2$, regulation of the Na$^+$–Ca^{2+} exchanger describes the stimulatory effect of nontransported, cytoplasmic Ca^{2+} on Na$^+$–Ca^{2+} exchange activity (127, 132, 170, 217, 227). First identified in the giant axon from squid (65), this regulatory mechanism appears to operate in all characterized Na$^+$–Ca^{2+} exchangers (123, 143, 202). Whole-cell current measurements from cardiac myocytes have established that sub-micromolar cytoplasmic Ca^{2+} is required to observe Na$^+$–Ca^{2+} exchange currents (169, 170, 227). This stimulatory effect of cytoplasmic Ca^{2+} is also evident in fluorometric, electrophysiological, and radioisotopic flux studies of the cloned cardiac exchanger expressed in a variety of different cell types (47, 54, 94, 202, 219, 320). Moreover, giant excised patch experiments have provided detailed characterization of this regulatory mechanism in both cardiac myocytes and *Xenopus* oocytes expressing NCX1.1 (127, 132, 219). In reasonable agreement among all studies is the existence of this mechanism as a means of activating cardiac Na$^+$–Ca^{2+} exchangers. However, the regulatory Ca^{2+} affinities producing a stimulatory response differ widely between experimental preparations. For example, Miura and Kimura (227) reported a K$_m$ value of 22 nM Ca$_i^{2+}$ for activating the exchanger in guinea pig myocytes. Saturation of this effect occurred at 50 nM Ca^{2+}. Similarly, Condrescu et al. (54) observed stimulation of exchange activity in the 20–50 nM range. In contrast, results from giant excised patch experiments are typically three- to fourfold higher. Apparent affinities for Ca^{2+} regulation typically range from 100 to 300 nM from giant excised patch camp studies (127, 219, 312).

While these disparities in the affinities or the K_m for regulatory Ca^{2+} are relatively small, this issue is especially important for understanding the role of Ca^{2+} regulation of Na^+–Ca^{2+} exchange in cardiac myocytes. That is, if the lower values obtained from whole-cell measurements are accepted, then activation through this mechanism would be essentially saturated, even at diastolic Ca^{2+} levels. On the other hand, if values obtained from giant excised patch-clamp experiments are correct, then activation through Ca^{2+}-dependent regulation is ideally poised to operate between anticipated diastolic and systolic Ca_i^{2+} values. Therefore, Ca^{2+} regulation could conceivably represent a major mechanism, which senses time-averaged changes in intracellular Ca^{2+} and couples Ca^{2+} entry and efflux. Clearly, this is an attractive possibility, although much additional evidence is required to support this hypothesis. One possible explanation for the differences observed between cell-based and excised-patch measurements may be the difficulties involved in examining a large range of intracellular Ca^{2+} concentrations in cells. Cellular preparations tend to show high affinity Ca^{2+} regulation below 100 nM. However, it may be difficult or impossible to evaluate higher intracellular Ca^{2+} levels (e.g. 10–30 μM) in most intact cell systems, and particularly in cardiac myocytes. Thus, the additional activation of Na^+–Ca^{2+} exchange by higher concentrations of intracellular Ca^{2+} concentrations (not typically achievable in whole-cell systems) may simply be missed. This limitation does not occur in excised patches.

Interestingly, the Na^+–Ca^{2+} exchanger from *Drosophila* (called CALX or DroNCX) exhibits an opposite response to regulatory Ca^{2+}. That is, cytoplasmic Ca^{2+} inhibits the activity of the *Drosophila* Na^+–Ca^{2+} exchanger (81, 143). All characterized mammalian exchangers are stimulated by regulatory Ca^{2+}. While not germane to the discussion of cardiac Na^+–Ca^{2+} exchange, this anomalous response highlights the natural diversity of this regulatory mechanism. Furthermore, alternatively spliced CALX and NCX1 Na^+–Ca^{2+} exchangers exhibit unique Ca^{2+} regulatory mechanisms (82, 251). Thus, while we do not know the role of Ca^{2+} regulation, this process has been highly conserved and is also modified by alternative splicing. These results lend credence to the notion that ionic regulation of Na^+–Ca^{2+} exchange serves a physiological role (awaiting discovery).

There is considerable interaction between the ionic regulatory mechanisms. Most prominent is the ability of regulatory Ca^{2+} to alleviate the Na^+-dependent inactivation process (132). At higher regulatory Ca^{2+} concentrations (e.g. 10–30 μM), Na_i^+-dependent inactivation is largely eliminated. Experimental and theoretical studies have revealed the regulatory Ca^{2+} accelerates recovery from, and reduces entry into, the Na_i^+-dependent inactive state (132). Furthermore, all mutants targeting the Na_i^+-dependent inactivation mechanism have influenced the behavior of Ca_i^{2+} regulation (218). Similarly, mutants targeting the regulatory Ca^{2+} binding site have exhibited altered Na_i^+-dependent inactivation (219). Complicating this issue even further, alternatively spliced variants of NCX1 show unique ionic regulatory profiles (82). Most dramatically, the kidney isoform (NCX1.3) does not exhibit any interaction between Na^+-dependent and Ca^{2+} dependent regulation. These results indicate that the alternative splicing region plays some role in tailoring ionic regulatory properties.

Structure–Function Relationships of Ionic Regulation

The XIP Region The XIP region of the canine cardiac Na^+–Ca^{2+} exchanger refers to amino acids, 219–238 (199, 218). Current topological modeling indicates that this region occurs on the N-terminus side of the large cytoplasmic loop, almost immediately after transmembrane segment 5. From structure–function studies, it is clear that the XIP region plays a prominent role in Na_i^+-dependent (or I_1) inactivation. Mutations or deletions of specific amino acids within the XIP region have been shown to accelerate or eliminate Na_i^+-dependent inactivation in the canine Na^+–Ca^{2+} exchanger (218). For example, mutation F223E in NCX1.1 leads to a sixfold increase in the rate of current inactivation. In contrast, Na_i^+-dependent inactivation is completely abolished for the NCX1.1 mutant K229Q. Several additional mutations within this region exhibit similar phenotypes (218).

The XIP region is well conserved throughout the exchanger family (82). While equivalent function has not been established for NCX2 and NCX3, the XIP region serves a similar functional role in the *Drosophila* Na^+–Ca^{2+} exchanger, CALX1.1. Analogous mutations to those identified for NCX1.1 produced similar consequences to the Na_i^+-dependent inactivation process (82). Thus, despite an opposite response to regulatory Ca^{2+}, Na_i^+-dependent inactivation appears similar for both NCX1 and CALX exchangers. Based on these results, it seems quite likely that the XIP region will be found to serve a similar functional role in most, if not all, Na^+–Ca^{2+} exchangers.

The mechanism of inhibition by exogenous or endogenous XIP remains unknown. Presumably, exogenous XIP (discussed below) simply mimics the inactivation process mediated by the endogenous XIP region, although there is no experimental evidence supporting this notion. As the role of Na$^+$-dependent inactivation of Na$^+$–Ca^{2+} exchange remains entirely unknown, it is equally difficult to envisage how alterations in this mechanism would influence cardiac excitation–contraction coupling. The use of transgenic animals expressing mutant Na$^+$–Ca^{2+} exchangers specifically targeting this inactivation process may shed light on this subject.

The Regulatory Ca^{2+} Binding Site Based on the initial structure–function studies of the cardiac Na$^+$–Ca^{2+} exchanger, the large cytoplasmic loop (loop f) was implicated in all ionic regulatory mechanisms (220). The high affinity regulatory Ca^{2+} binding site was subsequently identified in canine NCX1.1 using the ^{45}Ca^{2+}-overlay technique (194). Fusion proteins expressing portions of the large cytoplasmic loop (loop f) were examined for their ability to bind ^{45}Ca^{2+}. A span of 138 amino acids was identified (amino acids 371–508) as the Ca^{2+} binding domain. Calcium binding was cooperative with an estimated $K_{0.5}$ ranging from 0.3 to 3 μM. Two highly acidic sequences were identified within this segment, each possessing three consecutive aspartic acid residues. Decreases in Ca^{2+} binding affinity were observed upon mutations of the aspartic acid residues within these clusters (194).

The regulatory Ca^{2+} binding was further examined by combining mutagenesis with electrophysiological analysis using the giant excised patch technique (219). In this study, several mutations were examined within the identified regulatory Ca^{2+} binding domain. Four specific aspartic acid residues were identified (at positions 447, 448, 498, and 500) which, upon mutation, led to a reduction in the affinity for functional Ca^{2+} regulation. Regulation was assessed primarily for outward (i.e. reverse) Na$^+$–Ca^{2+} currents. However, the ability to study mutants with low-affinity Ca^{2+} regulation was also used to demonstrate Ca^{2+}-dependent regulation of inward Na$^+$–Ca^{2+} exchange currents. This study also revealed that transport properties and the kinetics of Ca^{2+}-dependent regulation were altered in several mutant exchangers (219).

The high affinity regulatory Ca^{2+} binding site is highly conserved among different Na$^+$–Ca^{2+} exchangers, particularly if the acidic clusters within this region are compared. While mutagenesis of this region has only been examined for NCX1.1 (194, 219) and CALX (81), it appears that the regulatory Ca^{2+} binding site serves a similar role in both exchangers. Analogous mutations in CALX led to similar reductions in affinity for functional Ca^{2+} regulation (81). Considering that these two exchangers exhibit opposite responses to regulatory Ca^{2+} (i.e. NCX1 is stimulated whereas CALX is inhibited), this result is somewhat surprising. However, if the regulatory Ca^{2+} binding site serves a similar role in these divergent exchangers, it seems quite likely that this role will have been retained throughout the NCX family. Functional Ca^{2+} regulation has been demonstrated for all NCX1, NCX2, and NCX3 exchangers examined to date (202). The results obtained for structure–function analysis of NCX1.1 and CALX, indicate that although a common regulatory Ca^{2+} binding site is employed, transduction of this signal differs between the two exchangers. Through chimeric analysis of NCX1 and CALX exchangers, functional interconversion of these opposite regulatory responses was partially accomplished (81). Further analysis of this type may provide insight into the transduction mechanism of the regulatory Ca^{2+} binding signal.

Regulation by Phosphorylation

Regulation of the cardiac Na$^+$–Ca^{2+} exchanger by phosphorylation remains a poorly understood and controversial issue. This regulatory mechanism was first described for the Na$^+$–Ca^{2+} exchanger in squid axon and has been extensively characterized in this tissue, primarily by DiPolo, Beauge, and coworkers (for recent reviews, see references 69, 74, 76). This review focuses primarily on results for mammalian exchangers. Direct evidence for phosphorylation of the smooth muscle Na$^+$–Ca^{2+} exchanger was reported by Iwamoto et al. (154). Shortly thereafter, similar results were obtained for the cardiac Na$^+$–Ca^{2+} exchanger (152). In these studies, Na$^+$–Ca^{2+} exchange activity was upregulated in response to protein kinase C (PKC:)–dependent phosphorylation, and phosphopeptide analyses revealed multiple phosphorylation sites on both exchangers, exclusively on serine residues. Prolonged exposure to phorbol 12-myristate 13-acetate (PMA) abolished the stimulatory effects of specific growth factors on Na$^+$–Ca^{2+} activity in both smooth muscle and cardiac cells (152, 154). In a subsequent study, these investigators examined all three NCX isoforms and determined that the stimulatory effects of PMA or platelet-derived growth factor-BB did not require direct phosphorylation of these proteins (150). Using site-specific mutagenesis, a mutant NCX1 exchanger was constructed where all identified phosphorylation sites (Ser-249, Ser-250, and Ser-357) were replaced with alanine. This exchanger still exhibited responsiveness to PMA, whereas deletion of the large cytoplasmic loop eliminated PKC-dependent regulation for both NCX1 and NCX3. Thus, the mechanisms underlying the stimulatory effects of PKC-mediated phosphorylation on the cardiac exchanger remain unknown.

Protein kinase A–dependent stimulation has been

demonstrated for specific alternatively spliced variants of the mammalian NCX1 exchanger. In particular, NCX1.4, which is preferentially found in neuronal cells and expresses the AD exons, was stimulated approximately 40% upon PKA activation. In contrast, no equivalent stimulation was observed for NCX1.3, which expresses the BD exons and which showed prominent expression in astrocytes (120). PKA-dependent regulation of the frog Na^+-Ca^{2+} exchanger has also been demonstrated; in this case, however, inhibition of Na^+-Ca^{2+} exchange activity is observed (93, 294). In this series of studies cyclic AMP did not alter the activity of the canine NCX1.1 exchanger. The frog exchanger contains a unique 9 amino acid exon, not present in mammalian exchangers, which could account for the observed functional consequences of β-adrenergic stimulation (294). Elimination of this exon, which confers a nucleotide binding motif (P-loop), in the frog exchanger resulted in loss of cAMP responsiveness. More recent investigations have shown that a mutant NCX1.1 exchanger, for which the P-loop had been inserted, gains sensitivity to cAMP (119). Studies in shark myocytes have revealed that cAMP suppresses Ca^{2+} influx via the Na^+-Ca^{2+} exchanger but enhances Ca^{2+} efflux.

Using the giant excised patch-clamp technique, Collins et al., examined the mechanism of ATP-mediated stimulation of Na^+-Ca^{2+} exchange currents (53). Based on the examination of a large number of kinase inhibitors, phosphatases, and phosphatase inhibitors, no evidence was found to indicate that the stimulatory effect of ATP was mediated by a Ca_i^{2+}-dependent mechanism or that it involved protein kinases. This study examined outward Na^+-Ca^{2+} exchange currents exclusively. More recently, in a study of the bovine cardiac exchanger expressed in Chinese hamster ovary cells, Condrescu et al. (56) identified pronounced effects of the phosphatase inhibitors, calyculin A and okadaic acid. Both of these agents markedly inhibited reverse Na^+-Ca^{2+} exchange activity, equivalent to outward currents in patches. In contrast, the effects were marginal or absent on forward exchange activity. The inhibitory effects of calyculin A and okadaic acid were still observed when examined on a mutant exchanger, devoid of the majority of the intracellular loop (420 amino acids deleted). Thus, the authors suggested that this inhibition was unlikely to involve direct phosphorylation of the exchanger (231). These strikingly different results, however, highlight the complexity of investigating phosphorylation–dependent Na^+-Ca^{2+} exchange regulation. Adding to this complexity, prolonged PKC and PKA activation have been demonstrated to produce marked downregulation of Na^+-Ca^{2+} exchange expression levels (300, 301).

Regulation by PIP_2

The mechanism underlying the stimulatory effects of ATP on the cardiac exchanger has recently been ascribed to the phosphorylation of phosphatidylinositol (PI) to produce phosphatidylinositol-4,5-bisphosphate (PIP_2) (130). Evidence supporting this mechanism was obtained from giant excised patch-clamp experiments in which outward Na^+-Ca^+ exchange currents from cardiac membrane patches were examined. The stimulatory effects of ATP were eliminated by a PI-specific phospholipase C and could be restored upon PI application to the membrane. A PIP_2-specific phospholipase reversed the stimulatory effects of ATP, as did aluminum, which binds to PIP_2 with high affinity. Mechanistically, stimulation of Na^+-Ca^{2+} exchange current by ATP (and therefore PIP_2) occurs through the elimination of the Na_i^+-dependent inactivation mechanism.

The interaction of PIP_2 and the XIP peptide has recently been demonstrated (121). Iodinated XIP bound with high affinity to immobilized phospholipid vesicles containing low PIP_2 concentrations. The authors then examined the functional responses to PIP_2 in exchangers bearing mutations in the XIP region. Irrespective of whether the XIP mutations led to an elimination or acceleration of Na_i^+-dependent inactivation, the functional response to PIP_2 (or PIP_2 antibodies) was eliminated.

These data suggest the intriguing possibility that PIP_2 may serve as an important physiological regulator of Na^+-Ca^{2+} exchange activity. As yet, the role for Na_i^+-dependent inactivation of Na^+-Ca^{2+} exchange remains unknown. Difficulties in conceptualizing a physiological role are based largely on the fact that intracellular Na^+ is unlikely to achieve the levels necessary to induce Na_i^+-dependent inactivation. While these two studies offer little to alleviate this concern (i.e. PIP_2 eliminates an inactivation process induced by very high Na_i^+), they provide additional evidence suggesting that Na_i^+-independent inactivation is physiologically relevant. It now seems essential to investigate the operation of this proposed mechanism in intact cardiac myocytes.

Regulation by pH

The activity of the Na^+-Ca^{2+} exchanger is markedly influenced by pH. For example, in the squid axon, a 50% decrease in Na^+-Ca^{2+} exchange activity was observed upon acidification of the internal environment from pH 7.3 to pH 6.8. In contrast, a fourfold increase in activity occurred upon intracellular alkalinization to pH 8.8. No effect on Na^+-Ca^{2+} exchange activity was observed upon alkalinization of the external environment to pH 9.0 (66). Similarly, studies in cardiac sarcolemmal vesicles demonstrated complex effects of pH on Na$^+$-Ca^{2+} exchange activity (258). A sigmoidal relationship between pH and Na$_i^+$-dependent Ca^{2+} uptake was obtained which was partially competitive with Ca^{2+}.

The effects of pH on Na$^+$–Ca^{2+} exchange have also been characterized in guinea pig myocytes using the giant excised patch technique (77, 78). Directionally similar responses to those noted above were obtained, although the investigators were able to provide greater mechanistic insight into the process. For example, the effects of pH were largely eliminated upon proteolysis of the exchanger with α-chymotrypsin, implicating Na$^+$–Ca^{2+} exchange regulatory mechanisms in this process. Furthermore, proton block of the exchanger could be separated into two relatively discrete components. One component, described as a rapid primary block, was evident irrespective of whether Na$^+$ was present. The secondary block occurred more slowly and was observed only in the presence of Na$^+$ (77). Subsequent modeling of these responses has implicated the Na$_i^+$-dependent inactivation mechanism in the modulatory effects of pH$_i$ (78).

Cytoskeletal Interactions

The Na$^+$–Ca^{2+} exchanger has been demonstrated to bind ankyrin with high affinity (200). Ankyrins are thought to serve as links between the spectrin-based cytoskeletal system and various membrane proteins (18). The functional importance of the interaction between the Na$^+$–Ca^{2+} exchanger and ankyrin is unknown but may serve to localize the exchanger to its appropriate sarcolemmal location (45). Reeves and coworkers demonstrated an inhibition of Na$^+$–Ca^{2+} exchange activity in Chinese hamster ovary cells in response to cytochalasin D treatment or ATP depletion, both of which produced a breakdown in the actin cytoskeleton (55). In addition, interactions have been identified between mitochondrial Ca^{2+} uptake and Na$^+$–Ca^{2+} exchange activity based on results using nocodazole, an agent that depolymerizes microtubules (254).

PHARMACOLOGY OF Na$^+$–Ca^{2+} EXCHANGE

The Exchanger Inhibitory Peptide, XIP

The inhibitory actions of the 20 amino acid XIP peptide on Na$^+$–Ca^{2+} exchange were first described in 1991 by Li et al. (199), shortly after the cloning of the cardiac exchanger (241). The amino acid sequence of XIP, RRLLFYKYVYKRYRAGKQRG, duplicates that of amino acids 219–238 on the canine NCX1.1 exchanger. This region was originally identified based on its similarity to a calmodulin-binding domain (241). When applied to the cytoplasmic face of the exchanger, the synthetic XIP peptide was found to be a potent inhibitor [50% inhibitory concentration (IC$_{50}$) of 0.15–1.5 μM] of Na$^+$–Ca^{2+} exchange in several systems, including cardiac sarcolemmal vesicles and excised sarcolemmal membrane patches (122, 199), cardiac myocytes (38, 49, 174), and excised membrane patches from *Xenopus* oocytes expressing various Na$^+$–Ca^{2+} exchangers (143, 198). The corresponding XIP sequences of NCX1, NCX2, and NCX3 are highly conserved (202). Peptides based on these sequences (called XIP1, XIP2, and XIP3 corresponding to the exchanger isoforms from which they where derived) were all shown to be active inhibitors of NCX1. Inhibitory potency against NCX1 activity was greatest for XIP1 and somewhat reduced for the other peptides (202). These investigators also found prominent effects of the experimental system employed in this assay. While all experiments examined Na$^+$-dependent ^{45}Ca^{2+} uptake, inhibitory potency was greatest in sarcolemmal membrane vesicles or for the reconstituted exchanger in proteoliposomes containing 55% phosphatidylcholine–25% phosphatidylscrine–20% cholesterol. The inhibitory potency was greatly reduced in membrane vesicles from baby hamster kidney (BHK) cells expressing NCX1 or upon reconstitution in asolectin (202).

The XIP peptide has been analyzed extensively with respect to residues essential for its inhibitory actions (122, 331, 332). In general, maximal inhibitory potency requires the full length of this 20 amino acid peptide. Truncations from either end led to a reduction in inhibitory potency. The interaction of XIP with its target site involves a combination of electrostatic and hydrophobic interactions. Charge neutralization at either arginine 12 or 14 led to a prominent reduction in potency in one study (122) whereas these residues were considered less essential by Xu et al. (331), who determined that at least one lysine residue (located at positions 7, 11, and 17) was critical for inhibition (331). Interestingly, arginine 12 and 14 were also found to be non-essential for inhibition of the plasma membrane Ca^{2+} pump (332). He et al. (122) also demonstrated the involvement of several aromatic residues in the inhibitory effects of XIP, including tyrosine 6, phenylalanine 5, and tyrosine 8. While there is some disagreement as to the specific roles of particular amino acid residues of XIP, it is interesting to compare these studies with the results obtained from structure–function analysis of the endogenous XIP region. In NCX1.1, mutations F223E (equivalent to phenylalanine 5), K225Q (equivalent to lysine 7), Y226T (equivalent to tyrosine 6), and R230Q (equivalent to arginine 12), all led to an acceleration of Na$_i^+$-dependent inactivation (218). In contrast, K229Q (equivalent to lysine 11) completely eliminates the inactivation process. These results tend to corroborate the findings from both groups of investigators (122, 331, 332).

XIP is a reasonably specific inhibitor of Na^+–Ca^{2+} exchange although cross-reactivity has been demonstrated with sarcolemmal Ca^{2+}-ATPases and presumably will occur with other calmodulin-regulated enzymes as well (89, 90). This cross-reactivity, combined with the requirement for intracellular application, limits the widespread utilization of XIP in studies of cardiac Na^+–Ca^{2+} exchange function. However, results obtained with the XIP peptide have necessitated the reevaluation of much previous work. Previously, it was assumed that measurements of Na^+–Ca^{2+} exchange activity in vesicular preparations were derived from a mixed vesicle population (i.e. equal numbers of inside-out and outside-out vesicles). Studies using the XIP peptide revealed nearly complete inhibition of exchange activity in sarcolemmal vesicles, whereas extracellular application of XIP to intact cells was largely ineffective. This finding led to the conclusion that only inside-out vesicles contribute to Na^+–Ca^{2+} exchange activity measurements in mixed-vesicle populations (199). Considering the differences in Ca^{2+} affinities of the exchanger at the intracellular (μM) and extracellular (mM) transport sites, this interpretation seems reasonable.

Other Peptide Inhibitors

Several other peptides have been identified as relatively potent and specific inhibitors of the Na^+–Ca^{2+} exchanger. For example, based on earlier work demonstrating an inhibitory effect of opiate agonists and antagonists on Na^+–Ca^{2+} exchange (165), Khananshvili et al. (164) demonstrated that the molluscan cardioexcitatory peptide Phe-Met-Arg-Phe (FMRF)-amide, and various analogues could inhibit Na^+–Ca^{2+} exchange activity in sarcolemmal vesicles. Subsequently, this group of investigators proceeded to identify a series of small cyclic hexapeptides [e.g. Phe-Arg-Cys-Arg-Cys-Phe (FRCRCF)-amide, myristyl-FRCRCF-amide] with inhibitory actions (166). When studied in rabbit ventricular myocytes, complete inhibition of Na^+–Ca^{2+} activity was observed with 1 μM pipette FRCRCF-amide and a K_D of 22.7 nM was reported (136). A cell permeant analog, myristyl-FRCRCF-amide, was subsequently found to inhibit Na^+–Ca^{2+} exchange in rabbit myocytes with reduced potency (57). The inhibitory potency of FRCRCF-amide has not been reproducible in another laboratory, which reported that, inhibition of Na^+–Ca^{2+} exchange activity mediated by NCX1, NCX2, and NCX3 ranged from 32% to 41% with 50 μM FRCRCF-amide (202). Clearly, additional studies using these peptides are required to establish their utility as Na^+–Ca^{2+} exchange inhibitors.

KB-R7943

The compound, KB-R7943 (formerly No. 7943), has become increasingly employed as a tool to investigate Na^+–Ca^{2+} exchange function. This sulphonylurea derivative, 2-[-2-[4-(4-nitrobenzyloxy)-phenyl]ethyl]isothiourea methanesulfonate, was first described in 1996 (151, 327) as a selective inhibitor of the reverse mode of Na^+–Ca^{2+} exchange transport. Since these original descriptions, several controversial aspects have emerged regarding the mechanism of action of KB-R7943. In general, its inhibitory mechanism is poorly understood. Despite this uncertainty, KB-R7943 has been shown to provide substantial protection against a wide array of cellular injury models, particularly in heart. Furthermore, it seems clear that the increasing use of this compound will provide insight into the physiological and pathophysiological role of Na^+–Ca^{2+} exchange. Mechanistic studies targeting the inhibitory actions of KB-R7943 are also likely to contribute to our understanding of Na^+–Ca^{2+} exchange function, in general.

Before describing the controversies surrounding the actions of KB-R7943, it is important to emphasize the reasons underlying the high level of interest associated with this compound. First, a selective inhibitor would be an extremely powerful scientific tool with which to investigate Na^+–Ca^{2+} exchange function. At present, pharmacological tools to modify Na^+–Ca^{2+} exchange transport are extremely limited. Selective inhibition of a specific transport mode of Na^+–Ca^{2+} exchange is even more attractive. Clearly, the selectivity of KB-R7943 for Na^+–Ca^{2+} exchange over other ion-transport pathways is not ideal, and numerous other ion channels are inhibited by this agent. However, until more selective agents become available, KB-R7943 shows great promise as an experimental tool for evaluating the consequences and benefits of inhibiting Na^+–Ca^{2+} exchange.

At present, there is no consensus regarding the inhibitory mechanism(s) of KB-R7943 with respect to selectivity for transport modes, potency, mode of action, and isoform specificity. In the original two reports describing the effects of KB-R7943, a preferential inhibition of reverse mode Na^+–Ca^{2+} exchange was observed and similar potencies were reported (151, 327). That is, reverse mode Na^+–Ca^{2+} exchange was inhibited with IC_{50} ranging from 0.3 to 2.4 μM whereas the IC_{50} for forward mode exchange were approximately 10–50-fold higher. The mechanism of inhibition was reported to be noncompetitive with respect to Na^+ and

Ca^{2+} in one study (151), whereas KB-R7943 was found to be a competitive antagonist with extracellular Ca^{2+} in two other consecutive reports (326, 327). More recently, Kimura et al. (171) reported that bi-directional block of Na^+-Ca^{2+} exchange was direction-independent. In their study, Na^+-Ca^{2+} exchange currents were activated in myocytes using voltage ramps under constant ionic conditions. Differential inhibition of Na^+-Ca^{2+} exchanger isoforms by KB-R7943 was observed in one study where NCX3 exhibited threefold greater sensitivity (153). This study evaluated NCX1, NCX2, and NCX3 exchangers expressed in CCL-39 fibroblasts using Na_i^+-dependent $^{45}Ca^{2+}$ uptake. Half-maximal inhibitory potencies (IC_{50}) ranged from 4.9 to 1.5 μM for the three isoforms. In contrast, Linck et al. (202) examined the same isoforms in BHK cells and did not observe differential selectivity of KB-R7943. In addition, the potency of KB-R7943 was found to be far less than in previous reports. At 10 μM KB-R7943, inhibition ranged from 30% to 45%. This study employed Na^+ gradient–dependent $^{45}Ca^{2+}$ uptake into membrane vesicles isolated from the transfected cells. The reasons for these differences are unknown.

Despite uncertainties concerning its mechanism of action, KB-R7943 has been used extensively to assess the role of reverse Na^+-Ca^{2+} exchange in several pathophysiological models. Surprisingly, the results have been very encouraging and largely unanimous in demonstrating beneficial effects of this agent. In their first report of KB-R7943, Iwamoto et al., demonstrated protection against the Ca^{2+} paradox model of injury in guinea pig myocytes (151). In guinea pig papillary muscles, 10 μM KB-R7943 was shown to offer protection against reoxygenation-induced injury (231). KB-R7943 has been shown to be protective against ischemia-reperfusion injury in perfused rat hearts (237) and in reoxygenation injury in isolated rat myocytes (178). Calcium overload due to metabolic inhibition was suppressed by KB-R7943 in guinea pig myocytes (246). Furthermore, ouabain-induced arrhythmias were suppressed both in vivo and in vitro in guinea pig by KB-R7943 (325). With ^{23}Na nuclear magnetic resonance spectroscopy, KB-R7943 was shown to reduce the recovery rate of intracellular Na^+ levels during reperfusion, highlighting the role of reverse Na^+-Ca^{2+} exchange in this process (147). This agent also suppressed the propagation of hypercontracture in rat myocyte cell pairs, where Na^+ passage through gap junctions was reported to mediate the cell-to-cell propagation of injury (276). In one report, KB-R7943 failed to produce beneficial efforts on ischemia-reperfusion-induced arrhythmias in anaesthetized rats (213).

KB-R7943 has come to be used more and more as a tool for assessing the contribution of reverse Na^+-Ca^{2+} exchange under physiological and pathophysiological conditions. For example, KB-R7943 has been used to establish a role for Na^+-Ca^{2+} exchange in rat peritoneal mast cells (267) and pancreatic islet cells exhibiting a glucose-mediated Ca_i^{2+} increase (337). Studies in rat hepatocytes employed KB-R7943 to examine the mechanism of PKC-mediated Na^+-Ca^{2+} exchange stimulation (146). Na^+-Ca^{2+} exchange has also been implicated in the reversible osmotic opening of the blood–brain barrier based on the responses to KB-R7943 (236). The cardiac inotropic efforts produced by endothelin-1 (335) and angiotensin II (100) employed KB-R7943 to establish the role of Na^+-Ca^{2+} exchange in these responses. The contribution of Na^+-Ca^{2+} exchange in contraction and relaxation of failing human ventricular myocytes was evaluated using KB-R7943 (64, 103). This agent has also been shown to produce beneficial effects in noncardiac models of Ca_i^{2+}-mediated injury. In rat hippocampal slices subjected to hypoxic–hypoglycemic injury, KB-R7943 significantly protected CA1 neurons (172). Partial protection was observed in an oxygen and glucose deprivation model in rat striatal neurons (42). Acute renal failure in rats induced by an ischemia–reperfusion model of kidney injury was suppressed by KB-R7943 (176).

A recent study employing KB-R7943 as a selective blocker of reverse exchange demonstrated that this transport mode is unlikely to be important for normal excitation–contraction coupling in rat (280). KB-R7943 did not influence steady-state twitches, Ca^{2+} transients, sarcoplasmic reticulum (SR) Ca^{2+} load, or post-rest potentiation. However, KB-R7943 did reduce many of the toxic manifestations of strophanthidin treatment, including the abolition of spontaneous Ca^{2+} oscillations and a reduction in diastolic Ca^{2+} levels. Despite this action, KB-R7943 did not abolish the inotropic effects of strophanthidin (280).

In summary, while the inhibitory mechanism of KB-R7943 remains largely unknown, it is clearly beneficial in a variety of injury models in which Ca_i^{2+}-overload has been implicated. Furthermore, this agent may prove useful toward investigating the transport mechanism of Na^+-Ca^{2+} exchange, as well as the physiological role of different Na^+-Ca^{2+} exchange transport modes. The widespread use of KB. R7943, in spite of its limitations, attests to the need for specific inhibitors of this transport system.

Other Inhibitors

A large number of compounds have been reported to exert inhibitory effects on the cardiac Na^+-Ca^{2+} exchanger. In general, all of these substances exert modest effects and/or lack specificity. Therefore, their use and utility in investigating Na^+–Ca^{2+} exchange has been limited. This topic has recently been reviewed in detail (34) and is not reiterated here.

STUDIES IN TRANSGENIC MICE

Transgenic mice have become a common model for investigating physiological properties of Na^+–Ca^{2+} exchange function. To date, these studies have been restricted to investigating the consequences of over-expressing the wild-type NCX1.1 exchanger (3, 16, 62, 222, 308, 336) or a deletion mutant of NCX1.1, called Δ680–685 (222), driven by the cardiospecific α-myosin heavy chain (α-MHC) promoter. In all of these study, Na^+–Ca^{2+} exchange activity or levels were increased approximately 2–9-fold above background, depending on the parameter used for assessment. Surprisingly, the consequences of this maneuver appear to be relatively subtle. While differences have been identified, the physiological alterations are relatively minor.

In the first reported study investigating over-expression of NCX1.1 (3), the major changes included a 3–4-fold increase in the Na^+–Ca^{2+} exchange current induced by caffeine application and a 2.5-fold increase in the decay rate of the Ca_i^{2+} transient and associated I_{NaCa}. Furthermore, release of SR Ca^{2+} by reverse exchange (upon depolarization to +80 mV) was observed in only a fraction of myocytes from transgenic mice, and never from control mice. The investigators concluded that the primary consequences of over-expression were manifest as changes in Ca^{2+} efflux, as opposed to increasing Ca^{2+} entry via reverse exchange. Furthermore, over-expression of the exchanger did not appear to alter intracellular Ca^{2+} handling or conventional Ca^{2+}-induced Ca^{2+} release (3).

Subsequent studies employing transgenic mice have been generally consistent with respect to the observation of enhanced Ca^{2+} efflux via the exchanger. However, one report suggests that augmented reverse exchange is a prominent consequence of Na^+-Ca^{2+} exchange over-expression. Specifically, Yao et al. (336) reported that electrically stimulated Ca_i^{2+} transients were maintained in the presence of nifedipine, indicating that SR Ca^{2+} release could be triggered by reverse exchange in transgenic mice. Neither Na_i^+ levels nor Ca^{2+} channel current density was altered in this preparation and no evidence was found to suggest alterations in the Ca^{2+}-ATPase from the sarcoplasmic reticulum (336). The inotropic responsiveness to the Na^+ channel agonist, BDF 9148, was shown to be increased in transgenic mice over-expressing NCX1.1 (16). This result is interesting from a clinical perspective, as increases in Na^+–Ca^{2+} exchange levels, as well as increased sensitivity to BDF 9148, have been reported during heart failure (95). This study did not attempt to distinguish between the consequences of forward vs. reverse exchange but did confirm that major sarcoplasmic reticulum proteins (calsequestrin, phospholamban, and the SR Ca^{2+}-ATPase) were unchanged.

In contrast to the above studies, which did not provide evidence for changes in SR calcium handling, Terracciano et al. (308) observed a prominent increase in both the SR Ca^{2+} load (69% greater) and the ability of the SR to mediate Ca^{2+} uptake in the absence of Na^+–Ca^{2+} exchange. These investigators did not detect changes in SR Ca^{2+} handling proteins (i.e. SERCA2a, phospholamban, and calsequestrin), consistent with the above reports. The time to peak of the Ca^{2+} transient was faster in transgenic mice, consistent with an augmented SR Ca^{2+} load. However, this result differs from the report by Yao et al. (336), in which a delayed time to peak of the Ca^{2+} transient was observed.

The study by Cross et al. (62) demonstrated a gender-specific consequence of Na^+–Ca^{2+} exchange over-expression. Specifically, male transgenic mice had greater susceptibility than wild-type males to ischemia–reperfusion injury. In contrast, the response to this insult did not differ between female transgenic mice and female controls. After bilateral ovariectomy, the response of hearts from female transgenic mice became similar to that of male transgenics, implicating a role for female hormones (e.g. estrogen) in this protective effect. Gender distinctions were not examined in any other reports.

The role of ionic regulation of Na^+–Ca^{2+} exchange was examined by comparing the response of transgenic animals over-expressing NCX1.1 and the NCX1.1. deletion mutant, Δ680–685 (222). This deletion mutant lacks Ca^{2+}-dependent (I_2) regulation and Na_i^+-dependent (I_1) regulation is greatly reduced. Electrophysiological analyses using the giant excised patch technique provided clear evidence that over-expression of the mutant exchanger could overwhelm the native ionic regulatory processes. Ionic regulation was not altered in transgenic mice over-expressing NCX1.1, compared to controls. Post-rest potentiation was used to investigate the competition between Na^+–Ca^{2+} exchange and the sarcoplasmic reticulum for cytosolic Ca^{2+} removal. At all frequencies and rest intervals examined, an augmentation of post-rest potentiation was observed in papillary muscles from transgenic mice over-expressing the Δ680–685 mutant exchanger. Thus, ionic regulation of Na^+–Ca^{2+} exchange does appear to serve a role in cardiac excitation–contraction coupling.

To date, studies of Na^+–Ca^{2+} exchange using transgenic animals have not contributed greatly to our understanding of physiological Na$^+$–Ca^{2+} exchange function. While experimental protocols have provided evidence for enhanced exchange activity, the consequences of this intervention have been relatively modest. Surprisingly, there do not appear to be major compensatory changes in proteins involved in sarcoplasmic reticulum Ca^{2+} handling. In contrast, over-expression of phospholamban in transgenic mice results in a dramatic increase (nearly fourfold) in Na$^+$–Ca^{2+} exchange protein levels (138). One possible explanation for the relatively innocuous consequences of exchanger over-expression is that Na$^+$-Ca^{2+} exchangers may normally be present in large excess over the number required for physiological cardiac function. Therefore, adding to this excess by over-expression of wild-type exchangers might be relatively benign, provided that their normal regulatory properties are retained. Continued examination of mutant exchangers using this approach should provide insight into specific regulatory mechanisms.

ADENOVIRAL TRANSFECTION OF Na$^+$–Ca^{2+} EXCHANGE PROTEINS

Studies employing adenoviral transfection of the Na$^+$–Ca^{2+} exchanger in cardiac myocytes have recently appeared. In two abstract reports, the consequences of over-expressing the Na$^+$–Ca^{2+} exchanger by this method were very pronounced (19, 307). Most transfected cells failed to exhibit a caffeine-induced inward Na$^+$–Ca^{2+} exchange current, indicating near complete depletion of SR Ca^{2+}. Furthermore, cell shortening was reduced more than 50% in transfected cells. These data demonstrate the profound consequences of skewing the competition for Ca^{2+} removal to favor Na$^+$–Ca^{2+} exchange over SR Ca^{2+} uptake. Furthermore, they suggest that massive over-expression of Na$^+$–Ca^{2+} exchange per se is unlikely to produce a positive inotropic response. In general, it may prove difficult to titrate the levels of Na$^+$–Ca^{2+} exchange over-expression using this approach. However, if this can be accomplished, the adenoviral transfection technique could provide a rapid and effective means to examine both wild-type and mutant Na$^+$–Ca^{2+} exchangers.

ANTISENSE OLIGONUCLEOTIDES

The use of antisense oligonucleotides (AS-ODN) to investigate Na$^+$–Ca^{2+} exchange function has increased (205, 298) and a review of this topic has recently appeared (286). Overall, this approach has provided a convincing demonstration of the importance of Na$^+$–Ca^{2+} exchange in mediating cardiac relaxation (205, 286). Following a 48 hour treatment with AS-ODN targeting the Na$^+$–Ca^{2+} exchanger in cardiac myocytes, current measurements of reverse and forward mode Na$^+$–Ca^{2+} exchange were essentially abolished. Ca$^{2+}_i$ transients were induced by flash photolysis of caged Ca^{2+} in these studies. After treatment with AS-ODN and impairment of SR function, the decay of the Ca^{2+} transient was severely reduced in these myocytes, illustrating the lack of parallel pathways for transsarcolemmal Ca^{2+} removal. This approach has also revealed a role for Na$^+$–Ca^{2+} exchange in modulating the spontaneous beating frequency of cultured cardiac myocytes (306). The use of AS-ODN knockdown of Na$^+$–Ca^{2+} exchange has been used in a number of other cell types with similar functional consequences to Ca^{2+} homeostasis (299, 318, 330). While the use of AS-ODN affords the opportunity to modulate Na$^+$–Ca^{2+} exchange levels, at present, it seems unlikely to provide the stability required to assess the consequences of graded reductions. However, in the absence of specific pharmacological tools, improvements in this approach may prove to be useful in the near future. To date, no studies have reported knockout of the Na$^+$–Ca^{2+} exchanger in transgenic animals. The results obtained using AS-ODN suggest that the creation of a knockout would almost certainly be lethal in the embryonic stage.

FREQUENCY-DEPENDENT BEHAVIOR OF Na$^+$–Ca^{2+} EXCHANGE

Advances in electrophysiological approaches have greatly facilitated the investigation of Na$^+$–Ca^{2+} exchange proteins. As already indicated, the giant excised patch technique has vastly improved our ability to study transport and kinetic features for both native and cloned exchangers. While elementary current events, analogous to single-channel recordings, have eluded detection, the kinetic features of regulation are completely amenable to investigation. In fact, ionic regulatory mechanisms are surprisingly slow. Specifically, Na$_i^+$-dependent inactivation develops with a time course of seconds (127). Ca^{2+}-dependent regulation can proceed within solution switching time (eg. 100 msec) or develop over a time course of seconds when steady-state currents are examined (127, 132, 219). While alternative splicing has been demonstrated to alter the kinetic features of ionic regulation (81, 251, 252), there is no information concerning the significance of these different regulatory profiles.

We have recently begun to investigate ionic regulatory properties of Na$^+$–Ca^{2+} exchange at near physiological frequencies (142). The intent of this work has been to establish how ionic regulation might be expected to behave under more physiological conditions.

Interestingly, alternatively spliced Na^+–Ca^{2+} exchangers (NCX1.1, NCX1.3, and NCX1.4) show unique frequency-dependent profiles. Continued efforts along these lines may provide additional insight into how ionic regulation is kinetically tuned to be appropriate for tissue-specific Ca^{2+} homeostasis requirements. Ultimately, however, a role for these processes remains to be identified.

DEVELOPMENTAL CHANGES

The activity and levels of Na^+–Ca^{2+} exchange are developmentally regulated in cardiac muscle. In general, these developmental changes coincide with progressive maturation of the t-tubular system and the sarcoplasmic reticulum. In neonates, both transverse tubules and the sarcoplasmic reticulum are poorly developed. Consequently, excitation–contraction coupling occurs largely via transsarcolemmal Ca^{2+} fluxes. For example, Cohen and Lederer (52) demonstrated that ryanodine abolished contractions in adult rat myocytes but had no effect on neonatal myocytes. Furthermore, prominent interaction was observed between Ca^{2+} currents and SR function in adult myocytes, whereas these affects were absent or greatly reduced in neonatal myocytes. Ca^{2+} current density has been reported to be greater in rat neonatal myocytes than in adult cells (52), although opposite results have been observed in rabbit myocytes (328). Regardless of these differences, there is consensus that neonatal cardiac cells initially depend upon transsarcolemmal Ca^{2+} fluxes (i.e. Ca^{2+} channels and Na^+–Ca^{2+} exchange) for excitation–contraction coupling. As the T-tubules and sarcoplasmic reticulum rapidly develop, reliance on intracellular Ca^{2+} stores becomes more prominent (5, 48, 107, 161). In a study examining old (24 months) and senescent (34 months) hearts in mice, Na^+–Ca^+ exchange levels were found to be considerably lower than those from adults (5 months) (201).

Na^+–Ca^{2+} exchange has been shown to be particularly prominent in late fetal life and early neonatal life based on the assessment of sarcolemmal Na^+–Ca^{2+} exchange activity and protein levels (7). Furthermore, Na^+–Ca^{2+} exchange mRNA levels were found to be 6–8-fold higher in rat (postnatal day 1) and rabbit myocytes (gestational day 29) than in myocytes from adults of either species (36). Na^+–Ca^{2+} exchange current density measurements revealed similar developmental changes in rabbit and guinea pig myocytes (8). Furthermore, neonatal rabbit myocytes were found to rely more heavily than adult cells on Na^+–Ca^{2+} exchange for intracellular Ca^{2+} removal during cardiac relaxation. Wetzel et al. (329) proposed that reverse Na^+–Ca^{2+} exchange may play a prominent role in providing intracellular Ca^{2+} to support cardiac contractions in neonatal rabbit cells. This idea has received additional support in a recent study by Haddock et al. (107). Here, newborn and adult rabbit ventricular myocytes were studied using confocal microscopy to evaluate subsarcolemmal and cell center Ca^{2+} transients as well as Ca^{2+} sparks. The investigators found that subsarcolemmal Ca^{2+} increased more quickly than cell center Ca^{2+} in newborn myocytes. In contrast, adult myocytes showed similar increases of Ca^{2+} at both locations. Immunolabeling studies demonstrated overlapping distributions for ryanodine receptors and Na^+–Ca^{2+} exchange in adult cells, but not in neonatal cells. Calcium sparks were observed primarily at the periphery of neonatal cells and the absence of t-tubules was confirmed using confocal sarcolemmal imaging. These experimental data were supported with a mathematical model demonstrating that Ca^{2+} fluxes via the exchanger were sufficient to account for both contraction and relaxation, even in the absence of sarcoplasmic reticulum and sarcolemmal Ca^{2+} channel function (107).

A major therapeutic opportunity appears to exist if information concerning the role of Na^+–Ca^{2+} exchange in neonatal cardiac excitation–contraction coupling could be used to improve myocardial preservation during pediatric cardiac surgery. Deep hypothermic circulatory arrest is commonly employed during surgery (177, 317) as an adjunct to pharmacological cardioplegia (9, 230). Furthermore, cardiac inotropic support is commonly used postoperatively. If the neonate represents a unique case of cardiac excitation–contraction coupling, with a prominent reliance on Na^+–Ca^{2+} exchange, then it would seem particularly worthwhile to reevaluate existing cardioplegic strategies in light of this information.

SPECIES DIFFERENCES

The relative levels of Na^+–Ca^{2+} exchange activity across species remain controversial. For example, using whole-cell current and fluorescence measurements, Sham et al. (292) found a rank order of Na^+–Ca^{2+} exchange activity (current densities in pA/pF are indicated in brackets) as follows: hamster (2.27) > guinea pig (1.06) ≥ human (0.54) ≥ rat (0.20). More recently, Su et al. (305) proposed a rank order of mouse (∼1.3) > rat (∼1.05) > rabbit (∼0.8) > dog (∼0.7) > human (∼0.6) based on whole-cell Na^+–Ca^{2+} exchange current measurements activated by removal of extracellular Na^+. The data with respect to rat myocytes are the most discordant. While the approaches used to obtain estimates of Na^+–Ca^{2+} exchange activity differed between these studies, the two approaches were internally consistent. At present, there is no obvious reason for the reported differences.

PATHOPHYSIOLOGICAL ALTERATIONS IN Na$^+$-Ca^{2+} EXCHANGE

Contribution of Na$^+$–Ca^{2+} Exchange to Cardiac Injury

Altered Na$^+$–Ca^{2+} exchange function and levels have been implicated in a variety of cardiac injury and disease models. A representative, rather than comprehensive, description is provided here, as this topic could easily constitute a separate review. Underlying the interest in this area is the consensus view that Na$^+$–Ca^{2+} exchange is a primary Ca^{2+} efflux pathway in cardiac myocytes and also has the ability to serve as a Ca^{2+} entry mechanism. Consequently, any malfunction of the Na$^+$–Ca^{2+} exchanger would be expected to result in serious disruption of Ca^{2+} homeostasis (228). As already mentioned, the Na$^+$–Ca^{2+} exchange system may remove the same amount of Ca^{2+} entering a myocyte on a beat-to-beat basis. Any imbalance would lead to Ca^{2+} overload or depletion, irrespective of other internal Ca^{2+} sequestration mechanisms. Furthermore, even if net transsarcolemmal Ca^{2+} flux balance was preserved, alterations in Na$^+$–Ca^{2+} exchange activity could presumably alter the nature of Ca^{2+} transients (27, 32), action potential characteristics (17, 30, 155, 156, 195, 209, 232, 233, 247, 248), and diastolic Ca^{2+} levels (32, 168, 229), and could contribute to arrythmogenic transient inward currents (83, 204).

Ischemic and hypoxic injury of cardiac muscle is associated with a prominent acidification of the cell interior as metabolism switches to glycolytic pathways (6, 262). Upon reperfusion, the Na$^+$/H$^+$ countertransporter contributes to the restoration of cellular pH with a consequent elevation of intracellular Na$^+$ (43, 159, 160, 214). In addition, intracellular Na$^+$ increases directly as a consequence of ischemia, independent of events occurring during reperfusion (147). With respect to Na$^+$–Ca^{2+} exchange activity, this increase in intracellular Na$^+$ produces two major consequences: First, the ability to extrude Ca^{2+} from myocytes is compromised since the driving force (i.e., the Na$^+$ electrochemical gradient) for Ca^{2+} efflux by forward exchange is reduced. Second, the ability of the exchanger to serve as a Ca^{2+} entry mechanism is enhanced, again due to thermodynamic considerations. The net consequence is an increase in intracellular Ca^{2+} levels, which, depending upon severity, can progress to Ca^{2+} overload and associated cellular toxicity (108, 207, 210, 213). The recent studies employing KB-R7943 (described above) highlight the utility of blocking reverse Na$^+$–Ca^{2+} exchange in preventing this type of injury.

Alterations in Na$^+$–Ca^{2+} Exchange Levels

In failing human left ventricular myocytes, several reports have identified a tonic component of cardiac contraction that is mediated by reverse Na$^+$–Ca^{2+} exchange, and an important role for the Na$^+$–Ca^{2+} exchanger has been established in myocyte relaxation (31, 64, 103, 141, 221). Furthermore, alterations in Na$^+$–Ca^{2+} exchange protein, transcript, and activity levels have been identified in a variety of human cardiac diseases (112, 113). For example, Flesch et al. (95) showed increases in both protein and transcript levels for the Na$^+$–Ca^{2+} exchanger in hearts obtained from patients with idiopathic dilated cardiomyopathy and ischemic heart disease. Similarly, Studer et al. (303, 304) identified reciprocal changes in Na$^+$–Ca^{2+} exchange mRNA levels ($\sim$ 50% increases) and SR Ca^{2+}-ATPase mRNA levels ($\sim$ 50% decreases) in hearts with dilated cardiomyopathy and coronary artery disease. Transmural differences in NCX1 expression across the ventricular wall of failing human hearts have not been identified (in contrast to results for SERCA2a).

In contrast to the above reports, a recent study utilizing NYHA class IV hearts failed to detect a significant difference in Na$^+$–Ca^{2+} exchanger protein levels (289). This study, which examined dilated cardiomyopathy exclusively, identified significant reductions in ^{3}H-ouabain binding, and protein levels for the α1, α3, and β1 subunits of the Na$^+$,K$^+$-ATPase. The increased inotropic responsiveness to interventions elevating intracellular Na$^+$ were attributed to these alterations in Na$^+$ pump expression. Similarly, Komuro et al. failed to identify changes in NCX1 transcript levels in patients with end-stage heart failure (175). Hearts from patients exhibiting idiopathic dilated cardiomyopathy and coronary artery disease were studied in this group (175).

Numerous animal models of heart failure and hypertrophy have identified increases in Na$^+$–Ca^{2+} exchange levels or activity (111, 114, 137). In a rabbit model employing combined aortic constriction and insufficiency, total Na$^+$–Ca^{2+} exchange mRNA levels increased nearly threefold. Activity assessed electrophysiologically or by measurements of the exchange-mediated relaxation of caffeine-induced contractures was also significantly increased. Using a tachycardia-induced model of heart failure, O'Rourke et al. (250) demonstrated $\sim$100% increases in Na$^+$–Ca^{2+} exchange protein levels with similar increases in functional activity. These data appear to mimic the human heart failure condition and emphasize an important role for Na$^+$–

Ca^{2+} exchange as a compensatory mechanism for reduced function of the sarcoplasmic reticulum (261). However, while several lines of evidence suggest that Na^+–Ca^{2+} exchange levels are upregulated in heart failure, there is by no means, consensus on this issue. Furthermore, it is unclear whether an upregulation of Na^+–Ca^{2+} exchange would be advantageous to cardiac function. A great deal of work is required to clarify this issue and identify appropriate targets for intervention. Ultimately, our understanding of the role of Na^+–Ca^{2+} exchange alterations in disease requires considerably greater insight into its operation during physiological excitation–contraction coupling.

SUMMARY

It is interesting to compare our level of understanding of Na^+–Ca^{2+} exchange transport and regulation with that known for many ion channels. Whole-cell current measurements for ion channels are readily understood by considering that $I = Np_oi$. Many channels are easily quantified using highly specific labels. Alterations in channel activity, either physiologically or pharmacologically, often appear as a consequence of changing some characteristic of the opening probability (135). For Na^+–Ca^{2+} exchange, we have become reasonably good at measuring whole-cell currents. However, there is little consensus on the number of exchangers contributing to these signals or on the size of the elementary currents producing these signals. Furthermore, most studies do not even consider the possibility that the exchanger population contributing to these signals might be regulated (i.e. have a specific probability of being active). Thus, our level of sophistication for evaluating Na^+–Ca^{2+} exchange function is, comparatively, quite low.

Fundamental advances have occurred over the past decade in our understanding of the Na^+–Ca^{2+} exchange system, particularly at the molecular level. Moreover, alterations in Na^+–Ca^{2+} exchange activity and expression are known to occur in a variety of cardiac diseases. In fact, operation of the exchanger in its reverse transport mode may be a prominent mediator of cellular injury under specific pathophysiological conditions. Despite the high level of progress that has been made, there remains a chasm between molecular studies of Na^+–Ca^{2+} exchange and an integrated picture of its role in physiology and pathophysiology. While bridges across this chasm are slowly appearing, it seems that there is a great deal to be learned to seamlessly integrate this field. The next decade promises to be particularly exciting for investigations of the Na^+–Ca^{2+} exchange transport system.

REFERENCES

1. Anonymous. The effect of digoxin on mortality and morbidity in patients with heart failure. The Digitalis Investigation Group. *N. Engl. J. Med.* 336:525–533, 1997.
2. Abete, P. and M. Vassalle. Relation between Na^+-K^+ pump, Na^+ activity and force in strophanthidin inotropy in sheep cardiac Purkinje fibres. *J. Physiol. (Lond.)* 404:275–299, 1988.
3. Adachi-Akahane, S., L. Lu, Z. Li, J. S. Frank, K. D. Philipson and M. Morad. Calcium signaling in transgenic mice overexpressing cardiac Na^+-Ca^{2+} exchanger. *J. Gen. Physiol.* 109:717–729, 1997.
4. Adams, K. F., Jr. Clinical practice guidelines for heart failure. *Am. J. Manag. Care* 4:S329–S337, 1998.
5. Anderson, P. A. Maturation and cardiac contractility. *Cardiol. Clin.* 7:209–225, 1989.
6. Anderson, S. E., P. M. Cala, C. Steenbergen, R. E. London, and E. Murphy. Effects of hypoxia and acidification on myocardial Na and Ca. Role of Na-H and Na-Ca exchange. *Ann. N.Y. Acad. Sci.* 639:453–455, 1991.
7. Artman, M. Sarcolemmal Na^+-Ca^{2+} exchange activity and exchanger immunoreactivity in developing rabbit hearts. *Am. J. Physiol.* 263:H1506–H1513, 1992.
8. Artman, M., H. Ichikawa, M. Avkiran and W. A. Coetzee. Na^+/Ca^{2+} exchange current density in cardiac myocytes from rabbits and guinea pigs during postnatal development. *Am. J. Physiol.* 268 (*Heart Circ. Physiol.* 37):H1714–H1722, 1995.
9. Baker, E. J., G. N. Olinger and J. E. Baker. Calcium content of St. Thomas' II cardioplegic solution damages ischemic immature myocardium. *Ann. Thorac. Surg.* 52:993–999, 1991.
10. Baker, P. F., M. P. Blaustein, A. L. Hodgkin and R. A. Steinhardt. The influence of calcium on sodium efflux in squid axons. *J. Physiol. (Lond).* 200:431–458, 1969.
11. Barcenas-Ruiz, L., D. J. Beuckelmann and W. G. Wier. Sodium-calcium exchange in heart: membrane currents and changes in $[Ca^{2+}]_i$. *Science* 238:1720–1722, 1987.
12. Barry, W. H., Y. Hasin and T. W. Smith. Sodium pump inhibition, enhanced calcium influx via sodium-calcium exchange, and positive inotropic response in cultured heart cells. *Circ. Res.* 56:231–241, 1985.
13. Barry, W. H., C. A. Rasmussen, Jr., H. Ishida and J. H. Bridge. External Na-independent Ca extrusion in cultured ventricular cells. Magnitude and functional significance. *J. Gen. Physiol.* 88:393–411, 1986.
14. Bassani, R. A., J. W. Bassani and D. M. Bers. Relaxation in ferret ventricular myocytes: unusual interplay among calcium transport systems. *J. Physiol. (Lond.)* 476:295–308, 1994.
15. Bassani, R. A., J. W. Bassani and D. M. Bers. Relaxation in ferret ventricular myocytes: role of the sarcolemmal Ca ATPase. *Pflugers Arch.* 430:573–578, 1995.
16. Baumer, A. T., M. Flesch, H. Kilter, K. D. Philipson and M. Bohm. Overexpression of the Na^+-Ca^{2+} exchanger leads to enhanced inotropic responsiveness to Na^+-channel agonist without sarcoplasmic reticulum protein changes in transgenic mice. *Biochem. Biophys. Res. Commun.* 249:786–790, 1998.
17. Benardeau, A., S. N. Hatem, C. Rucker-Martin, B. Le Grand, L. Mace, P. Dervanian, J. J. Mercadier and E. Coraboeuf. Contribution of Na^+/Ca^{2+} exchange to action potential of human atrial myocytes. *Am. J. Physiol.* 271 (*Heart Circ. Physiol.* 40):H1151–H1161, 1996.
18. Bennett, V. Ankyrins. Adaptors between diverse plasma membrane proteins and the cytoplasm. *J. Biol. Chem.* 267:8703–8706, 1992.
19. Bernobich, E., K. Davia, H. K. Ranu, C. M. Terracciano, K. T. MacLeod, R. J. Hajjar and S. E. Harding. Adenovirus-mediated Na/Ca exchanger overexpression depresses contractile

function in adult rabbit cardiomyocytes. *Biophys. J.* 78:373A, 2000.
20. Bers, D. M. Mechanisms contributing to the cardiac inotropic effect of Na pump inhibition and reduction of extracellular Na. *J. Gen. Physiol.* 90:479–504, 1987.
21. Bers, D. M. *Excitation-Contraction Coupling and Cardiac Contractile Force.* London, UK: Kluwer Academic Publishers, 1991.
22. Bers, D. M., J. W. Bassani and R. A. Bassani. Competition and redistribution among calcium transport systems in rabbit cardiac myocytes. *Cardiovasc. Res.* 27:1772–1777, 1993.
23. Bers, D. M., J. W. Bassani and R. A. Bassani. Na-Ca exchange and Ca fluxes during contraction and relaxation in mammalian ventricular muscle. *Ann. N.Y. Acad. Sci.* 779:430–442, 1996.
24. Bers, D. M. and J. H. Bridge. Effect of acetylstrophanthidin on twitches, microscopic tension fluctuations and cooling contractures in rabbit ventricle. *J. Physiol. (Lond.)* 404:53–69, 1988.
25. Bers, D. M., J. H. Bridge and K. W. Spitzer. Intracellular Ca^{2+} transients during rapid cooling contractures in guinea-pig ventricular myocytes. *J. Physiol. (Lond).* 417:537–553, 1989.
26. Bers, D. M., D. M. Christensen and T. X. Nguyen. Can Ca entry via Na-Ca exchange directly activate cardiac muscle contraction? *J. Mol. Cell Cardiol.* 20:405–414, 1988.
27. Bers, D. M., W. J. Lederer and J. R. Berlin. Intracellular Ca transients in rat cardiac myocytes: role of Na-Ca exchange in excitation-contraction coupling. *Am. J. Physiol.* 258 (*Cell Physiol.* 27):C944–C954, 1990.
28. Bers, D. M. and E. Perez-Reyes. Ca channels in cardiac myocytes: structure and function in Ca influx and intracellular Ca release. *Cardiovasc. Res.* 42:339–360, 1999.
29. Bersohn, M. M., R. Vemuri, D. W. Schuil, R. S. Weiss and K. D. Philipson. Effect of temperature on sodium-calcium exchange in sarcolemma from mammalian and amphibian hearts. *Biochim. Biophys. Acta* 1062:19–23, 1991.
30. Bett, G., D. Noble, S. Noble, Y. Earm, W. K. Ho and I. S. So. Na-Ca exchange current during the cardiac action potential. *Adv. Exp. Med. Biol.* 311:453–454, 1992.
31. Beuckelmann, D. J., M. Nabauer and E. Erdmann. Intracellular calcium handling in isolated ventricular myocytes from patients with terminal heart failure. *Circulation* 85:1046–1055, 1992.
32. Beuckelmann, D. J. and W. G. Wier. Sodium-calcium exchange in guinea-pig cardiac cells: exchange current and changes in intracellular Ca^{2+}. *J. Physiol. (Lond.)* 414:499–520, 1989.
33. Blaustein, M. P., M. Juhaszova and V. A. Golovina. The cellular mechanism of action of cardiotonic steroids: a new hypothesis. *Clin. Exp. Hypertens.* 20:691–703, 1998.
34. Blaustein, M. P. and W. J. Lederer. Sodium/calcium exchange: its physiological implications. *Physiol. Rev.* 79:763–854, 1999.
35. Blaustein, M. P. and J. M. Russell. Sodium-calcium exchange and calcium-calcium exchange in internally dialyzed squid giant axons. *J. Membr. Biol.* 22:285–312, 1975.
36. Boerth, S. R., D. B. Zimmer and M. Artman. Steady-state mRNA levels of the sarcolemmal Na^+-Ca^{2+} exchanger peak near birth in developing rabbit and rat hearts. *Circ. Res.* 74:354–359, 1994.
37. Bouchard, R. A., R. B. Clark and W. R. Giles. Role of sodium-calcium exchange in activation of contraction in rat ventricle. *J. Physiol. (Lond.)* 472:391–413, 1993.
38. Bouchard, R. A., R. B. Clark and W. R. Giles. Regulation of unloaded cell shortening by sarcolemmal sodium-calcium exchange in isolated rat ventricular myocytes. *J. Physiol. (Lond.)* 469:583–599, 1993.
39. Bridge, J. H. Relationships between the sarcoplasmic reticulum and sarcolemmal calcium transport revealed by rapidly cooling rabbit ventricular muscle. *J. Gen. Physiol* 88:437–473, 1986.
40. Bridge, J. H., J. R. Smolley and K. W. Spitzer. The relationship between charge movements associated with I_{Ca} and $I_{Na\text{-}Ca}$ in cardiac myocytes. *Science* 248:376–378, 1990.
41. Bridge, J. H., K. W. Spitzer and P. R. Ershler. Relaxation of isolated ventricular cardiomyocytes by a voltage-dependent process. *Science* 241:823–825, 1988.
42. Calabresi, P., G. A. Marfia, S. Amoroso, A. Pisani and G. Bernardi. Pharmacological inhibition of the Na^+/Ca^{2+} exchanger enhances depolarizations induced by oxygen/glucose deprivation but not responses to excitatory amino acids in rat striatal neurons. *Stroke* 30:1687–1694, 1999.
43. Ch'en, F. F., R. D. Vaughan-Jones, K. Clarke and D. Noble. Modelling myocardial ischaemia and reperfusion. *Prog. Biophys. Mol. Biol.* 69:515–538, 1998.
44. Chen, F., G. Mottino, T. S. Klitzner, K. D. Philipson and J. S. Frank. Distribution of the Na^+/Ca^{2+} exchange protein in developing rabbit myocytes. *Am. J. Physiol.* 268 (*Cell Physiol.* 37): C1126–C1132, 1995.
45. Chen, F., G. Mottino, V. Y. Shin and J. S. Frank. Subcellular distribution of ankyrin in developing rabbit heart—relationship to the Na^+-Ca^{2+} exchanger. *J. Mol. Cell Cardiol.* 29:2621–2629, 1997.
46. Cheon, J. and J. P. Reeves. Site density of the sodium-calcium exchange carrier in reconstituted vesicles from bovine cardiac sarcolemma. *J. Biol. Chem.* 263:2309–2315, 1988.
47. Chernaya, G., M. Vazquez and J. P. Reeves. Sodium-calcium exchange and store-dependent calcium influx in transfected Chinese hamster ovary cells expressing the bovine cardiac sodium-calcium exchanger. Acceleration of exchange activity in thapsigargin-treated cells. *J. Biol. Chem.* 271:5378–5385, 1996.
48. Chin, T. K., W. F. Friedman and T. S. Klitzner. Developmental changes in cardiac myocyte calcium regulation. *Circ. Res.* 67: 574–579, 1990.
49. Chin, T. K., K. W. Spitzer, K. D. Philipson and J. H. Bridge. The effect of exchanger inhibitory peptide (XIP) on sodium-calcium exchange current in guinea pig ventricular cells. *Circ. Res.* 72: 497–503, 1993.
50. Choi, H. S. and D. A. Eisner. The effects of inhibition of the sarcolemmal Ca-ATPase on systolic calcium fluxes and intracellular calcium concentration in rat ventricular myocytes. *Pflugers Arch.* 437:966–971, 1999.
51. Choi, H. S. and D. A. Eisner. The role of sarcolemmal Ca^{2+}-ATPase in the regulation of resting calcium concentration in rat ventricular myocytes. *J. Physiol. (Lond.)* 515:109–118, 1999.
52. Cohen, N. M. and W. J. Lederer. Changes in the calcium current of rat heart ventricular myocytes during development. *J. Physiol. (Lond.)* 406:115–146, 1988.
53. Collins, A., A. V. Somlyo and D. W. Hilgemann. The giant cardiac membrane patch method: stimulation of outward Na^+-Ca^{2+} exchange current by MgATP. *J. Physiol. (Lond.)* 454:27–57, 1992.
54. Condrescu, M., G. Chernaya, V. Kalaria and J. P. Reeves. Barium influx mediated by the cardiac sodium-calcium exchanger in transfected Chinese hamster ovary cells. *J. Gen. Physiol.* 109: 41–51, 1997.
55. Condrescu, M., J. P. Gardner, G. Chernaya, J. F. Aceto, C. Kroupis and J. P. Reeves. ATP-dependent regulation of sodium-calcium exchange in Chinese hamster ovary cells transfected with the bovine cardiac sodium-calcium exchanger. *J. Biol. Chem.* 270:9137–9146, 1995.
56. Condrescu, M., B. M. Hantash, Y. Fang and J. P. Reeves. Mode-specific inhibition of sodium-calcium exchange during protein phosphatase blockade. *J. Biol. Chem.* 274:33279–33286, 1999.
57. Convery, M. K., A. J. Levi, D. Khananshvili and J. C. Hancox. Actions of myristyl-FRCRCFa, a cell-permeant blocker of the cardiac sarcolemmal Na-Ca exchanger, tested in rabbit ventricular myocytes. *Pflugers Arch.* 436:581–590, 1998.

58. Cook, O., W. Low and H. Rahamimoff. Membrane topology of the rat brain Na$^+$-Ca^{2+} exchanger". *Biochim. Biophys. Acta* 1371:40–52, 1998.
59. Cooper, C. B., R. J. Winkfein, R. T. Szerencsei and P. P. Schnetkamp. cDNA cloning and functional expression of the dolphin retinal rod Na-Ca+K exchanger NCKX1: comparison with the functionally silent bovine NCKX1. *Biochemistry* 38:6276–6283, 1999.
60. Cordeiro, J. M., S. Litwin and J. H. Bridge. Can NCX rapidly set the gain of EC coupling without directly triggering SR Ca release in heart? *Biophys. J.* 78:373A, 2000.
61. Crespo, L. M., C. J. Grantham and M. B. Cannell. Kinetics, stoichiometry and role of the Na-Ca exchange mechanism in isolated cardiac myocytes. *Nature* 345:618–621, 1990.
62. Cross, H. R., L. Lu, C. Steenbergen, K. D. Philipson and E. Murphy. Overexpression of the cardiac Na$^+$/Ca^{2+} exchanger increases susceptibility to ischemia/reperfusion injury in male, but not female, transgenic mice. *Circ.Res.* 83:1215–1223, 1998.
63. Diaz, M. E., A. W. Trafford, S. C. O'Neill and D. A. Eisner. Measurement of sarcoplasmic reticulum Ca^{2+} content and sarcolemmal Ca^{2+} fluxes in isolated rat ventricular myocytes during spontaneous Ca^{2+} release. *J. Physiol (Lond.)* 501:3–16, 1997.
64. Dipla, K., J. A. Mattiello, K. B. Margulies, V. Jeevanandam and S. R. Houser. The sarcoplasmic reticulum and the Na$^+$/Ca^{2+} exchanger both contribute to the Ca^{2+} transient of failing human ventricular myocytes. *Circ. Res.* 84:435–444, 1999.
65. DiPolo, R. Calcium influx in internally dialyzed squid giant axons. *J. Gen. Physiol.* 73:91–113, 1979.
66. DiPolo, R. and L. Beauge. The effect of pH on Ca^{2+} extrusion mechanisms in dialyzed squid axons. *Biochim. Biophys. Acta* 688:237–245, 1982.
67. DiPolo, R. and L. Beauge. In squid axons, ATP modulates Na$^+$-Ca^{2+} exchange by a Ca$^{2+}_i$-dependent phosphorylation. *Biochim. Biophys. Acta* 897:347–354, 1987.
68. DiPolo, R. and L. Beauge. Asymmetrical properties of the Na-Ca exchanger in voltage-clamped, internally dialyzed squid axons under symmetrical ionic conditions. *J. Gen. Physiol.* 95:819–835, 1990.
69. DiPolo, R. and L. Beauge. Regulation of Na-Ca exchange. An overview. *Ann. N. Y. Acad. Sci.* 639:100–111, 1991.
70. DiPolo, R. and L. Beauge. Effects of some metal-ATP complexes on Na$^+$-Ca^{2+} exchange in internally dialysed squid axons. *J. Physiol. (Lond.)* 462:71–86, 1993.
71. DiPolo, R. and L. Beauge. In squid axons the Ca$^{2+}_i$ regulatory site of the Na$^+$/Ca^{2+} exchanger is drastically modified by sulfhydryl blocking agents. Evidences that intracellular Ca$^{2+}_i$ regulatory and transport sites are different. *Biochim. Biophys. Acta* 1145:75–84, 1993.
72. DiPolo, R. and L. Beauge. Phosphoarginine stimulation of Na$^+$-Ca^{2+} exchange in squid axons-a new pathway for metabolic regulation?. *J. Physiol. (Lond.)* 487:57–66, 1995.
73. DiPolo, R. and L. Beauge. Differential up-regulation of Na$^+$-Ca^{2+} exchange by phosphoarginine and ATP in dialysed squid axons. *J. Physiol. (Lond.)* 507:737–747, 1998.
74. DiPolo, R. and L. Beauge. Metabolic pathways in the regulation of invertebrate and vertebrate Na$^+$/Ca^{2+} exchange. *Biochim. Biophys. Acta* 1422:57–71, 1999.
75. DiPolo, R. and H. Rojas. Effect of internal and external K$^+$ on Na$^+$-Ca^{2+} exchange in dialyzed squid axons under voltage clamp conditions. *Biochim. Biophys. Acta* 776:313–316, 1984.
76. DiPolo, R., H. Rojas and L. Beauge. Regulation of the Na/Ca exchanger. *Acta Cient. Venez.* 44:103–10, 1993.
77. Doering, A. E. and W. J. Lederer. The mechanism by which cytoplasmic protons inhibit the sodium-calcium exchanger in guinea-pig heart cells. *J. Physiol. (Lond.)* 466:481–499, 1993.
78. Doering, A. E. and W. J. Lederer. The action of Na$^+$ as a cofactor in the inhibition by cytoplasmic protons of the cardiac Na$^+$-Ca^{2+} exchanger in the guinea-pig. *J. Physiol. (Lond.)* 480:9–20, 1994.
79. Doering, A. E., D. A. Nicoll, Y. Lu, L. Lu, J. N. Weiss and K. D. Philipson. Topology of a functionally important region of the cardiac Na$^+$/Ca^{2+} exchanger. *J. Biol. Chem.* 273:778–783, 1998.
80. Durkin, J. T., D. C. Ahrens, Y. C. Pan and J. P. Reeves. Purification and amino-terminal sequence of the bovine cardiac sodium-calcium exchanger: evidence for the presence of a signal sequence. *Arch. Biochem. Biophys.* 290:369–375, 1991.
81. Dyck, C., K. Maxwell, J. Buchko, M. Trac, A. Omelchenko, M. Hnatowich and L. V. Hryshko. Structure-function analysis of CALX1.1, a Na$^+$-Ca^{2+} exchanger from *Drosophila*. Mutagenesis of ionic regulatory sites. *J. Biol. Chem.* 273:12981–12987, 1998.
82. Dyck, C., A. Omelchenko, C. L. Elias, B. D. Quednau, K. D. Philipson, M. Hnatowich and L. Hryshko. Ionic regulatory properties of brain and kidney splice variants of the NCX1 Na$^+$-Ca^{2+} exchanger. *J. Gen. Physiol.* 114:701–711, 1999.
83. Egdell, R. M. and K. T. MacLeod. Calcium extrusion during aftercontractions in cardiac myocytes: the role of the sodium-calcium exchanger in the generation of the transient inward current. *J. Mol. Cell Cardiol.* 32:85–93, 2000.
84. Egger, M. and E. Niggli. Regulatory function of Na-Ca exchange in the heart: milestones and outlook. *J. Membr. Biol.* 168:107–130, 1999.
85. Egger, M., A. Ruknudin, P. Lipp, P. Kofuji, W. J. Lederer, D. H. Schulze and E. Niggli. Functional expression of the human cardiac Na$^+$/Ca^{2+} exchanger in Sf9 cells: rapid and specific Ni^{2+} transport. *Cell Calcium* 25:9–17, 1999.
86. Egger, M., A. Ruknudin, E. Niggli, W. J. Lederer and D. H. Schulze. Ni^{2+} transport by the human Na$^+$/Ca^{2+} exchanger expressed in Sf9 cells. *Am. J. Physiol.* 276 (*Cell Physiol.* 45): C1184–C1192, 1999.
87. Eisner, D. A. and W. J. Lederer. Na-Ca exchange: stoichiometry and electrogenicity. *Am. J. Physiol.* 248 (*Cell Physiol.* 17):C189–C202, 1985.
88. Eisner, D. A., A. W. Trafford, M. E. Diaz, C. L. Overend and S. C. O'Neill. The control of Ca release from the cardiac sarcoplasmic reticulum: regulation versus autoregulation. *Cardiovasc. Res.* 38:589–604, 1998.
89. Enyedi, A. and J. T. Penniston. Autoinhibitory domains of various Ca^{2+} transporters cross-react. *J. Biol. Chem.* 268:17120–17125, 1993.
90. Enyedi, A., T. Vorherr, P. James, D. J. McCormick, A. G. Filoteo, E. Carafoli and J. T. Penniston. The calmodulin binding domain of the plasma membrane Ca^{2+} pump interacts both with calmodulin and with another part of the pump. *J. Biol. Chem.* 264: 12313–12321, 1989.
91. Evans, A. M. and M. B. Cannell. The role of L-type Ca^{2+} current and Na$^+$ current-stimulated Na/Ca exchange in triggering SR calcium release in guinea-pig cardiac ventricular myocytes. *Cardiovasc. Res.* 35:294–302, 1997.
92. Fabiato, A. Calcium-induced release of calcium from the cardiac sarcoplasmic reticulum. *Am. J. Physiol* 245 (*Cell Physiol.* 14): C1–C14, 1983.
93. Fan, J., Y. M. Shuba and M. Morad. Regulation of cardiac sodium-calcium exchanger by beta-adrenergic agonists. *Proc. Natl. Acad. Sci. U.S.A.* 93:5527–5532, 1996.
94. Fang, Y., M. Condrescu and J. P. Reeves. Regulation of Na$^+$/Ca^{2+} exchange activity by cytosolic Ca^{2+} in transfected Chinese hamster ovary cells. *Am. J. Physiol.* 275 (*Cell Physiol.* 44):C50–C55, 1998.
95. Flesch, M., R. H. Schwinger, F. Schiffer, K. Frank, M. Sudkamp, F. Kuhn-Regnier, G. Arnold and M. Bohm. Evidence for functional relevance of an enhanced expression of the Na$^+$-Ca^{2+} ex-

changer in failing human myocardium. *Circulation* 94:992–1002, 1996.
96. Frank, J. S., F. Chen, A. Garfinkel, E. Moore and K. D. Philipson. Immunolocalization of the Na$^+$-Ca^{2+} exchanger in cardiac myocytes. *Ann. N.Y. Acad. Sci.* 779:532–533, 1996.
97. Frank, J. S., G. Mottino, D. Reid, R. S. Molday and K. D. Philipson. Distribution of the Na$^+$-Ca^{2+} exchange protein in mammalian cardiac myocytes: an immunofluorescence and immunocolloidal gold–labeling study. *J. Cell Biol.* 117:337–345, 1992.
98. Fujioka, Y., M. Komeda and S. Matsuoka. Stoichiometry of Na$^+$-Ca^{2+} exchange in inside-out patches excised from guinea-pig ventricular myocytes. *J. Physiol. (Lond.)* 523 (Pt 2):339–351, 2000.
99. Fujioka, Y., S. Matsuoka, T. Ban and A. Noma. Interaction of the Na$^+$-K$^+$ pump and Na$^+$-Ca^{2+} exchange via [Na$^+$]$_i$ in a restricted space of guinea-pig ventricular cells. *J. Physiol. (Lond.)* 509:457–570, 1998.
100. Fujita, S. and M. Endoh. Influence of a Na$^+$-H$^+$ exchange inhibitor ethylisopropylamiloride, a Na$^+$-Ca^{2+} exchange inhibitor KB-R7943 and their combination on the increases in contractility and Ca^{2+} transient induced by angiotensin II in isolated adult rabbit ventricular myocytes. *Naunyn Schmiedebergs Arch. Pharmacol.* 360:575–584, 1999.
101. Furman, I., O. Cook, J. Kasir, W. Low and H. Rahamimoff. The putative amino-terminal signal peptide of the cloned rat brain Na$^+$-Ca^{2+} exchanger gene (RBE-1) is not mandatory for functional expression. *J. Biol. Chem.* 270:19120–19127, 1995.
102. Gabellini, N., A. Zatti, G. Rispoli, A. Navangione and E. Carafoli. Expression of an active Na$^+$/Ca^{2+} exchanger isoform lacking the six C-terminal transmembrane segments. *Eur. J. Biochem.* 239:897–904, 1996.
103. Gaughan, J. P., S. Furukawa, V. Jeevanandam, C. A. Hefner, H. Kubo, K. B. Margulies, B. S. McGowan, J. A. Mattiello, K. Dipla, V. Piacentino, S. Li and S. R. Houser. Sodium/calcium exchange contributes to contraction and relaxation in failed human ventricular myocytes. *Am. J. Physiol.* 277 (*Heart Circ. Physiol.* 46):H714–H724, 1999.
104. Giles, W. and Y. Shimoni. Slow inward tail currents in rabbit cardiac cells. *J. Physiol. (Lond.)* 417:447–463, 1989.
105. Goldhaber, J. I. Sodium-calcium exchange: the phantom menace. *Circ. Res.* 85:982–984, 1999.
106. Goldhaber, J. I., S. T. Lamp, D. O. Walter, A. Garfinkel, G. H. Fukumoto and J. N. Weiss. Local regulation of the threshold for calcium sparks in rat ventricular myocytes: role of sodium-calcium exchange. *J. Physiol. (Lond.)* 520:431–438, 1999.
107. Haddock, P. S., W. A. Coetzee, E. Cho, L. Porter, H. Katoh, D. M. Bers, M. S. Jafri and M. Artman. Subcellular Ca$^{2+}_i$ gradients during excitation-contraction coupling in newborn rabbit ventricular myocytes. *Circ. Res.* 85:415–427, 1999.
108. Haigney, M. C., H. Miyata, E. G. Lakatta, M. D. Stern and H. S. Silverman. Dependence of hypoxic cellular calcium loading on Na$^+$-Ca^{2+} exchange. *Circ. Res.* 71:547–557, 1992.
109. Hale, C. C., S. B. Kleiboeker, C. G. Carlton, M. J. Rovetto, C. Jung and H. D. Kim. Evidence for high molecular weight Na-Ca exchange in cardiac sarcolemmal vesicles. *J. Membr. Biol.* 106:211–218, 1988.
110. Hammes, A., S. Oberdorf-Maass, T. Rother, K. Nething, F. Gollnick, K. W. Linz, R. Meyer, K. Hu, H. Han, P. Gaudron, G. Ertl, S. Hoffmann, U. Ganten, R. Vetter, K. Schuh, C. Benkwitz, H. G. Zimmer and L. Neyses. Overexpression of the sarcolemmal calcium pump in the myocardium of transgenic rats. *Circ. Res.* 83:877–888, 1998.
111. Hanf, R., I. Drubaix, F. Marotte and L. G. Lelievre. Rat cardiac hypertrophy. Altered sodium-calcium exchange activity in sarcolemmal vesicles. *FEBS Lett.* 236:145–149, 1988.
112. Hasenfuss, G., M. Meyer, W. Schillinger, M. Preuss, B. Pieske and H. Just. Calcium handling proteins in the failing human heart. *Basic. Res. Cardiol.* 92 (Suppl 1):87–93, 1997.
113. Hasenfuss, G., H. Reinecke, R. Studer, B. Pieske, M. Meyer, H. Drexler and H. Just. Calcium cycling proteins and force-frequency relationship in heart failure. *Basic. Res. Cardiol.* 91(Suppl 2):17–22, 1996.
114. Hatem, S. N., J. S. Sham and M. Morad. Enhanced Na$^+$-Ca^{2+} exchange activity in cardiomyopathic Syrian hamster. *Circ. Res.* 74:253–261, 1994.
115. Haug-Collet, K., B. Pearson, R. Webel, R. T. Szerencsei, R. J. Winkfein, P. P. Schnetkamp and N. J. Colley. Cloning and characterization of a potassium-dependent sodium/calcium exchanger in *Drosophila*. *J. Cell Biol.* 147:659–670, 1999.
116. Hauptman, P. J., R. Garg and R. A. Kelly. Cardiac glycosides in the next millennium. *Prog. Cardiovasc. Dis.* 41:247–254, 1999.
117. Hauptman, P. J. and R. A. Kelly. Digitalis. *Circulation* 99:1265–1270, 1999.
118. Hayashida, Y., T. Yagi and S. Yasui. Ca^{2+} regulation by the Na$^+$-Ca^{2+} exchanger in retinal horizontal cells depolarized by L-glutamate. *Neurosci. Res.* 31:189–199, 1998.
119. He, L. P., N. M. Soldatov, L. Cleemann and M. Morad. Molecular determinants of cAMP regulation of recombinant Na$^+$-Ca^{2+} exchanger. *Biophys. J.* 78:373A, 2000.
120. He, S., A. Ruknudin, L. L. Bambrick, W. J. Lederer and D. H. Schulze. Isoform-specific regulation of the Na$^+$/Ca^{2+} exchanger in rat astrocytes and neurons by PKA. *J. Neurosci.* 18:4833–4841, 1998.
121. He, Z., S. Feng, Q. Tong, D. W. Hilgemann and K. D. Philipson. Interaction of PIP$_2$ with the XIP region of the cardiac Na/Ca exchanger. *Am. J. Physiol.* 278 (*Cell Physiol* 47):C661–C666, 2000.
122. He, Z., N. Petesch, K. Voges, W. Roben and K. D. Philipson. Identification of important amino acid residues of the Na$^+$-Ca^{2+} exchanger inhibitory peptide, XIP. *J. Membr. Biol.* 156:149–156, 1997.
123. He, Z., Q. Tong, B. D. Quednau, K. D. Philipson and D. W. Hilgemann. Cloning, expression, and characterization of the squid Na$^+$-Ca^{2+} exchanger (NCX-SQ1). *J. Gen. Physiol.* 111:857–873, 1998.
124. Hess, P., J. B. Lansman, B. Nilius and R. W. Tsien. Calcium channel types in cardiac myocytes: modulation by dihydropyridines and beta-adrenergic stimulation. *J. Cardiovasc. Pharmacol.* 8: S11–S21, 1986.
125. Hess, P., J. B. Lansman and R. W. Tsien. Different modes of Ca channel gating behaviour favoured by dihydropyridine Ca agonists and antagonists. *Nature* 311:538–544, 1984.
126. Hilgemann, D. W. Giant excised cardiac sarcolemmal membrane patches: sodium and sodium-calcium exchange currents. *Pflugers Arch.* 415:247–249, 1989.
127. Hilgemann, D. W. Regulation and deregulation of cardiac Na$^+$-Ca^{2+} exchange in giant excised sarcolemmal membrane patches. *Nature* 344:242–245, 1990.
128. Hilgemann, D. W. Unitary cardiac Na$^+$, Ca^{2+} exchange current magnitudes determined from channel-like noise and charge movements of ion transport. *Biophys. J.* 71:759–768, 1996.
129. Hilgemann, D. W. The cardiac Na-Ca exchanger in giant membrane patches. *Ann. N.Y. Acad. Sci.* 779:136–158, 1996.
130. Hilgemann, D. W. and R. Ball. Regulation of cardiac Na$^+$, Ca^{2+} exchange and K$_{ATP}$ potassium channels by PIP$_2$. *Science* 273:956–599, 1996.
131. Hilgemann, D. W., S. Matsuoka, G. A. Nagel and A. Collins. Steady-state and dynamic properties of cardiac sodium-calcium exchange. Sodium-dependent inactivation. *J. Gen. Physiol.* 100:905–932, 1992.
132. Hilgemann, D. W., A. Collins and S. Matsuoka. Steady-state

and dynamic properties of cardiac sodium-calcium exchange. Secondary modulation by cytoplasmic calcium and ATP. *J. Gen. Physiol.* 100:933–961, 1992.
133. Hilgemann, D. W. and C. C. Lu. Giant membrane patches: improvements and applications. *Methods Enzymol.* 293:267–280, 1998.
134. Hilgemann, D. W., D. A. Nicoll and K. D. Philipson. Charge movement during Na$^+$ translocation by native and cloned cardiac Na$^+$/Ca^{2+} exchanger. *Nature* 352:715–718, 1991.
135. Hille, B. *Ionic Channels of Excitable Membranes.* Sunderland, Massachusetts: Sinauer Associates Inc., 1984.
136. Hobai, I. A., D. Khananshvili and A. J. Levi. The peptide "FRCRCFa", dialysed intracellularly, inhibits the Na/Ca exchange in rabbit ventricular myocytes with high affinity. *Pflugers Arch.* 433:455–463, 1997.
137. Hobai, I. A. and B. O'Rourke. Enhanced Ca-activated Na/Ca exchange activity in canine pacing induced heart failure. *Biophys. J.* 78:373A, 2000.
138. Hoit, B. D., D. A. Tramuta, V. J. Kadambi, R. Dash, N. Ball, E. G. Kranias and R. A. Walsh. Influence of transgenic overexpression of phospholamban on postextrasystolic potentiation. *J. Mol. Cell Cardiol.* 31:2007–2015, 1999.
139. Horackova, M. and G. Vassort. Sodium-calcium exchange in regulation of cardiac contraction. *Recent Adv. Stud. Cardiac. Struct. Metab.* 11:137–141, 1976.
140. Horackova, M. and G. Vassort. Sodium-calcium exchange in regulation of cardiac contractility. Evidence for an electrogenic, voltage-dependent mechanism. *J. Gen. Physiol.* 73:403–424, 1979.
141. Houser, S. R. and E. G. Lakatta. Function of the cardiac myocyte in the conundrum of end-stage, dilated human heart failure. *Circulation* 99:600–604, 1999.
142. Hryshko, L. V., C. L. Elias, S. Shurraw, M. Trac, A. Omelchenko and M. Hnatowich. Frequency-dependent activity of alternatively spliced Na$^+$-Ca^{2+} exchangers. *Biophys. J.* 78:55A, 2000.
143. Hryshko, L. V., S. Matsuoka, D. A. Nicoll, J. N. Weiss, E. M. Schwarz, S. Benzer and K. D. Philipson. Anomalous regulation of the *Drosophila* Na$^+$-Ca^{2+} exchanger by Ca^{2+}. *J. Gen. Physiol.* 108:67–74, 1996.
144. Hryshko, L. V., D. A. Nicoll, J. N. Weiss and K. D. Philipson. Biosynthesis and initial processing of the cardiac sarcolemmal Na$^+$−Ca^{2+} exchanger. *Biochim. Biophys. Acta* 1151:35–42, 1993.
145. Hryshko, L. V., V. Stiffel and D. M. Bers. Rapid cooling contractures as an index of sarcoplasmic reticulum calcium content in rabbit ventricular myocytes. *Am. J. Physiol.* 257 (*Heart Circ. Physiol.* 26):H1369–H1377, 1989.
146. Ikari, A., H. Sakai and N. Takeguchi. Protein kinase C-mediated up-regulation of Na$^+$/Ca^{2+}-exchanger in rat hepatocytes determined by a new Na$^+$/Ca^{2+}-exchanger inhibitor, KB-R7943. *Eur. J. Pharmacol.* 360:91–98, 1998.
147. Imahashi, K., H. Kusuoka, K. Hashimoto, J. Yoshioka, H. Yamaguchi and T. Nishimura. Intracellular sodium accumulation during ischemia as the substrate for reperfusion injury. *Circ. Res.* 84:1401–1406, 1999.
148. Iwamoto, T., A. Uehara, T. Y. Nakamura, I. Imanaga and M. Shigekawa. Chimeric analysis of Na$^+$/Ca^{2+} exchangers NCX1 and NCX3 reveals structural domains important for differential sensitivity to external Ni^{2+} or Li$^+$. *J. Biol. Chem.* 274: 23094–23102, 1999.
149. Iwamoto, T., T. Y. Nakamura, Y. Pan, A. Uehara, I. Imanaga and M. Shigekawa. Unique topology of the internal repeats in the cardiac Na$^+$/Ca^{2+} exchanger. *FEBS Lett.* 446:264–268, 1999.
150. Iwamoto, T., Y. Pan, T. Y. Nakamura, S. Wakabayashi and M. Shigekawa. Protein kinase C–dependent regulation of Na$^+$/Ca^{2+} exchanger isoforms NCX1 and NCX3 does not require their direct phosphorylation. *Biochemistry* 37:17230–17238, 1998.
151. Iwamoto, T., T. Watano and M. Shigekawa. A novel isothiourea derivative selectively inhibits the reverse mode of Na$^+$/Ca^{2+} exchange in cells expressing NCX1. *J. Biol. Chem.* 271: 22391–22397, 1996.
152. Iwamoto, T., Y. Pan, S. Wakabayashi, T. Imagawa, H. I. Yamanaka and M. Shigekawa. Phosphorylation-dependent regulation of cardiac Na$^+$/Ca^{2+} exchanger via protein kinase C. *J. Biol. Chem.* 271:13609–13615, 1996.
153. Iwamoto, T. and M. Shigekawa. Differential inhibition of Na$^+$/Ca^{2+} exchanger isoforms by divalent cations and isothiourea derivative. *Am. J. Physiol.* 275 (*Cell Physiol.* 44):C423–C430, 1998.
154. Iwamoto, T., S. Wakabayashi and M. Shigekawa. Growth factor-induced phosphorylation and activation of aortic smooth muscle Na$^+$/Ca^{2+} exchanger. *J. Biol. Chem.* 270:8996–9001, 1995.
155. Janvier, N. C. and M. R. Boyett. The role of Na-Ca exchange current in the cardiac action potential. *Cardiovasc. Res.* 32:69–84, 1996.
156. Janvier, N. C., S. M. Harrison and M. R. Boyett. The role of inward Na$^+$-Ca^{2+} exchange current in the ferret ventricular action potential. *J. Physiol. (Lond)* 498:611–625, 1997.
157. Kappl, M. and K. Hartung. Rapid charge translocation by the cardiac Na$^+$-Ca^{2+} exchanger after a Ca^{2+} concentration jump. *Biophys. J.* 71:2473–2485, 1996.
158. Kappl, M. and K. Hartung. Kinetics of Na-Ca exchange current after a Ca^{2+} concentration jump. *Ann. N.Y. Acad. Sci.* 779: 290–292, 1996.
159. Karmazyn, M. The myocardial sodium-hydrogen exchanger (NHE) and its role in mediating ischemic and reperfusion injury. *Keio. J. Med.* 47:65–72, 1998.
160. Karmazyn, M., X. T. Gan, R. A. Humphreys, H. Yoshida and K. Kusumoto. The myocardial Na$^+$-H$^+$ exchange. Structure, regulation, and its role in heart disease. *Circ. Res.* 85:777–786, 1999.
161. Kaufman, T. M., J. W. Horton, D. J. White and L. Mahony. Age-related changes in myocardial relaxation and sarcoplasmic reticulum function. *Am. J. Physiol.* 259: (*Heart Circ. Physiol.* 28):H309–H316, 1990.
162. Khananshvili, D. Distinction between the two basic mechanisms of cation transport in the cardiac Na$^+$-Ca^{2+} exchange system. *Biochemistry* 29:2437–2442, 1990.
163. Khananshvili, D. Structure, mechanism, and regulation of the cardiac sarcolemma Na$^+$-Ca^{2+} exchanger. *Adv. Mol. Cell. Biol.* 23B:311–358, 1998.
164. Khananshvili, D., D. C. Price, M. J. Greenberg and Y. Sarne. Phe-Met-Arg-Phe-NH2 (FMRFa)-related peptides inhibit Na$^+$-Ca^{2+} exchange in cardiac sarcolemma vesicles. *J. Biol. Chem.* 268:200–205, 1993.
165. Khananshvili, D. and Y. Sarne. The effect of opiate agonists and antagonists on Na$^+$-Ca^{2+} exchange in cardiac sarcolemma vesicles. *Life Sci.* 51:275–283, 1992.
166. Khananshvili, D., G. Shaulov, E. Weil-Maslansky and D. Baazov. Positively charged cyclic hexapeptides, novel blockers for the cardiac sarcolemma Na$^+$-Ca^{2+} exchanger. *J. Biol. Chem.* 270:16182–16188, 1995.
167. Kieval, R. S., R. J. Bloch, G. E. Lindenmayer, A. Ambesi and W. J. Lederer. Immunofluorescence localization of the Na-Ca exchanger in heart cells. *Am. J. Physiol.* (*Cell Physiol.* 32) 263: C545–C550, 1992.
168. Kihara, Y., S. Sasayama, M. Inoko and J. P. Morgan. Sodium/calcium exchange modulates intracellular calcium overload

during posthypoxic reoxygenation in mammalian working myocardium. Evidence from aequorin-loaded ferret ventricular muscles. *J. Clin. Invest.* 93:1275–1284, 1994.
169. Kimura, J., S. Miyamae and A. Noma. Identification of sodium-calcium exchange current in single ventricular cells of guinea-pig. *J. Physiol. (Lond.)* 384:199–222, 1987.
170. Kimura, J., A. Noma and H. Irisawa. Na-Ca exchange current in mammalian heart cells. *Nature* 319:596–597, 1986.
171. Kimura, J., T. Watano, M. Kawahara, E. Sakai and J. Yatabe. Direction-independent block of bi-directional Na$^+$/Ca^{2+} exchange current by KB-R7943 in guinea-pig cardiac myocytes. *Br. J. Pharmacol.* 128:969–974, 1999.
172. Koch-Weser, J. Effect of rate changes on strength and time course of contraction of papillary muscle. *Am. J. Physiol.* 204:451–45, 1999.
173. Kofuji, P., W. J. Lederer and D. H. Schulze. Mutually exclusive and cassette exons underlie alternatively spliced isoforms of the Na/Ca exchanger. *J. Biol. Chem.* 269:5145–5149, 1994.
174. Kohomoto, O., A. J. Levi and J. H. Bridge. Relation between reverse sodium-calcium exchange and sarcoplasmic reticulum calcium release in guinea pig ventricular cells. *Circ. Res.* 74:550–554, 1994.
175. Komuro, I., K. E. Wenninger, K. D. Philipson and S. Izumo. Molecular cloning and characterization of the human cardiac Na$^+$/Ca^{2+} exchanger cDNA. *Proc. Natl. Acad. Sci. U. S. A.* 89:4769–4773, 1992.
176. Kuro, T., Y. Kobayashi, M. Takaoka and Y. Matsumura. Protective effect of KB-R7943, a novel Na$^+$/Ca^{2+} exchange inhibitor, on ischemic acute renal failure in rats. *Jpn. J. Pharmacol.* 81:247–251, 1999.
177. Kurth, C. D., J. M. Steven and S. C. Nicolson. Cerebral oxygenation during pediatric cardiac surgery using deep hypothermic circulatory arrest. *Anesthesiology* 82:74–82, 1995.
178. Ladilov, Y., S. Haffner, C. Balser-Schafer, H. Maxeiner and H. M. Piper. Cardioprotective effects of KB-R7943: a novel inhibitor of the reverse mode of Na$^+$/Ca^{2+} exchanger. *Am. J. Physiol.* 276 (*Heart Circ. Physiol* 45):H1868–H1876, 1999.
179. Langer, G. A. and T. L. Rich. Further characterization of the Na-Ca exchange-dependent Ca compartment in rat ventricular cells. *Am. J. Physiol.* 265 (*Cell Physiol.* 34):C556–C561, 1993.
180. Langer, G. A., S. Y. Wang and T. L. Rich. Localization of the Na/Ca exchange-dependent Ca compartment in cultured neonatal rat heart cells. *Am. J. Physiol.* 268 (*Cell Physiol.* 37):C119–C126, 1995.
181. Lauger, P. Voltage dependence of sodium-calcium exchange: predictions from kinetic models. *J. Membr. Biol.* 99:1–11, 1987.
182. Leblanc, N. and J. R. Hume. Sodium current-induced release of calcium from cardiac sarcoplasmic reticulum. *Science* 248:372–376, 1990.
183. Lederer, W. J., E. Niggli and R. W. Hadley. Sodium-calcium exchange in excitable cells: fuzzy space. *Science* 248:283, 1990.
184. Ledvora, R. F. and C. Hegyvary. Dependence of Na$^+$-Ca^{2+} exchange and Ca^{2+}-Ca^{2+} exchange on monovalent cations. *Biochim. Biophys. Acta* 729:123–136, 1983.
185. Lee, C. O. 200 years of digitalis: the emerging central role of the sodium ion in the control of cardiac force. *Am. J. Physiol.* 249 (*Cell Physiol.* 18):C367–C378, 1985.
186. Lee, C. O., P. Abete, M. Pecker, J. K. Sonn and M. Vassalle. Strophanthidin inotropy: role of intracellular sodium ion activity and sodium-calcium exchange. *J. Mol. Cell Cardiol.* 17:1043–1053, 1985.
187. Lee, S. L., A. S. Yu and J. Lytton. Tissue-specific expression of Na$^+$-Ca^{2+} exchanger isoforms. *J. Biol. Chem.* 269:14849–14852, 1994.
188. Levesque, P. C., N. Leblanc and J. R. Hume. Role of reverse-mode Na$^+$-Ca^{2+} exchange in excitation-contraction coupling in the heart. *Ann. N.Y. Acad. Sci.* 639:386–397, 1991.
189. Levesque, P. C., N. Leblanc and J. R. Hume. Release of calcium from guinea pig cardiac sarcoplasmic reticulum induced by sodium-calcium exchange. *Cardiovasc. Res.* 28:370–378, 1994.
190. Levi, A. J., P. Brooksby and J. C. Hancox. A role for depolarisation induced calcium entry on the Na-Ca exchange in triggering intracellular calcium release and contraction in rat ventricular myocytes. *Cardiovasc. Res.* 27:1677–1690, 1993.
191. Levi, A. J., P. Brooksby and J. C. Hancox. One hump or two? The triggering of calcium release from the sarcoplasmic reticulum and the voltage dependence of contraction in mammalian cardiac muscle. *Cardiovasc. Res.* 27:1743–1757, 1993.
192. Levi, A. J., G. R. Dalton, J. C. Hancox, J. S. Mitcheson, J. Issberner, J. A. Bates, S. J. Evans, F. C. Howarth, I. A. Hobai and J. V. Jones. Role of intracellular sodium overload in the genesis of cardiac arrhythmias. *J. Cardiovasc. Electrophysiol.* 8:700–721, 1997.
193. Levi, A. J., K. W. Spitzer, O. Kohmoto and J. H. Bridge. Depolarization-induced Ca entry via Na-Ca exchange triggers SR release in guinea pig cardiac myocytes. *Am. J. Physiol.* 266 (*Heart Circ. Physiol.* 35):H1422–H1433, 1994.
194. Levitsky, D. O., D. A. Nicoll and K. D. Philipson. Identification of the high affinity Ca^{2+}-binding domain of the cardiac Na$^+$-Ca^{2+} exchanger. *J. Biol. Chem.* 269:22847–22852, 1994.
195. Li, G. R. and S. Nattel. Demonstration of an inward Na$^+$-Ca^{2+} exchange current in adult human atrial myocytes. *Ann. N.Y. Acad. Sci.* 779:525–528, 1996.
196. Li, J. M. and J. Kimura. Translocation mechanism of cardiac Na-Ca exchange. *Ann. N. . Acad. Sci.* 639:48–60, 1991.
197. Li, X. F. and J. Lytton. A circularized sodium-calcium exchanger exon 2 transcript. *J. Biol. Chem.* 274:8153–8160, 1999.
198. Li, Z., S. Matsuoka, L. V. Hryshko, D. A. Nicoll, M. M. Bersohn, E. P. Burke, R. P. Lifton and K. D. Philipson. Cloning of the NCX2 isoform of the plasma membrane Na$^+$-Ca^{2+} exchanger. *J. Biol. Chem.* 269:17434–17439, 1994.
199. Li, Z., D. A. Nicoll, A. Collins, D. W. Hilgemann, A. G. Filoteo, J. T. Penniston, J. N. Weiss, J. M. Tomich and K. D. Philipson. Identification of a peptide inhibitor of the cardiac sarcolemmal Na$^+$-Ca^{2+} exchanger. *J. Biol. Chem.* 266:1014–1020, 1991.
200. Li, Z. P., E. P. Burke, J. S. Frank, V. Bennett and K. D. Philipson. The cardiac Na$^+$-Ca^{2+} exchanger binds to the cytoskeletal protein ankyrin. *J. Biol. Chem.* 268:11489–11491, 1993.
201. Lim, C. C., R. Liao, N. Varma and C. S. Apstein. Impaired lusitropy-frequency in the aging mouse: role of Ca^{2+}-handling proteins and effects of isoproterenol. *Am. J. Physiol.* 277 (*Heart Circ. Physiol..* 46):H2083–H2090, 1999.
202. Linck, B., Z. Qiu, Z. He, Q. Tong, D. W. Hilgemann and K. D. Philipson. Functional comparison of the three isoforms of the Na$^+$/Ca^{2+} exchanger (NCX1, NCX2, NCX3). *Am. J. Physiol.* 274 (*Cell Physiol.*) 43:C415-C423, 1998.
203. Lipp, P. and E. Niggli. Sodium current-induced calcium signals in isolated guinea-pig ventricular myocytes. *J. Physiol. (Lond.)* 474:439–446, 1994.
204. Lipp, P. and L. Pott. Transient inward current in guinea-pig atrial myocytes reflects a change of sodium-calcium exchange current. *J. Physiol. (Lond.)* 397:601–630, 1988.
205. Lipp, P., B. Schwaller and E. Niggli. Specific inhibition of Na-Ca exchange function by antisense oligodeoxynucleotides. *FEBS Lett.* 364:198–202, 1995.
206. Litwin, S., O. Kohmoto, A. J. Levi, K. W. Spitzer and J. H. Bridge. Evidence that reverse Na-Ca exchange can trigger SR calcium release. *Ann. N.Y. Acad. Sci.* 779:451–463, 1996.

207. Litwin, S. E. and J. H. Bridge. Enhanced Na$^+$-Ca^{2+} exchange in the infarcted heart. Implications for excitation-contraction coupling. *Circ. Res.* 81:1083–1093, 1997.
208. Litwin, S. E., J. Li and J. H. Bridge. Na-Ca exchange and the trigger for sarcoplasmic reticulum Ca release: studies in adult rabbit ventricular myocytes. *Biophys. J.* 75:359–371, 1998.
209. Liu, Q. Y. and M. Vassalle. Role of Na-Ca exchange in the action potential changes caused by drive in cardiac myocytes exposed to different Ca^{2+} loads. *Can. J. Physiol. Pharmacol.* 77:383–397, 1999.
210. Liu, X. K., R. M. Engelman, J. Iyengar, G. A. Cordis and D. K. Das. Amiloride enhances postischemic ventricular recovery during cardioplegic arrest. A possible role of Na$^+$-Ca^{2+} exchange. *Ann. N.Y. Acad. Sci.* 639:471–474, 1991.
211. Loo, T. W., C. Ho and D. M. Clarke. Expression of a functionally active human renal sodium-calcium exchanger lacking a signal sequence. *J. Biol. Chem.* 270:19345–19350, 1995.
212. Lopez-Lopez, J. R., P. S. Shacklock, C. W. Balke and W. G. Wier. Local calcium transients triggered by single L-type calcium channel currents in cardiac cells. *Science* 268:1042–1045, 1995.
213. Lu, H. R., P. Yang, P. Remeysen, A. Saels, D. Z. Dai and F. De Clerck. Ischemia/reperfusion-induced arrhythmias in anaesthetized rats: a role of Na$^+$ and Ca^{2+} influx. *Eur. J. Pharmacol.* 365:233–2399, 1999.
214. Matsuda, N., T. Mori, H. Nakamura and M. Shigekawa. Mechanisms of reoxygenation-induced calcium overload in cardiac myocytes: dependence on pH$_i$. *J. Surg. Res.* 59:712–718, 1995.
215. Matsuoka, S., T. Ehara and A. Noma. Reversal potential of the Na-Ca exchange current in the cardiac myocyte of the guinea pig. *Bimed. Res.* 9:149–152, 1988.
216. Matsuoka, S. and D. W. Hilgemann. Steady-state and dynamic properties of cardiac sodium-calcium exchange. Ion and voltage dependencies of the transport cycle. *J. Gen. Physiol.* 100:963–1001, 1992.
217. Matsuoka, S. and D. W. Hilgemann. Inactivation of outward Na$^+$-Ca^{2+} exchange current in guinea-pig ventricular myocytes. *J. Physiol. (Lond.)* 476:443–458, 1994.
218. Matsuoka, S., D. A. Nicoll, Z. He and K. D. Philipson. Regulation of cardiac Na$^+$-Ca^{2+} exchanger by the endogenous XIP region. *J. Gen. Physiol.* 109:273–286, 1997.
219. Matsuoka, S., D. A. Nicoll, L. V. Hryshko, D. O. Levitsky, J. N. Weiss and K. D. Philipson. Regulation of the cardiac Na$^+$-Ca^{2+} exchanger by Ca^{2+}. Mutational analysis of the Ca^{2+}-binding domain. *J. Gen. Physiol.* 105:403–420, 1995.
220. Matsuoka, S., D. A. Nicoll, R. F. Reilly, D. W. Hilgemann and K. D. Philipson. Initial localization of regulatory regions of the cardiac sarcolemmal Na$^+$-Ca^{2+} exchanger. *Proc. Natl. Acad. Sci. U.S.A.* 90:3870–3874, 1993.
221. Mattiello, J. A., K. B. Margulies, V. Jeevanandam and S. R. Houser. Contribution of reverse-mode sodium-calcium exchange to contractions in failing human left ventricular myocytes. *Cardiovasc. Res.* 37:424–431, 1998.
222. Maxwell, K., J. Scott, A. Omelchenko, A. Lukas, L. Lu, Y. Lu, M. Hnatowich, K. D. Philipson and L. V. Hryshko. Functional role of ionic regulation of Na$^+$/Ca^{2+} exchange assessed in transgenic mouse hearts. *Am. J. Physiol.* 277 (*Heart Circ. Physiol.* 46):H2212–H2221, 1999.
223. McDonald, T. F., S. Pelzer, W. Trautwein and D. J. Pelzer. Regulation and modulation of calcium channels in cardiac, skeletal, and smooth muscle cells. *Physiol. Rev.* 74:365–507, 1994.
224. Medford, R. M. Digitalis and the Na$^+$,K$^+$-ATPase. *Heart Dis. Stroke* 2:250–255, 1993.
225. Mejia-Alvarez, R., C. Kettlun, E. Rios, M. Stern and M. Fill. Unitary Ca^{2+} current through cardiac ryanodine receptor channels under quasi-physiological ionic conditions. *J. Gen. Physiol.* 113:177–186, 1999.
226. Milanick, M. A. and M. D. Frame. Kinetic models of Na-Ca exchange in ferret red blood cells. Interaction of intracellular Na, extracellular Ca, Cd, and Mn. *Ann. N.Y. Acad. Sci.* 639:604–615, 1991.
227. Miura, Y. and J. Kimura. Sodium-calcium exchange current. Dependence on internal Ca and Na and competitive binding of external Na and Ca. *J. Gen. Physiol.* 93:1129–1145, 1989.
228. Mochizuki, S. and C. Jiang. Na$^+$/Ca^{++} exchanger and myocardial ischemia/reperfusion. *Jpn. Heart J.* 39:707–714, 1998.
229. Mochizuki, S. and K. T. MacLeod. Effects of hypoxia and metabolic inhibition on increases in intracellular Ca^{2+} concentration induced by Na$^+$/Ca^{2+} exchange in isolated guinea-pig cardiac myocytes. *J. Mol. Cell Cardiol.* 29:2979–2987, 1997.
230. Mori, F., M. Miyamoto, H. Tsuboi, H. Noda and K. Esato. Clinical trial of nicardipine cardioplegia in pediatric cardiac surgery. *Ann. Thorac. Surg.* 49:413–417, 1990.
231. Mukai, M., H. Terada, S. Sugiyama, H. Satoh and H. Hayashi. Effects of a selective inhibitor of Na$^+$/Ca^{2+} exchange, KB-R7943, on reoxygenation-induced injuries in guinea pig papillary muscles. *J. Cardiovasc. Pharmacol.* 35:121–128, 2000.
232. Mullins, L. J. The generation of electric currents in cardiac fibers by Na/Ca exchange. *Am. J. Physiol.* 236 (*Cell Physiol.* 5): C103–C110, 1979.
233. Mullins, L. J. An electrogenic saga: consequences of sodium-calcium exchange in cardiac muscle. *Soc. Gen. Physiol. Ser.* 38:161–179, 1984.
234. Mullins, L. J. Is stoichiometry constant in Na-Ca exchange? *Ann. N.Y. Acad. Sci.* 639:96–98, 1991.
235. Nabauer, M., G. Callewaert, L. Cleemann and M. Morad. Regulation of calcium release is gated by calcium current, not gating charge, in cardiac myocytes. *Science* 244:800–803, 1989.
236. Nagashima, T., K. Ikeda, S. Wu, T. Kondo, M. Yamaguchi and N. Tamaki. The mechanism of reversible osmotic opening of the blood-brain barrier: role of intracellular calcium ion in capillary endothelial cells. *Acta Neurochir. Suppl. (Wien)* 70:231–233, 1997.
237. Nakamura, A., K. Harada, H. Sugimoto, F. Nakajima and N. Nishimura. Effects of KB-R7943, a novel Na$^+$/Ca^{2+} exchange inhibitor, on myocardial ischemia/reperfusion injury. *Nippon Yakurigaku. Zasshi.* 111:105–115, 1998.
238. Navanglone, A., G. Rispoli, N. Gabellini and E. Carafoli. Electrophysiological characterization of ionic transport by the retinal exchanger expressed in human embryonic kidney cells. *Biophys. J.* 73:45–51, 1997.
239. Nicoll, D. A., B. D. Quednau, Z. Qui, Y. R. Xia, A. J. Lusis and K. D. Philipson. Cloning of a third mammalian Na$^+$-Ca^{2+} exchanger, NCX3. *J. Biol. Chem.* 271:24914–24921, 1996.
240. Nicoll, D. A., L. V. Hryshko, S. Matsuoka, J. S. Frank and K. D. Philipson. Mutation of amino acid residues in the putative transmembrane segments of the cardiac sarcolemmal Na$^+$-Ca^{2+} exchanger. *J. Biol. Chem.* 271:13385–13391, 1996.
241. Nicoll, D. A., S. Longoni and K. D. Philipson. Molecular cloning and functional expression of the cardiac sarcolemmal Na$^+$-Ca^{2+} exchanger. *Science* 250:562–565, 1990.
242. Nicoll, D. A., M. Ottolia, L. Lu, Y. Lu and K. D. Philipson. A new topological model of the cardiac sarcolemmal Na$^+$-Ca^{2+} exchanger. *J. Biol. Chem.* 274:910–917, 1999.
243. Nicoll, D. A. and K. D. Philipson. Molecular studies of the cardiac sarcolemmal sodium-calcium exchanger. *Ann. N.Y. Acad. Sci.* 639:181–188, 1991.
244. Niggli, E. Strontium-induced creep currents associated with tonic contractions in cardiac myocytes isolated from guinea-pigs. *J. Physiol. (Lond)* 414:549–568, 1989.
245. Niggli, E. and W. J. Lederer. Molecular operations of the

sodium-calcium exchanger revealed by conformation currents. *Nature* 349:621–624, 1991.
246. Nishida, M., T. Urushidani, K. Sakamoto and T. Nagao. L-*cis* diltiazem attenuates intracellular Ca^{2+} overload by metabolic inhibition in guinea pig myocytes. *Eur. J. Pharmacol.* 385:225–230, 1999.
247. Noble, D., J. Y. LeGuennec and R. Winslow. Functional roles of sodium-calcium exchange in normal and abnormal cardiac rhythm. *Ann. N.Y. Acad. Sci.* 779:480–488, 1996.
248. Noble, D., S. J. Noble, G. C. Bett, Y. E. Earm, W. K. Ho and I. K. So. The role of sodium-calcium exchange during the cardiac action potential. *Ann. N.Y. Acad. Sci.* 639:334–353, 1991.
249. O'Neill, S. C., M. Valdeolmillos, C. Lamont, P. Donoso and D. A. Eisner. The contribution of Na-Ca exchange to relaxation in mammalian cardiac muscle. *Ann. N.Y. Acad. Sci.* 639:444–452, 1991.
250. O'Rourke, B., D. A. Kass, G. F. Tomaselli, S. Kaab, R. Tunin and E. Marban. Mechanisms of altered excitation-contraction coupling in canine tachycardia-induced heart failure, I: experimental studies. *Circ. Res.* 84:562–570, 1999.
251. Omelchenko, A., C. Dyck, M. Hnatowich, J. Buchko, D. A. Nicoll, K. D. Philipson and L. V. Hryshko. Functional differences in ionic regulation between alternatively spliced isoforms of the Na^+-Ca^{2+} exchanger from *Drosophila melanogaster*. *J. Gen. Physiol.* 111:691–702, 1998.
252. Omelchenko, A., C.L. Elias, M. Hnatowich and L. V. Hryshko. A unique form of Ca^{2+}_i-dependent regulation of the kidney Na^+-Ca^{2+} exchanger, NCX1.3. *Biophys. J.* 78:54A, 2000.
253. Omelchenko, A. and L. V. Hryshko. Current-voltage relations and steady-state characteristics of Na^+-Ca^{2+} exchange: characterization of the eight-state consecutive transport model. *Biophys. J.* 71:1751–1763, 1996.
254. Opuni, K. and J. P. Reeves. Feedback inhibition of sodium/calcium exchange activity by mitochondrial calcium accumulation. *Biophys. J.* 78:56A, 2000.
255. Ottolia, M., Z. Qiu and K. D. Philipson. Functional characterization of a "split" Na^+-Ca^{2+} exchanger. *Biophys. J.* 78:54A, 2000.
256. Peterson, B. Z., C. D. DeMaria, J. P. Adelman and D. T. Yue. Calmodulin is the Ca^{2+} sensor for Ca^{2+}-dependent inactivation of L-type calcium channels. *Neuron* 22:549–558, 1999.
257. Peterson, B. Z., J. S. Lee, J. G. Mulle, Y. Wang, M. de Leon and D. T. Yue. Critical determinants of Ca^{2+}-dependent inactivation within an EF-hand motif of L-type Ca^{2+} channels. *Biophys. J.* 78:1906–1920, 2000.
258. Philipson, K. D., M. M. Bersohn and A. Y. Nishimoto. Effects of pH on Na^+-Ca^{2+} exchange in canine cardiac sarcolemmal vesicles. *Circ. Res.* 50:287–293, 1982.
259. Philipson, K. D. and D. A. Nicoll. Molecular and kinetic aspects of sodium-calcium exchange. *Int. Rev. Cytol.* 137C:199–227, 1993.
260. Philipson, K. D. and D. A. Nicoll. Sodium-calcium exchange: a molecular perspective. *Annu. Rev. Physiol.* 62:111–133, 2000.
261. Pieske, B., M. Sutterlin, S. Schmidt-Schweda, K. Minami, M. Meyer, M. Olschewski, C. Holubarsch, H. Just and G. Hasenfuss. Diminished post-rest potentiation of contractile force in human dilated cardiomyopathy. Functional evidence for alterations in intracellular Ca^{2+} handling. *J. Clin. Invest.* 98:764–776, 1996.
262. Pike, M. M., M. Kitakaze and E. Marban. ^{23}Na-NMR measurements of intracellular sodium in intact perfused ferret hearts during ischemia and reperfusion. *Am. J. Physiol* 259 (*Heart Circ. Physiol.* 28):H1767–H1773, 1990.
263. Pitts, B. J. Stoichiometry of sodium-calcium exchange in cardiac sarcolemmal vesicles. Coupling to the sodium pump. *J. Biol. Chem.* 254:6232–6235, 1979.
264. Poon, S., S. Leach, X. F. Li, J. E. Tucker, P. P. Schnetkamp and J. Lytton. Alternatively spliced isoforms of the rat eye sodium/calcium+potassium exchanger NCKX1. *Am. J. Physiol.* 278. (*Cell Physiol.* 47):C651–C660, 2000.
265. Powell, T., A. Noma, T. Shioya and R. Z. Kozlowski. Turnover rate of the cardiac Na^+-Ca^{2+} exchanger in guinea-pig ventricular myocytes. *J. Physiol. (Lond.)* 472:45–53, 1993.
266. Powis, D. A., C. L. Clark and K. J. O'Brien. Lanthanum can be transported by the sodium-calcium exchange pathway and directly triggers catecholamine release from bovine chromaffin cells. *Cell Calcium* 16:377–390, 1994.
267. Praetorius, H. A., U. G. Friis, J. Praetorius and T. Johansen. Evidence for a Na^+/Ca^{2+} exchange mechanism in rat peritoneal mast cells. *Pflugers Arch.* 437:86–93, 1998.
268. Prinsen, C. F., R. T. Szerencsei and P. P. Schnetkamp. Molecular cloning and functional expression of the potassium-dependent sodium-calcium exchanger from human and chicken retinal cone photoreceptors. *J. Neurosci.* 20:1424–1434, 2000.
269. Quednau, B. D., D. A. Nicoll and K. D. Philipson. Tissue specificity and alternative splicing of the Na^+/Ca^{2+} exchanger isoforms NCX1, NCX2, and NCX3 in rat. *Am. J. Physiol.* 272 (*Cell Physiol.* 41):C1250–C1261, 1997.
270. Reeves, J. P. Na^+/Ca^{2+} exchange and cellular Ca^{2+} homeostasis. *J. Bioenerg. Biomembr.* 30:151–160, 1998.
271. Reeves, J. P. and C. C. Hale. The stoichiometry of the cardiac sodium-calcium exchange system. *J. Biol. Chem.* 259:7733–7739, 1984.
272. Reilander, H., A. Achilles, U. Friedel, G. Maul, F. Lottspeich and N. J. Cook. Primary structure and functional expression of the Na/Ca, K-exchanger from bovine rod photoreceptors. *EMBO J.* 11:1689–1695, 1992.
273. Reilly, R. F. and C. A. Shugrue. cDNA cloning of a renal Na^+-Ca^{2+} exchanger. *Am. J. Physiol.* 262 (*Renal Fluid Electrolyte Physiol.* 31):F1105–F1109, 1992.
274. Riaz, K. and A. D. Forker. Digoxin use in congestive heart failure. Current status. *Drugs* 55:747–758, 1998.
275. Rios, E. and M. D. Stern. Calcium in close quarters: microdomain feedback in excitation-contraction coupling and other cell biological phenomena. *Annu. Rev. Biophys. Biomol. Struct.* 26:47–82, 1997.
276. Ruiz-Meana, M., D. Garcia-Dorado, B. Hofstaetter, H. M. Piper and J. Soler-Soler. Propagation of cardiomyocyte hypercontracture by passage of Na^+ through gap junctions. *Circ. Res.* 85:280–287, 1999.
277. Ruknudin, A., C. Valdivia, P. Kofuji, W. J. Lederer and D. H. Schulze. Na^+/Ca^{2+} exchanger in *Drosophila*: cloning, expression, and transport differences. *Am. J. Physiol. (Cell Physiol.* 42) 273:C257–C265, 1997.
278. Sahin-Toth, M., D. A. Nicoll, J. S. Frank, K. D. Philipson and M. Friedlander. The cleaved N-terminal signal sequence of the cardiac Na^+-Ca^{2+} exchanger is not required for functional membrane integration. *Biochem. Biophys. Res. Commun.* 212:968–974, 1995.
279. Santana, L. F., A. M. Gomez and W. J. Lederer. Ca^{2+} flux through promiscuous cardiac Na^+ channels: slip-mode conductance. *Science* 279:1027–1033, 1998.
280. Satoh, H., K. S. Ginsburg, K. Qing, H. Terada, H. Hayashi and D. M. Bers. KB-R7943 block of Ca^{2+} influx via Na^+/Ca^{2+} exchange does not alter twitches or glycoside inotropy but prevents Ca^{2+} overload in rat ventricular myocytes. *Circulation* 101:1441–1446, 2000.
281. Schnetkamp, P. P. How does the retinal rod Na-Ca+K exchanger regulate cytosolic free Ca^{2+}?. *J. Biol. Chem.* 270:13231–13239, 1995.

282. Schnetkamp, P. P., D. K. Basu and R. T. Szerencsei. Na$^+$-Ca^{2+} exchange in bovine rod outer segments requires and transports K$^+$. *Am. J. Physiol.* 257 (*Cell Physiol.* 26):C153–C157, 1989.
283. Schnetkamp, P. P., D. K. Basu and R. T. Szerencsei. The stoichiometry of Na-Ca+K exchange in rod outer segments isolated from bovine retinas. *Ann. N.Y. Acad. Sci.* 639:10–21, 1991.
284. Schnetkamp, P. P. and R. T. Szerencsei. Intracellular Ca^{2+} sequestration and release in intact bovine retinal rod outer segments. Role in inactivation of Na-Ca+K exchange. *J. Biol. Chem.* 268:12449–12457, 1993.
285. Scholz, H. Pharmacological aspects of calcium channel blockers. *Cardiovasc. Drugs Ther.* 10:869–872, 1997.
286. Schwaller, B., M. Egger, P. Lipp and E. Niggli. Application of antisense oligodeoxynucleotides for suppression of Na$^+$/Ca^{2+} exchange. *Methods Enzymol.* 314:454–476, 2000.
287. Schwarz, E. and S. Benzer. The recently reported NIbeta domain is already known as the Calx-beta motif. *Trends. Biochem. Sci.* 24:260, 1999.
288. Schwarz, E. M. and S. Benzer. *Calx*, a Na-Ca exchanger gene of *Drosophila melanogaster*. *Proc. Natl. Acad. Sci. U.S.A.* 94:10249–10254, 1997.
289. Schwinger, R. H., J. Wang, K. Frank, J. Muller-Ehmsen, K. Brixius, A. A. McDonough and E. Erdmann. Reduced sodium pump α_1, α_3, and β_1-isoform protein levels and Na$^+$, K$^+$-ATPase activity but unchanged Na$^+$-Ca^{2+} exchanger protein levels in human heart failure. *Circulation* 99:2105–2112, 1999.
290. Sham, J. S., L. Cleemann and M. Morad. Gating of the cardiac Ca^{2+} release channel: the role of Na$^+$ current and Na$^+$-Ca^{2+} exchange. *Science* 255:850–853, 1992.
291. Sham, J. S., L. Cleemann and M. Morad. Functional coupling of Ca^{2+} channels and ryanodine receptors in cardiac myocytes. *Proc. Natl. Acad. Sci. U.S.A.* 92:121–125, 1995.
292. Sham, J. S., S. N. Hatem and M. Morad. Species differences in the activity of the Na$^+$-Ca^{2+} exchanger in mammalian cardiac myocytes. *J. Physiol. (Lond.)* 488:623–631, 1995.
293. Shi, S., B. Chang and S. R. Brunnert. Identification and cloning of a truncated isoform of the cardiac sodium-calcium exchanger in the BALB/c mouse heart. *Biochem. Genet.* 36:119–135, 1998.
294. Shuba, Y. M., T. Iwata, V. G. Naidenov, M. Oz, K. Sandberg, A. Kraev, E. Carafoli and M. Morad. A novel molecular determinant for cAMP-dependent regulation of the frog heart Na$^+$-Ca^{2+} exchanger. *J. Biol. Chem.* 273:18819–18825, 1998.
295. Sipido, K. R. Efficiency of L-type Ca^{2+} current compared to reverse mode Na/Ca exchange or T-type Ca^{2+} current as trigger for Ca^{2+} release from the sarcoplasmic reticulum. *Ann. N.Y. Acad. Sci.* 853:357–360, 1998.
296. Sipido, K. R., E. Carmeliet and A. Pappano. Na$^+$ current and Ca^{2+} release from the sarcoplasmic reticulum during action potentials in guinea-pig ventricular myocytes. *J. Physiol. (Lond.)* 489:1–17, 1995.
297. Sipido, K. R., M. Maes and F. Van de Werf. Low efficiency of Ca^{2+} entry through the Na$^+$-Ca^{2+} exchanger as trigger for Ca^{2+} release from the sarcoplasmic reticulum. A comparison between L-type Ca^{2+} current and reverse-mode Na$^+$-Ca^{2+} exchange. *Circ. Res.* 81:1034–1044, 1997.
298. Slodzinski, M. K. and M. P. Blaustein. Na$^+$/Ca^{2+} exchange in neonatal rat heart cells: antisense inhibition and protein half-life. *Am. J. Physiol.* 275 (*Cell Physiol.* 44):C459–C467, 1998.
299. Slodzinski, M. K. and M. P. Blaustein. Physiological effects of Na$^+$/Ca^{2+} exchanger knockdown by antisense oligodeoxynucleotides in arterial myocytes. *Am. J. Physiol.* 275 (*Cell Physiol.* 44):C251–C259, 1998.
300. Smith, L., H. Porzig, H. W. Lee and J. B. Smith. Phorbol esters downregulate expression of the sodium/calcium exchanger in renal epithelial cells. *Am. J. Physiol.* 269 (*Cell Physiol.* 38):C457–C463, 1995.
301. Smith, L. and J. B. Smith. Activation of adenylyl cyclase downregulates sodium/calcium exchanger of arterial myocytes. *Am. J. Physiol.* 269 (*Cell Physiol.* 38):C1379–C1384, 1995.
302. Soler-Soler, J. and G. Permanyer-Miralda. Should we still prescribe digoxin in mild-to-moderate heart failure? Is quality of life the issue rather than quantity? *Eur. Heart J.* 19 (Suppl P):26–31, 1998.
303. Studer, R., H. Reinecke, J. Bilger, T. Eschenhagen, M. Bohm, G. Hasenfuss, H. Just, J. Holtz and H. Drexler. Gene expression of the cardiac Na$^+$-Ca^{2+} exchanger in end-stage human heart failure. *Circ. Res.* 75:443–453, 1994.
304. Studer, R., H. Reinecke, R. Vetter, J. Holtz and H. Drexler. Expression and function of the cardiac Na$^+$/Ca^{2+} exchanger in postnatal development of the rat, in experimental-induced cardiac hypertrophy and in the failing human heart. *Basic Res. Cardiol.* 92 (Suppl 1):53–58, 1997.
305. Su, Z., J. H. Bridge, K. D. Philipson, K. W. Spitzer and W. H. Barry. Quantitation of Na/Ca exchanger function in single ventricular myocytes. *J. Mol. Cell Cardiol.* 31:1125–1135, 1999.
306. Takahashi, K., M. Azuma, J. Huschenbett, M. L. Michaelis and J. Azuma. Effects of antisense oligonucleotides to the cardiac Na$^+$/Ca^{2+} exchanger on calcium dynamics in cultured cardiac myocytes. *Biochem. Biophys. Res. Commun.* 260:117–121, 1999.
307. Terracciano, C. M., E. Bernobich, K. Davia, H. K. Ranu, K. T. MacLeod, R. J. Hajjar and S. E. Harding. Adenovirus-mediated Na/Ca exchanger overexpression reduces sarcoplasmic reticulum (SR) Ca content in adult rabbit cardiomyocytes. *Biophys. J.* 78:373A, 2000.
308. Terracciano, C. M., A. I. Souza, K. D. Philipson and K. T. MacLeod. Na$^+$-Ca^{2+} exchange and sarcoplasmic reticular Ca^{2+} regulation in ventricular myocytes from transgenic mice overexpressing the Na$^+$-Ca^{2+} exchanger. *J. Physiol. (Lond.)* 512:651–667, 1998.
309. Tessari, M. and H. Rahamimoff. Na$^+$-Ca^{2+} exchange activity in synaptic plasma membranes derived from the electric organ of *Torpedo ocellata*. *Biochim. Biophys. Acta* 1066:208–218, 1991.
310. Tibbits, G. F. and K. D. Philipson. Na$^+$-dependent alkaline earth metal uptake in cardiac sarcolemmal vesicles. *Biochim. Biophys. Acta* 817:327–332, 1985.
311. Tibbits, G. F., K. D. Philipson and H. Kashihara. Characterization of myocardial Na$^+$-Ca^{2+} exchange in rainbow trout. *Am. J. Physiol.* 262 (*Cell Physiol.* 31):C411–C417, 1992.
312. Trac, M., C. Dyck, M. Hnatowich, A. Omelchenko and L. V. Hryshko. Transport and regulation of the cardiac Na$^+$-Ca^{2+} exchanger, NCX1. Comparison between Ca^{2+} and Ba^{2+}. *J. Gen. Physiol.* 109:361–369, 1997.
313. Trosper, T. L. and K. D. Philipson. Effects of divalent and trivalent cations on Na$^+$-Ca^{2+} exchange in cardiac sarcolemmal vesicles. *Biochim. Biophys. Acta* 731:63–68, 1983.
314. Tsien, R. W., B. P. Bean, P. Hess, J. B. Lansman, B. Nilius and M. C. Nowycky. Mechanisms of calcium channel modulation by beta-adrenergic agents and dihydropyridine calcium agonists. *J. Mol. Cell Cardiol.* 18:691–710, 1986.
315. Tsoi, M., K. H. Rhee, D. Bungard, X. F. Li, S. L. Lee, R. N. Auer and J. Lytton. Molecular cloning of a novel potassium-dependent sodium-calcium exchanger from rat brain. *J. Biol. Chem.* 273:4155–4162, 1998.
316. Uehara, A., T. Iwamoto, M. Shigekawa and I. Imanaga. Whole-cell currents from the cloned canine cardiac Na$^+$/Ca^{2+} exchanger NCX1 overexpressed in a fibroblast cell CCL39. *Pflugers Arch.* 434:335–338, 1997.

317. Ungerleider, R. M. "Pediatric cardiac surgery". *Curr. Opin. Cardiol.* 7:73–84, 1992.
318. Van Eylen, F., C. Lebeau, J. Albuquerque-Silva and A. Herchuelz. Contribution of Na/Ca exchange to Ca^{2+} outflow and entry in the rat pancreatic beta-cell: studies with antisense oligonucleotides. *Diabetes* 47:1873–1880, 1998.
319. Varro, A., N. Negretti, S. B. Hester and D. A. Eisner. An estimate of the calcium content of the sarcoplasmic reticulum in rat ventricular myocytes. *Pflugers Arch.* 423:158–160, 1993.
320. Vazquez, M., Y. Fang and J. P. Reeves. Acceleration of sodium-calcium exchange activity during ATP-induced calcium release in transfected Chinese hamster ovary cells. *J. Gen. Physiol.* 109:53–60, 1997.
321. Velez, P., S. Gyorke, A. L. Escobar, J. Vergara and M. Fill. Adaptation of single cardiac ryanodine receptor channels. *Biophys. J.* 72:691–697, 1997.
322. Vites, A. M. and J. A. Wasserstrom. Ca^{2+} influx via Na-Ca exchange and I_{Ca} can both trigger transient contractions in cat ventricular myocytes. *Ann. N.Y. Acad. Sci.* 779:521–524, 1996.
323. Wasserstrom, J. A. New evidence for similarities in excitation-contraction coupling in skeletal and cardiac muscle. *Acta Physiol Scand.* 162:247–252, 1998.
324. Wasserstrom, J. A. and A. M. Vites. The role of Na^+-Ca^{2+} exchange in activation of excitation-contraction coupling in rat ventricular myocytes. *J. Physiol. (Lond.)* 493:529–542, 1996.
325. Watano, T., Y. Harada, K. Harada and N. Nishimura. Effect of Na^+/Ca^{2+} exchange inhibitor, KB-R7943 on ouabain-induced arrhythmias in guinea-pigs. *Br. J. Pharmacol.* 127:1846–1850, 1999.
326. Watano, T. and J. Kimura. Calcium-dependent inhibition of the sodium-calcium exchange current by KB-R7943. *Can. J. Cardiol.* 14:259–262, 1998.
327. Watano, T., J. Kimura, T. Morita and H. Nakanishi. A novel antagonist, No. 7943, of the Na^+/Ca^{2+} exchange current in guinea-pig cardiac ventricular cells. *Br. J. Pharmacol.* 119:555–563, 1996.
328. Wetzel, G. T., F. Chen and T. S. Klitzner. L- and T-type calcium channels in acutely isolated neonatal and adult cardiac myocytes. *Pediatr. Res.* 30:89–94, 1991.
329. Wetzel, G. T., F. Chen and T. S. Klitzner. Na^+/Ca^{2+} exchange and cell contraction in isolated neonatal and adult rabbit cardiac myocytes. *Am. J. Physiol.* 268 (*Heart Circ. Physiol.* 33): H1723–H1733, 1995.
330. White, K. E., F. A. Gesek, R. F. Reilly and P. A. Friedman. NCX1 Na/Ca exchanger inhibition by antisense oligonucleotides in mouse distal convoluted tubule cells. *Kidney Int.* 54:897–906, 1998.
331. Xu, W., H. Denison, C. C. Hale, C. Gatto and M. A. Milanick. Identification of critical positive charges in XIP, the Na/Ca exchange inhibitory peptide. *Arch. Biochem. Biophys.* 341:273–279, 1997.
332. Xu, W., C. Gatto and M. A. Milanick. Positive charge modifications alter the ability of XIP to inhibit the plasma membrane calcium pump. *Am. J. Physiol.* 271 (*Cell Physiol.* 40):C736–C741, 1996.
333. Xue, X. H., C. L. Elias, A. Omelchenko, L. V. Hryshko and G. F. Tibbits. Temperature dependence of cardiac Na^+-Ca^{2+} exchanger: comparison of canine (NCX1) and salmonid (NCX-TR1) isoforms. *Biophys. J.* 78:54A, 2000.
334. Xue, X. H., L. V. Hryshko, D. A. Nicoll, K. D. Philipson and G. F. Tibbits. Cloning, expression, and characterization of the trout cardiac Na^+/Ca^{2+} exchanger. *Am. J. Physiol.* 277:C693–C700, 1999.
335. Yang, H. T., K. Sakurai, H. Sugawara, T. Watanabe, I. Norota and M. Endoh. Role of Na^+/Ca^{2+} exchange in endothelin-1-induced increases in Ca^{2+} transient and contractility in rabbit ventricular myocytes: pharmacological analysis with KB-R7943. *Br. J. Pharmacol.* 126:1785–1795, 1999.
336. Yao, A., Z. Su, A. Nonaka, I. Zubair, L. Lu, K. D. Philipson, J. H. Bridge and W. H. Barry. Effects of overexpression of the Na^+-Ca^{2+} exchanger on $[Ca^{2+}]_i$ transients in murine ventricular myocytes. *Circ. Res.* 82:657–665, 1998.
337. Yoshihashi, K. and Y. Habara. Contribution of Na^+/Ca^{2+} exchanger to glucose-induced $[Ca^{2+}]_i$ increase in rat pancreatic islets. *Jpn. J. Physiol.* 49:71–80, 1999.
338. Zoghbi, M. E., P. Bolanos, C. Villalba-Galea, A. Marcano, E. Hernandez, M. Fill and A. L. Escobar. Spatial Ca^{2+} distribution in contracting skeletal and cardiac muscle cells. *Biophys. J.* 78:164–173, 2000.

11. Regulation of cardiac contraction by calcium

RICHARD L. MOSS | *Department of Physiology, and the University of Wisconsin Cardiovascular Research Center, University of Wisconsin Medical School, Madison, Wisconsin*

SCOTT H. BUCK | *Department of Pediatrics, and the University of Wisconsin Cardiovascular Research Center, University of Wisconsin Medical School, Madison, Wisconsin*

CHAPTER CONTENTS

Contractile and Regulatory Proteins of the Cardiac Myofibril
  Myosin
    Myosin heavy chains
    Myosin light chains
  Actin
  Troponin
    Troponin C
    Troponin I
    Troponin T
  Tropomyosin
  C-protein
Mechanical Properties of Myocardium
  Isometric tension
  Shortening velocity
    Force–velocity relationship
    Power vs load curves
  Tension transients
    Transients in response to rapid changes in length
    Transients following photolysis of caged compounds
    Tension redevelopment following release and re-stretch
Regulation of Myocardial Contraction
  Tension
    Tension-pCa relationship
    Determinants of isometric tension
  Shortening velocity
    Effects of activation on velocity of shortening
    Agonist-induced changes in velocity
  Kinetics of tension development and relaxation
Conclusions

THE MYOCARDIAL TWITCH varies greatly on a beat-to-beat basis in terms of both amplitude and kinetics, which in turn are generally well-matched to the work the heart must do to pump blood under a wide range of conditions. While much of this variability can be explained on the basis of alterations in Ca^{2+} delivery to the myoplasm during excitation–contraction coupling, evidence now suggests that a variety of mechanisms match the kinetics of contractile protein interaction (83, 253) to the kinetics of the Ca^{2+} transient.

For example, a number of investigators, though not all, have found that the kinetics of protein interaction are accelerated as myoplasmic $[Ca^{2+}]$ is increased. Inotropic interventions such as β-adrenergic agonists appear to accelerate the kinetics of crossbridge cycling. Of potential interest in pathophysiological states, various physical factors such as myoplasmic pH or concentrations of energy substrate and products of ATP hydrolysis are known to differentially affect the extent and kinetics of crossbridge interaction with actin. The purpose of this chapter is to summarize in some detail the molecular processes mediating the regulation of myocardial contraction. To do this effectively, it will be necessary first to identify the primary molecular elements of the contractile and regulatory machinery, i.e., the components of the myofibril, then to discuss the ways by which contractile properties are assessed, and finally to synthesize an integrated view of the regulation of myocardial contraction. To limit the chapter's scope to a manageable amount of information, we will often cite previous reviews as likely first sources for readers who are interested in more detailed treatments of a topic. The reader should also consult chapters 6, 7, 8, 9, and 10.

Contraction of mammalian myocardium and of all vertebrate striated muscles results from cyclic interactions between the proteins myosin and actin, which in the intact muscle are formed into parallel arrays of overlapping thick and thin filaments (Fig. 11–1). In resting muscles, myosin crossbridges from the thick filament interact with actin weakly, or not at all, due to inhibitory effects of the regulatory proteins troponin and tropomyosin bound to the thin filament. Stimulation of living muscle, either by pacemaker cells in the conducting system of the heart or with applied electric current, results in an increase in myoplasmic Ca^{2+} concentration and subsequent activation of thin filaments due to binding of Ca^{2+} to troponin (Fig. 11–2). The detailed mechanisms of activation are not known, but

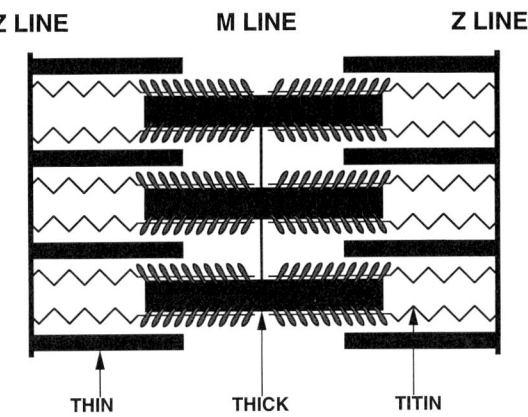

FIG. 11-1. Schematic representation of the spatial relationships of thick and thin filaments, titin, M-line, and Z-lines. Thick filaments are comprised primarily of myosin and a much smaller amount of C-protein. Thin filaments are comprised primarily of actin, troponin, and tropomyosin.

movement of tropomyosin is almost certainly required for crossbridge interaction to proceed. While involvement of Ca^{2+} in regulating contraction is widely accepted, most investigators now believe that the role of Ca^{2+} is complex. One view is that Ca^{2+} has a permissive role in regulation; i.e., the binding of Ca^{2+} to thin filament proteins allows crossbridges to bind to the thin filament and generate tension, but crossbridge binding exhibits positive cooperativity and thereby amplifies the effects of bound Ca^{2+}. In addition, the rate of crossbridge formation and therefore the rate of tension development appear to be regulated primarily by the proportions of crossbridges that are strongly bound; i.e., the rate of interaction becomes faster as the number of strongly bound crossbridges increases.

CONTRACTILE AND REGULATORY PROTEINS OF THE CARDIAC MYOFIBRIL

Myosin

The mechanoenzyme myosin is the major protein of the thick filament and constitutes the majority of cardiac myofibrillar protein mass. Each myosin molecule is ~170 nm in length, has molecular weight of ~525 kDa, and is comprised of six subunits, including two heavy chains (~220 kDa), two essential light chains (~21 kDa), and two regulatory light chains (~19 Kda) (76). The COOH-terminal region of the myosin heavy chain dimer is a coiled-coil α-helical rod approximately 150 nm in length, and these assemble to form the thick filament backbone. The dimeric heavy chains separate near the amino-terminal end of the molecule to form two globular head regions, each head containing a Mg-ATP binding and hydrolysis site, an actin binding site, and one of each type of myosin light chain.

Each thick filament is ~1.6 μm long and 10–15 nm in diameter and is comprised of ~300 myosin molecules. Myosin molecules are oriented in the thick filament in an anti-parallel manner, such that half of the myosin heads are directed toward one end of the sarcomere and the other half to the other end, with a bare area in the middle region where M-line proteins anchor the thick filaments into the sarcomeric lattice. In cross-section, myosin heads emerge from the long axis of the thick filament every 14.3 nm in a helical repeat-

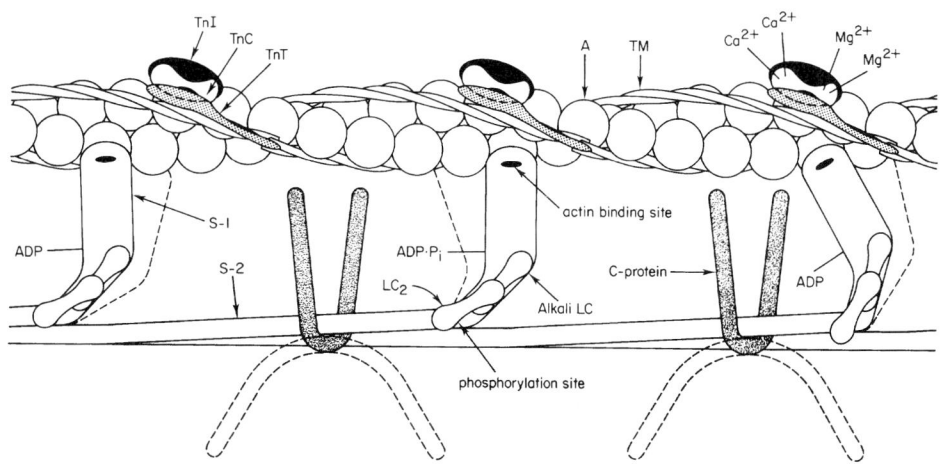

FIG. 11-2. Schematic diagram of thick and thin filaments drawn approximately to scale. A-actin, Tm-tropomyosin, Tn-troponin, LC_2-regulatory light chain (myosin light chain$_2$), Alkali LC-essential light chain (myosin light chain$_1$). C-protein (myosin binding protein C) is drawn in two different configurations because its position in the thick filament is not known (249).

ing pattern, each myosin head emerging at an angle of 40° relative to its predecessor resulting in an inter-head distance of 43 nm (210).

Treatment of myosin with trypsin cleaves the molecule into two fragments: light meromyosin (~160 kDa) derived from the coiled-coil tail, which exhibits solubility characteristics similar to native myosin, and heavy meromyosin (~360 kDa), consisting of the myosin heads and a coiled-coil rod-shaped subfragment (subfragment 2, or S2). Further proteolysis of heavy meromyosin with papain removes subfragment 2 and yields free subfragment 1 (S1, ~120 kDa), which consists of the myosin heavy chain heads and associated myosin light chains. The cleavage sites at which myosin is proteolyzed into light and heavy meromyosin, and subsequently into S1 and S2, are flexible hinge regions of the myosin molecule (76, 136), with the regulatory myosin light chain being located in the vicinity of the junction between S1 and S2.

Myosin Heavy Chains. The myosin heavy chains (MHC) and myosin light chains (MLC) are both encoded by highly conserved multi-gene families and are expressed in muscle as multiple isoforms. The myosin heavy chains found in the myofibrils of mammalian striated muscles are all isoforms of myosin II, and to date as many as 10 isoforms have been identified. In striated muscles of the rat, which is probably the most extensively studied species with respect to MHC diversity, the following MHCs have been described: cardiac α and β, skeletal slow type I (which is the same gene product as cardiac β), embryonic, neonatal, and three fast MHCs—types IIa, IIb, and IIx (or IId). A detailed description of the myosin heavy chain and light chain families can be found in extensive reviews by Swynghedauw (267), Pette and Staron (221), and Schiaffino and Reggiani (241). Because myosin is the most abundant of the myofibrillar proteins, and because it contains both the actin binding site and the myosin ATPase site, isoforms of MHC have figured prominently in studies of determinants of contractile properties of cardiac muscle (reviewed in 299).

In the cardiac ventricles of most species, including humans, three myosin heavy chain isoforms have been identified on the basis of electrophoretic mobility under non-denaturing conditions: V1, V2, and V3. V1 consists of a homodimer of the α myosin heavy chain (αα), V2 is a αβ heterodimer, and V3 is a ββ homodimer. The α and β myosin heavy chains are produced by closely linked genes on chromosome 3 in mouse and chromosome 14 in human. β-MHC is most abundant in utero until late fetal life. In small animals, α-MHC expression increases shortly before birth and becomes predominant throughout perinatal and adult life. In contrast, in large animals such as human, α-MHC is transiently predominant only shortly after birth while β-MHC predominates in the adult. Thyroid hormone and exercise increase α-MHC expression and decrease β-MHC expression; conversely, hypothyroidism, aging and work overload decrease α-MHC expression and increase β-MHC expression (155, 156, 267).

Despite 93% amino acid identity and 95% homology (176), α-MHC and β-MHC exhibit dramatically different enzymatic and mechanical activities. As originally described by Bárány (17), there is a positive correlation between the maximum velocity of shortening and the actin-activated ATPase activity of myosin. In keeping with this notion, shortening velocity for contractile systems comprised of V1 myosin is greater than velocities for those with V3 myosin, and in in vitro studies of isolated proteins, actin-activated and calcium-stimulated ATPase activities are about three times greater for V1 myosin than for V3 myosin (96, 152). Similarly, the economy of ATP utilization by V3 myosin is twice that of V1 (7, 98). Recently, ATPase activity, actin filament sliding velocity and force per myosin head of V1 and V3 were compared. Actomyosin ATPase activity per V1 myosin head was nearly twice that of V3, and V1 myosin demonstrated threefold faster actin filament sliding velocities than V3 myosin; however, the average force per myosin head for V3 was twice that for V1 (281).

The elaboration of a high-resolution x-ray crystallographic structure of skeletal muscle myosin S1 in the early 1990s (225, 226) and recent kinetic, genetic, crosslinking, and in vitro motility studies have led to remarkable new insights into the structure and function of the actin and nucleotide binding sites on the myosin heads, and of the regulatory and essential light chains and their interactions with S1 (76). Space-filling models (Fig. 11–3) have revealed the three major regions of the myosin head: a 25 kDa NH_2-terminal nucleotide binding region, a central 50 kDa segment that includes the actin binding domain ~4 nm from the nucleotide binding site, and a 20 kDa COOH-terminal region that in intact myosin continues to the thick filament. As described by Geeves and Holmes (76), current models include crossbridges as swinging lever arms in which small rotational movements (~0.5 nm) of the 50 kDa segment are translated into larger movements of the C-terminal region by the converter domain, resulting in displacement of the actin filament.

The light chains are wrapped around the α-helical "neck" region of S1 and overlap the flexible hinge region between the globular head and tail portions of S1. These structural relationships suggest that the light chains may stabilize the α-helical region of the head during force generation, thus allowing transmission of force to the thick filament backbone and to the thin filament. By making this part of S1 more rigid, the light

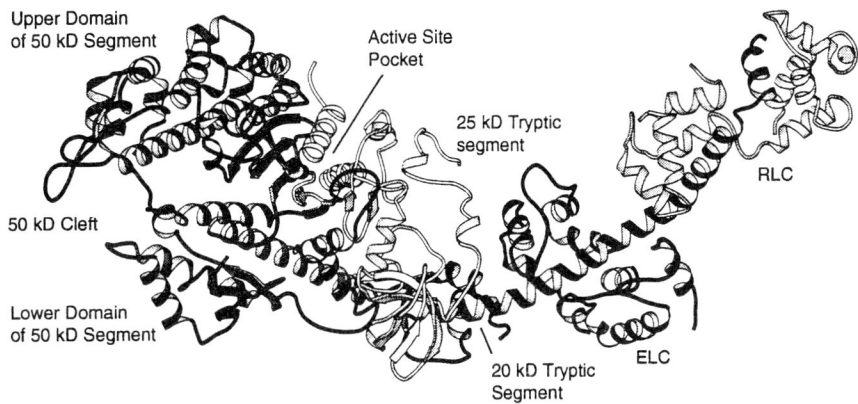

FIG. 11–3. Ribbon representation of chicken gizzard skeletal muscle myosin subfragment-1 looking into the narrow cleft that splits the central segment of the heavy chain. The heavy chain is displayed in different shades of gray to delineate the NH$_2$-terminal, central, and COOH-terminal fragments that extend from residues Asp 4 Glu 204, Gly 216 Tyr 626, and Gln 647 Lys 843, respectively. These segments are separated by disordered loops in the x-ray structure and were previously identified by mild tryptic cleavage of the myosin head as the 25, 50, and 20 kDa fragments, respectively 15, 192). These tryptic fragments are not independent folding domains; however, they are convenient for identifying large segments of the structure. Regulatory and essential light chains are labeled RLC and ELC, respectively.

chains might also act to amplify conformational changes that occur in other parts of S1 during the crossbridge cycle. Consistent with this notion, skeletal muscle myosins that are expressed with truncated neck lengths move actin filaments at reduced velocities and generate less force than myosins with full-length necks (159, 276, 278, 280).

A striking feature of the high-resolution model of S1 is the presence of a long narrow cleft dividing the 50 kDa segment into upper and lower domains. Expansion and closure of this cleft are thought to be integral elements of the communication between the nucleotide and actin binding sites. Most recently it has been demonstrated that P$_i$ released by cleavage of ATP leaves the nucleotide binding pocket via this cleft (so-called backdoor enzyme), so that ADP remains bound until the mechanical movement phase of the crossbridge cycle is complete (227, 309). The importance of cross-talk between the actin and nucleotide binding sites was demonstrated by Uyeda et al. (279) using chimeras of myosin from the slime mold *Dictyostelium*, in which myosin isoform-specific sequences of the actin binding domain were inserted between highly conserved sequences. Despite the fact that the ATP-binding sites were unaltered in these chimeras, their ATPase activities were found to differ, thereby demonstrating the importance of sequence substitution in the actin binding domain.

Mutations of the β-MHC gene (chromosomal locus 14q1) have been shown to be among the most common genetic defects in patients with familial hypertrophic cardiomyopathy (26, 39, 167). With an estimated prevalence of 0.1–2 per 1,000 population, *f*amilial *h*ypertrophic *c*ardiomyopathy (FHC) is inherited as an autosomal dominant disease and is characterized by hypertrophy that predominantly involves the interventricular septum. The clinical course of the disease is markedly variable, ranging in severity from minimal left ventricular outflow obstruction and symptoms to sudden cardiac death that has the highest incidence among younger patients. Approximately 40 different mutations of the β-MHC gene have been associated with FHC, and a correlation between genotype and phenotype (including risk of sudden death) has been observed in many cases (60). The mutations appear to be clustered primarily around specific regions in the myosin head: at or near the nucleotide binding site, adjacent to the converter region, close to the interface with the essential light chain, and much less frequently in the myosin rod. This distribution of mutations suggests that in FHC there are disturbances of regions critical to force transduction. Cuda and co-workers isolated β-MHC protein from skeletal muscle of patients with FHC (45) and subsequently showed that the velocity of contraction was significantly less than that of β-MHC from skeletal muscle of unaffected individuals (46). To date, nearly all β-MHC defects studied have been associated with decreased velocity, with the exception of replacement of Arg by Gln at residue 719 (26). Of potential importance, mapping of myosin S1 structure predicts that this residue resides at the interface of β-MHC and the essential light chain, i.e., LC$_1$ (123). More recently, Tyska et al. (277) have reported that myosin from transgenic mice expressing cardiac α-MHC with the R403Q mutation associated with FHC in humans actually has a faster in vitro motility than control myosin, suggesting that the mutation speeds kinetics and increases energy utilization by myocardium. While this is a potentially plausible mechanism for development of hypertrophy, it is unclear at present why results of this study differ from earlier work in which β-MHCs with the R403Q mutation were found to have slower than normal contraction kinetics (22, 142, 202).

Myosin Light Chains. In adult cardiac muscles, there are ventricular and atrial isoforms of the myosin light chains, i.e., the essential light chain (LC_1) is expressed as either the ventricular (LC_{1v}) or atrial (LC_{1a}) isoform, and the regulatory light chain (RLC or LC_2) is either the ventricular (LC_{2v}) or the atrial (LC_{2a}) isoform. From relatively more numerous studies on skeletal muscles, it is evident that the rate of crossbridge cycling assessed by mechanical V_{max} differs when essential light chain or regulatory light chain content varies. Recently, electrophoretic analysis suggests the existence of two ventricular RLC isoforms in human heart—these RLCs have identical molecular weights and different isoelectric points, but at present the functional significance of these variations is unknown (188).

Lowey et al. (159) have studied the possible roles of skeletal muscle essential light chains and the regulatory light chain (i.e., RLC or LC_2) in shortening, but did so by assessing the rate of movement of actin filaments in an in vitro motility assay (reviewed in 158). In these experiments, sliding velocity was measured in the presence of native myosin, myosin devoid of light chains, and light chain–depleted myosins that were reconstituted with essential light chains, regulatory light chain, or both. Velocity was slowest with light chain–deficient myosin, i.e., ~9% of control obtained in the presence of native myosin. Addition of RLC to light chain–deficient myosin increased V_{max} to ~17% of control. Addition of essential light chains increased V_{max} to ~35% of control, which is consistent with earlier findings that partial extraction of RLC significantly reduces V_{max} in skinned fibers (110, 197). Addition of both RLC and essential light chains resulted in virtually complete recovery of velocity to control values. These authors interpreted their results in terms of a model in which the myosin light chains play a critical role in transmitting force and movement from thick to thin filaments. Such a model is consistent with the notion advanced by Rayment et al. (225) that the light chains impart mechanical rigidity to the α-helical portion of myosin S1. At the same time, it is possible that extraction of one or both light chains reduces actin-activated ATPase activity, an idea that has not been systematically tested at physiological ionic strength. Most biochemical studies done at low ionic strength have observed no significant effects on ATPase activity due to light chain removal, although it should be noted that Margossian (163, 164) has reported a 50% reduction in actin-activated ATPase activity in LC_2-deficient myosins from skeletal and cardiac muscles when compared to control.

Regulatory light chains. There is increasing evidence that myosin RLC, which is also called LC_2 or P-light chain, plays an important role in determining mechanical properties, at least in fast-twitch skeletal muscle fibers (194). For example, partial extraction of RLC from rabbit skinned skeletal muscle fibers results in an increase in the Ca^{2+} sensitivity of tension (110), an increase in the rate of tension development at low levels of Ca^{2+} (183), and a decrease in maximum velocity of shortening (110, 197). While the mechanisms underlying the effects of RLC removal are not yet known, biochemical experiments showed that removal reduced the actin-activated ATPase of myosins from both heart (163) and skeletal muscles (164), which is consistent with a decrease in mechanical V_{max}. Thus, it is likely that RLC modulates the rate of crossbridge dissociation from actin. Further evidence in support of this idea has been obtained using an in vitro motility assay in which RLC-deficient myosin moved thin filaments at significantly lower velocities than did RLC-replete myosin (159).

The dramatic effects on mechanical properties of fast-twitch muscles due to RLC removal raises the interesting possibility that various isoforms of RLC, e.g., atrial vs ventricular, confer different mechanical properties to the myocardium in which the isoforms are expressed. While it is evident that cardiac and fast skeletal muscles have distinct mechanical behaviors, the contributions of RLC isoforms to these differences are not yet known. One possible clue is the finding by Larsson and Moss (143) that human type II fibers expressing both fast and slow isoforms of RLC had significantly lower V_{max} values than fibers expressing only the fast isoform. In living myocytes from mouse hearts, transgenic expression of ventricular RLC in atrial cells increased the extent and rate of myocyte shortening, i.e., the crossbridge cycling kinetics became more similar to the kinetics observed in ventricular myocytes (220). The idea that in heart muscle the RLC is an important determinant of the kinetics of contraction has gained further support in studies on skinned cells from the same animal model (35).

Cardiac RLC, like skeletal RLC and smooth muscle RLC, is phosphorylated by a Ca^{2+}, calmodulin-dependent myosin light chain kinase (reviewed in 261). In skeletal muscle, phosphorylation of RLC increases the extent and rate of force development and the Ca^{2+}-sensitivity of isometric tension, all of which have been attributed to an increase in f_{app}, the rate constant governing the transition from non-force-generating to force-generating states in the crossbridge cycle (180, 89; 265). Possible mechanisms for this effect include direct effects of phosphorylation on one or more kinetic transitions or alterations in crossbridge availability to actin due to charge-induced movements of the crossbridge heads away from the thick filament backbone and closer to the thin filament (150, 261, 308).

While phosphorylation of RLC in skeletal muscle appears to contribute to post-tetanic potentiation, it has been difficult in intact cardiac muscle to relate changes in contractile properties to levels of RLC phosphorylation, due primarily to slow rates of phosphorylation and dephosphorylation (261). However, in exercising rats, a positive correlation was found between the rate of left ventricle pressure development and the level of RLC phosphorylation (65). Subsequently, in an isolated Langendorff rat heart preparation, RLC phosphorylation was found to be regulated in a frequency-dependent manner at physiologically relevant rates (187). Morano et al. (190) subsequently assessed the rate of tension development (k_{td}) after photolytic release of ATP in skinned bundles of atrial and ventricular myocardium from pig hearts. In ventricular myocardium, increased RLC phosphorylation resulted in an increase in K_{td}, which the authors interpreted as indicating that cardiac RLC phosphorylation increases the rate of crossbridge attachment, similar to the case in skeletal muscle. As evidence of the likely importance of RLC function in living heart, Sanbe et al. (238) observed severe hypertrophy of the atria and valvular dysfunction in transgenic mouse hearts expressing a non-phosphorylatable RLC.

Essential light chains. The roles played by the essential light chains of myosin in muscle contraction are not well understood. Recent x-ray studies (226) of the essential light chain, as well as the RLC, in association with myosin subfragment 1 (S1) yielded potentially important structural information about the light chains. The essential light chain and, to a lesser degree, the RLC were found in close association with the α-helical portion of S1, suggesting the possibility that one or both of these light chains provide mechanical stabilization of the myosin head during force development. Other evidence suggests that the essential light chains influence the rate of interaction of myosin with actin, which implies that the light chain has a role in addition to mechanically stabilizing S1. A few studies combining mechanical and biochemical approaches strongly suggest that there is a close association between V_{max} and natural variations in essential light chain content of fast-twitch muscle fibers (241).

Another possibility suggested by the work of Sweeney and colleagues (260) is that the N-terminus of the essential light chain actually interacts electrostatically with actin, thereby slowing shortening velocity. This conclusion was based on experiments in which effects on shortening velocity due to various isoforms of essential light chains having variable N-terminal domains and mutant proteins in which charged amino acids were replaced with neutral residues were assessed in skinned skeletal muscle fibers. At present, the implications of these findings for cardiac function under normal or pathophysiological conditions are not known, but it is evident that changes in the essential light chain could have important functional consequences. Consistent with this point of view, Fewell et al. (63) reported that crossbridge cycling kinetics were accelerated by transgenic expression of the atrial isoform of the essential light chain in mouse ventricles. Interestingly, in some congenital heart defects there is increased expression of the atrial essential light chain in the ventricle (191), although it is unclear how this might contribute to or compensate for the mechanical dysfunctions of these disorders.

Additional studies have suggested that myosin light chain expression or content in heart may be altered in some pathological conditions. In human myopathic hearts, Margossian et al. (165) described a reduction in RLC content relative to LC_1, which was attributed to the presence of an active protease in myopathic hearts. However, Morano and colleagues (189, 191) reported no changes in the $RLC:LC_1$ ratio in failing hearts, nor in hearts of patients with congenital heart disease, but they did observe expression of atrial LC_1 (up to 17% of total LC_1 content) in ventricular myocardium from patients with congenital heart disease. When force-velocity characteristics were determined in ventricular skinned myocardium, they found a positive correlation between V_{max} and the amount of atrial LC_1 that was expressed (191). To explain these results, Morano (188) has proposed that the atrial essential light chain is less restrictive to movement of the myosin head than is the ventricular essential light chain, which would allow increased crossbridge mobility, crossbridge cycling, and force generation.

In an animal model of postischemic heart failure and hypertrophy, Liu et al. (153) reported that eight weeks after left coronary artery ligation, RLC phosphorylation was significantly increased in the right ventricle (by 60%) and interventricular septum (by 30%), but significantly reduced (by 50%) in the viable left ventricle. Bottinelli and colleagues (27) found that maximum shortening velocities assessed from force-velocity curves (V_{max}) and with the slack test (V_o) were significantly greater in atrial tissue than in ventricular tissue from hyperthyroid rat hearts. Because Ca^{2+}-stimulated ATPase activity and Ca-Mg-dependent ATPase activity were equal due to identical myosin heavy chain composition, the observed differences in velocity were attributed to an influence of myosin light chain isoform expression upon velocity. Finally, in a transgenic mouse model in which endogenous atrial RLC was replaced with ventricular RLC, unloaded velocity of shortening (V_o) of atrial cells expressing ventricular RLC was increased, suggesting that crossbridge kinetics are influenced by the RLC isoform expressed in myocardial cells (35). These findings agree well with previous results obtained from electrically stimulated living myocytes from the same animal model of altered RLC expression (220).

Actin

Actin is the primary protein of the thin filament and is notable for its ability to activate myosin ATPase activity. Actin exists in vitro in two states: as globular monomeric actin (G-actin, 42 kDa) and as filamentous polymeric actin (F-actin). Actin monomers have a mean diameter of ~5.5 nm and have a complex morphology of four subdomains surrounding a binding pocket for a divalent cation and nucleotide (83); F-actin is comprised of G-actin monomers that are assembled into a double helix of 7 actin monomer pairs per half turn, with an internodal distance of ~38.5 nm (reviewed in ref. 210). There are approximately 380 actin monomers per thin filament occurring with the ratio of 7:1:1 of actin monomers:troponin:tropomyosin. Actin is expressed in all eukaryotic cells and is very highly conserved; e.g., smooth muscle actin differs from skeletal actin by just 6 of 375 residues (237). In heart, the expression of α-skeletal actin and α-cardiac actin is developmentally regulated and species dependent. In hearts from newborn rats, approximately 60% of actin is α-cardiac actin and the remainder is α-skeletal actin, which decreases to less than 5% by 2 months of age (243). In human heart, approximately 20% of actin in utero is α-skeletal actin, which increases to 50%–60% by adulthood (100, 243). Furthermore, actin isoform expression in heart is influenced by pathological conditions. For example, expression of skeletal α-actin in heart increases twofold in spontaneously hypertensive rats as compared to normotensive controls (25).

There is now evidence that actin isoforms influence the regulation of contraction. For example, the concentration of actin required to activate specific myosin isozymes to half-maximal ATPase activity varies over a 2–4-fold range depending on which isoform of actin is used with particular isomyosins (237). More recently, in BALB/c mice exhibiting variable expression of α-skeletal in heart, a positive correlation was found between indices of contractility (dP/dt, time to peak tension) and α-skeletal actin content, which is remarkable in view of the fact that α-skeletal and α-cardiac actins differ by changes in just four neutral amino acid residues (100).

Troponin

Troponin is the Ca^{2+} binding protein of the thin filament of striated muscle, and was initially described by Ebashi and Kodama (53) as tropomyosin aggregation-promoting factor and subsequently as the Ca^{2+} binding element in the activation of muscle contraction. Later, Greaser and Gergely (89) showed that troponin is comprised of three subunits: a 24 kDa inhibitory subunit (TnI) that prevents contraction in the absence of Ca^{2+}, an 18.4 kDa calcium-binding subunit (TnC), and a 34 kDa subunit (TnT) that binds other troponin subunits and to tropomyosin. The troponin complex is distributed along the thin filament at approximately 40 nm intervals, so that each troponin complex is associated with one tropomyosin molecule and seven actins (reviewed in 253).

According to the classic steric blocking model of regulation, in the relaxed heart, myoplasmic Ca^{2+} is low, so that the Ca^{2+}-specific binding site on TnC is unoccupied. Under these conditions, the affinity of TnI for actin is high, which causes the thin filament to assume a conformation in which the myosin binding sites of actin are blocked by tropomyosin and perhaps by one or more subunits of troponin. In the presence of Ca^{2+}, there is a change in conformation of TnC, which results in increased affinity of TnC for the inhibitory region of TnI and functional dissociation of TnI from actin. The dissociation of TnI from actin allows tropomyosin to move toward the groove between the strands of actin monomers comprising the thin filament. This movement is thought to allow strong binding of myosin to sites on actin and ultimately leads to activation of actomyosin Mg-ATPase and muscle contraction (reviewed in 57, 273). As recently reviewed (83, 253), simple steric blocking models appear to be inadequate to completely describe regulation. For example, x-ray diffraction studies of isolated thin filaments suggest the existence of distinct positions of tropomyosin that are consistent with a three-state model of regulation—relaxed muscle includes blocked and closed states in which crossbridges are weakly bound, and active muscle includes an open state in which myosin can bind to actin and isomerize into strong-binding, force-generating states (147, 175). According to this model, the transition from blocked to closed states is favored by Ca^{2+} binding to TnC, and the transition from closed to open states is favored by strong binding of crossbridges to actin. Such a model has gained support from recent studies in which deletions of domains within tropomyosin have been found to reduce the positive cooperative effects of myosin S1 on tropomyosin–actin binding (141).

Troponin C. The cardiac isoform of TnC is virtually identical to the slow-twitch skeletal muscle isoform (282), but differs from the fast-twitch isoform in its capacity to bind Ca^{2+} (144, 296). Both isoforms of troponin C are dumbbell-shaped in that they each contain two globular regions separated by a 9-turn, 31-amino acid α-helix. Cardiac TnC and fast skeletal TnC have two high-affinity divalent cation binding sites (sites III and IV) in the COOH terminal globular domain, and these sites have greater affinity for Ca^{2+} than for Mg^{2+} (223). However, these sites are normally occupied by Mg^{2+} due to the relatively low concentration of Ca^{2+} in resting muscle. Based on their ability to extract TnC from myofibrils using a chelator of divalent cations, Zot and Potter (314) concluded that occupancy of the high-affinity sites on TnC stabilizes the association of TnC with the remainder of the troponin complex.

The two binding sites (I and II) in the NH_2-terminal domain are low-affinity Ca^{2+}-specific sites. In contrast to the case in skeletal muscle in which both low-affinity Ca^{2+}-specific sites of TnC are functional, site I in cardiac TnC is nonfunctional due to substitution of aspartic acid residues with leucine and alanine; thus, only site II functions as a low-affinity, Ca^{2+}-specific binding site (reviewed in 218, 253, 272). The low-affinity, Ca^{2+}-specific binding sites on TnC are commonly believed to regulate contraction such that Ca^{2+} binding to these sites activates the thin filament for interactions with myosin S1. There is good evidence that Ca^{2+} binding to TnC is increased by strongly bound cycling crossbridges in cardiac muscle, to a greater extent than in skeletal muscle (105), implying that in cardiac muscle there is strong coupling between S1 binding to actin, Tm movement, and TnT-TnI-TnC interactions (reviewed in 83).

Troponin I. The troponin I subunit (TnI) of troponin inhibits actin–myosin interaction in solution. The mature cardiac isoform, cTnI, contains two adjacent serines (Ser 32 and Ser 33) in the NH_2-terminal portion, which are absent from skeletal muscle RLC (310; reviewed in 253, 272). Presumably by modulating TnI-TnC interactions, phosphorylation of these serines in cTnI reduces the affinity of TnC for Ca^{2+} (230), thereby decreasing the Ca^{2+} sensitivity of the contractile proteins. Phosphorylation of TnI is thought to account, at least in part, for the lusitropic response (enhanced relaxation) of the heart to β-adrenergic stimulation (252). Consistent with this idea, Wattanapermpool et al. (293) reported that replacement of endogenous cTnI with a truncated cTnI lacking the 32- amino acid NH_2-terminus domain eliminated the effect of protein kinase A to reduce the Ca^{2+} sensitivity of tension. Thus, phosphorylation of cTnI at serine residues in the unique amino terminal extension is both necessary and sufficient to account for the decrease in myofilament Ca^{2+}-sensitivity associated with β-adrenergic stimulation.

Ca^{2+} calmodulin-dependent protein kinase and protein kinase C can also phosphorylate cTnI, resulting in reduced Ca^{2+}-dependent actomyosin Mg-ATPase activity (208, 253, 285). However, the functional role and significance of these phosphorylations are not presently known.

Troponin T. The third subunit of troponin, troponin T (TnT), is an asymmetric molecule that binds to other troponin subunits and to tropomyosin. Multiple TnT isoforms are generated during development by alternative splicing from a single TnT gene in avian (78), rabbit (170, 206), rat (124, 125, 241), and human (9, 10) heart muscles. Distinct variants of TnI are also expressed in fetal and mature hearts (21, 50, 86, 118, 166, 203, 239, 241). Isoform switching of cardiac TnC during development has not been observed, so that changes in cardiac thin filament function are thought to reside in isoform switching of TnI and/or TnT.

Several lines of evidence point to a role for TnT isoforms in modulating Ca^{2+} sensitivity of contraction in heart muscle. Utilizing reconstituted purified contractile proteins, Tobacman and Lee (274) demonstrated that calcium activation of ATPase activity differed depending on which of two TnT isoforms was present. Subsequently, McAuliffe et al., (170) showed that skinned cardiac fibers from ventricular strips isolated from 5-day-old rabbits were more sensitive to Ca^{2+} than fibers from 22-day-old rabbits, an effect that was attributed to differences in TnT isoform expression at the different ages. In longitudinal studies of TnT expression in developing rabbit heart, five TnT isoforms were resolved (8), and it was subsequently shown that the pCa_{50} for developed tension varied with TnT isoform composition (206).

Expression of TnT isoforms may also be altered in myocardial disease. Pagani and co-workers (212) demonstrated that left ventricular myofibrillar Mg-ATPase activity was reduced in end-stage human heart failure, while myosin Mg-ATPase was not reduced, suggesting that changes in myofibrillar Mg-ATPase may be due to alterations in isoform expression of myofibrillar regulatory proteins. Subsequent studies demonstrated that of the four TnT isoforms expressed in human fetal heart, the two with the fastest electrophoretic mobilities (TnT_1 and TnT_2) are expressed in normal and failing adult heart as well; however, in patients with heart failure, a greater percentage of total TnT was the TnT_2 isoform (9). An inverse relationship was observed between ATPase activity and expression of TnT_2. More recently, Wolff and colleagues (304) reported that a fetal TnT isoform was expressed in seven of eight failing human hearts but not in control hearts; however, Ca^{2+} sensitivity of isometric tension did not correlate with the amount of fetal TnT present but was instead related to alterations in basal β-adrenergically mediated phosphorylation of myofibrillar regulatory proteins (304). In another model of diseased myocardium, Akella et al. (1) reported alterations in TnT isoform distribution and in Ca^{2+} sensitivity of tension at long and short sarcomere lengths (1.9 and 2.4 μm) in cardiac trabeculae from diabetic rats. These authors related the greater length dependence of Ca^{2+} sensitivity in the diabetic heart to changes in expression of TnT. Finally, mutations of the cardiac troponin T gene (locus 1q3) have been associated with FHC in approximately 15% of affected families (167, 270, 290). These mutations have been characterized by relatively mild or subclinical hypertrophy but with a high incidence of sudden death (290).

Evidence points as well to a role for TnI isoforms in modulating the Ca^{2+} sensitivity of contraction. In contrast to the case for TnT, alternate isoforms of TnI are encoded by different genes (203, 240). The major TnI isoform expressed in fetal heart is identical to that expressed in slow-twitch skeletal muscle, but with maturation and under the influence of changes in thyroid hormone status (50), the quantity of ssTnI decreases and the amount of cTnI increases (21, 50, 86, 118, 166, 203, 239, 240). Accumulation of cTnI and disappearance of ssTnI proceeds along a caudorostral direction in the heart, decreasing immediately after birth in the atria and only later in ventricular tissue (86). In intact cardiac muscle, there is an initial fall in developed tension in response to acidosis, which is more pronounced in mature than in immature hearts (251). The response of membrane-permeabilized skinned ventricular strips to acidosis differs as well: the pCa_{50} of the tension–pCa relationship decreased by 0.61 pCa units in strips from mature heart but by only 0.26 pCa units in immature strips, an effect that was attributed to differences in TnI isoform expression. The molecular basis for greater sensitivity to acidosis in adult myocardium is discussed in detail later, under Myocardial Acidosis, as part of Determinants of isometric tension.

Tropomyosin

The thin filament protein tropomyosin is believed by most investigators to assume a position in the thin filament (146) that in the absence of Ca^{2+} bound to Tn either blocks or retards binding of crossbridges to actin. Tropomyosin is a flexible, filamentous dimeric molecule that is ~42 nm in length and is comprised of two α-helical coiled-coil monomeric chains (each ~33 kDa mol wt) that are linked by a single disulfide bond. Tm isoform expression appears to influence the flexibility of Tm (38), which may in turn influence the coupling between S1 binding and Ca^{2+} binding. Tropomyosin assembles as either a homodimer or a heterodimer containing either or both of two isoforms, α and β, that are 88% homologous (205). Different proportions of the two isoforms are found in fast and slow skeletal muscles and in heart muscle. Cardiac tropomyosin in small mammals is typically comprised of the αα homodimer; in large mammals, including humans, ~20% of tropomyosin in the heart is the β-isoform.

Tropomyosin binds stoichiometrically to actin in the thin filament in a ratio of 1 Tm to 7 actin monmers. Tropomyosin resides in each of the two grooves between the actin strands of the thin filament, and each Tm overlaps adjacent Tm molecules in head-to-tail fashion. A single troponin complex binds to each Tm molecule in anti-parallel fashion, such that the NH_2-terminal tail portion of troponin T binds to the head-tail overlap region of tropomyosin, and troponin C/troponin I bind to amino acids within residues 150–180 of tropomyosin.

Recent work has demonstrated potentially important functional consequences of alterations in tropomyosin isoform expression. Using a transgenic mouse line exhibiting a 34-fold increase in β-tropomyosin expression, i.e., control mice expressed virtually all α-tropomyosin whereas transgenic animals expressed ~60% β-tropomyosin, Muthucamy and colleagues (205) found no differences in the ultrastructure of transgenic hearts but observed that isolated perfused transgenic hearts had slower rates of relaxation and prolonged half-times of relaxation relative to controls. However, this observation in intact hearts seems to be inconsistent with results of experiments in solution (271) in which thin filaments reconstituted with αα tropomyosin homodimers had greater Ca^{2+} sensitivity of release of troponin inhibition than did αβ heterodimers or ββ homodimers. Also, αα and αβ dimers exhibited stronger binding to the TM binding domain of TnT than did ββ, and αα homodimers in a reconstituted Ca^{2+} regulated troponin-tropomyosin-actomyosin S1 ATPase system were associated with higher activities than were ββ or αβ dimers.

Mutations of the α-tropomyosin gene (locus 15q2) have recently been shown to be the primary genetic defect in familial hypertrophic cardiomyopathy in approximately 3% of affected individuals (167, 270, 291). Similar to cases in which defects in cardiac troponin T account for FHC, mutations of the α-tropomyosin gene have been associated with a high incidence of sudden death (291).

C-Protein

C-protein was first described by Offer et al. (209) as a protein that co-purified with myosin, and since that time considerable additional work has been done to elucidate the structure and function of the protein (300). C-protein (also called myosin binding protein-C, ~130 kDa mol wt), exists as isoforms specific to fast skeletal, slow skeletal, and cardiac muscles (75). Cardiac C-protein is encoded on a different chromosome than the skeletal isoforms, and has several unique features: an additional immunoglobulin repeat at the N-terminus, phosphorylation sites in the linker between the C1 and C2 domains, and an additional 28-residue loop in the C5 domain (300). C-protein has a relatively high-affinity myosin binding site near its COOH-terminus and appears to participate in assembly of thick filament proteins (242). Other physiological functions of this protein are not well understood. For example, actomyosin ATPase activity of cardiac myosin increases slightly in the presence of C-protein (306), but the physiological significance of this phenomenon is not known. However, because this effect on ATPase activity does not occur in the absence of the RLC, it appears that C-protein and RLC may influence ATPase activity in concert (300). Partial extraction of C-protein from skinned myocardial preparations increases isometric tension at sub-maximal [Ca^{2+}] but has no effect on maximum tension, which suggests that C-protein modulates the activation process in cardiac muscle, possibly by constraining the movement of myosin heads (109). Finally, adrenergic stimulation results in incorporation of as many as 3 moles phosphate per mole cardiac C-protein, which is localized to sites in the NH_2-terminus of the molecule (75). Again, the significance of this energetically expensive phenomenon is not understood, since phosphorylation of C-protein has been shown to be insufficient to alter reconstituted actomyosin Mg-ATPase activity (74) or to alter myofibrillar Ca^{2+} sensitivity (293). However, there is evidence to suggest that C-protein phosphorylation promotes myosin head movement away from the thick filament backbone and reduces flexibility of crossbridge heads (294). Thus, C-protein phosphorylation might affect total force developed by myocardium or the kinetics of the actomyosin ATPase (300), but definitive studies of this possibility have not yet been done.

In the past few years, several mutations of the cardiac C-protein gene on chromosome 11 have been identified in some patients with FHC (26, 290). In most cases, these mutations were predicted to disrupt the high-affinity myosin binding domain in the COOH terminus of C-protein. Consistent with this idea, transgenic mice expressing C-protein lacking the myosin binding domain exhibited significant changes in cardiac structure and depression of dynamic mechanical properties (307). Also, several of the mutations in β MHC that cause familial hypertrophic cardiomyopathies also appear to disrupt the interaction of myosin with C-protein (91).

MECHANICAL PROPERTIES OF MYOCARDIUM

Contractile properties of living myocardium can be assessed using multi-cellular and single-cell preparations isolated from the atria or ventricles of virtually any vertebrate heart. Mechanical measurements on these preparations yield information about the regulation of crossbridge interaction with actin, the rate of crossbridge cycling, and the kinetics of chemical and mechanical transitions between specific states in the interaction cycle (Fig. 11–4). Even relatively simple mechanical properties such as tension and shortening velocity provide important information about the distributions of crossbridges among weakly and strongly bound states and the kinetics of transitions between these states. To facilitate discussion of the regulation of contraction in myocardium, this part of the chapter considers the molecular mechanisms of mechanical behavior and the kinds of information that mechanical measurements provide. Of the approaches discussed here, only tension and shortening velocity have been widely used to probe mechanisms of regulation of mechanical function in myocardium.

Isometric Tension

Tension developed by myocardium is directly related to the number of crossbridges in strongly bound tension-generating states. Biochemically, these states appear to be those in the crossbridge cycle closely associated with or subsequent to the dissociation of inorganic phosphate (P_i) from the A.M.ADP.P_i complex (Fig. 11–4), since P_i release has been shown to be kinetically coupled to tension generation in skinned skeletal muscle fibers (185, 286) and in skinned myocardium (12: see also Chapter 6). Since the interaction of myosin with actin in muscle is regulated by Ca^{2+}, the number of crossbridges bound to actin, and consequently the tension, varies with the concentration of Ca^{2+} bathing the myofilaments. In living myocardium, a single, supra-threshold stimulus transiently increases myoplasmic Ca^{2+} to levels that are usually

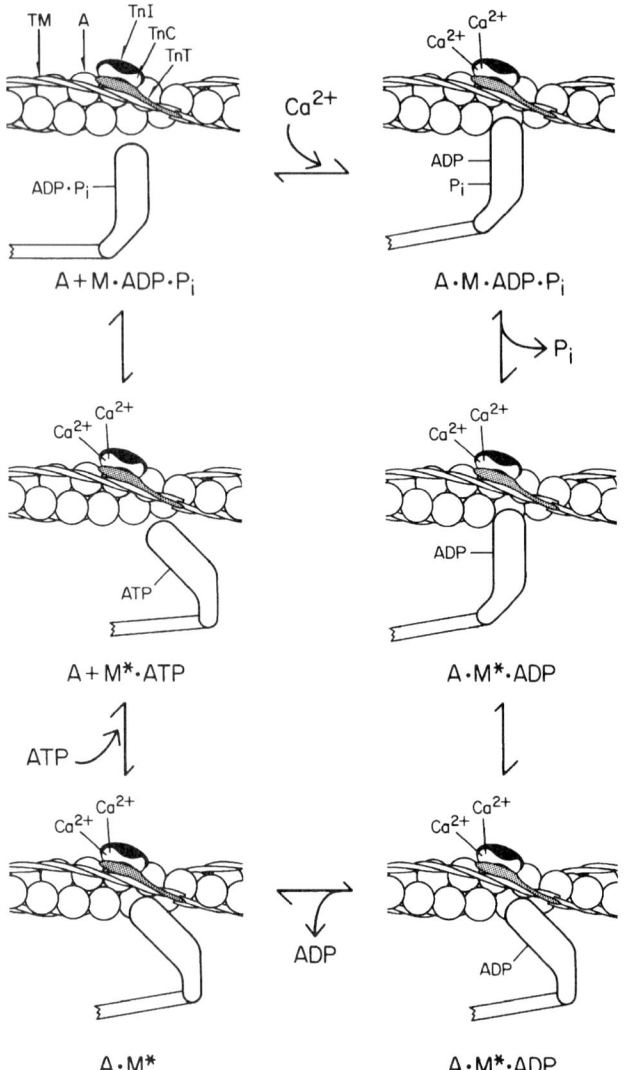

FIG. 11–4. Crossbridge interaction cycle. A-actin, M-myosin, P_i-inorganic phosphate, M*-myosin that has undergone the transition to the force-generating state.

insufficient to saturate Ca^{2+} binding sites on the thin filament. Also, at physiological temperatures, the Ca^{2+} transient is too brief to allow crossbridges to achieve a steady-state distribution between force-generating and non-force-generating states. Because of these two factors, peak twitch tension is usually less than the maximum the muscle would otherwise be capable of developing. For example, in the presence of extracellular Ba^{2+}, it is possible to maintain a steady contracture with tetanic stimulation, and under these conditions tension ultimately reaches a steady maximum (e.g., 112).

In skinned muscle preparations, the membrane is permeabilized or removed physically to directly expose the myofilaments to the bathing solution. Activation of contraction requires addition of Ca^{2+} to a bathing medium that already contains Mg-ATP, a Ca^{2+} buffer such as EGTA, a pH buffer, and physiological salts (reviewed in 194). The steady isometric tension developed by skinned muscle preparations represents a steady-state distribution of crossbridges between strongly and weakly bound states, and the number of strongly bound bridges (and therefore the tension) can be varied from near zero to maximal by adding various amounts of Ca^{2+} to this solution. The results of studies such as these are usually plotted as a tension–pCa relationship in which absolute isometric tension or relative tension (tension as a fraction of maximal) measured at each $[Ca^{2+}]$ is plotted against pCa, which is $-\log[Ca^{2+}]$. A Hill plot linearization of these data (247) yields several important variables: the pCa_{50} is the pCa at which tension is half-maximal and is taken as an index of Ca^{2+} sensitivity of tension; the slope of the Hill plot is the Hill coefficient, which is taken to indicate the degree of apparent cooperativity in the activation of tension. These characteristics of the tension–pCa relationship are discussed later, under Tension in the section title Regulation of Myocardial Contraction.

Shortening Velocity

Force-Velocity Relationship. When the load on a muscle is less than its isometric tension-generating capability, the muscle shortens and lifts the load at a velocity that varies inversely with the size of the load. In intact muscle, the shape of the force–velocity relationship is generally hyperbolic (Fig. 11–5) and can thus be described by the equation, $(P + a)(V + b) = $ constant, in which a and b define the asymptotes of the hyperbola (102, 130, 302).

While a hyperbola is usually a good approximation of the force–velocity relationship, velocity points at loads near zero or near maximum deviate from a hyperbola, at least in skeletal muscles: points near zero load generally lay above the hyperbola fitted to intermediate loads (e.g., 42, earlier work discussed in 302), as do points at loads near the steady isometric tension (e.g., 55). Nonetheless, a fitted hyperbola provides a means for describing the curvature of the force–velocity relationship and extrapolation of the fitted curve to zero load provides an estimate of unloaded shortening velocity, V_{max}. If the load on a muscle is greater than P_o, the muscle will actually lengthen at a low velocity (130). Thus, the load that can be lowered by a muscle is considerably greater than the load that can be lifted or held isometrically. The velocity of lengthening increases gradually until the load is equivalent to about $2 \times P_o$, above which velocity increases rapidly. The basis for the sudden increase in velocity of lengthening is not known, but this mechanism presumably provides

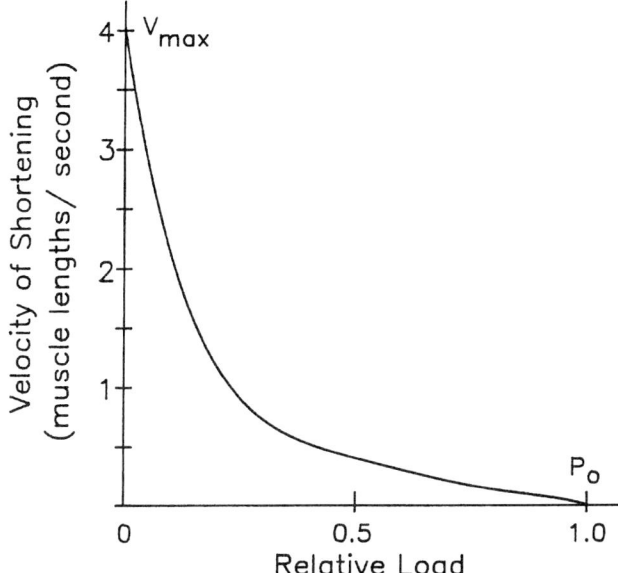

FIG. 11–5. Velocity of shortening as a function of relative load. V_{max} = maximum velocity of shortening, P_o = maximum isometric tension.

protection against muscle injury due to very large loads.

Mechanical V_{max} in a variety of skeletal muscles appears to be directly related to the V_{max} of actin-activated myosin ATPase activities of proteins from the same muscles (17). Based on a correlation between shortening velocity and rate of ADP release in a variety of muscles, Siemankowski et al. (248) have suggested that maximum shortening velocity is limited by the rate of ADP dissociation from the crossbridge, which effectively controls detachment of the crossbridge from actin. Consistent with this idea, Huxley's (119) two-state model of contraction predicts that V_{max} should be exquisitely sensitive to detachment rate, because crossbridges that remain bound after completing their power strokes will ultimately become a load on the muscle as shortening continues and thereby limit V_{max}. In Huxley's model, crossbridges that are slow to detach (due to slow rates of ADP dissociation) will ultimately become compressed as thick and thin filaments continue to slide past one another, giving rise to a restoring force that opposes contraction and slows velocity.

Maximum shortening velocity and the force–velocity relationship are frequently used to characterize functional differences in cardiac muscles due to alternate expression of myosin isoforms. When experimental conditions such as temperature and sarcomere length are equivalent, V_{max} provides an assessment of the relative rates of ADP release from different myosin isoforms complexed with actin; however, V_{max} can also vary with experimental conditions, and these must be taken into account when comparisons are made. In addition, while V_{max} and actin-activated ATPase activity are well correlated in muscles of different types and from different sources (17), these properties should not necessarily be interpreted as probing the same transition in the crossbridge interaction cycle. Many investigators believe that ATPase activity, which is a manifestation of crossbridge turnover rate, is limited by the rate of ATP hydrolysis while the crossbridge is dissociated from actin. Also, the rate of ADP dissociation during shortening is probably different than in isometric contractions, because the mean mechanical strain is less than in isometric contractions and many rate constants of the interaction cycle appear to be strain dependent (119).

Power vs Load Curves. In performing work against a load, muscles generate power, which is work per unit time and is estimated by multiplying force × velocity. Since force and velocity are inversely related, the product of the two will be greatest at an intermediate load, which turns out to be about 0.3 P_o. At this peak of the power curve, skeletal muscle is working most efficiently since 40%–45% of the chemical energy is converted to mechanical work.

Several investigators have characterized the ability of muscles to perform work by transforming force-velocity data to power-load curves (Fig. 11–6). Because power reaches a maximum in the mid-ranges of both force and velocity in muscles, and because velocity varies rather slowly with load in this range, some investigators (34, 233, 244) have suggested that maximum power output is a more reliable index of dynamic mechanical properties of a muscle than is V_{max}. Since V_{max} is usually estimated by extrapolating the steep part of the force–velocity curve to zero load, small errors in estimating loads near zero can have dramatic effects on estimates of values for V_{max}. In addition, maximum power provides a measure of mechanical properties of muscles operating under physiological loads. Muscles in vivo do not generally operate at either extreme of the force–velocity curve, i.e., at V_{max} or P_o, where power is zero, but instead operate at intermediate forces and velocities where power is close to its maximum.

Brooks et al. (34) measured maximum power outputs from fast-twitch and slow-twitch muscles of mice and determined that while isometric tension did not differ between the two types of muscles, fast-twitch muscles had significantly greater maximum power output than did slow-twitch muscles. Further studies have found that the relative velocity (V/V_{max}) at which maximum power is attained is a key parameter in defining the mechanical properties of a muscle. Rome et al. (231) determined that in swimming carp, both slow

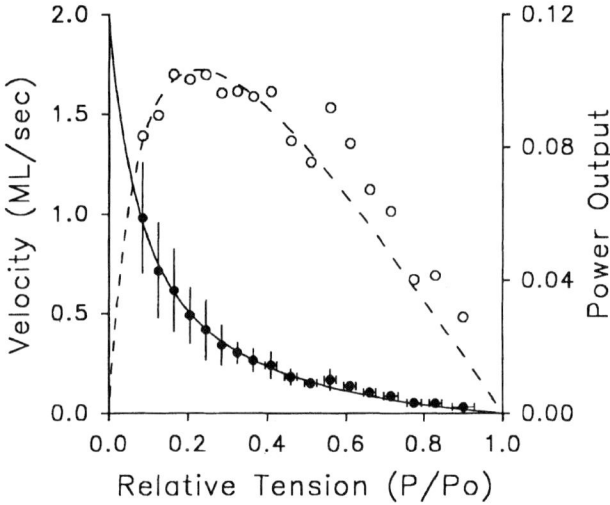

FIG. 11–6. Cumulative force-velocity (●) and power-load (★) relationships obtained from eight single skinned cardiac myocytes. Data points in the force–velocity relationship are means ± S.D. Mean force–velocity data were fit using the normalized form of the Hill equation:

$$\frac{V}{V_{max}} = \frac{(1-P)}{P_o} / [1 + \frac{P}{P_o}]\frac{P_o}{a}$$

where V_{max} and P_o are maximum velocity of shortening and isometric force, respectively.

and fast muscles operate at approximately the same V/V_{max}, although the absolute velocities differ considerably in the two muscle types. Rome et al. further determined that this value of V/V_{max} corresponded to the velocity at which maximum power was generated. Subsequent studies (232–234) indicated that muscles operate within the same narrow range of V/V_{max}, independent of temperature, suggesting that this ratio is an important constraint in defining the operation of muscles in vivo. Such a constraint raises the possibility that changes in muscle contractile proteins that are observed during development or in response to changing functional demands may be an adaptive response to shift shortening velocity, so that the muscle continues to operate in the range of V/V_{max} at which power output is maximal.

To date, power–load curves have not been extensively characterized in any muscle type with respect to possible sensitivity of peak power to Ca^{2+}, pH, or other determinants of shortening velocity. Ford et al. (70) investigated possible changes in normalized peak power in skinned skeletal muscle with changes in $[Ca^{2+}]$, and found the peak to be unaltered when activation was lowered from P_o to ~0.5 P_o by reducing $[Ca^{2+}]$. This result suggests that the maximum rate at which a muscle can do work does not vary with $[Ca^{2+}]$, at least when changes in tension-generating capability are taken into account. However, subsequent measurements on skinned cardiac myocytes showed that the relative load for maximum power output increased from 0.29 P_o to 0.34 P_o when $[Ca^{2+}]$ was reduced from maximal to half-maximal (173). Such an increase in power would tend to maintain the work capacity of myocardium at lower levels of activation.

Tension Transients

Tension transients in response to mechanical perturbations and rapid changes in solution composition provide information about specific transitions in the crossbridge interaction cycle. Transients have provided important information regarding mechanisms of contraction, but the reader should also be aware that measurements from force transients are subject to artifact if there is significant compliance at the points of attachment to the experimental apparatus. If the ends are compliant, rates of rise of tension are slowed as the compliant ends are extended by the actively contracting middle region of the fiber (see review in 194). For this reason, assessment of tension transients is best done in a mechanical system that allows monitoring and precise control of sarcomere length during the mechanical measurement. Most work using these approaches has been done in skeletal muscle preparations, although data from myocardial preparations have begun to appear.

Transients in Response to Rapid Changes in Length. Following rapid reductions in length complete within 1 ms, skeletal muscle fibers exhibit isometric force transients (Fig. 11–7) that include a phase thought to represent the force-generating transition(s) of the crossbridge interaction cycle (69, 120). When a step decrease in length is applied to a muscle fiber, tension decreases by an amount that is proportional to the length change, suggesting that the reduction in tension is due to recoil of elastic structures in the crossbridge. This phase of the transient is followed a phase of rapid recovery of force in which crossbridges remain strongly bound to actin and presumably undergo mechanical and/or chemical transitions to higher force-generating states. Further evidence suggests that this phase of tension recovery is coincident with a conformational change of the crossbridge inferred from high time resolution x-ray diffraction patterns obtained during the transients (122). The third phase of recovery is a transient pause, plateau, or reversal in recovery that is believed to be due to crossbridge detachment. In the final slow phase of recovery, crossbridges bind or re-bind, and force attains a new steady-state level.

If the length step applied to the muscle is sufficiently rapid (~0.2 ms), it is possible to record phase 1 of the

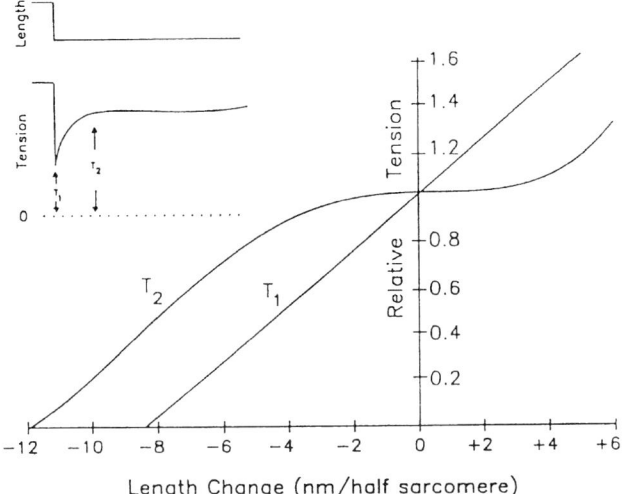

FIG. 11–7. Tension transient following rapid change in length of a single muscle fiber. Coincident with length change, tension decreases to a minimum (T_1), which represents recoil of an elastic part of the crossbridge due to relative sliding of thick and thin filaments. Once the length change is complete, tension recovers to an intermediate value, T_2, without detachment of the crossbridge from actin. This phase of force recovery is thought to be due to rotation of crossbridge heads. Thus, the total working distance of a crossbridge without detaching and reattaching is equivalent to the smallest imposed length changes (~12 nm/half-sarcomere) for which T_2 is zero. [Idealized diagram based on data from Ford, et al. (69).]

transient with minimal contributions from phase 2, the phase of rapid recovery (69). Assessment of phase 1 under these conditions suggests that elastic elements of the crossbridge are strained ~4 nm in the process of isometric force generation. The distance over which myosin interacts with actin during a single cycle is at least twice this amount, since rapid recovery to phase 3 is observed even when a step decrease of ~10 nm is applied to the fiber. To date, there is no evidence that the working stroke or interaction distance of crossbridges varies with myofibrillar protein composition, although it is likely that the rates of tension change in various phases of the isometric tension transients are myosin isoform dependent.

Transients Following Photolysis of Caged Compounds. In investigating molecular mechanisms by which protein isoforms influence contractile properties of muscle, rapid changes in solution composition would provide a means to probe specific transitions within the crossbridge interaction cycle. For example, by rapidly changing the concentration of P_i it is possible to assess the kinetics of crossbridge transitions associated with force development. These kinds of experiments were initially performed in fast-twitch muscle fibers of the rabbit by rapidly releasing compounds of interest from chemical cages, which make the compounds inert and therefore unreactive to the contractile proteins (reviewed in 116). Ca^{2+}, P_i, and nucleotides such as ATP and ADP can be chemically caged as part of photolabile compounds. Exposing these compounds in solution to intense U.V. light ($\lambda = 347$ nm) results in photolysis of the chemical cage and release of the compound of interest. In this way, sudden increases in the concentration of a variety of compounds can be achieved, thereby perturbing the transition in the cycle in which the compound participates as a reactant or product. Photorelease of compounds is accompanied in every instance by a mechanical force transient, which allows inferences about the role of the underlying transition in force generation. Again using P_i as an example, caged compounds have been employed to determine (1) that P_i release is associated with force development in muscle (116), (2) that P_i release is a two-step process involving an isomerization of the actomyosin–nucleotide complex either before or after P_i release (47, 185, 286, 312), and (3) that the rate of P_i release is crossbridge strain dependent (114). Qualitatively similar results have been obtained in skinned myocardium (12, 66). Numerous experiments have been done to probe other aspects of the crossbridge interaction cycle, including the ADP release step using caged ADP (47, 160), dissociation of rigor cross-bridges from actin using caged ATP (80, 81), and the rates of activation of using caged Ca^{2+} (reviewed in 13, 83). Similarly, the kinetics of activation and relaxation have been studied in skinned myocardium using caged ATP (168) and caged Ca^{2+} (11).

Tension Redevelopment Following Release and Restretch. The rate at which force is developed during the onset of contraction is considerably faster in fast-twitch muscles than in slow-twitch muscles. The faster rate could be due to faster delivery of Ca^{2+} to the myoplasm during excitation–contraction coupling and/or to faster transitions of crossbridges to force-generating states once Ca^{2+} is bound by the thin filaments. One way to distinguish between these possibilities is to attempt to change [Ca^{2+}] rapidly in the vicinity of the myofilaments in skinned fibers (see discussion of caged compounds below) and then record the rate of tension development. An alternative approach is to maintain the skinned fiber in a steady Ca^{2+}-activated state, and then apply a mechanical perturbation that disrupts formed crossbridges and reduces force to near zero. The subsequent redevelopment of force would then represent the transition from non-force-generating to force-generating states without limitations due to diffusion of Ca^{2+}, as would be expected in excitation–contraction coupling in living fibers. Brenner (31) has developed a very effective protocol to study the force-generating transition in steadily Ca^{2+} activated skinned muscle preparations (Fig. 11–8): The muscles are released, allowed to shorten under no load for a distance that requires several cycles of interaction of crossbridges with actin, and then restretched to the original length to break most of the crossbridges still bound to actin. Force at the end of re-stretch is zero or nearly zero, because all or most crossbridges are in detached, weakly bound states. The subsequent recovery of active force results from the transition of weakly bound crossbridges into strongly bound force-generating states. In most cases, the record of force redevelopment can be fit with a single exponential of the following form: tension = $C(1 - e^{-kt})$, in which C is steady isometric force and k is the rate constant of force redevelopment, k_{tr}. Using a simple two-state model for crossbridge interaction, $A + M \rightleftharpoons AM$, in which the formation of the force-generating AM complex is regulated by rate constant f and dissociation of the complex is regulated by rate constant g, Brenner and Eisenberg (31a) assumed that k_{tr} was the sum of f and g. This is an especially useful way to interpret k_{tr}, since force and ATPase activity can also be expressed in terms of these rate constants. Assuming this model, it is then possible by measuring combinations of force, k_{tr} and ATP activity to assess the effects of various experimental perturbations on one or both rate constants. For example, measurements that showed k_{tr} was Ca^{2+} dependent were interpreted as showing that Ca^{2+} had this effect primarily by altering f, the rate constant of the non-force-generating to force-generating transition(s).

A simple two-state crossbridge model does not account for all experimental results. For example, the Ca^{2+} sensitivity of the force-generating transition inferred by Brenner implies that k_{tr} should be P_i dependent, which it is (286), and that the rate constant of tension change (k_{Pi}) upon photolysis of caged P_i might vary with $[Ca^{2+}]$, which it does (286). However, k_{Pi} shows only a threefold sensitivity to Ca^{2+}, which is not sufficient to account for the approximate 20-fold regulation of ATPase activity during activation of contraction (151); and in any case, k_{tr} is substantially smaller than k_{Pi} suggesting that k_{tr} is dominated by a process not probed by P_i. Homsher and Millar (116) proposed that during the measurement of k_{tr}, dissociation of strongly bound crossbridges from actin results in cooperative inactivation of the thin filament, which is not the case in measurements of k_{Pi}. Thus, the lower value of k_{tr} might be due to cooperative reactivation of thin filament as strongly bound crossbridges re-form. This idea was tested in experiments in which k_{tr} was measured before and after application of an analogue of strongly bound crossbridges to skinned skeletal muscle fibers (259). N-ethyl maleimide conjugated myosin S1 (NEM-S1) binds strongly to thin filaments and has previously been shown to cooperatively activate actin-activated ATPase activity (298). Application of NEM-S1 to skinned fibers increased k_{tr} to maximal values even at very low concentrations of Ca^{2+} (259), suggesting that strongly bound crossbridges activate kinetic transitions in the crossbridge interaction cycle. On the other hand, even in the presence of NEM-S1 the maximum value of k_{tr} was no greater than that obtained in the presence of saturating $[Ca^{2+}]$. Thus, the basis for differences between maximum values of k_{tr} and k_{Pi} are still uncertain, although it seems likely that a step prior to P_i release, such as crossbridge binding to the thin filament or an isomerization, limits k_{tr} but not k_{Pi}.

Studies of k_{tr} have also been done in skinned preparations of myocardium (e.g., 94, 304), although results to date have been inconsistent with respect to possible effects of activation on the kinetics of force

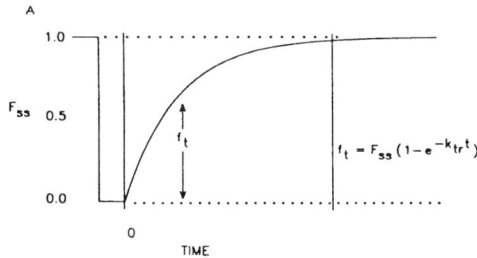

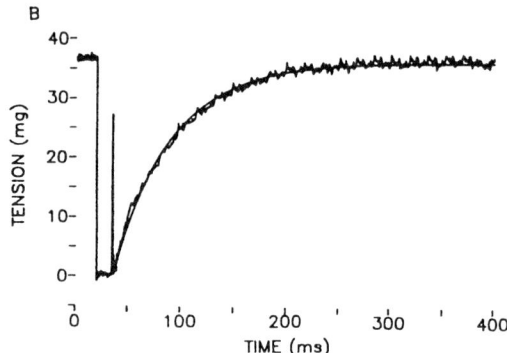

FIG. 11–8. Determination of k_{tr} in rabbit skinned psoas fibers. *A:* Schematic diagram of an experimental record showing the measured variables and the equation used for determining k_{tr}. Once a fiber was steadily activated in a Ca^{2+}-containing solution and tension was constant (F_{ss}), the fiber was slackened and tension was reduced to zero. Following a period of unloaded shortening, the fiber was rapidly re-extended to its original length, thereby straining attached crossbridges and transiently increasing tension. The strained crossbridges then rapidly dissociated from actin, reducing tension to zero. The subsequent time-course of tension recovery represents the redistribution of crossbridges from non-tension-generating to tension-generating states. *B:* Actual record obtained during an experimental measurement of k_{tr} at 15°C. The solid line is a computer-fitted curve for which k_{tr} was 18 s1. Sarcomere length was kept constant (± 0.5 nm) by controlling the position of the first-order line of a laser diffraction pattern obtained from the fiber. [From Metzger et al. (180).]

development. These results are discussed in detail in a later section, Kinetics of Force Development.

REGULATION OF MYOCARDIAL CONTRACTION

Tension

Tension–pCa Relationship. Regulation of contraction in cardiac muscle involves Ca^{2+} binding to troponin, which through a series of events involving troponin I, troponin T, and tropomyosin (Tm) disinhibits the thin filament (reviewed in 272). The mechanism of activation almost certainly involves movement of Tm to allow crossbridge interaction to proceed. However, it is not clear whether myosin crossbridges in relaxed muscle are sterically blocked from binding actin (97, 121) or, as now seems more likely, can be weakly bound to actin (32) but blocked from the transition to force-generating states (37, 57, 148). While the requirement for Ca^{2+} in activating contraction is widely recognized, the mechanisms mediating activation are complex and only partly understood (see also Chapter 9). As $[Ca^{2+}]$ in Mg-ATP-containing solutions is raised, isometric tension in skinned muscle preparations increases sigmoidally and reaches a plateau at about 10 μM Ca^{2+}, which as described earlier in this review comprises the tension–pCa relationship. The pCa_{50} (pCa = -log$[Ca^{2+}]$) for isometric tension defines the Ca^{2+} sensitivity of tension, which is similar in skinned skeletal muscle and skinned myocardium when measurements are made at the same sarcomere length (SL) and temperature and in identical solutions. In both muscle types, several factors are believed to contribute to Ca^{2+} sensitivity of tension (reviewed in 13): osmotic compression, increased SL, increased pH, increased [ADP], or reduced $[P_i]$ all increase the Ca^{2+} sensitivity of tension. The increase in pCa_{50} in each of these cases is thought to result from increased cooperative activation of tension as a result of greater numbers of crossbridges strongly bound to the thin filament. At present, much work is aimed at determining mechanisms of cooperativity in the activation of contraction and ways that these mechanisms may differ in heart and skeletal muscles. This problem has profound significance for understanding regulation in the two muscle types, since twitch contractions in skeletal muscle tend to be explosive, all-or-none events while cardiac twitches may be subtly graded on a beat-to-beat basis. Although some differences in twitch kinetics can be accounted for by differences in the time course of Ca^{2+} delivery and reuptake, the responsiveness of the contractile proteins to Ca^{2+} in the myoplasm undoubtedly contributes to the twitch characteristics of each muscle.

Tension–pCa relationships in fast-twitch skeletal muscle fibers are typically much steeper than those from myocardial preparations (13a, 266), a phenomenon that has frequently been interpreted as showing greater cooperativity of tension development in skeletal muscles. However, it is possible that differences in the isoforms of one or more regulatory proteins in the two muscles account for their apparent differences in Ca^{2+} responsiveness. Fast-twitch TnC has two low-affinity Ca^{2+} binding sites, while cardiac TnC has just one (reviewed in 88, 272). The significance of this difference is not well understood, but it may contribute to the differing slopes of the tension–pCa relationships in the two muscles. In one set of experiments using skinned myocardium, replacement of endogenous cardiac TnC with skeletal TnC resulted in an increase in the steepness of the tension–pCa relationship cardiac muscle, suggesting that TnC has an important role in determining the form of the tension–pCa relationship. However, in the converse experiment, stoichiometric replacement of endogenous fast TnC in skinned psoas fibers with cardiac TnC had no effects on either the Ca^{2+} sensitivity of tension or the slope of the tension–pCa relationship (201). The implication of this finding is that fast and cardiac isoforms of TnC do not account for differences in the form or midpoint of the tension–pCa relationships in these two muscles. Therefore, at this time, there is not a clear consensus about the role of TnC isoforms in determining the steepness of the tension–pCa relationships in muscles of different type. In any case, such experiments do not eliminate the possibility that the steepness of the relationship is related to interactions of other subunits of troponin (TnT or TnI) with TnC.

Tension–pCa relationships measured in skeletal and cardiac muscles are usually asymmetrical in that they are steeper at low $[Ca^{2+}]$ than at high $[Ca^{2+}]$ (194). The steepness evident at low $[Ca^{2+}]$ has generally been interpreted to mean that activation of contraction involves a high degree of molecular cooperativity among subunits of the thick and thin filaments, an inference that is supported by data from a variety of sources. From biochemical studies of myosin, regulated actin, and micromolar Mg-ATP in solution, rigor crossbridges bound to the thin filament appear to activate the filament to allow interaction with nucleotide-bound crossbridges (30). Consistent with this idea, skinned fibers develop substantial tensions in 1 μM Mg-ATP even when Ca^{2+} is absent (131) and slowly shorten under these same conditions (199). Brandt et al. (28) suggested that the steepness of the tension–pCa relationship at millimolar Mg-ATP actually involves sustained activation of regions of the thin filament due to bound crossbridges, which have much longer half-times for dissociation from actin than does Ca^{2+} from TnC.

The shape of the tension–pCa relationship may also be influenced by marked cooperativity in Ca^{2+} binding to the thin filament. Using isolated cardiac thin filaments, Tobacman and colleagues (273, 275) have shown that there is cooperativity of Ca^{2+} binding to the regulatory sites of TnC, most likely as a consequence of short-range intermolecular interactions. Using skeletal muscle proteins, Grabarek et al. (87) observed independent binding of Ca^{2+} to the two low-affinity sites of skeletal fast-twitch TnC in solution; however, Ca^{2+} binding to TnC exhibited positive cooperativity in regulated thin filaments, and this was enhanced when S1 was bound to actin. In this regard, both rigor (30) and cycling (93, 229) crossbridges increase the affinity of fast skeletal TnC for Ca^{2+}. In cardiac muscle, Ca^{2+} binding affinity of cardiac TnC is also increased by rigor (217) and cycling (105) crossbridges (reviewed in 72).

Further experiments, in which partial extraction of TnC reduced Ca^{2+} sensitivity of tension (29, 198, 266) and extraction of whole troponin increased Ca^{2+} sensitivity (196), also strongly suggest that Ca^{2+} binding to TnC is influenced by the state of activation of other regions of the same thin filament.

The regulatory subunits that mediate cooperativity within the thin filament are not known for certain, although it is likely that tropomyosin (Tm) is involved (reviewed in 272). Such cooperativity is a key element in some models of regulation (e.g., 104) in accounting for Ca^{2+}-dependent variations in tension. Head-to-tail polymerization of Tm within the thin filament (161) could provide a means for cooperative interactions between functional groups. In a test of this idea, Walsh et al. (287) found that the response of regulated actin-activated myosin ATPase to Ca^{2+} was unaffected by removal of regions of overlap between adjacent Tm molecules. However, Pan et al. (215) subsequently found that removal of head-to-tail overlap of Tm molecules reduced the cooperativity of S1 · ADP binding to reconstituted thin filaments, and they concluded that overlap of adjacent Tm is necessary for near-neighbor interactions. The difference in results between the two studies may be due to the low ionic strength of the assay system (-20 mM) used by Walsh et al. and their low ratios (1:100) of myosin relative to actin.

Thus far, the role of Tm overlap in the apparent cooperativity of tension development has not been studied directly—i.e., in force-generating muscle preparations—because it has not been feasible to disrupt overlap in intact filament lattices and still retain function. Nonetheless, it is evident that Tm does contribute to cooperativity in the activation mechanism in cardiac muscle. In myocytes from transgenic mice, overexpression of the β isoform of tropomyosin, which increased thin filament β Tm content of ~60% of the total, increased the Ca^{2+} sensitivity and apparent cooperativity of tension development as compared to control myocytes expressing nearly 100% α Tm (305). These results suggest that the isoform of Tm present in the thin filament influences the degree of cooperation in Ca^{2+} binding or crossbridge binding or both.

Another protein with possible roles in thin filament cooperativity is troponin T (TnT), which consists of a globular head (T_2) and an extended tail region (T_1) (68). To investigate whether Tn influenced the cooperative binding of S1 to regulated thin filaments, Williams and Greene (297) compared the effects of Tm and Tm-Tn on the binding of S1 to actin and found that Tn had no effect on the binding of S1 to regulated actin in the presence of Ca^{2+}. However, in the absence of Ca^{2+}, Tn-Tm conferred pronounced cooperativity to actin · S1 binding indicating that the major effect of Tn on the binding of S1 to regulated actin is to increase cooperativity in the absence of Ca^{2+}. With respect to TnT, the T_1 domain is long enough to extend to the region of overlap between adjacent Tm molecules (68). Interactions of T_1 with the NH_2-terminus of Tm seem to be relatively weak (33), whereas interactions with the COOH-terminus are strong. Thus, TnT may influence the interaction of overlapping Tm molecules by its binding to the COOH-terminus of its associated Tm, with little direct interaction with the adjacent Tm. However, removal of the NH_2-terminal 45 residues of TnT does not alter the apparent cooperativity in Ca^{2+} activation of the actomyosin S1 ATPase (216) and had little effect on Tm-Tm interactions (103). Nonetheless, the Ca^{2+} sensitivities of actomyosin ATPase (274) and tension (206) vary depending on the cardiac TnT isoforms that are present.

Fast-twitch and cardiac muscles appear to differ with respect to cooperative mechanisms of activation, since tension–pCa relationships are generally steeper in fast-twitch muscles. Such differences may be a manifestation of different Ca^{2+} binding properties mediated by muscle-specific isoforms of thin filament regulatory proteins, as discussed above. On the other hand, the differences may result from muscle-specific differences in responsiveness to strong binding of myosin crossbridges to the thin filament. Recent experiments support the second interpretation (259): Infusion of N-ethylmaleimide S1, a strong-binding derivative of myosin S1 (298), increased the Ca^{2+} sensitivity of tension and reduced the slope of the tension–pCa relationship in fast-twitch skeletal muscle from rabbit. Qualitatively similar results have been obtained in skinned myocardial preparations (66). However, the effects of a given concentration of NEM-S1 were greater in cardiac muscle, indicating that cardiac muscles are more responsive to strong-binding crossbridges. Thus, as was suspected from the greater steepness of the tension–pCa relationship, fast-twitch muscles are more highly cooperative in the sense that it takes a greater number of strongly bound crossbridges to cooperatively activate further binding of crossbridges to the thin filament.

Based on primarily biochemical measurements using skeletal muscle proteins, Geeves and colleagues (77, 175) have proposed a model of regulation that accounts for much of the data discussed above. In this scheme, the thin filament in the absence of Ca^{2+} is in a "closed" state in which crossbridges are blocked from binding to thin filament sites. However, when Ca^{2+} binds to the thin filament, it enters an "open" state in which crossbridges may bind, but the extent and rate of rate of binding depend upon the numbers of crossbridges that bind; i.e., this system exhibits positive cooperativity. In a scheme such as this, Ca^{2+} might be viewed as a permissive regulator of crossbridge binding, but the total number of crossbridges that ultimately bind to actin depends both on the concentration of Ca^{2+} and crossbridge-induced facilitation of further crossbridge binding. In this regard, it is interesting to note that even under rigor conditions, Ca^{2+} and rigor-S1 interact to determine the extent of crossbridge binding to the thin filament. Using skeletal myofibrils, Swartz et al. (258) showed that in the absence of Ca^{2+}, small amounts of fluorescent rigor S1 applied exogenously bound solely to thin filaments in the region of thick–thin filament overlap, which is consistent with the notion that the endogenous rigor complexes activated the thin filament locally in the overlap region. However, as the concentration of fluorescent S1 (and therefore of rigor S1) was increased, binding extended into the non-overlap region. Finally, in the presence of Ca^{2+}, fluorescent S1 was evident primarily in the non-overlap region, suggesting that Ca^{2+} binding to the thin filament permitted binding of the exogenous rigor S1 even when applied at low concentrations. Such results point strongly to a model of regulation involving both Ca^{2+} and myosin head binding to the thin filament. A review by Lehrer (147) provides an excellent synthesis of the data and concepts that are critical to such a model.

Determinants of Isometric Tension. Besides Ca^{2+} and strongly bound crossbridges, a variety of other factors can affect the distribution of crossbridges between weakly and strongly bound states and thus appear to have important effects on myocardial performance in both normal and pathophysiological states. For example, decreased pH reduces maximum Ca^{2+} activated tension in skinned myocardium, an effect that is much greater in cardiac muscle than in skeletal muscle (discussed below). Other factors, such as alterations in $[P_i]$ or [ADP] also affect tension development, presumably by direct or indirect effects on the equilibrium constant for the P_i release step in the crossbridge interaction cycle. The primary mechanisms thought to underlie changes in the regulation of myocardial contraction in vivo are discussed below.

Stimulus frequency. For over a century, scientists have known that myocardium from most mammalian species (rat is a major exception) exhibits a so-called positive staircase in which tension increases with stimulus frequency. Measurements of Ca^{2+} transients during a single twitch suggest that the amount of Ca^{2+} released to the myoplasm is not sufficient to saturate troponin C (58), the Ca^{2+} binding subunit of troponin. Thus, the most likely explanation for the positive staircase is that more Ca^{2+} is released to the myoplasm during E-C coupling at high frequencies of stimulation, presumably as a result of an increase in the Ca^{2+} content of the sarcoplasmic reticulum. Such an increase might be expected when the interbeat interval decreases because cellular Ca^{2+} extrusion processes may be too slow to effectively remove all the Ca^{2+} that enters the cell during the preceding action potential(s). In addition, prolongation of the Ca^{2+} transient at higher frequencies would presumably allow a greater number of crossbridges to assume strongly bound states.

Myocardial cell length. Cardiac output varies as a result of changes in beat frequency and in stroke volume. Stroke volume in turn depends upon several factors such as end-diastolic volume, the afterload against which the heart must work, and the contractile state of the myocardium (see chapter 20) One of the earliest descriptions of cardiac function was the relationship between cardiac output and end-diastolic pressure (254), i.e., the Frank-Starling relationship. When venous return to the heart increases, end-diastolic volume and stroke volume both increase, presumably due to the increased length of individual myocardial cells. Consequently, studies of mechanisms underlying the Frank-Starling relationship often involve measurements of length-dependent contractile behaviors using isolated myocardial strips or single myocardial cells (reviewed in 3, 138). As an example, twitch tension in cardiac muscle decreases rapidly when length is reduced from the optimum (2, 128, 132, 137, 269). Several plausible mechanisms have already emerged from this kind of study, but there is still no clear consensus as to the predominant mechanisms underlying the relationship or the degree to which a given mechanism may contribute. Based on length-dependent changes in tetanic tension in skeletal muscles (84), alterations in overlap of thick and thin filaments alone should account for less than 20% of the increase in cardiac performance when myocyte length is increased in the physiological range. There is evidence from living myocardium that tension declines at short lengths because of a progressive decrease in the amount of Ca^{2+} released from the sarcoplasmic reticulum (4, 5), an internal load that arises as heart muscle shortens and thereby opposes contraction (48, 99, 269), and/or a reduction in Ca^{2+} sensitivity of myofibrillar proteins (4). Excellent reviews of these and related topics are available (72, 138).

Using skinned myocardial preparations, most investigators have found that as muscle length is varied, maximal isometric tension varies with sarcomere length in a manner very similar to that observed in tetanically stimulated skeletal muscle fibers. At sarcomere lengths less than about 2.5–2.6 μm, which correspond to the longest working length of myocardium in vivo, the basis for length-dependent variations in maximum tension are generally well understood as being due to alterations in the amount of overlap of thick and thin filaments and resulting changes in the numbers of crossbridges interacting with actin (discussed in 302). As sarcomere length is reduced from 2.5 μm to about 2.2 μm, isometric tension at each length is maximal because the number of crossbridges interacting with actin is unchanged even though the amount of overlap of thick and thin filaments increases. As length is reduced below ~2.2 μm, tension progressively decreases, presumably as a result of overlap of thin filaments from opposite sides of the sarcomere, which results in a force that opposes contraction or a decrease in the number of crossbridges interacting with actin. At very short lengths, i.e., less than ~1.7 μm, tension falls dramatically as a consequence of structural interference with contraction, but these lengths are not reached under physiological conditions.

While it is interesting to note that the isometric length–tension relationship is similar in maximally activated skinned skeletal and heart muscle preparations, living myocardium does not achieve sustained maximal contractions, primarily because of to the transient nature of the increase in myoplasmic $[Ca^{2+}]$ during a twitch. As described earlier, under these circumstances, crossbridges will not achieve a steady-state distribution between weakly and strongly bound states, and for this reason alone, tension will be less than maximal. Also, when isometric tension is measured at lengths less than optimal for tension development, some fraction of the twitch time course is consumed by shortening to the isometric length, an effect that will be greater as isometric length is reduced. Based on these two factors, one would predict that isometric twitch tension in myocardium would decrease far more rapidly as length is reduced than does tetanically stimulated skeletal muscle. In fact, length–twitch tension relationships are very steep in both cardiac (128, 137) and skeletal (43) muscles.

Studies on skinned myocardial preparations have provided additional insights into possible mechanisms of decreased twitch tension at short sarcomere lengths. Several investigators have shown that the isometric tension–pCa ($-\log[Ca^{2+}]$) relationship in skinned myocardium shifts to higher $[Ca^{2+}]$ when sarcomere length is reduced; i.e., the Ca^{2+} sensitivity of tension decreases at short lengths, meaning that more Ca^{2+} is required to achieve a given level of isometric tension. The molecular basis for this phenomenon has engaged several research laboratories in recent years, leading to the major conclusion that Ca^{2+} sensitivity is reduced as lateral separation of thick and thin filaments increases at short lengths. Different laboratories (172, 289) have observed that the decrease in Ca^{2+} sensitivity can be reversed by adding osmotically active, high molecular weight polymers to the bathing solution, which compresses cell diameter to values similar to that observed at the optimal length for tension development. At present, there appear to be two possible explanations for the effects of lattice spacing on Ca^{2+} sensitivity of tension, both involving a reduction in the probability of crossbridge binding at short lengths. One possibility is that the affinity of TnC for Ca^{2+} is reduced as a consequence of fewer crossbridges strongly bound to the thin filament. In fact, Fuchs and colleagues have shown that the amount of Ca^{2+} bound to the thin filaments of skinned cardiac muscle decreases as length is reduced (72, 105, 106, 288). Another possibility is a reduction in the positive cooperativity of crossbridge binding to the thin filament at short lengths (172, 289). In support of this idea, Fitzsimons and Moss (66) have shown that application of a non-tension-generating derivative of myosin S1 (i.e., NEM-S1) to rat skinned ventricular myocytes eliminated the length-dependence of Ca^{2+} sensitivity of tension; i.e., strong binding of myosin heads (NEM-S1) to the thin filament evidently induced greater cooperative activation of the thin filament at short lengths, so that the apparent Ca^{2+} sensitivity of tension was similar at both short and long lengths.

Another idea that has been proposed as a mechanism for length-dependent Ca^{2+} sensitivity is the possibility that the cardiac isoform of troponin C has special length-sensing properties, such that binding affinity is reduced at short length (13a). This idea was based on the finding that replacement of endogenous cTnC with exogenous sTnC reduced the length-dependent shift of the tension–pCa relationship in skinned myocardium. While Fuchs's work has clearly demonstrated that Ca^{2+} binding in myocardium is length dependent, the idea that cardiac TnC acts as a length sensor has not been supported by results from a number of subsequent investigations. Moss and colleagues showed no change in length-dependence of Ca^{2+} sensitivity in skinned skeletal muscle fibers in which endogenous sTnC was replaced with cTnC (201) or in skinned cardiac myocytes from transgenic mice over-expressing sTnC in the ventricles (172). In addition, Fuchs and Wang (73) showed that skinned soleus muscle fibers, which have the same isoform of TnC as myocardium, exhibited no length dependence of Ca^{2+} binding. Evidently, the length dependence of Ca^{2+} binding observed by Fuchs is the result of some other mechanism; e.g., the reduced number of crossbridges at short length might induce a decrease in Ca^{2+} binding to TnC.

Myocardial acidosis. Investigators have long recognized that myocardial contraction is sensitive to intracellular acidosis. Perturbations of acid-base balance resulting in acidosis occur in various physiological and pathological conditions, including at the time of birth (135), during intense exercise (149), and accompanying cardiac ischemia (145, 211). The effects of acidosis upon excitation-contraction coupling in heart are many, and include decreased ligand binding to β-adrenergic receptors (186), perturbations of intracellular Ca^{2+} regulation (145, 211, 253), and decreased responsiveness of the contractile apparatus to Ca^{2+} (59, 79, 253).

Despite the fact that acidosis induces an increase in intracellular $[Ca^{2+}]$, acidosis causes a dramatic reduction in twitch tension (117, 145, 169, 211). In permeabilized cardiac preparations, acidosis decreases both maximal tension at saturating Ca^{2+} and Ca^{2+}-sensitivity of submaximal tension (52, 54, 59, 79, 253). Mechanisms underlying the reductions in maximal force and Ca^{2+} sensitivity of tension in acidosis are complex but likely involve (*1*) reductions in numbers of bound crossbridge due to direct effects of increased $[H^+]$ on force-generating transitions, (*2*) cooperative inactivation of the thin filament due to reduced numbers of crossbridges, (*3*) slowed kinetics of crossbridge interaction (179), and (*4*) reduced Ca^{2+} binding to TnC as a consequence of the reduction in crossbridge number (93, 313).

Many of the effects of acidosis involve the proteins of the thin filament regulatory strand (reviewed in 253). For example, Blanchard and Solaro (23) demonstrated that the affinity of cardiac troponin C for Ca^{2+} decreased as pH was reduced from 7.0 to 6.5. Subsequently, using TnC labeled with fluorescent probes as reporters of Ca^{2+} binding, El-Saleh et al. (56) reported in skeletal muscle and Solaro et al. (250) in cardiac muscle that acidosis-induced decreases in affinity for Ca^{2+} were amplified when TnC was complexed with TnI or with TnT-TnI, which was thought to involve pH-related effects on TnI affinity for TnC. That TnI has an integral role in mediating sensitivity to acidosis was suggested by observations that newborn heart expressing ssTnI and cTnC is less sensitive to acidosis than adult heart expressing cTnI and cTnC (78, 79, 166, 251). Such relative insensitivity to acidosis would be advantageous at the time of birth, when systemic acidosis is common (18, 82, 135).

The role of TnI was further investigated in studies (292) comparing the effects of acidic pH on Ca^{2+} activation of force in chemically skinned preparations of adult rat trabeculae and soleus fibers, which express the same cTnC isoform. Compared to soleus fibers, trabeculae demonstrated greater suppression of tension and a greater reduction in Ca^{2+} sensitivity of tension when pH was decreased from 7.0 to 6.2, indicating that the differential effects of acidosis between soleus fibers and trabeculae are due primarily to the different isoforms of TnI expressed in these muscles. Recently, Guo et al., (92) synthesized a truncated cTnI that was missing the 32 residue amino-terminal extension that is present in cTnI but absent in skeletal TnI, and that includes serine residues essential for β-adrenergic mediated shifts in Ca^{2+} sensitivity. The effect of acidosis on the Mg-ATPase–pCa relationship measured in reconstituted myofibrils was the same whether cTnI or truncated cTnI was present, indicating that domains outside the amino-terminal extension are important with respect to differences in effects of acidic pH upon Ca^{2+} activation of cardiac and skeletal myofilaments. Using chimeric analysis of troponin I domains in cardiac muscle, Westfall et al. (295) have concluded that a carboxy-terminal portion of cardiac TnI confers sensitivity to alterations in pH.

Investigations have also been undertaken to determine possible roles of TnC isoforms in determining the responses of Ca^{2+}-activated tension to acidosis. Using transgenic animals that expressed fast skeletal TnC in the heart, Metzger et al. (184) found that the pCa_{50} shifted by 0.90 ± 0.04 pCa units when pH was reduced from 7.0 to 6.2, while control cTnC-expressing hearts exhibited a shift of 1.27 ± 0.03 pCa units. In a reciprocal experiment, there was a greater acidosis-induced shift in pCa_{50} in skinned skeletal muscle fibers following extraction of the endogenous sTnC and reconstitution with purified cTnC. These results show clearly that the isoform of TnC plays a significant role in determining the greater sensitivity of cardiac muscle to acidosis. Ball et al. (16) subsequently demonstrated that isoform-specific interactions between TnI and TnC were at least in part responsible for the differential responses of skeletal and cardiac myofilaments to acidosis. Similar conclusions were reached by Palmer and Kentish (214) in comparative studies of the effects of acidosis on isometric tension in skinned skeletal and cardiac muscles, and it is now clear that other protein elements of the myofibril contribute to the responsiveness to acidosis (178, 179). Ding et al. (51) used a stepwise exchange protocol to replace endogenous cTnC in cardiac trabeculae with skeletal/cardiac TnC chimeras and endogenous cTnI with fast-twitch skeletal TnI. Based on the responses of the modified trabeculae to acidosis, these authors concluded that approximately 30% of the difference in response to acidosis between cardiac and skeletal muscles is mediated by TnC (involving cTnC residues 1–41) and about 65% by TnI.

The mechanisms of myofibrillar responses to acidosis also appear to involve effects on crossbridge mechanical properties and kinetics of interaction with actin. In skeletal muscle, acidosis has been shown to decrease the number of crossbridges and to reduce the force developed by each crossbridge bound to actin (181). Recently, Mayoux et al. (169) reported similar effects in rat myocardium: both tension and stiffness decreased in response to acidosis, but tension decreased to a greater extent, indicating that in myocardium acidosis decreases both the number of bound crossbridges and the force per crossbridge. Interestingly, alkalinization (pH 7.4) had the expected effect of increasing the number of crossbridges but surprisingly had no apparent effect on the force per crossbridge (169). Recent observations of the effects of respiratory, inorganic, and lactic acidosis upon left ventricular function in isolated rabbit hearts are consistent with the idea that acidosis reduces the transition of crossbridges from an attached non-force-generating state to an attached force-generating state, and that it also reduces the effects of bound crossbridges to cooperatively recruit crossbridges from the non-cycling pool into the cycling pool (19).

Differential effects of acidosis on crossbridge kinetics in cardiac and skeletal muscle fibers have been recently reported. Acidosis reduces the rate of crossbridge cycling in skeletal muscle fibers at submaximal but not maximal concentrations of Ca^{2+} (182). However, no effects of acidosis on cycling rate have been observed in myocardium (169). Furthermore, the unloaded velocity of shortening of skinned skeletal muscle fibers was reduced by acidosis (40, 44, 179), but no changes in V_{max} were observed in cardiac trabeculae once effects of acidosis on the contributions of internal load were taken into account (228). At present, there is no explanation for these differences in responsiveness of skeletal and cardiac muscles to acidosis, but one possibility is that cardiac and skeletal isoforms of myosin respond differently to reduced pH. Thus, any changes in isoform expression in vivo would be expected to affect protein–protein interactions within the troponin complex and to significantly alter Ca^{2+} binding.

In an attempt to define which myofilament proteins are responsible for the greater resistance to acidosis in immature heart, experiments were done in which troponin-tropomyosin (Tn-Tm) were extracted from the thin filaments of adult and immature cardiac myofibrils and subsequently replaced with Tn-Tm from adult hearts (166). In this work, the immature regulatory proteins were found to be relatively insensitive to acidic pH, since reconstitution of immature myofibrils with adult Tn-Tm increased their sensitivity to acidosis. Based on these results the authors suggested that ssTnI in the immature heart binds to cTnC with affinity that is different from that of cTnI and that ssTnI-cTnC binding is affected less by reduced pH than is cTnI-cTnC.

Products of ATP hydrolysis. There are several pathological conditions, such as chronic hypoxia, in which myocardial contraction may be depressed or slowed as a result of accumulation of the products of ATP hydrolysis, i.e., ADP, P_i and H^+. Even in the transiently ischemic heart, there is evidence that the phosphorylation potential (284) of the myocardial cell, calculated on the basis of the creatine kinase reaction as $[ATP]/([ADP] \cdot [P_i])$ or $[CrP]/([Cr] \cdot [Pi]) \times [H^+]/K_{eq}$, is substantially reduced and this has been associated with depression of myocardial contractility (reviewed in 6). While much work needs to be done to address the specific in vivo effects of each of these metabolites, there is considerable evidence from skinned myocardial preparations that changes in pH, [ADP], or $[P_i]$ affect the force of myocardial contraction. For example, increases in $[P_i]$ depress maximum force and reduce the Ca^{2+} sensitivity of isometric tension in both skeletal muscle (e.g., 178, 182) and cardiac (e.g., 86;) muscle (12, 132). Given that P_i release is associated with the force-generating step in the crossbridge cycle (47, 101, 185, 219, 286), an increase in $[P_i]$ would be expected to reduce the number of force-generating crossbridges, which would account for the observed decreases in both force and Ca^{2+} sensitivity. On the other hand, increases in [ADP] would be expected to result in accumulation of crossbridges in strongly bound, force-generating states and should therefore have opposite effects on tension and Ca^{2+} sensitivity, which has been observed in skeletal muscle (160).

Myocardial stunning is a syndrome of reversible postischemic contractile dysfunction (24) that seems to involve changes in myofibrillar Ca^{2+} sensitivity. Stunning is characterized by depressed contractility lasting up to several days despite restoration of normal or near-normal coronary flow and despite the absence of evidence of irreversible tissue damage. The pathogenesis of myocardial stunning remains unclear; however, generation of oxygen-derived free radicals and alterations of calcium homeostasis and calcium responsiveness have been proposed (24). Recent experimental evidence favors altered myofilament calcium sensitivity as a mechanism of stunning. Among ventricular myofilament proteins, α-actinin, troponin I (TnI), and myosin light chain 1 (essential light chain) appear most susceptible to degradation with ischemia/reperfusion injury (283). In subsequent studies, progressive degradation of TnI was correlated with duration of ischemia prior to reperfusion (174). A transgenic mouse line was then established in which TnI was truncated, mimicking the TnI degradation product observed following ischemia-reperfusion (TnI$_{1-193}$). With low-level expression of truncated TnI (9%–17% of native TnI expression), mice demonstrated cardiac chamber enlargement, diminished contractility, and reduced myofilament calcium sensitivity, recapitulating the phenotype of stunned myocardium (204). These results suggest that TnI proteolysis is integral to the pathogenesis of stunning, at least in small animal models of stunning; however, the mechanism by which truncated TnI decreases force and Ca^{2+} sensitivity is presently unknown.

Inotropic agonists. A variety of chemical agents have pronounced effects on the tension-generating capabilities of myocardium, most notably α and β adrenergic agonists, but also agents that activate purinergic and opioid receptors, among several others. In most instances, these agonists have multiple targets within the myocardial cell, including effects on trans-sarcolemmal ion fluxes and on the rate of release and reuptake of Ca^{2+} from the sarcoplasmic reticulum, as well as effects directly upon contractile and regulatory proteins. Thus, when considering the possible mechanisms of action of a particular agonist, it may be difficult to determine the contributions of the several elements of the E-C coupling cascade. For example, from the work of Endoh and Blinks (58), in which force and intracellular [Ca^{2+}] were measured in the same living myocardial preparations, application of α-adrenergic agonists increased force both by increasing the amount of Ca^{2+} released to the myoplasm and increasing the Ca^{2+}-sensitivity of tension. Studies on skinned myocardial preparations in which [Ca^{2+}] was well buffered and the sarcoplasmic reticulum was disrupted with detergents showed that treatment with β agonists prior to skinning reduced the Ca^{2+} sensitivity of tension but had no effect on maximum tension (301, 257). Such effects are almost certainly mediated by phosphorylation of troponin I, since *(1)* troponin I is phosphorylated as a result of β-agonist application, *(2)* the effects on sensitivity are mimicked by treatment of skinned preparations with protein kinase A (107, 257), and *(3)* PKA has nearly no effect on Ca^{2+} sensitivity of tension in cardiac preparations from transgenic mice that almost completely express the slow skeletal isoform of TnI, which lacks the serine residues that are phosphorylated in cardiac TnI (213). In fact, both serine 22 and serine 23 of mouse TnI must be phosphorylated in order to observe the decrease in Ca^{2+} binding affinity (311), which would explain the β-adrenergic-induced decrease in Ca^{2+}-sensitivity of tension. Such phosphorylations are also required for the observed effects of PKA treatment to accelerate the rate of relaxation of skinned myocardial preparations (310). Of interest in this regard, transgenic mice over-expressing slow skeletal TnI (which lacks the PKA phosphorylation sites of cardiac TnI), exhibited slowed rates of relaxation and nonresponsiveness to PKA stimulation (62).

While the effects of β-adrenergic stimulation and activation of PKA are relatively well studied in myocardium, much less is known about the specific effects of other inotropic agents on myocardium or mechanisms of action at the level of the myofibrillar proteins. For example, activation of the α-adrenergic pathway has positive inotropic effects which at least partly involve changes in the myofilaments mediated by protein kinase C. However, work on the specific molecular targets of PKC has only just begun, and in any case, there do not appear to be any effects of α-adrenergic agonists on the Ca^{2+} sensitivity of tension (255). Treatment of rat cardiac myocytes with phenylephrine prior to skinning had no effect on either maximum tension or tensions at submaximal concentrations of Ca^{2+}. The α-adrenergic pathway and others are receiving increasing attention from investigators in the field, and new perspectives should rapidly evolve in the next several years.

Roles of thick filament accessory proteins. There is increasing evidence that myosin binding protein C, also called C-protein, (108, 109) and myosin RLC (110), proteins associated with the thick filament, influence the Ca^{2+} sensitivity of tension, at least in skeletal muscles. Partial extraction of either protein increases the Ca^{2+} sensitivity of tension in skinned skeletal muscle fibers. This result has been explained in terms of effects of each of these proteins to influence the flexibility of the myosin molecule, thereby regulating the availability of crossbridges to actin and the number of crossbridges that are strongly bound. However, it is not yet known whether these proteins have roles in determining the rate or amount of tension developed in vivo.

A current issue with respect to possible roles of C-protein in modulating cardiac contraction is whether phosphorylation of C-protein in response to β-adrenergic or other agonists, influences the regulation or kinetics of crossbridge interaction (reviewed in 300). As pointed out by Winegrad (300), the difficulty in studies of this type is that receptor agonists invariably affect the levels of phosphorylation of other contractile and regulatory proteins, making it difficult to specifically ascribe a response to the phosphorylation of C-protein. The complicated responses to agonist binding point to the need for making specific mutations in myofibrillar proteins to begin to understand the role that each plays in inotropic responses. In this regard, Fenske et al. (62) observed that myocytes from transgenic mice expressing slow skeletal TnI, which lacks two PKA-dependent phosphorylation sites present in cardiac

TnC, were unresponsive to PKA in terms of force or shortening velocity. This result might be taken to suggest that phosphorylation of TnI is sufficient to account for PKA effects on myofibrillar function, although it is possible that C-protein phosphorylation influences other mechanical properties (e.g., kinetics of force development) or that phosphorylation of TnI must occur in order for the effects of C-protein phosphorylation to be evident.

Shortening Velocity

Effects of Activation on Velocity of Shortening. The possibility that Ca^{2+} influences the velocity of muscle shortening was for many years a controversial idea, since some investigators found that reductions in $[Ca^{2+}]$ reduced V_{max} in skeletal muscle (126) while other investigators found no change (222, 268). In this regard, Huxley's 1957 model predicted that activation should not affect V_{max}, since V_{max} was not thought to vary with numbers of interacting crossbridges but instead was determined by the rate of crossbridge dissociation, i.e., when a muscle is shortening at V_{max} the proportions of crossbridges with strains greater than 1.0 or less than 1.0 would be equal and external force developed by the muscle would be zero. More recent work (61, 193) clearly shows that $[Ca^{2+}]$ has a profound effect on V_{max} and also provides an explanation for the earlier discrepancies. At levels of Ca^{2+} that were saturating with respect to isometric tension, shortening velocity was high and was constant during the time-course of shortening (Fig. 11–9). However, at submaximal levels of Ca^{2+}, shortening was biphasic: there was an initial phase of high-velocity shortening, followed by a linear phase of low-velocity shortening. V_{max} in the high-velocity phase did not vary with $[Ca^{2+}]$ unless the isometric tension-generating capability of the fiber was less than 0.3 P_o. On the other hand, V_{max} in the low-velocity phase decreased with $[Ca^{2+}]$ over the entire range studied. Thus, in previous studies, if V_{max} was measured at moderate levels of Ca^{2+} (i.e., >0.3 P_o) or soon after changes in load (222, 268), no effect of Ca^{2+} would be seen. However, if V_{max} was assessed at low levels of activation or at longer times after a change in load or length, a clear reduction would be evident. Based on biochemical results (248), it seems likely that the reduction in high-velocity V_{max} at low levels of Ca^{2+} is due to slowing of ADP release.

The mechanism of activation dependent changes in V_{max} is incompletely understood (reviewed in 83, 194), although most features of results to date can be explained by either of two models. In either case, the Ca^{2+} sensitivity of the high-velocity phase is probably due to reduced rates of ADP dissociation at low $[Ca^{2+}]$, which has been observed in proteins in solution

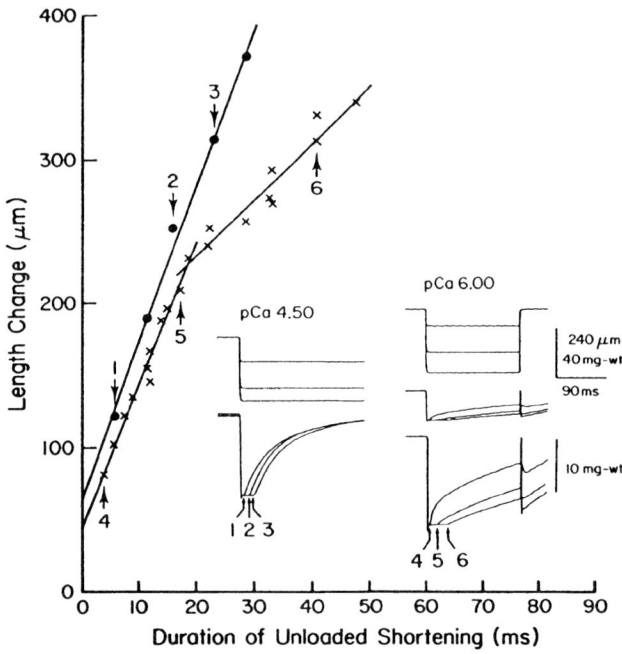

FIG. 11–9. Slack test plots from a skinned skeletal fiber at maximal (pCa 4.5, ●) and submaximal (pCa 6.0, ×) levels of activation. The insets show original recordings of length (*upper*) and tension (*lower*) at each pCa. The *arrows* indicate the time points at which tension redevelopment commenced, and the *numbers* indicate the corresponding points on the plots. [From Moss (193).]

(235). Subsequent studies of sliding velocities of regulated thin filaments in in vitro motility assays (85, 113, 115) suggest that velocity is maximal as long as a critical fraction (about 20%) of total crossbridges is bound to the thin filament, but that velocity progressively decreases as the number of crossbridges is reduced below this number by lowering the $[Ca^{2+}]$.

The low-velocity phase of shortening is less clearly understood. One possibility to explain this phase (193) is that in partially activated fibers, crossbridges are bound to the thin filament in zones of transition between fully active and fully inactive functional groups. However, because of the partial blocking position of Tm, these crossbridges are unable to attain a state (i.e., with no nucleotide bound) from which they could dissociate in the presence of ATP. As the muscle shortens, these crossbridges eventually constitute an internal load that retards further shortening (Fig. 11–10). Low-velocity V_{max} would be expected to decrease as $[Ca^{2+}]$ is reduced, since the proportion of crossbridges that are long-lived should increase. Alternatively, as the muscle shortens, the number of crossbridges interacting with the thin filament decreases (119, 127). Reductions in the number of strongly bound crossbridges reduce the kinetics of interaction of crossbridges with the thin filament (259) and thus might be expected to reduce

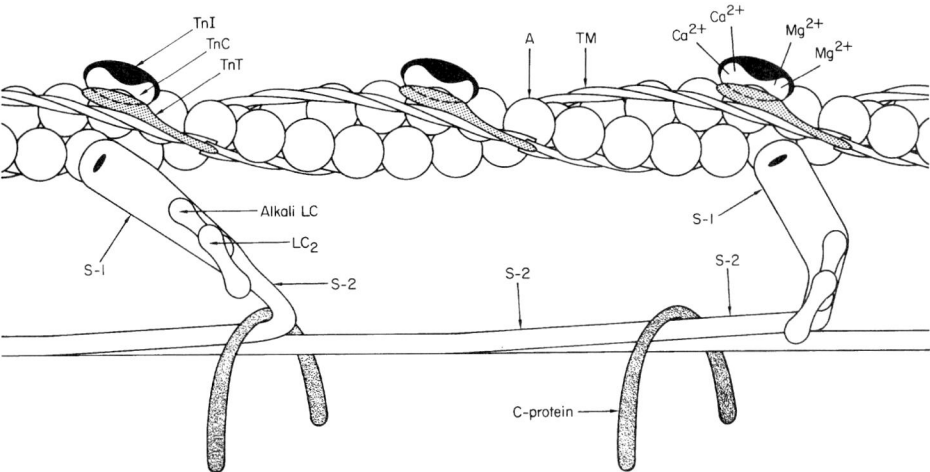

FIG. 11–10. Schematic representation of thick and thin filaments showing possible mechanisms for slowing of V_{max} at low levels of activation. Left: Representation of a slowly cycling cross-bridge proposed to exist at low levels of activation, that has been carried beyond the normal configuration as a result of shortening. Further sliding of the thick and thin filaments beyond this point would be impaired by stretch of S-2 and the overall rate of shortening would be slowed. Right: Cross-bridge in the normal force-generating configuration. If this cross-bridge is long-lived, continued shortening would result in a configuration similar to A. However, if this is a normally cycling cross-bridge, further will cause compressive strain of S-2 and detachment from actin before S-2 buckles. In both cases, the accumulation of compressively strained or buckled cross-bridges presumably depends on the rate of ADP dissociation from the A.M.ADP complex prior to the cross-bridge detachment step. [From Hofmann et al. (108).]

shortening velocity. This second model does not provide a simple explanation for the two phases of shortening at low levels of activation, although it is possible that the number of strongly interacting crossbridges decreases gradually as shortening proceeds, and the state of activation of the thin filament is reduced only when the number of crossbridges is less than a threshold value. If this were the case, shortening velocity would initially be high and would slow only when numbers of strongly bound crossbridges were sufficiently reduced. Consistent with this idea, application of NEM-S1 to skinned skeletal muscle fibers increases velocity in the low-velocity phase to values approaching those in the high-velocity phase (Swartz and Moss, unpublished results). Results obtained by Metzger (178) certainly argue for an effect of crossbridge number on shortening velocity, but more in terms of the mechanical load that crossbridges may introduce once they have completed their working stroke. In Metzger's experiments, increases in P_i increased V_{max} in the low-velocity phase, while increases in Mg-ADP slowed V_{max}—both effects could be manifestations of alterations in the number of A · M · ADP crossbridges bound to the thin filament. Such results are not consistent with the idea that slowing of velocity at low levels of activation is entirely a phenomenon of thin filament activation, since an increase in $[P_i]$ should reduce the numbers of crossbridges bound and presumably thereby reduce the level of thin filament activation and slow velocity, while increases in [Mg-ADP] should have opposite effects.

Following on this discussion, the question arises as to whether there are effects of activation on shortening velocity in mammalian myocardium. In living myocardium, shortening velocity is usually reduced under conditions that reduce the amplitude of the twitch, e.g., reductions in extracellular $[Ca^{2+}]$ (reviewed in 71). Such effects may be due to mechanisms like the one described above for submaximally activated skeletal muscle fibers or it is possible that maximum shortening velocity is reduced due to the presence of relatively large internal loads in cardiac muscle (48, 99). In the latter case, as the level of Ca^{2+} activation was reduced, thereby decreasing the force-generating capability of myocardium, a fixed internal load would become an increasingly large fraction of the force-generating capability. Consequently, maximum velocity would decrease. At this stage, the relative roles of internal loads and Ca^{2+} regulatory mechanisms in determining V_{max} are unknown, although effects of reduced activation to depress shortening velocity have been observed in single cardiac myocytes shortening under fixed loads (266). One potential artifact in measuring shortening velocity of skinned preparations is that uncorrected end-compliance will result in progressive slowing of velocity as the preparation shortens, an effect that increases as the level of activation is reduced (245). One way to address such a possibility is to improve the stiffness of end connections to skinned myocardial preparations. In experiments in which end compliances were reduced by improved physical attachments to skinned myocytes, no slowing of velocity under load was observed during maximal activations, but slower maximal velocities and progressive slowing during the time course of shortening were observed when [Ca^{2+}] was reduced to submaximal levels (173). Subsequent work has shown that application of NEM-S1 to skinned myocytes eliminates the progressive slowing at low levels of activation (McDonald and Moss, unpublished). Such an observation is certainly consistent with the idea that there are activation-dependent internal loads such as long-lived crossbridges that slow velocities when [Ca^{2+}] is low, but it also suggests the possibility of progressive cooperative inactivation of the thin filaments during low-activation shortening. Because activation of the thin filament is a highly cooperative process involving binding of both Ca^{2+} and crossbridges, one could envision a mechanism in which the reduction in number of crossbridges that occurs during shortening would cooperatively reduce the state of activation of the thin filament, which would lead to a further reduction in crossbridge number, and so forth. A recent review by Gordon et al. (83) includes an elegant discussion of this and other mechanisms.

Agonist-Induced Changes in Velocity. Positive inotropic interventions such as β-adrenergic stimulation can result in increases in shortening velocity in mammalian myocardium (reviewed in 71), although such effects have not always been observed (41, 49, 269). Studies on skinned myocytes indicate that treatment with β-adrenergic agonists prior to rapid skinning results in an increase in maximum shortening velocity as measured with the slack test method (257). These effects can be mimicked by direct application of PKA to skinned cells that were previously untreated with β-agonist, suggesting that phosphorylation of one or more myofibrillar proteins is responsible for the increase in maximum shortening velocity. While the precise molecular basis for this effect is unknown, an increase in shortening velocity would be advantageous during β-adrenergic stimulation, because the rate of work production (i.e., maximum power) by the heart would be increased.

It is now evident that shortening velocity is altered by other pharmacologic interventions, e.g., α-adrenergic (phenylephrine) stimulation (256) or purinergic (N^6-cyclopentyladenosine) stimulation (255) of rat cardiac myocytes prior to skinning resulted in a reduction in maximum shortening velocity. The mechanisms of these effects are not known for certain in every case, although it is evident that PKC-induced phosphorlyations of TnI reduces the maximum Ca^{2+}-stimulated myosin ATPase (207), which is consistent with the decreases in shortening velocity described by Strang and colleagues. The adaptive advantage of the reduction in shortening velocity is not known, but one possibility that should be considered is that such a response may be a secondary effect of protein phosphorylations, which have primary effects on other physiological variables such as the Ca^{2+} sensitivity of tension or the kinetics of tension development. Further work will be required to address each of these possibilities.

Kinetics of Tension Development and Relaxation

There is considerable experimental evidence that the *rate* of tension development is activation dependent, at least in skeletal muscles. Mechanical protocols to reduce active tension to near zero result in a timecourse of tension recovery that slows as [Ca^{2+}] is reduced (31, 180). Thus, the rate constant of tension recovery (k_{tr}) in these experiments is Ca^{2+} dependent. Because tension recovery results from a redistribution of crossbridges from weakly bound into tension-generating states, Ca^{2+} dependence is taken to indicate that Ca^{2+} influences rate constants (primarily f in Huxley's 1957 model [119]) in the crossbridge cycle.

Studies have been done to address the basis for activation dependence of k_{tr}, although at this time, the precise molecular mechanisms involved are unknown. Recently, activation dependence of contraction kinetics has been modelled primarily by coupling Ca^{2+} binding to Tn with the regulation of crossbridge cycling (139, 140), with the result that it was possible to account for Ca^{2+}-dependent variations in contractile properties. However, this approach does not yet include near-neighbor cooperative mechanisms involving crossbridges, and these appear to be important in the regulation of static and dynamic mechanical properties of heart and skeletal muscle. For example, in skinned skeletal muscle fibers, infusion of N-ethylmaleimide-modified myosin S1 increased the Ca^{2+} sensitivity of isometric tension and increased k_{tr} to maximal values at all levels of Ca^{2+} activation (259). Similar results have been obtained in rat skinned myocardium (Fitzsimons and Moss, unpublished results). These results imply that in both cardiac and skeletal muscle, strong binding of crossbridges cooperatively activates the thin filament to allow further crossbridge binding and is also essential for maximal activation of the kinetic transitions associated with force development. A recent model proposed by Campbell (36) is one example of how to take these cooperative mechanisms into account when describing activation of cardiac contraction. In his scheme, crossbridges are either in a cycling pool (capable of interacting with actin and generating force) or a non-cycling pool (blocked from interacting with actin). The non-cycling pool is large at low [Ca^{2+}] and small at high [Ca^{2+}] (and conversely for the cycling pool). According to Campbell, at high [Ca^{2+}] the rate of rise of force is maximal, or nearly so, because most or all thin filaments sites bind Ca^{2+}, which recruits all crossbridges to the cycling pool. At low [Ca^{2+}], the rate of rise of force is slowed because Ca^{2+} binds to only a few thin filament sites, i.e., the cycling pool is initially small. However, the binding of these crossbridges to the thin filament has an activating effect that recruits more crossbridges from the non-cycling pool into the cycling pool. Subsequent binding of additional crossbridges to actin will further recruit crossbridges into the cycling pool, and so forth. Thus, the slow rate of activation at low [Ca^{2+}] is in this model a consequence of the time taken for progressive cooperative recruitment of crossbridges into strongly bound states. This and other models of regulation have recently been reviewed by Gordon, et al. (83).

While it is now widely accepted that k_{tr} in skeletal muscle varies with [Ca^{2+}], there is controversy about whether this is also the case in cardiac muscle. Hancock, et al. (94) reported that the rate of tension redevelopment following rapid release of segment length-clamped living papillary muscles from ferret did not change when the level of activation was varied by increasing extracellular [Ca^{2+}] from 1.25 to 13 mM. On the other hand, Wolff et al. (304) found as much as a fivefold variation in k_{tr} in rat skinned trabeculae as the level of activation was varied from maximal to very low levels by changing the free [Ca^{2+}]. One possibility to explain the difference in results is that the protocol used on the living papillary muscles did not involve re-stretch following the release, so that a greater number of strongly bound crossbridges were bound at the onset of tension redevelopment. This is potentially very important because in skeletal muscle k_{tr} increases dramatically as the numbers of strongly bound crossbridges increase (259). However, subsequent experiments by Hancock et al. (95), using skinned preparations, still revealed no variation in k_{tr} with level of Ca^{2+} activation, even when re-stretch was applied immediately before the period of tension redevelopment. In contrast, more recent studies in which activation was induced by flash photolysis of caged Ca^{2+} have provided further evidence that the rate of force development is activation dependent in skinned myocardium (66). Furthermore, Baker et al. (14) have found that k_{tr} measured in living, tetanically stimulated myocardium varied approximately fivefold when steady tension was varied from high to low by adjusting extracellular [Ca^{2+}].

Activation-dependence of the rate of rise of force almost certainly includes cooperative effects of crossbridge binding, as discussed above for skeletal muscle. In support of this idea, application of NEM-S1 accelerated the rate of rise of force in cardiac muscle, increasing k_{tr} at low levels of Ca^{2+} to near-maximal values. Additional studies on transgenic mice expressing 60% β tropomyosin/40% α tropomyosin (Tm) in place of the 100% α Tm normally expressed in myocardium reported that twitch kinetics measured in free-floating transgenic myocytes were slowed compared to control (305). Measurements of force and ATPase activity in the same preparations suggested that the rates of crossbridge cycling were unchanged in the transgenics relative to control, but the Ca^{2+} sensitivity of force and the steepness of the force–pCa relationship were increased. From these results, the authors concluded that the apparent cooperativity of activation was increased by the expression of β Tm, and this, in turn, caused a slowing of both the rate of rise of force (see discussion vis à vis Campbell's 1997 model (36), above) and the rate of relaxation. The latter phenomenon was presumably due to an effect of β Tm to enhance the activating effects on the thin filament due to crossbridge binding, which in the presence of low [Ca^{2+}] in relaxing muscle would tend to facilitate the re-binding of crossbridges that detach and thereby slow the rate of relaxation (discussed in 195).

There is strong experimental evidence from several laboratories in support of the idea that crossbridge cycling rate is also modulated by β-adrenergic stimulation. Hoh et al. (112) and Berman et al. (20) showed that β-adrenergic agonists increased the rate of crossbridge cycling by nearly 50% in steadily activated living heart muscle during barium contracture. The fact that dibutyryl cyclic AMP mimicked this effect in living heart muscle strongly suggests that the increased cycling rate results from phosphorylation of myofibrillar proteins (111). Zhang et al. (310) also showed that the rate of myocardial relaxation is sped by PKA-mediated phosphorylation of TnI. All of these findings are consistent with the idea that crossbridge cycling rate is faster during β-adrenergic stimulation, presumably as a result of myofibrillar protein phosphorylations. Such results imply that thin filament regulatory proteins can modulate the rate of crossbridge cycling, suggesting the need for future studies to investigate possible effects of variable expression of cardiac regulatory proteins on contraction kinetics.

CONCLUSIONS

The regulation of force production and shortening velocity in myocardium is a complex process that is influenced by a number of physical factors and second messenger pathways in the myocardial cell. In considering mechanisms of altered force production in vivo in response to circulatory demand or as part of disease processes, it is important to recognize that activation of the thin filament not only involves Ca^{2+} binding to regulatory proteins but also depends on the number of crossbridges bound to actin; i.e., strongly bound crossbridges facilitate further binding of crossbridges and increase both the rate of interaction of myosin with actin and the apparent binding affinity of troponin C for Ca^{2+}. Thus, inotropic interventions or disease processes that increase or reduce the number of strongly bound crossbridges will have a wide range of effects on crossbridge interaction.

Much of this review has dealt with mechanisms of alterations in Ca^{2+} sensitivity of isometric tension, which provides an index of the apparent Ca^{2+} binding affinity of troponin C. Besides characterizing an important property of the main Ca^{2+} binding protein in the myofilament, knowledge of the Ca^{2+} sensitivity of tension provides valuable insights into mechanisms of altered contractile function under a variety of conditions. However, it is important to note that depressed contractile function—e.g., reduced twitch force—does not necessarily imply that the Ca^{2+} sensitivity of tension is reduced. For example, depressed contraction could be the result of similar proportional decreases in the rate constants of crossbridge attachment and detachment, in which case the steady-state tension tension at any given $[Ca^{2+}]$ would not be altered but the rate of attainment of steady-state tension would be slowed. Thus, in considering the basis for changes in contractile performance, it is necessary to make both steady-state and transient contractile measurements in order to differentiate between effects involving changes in Ca^{2+} binding affinity and those involving changes in crossbridge interaction kinetics.

Discussion has also focused on roles played by activation of membrane-bound receptors in modulating contractile properties. This is an area in which there is still much to be learned, because even in the most studied system, i.e., β-adrenergic stimulation, consensus has only recently been achieved concerning the involvement of phosphorylation sites on TnI in mediating the observed decrease in Ca^{2+} sensitivity of tension. Even here, there is no detailed understanding of the basis for β-agonist–induced alterations in crossbridge cycling kinetics or whether mechanical V_{max} is altered during β stimulation. Nonetheless, studies to date have shown that various agonists have multiple effects on Ca^{2+} sensitivity of tension and the kinetics of crossbridge interaction, which makes this a potentially fruitful area for continued investigation. One important consideration in studies of this type is that agonists frequently have effects on Ca^{2+} entry into the myocardial cell and release from intracellular stores. Changes in myocardial twitch properties would be expected just on the basis of alterations in the intracellular Ca^{2+} transient. Thus, in addressing mechanisms of agonist-induced inotropy, it is important to distinguish the roles of altered Ca^{2+} delivery, altered Ca^{2+} binding, and Ca^{2+} independent processes. In the case of β-adrenergic stimulation, for example, alterations in the Ca^{2+} transient are similar to changes in twitch time course, but agonist induced stimulation of crossbridge kinetics and a decrease in Ca^{2+} sensitivity of tension appear to match interaction kinetics to the Ca^{2+} transient. Also, accelerated crossbridge kinetics increase the ability of the myocardium to generate power.

Finally, it is possible that any or all of the regulatory mechanisms discussed in this chapter may come to play in myocardial pathophysiology. Because of this, there is a need for systematic cellular and molecular studies of myocardial function to determine not only process that is impaired in a pathophysiolgical state but also the molecular basis for observed functional deficiencies. Such studies represent an imporant emerging field, because work on the molecular basis of myocardial regulation has just recently begun, and so far, little is known about the myofibrillar mechanisms of myocardial diseases.

REFERENCES

1. Akella, A. B., X.-L. Ding, R. Cheng and J. Gulati. Diminished Ca^{2+} sensitivity of skinned cardiac muscle contractility coincident with troponin T-band shifts in the diabetic rat. *Circ. Res.* 76:600–606, 1995.
2. Allen, D. G., B. R. Jewell and J. W. Murray. The contribution of activation processes to the length-tension relation of cardiac muscle. *Nature* 248:606–607, 1974.
3. Allen, D. G., and J. C. Kentish. The cellular basis of the length-tension relation in cardiac muscle. *J. Mol. Cell. Cardiol.* 17:821–840, 1985.
4. Allen, D. G., and S. Kurihara. The effects of muscle length on intracellular Ca^{2+} transients in mammalian cardiac muscle. *J. Physiol.* 327:79–94, 1982.
5. Allen, D. G., C. G. Nichols and G. L. Smith. The effects of changes in muscle length during diastole on the calcium transient in ferret ventricular muscle. *J. Physiol.* 406:359–370, 1988.
6. Allen, D. G., and C. H. Orchard. Myocardial contractile function during ischemia and hypoxia. *Circ. Res.* 60:153–168, 1987.
7. Alpert, N. R., and L. A. Mulieri. Increased myothermal economy of isometric force generation in compensated cardiac hypertrophy induced by pulmonary artery constriction in the rabbit. *Circ. Res.* 50:491–500, 1982.
8. Anderson, P. A. W., G. E. Moore and R. N. Nassar. Developmental changes in the expression of rabbit left ventricular troponin T. *Circ. Res.* 63:742–747, 1988.
9. Anderson, P. A. W., N. N. Malouf, A. E. Oakeley, E. D. Pagani and P. D. Allen. Troponin T isoform expression in humans. A comparison among normal and failing adult heart, fetal heart, and adult and fetal skeletal muscle. *Circ. Res.* 69:1226–1233, 1991.
10. Anderson, P. A. W., A. Greig, T. M. Mark, N. N. Malouf, A. E. Oakeley, R. M. Ungerleider, P. D. Allen and B. K. Kay. Molec-

ular basis of human cardiac troponin T isoforms expressed in the developing, adult, and failing heart. *Circ. Res.* 76:681–686, 1995.

11. Araujo, A. and J. W. Walker. Kinetics of tension development in skinned cardiac myocytes measured by photorelease of Ca^{2+}. *Am. J. Physiol.* 267 (*Heart Circ. Physiol.* 36):H1643–H1653, 1994.

12. Araujo, A. and J. W. Walker. Phosphate release and force generation in cardiac myocytes investigated with caged phosphate and caged calcium. *Biophys. J.* 70:2316–2326, 1996.

13. Ashley, C., I. P. Mulligan and T. J. Lea. Ca^{2+} and activation mechanisms in skeletal muscle. *Qt. Rev. Biophys.* 24:1–73, 1991.

13a. Babu, A., E. Sonnenblick and J. Gulati. Molecular basis for the influence of muscle length on myocardial performance. *Science* 240:74–76, 1988.

14. Baker, A. J., V. M. Figueredo, E. C. Keung and S. A. Camacho. Ca^{2+} regulates the kinetics of tension development in intact cardiac muscle. *Am. J. Physiol.* 275 (*Heart Circ. Physiol.* 44): H744–H750, 1998.

15. Balint, M., F. A. Sreter, I. Wolf, B. Nagy and J. Gergely. The substructure of heavy meromyosin, the effect of Ca and Mg^{2+} on the tryptic fragmentation of heavy meromyosin. *J. Biol. Chem.* 250:6168–6177, 1975.

16. Ball, K. L., M. D. Johnson and R. J. Solaro. Isoform specific interactions of troponin I and troponin C determine pH sensitivity of myofibrillar Ca^{2+} activation. *Biochemistry* 33:8464–8471, 1994.

17. Barany, M. ATPase activity of myosin correlated with speed of muscle shortening. *J. Gen. Physiol.* 50:197–217, 1967.

18. Berg, T. G., and W. F. Rayburn. Umbilical cord length and acid-base balance at delivery. *J. Reprod. Med.* 40:9–12, 1995.

19. Berger, D. S., S. K. Fellner, K. A. Robinson, K. Vlasica, I. E. Godoy and S. G. Shroff. Disparate effects of three types of extracellular acidosis on left ventricular function. *Am. J. Physiol.* 276 (*Heart Circ. Physiol.* 45):H582–H594, 1999.

20. Berman, M. R., J. N. Peterson, D. T. Yue and W. C. Hunter. Effect of isoproterenol on force transient time course and on stiffness spectra in rabbit papillary muscle in barium contracture. *J. Mol. Cell. Cardiol.* 20:415–426, 1988.

21. Bhavsar, P. K., G. K. Dhoot, D. V. E. Cumming, G. S. Butler-Browne, M. H. Yacoub and P. J. R. Barton. Developmental expression of troponin I isoforms in fetal human heart. *FEBS Lett.* 292:5–8, 1991.

22. Blanchard, E., C. Seidman, J. G. Seidman, M. LeWinter and D. Maughan. Altered crossbride kinetics in the $\alpha MHC^{403/+}$ mouse model of familial hypertrophic cardiomyopathy. *Circ. Res.* 84: 475–483, 1999.

23. Blanchard, E. M., and R. J. Solaro. Inhibition of the activation and troponin calcium binding of dog cardiac myofibrils by acidic pH. *Circ. Res.* 55:382–391, 1984.

24. Bolli, R. and E. Marban. Molecular and cellular mechanisms of myocardial stunning. *Physiol. Rev.* 79:609–634, 1999.

25. Boluyt, M. O., L. O'Neill, A. L. Meredith, O. H. L. Bing, W. W. Brooks, C. H. Conrad, M. T. Crow and E. G. Lakatta. Alterations in cardiac gene expression during the transition from stable hypertrophy to heart failure. *Circ. Res.* 75:23–32, 1994.

26. Bonne, G, L. Carrier, P. Richarde, B. Hainique and K. Schwartz. Familial hypertrophic cardiomyopathy. From mutations to functional defects. *Circ. Res.* 83:580–593, 1998.

27. Bottinelli, R., M. Canepari, V. Cappelli and C. Reggiani. Maximum speed of shortening and ATPase activity in atrial and ventricular myocardia of hyperthyroid rat. *Am. J. Physiol.* 269: C785–C790, 1995.

28. Brandt, P. W., M. S. Diamond, J. S. Rutchik and F. H. Schachat. Co-operative interactions between troponin-tropomyosin units extend the length of the thin filament in skeletal muscle. *J. Mol. Biol.* 195:885–886, 1987.

29. Brandt, P. W., M. S. Diamond and F. H. Schachat. The thin filament of vertebrate skeletal muscle co-operatively activates as a unit. *J. Mol. Biol.* 180:379–384, 1984.

30. Bremel, R. D., and A. Weber. Cooperation within actin filaments in vertebrate skeletal muscle. *Nature [New Biol.]* 238:97–101, 1972.

31. Brenner, B. The cross-bridge cycle in muscle. *Basic Res. Cardiol.* 81:1–15, 1986.

31a. Brenner, B., and E. Eisenberg. Rate of force generation in muscle: correlation with actomyosin ATPase activity in solution. *Proc. Natl. Acad. Sci. U.S.A.* 83:3542–3546, 1986.

32. Brenner, B., M. Schoenberg, J. M. Chalovich, L. E. Greene and E. Eisenberg. Evidence for cross-bridge attachment in relaxed muscle at low ionic strength. *Proc. Natl. Acad. Sci. U.S.A.* 79: 7288–7291, 1982.

33. Brisson, J. B., K. Golosinska, L. B. Smillie and B. D. Sykes. Interaction of tropomyosin and troponin T: a proton nuclear magnetic resonance study. *Biochemistry.* 25:4548–4555, 1986.

34. Brooks, S. V., J. A. Faulkner and D. A. McCubbrey. Power outputs of slow and fast skeletal muscles of mice. *J. Appl. Physiol.* 68:1282–1285, 1990.

35. Buck, S. H., P. J. Konyn, J. Palermo, J. Robbins and R. L. Moss. Altered kinetics of contraction of atrial cells expressing ventricular myosin regulatory light chain. *Am. J. Physiol.* 276 (*Heart Circ. Physiol.* 45):H1167–H1171, 1996.

36. Campbell, K. Rate constant of muscle force redevelopment reflects cooperative activation as well as cross-bridge kinetics. *Biophys. J.* 72:254–262, 1997.

37. Chalovich, J. M. and E. Eisenberg. Inhibition of actomyosin ATPase activity by troponin without blocking binding of myosin to actin. *J. Biol. Chem.* 257:2432–2437, 1982.

38. Chandy, I. K., J. C. Lo and R. C. Ludescher. Differential mobility of skeletal and cardiac tropomyosin on the surface of F-actin. *Biochemistry* 38:9286–9294, 1999.

39. Charron, P., O. Dubourg, M. Desnos, R. Isnard, A. Hagege, G. Bonne, L. Carrier, F. Tesson, J. B. Bouhour, J.-C. Buzzi, J. Feingold, K. Schwartz and M. Komajda. Genotype-phenotype correlations in familial hypertrophic cardiomyopathy. *Eur. Heart J.* 19:139–145, 1998.

40. Chase, P. B., and M. J. Kushmerick. Effects of pH on contraction of rabbit fast and slow skeletal muscle fibers. *Biophys. J.* 53: 935–946, 1988.

40a. Chiu, Y., E. W. Ballou and L. E. Ford. Internal viscoelastic loading in cat papillary muscle. *Biophys. J.* 40:109–20, 1982.

41. Chiu, Y. C., K. R. Walley and L. E. Ford. Comparison of the effects of different inotropic interventions on force, velocity and power in rabbit myocardium. *Circ. Res.* 65:1161–1171, 1989.

42. Claflin, D. R., and J. A. Faulkner. The force-velocity relationship at high shortening velocities in the soleus muscle of the rat. *J. Physiol. (Lond.)* 411:627–637, 1989.

43. Close, R. I. The relations between sarcomere length and characteristics of isometric twitch contractions of frog sartorius muscles. *J. Physiol. (Lond.)* 220:745–762, 1972.

44. Cooke, R., K. Franks, G. B. Luciani and E. Pate. The inhibition of rabbit skeletal muscle contraction by hydrogen ions and phosphate. *J. Physiol. (Lond.)* 395:77–97, 1988.

45. Cuda, G., L. Fananapazir, W.-S. Zhu, J. R. Sellers and N. D. Epstein. Skeletal muscle expression and abnormal function of β-myosin in hypertrophic cardiomyopathy. *J. Clin. Invest.* 91: 2861–2865, 1993.

46. Cuda, G., J. R. Sellers, N. D. Epstein, and L. Fananapazir. In-vitro motility activity of β-cardiac myosin depends on the nature of the β-myosin heavy chain gene mutation in hypertrophic cardiomyopathy. *Circulation* 88:I-343, 1993.

47. Dantzig, J. A., Y. E. Goldman, J. Lacktis, N. C. Millar and E. Homsher. Reversal of the cross-bridge force-generating transition by photogeneration of phosphate in rabbit psoas muscle fibers. *J. Physiol. (Lond.)* 451:247–278, 1992.
48. de Tombe, P. P. and H. E. D. J. ter Keurs. An internal viscous element limits unloaded velocity of sarcomere shortening in rat myocardium. *J. Physiol. (Lond.)* 454:619–42, 1992.
49. de Tombe, P. P. and H. E. D. J. ter Keurs. Lack of effect of isoproterenol on unloaded velocity of sarcomere shortening in rat cardiac trabeculae. *Circ. Res.* 68:383–391, 1991.
50. Dieckman, L. J., and R. J. Solaro. Effect of thyroid status on thin-filament Ca^{2+} regulation and expression of troponin I in perinatal and adult rat hearts. *Circ. Res.* 67:344–351, 1990.
51. Ding, X.-L., A. B. Akella and J. Gulati. Contributions of troponin I and troponin C to the acidic pH-induced depression of contractile Ca^{2+} sensitivity in cardiotrabeculae. *Biochemistry* 34:2309–2316, 1995.
52. Donaldson, S. K. B., and L. Hermansen. Differential, direct effects of H^+ on Ca^{2+}-activated force of skinned fibers from the soleus, cardiac, and adductor magnus muscles of rabbits. *Pflugers Arch.* 376:55–65, 1978.
53. Ebashi, S. and A. Kodama. A new protein factor promoting aggregation of tropomyosin. *J. Biochem.* 58:107–198, 1965.
54. Ebus, J. P., G. J. M. Stienen and G. Elzinga. Influence of phosphate and pH on myofilament ATPase activity and force in skinned cardiac trabeculae from rat. *J. Physiol. (Lond.)* 476:501–516, 1994.
55. Edman, K. A. P. Double-hyperbolic force-velocity relation in frog muscle fibres. *J. Physiol. (Lond.)* 404:301–321, 1988.
56. El-Saleh, S. C., and R. J. Solaro. Troponin I enhances acidic pH-induced depression of Ca^{2+} binding to the regulatory sites in skeletal troponin C. *J. Biol. Chem.* 263:3274–3278, 1988.
57. El-Saleh, S., K. D. Warber and J. D. Potter. The role of tropomyosin-troponin in the regulation of skeletal muscle contraction. *J. Muscle Res. Cell Motil.* 7:387–404, 1986.
58. Endoh, M. and J. R. Blinks. Actions of sympathomimetic amines on the Ca^{2+} transients and contractions of rabbit myocardium: reciprocal changes in myofibrillar responsiveness to Ca^{2+} mediated through α and β-adrenoceptors. *Circ. Res.* 62:247–265, 1988.
59. Fabiato, A., and F. Fabiato. Effects of pH on the myofilaments and the sarcoplasmic reticulum of skinned cells from cardiac and skeletal muscles. *J. Physiol. (Lond.)* 276:233–255, 1978.
60. Fananapazir, L. and N. D. Epstein. Genotype-phenotype correlations in hypertrophic cardiomyopathy. *Circulation* 89:22–32, 1994.
61. Farrow, A. J., G. H. Rossmanith and J. Unsworth. The role of calcium ions in the activation of rabbit psoas muscles. *J. Muscle Res. Cell Motil.* 9:261–274, 1988.
62. Fentzke, R. C., S. H. Buck, J. R. Patel, H. Lin, B. M. Wolska, M. O. Stojanovic, A. F. Martin, R. J. Solaro, R. L. Moss and J. M. Leiden. Impaired cardiomyocyte relaxation and diastolic function in transgenic mice expressing slow skeletal troponin I in the heart. *J. Physiol. (Lond.)* 517:143–158, 1999.
63. Fewell, J. G., T. E. Hewett, A. Sanbe, R. Klevitsky, E. Hayes, D. Warshaw, D. Maughan and J. Robbins. Functional significance of cardiac myosin essential light chain isoform switching in transgenic mice. *J. Clin. Invest.* 101:2630–2639, 1998.
64. Fitts, R. Cellular mechanisms of muscle fatigue. *Physiol. Rev.* 74:49–94, 1994.
65. Fitzsimons, D. P., P. W. Bodell and K. M. Baldwin. Phosphorylation of rodent cardiac myosin light chain 2: effects of exercise. *J. Appl. Physiol.* 67:2447–2453, 1989.
66. Fitzsimons, D. P., and R. L. Moss. Strong binding of myosin modulates length-dependent Ca^{2+} activation of rat ventricular myocytes. *Circ. Res.* 83:602–607, 1998.
67. Fitzsimons, D. P., J. R. Patel and R. L. Moss. Role of myosin heavy chain composition in kinetics of force development and relaxation in rat myocardium. *J. Physiol. (Lond.)* 513:171–183, 1998.
68. Flicker, P. F., G. Phillips and C. Cohen. Troponin and its interactions with tropomyosin. *J. Mol. Biol.* 162:495–501, 1982.
69. Ford, L. E., A. F. Huxley and R. M. Simmons. Tension responses to sudden length change in stimulated frog muscle fibres near slack length. *J. Physiol. (Lond.)* 269:441–51, 1977.
70. Ford, L. E., K. Nakagawa, J. Desper and C. Y. Seow. Effect of osmotic compression on the force-velocity properties of glycerinated rabbit skeletal muscle cells. *J. Gen. Physiol.* 97:73–88, 1991.
71. Fozzard, H. A. Cellular basis for inotropic changes in the heart. *Am. Heart J.* 116:230–235, 1988.
72. Fuchs, F. Mechanical modulation of the Ca^{2+} regulatory protein complex in cardiac muscle. *News Physiol. Sci.* 10:6–12, 1995.
73. Fuchs, F. and Y.-P. Wang. Force, length, and Ca^{2+}-troponin C affinity in in skeletal muscle. *Am. J. Physiol.* 261 (*Cell Physiol.* 30):C787–C792, 1991.
74. Garvey, L., E. Kranias and R. J. Solaro. Phosphorylation of C protein, troponin I, and phospholamban in isolated rabbit hearts. *Biochem. J.* 249:709–714, 1988.
75. Gautel, M., O. Zuffardi, A. Freiburg and S. Labeit. Phosphorylation switches specific for the cardiac isoform of myosin binding protein-C: a modulator of cardiac contraction? *EMBO J.* 14:1952–1960, 1995.
76. Geeves, M. A. and K. C. Holmes. Structural mechanism of muscle contraction. *Annu. Rev. Biochem.* 68:687–728, 1999.
77. Geeves, M. A. and S. S. Lehrer. Dynamics of the muscle thin filament regulatory switch: the size of the cooperative unit. *Biophys. J.* 67:273–282, 1994.
78. Godt, R. E., R. T. H. Fogaça and T. M. Nosek. Changes in force and calcium sensitivity in the developing avian heart. *Can. J. Physiol. Pharmacol.* 69:1692–1697, 1991.
79. Godt, R. E., and T. M. Nosek. Changes of intracellular milieu with fatigue or hypoxia depress contraction of skinned rabbit skeletal and cardiac muscles. *J. Physiol. (Lond.)* 412:155–180, 1989.
80. Goldman, Y. E., M. G. Hibberd and D. R. Trentham. Relaxation of rabbit psoas muscle fibers from rigor by photochemical generation of ATP. *J. Physiol. (Lond.)* 354:577–604, 1984.
81. Goldman, Y. E., M. G. Hibberd and D. R. Trentham. Initiation of active contraction by photogeneration of ATP in rabbit psoas muscle fibers. *J. Physiol. (Lond.)* 354:605–624, 1984.
82. Goodlin, R. C., W. L. Freedman, J. G. McFee and S. D. Winter. The neonate with unexpected acidemia. *J. Reprod. Med.* 39:97–100, 1994.
83. Gordon, A. M., E. Homsher and M. Regnier. Regulation of contraction in striated muscle. *Physiol. Rev.* 80:853–924, 2000.
84. Gordon, A. M., A. F. Huxley and F. J. Julian. The variation in isometric tension with sarcomere length in vertebrate muscle fibres. *J. Physiol.* 184:170–192, 1966.
85. Gordon, A. M., M. A. LaMadrid, Y. Chen, Z. Luo and P. B. Chase. Calcium regulation of skeletal muscle thin filament motility in vitro. *Biophys. J.* 72:1295–1307, 1997.
86. Gorza, L., S. Ausoni, N. Merciai, K. E. M. Hastings and S. Schiaffino. Regional differences in troponin I isoform switching during rat heart development. *Dev. Biol.* 156:253–264, 1993.
87. Grabarek, Z., J. Grabarek, P. C. Leavis and J. Gergely. Cooperative binding to the Ca^{2+}-specific sites of troponin C in regulated actin and actomyosin. *J. Biol. Chem.* 258:14098–14102, 1983.
88. Grabarek, Z., T. Tao and J. Gergely. Molecular mechanism of troponin C function. *J. Muscle Res. Cell Motil.* 13:383–93, 1992.

89. Greaser, M. L., and J. Gergely. Reconstitution of troponin activity from three troponin components. *J. Biol. Chem.* 246: 4226–4233, 1971.

90. Greaser, M. L., R. L. Moss and P. J. Reiser. Variations in contractile properties of single muscle fibers in relation to troponin T isoforms and myosin light chains. *J. Physiol. (Lond.)* 406: 85–98, 1988.

91. Gruen, M. and M. Gautel. Mutations in β-myosin S2 that cause familial hypertrophic cardiomyopathy (FHC) abolish the interaction with the regulatory domain of myosin-binding protein-C. *J. Mol. Biol.* 286:933–949, 1999.

92. Guo, X., J. Wattanapermpool, K. A. Palmiter, A. M. Murphy and R. J. Solaro. Mutagenesis of cardiac troponin I. *J. Biol. Chem.* 269:15210–15216, 1994.

93. Guth, K., and J. D. Potter. Effect of rigor and cycling crossbridges on the structure of troponin C and the Ca^{2+} affinity of the Ca^{2+}-specific regulatory sites in skinned rabbit psoas fibers. *J. Biol. Chem.* 262:13627–13635, 1987.

94. Hancock, W. O., D. A. Martyn and L. L. Huntsman. Ca^{2+} and segment length dependence of isometric force kinetics in intact ferret cardiac muscle. *Circ. Res.* 73:603–611, 1993.

95. Hancock, W. O., D. A. Martyn, L. L. Huntsman and A. M. Gordon. Influence of Ca^{2+} on force redevelopment kinetics in skinned rat myocardium. *Biophys. J.* 70:2819–2829, 1996.

96. Harris, D. E., S. S. Work, R. K. Wright, N. R. Alpert and D. M. Warshaw. Smooth, cardiac and skeletal muscle myosin force and motion generation assessed by cross-bridge mechanical interactions in vitro. *J. Muscle Res. Cell Motil.* 15:11–19, 1994.

97. Haselgrove, J. C. X-ray evidence for a conformational change in the actin-containing filament of vertebrate striated muscle. *Cold Spring Harb. Symp. Quant. Biol.* 37:341–352, 1973.

98. Hasenfuss, G., L. A. Mulieri, E. M. Blanchard, C. Holubarsch, B. J. Leavitt, F. Ittleman and N. R. Alpert. Energetics of isometric force development in control and volume-overloaded human myocardium. *Circ. Res.* 68:836–846, 1991.

99. Helmes, M., K. Trombitas and H. Granzier. Titin develops restoring forces in rat cardiac myocytes. *Circ. Res.* 79:619–626, 1996.

100. Hewett, T. E., I. L. Grupp, G. Grupp and J. Robbins. α-Skeletal actin is associated with increased contractility in the mouse heart. *Circ. Res.* 74:740–746, 1994.

101. Hibberd, M. G., J. A. Dantzig, D. R. Trentham and Y. E. Goldman. Phosphate release and force generation in skeletal muscle fibers. *Science* 228:1317–1319, 1985.

102. Hill, A. V. The heat of shortening and the dynamic constants of muscle. *Proc. R. Soc. B* 126:136–195, 1938.

103. Hill, L. E., J. P. Meghan, C. A. Butters and L. S. Tobacman. Analysis of troponin-tropomyosin binding to actin. *J. Biol. Chem.* 267:16106–16113, 1992.

104. Hill, T. L., E. Eisenberg and L. Greene. Alternate model for cooperative equilibrium binding of myosin S1-nucleotide complex. *Proc. Natl. Acad. Sci. U.S.A.* 80:60–64, 1983.

105. Hofmann, P. A., and F. Fuchs. Evidence for a force-dependent component of calcium binding to cardiac troponin C. *Am. J. Physiol.* 253:C541–C546, 1987.

106. Hofmann, P. A., and F. Fuchs. Bound calcium and force development in skinned cardiac bundles: effect of sarcomere length. *J. Mol. Cell. Cardiol.* 20:667–677, 1988.

107. Hofmann, P. A., and J. H. Lange III. Effects of phosphorylation of troponin I and C-protein on isometric tension and velocity of unloaded shortening in skinned single cardiac myocytes from rats. *Circ. Res.* 79:718–726, 1994.

108. Hofmann, P. A., M. L. Greaser and R. L. Moss. C-protein limits shortening velocity of rabbit skeletal muscle fibres at low levels of Ca^{2+} activation. *J. Physiol. (Lond.)* 439:701–715, 1991.

109. Hofmann, P. A., H. C. Hartzell and R. L. Moss. Alterations in Ca^{2+} sensitive tension due to partial extraction of C-protein from rat skinned cardiac myocytes and rabbit skeletal muscle fibers. *J. Gen. Physiol.* 97:1141–1163, 1991.

110. Hofmann, P. A., J. M. Metzger, M. L. Greaser and R. L. Moss. The effects of partial extraction of light chain 2 on the Ca^{2+} sensitivities of isometric tension, stiffness and velocity of shortening. *J. Gen. Physiol.* 95:477–498, 1990.

111. Hoh, J. F. Y., G. H. Rossmanith and A. M. Hamilton. Effects of dibutyryl cyclic AMP, ouabain, and xanthine derivatives on crossbridge kinetics in rat cardiac muscle. *Circ. Res.* 68:702–713, 1991.

112. Hoh, J. F. Y., G. H. Rossmanith, L. J. Kwan and A. M. Hamilton. Adrenaline increases the rate of cycling of crossbridges in rat cardiac muscle as measured by pseudo-random binary noise-modulated perturbation analysis. *Circ. Res.* 62:452–461, 1988.

113. Homsher, E., B. Kim, A. Bobkova and L. S. Tobacman. Calcium regulation of thin filament movement in an in vitro motility assay. *Biophys. J.* 70:1881–1892, 1996.

114. Homsher, E., and J. Lactis. The effect of shortening on the phosphate release step of the actomyosin ATPase. *Biophys. J.* 53:564a, 1988.

115. Homsher, E., D. M. Lee, C. Morris, D. Pavlov and L. S. Tobacman. Regulation of force and unloaded sliding speed in single thin filaments: effects of regulatory proteins and calcium. *J. Physiol. (Lond.)* 524:233–243, 2000.

116. Homsher, E., and N. C. Millar. Caged compounds and striated muscle contraction. *Ann. Rev. Physiol.* 52:875–896, 1990.

117. Hongo, K., E. White and C. H. Orchard. The effect of mechanical loading on the response of rat ventricular myocytes to acidosis. *Exp. Physiol.* 80:701–712, 1995.

118. Hunkeler, N. M., J. Kullman and A. M. Murphy. Troponin I isoform expression in human heart. *Circ. Res.* 69:1409–1414, 1991.

119. Huxley, A. F. Muscle structure and theories of contraction. *Prog. Biophys. Biophys. Chem.* 7:255–318, 1957.

120. Huxley, A. F. and R. M. Simmons. Proposed mechanism of force generation in striated muscle. *Nature* 233:533–538, 1971.

121. Huxley, H. E. Structural changes in actin- and myosin-containing filaments during contraction. *Cold Spr. Harb. Symp. Quant. Biol.* 37:361–376, 1973.

122. Irving, M., V. Lombardi, G. Piazzesi and M. A. Ferenczi. Myosin head movements are synchronous with the elementary force-generating process in muscle. *Nature* 357:156–158, 1992.

123. Jiang, H., A. Chang, K. Poetter, N. D. Epstein, L. Fananapazir, and J. R. Sellers. Increased speed of actin movement by mutant cardiac Myosin from patients with familial hypertrophic cardiomyopathy. *Biophys. J.* 70: A3, 1996.

124. Jin, J.-P. and J. J.-C. Lin. Rapid purification of mammalian cardiac troponin T and its isoform switching in rat hearts during development. *J. Biol. Chem.* 263:7309–7315, 1988.

125. Jin, J. P., Q.-Q. Huang, H.-I. Yeh and J. J.-C. Lin. Complete nucleotide sequence and structural organization of rat cardiac troponin T gene. *J. Mol. Biol.* 227:1269–1276, 1992.

126. Julian, F. J. The effect of calcium on the force-velocity relation of briefly glycerinated frog muscle fibres. *J. Physiol. (Lond.)* 218:117–145, 1971.

127. Julian, F. J. and M. R. Sollins. Sarcomere length-tension relations in living rat papillary muscle. *Circ. Res.* 37:299–308, 1975.

128. Julian, F. J., M. R. Sollins and R. L. Moss. Absence of a plateau in length-tension relationship of rabbit papillary muscle when internal shortening is prevented. *Nature* 260:340–342, 1976.

129. Kahn, S. N., G. S. Ahmed, A. M. Abutaleb and M. A. Hathal. Is the determination of umbilical cord arterial blood gases necessary in all deliveries? *J. Perinatol.* 15:39–42, 1995.
130. Katz, B. Relation between force and speed in contraction. *J. Physiol. (Lond.)* 96:45–64, 1939.
131. Kawai, M. and P. W. Brandt. Two rigor states in skinned crayfish single muscle fibers. *J. Gen. Physiol.* 68:267–280, 1976.
132. Kentish, J. C. The effects of inorganic phosphate and creatine phosphate on force production in skinned muscles from rat ventricle. *J. Physiol. (Lond.)* 370:585–604, 1986.
133. Kentish, J. C., H. E. D. J. ter Keurs, L. Ricciardi, J. J. J. Bucx and M. I. M. Noble. Comparison between the sarcomere length-force relations of intact and skinned trabeculae from rat right ventricle: Influence of calcium concentration on these relations. *Circ. Res.* 58:755–768, 1986.
134. Kentish, J. C. and G. J. M. Stienen. Differential effects of length on maximum force production and myofibrillar ATPase activity in rat skinned cardiac muscle. *J. Physiol. (Lond.)* 475:175–184, 1994.
136. Knight, P. J. Dynamic behaviour of the head-tail junction of myosin. *J. Mol. Biol.* 255:269–274, 1996.
137. Krueger, J. W. and G. H. Pollack. Myocardial dynamics during isometric contraction. *J. Physiol. (Lond.)* 251:627–643, 1975.
138. Lakatta, E. G. Length modulation of muscle performance: Frank-Starling Law of the Heart. In *The Heart and Cardiovascular System*, 2nd ed., edited by H. A. Fozzard, et al. New York: Raven Press, pp. 1325–1352, 1991.
139. Landesberg, A., and S. Sideman. Coupling calcium binding to troponin C and cross-bridge cycling in skinned cardiac cells. *Am. J. Physiol.* 266 (*Heart Circ. Physiol.* 35):H1260–H1271, 1994.
140. Landesberg, A., and S. Sideman. Mechanical regulation of cardiac muscle by coupling calcium kinetics with cross-brige cycling: a dynamic model. *Am. J. Physiol.* 267:H779–H795, 1994.
141. Landis, C., N. Back, E. Homsher and L. S. Homsher. Effects of tropomyosin internal deletions on thin filament function. *J. Biol. Chem.* 274:31279–31285, 1999.
142. Lankford, E. B., N. D. Epstein, L. Fananapazir and H. L. Sweeney. Abnormal contractile properties of muscle fibers expressing β-myosin heavy chain mutations in patients with hypertrophic cardiomyopathy. *J. Clin. Invest.* 95:1409–1414, 1995.
143. Larsson, L., and R. L. Moss. Maximum velocity of shortening in relation to myosin isoform composition in single fibres from human quadriceps and soleus muscles. *(Lond.) J. Physiol.* 472:595–614, 1993.
144. Leavis, P. C. and E. L. Kraft. Calcium binding to cardiac troponin C. *Arch. Biochem. Biophys.* 186:411–415, 1978.
145. Lee, J. S., and D. G. Allen. Mechanisms of acute ischemic contractile failure of the heart. *J. Clin. Invest.* 88:361–367, 1991.
146. Lehman, W., P. Vibert, P. Uman and R. Craig. Steric blocking by tropomyosin visualized in relaxed vertebrate muscle thin filaments. *J. Mol. Biol.* 251:191–196, 1995.
147. Lehrer, S. S. The regulatory switch of the muscle thin filament: Ca^{2+} or myosin heads? *J. Mus. Res. Cell Motil.* 15:232–236, 1994.
148. Lehrer, S. S. and M. A. Geeves. The muscle thin filament as a classical cooperative/allosteric regulatory system. *J. Mol. Biol.* 277:1081–1089, 1998.
149. Leitch, S. P., and D. J. Paterson. Role of Ca^{2+} in protecting the heart from hyperkalemia and acidosis in rabbit: implications for exercise. *J. Appl. Physiol.* 77:2391–2399, 1994.
150. Levine, R. J. C., R. W. Kensler, Z. Yang and H. L. Sweeney. Myosin regulatory light chain phosphorylation and the production of functionally significant changes in myosin head arrangement on striated muscle thick filaments. *Biophys. J.* 68:224s, 1995.
151. Levy, R. M., Y. Umazume and M. J. Kushmerick. Ca^{2+} dependence of tension and ADP production in segments of chemically skinned muscle fibers. *Biochim. Biophys. Acta* 430:352–365, 1976.
152. Litten R. Z., III, B. J. Martin, R. B. Low and N. R. Alpert. Altered myosin isozyme patterns from pressure-overloaded and thyrotoxic hypertrophied rabbit hearts. *Circ. Res.* 50:856–864, 1982.
153. Liu, X., Q. Shao and N. S. Dahalla. Myosin light chain phosphorylation in cardiac hypertrophy and failure due to myocardial infarction. *J. Mol. Cell. Cardiol.* 27:2613–2621, 1995.
154. Lombardi, V., G. Piazzesi and M. Linari. Rapid regeneration of the actin-myosin power stroke in contracting muscle. *Nature* 355:638–641, 1992.
155. Lompré, A. M., J. J. Mercadier, C. Wisnewsky, P. Bouveret, C. Pantaloni, A. D'Albis, and K. Shwartz. Species- and age-dependent changes in the relative amounts of cardiac myosin isoenzymes in mammals. *Dev. Biol.* 84:286–290, 1981.
156. Lompré, A. M., B. Nadal-Ginard and V. Mahdavi. Expression of the cardiac ventricular α- and β-myosin heavy chain genes is developmentally and hormonally regulated. *J. Biol. Chem.* 259:6437–6446, 1984.
157. Lowey, S., and D. Risby. Light chains from fast and slow muscle myosins. *Nature* 234:81–85, 1971.
158. Lowey, S., and K. M. Trybus. Role of skeletal and smooth muscle myosin' light chains. *Biophys. J.* 68:120s–127s, 1995.
159. Lowey, S., G. S. Waller and K. M. Trybus. Skeletal muscle myosin light chains are essential for physiological speeds of shortening. *Nature* 365:454–456, 1993.
160. Lu, Z., R. L. Moss and J. W. Walker. Tension transients initiated by photo-generation of MgADP in skinned skeletal muscle fibers. *J. Gen. Physiol.* 101:867–888, 1993.
161. Mak, A. S. and L. B. Smillie. Structural interpretation of the two-site binding of troponin on the muscle thin filament. *J. Mol. Biol.* 149:541–550, 1981.
162. Manning, D. R. and J. T. Stull. Myosin light chain phosphorylation-dephosphorylation in mammalian skeletal muscle. *Am. J. Physiol.* 242:C234–C241, 1982.
163. Margossian, S. S. Reversible dissociation of dog cardiac myosin regulatory light chain 2 and its influence on ATP hydrolysis. *J. Biol. Chem.* 260:13747–13754, 1985.
164. Margossian, S. S., A. K. Bhan and H. S. Slayter. Role of the regulatory light chains in skeletal muscle actomyosin ATPase and minifilament formation. *J. Biol. Chem.* 258:13359–13369, 1983.
165. Margossian, S. S., H. D. White, J. B. Caulfield, P. Norton, S. Taylor, and H. S. Slayter. Light chain 2 profile and activity of human ventricular myosin during dilated cardiomyopathy. *Circulation* 85:1720–1733, 1992.
166. Martin, A. F., K. Ball, L. Gao, P. Kumar and R. J. Solaro. Identification and functional significance of troponin I isoforms in neonatal rat heart myofibrils. *Circ. Res.* 69:1244–1252, 1991.
167. Martin, A. J. and R. Roberts. Recent advances in the molecular genetics of hypertrophic cardiomyopathy. *Circulation* 92:1336–1347, 1995.
168. Martin, H. and R. J. Barsotti. Relaxation from rigor of skinned trabeculae of the guinea pig by laser flash photolysis of caged ATP. *Biophys. J.* 66:1115–1128, 1994.
169. Mayoux, E., N. Coutry, P. Lechêne, F. Marotte, C. Hoffman and R. Ventura-Clapier. Effects of acidosis and alkalosis on mechanical properties of hypertrophied rat heart fiber bundles. *Am. J. Physiol.* 266:H2051–H2060, 1994.
170. McAuliffe, J. J., L. Gao and R. J. Solaro. Changes in myofibrillar activation and troponin C Ca^{2+} binding associated with

troponin T isoform switching in developing rabbit heart. *Circ. Res.* 66:1204–1216, 1990.
171. McDonald, K. S., L. J. Field, M. S. Parmacek, M. Soonpaa, J. M. Leiden and R. L. Moss. Length dependence of Ca^{2+} sensitivity of tension in mouse cardiac myocytes expressing skeletal troponin C. *J. Physiol.* 483:131–139, 1995.
172. McDonald, K. S. and R. L. Moss. Osmotic compression of single cardiac myocytes eliminates the reduction of Ca^{2+} sensitivity of tension at short sarcomere length. *Circ. Res.* 77:199–205, 1995.
173. McDonald, K. S., M. R. Wolff and R. L. Moss. Force-velocity and power-load curves in rat skinned cardiac myocytes. *J. Physiol. (Lond.)* 511:519–531, 1998.
174. McDonough J. L., D. K. Arrell and J. E. Van Eyk. Troponin I degradation and covalent complex formation accompanies myocardial ischemia/reperfusion injury. *Circ. Res.* 84:9–20, 1999.
175. McKillop, D. F. A. and M. A. Geeves. Regulation of the interaction between actin and myosin subfragment 1: evidence for three states of the thin filament. *Biophys. J.* 65:693–701, 1993.
176. McNally, E. M., R. Kraft, M. Bravo-Zehnder, D. A. Taylor and L. A. Leinwand. Full-length rat alpha and beta cardiac myosin heavy chain sequences. *J. Mol. Biol.* 665–671, 1989.
177. Metzger, J. M. Effects of troponin C isoforms on pH sensitivity of contraction in mammalian fast and slow skeletal muscle fibres. *J. Physiol. (Lond.)* 492:163–172, 1996.
178. Metzger, J. M. Effects of phosphate and ADP on shortening velocity during maximal and submaximal calcium activation of the thin filament in skeletal muscle fibers. *Biophys. J.* 70:409–417, 1996.
179. Metzger, J. M., and R. L. Moss. Greater hydrogen ion-induced depression of tension and velocity in skinned single skeletal fibres of rat fast than slow muscles. *J. Physiol. (Lond.)* 393:727–742, 1987.
180. Metzger, J. M., M. L. Greaser and R. L. Moss. Variations in cross-bridge attachment rate with phosphorylation of myosin. *J. Gen. Physiol.* 93:855–883, 1989.
181. Metzger, J. M. and R. L. Moss. Effects on isometric tension and stiffness due to reduced pH in mammalian fast- and slow-twitch skinned skeletal muscle fibres. *J. Physiol. (Lond.)* 428:737–750, 1990.
182. Metzger, J. M. and R. L. Moss. pH modulation of the kinetics of a Ca^{2+} sensitive cross-bridge state transition in mammalian single skeletal muscle fibers. *J. Physiol. (Lond.)* 428:751–764, 1990.
183. Metzger, J. M. and R. L. Moss. Myosin light chain 2 modulates calcium sensitive cross-bridge transitions in vertebrate skeletal muscle. *Biophys. J.* 63:460–468, 1992.
184. Metzger, J. M., M. S. Parmacek, E. Barr, K. Pasyk, W.-I. Lin, K. L. Cochrane, L. J. Field and J. M. Leiden. Skeletal troponin C reduces contractile sensitivity to acidosis in cardiac myocytes from transgenic mice. *Proc. Natl. Acad. Sci. U.S.A.* 90:9036–9040, 1993.
185. Millar, N. C. and E. Homsher. The effect of phosphate and calcium on force generation in glycerinated rabbit skeletal muscle fibers. *J. Biol. Chem.* 265:20234–20240, 1990.
186. Modest, V., and J. F. Butterworth. Effect of pH and lidocaine on β-adrenergic receptor binding. *Chest* 108:1373–1379, 1995.
187. Moore, R. L., T. I. Musch and J. Y. Cheung. Modulation of cardiac contractility by myosin light chain phosphorylation. *Med. Sci. Sports Exerc.* 23:1163–1169, 1991.
188. Morano, I. Tuning the human heart molecular motors by myosin light chains. *J. Mol. Med.* 77:544–555, 1999.
189. Morano, I., K. Hädicke, S. Grom, A. Koch, R. H. G. Schwinger, M. Böhm, S. Bartel, E. Erdmann and E.-G. Krause. Titin, myosin light chains and C-protein in the developing and failing human heart. *J. Mol. Cell. Cardiol.* 26:361–368, 1994.
190. Morano, I., Ä. Österman and A. A. Arner. Rate of active tension development from rigor in skinned atrial and ventricular cardiac fibres from swine following photolytic release of ATP from caged ATP. *Acta Physiol. Scand.* 154:343–353, 1995.
191. Morano, M., U. Zacharzowski, M. Maier, P. E. Lange, V. Alexi-Meskishvili, M. Haase and I. Morano. Regulation of human heart contractility by essential myosin light chain. *J. Clin. Invest.* 98:467–473, 1996.
192. Mornet, D., P. Pantel, E. Audemard, R. Kassab. The limited tryptic cleavage of chymotryptic S1: an approach to the characterisation of the actin site in myosin heads. *Biochem. Biophys. Res. Commun.* 89:925–932, 1979.
193. Moss, R. L. Variations in maximum shortening velocity in skinned skeletal muscle fibers due to changes in thin filament activation with Ca^{2+} and by partial extraction of troponin-C. *J. Physiol. (Lond.)* 377:487–505, 1986.
194. Moss, R. L. Ca^{2+} regulation of mechanical properties of striated muscle: mechanistic studies using extraction and replacement of regulatory proteins. *Circ. Res.* 70:865–884, 1992.
195. Moss, R. L. Plasticity in the dynamics of myocardial contraction. Ca^{2+}, crossbridge kinetics, or molecular cooperation. *Circ. Res.* 84:862–865, 1999.
196. Moss, R. L., J. D. Allen and M. L. Greaser. The effects of partial extraction of whole troponin complex upon the tension-pCa relation in rabbit skeletal muscle. *J. Gen. Physiol.* 87:761–774, 1986.
197. Moss, R. L., G. G. Giulian and M. L. Greaser. Mechanical effects accompanying the removal of myosin LC_2 from skinned skeletal muscle fibres. *J. Biol. Chem.* 257:8588–8591, 1982.
198. Moss, R. L., G. G. Giulian and M. L. Greaser. The effects of partial extraction of TnC upon the tension-pCa relation in mammalian skeletal muscle. *J. Gen. Physiol.* 86:585–600, 1985.
199. Moss, R. L. and R. A. Haworth. The effects of low levels of MgATP upon the mechanical properties of skinned skeletal muscle fibers of the rabbit. *Biophys. J.* 45:733–742, 1984.
200. Moss, R. L., M. R. Lauer, G. G. Giulian and M. L. Greaser. Altered Ca^{2+} dependence of tension development in skinned skeletal muscle fibers following modification of troponin by partial substitution with cardiac TnC. *J. Biol. Chem.* 261:6096–6099, 1986.
201. Moss, R. L., L. O. Nwoye and M. L. Greaser. Substitution of cardiac troponin-C into rabbit muscle does not alter the length dependence of Ca^{2+} sensitivity of tension. *J. Physiol. (Lond.)* 440:273–289, 1991.
202. Moss, R. L. and J. Sant'Ana Periera. Enhanced myosin function due to a point mutation causing a familial hypertrophic cardiomyopathy. *Circ. Res.* 86:720–722, 2000.
203. Murphy, A. M., L. Jones III, H. F. Sims and A. W. Strauss. Molecular cloning of rat cardiac troponin I and analysis of troponin I isoform expression in developing rat heart. *Biochemistry* 30:707–712, 1991.
204. Murphy, A. M., H. Kogler, D. Georgakopolous, J. L. McDonough, D. A. Kass, J. E. Van Eyk and E. Marban. Transgenic mouse model of stunned myocardium. *Science* 287:488–491, 2000.
205. Muthuchamy, M., I. L. Grupp, G. Grupp, B. A. O'Toole, A. B. Kier, G. P. Boivin, J. Neumann and D. F. Wieczorek. Molecular and physiological effects of overexpressing striated muscle β-tropomyosin in the adult murine heart. *J. Biol. Chem.* 270:30593–30603, 1995.
206. Nassar, R., N. N. Malouf, M. B. Kelly, A. E. Oakeley and P. A. W. Anderson. Force-pCa relation and troponin T isoforms of rabbit myocardium. *Circ. Res.* 69:1470–1475, 1991.

207. Noland, T. A. Jr., X. Guo, R. L. Raynor, N. M. Jideama, V. Averyhart-Fullard, R. J. Solaro and J. F. Kuo. Cardiac troponin I mutants: phosphorylation by protein kinases C and A and regulation of Ca^{2+} stimulated MgATPase of reconstituted actomyosin S-1. *J. Biol. Chem.* 270:25445–25454, 1995.

208. Noland, T. A. Jr., and J. F. Kuo. Protein kinase C phosphorylation of cardiac troponin I and troponin T inhibits Ca^{2+}-stimulated MgATPase activity in reconstituted actomyosin and isolated myofibrils, and decreases actin-myosin interactions. *J. Mol. Cell. Cardiol.* 25:53–65, 1993.

209. Offer, G., C. Moos and R. Starr. A new protein of the thick filaments of vertebrate skeletal myofibrils. *J. Mol. Biol.* 74:653–676, 1973.

210. Opie, L. H. Myocardial contraction and relaxation. In: *The Heart Physiology and Metabolism*. New York: Raven Press, 1991:176–194.

211. Orchard, C. H., and J. C. Kentish. Effects of changes of pH on the contractile function of cardiac muscle. *Am. J. Physiol.* 258 (*Cell Physiol.* 27):C967–C981.

212. Pagani, E. D., A. A. Alousi, A. M. Grant, T. M. Older, S. W. Dziuban and P. D. Allen. Changes in myofibrillar content and Mg-ATPase activity in ventricular tissues from patients with heart failure caused by coronary artery disease, cardiomyopathy, or mitral insufficiency. *Circ. Res.* 63:380–385, 1988.

213. Palmiter, K., R. J. Solaro, X. Guo, R. Fentzke, K. Barton, C. Clendenin and J. M. Leiden. Exchange of slow skeletal troponin I (ssTnI) for cardiac troponin I (cTnI) in transgenic mouse hearts increases myofilament calcium senstivity at acidic pH. *Biophys. J.* 70:A171, 1996.

214. Palmer, S., and J. C. Kentish. The role of troponin C in modulating the Ca^{2+} sensitivity of mammalian skinned cardiac and skeletal muscle fibres. *J. Physiol. (Lond.)* 480:45–60, 1994.

215. Pan, B.-S., A. M. Gordon and Z. Luo. Removal of tropomyosin overlap modifies cooperative binding of myosin S-1 to reconstituted thin filaments of rabbit striated muscle. *J. Biol. Chem.* 264:8495–8495, 1989.

216. Pan, B.-S., A. M. Gordon and J. D. Potter. Deletion of the first 45 NH_2-terminal residues of rabbit skeletal troponin T strengthens binding to immobilized tropomyosin. *J. Biol. Chem.* 266:12432–12438, 1991.

217. Pan, B.-S. and R. J. Solaro. Calcium-binding properties of troponin C in detergent-skinned heart muscle fibers. *J. Biol. Chem.* 262:7839–7849, 1987.

218. Parmacek, M. S., and J. Leiden. Structure, function, and regulation of troponin C. *Circulation* 84:991–1003, 1991.

219. Pate, E. and R. Cooke. Addtion of phosphate to active muscle probes actomyosin states within the power stroke. *Pflugers Arch.* 414:73–81, 1989.

220. Pawloski-Dahm, C. M., G. Song, D. L. Kirkpatrick, J. Palermo, J. Gulick, G. W. Dorn, II, J. Robbins and R. A. Walsh. Effects of total replacement of atrial myosin light chain-2 with the ventricular isoform in atrial myocytes of transgenic mice. *Circulation* 97:1508–1513, 1998.

221. Pette, D., and R. S. Staron. Cellular and molecular diversities of mammalian skeletal muscle fibers. *Rev. Physiol. Biochem. Pharmacol.* 116:1–76, 1990.

222. Podolin, R. A. and L. E. Ford. Influence of partial activation on force-velocity properties of frog skinned muscle fibers. *J. Gen. Physiol.* 87:607–631, 1986.

223. Potter, J. D. and J. Gergely. The calcium and magnesium binding sites on troponin and their role in the regulation of myofibrillar adenosine triphosphatase. *J. Biol. Chem.* 250:4628–4633, 1975.

224. Rayment, I, H. M. Holden, J. R. Sellers, L. Fananapazir, and N. D. Epstein. Structural interpretation of the mutations in the β-cardiac myosin that have been implicated in familial hypertrophic cardiomyopathy. *Proc. Natl. Acad. Sci. U.S.A.* 92:3864–3868, 1995.

225. Rayment, I., H. M. Holden, M. Whitaker, C. B. Yohn, M. Lorenz, K. C. Holmes and R. A. Milligan. Structure of the actin-myosin complex and its implications for muscle contraction. *Science* 261:58–65, 1993.

226. Rayment, I., W. R. Rypniewski, K. Schmidt-Base, R. Smith, D. R. Tomchick, M. M. Benning, D. A. Winkelman, G. Wesenberg and H. M. Holden. Three-dimensional structure of myosin subfragment-1: a molecular motor. *Science* 261:50–58, 1993.

227. Rayment, I., C. Smith and R. G. Yount. The active site of myosin. *Ann. Rev. Physiol.* 58:671–702, 1996.

228. Ricciardi, L., J. J. J. Bucx, and H. E. D. J. ter Keurs. Effects of acidosis on force-sarcomere length and force-velocity relations of rat cardiac muscle. *J. Cardiovasc. Res.* 20:117–123, 1986.

229. Ridgway, E. B. and A. M. Gordon. Muscle calcium transient: effect of post-stimulus length changes in single fibers. *J. Gen. Physiol.* 83:75–103, 1984. Robbins, J., T. Horan, J. Gulick and K. Kropp. The chicken myosin heavy chain family. *J. Biol. Chem.* 261:6606–6612, 1986.

230. Robertson, S. P., J. D. Johnson, M. J. Holroyde, E. G. Kranias, J. D. Potter and R. J. Solaro. The effect of troponin I phosphorylation on the Ca^{2+}-binding properties of the Ca^{2+}-regulatory site of bovine cardiac troponin. *J. Biol. Chem.* 257:260–263, 1982.

231. Rome, L. C., R. P. Funke, R. M. Alexander, G. Lutz, H. Aldridge, F. Scott and M. Freadman. Why animals have different fiber types. *Nature* 335:824–827, 1988.

232. Rome, L. C., R. P. Funke and R. M. Alexander. The influence of temperature on muscle velocity and sustained performance in swimming carp. *J. Exp. Biol.* 154:163–178, 1990.

233. Rome, L. C., and S. L. Lindstedt. Mechanical and metabolic design of the muscular system in vertebrates. In: *Handbook of Physiology, Comparative Physiology*, edited by W. H. Dautzler. New York: Oxford University Press for the American Physiological Society; Section 13, Vol. II, Chapt. 23, 1997:1587–1651.

234. Rome, L. C., and A. A. Sosnicki. The influence of temperature on mechanics of red muscle in carp. *J. Physiol. (Lond.)* 427:151–169, 1990.

235. Rosenfeld, S. S., and E. W. Taylor. Kinetic studies of calcium binding to regulatory complexes from skeletal muscle. *J. Biol. Chem.* 260:252–261, 1985.

236. Rosenfeld, S. S. and E. W. Taylor. The mechanism of regulation of actomyosin subfragment 1 ATPase. *J. Biol. Chem.* 262:9984–9993, 1987.

237. Rubenstein, P. A. The functional importance of multiple actin isoforms. *Bioessays* 12:309–315, 1990.

238. Sanbe, A., J. G. Fewell, J. Gulick, H. Osinska, J. Lorenz, D. G. Hall, L. A. Murray, T. R. Kimball, S. A. Witt and J. Robbins. Abnormal cardiac structure and function in mice expressing nonphosphorylatable cardiac regulatory myosin light chain 2. *J. Biol. Chem.* 274:21085–21094, 1999.

239. Sasse, S., N. J. Brand, P. Kyprianou, G. K. Dhoot, R. Wade, M. Arai, M. Periasamy, M. H. Yacoub and P. J. R. Barton. Troponin I gene expression during human cardiac development and in end-stage heart failure. *Circ. Res.* 72:932–938, 1993.

240. Schiaffino, S., L. Gorza and S. Ausoni. Troponin isoform switching in the developing heart and its functional consequences. *Trends Cardiovasc. Med.* 3:12–17, 1993.

241. Schiaffino, S., and C. Reggiani. Molecular diversity of myofibrillar proteins: gene regulation and functional significance. *Physiol. Rev.* 76:371–423, 1996.

242. Schultheiss, T., Z. Lin, M.-H. Lu, J. Murray, D. A. Fischman, K. Weber, T. Masaki, M. Imamura and H. Holtzer. Differential

distribution of subsets of myofibrillar proteins in cardiac non-striated and striated myofibrils. *J. Cell. Biol.* 110:1159–1172, 1990.
243. Schwartz, K., L. Carrier, C. Chassagne, C. Wisnewsky and K. R. Boheler. Regulation of myosin heavy chain and actin isogenes during cardiac growth and development. *Symp. Soc. Exp. Biol.* 46:265–275, 1992.
244. Seow, C. Y., and L. E. Ford. Shortening velocity and power output of skinned muscle fibers from mammals having a 25,000-fold range of body mass. *J. Gen. Physiol.* 97:541–560, 1991.
245. Seow, C. Y., and L. E. Ford. Contribution of damped passive recoil to the measured shortening velocity of skinned rabbit and sheep muscle fibres. *J. Muscle Res. Cell Motil.* 13:295–307, 1992.
246. Sheng, Z., W. L. Strauss, J.-M. Francois and J. D. Potter. Evidence that both Ca^{2+}-specific sites of skeletal muscle TnC are required for full activity. *J. Biol. Chem.* 265:21554–21560, 1990.
247. Shiner, J. S., and R. J. Solaro. The Hill coefficient for the Ca^{2+} activation of striated muscle contraction. *Biophys. J.* 46:541–543, 1982.
248. Siemankowski, R. F., M. O. Wiseman and H. D. White. ADP dissociation from acto-S1 is sufficiently slow to limit unloaded shortening velocity in muscle. *J. Biol. Chem.* 260:658–662, 1985.
249. Solaro, R J. In: *Protein Phosphorylation in Heart Muscle.* CRC Press, Boca Raton, FL, 1986:129–156.
250. Solaro, R. J., S. C. El-Saleh and J. C. Kentish. Ca^{2+}, pH and the regulation of cardiac myofilament force and ATPase activity. *Mol. Cell. Biochem.* 89:163–167, 1989.
251. Solaro, R. J., J. A. Lee, J. C. Kentish and D. G. Allen. Effects of acidosis on ventricular muscle from adult and neonatal rats. *Circ. Res.* 63:779–787, 1988.
252. Solaro, R. J., A. J. G. Moir and S. V. Perry. Phosphorylation of troponin I and the inotropic effect of adrenaline in the perfused rabbit heart. *Nature* 262:615–617, 1976.
253. Solaro, R. J. and H. M. Rarick. Troponin and tropomyosin. Proteins that switch on and tune in the activity of cardiac myofilaments. *Circ. Res.* 83:471–480, 1988.
254. Starling, E. H. *Linacre Lecture on the Law of the Heart: 1915.* Longmans, London, 1918.
255. Strang, K. T., R. M. Mentzer and R. L. Moss. Slowing of shortening velocity of rat cardiac myocytes by adenosine receptor stimulation regardless of β-adrenergic stimulation. *J. Physiol. (Lond.)* 486:679–688, 1995.
256. Strang, K. T. and R. L. Moss. α_1-Adrenergic receptor stimulation decreases maximum shortening velocity of skinned single ventricular myocytes from rats. *Circ. Res.* 77:114–120, 1995.
257. Strang, K. T., N. K. Sweitzer, M. L. Greaser and R. L. Moss. β-Adrenergic receptor stimulation increases unloaded shortening velocity (V_o) of rat skinned single ventricular myocytes. *Circ. Res.* 74:542–549, 1994.
258. Swartz, D. R., M. L. Greaser and B. B. Marsh. Regulation of binding of subfragment 1 in isolated rigor myofibrils. *J. Cell Biol.* 111:2989–3001, 1990.
259. Swartz, D. R. and R. L. Moss. Influence of a strong-binding myosin analog on calcium sensitive mechanical properties of skinned skeletal muscle fibers. *J. Biol. Chem.* 267:20497–20506, 1992.
260. Sweeney, H. L. Function of the N terminus of the myosin essential light chain of vertebrate striated muscle. *Biophys. J.* 68:112s–119s, 1995.
261. Sweeney, H. L., B. F. Bowman and J. T. Stull. Myosin light chain phosphorylation in vertebrate striated muscle: regulation and function. *Am. J. Physiol.* 264 (*Cell Physiol.* 33):C1085–1095, 1993.
262. Sweeney, H. L. and M. J. Kushmerick. Myosin phosphorylation in permeabilized rabbit psoas fibers. *Am. J. Physiol.* 249 (*Cell Physiol.* 18):C362–365, 1985.
263. Sweeney, H. L., M. J. Kushmerick, K. Mabuchi, F. A. Sreter and J. Gergely. Myosin alkali light chain and heavy chain variations correlate with altered shortening velocity of isolated skeletal muscle fibers. *J. Biol. Chem.* 263:9034–9039, 1988.
264. Sweeney, H. L. and J. T. Stull. Phosphorylation of myosin in permeabilized mammalian cardiac and skeletal muscle cells. *Am. J. Physiol.* 250 (*Cell Physiol.* 19):C657–660, 1986.
265. Sweeney, H. L. and J. T. Stull. Alteration of cross-bridge kinetics by myosin light chain phosphorylation: implications for regulation of actin-myosin interaction. *Proc. Natl. Acad. Sci. U.S.A.* 87:414–18, 1990.
266. Sweitzer, N. K. and R. L. Moss. The effect of altered temperature on Ca^{2+} sensitive force in skinned single cardiac myocytes—Evidence for force dependence of thin filament activation. *J. Gen. Physiol.* 96:1221–1245, 1990.
267. Swynghedauw, B. Developmental and functional adaptation of contractile proteins in cardiac and skeletal muscles. *Physiol. Rev.* 66:710–771, 1986.
268. Teichholz, L. E. and R. J. Podolsky. The relation between calcium and contraction kinetics in skinned muscle fibres. *J. Physiol. (Lond.)* 211:19–35, 1970.
269. ter Keurs, H. E. D. J., J. J. J. Bucx, P. P. de Tombe, P. Backx and T. Iwazumi. The effects of sarcomere length and Ca^{++} on force and velocity of shortening in cardiac muscle. In *Molecular Mechanisms of Muscle Contraction*, H. Sugi and G. H. Pollack, eds. New York: Plenum Publishing Corporation, 1988:581–591.
270. Thierfelder, L., H. Watkins, C. MacRae, R. Lamas, W. McKenna, H. P. Vosberg, J. G. Seidman and C. E. Seidman. α-Tropomyosin and cardiac troponin T mutations cause familial hypertrophic cardiomyopathy: a disease of the sarcomere. *Cell* 77:701–712, 1994.
271. Thomas, L. and L. B. Smilie. Comparison of the interaction and functional properties of dephosphorylated hetero- and homodimers of rabbit striated muscle tropomyosins. *Biophys. J.* 66:A310, 1994.
272. Tobacman, L. S. Thin filament-mediated regulation of cardiac contraction. *Annu. Rev. Physiol.* 58:447–481, 1996.
273. Tobacman, L. S., and C. A. Butters. Thin filament activation is not proportional to TnC regulatory site Ca^{2+} binding. Studies of cardiac thin filaments containing mixtures of TnC and regulatory site mutant TnC. *Biophys. J.* 70:A25, 1996.
274. Tobacman, L. S., and R. Lee. Isolation and functional comparison of bovine cardiac troponin T isoforms. *J. Biol. Chem.* 262:4059–4064, 1987.
275. Tobacman, L. S., and D. Sawyer. Calcium binds cooperatively to the regulatory sites of the cardiac thin filament. *J. Biol. Chem.* 265:931–939, 1990.
276. Trybus, K. M., G. S. Waller and T. A. Chatman. Coupling of ATPase activity and motility in smooth muscle myosin is regulated by the regulatory light chain. *J. Cell Biol.* 124:963–969, 1994.
277. Tyska, M. J., E. Hayes, M. Giewat, C. E. Seidman, J. G. Seidman and D. M. Warshaw. Single-molecule mechanics of R403Q cardiac myosin isolated from the mouse model of familial hypertrophic cardiomyopathy. *Circ. Res.* 86:737–744, 2000.
278. Uyeda, T. Q. P., and J. A. Spudich. A functional recombinant myosin II lacking a regulatory light chain-binding site. *Science* 262:1867–1870, 1993.
279. Uyeda, T. Q. P., K. M. Ruppel and J. A. Spudich. Enzymatic activities correlate with chimaeric substitutions at the actin-binding face of myosin. *Nature* 368:567–569, 1994.

280. Van Buren, P., G. S. Waller, D. E. Harris, K. M. Trybus, D. M. Warshaw and S. Lowey. The essential light chain is required for full force production by skeletal muscle myosin. *Proc. Natl. Acad. Sci. U.S.A.* 91:12403–12407, 1994.

281. Van Buren, P., D. E. Harris, N. R. Alpert and D. M. Warshaw. Cardiac V_1 and V_3 myosins differ in their hydrolytic and mechanical activities in vitro. *Circ. Res.* 77:439–444, 1995.

282. van Eerd, J. P. and K. Takahashi. Amino acid sequence of bovine cardiac troponin-C. Comparison with rabbit skeletal troponin-C. *Biochem. Biophys. Res. Comm.* 64:122–127, 1975.

283. Van Eyk, J. E., F. Powers, W. Law, C. Larue, R. S. Hodges and R. J. Solaro. Breakdown and release of myofilament proteins during ischemia and ischemia/reperfusion in rat hearts. Identification of degradation products and effects on the pCa-force relation. *Circ. Res.* 82:261–271, 1998.

284. Veech, R. L., J. W. Lawson, N. W. Cornell and H. A. Krebs. Cytosolic phosphorylation potential. *J. Biol. Chem.* 254:6538–6547, 1979.

285. Venema, R. C., and J. F. Kuo. Protein kinase C-mediated phosphorylation of troponin I and C-protein in isolated myocardial cells is associated with inhibition of myofibrillar actomyosin MgATPase. *J. Biol. Chem.* 268:2705–2711, 1993.

286. Walker, J. W., Z. Lu and R. L. Moss. Effects of Ca^{2+} on the kinetics of phosphate release in skeletal muscle fibers. *J. Biol. Chem.* 267:2459–2466, 1992.

287. Walsh, T. P., C. Trueblood, R. Evans and A. Weber. Removal of tropomyosin overlap and the co-operative response to increasing calcium concentrations of the acto-subfragment-1 ATPase. *J. Mol. Biol.* 182:265–269, 1984.

288. Wang, Y.-P. and F. Fuchs. Length, force and Ca^{2+}-troponin C affinity in cardiac and slow skeletal muscle. *Am. J. Physiol.* 266 (Cell Physiol. 35):C1077–C1082, 1994.

289. Wang, Y.-P. and F. Fuchs. Osmotic compression of skinned cardiac and skeletal muscle bundles: effects on force generation, Ca^{2+} sensitivity and Ca^{2+} binding. *J. Mol. Cell. Cardiol.* 27:1235–1244, 1995.

290. Watkins, H., D. Conner, L. Thierfelder, J. A. Jarcho, C. MacRae, W. McKenna, B. J. Maron, J. G. Seidman and C. E. Seidman. Mutations in the cardiac myosin binding protein-C gene on chromosome 11 cause familial hypertrophic cardiomyopathy. *Nature Genet.* 11:434–437, 1995.

291. Watkins, H., W. McKenna, L. Thierfelder, H. J. Suk, R. Anan, A. O'Donoghue, P. Spirito, A. Matsumori, C. S. Moravec, J. G. Seidman and C. E. Seidman. Mutations in the genes for cardiac troponin T and α-tropomyosin in hypertrophic cardiomyopathy. *N. Engl. J. Med.* 332:1058–1064, 1995.

292. Wattanapermpool, J., P. J. Reiser and R. J. Solaro. Troponin I isoforms and differential effects of acidic pH on soleus and cardiac mMyofilaments. *Am. J. Physiol.* 268:C323–C330, 1995.

293. Wattanapermpool, J., X. Guo and R. J. Solaro. The unique amino-terminal peptide of cardiac troponin I regulates myofibrillar activity only when it is phosphorylated. *J. Mol. Cell. Cardiol.* 27:1383–1391, 1995.

294. Weisberg, A. and S. Winegrad. Relation between crossbridge structure and actomyosin ATPase activity in rat heart. *Circ. Res.* 83:60–72, 1998.

295. Westfall, M. V., F. P. Albayya, I. I. Turner and J. M. Metzger. Chimera analysis of troponin I domains that influence Ca^{2+}-activated myofilament tension in adult cardiac myocytes. *Circ. Res.* 86:470–477, 2000.

296. Wilkinson, J. M. Troponin C from rabbit slow skeletal and cardiac muscle is the product of a single gene. *Eur. J. Biochem.* 103:179–188, 1980.

297. Williams, D. L., and L. E. Greene. Comparison of the effects of tropomyosin and troponin-tropomyosin on the binding of myosin subfragment 1 to actin. *Biochemistry* 22:2770–2774, 1983.

298. Williams, D. L., L. E. Greene and E. Eisenberg. Cooperative turning on of myosin S1 ATPase activity by the troponin-tropomyosin-actin complex. *Biochemistry* 27:6987–6993, 1988.

299. Winegrad, S. How actin-myosin interactions differ with different isoforms of myosin. *Circ. Res.* 82:1109–1110, 1998.

300. Winegrad, S. Cardiac myosin binding protein C. *Circ. Res.* 84:1117–1126, 1999.

301. Winegrad, S., A. Weisberg, L. E. Lin and G. McClellan. Adrenergic regulation of myosin adenosine triphosphatase activity. *Circ. Res.* 58:83–95, 1986.

302. Woledge, R. C., N. A. Curtin and E Homsher. *Energetic Aspects of Muscle Contraction* London: Academic Press, 1985: 47–71.

303. Wolff, M. R., S. H. Buck, S. W. Stoker, M. L. Greaser and R. M. Mentzer. Myofibrillar calcium sensitivity of isometric tension is increased in human dilated cardiomyopathies. *J. Clin. Invest.* 98:167–176, 1996.

304. Wolff, M. R., K. S. McDonald and R. L. Moss. The rate of tension development in cardiac muscle varies with level of activator calcium. *Circ. Res.* 76:154–160, 1995.

305. Wolska, B. M., R. S. Keller, C. C. Evans, K. A. Palmiter, R. M. Philips, M. Muthuchamy, J. Oehlenschlager, D. F. Wieczorek, P. P. deTombe and R. J. Solaro. Correlation between myofilament response to Ca^{2+} and altered dynamics of contraction and relaxation in transgenic cardiac cells that express β-tropomyosin. *Circ. Res.* 84:745–751, 1999.

306. Yamamoto, K., and C. Moos. The C-proteins of rabbit red, white, and cardiac muscles. *J. Biol. Chem.* 258:8395–8401, 1983.

307. Yang, Q., A. Sanbe, H. Osinska, T. E. Hewett, R. Klevitsky and J. Robbins. In vivo modeling of myosin binding protein C familial hypertrophic cardiomyopathy. *Circ. Res.* 85:841–847, 1999.

308. Yang, Z., and H. L. Sweeney. Restoration of phosphorylation-dependent regulation to the skeletal muscle myosin regulatory light chain. *J. Biol. Chem.* 270:24646–24649, 1995.

309. Yount, R. G., D. Lawson and I. Rayment. Is myosin a "back door" enzyme? *Biophys. J.* 44s–49s, 1995.

310. Zhang, R., J. Zhao, A. Mandveno and J. D. Potter. Cardiac troponin I phosphorylation increases the rate of cardiac muscle relaxation. *Circ. Res.* 76:1028–1035, 1995.

311. Zhang, R., J. Zhao and J. D. Potter. Phosphorylation of both serine residues in cardiac troponin I is required to decrease the Ca^{2+} affinity of cardiac troponin C. *J. Biol. Chem.* 270:30773–30780, 1995.

312. Zhao, Y., and M. Kawai. Kinetic and thermodynamic studies of the cross-bridge cycle in rabbit psoas muscle fibers. *Biophys. J.* 67:1655–1668, 1994.

313. Zot, A. S., and J. D. Potter. Reciprocal coupling between troponin C and myosin crossbridge attachment. *Biochemistry* 28:6751–6756, 1989.

314. Zot, H. G. and J. D. Potter. A structural role for the Ca^{2+}-Mg^{2+} sites on troponin-C in muscle contraction. *J. Biol. Chem.* 257:7678–7683, 1982.

12. Normal and abnormal conduction in the heart

ANDRÉ G. KLÉBER | *Department of Physiology, University of Bern, Bern, Switzerland*

MICHIEL J. JANSE | *Laboratory for Experimental Cardiology, University of Amsterdam, Amsterdam, The Netherlands*

VLADIMIR G. FAST | *Department of Physiology, University of Bern, Bern, Switzerland*

CHAPTER CONTENTS

Basic Mechanisms of Cardiac Impulse Propagation
    The continuous cable
        Passive spread of current in a cable
        Impulse propagation in a cable
    Two-dimensional propagation and wavefront curvature
        Curved wavefronts and the "liminal area" concept
    Structural determinants of anisotropic and discontinuous conduction
    Propagation in discontinuous structures
        Wavefront propagation toward a resistive discontinuity and wavefront collision
        Wavefront dispersion and wavefront propagation from a high- to a low-impedance region
        Effects of periodically spaced resistive obstacles on propagation
        Interaction between active membrane properties and discontinuities in tissue architecture
    Discontinuous propagation in a cell chain and a cell strand
    Anisotropic propagation
        Macroscopic electrical anisotropy
        Anisotropic propagation in simulated and cultured cellular networks
    The electrical resistance of the extracellular space
    The bidomain behavior of cardiac tissue
        The virtual electrode effect
        The bidomain nature of myocardium and interaction with surrounding fluid
The Activation of the Whole Heart—From the Sinus Node to the Ventricles
    The sinus node—spread of excitation from the sinoatrial node to the atrium
    Atrial activation
    The atrioventricular junction
    Activation of the ventricles
Disturbances of Impulse Conduction and Conduction Block
    The safety factor of propagation
    Effects of changes in resting membrane potential and inhibition of Na^+ channels on conduction velocity
    Conduction slowing and block: the role of Ca^{++} inward current
    Conduction slowing and discontinuous conduction
        Cell-to-cell uncoupling
        Fiber branching
    Mechanisms of unidirectional block
        Tissue vulnerability: interference of local excitation or propagation with the refractory tail of the preceding wave
        Unidirectional block: dependence on tissue geometry
        Unidirectional block in anisotropic tissue: dependence on resistive tissue barriers and on the bidomain behavior
Circulating Excitation, Re-entry, and Spiral Waves
    Anatomic re-entry
    Functional re-entry—the leading circle concept
    Spiral wave re-entry
        Initiation of spiral waves
        Dynamics of spiral waves
        Spiral waves in anisotropic and microscopically discontinuous media
        Spiral waves in three dimensions
    Transition from functional to anatomic re-entry. Anchoring of spiral waves
        Anisotropic re-entry

AFTER INITIATION IN THE SINOATRIAL NODE, the cardiac electrical impulse spreads rapidly over the atria, the atrioventricular node, the specific ventricular conducting system, and both ventricles to produce synchronized excitation of the working myocardium. The basic biophysical properties underlying impulse propagation are common to nerve tissue, skeletal muscle, and cardiac muscle. These tissues can be considered reaction-diffusion systems that are able to generate a local regenerative reaction (action potential) in response to a suprathreshold current stimulus. The resulting voltage difference between the excited tissue and resting tissue drives local circuit currents that excite the resting tissue thereby supporting spread of excitation in a wavelike manner (see Fig. 12–1). The main factors governing propagation are (*1*) the properties of the ionic channels, (*2*) the "passive" electrical properties of the tissue, and for the case of two- or three-dimensional media, (*3*) the curvature of the excitation wave. In atrial myocardium, ventricular myocardium, and the specific ventricular conduction system, the

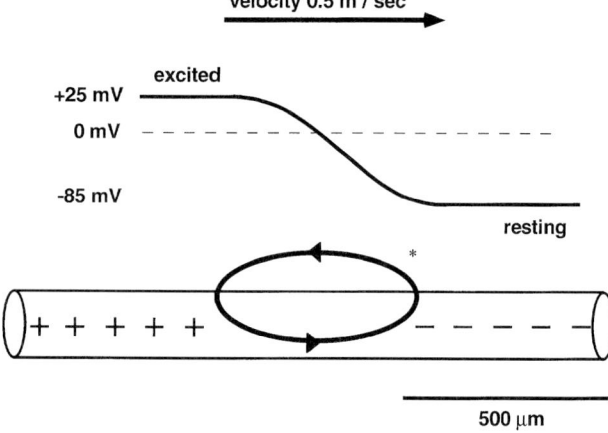

FIG. 12–1. Schematic presentation of electrical propagation. The scheme depicts an excitable cylindrical structure conducting the action potential from left to right at a velocity of 0.5 m/sec. The change in membrane potential along the axis of the cylinder corresponding to the action potential upstroke is plotted above the cylinder. The inside of the cylinder is negatively charged at its resting potential. The inside of the excited segment is charged positively. This potential difference drives the axial or local circuit current, as symbolized by the closed loop. The local circuit current depolarizes the membrane to the threshold for excitation at the site marked with an asterisk. In such a way a new segment of the membrane gets excited and excitation propagates from left to right.

main current responsible for the initial phase of the action potential and for delivering local current to propagation is carried by Na^+ ions. In the cells of the sinoatrial (SA) and atrioventricular (AV) node a major contribution is made by Ca^{2+} ions. In tissue with high degrees of electrical uncoupling or geometrical discontinuity flow of Ca^{2+} inward current becomes necessary to maintain propagation (2, 3). To analyze the participation of the various membrane ionic currents in the propagation process, computer simulations are necessary (3–9). In addition to the differences in distribution of ionic channels, the various regions of the heart differ with respect to the passive electrical properties, which depend on cell morphology, the type and distribution of gap junctions, and the arrangement of cells into strands and layers. As a result, the values of conduction velocity vary between approximately 0.05 m/sec, the lowest value found in the AV node, to approximately 3.5 m/sec, the highest value observed in the His/Purkinje system, as summarized in Table 12–1.

The first part of this chapter describes the basic mechanisms of propagation. Starting from the simple case of a linear conducting structure, the mechanism of passive electrical current flow and of impulse conduction is described. Subsequently, the effects of structural discontinuities and the anisotropic alignment of cells, which are typical for cardiac tissue, are discussed. In the second part, the process of cardiac excitation is

TABLE 12–1. *Conduction Velocity in Various Regions of the Heart*

Tissue	θ_L (m/sec)	θ_T (m/sec)	Source
Sinus node	0.03		Hariman et al. 1980 (159)
Bachmann's bundle	1.00		Horiba, 1963 (428)
	1.30		Wagner et al. 1966 (429)
	3.00	0.1	Goodman et al. 1971 (174)
	1.07		Spach et al. 1985 (430)
	1.44		Kirchhof et al. 1991 (431)
Average	1.56		
Crista terminalis	1.50		Horibe, 1961 (432)
	0.80	0.09	Hogan & Davis, 1971 (433)
	1.02		Goodman et al. 1971 (174)
	1.05		Spach et al. 1981 (93)
Average	1.09		
Atrial muscle	0.80		Brendel et al. 1950 (434)
	0.60		Yamada et al. 1965 (170)
	0.40		Wagner et al. 1966 (429)
	0.43		Hogan & Davis, 1971 (433)
	0.79		Goodman et al. 1971 (174)
	0.57		Frame et al. 1987 (435)
Average	0.60		
AV node	0.05		Hoffman & Cranefield, 1960 (258)
Purkinje fibers	2.00		Draper & Weidmann, 1951 (436)
	2.50		Trautwein et al. 1953 (437)
	3.50		Hoffman et al. 1959 (438)
	2.48		Draper & Mya-Tu, 1959 (439)
	2.01		Sakamoto & Goto, 1970 (425)
	1.95		Cranefield et al. 1971 (300)
	1.76		Rosen et al. 1981 (440)
	2.04		Pressler et al. 1982 (441)
Average	2.28		
Ventricular muscle	0.60	0.14	Sano et al. 1959 (442)
	0.48	0.16	Clerc, 1976 (90)
	0.58	0.25	Roberts et al. 1979 (105)
	0.50	0.17	Spach et al. 1981 (93)
	0.57	0.24	Roberts & Scher, 1982 (443)
	0.54	0.25	Spear et al. 1983 (444)
	0.55	0.25	Tsuboi et al. 1985 (445)
	0.50	0.21	Kléber et al. 1986 (287)
	0.60	0.19	Kadish et al. 1986 (103)
	0.56	0.24	Balke et al. 1988 (446)
	0.61	0.19	Kadish et al. 1988 (422)
	0.60	0.17	Quinteiro et al. 1990 (447)
	0.61	0.25	Boersma et al. 1991 (420)
Average	0.56	0.21	

Abbreviations: θ_L: longitudinal velocity; θ_T: transverse velocity.

followed from its initiation at the sinoatrial node to its extinction at the epicardial surface of the ventricles. The third part of this chapter treats the mechanisms that underlie the changes in cardiac propagation and the formation of conduction block The fourth and last part focuses on the biophysical laws underlying circulating excitation with re-entry, which is one of the key mechanisms of cardiac arrhythmias.

BASIC MECHANISMS OF CARDIAC IMPULSE PROPAGATION

The Continuous Cable

The "continuous electrical cable" represents a simple model relating ionic channel function and resistive tissue properties to propagation in excitable tissue. In this approach, resistive elements of the cytoplasm and the intercellular connections (gap junctions) are lumped together into a single intracellular resistive space forming an electrical continuum. The extracellular resistance is either added to the intracellular resistor or represented by a separate resistor.

Passive Spread of Current in a Cable. The passive electrical properties of the tissue, which determine its behavior during flow of *subthreshold current*, can be analyzed with the help of *linear cable theory* where the membrane resistor is taken as constant (Fig. 12-2) (10). Linear cable theory was originally introduced to biology to describe the spread of electrical current in nerve (11). It has also provided major information about the electrical interactions between cardiac cells. The application of linear cable theory to experiments in the specific ventricular conducting system and in ventricular muscle, together with experiments analyzing diffusion of $^{43}K^+$ (12), demonstrated that normal cells are coupled by low-resistance junctions (13, 14). If a subthreshold current pulse is applied to such a system intracellularly or extracellularly, the current will distribute along the cable according to the respective values of the transmembrane and intra- and extracellular resistors (Fig. 12-2). At steady state, the transmembrane voltage decays exponentially from a point P of current injection. The space constant of the voltage decay, λ, is a useful parameter to characterize electrotonic interaction between adjacent excitable structures. In a one-dimensional cable of infinite length, it is defined as the point where the membrane voltage is reduced to 1/e or 37% of the membrane voltage at the site of current injection.(10). Formally, $\lambda^2 = r_m/(r_o + r_i)$, whereby r_m corresponds to membrane resistance, r_o and r_i are the longitudinal resistances of the extra- and intracellular spaces, respectively. Given a value for

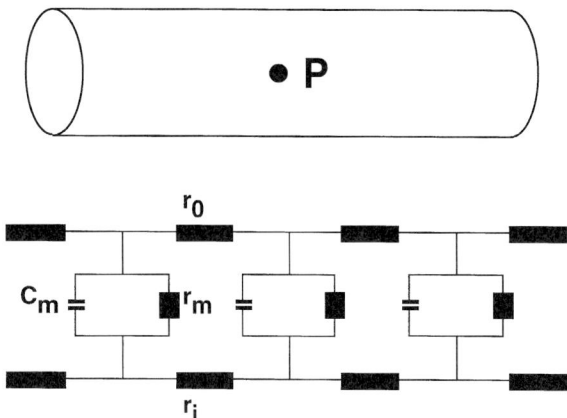

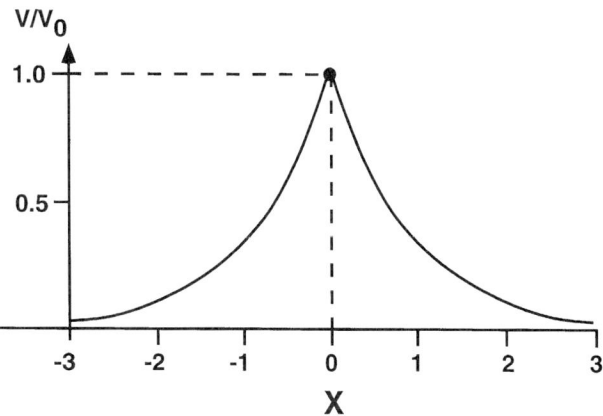

FIG. 12-2. Electrical cable. *Top:* Cylindrical structure of cell membrane enveloping the intracellular medium. Point P marks the site of current injection, as explained in bottom panel. *Middle:* Equivalent electrical circuit. The extra- and intracellular spaces are represented by the resistances r_o and r_i, respectively. The membrane is represented by a parallel circuit of membrane capacitance, c_m, and membrane resistance, r_m. *Bottom:* Decrease of relative membrane voltage, V/V_o, during injection of intracellular current in a cable of infinite length. The voltage drops exponentially from the site of current injection at point P (X = 0), from the initial value V_o. The distance on the abscissa is given in the relative unit X, which corresponds to the distance x scaled by the space constant λ (X = x/λ).

membrane resistance, λ will be a measure of both intracellular resistance and extracellular resistance in series and be affected by processes like electrical cell-to-cell uncoupling. While the decrease of electrotonic potential can be simulated by a simple exponential in a one-dimensional cable of infinite length, the decay of electrotonic potential is more complex in linear cables with sealed or open ends, and in two- and three-dimensional structures (10, 13). With circular (two-dimensional) or spherical (three-dimensional) point injection of electrotonic current, the decay of electrotonic potential at steady state follows a zero-order Bessels function and an Error function, respectively (10). Although the space constant of electrotonic decay is not formally defined for these functions, the same definition of λ has been applied to determine λ in two-dimensional tissue, such as atrium (15), cell cultures (16), and simulated layers of excitable elements (4). In cardiac Purkinje fibers, point injection of current led to a biphasic decrease of transmembrane voltage. This suggested that the spread of electrotonic current was spherical close to the injection site and parallel to the fiber at remote sites (17). Values for λ in heart have been reported to vary from about 0.15 mm to 2.2 mm (Table 12–2), indicating that the constant of electrotonic interaction exceeds the average length of a single cell. Linear cable theory predicts values for intracellular resistivities to be 150–500 Ωcm (Table 12–2) which are several times higher than the specific resistance of normal iso-osmotic extracellular solution (51–71 Ωcm) (14, 18). These relatively high values indicate that the resistivity of the cytoplasm is higher than that of normal intra- or extracellular electrolyte solution, and that normal intercellular connections (gap junctions) form resistive obstacles during propagation.

Impulse Propagation in a Cable. To analyze propagation of the action potential in cardiac muscle, the linear cable model shown in Figure 12–2 is modified by replacing the fixed membrane resistor with a variable resistor (Fig. 12–3). The voltage- and time-dependent values of this resistor are selected to simulate current flow through specific ionic channels (I_{ion}). In ventricular muscle, I_{ion} during the upstroke is dominated by the rapid inward sodium current. In addition to I_{ion}, changes in V_M during propagation are dependent on the flow of axial current, I_A. The change in axial current equals the current flowing into or from the membrane, I_M. In the early phase of the action potential, i.e. before Na$^+$ channels are activated, a fraction of the axial current flows into the membrane (positive I_M) and brings V_M to threshold. Subsequently, I_{ion} becomes activated. In this later phase, I_{ion} (i) flows into the membrane capacitance to change V_M and (ii) contributes to further flow of axial current. This contribution causes the transmembrane current, I_M to change direction. In such a way, new axial current is generated which will, in turn, excite the next segment of the cable. The relation between flow of depolarizing inward current and dV/dt_{max} during impulse propagation is different from the situation where tissue is uniformly excited ("space clamped" action potential). In tissue with uniform voltage distribution, electrotonic axial current

TABLE 12–2. *Space Constants and Resistivities of the Intracellular Space in Cardiac Tissues*

Experiment	λ (μm)*	Ri (Ωcm)	Source (Reference)
Rabbit SA node	465	—	Bonke, 1973 (423)
Rabbit crista terminalis	1000	—	Bonke, 1973 (424)
Rabbit atrial trabeculae	650	—	Bonke, 1973 (424)
Rat atrium	130	—	Woodbury & Crill, 1961 (15)
Dog atrium	1240	—	Sakamoto & Goto, 1970 (425)
Rabbit AV node (AN-layer)	400	—	Baukauskas & Veteikis, 1977 (238)
Rabbit AV node (N-layer)	223	—	Baukauskas & Veteikis, 1977 (238)
Rabbit AV node (NH-layer)	621	—	Baukauskas & Veteikis, 1977 (238)
Rabbit AV node (N-layer)	430	—	De Mello, 1977(239)
Rabbit AV node (entire node)	692	—	Kokubun et al., 1982(241)
Sheep Purkinje fiber	1940	154	Weidmann, 1952(13)
Sheep Purkinje fiber (resting)	2120	298	Pressler, 1984(17)
Sheep Purkinje fiber (paced)	1410	214	Pressler, 1984(17)
Rabbit ventricle	300–600	—	Tille, 1966(426)
Sheep ventricle	960	470	Weidmann, 1970(14)
Rat heart (tissue culture)	362	502	Jongsma & van Rijn, 1972(16)
Guinea pig ventricle	580	250	Daut, 1982(427)
Arterially perfused rabbit papillary muscle	357	166	Kléber & Riegger, 1986(32)

λ = space constant of voltage decay.

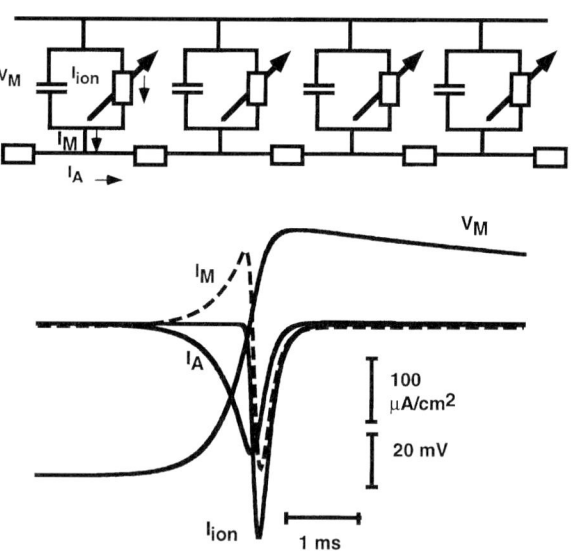

FIG. 12–3. Relation between the change in transmembrane potential, V_M, flow of ionic current, I_{ion}, flow of membrane current, I_M, and axial or local circuit current, I_A, in a continuous linear structure. The cell membrane is symbolized by a parallel circuit consisting of a capacitance and a changing resistance corresponding to a time- and voltage-dependent ionic conductance. The cell interior is symbolized by an internal resistance. Simulation using the Luo-Rudy model (7). Note that there is *axial or local circuit* current flow during the early phase of the action potential, which provides the transmembrane current for excitation, I_M. Once the threshold is reached and Na$^+$ channels are activated, the Na$^+$ inward current contributes to axial current (see text).

is zero, and consequently the current flowing through membrane channels is used to change the charge on the membrane capacitance, C. As a result, the maximal upstroke velocity dV/dt_{max} of the action potential is a direct measure for the maximal depolarizing inward current, I ($I = C \times dV/dt_{max}$) (19). In a continuous model of a propagation, the relation between dV/dt_{max} and maximal ionic current flow is no longer preserved, and maximal flow of I_{Na} occurs late in the action potential, after the time of dV/dt_{max} (20). Nevertheless, the changes in dV/dt_{max} can still be taken as an indirect parameter for changes in ionic current flow (21). The theory of impulse propagation in a *continuous* electrical medium states that changes in ionic depolarizing current flow and changes in r_o or r_i have independent effects on propagation velocity, θ. Formally, θ is proportional to the square root of the maximal upstroke velocity, dV/dt_{max}, and independently, inversely proportional to the square root of $(r_o + r_i)$ (21–23):

$$\theta^2 \sim \frac{dV}{dt_{max}} \text{ and } \theta^2 \sim \frac{1}{(r_o + r_i)}$$

It is evident from structural studies (24, 25) and from computer simulations of propagation in discontinuous structures (26–29) that representation of cardiac tissue by a continuous intracellular space is an oversimplification. Nevertheless, the application of linear cable theory to experimental results has proven useful to assess the effects of Na$^+$ channel blockers (30) and changes in the extra- and intracellular resistance on macroscopic propagation in pathophysiological settings (18, 31–33). However, the application of this theory is limited to electrically well-coupled cellular networks with a small amount of connective tissue—e.g. papillary muscles—and to the process of propagation along the main axis of cardiac strands. During the process of electrical cell-to-cell uncoupling or during transverse conduction, when the discontinuous nature of cardiac tissue becomes more prominent, application of the continuous cable model is not valid.

Two-Dimensional Propagation and Wavefront Curvature

Analysis of the mechanisms of propagation in two- and three-dimensional tissue has shown that in addition to the passive and active properties of the excitable medium, a third factor—the geometry of the excitation wavefront—may modulate propagation velocity (34–38). Wavefront curvature may be crucial for centrifugal propagation of a wave from the site of a point stimulus, for the formation of conduction block, and for defining the period and the dynamic behavior of spiral waves, which are responsible for some types of cardiac arrhythmias, as explained in the fourth part of this chapter.

The basic mechanism relating wavefront curvature to velocity of propagation, θ, in an excitable medium is illustrated in Figure 12–4. In the case of a flat wavefront (panel A), conduction velocity is equal to the steady-state velocity in a one-dimensional strand (θ_0). As previously mentioned, the steady-state velocity, θ_0, is solely determined by the passive and active properties of excitable tissue (10, 21). When the excitation front is curving outward (convex) the conduction velocity is lower than θ_0. This is so because the local excitatory current supplied by the cells at the front of a convex wave distributes over a larger membrane area downstream. An opposite process takes place when the excitation front is curving inward (concave). In this case, excitatory current converges in the front of the propagating wave, producing a more rapid membrane depolarization. As a result, conduction velocity of a concave wavefront is larger than θ_0. The degree of wavefront bending is characterized by the local curvature, ρ, which can be defined as the negative reciprocal of the local radius of curvature, r:

$$\rho = \frac{-1}{r}$$

A quantitative description of the dependence of conduction velocity on curvature in a continuous isotropic two-dimensional excitable medium can be obtained analytically for small values of r. It was shown (36) that in such conditions the velocity, θ, is given by the following equation:

$$\theta = \theta_0 + D\rho$$

The coefficient D is determined by the passive properties of the medium. For a continuous isotropic model

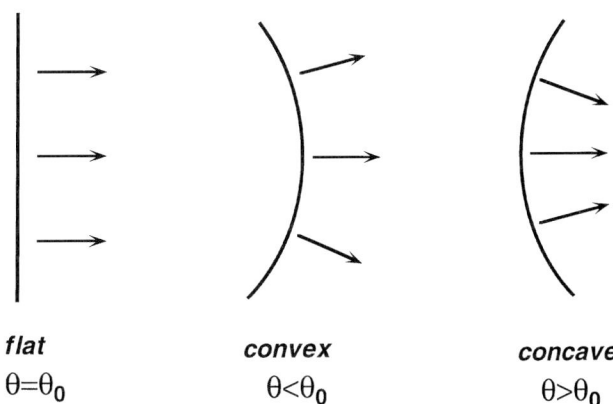

flat   *convex*   *concave*
$\theta = \theta_0$ $\theta < \theta_0$ $\theta > \theta_0$

FIG. 12–4. Schematic presentation of the effect of wavefront curvature on conduction. *Left:* A flat wavefront propagates at a basic velocity θ_0. Arrows denote direction of flow of local circuit current. *Middle:* Convex wavefront with dispersion of local current, resulting velocity θ is smaller than θ_0. *Right:* Concave wavefront with conversion of local current, resulting velocity θ is larger than θ_0.

representing the electrical structure of cardiac muscle, D is equal to $1/C_m S_v R_i$ where C_m is the specific membrane capacitance, S_v is the cell surface-to-volume ratio, and R_i is the intracellular resistivity. Direct experimental evidence that wavefront curvature affects propagation of waves initiated from small stimulating electrodes was recently obtained by Knisley and Hill (39). They investigated impulse conduction in two-dimensional strips of epicardial tissue stimulated either by a bipolar electrode or by a linear array of bipolar electrodes as shown on Figure 12–5. Optical mapping of activation spread with a laser scanning technique demonstrated that stimulation with a single electrode resulted in elliptical excitation spread, while stimulation with the linear array produced a nearly flat activation front. As a result of the increased wavefront curvature, the velocity of the elliptical propagation was significantly smaller than the velocity of the flat wavefront. The dispersion of local current at the head of the longitudinal wavefront during elliptical spread is also reflected by a decrease in the maximal upstroke velocity of the transmembrane action potential (dV/dt_{max}) with respect to planar propagation (see below).

Curved Wavefronts and the "Liminal Area" Concept.

The inability of excitable tissue to support propagation of waves with a very high curvature suggests that, during spread of excitation from a focus, a critical amount of cells encompassed within the nucleus of excitation with a critical radius r_c must be excited to get a propagated response. A similar requirement has long been recognized and formulated in the concept of "liminal length" for one-dimensional excitable strands (10, 40–42). The "liminal length" was defined as the length of an excited strand segment necessary to produce the local current required for a propagated response. Accordingly, in two-dimensional tissue this critical amount of cells is characterized by a "liminal area" (43). The liminal area was calculated in a 2-dimensional computer model by Ramza et al. (44), who studied impulse initiation produced by a point current injection in a continuous, isotropic model described by the Beeler-Reuter (5) ionic kinetics. The liminal area necessary to generate sufficient inward current during stimulation was determined as a function of the maximal sodium conductance (g_{Namax}). At a level of excitability estimated to correspond to the adult ventricular myocardium, the radius of the liminal area was 200–250 μm. Experimentally, the liminal area was estimated from measurements of stimulation threshold as a function of electrode size by Lindemans and co-workers (Fig. 12–6); (43, 45). Stimulation current was applied to canine epicardium via disk electrodes with radii varying between 0.01 to 9 mm. It was found that the current threshold was independent of the electrode size when the disk radius was less than 0.2 mm and was proportional to the electrode radius to the power 1.5 when the radius was larger than 0.4 mm. Such a behavior was explained by the fact that, with small electrodes, all current passed through the liminal area and, therefore, the current density at the edge of the liminal area was independent of electrode size. With

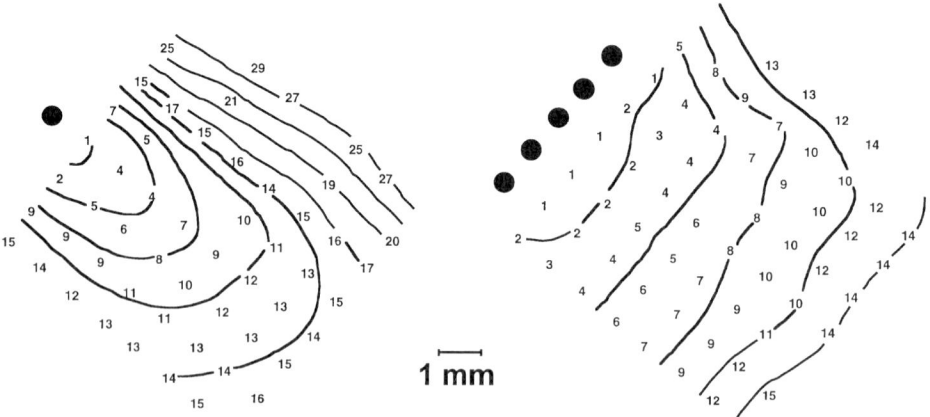

FIG. 12–5. Effect of point stimulation (*left panel*) versus linear stimulation (*right panel*) on activation spread. Stimulation with a single electrode (point stimulation) produces a convex excitation front. Stimulation with a line of electrodes (line stimulation) produces an almost flat excitation front. Numbers denote activation times in milliseconds relative to the earliest activation. The interval between isochrones is 3 msec. Average longitudinal velocity of curved wave is 13% lower than of flat wave. [Reproduced from reference 39 with permission.]

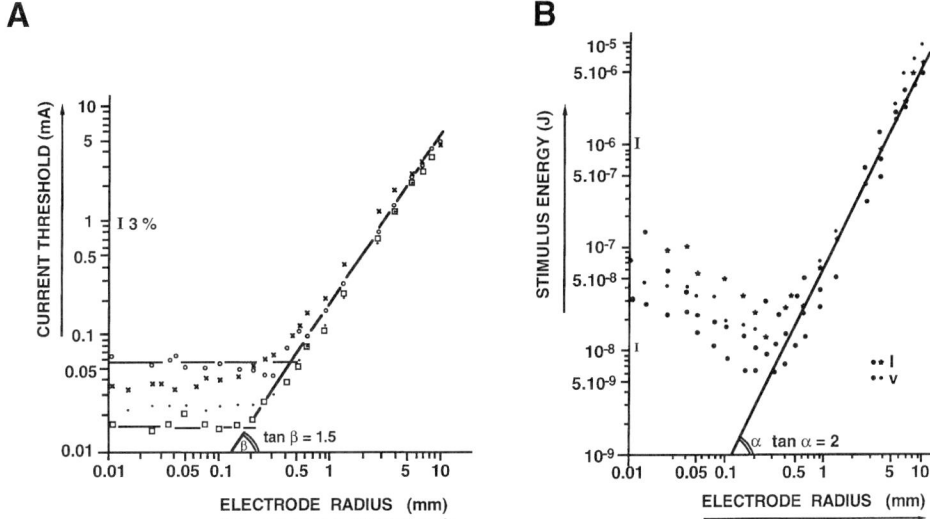

FIG. 12-6. Effect of the radius of a circular stimulation electrode on current threshold (*panel A*) and stimulus energy (*panel B*): Epicardial stimulation of the canine heart. At an electrode size below 0.1–0.4 mm, the current threshold is independent of electrode size; above this radius, which corresponds approximately to the radius of the liminal area, current threshold increases with increasing electrode size. The stimulus energy is lowest at the electrode radius which corresponds to the radius of the liminal area. [Reproduced from references 43 and 45 with permission.]

large electrodes, more current had to be provided to maintain a constant stimulatory current density as the electrode surface area increased. From these measurements, the radius of the liminal area was found to be approximately 0.3 mm, i.e. close to the value given above. As pointed out by Lindemans and Zimmerman (45) and by Winfree (46), the dependence of the excitation threshold on the electrode diameter is also of practical importance, because an electrode of the size corresponding to the liminal area requires the lowest stimulation energy.

Structural Determinants of Anisotropic and Discontinuous Conduction

The anisotropic and discontinuous architecture of the heart is important for our understanding of both normal propagation and the activation pattern in certain forms of re-entrant arrhythmias. Structural anisotropy and discontinuity may occur at different levels. Figure 12-7 shows an isolated single cell forming the basic element of the anisotropic cardiac structure. In canine ventricular tissue, cells have an elongated form with an average length of 122 μm and an average width of 23 μm (47, 48). Comparison of individual cells among species and different regions of the heart shows a relatively large variability in size with a consistent length to width ratio (34, 48). In addition to cell shape, anisotropy is further determined by the connectivity (number of cells connected to an individual myocyte) and the arrangement and density of intercellular connections. Different connectivities between cells in two different cardiac regions and in tissue healed from infarction are given in Table 12-3. While normal ventricular cells show a relatively high degree of connectivity and lateral coupling, regions such as atrial crista terminalis exhibit a marked end-to-end connectivity with sparse lateral coupling (48–50). This difference in microscopic structure is reflected in different degrees of functional anisotropy (see below).

In addition to the pattern of intercellular connections, different regions of the heart express different connexins (Table 12-4). Although the cardiac connexins have been well characterized with respect to their individual electrical properties and ion selectivity, the contribution of the individual connexins to the propagation process, and especially the reason for co-expression and co-localization of connexins in cardiac tissue, is not well understood (50, 51). Connexin43 (Cx43) is the most abundant protein in heart and in many other organs. Expression of Cx43 seems to be mostly restricted to ventricle, atrium and the specific ventricular conducting system (51–56). The presence of Cx43 is disputed in the sinoatrial node and in the atrioventricular node. In most species, except for rabbit and hamster (57, 58), it has not been detected in the node (51, 54, 55). As discussed by Opthof, some of these discrepancies might be related to technical difficulties involved in connexin detection in nodal tissues (59). Moreover, gap junction distribution appears to be

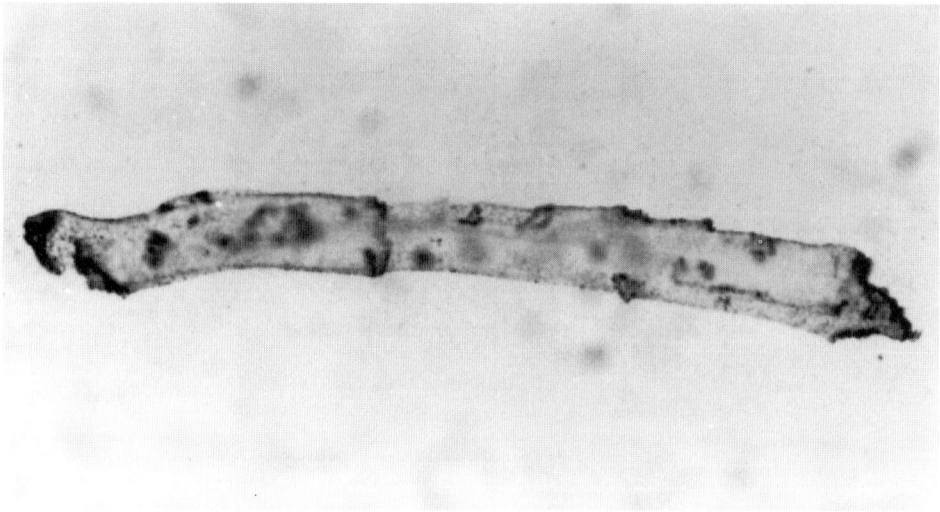

FIG. 12–7. Isolated myocyte: Micrograph of immunostained, paraformaldehyde-fixed disaggregated canine myocyte. Immunostaining of connexin43 reveals a pattern that conforms precisely to the distribution of intercellular gap junctions. [Reproduced from reference 49 with permission.]

inhomogeneous in the SA node. A recent analysis of gap junction expression in cells of the canine SA node has shown that approximately 55% of SA cells expressed only Cx40, while 30%–35% expressed the three connexins, Cx40, Cx45, and Cx43, the latter cells being arranged into strands that were confined to the border adjacent to the atrium (60). Expression of connexin45 appears to occur in most myocytes (61). Connexin40, which has a high single-channel conductance, is most abundantly expressed in tissue with high propagation velocities (His-Purkinje system, atrial bundles), but it is also found in nodal tissue (48, 51, 53, 61–63). While adult myocardial tissue exhibits a discrete distribution of gap junctions along the cell perimeter with relatively small junctions along the lateral borders and larger junctions at the cell poles (48, 64), neonatal tissue in culture (34) and in vivo (53) and remodeled tissue in peri-infarction areas (65) show a more regularly distributed alignment of gap junctions of about equal size. Remodeling of gap junctions also occurs in early and later stages of ventricular hypertrophy (66) and can be induced within relative short time periods in culture by cyclic adenosine monophosphate (cAMP), a mediator of left ventricular hypertrophy (67) and mechanical stretch (68).

The arrangement of the elongated cells to form compact tissue involves various levels of structural discontinuity. A first step consists in the formation of small cell bundles with narrow interstitial clefts. These bundles are organized within fascicles and separated by larger spaces containing the microvasculature and connective tissue (24). Several fascicles together may form distinct muscle sheets or bundles in which the individual fibers are arranged in parallel (24). A recent morphometric analysis of canine ventricular tissue has revealed a laminar structure that is prominent in the mid-intramural layers (Fig. 12–8; 25). Stacks of rotating connective lamina appear to separate fiber layers comprising an average number of 4.5 cells in width. The cell layers formed in such a way are interconnected

TABLE 12–3. *Connectivity of Cells in Cardiac Tissue*

		Left Ventricle	Crista Terminalis	Infarct Border Zones
I		3.3 ± 1.5 (29)	0.8 ± 0.5 (12)	0.6 ± 0.6 (9)
II		2.0 ± 0.8 (18)	0.7 ± 0.7 (11)	1.9 ± 1.4 (29)
III		2.1 ± 1.0 (19)	1.1 ± 0.7 (17)	1.2 ± 0.8 (19)
IV		3.9 ± 1.1 (34)	3.8 ± 1.1 (60)	2.8 ± 0.8 (43)
Total cells connected to each myocyte		11.3 ± 2.2 CELLS	6.4 ± 1.7 CELLS	6.5 CELLS

Reproduced from references 48 and 49 with permission.

TABLE 12–4. *Structural and Molecular Features of Canine Cardiac Gap Junctions*

Cardiac Tissue	Gap Junction Structure		Connexin Phenotype		
	Size	Number	Cx40	Cx43	Cx45
Sinus node	Small	Few	Scant	Absent	Scant
AV node and proximal bundle branches	Small	Few	Scant	Absent	Scant
Distal His bundle and proximal bundle branches	Large	Moderate	Abundant	Abundant	Moderate
Right atrium	Large	Many	Abundant	Abundant	Moderate
Ventricle	Moderate	Many	Scant	Abundant	Moderate

Reproduced from reference 51 with permission.

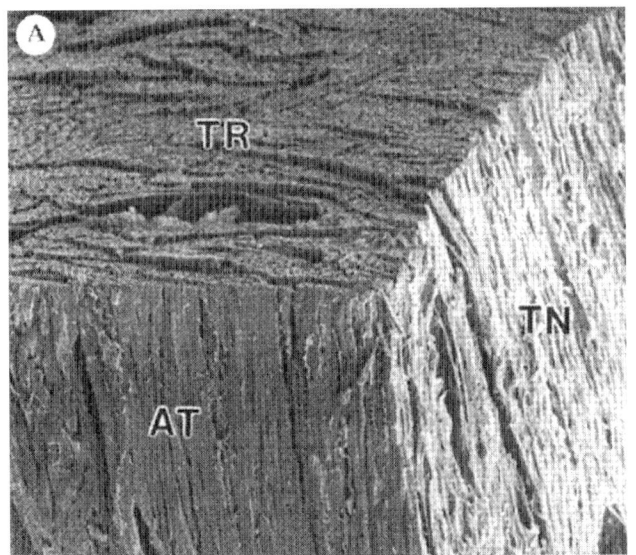

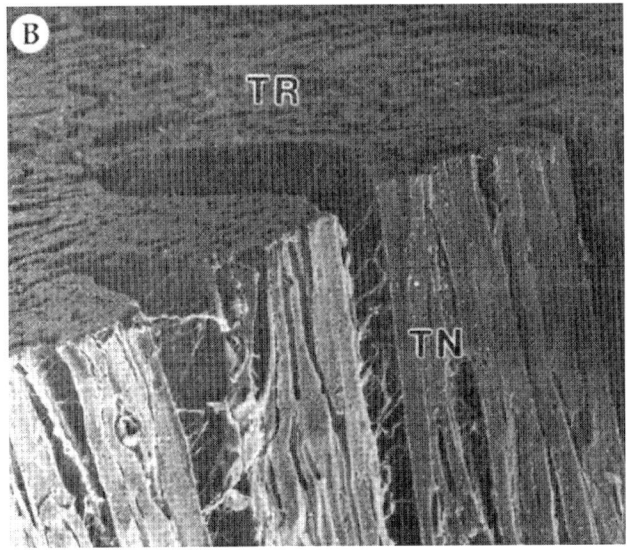

FIG. 12–8. Laminar organization of ventricular myocardium. Micrographs of tangential surface of a ventricular specimen showing layered organization of myocytes, branching of layers (*arrow*) and collagen fibers between adjacent sheets. [Reproduced from reference 25 with permission.]

approximately every 1–2 mm by smaller cell bridges. The relation between the cellular and the connective tissue matrix is known to undergo changes with age, hypertrophy, and infarction. In all these conditions, the specific effects of remodeling on the propagation of the electrical impulse need to be considered specifically. In conclusion, relating cardiac structure to function involves consideration of both a macroscopic *order* defined by fibers, bundles, and fascicles, and microscopic *variability* of individual cells shapes and cell-to-cell connections. As discussed below, propagation through anisotropic tissue is determined by the interactions between these various levels of structural complexity.

Propagation in Discontinuous Structures

The subsequent paragraphs describe the influence of gap junctions, tissue anisotropy and macroscopic tissue discontinuities on the cardiac propagation process. Although each of these structural elements specifically affects impulse propagation and action potential shapes, the underlying biophysical events, although they occur at different spatial and temporal scales, are very similar to each other. The discussion in the following paragraph is intended to facilitate subsequent detailed discussion of findings in experimental and simulation studies.

Wavefront Propagation Toward a Resistive Discontinuity and Wavefront Collision. If subthreshold current is injected into a cable close to a sealed end at a site x, the electrical charge at that site will be prevented from flowing across the seal and will accumulate locally in the membrane capacitance. Formally, this is equivalent to "reflection" of the electrotonic current at the sealed end. The reflected current will affect the amount and time course of the change in membrane potential at the site (4, 10, 13). Analogous to the effect of injected subthreshold current, the electrotonic current generated by a *propagating wavefront* and reflected by an obstacle is expected to affect (i) the velocity, (ii) the action potential shape, and (iii) the amplitude and time course of activated ionic currents. The reflection can be total or partial. Partial reflection occurs with a local increase in tissue impedance or with a decreasing diameter.

Very similar events take place at a site of collision of two wavefronts. In this situation, accumulation of electrotonic current does not originate from reflection, but from the opposite wavefront approaching the collision site. Figure 12–9 shows results from a simulation of a cardiac excitation wave approaching the sealed end of a cable or colliding with a second wavefront of opposite velocity (20). At the collision site, there is a shape change of the action potential with a twofold increase of dV/dt_{max} during steady-state propagation. The concomitant maximal flow of inward Na^+ current and the total inward charge flow is decreased. This increase is explained by the rapid and large flow of electrotonic current into the local membrane capacitance. With respect to steady-state propagation, the electrotonic current will depolarize the membrane more rapidly and thereby decrease the electrochemical driving force for Na^+ current, and consequently, Na^+ current flow. As a consequence, the *increase* in the upstroke velocity can be associated with a *decrease* in local depolarizing ionic current and is inverse to the relationship between dV/dt_{max} and inward Na^+ current in a continuous cable. In addition to the changes illustrated in Figure 12–9, the tissue before a sealed end or a collision site gets activated more rapidly. This and results analogous to those shown in Figure 12–9 have been published in the reports of several studies (4, 26, 69). While wavefronts colliding or approaching a sealed end lead to identical local changes in transmembrane potential and Na^+ inward current, the shapes of the extracellular unipolar electrograms during wavefront collision differ from the shapes occurring with wavefront extinction at a sealed end (20, 70).

Wavefront Dispersion and Wavefront Propagation from a High- to a Low-Impedance Region. If a wavefront propagates through a transition between a region of high internal resistance to a region with low internal resistance or—in analogy-across a site with an increase in the diameter of the excitable medium, there is a mismatch between the local current supplied by the wavefront and the load ahead of the wavefront (69, 71–73). In either case, less local current is flowing into a unit membrane area downstream than during steady-state propagation. The consequences of this mismatch for the change in conduction velocity, dV/dt_{max}, and Na^+ inward current flow are shown from a study simulating impulse transmission at an abrupt geometrical expansion of tissue (Fig. 12–10). A transient decrease in conduction velocity is associated with a decrease in local

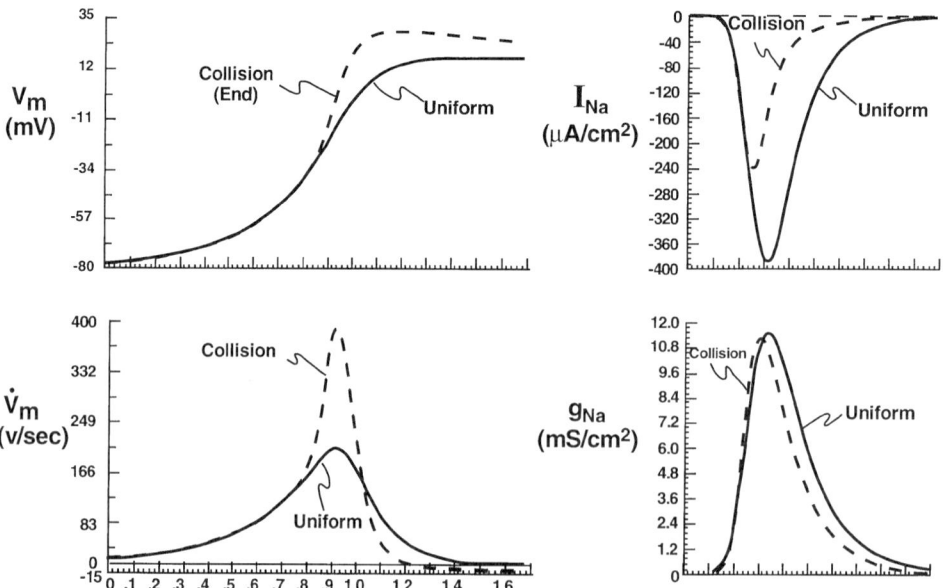

FIG. 12–9. Simulation of the effect of wavefront collision on the upstroke of the transmembrane action potential and the Na^+ inward current. The values computed during uniform conduction (*solid lines*) are compared to the values computed at a collision site (*dashed lines*). *Left top*: Change of membrane potential, V_M, during action potential upstroke. *Left bottom*: maximal upstroke velocity of transmembrane action potential in Volts/sec. *Right top*: Na^+ inward current, I_{Na}. *Right bottom*: time course of Na^+ conductance, g_{Na}. [Reproduced from reference 20 with permission.]

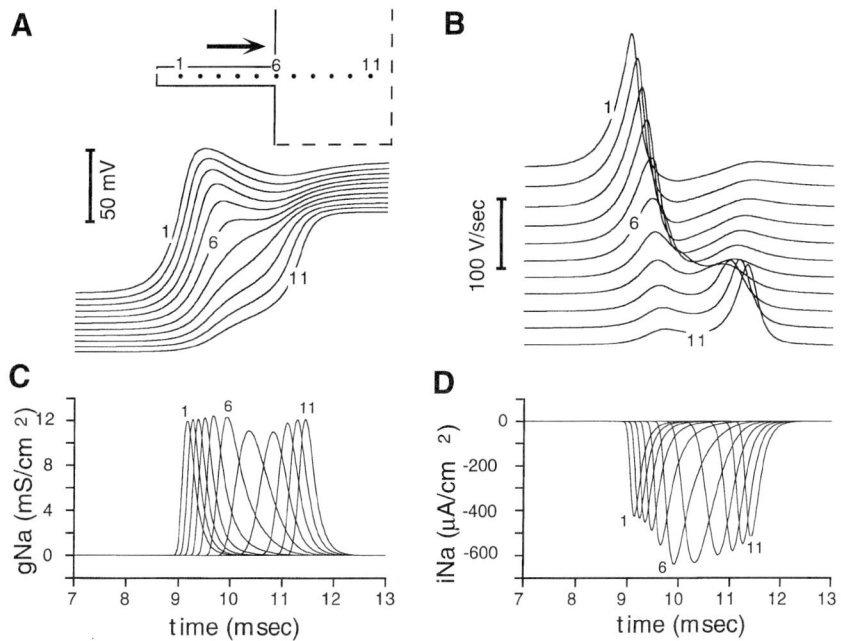

FIG. 12-10. Simulation of the effect of wavefront dispersion on the upstroke of the transmembrane action potential and the Na$^+$ inward current. A: Inset shows simulated two-dimensional strand of excitable tissue emerging into a large area. Signals on panels A–D are simulated from sites 1–11 shown on the inset. Action potential upstrokes show a double component, which is most prominent at the expansion site. B: First time derivatives dV/dt from action potential upstrokes shown on panel A. C: Time course of Na$^+$ conductance, g_{Na}. D: Time course of Na$^+$ inward current, I_{Na}. Note increase of I_{Na} at expansion site, associated with a decrease of dV/dt$_{max}$. [Reproduced from reference 72 with permission.]

dV/dt$_{max}$ *below the steady-state value*, and an increase in the amount of locally activated inward Na$^+$ current. This corresponds to the inverse situation shown in Figure 12–9. It is explained by the fact that the relatively large amount of electrotonic current flowing from the site of current-to-load mismatch downstream decreases the portion of electrotonic current flowing into the local membrane capacitance. In this case, there is no interference with local activation of Na$^+$ inward current, and this current can fully activate.

Effects of Periodically Spaced Resistive Obstacles on Propagation. Although some of the important features of discontinuous conduction can be explained by the two basic mechanisms just discussed, the consequences of periodically spaced resistive obstacles on local propagation delays, dV/dt$_{max}$ and ionic current flow, are more complex. This was elegantly shown in a study by Joyner in 1982 (69). In this computer simulation, membrane elements were joined by resistors to represent a linear discontinuous cable. Within this cable a variable number, N, of elements, linked by a resistor of low and constant value, were periodically separated by a resistor R$_i'$ of higher value (Fig. 12–11). This arrangement allowed change in the degree of discontinuity independent of the effective or overall longitudinal resistance. For the same value of effective longitudinal resistance, a low degree of discontinuity was defined as a relatively low R$_i'$ combined with a small N, a high degree of discontinuity was defined as a high R$_i'$ combined with a large N. Figure 12–11 shows that increasing the degree of discontinuity (lower panel A to C) decreased conduction velocity (θ), as demonstrated by the increase in the delay between the two action potential upstrokes. Importantly, the relationship between the change in conduction velocity dV/dt$_{max}$, and effective longitudinal resistance was more complex than predicted by simple additive effects of single resistive obstacles. This is because, at appropriate spacing, the events occurring at a given resistive barrier were affected by the neighboring barriers. This is shown in Figure 12–12, which depicts the changes in Θ as a function of effective or total longitudinal resistance (R$_i$). In the case of a relatively low degree of discontinuity (upper curve A, low value of R$_i'$), decreasing the number of elements between the resistors R$_i'$ was associated with an increase of the effective or overall resistance R$_i$, and concomitantly, with a decrease in velocity. This decrease was qualitatively similar to the decrease of conduction velocity in a continuous cable

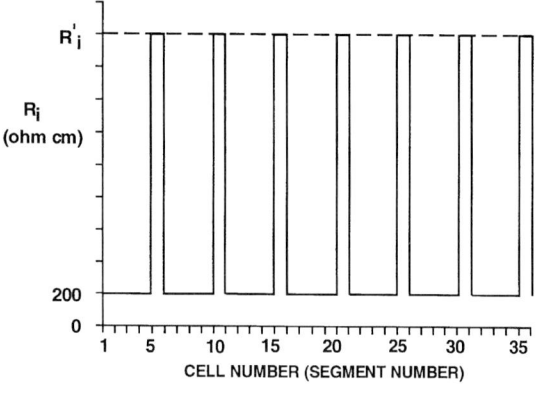

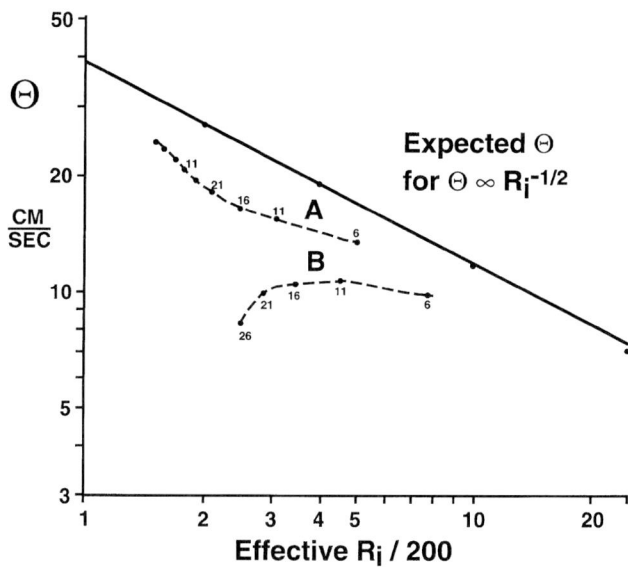

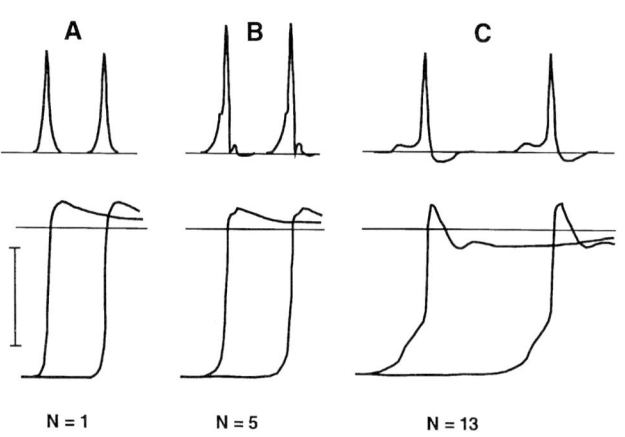

FIG. 12–11. Effects of resistive discontinuities on propagation. *Top:* A row of simulated excitable elements (abscissa denotes element number) is separated by resistors. A number N of elements is connected by resistors of low value (200 Ω cm). Each group of N elements is connected to the next group by a single resistor, R'_i, of high value. Discontinuity at a constant value of effective longitudinal resistance can be changed by the simultaneous increase of N and R'_i. *Bottom:* Propagation along the simulated row of excitable elements, as illustrated by the time course of dV/dt_{max} (*upper trace*) and the action potential upstroke (*lower trace*). The degree of discontinuity is increased from panel A to C, while the value of effective or total longitudinal resistance is kept constant. Note increasing delay between the two action potential upstrokes, and the discontinuous upstroke in C. [Reproduced from reference 69 with permission.]

FIG. 12–12. Effects of resistive discontinuities on conduction velocity, θ. Propagation velocity is simulated in the model shown in the upper panel of Figure 12–11 as a function of the overall or effective resistance R_i (expressed as a fraction of the low value resistance of 200 Ωcm shown in Fig. 12–11, $R_i/200$) The *solid line* depicts the decrease of θ in a continuous cable where $θ^2 \sim R_i$. In *curve A*, the value for the high resistor, R'_i, is 5000 Ωcm, the numbers on the curve denote the number of elements N. In *curve B*, the degree of discontinuity is higher, because R'_i is 10,000 Ωcm. Note that in curve B, θ decreases above N = 16 and conduction block occurs when N >26 (see text). [Reproduced from reference 69 with permission.]

("inverse square root relationship," corresponding to the straight line in Fig. 12–12). In this case, there was minor interaction between sequential resistive barriers, and decreasing N simply increased the number of high resistors for a given segment length and therefore the number of local delays per unit length. This situation is basically different for curve B, depicting the situation where the value of the high resistor R'_i was doubled with respect to curve A. Curve B shows that conduction velocity *decreased* with increase in the number of elements, and eventually got blocked. In this seemingly paradoxical situation, block occurred at a low value of overall resistance R_i, and conduction, albeit slow, was preserved at higher values of R_i. It was explained by the fact that the resistor R'_i was so high that the current driven through by the excitation wavefront did not suffice to excite the elements after the obstacle if the load was too high (large N). If the next resistive obstacle was brought nearer (decrease in N), then the impedance load decreased and the current flowing through R'_i was confined to excite a smaller number of patches. In other words, the fact that the resistive obstacles were placed nearer to each other prevented formation of conduction block (71).

The changes in the maximal upstroke velocity, dV/dt_{max}, in the case of repetitive high resistive obstacles taken from the same study (69) are shown in Figure 12–13. In these simulations, the value of the high resistance R'_i was kept constant and N was varied. For comparison, the value for dV/dt_{max} was plotted for propagation in a continuous cable for the cases of either a high or a low uniform resistance (cf. Fig. 12–11). With a large N (corresponding to a long segment length between the high resistors) there was no interaction between the two resistive obstacles, and consequently dV/dt_{max} decreased after and increased before the ob-

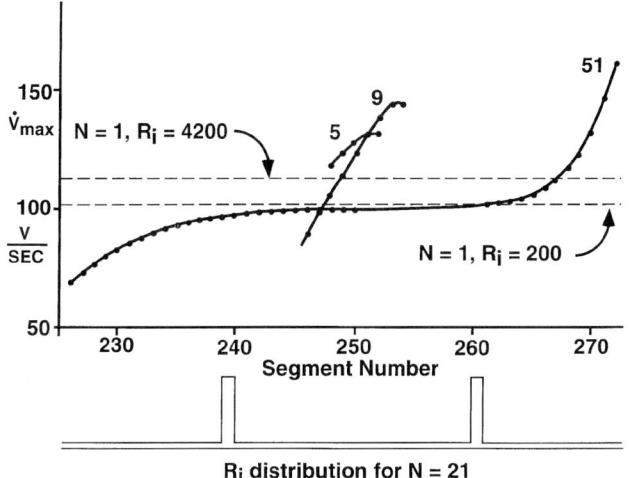

FIG. 12–13. Effects of resistive discontinuities on the maximal upstroke velocity of the transmembrane action potential, dV/dt_{max} (simulated in the model shown in the upper panel of Fig. 12–11). As a control, the dashed lines depict the dV/dt_{max} values for continuous cables (*upper line* $R_i = 200$ Ωcm, lower line $R_i = 4200$ Ωcm). In all solid curves shown, the value of the high resistor is set to $R'_i = 4200$ Ωcm, and the curves differ with respect to their numbers of elements N. The curves are shown for N = 5, N = 9, and N = 51. With N = 51, there is dispersion of local current beyond the first resistive obstacle with a decrease of dV/dt_{max}, and collision before the next resistive obstacle (from N 40 to 51) with an increase in dV/dt_{max}. With a small number of N (5), the effect of dispersion and collision is minor and all of the dV/dt_{max} values are above the upper dashed line. This is due to the almost simultaneous excitation of all elements, similar to the situation of a space-clamped action potential. N = 9 corresponds to an intermediate situation. [Reproduced from reference 69 with permission.]

stacles, as expected from the mechanisms explained for a single discontinuity (cf. Figs. 12–9 and 12–10). With a very short segment length, however, the average dV/dt_{max} was always higher than *both* steady-state values. This was explained by an almost simultaneous, isopotential excitation of the patches in the whole segment, with minimal electrotonic charge exchange between the elements of a given segment. In this case, the conduction delays were confined to the high resistance region. For heart tissue, this situation, which may occur with high degrees of resistive or geometrical discontinuity, has been termed "saltatory conduction" by Spach et al. (74). A similar result was obtained in a simulation study by Henriquez and Plonsey (75).

Interaction Between Active Membrane Properties and Discontinuities in Tissue Architecture. The discussion of the effects of resistive barriers or sites of current-to-load mismatch on the shape of the action potential upstroke and flow of sodium inward current (cf. Figs. 12–9 and 12–10) has shown that discontinuities in tissue architecture affect the amount of local inward current flow. This interaction is not only confined to inward Na^+ current; tissue discontinuities may also determine the type of depolarizing ionic current involved in conduction and modify the driving force for propagation. This was shown in a computer simulation of propagation in a cell chain (see later under Cell-to-Cell Uncoupling; Fig. 12–40) (3), and in an experimental model discussed to investigate action potential transfer between two cells ("driver" cell and "follower" cell) coupled by a (simulated) resistor (76, 77). If a large coupling resistor is selected, this experimental arrangement can be taken as a simple model for highly discontinuous action potential transfer between two excitable regions. In the presence of a large coupling resistance and, consequently, a large conduction delay between the two cells, two factors appeared to have a major influence on propagation through the resistive obstacle: First, the fact that *early repolarization* was involved in driving excitatory current through the coupling resistor suggested that the L-type Ca^{++} current contributed to action potential transfer. This was confirmed by an increase in the delay upon the application of nifedipine (78, 79). An analogue observation, (discussed later, under Mechanisms of Unidirectional Block, cf. Fig. 12–48) was recently made at abrupt tissue expansions in patterned cell cultures (80). Second, because of the decreased electrotonic coupling, early repolarization of the driver cell was faster than during control. This fast early repolarization of the driver cell was responsible for the electrotonic driving force already being decreased at the time the follower cell was reaching threshold.

Discontinuous Propagation in a Cell Chain and a Cell Strand

Representation of heart tissue as a continuous electrical medium, as illustrated in Figures 12–1 through 12–3, ignores the fact that individual cells are interconnected via gap junctional resistors at a microscopic level. A comparison of propagation in a continuous cable with propagation in a chain of cells was made by Rudy and Quan (26, 81) and by Henriquez and Plonsey (75). In contrast to the simulations by Joyner et al. (69), which treated the problem of discontinuous propagation in general, these studies specifically addressed propagation in cell chains. Individual cells were connected to form a chain by single resistors representing gap junctions. During simulation of physiological propagation (conduction velocity 50 cm/sec), the conduction delay imposed by a cellular interconnection (assumed gap junction length 80 Å) was equal to the delay across the cytoplasm of a whole cell (cell length 100 μm) reflecting the high local resistivity of a gap junction (81). There was a close fit between the discontinuous cellular model and the continuous model when comparing the decrease of conduction velocity with moderate cell-to-cell uncoupling (Fig. 12–14). The different behavior of the discrete cellular model became manifest when coupling resistance was increased about *fivefold above normal* (26). Beyond that level, the decrease in conduction velocity was larger in the discontinuous, structure than in the continuous structure.

Increasing the degree of discreteness of the electrical network produced a marked delay of action potential transfer between cells. Within an individual cell, the excitation process became more synchronous with a decrease in cytoplasmic excitation time and almost simultaneous excitation of all cellular membrane sites (81). Because there was almost synchronous excitation within one cell (81), the action potentials elicited in such an uncoupled state closely resembled a space clamped action potential, i.e. an action potential where the generated ionic current is mostly used to discharge local membrane capacitance and only a small amount of ionic current at the cell end is used to excite the next cell. This mechanism, which is in accordance with the typical behavior of a discontinuous structure (Fig. 12–13), also explained the transient increase in dV/dt_{max} with partial electrical uncoupling, as depicted in Figure 12–15. It illustrates that with increasing discontinuity, dV/dt_{max} is not a simple function of ionic inward current flow but becomes dependent on the resistive properties of the excitable network. In addition to the changes in the action potential upstroke, there was a *prolongation* of the foot of the transmembrane action potential, and accordingly an increase in the time constant of the initial change in transmembrane potential, τ_{foot}.

Experimentally, the effects of discontinuities introduced by single cell-to-cell connections on propagation were estimated in cultures of neonatal rat myocytes (82, 83). With a technique similar to those reported earlier for the fabrication of synthetic cardiac strands, (84–86), patterned myocyte cell growth was produced in culture dishes (87). Cell chains one or several myocytes in width were obtained and action potential upstrokes were measured as the fluorescence change of a voltage-sensitive dye (88). Figure 12–16 shows the results from measurements in a single cell chain. The average conduction time between two measuring points including an intercellular connection was 118 μsec, and the average conduction time between points including the cytoplasmic spaces alone was 38 μsec (83). Subtraction of these two times yielded a delay across the cell-to-cell connection of 80 μsec or 50% of overall conduction time, in close accordance with the simulated values indicated above (81).

In all regions of the heart, cells are coupled longitudinally and laterally to form cell strands and other structures. As shown in computer simulations and in experiments on cultured neonatal rat myocytes (83) the degree of conduction discontinuity in cell strands is smaller than in single cell chains. In cell cultures, ap-

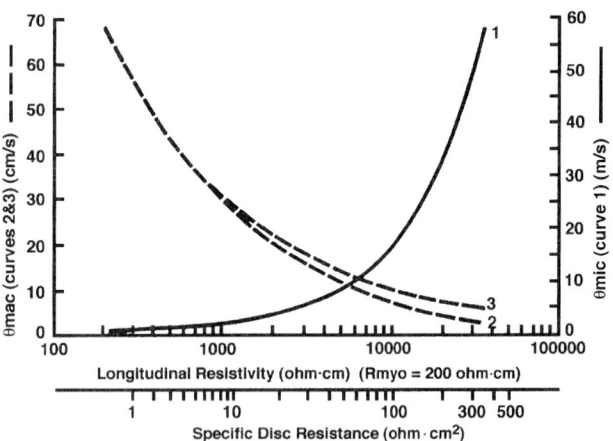

FIG. 12–14. Simulated cell chain. Comparison of continuous with discontinuous conduction with decreasing cell-to-cell coupling. Effects of variations in axial (longitudinal) resistance on microscopic velocity (θmic, curve 1) and on average macroscopic velocity (θmac, curve 2). The microscopic velocity corresponds to the velocity *inside* a cell. The case of a continuous structure is shown for comparison on curve 3 and follows the inverse square root relation of continuous cable theory. The effective longitudinal resistance is changed by varying the disk resistance while the myoplasm resistance is kept constant at 200. Both effective longitudinal resistivity and the corresponding disk resistance are indicated. [Reproduced from reference 26 with permission.]

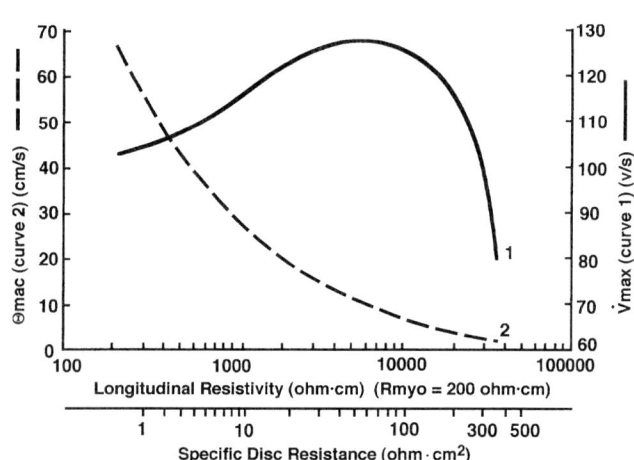

FIG. 12–15. Simulated chain of cells. Changes of maximal upstroke velocity with decreasing cell-to-cell coupling. Conduction velocity θ (*dashed line*) and dV/dt_{max} (*solid line*) are plotted as a function of the increasing effective resistance or the specific disk resistance (coupling resistance between simulated cells). There is a transient increase of dV/dt_{max} with increasing cell-to-cell uncoupling and decreasing velocity of propagation. [Reproduced from reference 26 with permission.]

position of lateral cell chains to a strand of 5–6 cells in width causes the cytoplasmic conduction times to increase and the intercellular conduction times to decrease. In the experiments shown in Figure 12–17, the presence of lateral coupling reduced the conduction delay (in % of total activation time) across gap junctions from the 50% measured in the single chains to 22%. These experiments showed that longitudinal propagation in a network with lateral coupling is more continuous than predicted by the presence of gap junctions at the cell ends alone. This process of smoothing or "lateral averaging," which has also been demonstrated for the flow of subthreshold current in a computer model (89) is explained by electrotonic current flow through the lateral junctions, which partially cancels the effect of the longitudinal discontinuities. Since this process is dependent on the degree of lateral coupling, it will be of relevance in relatively well-coupled tissue, such as ventricular myocardium (47, 49). Tissue with prominent end-to-end coupling and sparse lateral coupling (48) such as atrial crista terminalis, will show a high degree of longitudinal dissociation and discontinuity. In a computer simulation of propagation in a cellular network with an anisotropy ratio 3.2, i.e. higher than in the patterned cell cultures, the effect of lateral averaging was still observed (29).

Anisotropic Propagation

Macroscopic Electrical Anisotropy. It has long been known that conduction velocity, Θ, in atrial and ventricular tissue is dependent on the relation between the direction of the propagating wave and the alignment of the muscular tissue. As a consequence, macroscopic spread of excitation elicited by point stimuli of small strength follows in general an elliptical pattern (cf. Fig. 12–5). As shown in Table 12–1, values reported for longitudinal and transverse conduction velocity indicate a very high degree of anisotropy in the atria (ratio Θ_l / Θ_t of 10–15) and a lower degree of anisotropy in ventricular tissue (average ratio Θ_l / Θ_t of 2.7).

In the simplest possible model, where the intracellular space in both the *longitudinal and transverse* directions is represented as an electrical continuum, the explanation for this difference is given by the different intra- and extracellular resistivities in longitudinal versus transverse direction. Thus an approximately ninefold higher intracellular transverse than longitudinal resistivity was measured in guinea pig papillary muscles. This was in accordance with a threefold higher longitudinal than transverse Θ, and with the "square-root" relationship between intracellular resistance and Θ, as theoretically predicted from a continuous model (90). In such a model, owing to the difference in average spacing of cell borders and gap junctions in the longitudinal versus the transverse direction, the higher lumped transverse resistance would slow down transverse propagation compared to longitudinal propagation. Indeed the average spacing of cell borders seems to be a major determinant of conduction velocity, as recently suggested by a simulation study that demonstrated a marked dependence of conduction velocity on cell size (91). However, the propagation process in anisotropic tissue is not adequately represented by a simple continuous model (92). Thus, the upstroke velocity of the action potential generated by a given transmembrane site changed with the changing direction of impulse spread (93). Also, the time course of the initial portion of the transmembrane action potential (τ_{foot}) was direction-dependent (93). These findings indicated either a direction-dependent difference in the local activation of ionic depolarizing current, a direction-dependent difference in the flow of electrotonic current flowing into or from this membrane site, or both. In further work, it was found by analysis of action potential upstrokes and extracellular electrograms, that in some tissue, especially in aged myocardium, transverse but not longitudinal conduction was discontinuous (94). This led to the subdivision of functional anisotropy into "discontinuous and continuous anisotropic conduction," with the attribution of a distinctly different behavior to each type (95).

Anisotropic Propagation in Simulated and Cultured Cellular Networks. Anisotropic conduction at a microscopic level has been studied either by computer simulation (26–29, 81, 96) or in experiments carried out in cell cultures (34, 83, 97). A simulated network representing the stochastic distribution of cell shapes and gap junctional resistors at the cell perimeter (29), and which was derived from cellular morphology present in subepicardial muscle layers in the canine heart (47), was constructed by Spach and Heidlage (29). In this cellular pattern, a single cell was represented by multiple membrane patches with several patches, being aligned in longitudinal and transverse direction. According to their morphologic appearance and density, gap junctions were simulated as resistors of different magnitude. For both transverse and longitudinal propagation, the sequential activation of the membrane patches yielded the profiles of activation time at subcellular resolution. The major finding was that propagation in such networks was discontinuous at the cellular and subcellular level in accordance with the stochastic variability in cell structure and the distribution of the intercellular junctions (Fig. 12–18). The stochastic distribution of structural discontinuities surrounding a given cell led to a corresponding variability in electrotonic interaction. Consequently, the patterns of isochrones and dV/dt_{max} within a given cell during

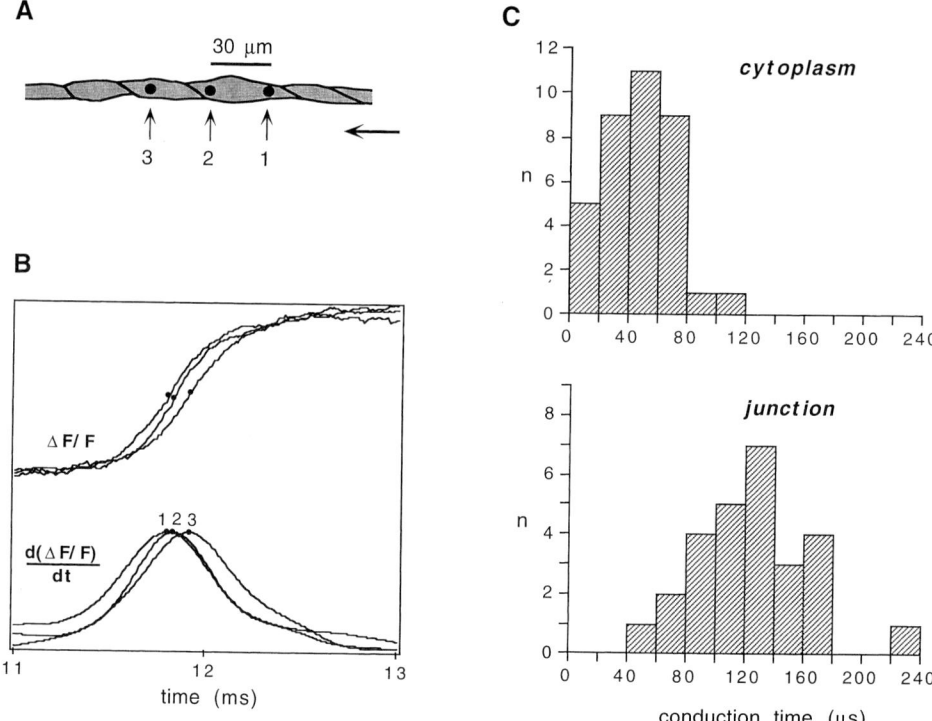

FIG. 12–16. Experimental determination of conduction in a single cell chain. A: Reproduction of the microscopic appearance of a cultured cell chain. Dots and numbers denote positions of three light-sensitive diodes (6.5 μm in diameter) separated by a distance of 30 μm. B: Optical recording of action potential upstrokes from diodes 1–3, measured as fluorescence change ΔF/F of a voltage-sensitive dye (upper traces) and the first time derivatives (lower traces). Numbers 1–3 denote times of local activation. Note that the conduction delay across the cell border (2–3) is larger than delay within the cytoplasm (1–2). C: Histograms of cytoplasmic (upper graph) and junctional (lower graph) conduction times. The difference between the mean conduction times amounts to approximately 80 μsec and reflects the mean conduction time across the end-to-end cell junctions. [Reproduced from reference 83 with permission.]

longitudinal or transversal spread were not the simple mirror images of the patterns during propagation in the opposite direction. As a common rule, intracellular locations that corresponded to entry sites of local microcircuit currents, where there was dispersion of current beyond the gap junctions, showed local conduction slowing. Conversely, sites where wavefronts collided with another wavefront or approached a resistive obstacle (cell end) showed local acceleration of the impulse. In the model study by Spach and Heidlage there was a close correlation between subcellular arrangement of isochrones, dV/dt_{max}, and local Na$^+$ inward charge movement. This is illustrated in Figure 12–19 for longitudinal and transverse propagation. In accordance with the mechanisms underlying propagation in discontinuous structures, there was an inverse relationship between local propagation velocity and dV/dt_{max} on one hand and local Na$^+$ inward charge movement on the other. The highest values for dV/dt_{max} were observed at collision sites which occasionally occurred in the transverse direction. The occurrence of subcellular microcollisions during transverse propagation was recently confirmed by experiments using high-resolution multisite optical mapping of transmembrane potential in anisotropic cell cultures (34). Like the mechanism explained in Figure 12–11, the small traverse cell diameters in combination with the relatively high resistances attributed to the lateral gap junctions produced large conduction delays at the lateral junctions, and inversely, fast intracellular activation during transverse conduction. The simulated undulating behavior of dV/dt_{max} during transverse and longitudinal spread, which was also shown in an other simulation study (27), produced an overlap of dV/dt_{max} values, the lowest values during transverse spread being lower than the highest values during longitudinal spread. In accordance with experimental results,(29, 98) dV/dt_{max} varied not only upon the change from longitudinal to transverse spread, but changing the transverse or longitudinal activation front by 180° altered the value of dV/dt_{max} as well.

Whether or not cellular and subcellular propagation

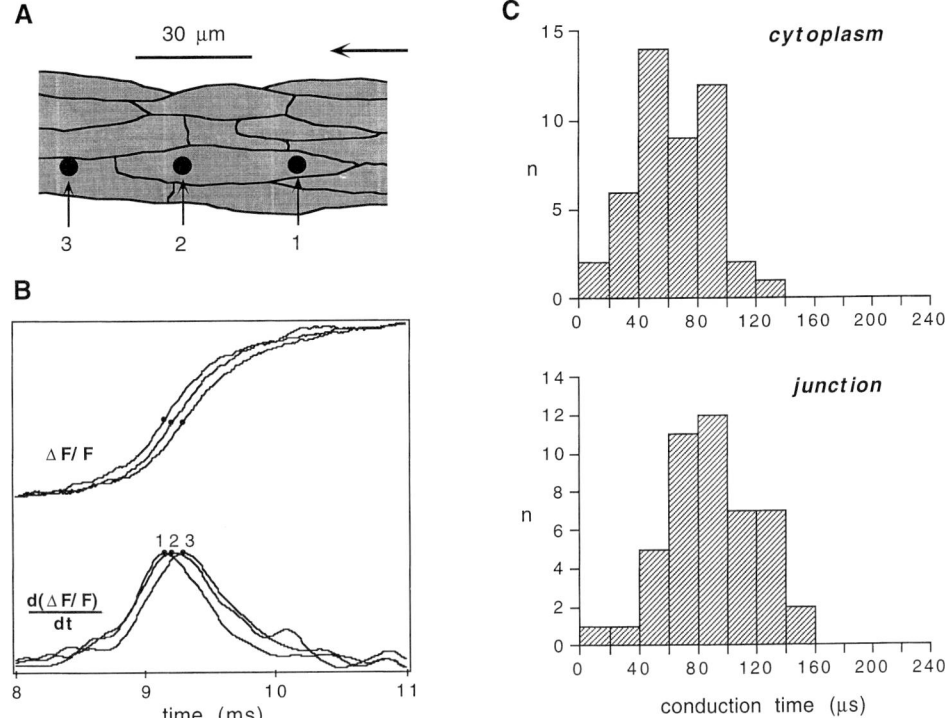

FIG. 12–17. Experimental determination of conduction in a cell strand. A: Reproduction of the microscopic appearance of a cultured cell strand (4–5 cells in width). Dots and numbers denote positions of three light-sensitive diodes (6.5 μm in diameter) separated by a distance of 30 μm. B: Optical recording of action potential upstrokes from diodes 1–3, measured as fluorescence change ΔF/F of a voltage-sensitive dye (*upper traces*) and the first time derivatives (*lower traces*). Numbers 1–3 denote times of local activation. C: Histograms of cytoplasmic (*upper graph*) and junctional (*lower graph*) conduction times. With respect to the measurements shown in Figure 12–16 the mean cytoplasmic conduction time has increased from 38 μsec to 60 μsec and the mean junctional conduction time has decreased from 118 μsec to 80 μsec. This is explained by electrotonic current flow through lateral gap junctions ("lateral averaging"; see text). [Reproduced from reference 83 with permission.]

in situ is discontinuous to the extent shown in the computer simulations and cell culture experiments depends on the difference in cell-to-cell connectivity between three-dimensional tissue in vivo and the two-dimensional simulation models or cell cultures. Comparison of morphometrically determined connectivity in two-dimensional slices of dog ventricle with connectivity in three-dimensions suggests that conduction discontinuities will be significantly less prominent in three-dimensional cellular networks in situ. Thus, in canine ventricular myocardium a given myocyte is connected to 5.2 other myocytes in one plane (two-dimensions) and to 11.3 other myocytes in three dimensions (Table 12–3); (34, 48). At present, simulating a fully comprehensive link between the function of individual ionic channels, transporters, pumps, connexins and microscopic propagation is limited by the lack of knowledge about (*1*) the role of subcellular clustering of membrane channels, and as mentioned, (*2*) the contribution of the different types and connexins to cellular electrotonic interaction. It has been shown in atrial tumor cells that K^+ channels encoded by the kv1.5 gene (99) and Na^+ channels (100–102) are preferentially clustered in the surface membrane at locations of gap junctions. It is important to note that the notion of normal conduction in a cellular network being "discontinuous" is eventually a matter of scale, i.e. of the relation between size and spacing of resistive obstacles and the resolution of the mapping system. Thus, assessment of physiological propagation with a distance between measuring sites > 30 μm in anisotropic myocyte cultures showed a homogeneous spread of propagation (34, 97).

A question that remains a matter of dispute is whether the higher (average) dV/dt_{max} values and the lower τ_{foot} during transverse versus longitudinal propagation, as observed in situ, stem mainly from the electrical properties of the anisotropic cellular network, or whether they are due to other factors related to tissue anisotropy. Such factors may include (*1*) the presence of the dis-

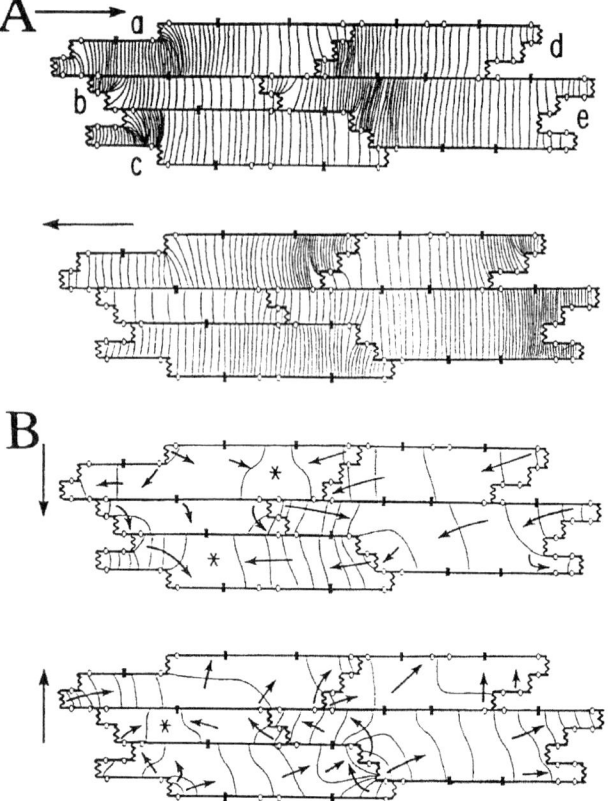

FIG. 12–18. Propagation in a cellular network, simulation of intracellular excitation sequences. *A, longitudinal conduction:* Conduction from left to right is depicted on the upper trace, conduction from right to left is depicted on the lower trace. Isochrone lines are separated by 4 μsec. *B, transverse conduction:* Conduction from top to bottom is shown on the *upper trace*, propagation from bottom to top is depicted on the *lower trace*. Intracellular isochrones are separated by 3 μsec. During longitudinal propagation, there is a crowding of isochrones (slow propagation) at the beginning of propagation in the individual cells and acceleration of propagation toward the end of the cells. During transverse propagation, the arrows indicate preferential longitudinal propagation spread, with microcollisions occurring occasionally (asterisk). [Reproduced from reference 29 with permission.]

continuities introduced by the connective tissue separations and microvessels (2) the effect of wavefront curvature, and (3) the bidomain nature of cardiac tissue (see below). While dV/dt_{max} has been shown to be on average 30% higher in transverse versus longitudinal direction in situ, (29, 93, 98, 103, 104) differences were small in simulated or absent in cultured cellular networks at comparable degrees of anisotropy. In anisotropic networks of cultured myocytes (anisotropic velocity ratio 1.9–2.3) microscopic variability of dV/dt_{max} was present during transverse and longitudinal flat wave propagation but the average values were not different (34, 97). In the simulation study by Spach and Heidlage (anisotropic velocity ratio 3.2), the average transverse dV/dt_{max} was higher by only 11% than longitudinal dV/dt^{max} (29). As discussed later, under The Bidomain Behavior of Cardiac tissue, the direction-dependent changes in dV/dt_{max} can partially be attributed to the bidomain behavior, while the explanation of direction-dependence of $τ_{foot}$ seems more complex.

The Electrical Resistance of the Extracellular Space

In many of the experimental and theoretical studies on cardiac propagation, the resistive properties of the extracellular space are not considered separately from the intracellular resistance. This simplification is probably justified only for isolated thin tissue superfused with a large conducting bulk solution. As already mentioned, dense intramural myocardial tissue consists of cell bundles separated by narrow extracellular clefts carrying lamina of connective tissue and the microvascular tree, i.e. structures supposed to have a high electrical resistance (24, 25). Measurements of intra- and extracellular resistances have been performed in superfused and perfused heart specimens (14, 31, 32, 90). If an arterially perfused muscle specimen of defined geometry (cylindrical papillary muscle) is placed in an electrical insulator, subthreshold current, flowing longitudinally through the muscle cylinder, will distribute in both the extra cellular and intracellular compartments. According to cable theory (14), the change in extracellular or intracellular voltage along the muscle divided by the amount of injected current, is equal to the resistance of the tissue, r_t, which in turn consists of the extra- and intracellular resistances (r_i and r_o) in parallel, $1/r_t = 1/r_i + 1/r_o$. Both these resistances are also the main series resistances within the loop of local circuit current during propagation of an action potential. During propagation they form a voltage divider, which separates the amplitude of the transmembrane potential into an intracellular and an extracellular component. Thus, both r_i and r_o can be determined from the assessment of r_t, the transmembrane action potential and the amplitude of the bipolar electrogram. As can be seen from Figure 12–20, the amplitude of the extracellular wavefront (and accordingly of the intracellular wavefront) is about 50% of the amplitude of the transmembrane action potential (31, 32). This division of the electrical driving force into two equal parts signifies that the intracellular and extracellular longitudinal resistances are of about *equal magnitude*. This high value of extracellular resistance, which is also observed in the left ventricle in situ (105, 106), predicts that changes in extracellular resistance are expected to affect propagation velocity to a similar extent as changes in cellular coupling. So far, changes in extracellular resistance have been shown to affect conduction velocity in the case of interstitial swelling (18), which produces a

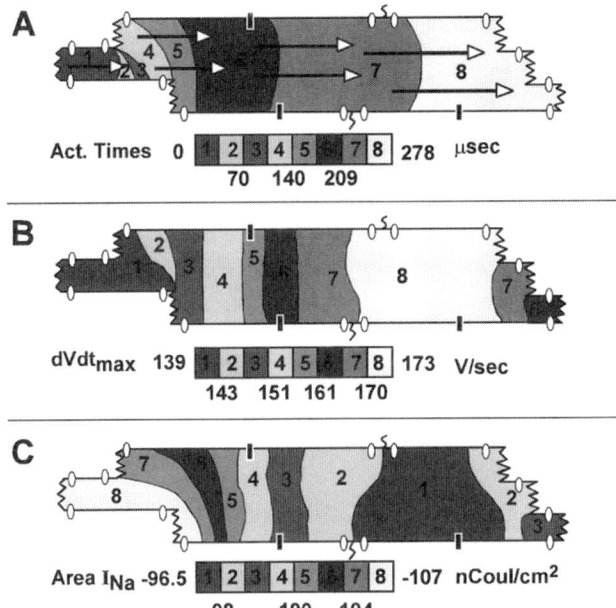

FIG. 12–19. Simulation of intracellular excitation sequences (A), intracellular distributions of dV/dt$_{max}$ (B) and inward Na$^+$ charge movements during excitation (C) in an anisotropic cellular network. The left graphs correspond to longitudinal propagation from left to right and the right graphs correspond to transverse propagation from top to bottom. Note the close correspondence between the isochrone spacing, dV/dt$_{max}$ and inward Na$^+$ charge movement during both transverse and longitudinal propagation: The dV/dt$_{max}$ is relatively low where excitation is slow and vice versa. By contrast the locations of slow activation and low dV/dt$_{max}$ correspond to large inward Na$^+$ charge movements and vice versa. [Reproduced from reference 29 with permission.]

decrease of extracellular resistance with a concomitant increase in propagation velocity, with the collapse of the vascular space following coronary occlusion (31, 32) and during acute ischemia (31).

The high-resistance value of the intramural extracellular space in ventricular tissue is also important for our understanding of the propagation process at the boundary between the conducting subendocardial muscle layers and the bulk conductor made up by the ventricular cavity fluid. Since the resistance for the local circuit currents is smaller at the boundary to a bulk conductor than in the depth of the tissue, owing to the smaller extracellular resistance of the bulk solution, the propagation velocity in a cylindrical muscle soaked in a volume conductor will increase with decrease in the fiber radius (107). Similarly, the conduction velocity at the surface of a tissue slab soaked in a tissue bath will increase with decreasing slab thickness (108–111). Importantly, the interaction between the low resistance of the volume conductor and the higher intramural extracellular resistance will produce a concave shape of the wavefront in the transmural direction, and this will affect the action potential upstroke. The results from the study of Suenson (107), which first brought attention to the electrical phenomena occurring at the boundary between compact ventricular tissue and a large volume of superfusate fluid is shown in Figure 12–21. In this

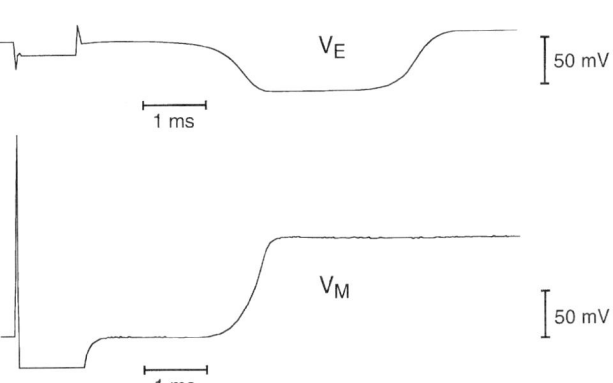

FIG. 12–20. Ratio of extracellular to intracellular resistance in compact ventricular tissue. The amplitude of the bipolar extracellular electrogram (upper trace, V$_E$) and the amplitude of the action potential upstroke (lower trace, V$_M$) are shown from an isolated, arterially-perfused papillary muscle. The signals are measured in a muscle which is surrounded by an electrical insulator. The ratio of V$_E$/(V$_M$ − V$_E$) which is approximately 1, corresponds to the ratio of extracellular: intracellular resistance, r$_e$/r$_i$. This demonstrates that the extracellular resistance in compact ventricular tissue is of approximately the same magnitude is the resistance of the intracellular space (including the gap junctions). [Reproduced from reference 32 with permission.]

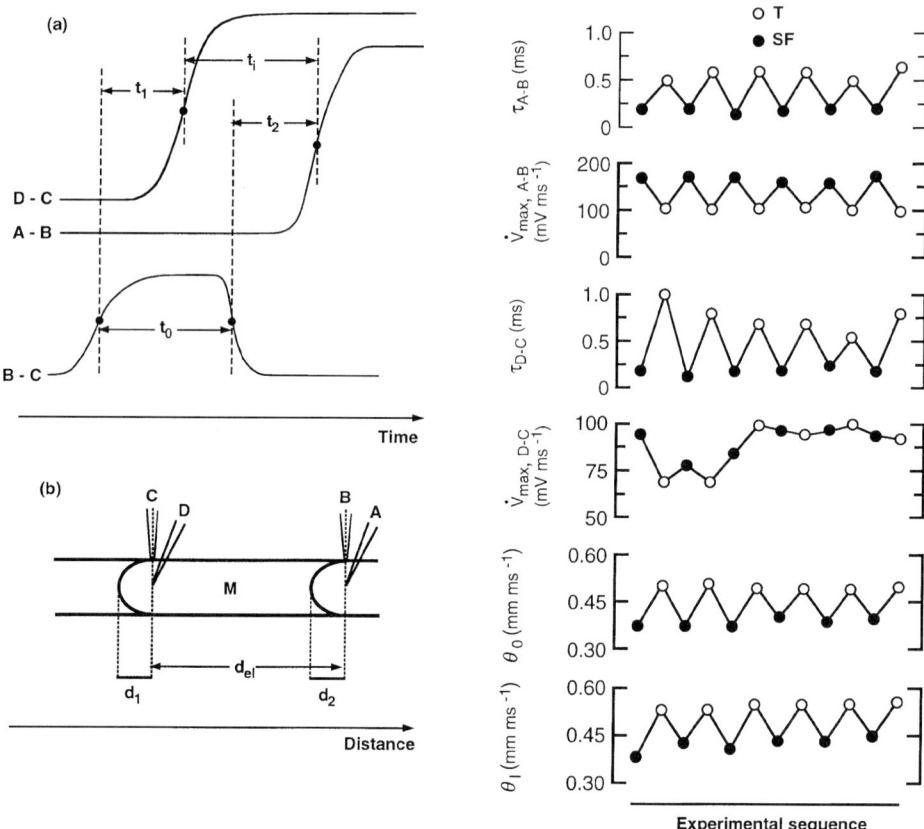

FIG. 12–21. Effect of superfusion fluid on conduction velocity, θ, the maximal upstroke velocity of the transmembrane action potential dV/dt_{max}, and the time constant of the initial rise of the action potential, τ_{foot}. *Panels (a) and (b)* show action potentials measured at two sites along a cylindrical papillary muscle, between electrodes D and C, (D-C), and between electrodes A and B, (A-B). The bipolar extracellular electrogram is measured between the extracellular electrodes c and b, (b-c). The muscle is either soaked in a large bulk solution (SF, *closed circles*) or covered only by a thin fluid layer (T, *open circles*). Panel (b) illustrates the curved wavefronts measured in the presence of the large bulk solution during propagation from left to right. Traces on the right correspond from top to bottom: τ_{a-b}, $dV/dt_{max, a-b}$, τ_{d-c}, $dV/dt_{max\ d-c}$, θ_o (conduction velocity at the surface) and θ_i (conduction velocity in the core of the fiber). Increasing the thickness of the fluid layer (electrical shunting, transition from T to SF) produces (*1*) an increase of θ_o and θ_i; (*2*) an increase of τ_{a-b} and τ_{d-c}; (*3*) a decrease of dV/dt_{max}. [Reproduced from reference 107 with permission.]

experiment conduction velocity, Θ, in the depth and the surface of a cylindrical papillary muscle, dV/dt_{max} and the time course of the initial part of the action potential upstroke (represented by the time constant τ_{foot}) were determined in the absence and the presence of a large bulk superfusate. Adding a large bulk superfusate and decreasing extracellular resistance decreased Θ, dV/dt_{max}, and τ_{foot}. These alterations were explained by the change of the propagation wavefront from a planar shape (absence of superfusate) to a concave shape (presence of superfusate). At the surface of the muscle, this transition to a curved wavefront increased the amount of local circuit current flow at the expense of the current responsible for the discharge of the membrane capacitance with a reduction in dV/dt_{max}, and τ_{foot} (cf. Fig. 12–3); (108–111).

The Bidomain Behavior of Cardiac Tissue

Excitation of tissue by a propagating wavefront and excitation by intra- and extracellular electrodes involves flow of local circuit currents in a loop including the extra- and intracellular domains. As mentioned, the resistance of the extracellular space, hosting connective tissue and blood vessels is not only responsible for the production of the extracellular field and the electrocardiogram, but it forms part of the resistance limiting the speed of propagation. While the effect of extracellular resistance is easily predictable for one-dimensional waves or two-dimensional flat wavefronts (cf. Fig. 12–21), the combination of the bidomain nature with anisotropy has complex effects on propagation (*1*) in the case where excitation emerges from a point source and

(2) if anisotropic tissue is immersed in a bulk solution that acts as a electrical shunt. The reason for this complexity appears to relate to the differences in electrical conductivities between the extra- and intracellular domains and/or the superfusate.

The Virtual Electrode Effect. The scarce experimental data providing quantitative information about the conductivity values in cardiac tissue (90) suggest that for ventricular tissue the ratio of extracellular resistivity in a longitudinal (l) direction of the cellular strands to transverse (t) resistivity, $R_{e,t}:R_{e,l}$ equals approximately 2.5, while the corresponding ratio of intracellular resistivities, $R_{i,t}:R_{i,l}$ is approximately 8.9. The resulting change in transmembrane potential close to a unipolar extracellular stimulation electrode during application of stimulatory current is shown in Figure 12–22. In this study (112), intracellular, extracellular, and transmembrane potentials were simulated during spread of extracellularly injected current. In a model with equal ratios of anisotropy ($R_{i,l} : R_{e,l} = R_{i,t} : R_{e,t}$) there was, as expected, an elliptical arrangement of isopotential lines, decreasing monotonically with increasing distance from the simulation site and a monotonically decreasing change in membrane potential. In the presence of anisotropy ratios assumed to reflect ventricular tissue in vivo, there was a local hyperpolarization along the L-axis and depolarization along the T-axis. Experimental confirmation of the theoretically predicted transmembrane distribution during various types of local stimuli was obtained by multielectrode mapping (113) and by multisite optical recordings of transmembrane voltage (114–116).

The consequences of the voltage distribution shown in Figure 12–22 for excitation have been investigated in several experimental and theoretical studies. During point stimulation, threshold requirements for stimulation are determined by the relation between electrode size and liminal area. At threshold, the sites at which propagation is initiated are located at the circumference of the liminal area, which has been estimated to be approximately 0.3–0.4 mm in radius. (43, 45). Increasing stimulus strength beyond threshold displaces the sites of impulse initiation remote from the electrode. The area circumscribed by these sites has been termed "virtual electrode" (117). In accordance with the voltage distribution shown in Figure 12–22 it assumes a dog-bone shape in the case of cathodal-make excitation (Fig. 12–23). The dogs bone shape first appears at stimulation strengths of approximately double threshold intensity. It gets more distinct with increasing stimulus strength and anisotropy. The size and shape of the virtual electrode can lead to an earlier activation of relatively remote sites along the transversal axis and a later activation of sites closer to the electrode along

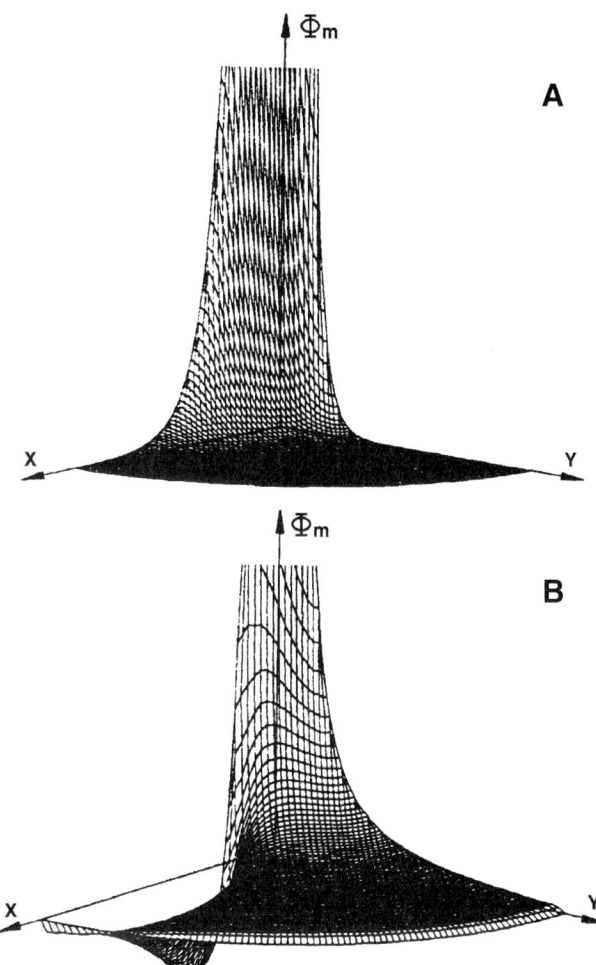

FIG. 12–22. Three-dimensional plot of simulated transmembrane voltage (Φm) after application of a point stimulus to two-dimensional anisotropic tissue. The X-axis corresponds to the longitudinal direction of the fibers, the Y-axis to the transversal direction of the fibers. *Panel A:* Simulation of anisotropy with equal ratios of extracellular to intracellular conductivities. *Panel B:* Longitudinal conductivity ratio (σ_{ex}/σ_{ix}) $8 \times 10^{-4}:2 \times 10^{-4}$; conductivity ratio ($\sigma_{ey}/\sigma_{iy}$) $2 \times 10^{-4}:2 \times 10^{-5}$. Note that with an equal anisotropic ratio there is a drop of Φm with distance from current injection and a elliptical shape of Φm distribution in the x/y plane. In Panel B, which corresponds to the simulation using experimentally determined values of intra- and extracellular conductivities, there is a hyperpolarization of Φm in the X (longitudinal) and a depolarization in the Y (transverse) directions. [Reproduced from reference 112 with permission.]

the longitudinal axis. As a consequence, sites close to the electrodes on the longitudinal axis can get activated from sites excited earlier by transversal excitation, and extracellular electrograms can acquire a "discontinuous" configuration. The shape of virtual electrodes has been considered important for explaining excitation following large extracellular shocks.

The Bidomain Nature of Myocardium and Interaction with Surrounding Fluid. The experiments of Suenson

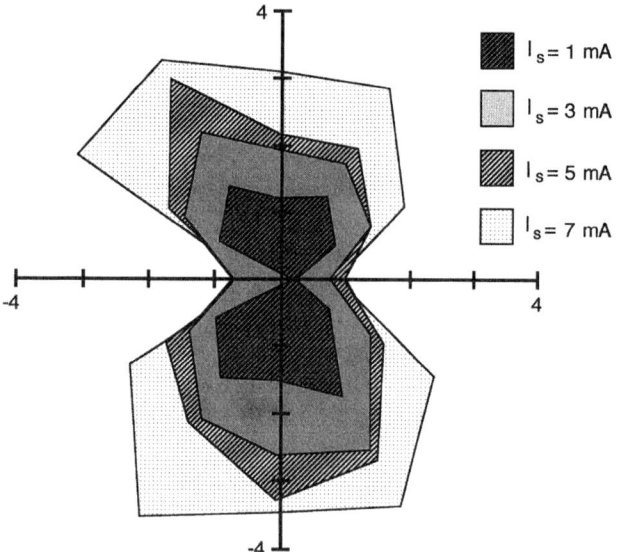

FIG. 12-23. Dog-bone shape of virtual electrode. Plots showing the shape of virtual electrodes caused by stimuli from 1–7 mA. The horizontal axis corresponds to the longitudinal direction of the anisotropic subepicardial layer of a dog, the vertical axis corresponds to the transverse fiber direction. Note that upon application of a central cathodal stimulus, the line where excitation starts to propagate, i.e. the virtual electrode, has a dog bone shape with a very large extension of the electrode in the transverse direction. [Reproduced from reference 113 with permission.]

(Fig. 12-21) demonstrated that bathing fluid surrounding compact ventricular tissue exerts a significant influence on Θ, dV/dt_{max}, and τ_{foot}. A large bulk of fluid is not only present adjacent to subendocardial muscle layers in vivo but, in addition, in all experimental studies involving superfusion of cardiac tissue to maintain ionic and metabolic steady state. The results of Suenson initiated several theoretical studies aimed to investigate the interaction between tissue anisotropy and electrical shunting by a bulk solution (108–111, 118–120) The results of simulations comparing dV/dt_{max} and the initial portion of the transmembrane action potential in anisotropic tissue in the absence and the presence of a bath solution is illustrated in Figure 12-24. If the model consisted of a bidomain structure with unequal anisotropy alone, the transmembrane action potential upstrokes were identical with respect to dV/dt_{max} and τ_{foot} during propagation in the longitudinal and the transversal direction or at intermediate angles. Introduction of a bath solution that was in electrical contact with the tissue into the model produced an increase of dV/dt_{max} in transversal direction and a decrease in the longitudinal direction, as well as a faster initial loading of the membrane capacitance during transversal propagation. These results not only quantitatively simulated most of the direction-dependent differences in dV/dt_{max} ob-

served experimentally, but they also accounted for the experimentally observed changes in τ_{foot} in superficial cell layers.

In a recent study, Spach et al. have shown that direction-dependence of the early rise (τ_{foot}) of the transmembrane action potential is also explained by capacitive loading of microvessels by local current flow during propagation (121). To what extent and at what site in the heart the relative role of one of the two suggested mechanisms will predominate is still a matter of dispute (122).

THE ACTIVATION OF THE WHOLE HEART—FROM THE SINUS NODE TO THE VENTRICLES

The Sinus Node—Spread of Excitation from the Sinus Node to the Atrium

The morphological sinus node, first described by Keith and Flack in 1907 (123), lies at the junction of the superior vena cava and the right atrium, close to the crest of the atrial appendage. Two types of myocytes are found within the sinus node (124–127). The cells in the center of the node are arranged in a complex interdigitating manner, interspersed with connective tissue. Individual central nodal cells contain very few myofilaments. The organized intracellular structures of central, or "typical" nodal cells (myofilaments, mitochondria, nuclei, and sarcoplasmic reticulum tubules) occupy only 50% of the cell volume, whereas in atrial cells these structures comprise 90% of total cell volume. The second type of myocyte, the transitional cell, is truly transitional in that it changes gradually from the central, typical nodal cell to an atrial myocyte. Gradually, the number of myofilaments increases, and their arrangement becomes more organized, as the transitional cells are localized, closer to the atrial cells. In some species, such as the rabbit, the zone of transitional cells is large, in others, such as the dog or the pig, it is narrow. The boundary between the transitional zone and the working atrial myocardium is morphologically not sharply defined. Studies in which immunohistochemical staining techniques were used showed a sharp boundary between nodal and atrial cells, however. Nodal cells were characterized by the fact that they reacted with a monoclonal antibody against bovine Purkinje fibers and did not react to an antibody against connexin43. Atrial cells, on the other hand did not react to the antibody against Purkinje cells, but did react with the Cx43 antibody (54). However, since no electrophysiologic measurements were made, and no morphological studies were performed to quantify the number of intracellular organelles and filaments, no certainty exists whether some cells de-

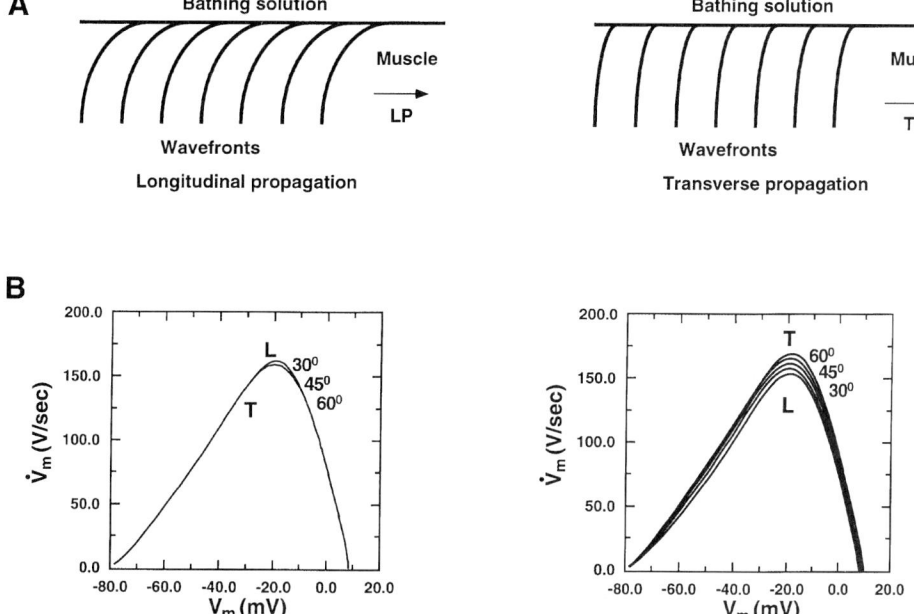

FIG. 12–24. Interaction between an anisotropic medium and a bathing solution. *A:* Deviation of the isochrones of a wave propagating in the longitudinal direction (*left side*) and a wave propagating in the transverse direction (*right side*). Note that due to the anisotropy-dependent differences in intra- and extracellular conductivities, wavefront bending in the longitudinal direction is significantly more expressed. In the absence of a bulk conductor, both longitudinal and transverse wavefronts are flat (not shown). *B:* Phase plane plots of dV/dt_{max} versus membrane potential in a model with unequal anisotropy. Superimposed are phase plane plots of action potentials propagating in the longitudinal direction (L), at angles of 30°, 45°, and 60° from the longitudinal direction and in the transverse direction (T). *On the left hand side,* the bathing fluid was absent. Note that all the traces almost superimpose. *On the right hand side,* a bathing fluid has been added to the boundary of the tissue. In this case there is a marked direction dependence of both the initial portion of the action potential of and of dV/dt_{max}. [Reproduced from references 109, 120 with permission.]

fined as atrial by immunohistochemical criteria might not be transitional according to other criteria.

A striking feature of the sinus node is the presence of abundant connective tissue surrounding the nodal cells (128–131). The amount of connective tissue in the human sinus node has been reported to increase with age. In young individuals approximately 50% of the volume of the sinus node is occupied by myocytes. By 70 years of age, the proportion of the node occupied by myocytes may be as low as 10% (132). There are marked species differences regarding the amount of collagen in the sinus node. In cats 75% to 95% of the volume may consist of collagen; in pigs 75%, and in guinea pigs, 50% (129–131). Attempts to document an increase in connective tissue with age in various animal species yielded variable results. Thus, the relative volume of collagen in the SA node was found to remain constant both in cats and humans once adulthood was reached. No consistent relationship between the amount of collagen and sino-atrial conduction time could be established (133).

The first combined electrophysiological and morphological studies on the pacemaker of the heart were performed in 1910 (134, 135). The site of origin of the heartbeat was determined by searching for the site of primary extracellular negativity, which was found on the epicardial surface of the canine right atrium in the sulcus terminalis near the vena cava superior. This site of "primary negativity" coincided with the site of the histologic sinus node. Transmembrane potentials from pacemaker cells were first recorded from the sinus venosus of the frog heart in 1952 (136) and in 1955 from the sinus node in mammalian hearts (137). These studies revealed the most characteristic electrophysiological feature of pacemaking cells: spontaneous diastolic depolarization of the membrane potential. A number of ionic currents are involved in normal pacemaking: first an inward current carried by sodium ions, called I_f, which is activated after repolarization; second, a decay in outward current I_K carried by potassium ions following repolarization; third, the slow calcium inward current which is activated as the membrane depolarizes. (138–141). In 1963 Trautwein and Uchizono (142) determined the ultrastructure of cells very close (i.e. less than 1 mm) to cells from which typical pacemaker potentials were recorded, and in 1978, direct identification of the cell from which pacemaker potentials had been obtained was made (143). Not unexpectedly, pacemaker potentials originated from nodal cells.

The most complete correlation between structure and spread of excitation in the sinus node is provided by the studies of Masson-Pévet et al. and of Bleeker et al. (125, 126). Their findings are in agreement with those of other mapping studies (144–147). Multiple microelectrode recordings were made from isolated, superfused rabbit heart preparations, resulting in maps depicting the spread of excitation during spontaneous sinus beats, as shown on Figure 12–25. Dominant pacemaker cells, i.e. those with the earliest action potential upstrokes, the fastest rate of diastolic depolarization, the slowest rate of rise of the action potential, and a gradual transition from diastolic to systolic depolarization, comprise a small area of about 0.3 mm square containing about 5000 cells that fire synchronously. Ultrastructural reconstruction showed that this dominant group of pacemaker cells was part of a larger group consisting of typical nodal cells. Gap junctions, although less frequent than in transitional cells or atrial cells, were found in every cell contour in ultrathin sections. It was estimated that every cell in the pacemaker center was coupled to other cells with at least 100 gap junctions (125). This is far in excess of what is needed to ensure synchronization of diastolic depolarization (148, 149). These findings are apparently in contrast with more recent studies in which the sinus node failed to react with antibodies against connexin43 (54, 56), although in other studies nodal cells did show a reaction (58). There are as yet insufficient data to demonstrate that there is a gradual increase in gap junctions throughout the zone of transitional cells towards the atrium. Still, the degree of electrotonic interaction between atrial and nodal cells plays a crucial role in the functioning of the sinus node. Pacemaker activity in peripheral transitional cells is suppressed because they are coupled to atrial cells, which do not have the capacity for spontaneous diastolic depolarization in normal conditions. Because the constant diastolic resting membrane potential of atrial cells is more negative than the maximum diastolic potential of transitional nodal cells, an electrotonic current flows from atrial to transitional cells, tending to hyperpolarize the latter, thereby suppressing diastolic depolarization. When transitional cells are isolated from the surrounding atrium, their intrinsic pacemaking rate is actually higher than that from the centrally located "dominant" pacemaker (131, 150, 151). Computer simulations (152) have indicated that a critical degree of electrical coupling between atrial and nodal cells, as well as a gradual decrease in coupling resistance from central nodal cells toward the atrium, is necessary for the small group of dominant pacemakers to activate the atrium. When coupling resistance is too low, electrotonic current from the large mass of surrounding atrial tissue will suppress diastolic depolarization. When coupling resistance is too high, the current provided by the small group of dominant pacemaker cells firing synchronously will not be sufficient to depolarize atrial cells to threshold.

As shown in Figure 12–25, conduction from the center of the node towards the crista terminalis occurs preferentially in an oblique cranial direction. This preferential conduction could be explained by the tissue architecture, conduction being faster in areas where fibers were arranged in parallel. In the isolated rabbit heart preparation, conduction block occurs towards the interatrial septum. This is not due to an absence of gap junctions, but to a reduced excitability of cells in this region (153).

Alterations in the activity of the autonomic nervous

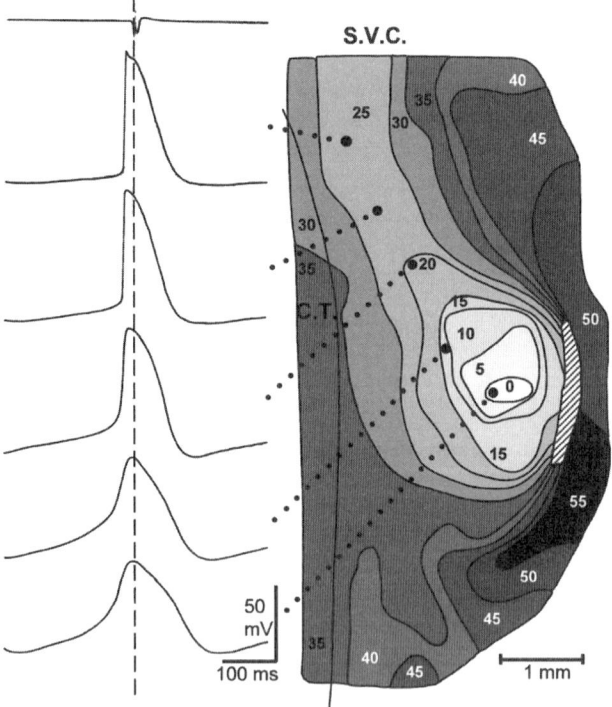

FIG. 12–25. Isochronal map of excitation spread from the sinoatrial node. Tones depict excitation intervals in steps of 5 msec, numbers correspond to activation times in msec. Configuration of action potentials is shown along the pathway of conduction from the sinus node to the atrium. The dashed line indicates the beginning of the atrial electrogram used as time reference. Toward the periphery, action potentials show an increase in amplitude and dV/dt_{max} and a decrease in rate of diastolic depolarization. The area in which two component action potentials were recorded is hatched in the activation map. [Reproduced with permission 126.]

system do not only cause changes in sinus rhythm because of their effects on transmembrane currents, they also produce shifts in pacemaker sites. Under the influence of acetylcholine, the dominant pacemaker site in isolated hearts shifts away from the central area of the node toward transitional cells in the cauda of the node; adrenalin induces a pacemaker shift to a more inferior site (154–156).

Identification of pacemaking areas has also been performed by recording of extracellular potentials in canine hearts and in the human heart during cardiac surgery (157–160). The extracellular electrogram from the sinus node shows two deflections of low amplitude and frequency, which precede the high-frequency deflections caused by activity of atrial tissue: a "diastolic slope," corresponding to diastolic depolarization and an "upstroke slope," corresponding to phase zero, or systolic, depolarization. Areas functioning as active pacemakers were characterized by the presence of both the diastolic and upstroke slopes. In the canine heart these were found in an area 4 mm square. The area showing only diastolic slopes was much larger. Asynchronous activity of several pacemaking groups was recorded, suggesting that, despite strong coupling within one group of pacemaking cells, intergroup coupling may not be strong. As in the isolated rabbit heart, the spread of excitation from the canine sinus node was more rapid along the axis of the sulcus terminalis than in other directions. Earliest atrial activation occurs simultaneously over a relatively broad area of 8 mm square. Earliest right atrial activation could result from impulses arising from more than one automatic group in the sinus node. As already mentioned, in the classical studies of Lewis et al. and of Wybauw (134, 135), the site of pacemaking was determined by the site of primary negativity. Later studies (161, 162) found that in the region of primary negativity, several low-voltage deflections preceded the large, negative deflection. In a study in which both microelectrode recordings and extracellular recordings were used, two sources for these fragmented, low-voltage deflections were found (163). Activity within the transitional zone was responsible for the complex waveforms preceding the main complex; propagation of independent wavefronts in different layers of the crista terminalis resulted in multiple deflections occurring after the inscription of the primary negative wave. Studies by Boineau and coworkers showed that in the canine heart, impulses were simultaneously initiated from up to three atrial sites separated by more than 1 cm. Multiple depolarization waves originated from these sites, merging into a common wavefront after 10–15 msec. Changes in heart rate were associated with changes in the sites of origin (164–166). It was argued that these findings should be explained by a multicenter pacemaker model, and that the system of atrial pacemakers is much larger than the sinus node, extending both craniocaudally and mediolaterally. At extreme heart rates, extranodal pacemakers could dominate the pacemakers in the sinus node. Thus, whereas in isolated preparations, the site of the dominant pacemaker is constant, in the heart in vivo, considerable pacemaker shifts may occur and the earliest activated atrial areas may shift as well.

Atrial Activation. Lewis, who was the first to map the spread of excitation in the atria, described this process as follows: "the excitation wave in the auricle may be likened to the spread of fluid poured upon a flat surface, its edges advancing as an ever widened circle, until the whole surface is covered: such variation as exists in the rate of travel along various lines in the auricle is fully accounted for by the simple anatomical arrangements of the tissue" (167). From Figure 12–26 depicting isochrone lines on the epicardial surface of the right atrium of a canine heart, it is evident that the isochrones deviate along the crista terminalis, indicating preferential conduction through that muscle bundle. Figures 12–27 and 12–28 show that the right atrium is a "bag full of holes". The orifices of the superior and inferior vena cava, the ostium of the coronary sinus, and the fossa ovalis divide the atrial myocardium into muscular bands. Owing to the architecture of the right atrium, only a limited number of routes are available for conduction of the impulse from sinus node to atrioventricular node. In 1926, Rothberger and Scherf

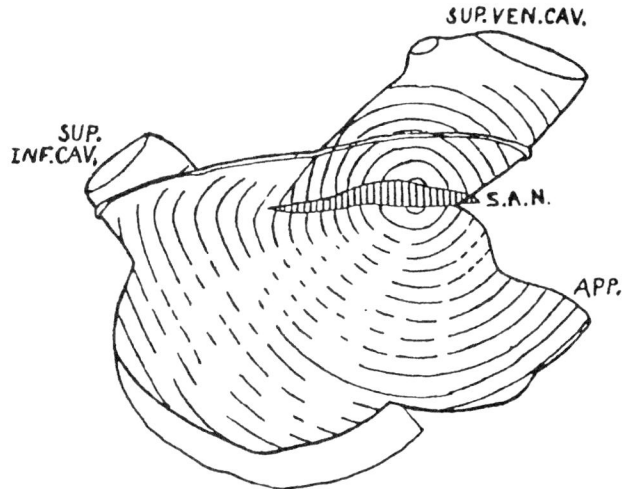

FIG. 12–26. Spread of excitation in the right atrium. Isochronal map of the spread of excitation from the sinoatrial node (S. A. N.) over the epicardial surface of the right atrium made by Thomas Lewis in 1915. Although in general spread of activation is depicted as being radial, the isochrones deviate over the crista terminalis, indicating preferential conduction in that region. [Reproduced with permission from reference 448.]

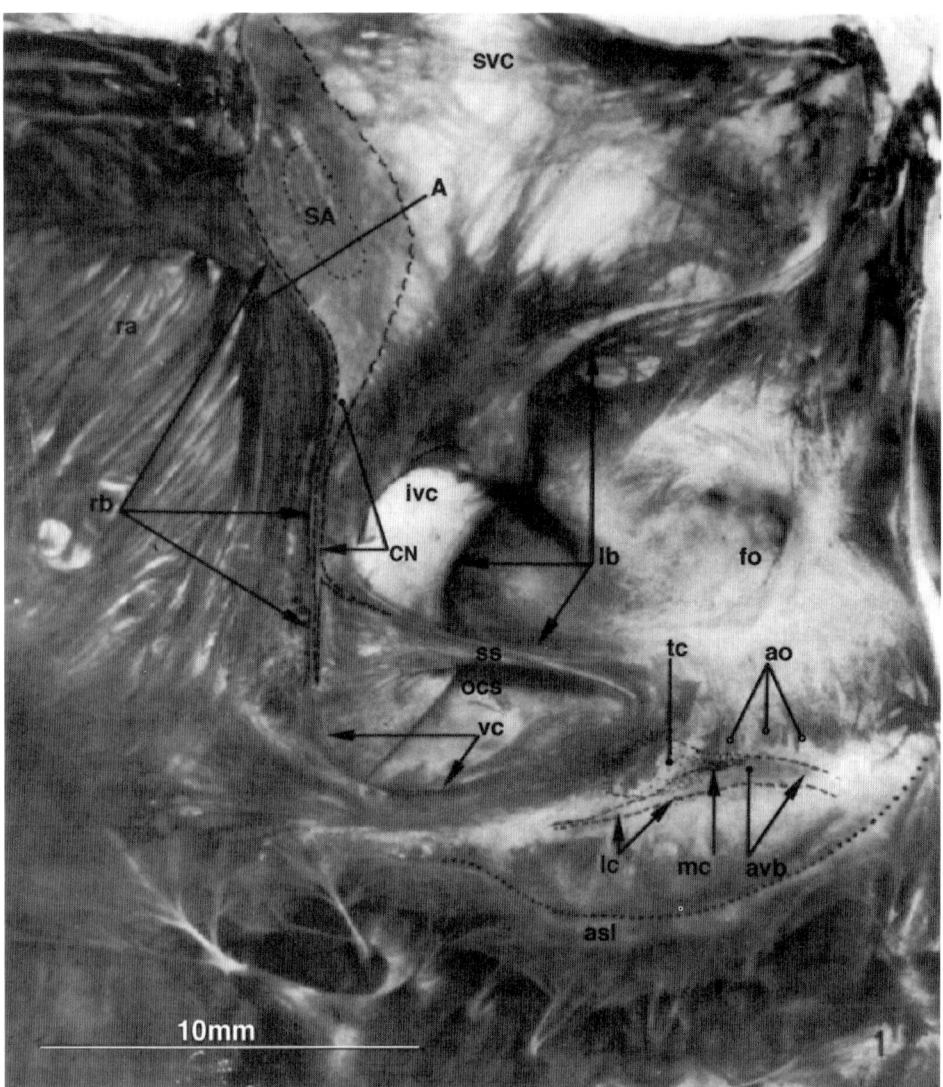

FIG. 12-27. Anatomy of the rabbit right atrium. The contrast of the preparation has been enhanced by supravital staining with methylene blue: *ct*, cut ends of the crista terminalis; *ra*, right auricle; *fo*, fossa ovalis; *SVC*, superior vena cava; *ivc*, inferior vena cava; *ocs*, ostium of the coronary sinus; *vc*, valve of the coronary sinus; *ss*, sinus septum; *asl*, attachment of the septal tricuspid leaflet (marked by a dotted line); *SA*, sinoatrial node (the letters inside surrounded by a dotted line indicate the approximate area of the compact node consisting of typical nodal cells); *CN*, cauda of the sinoatrial node; *rb*, right branch of the sinoatrial right bundle; *lb*, left (septal) branch of the sinoatrial ring bundle; *tc*, transitional cell zone of the atrioventricular node; *mc*, midnodal cells; *lc*, lower nodal cells; *avb*, atrioventricular bundle; *ao*, atrial overlay fibers. [Reproduced with permission from reference 449.]

(168) emphasized that the excitatory wave from the atrium can use two main routes to excite the atria: the interauricular band (Bachmann's bundle), which connects the sinus node area to the left atrium, and the crista terminalis which runs down the right atrium and also through the interatrial septum toward the AV node. They also observed that following interruption of one or both of these main pathways, P-wave morphology in the electrocardiogram altered, but, owing to the numerous other connections of the sinus node to the atrial myocardium, the atria could still be activated. From the many subsequent studies in which atrial activation was mapped (144, 169–177), it emerged that internodal conduction followed routes indicated by gross anatomical landmarks. The crista terminalis and the anterior limbus of the fossa ovalis are the main routes for preferential conduction between the sinus node and the atrioventricular node, and these prominent muscle bands provide a dual input into the AV node. A similar activation sequence as that shown

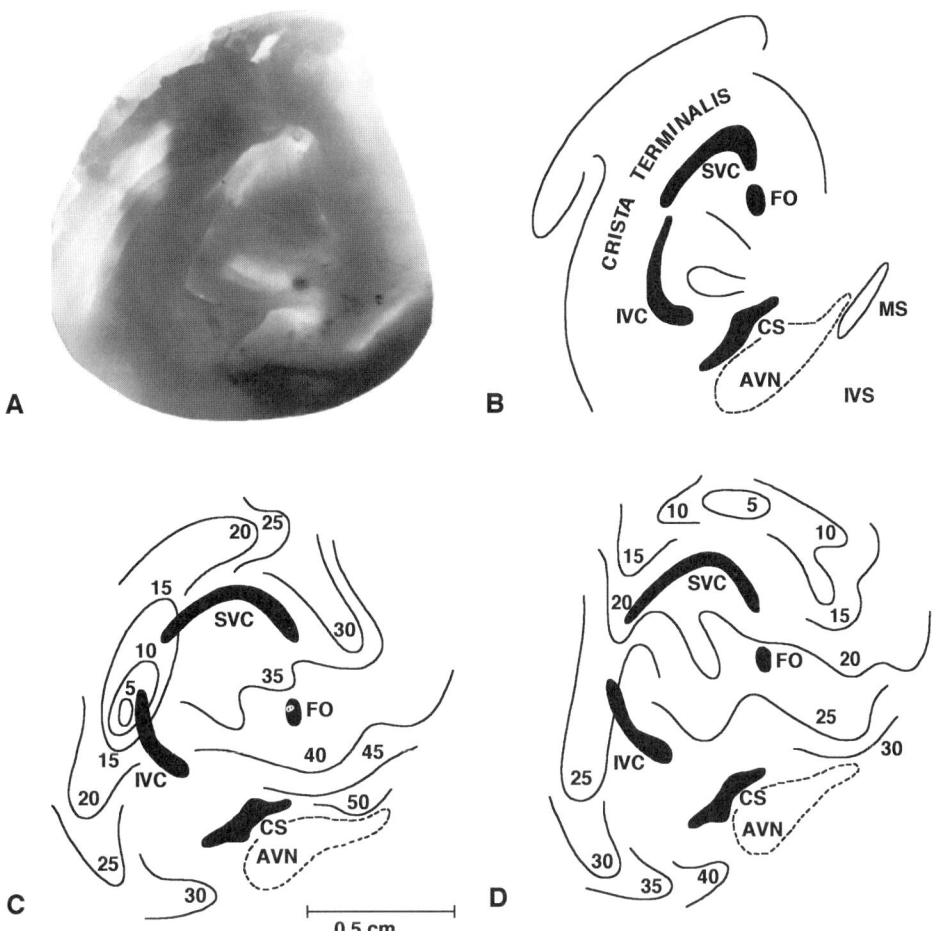

FIG. 12–28. Activation sequence in the right atrium. *A:* A photograph of the right atrium of a rabbit: the activation sequence has been mapped using a tenfold microelectrode assembly, with which 280 different atrial cells have been impaled during the course of the experiment. The specimen was opened by an incision along the lateral margin of the tricuspid valve, and pinned out in order not to interrupt the internodal tissues. After the experiment, the preparation was fixed before being photographed. The specimen is illuminated from behind to illustrate the thick and thin parts of the myocardium. *B:* A diagrammatic representation, in which the abbreviations are as follows: *SVC*, superior vena cava; *IVC*, inferior vena cava; *FO*, fossa ovalis; *CS*, coronary sinus; *AVN*, atrioventricular node; *MS*, membranous septum; *IVS*, interventricular septum; *C* and *D:* Activation maps made according to photographs taken while the preparation was in the tissue bath—hence the slight differences in shape when compared to the fixed specimen. The preparation was beating spontaneously for the construction of (C); in (D), the preparation was paced through an electrode placed above the ostium of the SVC. In both instances, the activation sequence, indicated by isochrone lines separating areas activated within 5 msec intervals, follows the thicker muscle bundles. These are the crista terminalis, the septal branch of the crista, and the thick muscle ridge between IVC and FO. The AV node receives a dual input. The localization of the pacemaker determines the dominant input. In *C*, during spontaneous sinus rhythm, the AV node is reached earliest by the posterior route. In *D* during driving from the SVC, the anterior limbus activates the AV node earlier. [Reproduced with permission from reference 176.]

in Figure 12–28 for the isolated rabbit heart was found during surgery in the human heart (177). Here also, the AV node receives a dual input. In most patients, the anterior septal input was activated some 10 msec prior to the posterior input via the crista terminalis (cf. Fig. 12–28D). In patients with a low crista terminalis pacemaker (cf. Fig. 12–28C), the atrioventricular node was activated via the crista terminalis 15–20 msec before activation of the anterior input. The importance of these dual inputs for atrioventricular nodal reentry is discussed later, under CIRCULATING EXCITATION, REENTRY AND SPIRAL WAVES.

From the time the sinus node and AV node were discovered, there has been a controversy regarding the questions of whether specialized internodal pathways connect both nodes and are responsible for preferential conduction along such pathways, or whether spread of excitation occurs through "ordinary" atrial myocardium. With reference to an earlier review (176), it is our view that morphologically discrete tracts of specialized cells that connect SA node to AV node have yet to be demonstrated. It is possible that single, morphologically "specialized" cells are scattered between ordinary atrial cells, and one paper describes five different species of such specialized atrial cells (178). Their role in determining conduction between the nodes is unclear. It is true that action potentials of different configuration can be recorded in the atrium, one with a distinct plateau and one without a plateau. In one study in which the very cells from which transmembrane potentials had been recorded were histologically and ultrastructurally identified, both types of action potentials were found to originate from ordinary atrial cells (179). This finding does not rule out the possibility that morphologically nonspecialized cells may produce "specialized" action potentials. However, differences in cellular coupling may explain why some atrial cells have long action potentials with a plateau and others have short, triangular action potentials. In a large bundle of well coupled fibers arranged in parallel, electrotonic current flow from depolarized cells upstream tends to prolong the action potentials downstream. This electrotonic current may not be present to the same degree in structures where cells are poorly coupled, or in cells close to the boundaries of the atrium. At this time, the controversy regarding specialized atrial pathways seems largely semantic. In our view, the preferential conduction of the atrial impulse along certain routes can adequately be explained by the architecture of the atria and the orientation of normal atrial cells.

During sinus rhythm, the left atrium is activated via the interatrial band (Bachmann's bundle). A typical feature of left atrial activation is that different wavefronts simultaneously proceed in multiple directions and that wavefronts frequently collide (171). In a study on atrial activation of the horse, it was said that the explanation for the "chaotic pattern of left atrial activation may be that the two great pulmonary veins break the left atrial surface into discontinuous islets in which no general front of depolarization can develop" (172). The major portion of the left atrium depolarizes after right atrial excitation has been completed. The last parts to be activated are the left atrial appendage and the posteroinferior part near the left inferior pulmonary vein. In the canine heart, atrial activation is completed in approximately 60 msec, in the isolated human heart after 90–100 msec (169, 171, 173).

During retrograde atrial activation, studied while pacing the ventricles at a rate higher than the sinus rate, the pattern of left atrial excitation is similar to that during sinus rhythm (173, 174, 180–182). The retrograde wavefront quickly spreads up the interatrial septum to emerge very early at Bachmann's bundle. Activation then proceeds over this bundle to activate the left atrium in much the same way as during sinus rhythm. When the atrium is paced from the posteroinferior left atrium or from a site just posterior to the ostium of the coronary sinus, Bachmann's bundle is activated late, and P-waves in leads I, III, and avF were negative. When Bachmann's bundle was activated early, as during ventricular pacing or pacing from an atrial site anterior to the coronary sinus, P-waves were positive (180, 182). The time of arrival of a retrograde wavefront at Bachmann's bundle is therefore critical in determining the polarity of a "retrograde" P wave.

The Atrioventricular Junction. The anatomical and histologic arrangement of the specialized atrioventricular junctional area is very complex (183). The atrial components of the junction are contained within the triangle of Koch, as shown for the human heart in Figure 12–29. The triangle is delimited by the tendon of Todaro, the attachment of the septal leaflet of the tricuspid valve, and by the ostium of the coronary sinus. Atrial fibers impinge upon the triangle of Koch from four main areas, as schematically shown in Figure 12–30. The first input is beneath the floor of the coronary sinus in the posterior part of the triangle, the second is from the anterior atrial wall in front of the fossa ovalis, the third is from the sinus septum, the musculature between the coronary sinus and the fossa ovalis. A fourth input, which is almost always neglected, involves the left side of the atrial septum. As emphasized by Scherf and Cohen (184) the atrioventricular node is an interatrial rather than a right atrial structure. In 1906, Tougher described a spindle-shaped compact network of small cells in the anterior part of Koch's triangle (185). These cells were connected via *Knotenpunkte* in which four or five fibers were often joined together. It was this characteristic that prompted him "for simplicity's sake" to call this compact network *Knoten* (node). Nowadays, this part of the AV junction is usually called the compact node. Tawara emphasized that there is a large variability between species: "the network in the human is relatively small, but it may in individual cases be very different" (p. 150). In studies performed in rabbit hearts, these cells have also been named midnodal cells: small, spherical, tightly packed cells without much connective tissue between them (186). In the human heart, the compact node often divides into two strands that run posteriorly toward the attachments of the leaflets of the mitral and tricuspid valves. The compact node is surrounded by transitional cells. Although

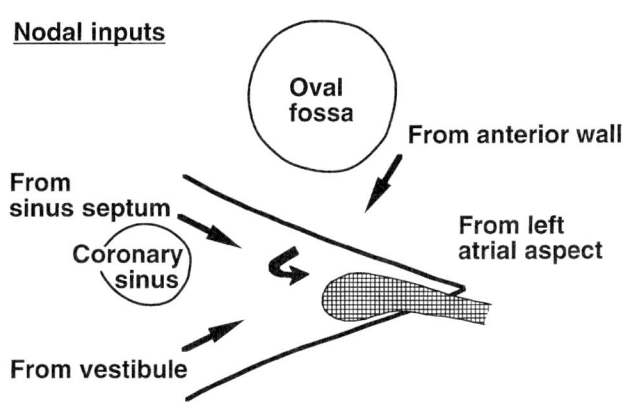

FIG. 12–30. Propagation toward the AV node. Arrows indicate the four areas from which atrial fibers approach the specialized AV junctional area. The fourth area, indicated by the curved arrow, is from the left atrial aspect of the septum. [Reproduced with permission from reference 183.]

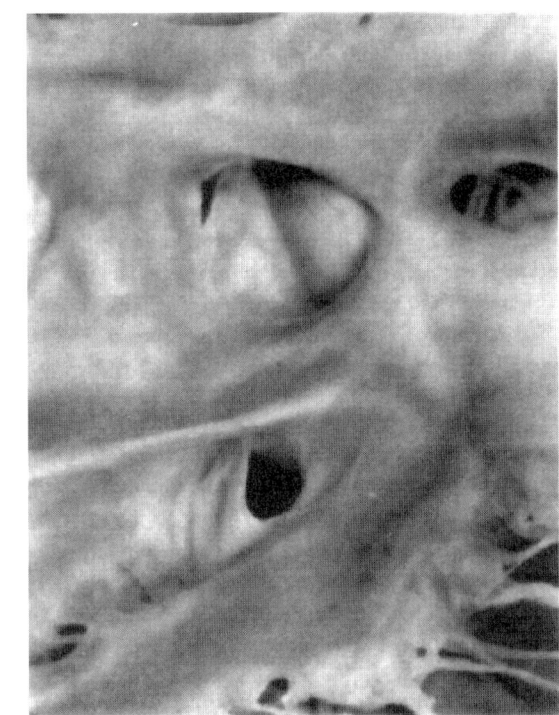

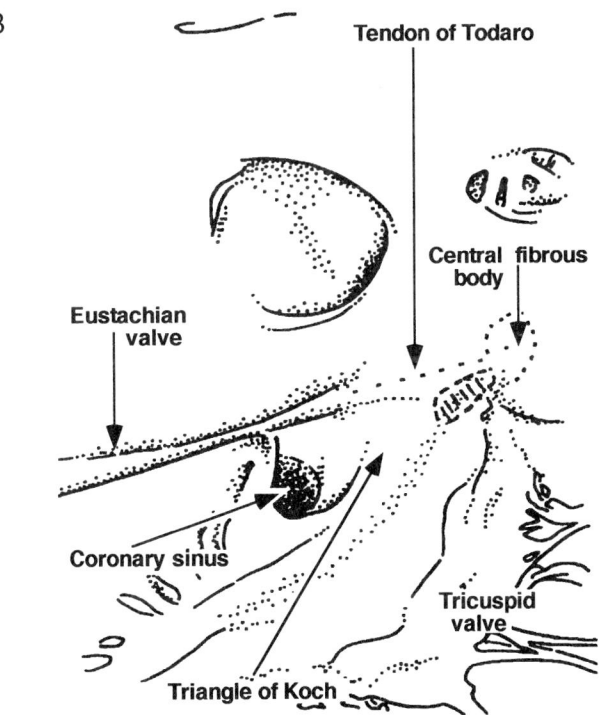

FIG. 12–29. Anatomy of the AV junction. *A*: Photograph and *B* sketch of a normal human heart showing the anatomical landmarks of the triangle of Koch. The approximate site of the compact AV node is indicated by the stippled area adjacent to the central fibrous body. [Reproduced with permission from reference 183.]

Tawara did not use the term transitional cell, he wrote that between the compact node and the atrial musculature "the cells are very small. They do not form a complicated network, but course more or less parallel to the posterior part. They are joined into several small bundles, separated by strands of connective tissue, which in this area is abundant" (p. 136). "These bundles are connected to atrial muscle. . . . these connections are so gradual that no sharp boundaries can be detected. . . . Either single cells become gradually larger and change inconspicuously into atrial fibers, or several small bundles gradually join into a broader bundle which then merges with atrial muscle" (p. 137).

Similar descriptions were given by later authors (186, 187). There is room for confusion when speaking about the atrioventricular (AV) node because some authors mean by this the compact node only, others the whole area occupied by compact node and transitional cells. It is of interest to note that Tawara was unable to determine precisely where the atrium ended and the specialised AV nodal region begins, because of the gradual change from atrial to transitional cells, as were subsequent investigators (186, 188, 189). Perhaps terms like "AV nodal area" or "specialized AV junctional area" are to be preferred over "AV node." Some atrial fibers from the anterior wall pass directly across the compact node as so-called overlay fibers and run down into the attachment of the septal leaflet of the tricuspid valve. The transitional cells are the continuation of the four atrial approaches. When traced anteriorly, the compact node, without any perceptible change in cellular configuration, enters the central fibrous body. This point marks the transition from the compact node to the penetrating atrioventricular bundle, or bundle of His. In the rabbit heart, the midnodal cells of the compact node make contact with larger, so-called lower nodal cells, which are arranged in parallel and continue anteriorly as the penetrating AV bundle. Tawara noted that at the point of entry in the central fibrous body, typical nodal cells were interspersed with larger His bundle cells. Again, on a histologic basis he could not tell where the AV node ended and the His bundle began. "I set the boundary at the site where this system penetrates into the membranous septum" (p. 127; all quotations from Tawara are in our translation).

As in the sinus node, intercellular connections in the AV node are scarce. Classical intercalated disks were not observed in several species (190–192). However, desmosomes, fasciae adherentes, and gap junctions often appear as a junctional complex (191, 192). The length and percentage of the plasma membrane occupied by these junctions decease progressively from transitional cells to superficial cells of the midnodal area and then increase progressively from deep midnodal cells to the AV bundle (191).

Correlation between cellular electrophysiology and structure. Based on the characteristics of transmembrane potentials recorded with microelectrodes in isolated superfused preparations of rabbit hearts, Paes de Carvalho and de Almeida divided the AV nodal area into three zones, and since then, their terms AN (atrionodal), N (nodal), and NH (nodal-His) cells or zones have been widely used (188). N cells had action potentials with low amplitudes and upstroke velocities, the AN zone was a transitional zone between fast conducting atrial tissue and the slowly conducting N zone, and the NH zone was a transitional zone between the N zone and the His bundle, where conduction became rapid and action potential upstroke velocity was high. Billette (193) refined this classification based on action potential configuration, activation times and changes during premature atrial stimulation (see Fig. 12–31). He distinguished between AN, ANCO (AN cells with an action potential upstroke that had two components), ANL (late AN), N, NH, and H (His bundle) cells. The timing of the upstroke of AN cells with respect to an atrial potential did not change during atrial premature stimulation. ANCO cells had a similar timing, but a lower action potential upstroke velocity and a notch on the upstroke. Late AN cells had a still lower upstroke velocity, but the lowest values were found in the N cells, which also had low resting membrane potentials. During premature atrial stimulation, action potential amplitude of the N cells markedly decreased and the response dissociated into two components. Activation times of the first component were linked to those of AN, ANCO, and ANL cells, all of which increased, if at all, only slightly with premature stimulation. In contrast, activation of the NH cells markedly increased with prematurity, and the upstroke of NH cell action potentials was linked to the second component of the N potentials.

Several studies have attempted to localize the tip of the recording microelectrode in isolated rabbit preparations and to correlate cellular electrophysiology to structure (179, 194–196). In general, it can be said that AN potentials were recorded from transitional cells and NH potentials from the tract of lower nodal cells in continuity with the His bundle. N potentials were recorded from the central AV node, and could originate both from transitional cells and from cells in the beginning of the AV bundle. In a recent study in isolated, arterially perfused canine and porcine hearts, (197) it was found that cells with N type action potentials were not confined to the triangle of Koch, but extended along both AV orifices. These cells had low resting membrane potentials between −55 and −65 mV, a maximum upstroke velocity lower than 5 V/sec, a low action potential amplitude between 45 and 65 mV, and they responded to the administration of adenosine by a further reduction of action potential amplitude and upstroke velocity. Histologically, these cells were similar to atrial cells, but they lacked Cx43. This study raises questions about how to define the AV nodal region. It cannot be defined as the region where AN-, and N-types of action potentials are found, because cells with similar action potentials are present around the entire tricuspid and mitral annuli. Nor does it appear that light microscopy is accurate in defining this region, because cells similar to atrial cells may have nodal type action potentials.

It must be emphasized that almost all studies employing microelectrodes have been performed in isolated, superfused rabbit heart preparations. In such preparations, hypoxic cell damage may be present at depths below 100 to 150 µm (143), and it is possible that this influences the electrophysiologic characteristics of more superficial cells.

Activation patterns of the AV nodal area. Mapping the spread of excitation in the triangle of Koch by extracellular recordings is very difficult, because the rate of change in the extracellular potentials may be very slow, because extracellular potentials may have multiple deflections, and because activation of the central AV nodal area is a three-dimensional event where slow, low-amplitude action potentials in deep layers may not generate extracellular potentials of sufficient amplitude to be recorded by surface electrodes. There are only two studies in which intra-cellular and extracellular recordings have been made simultaneously, and their results with respect to the cause of extracellular potentials with double components differ. In a study on superfused rabbit and canine preparations (175), where extracellular waveforms with multiple deflections were

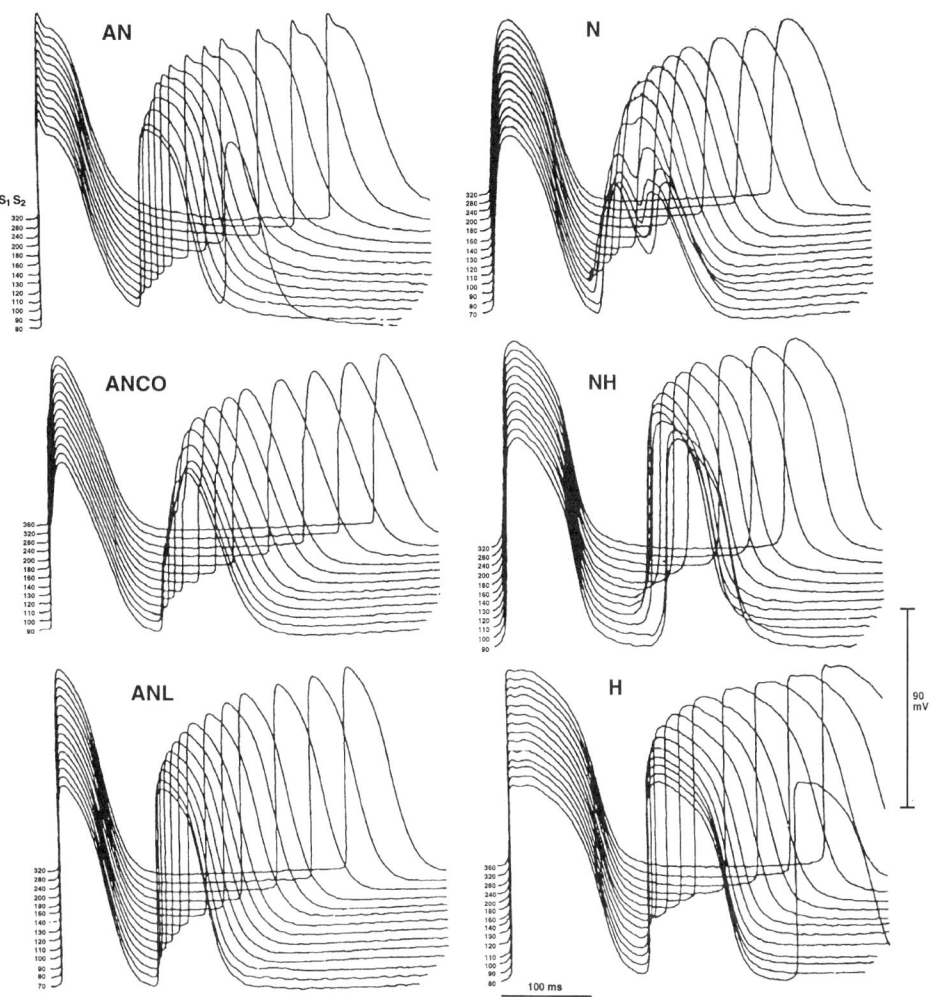

FIG. 12-31. Action potential characteristics in the AV node: Action potentials of six types of AV nodal cells during periodic premature stimulation of the right atrium. Each section was obtained by superimposing (in decreasing order of coupling stimulation intervals [numbers at left in msec]) tracings corresponding to last basic and premature beat. Baseline of each subsequent tracing was shifted downward to help distinguish potentials. Action potential after premature potential in lower trace in *AN* (atrionodal) and *H* (His) was caused by an atrial re-entrant beat. Note double components in *N* (nodal) cell of early premature responses. *ANL*, late AN cells; *ANCO*, AN cells with action potential upstroke with two components. [Reproduced with permission from reference 193.]

found at the posterior approach to the AV node, the initial rapid deflection corresponded to the action potential upstroke of superficial atrial cells, the second, usually slower deflection originated from underlying nodal cells. In a study on arterially, blood-perfused canine and porcine hearts, the initial rapid deflection originated from deep atrial cells, the second slow deflection from more superficial nodal cells (198).

Activation maps based on microelectrode recordings are only available for the superfused rabbit heart preparation (188, 193, 199–202). Figure 12-32 shows such a map, where each circle indicates a site where a transmembrane potential was recorded. The activation sequence is depicted in 20 msec intervals, with time zero being the activation time of a site close to the sinus node. The main features of the activation sequence are (1) there is a dual input into the AV nodal region, a posterior one via the crista terminalis and an anterior one in front of the ostium of the coronary sinus; (2) in the central part of Koch's triangle, the activation pattern is complex and isochronal lines cannot be drawn. This is so in part because at one location superficial cells may be excited up to 40 msec earlier than deeper cells. The speed of propagation is slow; it takes some 60 msec to cover a distance of about 1 mm, which corresponds to a conduction velocity in the order of 1.7 cm/sec.; (3) in the last part to be activated (at 90 to 110 msec), activation is rapid and synchronous.

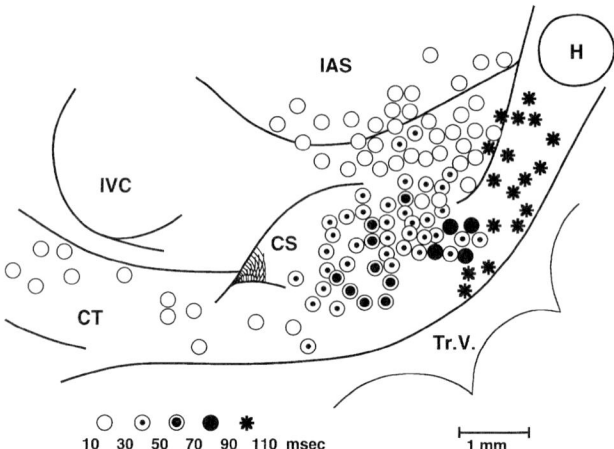

FIG. 12–32. Activation of the AV node. Map showing sequence of normal antegrade conduction of rabbit AV node. Symbols indicate position of AV nodal cells from which action potentials were recorded and also in which 20 msec interval these cells were activated. Note dual input into AV node. *CT*, crista terminalis; *IAS*, interatrial septum; *CS*, ostium of coronary sinus; *Tr. V.*, tricuspid valve; *H*, position of extracellular electrode on His bundle. [Reproduced with permission from reference 200.]

There is a sharp demarcation between cells activated early and cells activated late. The anterior input does not bypass the central node but curves posteriorly to merge with the posterior input.

One feature not apparent from Figure 12–32 is the existence of "dead-end pathways." These consist of cells that do not participate in transmitting the impulse from atria to ventricles and vice versa. They can be identified by expressing their moment of excitation as a percentage of the atrium-His bundle and His bundle-atrium conduction time during anterograde and retrograde conduction, respectively. The sum of these times for a cell in the nodal mainstream is around 100%. For dead-end pathway cells, this sum far exceeds 100%, indicating that they are activated "too late" in both modes of conduction. One type of dead-end pathway consists of atrial overlay fibers terminating in the base of the septal leaflet of the tricuspid valve, another dead-end pathway branches off the central node and extends posteriorly along the tricuspid orifice (194, 201).

It is now customary to equate the posterior and anterior inputs to the so-called slow and fast AV nodal pathways, which are thought to underlie AV nodal reentrant tachycardia (for reviews see (183, 203, 204). The evidence for the existence of slow and fast pathways stems from a number of observations. As early as 1913, Mines described what he called a reciprocating rhythm after electrical stimulation of the "auricle-ventricle preparation" of the electric ray. He reasoned that the AV connection had two divisions with a slight difference in the rate of recovery. A premature stimulus delivered to the ventricle "should spread up to the auricle by that part of the A-V connection having the quicker recovery process and not by the other part. In such a case, when the auricle would be excited by this impulse, the other portion of the A-V connection would be ready to take up the transmission again back to the ventricle. Provided the transmission in each direction was slow, the chamber at either end would be ready to respond (its refractory phase being short) and thus the condition once established would tend to continue, unless upset by the interpolation of a premature systole" (205). A similar explanation was given two years later by White, who described a clinical case where, during AV dissociation, idioventricular beats were sometimes conducted back to the atria, and the retrograde inverted P wave was followed by a narrow QRS complex (206). In 1926, Scherf and Shookhoff studied reciprocating rhythms in dogs and introduced the term "longitudinal dissociation" (207). Rosenblueth in 1958 introduced the term "ventricular echo," and Moe at al. in 1956 suggested "dual AV transmission" (208, 209). Reciprocation in the other direction, where an atrial premature impulse turns back in the AV node to reexcite the atria as an echo was also described (210). When catheters were used for intracardiac recording and stimulation in patients, many studies reported on the induction of both atrial and ventricular echoes by premature stimulation in hearts without apparent AV conduction abnormalities, so that functional longitudinal dissociation was considered to be a property of the normal AV node (210–214). Animal studies supported this conclusion (208, 215, 216). In some animal studies, it was possible, if only occasionally, to induce repetitive reciprocation leading to reentrant tachycardia (217–220), but in humans with normal AV nodal function this was not observed. In patients with spontaneous AV nodal re-entrant tachycardias, this arrhythmia could easily be induced by premature stimulation (211, 214, 221). A key factor thought to indicate the presence of dual AV nodal pathways is the so-called discontinuity in the AV conduction curve during premature atrial stimulation, which can be demonstrated both in individuals without spontaneous tachycardias (222, 223) and in patients with tachycardias (224). During atrial premature stimulation, the interval between the premature atrial response and subsequent His bundle deflection (the A2–H2 interval) gradually prolongs with increasing prematurity, until at a certain coupling interval it abruptly increases and then continues to increase gradually. The explanation is that with moderate prematurity AV conduction proceeds over a fast pathway that has a long refractory period; when at a certain coupling interval the fast pathway is refractory, AV conduction now occurs via the slow pathway having a shorter refractory period, hence the abrupt "jump" in the AV conduction curve. Presumably, the same pathways are used for both "atrio-ventricular" and for "ventriculo-atrial" conduction. During ventricular stimulation, the atrial exits of slow and fast pathways in humans roughly correspond to the posterior and anterior inputs found in animal experiments (225, 226). These findings form the basis for the successful surgical or catheter ablation of either fast or slow pathway to cure AV nodal re-entrant tachycardias (227–230). There are as yet insufficient data to link clinical experience to mapping experiments in animals. There is evidence that more than two AV nodal pathways may exist (for review see (203). The possibility exists that the tissue in the posterior approach to the compact AV node, having "nodal" electrophysiological properties and histologically resembling atrial cells, is the substrate of the slow pathway (197). No anatomical abnormalities have been detected in the AV nodal region of patients with proven dual AV nodal pathways (231), and it is as yet unknown which features distinguish hearts with "normal" dual AV pathways and hearts with "abnormal" dual AV pathways that are prone to sustained re-entry.

In isolated hearts, it was demonstrated that the re-entrant pathway during ventricular echo beats was confined to the compact node. In these hearts, there was no "jump" in the VA conduction curve during premature stimulation of the ventricle or the right bundle branch (232). It is, however, by no means certain that in sustained AV nodal re-entry the same re-entrant circuit is used as for single ventricular echo beats. In the rabbit heart, a posterior nodal extension has been described that forms a cycle length-dependent slow pathway with a shorter refractory period than that of the compact node (233). Single atrial echo beats in the isolated superfused rabbit hearts preparation could reproducibly be induced, and perinodal activation was involved in the re-entrant circuit. Ablation of the posterior nodal extension abolished reentry (234). In a recently published book (235), Zipes described the AV node in terms of Winston Churchill: "a riddle wrapped in a mystery inside an enigma" (236). In that book, dual pathway electrophysiology is reviewed by Mazgalev and Tschou (237). It was emphasized that there were no specialized atrionodal tracts and that fast and slow pathways are not cable-like structures similar to the right bundle branch. Rather, "the nonuniform anisotropy of the atrial approaches, the specific architecture of the triangle of Koch, the presence of two or more conduction layers with different functional properties, and the overall functional heterogeneity of the AV node are factors that may contribute to the formation of distinct and interacting wavefronts of propagation" (237).

Factors that cause AV nodal delay. There is no single factor responsible for the slowing of the cardiac impulse as it traverses the AV nodal area. Various geometrical factors, such as the small size of AV nodal cells, the paucity of intercellular connections, and the complex network of small bundles separated by connective tissue where summation and collision of impulses occur, play a role in addition to the role of the calcium inward current, which is the dominant current depolarizing nodal cells.

Conduction velocity in a linear cable is proportional to the square root of fiber diameter. Given a fiber diameter of Purkinje fibers of 50 µm, and of 7 µm for an AV nodal cell, the ratio of conduction velocities of both tissues would be 2.7, if fiber diameter were the only determinant. In fact, the ratio is much larger, conduction velocity in Purkinje fibers being in the order of meters per second, and that in the N zone being less than 5 cm/sec. Several studies have attempted to determine space constants in the AV node (238–241). In general, data were analyzed by assuming that the node had a negligible extracellular resistance and behaved as a cable. Sometimes, a more complex analysis was used, based on a two-dimensional regular lattice (239) or a two-dimensional model of anisotropic syncytium (238). Given the complex three-dimensional structure of the AV nodal region, it is clear, as the authors themselves realized, that the analysis is based on oversimplification of tissue geometry. Nevertheless, the values reported for the AN zone (ranging from 210 µm to 690 µm) and the N zone (176 µm ± 55 µm) are lower than those reported for other cardiac tissues. Measurements have almost always been made in superfused preparations where the large volume of extracellular fluid acts as an extracellular shunt resistance. In densely packed tissue, extracellular resistance has a value similar to intracellular resistance, and the space constant of arterially perfused papillary muscle is 357 µm, as compared to 528 µm in superfused tissue (32). It may therefore be assumed that in the intact heart, the space constant of the densely packed compact node, where extracellular resistance is certainly not zero, is much smaller than the values quoted above. It is therefore not possible to quantify the effect of the high coupling resistance on conduction velocity in the AV node. Assuming that extracellular resistance in the compact node is similar to that in arterially perfused ventricular muscle, and that intracellular resistance is higher by a factor of ten, conduction velocity in the node would be about three times less than that in ventricular muscle, i.e. in the order of 20 cm/sec, which is still about ten times that of the lowest values found in the N zone.

Summation of impulses, arriving more or less simultaneously over converging pathways, appears to play an important role in AV conduction (242–245).

Figure 12-33 shows microelectrode recordings from the AV node of a Langendorff, blood-perfused canine heart. Premature stimuli with the same coupling interval were applied alternatively to the posterior and anterior inputs. The premature impulse from the anterior input was blocked, while the one from the posterior input was conducted to the His bundle. Because the impulses arrived at the same moment at the cells recorded from, whether the anterior or the posterior input was stimulated, the level of excitability of the cells involved must have been the same in both situations. Apparently, the wavefront arriving via the anterior input provided less stimulating current than the posterior input. This may be equivalent to the concept that the anterior ("fast") pathway has a longer refractory period than the posterior ("slow") pathway.

Another example where AV nodal conduction delay was apparently caused by a combination of reduced excitability in the N zone and lack of summation of impulses traveling in anterior and posterior inputs is given in Figure 12-34 (200). Three action potentials were simultaneously recorded from the AV nodal area of an isolated rabbit heart preparation. The atrium was regularly stimulated at a cycle length of 192 msec, which produced a peculiar type of Wenckebach block, in which the conduction time of the second beat alternated between 140 msec and 160 msec in subsequent cycles of 3:2 block, while conduction time of the first beat of each cycle remained constant (120 msec). In the second cycle, the action potential of cell b occurred much later than that of cell a (while during the first cycle both cells were excited almost simultaneously), and activation of cell c was delayed and its upstroke was slower and more slurred than during the second beat of the first cycle. The diagram offers a tentative explanation. The impulse in the anterior input failed to reach the junction of both inputs. As a consequence, the wavefront arriving over the posterior input had to distribute excitatory current both to the distal common pathway (cell c), and in a retrograde direction to the anterior input (cell b). This led to retrograde propagation in the anterior input and to re-excitation of the atrium as an echo beat, as well as to delayed activation of cell c and the His bundle.

While there is no controversy about the notion that the calcium inward current plays a dominant role in depolarizing AV nodal cells, the question of whether N cells have no fast sodium channels at all, or whether they are merely inactivated by the low resting membrane potential has not been settled. Observations supporting the concept that N cells have no sodium channels are the following: (1) application of hyperpolarizing current to N cells did not cause an increase in the maximum upstroke velocity, or even decreased it (246, 247); (2) verapamil, D 600, and manganese ions suppressed action potentials in the N zone (248-250), whereas tetrodotoxin was without effect (248, 250, 251). There are, however other observations indicating that the action potential upstroke is due to a mixture of fast sodium current and slow calcium current, and that the relative contribution of the sodium current diminishes as one approaches the N zone. Thus, in several studies in intact preparations, hyperpolarizing currents did increased action potential amplitude and upstroke velocity in N cells (252, 253). Also, action potential upstrokes in AN and N cells often have two components, of which the first is depressed by tetrodotoxin, the second by magnesium ions (254). Voltage-clamp studies on very small pieces dis-

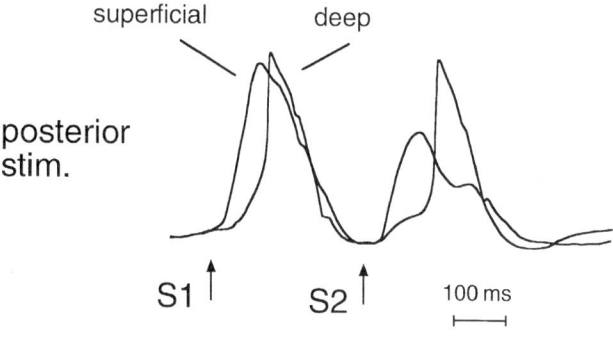

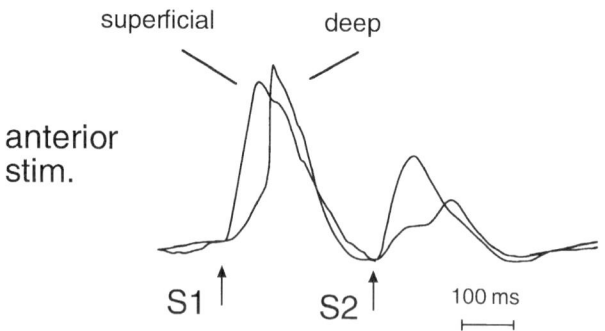

FIG. 12-33. Conduction in the AV node. Two simultaneously recorded transmembrane potentials from the AV node of a Langendorff blood-perfused canine heart at a superficial and a deep site at the same location. The atrium was paced at a basic cycle length of 600 msec, and a premature stimulus S_2 was applied at a coupling interval of 300 msec, either at the posterior input ("slow pathway," *upper panel*) or at the anterior input ("fast pathway," *lower panel*). Note double components, especially during premature stimulation, where the action potential of the superficial cell causes a slow prepotential in the deeper cell which during posterior stimulation is large enough to cause an action potential that is propagated to the His bundle (not shown), but that fails to reach threshold during antegrade stimulation. [Retraced from unpublished recordings by J. M. T. de Bakker.]

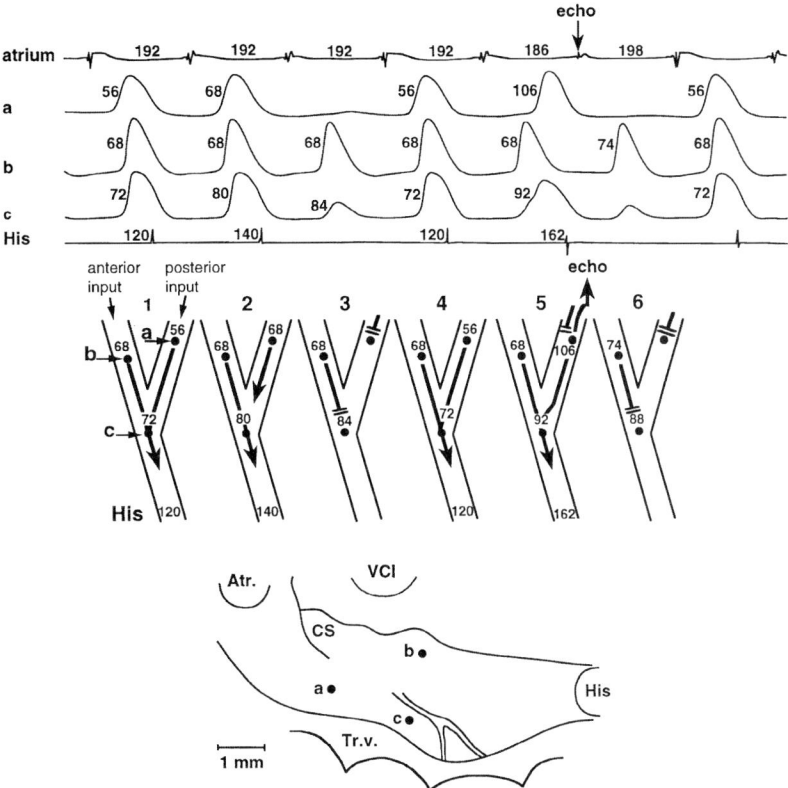

FIG. 12-34. Abnormal Wenckebach phenomenon. Three simultaneously recorded action potentials in posterior input (*cell a*), in anterior input (*cell b*), and in junctional area of these two inputs (*cell c*). Note the difference in timing and configuration of the action potentials of cells a and c and of the His bundle complex during the first and fifth beats. *Double bars* indicate block. Numbers are activation times in msec. *Atr.*, recording electrode on crista terminalis from which the electrogram in the upper trace was recorded. *His*, position of electrode recording electrogram of His bundle (*lower trace*). [Reproduced with permission from reference 200.]

sected from the AV node showed that hyperpolarization restored the availability of fast sodium channels (241).

As mentioned earlier, recovery from inactivation of the slow calcium inward current is slow in cells with low resting membrane potentials and may lag behind completion of repolarization (255). This may be an important factor in causing cycle-length-dependent conduction delay in the AV node. Figure 12–35 shows selected action potentials from the AV nodal area during application of five successive premature atrial stimuli at progressively shorter coupling intervals (199). The key feature of these recordings is that with prolongation of the atrium-His bundle conduction time, the action potential upstrokes of the cells in the N region separate into two components. The first component coincides with the upstroke of the latest activated AN cells, just proximal to the N cells; the second component, with the upstroke of earliest activated NH cells, just distal to the N zone. No action potentials were recorded with upstrokes occurring in between these two components. The cycle-length-dependent delay occurred within the small N zone, and instead of being caused by a progressive slowing of continuous propagation, it appeared due to a local discontinuity of conduction. The ladder diagrams used in clinical electrocardiology should therefore be changed, as shown in Figure 12–36, to indicate the saltatory nature of the cycle-length-dependent conduction delay. The explanation given by Billette et al. was that the excitability of the N cells progressively diminished at short cycle lengths, so that at very short cycles the N cells acted as a purely passive barrier between late AN cells and early NH cells, capable only of transmitting electrotonic currents that would slowly bring the early NH cells to threshold. An alternative factor to consider is the role of tissue geometry. Very similar action potentials were found in computer simulation's in which premature impulses arrived over a narrow strand inserting into a large tissue mass (72, 256). A particular role in AV-nodal conduction may be played by the so-called dead-end pathways, as described earlier (see Fig. 12–

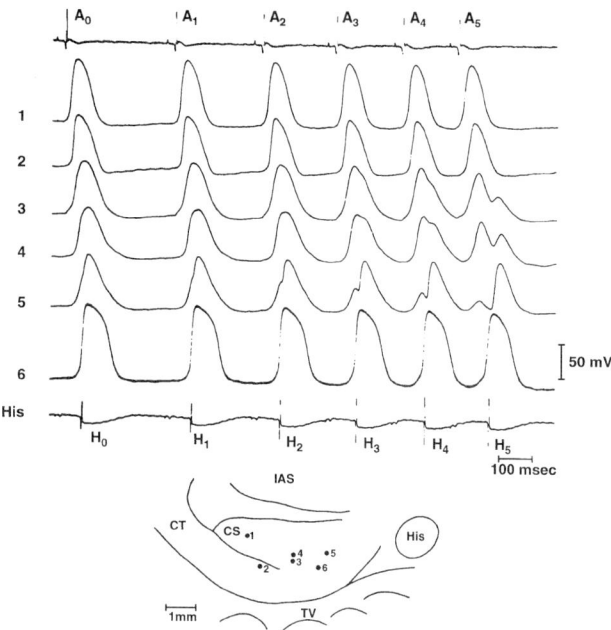

FIG. 12-35. Cycle length dependence of AV-nodal conduction. Action potentials illustrating dependency of first and second component in N cells upon late AN and early NH potentials. Signals 1 and 2 were recorded from AN cells, signals 3, 4, and 5 from N cells, and signal 6 from an NH cell. *Inset* shows position of cells. First component is largest in N cells close to AN zone; second component is largest in cells close to NH cells. Note that second component occurs later than upstrokes of action potentials in cell 6. Note also that duration of prepotential in cell 6 increases progressively in successive activation and that level at which prepotential breaks into a fast upstroke remains constant in all cycle lengths. Cells 4, 5, and 6 were recorded simultaneously. Cells 1, 2, and 3 were recorded separately, approximately 3 min earlier. [Reproduced with permission from reference 199.]

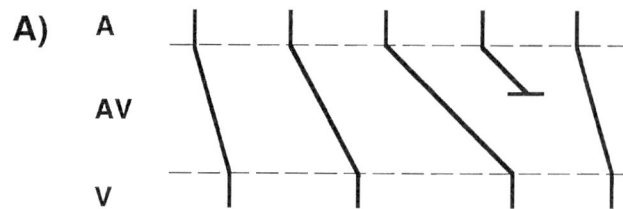

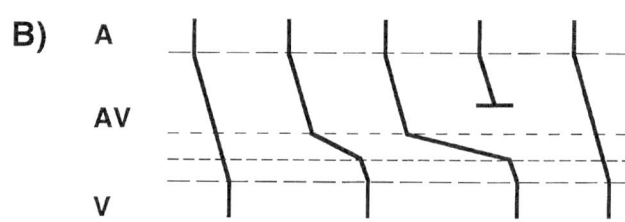

FIG. 12-36. Cycle length dependence of AV nodal conduction. *A*: Classical ladder diagram used in electrocardiography to depict cycle length-dependent conduction delay in the AV junction, in this case during a 4:3 Wenkenbach phenomenon. *B*: Modification of the ladder diagram to express saltatory nature of the cycle length-dependent conduction delay.

32). The effects of such pathways, i.e. blindly ending extensions of the N-region, on propagation was recently shown in patterned cell cultures (2). It was demonstrated that such pathways reduce propagation velocity of action potentials carried by $I_{Ca,L}$ from approximately 15 cm/sec in linear strands to approximately 2–4 cm/sec.

Activation of the Ventricles. In the mammalian heart, the impulse that has passed through the AV node reaches the ventricular myocardium by way of the specialized conduction system, consisting of the His bundle, the main right and left bundle branches, their fascicles, and the peripheral Purkinje network, which at discrete sites—the Purkinje–ventricular muscle junctions—is in contact with the ventricular myocardium. Proximal to the Purkinje–muscle junctions, the specialized conduction system has no functional connections to the ventricular myocardium because it is isolated from it by a thin collagenous sheet (257). Conduction velocity in the bundle branches is high, in the order of 2 m/sec (258).

There is a large variability in the distribution of the main branches of the specialized conduction system, both between species and between individual hearts within a given species. (259, 260). It is often assumed that the main left bundle branch in its course below the membranous part of the interventricular septum splits into two divisions: the anterior and posterior fascicles. As shown in Figure 12-37 (259), in a number of hearts there is a more or less separate middle fascicle occupying the left midseptal area. This "septal fascicle" was first described in 1906 by Tawara for the human heart. In isolated, Langendorff-perfused human hearts, three distinct areas of initial myocardial activation have been found that correspond to the transition of these three fascicles into the peripheral Purkinje network (173), see Plate 10.

Because of the many connections between the main branches of the left-sided conduction system, only extensive lesions result in complete conduction block in the left bundle branch system (261). Depending on the extent of the lesions, and the pre-existing anatomy of the conduction system, many conduction disturbances exist, and they have not been completely explored (262). In clinical electrocardiography, a distinction is made between complete bundle branch block, incomplete bundle branch block, and fascicular block (263).

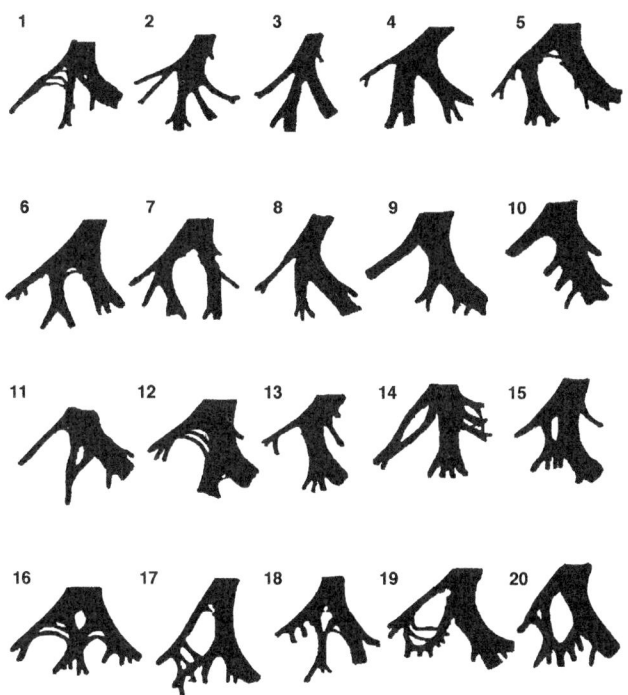

FIG. 12–37. Division of the left bundle branch. An illustration of the variation in the structure of the divisions of the left bundle branch in 20 different hearts. [Reproduced with permission from reference 259.]

The Purkinje–ventricular muscle junction. The junctions between the terminal Purkinje fibers and ventricular muscle (PV junctions) are electrophysiologically defined as sites where unipolar extracellular electrograms show a completely negative muscle deflection that is preceded by 2–5 msec by a Purkinje spike (264). At nonjunctional sites where both Purkinje and muscle deflections are found, the muscle deflection is characterized by initial positivity ("R wave"). Unidirectional block has been demonstrated to occur at PV junctions, where conduction is maintained from ventricular muscle to Purkinje fibers but fails in the opposite direction (265, 266). Mendez et al. (1970) proposed the "funnel" hypothesis to explain the PV delay, in which the "narrow portion would correspond to a terminal Purkinje fiber whose conical part would be composed of a progressively increasing number of interconnected muscle fibers" (266). In this view, the Purkinje network is seen as a branching cable, and at the PV junction the "terminal" Purkinje fiber has to provide excitatory current to a three-dimensional mass of myocardium. Joyner and co-workers (71, 264, 265, 267), using both computer simulations and extensive intracellular and extracellular recordings of endocardial activation, suggested that the Purkinje network is better represented by a two-dimensional sheet that is coupled at discrete sites to the deeper muscle mass. If coupling resistance at these sites is too low, the load that the large muscle mass imposes on the Purkinje sheet would prevent activation of the muscle. If coupling resistance is too high, the Purkinje network could not deliver sufficient excitatory current to activate the muscle. A certain resistive barrier between the two tissues allows rapid propagation in the Purkinje layer over the endocardial surface to synchronize ventricular activation, facilitates ventricular activation, and maintains a longer action potential duration in the Purkinje layer as compared to ventricular muscle (69, 71). Microelectrode studies by Alanis and co-workers (69, 71, 268, 269) suggested that the delay between Purkinje fiber and ventricular muscle was not due to slow conduction but to a "stop of the impulse in this region" (268). Action potentials recorded from PV junctional sites can be typical for Purkinje cells or ventricular muscle, or they can show upstrokes with multiple components. These latter action potentials were thought to arise from "transitional" cells (268–270). Early attempts to identify these transitional cells morphologically indicated that they are distinguished from both Purkinje and muscle fibers by having a smaller diameter (270, 271). In a more recent study, microelectrode recordings from the three different cell types at PV junctions in isolated superfused preparations of rabbit and pig hearts were obtained, and the cells recorded from were retrieved microscopically (272). Examples of extracellular recordings at PV junctions and of intracellular recordings of Purkinje fibers and transitional cells at these sites are shown in Figure 12–38. The interval between Purkinje and muscle deflection in the extracellular recording is not always isoelectric; sometimes distinct deflections caused by activity of transitional cells can be seen. The upstroke of the action potential of transitional cells typically shows a slow foot and a dissociation into two or more components. This feature is consistent with the view that propagation at the junction is discontinuous and is compatible with the existence of one or several resistive barriers between Purkinje and muscle. Transitional cells in the rabbit heart are thin, broad, bandlike cells (30–35 μm by 3–5 μm) arranged in one or two sheets in the subendocardium between the Purkinje layer and the ventricular mass. Transitional cells are coupled via short, thin strands to both Purkinje and ventricular muscle cells. Distances between Purkinje–transitional cell coupling sites and transitional cell–ventricular muscle coupling sites varied between 100 μm and 1000 μm. This arrangement is schematically depicted in Figure 12–39. This anatomical arrangement is in line with the concept of Joyner and co-workers, with one difference: In their concept, the transitional cell forms the high-resistance barrier between the sheet

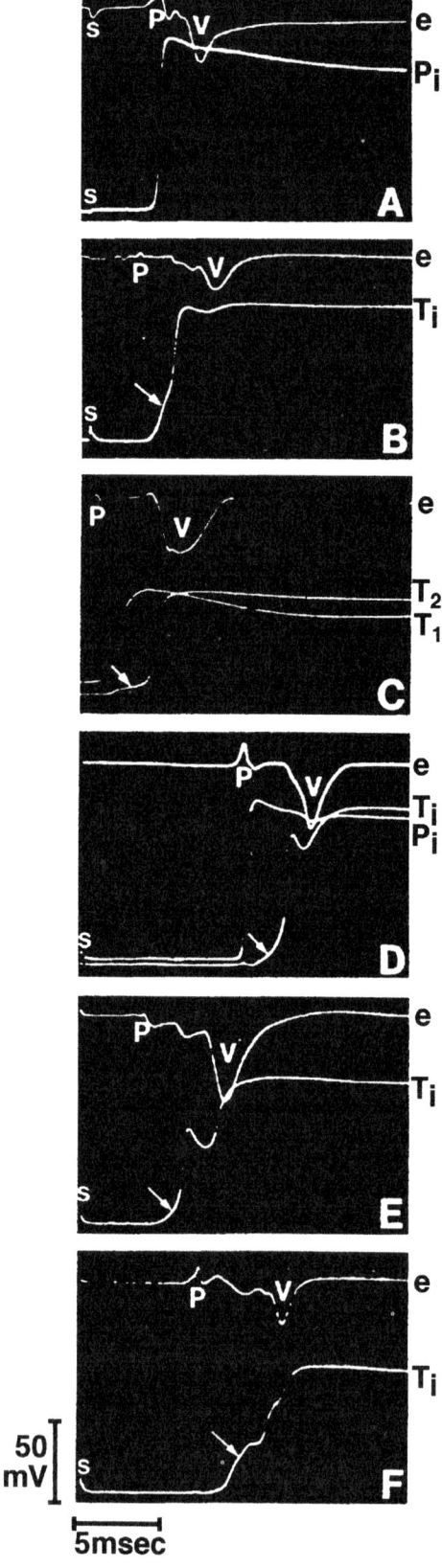

of Purkinje fibers and the ventricular muscle mass. In this structure the connections between the Purkinje fiber sheet and the sheet of transitional cells would be one resistive barrier; the thin connections between the transitional cells and the ventricular muscle mass would be a second barrier. Another type of PV coupling was observed frequently in the pig heart, but only rarely in the rabbit. Here, a short linear segment of small transitional cells connected large-diameter Purkinje cells to ventricular muscle cells. This arrangement would be compatible with the "funnel" hypothesis.

Left ventricular activation. After activation of the subendocardial myocardium by the specialized conducting system, excitation of the left ventricular wall in human and canine hearts occurs by myocardial conduction in an endocardial-to-epicardial direction, with a more or less concentric arrangement of isochrones (173, 273); see Plate 10. Epicardial breakthrough in the human left ventricle occurs almost simultaneously in anterior and posterior paraseptal areas located halfway between apex and base, after about 30 msec following onset of myocardial activation. Initial myocardial activation occurs on the endocardial surface of the septum, at anterior, midseptal, and posterior sites. The septum is largely activated in a left-to-right direction, although a small part of its structure is activated in the opposite direction by a wavefront originating at the lower right septal surface. The basal portions of the septum, particularly the posterior parts, are devoid of Purkinje fibers and are the last to be depolarized in the normal human heart. The papillary muscles are activated via false tendons, consisting mainly of Purkinje fibers, that run through the ventricular cavity from the septal surface to the apex of the anterior and posterior papillary muscles. From there, activation proceeds over the sheet of Purkinje fibers to excite the papillary muscles via the PV junctions at their base, nearly synchronous with the

FIG. 12–38. Propagation across the Purkinje–muscle junction. Intracellular and extracellular recordings at Purkinje–ventricular muscle junctional sites. *A:* Action potential of a Purkinje fiber (P_i), coinciding with the Purkinje (P) deflection preceding the all-negative ventricular muscle (V) deflection in the extracellular electrogram (e). s, Stimulus artifact. *B:* Action potential of a transitional cell (T_i), with an early slow component (arrow). *C: Simultaneous* intracellular recordings of an early (T_{1i}) and a late (T_{2i}) transitional cell. The latter could also be classified as an early ventricular cell that is electrotonically influenced from the transitional cells, giving rise to the long, slow foot (arrow). *D:* Simultaneous intracellular recordings of a Purkinje fiber and a transitional cell with a slow foot (arrow) and an inherent low amplitude that is heightened on activation of the ventricular mass. *E:* Intracellular recording from a transitional cell that coincides with a small deflection in the extracellular electrogram during the Purkinje fiber–ventricular muscle delay period. *F:* Intracellular recording of a transitional cell with multiple components during the upstroke (arrow). Panels A–C derive from rabbit hearts, and panels D–F derive from pig hearts. [Reproduced with permission from reference 272.]

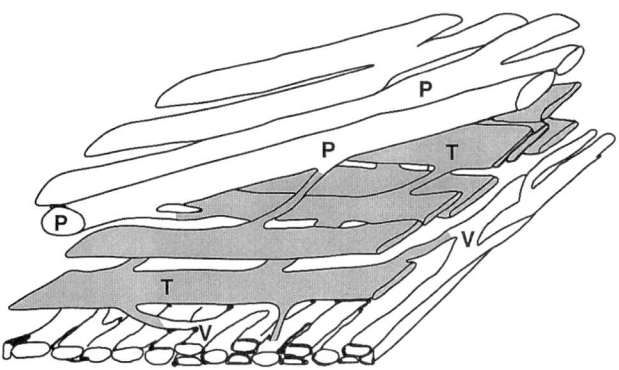

FIG. 12–39. Structure of the Purkinje–muscle junction. Schematic representation of the structure of a rabbit Purkinje fiber–ventricular muscle junction. P, Purkinje fibers; T, transitional cells; V, ventricular myocardium. [Reproduced with permission from reference 272.]

onset of depolarization at the initially activated left septal areas.

The myocardium of the left ventricular wall consists of discrete muscle layers that follow a curving radial path from the subendocardium to the subepicardium (25). These layers consist of a uniformly connected array of myocytes stacked four cells deep. Branches consisting of one to two cells connect adjacent layers. The extent of coupling between adjacent layers varies throughout the wall, with a progressive reduction in coupling from subepicardial to midmural layers. To what extent the laminar organization of the ventricular wall affects propagation is unclear. Intramural recordings, utilizing needles with multiple electrode terminals at distances of 1 mm, have not revealed discontinuities in the spread of excitation from subendocardium to subepicardium (173). On a microscopic scale, one might suppose that the pathway of activation is convoluted, if the muscle layers are electrically insulated and make contact only via direct muscle branches. It is possible that the structural anisotropy of ventricular myocardium may lead to irregular patterns of propagation when coupling between muscle layers becomes impaired, but direct evidence for this is lacking.

Right ventricular activation. The right bundle branch, in its course on the right endocardial surface of the interventricular septum, ends at the base of the anterior papillary muscle, where it gives off branches to the lower right anterior surface of the septum, to the free right ventricular wall at the pretrabecular area, and to the subendocardial Purkinje network of the right ventricular free wall (25, 274). As shown in Plate 10, initial right ventricular activation occurs near the base of the papillary muscle and the overlying free wall. From here, activation proceeds in a right-to-left direction in the interventricular septum, and tangentially toward the epicardium of the right ventricular free wall. Right ventricular epicardial breakthrough occurs approximately 25 msec after the onset of left septal depolarization, some 10 msec before activation reaches the left epicardial surface. In human and canine hearts, Purkinje activity is absent in the superior two-thirds of the right septal surface. The last parts of the right ventricle to be activated are the outer layers of the outflow tract and the crista supraventricularis, which are activated from the top of the interventricular septum (173).

DISTURBANCES OF IMPULSE CONDUCTION AND CONDUCTION BLOCK

The Safety Factor of Propagation

Intuitively, the safety factor of propagation, (SF) should indicate how much the basic electrical parameters involved in propagation can change until propagation block occurs. Shaw and Rudy (3) have recently proposed a definition which is based on earlier formulations by Delgado et al. (104) and Leon and Roberge (27). According to this definition, SF is described by a ratio of electrical charges: the charge generated by a given excited cell or tissue segment divided by the charge required to bring the same cell or threshold to excitation. With this definition, propagation is safe if SF > 1. The equation describing the safety factor is:

$$SF = \frac{\int_A I_c * dt + \int_A I_{out} * dt}{\int_A I_{in} * dt}$$

where, according to Figure 12–3, I_c is the capacitive current of the cell or tissue segment in question, I_{out} is the axial current delivered by the excited segment to the next segment *downstream*, and I_{in} is the axial current that enters the cell or tissue segment in question from the driving cells or segments *upstream*. Thus the sum of the integrals in the *numerator*, which are taken during the time, A, the cell or segment in question is involved in propagation ($I_M \neq 0$ in Fig. 12–3), is equal to the charge produced by the excited cell or membrane, while the integral in the *denominator* of the equation is equal to the charge required to bring the given cell or segment to threshold. Accordingly, the fraction of SF which is > 1 can be taken as a measure for propagation safety, i.e. the so-called *margin of safety*. Although depolarizing inward currents, such as I_{Na}, and electrical cell-to-cell coupling resistance do not appear as direct parameters in the above equation, their effect to change SF can be computed by an appropriate model of excitable tissue, as illustrated in Fig-

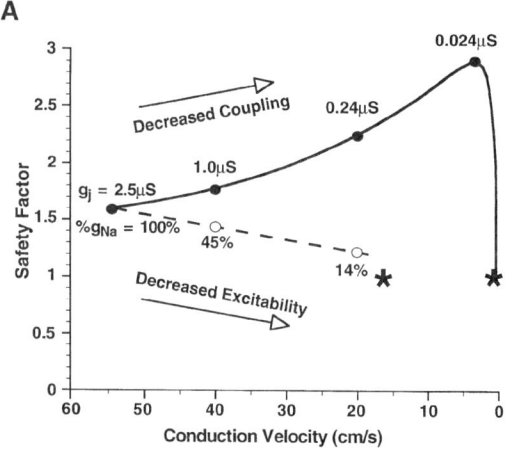

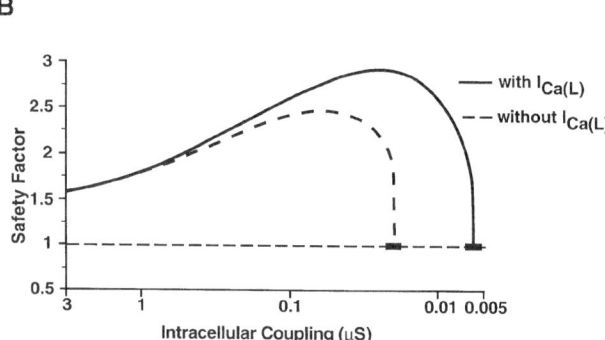

FIG. 12–40. Safety factor of propagation. Results of computer simulation of propagation in a cell chain. The cells are separated by a simulated gap junction resistor. *A:* Safety factor of propagation, SF, as a function of propagation velocity. *Dashed line:* Change of SF with a decrease of excitability. *Solid line:* Change of SF with decreasing conductance (increasing resistance) between cells. *B:* Change of SF as a function of propagation velocity in the absence and presence of $I_{Ca,L}$. Note that very low conduction velocities can only be achieved with flow of $I_{Ca,L}$. (See text.) [Reproduced with permission from reference 3.]

ure 12–40 and discussed in the subsequent paragraphs. In the original definition, the safety factor for propagation was calculated for one cell that was located within a simulated chain of single cells, which all were exposed to the same test conditions (e.g. changes in maximum Na$^+$ channel conductance or gap junctional conductance). Recently, the concept of the safety factor for propagation was extended to inhomogeneous tissue structures (275).

Effects of Changes in Resting Membrane Potential and Inhibition of Na$^+$ Channels on Conduction Velocity

It has long been known that depolarization of the resting membrane ultimately blocks propagation. In heart tissue, the effects of depolarization of the resting membrane on propagation velocity are complex. This complexity results from the fact that changes in resting potential affect both the excitability, i.e. the charge needed to reach the threshold for activation of Na$^+$ channels, and the number of available Na$^+$ channels, i.e. the driving force for propagation. Activation of other ionic conductances may play an additional role, especially at very low levels of resting potential. The effects of resting membrane potential on conduction have been assessed in three different ways: (*1*) By variation of extracellular potassium, [K$^+$]$_o$, (*2*) during repolarization of the preceding action potential, and (*3*) during spontaneous diastolic or "phase 4" depolarization.

In the specific ventricular conducting system, atrial tissue and working ventricular myocardium, elevating extracellular potassium, [K$^+$]$_o$ and displacing membrane potential from very negative values into the normal range resulted in a significant increase of propagation velocity, Θ (276–278). In Purkinje fibers, increasing [K$^+$]$_o$ from 2.7 mmoles/liter to 4 mmoles/liter produced an increase in Θ from 3.5 m/sec to 4.1 m/sec. However, a further elevation of [K$^+$]$_o$ was associated with a decrease in Θ. The increase in Θ was explained by the fact that shifting membrane potential to more positive values decreased the voltage difference between resting potential and threshold for excitation. This effect dominated over the decrease in membrane resistance, which was also associated with K$^+$-induced depolarization (276). Conduction slowing at [K$^+$]$_o$ 4 mmoles/liter was explained by increasing inactivation of Na$^+$ channels (19). During repolarization from the preceding action potential, the changes in excitability and conduction velocity in Purkinje fibers were found to be different from ventricular muscle (Fig. 12–41) (279, 280). At low [K$^+$]$_o$ (2.7 mmoles/liter) in Purkinje fibers, there was a time window during repolarization when excitability and Θ increased to its highest level before decreasing to diastolic steady state. In analogy to the phase of supernormal excitability, this phase was termed period of *supernormal conduction*. Supernormal conduction was not found in ventricular muscle at [K$^+$]$_o$ = 2.7 mmoles/liter and was absent in both Purkinje tissue and ventricular muscle at [K$^+$]$_o$ = 5 mmoles/liter. The difference between Purkinje and ventricular tissue was explained by a different time course of recovery from Na$^+$ current inactivation with ongoing repolarization. The dependence of conduction velocity on the take-off potential during spontaneous phase 4 depolarization is a further important consequence of the change in excitability with changing resting potential (281). Figure 12–42 illustrates the inverse relation between conduction time, taken as a relative measure of conduction velocity, and dV/dt$_{max}$ of the action potential upstroke with progressing phase 4

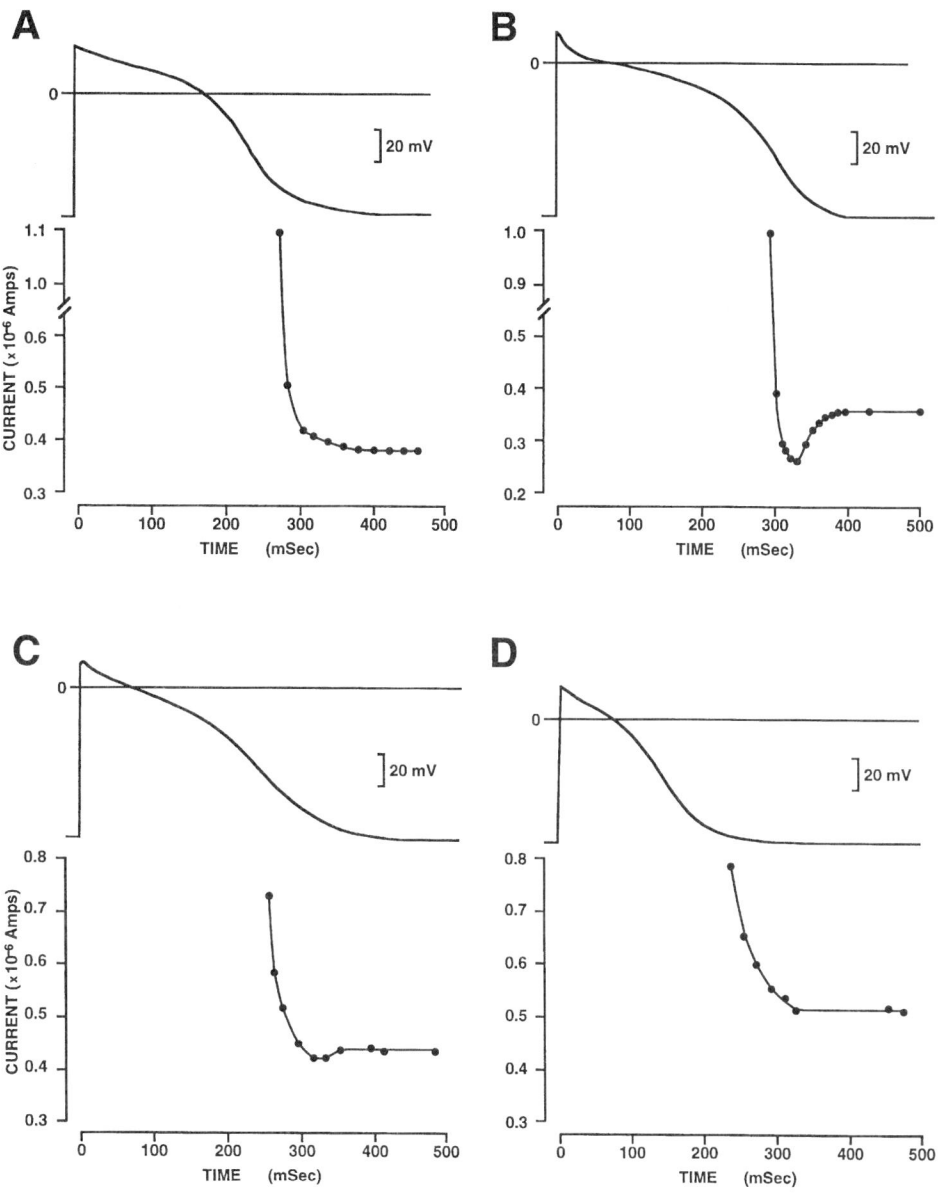

FIG. 12–41. Supernormal excitability and conduction. A, B: Transmembrane action potentials. C, D: Strength interval curves. Time scale is identical for both traces. A: Recording from the His bundle. B: Recording from a Purkinje fiber running freely in a false tendon. C: Recording from a transitional type Purkinje fiber. D: Recording from a ventricular cell. The supernormal phase of excitability in B is associated with a supernormal conduction. [Reproduced with permission from reference 279.]

depolarization. While dV/dt_{max} decreased with spontaneous depolarization (because of the increasing inactivation of Na^+ channels) excitability increased, and concomitantly, conduction velocity increased. The change in excitability was due in part, as mentioned, to the take-off potential approaching threshold for excitatory Na^+ current flow, to the change in membrane conductance, which is known to decrease with ongoing phase 4 depolarization (282). In clinical and experimental settings, propagation block during phase 4 depolarization (*bradycardia-dependent block*) has been described (283, 284). The theoretical explanation of this observation, which is in apparent contrast to the experimental results depicted in Figure 12–42 is controversial. Singer et al., (285) showed that block during late spontaneous diastolic depolarization occurred if the take-off potential was shifted to levels more positive than −65 mV. They proposed that the degree of inactivation of the inward current depended upon successful propagation or block in this situation.

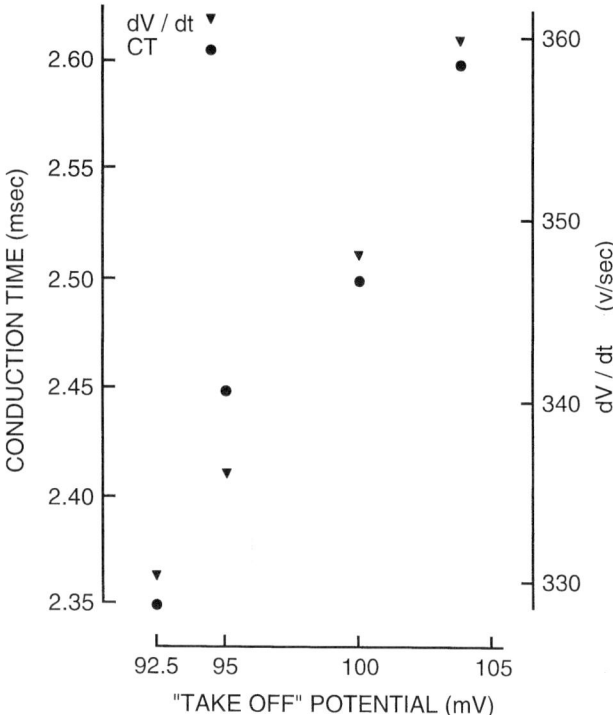

FIG. 12–42. Relationship of excitability to conduction velocity during phase-4 depolarization. Conduction time along a fixed distance of a Purkinje strand and maximal upstroke velocity of the transmembrane action potential, dV/dt_{max} of a Purkinje fiber are plotted as a function of the "take-off" potential during spontaneous phase 4 depolarization ranging from 92.5 to 105 mV. Note that with ongoing spontaneous depolarization (decrease of "take-off" potential") there is a decrease of conduction time corresponding to an increase in conduction velocity and a decrease of dV/dt_{max}. [Reproduced with permission from reference 281.]

increasing $[K^+]_o$ is depicted in Figure 12–43 from measurements carried out in Langendorff-perfused porcine hearts (287). Between $[K^+]_o$ of 4.5 mmoles/liter and 8 mmoles/L, Θ increased slightly and subsequently decreased until propagation block occurred at approximately 40 cm/sec in the longitudinal direction, i.e. at a level of about 50% of the initial value. The occurrence of conduction block at elevated $[K^+]_o$ (approximately 12–15 mmoles/liter, ([30, 287]) involves, in addition to the voltage-dependent inactivation of Na^+ channels, other ionic conductances. This voltage-independent effect was first described in isolated guinea pig papillary muscles (288) and later more closely investigated in isolated rabbit ventricular myocytes (289). It produces a significantly greater depression of dV/dt_{max} of the transmembrane potential upstroke than anticipated from Na^+ channel inactivation alone and is due to an increase in conductance of the inward rectifier K^+ channel, g_{K1}. It is confined to ventricular tissue and not observed in atrial cells (289). In the setting of myocardial ischemia or hypoxia, activation of ATP-sensitive K^+ channels (290) is likely to add to the voltage-independent decrease in dV/dt_{max} and to the decrease in propagation velocity.

As illustrated in Figure 12–43, inactivation of Na^+ channels by elevation of $[K^+]_o$ produced a decrease of conduction velocity, and subsequently, an abrupt transition from conducted impulses to block at relatively high values of Θ (approximately 50% of control). Similarly, partial blockade of Na^+ channels by tetrodotoxin led to minimal conduction velocities of about

Such low take-off potentials at the end of phase 4 were encountered in *partially damaged* cells of the specific ventricular conducting system (hypoxia, mechanical stretch, presence of cardiac steroids). A later study, however, showed that spontaneous phase 4 depolarization was not a prerequisite for the occurrence of bradycardia-dependent block, and that cycle- and time-dependent changes in excitability of depolarized Purkinje fibers could explain this phenomenon (286).

While the relation between conduction velocity and resting or take-off potential appears to be complex in the range between −90mV and −70mV, voltage-dependent inactivation of Na^+ channels and the concomitant decrease of conduction velocity dominate at potentials more positive than −70 mV. Such changes are e.g. observed in acute myocardial ischemia, when the resting potential (associated with cellular loss of K^+ and extracellular K^+ accumulation) can change from about 80 mV to −50 mV within a few minutes after arrest of coronary flow. The change of Θ with

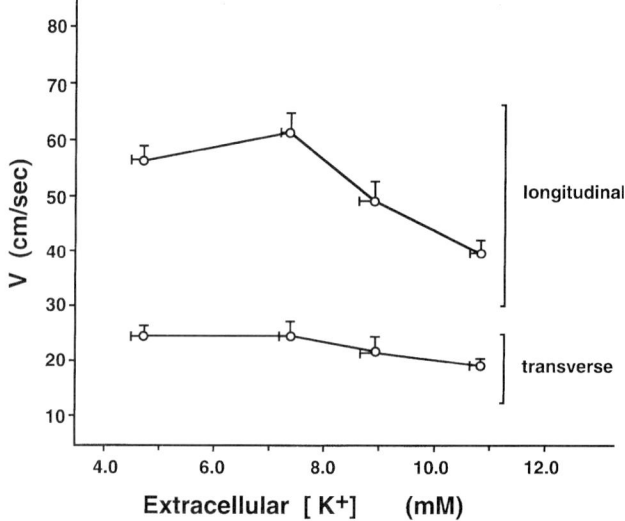

FIG. 12–43. Change of longitudinal and transverse conduction velocity with increasing extracellular potassium concentration, $[K^+]_o$. Measurements were made in an isolated perfused porcine heart. Note that propagation blocks at a $[K^+]_o$ of 11 mM. [Reproduced with permission from reference 287.]

25 cm/sec in guinea pig papillary muscles (30). Blockade of Na$^+$ channels is also a major mechanism of action of antiarrhythmic drugs (291). In normoxic guinea-pig papillary muscle, there was a linear relation between the decrease in dV/dt$_{max}$ and Θ^2 for a variety of drugs applied (lidocaine, procainamide, quinidine); (30). As with elevated [K$^+$]$_o$ and TTX, conduction block occurred abruptly at velocities of 45%–60% of the normal value; i.e. very slow conduction was never observed in presence of Na$^+$ channel blockade. Thus, beat-to-beat transition from relatively fast propagation to block seems to be a typical consequence of Na$^+$ channel inhibition or inactivation. In pathological settings (ischemia, hyperkalemia) this type of conduction block is the main determinant of circus movement reentry which is responsible for ventricular tachycardia and fibrillation (292). The relatively high velocity of the conducted action potentials produces relatively large circus movements (several millimeters internal diameter), and the abrupt transitions between block and propagation are responsible for the beat-to-beat changes in the excitation patterns during these arrhythmias (293). In agreement with these results, critical inhibition of I$_{Na}$ produced a beat-to-beat transition from propagation at a relatively high velocity to block in computer simulations of propagation, as illustrated in Figure 12–40; (3).

Refractoriness of cardiac tissue is due to the fact that the recovery of Na$^+$ and Ca^{++} channels from inactivation is voltage- and time-dependent. In normal tissue the value of membrane potential during repolarization is the main determinant of the amount of available Na$^+$ channels. This is because—in normal tissue—the time constant of recovery from inactivation is so fast that adaptation to the changing membrane potential is almost instantaneous. In depolarized tissue, the recovery time constant gets markedly prolonged, and consequently, recovery from inactivation no longer follows the time course of repolarization but instead becomes time dependent. This was first shown by Erich Schütz in 1936 who measured the recovery of the amplitude of so-called injury potential in hearts perfused at elevated [K$^+$]$_o$ and low pH (294). Later this phenomenon was systematically analyzed in voltage clamp experiments by Gettes and Reuter (255) as illustrated in Figure 12–44. While action potential amplitude and dV/dt$_{max}$ fully recover by the end of repolarization of a normal action potential, the relative refractoriness markedly extends into the phase of post repolarization in tissue depolarized by elevation of [K$^+$]$_o$. This effect is even enhanced by additional acidification, hypoxia or ischemia (295–297). In these situations, the absolute refractory period can outlast the duration of the preceding action potential (post-repolarization refractoriness [292]) and the subsequent relative refractory period gets pro-

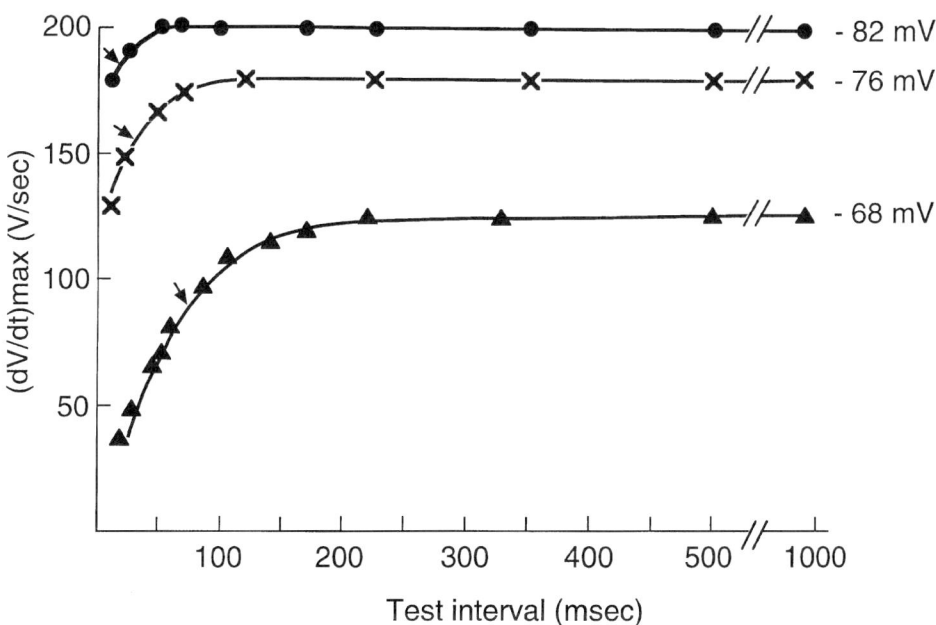

FIG. 12–44. Recovery of maximal upstroke velocity of the action potential, dV/dt$_{max}$. Action potentials were elicited at different times in the wake of the preceding action potential. Time 0 denotes the beginning of the preceding action potential. The curves depict the recovery curves of dV/dt$_{max}$ with increasing time measured at different resting potentials. Note that recovery from activation becomes delayed with depolarization. [Reproduced with permission from reference 255.]

longed as well. As a consequence of this prolongation, the interval after a preceding action potential, during which there is a gradual change in action potential amplitude and propagation velocity, may correspond to the excitation intervals present during slightly elevated sinus rhythm or after ventricular premature beats. Therefore, slight increases in basic rhythm or premature impulses may induce *rate-dependent* conduction block, conduction slowing, and re-entry in partially depolarized tissue (287, 292).

Conduction Slowing and Block: The Role of Ca^{++} Inward Current

Action potentials carried by the slow inward Ca^{++} current occur physiologically in the AV node. In other tissue, such as the SA node (298) and partially in ventricular cells, Ca^{++} current can contribute to various extents to the action potential upstroke. In rat ventricular myocytes, L-type Ca^{++} channels prevail at birth and then subsequently diminish in density with ongoing development to the adult phenotype (299). Besides its dominating role for explaining slow propagation through the AV junction, Ca^{++}-dependent propagation was invoked in the explanation of circus movement re-entry occurring across tissue zones with depressed Na^+ inward current (300–302). The special interest in the involvement of Ca^{++}-dependent propagation in circus movement resides in the fact that the dimensions of a re-entrant circuit is scaled by propagation velocity (see below). Therefore, low propagation velocities, as present during propagation of Ca^{++}-dependent action potentials may explain re-entry in very small volumes of tissue. Although the Ca^{++} inward current can contribute to slow propagation, very slow conduction (< 10 cm/sec) as encountered in the central part of the AV node or in pathophysiological settings requires further alterations in electrical cell-to-cell coupling or in tissue geometry, as discussed in the paragraphs below. This is suggested from the observation that Ca^{++}-dependent propagation induced by epinephrine (287) in perfused porcine hearts or spontaneous Ca^{++}-dependent propagation in neonatal rat tissue (presence of TTX to inhibit Na^+ inward current (80) produced conduction velocities of approximately 15 cm/sec, i.e. values that are higher than the velocity observed in the AV node. The ability of the AV junction to slow conduction of premature atrial impulses, or to block them, is to a large extent related to the slow recovery from excitability of the Ca^{++} current–dependent N cells. Very similarly to the behavior of the Na^+ channels at depolarized membrane potentials (see above), recovery of Ca^{++} inward current from inactivation shows a marked dependence on the preceding excitation interval (255).

Conduction Slowing and Discontinuous Conduction

Cell-to-Cell Uncoupling. The closure of gap junctions and the consequent electrical cell-to-cell uncoupling eventually leads to block of propagation. While a large number of studies have investigated the dependence of gap junctional conductance on activities of ions, metabolites and drugs, no experimental studies have been carried out that would quantitatively correlate the decrease of gap junctional resistance, r_i, to the decrease in propagation velocity, θ. The difficulty for obtaining such information resides in the fact that the measurement of electrical resistance, r_i, between cells requires the voltage-clamp technique, a method that excludes action potential propagation (303). Weingart and Maurer (304) compared r_i to the time of action potential transfer in a pair of isolated guinea pig cells by measuring r_i in the voltage-clamp mode and action potential transfer in a current-clamp mode. They found that the transfer time was too short to be detected when r_i was within the range of normal. By contrast, cell-to-cell delays of approximately 25 msec were measured when r_i had risen to values between 155 and 375MΩ, i.e. to about 200 times normal, and block of action potential transmission occurred at r_I > 750MΩ. Because cardiac tissue represents a complex network of changing resistive loads, it is difficult to extrapolate these data quantitatively to changes in propagation velocity. Computer simulation studies (cf. Fig. 12–14) correlating the decrease of θ in a simulated cell chain to increasing r_i suggest that the margin of safety for conduction remains large with ongoing uncoupling. Thus, in the simulation study by Rudy and Quan (26) r_i had to increase about a 100-fold until conduction block occurred. With a normal excitability of the simulated cells, minimal θ values of a few cm/sec were obtained before occurrence of conduction block (26). This indicates that minimal propagation velocities present with advanced cell-to-cell uncoupling are significantly lower that the velocities produced by Ca^{++}-dependent action potentials or with partial inhibition of Na^+-channels, and can amount to only a few centimeters per second, a result that has recently been confirmed in an experimental study (305). Simulations by Shaw and Rudy (3) have shown a close interaction between the advanced stage of cell-to-cell uncoupling and the role of $I_{Ca,L}$ to maintain propagation (Fig. 12–40, lower panel). With advanced cell-to-cell uncoupling, excitation of cells occurs almost simultaneously, while the conduction delays—causing the low propagation velocity—are confined to the gap junctions. As a consequence, the driver cell will already be depolarized to its *plateau phase* when the driven cell downstream is about to reach threshold for excitation. Therefore flow of $I_{Ca,L}$ is necessary to support the axial current required for excitation downstream; i.e. the success of propagation becomes $I_{Ca,L}$-dependent. In pathological settings, uncoupling can contribute to the disturbances of impulse propagation, and rapid uncoupling has been shown to characterize anoxia and acute ischemia (31, 33, 306, 307). Ventricular tachycardias and ventricular fibrillation during acute myocardial ischemia (type IB arrhythmias [308]) have been shown to be correlated with the onset of electrical uncoupling (309).

Fiber Branching. Kucera et al. (2) have demonstrated that the propagation behavior of branching tissue is very similar to tissue with a very low degree of cell-to-cell coupling. In synthetic tissue consisting of a main strand and several blindly ending side branches of various lengths (with a narrow interbranch interval), conduction velocities were significantly lower than in linear strands. If the propagation was driven by $I_{Ca,L}$ (in presence of Na$^+$ inhibition), safe conduction was observed at velocities of <1 cm/sec, i.e. in a range very similar to the values observed with advanced cell-to-cell uncoupling. Two mechanisms determined propagation. First, current-to-load mismatch at the branching points was responsible for conduction slowing and the marked conduction delays between the branch points. Second, the simultaneous activation of the initial portions of the side branches, which provided local excitatory current from a large cell area to a small tissue portion downstream, was responsible for the *safe* propagation of the impulse to the next branching point. The striking similarity of this conduction behavior to the increased conduction safety in partially uncoupled tissue (see Fig. 12–41) may explain some important observations made in the normal AV node and in highly fibrotic tissue, i.e. in infarct scars and the atria during chronic fibrillation. In the normal AV node, the so-called dead-end pathways are likely to contribute to slow AV-nodal propagation. In tissue showing marked fibrosis, conduction may not only be very slow but also "safe," i.e. more resistant to blockers of depolarizing current (I_{Na}) than normal tissue. This may partially explain the resistance of chronic atrial fibrillation to antiarrhythmic therapy.

Mechanisms of Unidirectional Block

Unidirectional conduction block is a prerequisite for the occurrence of re-entry (205). As a fundamental principle, formation of unidirectional block requires local asymmetry in excitability, in electrical cell-to-cell coupling, in the shape of a propagating wavefront, and/or in macroscopic tissue structure. While most of these criteria are ultimately determined by structural features, it is important to note that asymmetry may be functional and transient in nature, if occurring in the wake of a preceding excitation wave.

Tissue Vulnerability: Interference of Local Excitation or Propagation with the Refractory Tail of the Preceding Wave. Interaction between an excitation wave with the refractory tail of another wave may be important in several conditions: (*1*) If an external stimulus excites tissue during the period of relative refractoriness, (*2*) if a spontaneous premature beat interacts with the refractory tail of a preceding wave, and (*3*) if one wavefront hits the refractory tail of another wavefront, e.g. during multiple wavelet re-entry. Interaction of a premature impulse with the wake of a preceding excitation wave has been investigated in computer simulations (310–313) and is illustrated in Figure 12–45. Establishment of unidirectional block during repolarization from the preceding action potential occurs within a critical window of vulnerability. This window can be characterized by a critical time period, a critical range of membrane potentials, or a critical zone within the refractory tail. Stimulation before the period of vulnerability leads to bi-directional block; stimulation afterwards, to bidirectional conduction. When a premature impulse falls into the window of vulnerability, it propagates in a retrograde direction initially with low velocity until, at a critical distance from the site of stimulation, the Na$^+$ channels have fully recovered from inactivation. In the anterograde direction, propagation becomes decremental and eventually blocks because of failure of Na$^+$ channel activation. Importantly, the spatial and temporal extension of the vulnerability window depends on the availability of the Na$^+$ channels, on cell-to-cell coupling (312) and on depolarizing K$^+$ currents (310). As mentioned by Starmer, (310) vulnerability becomes smaller with decreasing cell-to-cell coupling and with action potential prolongation in the presence of K$^+$ channel inhibition. This decrease might contribute to the antiarrhythmic effect of K$^+$ channel inhibitors. By contrast vulnerability increases with decreasing Na$^+$ conductance, i.e. with inhibition of Na$^+$ channels. This mechanism might partially explain pro-arrhythmic effects observed with the application of Na$^+$ channel blockers.

Although intrinsic heterogeneity in excitability or in local distribution of refractory periods is *not necessary* for unidirectional block and re-entry to occur, any of these conditions adds to the formation of unidirectional block (312). Local dispersion of refractory periods is a normal feature of ventricular myocardium. In the normal ventricles, the differences between the shortest and longest refractory periods amount to approximately 40 msec (314, 315). By lowering local temperature, large local dispersions in refractory peri-

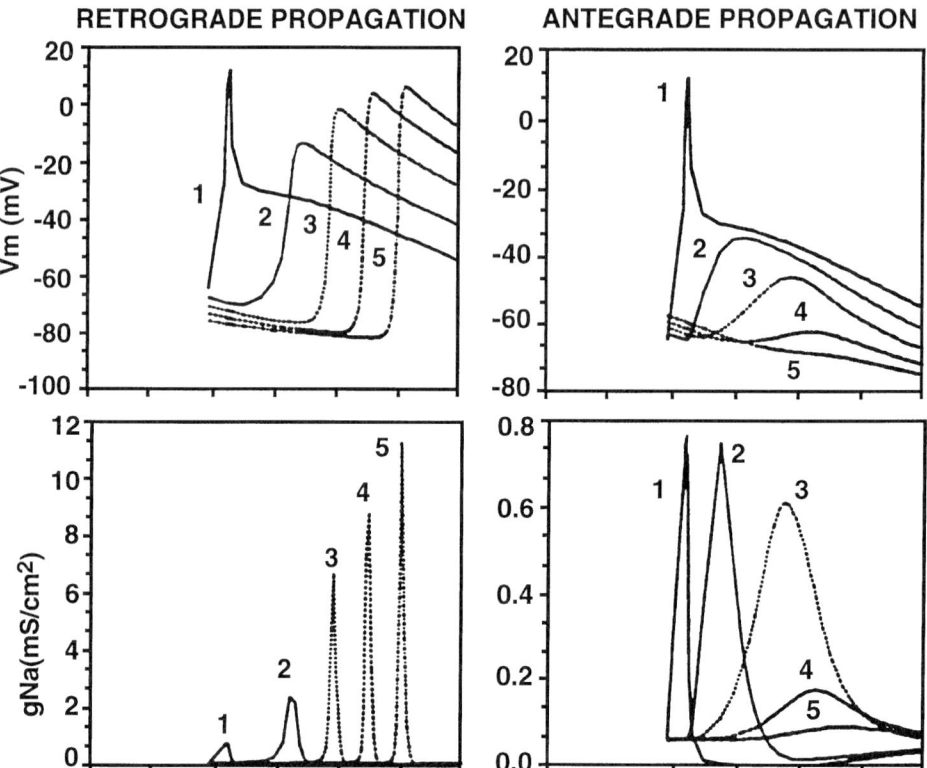

FIG. 12–45. Unidirectional block in the wake of the preceding wavefront. Transmembrane potentials (V_m) and sodium channel conductance (gNa) computed after application of a premature stimulus (cell 1) in the wake of propagating action potential. In the antegrade direction (*right panel*) recordings were taken from cells 0.5 mm apart. In the retrograde direction (*left panel*) traces were recorded from cells 1 mm apart. At the time of premature stimulation, membrane excitability at cell 1 was less than 10% of the maximum excitability (compare gNa curves 1 and 5 on the left panel). In the retrograde direction, the action potential propagated a distance of 4 mm before reaching the region of fully excitable membrane. In the antegrade direction, membrane excitability gradually decreased and propagation extinguished. Note different gNa scales in the left and right panels. [Reproduced with permission from reference 312.]

ods can be produced, and re-entrant arrhythmias can be elicited by premature stimulation in this condition (316, 317). Further experimental interventions that lead to increased dispersion in refractoriness are (*1*) stimulation of sympathetic nerves, (*2*) application of chloroform, cardiac steroids, or high doses of quinidine, and (*3*) ischemia (315). A single premature stimulus, applied at the site of the shortest refractory period, induced unidirectional block and repetitive activity in the canine ventricle when the refractory periods varied between 95 and 145 msec (316). Assessment of local differences between refractory periods is not sufficient to postulate an increased probability for the occurrence of unidirectional block, however. As discussed by Allessie et al. (318), such differences have to extend over a critical area or volume of tissue, and consequently, to produce a refractory area or volume of critical size.

Occurrence of asymmetrical unidirectional block in a region of depressed excitability was postulated as early as 1895 by Engelmann, who locally applied cold and poison to the sartorius muscle of the frog (319). Subsequently, various techniques have been used to locally produce depression of excitability and conduction block (hyperkalemia, (300, 320) focal cooling (321, 322), crushing (320–322) application of depolarizing current). In a classical work, Schmitt and Erlanger provided a scheme for production of unidirectional block in a strip of turtle heart, which was subjected locally to pressure injury and elevated $[K^+]_o$ (320–322). The relevance of an asymmetric decrease of excitability for the generation of unidirectional block is shown in Figure 12–46 from experiments using local cooling or crushing. The asymmetry in these experiments led to an abrupt rise in the threshold for excitation in one direction and to a more gradual rise in the other. In between the transitional zones, an inexcitable gap was located. An impulse traveling in a retrograde direction

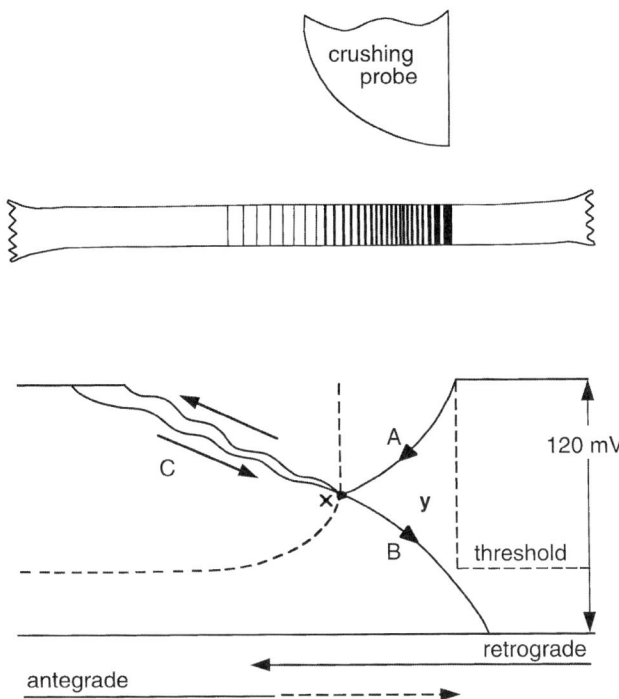

FIG. 12-46. Unidirectional block with asymmetric depression of excitability. *Top:* Injury is produced by a crushing probe. The line spacing on the Purkinje fiber indicates increasing degree of injury. *Bottom:* The influence of injury on the excitability threshold is illustrated. The amplitudes of the anterograde wavefront (C-x-B) are compared to the amplitudes of the retrograde wavefront (A-x-C). At y, the transition between normal cells and inexcitable, injured cells is abrupt. C represents decremental or augmental conduction, depending on direction, through a transitional zone of partial injury; x represents the point of transition between partially excitable cells and inexcitable cells (x-y). A and B represent electrotonic transmission through inexcitable cells. The retrograde wave succeeds in conducting across, and the anterograde wave front fails. [Reproduced with permission from reference 322.]

and encountering an abrupt transition to the inexcitable gap transmitted the impulse electrotonically across this gap, if the gap length was below a critical value. By contrast, the impulse was not transmitted across the same gap during conduction from the other direction, because the gradual decrease of excitability on the other side of the gap diminished the amplitude and consequently the driving force for electrotonic transmission. Thus, conduction failed when the wavefront encountered the least depressed site first, and was successful in the direction it encountered the most depressed site first. Engelmann concluded in 1896 that impulses are conducted more easily from rapidly conducting tissue to slowly conducting tissue than in the reverse direction, a suggestion which most likely anticipated the described mechanism (323).

Unidirectional Block: Dependence on Tissue Geometry.

When a thin cell strand inserts into a large muscle mass, local circuit currents produced by a relatively small amount of excitable membrane area have to exert an excitatory effect on a larger membrane area downstream (*current-to-load mismatch*). Unidirectional block preferentially occurs at sites of current-to-load mismatch, if the strength of the wavefront in the smaller structure does not suffice to excite the larger structure. In the reverse direction, local circuit current produced by the larger structure will be sufficient to excite the smaller structure. Physiologically this mechanism is likely to affect propagation across Purkinje fiber–muscle junctions (266, 270), the branching trabecular structure of the atria (93, 324), and possibly in the AV node (243). Furthermore, structures predicting current-to-load mismatch have been described in the midmural portion of the left ventricle (25). In pathological settings, this situation is likely to occur in surviving myocardial strands in infarct scars (325). In the presence of elevated $[K^+]_o$, when the Na^+ channels are partially or fully inactivated, unidirectional block has been demonstrated at Purkinje fiber-muscle junctions (266). The dependence of unidirectional block on tissue geometry, tissue excitability and cell-to-cell coupling has been investigated in computer simulations and in patterned cell cultures (72, 73, 326). In a study using a technique to pattern neonatal rat cardiomyocytes (87), small cell strands were grown in such a way that they emerged into a large cell area of varying geometry. In accordance with the mechanism of current-to-load mismatch, anterograde conduction delays became large when the strand emerged into area that extended behind the insertion point and provided a maximal sink for the excitatory current produced in the strand. Conversely, the delay became smaller when the strand gradually widened before merging with the large area (so-called funnel). In a computer simulation, the minimal strand diameter that was able to excite a large area was estimated to amount to approximately 200 μm in absence of a funnel, while a small funnel (as consistently present in patterned cell cultures) decreased this minimal strand width to between 30 μm and 50 μm, (73), in close accordance with results obtained in cell cultures (72) cultures (72).

A marked discontinuity in tissue geometry not only may cause unidirectional block, it may also determine the types of inward currents involved in impulse transmission. This is illustrated in Figure 12–47, which depicts a site of current-to-load mismatch produced in patterned cell cultures. If the pattern is grown in such a way that the delays at the transition to the large area is minor (<2msec), inhibition of the Na^+ inward current by TTX in the small strand produces unidirectional block, while inhibitors of the L-type Ca^{++} channel current have no effect. If a smaller strand width is selected, and accordingly the conduction delay caused

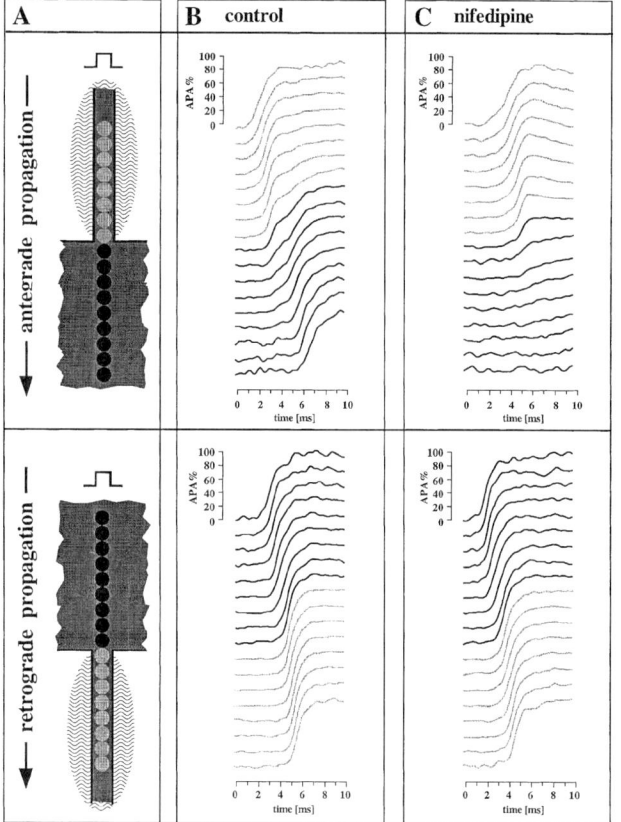

FIG. 12–47. Unidirectional block at a geometrical tissue expansion: The role of Ca^{++}–inward current. *A:* Schematic representation of a cultured cell monolayer with geometrical expansion and overlaid photodiodes during antegrade (*upper panel*) and retrograde (*lower panel*) conduction. *B* and *C:* Action potential upstrokes recorded using a voltage-sensitive dye in control conditions (*B*) and after administration of 5 μM nifedipine. In control conditions, the antegrade propagation was characterized by biphasic upstrokes and local slowing of conduction at the expansion (*B*). The blockage of Ca^{++} current with nifedipine produced antegrade conduction block (*C*). The retrograde propagation was successful in both cases. [Reproduced with permission from reference 80.]

by the change in tissue geometry is larger (> 2 msec) block is induced by inhibition of the L-type Ca^{++} channels. If patterns with a very small strand width are selected, where unidirectional block is present during normal conditions, this block can be reversed by an enhancer of the L-type Ca^{++} channel current. The explanation for this phenomenon is given by the fact that delays > 2 msec imposed by the discontinuous tissue geometry require inward current flowing during early plateau and not during the action potential upstroke for successful propagation (80), much like the resistive discontinuities described above (3, 78). The flow of electrotonic current from the small source into the large sink in case of geometrical discontinuities is also influenced by cell-to-cell coupling. While, in linear structures, cell-to-cell coupling induces conduction slowing and block, partial cell-to-cell uncoupling or a resistive barrier is predicted to reduce the load of the current sink and to reverse unidirectional block to bidirectional conduction in case of geometrical current-to-load mismatch (Plate 11; 73, 327). This indicates that a combination of a cellular network with macroscopic tissue geometries (interstitial clefts) produces a system with complex interactions between ionic currents, cell-to-cell coupling, and local conduction.

Unidirectional Block in Anisotropic Tissue: Dependence on Resistive Tissue Barriers and on the Bidomain Behavior. Resistive barriers formed by connective tissue sheets and blood vessels are a normal anatomical feature of both atrial and ventricular muscle. They increase with age and in myocardial infarction or heart failure. Since such small anatomical obstacles are typically oriented in parallel to cardiac strands, the electrophysiological effects of these discontinuities are also anisotropic; i.e. they are unmasked preferentially during transverse propagation. During transverse impulse spread these resistive barriers become manifest as discontinuities in action potential upstrokes or in the intrinsic deflection of unipolar electrograms. They can be visible in original tracings (324) or be unmasked only in the first and second time derivatives of the signals (94). Spach *et al.* (95) used the observation that discontinuities in extracellular electrograms were present in some recordings or preparations but not in others to functionally classify anisotropic tissue as being *continuous* or *discontinuous*.

In 1981 Spach et al. showed that premature impulses generated by point stimulation in atrial trabeculae, which were blocked earlier in the longitudinal direction than in the transverse direction to the fiber axis, elicited circus movement reentry (93). This finding was important because it attributed an intrinsic arrhythmogenic substrate to physiological tissue architecture. As shown in Figure 12–48 (74, 328), impulses traveling in either the longitudinal or the transverse direction were blocked at the same premature interval in tissue devoid of major discontinuities. By contrast, longitudinal conduction was blocked at an earlier prematurity interval than transverse conduction in atrial trabeculae exhibiting discontinuous conduction. This and the observation of direction dependency of dV/dt_{max} were taken to postulate a basically different mechanism for longitudinal conduction than for transverse conduction. The later studies investigating the role of resistive barriers in the formation of unidirectional conduction in anisotropy have produced controversial results, however, and the discrepancies have not yet been fully elucidated. In human and atrial tissue with high degrees of discontinuous anisotropy (anisotropy velocity ratios >3), anisotropy-dependent, preferential conduction

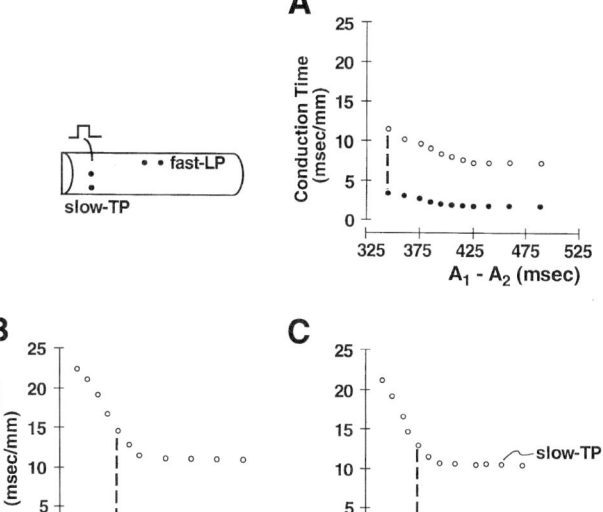

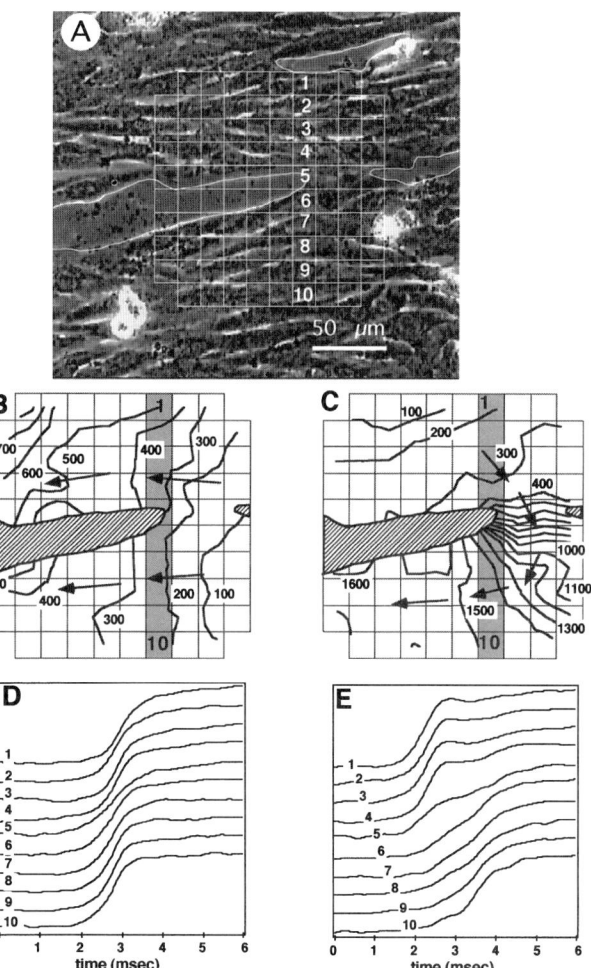

FIG. 12–48. Unidirectional block in anisotropic tissue. Anisotropic conduction time curves obtained in human and canine atrial bundles. *A:* Uniform anisotropic pectinate muscle of a 12-year-old child. *B:* Non-uniform anisotropic pectinate muscle of a 62-year-old man. *C:* Non-uniform anisotropic muscle (christa terminalis) of an adult dog. In each preparation conduction times (msec per mm interelectrode distance) were obtained from analyzing the unipolar extracellular electrogram of two electrode pairs. As shown in the *inset*, the two electrode pairs were placed in longitudinal and transverse directions, respectively. *Solid circles* represent longitudinal propagation, *open circles* represent transverse propagation. Each preparation was stimulated at a basic rate, and premature action potentials were introduced at variable intervals, A_1–A_2. In the uniform anisotropic bundle (*A*) conduction times became longer with the shortening of the A_1–A_2 intervals, block occurred in both directions at the same interval. In the non-uniform cases (*B* and *C*), block occurred in the longitudinal direction at a premature interval of 325 and 310 msec, respectively. At this prematurity, transverse propagation was still preserved. [Reproduced from reference 74 with permission.]

ically oriented resistive obstacles in the formation of unidirectional conduction slowing and block was suggested from two experimental studies in which the resistive barriers were produced in cell cultures and in superfused epicardial tissue slices. An experiment showing the effect of a microscopic obstacle, oriented in parallel to the main axis of the cells, is shown in Figure 12–49 (34). This obstacle, which had a length of approximately 150 µm, exerted only minor effects

FIG. 12–49. Effect of microscopic resistive barriers on propagation. *A:* A phase-contrast image of a cell culture (neonatal rat myocytes) with the overlaid diode array. Action potential upstrokes are measured at each diode location. The numbers 1–10 on the diode array correspond to the locations of the signals shown in *D* and *E*. In *D* and *C*, the location of these signals is indicated by the gray area. Two clefts in the central area (outlined in white in *A*) form an narrow isthmus of 40 µm. Activation maps of longitudinal and transverse conduction are shown in *B* and *C* respectively. Note slowing and deviation of the wavefront at the isthmus. Numbers denote separation of isochrones by 100 µsec. Selected recordings of action potential upstrokes during longitudinal and transverse conduction are shown in *D* and *E*, respectively. Discontinuities in the action potential upstrokes occur at the expansion site during transverse propagation. [Reproduced from reference 34 with permission.]

block in the longitudinal direction was a consistent finding (104, 329, 330) In subepicardial layers of porcine hearts (anisotropy velocity ratios <3), under conditions of reduced excitability, unidirectional block upon premature stimulation was independent of fiber direction, however (287). Even more controversial, unidirectional block was found to occur preferentially in transverse direction in other studies (104, 329, 330).

Anisotropically oriented obstacles can form pivoting points, around which the excitatory waves have to turn (331), or they may form narrow gates, or "isthmuses" which allow transmission of excitation waves from one excitable region to than other (34, 332). In all these situations, the wavefront encounters a resistive obstacle and spreads from the edges of this obstacle into the surrounding medium. An important role of anisotrop-

on the shape of the transmembrane action potential and the arrangement of isochrones during longitudinal propagation. During transverse spread, local activation slowed behind the obstacle and the action potential upstrokes were discontinuous. Both the local conduction slowing and the discontinuity in action potential upstroke were attributed to current-to-load mismatch at the isthmus between the large extracellular cleft. In cell cultures, localized conduction slowing with wavefront deviation was also shown at locations of myocytes with decreased expression of gap junctions and of nonmyocyte cells which are electrically coupled to myocytes (34). In another type of experiment, excitable cardiac tissue was cut in two parts with a narrow bridge or isthmus between these parts left intact (Fig. 12–50) (332, 333). The critical isthmus width at which unidirectional block occurred was dependent on the frequency of stimulation and varied from a few hundreds of micrometers at low stimulation rates to several millimeters at high stimulation rates. Unidirectional block never occurred at the location of the isthmus, but the impulses always propagated for a short distance through the gate. Simulations of excitation in the presence of an isthmus (332) or at geometrical expansions (73) have explained this phenomenon by *the critical curvature of the wavefront* beyond the gate or expansion. At a critical radius of curvature, the dispersion of local excitatory current was too large for excitation to occur. This indicates that wavefront curvature is an important determinant not only of conduction velocity but also of conduction block.

Recent studies have suggested that a particular type of block and re-entry may be related to the *bidomain behavior of anisotropic tissue*. Application of *very large premature cathodal point stimuli* during the relative refractory period of the preceding action potential produced block in the transverse direction and conduction in the longitudinal direction, followed by re-entry (334). It was assumed that, during the basic stimulus, hyperpolarization of the sites located on the longitudinal axis (112) would locally shorten the refractory period and increase the excitability of the membrane area located on the longitudinal axis relative to the sites located on the transversal axis (335). Circus movement attributed to virtual electrode effects was also observed after application of large defibrillation shocks (336).

CIRCULATING EXCITATION, RE-ENTRY, AND SPIRAL WAVES

At the completion of normal cardiac activation, the electrical wave becomes extinct at the boundaries of the excitable tissue, and subsequent excitation has to originate from a pacemaker impulse. In pathological settings, excitation waves can be blocked in circumscribed areas, rotate around these zones, and re-enter the site of original excitation in repetitive cycles. This mechanism is known to be responsible for a number of clinically important tachyarrhythmias. According to the nature of the area of block around which the wave propagates, circus movement re-entry has been classified into *anatomic* and *functional* re-entry. Although this separation is useful for the explanation of the basic rules characterizing circulating excitation, the area of block in re-entrant circuits is often composed of both anatomical and functional elements.

Anatomic Re-entry

A first indication that circus movement can occur in excitable tissue was provided by Mayer in experiments on the jellyfish (337, 338). He cut rings from the subumbrella tissue and stimulated them at some point. Appropriately timed stimuli induced unidirectional block with a single wave of contraction propagating in only one direction. The wave circled around the central hole, and returned to and re-excited the site of initiation. Wave rotation could continue for many days at a constant rate, and the location of wave initiation did not play any role in the maintenance of circulating excitation. Mayer proved this by removing the site where the wave originated from the rest of the tissue without

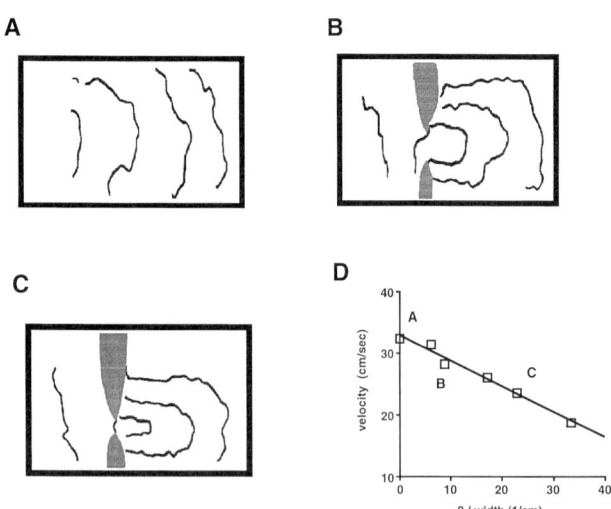

FIG. 12–50. Unidirectional conduction block at an "isthmus." Wave propagation across a narrow tissue isthmus in an isolated ventricular preparation of sheep heart. *A:* Map of activation spread before an isthmus was produced. *B:* Activation spread in the same preparation with the isthmus 2.26 mm wide. The isthmus was produced by two tissue cuts (gray zones). *C:* Activation spread after the isthmus was reduced to 0.88 mm. *D:* Local conduction velocity measured across the isthmus as a function of isthmus width. [Reproduced with permission from reference 332.]

observing termination of wave rotation. Mayer himself did not consider such a circus movement as a cause for cardiac arrhythmias, because he assumed the heart to be constructed in such a way as to make re-entrant excitation impossible. However, his experiments inspired Mines to investigate circus movement in cardiac muscle (205, 339). Mines reproduced Mayer's observations using ring-like preparations of atrial and ventricular tissue from various animals and suggested that circus movement would be responsible for cardiac tachyarrhythmias in humans. He predicted re-entrant excitation to occur in hearts with accessory atrioventricular (AV) connections. This prediction was confirmed many years later in patents with Wolff Parkinson-White syndrome syndrome (340–343).

Mines defined one of the basic requirements for initiation of re-entrant excitation—the establishment of unidirectional conduction block. Also, he realized that the initiation and maintenance of re-entry were dependent on both conduction velocity and refractory period. He noted that "if the rate of propagation is rapid as compared to the duration of the wave, the whole circuit will be in the excited state at the same time, and the excitation wave will die out." However, when "the wave is slower and shorter . . . , the excited state will have passed off at the region where the excitation started. . . . Under these circumstances, the wave of excitation may spread a second time over the same tract of tissue." The basic properties of anatomic re-entry according to Mines are illustrated in Figure 12–51. In this type of re-entry, the excitation wave propagates around a relatively large unexcitable obstacle so that the revolution time exceeds the absolute and the relative refractory periods, and therefore, the re-entrant circuit contains a fully excitable gap. Because of the fully excitable gap, wave rotation is stable, persisting at a constant rate for hours. The existence of an excitable gap within the re-entrant circuit also implies that impulses originating outside the re-entrant circuit can penetrate into the circuit to influence the re-entrant rhythm. Figure 12–52 (344) shows schematically the effects of a single premature impulse on a re-entrant circuit exhibiting an excitable gap. In the case shown in panel A, the premature impulse enters the re-entrant circuit at the end of the relative refractory period and propagates in both the antegrade and the retrograde directions. In the retrograde direction, the premature wave collides with the circulating wavefront and both waves annihilate. In the antegrade direction, the premature wave continues to propagate (panel B). As a result, the arrhythmia is reset, i.e. propagation continues to circulate with the former frequency but with a phase shift caused by the penetrating impulse. When, as shown in panel C, the premature impulse enters the re-entrant circuit early enough in the relative refractory

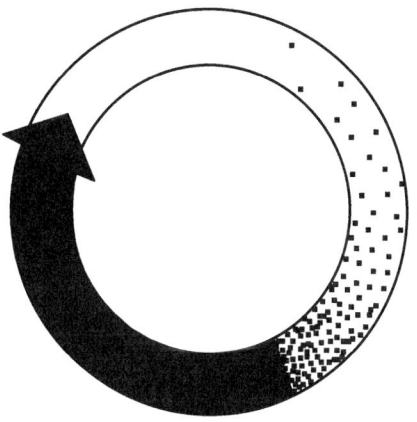

1. Length of circular pathway determined by perimeter of anatomic obstacle

2. Length of circular pathway fixed

3. Excitable gap between crest and tail of the impulse (white part of circuit)

4. Impulse can not shortcut the circuit

5. Revolution time inversely related to conduction velocity

FIG. 12–51. Circus movement re-entry around a large anatomical obstacle. [Reproduced with permission from reference 350.]

period, it fails to propagate in the antegrade direction because it encounters absolutely refractory tissue. In the retrograde direction, it meets increasingly recovered tissue and is able to propagate until it meets the circulating wave and terminates the arrhythmia (panel D). When the heart is paced at a regular rate that is faster than the rate of the wave rotation, the situation depicted in Panels A and B may be perpetuated: every paced impulse blocks the circulating wave front but also enters the anterograde pathway and maintains the circulating wave. The heart, therefore, follows the pacing rate, but on stopping the pacing, the original rhythm resumes. This phenomenon is called "transient entrainment" (345–349). The existence of a long re-entrant circuit with an excitable gap also means that the revolution time, and therefore, the frequency of the arrhythmia, is insensitive to changes in tissue refractory period. Thus, it was found in long ring-shaped preparations of rabbit atrial tissue that shortening of the tissue refractory period by carbamylcholine did not affect revolution time, while reduction of conduction velocity by tetrodotoxin caused slowing of wave rotation (350).

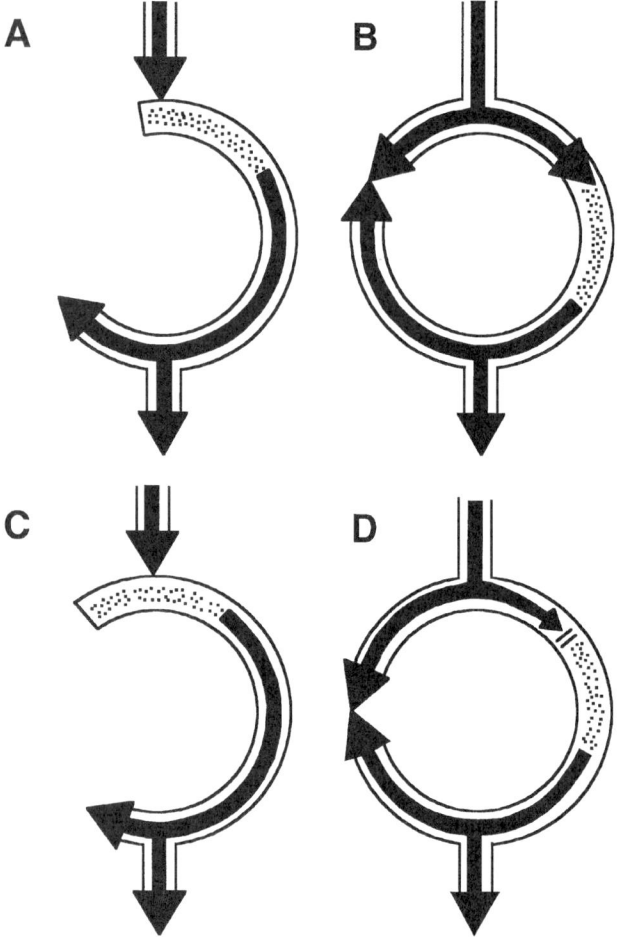

FIG. 12–52. Effect of a premature impulse entering a re-entrant circuit. The black and dotted areas show the absolute and relative refractory periods, respectively. In *A* and *B*, a premature impulse enters the circuit at the end of the relative refractory period and spreads in two directions. In the retrograde direction, the premature wave is annihilated by the circulating wave; in the anterograde direction, the premature impulse advances, resetting the tachycardia. In *C* and *D*, the premature impulse reaches the circuit closer to the state of absolute refractoriness. The impulse annihilates the retrograde wave and fails to propagate in the anterograde direction thereby terminating the tachycardia. [Reproduced with permission from reference 219.]

Likewise, a moderate lengthening of the refractory period is expected to cause no effect on wave rotation, provided that an excitable gap persists. Therefore, arrhythmias based on this mechanism are expected to be resistant to antiarrhythmic drugs that lengthen the refractory period.

When the length of re-entrant circuit is smaller than the excitation wavelength, as defined by the product of conduction velocity and the fully refractory period, the front of the circulating wave is located within its own refractory tail, and a fully excitable gap is no longer present. The behavior of this type of re-entry differs from the situation where a fully excitable gap is present, because of interaction between the front of the wave and the refractory tail. Conduction velocity becomes smaller when the excitation wavefront gets closer to the absolute refractory zone (351). Therefore, changing the duration of refractoriness at a given length of the anatomical pathway affects conduction velocity and revolution time of the circuit. Thus, shortening the duration of the action potential and refractoriness by stimulation of muscarinic receptors reduced the cycle length of atrial tachycardias (352). In re-entrant circuits exhibiting a partially excitable gap, it is less likely that an electrical impulse originating outside the re-entrant circuit may penetrate it. In stable, anatomically defined atrial tachycardia in dogs, a single premature stimulus applied outside of the circuit could reset the tachycardia (352). However, the impulse penetrating into the re-entrant circuit propagated more slowly than the tachycardia impulse, suggesting that the penetration occurred into the relative refractory zone where excitability had not completely recovered. The lack of a fully excitable gap is likely to explain the resistance of type II rapid atrial flutter to high-frequency electrical stimulation in patients (353).

Anatomical re-entry in which there is an interaction between the head and the tail of the rotating wave can be intrinsically unstable. Several mechanisms may contribute to this instability. First, instability may arise from the dependence of conduction velocity on the excitation interval. A wavefront penetrating into the partially refractory tail slows down. As the velocity decreases, the wavefront retreats from the refractory tail and propagates in a more recovered medium. Consequently, the velocity increases and the wavefront impinges on the refractory tail again. Sequential slowing and acceleration of the wave lead to oscillations of the tachycardia cycle length. Simson et al. investigated this type of instability in computer simulations and in an experimental model of a re-entrant circuit involving the AV node and a bypass tract (354). During wave rotation, they observed oscillations in cycle length that could either dampen or increase in amplitude. In the latter case conduction got eventually blocked. The stability of rotation was critically dependent on the steepness of the AV nodal recovery curve (dependence of AV nodal conduction time on excitation interval) and on the length of the re-entrant circuit. When the circuit was short, the re-entrant tachycardia operated in the range of the recovery curve where AV nodal conduction time was sensitive to changes in cycle length. In this case a small initial perturbation in the cycle length caused a large change in the AV nodal conduction time, which translated into a larger change in the cycle length during the next re-entrant beat. In such a way, small initial perturbations in the cycle length amplified with time, causing termination of reentry. During these oscillations, short and long intervals alternated and termination followed a critically short cycle length. In the case of a long circuit, perturbations of cycle length produced dampened oscillations which finally settled to a stable rotation.

The second source of instability in an anatomic reentrant circuit is the dependence of the action potential duration and the refractory period on the preceding diastolic intervals (restitution dependence). In a re-entrant circuit, action potential duration and diastolic interval are mutually dependent (diastolic interval = cycle length − action potential duration) at any given cycle length. If action potential duration gets prolonged during a re-entry cycle, then the subsequent, reduced diastolic interval can cause shortening of action potential during the following cycle and the diastolic interval will increase again. Oscillations in action potential and refractoriness may cause changes in conduction velocity and in the rotation period. Like the instability related to the rate dependence of conduction velocity (see above), the oscillations of action potential duration can either dampen or increase in amplitude (355). The transition from one regime to the other was determined by the slope of the restitution dependence: when the slope was greater than 1, re-entry was unstable (355). In real tissue, oscillations of conduction velocity and action potential duration may interact in a complex way. In addition they can occur at more than one site within the anatomically defined pathway. As a result, oscillations in such circuits may be complex and can include periodic and aperiodic regimes (355, 356). Frame et al. (357) investigated circus movement propagating around the tricuspid orifice in preparations of canine atrial tissue. They found that unstable tachycardias often exhibited spontaneous irregular oscillations of cycle length, diastolic interval, action potential duration, and conduction velocity. The variations in diastolic interval and action potential duration tended to be much larger than the changes in cycle length and conduction velocity. In several cases they observed unstable tachycardias with no cycle length variation. Termination of re-entry usually occurred at a short cycle length typical for the oscillatory behavior of conduction velocity, but occasionally it happened after a long cycle or with stable cycle length. In these latter cases, instability and termination of re-entry were presumably caused by oscillations in action potential duration and refractoriness.

Functional Re-entry—the Leading Circle Concept

In functional re-entry, the excitation wave propagates around a central area with functional conduction block. The hypothesis that re-entry can occur without involvement of an anatomic obstacle was first proposed by Garrey in 1924 (358). Only 50 years later, with the development of the multielectrode mapping technique, the experimental proof that such a re-entry can occur was provided by Allessie et al. (318, 350, 359). They induced a rapid tachycardia in isolated preparations of rabbit atrial tissue by application of a critically timed premature stimulus. Figure 12–53 shows an activation map during regular pacing (basic beat), during the premature beat that initiated the tachycardia, and during the first cycle of tachycardia (359). Also shown is a distribution of refractory periods measured during regular basic rhythm. No anatomic obstacle was detected on the map of the basic beat, i.e. the excitation propagated in all directions from the central stimulating electrode. The premature wave propagated into the areas with shorter refractory periods and was blocked in the direction where refractory periods were longer. The line of conduction block extended across the center of the preparation along a distance of approximately 5 mm. Excitation propagated in two directions around the line of block and the two wavefronts merged behind the line of block. At that time, the tissue proximal to the site of block had recovered from the premature excitation and could be re-excited by the merged wavefront. The original area of conduction block broke up into two new areas, and two wavefronts propagated around them in opposite directions, clockwise, the other counterclockwise. Subsequently, one wave became extinct at the border of the preparation, leaving only a single re-entrant circuit. Arrhythmias induced in such a way were often short-lived, terminating spontaneously after one or several beats, or more stable, lasting for many seconds. Figure 12–54 shows an activation map during stable tachycardia, together with recordings of membrane potential from the center of the re-entrant circuit. Intracellular recordings were made from seven sites located on a straight line through the zone of functional conduction block. Recordings obtained from one side of the central area (traces A, 1, 2, and 3) demonstrate a gradual decrease of the amplitude, rate of rise, and duration of the action potentials. The recording from fiber 3 demonstrates double potentials where the larger voltage deflection is caused by the wavefront propagating from left to right and the smaller voltage deflection is caused by the electrotonic influence of the same wavefront propagating half a cycle length later from left to right. The same sequence of events occurs on the opposite side of the circuit (traces D, 5, and 4). The stable tachycardias could be reset or terminated by a properly timed stimulus delivered from an electrode located close to the central re-entrant circuit, which indicated the presence of a partially excitable gap (359).

After the pioneering experiments of Allessie and co-

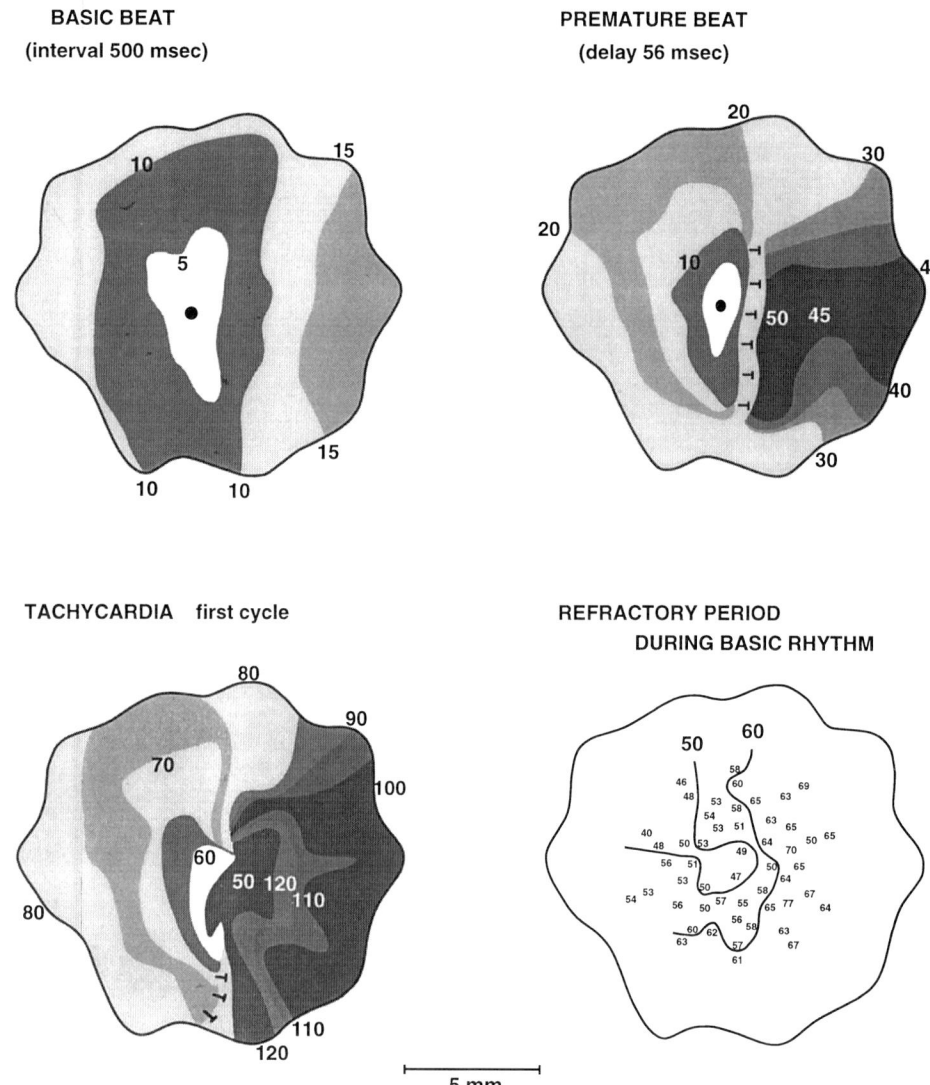

FIG. 12-53. Initiation of functional re-entry by premature stimulation in an isolated preparation of rabbit atrial muscle. *A:* Isochronal activation map of basic beat (interval 500 msec). *Dots* indicate sites of stimulation. Activation times (msec) are given relative to the stimulus onset. *B:* Map of premature beat (interval 56 msec). *T bars* indicate conduction block. *C:* First cycle of tachycardia. *D:* Refractory periods measured during basic rhythm (in msec). [Reproduced with permission from reference 318.]

workers in atrial muscle, functional re-entrant circuits with activation patterns of varying complexity were observed in both atrial and ventricular muscle. It was found that circulating waves often appear in pairs, whereby two wavefronts rotate in opposite directions. This type of activation pattern was called "figure-8" re-entry (360–362). Because the functional re-entrant circuits are not tied to anatomic structures, they can change their location and size. The activation can become even more complex when several rotating wavefronts are present in cardiac muscle (so called random re-entry [363]). Thus, multiple re-entrant circuits were observed during stable atrial fibrillation (364) and during ventricular fibrillation in ischemic hearts (365).

To explain the properties of a single functional re-entrant circuit, Allessie et al. formulated the concept of the "leading circle" re-entry (350). It was postulated that during wave rotation in a tissue without unexcitable obstacles, the wavefront impinges on its refractory tail and travels through partially refractory tissue. The interaction between the wavefront and the refractory tail determines the properties of functional re-entry. The leading circle was defined as "the smallest possible pathway in which the impulse can continue to circu-

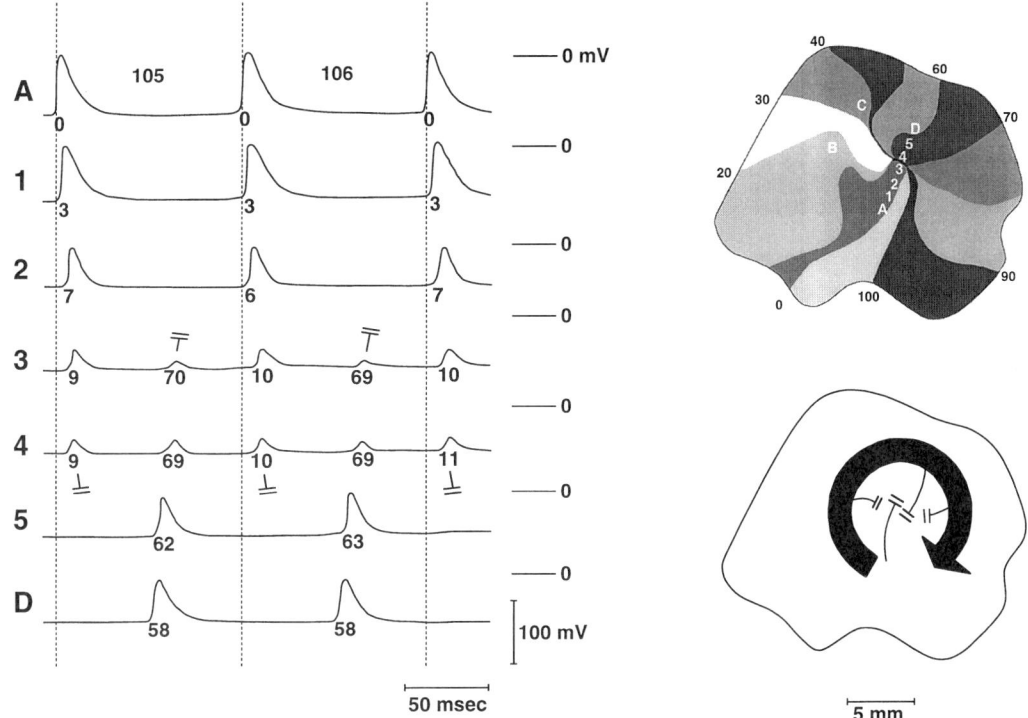

FIG. 12–54. Functional re-entry and tachycardia. Activation map (*right*) and action potential recordings (*left*) obtained during steady-state tachycardia. Cells in the central area of the re-entrant circuit show double potentials of low amplitude (traces 3 and 4). *Lower right:* Schematic representation of the activation pattern. Double bars indicate conduction block. [Reproduced with permission from reference 350.]

late," and "in which the stimulating efficacy of the wavefront is just enough to excite the tissue ahead which is still in its relative refractory phase" (350). Because the wavefront propagates through partially refractory tissue, the conduction velocity is reduced. The velocity value and the length of the circuit depend on the excitability of the partially refractory tissue and on the stimulating efficacy of the wavefront, which is determined by the amplitude and the upstroke velocity of the action potential. The revolution time is confined to the relative refractory period, and no fully excitable gap exists according to this mechanism.

The leading circle mechanism takes into consideration those parameters of impulse conduction that determine propagation in a one-dimensional tissue. The concept was a major breakthrough in the understanding of the mechanisms of re-entrant excitation. However, it recently became evident that these considerations alone do not fully describe wave rotation in two- and three-dimensional tissues. As has been discussed in previous sections, propagation of two- and three-dimensional waves depends on wavefront curvature. A mechanism of wave rotation which additionally takes into account the curvature dependence was developed in studies of rotating waves known in literature as "spiral waves."

Spiral Wave Re-entry

The notion of spiral waves appeared in the generic theory of excitable media to describe rotating waves of excitation in a variety of excitable systems of biological, chemical, and physical origin. One of the most extensively studied examples is the Belousov-Zhabotinsky (BZ) reaction. In this reaction, malonic acid is reversibly oxidized by bromate in the presence of ferroin. In this process, ferroin changes in color from red to blue and then back to red, which allows the visual observation of the reaction. Figure 12–55A demonstrates a rotating wave in a thin two-dimensional layer of the Belousov-Zhabotinsky (BZ) reaction (366). In the center of the rotating wave (core) the tip of the wave moves along a complex trajectory and radiates waves into the surrounding medium. Since the velocity of a convex wavefront can not exceed the speed of the flat wave, θ_0, the rotating wave has to acquire the shape of a spiral, hence the name "spiral wave." Other names used in the literature include "vortices" and "reverber-

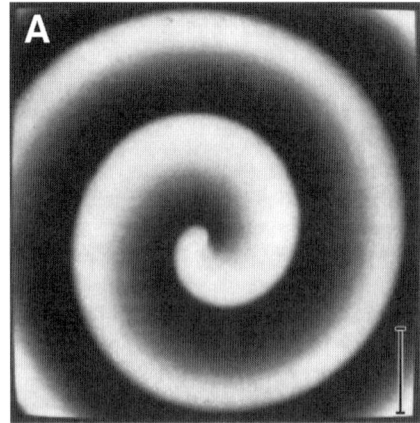 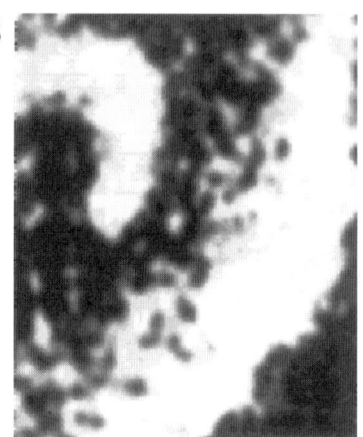

FIG. 12–55. Spiral waves. Spiral waves in chemical Belousov-Zhabotinsky reaction (*A*) and in an isolated preparation of canine epicardial muscle (*B*). [Reproduced with permission from references 366 and 376.]

ators." In some cases a term "rotor" was used to refer to the core of a spiral wave. Besides the Belousov-Zhabotinsky reaction, (367) spiral waves were also found in other excitable media including neural tissue (depression waves in the retina [368] and cerebral cortex [369]), intracellular calcium signaling systems (*Xenopus laevis* oocytes (370), cardiac myocytes [371]), and amoebae colonies (372).

In the heart, spiral waves have been implicated in the generation of cardiac arrhythmias for a long time (367, 373–375). However the first experimental observation of rotating waves in atrial muscle (cf. Fig. 12–53 and 12–54) revealed no obvious spiral pattern of activation. The lack of spiral shape in the experiments of Allessie et al. (318, 350, 359) might be due to two reasons: (*1*) the diameter of the preparation in these experiments, about 2 cm, was close to the wavelength of excitation. Therefore, there was room for only the central portion of the rotating wave, and the spiral shape was not prominent on this scale. (*2*) The spiral shape might have been further masked by electrophysiological heterogeneities present in atrial muscle. Provided that the size of the preparation is large and/or the excitation wavelength is small, the wavefront will inevitably acquire a spiral shape. Indeed, rotating waves with the spiral shape were observed recently in preparations of sheep ventricular muscle (376). Figure 12–55*B* shows an optical image of transmembrane potential distribution obtained using a voltage-sensitive dye. These preparations were highly anisotropic with low conduction velocity and, therefore, had a short wavelength of excitation in the transverse direction. Because of the short wavelength, there was enough place for the wave to curl and to assume a distinct spiral shape.

Initiation of Spiral Waves. The starting event in the initiation of spiral wave re-entry is formation of a free wave break (or so-called phase singularity [377]). This can be achieved in several different ways. The classical and most extensively investigated mechanism depends on the delivery of a critically timed premature stimulus to an area of tissue that exhibits gradients in refractoriness. As explained in the paragraph on unidirectional conduction block, such gradients may be due to spatial differences in intrinsic electrical properties (318, 362, 378), or they may arise from the passage of another wavefront (312, 313, 373). As shown in Figure 12–56, Selfridge induced a flat propagating wave by stimulation from one location and then delivered a premature stimulus at another location over a rectangular area that overlapped with the refractory tail of the propagating wave (panel A). The newly excited wavefront could propagate in the retrograde (from right to left) and in the upward directions, but not in the antegrade direction because the tissue ahead in this direction was still refractory. Therefore, a wave break was formed at the upper edge of the excited area which propagated first in the vertical direction and then, when the refractory tissue ahead recovered from the previous excitation, in the antegrade and downward directions as well (panel B). After recovery of the directly excited rectangular area, the wavefront made a complete turn (panels C, D, and E) and formed a spiral wave (panel F).

Cardiac tissue is usually stimulated by extracellular electrodes that produce gradients in the extracellular electrical field. It has been predicted theoretically (1) and shown experimentally (379) that strong electrical fields overlapping with the refractory tails of propagating waves can produce breaks of excitation waves

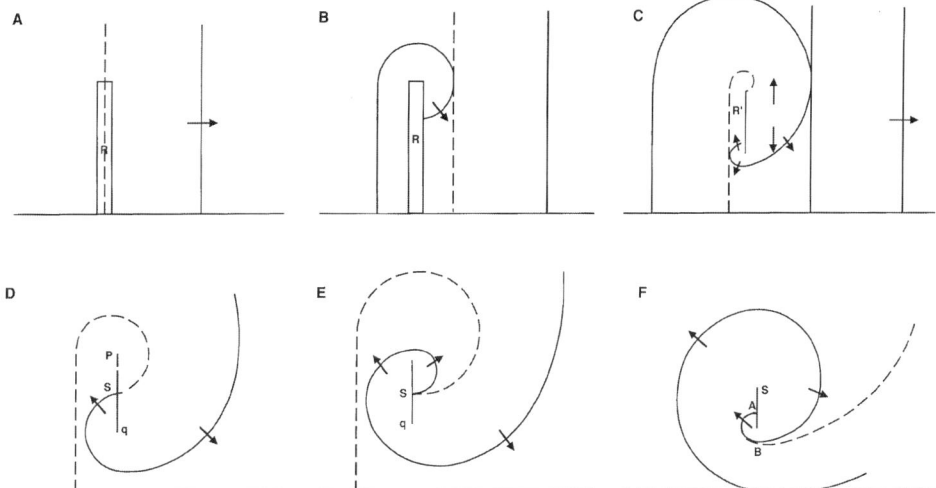

FIG. 12–56. Initiation of spiral wave in a simple model of cardiac excitation. A rectangular area R is excited overlapping the absolutely refractory tail of a propagating wave (*A*). The premature wave propagates in the retrograde direction (right to left) but blocks in the anterograde direction, forming a wave break that turns around the refractory area R (*B*). When the area R recovers, the excitation wave short-circuits this area (*C*) and forms a spiral wave rotating around a linear line of block (*D–F*). [Reproduced with permission from reference 373).]

and initiate re-entry. Called "cross-field" stimulation, this method is now routinely used to initiate re-entrant excitation (376, 380). The mechanism of cross-field stimulation is demonstrated in Figure 12–57. In this experiment, the epicardial surface of a healthy canine heart was stimulated first by a linear electrode array, S1, to induce a flat propagating wave. As shown in panel A, both the wavefront and the refractory tail were rectilinear and running parallel to each other, indicating absence of heterogeneities in refractory periods. After some delay, an electrical shock was applied via a separate electrode, S2, oriented perpendicular to the S1 electrode. Electrical field gradients created by the S2 shock are shown in panel B. Panel C demonstrates the pattern of re-entry initiation when the S2 shock was applied 190 msec after the S1 stimulus. Earliest propagated activity was detected in the upper part of the mapping area at a distance of approximately 20 mm away from the shock electrode. This activity propagated in the counterclockwise direction around the zone of functional conduction block (thin hatched area) and initiated re-entry. Panel D schematically shows the mechanism of re-entry initiation. According to this mechanism, the S2 shock directly activates the tissue in the wake of the propagating wave. Because the stimulating efficacy of the S2 shock depends on tissue recovery from the previous excitation and the shock strength decreases with distance, a variable amount of tissue is excited by the shock. Near the S2 electrode, the shock directly excites all relatively refractory tissue. In the periphery, the S2 shock gradient is small and excites only the tissue that has fully recovered from the previous excitation. In this area, the directly excited tissue faces relative refractory tissue on the left side and, therefore, excitation is able to propagate from left to right. At the junction of the two areas a wave break is created which initiates the circus movement.

Spiral waves may further be initiated if wavefronts detach from sharp unexcitable obstacles. Figure 12–58 demonstrates wave propagation around a thin obstacle in a computer model of an excitable medium. The ionic currents in this model are described by the Luo-Rudy kinetics (7) with maximal sodium conductance reduced to approximately 30% of its nominal value. Panel A shows the snapshot of the sodium current distribution; times of local activation taken at the peak of the sodium current were used to construct the isochronal activation map shown in panel B. The wave was initiated at the upper left edge of the medium and propagated from left to right. After the wave reached the end of the obstacle, the front detached and started to move freely. This detachment took place because the *strong curvature* at the tip of the wave excluded an abrupt turn around the sharp edge. The tip moved along a circular trajectory and the area circumnavigated by the tip remained at rest. The radius of this pivoting trajectory, r_p, is important for the understanding of wave detachment. In tissue with normal excitability r_p is very small, much smaller than the wavelength of excitation.

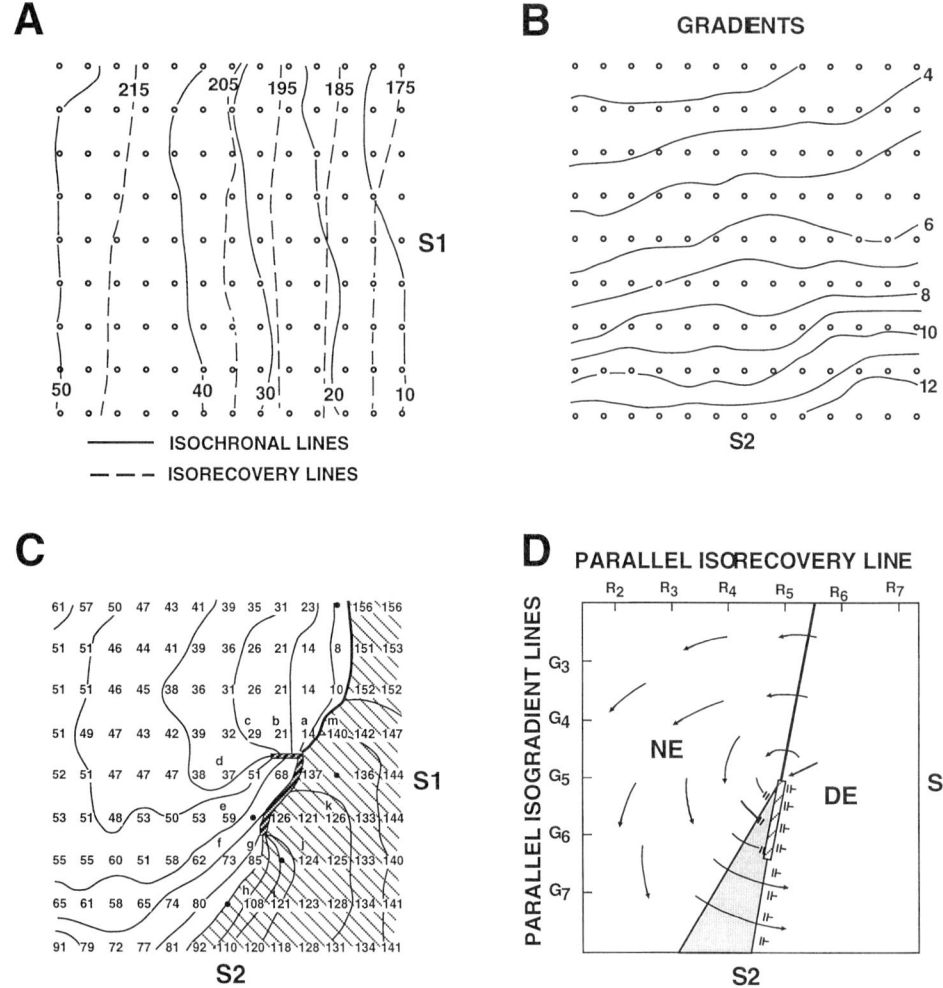

FIG. 12–57. Initiation of a spiral wave by cross-field stimulation in canine right ventricular myocardium. *A:* Isochronal maps of activation and repolarization during wave propagation induced by stimulation (S1) from a line of eight epicardial pacing sites. Solid lines depict isochronal activation lines; dashed lines depict isorecovery lines. Numbers indicate time in msec. *B:* Gradients of extracellular potential (in V/cm) produced by a unipolar cathodal shock (S2) of 150 V from a mesh electrode at the bottom. *C:* Pattern of activation spread following sequential application of S1 stimulus from the right and S2 shock from the bottom. The S1–S2 interval was 191 msec and the S2 strength was 150 V. Activation times (msec) are measured from the start of the 3 msec S2 shock. The heavy solid line represents the transition between successive activation maps. Isochrones are drawn at 10 msec intervals. The hatched line represents a zone of conduction block. The double-headed arrow indicates the mean epicardial fiber orientation in the area of conduction block. The hatched area indicates the region assumed to be directly excited by the S2 shock field. Earliest post-shock activation occurs distant from the S2 site, with no early activation wavefronts conducting away from the directly excited region located between the S2 site and the critical point. A counterclockwise re-entrant circuit is formed around the region containing the critical point and the block line. The potential gradient equals 5.8 V/cm, and the pre-shock interval equals 171 msec at the critical point (critical refractory period = 169 msec). *D:* Schematic representation of the re-entry initiation by cross-field stimulation. The row of pacing wires (S1) on the right creates parallel isorecovery lines (R_7 through R_2), with R_7 the least refractory and R_2 the most refractory. The S2 from the bottom creates parallel isogradient lines (G_7 through G_3), with G_7 the largest potential gradient and G_3 the weakest. The S2 shock produces direct excitation (DE), graded response (GR), or neither effect (NE). Activation fronts propagate from only one part of the directly excited area, not from the directly excited region abutting the area of graded response, thus forming a zone of unidirectional conduction block. [Reproduced with permission from reference 379.]

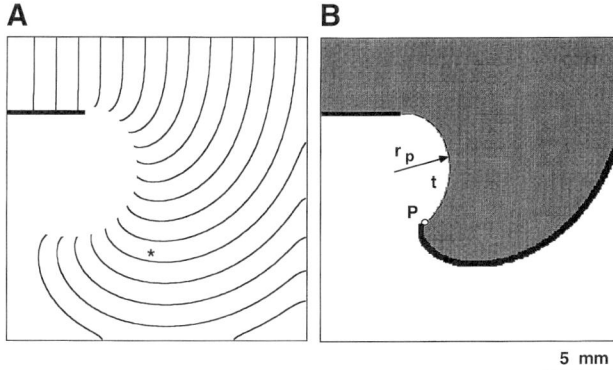

FIG. 12–58. Initiation of a spiral wave at a pivoting point. Formation of a free wave break after wavefront detachment from the sharp edge of an inexcitable obstacle. Computer model with Luo-Rudy ionic kinetics. The maximal sodium conductance was reduced to 6.6 mS/cm^2. A: Isochronal map of activation spread with an interval of 5 msec. B: Snapshot of activation at the moment marked by the asterisk in A. Black indicates the excited area defined by the activation of inward Na$^+$ current. Gray indicates the area in the refractory state as defined by Na$^+$ current inactivation. Point P marks the wave tip, defined as a point where excited, refractory, and resting states meet. The dashed line t shows the trajectory of the wave tip with the radius r$_p$ [Reproduced with permission from reference 34.]

Therefore, the tissue is still refractory when the wavefront tip returns to the obstacle. However, r$_p$ rapidly increases with the reduction of tissue excitability. In this case the pivoting radius, which is closely related to the minimal radius of curvature, can become so large that the returning wavefront encounters excitable tissue and detaches from the pivoting point. Formally this criterion is met when the pivoting trajectory gets longer than the wavelength of excitation (r$_p$ × 2π > λ). Formation of spiral waves at a sharp obstacle was described in a computer model (381) and in the experiments on the chemical Belousov-Zhabotinsky reaction (382). In cardiac tissue, wave propagation around an unexcitable obstacle was recently investigated in two studies. In the work of Girouard et al. (331) long linear unexcitable obstacles were created on the epicardial surface of rabbit myocardium with a laser beam. Since excitability was normal, no detachment of the wavefront from the obstacle took place. Nevertheless, wavefront curvature produced a significant slowing of conduction when the wave turned around the obstacle. In another study, narrow obstacles were created on the epicardial surface of sheep ventricular muscle with sharp cuts (332). As in the work by Girouard et al., no detachment of the wavefront was found under control physiological conditions. However, reduction of tissue excitability caused by application of tetrodotoxin or by stimulation at high rates, caused detachment of wavefronts from sharp obstacles and initiation of spiral waves.

Dynamics of Spiral Waves. *In anatomic re-entry*, interaction between the head and the tail of the wavefront was shown to cause complex oscillatory behavior of rotation periods, while the location of the re-entrant circuit, because of its anatomical nature, remained fixed. *In functional re-entry*, mutual dependence and interaction between electrophysiological parameters and the excitation rate during re-entrant activity may further result in complex and unstable *movements* of spiral waves. Three main types of instabilities were distinguished in computer simulations and experiments. In the first, the dynamic interaction between the wavefront and the wave tail during spiral wave rotation in a homogeneous medium resulted in the "meandering" of the tip or center of the spiral waves. In the second, the wavefront–tail interaction caused spontaneous break-up and multiplication of spiral waves. In the third, heterogeneities in electrophysiological tissue parameters produced spiral wave drift.

Meandering. Figure 12–59 demonstrates the dynamics of spiral wave rotation in computer models of homogeneous excitable media. Results obtained with two different models are presented. The first model (panels A–C) uses so-called cellular automata to represent excitable properties of the medium. In this

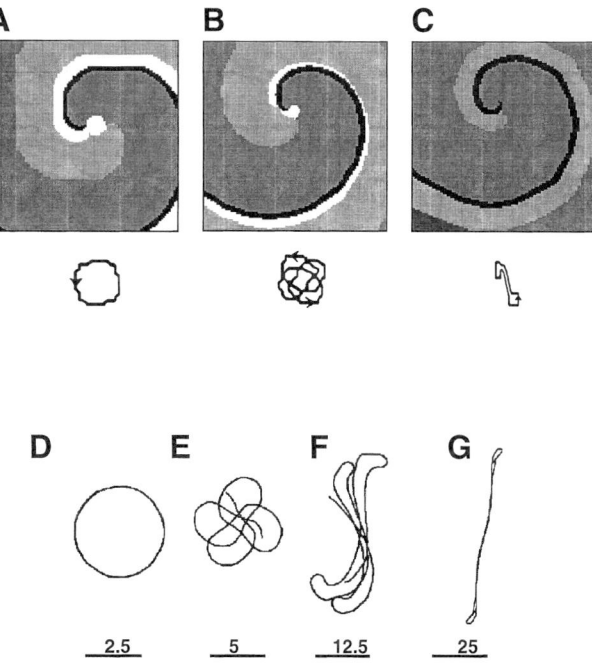

FIG. 12–59. Dynamics of spiral wave rotation in mathematical models of cardiac excitation. A–C: Cellular automata model. Spiral wave rotation changes from circular (A) to meandering (B), and then to Z-type (C) with increasing excitability. D–G: FitzHugh-Nagumo model. The same types of rotation are observed when the wavelength of excitation is increased. [Reproduced with permission from references 450 and 383.]

model, excitable elements are described by four states (excited, absolute refractory, relative refractory, and resting) and formal rules determine the transition from one state to another (383). The integrative properties of excitable media such as excitability and the durations of the absolute and relative refractory periods are set as model parameters and can be easily monitored during spiral wave rotation. The second model (panels D–G) describes excitable dynamics by means of partial differential equations (FitzHugh-Nagumo type, FHN) (384). Both models reproduce qualitatively the dependence of conduction velocity on excitation interval and wavefront curvature. Panel A illustrates the simplest type of spiral wave rotation when the excitability in the model was very low. In this case, the critical radius of curvature of the wavefront tip, r_c, and therefore the pivoting radius of the wave tip, r_p, were relatively large. By contrast, the wavelength of excitation (λ) given by product of the velocity of propagation θ and the refractory period R ($\lambda = \theta * R$) was short as a result of the small θ. Under these conditions, the length of the pivoting trajectory ($2\pi r_p$) was larger than λ, and, therefore, propagation of the excitation wavefront was not affected by the refractory tail. The only constraint on the wavefront propagation was imposed by the curvature at its tip. Because the wavefront curvature could not exceed the critical curvature, r_c, the wave tip did not extend toward the center of the rotation but followed a circular trajectory (panel A, bottom). The wave rotated rigidly around a circular area that remained at rest. In addition, there was a zone in the resting state between the wave front and the wave tail, i.e. the spiral wave contained a fully excitable gap.

At a higher level of excitability, when the length of the pivoting trajectory became comparable to the wavelength of excitation ($2\pi r_p \approx \lambda$), the front of the excitation wave started to interact with its own refractory tail, as shown at the top of panel B. This interaction resulted in the loss of rotation stability which is best seen on the 'meandering' trajectory of the wave tip shown on panel B (bottom). The unstable rotation was explained by the fluctuations of the wavefront velocity caused by sequential intrusion and retraction of the wavefront within the wave tail. Such a meandering movement of spiral waves was first observed in the BZ reaction (1, 385) and was extensively investigated in a variety of mathematical models (38, 384, 386–391).

When excitability was further increased and the wavelength became larger than the length of the pivoting trajectory ($\lambda > 2\pi r_p$), the interaction between the wavefront and the refractory wave tail became stronger. Panel C (top) shows that, in this case, the wavefront penetrated deeper into the wave tail and there was no longer a fully excitable gap. A part of the wave tip trajectory acquired a linear shape. The linear part was formed when the tip of the spiral wave moved along its refractory tail, which served as a zone of functional conduction block. At the end of the linear part the wave tip made a turn and propagated in the opposite direction. As a result, the wave tip trajectory was composed of the linear portion and two circular parts at the ends of the linear portion, thus resembling a letter "Z", as shown in panel C (bottom). The size of the circular part in such a trajectory depends on the pivoting radius, while the length of the linear portion depends on the wavelength of excitation. An increase of the ratio λ/r_p increases the linear part of the trajectory and decreases the circular part. In the extreme case of a negligibly small r_p, the wave tip follows a linear trajectory (not shown). The shapes of spiral wave rotation observed in the cellular automata model were also found in the FHN model (panels D–G), indicating that they are a general feature of spiral waves and are model-independent.

To predict the type of spiral wave rotation in cardiac muscle, one needs to compare the excitation wavelength λ with the length of the pivoting trajectory ($2 p r_p$). The normal wavelength value in cardiac muscle is approximately 2 cm during sustained wave rotation ($\theta = 20$ cm/sec, refractory period = 0.1 sec). The value of the pivoting radius has not yet been measured yet. Estimation of this parameter in computer models and experiments with wavefront detachment from a sharp unexcitable obstacle (see above) suggests, that it is much smaller than l, however. Therefore, for cardiac tissue in a normal state of cell-to-cell coupling and with normal excitability, the trajectory of the tip is expected to assume the linear ƻ shape (Fig. 12–59 C, F, and G). Indeed, mapping experiments in myocardium have shown that the zone of functional conduction block often has a linear shape (350, 351, 379, 392). Under conditions of reduced excitability, the contribution of curvature dependence may become more pronounced and in such a case, "meandering" or even circular movement of spiral waves can be anticipated (Fig. 12–57 A, B, D, and E). Such meandering of spiral wave rotation has been implicated in the mechanism of polymorphic arrhythmias (391, 393).

Break-up and multiplication. The mechanism of the spiral wave meandering illustrated in Figure 12–59 was related mainly to the dependence of conduction velocity on the excitation interval, i.e. the degree of penetration of the wavefront into the partially refractory tail of the preceding wave. By contrast, the dependence of the refractory period and the action potential duration on the diastolic interval or the restitution dependence (see earlier, under Anatomical Re-entry) was absent in the cellular automata model and relatively weak in the FHN model. More realistic ionic models of cardiac excitation exhibit rather strong restitution dependence. Computer simulations in these models have shown that spiral waves can undergo more complex transformations including spontaneous break-up and multiplication of wavefronts. Using the Beeler-Reuter model (5), it was found that a single spiral wave could spontaneously break up soon after initiation and generate multiple excitation wavelets (394, 395). This effect was observed at nominal values of model parameters but it was absent when sodium conductance was reduced (389) or when calcium current dynamics became accelerated (396). The effect of spontaneous break-up into multiple waves was also reported for more precise models of cardiac excitation such as the Luo-Rudy model (397, 398) as well as for several generic models of excitable media (399–401). Analysis of the conditions for the spiral wave break-up in computer models indicated that, like instabilities in anatomical re-entry, the spiral wave break-up was promoted by an increase in the slope of the restitution dependence (397, 402). Based on theoretical studies it has been suggested that such spontaneous wave break-up due to steep restitution dependence is responsible for the transition from ventricular tachycardia to ventricular fibrillation. This hypothesis was supported by the data from experiments in canine ventricles where large values of the restitution dependence slope (>1) were measured during fibrillation (403). Furthermore, application of drugs that reduced the slope of the restitution dependence also prevented the induction of ventricular fibrillation or converted fibrillation into periodic rhythm (404).

Drift in media with heterogeneity in refractoriness. In addition to the meandering and the break-up instabilities that can occur in a homogenous tissue, spiral wave instability may result from the electrophysiological heterogeneity of cardiac tissue. It was shown both in computer simulations (405, 406) and in experiments (378, 407) that heterogeneities in refractory period can cause drift of spiral waves, and eventually, termination. The first experimental observation of spiral wave drift in cardiac muscle was reported by Fast and Pertsov (407). In this work spiral waves were initiated in isolated two-dimensional preparations of rabbit ventricular epicardium. Preparations were placed in a chamber with two compartments divided by a thin rubber barrier (shown by a dashed line on Figure 12–60). The bottom part of the preparation was perfused with a solution containing quinidine to prolong the refractory period, while the upper part was perfused with normal Tyrode's solution. As shown in panel A, premature stimulation from the top area (with the short refractoriness) induced conduction block at the border between the two compartments and the formation of a spiral wave rotating in a counterclockwise direction. Wave rotation lasted for 3.5 cycles. After initiation the spiral wave moved along the border of heterogeneity perpendicular to the gradient of refractoriness (panel B). The trajectory of the wave tip during the whole arrhythmia illustrates that the spiral wave continued to drift until it became extinct at the border of the preparation (panel C). The drift velocity amounted to about one-fifth of the propagation velocity. Its direction was determined by the direction of wave rotation and the gradient of refractoriness. When a spiral wave with a clockwise rotation was initiated, it drifted in the opposite direction.

Because of the drift of a spiral wave, the frequency of excitation at a given measurement site depends on the location of this site relative to the moving spiral. Figure 12–60D shows excitation intervals measured during spiral wave drift at various tissue locations. The measuring sites were distributed along the boundary of heterogeneity which determined the direction of the drift. Because of the drift, the sites located in front of the drifting spiral wave were excited significantly faster than the sites located behind it. This effect is known in the theory of electromagnetic and acoustic waves as the *Doppler effect*. The difference in excitation intervals measured ahead of and behind the spiral wave amounted to 30%. Drift of spiral waves and the Doppler effect were also observed in isolated preparations of sheep ventricular muscle (376, 408). In this case, no artificial heterogeneity in refractoriness was created and the spiral wave drift was likely to be a result of intrinsic spatial gradients of electrophysiologic properties. The Doppler effect and the coexistence of different excitation frequencies within the same preparation were used to explain one of the possible mechanisms underlying the ECG pattern during ventricular tachycardias (*torsades de pointes* [408, 409]) and fibrillation (393, 410).

Spiral Waves in Anisotropic and Microscopically Discontinuous Media. Cardiac muscle is different in several important aspects from the generic excitable media typically considered in the theory of spiral waves. These differences include tissue anisotropy and discontinuities in tissue structure. In absence of discontinuities, the results obtained for isotropic models can be directly extended to anisotropic tissue. In such a case, the effect of anisotropy is formally equivalent to geometrical scaling. The dimensions in the transverse direction are thereby reduced by a factor, f, which equals the square root of the ratio between resistivities in the transverse and the longitudinal directions [$f = (r_t/r_l)^{1/2}$]. Computer simulations have shown that introducing anisotropy in such a way changes neither the period of spiral wave rotation nor the duration of the excitable gap (408).

The effect of tissue discontinuities on spiral wave ro-

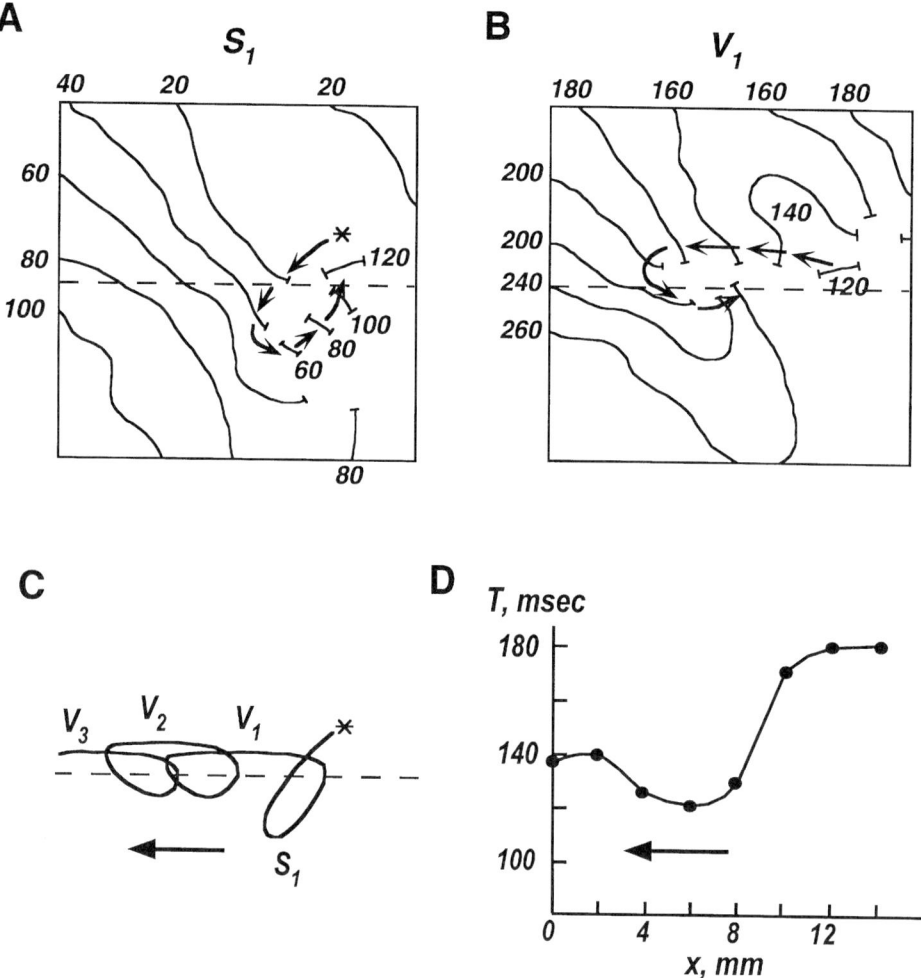

FIG. 12-60. Drift of a spiral wave and the Doppler effect. *A* and *B:* Isochronal activation maps showing initiation (*A*) and the first rotation cycle (*B*) of a spiral wave in an isolated preparation of epicardial muscle. A stepwise inhomogeneity in refractory period was created by separate superfusion of two parts of the preparation with normal and quinidine-containing solutions. Dashed line shows the border of inhomogeneity with larger refractoriness in the upper part. The asterisk shows the location of the stimulation electrode. *C:* Trajectory of the spiral wave tip during initiation (S_1) and three subsequent cycles of spiral wave rotation (V_1–V_3). *D:* Excitation intervals measured along the border of inhomogeneity during spiral wave drift (cycle V_2). Because of the drift, excitation intervals in front of the spiral wave are significantly shorter than intervals behind the spiral wave (Doppler effect). [Reproduced with permission from reference 407.]

tation depends on their dimensions, shapes, and distribution pattern. Myocardium contains electrical discontinuities at different levels of tissue architecture. The smallest discontinuities, created by cell borders and nonuniform pattern of gap junction distribution, were reproduced in a computer model in the study by Leon et al. (395). They simulated spiral waves in a medium composed of a set of parallel, continuous, and uniform cables transversely interconnected by a brick-wall arrangement of fixed resistors separated by a distance of 100 μm. In this model, longitudinal propagation was continuous, whereas transverse propagation exhibited discontinuous features. On a qualitative level, spiral wave rotation in this model was similar to the behavior observed in electrically continuous models, which suggests that small-scale discontinuities compatible with the cellular structure at normal levels of intercellular coupling do not significantly alter spiral wave rotation and movement. This may be different in tissues with more sparse intercellular coupling, in tissues where coupling is impaired, or in tissue with increased fibrosis. In this case, predictions based on models of generic continuous excitable media may not be valid anymore (see below).

Spiral Waves in Three Dimensions. Representation of the myocardium as a two-dimensional excitable medium may be valid for thin myocardial tissue such as atrial muscle (350) or surviving subepicardial muscle layers (411, 412). However, in other preparations such as intact left ventricular wall, the three-dimensional structure of cardiac muscle must be taken into account. Analogues of spiral waves in three dimensions are called *scroll waves*. In a three-dimensional medium, the front of a scroll wave is characterized by a filament, in analogy to the tip of a spiral wave in two-dimensions. The simplest case of a scroll wave is an extension of a two-dimensional spiral wave into the third dimension. Provided that cardiac tissue is homogeneous and the scroll filament is a straight line, the behavior of such a wave is equivalent to the behavior of a two-dimensional spiral wave. The behavior of a scroll wave may change when muscle properties vary with depth or when the scroll wave filament gets bent or twisted. The specific three-dimensional effects related to scroll wave rotation were extensively investigated in computer models. A brief review of these data has been published recently (413). One of the effects specific to three-dimensional media is the rotation of scroll waves with filaments which are bent or closed to form rings. These scroll waves are intrinsically unstable and can terminate spontaneously (414). Another theoretical possibility is a persistent, twisted rotation of a scroll wave. Such a movement results in a fibrillation-like activation pattern when projected to the surface of the medium (415). The experimental verification of these effects in cardiac muscle is still lacking due to the inability to map three-dimensional activation spread with sufficiently high spatial resolution.

Transition from Functional to Anatomic Re-entry. Anchoring of Spiral Waves

One of the discrepancies between the theoretical predictions and the experimental results relates to the stability of re-entrant circuits. In many of the experimentally induced tachycardias, the initial transition from a normal propagation pattern during a basic beat to functional re-entrant excitation is caused by a premature wave propagating through tissue with heterogeneous refractoriness. According to the mechanisms of spiral wave instability described above, including meandering and heterogeneity-dependent drift, such waves should be unstable. However, mapping experiments have shown that such re-entrant circuits are often stable, rotating rigidly around a fixed core. This discrepancy can be explained by stabilizing effects of small localized discontinuities in tissue structure which create inexcitable obstacles (376). Stabilization may occur at the beginning of tachycardia. Alternatively, the tachycardia may be initiated first as a functional re-entrant circuit, drift until it meets a resistive barrier, and stabilize at such a discontinuity, thereby changing from functional into anatomic or combined functional-anatomic re-entry. Figure 12–61 shows an example of the anchoring of an initially drifting spiral wave (380). Electrical activity in this case is represented in the form of a time-space plot (panel B) where signals from all measuring points are projected into a single line that is displayed as a function of time (see reference 376 for details). In such diagrams, a

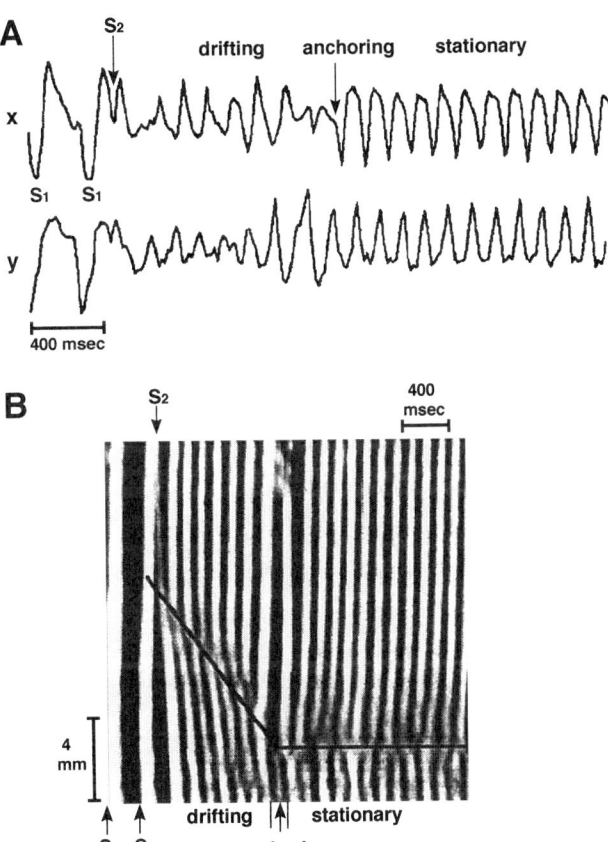

FIG. 12–61. Anchoring of a spiral wave. *A*: Electrocardiographic recordings showing that premature stimulation (S_2) produced polymorphic arrhythmic activity followed by a transition to sustained monomorphic tachycardia. *B*: Time-space plot of activation spread obtained from video-imaging of transmembrane potential (voltage-sensitive dye). In these plots, the activity from the whole image is projected onto a single direction (vertical axis) and displayed as a function of time. White bands show a planar wave propagation while *branching* of bands indicates the presence of a spiral wave induced by the S_2 stimulus. As detected from the movement of the branching point, which marks the center of the spiral, the spiral drifted during the first seven cycles and became stationary thereafter. [Reproduced with permission from reference 380.]

propagating wave is represented by a narrow band and the location of the spiral wave core is equivalent to the point of band branching. Initially the spiral wave drifted in a downward direction as shown by the straight line. After eight cycles of rotation, the spiral wave was anchored and became stationary. In most cases of stable rotation a band of connective tissue or a small branch of the coronary artery was identified as the site of anchoring.

Anisotropic Re-entry. The role of tissue anisotropy in re-entrant excitation was investigated in several experimental models of anisotropic tissue including a surviving layer of epicardial muscle overlaying a healed infarct in the canine heart (349, 360–362, 416–419) and a two-dimensional preparation of ventricular muscle produced by cryodestruction of intramural muscle layers in Langendorff-perfused hearts (347, 411, 420). Either short-lived or sustained tachycardias could be initiated by premature stimulation in these preparations without involvement of gross anatomical obstacles. Re-entrant activation patterns with double (Fig. 12-8) or single re-entrant circuits were typically found on the epicardial surface. During sustained tachycardias, the location of re-entrant circuits was stable and the line of block was typically oriented along the fiber axis. A relatively large excitable gap was present within the re-entrant circuits.

From these studies, a specific mechanism for "anisotropic re-entry" was postulated (412, 421). The main distinctive features of this mechanism are (1) the stability of wave rotation and (2) the presence of an excitable gap. Considerations of the basic features of functional and anatomic re-entry indicate that "anisotropic re-entry" can be considered a mixed form of the two mechanisms. Indeed, like the spiral wave mechanism, the existence of an excitable gap in the "anisotropic re-entry" can be explained by the dependence of conduction velocity on curvature. At the pivoting points the pronounced curvature leads to local slowing of propagation. The stability of anisotropic re-entry is likely to be caused by the small unexcitable obstacles on the epicardial surface. Such obstacles can be present even in healthy muscle (blood vessels, connective tissue [24, 25]) and they increase after myocardial infarction due to tissue necrosis (416, 417). The electrophysiological mapping of basic propagation, which was normally employed to detect unexcitable obstacles, may underestimate their presence and their dimensions because thin, longitudinally oriented obstacles or disruptions between neighboring fibers produce little distortions on activation maps (422). As discussed, such obstacles can anchor and stabilize wave rotation during anisotropic re-entry.

This work was supported by the Swiss National Science Foundation, the Swiss Heart Foundation and the Scientific Durrer Foundation. We would thank Mrs. Lilly Lehmann for invaluable help with the illustrations.

REFERENCES

1. Winfree, A. T. *When Time Breaks Down*. Princeton, N.J.: Princeton University Press, 1987.
2. Kucera, J. P., A. G. Kleber, and S. Rohr. Slow conduction in cardiac tissue: II. effects of branching tissue geometry. *Circ. Res.* 83:795–805, 1998.
3. Shaw, R. M., and Y. Rudy. Ionic mechanisms of propagation in cardiac tissue. Roles of the sodium and L-type calcium currents during reduced excitability and decreased gap junction coupling. *Circ. Res.* 81:727–741, 1997.
4. Joyner, R. W., F. Ramon, and J. W. Moore. Simulation of action potential propagation in an inhomogeneous sheet of coupled excitable cells. *Circ. Res.* 36:654–661, 1975.
5. Beeler, G. W., and H. Reuter. Reconstruction of the action potential of ventricular myocardial fibres. *J. Physiol. (Lond.)* 268:177–210, 1977.
6. Ebihara, L., and E. A. Johnson. Fast sodium current in cardiac muscle. A quantitative description. *Biophys. J.* 32:779–790, 1980.
7. Luo, C. H., and Y. Rudy. A model of the ventricular cardiac action potential—depolarization, repolarization, and their interaction. *Circ. Res.* 68:1501–1526, 1991.
8. Luo, C. H., and Y. Rudy. A dynamic model of the cardiac ventricular action potential. 1. Simulations of ionic currents and concentration changes. *Circ. Res.* 74:1071–1096, 1994.
9. Noble, D. The development of mathematical models of the heart. *Chaos Solitons and Fractals.* 5:321–333, 1995.
10. Jack, J. J. B., D. Noble, and R. W. Tsien. *Electric Current Flow in Excitable Cells*. Oxford: Clarendon Press, 1975.
11. Hodgkin, A. L., and W. A. H. Rushton. The electrical constants of crustacean nerve fibers. *Proc. R. Soc. (Lond.)* B133:444–479, 1946.
12. Weidmann, S. The diffusion of radiopotassium across intercalated disks of mammalian cardiac muscle. *J. Physiol. (Lond.)* 187:323–342, 1966.
13. Weidmann, S. The electrical constants of Purkinje fibres. *J. Physiol. (Lond.)* 118:348–360, 1952.
14. Weidmann, S. Electrical constants of trabecular muscle from mammalian heart. *J. Physiol. (Lond.)* 210:1041–1054, 1970.
15. Woodbury, J. W., and W. E. Crill. On the problem of impulse conduction in the atrium. In: *Nervous Inhibition*, edited by L. Florey. New York: Plenum Press, 124–135, 1961.
16. Jongsma, H. J. and H. E. van Rijn. Electrotonic spread of current in monolayer cultures of neonatal rat heart cells. *J. Membr. Biol.* 9:341–360, 1972.
17. Pressler, M. L. Cable analysis in quiescent and active sheep Purkinje fibres. *J. Physiol. (Lond.)* 352:739–757, 1984.
18. Fleischhauer, J., L. Lehmann, A. G. Kléber. Electrical resistances of interstitial and microvascular space as determinants of the extracellular electrical field and velocity of propagation in ventricular myocardium. *Circulation* 92:587–594, 1995.
19. Weidmann, S. The effect of the cardiac membrane potential on the rapid availability of the sodium-carrying system. *J. Physiol. (Lond.)* 127:213–224, 1955.
20. Spach, M. S., and J. M. Kootsey. Relating the sodium current and conductance to the shape of transmembrane and extracellular potentials by simulation: effects of propagation boundaries. *IEEE Trans. Biomed. Eng.* 32:743–755, 1985.
21. Walton, M. K., and H. A. Fozzard. The conducted action poten-

tial: models and comparison to experiments. *Biophys. J.* 44:9–26, 1983.
22. Hodgkin A. L. A note on conduction velocity. *J. Physiol. (Lond.)* 125:221–224, 1954.
23. Tasaki I. and S. Hagiwara. Capacity of muscle fiber membrane. *Am. J. Physiol.* 188:423–429, 1957.
24. Sommer, J. R., and B. Scherer. Geometry of cell and bundle appositions in cardiac muscle: light microscopy. *Am. J. Physiol.* 248 (*Heart Circ. Physiol.* 17):H792–H803, 1985.
25. Le Grice, I. J., B. H. Smaill, L. Z. Chai, S. G. Edgar, J. B. Gavin, and P. J. Hunter. Laminar structure of the heart: ventricular myocyte arrangement and connective tissue architecture in the dog. *Am. J. Physiol.* 269 (*Heart Circ. Physiol.* 38):H571–H582, 1995.
26. Rudy, Y., and W. Quan. A model study of the effects of the discrete cellular structure on electrical propagation in cardiac tissue. *Circ. Res.* 61:815–823, 1987.
27. Leon, L. J., and F. A. Roberge. Directional characteristics of action potential propagation in cardiac muscle. A model study. *Circ. Res.* 69:378–395, 1991.
28. Muller-Borer, B. J., D. J. Erdman, and J. W. Buchanan. Electrical coupling and impulse propagation in anatomically modeled ventricular tissue. *IEEE Trans. Biomed. Eng.* 41:445–454, 1994.
29. Spach, M. S., and J. F. Heidlage. The stochastic nature of cardiac propagation at a microscopic level—electrical description of myocardial architecture and its application to conduction. *Circ. Res.* 76:366–380, 1995.
30. Buchanan, J. W., T. Saito, and L. S. Gettes. The effects of antiarrhythmic drugs, stimulation frequency, and potassium-induced resting membrane potential changes on conduction velocity and dV/dt_{max} in guinea pig myocardium. *Circ. Res.* 56:696–703, 1985.
31. Kléber, A. G., C. B. Riegger, and M. J. Janse. Electrical uncoupling and increase of extracellular resistance after induction of ischemia in isolated, arterially perfused rabbit papillary muscle. *Circ. Res.* 61:271–279, 1987.
32. Kléber, A. G., and C. B. Riegger. Electrical constants of arterially perfused rabbit papillary muscle. *J. Physiol. (Lond.)* 385:307–324, 1987.
33. Riegger, C. B., G. Alperovich, and A. G. Kléber. Effect of oxygen withdrawal on active and passive electrical properties of arterially perfused rabbit ventricular muscle. *Circ. Res.* 64:532–541, 1989.
34. Fast, V. G., B. J. Darrow, J. E. Saffitz, and A. G. Kléber. Anisotropic activation spread in heart cell monolayers assessed by high-resolution optical mapping: role of tissue discontinuities. *Circ. Res.* 79:115–127, 1996.
35. Keener, J. P. A geometrical theory for spiral waves in excitable media. *SIAM J. Appl. Math.* 46:1039–1056, 1986.
36. Zykov, V. S., and O. L. Morozova. Speed of spread of excitation in two-dimensional excitable medium. *Biofizika* 24:739–744, 1979.
37. Zykov, V. S. Analytical evaluation of the dependence of the speed of an excitation wave in a two-dimensional excitable medium on the curvature of its front. *Biophysics* 25:906–911, 1980.
38. Zykov, V. S. *Simulation of Wave Processes in Excitable Media.* Manchester, England: Manchester University Press, 1987.
39. Knisley, S. B., and B. C. Hill. Effects of bipolar point and line stimulation in anisotropic rabbit epicardium: assessment of the critical radius of curvature for longitudinal block. *IEEE Trans. Biomed. Eng.* 42:957–966, 1995.
40. Noble, D. The relation of Rushton "liminal length" for excitation to the resting and active conductances of excitable cells. *J. Physiol. (Lond.)* 226:573–591, 1972.

41. Fozzard, H. A., and M. Schoenberg. Strength-duration curves in cardiac Purkinje fibres: effects of liminal length and charge distribution. *J. Physiol. (Lond.)* 226:593–618, 1972.
42. Rushton, W. A. H. Initiation of the propagated disturbance. *Proc. R. Soc.*B124:210, 1937.
43. Lindemans, F. W., and J. J. D. van der Gon. Current thresholds and liminal size in excitations of heart muscle. *Cardiovasc. Res.* 12:477–485, 1978.
44. Ramza, B. M., R. W. Joyner, R. C. Tan, and T. Osaka. Cellular mechanism of the functional refractory period in ventricular muscle. *Circ. Res.* 66:147–162, 1990.
45. Lindemans, F. W., and A. N. E. Zimmerman. Acute voltage, charge, and energy thresholds as functions of electrode size for electrical stimulation of the canine heart. *Cardiovasc. Res.* 13:383–391, 1979.
46. Winfree, A. T. The electrical thresholds of ventricular myocardium. *J. Cardiovasc. Electrophysiol.* 1:393–410, 1990.
47. Hoyt, R. H., M. L. Cohen, and J. E. Saffitz. Distribution and three-dimensional structure of intercellular junctions in canine myocardium. *Circ. Res.* 64:563–574, 1989.
48. Saffitz, J. E., H. L. Kanter, K. G. Green, T. K. Tolley, and E. C. Beyer. Tissue-specific determinants of anisotropic conduction velocity in canine atrial and ventricular myocardium. *Circ. Res.* 74:1065–1070, 1994.
49. Luke, R., and J. Saffitz. Remodelling of ventricular conduction pathways in healed canine infarct border zones. *J. Clin. Invest.* 87:1594–1602, 1991.
50. Saffitz, J. E., M. D. Lloyd, B. J. Darrow, H. L. Kanter, J. G. Laing, and E. C. Beyer. The molecular basis of anisotropy: role of gap junctions. *J. Cardiovasc. Electrophysiol.* 6:498–510, 1995.
51. Davis, L. M., H. L. Kanter, E. C. Beyer, and J. E. Saffitz. Distinct gap junction protein phenotypes in cardiac tissues with disparate conduction properties. *J. Am. Coll. Cardiol.* 24:1124–1132, 1994.
52. Kanter, H., J. Saffitz, and E. Beyer. Cardiac myocytes express multiple gap junction proteins. *Circ. Res.* 70:438–444, 1992.
53. Gourdie, R., C. Green, N. Severs, and R. Thompson. Immuno-labelling patterns of gap junction connexins in the developing and mature rat heart. *Anat. Embryol.* 185:163–178, 1992.
54. Oosthoek, P. W., S. Viragh, A. E. M. Mayen, M. J. A. Vankempen, W. H. Lamers, and A. F. M. Moorman. Immunohistochemical delineation of the conduction system: 1. The sinoatrial node. *Circ. Res.* 73:473–481, 1993.
55. Oosthoek, P. W., S. Viragh, W. H. Lamers, and A. F. M. Moorman. Immunohistochemical delineation of the conduction system. 2. The atrioventricular node and Purkinje fibers. *Circ. Res.* 73:482–491, 1993.
56. Van Kempen, M. J. A., C. Fromaget, D. Gros, A. F. M. Moorman, and W. H. Lamers. Spatial distribution of connexin-43, the major cardiac gap junction protein-in the developing and adult rat heart. *Circ. Res.* 68:1638–1651, 1991.
57. Anumonwo, J. M. B., H. Z. Wang, E. Trabkajanik, B. Dunham, R. D. Veenstra, M. Delmar, and J. Jalife. Gap junctional channels in adult mammalian sinus nodal cells—immunolocalization and electrophysiology. *Circ. Res.* 71:229–239, 1992.
58. Trabka, Janik E., W. Coombs, L. F. Lemanski, M. Delmar, and J. Jalife. Immunohistochemical localization of gap junction protein channels in hamster sinoatrial node in correlation with electrophysiologic mapping of the pacemaker region. *J. Cardiovasc. Electrophysiol.* 5:125–137, 1994.
59. Opthof, T. Gap junctions in the sino-atrial node: immunohistochemical localization and correlation with activation pattern. *J. Cardiovasc. Electrophysiol.* 5:138–143, 1994.
60. Kwong, K. F., R. B. Schuessler, K. G. Green, J. G. Laing, E. C. Beyer, J. P. Boineau, and J. E. Saffitz. Differential expression of

gap junction proteins in the canine sinus node. *Circ Res.* 82:604–612, 1998.

61. Chen, S., L. M. Davis, L. M. Westphale, E. C. Beyer, and J. E. Saffitz. Expression of multiple gap junction proteins in human fetal and infant heart. *Pediatr. Res.* 36:561–566, 1994.

62. Bastide, B., L. Neyses, D. Ganten, M. Paul, and K. Willecke. Gap junction protein connexin40 is preferentially expressed in vascular endothelium and conductive bundles of the rat myocardium and is increased under hypertensive conditions. *Circ. Res.* 73:1138–1149, 1993.

63. Gros, D., T. Jarryguichard, I. Tenvelde, A. De Maziere, M. J. A. Van Kempen, J. Davoust, J. P. Briand, A. F. M. Moorman, and H. J. Jongsma. Restricted distribution of connexin40, a gap junctional protein, in mammalian heart. *Circ. Res.* 74:839–851, 1994.

64. Dolber, P. C., E. C. Beyer, J. L. Junker, and M. S. Spach. Distribution of gap junctions in dog and rat ventricle studied with a double-label technique. *J. Mol. Cell. Cardiol.* 24:1443–1457, 1992.

65. Smith, J. H., C. R. Green, N. S. Peters, S. Rothery, and N. J. Severs. Altered patterns of gap junction distribution in ischemic heart disease—an immunohistochemical study of human myocardium using laser scanning confocal microscopy. *Am. J. Pathol.* 139:801–821, 1991.

66. Peters, N. S. New insights into myocardial arrhythmogenesis: distribution of gap-junctional coupling in normal, ischaemic and hypertrophied human hearts. *Clin. Sci.* 90:447–452, 1996.

67. Darrow, B. J., V. G. Fast, A. G. Kléber, E. C. Beyer, and J. E. Saffitz. Functional and structural assessment of intercellular communication: increased conduction velocity and enhanced connexin expression in dibutyryl cAMP-treated cultured cardiac myocytes. *Circ. Res.* 79:174–183, 1996.

68. Zhuang, J., K. A. Yamada, J. E. Saffitz, and A. K. Kléber. Pulsatile stretch remodels cell-to-cell communication in cultured myocytes. *Circ. Res.* 87:316–322, 2000.

69. Joyner, R. W. Effects of the discrete pattern of electrical coupling on propagation through an electrical syncytium. *Circ. Res.* 50:192–200, 1982.

70. Spach, M. S., R. C. Barr, G. S. Serwer, E. A. Johnson, and J. M. Kootsey. Collision of excitation waves in the dog Purkinje system: extracellular identification. *Circ. Res.* 24:499–511, 1971.

71. Joyner, R. W., R. Veenstra, D. Rawling, and A. Chorro. Propagation through electrically coupled cells. Effects of a resistive barrier. *Biophys. J.* 45:1017–1025, 1984.

72. Fast, V. G., and A. G. Kléber. Cardiac tissue geometry as a determinant of unidirectional conduction block: assessment of microscopic excitation spread by optical mapping in patterned cell cultures and in a computer model. *Cardiovasc. Res.* 29:697–707, 1995.

73. Fast, V. G., and A. G. Kléber. Block of impulse propagation at an abrupt tissue expansion: evaluation of the critical strand diameter in 2- and 3-dimensional computer models. *Cardiovasc. Res.* 30:449–459, 1995.

74. Spach, M. S, and M. E. Josephson. Initiating reentry: the role of nonuniform anisotropy in small circuits. *J. Cardiovasc. Electrophysiol.* 5:182–209, 1994.

75. Henriquez, C. S., and R. Plonsey. Effects of resistive discontinuities on waveshape and velocity in a single cardiac fibre. *Med. Biol. Eng. Comput.* 25:428–438, 1987.

76. Tan, R. C., and R. W. Joyner. Electrotonic influences on action potentials from isolated ventricular cells. *Circ. Res.* 67:1071–1081, 1990.

77. Joyner, R. W., H. Sugiura, and R. C. Tan. Unidirectional block between isolated rabbit ventricular cells coupled by a variable resistance. *Biophys. J.* 60:1038–1045, 1991.

78. Sugiura, H., and R. W. Joyner. Action potential conduction between guinea pig ventricular cells can be modulated by calcium current. *Am. J. Physiol.* 263 (*Heart Circ. Physiol.* 32):H1591–H1604, 1992.

79. Kumar, R R., and R. W. Joyner. Calcium currents of ventricular cell pairs during action potential conduction. *Am. J. Physiol.* 268 (*Heart Circ. Physiol.* 37):H2476–H2486, 1995.

80. Rohr, S., A. G. Kléber, and J. P. Kucera. Induction of very slow and discontinuous conduction by palmitoleic acid in linear strands of rat ventricular myocytes. *Biophys. J.* 70:A279, 1996.

81. Rudy, Y., and W. Quan. Propagation delays across cardiac gap junctions and their reflection in extracellular potentials: a simulation study. *J. Cardiovasc. Electrophys.* 2:299–315, 1991.

82. Rohr, S., and B. M. Salzberg. Discontinuities in action potential propagation along chains of single ventricular myocytes in culture : multiple site optical recording of transmembrane voltage (MSORTV) suggests propagation delays at the junctional sites between cells. *Biol. Bull. Mar. Biol. Lab.* 183:342–343, 1992.

83. Fast, V. G., and A. G. Kléber. Microscopic conduction in cultured strands of neonatal rat heart cells measured with voltage-sensitive dyes. *Circ. Res.* 73:914–925, 1993.

84. Purdy, J. E., M. Lieberman, A. E. Roggeveen, and R. G. Kirk. Synthetic strands of cardiac muscle. Formation and ultrastructure. *J. Cell Biol.* 55:563–578, 1972.

85. Lieberman, M., A. E. Roggeveen, J. E. Purdy, and E. A. Johnson. Synthetic strands of cardiac muscle: growth and physiological implication. *Science.* 175:909–911, 1972.

86. Horres, C. R., M. Lieberman, and J. E. Purdy. Growth orientation of heart cells on nylon monofilament: determination of the volume-to-surface ratio and intracellular potassium concentration. *J. Membr. Biol.* 34:313–329, 1977.

87. Rohr, S., D. M. Schölly, and A. G. Kléber. Patterned growth of neonatal rat heart cells in culture: morphological and electrophysiological characterization. *Circ. Res.* 68:114–130, 1991.

88. Rohr, S. Determination of impulse conduction characteristics at a microscopic scale in patterned growth heart cell cultures using multisite optical mapping of transmembrane voltage. *J. Cardiovasc. Electrophysiol.* 6:551–568, 1995.

89. Buchanan, J. W., and L. S. Gettes. Ionic environment and propagation. In: *Cardiac Electrophysiology: From Cell to Bedside*, edited by D. P. Zipes and J. Jalife, F. L. Orlando: W. B. Saunders; 149–156, 1990.

90. Clerc, L. Directional differences of impulse spread in trabecular muscle from mammalian heart. *J. Physiol. (Lond.)* 255:335–346, 1976.

91. Spach, M. S., J. F. Heidlage, P. C. Dolber, and R. C. Barr. Electrophysiological effects of remodeling cardiac gap junctions and cell size: experimental and model studies of normal cardiac growth. *Circ. Res.* 86:302–311, 2000.

92. Spach, M. S., and J. M. Kootsey. The nature of electrical propagation in cardiac muscle. *Am. J. Physiol.* 244 (*Heart Circ. Physiol.* 13):H3–H22, 1983.

93. Spach, M. S., W. T. I. Miller, D. B. Gezelowitz, R. C. Barr, J. M. Kootsey, and E. A. Johnson. The discontinuous nature of propagation in normal canine cardiac muscle. Evidence for recurrent discontinuities of intracellular resistance that affect the membrane currents. *Circ. Res.* 48:39–54, 1981.

94. Spach, M. S., and P. C. Dolber. Relating extracellular potentials and their derivatives to anisotropic propagation at a microscopic level in human cardiac muscle. Evidence for electrical uncoupling of side-to-side fiber connections with increasing age. *Circ. Res.* 58:356–371, 1986.

95. Spach, M. S., P. C. Dolber, and J. F. Heidlage. Properties of discontinuous anisotropic propagation at a microscopic level. *Ann. N.Y. Acad. Sci.* 591:62–74, 1990.

96. Cole, W. C., J. B. Picone, and N. Sperelakis. Gap junction uncoupling and discontinuous propagation in the heart. A com-

parison of experimental data with computer simulation. *Biophys. J.* 53:809–818, 1988.
97. Fast, V. G., and A. G. Kléber. Anisotropic conduction in monolayers of neonatal rat heart cells cultured on collagen substrate. *Circ. Res.* 75:591–595, 1994.
98. Spach, M. S., J. F. Heidlage, E. D. Darken, E. Hofer, K. H. Raines, and C. F. Starmer. Cellular dV/dtmax reflects both membrane properties and the load presented by ajoining cells. *Am. J. Physiol.* 263 (*Heart Circ. Physiol.* 32):H1885–H1863, 1992.
99. Mays, D. J., J. M. Foose, L. H. Philipson, and M. M. Tamkun. Localization of the Kv1.5 K^+ channel in explanted cardiac tissue. *J. Clin. Invest.* 96:282–292, 1995.
100. Rohr, S., R. Flückiger, and S. Cohen. Immunocytochemical localization of sodium and calcium channels in cultured neonatal rat ventricular myocytes. *Biophys J.* 76:A366, 1999 (abstract).
101. Petrecca, K., F. Amellal, D. W. Laird, S. A. Cohen, and A. Shrier. Sodium channel distribution within the rabbit atrioventricular node as analysed by confocal microscopy. *J Physiol (Lond.)* 501:263–274, 1997.
102. Cohen, S. A. Immunocytochemical localization of rH1 sodium channel in adult rat heart atria and ventricle. Presence in terminal intercalated disks. *Circulation* 94:3083–3086, 1996.
103. Kadish, A. H., J. F. Spear, J. H. Levine, and E. N. Moore. The effects of procainamide on conduction in anisotropic canine ventricular myocardium. *Circulation* 74:616–625, 1986.
104. Delgado, C., B. Steinhaus, M. Delmar, D. R. Chialvo, and J. Jalife. Directional differences in excitability and margin of safety for propagation in sheep ventricular epicardial muscle. *Circ. Res.* 67:97–110, 1990.
105. Roberts, D. E., L. T. Hersh, and A. M. Scher. Influence of cardiac fiber orientation on wavefront voltage, conduction velocity, and tissue resistivity in the dog. *Circ. Res.* 44:701–712, 1979.
106. Vander Ark, C. R., and E. W. Reynolds. An experimental study of propagated electrical activity in the canine heart. *Circ. Res.* 26:451–460, 1970.
107. Suenson, M. Interaction between ventricular cells during the early part of excitation in the ferret heart. *Acta Physiol. Scand.* 125:81–90, 1985.
108. Roth, B. J. Action potential propagation in a thick strand of cardiac muscle. *Circ. Res.* 68:162–173, 1991.
109. Henriquez, C. S., A. L. Muzikant, and C. K. Smoak. Anisotropy, fiber curvature, and bath loading effects on activation in thin and thick cardiac tissue preparations: Simulations in a three-dimensional bidomain model. *J. Cardiovasc. Electrophysiol.* 7:424–444, 1996.
110. Henriquez, C. S. Structure and volume conductor effects on propagation in cardiac tissue. In:. Durham, North Carolina, USA: Department of Biomedical Engeneering, Duke University; 1988.
111. Roth, B. J. The effect of a perfusing bath on the rate of rise of an action potential propagating through a slab of cardiac tissue. *Ann. Biomed. Eng.* 24:639–646, 1996.
112. Sepulveda, N. G., B. J. Roth, and J. P. Wikswo. Current injection into a two-dimensional anisotropic bidomain. *Biophys. J.* 55:987–999, 1989.
113. Wikswo, J. P., T. A. Wisialowski, W. A. Altemeier, J. R. Balser, H. A. Kopelman, and D. M. Roden. Virtual electrode effects during stimulation of cardiac muscle. Two-dimensional in vivo experiments. *Circ. Res.* 68:513–530, 1991.
114. Wikswo, J. P., S.-F. Lin, and R. A. Abbas. Virtual electrode effect in cardiac tissue: a common mechanism for anodal and cathodal stimulation. *Biophys. J.* 69:2195–2210, 1995.
115. Knisley, S. B. Transmembrane voltage changes during unipolar stimulation of rabbit ventricle. *Circ. Res.* 77:1229–1239, 1995.
116. Neunlist, M., and L. Tung. Optical recordings of ventricular excitability of frog heart by an extracellular stimulating point electrode. *PACE* 17:1641–1654, 1994.
117. Wikswo, J. P. Tissue ansiotropy, the cardiac bidomain, and the virtual cathode effect. In: *Cardiac Electrophysiology: From Cell to Bedside*, edited by D. Zipes and J. Jalife. Orlando, FL: W. B. Saunders; 348–361, 1990.
118. Plonsey, R., C. Henriquez, and N. Trayanova. Extracellular (volume conductor) effect on adjoining cardiac muscle electrophysiology. *Med. Biol. Eng. Comp.* 26:126–129, 1987.
119. Henriquez, C. S. Simulating the electrical behavior of cardiac tissue using the bidomain model. *Crit. Rev. Biomed. Eng.* 21:1–77, 1993.
120. Wu, J. The anatomical basis of anisotropic propagation in cardiac muscle. In:. Durham, North Carolina, USA: Department of Biomedical Engineering, Duke University, 1993.
121. Spach, M. S., J. F. Heidlage, P. C. Dolber, and R. C. Barr. Extracellular discontinuities in cardiac muscle: evidence for capillary effects on the action potential foot. *Circ. Res.* 83:1144–1164, 1998.
122. Spach, M. S., and R. C. Barr. Effects of cardiac microstructure on propagating electrical waveforms. [In Process Citation]. *Circ. Res.* 86:E23–E28, 2000.
123. Keith, A., and M. Flack. The form and nature of the muscular connections between the primary divisions of the vertebrate heart. *J. Anat. Physiol.* 41:172–189, 1907.
124. Tranum-Jensen, J. The fine structure of the sinus node: a survey. In: *The sinus node*, edited by F. J. M. Bonke. The Hague: Nijhoff; 149–165, 1978.
125. Masson-Pévet, M., W. K. Bleeker, A. J. C. Mackaay, L. N. Bouman, and J. M. Houtkooper. Sinus node and atrial cells from the rabbit heart: a quantitative electron microscopic description after electrophysiological localization. *J. Mol. Cell. Cardiol.* 11:555–568, 1979.
126. Bleeker, W. K., A. J. Mackaay, M. Masson-Pévet, L. N. Bouman, and A. E. Becker. Functional and morphological organization of the rabbit sinus node. *Circ. Res.* 46:11–22, 1980.
127. Opthof, T. The mammalian sinoatrial node. *Cardiovasc. Drugs Ther.* 1:573–597, 1988.
128. James, T. N. The sinus node. *Am. J. Cardiol.* 40:965–986, 1977.
129. Opthof, T., B. de Jonge, A. J. Mackaay, W. K. Bleeker, M. Masson-Pévet, H. J. Jongsma, and L. N. Bouman. Functional and morphological organization of the guinea-pig sinoatrial node compared with the rabbit sinoatrial node. *J. Mol. Cell Cardiol.* 17:549–564, 1985.
130. Opthof, T., B. de Jonge, M. Masson-Pévet, H. J. Jongsma, and L. N. Bouman. Functional and morphological organization of the cat sinoatrial node. *J. Mol. Cell Cardiol.* 18:1015–1031, 1986.
131. Opthof, T., B. de Jonge, H. J. Jongsma, and L. N. Bouman. Functional morphology of the pig sinoatrial node. *J. Mol. Cell Cardiol.* 19:1221–1236, 1987.
132. Davies, M. J. Pathology of atrial arrhythmias. In: M. J. Davies, R. H. Anderson, and A. E. Becker eds. *The Conduction System of the Heart*. London: Butterworths; 203–215, 1983.
133. Alings, A. M. W. The aging sino-atrial node. In: *University of Amsterdam*. Amsterdam, The Netherlands: University of Amsterdam; 1993.
134. Wybauw, R. Sur le point d'origine de la systole cardiaque dans l'oreillette droite. *Arch. Int. Physiol.* 10:78–89, 1910.
135. Lewis, T., B. S. Oppenheimer, and A. Oppenheimer. The site of origin of the mammalian heart beat: the pacemaker in the dog heart. *Heart* 2:147–169, 1910.
136. Trautwein, W., and K. Zink. Ueber Membran-und Aktionspo-

tentiale einzelner Muskelfasern des Kalt-und Warmblüterherzens. *Pflugers Arch.* 256:68–84, 1952.
137. West, T. C. Ultramicroelectrode recording from the cardiac pacemaker. *J. Pharmacol. Exp. Ther.* 115:283–290, 1955.
138. Yanagihara, K., and H. Irisawa. Inward current activated during hyperpolarization in the rabbit sinoatrial node cell. *Pflugers Arch.* 385:11–19, 1980.
139. DiFrancesco, D., and C. Ojeda. Properties of the current if in the sino-atrial node of the rabbit compared with those of the current iK, in Purkinje fibres. *J. Physiol. (Lond.)* 308:353–367, 1980.
140. Reuter, H. Ion channels in cardiac cell membranes. *Annu. Rev. Physiol.* 46:473–484, 1984.
141. DiFrancesco, D., A. Ferroni, M. Mazzanti, and C. Tromba. Properties of the hyperpolarizing-activated current (if) in cells isolated from the rabbit sino-atrial node. *J. Physiol. (Lond.)* 377:61–88, 1986.
142. Trautwein, W., and K. Uchizono. Electrophysiologic study of the pacemaker in the sino-atrial node of the rabbit heart. *Z. Zellforsch.* 61:96–109, 1963.
143. Janse, M. J., J. Tranum-Jensen, A. G. Kléber, and F. J. L. Van Cappelle. Techniques and problems in correlating cellular electrophysiology and morphology in cardiac nodal tissue. In: *The Sinus Node*, edited by F. J. M. Bonke. The Hague: Nijhoff; 183–194, 1978.
144. Sano, T., and S. Yamagishi. Spread of excitation from the sinus node. *Circ. Res.* 16:423–431, 1965.
145. Steinbeck, G., M. A. Allessie, F. I. M. Bonke, and W. E. J. P. Lammers. The response of the sinus node to premature stimulation of the atrium studied with microelectrodes in isolated atrial preparations of the rabbit heart. In: *The Sinus Node*, edited by F. I. M. Bonke. The Hague: Nijhoff; 245–257, 1978.
146. Bouman, L. N., A. J. C. Mackaay, W. K. Bleeker, and A. E. Becker. Pacemaker shifts in the sinus node. Effects of vagal stimulation, temperature and reduction of extracellular calcium. In: *The Sinus Node*, edited by F. I. M. Bonke. The Hague: Nijhoff; 245–257, 1978.
147. Bouman, L. N., and H. J. Jongsma. Structure and function of the SA node: a review. *Europ. Heart J.* 7:94–104, 1986.
148. Noble, D. Discussion on models of entrainment of cardiac cells by R. L. de Haan. In: *Cardiac Rate and Rhythm*, edited by L. N. Bouman and H. J. Jongsma. The Hague, Boston, New York: Martinus Nijhoff Publishers; 359–361, 1982.
149. Rook, M. B., B. de Jonge, and H. L. Jongsma. Gap junction formation and functional intercation between neonatal rat cardiocytes in culture. *J. Membr. Biol.* 118:179–192, 1990.
150. Kodama, I., and M. R. Boyett. Regional differences in the electrical activity of the rabbit sinus node. *Pflugers Arch.* 404:214–226, 1985.
151. Kirchhof, C. J., F. I. M. Bonke, M. A. Allessie, and W. E. J. P. Lammers. The influence of the atrial myocardium on impulse formation in the rabbit sinus node. *Pflugers Arch.* 410:198–203, 1987.
152. Joyner, R. W., and F. J. L. van Capelle. Propagation through electrically coupled cells. How a small SA node drives a large atrium. *Biophys. J.* 50:1157–1164, 1986.
153. Optho, T., W. K. Bleeker, M. Masson-Pévet, H. J. Jongsma, and L. N. Bouman. Little-excitable transitional cells in the rabbit sinoatrial node: a statistical, morphological and electrophysiological study. *Experientia* 39:1099–1101, 1983.
154. Meek, W. J., and J. A. E. Eyster. Experiments on the origin and propagation of the impulse in the heart. IV. The effect of vagal stimulation and cooling on the location of the pacemaker within the sino-atrial node. *Am. J. Physiol.* 34:368–383, 1914.
155. Bouman, L. N., E. D. Gerlings, P. A. Biersteker, and F. I. M. Bonke. Pacemaker shift in the sino-atrial node during vagal stimulation. *Pflugers Arch.* 302:255–267, 1968.
156. Mackaay, A. J. C., T. Opthof, W. K. Bleeker, H. J. Jongsma, and L. N. Bouman. Interaction of adrenaline and acetylcholine on sinus node function. In: *Cardiac Rate and Rhythm*, edited by L. N. Bouman and H. J. Jongsma. The Hague: Nijhoff; 507–523, 1982.
157. Cramer, M., M. Siegal, J. T. J. Bigger, and B. F. Hoffman. Characteristics of extracellular potentials recorded from the sinoatrial pacemaker of the rabbit. *Circ. Res.* 41:292–300, 1977.
158. Cramer, M., R. J. Hariman, R. Boxer, and B. F. Hoffman. Electrograms from the canine sinoatrial pacemaker recorded in vitro and in situ. *Am. J. Cardiol.* 42:939–946, 1978.
159. Hariman, R. J., B. F. Hoffman, and R. E. Naylor. Electrical activity from the sinus node region in conscious dogs. *Circ. Res.* 47:775–791, 1980.
160. Hariman, R. J., E. Krongrad, R. A. Boxer, F. O. Bowman, J. R. Malm, and B. F. Hoffman. Methods for recording electrograms from the sino-atrial node during cardiac surgery in man. *Circulation* 61:1024–1029, 1980.
161. Rijlant, P. The pacemaker of the mammalian heart. *J. Physiol. (Lond.)* 75:28P–29P, 1932.
162. Van der Kooi, M. W., D. Durrer, R. T. Van Dam, and L. H. Van der Tweel. Electrical activity in the sinus node and atrioventricular node. *Am. Heart J.* 51:684–700, 1956.
163. Masuda, M. O., and A. Paes de Carvalho. Sinoatrial transmission and atrial invasion during normal rhythm in the rabbit heart. *Circ. Res.* 37:414–421, 1975.
164. Boineau, J. P., R. B. Schuessler, C. R. Mooney, A. C. Wylds, C. B. Miller, R. D. Hudson, J. M. Borremans, and C. W. Brockus. Multicentric origin of the atrial depolarization wave: the pacemaker complex. Relation to dynamics of atrial conduction, P-wave changes and heart rate control. *Circulation* 58:1036–1048, 1978.
165. Boineau, J. P., C. B. Miller, R. B. Schuessler, W. R. Roeske, L. J. Autry, A. C. Wylds, and D. A. Hill. Activation sequence and potential distribution maps demonstrating multicentric atrial impulse origin in dogs. *Circ. Res.* 54:332–347, 1984.
166. Schuessler, R. B., J. P. Boineau, and B. I. Bromberg. Origin of the sinus impulse. *J. Cardiovasc. Electrophysiol.* 7:263–274, 1996.
167. Lewis T. *Lectures on the Heart*: New York: Paul H. Hoeber, London: Shaw and Sons, 1915.
168. Rothberger, C. G., and D. Scherf. Zur Kenntnis der Erregungsausbreitung vom Sinusknoten auf den Vorhof. *Z. Ges. Exp. Med.* 53:792–835, 1926.
169. Puech, P., M. Esclavissat, D. Sodi-Pallares, and F. Cineros. Normal auricular activation in the dog's heart. *Am. Heart J.* 47:174–191, 1954.
170. Yamada, K., M. Horiba, Y. Sakaida, M. Okajima, H. Horibe, H. Muraki, T. Kobayashi, A. Miyauchi, H. Oishi, A. Nonogawa, K. Ishikawa, and J. Toyama. Origination and transmission of impulse in the right auricle. *Jpn. Heart J.* 6:71–97, 1965.
171. Spach, M. S., T. D. King, R. C. Barr, D. E. Boaz, M. N., Morrow, and S. Herman-Giddens. Electrical potential distribution surrounding the atria during depolarization and repolarization in the dog. *Circ. Res.* 24:857–873, 1969.
172. Hamlin, R. L., D. L. Smetzer, T. Senta, and C. R. Smith. Atrial activation paths and P waves in horses. *Am. J. Physiol.* 219:306–313, 1970.
173. Durrer, D., R. T. Van Dam, G. E. Freud, M. J. Janse, F. L. Meijler, and R. C. Arzbaecher. Total excitation of the isolated humane heart. *Circulation* 41:895–912, 1970.
174. Goodman, D., A. B. M. van der Steen, and R. T. van Dam.

Endocardial and epicardial activation pathways of the canine right atrium. *Am. J. Physiol.* 220:1–11, 1971.
175. Spach, M. S., M. Lieberman, J. G. Scott, R. C. Barr, E. A. Johnson, and J. M. Kootsey. Excitation sequences of the atrial septum and the AV node in isolated hearts of the dog and rabbit. *Circ. Res.* 29:156–172, 1971.
176. Janse, M. J., and R. H. Anderson. Specialized internodal atrial pathways: fact or fiction? *Eur. J. Cardiol.* 2:117–136, 1974.
177. Wittig, J. H., M. R. de Leval, and G. Stark. Intraoperative mapping of atrial activation before, during and after the Mustard operation. *J. Thorac. Cardiovasc. Surg.* 73:1–13, 1977.
178. Sherf, L., and T. N. James. Fine structure of cells and their histologic organization within internodal pathways of the heart: clinical and electrocardiographic implications. *Am. J. Cardiol.* 44:345–369, 1979.
179. Tranum-Jensen, J., and M. J. Janse. Fine structural identification of individual cells subjected to microelectrode recording in perfused cardiac preparations. *J. Mol. Cell. Cardiol.* 14:233–247, 1982.
180. Moore, E. N., S. L. Jomain, J. H. Stuckey, J. W. Buchanan, and B. F. Hoffman. Studies on ectopic atrial rhythms in dogs. *Am. J. Cardiol.* 19:676–685, 1967.
181. Moore, E. N., J. Melbin, J. F. Spear, and J. D. Hill. Sequence of atrial excitation in the dog during antegrade and retrograde activation. *J. Electrocardiol.* 4:283–290, 1971.
182. Waldo, A. L., K. J. Vittikainen, and B. F. Hoffman. The sequence of retrograde atrial activation in the canine heart: correlation with positive and negative retrograde p waves. *Circ. Res.* 37:156–163, 1975.
183. Janse, M. J., R. H. Anderson, M. A. McGuire, and S. Y. Ho. "AV-nodal" reentry: Part I: "AV-nodal" reentry revisited. *J. Cardiovasc. Electrophysiol.* 4:561–572, 1993.
184. Scherf, D., and J. Cohen. *The Atrioventricular Node and Selected Cardiac Arrhythmias.* New York: Grune and Stratton; 1964.
185. Tawara, S. *Das Reizleitungssystem des Säugetierherzens. Eine anatomisch-histologissche Studie über das Atrioventrikularbündel und die Purkinjeschen Fäden.* Jena: Fischer; 1906.
186. Anderson, R. H. Histologic and histochemical evidence concerning the presence of morphologically distinct cellular zones within the rabbit atrioventricular node. *Anat. Rec.* 173:7–23, 1972.
187. Woods, W. T., L., Sherf, and T. N. James. Structure and function of specific regions in the canine atrioventricular node. *Am. J. Physiol.* 243 (*Heart Circ. Physiol.* 12): H41–H50, 1982.
188. Paes de Carvalho, A. and D. F. de Almeida. Spread of activity through the atrioventricular node. *Circ. Res.* 8:801–809, 1960.
189. Becker, A. E., and R. H. Anderson. Morphologyy of the human atrioventricular junctional area. In: H. J. J. Wellens, K. I., Lie M. J., Janse, eds. *The Conduction System of the Heart: Structure, Function and Clinical Implication,* edited by H. J. J. Wellens, K. I. Lie, and M. J. Janse. Philadelphia: Lea and Febiger; 263–286, 1976.
190. Kawamura, K., and T. N. James. Comparative ultrastructure of cellular junctions in working myocardium and the conduction system under normal and pathological conditions. *J. Mol. Cell. Cardiol.* 3:31–60, 1972.
191. Marino, T. A. The atrioventricular bundle in the ferret heart. A light and quantitative electron microscopic study. *Am. J. Anat.* 154:365–392, 1979.
192. Thaemert, J. C. Fine structure of the atrioventricular node as viewed in serial sections. *Am. J. Anat.* 136:43–66, 1973.
193. Billette, J. Atrioventricular nodal activation during premature stimulation of the atrium. *Am. J. Physiol.* 252 (*Heart Circ. Physiol.* 21):H163–H177, 1987.
194. Anderson, R. H., M. J. Janse, F. J. L. Van Capelle, J. Billette, A. E., Becker, and D. Durrer. A combined morphological and electrophysiological study of the atrioventricular node of the rabbit heart. *Circ. Res.* 35:909–922, 1974.
195. Nagata, F. An experimental study on the conduction of excitation in the A-V nodal region. *Jpn. Circ. J.* 30:1507–1527, 1966.
196. Takayasu, M., Y. Tateishi, H. Tamai, J. Kanazu, T. Nagata, and K. Kawamura. Conduction of excitation in the A-V nodal region. In: T. Sano, V. Mizuhira, and K. Matsuda, eds. *Electrophysiology and Ultrastructure of the Heart,* edited by J. Jans, V. Mizuhira, and K. Matsuda. New York: Grune and Stratton; 143–152, 1967.
197. McGuire, M. A., J. M. T. De Bakker, J. T. Vermeulen, A. F. Moorman, P. Loh, B. Thibault, J. L. M. Vermeulen, A. E. Becker, and M. J. Janse. Atrioventricular junctional tissue. Discrepancy between histological and electrophysiological characteristics. *Circulation* 94:571–577, 1996.
198. McGuire, M. A., J. M. T. De Bakker, J. T. Vermeulen, T. Opthof, A. E. Becker, and M. J. Janse. Origin and significance of double potentials near the atrioventricular node. Correlation of extracellular potentials, intracellular potentials, and histology. *Circulation* 89:2351–2360, 1994.
199. Billette, J., M. J. Janse, F. J. L. Van Capelle, R. H. Anderson, P., Touboul, and D. Durrer. Cycle-length-dependent properties of AV nodal activation in rabbit hearts. *Am. J. Physiol.* 231: 1129–1139, 1976.
200. Janse, M. J., F. J. L. Van Capelle, R. H. Anderson, P. Touboul, and J. Billette. Electrophysiology and structure of the atrioventricular node of the rabbit heart. In: *The Conduction System of the Heart,* edited by H. J. J. Wellens, K. I. Lie, and M. J. Janse. Leiden: Stenfert Kroese; 296–315, 1976.
201. Van Capelle, F. J. L., M. J. Janse, P. J. Varghese, G. E. Freud, C. Mater, and D. Durrer. Spread of excitation in the atrioventricular node of isolated rabbit hearts studied by multiple microelectrode recording. *Circ. Res.* 31:602–616, 1972.
202. Watanabe, Y., and L. S. Dreifus. Sites of impulse formation within the atrioventricular junction of the rabbit. *Circ. Res.* 22: 717–727, 1968.
203. McGuire, M. A., M. J. Janse, and D. L. Ross. "AV nodal" reentry: Part II: AV nodal, AV junctional, or atrionodal reentry? *J. Cardiovasc. Electrophysiol.* 4:573–586, 1993.
204. Akhtar, M., M. R. Jazayeri, J. Sra, Z. Blanck, S. Deshpande, and A. Dhala. Atrioventricular nodal reentry: clinical, electrophysiological, and therapeutic considerations. *Circulation* 88: 282–295, 1993.
205. Mines, G. R. On dynamic equilibrium in the heart. *J. Physiol.* (Lond.) 46:349–382, 1913.
206. White, P. D. A study of atrioventricular rhythm following auricular flutter. *Arch. Intern. Med.* 16:517–535, 1915.
207. Scherf, D., and C. Shookhoff. Experimentelle Untersuchungen ueber die "Umkehr-Extrasystole" (reciprocating beats). *Wien. Arch. Inn. Med.* 12:501–529, 1926.
208. Moe, G. K., J. B. Preston, and H. J. Burlington. Physiologic evidence for a dual A-V transmission system. *Circ. Res.* 4:357–375, 1956.
209. Rosenblueth A. Ventricular "echoes." *Am. J. Physiol.* 195:53–60, 1958.
210. Kistin, A. D. Atrial reciprocating rhythm. *Circulation* 32:687–707, 1965.
211. Puech, P. La conduction reciproque par le noeud de Tawara. Bases experimentales et aspects cliniques. *Ann. Cardiol. Angiol.* 19:21–40, 1970.
212. Schuilenburg, R. M., and D. Durrer. Atrial echo beats in the human heart elicited by induced atrial premature beats. *Circulation* 37:680–693, 1968.
213. Schuilenburg, R. M., and D. Durrer. Ventricular echo beats in

the human heart elicited by induced ventricular premature beats. *Circulation* 40:337–347, 1969.
214. Bigger J. T. and B. N. Goldreyer. The mechanism of supraventricular tachycardia. *Circulation* 42:673–688, 1970.
215. Mendez, C., J. Han, P. D. Garcia de Jalon, and G. K. Moe. Some characteristics of ventricular echoes. *Circ. Res.* 16:562–581, 1965.
216. Mignone, R. J., and A. G. Wallace. Ventricular echoes. Evidence for dissociation of conduction and reentry within the A-V node. *Circ. Res.* 19:638–649, 1966.
217. Mendez, C., and G. K. Moe. Demonstration of a dual AV nodal conduction system in the isolated rabbit heart. *Circ. Res.* 19:378–393, 1966.
218. Moe, G. K., W. Cohen, and R. L. Vick. Experimentally induced paroxysmal A-V nodal tachycardia in the dog. *Am. Heart J.* 65:87–92, 1963.
219. Janse, M. J., F. J. L. Van Capelle, G. E. Freud, and D. Durrer. Circus movement within the A-V node as a basis of supraventricular tachycardia as shown by multiple microelectrode recording in the isolated rabbit heart. *Circ. Res.* 28:403–414, 1971.
220. Wit, A. L., B. N. Goldreyer, and A. N. Damato. An in vitro model of paroxysmal supraventricular tachycardia. *Circulation* 43:862–875, 1971.
221. Coumel, P., C. Cabrol, A. Fabiato, R. Gourgon, and R. Slama. Tachycardie permanente par rythme reciproque. *Arch. Mal. Coeur Vaiss.* 60:1830–1864, 1967.
222. Casta, A., G. Wolff, A. Mehta, D. Tamer, O. L. Garcia, A. S. Pickoff, P. L. Ferrer, R. J. Sung, and H. Gelband. Dual atrioventricular nodal pathways. A benign finding in arrhythmia-free children with heart disease. *Am. J. Cardiol.* 46:1013–1018, 1980.
223. Denes, P., D. Wu, R. C. Dhingra, E. AmatyLeon, C. R. C. Wyndham, and K. M. Rosen. Dual A-V nodal pathways. A common electrophysiological response. *Br. Heart J.* 37:1069–1076, 1975.
224. Denes, P., D. Wu, R. C. Dhingra, R. Chuquimia, and K. Rosen. Demonstration of dual A-V nodal pathways in patients with paroxysmal supraventricular tachycardia. *Circulation* 48:549–555, 1973.
225. McGuire, M. A., J. P. Bourke, M. C. Robotin, I. C. Johnson, W. Meldrum-Hanna, G. R. Nunn, J. B. Uther, and D. L. Ross. High resolution mapping in Koch's triangle using sixty electrodes in humans with atrioventricular junctional (AV nodal) reentrant tachycardia. *Circulation* 88:2315–2328, 1993.
226. Sung, R. J., H. L. Waxman, S. Saksena, Z. Juma. Sequence of retrograde atrial activation in patients with dual atrioventricular nodal pathways. *Circulation* 64:1059–1067, 1981.
227. Ross, D. L., D. C. Johnson, A. R. Denniss, M. J. Cooper, D. A. Richards, and J. B. Uther. Curative surgery for atrioventricular junctional ("AV nodal") reentrant tachycardia. *J. Am. Coll. Cardiol.* 6:1383–1392, 1985.
228. Jackman, W. M., K. J. Beckman, J. H. McClelland, X. Wang, K. J. Friday, C. A. Roman, K. P. Moulton, N. Twidale, A. Hazlitt, M. I. Prior, J. Oren, E. D. Overholt, and R. Lazzara. Treatment of supraventricular tachycardia due to atrioventricular nodal reentry by radiofrequency ablation of slow-pathway conduction. *N. Engl. J. Med.* 327:313–318, 1992.
229. Haissaguerre, M., F. Gaita, B. Fischer, D. Commenges, P. Montserrat, P. d'Ivernois, P. Lemetayer, and J. Warin. Elimination of atrioventricular nodal reentrant tachycardia using discrete slow potentials to guide application of radiofrequency energy. *Circulation* 85:2162–2175, 1992.
230. Cox, J. L., W. L. Holman, and M. E. Cain. Cryosurgical treatment of atrioventricular node reentrant tachycardia. *Circulation* 76:1329–1336, 1987.
231. Ho, S. Y., J. M. McComb, C. D. Scott, and R. H. Anderson. Morphology of the cardiac conduction system in patients with electrophysiologically proven dual atrioventricular pathways. *J. Cardiovasc. Electrophysiol.* 4:504–512, 1993.
232. Loh, P., J. M. de Bakker, M. Hocini, B. Thibault, R. N. Hauer, and M. J. Janse. Reentrant pathway during ventricular echoes is confined to the atrioventricular node : high-resolution mapping and dissection of the triangle of Koch in isolated, perfused canine hearts. *Circulation* 100:1346–1353, 1999.
233. Medkour, D., A. E. Becker, K. Khalife, and J. Billette. Anatomic and functional characteristics of a slow posterior AV nodal pathway: role in dual-pathway physiology and reentry. *Circulation* 98:164–174, 1998.
234. Lin, L. J., J. Billette, K. Khalife, K. Martel, J. Wang, and D. Medkour. Characteristics, circuit, mechanism, and ablation of reentry in the rabbit atrioventricular node. *J. Cardiovasc. Electrophysiol.* 10:p954–964, 1999.
235. Mazgalev, T., and P. Tschou. *Atrial-AV nodal electrophysiology: a view from the millenium.* Armonk, NY: Futura Publishing Company; 2000.
236. Zipes, D. The atrioventricular node: a riddle wrapped in a mistery inside an enigma. In: T., Mazgalev, P., Tschou eds. *Atrial-AV Nodal Electrophysiology: A View from the Millennium.* Armonk, NY: Futura Publishing Company; 2000.
237. Mazgalev, T., and P. Tschou. The AV nodal dual pathway electrophysiology: still a controversial concept. In: *Atrial-AV Nodal Electrophysiology: A View from the Millennium*, edited by J. Mazgalev and P. Tschou. Armonk, NY: Futura Publishing Company; 2000.
238. Bukauskas F. F., and R. P. Veteikis. Passive electrical properties of the atrioventricular region of the rabbit heart. *Biofizika* 22:499–504, 1977.
239. De Mello, W. C. Passive electrical properties of the atrioventricular node. *Pflugers Arch.* 371:135–139, 1977.
240. Ikeda, N., J. Toyama, T. Shimizu, I. Kodama, and K. Yamada. The role of electrical uncoupling in the genesis of atrioventricular conduction disturbance. *J. Mol. Cell Cardiol.* 12:809–826, 1980.
241. Kokubun, S., M. Nishimura, A. Noma, and H. Irisawa. Membrane currents in the rabbit atrioventricular node cell. *Pflugers Arch.* 393:15–22, 1982.
242. Cranefield, P. F., B. F. Hoffman, and A. Paes de Carvalho. Effects of acetylcholine on single fibers of the atrio-ventricular node. *Circ. Res.* 7:19–23, 1959.
243. Janse, M. J. Influence of the direction of the atrial wave front on A-V nodal transmission in isolated hearts of rabbits. *Circ. Res.* 25:439–449, 1969.
244. Mazgalev, T., L. S. Dreifus, H. Iinuma, and E. L. Michelson. Effects of the site and timing of atrio-ventricular nodal input on atrio-ventricular conduction in the isolated perfused rabbit heart. *Circulation* 70:748–759, 1984.
245. Zipes, D. P., C. Mendez, and G. K. Moe. Evidence for summation and voltage dependency in rabbit atrioventricular nodal fibers. *Circ. Res.* 32:170–177, 1973.
246. Hoffman, B. F. Physiology of atrioventricular transmission. *Circulation* 24:506–517, 1961.
247. Mendez, C. Characteristics of impüulse propagation in the mammalian atrioventricular node. In: *Normal and Abnormal Conduction in the Heart*, edited by A. Paes de Carvalho, B. F. Hoffman, and M. Lieberman. Mount Kisco, NY: Futura; 363–377, 1982.
248. Noma, A., H. Irisawa, S. Kokobun, H. Kotake, M. Nishimura, and Y. Watanabe. Slow current systems in the A-V node of the rabbit heart. *Nature* 285:228–229, 1980.
249. Wit, A. L., and P. F. Cranefield. Effect of verapamil on the sinoatrial and atrioventricular nodes of the rabbit and the mech-

anism by which it arrests reentrant atrioventricular tachycardias. *Circ. Res.* 35:413–425, 1974.
250. Zipes, D. P. and C. Mendez. Action of manganese ions and tetrodotoxin on atrioventricular nodal transmembrane potentials in isolated rabbit hearts. *Circ. Res.* 32:447–454, 1973.
251. Akiyama, T., and H. A. Fozzard. Ca and Na selectivity of the active membrane of rabbit AV nodal cells. *Am. J. Physiol.* 236 (*Cell Physiol.* 5):C1–C8, 1979.
252. Van Capelle, F. J., and M. J. Janse. Influences of geometry on the shape of the propagated action potential. In: *The Conduction System of the Heart*, edited by H. J. J. Wellens, K. I. Lie, and M. J. Janse. Leiden: Stenfert Kroese; 316–335, 1976.
253. Shigeto, N., and H. Irisawa. Slow conduction in the atrioventricular node of the cat: a possible explanation. *Experientia* 28: 1442–1443, 1972.
254. Ruiz-Ceretti, I., and A. Ponce Zumino. Action potential changes under varied (Na^+) and (Ca^{2+}) indicating the existence of two inward currents in cells of the rabbit atrioventricular node. *Circ. Res.* 39:326–336, 1976.
255. Gettes, L. S. and H. Reuter. Slow recovery from inactivation of inward currents in mammalian myocardial fibres. *J. Physiol. (Lond.)* 240:703–724, 1974.
256. Maglaveras, N., F. J. L. van Cappelle, J. M. T. de Bakker, C. Pappas, and M. J. Janse. Activation delay in healed myocardial infarction: a comparison between model and experiment. *Am. J. Physiol.* 269 (*Heart Circ. Physiol.* 38):H1441–1449, 1995.
257. Truex, R. C. Comparative anatomy and functional considerations of the cardiac conduction system. In: A. Paes de Carvalho, W. C. de Mello, and B. F. Hoffman, eds. *The Specialized Tissues of the Heart*, edited by A. Paes de Carvalho, W. C. de Mello, and B. F. Hoffman. Amsterdam: Elsevier; 22–43, 1961.
258. Hoffman, B. F., and P. F. Cranefield. *Electrophysiology of the Heart*. New York: McGraw-Hill; 1960.
259. Demoulin, G. C., and H. E. Kulbertus. Histopathological examination of concept of left hemiblock. *Br. Heart J.* 34:807–814, 1972.
260. Truex, R. C., and M. Q. Smythe. Comparative morphology of the cardiac conduction tissue in animals. *Ann. N.Y. Acad. Sci.* 127:19–33, 1965.
261. Myerburg, R. J., K. Nilsson, and H. Gelband. Physiology of canine intraventricular conduction and endocardial excitation. *Circ. Res.* 30:217–243, 1972.
262. Van Dam, T. T., and M. J. Janse. Activation of the heart. In: *Comprehensive Electrocardiology*, edited by P. W. MacFarlane, and T. D. Veitch Lawrie. New York: Pergamon Press; 101–128, 1988.
263. Rosenbaum, M. B., M. V. Elizari, and J. O. Lazzari. *The Hemibiocks: New Concepts of Intratriuvcular Conduction Based on Human Anatomical, Physiological and Clinical Studies*. Oldsmar: Tampa Tracings; 1970.
264. Veenstram, R. D., R. W. Joyner, and D. A. Rawling. Purkinje and ventricular activation sequences of canine papillary muscle. Effects of quinidine and calcium on the Purkinje-ventricular conduction delay. *Circ. Res.* 54:500–515, 1984.
265. Overholt, E. D., R. W. Joyner, R. D. Veenstra, D. Rawling, and R. Wiedmann. Unidirectional block between Purkinje and ventricular layers of papillary muscle. *Am. J. Physiol.* 247 (*Heart Circ. Physiol.* 16):H584–H595, 1984.
266. Mendez, C., W. J. Mueller, and X. Urguiaga. Propagation of impulses across the Purkinje fiber-muscle junctions in the dog heart. *Circ. Res.* 36:135–150, 1970.
267. Rawling, D. A., R. W. Joyner, and E. D. Overholt. Variations in the functional electrical coupling between the subendocardial Purkinje and ventricular layers of the canine left ventricle. *Circ. Res.* 57:252–261, 1985.
268. Alanis, J., D. Benitez, and G. Pilar. A functional discontinuity between the Purkinje and ventricular muscle cells. *Acta Physiol. Latino Am.* 11:171–183, 1961.
269. Alanis, J., and D. Benitez. Transitional potentials and the propagation of impulses through different cardiac cells. In: *Electrophysiology and Ultrastructure of the Heart*, edited by T. Sano, V. Misuhira, and K. Matsuda. New York: Grune & Stratton; 153–175, 1967.
270. Matsuda, K., A. Kamiyama, and T. Hoshi. Configuration of the transmembrane action potential of the Purkinje-ventricular fiber junction and its analysis. In: *Electrophysiology and Ultrastructure of the Heart*, edited by T. Sano, V. Misuhira, and K. Matsuda. New York: Grune & Stratton; 177–187, 1967.
271. Martinez-Palomo, A., J. Alanis, and D. Benitez. Transitional cardiac cells of the conductive system of the dog heart. Distinguishing morphological and electrophysiological features. *J. Cell Biol.* 47:1–17, 1970.
272. Tranum Jensen, J., A. A. Wilde, J. T. Vermeulen, and M. J. Janse. Morphology of electrophysiologically identified junctions between Purkinje fibers and ventricular muscle in rabbit and pig hearts. *Circ. Res.* 69:429–437, 1991.
273. Scher, A. M. and A. C. Young. Ventricular depolarization and the genesis of QRS. *Ann. N. Y. Acad. Sci.* 65:766–778, 1957.
274. Nagao, K., J. Toyama, I. Kodama, and K. Yamada. Role of the conduction system in the endocardial excitation spread in the right ventricle. *Am. J. Cardiol.* 48:864–870, 1981.
275. Wang, Y., Y. Rudy Action potential propagation in inhomogeneous cardiac tissue: safety factor considerations and ionic mechanism. *Am. J. Physiol.* 278 (*Heart Circ. Physiol.* 47): H1019–H1029, 2000.
276. Dominguez, G., and H. A. Fozzard. Influence of extracellular K^+ concentration on cable properties and excitability of sheep cardiac Purkinje fibers. *Circ. Res.* 26:565–574, 1970.
277. Han, J., A. M. Malozzi, and G. K. Moe. Transient ventricular conduction disturbances produced by intra-atrial injection of single doses of KCl. *Circ. Res.* 21:3–8, 1967.
278. Antoni, H., and T. Zerweck. Besitzen die sympathischen Übertragerstoffe einen direkten Einfluss auf die Leitungsgeschwindigkeit des Säugetiermyokards. *Pflugers Arch.* 293:310–330, 1967.
279. Spear, J. F., and E. N. Moore. Supernormal excitability and conduction in the His-Purkinje system of the dog. *Circ. Res.* 35:782–792, 1974.
280. Spear, J. F., and E. N. Moore. Supernormal conduction in the canine bundle of His and proximal bundle branches. *Am. J. Physiol.* 238 (*Heart Circ. Physiol.* 7):H300–H306, 1980.
281. Peon, J., G. R. Ferrier, and G. K. Moe. The relationship of excitability to conduction velocity in canine Purkinje tissue. *Circ. Res.* 43:125–135, 1978.
282. Weidmann, S. Effects of calcium ions and local anaesthetics on electrical properties of Purkinje fibers. *J. Physiol. (Lond.)* 129: 568–582, 1955.
283. Corrado, G., R. J. Levi, G. J. Nau, and M. B. Rosenbaum. Paroxysmal atrioventriculasr block related to phase 4 bilateral bundle branch block. *Am. J. Cardiol.* 33:553–556, 1974.
284. Elizari, M. V., G. J. Nau, R. J. Levi, J. O. Lazzari, M. S. Halpern, and M. B. Rosenbaum. Experimental production of rate-dependent bundle branch block in the canine heart. *Circ. Res.* 34:730–742, 1974.
285. Singer, D. H., R. Lazzara, and B. F. Hoffman. Interrelationships between automaticity and conduction in Purkinje fibers. *Circ. Res.* 21:537–558, 1967.
286. Jalife, J., C. Antzelevitch, V. Lamanna, and G. K. Moe. Rate-dependent changes in excitability of depressed cardiac Purkinje fibers as a mechanism of intermittent bundle branch block. *Circulation* 67:912–922, 1983.
287. Kléber, A. G., M. J. Janse, F. J. G. Wilms-Schopmann, A. A. M.

Wilde, and R. Coronel. Changes in conduction velocity during acute ischemia in ventricular myocardium of the isolated porcine heart. *Circ. Res.* 73:189–198, 1986.

288. Kishida, H., B. Surawicz, and L. T. Fu. Effects of K^+ and K^+-induced depolarization on $(dV/dt)_{max}$, threshold potential, and membrane input resistance in guinea pig and cat ventricular myocardium. *Circ. Res.* 44:800–814, 1979.

289. Whalley, D. W., D. J. Wendt, C. F. Starmer, Y. Rudy, and A. O. Grant. Voltage-independent effects of extracellular K^+ on the Na^+ current and phase 0 of the action potential in isolated cardiac myocytes. *Circ. Res.* 75:491–502, 1994.

290. Noma, A. ATP-regulated K channels in cardiac muscle. *Nature* 305:147–148, 1983.

291. Grant, A. O., C. F. Starmer, and H. C. Strauss. Antiarrhythmic drug action: blockade of inward sodium current. *Circ. Res.* 55:427–439, 1984.

292. Janse, M. J., and A. L. Wit. Electrophysiological mechanisms of ventricular arrhythmias resulting from ischemia and infarction. *Physiol. Rev.* 69:1049–1169, 1989.

293. Janse, M. J., and A. G. Kléber. Electrophysiological changes and ventricular arrhythmias in the early phase of regional myocardial ischemia. *Circ. Res.* 49:1069–1081, 1981.

294. Schütz, E. Elektrophysiologie des Herzens bei einphasischer Ableitung. *Ergebn. Physiol.* 38:493–620, 1936.

295. Moréna, H., M. J. Janse, J. W. T. Fiolet, W. J. G. Krieger, H. Crijns, and D. Durrer. Comparison of the effects of regional ischemia, hypoxia, hyperkalemia, and acidosis on intracellular and extracellular potentials and metabolism in the isolated porcine heart. *Circ. Res.* 46:635–646, 1980.

296. Downar, E., M. J. Janse, and D. Durrer. The effect of acute coronary artery occlusion on subepicardial transmembrane potentials in the intact porcine heart. *Circulation* 56:217–224, 1977.

297. Kodama, I., A. A. M. Wilde, M. J. Janse, D. Durrer, and K. Yamada. Combined effects of hypoxia, hyperkalemia and acidosis on membrane action potential and excitability of guinea-pig ventricular muscle. *J. Mol. Cell Cardiol.* 16:247–259, 1984.

298. Nakayama, T., Y. Kurachi, A. Noma, and H. Irisawa. Action potential and membrane currents of single pacemaker cells of the rabbit heart. *Pflugers Arch.* 402:248–257, 1984.

299. Gomez, J. P., J. E. Potreau, J. E. Branka, and G. Raymond. Developmental changes in Ca^{2+} current from newborn rat cardiomyocytes in primary culture. *Pflugers Arch.* 428:241–249, 1994.

300. Cranefield, P. F., H. O. Klein, and B. F. Hoffman. Conduction of the cardiac impulse. 1. Delay, block, and one-way block in depressed Purkinje fibers. *Circ. Res.* 28:199–219, 1971.

301. Cranefield, P. F., A. L. Wit, and B. F. Hoffman. Conduction of the cardiac impulse. 3. Characteristics of very slow conduction. *J. Gen. Physiol.* 59:227–246, 1972.

302. Wit, A. L., B. F. Hoffman, and P. F. Cranefield. Slow conduction and reentry in the ventricular conducting system. I. Return extrasystole in canine Purkinje fibers. *Circ. Res.* 30:1–10, 1972.

303. Weingart, R. Electrical properties of the nexal membrane studied in rat ventricular cell pairs. *J. Physiol. (Lond.)* 370:267–284, 1986.

304. Weingart, R., and P. Maurer. Action potential transfer in cell pairs isolated from adult rat and guinea pig ventricles. *Circ. Res.* 63:72–80, 1988.

305. Rohr, S., J. P. Kucera, and A. G. Kleber. Slow conduction in cardiac tissue: I. Effects of a reduction of excitability vs. a reduction in cell-to-cell coupling on microconduction. *Circ. Res.* 83:781–794, 1998.

306. Streit, J. Effects of hypoxia and glycolytic inhibition on electrical properties of sheep cardiac Purkinje fibers. *J. Mol. Cell. Cardiol.* 19:875–885, 1987.

307. Wojtczak, J. Contractures and increase in internal longitudinal resistance of cow ventricular muscle induced by hypoxia. *Circ. Res.* 44:88–95, 1979.

308. Kaplinsky, E., S. Ogawa, C. W. Balke, and L. S. Dreifus. Two periods of early ventricular arrhythmia in the canine acute myocardial infarction model. *Circulation* 60:397–403, 1979.

309. Smith, W. T., W. F. Fleet, T. A. Johnson, C. L. Engle, and W. E. Cascio. The 1b phase of ventricular arrhythmias in ischemic in situ porcine heart is related to changes in cell-to-cell coupling. *Circulation* 92:3051–3060, 1995.

310. Starmer, C. F., V. N. Biktashev, D. N. Romashko, M. R. Stepanov, O. N. Makarova, and V. I. Krinsky. Vulnerability in an excitable medium: analytical and numerical studies of initiating unidirectional propagation. *Biophys. J.* 65:1775–1787, 1993.

311. Quan, W., and Y. Rudy. Induced unidirectional block and reentry of cardiac excitation. *Proc. 9th Annu. Conf. IEEE Eng.* 1:210–211, 1987.

312. Quan, W., and Y. Rudy. Unidirectional block and reentry of cardiac excitation: a model study. *Circ. Res.* 66:367–382, 1990.

313. Van, Capelle F. J. L. and D. Durrer. Computer simulation of arrhythmias in a network of coupled excitable elements. *Circ. Res.* 47:453–466, 1980.

314. Janse, M. J., The effects of changes of heart rate on the refractory period of the heart. In:. Amsterdam: University of Amsterdam; 1971.

315. Han, J., and G. K. Moe. Nonuniform recovery of excitability of ventricular muscle. *Circ. Res.* 14:44–60, 1964.

316. Kuo, C. S., K. Munakata, C. P. Reddy, and B. Surawicz. Characteristics and possible mechanism of ventricular arrhythmia dependent on the dispersion of action potential durations. *Circulation* 67:1356–1367, 1983.

317. Wallace, A. G., and R. J. Mignone Physiologic evidence concerning the re-entry hypothesis for ectopic beats. *Am. Heart J.* 72:60–70, 1966.

318. Allessie, M. A., F. I. M. Bonke, and F. J. C. Schopman. Circus movement in rabbit atrial muscle as a mechanism of tachycardia. II. The role of nonuniform recovery of excitability in the occurrence of unidirectional block as studied with multiple microelectrodes. *Circ. Res.* 39:168–177, 1976.

319. Engelmann, T. W. Über die reziproke und irreziproke Reizleitung mit besonderer Beziehung auf das Herz. *Pflugers Arch.* 61:272–284, 1895.

320. Schmitt, F. O., and J. Erlanger. Directional differences in the conduction of the impulse through heart muscle and their possible relation to extrasystolic anf fibrillatory contractions. *Am. J. Physiol.* 87:326–347, 1928.

321. Downar, E., and M. B. Waxman. Depressed conduction and unidirectional block in Purkinje fibers. In: H. J. J. Wellens, K. I., Lie, and M. J. Janse. eds. *The Conduction System of the Heart*, Philadelphia: Lea & Febiger; 393–409, 1976.

322. Waxman, M. B., E. Downar, and R. W. Wald. Unidirectional block in Purkinje fibers. *Can. J. Physiol. Pharmacol.* 58:925–933, 1980.

323. Engelmann T. W. Versuche über die irreziproke Reizleitung in Muskelfasern. *Pflugers Arch.* 62:400–414, 1896.

324. Spach, M. S., W. T. Miller, P. C. Dolber, J. M. Kootsey, J. R. Sommer, and C. E. J. Mosher. The functional role of structural complexities in the propagation of depolarization in the atrium of the dog. Cardiac conduction disturbances due to discontinuities of effective axial resistivity. *Circ. Res.* 50:175–191, 1982.

325. De Bakker, J. M. T., F. J. L. Van Capelle, M. J. Janse, S. Tasseron, J. T. Vermeulen, N. Dejonge, and J. R. Lahpor. Slow conduction in the infarcted human heart—zigzag course of activation. *Circulation* 88:915–926, 1993.

326. Rohr, S., and B. M. Salzberg. Characterization of impulse prop-

agation at the microscopic level across geometrically defined expansions of excitable tissue: multiple site optical recording of transmembrane voltage (MSORTV) in patterned growth heart cell cultures. *J. Gen. Physiol.* 104:287–309, 1994.
327. Rohr, S., J. P. Kucera, V. G. Fast, and A. G. Kleber. Paradoxical improvement of impulse conduction in cardiac tissue by partial cellular uncoupling. *Science* 275:841–844, 1997.
328. Spach, M. S., P. C. Dolber, and J. F. Heidlage. Influence of the passive anisotropic properties on directional differences in propagation following modification of the sodium conductance in human atrial muscle. A model of reentry based on anisotropic discontinuous propagation. *Circ. Res.* 62:811–832, 1988.
329. Delmar, M., D. C. Michaels, T. Johnson, and J. Jalife. Effects of increasing intercellular resistance on transverse and longitudinal propagation in sheep epicardial muscle. *Circ. Res.* 60:780–785, 1987.
330. Schalij, M. J. Anisotropic conduction and ventricular tachycardia. In:. Maastricht, The Netherlands: Rijksuniversiteit Limburg; 1988.
331. Girouard, S. D., J. M. Pastore, K. R. Laurita, K. W. Gregory, and D. S. Rosenbaum. Optical mapping in a new guinea pig model of ventricular trachycardia reveals mechanisms for multiple wavelengths in a single reentrant circuit. *Circulation* 93:603–613, 1996.
332. Cabo, C. A. M. Pertsov, W. T. Baxter, J. M. Davidenko, R. A. Gray, and J. Jalife. Wave-front curvature as a cause of slow conduction and block in isolated cardiac muscle. *Circ. Res.* 75:1014–1028, 1994.
333. De la Fuente, D., B. Sasyniuk, and G. K. Moe. Conduction through a narrow isthmus in isolated canine atrial tissue. A model of the W-P-W syndrome. *Circulation* 44:803–809, 1971.
334. Lin, S. F., B. J. Roth, D. S. Echt, and J. P. Wikswo. Complex dynamics following unipolar stimulation during the vulnerable phase. *Circulation* 94:I–174, 1996.
335. Saypol, J. M., and B. J. Roth. A mechanism for anisotropic reentry in electrically active tissue. *J. Cardiovasc. Electrophysiol.* 3:558–566, 1992.
336. Efimov, I. R., Y. N. Cheng, W. D. Van, T. N. Mazgalev, and P. J. Tchou. Virtual electrodes induced phase singularity: a basic mechanism of defibrillation failure. *Circ Res.* 82:918–925, 1998.
337. Mayer, A. G. Nerve conduction and other reactions in Cassiopea. *Am. J. Physiol.* 39:375–393, 1916.
338. Mayer, A. G. Rhythmical pulsation in scyphomedusae. II. In: *Papers from the Marine Biological Laboratory at Tortugas.* Washington; 115–131, 1908.
339. Mines, G. R. On circulating excitations in heart muscles and their possible relation to tachycardia and fibrillation. *Trans. R. Soc. Can. Sect. IV:*43–52, 1914.
340. Durrer, D., and J. P. Roos. Epicardial excitation of the ventricles in a patient with Wolff-Parkinson-White syndrome (type B). *Circulation* 35:15–21, 1967.
341. Durrer, D., L. Schoo, R. M. Schuilenburg, and H. J. J. Wellens. The role of premature beats in the initiation and termination of supraventricular tachycardia in Wolff-Parkinsin-White syndrome. *Circulation* 36:644–662, 1967.
342. Holzmann, M., and D. Scherf. Über Elektrokardiogramme und verkürzter Vorhof-Kammerdistanz und positiven P-Zacken. *Z. Klin. Med.* 121:404–410, 1932.
343. Wolff, L., J. Parkinson, and P. D. White. Bundle branch block with short PR-interval in healthy young people prone to paroxysmal tachycardia. *Am. Heart J.* 5:685–692, 1930.
344. Janse, M. J. Reentrant arrhythmias. In: *The Heart and Cardiovascular System*, 2nd Edition, edited by H. A. Fozzard. New York: Raven Press; 2055–2094, 1992.
345. MacLean, W. A. H., V. J. Plumb, and A. L. Waldo. Transient entrainment and interruption of ventricular tachycardia. *PACE* 4:358–365, 1981.
346. Arenal, A., J. Almendral, D. San Román, J. L. Delcan, and M. E. Josephson. Frequency and implications of resetting and entrainment with right atrial stimulation in atrial flutter. *Am. J. Cardiol.* 70:1292–1298, 1992.
347. Boersma, L., J. Brugada, C. Kirchhof, and M. Allessie. Entrainment of reentrant ventricular tachycardia in anisotropic rings of rabbit myocardium—mechanisms of termination, changes in morphology, and acceleration. *Circulation* 88:1852–1865, 1993.
348. Frazier, D. W. and M. S. Stanton. Resetting and transient entrainment of ventricular tachycardia. *Pacing Clin. Electrophysiol.* 18:1919–1946, 1995.
349. Waldecker, B., J. Coromilas, A. E. Saltman, S. M. Dillon, and A. L. Wit. Overdrive stimulation of functional reentrant circuits causing ventricular tachycardia in the infarcted canine heart—resetting and entrainment. *Circulation* 87:1286–1305, 1993.
350. Allessie, M. A., F. I. M. Bonke, and F. J. C. Schopman. Circus movement in rabbit atrial muscle as a mechanism of tachycardia. III. The "leading circle" concept: a new model of circus movement in cardiac tissue without the involvement of an anatomical obstacle. *Circ. Res.* 41:9–18, 1977.
351. Smeets, J. L. R. M., M. A. Allessie, L. W. J. E. P., F. I. M. Bonke, and J. Hollen. The wavelength of the cardiac impulse and reentrant arrhythmias in isolated rabbit atrium. The role of heart rate, autonomic transmitters, temperature, and potassium. *Circ. Res.* 58:96–108, 1986.
352. Frame, L. H., R. L. Page, and B. F. Hoffman. Atrial reentry around an anatomic barrier with a partially refractory excitable gap. A canine model of atrial flutter. *Circ. Res.* 58:495–511, 1986.
353. Baeriswyl, G., M. Zimmermann, and R. Adamec. Efficacy of rapid atrial pacing for conversion of atrial flutter in medically treated patients. *Clin. Cardiol.* 17:246–250, 1994.
354. Simson, M. B., J. F. Spear, E. N. Moore. Stability of an experimental atrioventricular reentrant tachycardia in dogs. *Am. J. Physiol.* 240 (*Heart Circ. Physiol.* 9):H947-H953, 1981.
355. Vinet, A., and F. A. Roberge. The dynamics of sustained reentry in a ring model of cardiac tissue. *Ann. Biomed. Eng.* 22:568–591, 1994.
356. Ito, H., and L. Glass. Theory of reentrant excitation in a ring of cardiac tissue. *Physica D.* 56:84–106, 1992.
357. Frame, L. H., and M. B. Simson. Oscillations of conduction, action potential duration, and refractoriness. A mechanism for spontaneous termination of reentrant tachycardias. *Circulation* 78:1277–1287, 1988.
358. Garrey, W. E. Auricular fibrillation. *Physiol. Rev.* 4:215–250, 1924.
359. Allessie, M. A., F. I. M. Bonke, and F. J. C. Schopman. Circus movement in rabbit atrial muscle as a mechanism of tachycardia. *Circ. Res.* 33:54–62, 1973.
360. El-Sherif, N., R. Mehra, W. B. Gough, and R. H. Zeiler. Reentrant ventricular arrhythmias in the late myocardial infarction period. Interruption of reentrant circuits by cryothermal techniques. *Circulation* 68:644–656, 1983.
361. El-Sherif, N., A. Smith, and K. Evans. Canine ventricular arrhythmias in the late myocardial infarction period: epicardial mapping of reentrant circuits. *Circ. Res.* 1981:255–265, 1981.
362. Gough, W. B., R. Mehra, M. Restivo, R. H. Zeiler, and N. El-Sherif. Reentrant ventricular arrhythmias in the late myocardial infarction period in the dog. 13. Correlation of activation and refractory maps. *Circ. Res.* 57:432–442, 1985.
363. Hoffman, B. F., and M. R. Rosen. Cellular mechanisms for cardiac arrhythmias. *Circ. Res.* 49:1–15, 1981.

364. Allessie, M. A., W. J. E. P., Lammers, F. I. M., Bonke, and J. Hollen. Experimental evaluation of Moe's multiple wavelet hypotheis of atrial fibrillation. In: *Cardiac Arrhythmias*, edited by D. P., Zipes and J. Jalife. New York: Grune & Stratton; 265–276, 1985.
365. Janse, M. J., F. J. L. Van Capelle, H. Morsink, A. G. Kléber, F. J. G. Wilms-Schopman, R. Cardinal, C. Naumann d'Alnoncourt, and D. Durrer. Flow of "injury" current and patterns of excitation during early ventricular arrhythmias in acute regional myocardial ischemia in isolated porcine and canine hearts. Evidence for 2 different arrhythmogenic mechanisms. *Circ. Res.* 47:151–165, 1980.
366. Müller, S. C., T. Plesser, B. Hess. The structure of the core of the spiral wave in the Belousov-Zhabotinskii reaction. *Science* 230:661–663, 1985.
367. Winfree, A. T. Spiral waves of chemical activity. *Science* 175:634–636, 1972.
368. Gorelova, N. A. and J. Bures. Spiral waves of spreading depression in the isolated chicken retina. *J. Neurobiol.* 14:353–363, 1983.
369. Shibata, J. and J. Bures. Optimum topographical conditions for reverberating cortical spreading depression in rats. *J. Neurobiol.* 5:107–118, 1974.
370. Lechleiter, J., S. Girard, E. Peralta, and D. Clapham. Spiral calcium wave propagation and annihilation in *Xenopus laevis* oocytes. *Science* 252:123–126, 1991.
371. Lipp, P. and E. Niggli. Microscopic spiral waves reveal positive feedback in subcellular calcium signaling. *Biophys. J.* 65:2272–2276, 1993.
372. Tomchik, K. J. and P. N. Devreotes. Adenosine 3',5'—monophosphate waves in *Dictyostelium discoideum*: a demonstration by isotope dilution-fluorography. *Science* 212:443–446, 1981.
373. Selfridge, O. Studies of flutter and fibrillation. *Arch. Inst. Cardiologia de Mexico.* 18:177–187, 1948.
374. Balakhovsky, I. S. Several modes of excitation movement in ideal excitable tissue. *Biophysics* 10:1175–1179, 1965.
375. Gul'ko, F. B. and A. A. Petrov. Mechanism of the formation of closed pathways of conduction in excitable media. *Biophysics* 17:271–282, 1972.
376. Davidenko, J. M., A. V., Pertsov, R., Salomonsz, W., Baxter, and J. Jalife. Stationary and drifting spiral waves of excitation in isolated cardiac muscle. *Nature* 355:349–351, 1992.
377. Gray, R., A. Pertsov, and J. Jalife. Spatial and temporal organization during cardiac fibrillation. *Nature* 392:75–78, 1998.
378. Fast, V. G. and A. M. Pertsov. Shift and termination of functional reentry in isolated ventricular preparations with quinidine-induced inhomogeneity on refractory period. *J. Cardiovasc. Electrophysiol.* 3:255–265, 1992.
379. Frazier, D. W., P. D. Wolf, J. M. Wharton, A. S. L. Tang, W. M. Smith, and R. E. Ideker. Stimulus-induced critical point. Mechanism for electrical initiation of reentry in normal canine myocardium. *J. Clin. Invest.* 83:1039–1052, 1989.
380. Davidenko, J. M. Spiral wave activity: a possible common mechanism for polymorphic and monomorphic ventricular tachycardias. *J. Cardiovasc. Electrophysiol.* 4:730–746, 1993.
381. Pertsov, A. M., A. V. Panfilov, and F. U. Medvedeva. Instabilities of autowaves in excitable media associated with critical curvature phenomenon. *Biofizika* 28:100–102, 1983.
382. Agladze, K., J. P. Keener, S. C. Muller, and A. Panfilov. Rotating spiral waves created by geometry. *Science* 264:1746–1748, 1994.
383. Fast, V. G., I. R. Efimov, and V. I. Krinsky. Transition from circular to linear rotation of a vortex in an excitable cellular medium. *Physics Lett. A* 151:157–161, 1990.
384. Krinsky, V. I., I. R. Efimov, and J. Jalife. Vortices with linear cores in excitable media. *Proc. R. Soc. London Ser. A.* 437:645–655, 1992.
385. Winfree, A. T. Scroll-shaped waves of chemical activity in three dimensions. *Science* 181:937–939, 1973.
386. Zykov, V. S. Cycloid circulation of spiral waves in excitable medium. *Biophysics* 31:940–944, 1986.
387. Lugosi, E. Analysis of meandering in Zykov kinetics. *Physica D* 40:331–337, 1989.
388. Gerhardt, M., H. Schuster, and J. J. Tyson. A cellular automaton model of excitable media. II. Curvature, dispersion, rotating waves and meandering waves. *Physica D* 46:392–415, 1990.
389. Efimov, I., V. Krinsky, and J. Jalife. Dynamics of rotating vortices in the Beeler-Reuter model of cardiac tissue. *Chaos, Solitons & Fractals* 5:513–526, 1995.
390. Holden, A. V. and H. Zhang. Characteristics of atrial re-entry and meander computed from a model of a rabbit single atrial cell. *J. Theor. Biol.* 175:545–551, 1995.
391. Starmer, C. F., D. N. Romashko, R. S. Reddy, Y. I. Zilberter, J. Starobin, A. O. Grant, and V. I. Krinsky. Proarrhythmic response to potassium channel blockade: numerical studies of polymorphic tachyarrhythmias. *Circulation* 92:595–605, 1995.
392. El-Sherif, N. Reentrant mechanisms in ventricular arrhythmias. In: *Cardiac Electrophysiology: From Cell to Bedside*, edited by D. P. Zipes and J. Jalife. Philadelphia: W. B. Sounders; 567–582, 1995.
393. Gray, R. A., J. Jalife, A. Panfilov, W. T. Baxter, C., Cabo, J. M., Davidenko, and A. M. Pertsov. Nonstationary vortexlike reentrant activity as a mechanism of polymorphic ventricular tachycardia in the isolated rabbit heart. *Circulation* 91:2454–2469, 1995.
394. Courtemanche, M. and A. T. Winfree. Two dimensional rotating depolarization waves in a modified Beeler-Reuter model of cardiac cell activity. In: *Science at the John von Neumann National Supercomputer Center*, edited by G. Cook. Princeton, NJ: Consortium for Scientific Computing, 79–86, 1990.
395. Leon, L. J., F. A. Roberge, and A. Vinet. Simulation of two-dimensional anisotropic cardiac reentry: effects of the wavelength on the reentry characteristics. *Ann. Biomed. Eng.* 22:592–609, 1994.
396. Courtemanche, M. Complex spiral wave dynamics in a spatially distributed ionic model of cardiac activity. *Chaos* 6:579–600, 1996.
397. Qu, Z., J. N. Weiss, A Garfinkel. Cardiac electrical restitution properties and stability of reentrant spiral waves: a simulation study. *Am J Physiol.* 276 (*Heart Circ. Physiol.* 45):H269–283, 1999.
398. Cao, J. M., Z. Qu, Y. H. Kim, T. J. Wu, A. Garfinkel, J. N. Weiss, H. S. Karagueuzian, and P. S. Chen. Spatiotemporal heterogeneity in the induction of ventricular fibrillation by rapid pacing: importance of cardiac restitution properties. *Circ. Res.* 84:1318–1331, 1999.
399. Ito, H. and L. Glass. Spiral breakup in a new model of discrete excitable media. *Phys. Rev. Lett.* 66:671–674, 1991.
400. Karma, A. Spiral breakup in model equations of action potential propagation in cardiac tissue. *Phys. Rev. Lett.* 71:1103–1106, 1993.
401. Panfilov, A. and P. Hogeweg. Spiral breakup in a modified Fitzhugh-Nagumo model. *Phys. Lett. A.* 176:295–299, 1993.
402. Karma A. Electrical alternans and spiral wave breakup in cardiac tissue. *Chaos* 4:461–472, 1994.
403. Koller, M. L., M. L. Riccio, and R. F. Gilmour, Jr. Dynamic restitution of action potential duration during electrical alternans and ventricular fibrillation. *Am J Physiol.* 275 (*Heart Circ. Physiol.* 44):H1635–1642, 1998.
404. Riccio, M. L., M. L. Koller, and R. F. Gilmour, Jr. Electrical

restitution and spatiotemporal organization during ventricular fibrillation. *Circ. Res.* 84:955–963, 1999.
405. Panfilov, A. V. and B. N. Vasiev. Vortex initiation in a heterogeneous excitable medium. *Physica D* 49:107–113, 1991.
406. Fast, V. G. and I. R. Efimov. Stability of vortex rotation in an excitable cellular medium. *Physica D* 49:75–81, 1991.
407. Fast, V. G. and A. M. Pertsov. Drift of a vortex in the myocardium. *Biophysics* 35:489–494, 1990.
408. Pertsov, A. M., J. M. Davidenko, R. Salomonsz, W. T. Baxter, and J. Jalife. Spiral waves of excitation underlie reentrant activity in isolated cardiac muscle. *Circ. Res.* 72:631–650, 1993.
409. Abildskov, J. A. and R. L. Lux. The mechanism of simulated torsade de pointes in a computer model of propagated excitation. *J. Cardiovasc. Electrophysiol.* 2:224–237, 1991.
410. Jalife, J. and R. Gray. Drifting vortices of electrical waves underlie ventricular fibrillation in the rabbit heart. *Acta. Physiol. Scand.* 157:123–131, 1996.
411. Schalij, M. J., W. E. J. P. Lammers, P. L. Rensma, and M. A. Allessie. Anisotropic conduction and reentry in perfused epicardium of rabbit left ventricle. *Am. J. Physiol.* 263 (*Heart Circ. Physiol.* 32):H1466–H1478, 1992.
412. Wit, A. L. and S. M. Dillon. Anisotropic reentry. In: *Cardiac Electrophysiology. From Cell to Bedside*, edited by D. P. Zipes and J. Jalife. Philadelphia: W. B. Saunders, 353–364, 1990.
413. Pertsov, A. M., J. Jalife. Three-dimensional vortex-like reentry. In: *Cardiac Electrophysiology: From Cell to Bedside*, edited by D. P. Zipes and J. Jalife. Philadelphia: W. B. Saunders; 403–409, 1995.
414. Panfilov, A. V. and A. M. Pertsov. Vortex rings in a three-dimensional medium described by reaction-diffusion equations. *Doklady AN SSSR* 274:58–60, 1984.
415. Winfree, A. T. Electrical turbulence in three-dimensional heart muscle. *Science* 266:1003–1006, 1994.
416. Dillon, S. M., M. A. Allessie, P. C. Ursell, and A. L. Wit. Influences of anisotropic tissue structure on reentrant circuits in the epicardial border zone of subacute canine infarcts. *Circ. Res.* 63:182–206, 1988.
417. Ursell, P. C., P. I. Gardner, A. Albala, J. J. J. Fenoglio, and A. L. Wit. Structural and electrophysiological changes in the epicardial border zone of canine myocardial infarcts during infarct healing. *Circ. Res.* 56:436–451, 1985.
418. Restivo, M., H. Yin, E. B. Caref, A. I. Patel, G. Ndrepepa, M. J. Avitable, M. A. Assadi, N. Isber and N. Elsherif. Reentrant arrhythmias in the subacute infarction period: the proarrhythmic effect of flecainide acetate on functional reentrant circuits. *Circulation* 91:1236–1246, 1995.
419. El-Sherif, N., H. Yin, E. B. Caref, and M. Restivo. Electrophysiological mechanisms of spontaneous termination of sustained monomorphic reentrant ventricular tachycardia in the canine postinfarction heart. *Circulation* 93:1567–1578, 1996.
420. Boersma, L, J. Brugada, M. J. Schalij, C. Kirchhof, and M. Allessie. The effects of K⁺ on anisotropic conduction in sheets of perfused rabbit ventricular epicardium. *J. Cardiovasc. Electrophysiol.* 2:492–502, 1991.
421. Wit, A. L., S. M. Dillon, and J. Coromilas. Anisotropic reentry as a cause of ventricular tachyarrhythmias in myocardial infarction. In: *Cardiac Electrophysiology: From Cell to Bedside*, edited by D. P. Zipis and J. Jalife. Philadelphia: W. B. Saunders; 511–526, 1995.
422. Kadish, A., M. Shinnar, E. N. Moore, J. H. Levine, C. W. Balke, and J. F. Spear. Interaction of fiber orientation and direction of impulse propagation with anatomic barriers in anisotropic canine myocardium. *Circulation* 78:1478–1494, 1988.
423. Bonke, F. I. M. Electrotonic spread in the sinoatrial node of the rabbit heart. *Pflugers Arch.* 339:17–23, 1973.
424. Bonke, F. I. M. Passive electrical properties of atrial fibers of the rabbit heart. *Pflugers Arch.* 339:1–15, 1973.
425. Sakamoto, Y., and M. Goto. A study of the membrane constant in the dog myocardium. *Jpn. J. Physiol.* 20:30–41, 1970.
426. Tille, J. Electronic interaction between muscle fibers in the rabbit ventricle. *J. Gen. Physiol.* 50:189–202, 1966.
427. Daut, J. The passive electrical properties of Guinea-pig ventricular muscle as examined with a voltage-clamp technique. *J. Physiol. (Lond.)* 330:221–242, 1982.
428. Horiba, M. Stimulus conduction in atria studied by means of intracellular microelectrode. Part I. That in Bachmann's bundle. *Jpn. Heart. J.* 4:333–345, 1963.
429. Wagner, M. L., R. Lazzara, R. M. Weiss, and B. F. Hoffman. Specialized conducting fibers in the interatrial band. *Circ. Res.* 18:502–518, 1966.
430. Spach, M., and P. C. Dolber. The relation between discontinuous propagation in anisotropic cardiac muscle and the "vulnerable period" of reentry. In: *Cardiac Electrophysiology*, edited by D. P. Zipes and J. Jalife. New York: Grune and Stratton; 241–252, 1985.
431. Kirchhof, C., M. Wijffels, J. Brugada, J. Planellas, and M. Allessie. Mode of action of a new class IC drug (ORG 7797) against atrial fibrillation in conscious dogs. *J. Cardiovasc. Pharmacol.* 17:116–124, 1991.
432. Horibe, H. Studies on the spread of the right atrial activation by means of intracellular microelectrode. *Jpn. Circ. J.* 25:583–593, 1961.
433. Hogan, P. M. and L. D. Davis. Electrophysiological characteristics of canine atrial plateau fibers. *Circ. Res.* 28:62–73, 1971.
434. Brendel, W., W. Raule and W. Trautwein. Leitungsgeschwindigkeitund Erregungsausbreitung in den Vörhofendes Hundes. *Pflugers Arch.* 253:106–113, 1950.
435. Frame, L. H., R. L. Page, P. A. Boyden, J. J. Fenoglio, and B. F. Hoffman. Circus movement in the canine atrium around the tricuspid ring during experimental atrial flutter and during reentry in vitro. *Circulation* 76:1155–1175, 1987.
436. Draper, M. H., and S. Weidmann. Cardiac resting and action potentials recorded with an intracellular electrode. *J. Physiol. (Lond.)* 115:74–94, 1951.
437. Trautwein, W., U. Gottstein, and K. Federschmidt. Der Einfluss der Temperatur auf den Actionsstrom des excidierten Purkinje-Fadens, gemessen mit einer intracellulären Elektrode. *Pflugers Arch.* 258:243–260, 1953.
438. Hoffman, B. F., P. F. Cranefield, and J. H. Stuckey, et al. Direct measurement of conduction velocity in *in situ* specialized conduction system of mammalian heart. *Proc. Soc. Exp. Biol. Med.* 102:55–57, 1959.
439. Draper, M. H., and M. Mya-Tu. A comparison of the conduction velocity in cardiac tissues of various mammals. *Q. J. Exp. Physiol.* 44:91–109, 1959.
440. Rosen, M. R., M. J. Legato, and R. M. Weiss. Developmental changes in impulse conduction in the canine heart. *Am. J. Physiol.* 240 (*Heart Circ. Physiol.* 9):H546-H554, 1981.
441. Pressler, M. L., V. Elharrar, and J. C. Bailey. Effects of extracellular calcium ions, verapamil, and lanthanum on active and passive properties of canine cardiac Purkinje fibers. *Circ. Res.* 51:637–651, 1982.
442. Sano, T., N. Takayama, and T. Shimamoto. Directional difference of conduction velocity in the cardiac ventricular syncytium studied by microelectrodes. *Circ. Res.* VII:262–267, 1959.
443. Roberts, D. E., and A. M. Scher. Effect of tissue anisotropy on extracellular potential fields in canine myocardium in situ. *Circ. Res.* 50:342–351, 1982.
444. Spear, J. F., E. L. Michelson, and E. N. Moore. Cellular electrophysiologic characteristics of chronically infarcted myocar-

dium in dogs susceptible to sustained ventricular tachyarrhythmias. *J. Am. Coll. Cardiol.* 1:1099–1110, 1983.
445. Tsuboi, N., I. Kodama, J. Tayama, and K. Yamada. Anisotropic conduction properties of canine ventricular muscles. *Jpn. Circ. J.* 49:487–498, 1985.
446. Balke, C. W., M. D. Lesh, J. F. Spear, A. Kadish, J. H. Levine, and E. N. Moore. Effects of cellular uncoupling on conduction in anisotropic canine ventricular myocardium. *Circ. Res.* 63: 879–892, 1988.
447. Quinteiro, R. A., M. O. Biagetti, E. de Forteza. Relationship between V_{max} and conduction velocity in uniform anisotropic canine ventricular muscle: differences between the effects of lidocaine and amiodarone. *J. Cardiovasc. Pharmacol.* 16:931–939, 1990.
448. Lewis, T. *The Mechanism and Graphic Registration of the Heart Beat.* London: Shaws & Sons, 1920.
449. Tranum-Jensen, J. The fine structure of the atrial and atrio-ventricular (AV) junctional specialized tissues of the rabbit heart. In: *The Conduction System of the Heart*, edited H. J. J. Wellens, K. I. Lie, and M. J. Janse. Leiden: Stenfert Kroese, 1976.
450. Krinsky, V. I., I. R. Efimov. Vortices with linear cores in mathematical models of excitable media. *Physica A* 188:55–60, 1992.

13. The cardiac ventricular action potential

YORAM RUDY

Departments of Biomedical Engineering, Physiology & Biophysics, and Medicine, and the Cardiac Bioelectricity Research and Training Center, Case Western Reserve University, Cleveland, Ohio,

CHAPTER CONTENTS

Fundamental Principles
The Ventricular Cell Is a Complex Interactive System
Ionic Basis of the Action Potential
   The normal action potential
   The premature action potential and adaptation to rate
Heterogeneity of Ventricular Action Potentials
Abnormal Repolarization. Example—Early Afterdepolarizations
Effects of Ionic Concentrations on the Action Potential. Example—Sodium Overload
Pathological Action Potential Changes. Example—Acute Ischemia
Epilogue

THE ABILITY OF CARDIAC MUSCLE TO GENERATE PROPAGATING ELECTRICAL IMPULSES (action potentials) classifies it in the category of excitable tissues, together with skeletal muscle and nerve. The process of cardiac excitation involves generation of the action potential (AP) by individual cells and its conduction from cell to cell through intercellular gap junctions. The resulting propagating wave of electrical activation triggers contraction of the heart and synchronizes its blood pumping action. At the cellular level, the electrical AP triggers mechanical contraction by inducing a transient increase of the intracellular calcium concentration which, in turn, carries the contraction message to the contractile elements of the cell, a process known as excitation–contraction coupling. Similar to other excitable cells, the excitatory process that generates the ventricular AP is dominated by a single membrane mechanism (activation of sodium channels in the case of ventricular myocytes). However, in distinction from nerve and skeletal muscle, the cardiac ventricular AP is characterized by long plateau and repolarization phases that provide control of mechanical contraction and prevent premature arrhythmogenic excitation. Clearly, the plateau plays an important functional role in cardiac excitation and contraction. As will be demonstrated throughout this chapter, the plateau and repolarization phases involve many interacting processes that provide for precise control and modulation of the AP time course and duration. The objective of this chapter is to explore the ionic mechanisms that participate in the generation of the ventricular AP and determine its properties. The chapter also serves to illustrate the complexity of the cellular processes that underlie the cardiac AP and the high degree of synthesis and integration that takes place at the level of the single cardiac cell. Ion channels are also discussed elsewhere in this book, especially in chapters 12, 14, 17, and 18.

FUNDAMENTAL PRINCIPLES

Action potentials are generated by the movement of ions across the cell membrane, a process that displaces charge on the membrane capacitance (C_m) and changes the membrane potential (V_m) according to the following relationship (60):

$$\frac{dV_m}{dt} = \left(\frac{-1}{C_m}\right) * I_{ion} \qquad (1)$$

Eq. (1) assumes space-clamp conditions and absence of external stimulation.

I_{ion} is the total transmembrane ionic current, carried through ion-selective protein channels and exchange mechanisms. Note that the rate of change of V_m, given by dV_m/dt, is proportional to I_{ion}. By convention, a negative I_{ion} represents the inward flow of positive charge; it produces a positive dV_m/dt which elevates (depolarizes) the membrane potential. A positive I_{ion} is an outward current; it produces a negative dV_m/dt and reduces (repolarizes) the membrane potential.

In general, I_{ion} is the net result of several inward and outward currents that are carried by different ions and exhibit very different magnitudes, voltage dependence, and time course of activation and inactivation. It is the dynamic interplay between these currents that determines the morphology and properties of the action potential. Typically, each ion channel current can be represented by its conductance (g_i) times a driving force ($V_m - E_i$):

$$I_i = g_i (V_m - E_i) \qquad (2)$$

E_i, the reversal potential, is determined by the transmembrane concentration gradients and relative permeabilities of the permeant ions through this selective channel. Conductance may depend on membrane potential, on time, and on intracellular and extracellular concentrations of certain ions, as well as other factors.

THE VENTRICULAR CELL IS A COMPLEX INTERACTIVE SYSTEM

The single myocyte is the building block of cardiac tissue. Figure 13–1 is a schematic diagram of a ventricular cell and its electrophysiological components. It also describes a mathematical model of the cell (the Luo-Rudy [LRd] model) that will be used extensively throughout this chapter (45, 88, 89, 120, 136, 137, 151). This model is a general mammalian ventricular cell model, based mainly on single-cell and single-channel data from the guinea pig. Included in the model are the membrane ionic channel currents, as well as ionic pumps and exchangers. In addition, processes that regulate dynamic ionic concentrations are represented. These include concentrations of sodium, potassium, and calcium ions. Importantly, the model simulates the intracellular calcium transient that is generated by calcium-induced-calcium-release (CICR) from the sarcoplasmic reticulum (SR) during an action potential (46, 89), or generated by spontaneous SR Ca^{2+} release under conditions of calcium overload (22, 128). (See also chapters 9 and 11) Important properties that are represented in the model include the following (parameters are defined in the legend to Figure 13–1): (1) I_{Na} is characterized by fast activation and by fast and slow inactivation processes (11, 50, 51, 73, 76, 97, 118). (2) $I_{Ca(L)}$ is inactivated by both voltage-dependent and Ca^{2+}-dependent processes. The Ca^{2+}-induced inactivation is the faster process, whereas voltage-induced inactivation is slow (55, 57, 59, 69, 77, 81, 93, 102, 122, 125, 148). (3) The model accounts for the two components of the delayed rectifier potassium current, I_{Kr} (rapid) and I_{Ks} (slow) (27, 61, 92, 114, 151). (4) The conductances of I_{K1}, I_{Kr}, and $I_{K(ATP)}$ increase with extracellular potassium concentration, $[K^+]_o$ (66, 74, 113, 115). (5) The conductance of I_{Ks} increases with intracellular calcium concentration, $[Ca^{2+}]_i$ (132, 104). (6) I_{to} is not found in guinea pig ventricular myocardium; it is prominent in epicardium of certain other species (21, 30, 48, 52, 82, 83, 84, 100, 144).

Figure 13–1 serves to illustrate the complex, highly interactive cellular environment, where the various ionic currents interact with changing ionic concentrations and varying transmembrane voltage. In addition to various regulatory mechanisms, the dynamically changing environment modulates the behavior of ion channels. An example is shown in Figure 13–2. In this scheme, $I_{Ca(L)}$ induces Ca^{2+} release from the SR through the CICR mechanism. The released Ca^{2+} in the myoplasm, in turn, modulates several ionic currents, including $I_{Ca(L)}$ itself. It activates the sodium–calcium exchanger (I_{NaCa}) to extrude calcium from the cell, it increases the conductance of the slow delayed rectifier potassium current (I_{Ks}), and it contributes to $I_{Ca(L)}$ inactivation through the Ca^{2+}-dependent inactivation process. It should be recognized that the function of most cellular components is studied experimentally in isolation, away from the physiological environment of the cell (e.g., cloned ion channels in expression systems). The mathematical model of Figure 13–1 will be used in this chapter to "reinstitute" these components into the interactive cellular environment in order to study their role in the integrated behavior of the cell during action potential generation.

IONIC BASIS OF THE ACTION POTENTIAL

The Normal Action Potential

As stated earlier, the AP is generated by a dynamic interplay between different ion channels, pumps, and exchangers. It is the integrated cellular behavior that determines the AP properties and AP response to different physiological and pathological conditions. In Figure 13–3 we use the cell model of Figure 13–1 to describe the role played by various currents in generating the AP and in determining its duration and morphology. The AP and calcium transient are shown, together with selected ionic currents during the AP. Once the cell is excited by a suprathreshold stimulus, the fast inward sodium current, I_{Na}, activates and depolarizes the membrane at a very fast rate (maximum dV_m/dt of 393 volts/sec), generating the fast upstroke of the AP and quickly inactivating. Subsequently (when V_m depolarizes to about -25 mV) the inward $I_{Ca(L)}$ activates and provides a depolarizing current that supports the AP plateau against the repolarizing action of the outward currents I_{Kr} and I_{Ks}. $I_{Ca(L)}$ displays a "spike and dome" morphology during the AP (see also 35, 89). It reaches its early peak value of -4.92 $\mu A/\mu F$ in 2.74 msec, whereas I_{Na} reaches its (two orders of magnitude larger) peak value of -391 $\mu A/\mu F$ in 1 msec, a time when $I_{Ca(L)}$ is still very small (only -0.84 $\mu A/\mu F$). Therefore, the early spike of $I_{Ca(L)}$ contributes very little to the rising phase of the normal ventricular AP; it plays an important role in triggering calcium release from the SR to generate the calcium transient. It is the dome phase of $I_{Ca(L)}$ that maintains the AP plateau; it slowly declines as L-type Ca^{2+} channels inactivate. Both I_{Kr} and I_{Ks}

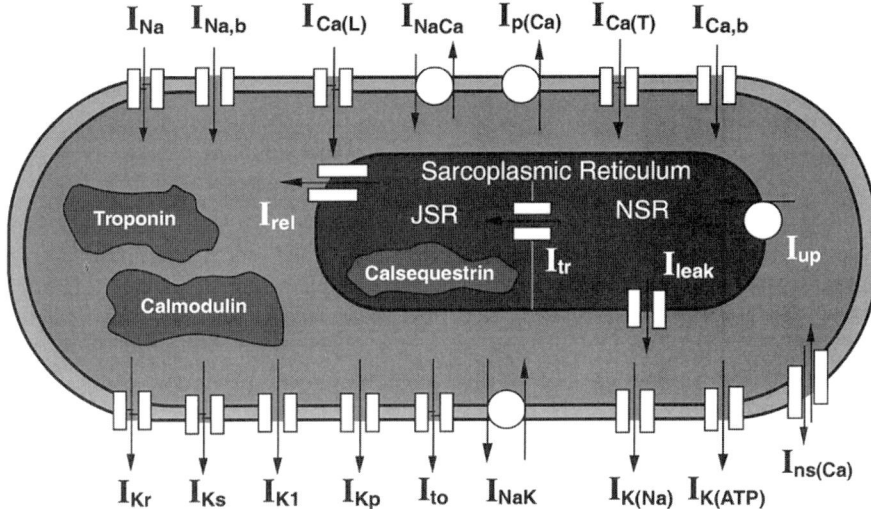

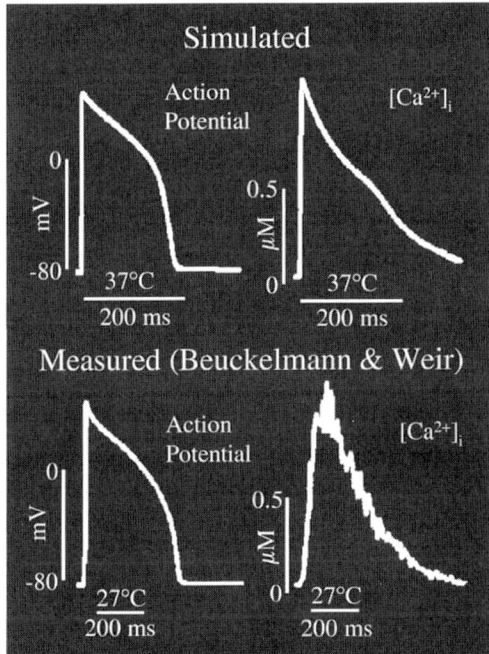

FIG. 13–1. *Top:* Schematic diagram of the dynamic Luo-Rudy (LRd) ventricular cell model. *Bottom:* Action potential and calcium transient, [Ca^{2+}]$_i$, simulated by the model are shown in comparison with experimental data from Beuckelmann and Wier (13). Note that simulations are conducted at 37°C and experiments at 27°C and are shown on different scales (200 ms bars). The scales become identical, and the close similarity of simulated and measured data is preserved when the appropriate Q$_{10}$ is used to correct for the temperature difference. Definitions: I$_{Na}$, fast sodium current; I$_{Ca(L)}$, calcium current through L-type calcium channels; I$_{Ca(T)}$, calcium current through T-type calcium channels (6, 36, 134); I$_{to}$, transient outward current; I$_{Kr}$, rapid delayed rectifier potassium current (21); I$_{Ks}$, slow delayed rectifier potassium current; I$_{K1}$, inward rectifier potassium current (74); I$_{Kp}$, plateau potassium current (also known as ultra-rapid current, I$_{kur}$) (5, 147); I$_{K(ATP)}$, ATP-sensitive potassium current (66, 103, 105, 120); I$_{K(Na)}$, sodium-activated potassium current (45, 67, 86, 140); I$_{ns(Ca)}$, nonspecific calcium-activated current (activated under conditions of calcium overload) (43); I$_{Na,b}$, sodium background current; I$_{Ca,b}$, calcium background current; I$_{NaK}$, sodium-potassium pump current; I$_{NaCa}$, sodium–calcium exchange current; I$_{p(Ca)}$, calcium pump in the sarcolemma (24); I$_{up}$, calcium uptake from the myoplasm to network sarcoplasmic reticulum (NSR) (130); I$_{rel}$, calcium release from juncitonal sarcoplasmic reticulum (JSR) (94); I$_{leak}$, calcium leakage from NSR to myoplasm; I$_{tr}$, calcium translocation from NSR to JSR (149). Calmodulin and troponin represent calcium buffers in the myoplasm. Calsequestrin is a calcium buffer in the JSR. (Details of the LRd model can be found in references 45, 88, 89, 120, 136, 137, 151). The model code can be downloaded from the Research Section of www.cwru.edu/med/CBRTC. [Experimental data are adapted from reference (13), with permission.]

gradually increase during the AP plateau, shifting the balance of currents in the outward direction and repolarizing the membrane toward its rest potential. I$_{NaCa}$ is initially a relatively small outward current (it operates in its "reverse mode" to extrude Na$^+$ and bring in Ca^{2+} with a stoichiometry of 3Na$^+$:1Ca^{2+}) (12, 14–16, 18, 32, 44, 49, 71, 75, 95, 96, 98, 99, 110). It then reverses direction and operates in its "direct mode" to extrude Ca^{2+}, becoming a significant inward current that slows the rate of repolarization during the late phase of the AP and prolongs its duration (9, 35, 40, 42). Finally, there is a large increase of I$_{K1}$ that together with I$_{Kr}$ and I$_{Ks}$ repolarizes the membrane back to its rest potential. Note that I$_{NaK}$ (a time-independent electrogenic process with 3Na$^+$:2K$^+$ stoichiometry) (34, 51, 53, 101) increases during the AP plateau (partly

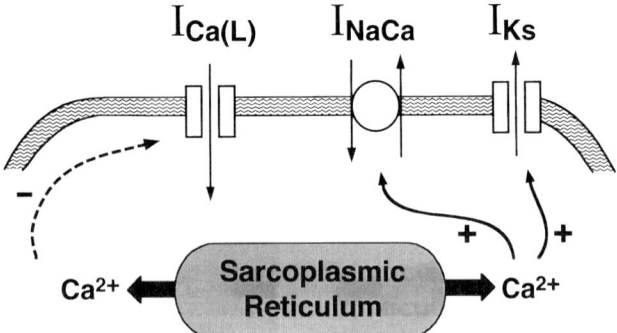

FIG. 13–2. Example of interactive processes in a single ventricular myocyte. $I_{Ca(L)}$ triggers Ca^{2+} release from the sarcoplasmic reticulum (SR). Ca^{2+}, in turn, activates I_{NaCa} and augments I_{Ks} (+ indicates a positive, enhancing effect). Ca^{2+} also acts to inactivate $I_{Ca(L)}$ in a "negative feedback" process (indicated by −). Ca^{2+} has multiple other actions, not shown in the scheme. [From reference 109 with permission.]

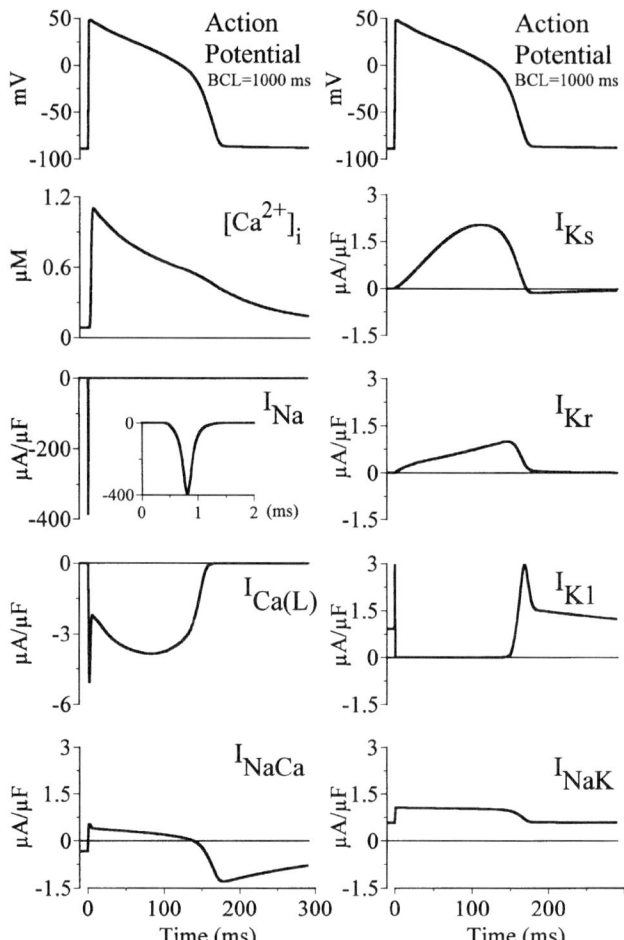

FIG. 13–3. Major ionic currents during the action potential (AP). Shown are the AP (repeated at top of both columns for reference), the calcium transient (free calcium in the myoplasm during the AP, $[Ca^{2+}]_i$), and selected ionic currents that determine the AP morphology (current symbols are defined in Figure 13–1). I_{Na} is also shown on an expanded time scale (*inset*). All quantities are simulated using the LRd model. The cell has reached steady state during pacing at a constant BCL of 1000 ms. (BCL is basic cycle length, the interval between pacing stimuli). Note that I_{to} (which is absent from guinea pig myocardium and is prominent in epicardium of certain species) is not included in this simulation. Its role will be considered in the context of AP heterogeneity (Fig. 13–9). [Compiled from references (89 and 151), with permission.]

because of its voltage dependence) as it operates to extrude Na^+ ions that entered the cell during the AP upstroke.

Figure 13–4 highlights the repolarizing outward potassium currents I_{Kr}, I_{Ks}, I_{K1}, and I_{Kp} (also known as I_{Kur}, the ultra-rapid K^+ current). In panel B, I_{Kr}, the rapid delayed rectifier, increases faster than I_{Ks} at the very beginning of the AP. It does not, however, attain a large magnitude because its fast inactivation at depolarized potentials results in strong inward rectification. During the slow repolarization of the plateau, I_{Kr} increases slowly because of the decreased inward rectification at less positive potentials. Compared with I_{Kr}, I_{Ks} is slower to increase (due to its slower activation kinetics) but attains a much larger magnitude during most of the plateau, reflecting the greater density of the I_{Ks} channels in the membrane. It is the major repolarizing current during the plateau phase. During the fast repolarization phase that follows the plateau, the I_{Kr} and I_{Ks} traces crossover, and I_{Kr} is larger than I_{Ks}, especially near the end of repolarization. This is due to the different driving forces of these currents. I_{Kr} is purely selective to K^+ ions. Its reversal potential is −95.86 mV at $[K^+]_o$ of 4 mmol/liter, which is more negative than the rest potential. I_{Ks} channels are permeable to both K^+ and Na^+. At $[K^+]_o$ = 4 mmol/liter the I_{Ks} reversal potential is −83.26 mV. Therefore, during late repolarization as V_m approaches its value at rest, the greater driving force on I_{Kr} is sufficient to cause the crossover, with the magnitude of I_{Kr} exceeding that of I_{Ks}. At this late phase, however, the larger peak of I_{K1} (Fig. 13–4 D, 200 msec) is much greater than either I_{Kr} or I_{Ks} and dominates the fast final repolarization to rest. Note that I_{Kp} (Fig. 13–4 C), the ultra-rapid plateau current, activates almost instantaneously. Its magnitude is larger than that of I_{Ks} only during the very early plateau phase, when it contributes to early repolarization, but is much smaller than I_{Ks} during most of the plateau.

The Premature Action Potential and Adaptation to Rate

When a cell is excited prematurely, at a short coupling interval from a previous AP, many of the ion channels have not yet returned to their steady-state conditions. As a result, the premature AP is generated by ionic

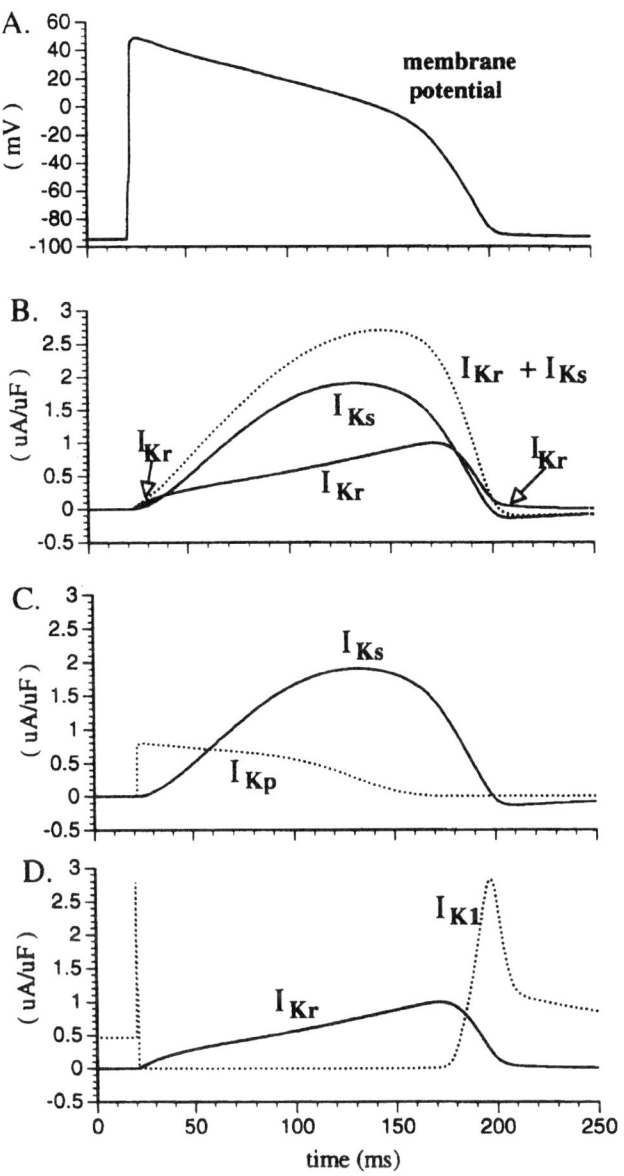

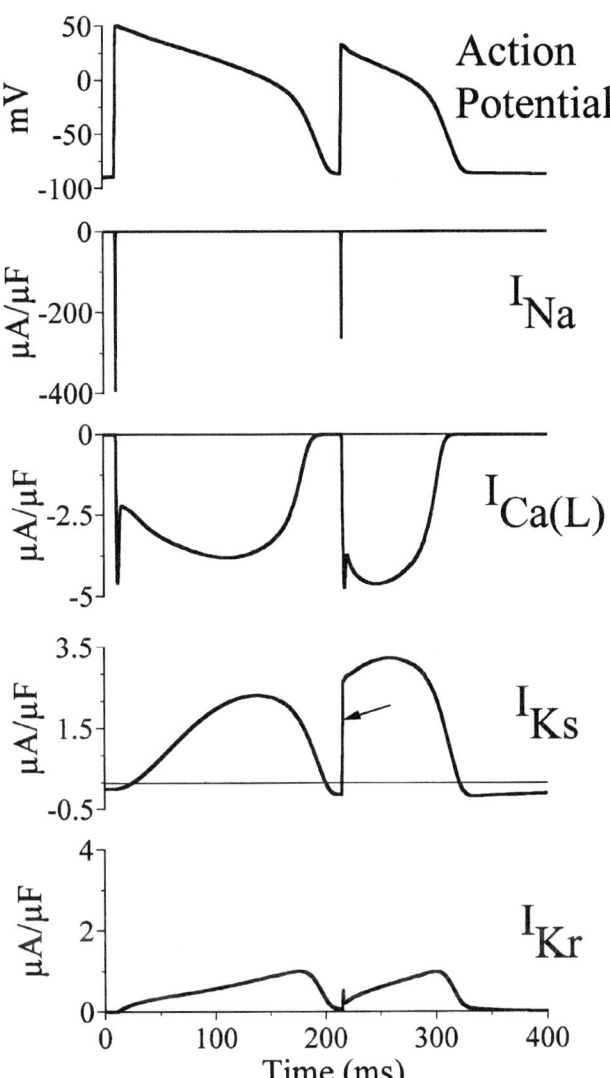

FIG. 13–4. Repolarizing outward potassium currents during the action potential. I_{Kr} and I_{Ks} are the rapid and slow delayed rectifier currents, respectively. Their sum constitutes I_K ($I_K = I_{Kr} + I_{Ks}$), originally termed the delayed rectifier K^+ current. I_{K1}, the inward rectifier, is time-independent. I_{Kp}, the plateau current, is also known as the ultra-rapid K^+ current I_{Kur}. From reference 151, with permission.

FIG. 13–5. Membrane potential and selected ionic currents during a fully recovered and a premature action potential. The premature AP is stimulated 15 msec after return of the previous AP to rest potential.

currents that are not fully recovered. Figure 13–5 shows a fully recovered AP followed by a premature AP that was stimulated 15 msec after the return of V_m to its rest value. Selected ionic currents during the two APs are also shown. Note that peak I_{Na} is reduced from −391 µA/µF to −261 µA/µF because of incomplete recovery from inactivation of the sodium channels. The result is a slower upstroke of the AP (maximum dV_m/dt is reduced from 393 volts/sec to 263 volts/sec) to a lower peak potential. The most obvious effect of the premature excitation is a major shortening of the action potential duration (APD is reduced from 190 to 105 msec). This shortening is caused mostly by the large magnitude of I_{Ks} during the premature AP due to residual activation (incomplete deactivation) of this slowly deactivating current from the previous AP. As a result of the large residual conductance, I_{Ks} exhibits an instantaneous jump (*arrow* in Fig. 13–5) upon AP depolarization, providing a large repolarizing current starting from the early plateau phase that shortens APD. There is also a small increase in early I_{Kr}, which increases the rate of early repolarization. Interestingly, $I_{Ca(L)}$ is increased during the plateau by an increased driving force (lower AP potential) and reduced Ca^{2+}-dependent inactivation second-

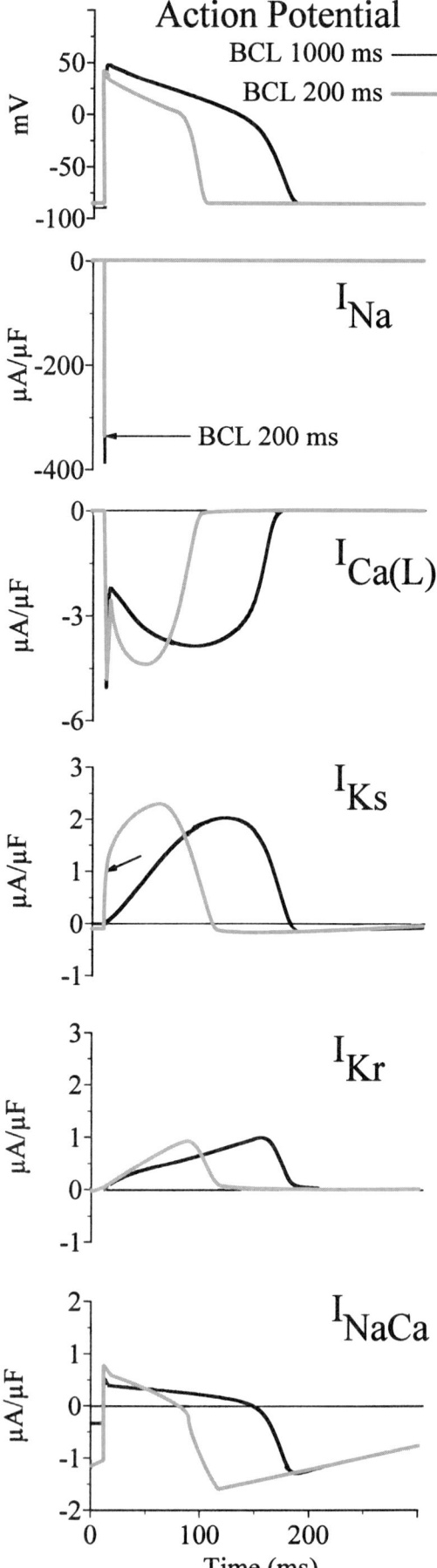

ary to a smaller calcium transient (not shown). Despite this increase of a particular inward current, the net dynamic balance of currents shifts in the outward direction to accelerate repolarization and shorten APD.

Shortening of the APD also occurs when the steady-state rate of periodic excitation (pacing) is increased, a process known as adaptation. Figure 13–6 shows APs during slow pacing at a basic cycle length (BCL) of 1000 msec and during fast pacing at a BCL of 200 msec. Selected ionic currents during the AP are also shown. Like a premature AP, residual activation during fast pacing (insufficient time for complete deactivation between beats) results in an instantaneous jump of I_{Ks} (arrow in Fig. 13–6) upon depolarization and a large current magnitude that shortens APD relative to that during slow pacing. In addition, plateau I_{NaCa} is somewhat enlarged in the outward direction ("reverse mode") because of $[Na^+]_i$ accumulation at the fast rate, contributing to the adaptation process and APD shortening.

HETEROGENEITY OF VENTRICULAR ACTION POTENTIALS

Electrophysiological heterogeneity is an important property of ventricular myocardium (see also Chapter 17). Variability of protein expression and/or electrophysiologic function has been reported for several ion channels (8, 17, 41, 83–85, 100, 136, 138, 141, 144). An important and extensively studied example is the heterogeneity of I_{Ks} across the ventricular wall, giving rise to a subpopulation of cells (mid-myocardial, M-cells) that display a longer APD with a steeper rate adaptation than other (epicardial or endocardial) cell types (1–3, 37, 123, 124). The underlying ionic basis for the unique repolarization properties of the M-cells is a lower density of I_{Ks} channels (85). This observation is not surprising in view of the important role of I_{Ks} in AP repolarization and in APD adaptation, as described in the previous section.

Figure 13–7 (136) shows simulated APs (paced at BCL = 2000 msec) for the three cell types, differing in the density of I_{Ks} (I_{Ks}: I_{Kr} density ratios are 23:1, 15:1, and 7:1 in epicardial, endocardial, and M-cells, respectively with I_{Kr} density the same in all cell types). The associated I_{Kr} and I_{Ks} are also shown. APD of the M-cell is longer than that of the other cell types. I_{Ks} is significantly smaller in the M-cell, starting from the

FIG. 13–6. Action potentials and selected ionic currents at slow (BCL = 1000 msec, black line) and fast (BCL = 200 msec, gray line) pacing rates.

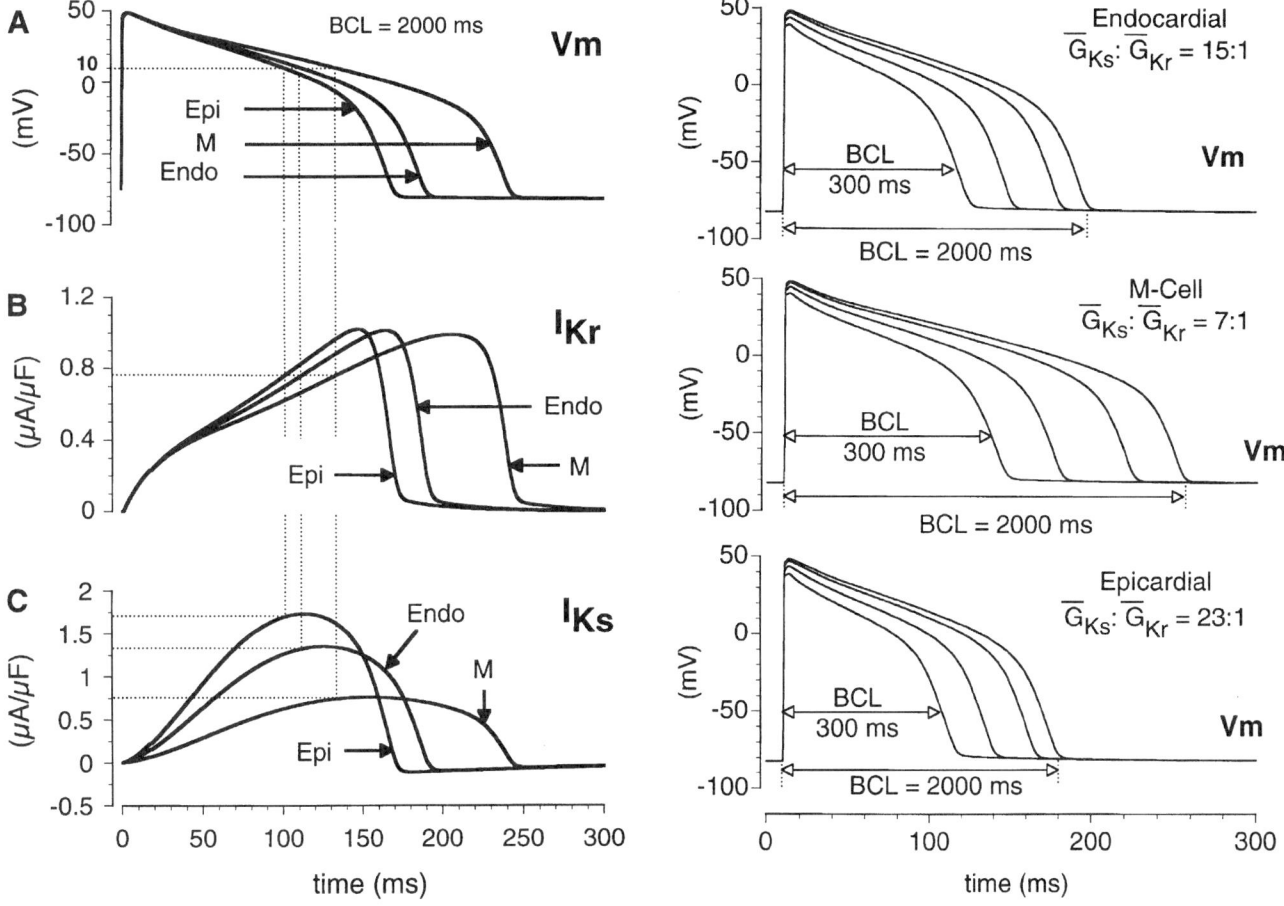

FIG. 13–7. Heterogeneity of APD in three cell types in relation to I_{Kr} and I_{Ks}. A: Simulated APs of the three cell types at BCL of 2000 msec. B: Corresponding I_{Kr}. C: Corresponding I_{Ks}. *Dotted lines* denote magnitudes of I_{Kr} and I_{Ks} at membrane potential of 10 mV. Epi, epicardial; M, midmyocardial; Endo, endocardial. [From reference 136, with permission.]

FIG. 13–8. Rate dependence of APD in the three cell types. M-cells prolong their APD dramatically compared with epicardial and endocardial cells with slowing of rate. APs at progressively decreasing rate (BCL = 300, 500, 1000, and 2000 msec) are shown for each cell type. [From reference 136, with permission.]

early phase of the AP, and attains a much smaller peak magnitude during the course of the AP. The M-cell I_{Kr} appears to be somewhat smaller during the AP plateau. However, this merely reflects the different time course of the AP in this cell. Thus, reduced I_{Ks} in M-cells is the major cause for their longer APD at slow rates.

Figure 13–8 (136) shows simulated APs for the three cell types for a wide range of BCLs. During fast pacing (BCL = 300 msec), the three cells display relatively short APs of similar durations (APD = 105, 113, and 135 msec for epicardial, endocardial, and M-cells, respectively). With slowing of pacing rate, the APD of the M-cell is prolonged much more than that of the epicardial or endocardial cells, demonstrating a steeper dependence of APD on rate (greater adaptation). At BCL = 2000 msec, the APD of epicardial, endocardial, and M-cells is 168, 188, and 240 msec, respectively. As explained in the previous section, shortening of APD at fast rates (the adaptation process) results mostly from incomplete deactivation of I_{Ks} between beats (reflecting its slow deactivation kinetics), with an added contribution from I_{NaCa}, which increases in the outward direction because of the rise of $[Na^+]_i$. The greater adaptation of M-cells reflects their smaller I_{Ks} density and a larger degree of residual I_{Ks} activation between beats. Because of their longer APD, there is less time for I_{Ks} deactivation between beats. As a result, there is greater residual activation and a greater relative increase of I_{Ks} in the M-cell upon BCL shortening. When BCL is decreased from 2000 to 300 msec, the percent increase of I_{Ks} is 128% in the M-cell but only 33% in the epicardial cell. I_{NaCa} also plays a role in the greater adaptability of M-cells. Because of the small I_{Ks} (and hence the small total repolarizing current) of the M-cell, the increase of outward I_{NaCa} at fast rates results in a large relative change of the total repolarizing current and participates significantly in APD shortening. It should be added that responsiveness to interventions that change the balance of currents during repolarization is a hallmark of the M-cells. Since such changes occur on the background of a relatively small total repolarizing current, they cause a significant relative change in this current and have a major effect on repolarization and APD. Such changes can be due to disease (e.g., the congenital long QT syndrome) (111) or as a result of channel modification by drugs (e.g., block of I_{Kr} by agents with class III antiarrhythmic action) (2, 121, 141).

Transmural heterogeneity also exists in the density of I_{to}, the transient outward current (30, 48, 52, 82, 84, 100, 144), which is not found in guinea pig ventricular myocardium but is prominent in the epicardium, but not endocardium, of other species. Figure 13–9 shows a simulated epicardial AP, the corresponding I_{to}, and a simulated endocardial AP (in which I_{to} is not expressed) for comparison. I_{to}, carried by K^+ ions, activates and inactivates rapidly (hence the term "transient"). It causes the fast, early repolarization phase that follows the AP upstroke (*arrow* in Fig. 13–9 *A*), and creates a prominent notch that gives the epicardial AP a "spike-and-dome" appearance. The extent of this I_{to}-induced early repolarization can indirectly affect the APD, since it affects the time course of other voltage-gated channels that determine the plateau and repolarization phases of the AP. For example, reduced V_m due to enhanced I_{to} acts to augment the driving force on $I_{Ca(L_s)}$ which, being an inward current, can prolong APD (a "paradoxical" effect given the repolarizing effect of I_{to}). The presence of I_{to} shifts the balance of currents in the outward (repolarizing) direction early during the AP. Consequently, a suppression of an inward current at this phase can cause premature repolarization and loss of the AP dome (87). Since I_{to} is prominent in epicardial cells, loss of the AP dome is likely to occur preferentially in the epicardium, resulting in a transmural V_m gradient that is reflected as ST-segment elevation in the electrocardiogram (ECG). An example is the Brugada syndrome, where an I_{Na} channel mutation leads to faster decay of the I_{Na} current leaving I_{to} unopposed (38). Indeed, this syndrome is associated with an ST-segment elevation in ECG leads V1 through V3 (19).

ABNORMAL REPOLARIZATION. EXAMPLE—EARLY AFTERDEPOLARIZATIONS

The delicate balance of inward and outward currents that determines the precise time course of the AP plateau can be disturbed during pathology or as a result of channel modification by drugs. An example is early afterdepolarizations (EADs) that develop from plateau potentials and can result in arrhythmic activity (63, 64, 90, 91, 108, 129, 150). EADs are associated with slow rates (bradycardia), the occurrence of a pause, and AP prolongation (31, 112, 137, 138). They can be induced experimentally by various pharmacological interventions that prolong APD (e.g., agents with class III antiarrhythmic action) (56, 137, 138, 139). They can also develop in conjunction with APD prolongation caused by various forms of the hereditary long QT syndrome (LQT) (4, 7, 68, 70, 111, 119, 137, 138, 143) (see also chapter 19). Because the plateau is controlled by a balance of depolarizing and repolarizing currents, APD prolongation can result from an increase of an inward current or a decrease of an outward current. Examples include the persistence of inward I_{Na} during the plateau in the LQT3 form of LQT (10, 26, 29, 39, 137), or

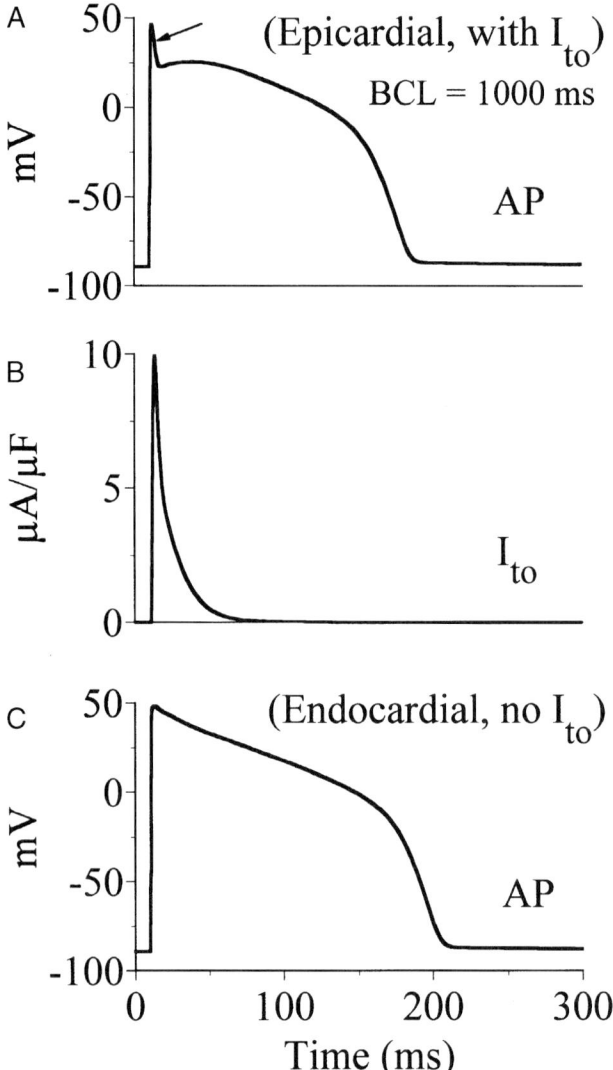

FIG. 13–9. Simulated epicardial AP (*A*) and the corresponding I_{to} (*B*). An endocardial AP, in which I_{to} is not expressed, is shown in *panel C* for comparison.

reduced I_{Kr} or I_{Ks} in LQT2 (33, 117) or LQT1 (127, 28), respectively.

Figure 13–10 (137) shows the last three APs in a train of forty beats (BCL = 500 ms) and an additional AP stimulated after a 1500 msec pause. Panel A is obtained under control conditions to simulate wild-type (WT) behavior. Panel B simulates LQT1 (70% reduction of I_{ks}). Panel C simulates LQT2 (40% reduction of I_{Kr}). Panel D is obtained for enhanced late I_{Na} to simulate LQT3. APs from epicardial cells and M-cells are shown in each panel. In control (panel A), the pause causes slight APD prolongation of epicardial cells and M-cells, but EADs do not develop. In all cases of the different LQT types (panels B–D) the post-pause AP of the M-cell develops EADs from a takeoff potential of −25 mV (in panel B the membrane potential repolarizes back to rest outside the scale shown in the figure).

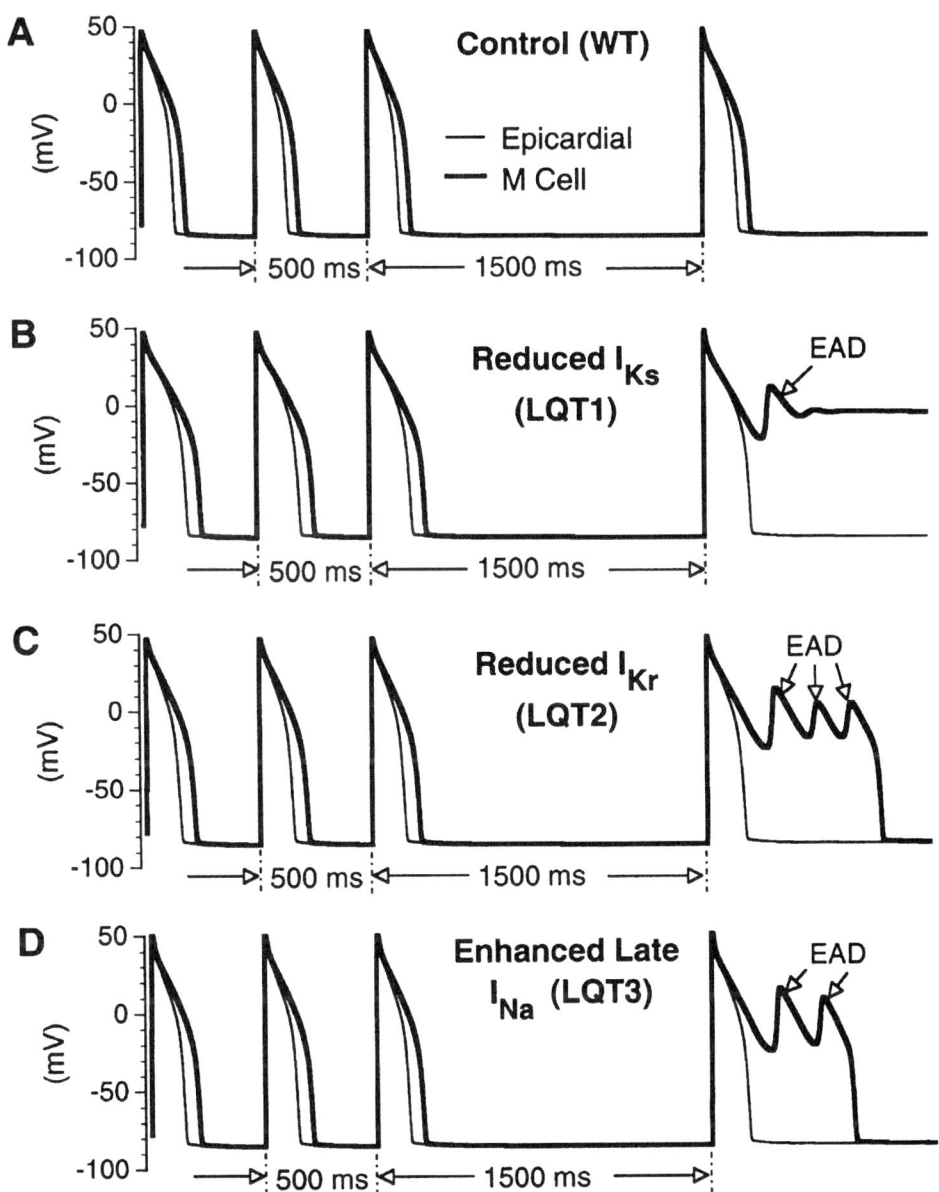

FIG. 13–10. Pause-induced early afterdepolarizations (EADs). Action potentials from epicardial and midmyocardial cells are overlaid for comparison. A: control conditions for wild-type (WT) ion channels. B: reduced I_{Ks} simulating LQT1. C: reduced I_{Kr} simulating LQT2. D: enhanced late I_{Na} simulating LQT3. The pause only causes slight prolongation of the APD of WT M-cell, but results in development of multiple EADs in the mutant M cells. [From reference 137, with permission.]

Figure 13–11A (137), shows the last pre-pause AP (thin line) and the post-pause AP (bold line) that develops plateau EADs in the case of LQT2 (reduced I_{Kr}). The corresponding L-type calcium current, $I_{Ca(L)}$, is shown in panel B. The pre- and post-pause data are overlaid to facilitate comparison. Decreased I_{Kr} (due to the LQT2 mutation) and deactivation of I_{Ks} during the pause reduce the repolarizing current during the post-pause AP and prolong its plateau (panel A). Prolongation of the plateau provides sufficient time (at the appropriate voltage) for the recovery from inactivation and reactivation of $I_{Ca(L)}$ (panel B) which, being an inward current, results in secondary membrane depolarization to generate the EADs. Note that in the absence of EADs (the pre-pause AP) $I_{Ca(L)}$ returns monotonically to zero. When $I_{Ca(L)}$ reactivation was prevented in the simulation during the post-pause AP, EADs did not develop. It should be emphasized that for all types of LQT in Figure 13–10, the EADs are caused by $I_{Ca(L)}$ reactivation. In other words, $I_{Ca(L)}$ is the depolarizing charge carrier that generates the EAD in all cases (90, 150). Interestingly, the defective mutant channels play only a secondary role in this process. They shift the delicate balance of currents during the plateau in the inward direction (LQT1 by reducing I_{Ks}, LQT2 by reducing I_{Kr}, and LQT3 by augmenting late I_{Na}). This shift prolongs the plateau, setting the stage for EAD generation by $I_{Ca(L)}$.

EFFECTS OF IONIC CONCENTRATIONS ON THE ACTION POTENTIAL. EXAMPLE—SODIUM OVERLOAD

The fact that ionic concentrations affect the reversal potential and modulate the conductance of certain ion channels (examples: I_{Kr} and I_{K1} conductances increase with increasing $[K^+]_o$, I_{Ks} conductance increases with increasing $[Ca^{2+}]_i$) implies that the cardiac AP morphology changes with variations of the ionic milieu. In particular, abnormal elevation of intracellular sodium and conditions of intracellular calcium overload are known to be associated with cardiac arrhythmias (31, 79, 145). Sodium overload can occur during conditions of metabolic compromise such as digitalis toxicity (58, 78) and chronic ischemia (131, 133). Intracellular sodium also accumulates with the fast stimulation rates that occur during tachycardia and fibrillation. In addition, sodium elevation can occur as a result of abnormal inactivation of I_{Na} that leads to a sustained current. Such inactivation can be due to channel modification by drugs (20), or by mutation, as occurs in LQT3 (10, 26, 29, 39, 137). Importantly, changes in $[Na^+]_i$ have a direct effect on the sodium–potassium pump (I_{NaK}) and the sodium–calcium exchanger (I_{NaCa}) which, because of their electrogenic properties, affect the action potential. Elevated $[Na^+]_i$ also augments the sodium-activated potassium current ($I_{K(Na)}$), which has been suggested to affect APD under

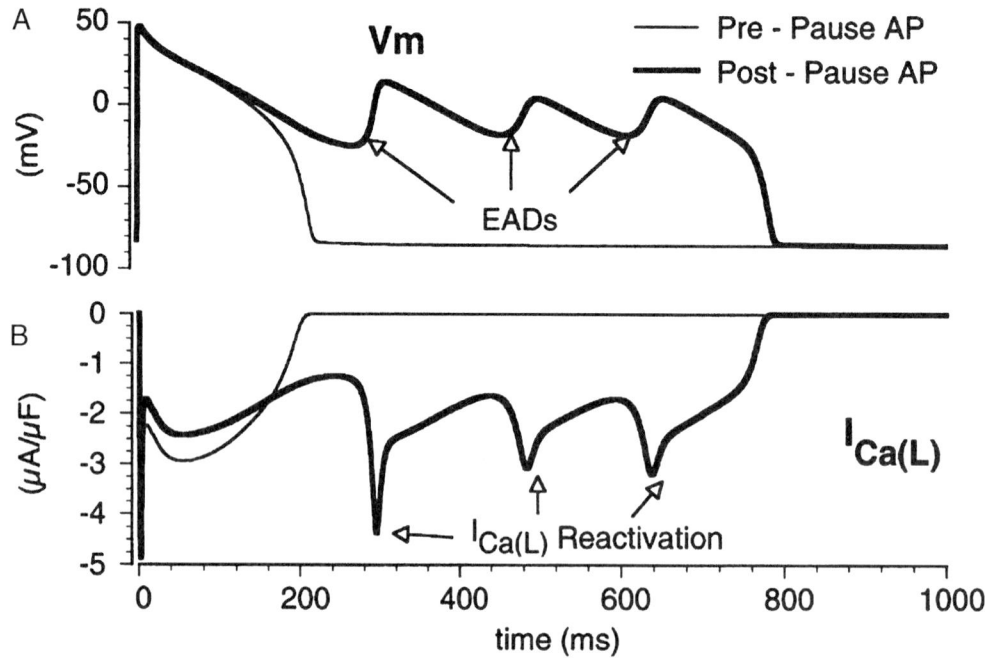

FIG. 13–11. Ionic mechanism of pause-induced EADs. A: The last pre-pause AP (*thin line*) and a post-pause AP developing plateau EADs (*bold line*). The *arrows* indicate the start of secondary membrane depolarization (EAD). B: Corresponding $I_{Ca(L)}$. Arrows indicate $I_{Ca(L)}$ reactivation, which generates the EADs. [From reference 137, with permission.]

conditions of Na⁺ overload (67, 79, 86, 116, 135, 140).

Figure 13–12 (45) shows simulated APs and ionic currents for control conditions ($[Na^+]_i$ = 10 mM) and for conditions of sodium overload ($[Na^+]_i$ = 20 mM). In this simulation, all conditions are identical for the two APs (the cell is paced until steady-state is achieved), except $[Na^+]_i$ is clamped to the assigned value (10 mM or 20 mM) just prior to the stimulus. This protocol permits examination of effects that are specifically due to $[Na^+]_i$ changes. As observed in Figure 13–12, AP changes brought about by $[Na^+]_i$ overload include slower upstroke, reduced maximum amplitude, reduced plateau potential, and shortened APD. Similar changes are observed experimentally.

Figure 13–12 relates the above changes to the underlying ionic currents. $[Na^+]_i$ accumulation reduces the driving force for I_{Na}. The smaller I_{Na} current (panel B) results in a slower AP upstroke and a lower peak amplitude (panel A). The elevated $[Na^+]_i$ drives I_{NaCa} and I_{NaK} in the outward direction (panels D and G), providing significantly greater repolarizing current during the early stages and throughout the AP, which results in a reduced plateau potential and shortened APD. While I_{Kr} shows no significant change (panel F), the reduced plateau potential slows I_{Ks} activation and decreases its driving force, resulting in a greatly reduced I_{Ks} current (panel E). Smaller I_{Ks} is typically associated with APD prolongation, but the enhanced I_{NaCa} and I_{NaK} more than compensate for this loss of repolarizing current. The "paradoxical" APD shortening, despite a reduced I_{Ks} serves to illustrate the complex dynamic interactions between various currents that determine the AP plateau and duration. $I_{K(Na)}$, the Na⁺-activated K⁺ current (panel H) is of small magnitude and its contribution to APD shortening is minimal.

PATHOLOGICAL ACTION POTENTIAL CHANGES. EXAMPLE—ACUTE ISCHEMIA

The major pathophysiological component conditions of acute myocardial ischemia are elevated extracellular potassium (hyperkalemia), acidosis, and anoxia (23, 120). These conditions cause the following electrophysiological changes: reduced membrane excitability, shortening of APD, and prolongation of recovery of excitability following an AP (54, 125, 146). The most important electrophysiological effect of anoxia is the activation of an ATP-sensitive potassium current, $I_{K(ATP)}$, which is increasingly more outward with decreasing levels of ATP (66, 103, 105, 106, 142). In addition, $I_{Ca(L)}$ exhibits ATP-dependence and decreases with reduced ATP availability (107). Hyperkalemia enhances the conductance of I_{K1}, I_{Kr}, and $I_{K(ATP)}$ (66, 74, 113–116). It also augments I_{NaK} in the direction of Na⁺ extrusion (an electrogenic outward current) and shifts the potassium reversal potential (E_K) in the positive direction. Acidosis causes a reduction of I_{Na} maximum conductance and a positive shift of its current-voltage relationship (65). It also reduces the maximum conductance of $I_{Ca(L)}$ (62) and causes a 2–5 mV depolarization of the resting membrane potential (72, 126).

In Figure 13–13 (120) the ischemic conditions listed above were incorporated in the LRd model. The AP and major ionic currents during acute ischemia are shown in the left panels and can be compared to those under control conditions (right panels). The ischemic AP displays an elevated (depolarized) rest potential, mostly as a result of $[K^+]_o$ elevation with small additional depolarization due to acidosis. I_{Na} is greatly reduced as a result of channel inactivation at the depolarized rest potential and due to the effects of acidosis. This reduction of I_{Na} translates into a slower upstroke and lower maximum amplitude of the ischemic AP. Importantly, as a consequence of the major I_{Na} suppres-

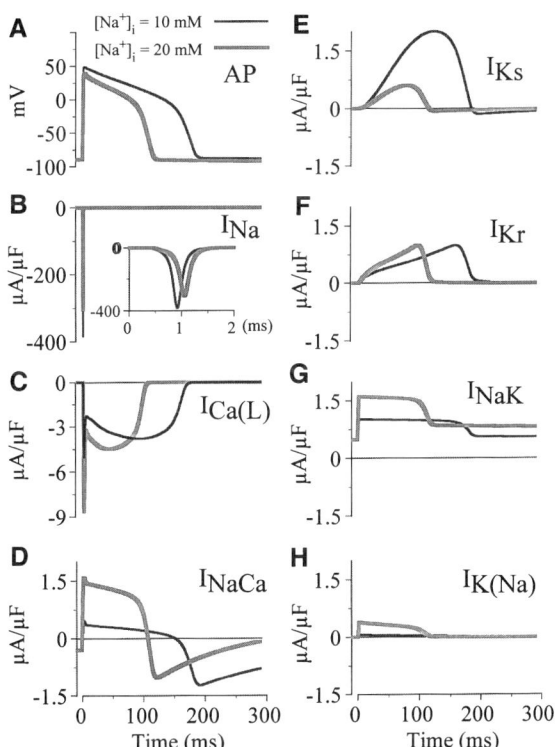

FIG. 13–12. Effect of elevated $[Na^+]_i$ on the action potential. Action potentials (AP) and selected corresponding ionic currents are shown for two different concentrations of intracellular Na⁺, $[Na^+]_i$ = 10 mM (control, *thin lines*) and $[Na^+]_i$ = 20 mM (high Na⁺, *thick lines*). Inset in B shows I_{Na} on an expanded time scale. $I_{K(Na)}$ is the Na⁺-activated K⁺ current that is augmented by Na⁺ overload. [Adapted from reference 45, with permission.]

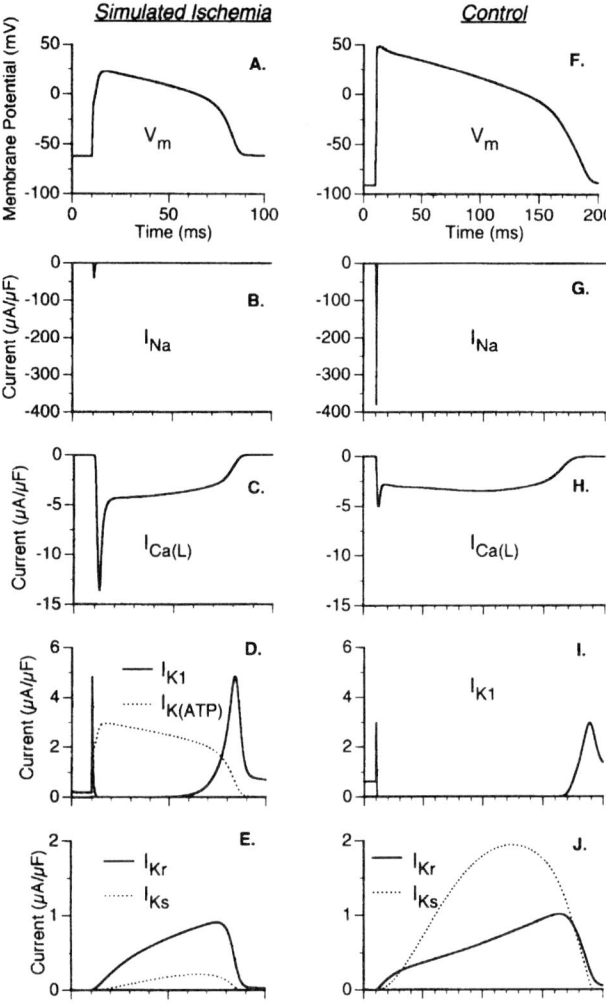

FIG. 13-13. Action potential (AP) and major ionic currents during acute ischemia. An ischemic AP (A) and the principal ionic currents (B–E) are shown for conditions of elevated $[K^+]_o$ = 12 mM, reduced pH=6.5, and reduced $[ATP]_i$ = 3 mM. A control, nonischemic AP (F) and corresponding ionic currents (G–J) are shown for comparison. [From reference 120, with permission.]

sion, $I_{Ca(L)}$ supports the last portion of the upstroke (at $V_m > 0$ mV). Note that $I_{Ca(L)}$ is increased during the ischemic AP despite the acidic depression of its maximum channel conductance. This increase reflects a greater driving force due to the lower plateau potential. I_{K1} is enhanced as a direct result of elevated $[K^+]_o$. Anoxia results in activation of $I_{K(ATP)}$, which contributes a repolarizing current during the entire AP and is the major contributor to the large degree of APD shortening (about 50%). I_{Kr} is relatively unchanged because of a balance between reduced driving force (depolarized E_K and reduced AP potential) and direct enhancement of its conductance by elevated $[K^+]_o$. I_{Ks} conductance is not enhanced by the elevated $[K^+]_o$. Therefore, the reduction in its driving force and slower activation at decreased plateau potentials are unopposed and lead to a significant reduction of I_{Ks} during the ischemic AP. An interesting and important pathophysiological phenomenon is the recruitment during abnormal conditions (in this case ischemia) of channels that are normally "dormant." The K(ATP) channels are present in the membrane with a very high density (similar to that of Na^+ channels) and "on demand" generate a large current that is sufficient to dominate the plateau and shorten APD despite the reduction of I_{Ks} (it takes only about 1% activation of $I_{K(ATP)}$ to shorten APD by 50%) (47, 103, 120).

EPILOGUE

In this chapter, we describe principles and ionic processes that underlie action potential generation and determine its properties. Using a mathematical model based on current information on ionic channels, we demonstrate through examples of normal and pathological behavior that the cell is a complex, highly interactive system and that the action potential is the integrated result of many component processes. Such "system design" is ideal for the precise control and adaptability that are necessary for normal physiological function and for the ability to adjust to various disease states. For example, the dependence of repolarization on a delicate balance between many currents provides for precise control of the action potential duration and its adaptation to rate changes during normal function. It also makes possible the major APD shortening by $I_{K(ATP)}$ activation under ishemic conditions. Such shortening may play a protective role during the ischemic insult (23).

The dependence of the AP on multiple ionic processes provides many potential targets for antiarrhythmic interventions, either by drugs or by molecular/genetic modification. In the case of genetic disorders, the mutant channel is not necessarily the only target for intervention. The LQT example in this chapter shows that while genetic mutations act to alter I_{Na} (in LQT3), I_{Kr} (in LQT2), or I_{Ks} (in LQT1) in such a way that APD is prolonged, it is another current ($I_{Ca(L)}$) that generates arrhythmogenic EADs in the three LQT variants. Therefore, if the objective of an intervention is to prevent EADs, $I_{Ca(L)}$ can be considered a target as well. Of course, the multiplicity of interacting processes that determine the AP also makes it difficult to predict the outcome of a particular intervention. It also makes the system more vulnerable since it increases the probability of altered function during pathology (there is a large number of components that can be affected by disease). Another complexity is added by the fact that the cell is not a fixed system; for example, it changes dynamically by regulating (up or down) the expression of ion channels during remodeling. Finally, it must be recognized that in the heart cells are not isolated but function in an ensemble, communicating with each other through gap junctions. The electric load on a cell can modify its action potential and modulate the ionic processes that determine its properties (136, 138).

This work was supported by grants RO1 HL-49054 and R37 HL-33343 from the National Institutes of Health—National Heart, Lung and Blood Institute, and by a Development Award from the Whitaker Foundation. Y. R. holds the M. Frank and Margaret C. Rudy Chair in Cardiac Bioelectricity.

My thanks to Gregory M. Faber, M.S., for his help in preparing the figures. Thanks also to Valeria Jurkovich and Brenda Hudson for their scretarial help in preparing the manuscript.

REFERENCES

1. Antzelevitch, C., G. Yan, W. Shimizu, A. Burashnikov. Electrical heterogeneity, the ECG, and cardiac arrhythmias. In: *Cardiac Electrophysiology: From Cell to Bedside*, edited by D. P. Zipes and J. Jalife. Philadelphia: W. B. Saunders, 1999:222–238.
2. Antzelevitch, C., S. Sicouri, S. H. Litovsky, et al. Heterogeneity within the ventricular wall: electrophysiology and pharmacology of epicardial, endocardial and M cells. *Circ. Res.* 69:1427–1449, 1991.
3. Anyukhovsky E. P., E. A. Sosunov, and M. R. Rosen. Regional differences in electrophysiologic properties of epicardium, midmyocardium, and endocardium: in vitro and in vivo correlations. *Circulation* 94:1981–1988, 1996.
4. Attali, B. Ion channels. A new wave for heart rhythms. *Nature* 384:24–25, 1996.
5. Backx, P. H. and E. Marban. Background potassium current active during the plateau of the action potential in guinea pig ventricular myocytes. *Circ. Res.* 72:890–900, 1993.
6. Balke, C. W., W. C. Rose, E. Marban, and W. G. Wier. Macroscopic and unitary properties of physiological ion flux through T-type Ca^{2+} channels in guinea-pig heart cells. *J. Physiol. (Lond.)* 456:247–265, 1992.
7. Barinaga, M. Tracking down mutations that can stop the heart. *Science* 281:32–34, 1998.
8. Barry, D. M. and J. M. Nerbonne. Myocardial potassium channels: electrophysiological and molecular diversity. *Annu Rev. Physiol.* 58:363–394, 1996.
9. Benardeau, A., S. N. Hatem, C. Ruecker-Martin, et al. Contribution of Na^+/Ca^+ exchange to action potential of human atrial myocytes. *Am. J. Physiol.* 271 (*Heart Circ. Physiol.* 40):H1151–H1161, 1996.
10. Bennett, P. B., K. Yazawa, N. Makita, and A. L. George, Jr. Molecular mechanism for an inherited cardiac arrhythmia. *Nature* 376:683–685, 1995.
11. Berman, M. F., J. S. Camardo, R. B. Robinson, and S. A. Siegelbaum. Single sodium channels from canine ventricular myocytes: voltage dependence and relative rates of activation and inactivation. *J. Physiol. (Lond.)* 415:503–531, 1989.
12. Bers, D. M., W. J. Lederer, and J. R. Berlin. Intracellular Ca transients in rat cardiac myocytes: role of Na-Ca exchange in excitation-contraction coupling. *Am. J. Physiol.* 258 (*Cell Physiol.* 27):C944–C954, 1990.
13. Beuckelmann, D. J. and W. G. Wier. Mechanism of release of calcium from sarcoplasmic reticulum of guinea-pig cardiac cells. *J. Physiol. (Lond.)* 405:233–255, 1988.
14. Beuckelmann, D. J. and W. G. Wier. Sodium-calcium exchange in guinea-pig cardiac cells, exchange current and changes in intracellular Ca^{2+}. *J. Physiol. (Lond.)* 414:499–520, 1989.
15. Blaustein, M. P. and W. J. Lederer. Sodium/calcium exchange: its physiological implications. *Physiol. Rev.* 79:763–854, 1999.
16. Blaustein, M. P., R. DiPolo, and J. P. Reeves. Sodium/calcium exchange. *Ann. N.Y. Acad. Sci.* 639:1–671, 1991.
17. Brahmajothi, M. V., M. J. Morales, K. A. Reimer, and H. C. Strauss. Regional localization of ERG, the channel protein responsible for the rapid component of the delayed rectifier, K^+ current in the ferret heart. *Circ. Res.* 81:128–135, 1997.
18. Bridge, J. H. B., J. R. Smolley, and K. W. Spitzer. The relationship between charge movements associated with I_{Ca} and I_{NaCa} in cardiac myocytes. *Science* 248:376–378, 1990.
19. Brugada, P. and J. Brugada. Right bundle branch block, persistent ST segment elevation and sudden cardiac death: a distinct clinical and electrocardiographic syndrome: a multicenter report. *J. Am. Coll. Cardiol.* 20:1391–1396, 1992.
20. Brill, D. M. and J. A. Wasserstrom. Intracellular sodium and the positive inotropic effect of veratridine and cardiac glycoside in sheep Purkinje fibers. *Circ. Res.* 58:109–119, 1986.
21. Campbell, D. L., R. L. Rasmusson, M. B. Comer, and H. C. Strauss. The cardiac calcium-independent transient outward potassium current: kinetics, molecular properties, and role in ventricular transient repolarization. In: *Cardiac Electrophysiology: From Cell to Bedside*, edited by D. P. Zipes and J. Jalife. Philadelphia: WB Saunders, 1995:83–96.
22. Capogrossi, M. C., M. D. Stern, H. A. Spurgeon, and E. G. Lakatta. Spontaneous Ca^{2+} release from the sarcoplasmic reticulum limits Ca^{2+}-dependent twitch potentiation in individual cardiac myocytes: a mechanism for maximum inotropy in the myocardium. *J. Gen. Physiol.* 91:133–155, 1988.
23. Carmeliet, E. Cardiac ionic currents and acute ischemia: from channels to arrhythmias. *Physiol. Rev.* 79:917–1017, 1999.
24. Caroni, P., M. Zurini, A. Clark, and E. Carafoli. Further characterization and reconstitution of the purified Ca-pumping ATPase of heart sarcolemma. *J. Biol. Chem.* 258:7305–7310, 1983.
25. Cascio, W. E., T. A. Johnson, and L. S. Gettes. Electrophysiologic changes in ischemic ventricular myocardium: I. Influence of ionic, metabolic and energetic changes. *J. Cardiovasc. Electrophysiol.* 6:1039–1062, 1995.
26. Chandra, R., F. Starmer, and A. O. Grant. Multiple effects of KPQ deletion mutation in gating of human cardiac Na^+ channels expressed in mammalian cells. *Am. J. Physiol.* 274 (*Heart Circ. Physiol.* 43):H1643–H1654, 1998.
27. Chinn, K. Two delayed rectifiers in guinea pig ventricular myocytes distinguished by tail current kinetics. *J. Pharmacol. Exp. Ther.* 264:553–560, 1993.
28. Chouabe C., N. Neyroud, P. Guicheney, et al. Properties of KvLQT1 K^+ channel mutations in Romano-Ward and Jervell and Lange-Nielsen inherited cardiac arrhythmias. *EMBO J.* 16:5472–5479, 1997.
29. Clancy, C. E. and Y. Rudy. Linking a genetic defect to its cellular phenotype in a cardiac arrhythmia. *Nature* 400:566–569, 1999.
30. Clark, R. B., R. A. Bouchard, E. Salinas-Stefanon, et al. Heterogeneity of action potential waveforms and potassium currents in rat ventricle. *Cardiovasc. Res.* 27:1795–1799, 1993.
31. Cranefield, F. P. and R. S. Aronson. *Cardiac Arrhythmias: The Role of Triggered Activity and Other Mechanisms.* Mt, Kisco, NY: Futura Publishing Company, 1988.
32. Crespo, L. M., C. J. Grantham, and M. B. Cannell. Kinetics, stoichiometry and role of the Na-Ca exchange mechanism in isolated cardiac myocytes. *Nature* 345:618–621, 1990.
33. Curran, M. E., I. Splawski, K. W. Timothy, et al. A molecular

basis for cardiac arrhythmia: *HERG* mutations cause long QT syndrome. *Cell* 80:795–803, 1995.
34. Daut, J. The energetics of the Na,K-pump in cardiac muscle. In: *Fortschritte der Zoologie, Luttgau (Hrsg): Volume 33, Membrane Control.* Stuttgart/New York: Gustav Fischer Verlag, 1986:419–427.
35. Doerr, T., R. Denger, A. Doerr, and W. Trautwein. Ionic currents contributing to the action potential in single ventricular myocytes of the guinea pig studied with action potential clamp. *Pflugers Arch.* 416:230–237, 1990.
36. Droogmans, G. and B. Nilius. Kinetic properties of the cardiac T-type calcium channel in the guinea-pig. *J. Physiol (Lond.)* 419:627–650, 1989.
37. Drouin, E., F. Charpentier, C. Gauthier, K. Laurent, and H. Le Marec. Electrophysiologic characteristics of cells spanning the left ventricular wall of human heart: evidence for presence of M cells. *J. Am. Coll. Cardiol.* 26:185–192, 1995.
38. Dumaine, R., J. A. Towbin, P. Brugada, M. Vatta, D. V. Nesterenko, V. V. Nesterenko, J. Brugada, R. Brugada, and C. Antzelevitch. Ionic mechanisms responsible for the electrocardiographic phenotype of the Brugada syndrome are temperature dependent. *Circ. Res.* 85:803–809, 1999.
39. Dumaine, R., Q. Wang, M. T. Keating, et al. Multiple mechanisms of sodium channel-linked long QT syndrome. *Circ. Res.* 78:916–924, 1996.
40. Earm, Y. E., W. K. Ho, and I. S. So. Inward current generated by Na-Ca exchange during the action-potential in single atrial cells of the rabbit. *Proc. R. Soc Lond. B. Biol. Sci.* 240:61–81, 1990.
41. Eddlestone, G. T., A. C. Zygmont, and C. Antzelevitch. Larger late sodium current contributes to the longer action potential of the M-cell in canine ventricular myocardium. *PACE* 19:569 (Abstract), 1996.
42. Egan, T. M., D. Noble, S. J. Noble, et al. Sodium-calcium exchange during the action-potential in guinea-pig ventricular cells. *J. Physiol.* 411:639–661, 1989.
43. Ehara, T., A. Noma, and K. Ono. Calcium-activated non-selective cation channel in ventricular cells isolated from adult guinea-pig hearts. *J. Physiol. (Lond.)* 403:117–133, 1988.
44. Eisner, D. A. and W. J. Lederer. Na-Ca exchange: stoichiometry and electrogenicity. *Am. J. Physiol.* 236 (Cell Physiol. 5):C189–C202, 1985.
45. Faber, G. M. and Y. Rudy. Action potential contractility changes in $[Na^+]_i$ overloaded cardiac myocytes: a simulation study. *Biophys. J.* 78:2392–2404, 2000.
46. Fabiato, A. Simulated calcium current can both cause calcium loading in and trigger calcium release from the sarcoplasmic reticulum of a skinned canine cardiac Purkinje cell. *J. Gen. Physiol.* 85:291–320, 1985.
47. Faivre, J. F. and I. Findlay. Action potential duration and activation of ATP-sensitive potassium current in isolated guinea-pig ventricular myocytes. *Biochim. Biophys. Acta* 1029:167–172, 1990.
48. Fedida, D. and W. R. Giles. Regional variations in action potentials and transient outward current in myocytes isolated from rabbit left ventricle. *J. Physiol. (Lond.)* 442:191–209, 1991.
49. Fedida, D., D. Noble, Y. Shimoni, and A. J. Spindler. Inward current related to contraction in guinea-pig ventricular myocytes. *J. Physiol. (Lond).* 385:565–589, 1987.
50. Fozzard, H. A. and D. A. Hanck. Structure and function of voltage-dependent sodium channels: comparison of brain II and cardiac isoforms. *Physiol. Rev.* 76:887–926, 1996.
51. Fozzard, H. A. and G. Lipkind. Ion channels and pumps in cardiac function. *Adv. Exp. Med. Biol.* 382:3–10, 1995.
52. Furukawa, T., R. J. Myerburg, N. Furukawa, et al. Differences in transient outward currents of feline endocardial and epicardial myocytes. *Circ. Res.* 67:1287–1291, 1990.
53. Gadsby, D. C. and M. Nakao. Steady-state current-voltage relationship of the Na/K pump in guinea pig ventricular myocytes. *J. Gen. Physiol.* 94:511–537, 1989.
54. Gettes, L. S. and W. E. Cascio. Effect of acute ischemia on cardiac electrophysiology. In: *The Heart and Cardiovascular System,* edited by H. A. Fozzard, R. B. Jennings, E. Haber, A. M. Katz, and H. E. Morgan. New York: Raven Press, 1992:2021–2054.
55. Grantham, C. J. and M. D. Cannell. Ca^{2+} influx during the cardiac action potential in guinea pig ventricular myocytes. *Circ. Res.* 79:194–200, 1965.
56. Habbab, M. A. and N. El-Sherif. Drug-induced torsades de pointes: role of early afterdepolarizations and dispersion of repolarization. *Am. J. Med.* 89:241–246, 1990.
57. Hadley, R. W. and W. J. Lederer. Ca^{2+} and voltage inactivate Ca^{2+} channels in guinea-pig ventricular myocytes through independent mechanisms. *J. Physiol. (Lond.)* 444:257–268, 1991.
58. Harrison, S. M., E. McCall, and M. R. Boyett. The relationship between contraction and intracellular sodium in rat and guinea-pig ventricular myocytes. *J. Physiol. (Lond).* 449:517–550, 1992.
59. Hess, P., J. B. Lansman, and R. W. Tsien. Calcium channel selectivity for divalent and monovalent cations, voltage and concentration dependence of single channel current in ventricular heart cells. *J. Gen. Physiol.* 88:293–319, 1986.
60. Hodgkin, A. L. and A. F. Huxley. A quantitative description of membrane current and its application to conduction and excitation in nerve. *J. Physiol. (Lond.)* 117:500–544, 1952.
61. Horie, M., S. Hayashi, and C. Kawai. Two types of delayed rectifying K^+ channels in atrial cells of guinea pig heart. *Jpn. J. Physiol.* 40:479–490, 1990.
62. Irisawa H. and R. Sato. Intra- and extracellular actions of proton on the calcium current of isolated guinea pig ventricular cells. *Circ. Res.* 59:348–355, 1986.
63. January, C. T., and J. M. Riddle. Early afterdepolarizations: mechanism of induction and block: a role of L-type Ca^{2+} current. *Circ. Res.* 64:977–989, 1989.
64. January, C. T., J. M. Riddle, and J. J. Salata. A model for early afterdepolarizations: induction with the Ca^{2+} channel agonist Bay K8644. *Circ. Res.* 62:563–571, 1988.
65. Kagiyama, Y., J. L. Hill, and L. S. Gettes. Interaction of acidosis and increased extracellular potassium on action potential characteristics and conduction in guinea pig ventricular muscle. *Circ. Res.* 51:614–623, 1982.
66. Kakei, M., A. Noma, and T. Shibasaki. Properties of adenosine-triphosphate-regulated potassium channels in guinea-pig ventricular cells. *J. Physiol. (Lond.)* 363:441–462, 1985.
67. Kameyama, M., M. Kakei, R. Sato, T. Shibasaki, H. Matsuda, and H. Irisawa. Intracellular Na^+ activates a K^+ channel in mammalian cardiac cells. *Nature* 309:354–356, 1984.
68. Kass, R. S. and M. P. Davies. The roles of ion channels in an inherited heart disease: molecular genetics of the long QT syndrome. *Cardiovasc. Res.* 32:443–454, 1996.
69. Kass, R. S. and M. C. Sanguinetti. Inactivation of calcium channel current in the calf cardiac Purkinje fiber: evidence for voltage- and calcium-mediated mechanisms. *J. Gen. Physiol.* 84:705–726, 1984.
70. Keating, M. T. and M. C. Sanguinetti. Molecular genetic insights into cardiovascular disease. *Science* 272:681–685, 1996.
71. Kimura, J., S. Miyamae, and A. Noma. Identification of sodium-calcium exchange current in single ventricular cells of guinea-pig. *J. Physiol. (Lond.)* 384:199–222, 1987.
72. Kléber, A. G. Resting membrane potential, extracellular potas-

sium activity, and intracellular sodium activity during acute global ischemia in isolated perfused guinea pig hearts. *Circ. Res.* 52:442–450, 1983.
73. Kunze, D. L., A. E. Lacerda, D. L. Wilson, and A. M. Brown. Cardiac Na currents and the inactivating, reopening, and waiting properties of single cardiac Na channels. *J. Gen. Physiol.* 86:691–719, 1985.
74. Kurachi, Y. Voltage-dependent activation of the inward-rectifier potassium channel in the ventricular cell membrane of guinea-pig heart. *J. Physiol. (Lond.)* 366:365–385, 1985.
75. Lagnado, L. and P. A. McNaughton. Electrogenic properties of the Na,Ca exchange. *J. Membr. Biol.* 113:177–191, 1990.
76. Lawrence, J. H., D. T. Yue, W. C. Rose, and E. Marban. Sodium channel inactivation from resting states in guinea-pig ventricular myocytes. *J. Physiol. (Lond.)* 443:629–650, 1991.
77. Lee, K. S., E. Marban, and R. W. Tsien. Inactivation of calcium channels in mammalian heart cells: joint dependence on membrane potential and intracellular calcium. *J. Gen. Physiol.* 364:395–411, 1985.
78. Levi, A. The effect of strophanthidin on action potential, calcium current and contraction in isolated guinea-pig ventricular myocytes. *J. Physiol. (Lond.)* 443:1–23, 1991.
79. Levi, A. J., G. R. Dalton, J. C. Hancox, J. S. Mitcheson, J. Issberner, J. A. Bates, S. J. Evans, F. C. Howarth, I. A. Hobai, and J. V. Jones. Role of intracellular sodium overload in the genesis of cardiac arrhythmias. *J. Cardiovasc. Electrophysiol.* 8:700–721, 1997.
80. Lipp, P. and M. D. Bootman. The physiology and molecular biology of cardiac Na/Ca exchange. In: *Cardiac Electrophysiology: From Cell to Bedside*, edited by D. P. Zipes and J. Jalife. Philadelphia: WB Saunders, 1999:41–51.
81. Lipp, P., S. Mechmann, and L. Pott. Effects of calcium release from sarcoplasmic reticulum on membrane currents in guinea pig atrial cardioballs. *Pflugers Arch.* 410:121–131, 1987.
82. Litovsky, S. H. and C. Antzelevitch. Transient outward current prominent in canine ventricular epicardium but not endocardium. *Circ. Res.* 62:116–126, 1988.
83. Litovsky, S. H. and C. Antzelevitch. Rate dependence of action potential duration and refractoriness in canine ventricular endocardium differs from that of epicardium: role of the transient outward current. *J. Am. Coll. Cardiol.* 14:1053–1066, 1989.
84. Liu, D. W., G. A. Gintant, and C. Antzelevitch. Ionic bases for electrophysiological distinctions among epicardial, midmyocardial, and endocardial myocytes from the free wall of the canine left ventricle. *Circ. Res.* 72:671–687, 1993.
85. Liu, D. W. and C. Antzelevitch. Characteristics of the delayed rectifier current (IKr and IKs) in canine ventricular epicardial, midmyocardial, and endocardial myocytes: a weaker IKs contributes to the longer action potential of the M cell. *Circ. Res.* 76:351–365, 1995.
86. Luk, H. N. and E. Carmeliet. Na^+-activated K^+ current in cardiac cells: rectification, open probability, block and role in digitalis toxicity. *Pflugers Arch.* 416:766–769, 1990.
87. Lukas, A. and C. Antzelevitch. Phase 2 reentry as a mechanism of initiation of circus movement reentry in canine epicardium exposed to simulated ischemia. The antiarrhythmic effects of 4-aminopyridine. *Cardiovasc. Res.* 32:593–603, 1996.
88. Luo, C. and Y. Rudy. A model of the ventricular cardiac action potential: depolarization, repolarization and their interaction. *Circ. Res.* 68:1501–1526, 1991.
89. Luo, C. and Y. Rudy. A dynamic model of the cardiac ventricular action potential: I. Simulations of ionic currents and concentration changes. *Circ. Res.* 74:1071–1096, 1994.
90. Luo, C. and Y. Rudy. A dynamic model of the cardiac ventricular action potential: II. Afterdepolarizations, triggered activity and potentiation. *Circ. Res.* 74:1097–1113, 1994.
91. Marban, E., S. W. Robinson, and W. G. Wier. Mechanisms of arrhythmogenic delayed and early afterdepolarizations in ferret ventricular muscle. *Clin. Invest.* 78:1185–1192, 1986.
92. Matsuura, H., T. Ehara, and Y. Imoto. An analysis of the delayed outward current in single ventricular cells of the guinea-pig. *Pflugers Arch.* 410:596–603, 1987.
93. McDonald, T. F., S. Pelzer, W. Trautwein, and D. J. Pelzer. Regulation and modulation of calcium channels in cardiac, skeletal, and smooth muscle cells. *Physiol. Rev.* 74:365–507, 1994.
94. Meissner, G. Sarcoplasmic reticulum ion channels. In: *Cardiac Electrophysiology: From Cell to Bedside*, edited by D. P. Zipes and J. Jalife. Philadelphia: W. B. Saunders, 1995:51–58.
95. Mechmann, S. and L. Pott. Identification of Na-Ca exchange current in single cardiac myocytes. *Nature* 319:597–599, 1986.
96. Mitchell, M. R., T. Powell, D. A. Terrar, and V. W. Twist. The effect of ryanodine, EGTA and low-sodium on action potentials in rat and guinea-pig ventricular myocytes: evidence for two inward currents during the plateau. *Br. J. Pharmacol.* 81:543–550, 1984.
97. Mitsuiye, T. and A. Noma. Exponential activation of the cardiac Na^+ current in single guinea-pig ventricular cells. *J. Physiol. (Lond.)* 453:261–277, 1992.
98. Mullins, L. J. A mechanism for Na/Ca transport. *J. Gen. Physiol.* 70:681–695, 1977.
99. Mullins, L. J. The generation of electric currents in cardiac fibers by Na/Ca exchange. *Am. J. Physiol.* 236 (*Cell Physiol.* 5):C103–C110, 1979.
100. Nabauer, M., D. J. Beuckelmann, P. Uberfuhr, and G. Steinbeck. Regional differences in current density and rate-dependent properties of the transient outward current in subepicardial and subendocardial myocytes of human left ventricle. *Circulation* 93:168–177, 1996.
101. Nakao, M. and D. C. Gadsby. [Na] and [K] dependence of the Na/K pump current-voltage relationship in guinea-pig ventricular myocytes. *J. Gen. Physiol.* 94:539–565, 1989.
102. Neely, A., R. Olcese, X. Wei, L. Birnbaumer, and E. Stefani. Ca^{2+}-dependent inactivation of a cloned cardiac Ca^{2+} channel α_1 subunit (α_{1C}) expressed in *Xenopus* oocytes. *Biophys. J.* 66:1895–1903, 1994.
103. Nichols, C. G., C. Ripoll, W. J. Lederer. ATP-sensitive potassium channel modulation of the guinea pig ventricular action potential and contraction. *Circ. Res.* 68:280–287, 1991.
104. Nitta, J., T. Furukawa, F. Marumo, T. Sawanobori, and M. Hiraoka. Subcellular mechanism for Ca^{2+}-dependent enhancement of delayed rectifier $K+$ current in isolated membrane patches of guinea pig ventricular myocytes. *Circ. Res.* 74:96–104, 1994.
105. Noma, A. ATP-regulated K^+ channels in cardiac muscle. *Nature* 305:147–148, 1983.
106. Noma, A. and T. Shibasaki. Membrane current through adenosine-triphosphate-regulated potassium channels in guinea-pig ventricular cells. *J. Physiol. (Lond.)* 363:463–480, 1985.
107. Ohya, Y. and N. Sperelakis. ATP regulation of the slow calcium channels in vascular smooth muscle cells of guinea pig mesenteric artery. *Circ. Res.* 64:145–154, 1989.
108. Priori, S. G. and P. B. Corr. Mechanisms underlying early and delayed afterdepolarizations induced by catecholamines. *Am. J. Physiol.* 258 (*Heart Circ. Physiol.* 27):H1796–H1805, 1990.
109. Priori, S. G., J. Barhanin, R. N. W. Hauer, W. Haverkamp, H. J. Jongsma, A. G. Kleber, W. J. McKenna, D. M. Roden, Y. Rudy, K. Schwartz, P. J. Schwartz, J. A. Towbin, and A. M. Wilde. Genetic and molecular basis of cardiac arrhythmias, Part III.

Circulation 99:674–681, 1999. (Also published in *Eur. Heart J.* 20:179–195, 1999.)
110. Reeves, J. P. and C. C. Hale. The stoichiometry of the cardiac sodium-calcium exchange system. *J. Biol. Chem.* 259:7733–7739, 1984.
111. Roden, D. M. and P. M. Spooner. Inherited long QT syndrome: a paradigm for understanding arrhythmogenesis. *J. Cardiovasc. Electrophysiol.* 10:1664–1683, 1999.
112. Rosen, M. R. The concept of afterdepolarizations. In: *Cardiac Electrophysiology: A Textbook*, edited by M. R. Rosen, M. J. Janse, A. L. Wit. Mount Kisco, NY: Futura, 1990:267–271.
113. Sakmann, B. and G. Trube. Conductance properties of single inwardly rectifying potassium channels in ventricular cells from guinea-pig heart. *J. Physiol. (Lond.)* 347:641–657, 1984.
114. Sanguinetti, M. C. and N. K. Jurkiewicz. Two components of cardiac delayed rectifier K^+ current: differential sensitivity to block by class III antiarrhythmic agents. *J. Gen. Physiol.* 96:195–215, 1990.
115. Sanguinetti, M. C. and N. K. Jurkiewicz. Role of external Ca^{2+} and K^+ in gating of cardiac delayed rectifier K^+ currents. *Pflugers Arch.* 420:180–186, 1992.
116. Sanguinetti, M. C. Na^+-activated and ATP-sensitive K^+ channels in the heart. In: *Potassium Channels: Basic Function and Therapeutic Aspects*, edited by T. J. Colatsky. New York: Alan R. Liss, Inc., 1990:85–109.
117. Sanguinetti, M. C., M. E. Curran, P. S. Spector, et al. Spectrum of HERG $K+$ channel dysfunction in an inherited cardiac arrhythmia. *Proc. Natl. Acad. Sci. U.S.A.* 93:2208–2212, 1996.
118. Scanley, B. E., D. A. Hanck, T. Chay, and H. A. Fozzard. Kinetic analysis of single sodium channels from canine cardiac Purkinje cells. *J. Gen. Physiol.* 95:411–447, 1990.
119. Schwartz, P. J., S. G. Priori, and C. Napolitano. Long QT syndrome. In: *Cardiac Electrophysiology: From Cell to Bedside*, edited by D. P. Zipes and J. Jalife. Philadelphia: W. B. Saunders, 1999:788–810.
120. Shaw, R. M. and Y. Rudy. Electrophysiologic effects of acute myocardial ischemia: a theoretical study of altered cell excitability and action potential duration. *Cardiovasc. Res.* 35:256–272, 1997.
121. Shimizu, W. and Anzelevitch, C. Sodium channel block with mexiletine is effective in reducing dispersion of repolarization and preventing torsades de pointes in LQT2 and LQT3 models of the long-QT syndrome. *Circulation* 96:2038–2047, 1997.
122. Shirokov, R., R. Levis, N. Shirokova, and E. Rios. Ca^{2+}-dependent inactivation of cardiac L-type Ca^{2+} channels does not affect their voltage sensor. *J. Gen. Physiol.* 102:1005–1030, 1993.
123. Sicouri, S., M. Quist, and C. Antzelevitch. Evidence for the presence of M cells in the guinea pig ventricle. *J. Cardiovasc. Electrophysiol.* 7:503–511, 1996.
124. Sicouri, S. and C. Antzelevitch. A subpopulation of cells with unique electrophysiological properties in the deep subepicardium of the canine ventricle: the M cell. *Circ. Res.* 68:1729–1741, 1991.
125. Sipido, K. R., G. Callewaert, and E. Carmeliet. Inhibition and rapid recovery of Ca^{2+} current during release from sarcoplasmic reticulum in guinea pig ventricular myocytes. *Circ. Res.* 76:102–109, 1995.
126. Skinner, R. B., Jr., and D. L. Kunze. Changes in extracellular potassium activity in response to decreased pH in rabbit atrial muscle. *Circ. Res.* 39:678–683, 1976.
127. Splawski, I., M. Tristanti-Firouzi, M. H. Lehmann, et al. Mutations in the *hminK* gene cause long QT syndrome and suppress IKs function. *Nat. Genet.* 17:338–340, 1996.
128. Stern, M. D., M. C. Capogrossi, and E. G. Lakatta. Spontaneous calcium release from the sarcoplasmic reticulum in myocardial cells, mechanisms and consequences. *Cell Calcium* 9:247–256, 1988.
129. Szabo, B., T. Kovacs, and R. Lazzara. Role of calcium loading in early afterdepolarizations generated by Cs^+ in canine and guinea pig Purkinje fibers. *J. Cardiovasc. Electrophysiol.* 6:796–812, 1995.
130. Tada, M., M. Shigekawa, M. Kadoma, and Y. Nimura. Uptake of calcium by sarcoplasmic reticulum and its regulation and functional consequences. In: *Physiology and Pathophysiology of the Heart*, edited by N. Sperelakis. Boston: Kluwer Academic Publishers, 1989:267–290.
131. Tani, M. and J. Neely. Na^+ accumulation increases Ca^{2+} overload and impairs function in anoxic rat heart. *J. Mol. Cell. Cardiol.* 22:57–72, 1990.
132. Tohse, N. Calcium-sensitive delayed rectifier potassium current in guinea pig ventricular cells. *Am. J. Physiol.* 258 (*Heart Circ. Physiol.* 27):H1200–H1207, 1990.
133. van Echteld, C., J. Kirkels, M. Eijgelshoven, P. van der Meer, and T. Ruigrok. Intracellular sodium during ischemia and calcium-free perfusion: a ^{23}Na NMR study. *J. Mol. Cell. Cardiol.* 23:297–307, 1991.
134. Vassort, G. and J. Alvarez. Cardiac T-type calcium current: pharmacology and roles in cardiac tissues. *J. Cardiovasc. Electrophysiol.* 5:376–393, 1994.
135. Veldkamp, M. W., J. Vereecke, and E. Carmeliet. Effects of intracellular sodium and hydrogen ion on the sodium activated potassium channel in isolated patches from guinea pig ventricular myocytes. *Cardiovasc. Res.* 28:1036–1041, 1994.
136. Viswanathan, P. C., R. M. Shaw, and Y. Rudy. Effects of IKr and IKs heterogeneity on action potential duration and its rate-dependence: A simulation study. *Circulation* 99:2466–2474, 1999.
137. Viswanathan, P. C. and Y. Rudy. Pause induced early afterdepolarizations in the long QT syndrome: A simulation study. *Cardiovasc. Res.* 42:530–542, 1999.
138. Viswanathan, P. C. and Y. Rudy. Cellular arrhythmogenic effects of the congenital and acquired long QT syndrome in the heterogeneous myocardium. *Circulation* 101:1192–1198, 2000.
139. Vos, M. A., S. C. Verduyn, A. P. Gorgels, G. C. Lipcsei, and H. J. J. Wellens. Reproducible induction of early afterdepolarizations and torsade de pointes arrhythmias by d-sotalol and pacing in dogs with chronic atrioventricular block. *Circulation* 91:864–872, 1995.
140. Wang, Z., T. Kimitsuki, and A. Noma. Conductance properties of the Na^+-activated K^+ channel in guinea-pig ventricular cells. *J. Physiol. (Lond.)* 433:241–257, 1991.
141. Weirich, J., R. Bernhardt, N. Loewen, et al. Regional- and species-dependent effects of K^+-channel blocking agents on subendocardium and mid-wall slices of human, rabbit, and guinea pig myocardium. *Pflugers Arch.* 431:R130 (Abstract), 1996.
142. Weiss, J. N., N. Venkatesh, and S. T. Lamp. ATP-sensitive K^+ channels and cellular K^+ loss in hypoxic and ischaemic mammalian ventricle. *J. Physiol. (Lond.)* 447:649–673, 1992.
143. Welsh, J. J. and T. Hoshi. Molecular cardiology. Ion channels lose the rhythm. *Nature* 376:640, 1995.
144. Wettwer E., G. J. Amos, H. Posival, and U. Ravens. Transient outward current in human ventricular myocytes of subepicardial and subendocardial origin. *Circ. Res.* 75:473–482, 1994.
145. Wier, W. and P. Hess. Excitation-contraction coupling in cardiac Purkinje fibers. Effects of cardiotonic steroids on the intracellular [Ca^{2+}] transient, membrane potential, and contraction. *J. Gen. Physiol.* 83:395–415, 1984.

146. Wit, A. L. and M. J. Janse. The ventricular arrhythmias of ischemia and infarction: electrophysiological mechanisms. Mt. Kisco, NY: *Futura Publishing Company*, 1992.
147. Yue, D. T. and E. Marban. A novel cardiac potassium channel that is active and conductive at depolarized potentials. *Pflugers Arch.* 413:127–133, 1988.
148. Yue, D. T., P. H. Backx, and J. P. Imredy. Calcium-sensitive inactivation in the gating of single calcium channels. *Science* 250: 1735–1738, 1990.
149. Yue, D. T., D. Burkhoff, M. R. Franz, W. C. Hunter, and K. Sagawa. Postextrasystolic potentiation of the isolated canine left ventricle: relationship to mechanical restitution. *Circ. Res.* 56:340–350, 1985.
150. Zeng, J. and Y. Rudy. Early afterdepolarizations in cardiac myocytes: mechanism and rate dependence. *Biophys. J.* 68:949–964, 1995.
151. Zeng, J., K. R. Laurita, D. S. Rosenbaum, and Y. Rudy. Two components of the delayed rectifer K^+ current in ventricular myocytes of the guina pig type: theoretical formulation and their role in repolarization. *Circ. Res.* 77:1–13, 1995.

14. Ion channels in the heart: cellular and molecular properties of cardiac Na, Ca, and K channels

BRONAGH HEATH — *Department of Pharmacology, College of Physicians & Surgeons, Columbia University, New York, New York*

KEVIN GINGRICH — *Department of Anesthesiology, University of Rochester School of Medicine and Dentistry, Rochester, New York*

ROBERT S. KASS — *Department of Pharmacology, College of Physicians & Surgeons, Columbia University, New York, New York*

CHAPTER CONTENTS

Calcium Channels
Sodium Channels
   Primary structure of the voltage-gated Na^+ channel
   Molecular pharmacology of Na^+ channels
   Molecular pharmacology of an inherited disease
Potassium Channels
   Voltage-dependent K^+ channels
      Transient outward K current, Ito
      Delayed rectifier K currents, I_K
      K channels and LQT
      Ultra-rapid K channel, IKur
   Inward rectifier K channels
      Cardiac inward rectifier, IK1
      Ach-activated K channel, IKACh
      ATP-sensitive K channels, IKATP
Summary

ELECTRICAL ACTIVITY IN THE HEART is generated by the summation of currents through multiple ion channels (74). The ventricular action potential is characterized by a long-lasting plateau period in which a balance is maintained between small inwardly and outwardly directed exchange and ion channel currents; small changes in this balance can have severe functional consequences. In the final decade of the twentieth century, a wealth of information accumulated on the molecular structures that form the protein pathways for ion conduction in heart and other excitable cells. In this chapter we review only three types of ion channels: calcium (L-type, T-type), sodium (Na^+), and potassium channels (K^+). It will provide an introduction to further discussions of ion channels in chapters 12, 13, 15, 17, and 18. We focus on the structural characteristics as well as the pharmacological properties of these channels. Figure 14–1 provides a schematic overview a of voltage-gated ion channels that includes potassium channels, calcium channels, sodium channels, and chloride channels (not discussed in this chapter).

CALCIUM CHANNELS

At least six types of voltage-gated calcium channels (N-, L-, P-, Q-, R-, and T-) have been identified based on their pharmacological and/or biophysical properties (14, 155). In the heart both T- and L-type channels contribute to cardiac electrophysiology, but L-type channels, the targets of organic calcium channel modulators and substrates for cyclic odenosine monophosphate cAMP-dependent protein kinase A and protein kinase C, are unique in their importance to the maintenance of calcium homeostasis because they can be under pharmacological and/or neuro/hormonal control (28, 53, 91, 136, 137, 155, 175). Skeletal muscle L-type calcium channels are heteromultimeric proteins consisting of α_1, β_2, and α_2/δ subunits (29, 52, 57), and it is likely that L-type calcium channels in other tissues are also multi-subunit proteins (1, 138, 148, 149). Figure 14–2 shows a comparison of putative subunit structure of skeletal and cardiac calcium channels as well as potential phosphorylation sites.

Functional roles of the auxiliary subunits have been studied by several groups with particular focus on the role of the $\beta 2$ subunit (49, 127, 141). When both α and β subunits of the L-type Ca^{2+} channel are co-expressed the kinetics of I_{Ca} are more nearly normal than when the α subunit is expressed alone (83, 86, 103, 158) and expression levels are enhanced (103). One role of the β subunit is thus thought to involve

A. Potassium Channel

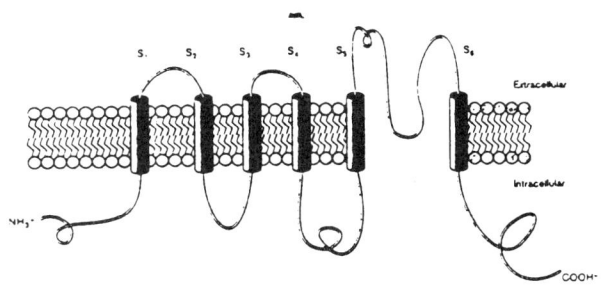

B. Na or Ca Channel

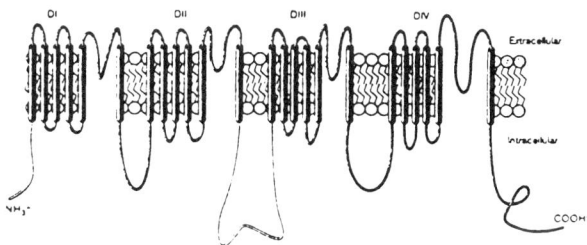

FIG. 14–1. Predicted topology for the α_1 subunit of voltage-gated potassium (A), and sodium or calcium (B) channels. [From Keating and Sanguinetti (128), with permission].

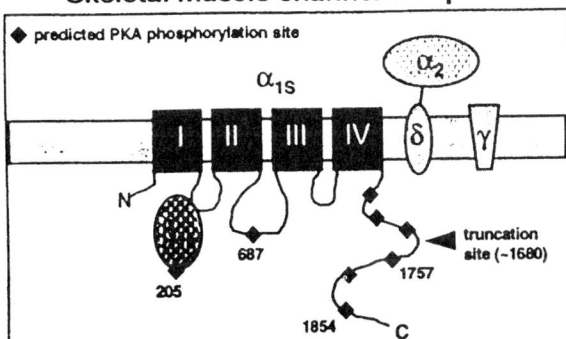
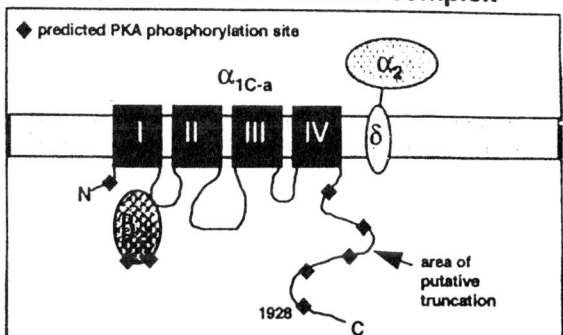

FIG. 14–2. Schematic representation of the subunit composition of L-type skeletal (*left*) and cardiac (*right*) calcium channels. Note that predicted PKA phosphorylation sites are indicated as *solid squares*. [From Hosey et al., (63) with permission.]

the targeting of the α1 subunit to the surface membrane. Similarly, α_2/δ subunits increase gating charge and ionic current of recombinant channel activity (7). The roles of auxiliary subunit in modulating native channel function continue to be an important area of investigation that will be significant in unraveling drug and neurohormonal modulation of L-type calcium channels (63).

L-type calcium channels inactivate in a voltage- and calcium-dependent manner (77, 173) and are the targets of the most extensively developed calcium channel pharmacology (73). Perhaps best studied is the marked modulation of L-type calcium channels by the β-adrenergic (β-AR) signaling cascade. Action potentials in the heart are sensitive to catecholamines. Exposure of isolated tissue to norepinephrine increases pacemaker activity (154), increases the height affects the duration of the ventricular action potential plateau (124), and increases the strength of contraction, all of which have been shown to be due, at least in part, to modulation of L-type channels by β-AR stimulation (17, 94, 97, 98, 123, 124).

L-type calcium channel activity is markedly enhanced by β-AR stimulation (83), but demonstrating the molecular basis of this modulation has been difficult in heterologous expression systems. Biochemical and electrophysiological evidence from single cell recordings has been provided to indicate that the enhanced activity depends on phosphorylation of a target protein by cAMP-dependent protein kinase A (112, 113, 140, 175, 177). Kinetic analysis of single-channel and whole-cell currents recorded from isolated myocytes has provided further evidence that two distinct sites are likely to be phosphorylated (112, 113, 169). Figure 14–3 shows the developmental change in β-AR sensitivity of cardiac calcium channels. More recent studies indicate that, in addition to key L-type channel subunits, anchoring proteins are needed to target protein kinase A to the channel subunit to be phosphorylated (50). This finding opens the possibility of specific targeting of channel proteins and other cellular proteins by signaling cascades such that receptor isoforms that stimulate similar signal cascades may target different ion channel proteins (2).

Because of the unique relationship between the entry of calcium both as a modulator of channel function

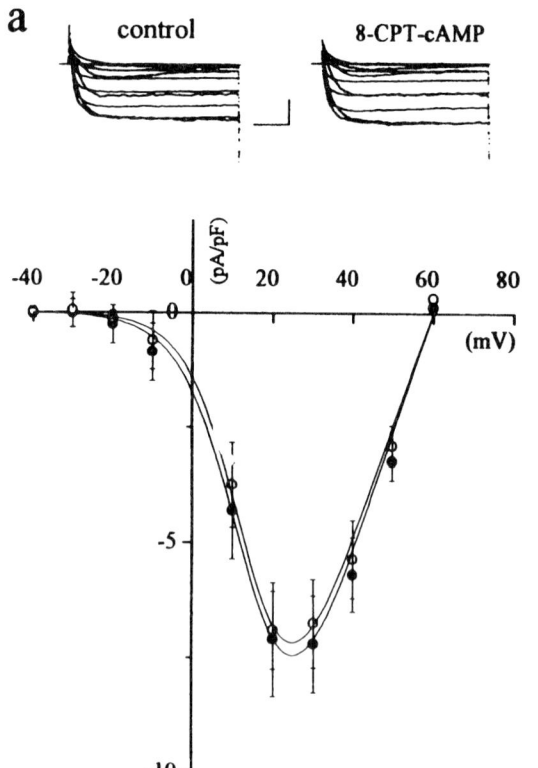
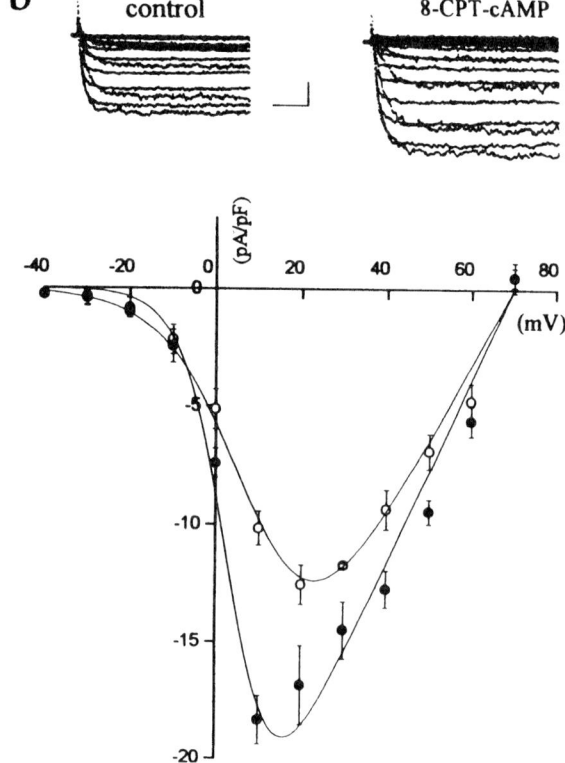

FIG. 14–3. The response of L-type calcium channels to β-AR stimulation changes with development. Response of currents measured in single murine embryonic cells to isoproterenol in early stage (*a*) and late stage (*b*) embryonic heart. The currents in the late, but not early, stage cells are enhanced by isoproterenol and this effect is due to an increase in intracellular cAMP. [From An et al., (3) with permission.]

(inactivation and current amplitude) as well as a modulator of intracellular processes (activation of contraction and modification of enzyme activity), understanding the role of the L-type calcium channel in controlling the cardiac action potential duration is key to understanding cardiac muscle physiology. Calcium entry has pronounced effects on the cardiac action potential. Early microelectrode recordings and voltage-clamp records indicated a close relationship between Ca-dependent changes in the action potential and in a slow inward current and contractile activation (11, 12, 21, 22, 98, 104, 122). The waveform of the action potential plateau depends on calcium entry in a tissue-specific manner (78, 79) suggesting strongly that calcium might affect other calcium-sensitive electrogenic pathways in addition to the calcium channel itself, a point substantiated by others (179) in later studies.

Calcium entry via L-type channels contributes the major source of calcium ions to load intracellular stores for subsequent release and activation of contractile proteins. The process linking calcium entry via sarcolemmal channels and release of calcium from the sarcoplasmic reticulum (SR) is thought to be due to calcium-induced calcium release from the SR due to rapid accumulation of calcium ions in a restricted space surrounding L-type calcium channel and ryanodine receptors (RYRs), the intracellular calcium channels of the SR (18, 92, 111, 171). This work does not rule out the interesting possibility that L-type calcium channels and RYRs are coupled with molecular bridges in heart as they are in skeletal muscle (32), a possibility presently under experimental investigation (93, 139).

Modulation of L-type Ca^{2+} channel activity by calcium channel antagonists has become a key clinical therapeutic approach to the management of hypertension and certain types of cardiac rhythm disturbances (73). Several more recent reports, however, have raised questions about the effectiveness and safety of some calcium channel antagonists in the treatment of hypertension (48), making it clear that an understanding of the precise molecular targets of this important drug family is crucial to improved therapeutic efficacy.

The drugs that have received the most attention belong to three distinct chemical classes: (1) phenylalkylamines (verapamil, D-600); (2) benzothiazepines [(+) cis diltiazem]; and (3) the 1–4, dihydropyridines (PN 200–110, nitrendipine, nifedipine, nisoldipine) (77). These drugs bind to distinct but allosterically coupled sites on the channel protein (sites 93 and 404). The α_1 subunit of the L-type calcium channel contains the binding sites for the three major classes of calcium channel modulators described above (30), and, when expressed in heterologous expression systems, is sufficient to encode channels with most of the biophysical and pharmacological properties of intact native channels (62, 95, 101, 167; Fig. 14–4). Studies of the molecular site(s) and mechanisms of action of calcium channel blockers have focused on the biochemical and biophysical role of the α_1 subunit and its relationship to modulation of native L-type channels.

Site-directed mutagenesis studies have revealed specific residues that form the binding domains for all three classes of drugs. Emerging from these studies is the consensus view that domains III and IV of the α_1 subunit are crucial to modulation of L-type Ca^{2+} channels, and that it is likely that multiple residues on the α_1 subunit interact in an allosteric manner to cause voltage-dependent modulation of channel gating (30). The most provocative model for the actions of these drugs has been developed by Catterall and his colleagues who have proposed a domain interface model (Fig. 14–5) for the mode of action of dihydropyridine derivatives (60). Most importantly, in this model, allosteric interactions between bound drug and two domains of the α1 subunit cause conformational changes in the channel that modify channel gating and control the entry of divalent ions.

T-type calcium channels have voltage-dependent kinetics, ion permeability, and pharmacological properties that distinguish them from L-type calcium channels. They are resistant to block by dihydropyridines, inactivate in voltage-dependent manner, and most importantly, activate at voltages much more negative than L-type calcium channels (10). Because of the voltage dependence of T-type channels and the relatively small size of T-channel current in the ventricle (9), direct activation of contractile proteins and/or calcium-induced release of calcium from the SR (16, 19) through this channel has not been considered a likely pathway. Nevertheless, Zhou and January (176) have provided evidence that contractions can, in fact, be initiated by T-type channels in cardiac Purkinje cells and that these T-channel–induced contractions have unique kinetic and pharmacological profiles. T-type channel activity has also been suggested to contribute to pacemaker activity in nodal cells (67), and this activity may be particularly important in the Purjinke fibers of the ventricle. The cloning of the neuronal T-type channel has opened the possibility of determining the molecular basis for these differences (115), and evidence based on antisense oligonucleotide technology has suggested that in cardiac atrial muscle, T-type channels may belong to the E class of calcium channel genes (116).

SODIUM CHANNELS

Voltage-gated Sodium (Na^+) channels are also integral membrane proteins (24) that not only control the movement of Na^+ and underlie the spread of excitation

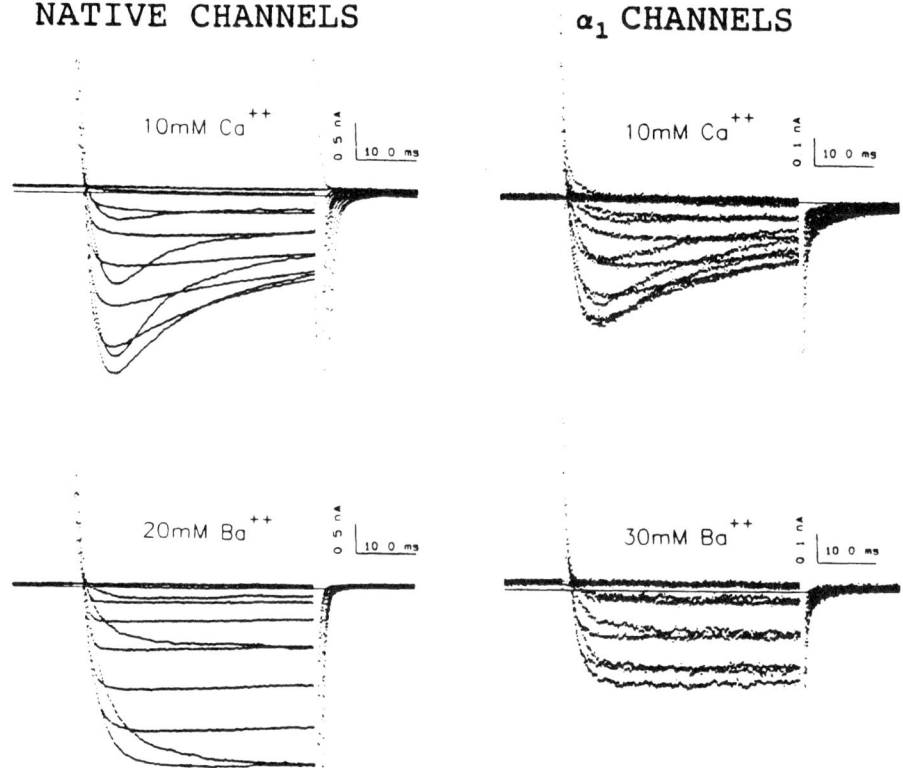

FIG. 14–4. Recombinant channels formed by α_1 subunits reconstitute voltage- and calcium-dependent properties of native channels. Recordings from mammalian cells transfected with cDNA encoding the α_1 subunit of smooth muscle L-type calcium channels (α_{1c-b}) (*right-hand panel*) compared with L-type channel activity measured in guinea pig ventricular myocytes (*left-hand panel*). The rows compare current when barium (*lower*) or calcium (*upper*) is the charge carrier. [From Welling et al., (167), with permission]

in ventricular and atrial muscle cells and in the Purkinje fiber network throughout the heart (75), but also can contribute so called "window" inward current that prolongs action potential duration (5). In most tissues the voltage-gated Na^+ channel is a heterotrimeric protein consisting of α (33 kDa), β_1 (36 kDa), and/or β_2 (33 kDa) subunits (23, 24, 31) but only the α subunit is needed for expression of recombinant channels, particularly for heart channels (108, 146, 147).

In heart, Na channel activity underlies the rapid spread of electrical impulses in specialized conducting tissue of the atria and ventricle (Purkinje fibers) as well as the working muscle of both atrial and ventricular tissue (74). Consequently, activity of cells can be indirectly read from the electrocardiogram: the QRS interval reflects conduction time through the ventricle and hence the number of available Na channels.

Prolongation of the QRS interval can occur when Na channel activity is reduced by drugs or cellular conditions. Although the role of Na^+ channel currents in impulse propagation is well-known, Na^+ channel activity can also contribute to duration of the ventricular action potential. The action potential is shortened in the presence of tetrodotoxin (TTX; a Na channel blocking toxin) or after sodium removal (34, 35, 58). This is so because there is a very small fraction of channels that fail to enter the absorbing inactivated state of the channel and thus create what has been referred to as a "window current" through TTX-sensitive Na. Most importantly, inherited mutations of the human Na channel can affect this property of the channel and promote a larger fraction of channels to reopen after inactivating. This produces enhanced inward current that prolongs the action potential in forms of the long QT syndrome linked to the gene that encodes the Na channel α subunit (74, 76; Fig. 14–6).

The selective pore of Na^+ channels is regulated by voltage-sensitive channel gates. According to Hodgkin and Huxley (61) at resting membrane potentials, Na^+ channels are in a resting state where the pore is closed by activation (*m*) gates. Membrane depolarization induces conformational changes (gating) that opens *m*-gates, resulting in conduction of Na^+ ions through the pore (permeation) and Na^+ current. Continued depo-

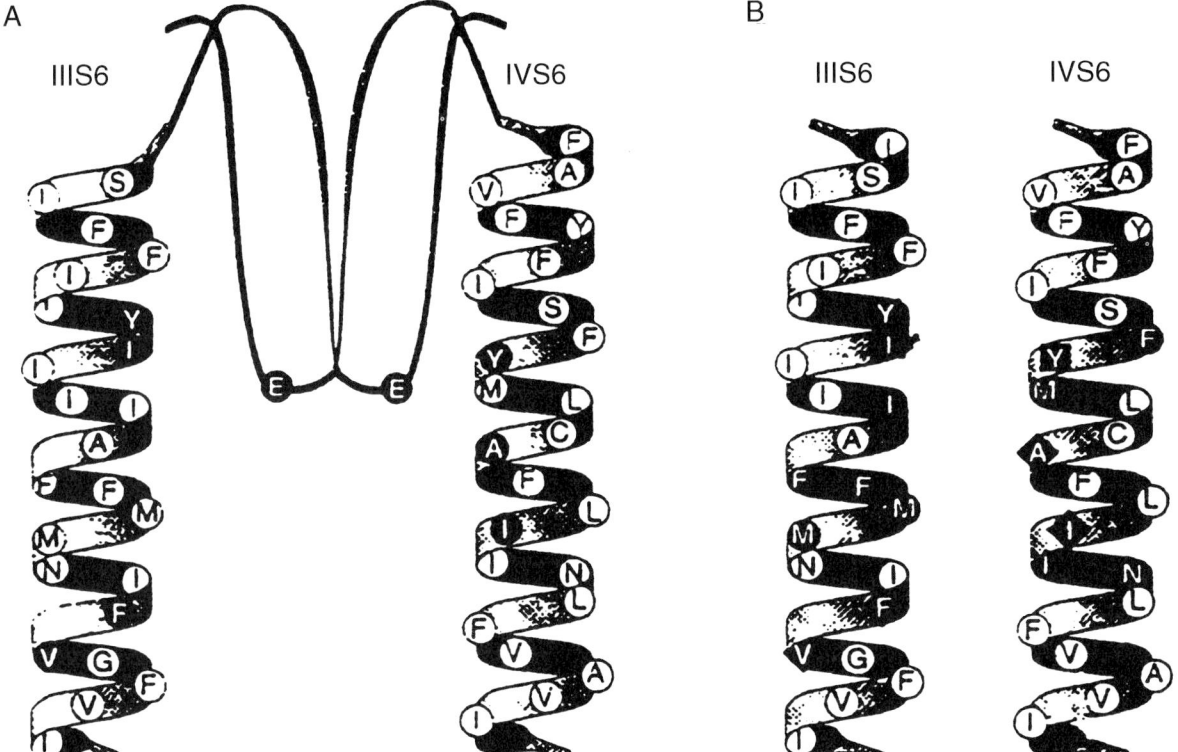

FIG. 14–5. Domain interface model of high-affinity phenylalkylamine block of L-type calcium channels. Location of pore region glutamates (A) and key amino acid residues in domains IIIS6 and IVS6 (*white symbols on black circles*) that, when mutated, disrupt block of channel activity by the charged phenylalkylamine (−)-D888. Proposed model to explain block of channels postulates that convergence of the pore region of domains III and IV with key residues of IIIS6 forms the binding site for this drug. [From Hockerman et al. (60a), with permission].

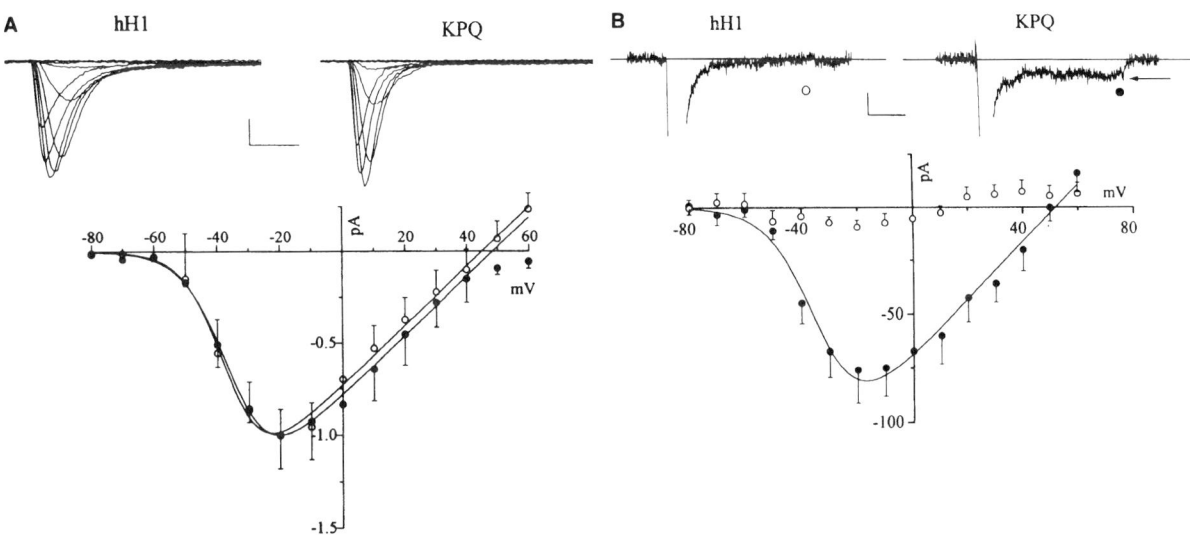

FIG. 14–6. An inherited deletion mutation (KPQ) of the human sodium channel α subunit (hH1) promotes maintained current in response to prolonged depolarization. Currents measured from cells transfected with wild-type (hH1) or mutant (KPQ) Na channel α subunits are shown for peak (*left*) and maintained (*right*) current. The KPQ mutation, which causes one form of the long QT syndrome, promotes additional maintained current (*right*), but does not affect peak currents. [From An et al. (3), with permission.]

larization triggers closure of an inactivation (*h*) gate, occlusion of the channel pore, and termination of the Na⁺ current. Membrane repolarization returns the channel to the resting state by shutting *m*-gates and opening the *h*-gate. Na⁺ channel gating is more complex than the fundamental workings detailed in this model (for a review see 14). However, the addition of a single state, slow inactivation, provides a satisfactory backdrop for considering binding and gating interactions relevant to LA action. Inactivation involves at least two kinetically distinct processes (fast and slow). Fast inactivation occurs after brief depolarizations, recovers at resting membrane potential rapidly (<20 msec), and is already represented in the model. Slow inactivation is triggered by long depolarizations and recovers slowly over seconds. A simple gating model that embodies these features is given in Scheme 1 with a resting closed state (R), an open conducting state (O), a fast inactivated state (I_F), and a slow inactivated state (I_S). Arrows represent gating transitions. Depolarization triggers transition from (R) to (O), and as depolarization continues, the channels rapidly transition to (I_F) and subsequently slow to (I_S). Upon membrane repolarization all states return to (R).

Local anesthetic drugs, like lidocaine and mexilitine block Na channels in a voltage-dependent manner. Investigation of the molecular basis for this action has provided valuable information about the structure and function of the Na channel with particular emphasis on channel gating. LA modulation of Na⁺ currents and underlying channel gating is commonly investigated using electrophysiological studies: both single channel and macroscopic current.

Our present understanding of LA action is founded on a number of seminal experimental observations that lead to hypotheses that account for tonic and phasic inhibition. Permanently charged, hydrophilic analogs of LAs (e.g. QX-314) are poorly membrane permeable, and only block Na⁺ currents when delivered intracellularly (145). In addition, QX-314 binding requires open channels, traverses 60% of the membrane electric field from the cytoplasmic channel mouth to reach its receptor, and does not prevent channel gating. However, extracellular QX-314 blocks cardiac channels, (la) probably by slow passage trough the pore and binding to an intrapore receptor (119a). Na⁺ currents recover rapidly from phasic inhibition induced by hydrophobic LAs compared with permanently charged analogs, suggesting that uncharged molecules leak out from closed channels. Reducing external pH slows recovery from phasic inhibition by tertiary amine LAs, suggesting that hydrogen ions can pass the Na⁺ channel selectivity filter and ionize the LA molecule (55). LAs enhance Na⁺ channel inactivation such that voltage-dependent recovery from inactivation is leftward shifted, hyperpolarization relieves inhibition, and recovery from inactivation is slow (134). These results led to the proposal of an intrapore LA receptor just inside of the Na⁺ channel selectivity filter involving hydrophobic and hydrophilic access routes (56).

Extending these concepts, Hille (56) proposed the Modulated Receptor Hypothesis. Here, a single LA receptor lies within the pore, between the selectivity filter and the channel gates. Receptor occupation leads to cessation of ion flow and promotion of inactivation. Uncharged molecules gain access through a hydrophobic transmembrane pathway. Charged molecules approach the receptor by an aqueous, hydrophilic pathway through the open cytoplasmic mouth (channel gates open) and the pore (see Fig. 14–1). Also, receptor affinity is modulated by channel state, where open and inactivated states bind drug avidly and resting states do not. Alternatively, Starmer et al. (144) proposed that state-dependent affinity of an intrapore receptor arises from a changeless receptor that is guarded by channel gates, a "guarded receptor." Here, receptor access is regulated by channel gates where open channels provide greater receptor access. Such state-dependent accessibility manifests as affinity modulation but with greater mechanistic parsimony.

With regard to long-lived blocked states underlying phasic inhibition, the Modulated Receptor Hypothesis holds that LA binding to the intrapore receptor promotes inactivation. Therefore, long-lived block arises from delayed recovery from inactivation because drug binding makes this state energetically favored. In contrast, for a guarded receptor, long-lasting block results when channel gates (*m* or *h*) close in open channels after the intrapore receptor is occupied by a LA molecule. This results in *channel gate trapping*, where the LA molecule cannot leave via its initial access (i.e. the pore and open cytoplasmic mouth). The channel then remains blocked until the LA molecule escapes slowly via the hydrophobic pathway, or the channel resumes the open conformation.

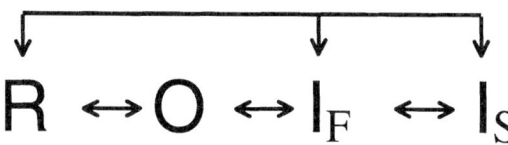

SCHEME 1. Simplified gating states for model Na channel. Transitions are allowed between rested (R), open (O), fast inactivated (IF) and slow inactivated (IS) states. Not indicated here are intermediate inactivated states of the channel as well as multiple open states. However, upper arrows indicate direct transitions between rested and inactivated states of the channel.

Primary Structure of the Voltage-Gated Na^+ Channel

The main functional component of the Na^+ channel is a 260 kDa α subunit that is associated with two smaller accessory β subunits (1 and 2) in rat brain, or a single β subunit in rat skeletal muscle and possibly in cardiac muscle (27). The sequence of the α subunit is highly conserved among nervous, cardiac, and skeletal tissues (36, 51), suggesting a common fundamental structure, in which the channel is arranged in the membrane as four homologous domains or repeats (I–IV). Each domain contains six α-helical transmembrane repeats S1–S6 (Scheme 2); see Fig. 14–1) (for a review, (see 26).

Each "extracellular" region between segment 5 and 6 of each of the four domains is called a "P-region" because each folds into the membrane to line the ion permeation "pore" that provides ion selectivity and a pathway across the membrane. This P-region contains the TTX binding site and the four amino acids (D or aspartic acid, E or glutamic acid, K or lysine, and A or alanine), one from each P-region, that create the canonical Na^+ selectivity filter. The stretch of intracellular amino acids between domains I and II (the "I–II linker") has been shown to contain virtually all of the consensus sequences for phosphorylation by PKA. The cardiac and neuronal α subunits both have long I–II linkers, while the α subunits from other tissues (e.g. skeletal muscle) have short I–II linkers.

Molecular Pharmacology of Na^+ Channels

Na^+ currents from neurons, cardiac and skeletal muscle display different electrophysiological and pharmacological properties, which is reproduced in channels expressed from genes encoding the corresponding tissue isoforms (51, 118, 126). The α subunit alone forms functional channels when expressed in *Xenopus* oocytes (25) with receptor sites for the diversity of pharmacological agents. For neuronal and skeletal muscle isoforms expressed in *Xenopus* oocytes, the $β_1$ subunit enhances expression, accelerates activation and inactivation, and alters the voltage dependence of inactivation (70). Thus, these isoforms require $β_1$-subunit coexpression in oocytes to replicate the function of native channels.

The general features of LA action, phasic and tonic inhibition, are shared by Na^+ currents of nervous tissue and skeletal muscle and cardiac muscle tissue. This indicates that fundamental structures mediating LA action are conserved and that observations made in any isoform will have general applicability. However, recent studies have revealed some isoform-specific differences in LA sensitivity (110), suggesting some degree of structural divergence.

Recent studies using expressed channels have begun to identify structural features involved in LA modulation of Na^+ channels (121). Ragsdale and colleagues (121) reported that mutations in the putative pore-lining S6 segment of domain IV modified block by LAs. Specifically, mutation of phenylalanine 1764 in rat brain IIA to alanine-induced insensitivity to block by etidocaine. LAs induced two kinetically distinct blocking modes, rapid and discrete, of single-channel in Na^+ channels lacking fast inactivation, consistent with binding to an intrapore receptor that results in open channel blockade. Furthermore, the homologous mutation in rat skeletal muscle isoform causes similar alteration of lidocaine block while selectively eliminating discrete blockade induced by QX-314. The results suggest that

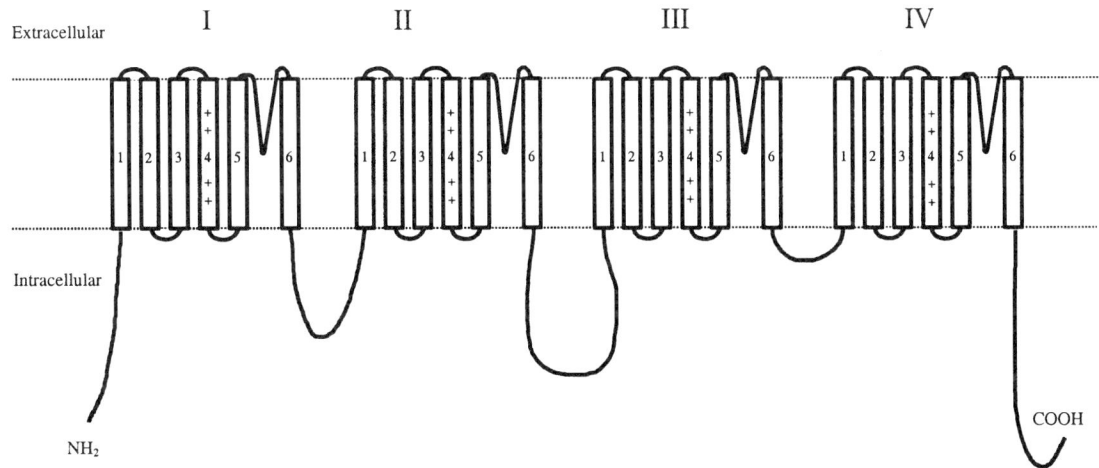

SCHEME 2. Schematic of sequence of voltage-gated Na channel alpha subunit. Note four homologous domains, each of which contains six helical transmembrane fragments. C- and N-termini are intracellular.

LA block involves binding to an intrapore receptor contributed to by phenyalanine 1764 and an essential binding configuration reported by discrete blockade. However, this region is also involved in fast inactivation such that interactions between drug binding and inactivation, thought to be involved in LA action, could also be affected. Makielski et al. (91) have shown that β_1 coexpression reduces the sensitivity of the cardiac α subunit to tonic and phasic inhibition by lidocaine. However, it must be pointed out that evidence for a direct modulatory role of the β_1 subunit in heart remains controversial.

Molecular Pharmacology of an Inherited Disease

The molecular basis of one form of the inherited cardiac rhythm disorder, the long QT syndrome (LQTS-3), has been shown to be caused by mutations in the gene encoding the α subunit of the human heart Na channel (163, 164; see also Chapter 19). These mutations cause abnormal channel inactivation such that a small fraction of channels no longer enters an absorbing inactivated state, but reopen after inactivating (13). As a result of the mutations, Na channel activity is maintained during the plateau phase of the ventricular action potential, providing an enhanced presence of window current. Hence the mutations promote delayed repolarization of the ventricle and account for the clinical phenotype: prolonged QT interval of the electrocardiogram (EKG).

The discovery of gene defects that changed the inactivation properties of human cardiac Na channels raised the possibility of applying a therapeutic strategy based on the particular gene defect. An and co-workers (3) using a mammalian expression system, found that for one LQT-3 mutant channel, the so-called KPQ deletion mutant channel maintained current during the cardiac action potential plateau phase was roughly twice as sensitive to lidocaine block as current generating the cardiac action potential upstroke (Fig. 14–7). Others found similar results (119, 161), and initial results in clinical trials have shown that the predictions based on recombinant channel pharmacology were being substantiated in carriers of this gene defect (Dr. A. Moss, personal communication). This work represented the first successful identification of an ion chan-

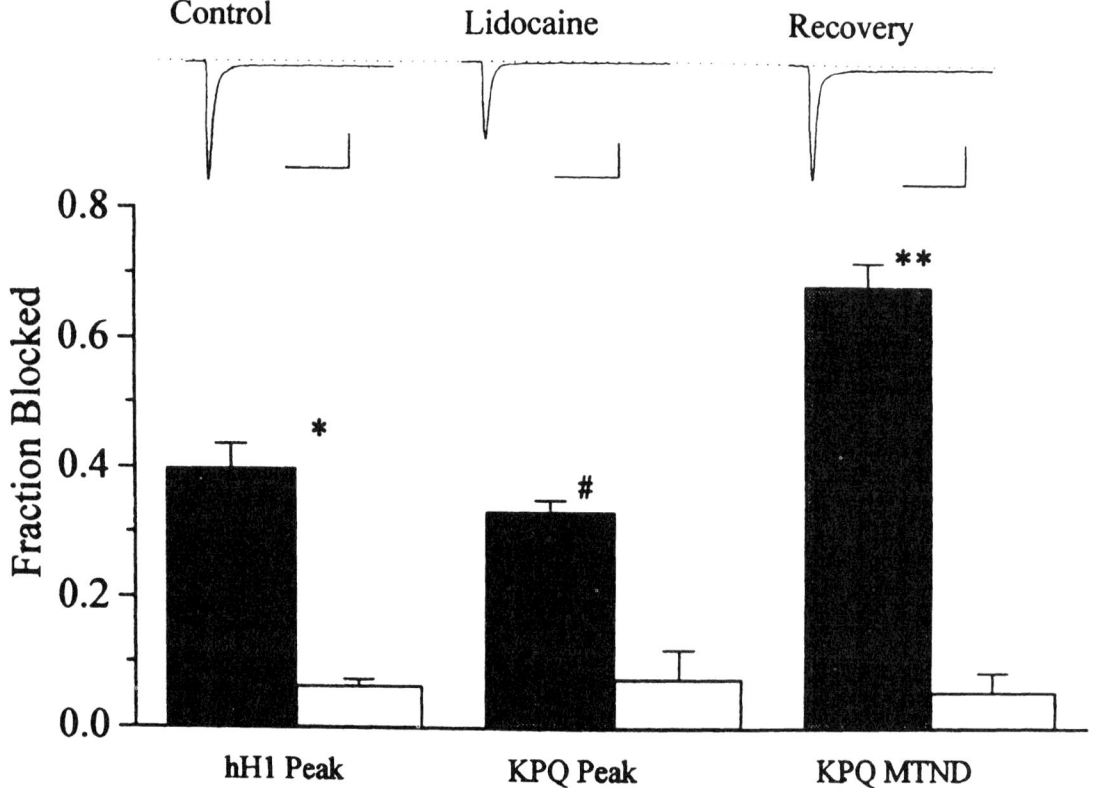

FIG. 14–7. The local anesthetic drug lidocaine blocks maintained current through mutant LQT-3 (KPQ) Na channels more potently than peak currents of either hH1 (wild-type) or KPQ channels. Plotted is the fraction of current blocked for each channel construct in response to 100 μM lidocaine. These results strongly suggested that this type of drug might be useful in specifically treating the inherited arrhythmia LQT-3 caused by this gene mutation. [From An et al. (3), with permission.]

nel property that is changed because of an inherited mutation and that, at the same time, could be targeted specifically by a pharmacological agent. Clearly more work needs to be done both in the discovery of other gene defects and in finding new and gene-specific drugs to correct the function consequences of the inherited mutations.

POTASSIUM CHANNELS

Potassium (K^+) channels regulate potassium ion movement across the cell membrane and are important in maintaining the electrical activity in most excitable cells because they control cellular resting potential and action potential duration.

Action potentials recorded from cardiac cells are characterized by their long duration and slow repolarization, quite unlike action potentials found in other electrically excitable cells such as nerve and skeletal muscle cells. This prolonged depolarization is important in regulating the strength and duration of the contraction of the heart. Outward current through potassium channels play important roles in influencing the morphology of the action potential in the heart: inward rectifier potassium current is important in controlling the resting membrane potential, and current through voltage-dependent potassium channels plays a major role in controlling the duration of the action potential in cardiac cells. Many potassium channels are the targets of neurotransmitters and hormones that influence heart rate and contractility through their action on many ion channels, including potassium channels.

Insights into potassium channel structure and function were made possible by the cloning of the *Shaker* gene from *Drosophila* (72), which codes for a variety of voltage-gated potassium channels. Typically, the α subunit of a potassium channel is homologous to a one of the four domains of Na or Ca channels, consistent with the association of four such subunits to form tetramers (88). From the amino acid sequence, hydrophobicity analysis has indicated that the α subunit consists of six putative transmembrane-spanning regions (S1–S6) with both N and C termini located intracellularly. Functions have been assigned to different parts of the α subunit based on pharmacological and mutagenesis experiments. In *Shaker* channels, the binding of charybdotoxin (CTX), a pore-blocking toxin was influenced by site-directed mutagensis in the linker region between S5 and S6, consistent with the hypothesis that this portion of the channel contributes to the pore region. Further evidence that this region forms part of the channel pore was provided by the localization of CTX binding, the external and internal block by tetraetaylammonium (TEA), single-channel conductance properties and channel selectivity to this region of the channel (89, 90, 96). Further experiments have suggested that the linker region between S5 and S6 (the H5- or P-region) forms part of the channel pore by folding back into the membrane as two antiparallel β sheets, and it seems likely that other parts of the channel protein are also involved in the formation of the pore. The S4 transmembrane region, which contains positively charged amino acids at every third position, was shown to function as the voltage sensor for Na channels; in potassium channels, mutagenesis experiments have shown this region to have the same function (68).

Inwardly rectifying potassium channels are also thought to be formed from tetramers, but the α subunit of these channels is likely to consists of only two membrane-spanning domains homologous to the S5 and S6 regions of the α-subunits of voltage-dependent channels (59, 82). Although these channels have no voltage-sensing S4 region, there is a region, denoted M0 by Ho et al., (59) with some homology to S4 and containing repeated charged residues.

There is an ever-increasing diversity of potassium channels, not only in the number of different channels that have been cloned, but through alternate splicing of genes (4), the heterotetramerization of α-subunits from the same and different subfamilies (117), and the modification of channel activity by association with additional non-pore-forming subunits. Many such accessory subunits, known as β subunits, have been cloned (41, 42, 54) and are believed to associate with the α subunit of potassium channels and modify their properties. For example, a β subunit cloned from human atria, Kvβ3, accelerated the inactivation of Kv1.4 channels when co-expressed in *Xenopus* oocytes. Recently, additional accessory proteins have been cloned: Kv5.1, Kv6.1, Kv8.1, and jShalγ1. Although these proteins are homologous to the pore-forming α subunit, they cannot generate electrical activity by themselves. Instead, they regulate the function of Kv2.1, Kv2.2 channels and channels from the Kv4 family.

Voltage-Dependent K^+ Channels

There are at least twenty different functional voltage-gated potassium channels cloned to date, divided into six subfamilies designated Kv1 (*Shaker*), Kv2 (Shab), Kv3 (Shaw), Kv4 (Shal), KvLQT1, and EAG. The paragraphs that follow outline the characteristics of the voltage-dependent potassium currents found in the heart and, where known, their molecular basis.

Transient Outward K Current, Ito. Ito was first identified in sheep Purkinje fibers, (47) and later in single cells (71). Subsequent work has shown that Ito can be separated into two components: one voltage-dependent and insensitive to calcium and one activated by calcium (81). These two currents can also be separated by their sensitivity to 4-AP: Ito1, the voltage-dependent current, is blocked by 4-AP, whereas Ito2, the ca-dependent current is insensitive to 4-AP. It is now generally accepted that Ito2 is carried predominantly by Cl−ions (178–181), and therefore only Ito1 will be described further here.

Ito1 is found in both atrial and ventricular cells and in a wide range of species including human, dog, cat, rat, ferret, rabbit, and mouse. It is characterized by a rapid activation and inactivation and is thought to cause a phase of early repolarization of the action potential, usually manifested as a "notch" during repolarization in cells expressing a prominent Ito such as Purkinje fibres. Regional differences in the density of Ito across the wall of the heart have been observed, with a much larger current density in epicardial and midmyocardial cells than in endocardial cells (43). Ito is illustrated in Figure 14–8.

Diverse transcripts for multiple types of K+ channel clones have been reported in heart, confounding the problem of unique identification of the molecular basis of cardiac K+ channel activity (15). An RNAse protection essay has revealed the presence of Kv 1.2, 1.4, 1.5 (*Shaker* family), 2.1 (Shab), and 4.2 (Shal) in the adult rat atria and ventricle(39). The molecular basis of the cardiac Ito1 is not entirely clear, but the most likely candidate genes are from the Kv4 family of voltage-dependent K channels. In the rat heart, Ito arises from a combination of Kv4.2 and Kv 4.3, which are expressed at different levels across the ventricular wall. For example the level of expression of Kv 4.2 varies across the ventricular wall in rat heart, as does the density of the current Ito. In contrast, expression levels of Kv 4.3 are uniform across the ventricular wall (39). In canine and human heart, Ito is thought to arise from Kv4.3 alone, and the pharmacology of this cloned channel is similar to the native Ito(40).

The fast inactivation of channels like Ito is thought to occur through "N-type" inactivation, a mechanism that involves the blocking of the pore from the inside by a cytoplasmic "ball" after the channel has opened. In some Kv channels, the amino terminus of the channel protein may form the blocking 'ball' (64, 100, 174).

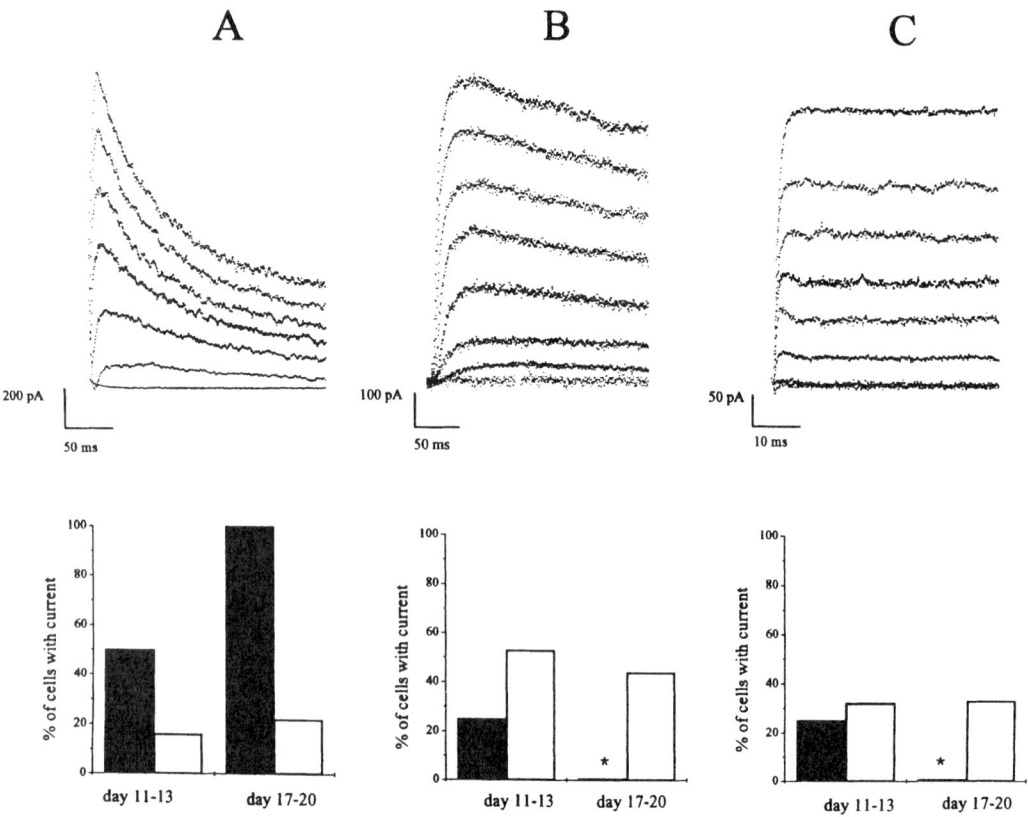

FIG. 14–8. Multiple potassium channels in the developing mouse heart. Patch-clamp recordings of murine embryonic ventricular cells reveals rapidly activating K channel current that inactivates rapidly (*A*), slowly (*B*), or not at all (*C*). These components in the mouse heart reflect Ito (left and center) and Iur (right). [From Davies et al. (37a), with permission.]

Cardiac Ito is blocked by 5 mM 4-AP and is insensitive to 5 mM TEA. The Kv4 family can be distinguished pharmacologically from Kv1.4 by its sensitivity to flecainide and heteropoda toxin peptides (131, 172).

Delayed Rectifier K currents, I_K. The delayed rectifier potassium current is a voltage- and time-dependent K current originally described in sheep cardiac Purkinje fibres (107). Two components of I_K have been separated on the basis of the activation kinetics: a rapidly activating current called I_{Kr} and a slowly activating component called I_{Ks} (132; see Fig. 14–9). I_{Kr} can also be separated pharmacologically by its sensitivity to block by class III antiarryhthmic drugs such as E4031 and dofetilide (20). The genes coding for these two channels have recently been cloned. I_{Kr} is thought to be formed by the ether-a-go-go (EAG) channel (130), originally cloned by screening a hippocampal library (166) and later cloned from the human heart and named HERG (Human Ether-a-go-go Related Gene; 37). I_{Ks} is thought to arise from the co-assembly of two proteins (8, 129): the min K protein, first cloned from the kidney (150), which is a small protein of about 130 amino acids with one putative transmembrane-spanning region, and KvLQT1, a recently cloned K$^+$ channel with the typical six transmembrane-spanning regions (162). The latter derives its name, KvLQT1, from its suspected role in the cardiac disorder long QT (LQT) syndrome.

I_{Kr} activates over a more negative range of voltages than I_{Ks} (V-half for I_{Kr} activation in guinea-pig is −21.5 mV and I_{Ks} is +15.7 mV and shows rectification at more positive potentials characterized by a negative slope conductance at voltages positive to 0 or +10 mV

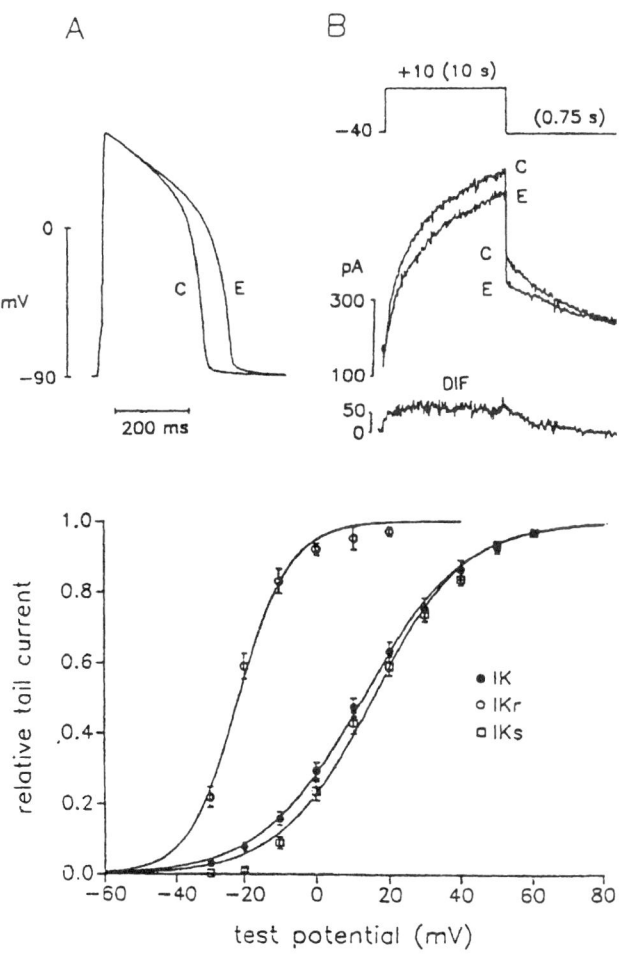

FIG. 14–9. Two components of delayed rectifier potassium current are revealed by differential sensitivity to block by class III antiarrhythmic agents, Action potentials and membrane currents recorded in the absence (*Curve C*) and presence (*Curve E*) of 5 μM E-4031. Difference currents (DIF) reveal the properties of the current blocked by the drug, which is called I_{Kr}. *Lower panel* shows the voltage-dependence of activation of total delayed rectifier current (IK) as well as the two components: I_{Kr} (*open circles*) and I_{Ks} (*open squares*). [From Sanguinetti and Jurkiewicz (132), with permission.]

(132). More recent studies have shown that this apparent inward rectification is caused by rapid C-type inactivation and could be abolished by mutation of one amino acid residue (S631A) in the outer mouth of the pore of HERG. Unlike C-type inactivation in other channels, HERG appears to be unique in possessing voltage-dependent inactivation (134, 142).

Cardiac I_{Ks} is regulated by the sympathetic nervous system. Stimulation of β-adrenoceptors enhances I_{Ks} through activation of cAMP-dependent protein kinase and probable phosphorylation of the channel protein (PKA). Regulation of I_{Ks} also occurs in the absence of β-adrenergic stimulation. Elevation of $[Ca^{2+}]_i$ above 10 nM enhanced I_{Ks} without altering the current voltage-dependency (80, 160). Noise analysis indicated that that elevated intracellular calcium increased the open probablility of the channels without changing the unit amplitude, estimated to be 0.21 pA at pCa 10 and 0.19 pA at pCa 7 (152). I_{Ks} is also regulated indirectly by calcium through activation of the calcium-dependent protein kinase (PKC) (153). Exposure of cardiac myocytes to phorbol esters such as 12-O-tetradecanoylphorbol-13-acetate enhanced I_K recorded from guinea-pig ventricular myocytes. PKC activation may be the mechanism through which α-adrenergic agonists like phenylephrine enhance I_K (159).

K channels and LQT. Mutations in both HERG and KvLQT1 genes are thought to give rise to some instances of LQT, an inherited cardiac disorder that causes syncope, seizures, and sudden death in otherwise healthy individuals (102). (See also chapter 19) Inherited forms of LQT can result from mutations in at least four different genes, which have been mapped to chromosomes 11p15.5 (LQT1), 7q35–36 (LQT2), 3p21–24 (LQT3) and 4q25–27 (LQT4)(76). Two of these genes code for potassium channels that are found in the heart; LQT1 is thought to underlie cardiac I_{Ks} (KvLQT1), and LQT2 is thought to underlie I_{Kr} (HERG). To date twelve mutations in KvLQT1 (138) and nine in HERG (128) have been identified, and it is likely that they cause some dysfunction of the potassium channels leading to abnormal repolarization in the heart. Most recently, mutations in minK have also been shown to be linked to LQT-2 (143).

Ultra-Rapid K Channel, IKur. First described in human atrial myocytes, the ultra-rapid K channel current is a depolarization-induced sustained potassium current that remains after Ito1 inactivation and can be distinguished from Ito1 on the basis of its voltage-dependent inactivation and by its much higher sensitivity to block by 4 Amino Pyridine (AP) (165; see Fig. 14–8). Block of this current by a low concentration of 4-AP (typically 50 μM) prolongs the cardiac action potential, demonstrating its role in the process of cardiac repolarization.

Expression of Kv1.5 results in a potassium current with many of the biophysical and electrophysiological properties of IKur in the heart (44). Thus seems likely that IKur results from current through the channel Kv1.5 (165), which has been cloned from rat and human heart (125, 151).

Inward Rectifier K Channels

Inwardly rectifying K channels represent a genetically diverse group of proteins that conduct K^+ more efficiently in the inward direction than in the outward direction. Three kinds of inwardly rectifying potassium current have been described in heart: the cardiac inward rectifier (IK1), the acetylcholine-sensitive current (IKACh), and the ATP-sensitive potassium current (IKATP). These channels play important roles in controlling membrane potentials, influencing repolarization, and maintaining vagal control of heart rate.

Cardiac Inward Rectifier, IK1. The cardiac inward rectifier potassium current is very important in maintaining the resting membrane potential and influencing phase 3 of repolarization of the cardiac action potential. It has been detected in atrial and ventricular myocytes and in Purkinje fibers but is not usually found in nodal tissue. IK1 is activated by hyperpolarization of the membrane and is characterized by inward rectification that, in general, allows very little current to pass through the channel at potentials positive to about −40 mV. Their high conductance at negative potentials allows cells to maintain a stable resting membrane potential (Fig. 14–10). The rectification of IK1 channels can result from block of the channels by intracellular Mg^{2+} (120, 157) and by polyamines (45, 85, 105).

At least six sub-families of inward rectifier K channels (Kir1–6) have been cloned to date from various tissues, and it is thought that channels from the Kir2 subfamily (Kir 2.1, 2.2 and 2.3) underlie the native cardiac IK1 channel (69, 168).

Ach-Activated K Channel, IKACh. IKACh channels are found in atrial and nodal cells and open in response to stimulation of m2 muscarinic receptors in the heart. Release of acetylcholine from vagal nerves in the heart activates IKACh channels, leading to a hyperpolarization of the membrane and a slowing of heart rate. These types of inwardly rectifying K^+ channels are believed to be directly coupled to the muscarinic receptors by a pertussis toxin–sensitive G protein (84).

Native IKACh channels are believed to be formed from heteromultimers of two potassium channel α subunits, a G protein–coupled inwardly rectifying K^+

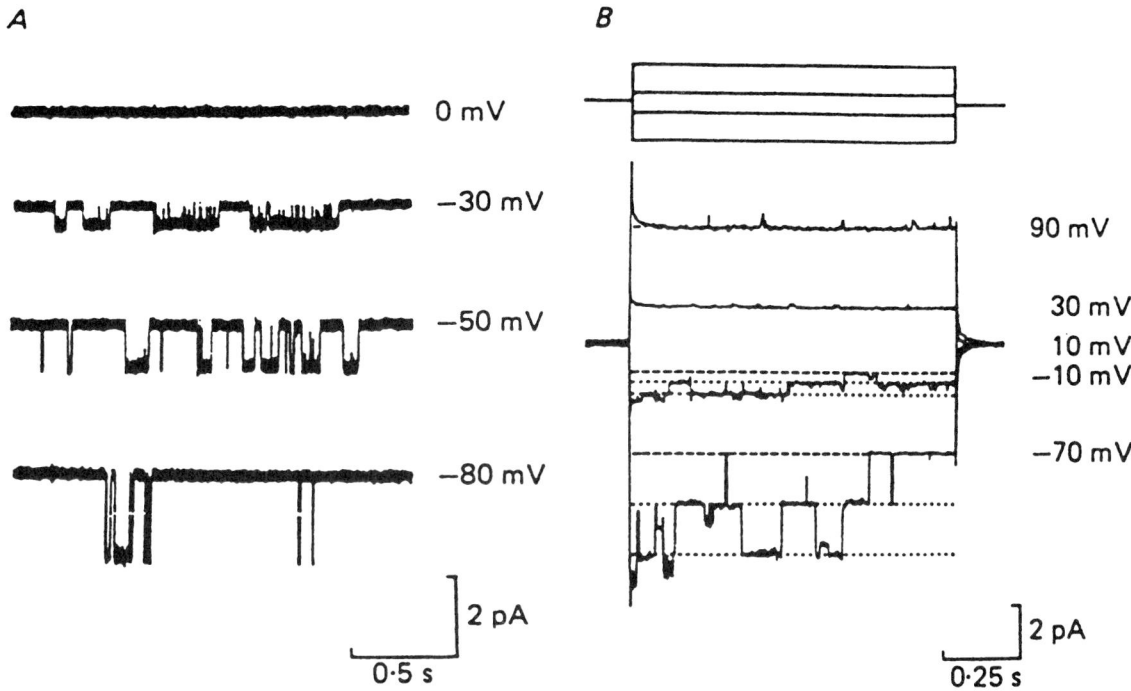

FIG. 14–10. Single-channel recordings from inward rectifier channels indicate that rectification (the tendency to pass more current in one direction than another) occurs at the single-channel level. [From Sakmann and Trube (127a), with permission.]

channel, GIRK (Kir 3.1) and a second cardiac inwardly rectifying K⁺ channel named CIR (Kir3.4)

ATP-Sensitive K Channels, IKATP. KATP channels were originally discovered in cardiac muscle and are characterized by an inhibition of channel opening when the ATP concentration at the cytoplasmic cell surface is increased (109; Fig. 14–11). These channels play an important role in a variety of cellular responses by linking the metabolic status of the cell to its membrane potential. They have been found in various other tissues, including pancreatic β cells, skeletal muscle, brain, and smooth muscle (38).

In the heart, KATP channels have been implicated in the shortening of the action potential duration and the cellular loss of K⁺ that occurs during various forms metabolic stress, including ischemia, hypoxia, and inhibition of glycolysis or oxidative phosphorylation (46).

It has been shown that the KATP channel in the heart is a heteromer, formed from a complex of at least two subunits: the K⁺ channel subunit Kir6.2, a member of the inward rectifier family (66), and the sulfonylurea receptor (SUR2A), a member of the ATP-binding cassette family (65). Co-expression of the cloned SUR2A and Kir6.2 produces a channel with the primary characteristics of the cardiac KATP channel (65).

The subunit of the KATP complex that confers ATP sensitivity is not clear. Kir6.2 associates with both SUR1 (cloned from pancreatic β cells (33) and SUR2A (cardiac cells; see ref. 33) to form IKATP channels with contrasting properties. The channel formed with SUR2A has a lower sensitivity to ATP and the sulphonylurea glibenclamide, and, unlike the channel formed with SUR1, is not activated by diazoxide. Therefore, it has been suggested that it is the SUR subunit that confers these properties on the IKATP channel (16). However, recent work showing that when Kir6.2 was expressed without SUR (as a truncated form) the channel demonstrated ATP sensitivity, consistent with the hypothesis that it is the Kir channel itself that is sensitive to the ATP concentration (156). Further support for this comes from the finding that co-expression of Kir6.1 with SUR2B, the smooth muscle isoform of SUR, fails to confer ATP sensitivity on this channel (170).

SUMMARY

This chapter gives a brief overview of the molecular and cellular properties of major Ca, K, and Na channel currents that are important in generating the electrical properties of the heart. This is an ever changing topic that, with the groundbreaking studies revealing linkage between mutations in cardiac ion channel genes and the inherited heart disease, LQT, is becoming increasingly important for clinical as well as basic scientists

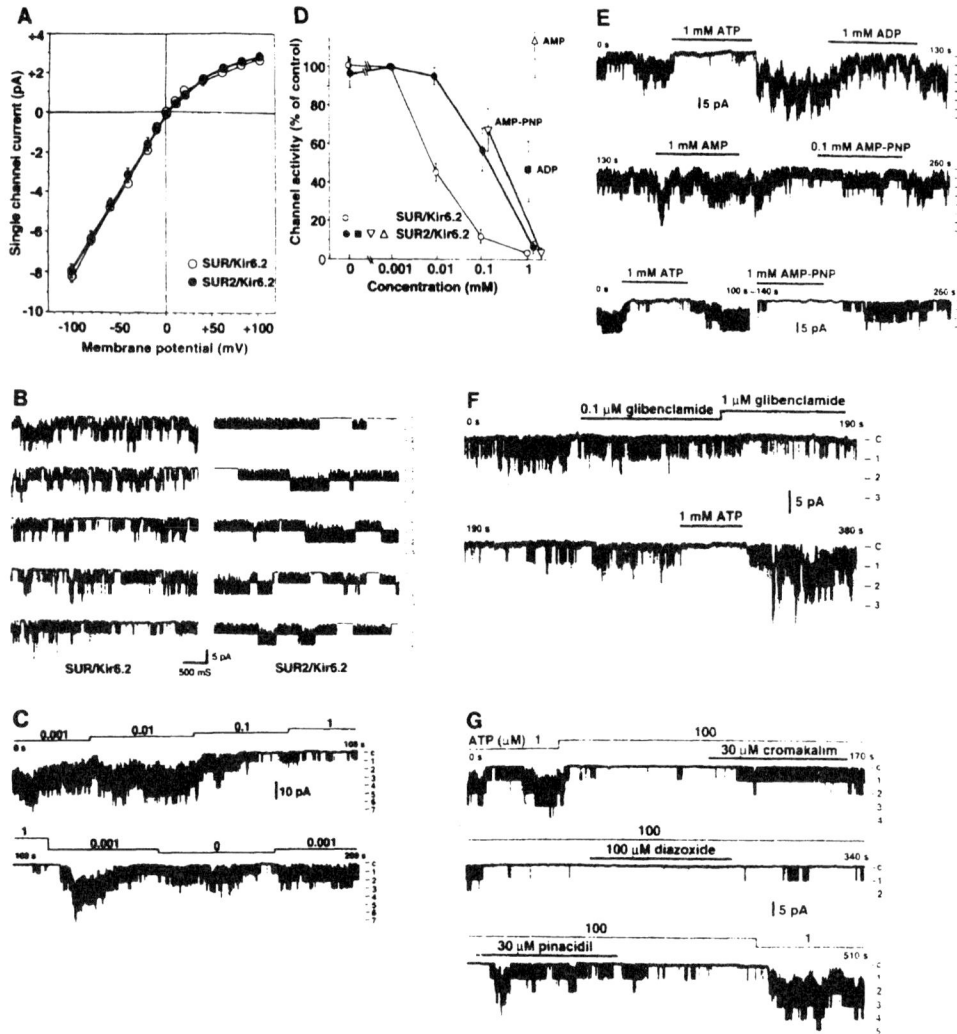

FIG. 14-11. Reconstitution of IKATP. Co-expression of inward rectifier subunit (Kir6.2) with, a the sulfonylurea receptor (SUR2A) encodes channel activity that demonstrates conductance, permeation, and ATP-sensitivity of native IKATP channels (from Inagaki et al (65), with permission.]

to understand. This chapter should provide a useful series of references relating both structural and pharmacological properties of these membrane ion channel proteins that will enable readers to pursue more specific and detailed descriptions for individual cases.

REFERENCES

1a. Alpert, L. A., H. A. Fozzard, D. A. Hanck, and J. C. Makielski. Is there a second external lidocaine binding site on mammalian cardiac cells? *Am. J. Physiol.* 257 (Heart Circ. Physiol.): H79–H84, 1989.
1. Ahlijanian, M. K., R. E. Westenbroek, and W. A. Catterall. Subunit structure and localization of dihydropyridine-sensitive calcium channels in mammalian brain, spinal cord, and retina. *Neuron* 4:819–832, 1990.
2. An, R.-H., B. Heath, W. J. Koch, R. J. Lefkowitz, and R. S. Kass. Targeting of cAMP-dependent increases In L-type Ca (I_{Ca}) over delayed K channel (I_{Ks}) activity by overexpression of the beta$_2$-adrenergic receptor in the developing mouse heart. *Biophys. J.* 74:A35(Abstract), 1998.
3. An, R. H., R. Bangalore, S. Z. Rosero, and R. S. Kass. Lidocaine block of LQT-3 mutant human Na channels. *Circ. Res.* 79, 103–108, 1996.
4. Attali, B., F. Lesage, P. Ziliani, E. Guillemare, E. Honore, R. Waldmann, M. G. Mattei, M. Lazdunski, and J. Barhanin. Multiple mRNA isoforms encoding the mouse cardiac Kv1–5 delayed rectifier K$^+$ channel. *J. Biol. Chem.* 268, 24283–24289, 1993.
5. Attwell, D., I. Cohen, D. Eisner, M. Ohba, and C. Ojeda. The steady state TTX-sensitive ("window") sodium current in cardiac Purkinje fibres. *Pflugers Arch.* 379, 137–142, 1979.
6. Balke, C. W., W. C. Rose, B. O'Rourke, R. Mejia-Alvarez, P. Backx, and E. Marban. Biophysics and physiology of cardiac calcium channels. *Circulation* 87 (Suppl. 7):VII49–VII53, 1993.
7. Bangalore, R., G. Mehrke, K. Gingrich, F. Hofmann, and R. S. Kass. Influence of the L-type Ca-channel $_2/\Delta$ subunit on ionic and gating current in transiently-transfected HEK 293 cells.

Am. J. Physiol. 270 (*Heart Circ. Physiol.* 39), H1521–H1528. 1996.
8. Barhanin, J., F. Lesage, E. Guillemare, M. Fink, M. Lazdunski, and G. Romey. K(V)LQT1 and ISK (MINK) proteins associate to form the i-ks cardiac potassium current. *Nature* 384:78–80, 1996.
9. Bean, B. P. (1985). Two kinds of calcium channels in canine atrial cells. Differences in kinetics, selectivity, and pharmacology. *Journal of General Physiology* 86, 1–30.
10. Bean, B. P. Classes of calcium channels in vertebrate cells. *Annu. Rev. Physiol.* 51:367–384, 1989.
11. Beeler, G. W., Jr. and H. Reuter. Membrane calcium current in ventricular myocardial fibres. *J. Physiol. (Lond.)* 207:191–209, 1970.
12. Beeler, G. W., Jr. and H. Reuter. The relation between membrane potential, membrane currents and activation of contraction in ventricular myocardial fibres. *J. Physiol. (Lond.)* 207:211–229, 1970.
13. Bennett, P. B., K. Yazawa, N. Makita, and A. L. George. Molecular mechanism for an inherited cardiac arrhythmia. *Nature* 376:683–685, 1995.
14. Birnbaumer, L., K. P. Campbell, W. A. Catterall, M. M. Harpold, F. Hofmann, W. A. Horne, Y. Mori, A. Schwartz, T. P. Snutch, T. Tanabe, et al. The naming of voltage-gated calcium channels. *Neuron* 13:505–506, 1994.
15. Brahmajothi, M. V., M. J. Morales, S. Liu, R. L. Rasmusson, D. L. Campbell, and H. C. Strauss. In situ hybridization reveals extensive diversity of K^+ channel mRNA in isolated ferret cardiac myocytes. *Circ. Res.* 78:1083–1089, 1996.
16. Bryan, J. and L. Aguilar-Bryan. The ABCs of ATP-sensitive potassium channels: more pieces of the puzzle. *Curr. Opin. Cell Biol.* 9:553–559, 1997.
17. Cachelin, A. B., J. E. De Peyer, S. Kokubun, and H. Reuter. Ca channel modulation by 8-bromocyclic AMP in cultured heart cells. *Nature* 304:462–464, 1983.
18. Cannell, M. B., H. Cheng, and W. J. Lederer. Spatial non-uniformities in $[Ca^{2+}]_i$ during excitation-contraction coupling in cardiac myocytes. *Biophys. J.* 67:1942–1956, 1994.
19. Cannell, M. B., H. Cheng, and W. J. Lederer. The control of calcium release in heart muscle. *Science* 268:1045–1049, 1995.
20. Carmeliet, E. Voltage- and time-dependent block of the delayed K^+ current in cardiac myocytes by dofetilide. *J. Pharmacol. Exp. Ther.* 262:809–817. 1992.
21. Carmeliet, E., P. Busselen, F. Verdonck, and J. Vereecke. Ca ions and excitation-contraction coupling in heart muscle. *Verh. K. Acad. Geneeskd. Belg.* 35:181–222, 1973.
22. Carmeliet, E. and P. P. van Bogaert. Strontium action potentials in cardiac Purkinje fibers. Reunion de Liège, Societé Belge de Physiologie et de Pharmacologie, 1969:134–135.
23. Catterall, W. and P. N. Epstein. Ion channels. [Review]. *Diabetologia* 35 (Suppl 2):S23–33, 1992.
24. Catterall, W. A. Structure and function of voltage-gated ion channels. [Review]. *Trends Neurosci.* 16:500–506, 1993.
25. Catterall, W. A. Molecular properties of a superfamily of plasma-membrane cation channels. [Review]. *Curr. Opin. Cell Biol.* 6:607–615, 1994.
26. Catterall, W. A. Ion channels in plasma membrane signal transduction. *J. Bioenerg. Biomembr.* 28:217–218, 1996.
27. Catterall, W. A. Molecular properties of sodium and calcium channels. *J. Bioenerg. Biomembr.* 28:219–230, 1996.
28. Catterall, W. A., T. Scheuer, W. Thomsen, and S. Rossie. Structure and modulation of voltage-gated ion channels. *Ann. N.Y. Acad. Sci.* 625:174–180, 1991.
29. Catterall, W. A., M. J. Seagar, and M. Takahashi. Molecular properties of dihydropyridine-sensitive calcium channels in skeletal muscle. *J. Biol. Chem.* 263:3535–3538, 1988.

30. Catterall, W. A. and J. Striessnig. Receptor sites for Ca channel antagonists. *TIPS* 13:256–262, 1992.
31. Catterall, W. A., V. Trainer, and D. G. Baden. Molecular properties of the sodium channel: a receptor for multiple neurotoxins. *Bull. Soc. Pathol. Exot.* 85:481–485, 1992.
32. Chu, A., M. Fill, M. L. Entman, and E. Stefani. Different Ca^{2+} sensitivity of the ryanodine-sensitive Ca^{2+} release channels of cardiac and skeletal muscle sarcoplasmic reticulum. *Biophys. J.* 59:102a–102a, 1991.
33. Chutkow, W. A., M. C. Simon, M. M. Le Beau, and C. F. Burant. Cloning, tissue expression and chromosomal localization of SUR2, the putative drug-binding subunit of cardiac, skeletal muscle, and vascular KATP channels. *Diabetes* 45:1439–1445, 1996.
34. Colatsky, T. J. Mechanisms of action of lidocaine and quinidine on action potential duration in rabbit Purkinje fibers. An effect on steady state sodium currents? *Circ. Res.* 50:17–27, 1982.
35. Coraboeuf, E., E. Deroubaix, and A. Coulombe. Effect of tetrodotoxin on action potentials of the conducting system in the dog heart. *Am. J. Physiol.* 236: (*Heart Circ. Physiol.* 5): H561–H567, 1979.
36. Cribbs, L. L., J. Satin, H. A. Fozzard, and R. B. Rogart, Functional expression of the rat heart I Na^+ channel isoform. Demonstration of properties characteristic of native cardiac Na^+ channels. *FEBS Lett.* 275:195–200, 1990.
37. Curran, M. E., I., Splawski, K. W., Timothy, G. M., Vincent, E. D. Green, and M. T. Keating. A molecular basis for cardiac arrhythmia: *HERG* mutations cause long QT syndrome. *Cell* 80: 795–803, 1995.
37a. Davies, M. P., R. H. An, P. Doevendans, S. Kubalak, K. R. Chien, R. S. Kass. Developmental Changes in Ionic Channel Activity in the Embryonic Murine Heart. American Heart Assoc., Inc. 1996.
38. Davis, N. W., N. B. Standen, and P. R. Stanfield. ATP-dependent potassium channels of muscle cells: their properties, regulation, and possible functions. *J. Bioenerg. Biomembr.* 23:509–535, 1991.
39. Dixon, J. E. and D. McKinnon. Quantitative analysis of potassium channel mRNA expression in atrial and ventricular muscle of rats. *Circulation Research* 75:252–260, 1994.
40. Dixon, J. E., W. Shi, H. S. Wang, C. McDonald, H. Yu, R. S. Wymore, I. S. Cohen, and D. McKinnon. Role of the Kv4.3 K^+ channel in ventricular muscle. A molecular correlate for the transient outward current. [Published erratum appears in *Circ. Res.* 1997 Jan, 80(1):147]. *Circ. Res.* 79:659–668, 1996.
41. England, S. K., V. N. Uebele, J. Kodali, P. B. Bennett, and M. M. Tamkun. A novel K^+ channel α-subunit (hKv 1.3) is produced via alternative mRNA splicing. *J. Biol. Chem.* 270:000–000, 1995.
42. England, S. K., V. N. Uebele, H. Shear, J. Kodali, P. B. Bennett, and M. M. Tamkun. Characterization of a voltage-gated K^+ channel α subunit expressed in human heart. *Proc. Natl. Acad. Sci. U.S.A.* 92:6309–6313, 1995.
43. Fedida, D. and W. R. Giles. Regional variations in action potentials and transient outward current in myocytes isolated from rabbit left ventricle. *J. Physiol. (Lond)* 442:191–209, 1991.
44. Fedida, D., B. Wible, Z. Wang, B. Fermini, F. Faust, S. Nattel, and A. M. Brown. Identity of a novel delayed rectifier current from human heart with a cloned K channel current. *Circ. Res.* 73:210–216, 1993.
45. Ficker, E., M. Taglialatela, B. A. Wible, C. M. Henley, and A. M. Brown. Spermine and spermidine as gating molecules for inward rectifier K^+ channels. *Science* 266:1068–1072, 1994.
46. Findlay, I. The ATP sensitive potassium channel of cardiac muscle and action potential shortening during metabolic stress. *Cardiovasc. Res.* 28:760–761, 1994.

47. Fozzard, H. A. and M. Hiraoka. The positive dynamic current and its inactivation properties in cardiac Purkinje fibres. *J. Physiol. (Lond.)* 234:569–586, 1973.
48. Furberg, C. D. and B. M. Psaty. Should dihydropyridines be used as first-line drugs in the treatment of hypertension—the con side. *Arch. Intern. Med.* 155:2157–2161, 1995.
49. Gao, T., T. S. Puri, B. L. Gerhardstein, A. J. Chien, R. D. Green, and M. M. Hosey. Identification and subcellular localization of the subunits of L-type calcium channels and adenylyl cyclase in cardiac myocytes. *J. Biol. Chem.* 272:19401–19407, 1997.
50. Gao, T., A. Yatani, M. L. Dell'Acqua, H. Sako, S. A. Green, N. Dascal, J. D. Scott, and M. M. Hosey. cAMP-dependent regulation of cardiac L-type Ca^{2+} channels requires membrane targeting of PKA and phosphorylation of channel subunits. *Neuron* 19:185–196, 1997.
51. Gellens, M. E., A. L. George, Jr., L. Q. Chen, M. Chahine, R. Horn, R. L. Barchi, and R. G. Kallen. Primary structure and functional expression of the human cardiac tetrodotoxin-insensitive voltage-dependent sodium channel. *Proc. Natl. Acad. Sci. U.S.A.* 89:554–558, 1992.
52. Gutierrez, L. M., R. M. Brawley, and M. M. Hosey. Dihydropyridine-sensitive calcium channels from skeletal muscle. I. Roles of subunits in channel activity. *J. Biol. Chem.* 266:16387–16394, 1991.
53. Gutierrez, L. M., X. L. Zhao, and M. M. Hosey. Protein kinase C–mediated regulation of L-type Ca channels from skeletal muscle requires phosphorylation of the alpha 1 subunit. *Biochem. Biophys. Res. Commun.* 202:857–865, 1994.
54. Heinemann, S. H., J. Rettig, F. Wunder, and O. Pongs. Molecular and functional characterization of a rat brain Kv beta 3 potassium channel subunit. *FEBS Lett.* 377:383–389, 1995.
55. Hille, B. Local anesthetics: hydrophilic and hydrophobic pathways for the drug-receptor reaction. *J. Gen. Physiol.* 69:497–515, 1977.
56. Hille, B. Local anesthetics: hydrophilic and hydrophobic pathways for the drug-receptor reaction. *J. Gen. Physiol.* 69:497–515, 1977.
57. Hille, B. *Ionic Channels of Excitable Membranes.* Sunderland, MA: Sinauer, 1992.
58. Hiraoka, M., K. Sawada, and S. Kawano. Effect of quinidine on plateau currents of guinea-pig ventricular myocytes. *J. Mol. Cell. Cardiol.* 18:1097–1106, 1986.
59. Ho, K., C. G. Nichols, W. J. Lederer, J. Lytton, P. M. Vassilev, M. V. Kanazirska, and S. C. Hebert. Cloning and expression of an inwardly rectifying ATP-regulated potassium channel. *Nature* 362:31–38, 1993.
60. Hockerman, G. H., B. Z. Peterson, B. D. Johnson, and W. A. Catterall. Molecular determinants of drug binding and action on L-type calcium channels. *Annu. Rev. Pharmacol. Toxicol.* 37:361–396, 1997.
60a. Hockerman, G. H., B. D. Johnson, M. R. Abbott, T. Scheuer, and W. A. Catterall. Molecular determinants of high affinity phenylalkylamine block of L-type calcium channels in transmembrane segment IIIS6 and the pore region of the alpha1 subunit. *J. Biol. Chem.* 272:18759–18765, 1997.
61. Hodgkin, A. L. and A. F. Huxley. A quantitive description of membrane current and its application to conduction and excitation in nerve. *J. Physiol.(Lond.)* 117:500–544, 1952.
62. Hofmann, F., M. Biel, E. Bosse, V. Flockerzi, P. Ruth, and A. Welling. Functional expression of cardiac and smooth muscle calcium channels. In *Ion Channels in the Cardiovascular System: Function and Dysfunction*, edited by A. M. Brown, W. A. Catterrall, G. J. Kaczorowski, P. S. Spooner, and H. C. Strauss. pp. Washington, DC: AAAS Press, 1993.
63. Hosey, M. M., A. J. Chien, and T. S. Puri. Structure and regulation of L-type calcium channels—a current assessment of the properties and roles of channel subunits. *Trends Cardiovasc. Med.* 6:265–273, 1996.
64. Hoshi, T., W. N. Zagotta, and R. W. Aldrich. Biophysical and molecular mechanisms of Shaker potassium channel inactivation [see comments]. *Science* 250:533–538, 1990.
65. Inagaki, N., T. Gonoi, J. P. Clement, C. Z. Wang, L. Aguilar-Bryan, J. Bryan, and S. Seino. A family of sulfonylurea receptors determines the pharmacological properties of ATP-sensitive K^+ channels. *Neuron* 16:1011–1017, 1996.
66. Inagaki, N., Y. Tsuura, N. Namba, K. Masuda, T. Gonoi, M. Horie, Y. Seino, M. Mizuta, and S. Seino. Cloning and functional characterization of a novel ATP-sensitive potassium channel ubiquitously expressed in rat tissues, including pancreatic islets, pituitary, skeletal muscle, and heart. *J. Biol. Chem.* 270:5691–5694, 1995.
67. Irisawa, H. and N. Hagiwara, Ionic current in sinoatrial node cells. *J. Cardiovascu. Electrophysiol.* 2:531–540, 1991.
68. Isacoff, E., D. Papazian, L. Timpe, Y. N. Jan, and L. Y. Jan, Molecular studies of voltage-gated potassium channels. *Cold Spring Harbor Symp. Quant. Biol.* 55:9–17, 1990.
69. Ishii, K., T. Yamagishi, and N. Taira. Cloning and functional expression of a cardiac inward rectifier K^+ channel. *FEBS Lett.* 338:107–111, 1994.
70. Isom, L. L., K. S. De Jongh, and W. A. Catterall. Auxiliary subunits of voltage-gated ion channels. *Neuron* 12:1183–1194, 1994.
71. Josephson, I. R., J. Sanchez-Chapula, and A. M. Brown. Early outward current in rat single ventricular cells. *Circ. Res.* 54:157–162, 1984.
72. Kamb, A., L. E. Iverson, and M. A. Tanouye. Molecular characterization of *shaker*, a Drosophila gene that encodes a potassium channel. *Cell* 50:405–413, 1987.
73. Kass, R. S. Dihydropyridine modulation of cardiovascular L-type calcium channels: molecular and cellular pharmacology. In *Ion Channels in the Cardiovascular System: Function and Dysfunction*, edited by P. M. Spooner, A. M. Brown, W. A. Catterall, G. J. Kaczorowski, and H. C. Strauss. Armonk, NY: Futura Publishing Co., 1994:425–440.
74. Kass, R. S. Ionic basis of electrical activity in the heart. In *Physiology and Pathophysiology of the Heart*, edited by N. Sperelakis, Norwell, MA: Kluwer Academic, 1994.
75. Kass, R. S. Molecular pharmacology of cardiac L-type calcuim channels. In *Handbook of Membrane Channels: Molecular and Cellular Physiology*, edited by C., Peracchia. Orlando, FL: Academic Press, 1994:187–198.
76. Kass, R. S. and M. P. Davies. The roles of ion channels in an inherited heart disease: molecular genetics of the long QT syndrome. *Cardiovasc. Res.* 32:443–454, 1996.
77. Kass, R. S. and M. C. Sanguinetti, Calcium channel inactivation in the cardiac Purkinje fiber. Evidence for voltage-and calcium-mediated mechanisms. *J. Gen. Physiol.* 84:705–726, 1984.
78. Kass, R. S. and R. W. Tsien. Multiple effects of calcium antagonists on plateau currents in cardiac purkinje fibers. *J. Gen. Physiol.* 66:169–192, 1975.
79. Kass, R. S. and R. W. Tsien. Control of action potential duration by calcium ions in cardiac purkinje fibers. *J. Gen. Physiol.* 67:599–617, 1976.
80. Kass, R. S. and S. E. Wiegers. The ionic basis of concentration-related effects of noradrenaline on the action potential of calf cardiac Purkinje fibres. *J. Physiol. (Lond.)* 322:541–558, 1982.
81. Kenyon, J. L. and J. L. Sutko. Calcium- and voltage-activated plateau currents of cardiac Purkinje fibers. *J. Gen. Physiol.* 89:921–958, 1987.
82. Kubo, Y., E. Reuveny, P. A. Slesinger, Y. N. Jan and L. Y. Jan. Primary structure and functional expression of a rat G-protein-

coupled muscarinic potassium channel [see comments]. *Nature* 364:802–806, 1993.
83. Lacerda, A. E., H. S. Kim, P. Ruth, E. Perez-Reyes, V. Flockerzi, F., Hofmann, L. Birnbaumer, and A. M. Brown. Normalization of current kinetics by interaction between the α 1 and β subunits of the skeletal muscle dihydropyridine-sensitive Ca^{2+} channel. *Nature* 352:527, 1991.
84. Logothetis, D. E., Y. Kurachi, J. Galper, E. J. Neer, and D. E. Clapham. The beta-gamma subunits of GTP-binding proteins activate the muscarinic K$^+$ channel in heart. *Nature* 325:321–326, 1987.
85. Lopatin, A. N., E. N. Makhina, and C. G. Nichols. Potassium channel block by cytoplasmic polyamines as the mechanism of intrinsic rectification. *Nature* 372:366–369, 1994.
86. Lory, P., G. Varadi, D. F. Slish, M. Varadi, and A. Schwartz. Characterization of beta subunit modulation of a rabbit cardiac L-type Ca^{2+} channel alpha 1 subunit as expressed in mouse L cells. *FEBS Lett.* 315:167–172, 1993.
87. Ma, J., L. M. Gutierrez, M. M. Hosey, and E. Rios. Dihydropyridine-sensitive skeletal muscle Ca channels in polarized planar bilayers. 3. Effects of phosphorylation by protein kinase C. *Biophys. J.* 63:639–647, 1992.
88. MacKinnon, R., R. W. Aldrich, and A. W. Lee. Functional stoichiometry of Shaker potassium channel inactivation. *Science* 262:757–759, 1993.
89. MacKinnon, R. and C. Miller. Mutant potassium channels with altered binding of charybdotoxin, a pore-blocking peptide inhibitor. *Science* 245:1382–1384, 1989.
90. MacKinnon, R. and G. Yellen, G. Mutations affecting TEA blockade and ion permeation in voltage activated K$^+$ channels. *Science* 250:276–279, 1990.
91. Makielski, J. C., J. T. Limberis, S. Y. Chang, Z. Fan and J. W. Kyle. Coexpression of beta 1 with cardiac sodium channel alpha subunits in oocytes decreases lidocaine block. *Mol. Pharmacol.* 49:30–39, 1996.
92. Marks, A. R. Intracellular calcium-release channels: regulators of cell life and death. *Am. J. Physiol.* 272 (*Heart Circ. Physiol.* 41):H597–H605, 1997.
93. McCall, E., L. V. Hryshko, V. M. Stiffel, D. M. Christensen, and D. M. Bers. Possible functional linkage between the cardiac dihydropyridine and ryanodine receptor: acceleration of rest decay by Bay K 8644. *J. Mol. Cell. Cardiol.* 28:79–93, 1996.
94. McDonald, T. F., S. Pelzer, W. Trautwein, and D. J. Pelzer. Regulation and modulation of calcium channels in cardiac, skeletal, and smooth muscle cells. *Physiol. Rev.* 74:365–507, 1994.
95. Mikami, A., K. Imoto, T. Tanabe, T. Niidome, Y. Mori, H. Takeshima, S. Narumiya and S. Numa. Primary structure and functional expression of the cardiac dihydropyridine-sensitive calcium channel. *Nature* 340:230–233, 1989.
96. Miller, C. Genetic manipulation of ion channels: a new approach to structure and mechanism. *Neuron* 2:1195–1205, 1989.
97. Morad, M. and E. L. Rolett. Relaxing effects of catecholamines on mammalian heart. *J. Physiol. (Lond.)* 224:537–558, 1972.
98. Morad, M. and W. Trautwein, The effect of the duration of the action potential on contraction in the mammalian heart muscle. *Pflügers Arch.* 299:66–82, 1968.
99. Morad, M. and W. Trautwein. The effect of the duration of the action potential on contractions in mammalian heart tissue. *Pflugers Arch* 299:66–82, 1968.
100. Morales, M. J., J. O. Wee, S. Wang, H. C. Strauss, and R. L. Rasmusson. The N-terminal domain of a K$^+$ channel beta subunit increases the rate of C-type inactivation from the cytoplasmic side of the channel. *Proc. Natl. Acad. Sci. U.S.A.* 93: 15119–15123, 1996.
101. Mori, Y., T. Friedrich, M.-S. Kim, A. Mikami, J. Nakai, P. Ruth, E. Bosse, F. Hofmann, V. Flockerzi, T., Furuichi, K. Nikoshiba, K., Imoto, T. Tanabe, and S. Numa. Primary structure and functional expression from complementary DNA of a brain calcium channel. *Nature* 350:398–402, 1991.
102. Moss, A. J. and J. L. Robinson. The long-QT syndrome: genetic considerations. *Trends Cardiovasc. Med.* 2:81–83, 1993.
103. Neely, A., X. Wei, R. Olcese, L. Birnbaumer, and E. Stefani. Potentiation by the beta subunit of the ratio of the ionic current to the charge movement in the cardiac calcium channel. *Science* 262:575–578, 1993.
104. New, W. and W. Trautwein. The ionic nature of slow inward current and its relation to contraction. *Pflügers Arch.* 334:24–38, 1972.
105. Nichols, C. G. and A. N. Lopatin. Inward rectifier potassium channels. *Annu. Rev. Physiol.* 59:171–191, 1997.
106. Nishimura, S., H. Takeshima, F. Hofmann, V. Flockerzi, and K. Imoto. Requirement of the calcium channel beta subunit for functional conformation. *FEBS Lett.* 324:283–286, 1993.
107. Noble, D. and R. W. Tsien. Outward membrane currents activated in the plateau range of potentials in cardiac Purkinje fibres. *J. Physiol. (Lond.)* 200:205–231, 1969.
108. Noda, M., H. Suzuki, S. Numa, and W. Stuhmer. A single point mutation confers tetrodotoxin and saxitoxin insensitivity on the sodium channel II. *FEBS Lett.* 259:213–216, 1989.
109. Noma, A. ATP-regulated K$^+$ channels in cardiac muscle. *Nature* 305:147–148, 1983.
110. Nuss, H. B., N. Chiamvimonvat, M. T. Perezgarcia, G. F. Tomaselli, and E. Marban. Functional association of the beta(1) subunit with human cardiac (HH1) and rat skeletal muscle (MU-1) sodium channel alpha subunits expressed in *Xenopus* oocytes. *J. Gen. Physiol.* 106:1171–1191, 1995.
111. Oh, S. T., E. Yedidag, J. L. Conklin, M. Martin, and K. Bielefeldt. Calcium release from intracellular stores and excitation-contraction coupling in intestinal smooth muscle. *J. Surg. Res.* 71:79–86, 1997.
112. Ono, K., H. A. Fozzard, and D. A. Hanck. Mechanism of cAMP-dependent modulation of cardiac sodium channel current kinetics. *Circ. Res.* 72:807–815, 1993.
113. Ono, K., H. A. Fozzard, and D. A. Hanck. Mechanism of cAMP-dependent modulation of cardiac sodium channel current kinetics. *Circ. Res.* 72:807–815, 1993.
114. Patlak, J. Molecular kinetics of voltage-dependent Na$^+$ channels. *Physiol. Rev.* 71:1047–1080, 1991.
115. Perez-Reyes, E., L. L. Cribbs, A. Daud, A. E. Lacerda, J., Barclay, M. P., Williamson, M. Fox, M. Rees, and J. H. Lee. Molecular characterization of a neuronal low-voltage-activated T-type calcium channel [see comments]. *Nature* 391:896–900, 1998.
116. Piedras-Renteria, E. S., C. C. Chen, and P. M. Best. Antisense oligonucleotides against rat brain alpha1E DNA and its atrial homologue decrease T-type calcium current in atrial myocytes. *Proc. Natl. Acad. Sci. U.S.A.* 94:14936–14941, 1997.
117. Po, S., S. Roberds, D. J. Snyders, M. M. Tamkun, and P. B. Bennett. Heteromultimeric assembly of human potassium channels: molecular basis of a transient outward current? *Circ. Res.* 72:1326–1336, 1993.
118. Pragnell, M., K. J. Snay, J. S. Trimmer, N. J. Maclusky, F. Naftolin, L. K. Kaczmarek, and M. B. Boyle. Estrogen induction of a small, putative K channel mRNA in rat uterus. *Neuron* 4: 807–812, 1990.
119. Priori, S. G., F. Cantu, and P. J. Schwartz. The long QT syndrome—new diagnostic and therapeutic approach in the era of molecular biology. *Schweiz. Med. Wochenschr.* 1727–1731, 1996.
119a. Qu, Y., J. Rogers, T. Tanada, T. Scheuer, and W. A. Catterall. Molecular determinants of drug access to the receptor site for

antiarrhythmic drugs in the cardiac Na$^+$ channel. *Proc. Natl. Acad. Sci. U.S.A.* 92:11839–11843, 1995.
120. Raab-Graham, K. F., C. M. Radeke, and C. A. Vandenberg. Molecular cloning and expression of a human heart inward rectifier potassium channel. *NeuroReport* 5:2501–2505, 1994.
121. Ragsdale, D. S., J. C. McPhee, T. Scheuer, and W. A. Catterall. Molecular determinants of state-dependent block of Na$^+$ channels by local anesthetics. *Science* 265:1724–1728, 1994.
122. Reuter, H. Slow inactivation of currents in cardiac Purkinje fibres. *J. Physiol.* 197:233–253, 1968.
123. Reuter, H. Calcium channel modulation by neurotransmitters, enzymes and drugs. *Nature* 301:569–574, 1983.
124. Reuter, H. and H. Scholz. The regulation of Ca conductance of cardiac muscle by adrenaline. *J. Physiol. (Lond.)* 264:49–62, 1977.
125. Roberds, S. L. and M. M. Tamkun. Cloning and tissue-specific expression of five voltage-gated potassium channel cDNAs expressed in rat heart. *Proc. Nat. Acad. Sci. U.S.A.* 88:1798–1802, 1991.
126. Rogart, R. B., L. L. Cribbs, L. K. Muglia, M. W. Kaiser, and D. D. Kephart. Molecular cloning of a putative tetrodotoxin-resistant rat heart Na channel isoform. *Proc. Natl. Acad. Sci. U.S.A.* 86:8170–8174, 1989.
127. Ruth, P., A. Rohrkasten, M., Biel, E., Bosse, S., Regulla, H. E. Meyer, V. Flockerzi, and F. Hofmann. Primary structure of the subunit of the DHP-sensitive calcium channel from skeletal muscle. *Science* 245:1115–1118, 1989.
127a. Sakmann B., and G. Trube. Voltage-dependent inactivation of inward rectifying single-channel currents in the guinea-pig heart cell membrane. *J. Physiol* 347:659–683, 1984.
128. Sanguinetti, M. C., M. E. Curran, P. S. Spector, and M. T. Keating. Spectrum of HERG K$^+$-channel dysfunction in an inherited cardiac arrythmia. *Proc. Nat. Acad. Sci. U.S.A.* 93:8796–8796, 1996.
129. Sanguinetti, M. C., M. E. Curran, A. Zou, J. Shen, P. S. X. A. D. Spector, and M. T. Keating. Coassembly of K(V)LQT1 and mink (isk) proteins to form cardiac I-KS potassium channel. *Nature* 384:80–83, 1996.
130. Sanguinetti, M. C., C., Jiang, M. E. Curran, and M. T. Keating. A mechanistic link between an inherited and an acquired cardiac arrhythmia: HERG encodes the I_{Kr} potassium channel. *Cell* 81:299–307, 1995.
131. Sanguinetti, M. C., J. H. Johnson, L. G. Hammerland, P. R. Kelbaugh, R. A. Volkmann, N. A. Saccomano, and A. L. Mueller. Heteropodatoxins: peptides isolated from spider venom that block Kv4.2 potassium channels. *Mole. Pharmacol.* 51:491–498, 1997.
132. Sanguinetti, M. C. and N. K. Jurkiewicz. Two components of cardiac delayed rectifier K$^+$ current. Differential sensitivity to block by class III antiarrhythmic agents. *J. Gen. Physiol.* 96:195–215, 1990.
133. Schneider, T., and F. Hofmann. The bovine cardiac receptor for calcium channel blockers is a 195-kDa protein. *Eur. J. Biochem.* 174:369–375, 1988.
134. Schonenherr, R., and S. H. Heinemann. Molecular determinants for activation and inactivation of HERG, a human inward rectifier potassium channel. *J. Physiol. (Lond.)* 493:635–642, 1996.
135. Schwarz, W., P. T. Palade, and B. Hille. Local anesthetics. Effect of pH on use-dependent block of sodium channels in frog muscle. *Biophys. J.* 20:343–368, 1977.
136. Sculptoreanu, A., E. Rotman, M., Takahashi, T. Scheuer, and W. A. Catterall. Voltage-dependent potentiation of the activity of cardiac L-type calcium channel alpha 1 subunits due to phosphorylation by cAMP-dependent protein kinase. *Proc. Natl. Acad. Sci. U.S.A.* 90:10135–10139, 1993.
137. Sculptoreanu, A., T. Scheuer, and W. A. Catterall. Voltage-dependent potentiation of L-type Ca^{2+} channels due to phosphorylation by cAMP-dependent protein kinase. *Nature* 364:240–243, 1993.
138. Shalaby, F. Y., P. C. Levesque, W. P. Yang, W. A. Little, M. L., Conder, T. Jenkins-west, and M. A. Blanar. Dominant-negative KvLQT1 mutations underlie the LQT1 form of long QT syndrome [see comments]. *Circulation* 96:1733–1736, 1997.
139. Sham, J. S., L. Cleemann, and M. Morad. Functional coupling of Ca^{2+} channels and ryanodine receptors in cardiac myocytes. *Proc. Natl. Acad. Sci. U.S.A.* 92:121–125, 1995.
140. Singer-Lahat, D., I. Lotan, M. Biel, V. Flockerzi, F. Hofmann, and N. Dascal. Cardiac calcium channels expressed in *Xenopus* oocytes are modulated by dephosphorylation but not by cAMP-dependent phosphorylation. *Receptors Channels* 2:215–226, 1994.
141. Singer, D., M., Biel, I., Lotan, V. Flockerzi, F. Hofmann, and N. Dascal. The roles of the subunits in the function of the calcium channel. *Science* 253:1553–1557, 1991.
142. Smith P. L., T. Baukrowitz, and G. Yellen. The inward rectification mechanism of the HERG cardiac potassium channel. *Nature* 379:833–836, 1996.
143. Splawski, I., M., Tristani-Firouzi, M. H. Lehmann, M. C. Sanguinetti, and M. T. Keating. Mutations in the hminK gene cause long QT syndrome and suppress IKs function. *Nat. Genet.* 17:338–340, 1997.
144. Starmer, C. F. and K. R. Courtney. Modeling ion channel blockade at guarded binding sites: application to tertiary drugs. *Am. J. Physiol.* 251 (*Heart Circ. Physiol.* 20):H848–H856, 1986.
145. Strichartz, G. Effects of tertiary local anesthetics and their quaternary derivatives on sodium channels of nerve membranes *Biophys. J.* 18:353–354, 1977.
146. Stuhmer, W., F. Conti, H., Suzuki, X., Wang, M., Noda, N., Yahagi, H. Kubo, and S. Numa. Structural parts involved in activation and inactivation of the sodium channel. *Nature* 339:597–603, 1989.
147. Suzuki, H., S., Beckh, H., Kubo, N., Yahagi, H., Ishida, T., Kayano, M. Noda, and S. Numa. Functional expression of cloned cDNA encoding sodium channel III. *FEBS Lett.* 228:195–200, 1988.
148. Takahashi, M. and W. A. Catterall. Dihydropyridine-sensitive calcium channels in cardiac and skeletal muscle membranes: studies with antibodies against the alpha subunits. *Biochemistry* 26:5518–5526, 1987.
149. Takahashi, M., M. J. Seagar, J. F. Jones, B. F. X. Reber, and W. Catterall, Subunit structure of dihydropyridine-sensitive calcium channels from skeletal muscle. *Proc. Natl. Acad. Sci. U.S.A.* 84:5478–5482, 1987.
150. Takumi, T., H. Ohkubo, and S. Nakanishi. Cloning of a membrane protein that induces a slow voltage-gated potassium current. *Science* 242:1042–1045, 1988.
151. Tamkun, M. M., K. M. Knoth, J. A. Walbridge, H. Kroemer, D. M. Roden, and D. M. Glover. Molecular cloning and characterization of two voltage-gated K$^+$ channel cDNAs from human ventricle. *FASEB J.* 5:331–337, 1991.
152. Toshe, N. Calcium-sensitive delayed rectifier potassium current in guinea pig ventricular cells. *Am. J. Physiol.* 258 (*Heart Circ. Physiol.* 27):H1200–H1207, 1990.
153. Toshe, N., M. Kameyama, and H. Irasawa. Intracellular Ca and PKC modulate K current in guinea pig heart cells. *Am. J. Physiol.* 253 (*Heart Circ. Physiol.* 22):H1321–H1324, 1987.
154. Tsien, R. W. Effects of epinephrine on the pacemaker potassium current of cardiac Purkinje fibers. *J. Gen. Physiol.* 64:293–319, 1977.
155. Tsien, R. W., P. T. Ellinor, and W. A. Horne. Molecular diver-

sity of voltage-dependent Ca^{2+} channels. *TIPS* 12:349–354, 1991.
156. Tucker, S. J., F. M. Gribble, C. Zhao, S. Trapp, and F. M. Ashcroft. Truncation of Kir6.2 produces ATP-sensitive K$^+$ channels in the absence of the sulphonylurea receptor. *Nature* 387:179–183, 1997.
157. Vandenberg, C. A. Inward rectification of a potassium channel in cardiac ventricular cells depends on internal magnesium ions. *Proc. Natl. Acad. Sci. USA* 84:2560–2564, 1987.
158. Varadi, G., P. Lory, D. Schultz, M. Varadi, and A. Schwartz. Acceleration of activation and inactivation by the subunit of the skeletal muscle calcium channel. *Nature* 352:159–162, 1991.
159. Walsh, K. B. and R. S. Kass. Regulation of a heart potassium channel by protein kinase A and C. *Science* 242:67–69, 1988.
160. Walsh, K. B. and R. S. Kass. Distinct voltage-dependent regulation of a heart-delayed I_K by protein kinases A and C. *Am. J. Physiol.* 261 (*Cell Physiol.* 30):C1081–C1090, 1991.
161. Wang, D. W., K. Yazawa, N. Makita, A. L. George, and P. B. Bennett. Pharmacological targeting of long QT mutant sodium channels. *J. Clin. Invest.* 99:1714–1720, 1997.
162. Wang, Q., M. E. Curran, I. Splawski, T. C. Burn, J. M. Millholland, T. J. Vanraay, J. Shen, K. W. Timothy, G. M. Vincent, T. Dejager, P. J. Schwartz, J. A. Towbin, A. J. Moss, D. L. Atkinson, G. M. Landes, T. D. Connors, and M. T. Keating. Positional cloning of a novel potassium channel gene—KVLQT1 mutations cause cardiac arrhythmias. *Nat. Genet.* 12:17–23, 1996.
163. Wang, Q., J. Shen, Z. Li, K. Timothy, G. M. Vincent, S. G. Priori, P. J. Schwartz, and M. T. Keating. Cardiac sodium channel mutations in patients with long QT syndrome, an inherited cardiac arrhythmia. *Hum. Mol. Genet.* 4:1603–1607, 1995.
164. Wang, Q., J. Shen, I. Splawski, D. Atkinson, Z. Li, J. L. Robinson, A. J. Moss, J. A. Towbin, and M. T. Keating. SCN5A mutations associated with an inherited cardiac arrhythmia, long QT syndrome. *Cell* 80:805–811, 1995.
165. Wang, Z., B. Fermini, and S. Nattel. Sustained depolarization-induced outward current in human atrial myocytes. Evidence for a novel delayed rectifier K$^+$ current similar to Kv1.5 cloned channel currents. *Circ. Res.* 73:1061–1076, 1993.
166. Warmke, J. W. and B. Ganetzky. A family of potassium channel genes related to eag in Drosophila and mammals. *Proc. Natl. Acad. Sci. U.S.A.* 91:3438–3442, 1994.
167. Welling, A., Y. W. Kwan, E. Bosse, V. Flockerzi, F. Hofmann, and R. S. Kass. Subunit-dependent modulation of recombinant L-type calcium channels: molecular basis for dihydropyridine tissue selectivity. *Circ. Res.* 73:974–980, 1993.
168. Wible, B. A., M. De Biasi, K. Majumder, M. Taglialatela, and A. M. Brown. Cloning and functional expression of an inwardly rectifying K$^+$ channel from human atrium. *Circ. Res.* 76:343–350, 1995.
169. Wiechen, K., D. T. Yue, and S. Herzig. Two distinct functional effects of protein phosphatase inhibitors on guinea-pig cardiac L-type Ca^{2+} channels. *J. Physiol. (Lond.)* 484:583–592, 1995.
170. Yamada, M., S. Isomoto, S. Matsumoto, C. Kondo, T. Shindo, Y. Horio, and Y. Kurachi. Sulphonylurea receptor 2B and Kir6.1 form a sulphonylurea-sensitive but ATP-insensitive K$^+$ channel. *J. Physiol. (Lond.)* 499:715–720, 1997.
171. Yamazawa, T., H. Takeshima, M. Shimuta, and M. Iino. A region of the ryanodine receptor critical for excitation-contraction coupling in skeletal muscle. *J. Biol. Chem.* 272:8161–8164, 1997.
172. Yeola, S. W. and D. J. Snyders. Electrophysiological and pharmacological correspondence between Kv4.2 current and rat cardiac transient outward current. *Cardiovasc. Res.* 33:540–547, 1997.
173. Yue, D. T., P. H. Backx, and J. P. Imredy. Calcium-sensitive inactivation in the gating of single calcium channels. *Science* 21:1735–1738, 1990.
174. Zagotta, W. N., T. Hoshi, and R. W. Aldrich. Restoration of inactivation in mutants of *Shaker* potassium channels by a peptide derived from ShB. *Science* 250:568–571, 1990.
175. Zhao, X. L., L. M. Gutierrez, C. F. Chang, and M. M. Hosey. The alpha 1-subunit of skeletal muscle L-type Ca channels is the key target for regulation by A-kinase and protein phosphatase-1C. *Biochemic. Biophys. Res. Commun.* 198:166–173, 1994.
176. Zhou, Z. and C. T. January. Both T- and L-type Ca^{2+} channels can contribute to excitation-contraction coupling in cardiac Purkinje cells. *Biophys. J.* 74:1830–1839, 1998.
177. Zong, X. G., J. Schreieck, G. Mehrke, A. Welling, A. Schuster, E. Bosse, V. Flockerzi, and F. Hofmann. L-type calcium channels, cAMP-dependent regulation of calcium channels, transient and stable expression of calcium channels, CHO cells, HEK 293 and cells. on the regulation of the expressed L-type calcium channel by cAMP-dependent phosphorylation. *Pflugers Arch.* 430:340–347, 1995.
178. Zygmunt, A. C. Intracellular calcium activates a chloride current in canine ventricular myocytes. *Am. J. Physiol.* 267 (*Heart Circ. Physiol.* 36):H1984–H1995, 1994.
179. Zygmunt, A. C., and W. R. Gibbons. Properties of the calcium-activated chloride current in heart. *J. Gen. Physiol.* 99:391–414, 1992.
180. Zygmunt, A. C., R. J. Goodrow, and C. Antzelevitch. Sodium effects on 4-aminopyridine-sensitive transient outward current in canine ventricular cells. *Am. J. Physiol.* 272 (*Heart Circ. Physiol.* 41):H1–H11, 1997.

15. Molecular analysis of voltage-gated K⁺ channel diversity and functioning in the mammalian heart

JEANNE M. NERBONNE | Department of Molecular Biology and Pharmacology, Washington University Medical School, St. Louis, Missouri

CHAPTER CONTENTS

Electrophysiological Diversity of Voltage-Gated Myocardial K⁺ Channel Currents
   Transient outward K⁺ currents, I_{to}
      $I_{to(fast)}$ ($I_{to,f}$)
      $I_{to(slow)}$ ($I_{to,s}$)
   Delayed rectifier K⁺ currents, I_K
      $I_{K(rapid)}$ (I_{Kr}) and $I_{K(slow)}$ (I_{Ks})
      $I_{K(ultra-rapid)}$ (I_{Kur})
      Other delayed rectifiers
   Cellular/regional heterogeneity in voltage-gated K⁺ current expression and properties
Molecular Determinants of Voltage-Gated Cardiac K⁺ Channels
   Voltage-gated K⁺ channel pore-forming α subunits
      Homologous voltage-gated (Kv) subfamilies
      Ether-A-Go-Go-related gene subfamily
      KvLQT1 subfamily
   Accessory subunits of voltage-gated K⁺ channels
      Minimal K⁺ channel subunits, minK, miRP1
      Accessory β subunits
      K⁺ channel associated proteins, KChAPs
      K⁺ channel interacting proteins, KChIPs
   Voltage-gated K⁺ channels and the cytoskeleton
Molecular Correlates of Functional Voltage-Gated K⁺ Channels
   Molecular genetics of cardiac delayed rectifier K⁺ currents, I_{Kr} and I_{Ks}
      ERG1 and MiRP1 underlie I_{Kr}
      KvLQT1 and minK underlies I_{Ks}
   Transgenic and targeted gene deletion approaches
      Kv4.2/Kv4.3 α subunits underlie $I_{to,f}$
      Kv1.4 underlies $I_{to,s}$
   Molecular correlates of other voltage-gated cardiac K⁺ currents
      Kv1.5 underlies human and rat I_{Kur}
      Kv1.5 and Kv2.1 contribute to mouse $I_{K(slow)}$
      Kv1.2 underlies rat atrial $I_{K,DTX}$
Functional Consequences of In Vivo Alterations in Voltage-Gated Myocardial K⁺ Channels
   QT prolongation
   Atrioventricular block
   Ventricular arrhythmia/tachycardia
   Pathophysiology
Summary, Conclusions, and Future Directions

DEPOLARIZATION-ACTIVATED, CA²⁺-INDEPENDENT OUTWARD K⁺ CURRENTS contribute to determining the heights and the durations of action potentials in cardiac cells, and several distinct types of voltage-gated K⁺ currents that subserve these functions have been identified (8, 18, 168). In many cardiac cells, transient outward currents, $I_{to,f}$ and $I_{to,s}$, and/or several distinct components of delayed rectification, including I_{Kr} ($I_{K(rapid)}$), I_{Ks} ($I_{K(slow)}$), and I_{Kur} ($I_{K(ultra\ rapid)}$), appear to be coexpressed. Nevertheless, there are clear and substantive differences in the expression patterns of the various voltage-gated K⁺ currents in cardiac cells isolated from different species, as well as in cells from different regions of the heart in the same species. Considerable evidence suggests that the differential expression of voltage-gated K⁺ currents contributes to determining the variations in action potential waveforms evident in different species and in different myocardial cell types (6, 7, 14, 18, 141). In spite of the differences in expression patterns, the time- and voltage-dependent properties and the pharmacological properties of the voltage-gated K⁺ (I_{to} and I_K) currents in different cardiac cell types (and species) are similar, suggesting that the molecular correlates of the underlying K⁺ channels are the same.

Importantly, there are marked and rather stereotyped changes in action potential waveforms and in the densities and/or the properties of voltage-gated K⁺ currents in the heart during normal development (152, 230), as well as in the damaged or diseased myocardium (13, 21, 25, 28, 31, 77, 103, 142, 143, 150, 155, 167, 195, 199, 207, 208, 245). In addition, voltage-gated K⁺ channels are important downstream targets for the actions of a variety of endogenous transmitters, hormones, and exogenous drugs that modulate cardiac functioning (8, 81). Thus, there has been considerable interest in defining the molecular correlates of voltage-gated myocardial K⁺ channels (18, 168) and in exploring the molecular mechanisms involved in the regulation and modulation of the expression and the properties of these channels.

A number of voltage-gated K⁺ channel (Kv) pore-forming (α) and accessory (β, minK, MiRP1) subunits have been identified in heart, and a sophisticated combination of in vivo and in vitro molecular genetic approaches has been exploited to define the relationships between these subunits and the various types of voltage-gated K⁺ channels in cardiac cells. Considerable progress has been made in defining the molecular correlates of functional voltage-gated myocardial K⁺ channels, and the results obtained to date suggest that distinct molecular entities underlie the electrophysiologically distinct types of voltage-gated K⁺ currents/channels in cardiac cells. This chapter begins with an overview of the electrophysiological diversity of the repolarizing voltage-gated K⁺ channel currents that have been identified in the mammalian myocardium, with an emphasis on heterogeneity and how the differential expression of voltage-gated K⁺ currents contributes to observed differences in action potential repolarization in different cardiac cell types. This section is followed by a review of the voltage-gated K⁺ (Kv) channel pore-forming (α) and accessory (β, minK, MiRP1) subunits that have been cloned from or shown to be expressed in the mammalian heart. The focus is then shifted to recent efforts aimed at defining the (Kv α and accessory) subunits that underlie the various functionally distinct types of myocardial voltage-gated K⁺ channel currents. The final sections of this chapter examine the functional consequences of in vivo manipulation of functional voltage-gated K⁺ channels and summarize likely future areas of research.

ELECTROPHYSIOLOGICAL DIVERSITY OF VOLTAGE-GATED MYOCARDIAL K⁺ CHANNEL CURRENTS

In the mammalian myocardium, the amplitudes and the durations of action potentials (Fig. 15–1) are de-

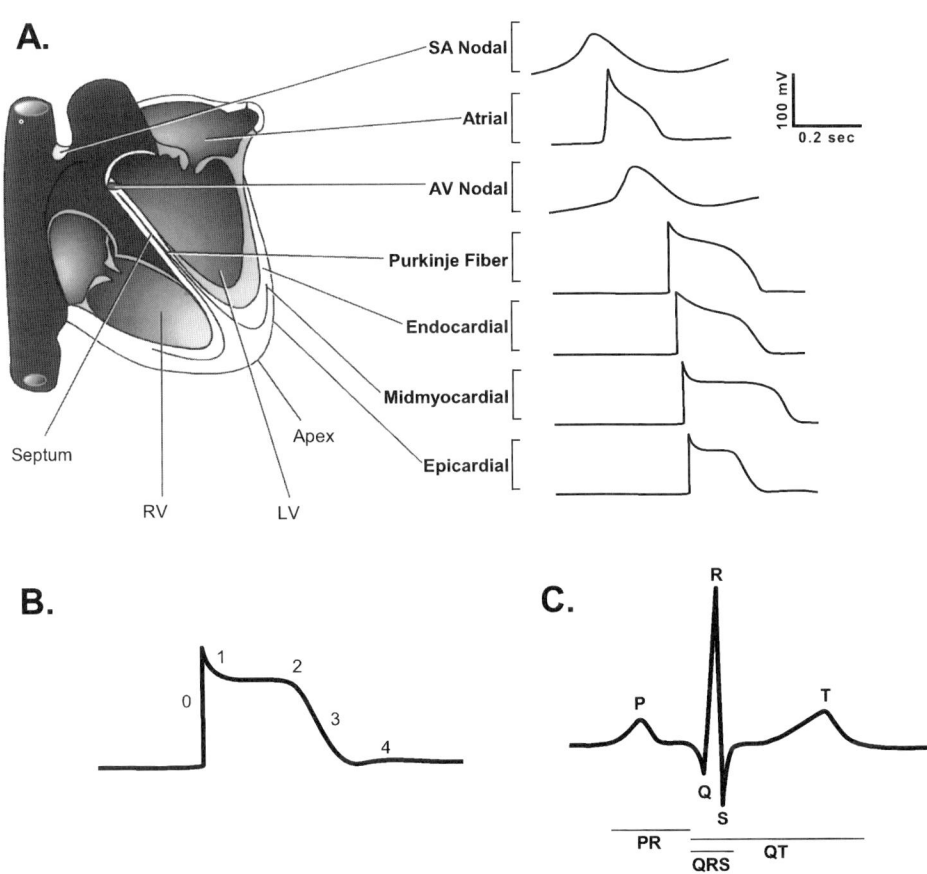

FIG. 15–1. Action potential waveforms and propagation in the mammalian myocardium. *A:* Schematic representation of action potential waveforms recorded in different regions of the human heart; action potentials are displaced in time to reflect the temporal sequence of propagation. *B:* Schematic of a ventricular action potential labeled as follows: (0) depolarization; (1) early (fast) repolarization, which results in the "notch"; (2) plateau phase; (3) late (slower) phase of repolarization; and, (4) afterhyperpolarization/return to the resting membrane potential. *C:* Configuration of a typical scalar electrocardiogram with the various deflections (P, Q, R, S, T) and intervals (PR, QRS, QT) marked; QT intervals, however, must be corrected for variations in heart rate (see text).

termined in large part by voltage-gated K⁺ channels. In most cardiac cells, two broad classes of voltage-gated K⁺ channel currents have been distinguished based on differences in time- and voltage-dependent properties and pharmacological sensitivities: (1) rapidly activating and inactivating transient, outward K⁺ currents I_{to}, and, (2) slowly inactivating outward K⁺ currents, referred to as I_K (Table 15–1). These currents play distinct roles in action potential repolarization: the transient currents, which activate and inactivate relatively rapidly, for example, underlie the early phase (1) of action potential repolarization (Fig. 15-1B), whereas the delayed rectifiers contribute to the latter phase (3) of membrane repolarization, back to the resting membrane potential (Fig. 15-1B). Nevertheless, these (I_{to} and I_K) are broad classifications, and there are multiple components of I_{to} and of I_K (Table 15–1) in cardiac cells with distinct properties and functional roles. In addition, there are marked differences in the densities of the various voltage-gated K⁺ currents in different species, as well as in different cell types in the same species, and these differences contribute to the regional differences in action potential waveforms recorded in the myocardium (Fig. 15–1A). The normal spread of electrical activity in the myocardium is readily detected in surface electrocardiographic (ECG) recordings, and the configuration of a typical scalar (human) ECG is illustrated in Figure 15–1C. The P wave corresponds to atrial depolarization and the QRS complex to ventricular depolarization; the T wave, in contrast, reflects repolarization (Fig. 15–1C). Importantly, there is a direct relationship between the surface ECG (Fig. 15–1C) and action potential waveforms (Fig. 15–1B): the rapid upstroke in phase 0, for example, corresponds to the beginning of the QRS complex, whereas the rapid phase 1 repolarization and the plateau phase (2) correspond to the ST segment; the late phase of repolarization (3) is reflected in the T wave. In addition, the

TABLE 15–1. *Voltage-Gated K⁺ Currents in the Mammalian Myocardium**

Current	Activation	Inactivation	Bloker†	Cell Type	Species
I_{to}					
$I_{to,f}$	Fast	Fast	mM 4-AP	Atrial	Dog, human, mouse, rat
			Flecainide	Ventricular	Cat, dog, ferret, human, mouse, rat
			HaTX	Purkinje	Sheep
			HpTX		
$I_{to,s}$	Fast	Slow	mM 4-AP	Atrial	Rabbit
				Ventricular	Ferret, human, mouse, rabbit, rat
				Purkinje	Rabbit
				Nodal	Rabbit
I_K					
I_{Kr}	Moderate	Fast	E-4031	Atrial	Dog, guinea pig, human, rat
			Dofetilide	Ventricular	Cat, dog, guinea pig, human,
			Lanthanum	Purkinje	Mouse, rabbit, rat
				Nodal	Rabbit
					Rabbit
I_{Ks}	Very slow	No	NE-10064	Atrial	Dog, guinea pig, human
			NE-10133	Ventricular	Dog, guinea pig, human
				Purkinje	Rabbit
				Nodal	Guinea pig, rabbit
I_{Kur}	Fast	No	μM 4-AP	Atrial	Dog, human, rat
I_{Kp}	Fast	No	Ba²⁺	Ventricular	Guinea pig
I_K	Slow	Slow	mM TEA	Ventricular	Rat
$I_{K(slow)}$	Fast	Slow	mM 4-AP	Atrial	Mouse
			mM TEA	Ventricular	Mouse
$I_{K(slow)}$ ($I_{K(DTX)}$)	Fast	Very slow	mM 4-AP	Atrial	Human, rat
			α-DTX		
I_{ss}	Slow	—	mM TEA	Atrial	Mouse, rat
			mM 4-AP	Ventricular	Dog, human, mouse, rat

*Voltage-gated K⁺ currents identified to date in adult cells from various species (see text). †4-AP = 4-aminopyridine; HaTX = hanatoxin; HpTX = heteropodatoxin; TEA = tetraethylammonium; α-DTX = α-dendrotoxin

durations of the various intervals reveal information about conduction times. The duration of the P wave, for example, reflects the intraatrial conduction time, and the duration of the QRS complex reflects the interventricular conduction time; the PR interval, therefore, reveals the AV conduction time and the total time for depolarization and repolarization is the QT interval (Fig. 15–1C). Alterations in action potential durations, conduction times, as well as in the normal propagation of activity through the myocardium, are therefore readily detected in ECG recordings.

Transient Outward K$^+$ Current Channels, I$_{to}$

Transient outward currents were first described in sheep Purkinje fibers and were thought to be carried primarily by Cl$^-$ (57, 61, 75). Subsequent work distinguished two transient outward current components, I$_{to1}$, which is Ca^{2+}-independent and 4-aminopyridine (4-AP)-sensitive, and I$_{to2}$, which is 4-AP-insensitive and Ca^{2+}-dependent (50, 107, 108). It is now clear that I$_{to2}$ is a Cl$^-$ selective conductance pathway (107, 108, 248, 249, 250) and, for this reason, (I$_{to2}$) is not discussed further here. The Ca^{2+}-independent, 4-AP-sensitive transient outward, current, I$_{to1}$, in contrast, is K$^+$ selective. Historically, Ca^{2+}-insensitive transient outward K$^+$ currents in different preparations have been referred to as I$_{to}$, I$_{to1}$, or I$_t$ and assumed to reflect the same conductance pathway (18, 41, 84, 152). It is now clear, however, that there are (at least) two distinct types of transient outward K$^+$ currents in cardiac cells, and that these are differently distributed (36, 223, 236). These will be considered separately here and referred to as I$_{to(fast)}$ (I$_{to,f}$) and I$_{to(slow)}$ (I$_{Ito,s}$), as suggested in Xu et al. (236).

I$_{to(fast)}$ (I$_{to,f}$). Rapidly activating and inactivating, transient outward K$^+$ currents that can be classified as I$_{to(fast)}$(I$_{to,f}$) have been characterized in considerable detail in cat (78), dog (118, 202), ferret (40), human (4, 110, 227, 228), mouse (22, 23, 236, 237), and rat (10, 89, 227, 232) ventricular myocytes, as well as in atrial cells from dog (243), rat (31, 33), human (4, 64, 69, 188, 209), mouse (29, 237), and guinea pig (219; Table 15–1). In contrast to the robust expression of I$_{to,f}$ in most species (Table 15–1), guinea pig ventricular myocytes reportedly lack I$_{to,f}$ (177, 178). A rapidly activating and inactivating (I$_{to,f}$-like) outward K$^+$ current is revealed in guinea pig ventricular cells, however, when extracellular Ca^{2+} is removed (96), suggesting that I$_{to,f}$ channels are present but are rendered nonfunctional by a Ca^{2+}-dependent mechanism(s).

The properties of I$_{to,f}$ in different cardiac cell types and species are similar in that activation, inactivation, and recovery from steady-state inactivation are all rapid (10, 33, 40, 110, 118, 202, 227, 228, 236, 243). The detailed properties of I$_{to,f}$ (and other voltage-gated K$^+$ currents) in mouse ventricular myocytes are shown for illustration purposes in Figure 15–2. The rapid activation (Fig. 15–2B) and inactivation (Fig. 15–2C) of I$_{to,f}$ suggest an important role in early (phase 1) repolarization and in determining the plateau potential. The fact that I$_{to,f}$ recovers rapidly from inactivation (Fig. 15–2D) also suggests that this current will play an important role in shaping action potentials over a wide range of heart rates (168). In addition, the rapid rate of recovery of I$_{to,f}$ from steady-state inactivation (Fig. 15–2D) can be exploited to distinguish I$_{to,f}$ and I$_{to,s}$ (36, 223, 236). These currents can also be distinguished pharmacologically using the *Heteropoda* toxins (36, 87, 181, 236). The fact that the time- and voltage-dependent properties and the pharmacological sensitivities of I$_{to,f}$ in different cardiac cells are similar suggested that the molecular correlates of functional I$_{to,f}$ channels are the same (18), and considerable evidence in support of this hypothesis has now been provided (see later, under Transgenic and Targeted Gene Deletion Approaches). Nevertheless, the detailed time- and voltage-dependent properties of I$_{to,f}$ do vary among cells. In both rat and human, for example, the rates of inactivation and recovery from steady-state inactivation of I$_{to,f}$ in ventricular and atrial myocytes are distinct (4, 10, 33, 209). Recent studies suggest that in the rat, these differences reflect differences in the Kv α subunit composition of atrial and ventricular I$_{to,f}$ channels (see later, under Transgenic and Targeted Gene Deletion Approaches). Although it seems unlikely that a similar mechanism underlies the differences in human atrial and ventricular I$_{to,f}$ kinetics, tissue-specific differences in alternative splicing or post-translational processing could be important.

I$_{to (slow)}$ (I$_{to,s}$). It has been recognized for some time that the properties of the transient outward K$^+$ currents in rabbit cardiocytes (51, 82, 84, 139) are quite different from those of I$_{to,f}$ (Table 15–1). The transient outward currents in rabbit cells are characterized by slow inactivation and slow recovery from steady-state inactivation (66, 82). In mouse ventricular myocytes, two transient outward K$^+$ currents have been distinguished (Figure 15–2): I$_{to,f}$, as described above, and a more slowly decaying (Figure 15–2C) transient K$^+$ current, referred to as I$_{to(slow)}$ or I$_{to,s}$ (236). Mouse ventricular I$_{to,s}$ also recovers from steady-state inactivation more slowly than I$_{to,f}$ (Fig. 15–2D) and is insensitive to the *Heteropoda* toxins (87, 88). In mouse right and left ventricles (Fig. 15–2A), I$_{to,f}$ and I$_{to,s}$ are differentially distributed (87, 88, 236): in cells isolated from the right ventricle or from the apex of the left ventricle, for example, only I$_{to,f}$ is present (Fig. 15–2A), whereas in cells

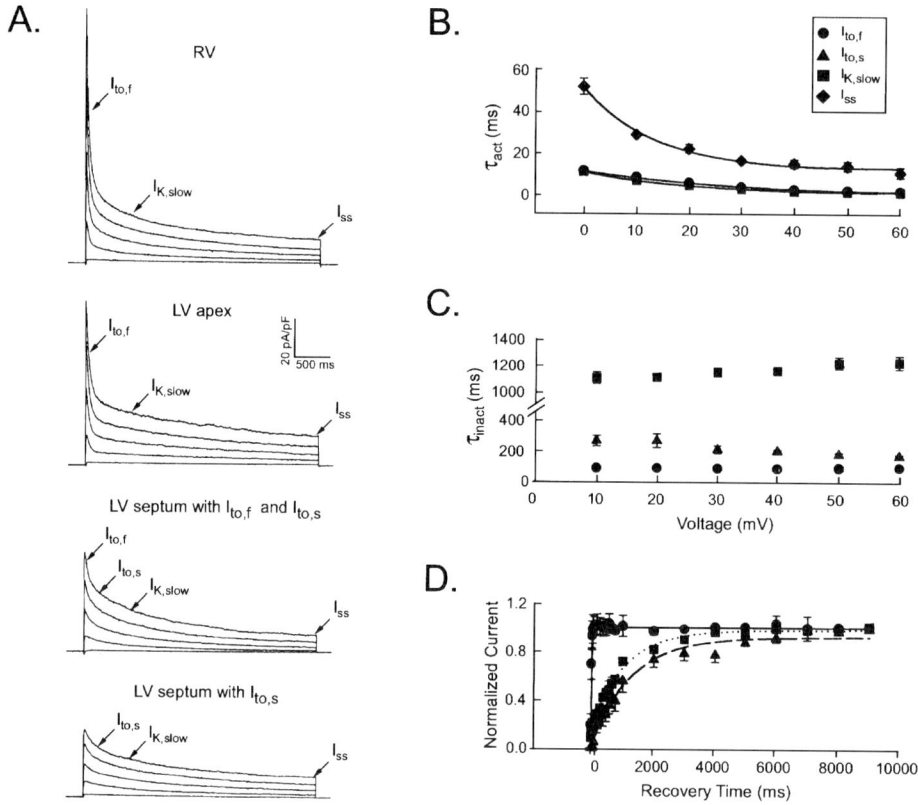

FIG. 15-2. Differential expression of the transient outward K$^+$ currents, $I_{to,f}$ and $I_{to,s}$ in mouse left ventricular myocytes. A: Whole-cell outward K$^+$ currents recorded from isolated adult C57BL6 mouse right ventricular (RV) myocytes and from left ventricular (LV) cells from the apex or septum; currents recorded in response to 4.5 sec depolarizing voltage steps from a holding potential of −70 mV to potentials between −20 and +60 mV in 20 mV increments are shown. As is evident, peak outward K$^+$ densities are highest in RV myocytes, and peak outward K$^+$ current densities are higher in cells from the apex than from septum. In addition, the decay phases of the currents are slower in LV septum, than LV apex or RV, cells. B: Mean ± SEM activation time constants, determined from single exponential fits to the rising phases of the currents, are plotted as a function of test potential; the solid lines represent the best single exponential fits to the data points and describe the voltage-dependence of current activation. The rates of activation of $I_{to,f}$, $I_{to,s}$ and $I_{K(slow)}$ in mouse ventricular myocytes are similar, whereas I_{ss} activates more slowly. C: Mean ± SEM inactivation time constants (determined from double or triple exponential fits to the decay phases of the outward currents) for $I_{to,f}$, $I_{to,s}$ and $I_{K(slow)}$ are plotted as a function of test potential. D: Mean ± SEM normalized recovery data for $I_{to,f}$, $I_{to,s}$ and $I_{K(slow)}$. The rates of recovery of $I_{to,f}$, $I_{to,s}$ and $I_{K(slow)}$ from steady-state inactivation were determined using a three-pulse protocol: cells were first depolarized to +50 mV for 5 sec (to inactivate the currents), hyperpolarized to −70 mV for varying times (to allow recovery) and subsequently depolarized to +50 mV (to assess the extent of recovery). The amplitudes of $I_{to,f}$, $I_{to,s}$ and $I_{K(slow)}$ evoked at +50 mV following each recovery period were then determined, and normalized to the current amplitudes evoked following the 10 sec recovery period. As is evident, $I_{to,f}$ recovers very rapidly from inactivation, whereas $I_{to,s}$ and $I_{K(slow)}$ recover slowly. [Figure produced from data in Xu et al. (23) and Guo et al. (87, 88).]

isolated from the left ventricular septum, $I_{to,s}$ is also expressed (Fig. 15-2A). In ≈20% of the (septum) cells, only $I_{to,s}$ is detected (Fig. 15-2A), whereas in the remaining ≈80% of the cells, both $I_{to,f}$ and $I_{to,s}$ (Fig. 15-2A) are expressed (87, 88, 236).

Distinct transient outward K$^+$ current components have also been reported in ferret, human, and rat ventricular myocytes (36, 144, 232). The rates of inactivation and recovery from steady-state inactivation of the transient outward currents in ferret (36) and human (144), for example, are significantly slower in endocardial cells than in epicardial cells. In ferret, there are also regional differences in the expression patterns of K$^+$ channel subunits, suggesting that the molecular correlates of the transient outward current in (ferret left ventricular) epicardial and endocardial cells are also distinct (36; also, see later, under Transgenic and Targeted Gene Deletion Approaches). The properties of the transient outward K⁺ currents in ferret (36) and human (144) epicardial and endocardial left ventricular myocytes are similar to those of mouse ventricular $I_{to,f}$ and $I_{to,s}$, respectively. For this reason, the ferret and human epicardial and endocardial transient outward K⁺ currents as now also referred to as $I_{to,f}$ and $I_{to,s}$, respectively (Table 15–1). The properties of the transient outward currents in rabbit cells are also similar to mouse ventricular $I_{to,s}$ (Table 15–1). Consistent with this classification, recent studies suggest that the molecular correlate of the slow transient outward K⁺ current in rabbit atrial myocytes and $I_{to,s}$ in mouse ventricle are the same (87, 223; see also, later, under Transgenic and Targeted Gene Deletion Approaches).

Delayed Rectifier K⁺ Currents, I_K

The detailed properties of delayed rectifier K⁺ currents have been characterized in myocytes isolated from canine (119, 202, 243, 244), feline (74, 79), guinea pig (16, 72, 92, 95, 177, 178, 215), human (117, 222), mouse (87, 236, 237, 247), rabbit (187, 211), and rat (10, 33, 162) heart. In most cells, multiple components of I_K (Table 15–1), with distinct kinetic and voltage-dependent properties and pharmacological sensitivities, are evident.

$I_{K\ (rapid)}$ (I_{Kr}) and $I_{K\ (slow)}$ (I_{Ks}). Two prominent components of I_K, referred to as I_{Kr} ($I_{K(rapid)}$) and I_{Ks} ($I_{K(slow)}$), were first distinguished in guinea pig atrial and ventricular myocytes (177–179). I_{Kr} activates and inactivates rapidly, displays marked inward rectification, and is selectively blocked by lanthanum and by several class III antiarrhythmics, including dofetilide, E-4031 and sotalol (177, 178). In contrast, no inward rectification is evident for I_{Ks}, and this conductance pathway is selectively attenuated by several class III antiarrhythmics, such as NE-10064 and NE-10133, that do not appear to affect I_{Kr} appreciably (38). At the microscopic level, I_{Kr} and I_{Ks} have also been distinguished: in symmetrical K⁺, the single-channel conductances of I_{Kr} and I_{Ks} channels are 10–13 and 3–5 pS, respectively (16, 95, 187, 211). Similar currents have been described in human atrial and ventricular myocytes (117, 220, 222), in canin (119, 210, 243), and rabbit (174, 211) ventricular cells and in canine Purkinje fibers (210). The time- and voltage-dependent properties (Table 15–1) suggest that I_{Kr} and I_{Ks} both contribute to the plateau and to the latter phase (3) of action potential repolarization (Fig. 15–1B). In some myocardial cells, however, only I_{Kr} or I_{Ks} is expressed. In guinea pig nodal cells, for example, only I_{Ks} is evident (9), whereas in feline (74), human (97), rat (162), ventricular myocytes and in rat atrial (162) and rabbit nodal (93, 98, 187) cells, only I_{Kr} is reported to be evident (Table 15–1). The detailed properties of the I_{Kr} and I_{Ks} currents, however, do vary somewhat in different preparations. Deactivation of I_{Kr} in rabbit atrioventricular nodal cells, for example, is significantly faster than in ventricular cells, an observation interpreted as suggesting differences in the underlying channel proteins (93).

$I_{K\ (ultra\text{-}rapid)}$ (I_{Kur}). In rat (32, 33), human (220, 221) and canine (243, 244) atrial myocytes, rapidly activating, non-inactivating K⁺ currents (Table 15–1) with time- and voltage-dependent properties quite different from I_{Kr} and I_{Ks} have also been described, and referred to as I_{ss} (steady-state), I_{sus} (*sus*tained), or I_{Kur} (*u*ltra-*r*apid). The similarities in the properties of the currents characterized in rat, human, and canine atrial myocytes, together with experimental findings demonstrating that the molecular correlates of the rat and human currents are the same (29, 68; see also later, under Molecular Correlates of Other Voltage-Gated Cardiac K⁺ Currents), however, suggests that these currents should all be referred to by the same name, I_{Kur} (Table 15–1). In guinea pig ventricular myocytes, a novel, 12–14 pS, K⁺-selective channel, referred to as I_{Kp}, has also been reported (242). I_{Kp} activates very rapidly on depolarization, does not inactivate and is sensitive to millimolar concentrations of Ba^{2+} (12). The properties of guinea pig I_{Kp} are very similar to the dog, human, and rat atrial currents, suggesting that I_{Kp} (Table 15–1) should probably also be referred to as I_{Kur}.

Other Delayed Rectifiers. In several cardiac cell types, additional components of I_K have been described (Table 15–1). In mouse ventricular and atrial myocytes, for example, two additional voltage-gated K⁺ currents, referred to as $I_{K(slow)}$ and I_{ss} (steady-state) have been identified (72, 87, 88, 123, 236, 237, 243). $I_{K(slow)}$ is a rapidly activating and slowly inactivating K⁺ current (Fig. 15–2) that is blocked effectively and selectively by micromolar concentrations of 4-AP (72, 123, 247), which do not affect $I_{to,f}$, $I_{to,s}$, or I_{ss} in the same cells (236, 237). The current, I_{ss}, remaining at the end of prolonged depolarizing voltage steps (Fig. 15–2A), in contrast, is slowly activating (Fig. 15–2B) and 4-AP insensitive (236, 237). Unlike $I_{to,f}$ and $I_{to,s}$, $I_{K,slow}$ and I_{ss} appear to be expressed in all mouse ventricular (Fig. 15–2A) and atrial myocytes (29, 87, 88, 236, 237).

In rat ventricular and atrial myocytes, there are also novel delayed rectifier K⁺ currents that have been referred to as I_K and $I_{K(slow)}$, respectively (Table 15–1), 10, 29, 32, 33). In addition to differences in inactivation kinetics, I_K and $I_{K(slow)}$ have distinct pharmacological properties: I_K, for example, is selectively blocked by tetraethylammonium (TEA; 10), whereas $I_{K(slow)}$ is blocked by millimolar concentrations of 4-AP (32, 33) and dendrotoxin (DTX; 206). Rat atrial $I_{K,slow}$ is distinct from mouse (atrial and ventricular) $I_{K,slow}$, which is DTX-insensitive (236). To make this point clearly, the slowly inactivating current in rat atrial myocytes is now referred to as $I_{K(DTX)}$ (Table 15–1). It also seems appropriate to suggest that, once the pore-forming α and accessory subunits contributing to the various types of voltage-gated K+ channels are determined, channel nomenclature might be changed to reflect the molecular composition(s) of the channels, rather than the kinetic or the pharmacological properties of the currents, as has been done in the past. For the present, however, the standard descriptions must remain (Table 15–1).

Cellular/Regional Heterogeneity in Voltage-Gated K+ Current Expression and Properties

Although the properties of $I_{to,f}$ (Table 15–1) in most cardiac cell types/species are similar, there are marked differences in current densities (see also Chapter 17). In rat and human, for example, $I_{to,f}$ density is higher in atrial, than in ventricular, myocytes (32, 33, 209). $I_{to,s}$ density is also significantly higher in rabbit atrial and Purkinje cells than in ventricular cells (51, 82). In the mouse, in contrast, the density of $I_{to,f}$ is greater in ventricular, than in atrial, myocytes (237). The density of $I_{to,f}$ also varies in sheep Purkinje fibers (212) and in different regions of the ventricles in canine (118, 120, 213), cat (79), ferret (36), human (144, 227), mouse (87, 236), and rat (47, 232) hearts. In canine and mouse myocardium, for example, $I_{to,f}$ density is significantly higher in right than in left ventricular myocytes (88, 213). In canine and human, $I_{to,f}$ density also varies through the thickness of the walls of the ventricles, being severalfold higher in epicardial and midmyocardial cells than in endocardial cells (120, 228). Differences in $I_{to,f}$ density are reflected in variations in action potential waveforms in Purkinje, ventricular, and atrial cells (14, 33, 47, 145, 212), most notably in the prominence of phase 1 repolarization (Fig. 15–1B).

In mouse, ferret, human, and rat ventricles, $I_{to,f}$ and $I_{to,s}$ are also differentially distributed (36, 87, 88, 144, 232, 236). As noted above, for example, $I_{to,s}$ is undetectable in myocytes isolated from right ventricle or from the apex of the left ventricle in the mouse (Fig. 15–2A), whereas cells from the septum express $I_{to,f}$ and $I_{to,s}$ or $I_{to,s}$ alone (187, 88, 236). The waveforms of the currents typically recorded in myocytes isolated from mouse right and left ventricles are shown in Figure 15–2A, illustrating the marked differences in peak outward K+ current densities, as well as the differential expression of $I_{to,f}$ and $I_{to,s}$. In contrast to $I_{to,f}$ and $I_{to,s}$, $I_{K(slow)}$ and I_{ss} are evident in all mouse ventricular (Fig. 15–2A; 87, 88, 236) and atrial (29a, 237) myocytes. Importantly, the kinetic properties of the currents ($I_{to,f}$, $I_{to,s}$, $I_{K(slow)}$, and I_{ss}) are similar in different cell types (Fig. 15–2B–D), suggesting that the molecular correlates of the underlying K+ channels are also the same (see later, under MOLECULAR CORRELATES OF FUNCTIONAL VOLTAGE-GATED K+ CHANNELS).

The densities of I_{Ks} and I_{Kr} in different myocardial cell types are also variable. In guinea pig, for example, I_{Ks} and I_{Kr} densities are two fold higher in atrial, than in ventricular, myocytes (178). In human ventricular myocytes and Purkinje fibers, however, I_{Kr} appears to be the major repolarizing K+ current (210). In canine heart, I_{Ks} density is higher in right, than in left ventricular, cells, whereas I_{Kr} densities are similar (213). I_{Ks} density is also higher in canine left ventricular epicardial and endocardial cells than in M-cells (119). In the guinea pig left ventricle, there are also regional differences in I_{Kr} and I_{Ks} expression (37, 126). In cells isolated from the (guinea pig) left ventricular free wall, for example, I_{Kr} density is higher in subepicardial, than in midmyocardial or subendocardial, myocytes (126). At the base of the (guinea pig) left ventricle, however, both I_{Kr} and I_{Ks} densities are significantly lower in endocardial, than in midmyocardial or epicardial cells (126). These differences in voltage-gated K+ current expression likely contribute importantly to the variations in action potential waveforms recorded in atrial and ventricular myocytes, as well as in cells isolated from different regions (apex versus base) and layers (epicardial, midmyocardial, and endocardial) of the atria and ventricles (Fig. 15–1), and to the normal spread of repolarization in the mammalian myocardium (6, 7, 14).

MOLECULAR DETERMINANTS OF VOLTAGE-GATED CARDIAC K+ CHANNELS

Voltage-Gated K+ Channel Pore-Forming α Subunits

Homologous Voltage-Gated (Kv) Subfamilies. The first voltage-gated K+ channel (Kv) pore-forming (α) subunit was cloned from the *Shaker* locus in *Drosophila* (105, 157, 165), and this was followed by the cloning of three homologous Kv α subunit subfamilies in *Drosophila*, referred to as *Shab*, *Shaw*, and *Shal* (39, 226). A number of vertebrate homologues were subsequently identified, and a terminology for referring to these subunits (44) has been adopted: K+ channel α subunit genes of the *Shaker*, *Shab*, *Shaw*, and *Shal* subfamilies are now referred to as Kv1.x, Kv2.x, Kv3.x, and Kv4.x, respectively (Table 15–2). In vertebrates, a number of members of each subfamily have been identified (48, 163, 166). Each of the Kv α subunit proteins has six transmembrane domains, a K+-selective pore region and a highly charged S4 domain (Fig. 15–3A) placing the Kv α subunits in the "S4 superfamily" of voltage-

TABLE 15–2. *Kvα Subunits: Relation to Functional Voltage-Gated Cardiac K⁺ Currents*

Family	Subunit	Activation*	Inactivation*	Blocker*†	Endogenous Current
Kv1 (*Shaker*)	Kv 1.1				
	Kv 1.2	Fast	Slow	4-AP, DTX	$I_{K(slow)}$(rat) ($I_{K,DTX}$)
	Kv 1.3				
	Kv 1.4	Fast	Slow	4-AP	$I_{to,s}$
	Kv 1.5	Fast	Slow	4-AP	I_{Kur}(human/rat) $I_{K(slow)}$(mouse)
	Kv 1.6				
	Kv 1.7	Fast	Fast	NTX	??
	Kv 1.8				
Kv2 (*Shab*)	Kv 2.1	Slow	Very slow	TEA, HaTx	$I_{K(slow)}$(mouse)
	Kv 2.2	Slow	Very slow	TEA	??
Kv3 (*Shaw*)	Kv 3.1	Fast	Slow	TEA	I_{Kur}(canine)
	Kv 3.2				
	Kv 3.3				
	Kv 3.4				
Kv4 (*Shal*)	Kv 4.1				
	Kv 4.2	Fast	Fast	4-AP, HaTx, HpTx	$I_{to,f}$
	Kv 4.3	Fast	Fast	4-AP, HpTx	$I_{to,f}$
Kv5	Kv 5.1	Coassemble with Kv2 subunits		—	??
Kv6–9					
egg family					
eag	eag				
elk	elk				
erg1	erg1	Moderate	Fast	E-4031	I_{Kr}(with mirp)
	erg2				
	erg3				
KvLQT1 family					
KCNQ1	KvLQT1	Very slow	Very, very slow	NE-10064	I_{Ks}(with mink)
KCNQ2					
KCNQ3					

*Properties determined for heterologously expressed subunits; detailed properties, however, do vary with expression system (see text).
☐ indicates cardiac expression; DTX = dendrotoxin; NTX = noxioustoxin; HaTX = hanatoxin; HpTX = heteropodatoxin.

gated ion channels (48, 99, 163, 166). In *Drosophila*, an important mechanism for generating functional K⁺ channel diversity is through alternative splicing (Fig. 15–3B) of transcripts (183). Although splicing (Fig. 15–3B) also occurs for some vertebrate Kv α subunits (48), considerably more diversity results from the presence of multiple members of each subfamily (Table 15–2). Importantly, heterologous expression of the various Kv α subunit cDNA/cRNA reveals voltage-gated K⁺-selective currents (Fig. 15–3C) with distinct time- and voltage-dependent properties. The fact that functional voltage-gated K⁺ channels comprise four α subunits

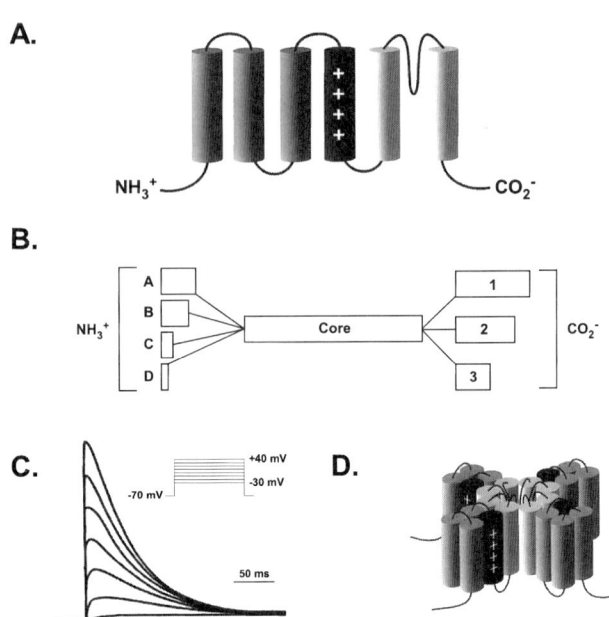

FIG. 15–3. Structure, expression and assembly of voltage-gated K$^+$ channel pore-forming (α) subunits. A: Voltage-gated K$^+$ channel α subunits are integral membrane proteins with six transmembrane domains, intracellular N- and C-termini, and a positively charged S4 region, placing them in the "S4 superfamily" of voltage-gated ion channels. B: Alternative splicing of Kv α subunits will give rise to proteins with novel N-and C-termini that produce voltage-gated K$^+$ currents with distinct properties. C: Voltage-gated outward K$^+$ currents are produced on heterologous expression of Kv α subunits. In some cases, such as Kv4.2 illustrated here, the currents are rapidly activating and inactivating. Outward K$^+$ currents with distinct time- and voltage-dependent properties are observed on heterologous expression of the various Kv1.x, Kv2.x, Kv3.x, and Kv4.x subfamily members. D: Schematic of a "functional" voltage-gated K$^+$ channel illustrating four Kv α subunits contributing to a K$^+$ selective pore.

(Fig. 15–3D) suggests that further diversity could arise through the formation of heteromultimeric channels between two or more Kv α subunit proteins in the same subfamily (52). Nevertheless, it has not been demonstrated directly to date that Kv α subfamily members coassemble in vivo to form functional heteromeric voltage-gated K$^+$ channels in the mammalian heart.

Several additional Kv α subunit subfamilies, Kv5.x through Kv9.x (Table 15–2), have also been identified (60, 94, 175). Although heterologous expression of these (Kv5.1, Kv6.1, Kv8.1, or Kv9.1) subunits alone does *not* reveal functional voltage-gated K$^+$ channels (42, 60, 94, 175), coexpression with Kv2.x (or Kv3.x) α subunits attenuates the amplitudes of the Kv2.x-(Kv3.x)-induced currents (175). These observations, together with sequence similarities (with the Kv2.x) subfamily), suggest that Kv5.1, Kv6.1, Kv8.1, and Kv9.1 may be more appropriately considered regulatory (Kv α) subunits of the Kv2.x subfamily (42) than distinct subfamilies (175). Of these subfamilies, to date only the Kv5.1 message has been shown to present in mammalian cardiac (ferret left ventricular) myocytes (35). The role of the Kv5.1 subunit (as well as subunits of the Kv6, Kv8, and Kv9 subfamilies) in the generation of functional cardiac K$^+$ channels, however, has not been explored directly. By analogy to the G protein–coupled inwardly rectifying K$^+$ channel (GIRK) pore forming α subunits (106), however, it certainly seems possible that the Kv5.x-Kv9.x subunits could be associated with other Kv (Kv2 or Kv3) α subunits in vivo and, further, that these subunits play roles in regulating post-translational processing and/or in the cell surface expression of functional voltage-gated K$^+$ channels. Further experiments aimed at testing this hypothesis directly are clearly warranted.

Ether-A-Go-Go-related Gene Subfamily. A homologous subfamily of the "S4 superfamily" of voltage-gated K$^+$ channel α subunit genes was revealed with the cloning of the *Drosophila ether-a-go-go (eag)* locus (225) and with the identification of the *eag*-like (ELK) and the *eag*-related (ERG) genes in mammals (224). The pore regions and the predicted membrane topologies of the *eag* (ELK and ERG) proteins are similar to the Kv α subunits (Fig. 15–3A). Importantly, ERG1 is the locus of mutations leading to one form of familial long QT syndrome, LQT2 (54), and heterologous expression of ERG1 reveals inwardly rectifying voltage-gated, K$^+$-selective currents (179, 201), similar to cardiac I_{Kr} (see later, under Molecular Genetics of Cardiac Delayed Rectifier K$^+$ Currents) Additional members of the ERG subfamily (ERG2 and ERG3) have been cloned from brain (Table 15–2), although these appear to be nervous system–specific and are not expressed in heart (186). Alternatively processed forms of ERG1, however, have been cloned from mouse and human heart cDNA libraries and postulated to contribute to cardiac I_{Kr} (112, 113, 121, 124). Biochemical evidence in support of this hypothesis, however, is lacking (162; see also, later, under Molecular Genetics of Cardiac Delayed Rectifier K$^+$ Currents).

KvLQT1 Subfamily. Another subfamily of voltage-gated K$^+$ channel α subunits was identified with the cloning of KvLQT1 (218), the locus of mutations in LQT1. Although heterologous expression of KvLQT1 alone reveals rapidly activating and noninactivating K$^+$ currents, coexpression with minK (see below) produces slowly activating K$^+$ currents that resemble cardiac I_{Ks} (17, 180). These findings were interpreted as suggesting that functional I_{Ks} channels are heteromeric (Fig. 15–4A), comprising the protein products of minK and KvLQT1 (17, 136, 180). Additional members of the

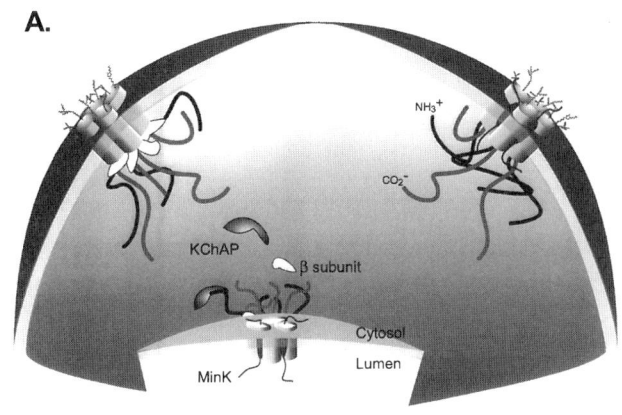

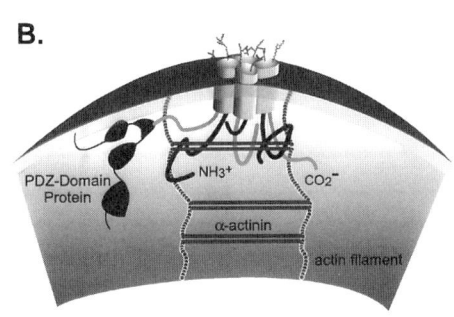

FIG. 15–4. Accessory subunits and the formation of functional voltage-gated K$^+$ channels. *A:* Putative membrane topology and subunit composition of voltage-gated K$^+$ myocardial channels with minK (miRP1) or accessory β subunits. Although Kv α and β subunits appear to associate in 1:1 ratios, the functional stoichiometry of minK- and KvLQT1-(or MiRP1-ERG1)-containing K$^+$ channels has not been defined. *B:* Representations of voltage-gated K$^+$ channel biogenesis and interactions with the cytoskeleton. Channel biosynthesis and assembly occur in the endoplasmic reticulum, and accessory β and regulatory KChAP (KChIP) subunits appear to play roles in mediating the biochemical maturation of functional voltage-gated K$^+$ channels, as well as in regulating the cell surface expression of these channels. In addition to associations with β subunits/minK and/or the KChAPs/KChIPs, it has recently been suggested that voltage-gated K$^+$ channel α subunits also interact directly with cytoskeletal proteins, including α-actinin-2 and PDZ-binding domain proteins that function to link the channels to the actin cytoskeleton.

KvLQT (KCNQ) subfamily, KCNQ2 and KCNQ3, have also been cloned from brain and identified as loci of mutations that lead to benign familial neonatal convulsions (26, 182, 216). Expression of either of these subunits in *Xenopus* oocytes produces slowly activating, non-inactivating K$^+$-selective currents that deactivate very slowly on membrane repolariztion (182, 216). The unique kinetic and pharmacological properties of the expressed currents led Wang and colleagues (216) to suggest that KCNQ2/KCNQ3 are the molecular correlates of functional neuronal M channels. Interestingly, the densities of the heterologously expressed K$^+$ currents are significantly higher when KCNQ2 and KCNQ3 are coexpressed than with the expression of either subunit alone, an observation interpreted as suggesting that functional M channels are heteromultimeric (216). Importantly, however, neither KCNQ2 nor KCNQ3 appears to be expressed in the heart (182, 216), suggesting that these subunits do not play roles in the generation of functional voltage-gated myocardial K$^+$ channels.

Accessory Subunits of Voltage-Gated K$^+$ Channels

Minimal K$^+$ Channel Subunits, minK, MiRP1. The potential for further functional voltage-gated K$^+$ channel diversity was revealed with the molecular cloning of minK (also called I_{sK}), which encodes a protein of 130 amino acids with a single membrane-spanning domain (73, 114, 140). Although heterologous expression of minK in *Xenopus* oocytes reveals voltage-gated K$^+$ channel currents (73, 85, 193, 218), subsequent work has revealed that the K$^+$ channels formed in oocytes injected with minK cRNA reflect coassembly (of minK) with the *Xenopus* homolog of KvLQT1 (Fig. 15–4A; 180). By itself, therefore, minK does not form functional voltage-gated K$^+$ channels. Rather, I_{sK} appears to coassemble with KvLQT1 to form functional cardiac I_{Ks} channels (17, 180; see also later, under Molecular Genetics of Cardiac Delayed Rectifier K$^+$ Currents). Similar to the heterogeneity in Kv α subunit proteins, it has been assumed that additional minK like peptides exist, and, recently, experimental support for this hypothesis has been provided with the identification of minK-related peptides like MiRP1 (1), that also associate with Kv α subunits to form functional voltage-gated K$^+$ channels.

Accessory β Subunits. Another type of voltage-gated K$^+$ channel accessory subunit was revealed with the biochemical identification (138) and subsequent molecular cloning (169), of low molecular weight ($\approx$45 kD) accessory β subunits in brain. Three homologous Kv β subunits, Kv $β_1$, Kv $β_2$, Kv $β_3$, have now been cloned, and alternatively spliced transcripts of Kv $β_1$ (Kv $β_{1.x}$) have been identified (48, 56, 166); of these, Kv $β_{1.2}$ and Kv $β_{1.3}$ are found in heart. In contrast to minK and MiRP1, the Kv β subunits are cytosolic (not integral membrane) proteins that interact with the intracellular domains of Kv α subunits in assembled voltage-gated K$^+$ channels in a 1:1 stoichiometry (48; Fig. 15–4A). Functional studies have revealed that β subunit coexpression can affect the time- and voltage-dependent properties of Kv α subunit-induced currents (2, 3, 43, 62, 63, 127, 137), as well as the cell-surface expression of functional voltage-gated K$^+$ channels (2, 3, 185). Because Kv α and β subunits coassemble in the endoplasmic reticulum (146), the observed increases in functional K$^+$ channel expression suggest that β subunits can affect channel assembly, processing, or stability and/or that they function as chaperon proteins (Fig. 15–4B).

Heterologous coexpression experiments and binding studies have suggested that Kv β$_1$ and Kv β$_2$ subunits interact only with the Kv 1 subfamily of α subunits (147, 166, 184), whereas Kv β$_3$ also interacts with Kv2 subfamily members (70). Coexpression of Kv β$_3$ with Kv2.1 (or Kv2.2) increases functional K$^+$ channel density without affecting the properties of the currents (70). Given the specificity in α subunit coassembly and in the associations between Kv1 (or Kv2) α subunits with Kv β subunits, it seems reasonable to suggest that there likely are additional Kv β subunits subfamilies, specific for the Kv3, Kv4, ERG, etc., subfamilies of Kv α subunits. It is important to emphasize that in spite of the presence and heterogeneity of accessory Kv β subunits and the clear specificity in Kv α–Kv β subunit interactions (in heterologous expression studies), the role of these (β) subunits in the generation of functional voltage-gated K$^+$ channels in the mammalian myocardium remains to be defined.

K$^+$ *Channel Associated Proteins, KChAPs.* Using a yeast two-hybrid screen, a novel K$^+$ channel regulatory protein, KChAP (for voltage-gated K$^+$ channel associated protein), was identified in heart (231). Sequence analysis of KChAP revealed a 574 amino acid protein with no transmembrane domains and no homology to Kv α or β subunits (231). Coexpression of KChAP with Kv2.1 (or Kv2.2) in *Xenopus* oocytes, however, markedly increases functional Kv2.x-induced current densities without measurably affecting the time- and/or the voltage-dependent properties of the currents (231). Like the effects of some Kv β subunits, therefore, KChAP influences functional Kv2.x channel cell surface expression, suggesting that KChAP functions as a chaperon protein (Fig. 15–4B). Yeast two-hybrid assays also revealed that KChAP interacts with the N-termini of Kv1.x α subunits, as well as with the C-termini of Kv β1.x subunits (231). In contrast to findings for Kv2.1, however, KChAP coexpression has no measurable effects on Kv1.5-induced currents in *Xenopus* oocytes (231). These results suggest either that KChAP and Kv1.5 do not associate in oocytes or, alternatively, that the interaction between KChAP and Kv1.5 is ineffective in influencing functional Kv1.5 K$^+$ channel expression. Biochemical experiments, using antibodies directed against KChAPs and Kv α subunits, will be required to define the in vivo partners of KChAP. In particular, it will be of interest to determine if there are additional Kv α subunits that interact with KChAP and if there are homologous, and perhaps subfamily-specific, KChAP homologues expressed in cardiac (and other) cells.

K$^+$ *Channel Interacting Proteins, KChIPs.* A yeast two-hybrid screen was also used to identify a distinct family of Kv channel interacting proteins (KChIPs) that bind to the (intracellular) N-terminus of Kv4 α subunits and modify the time- and voltage-dependent properties of the currents (5). Although three KChIPs have been identified in brain, only KChIP2 is detectable (at the message level) in heart (5). Sequence analysis revealed that the KChIPs share a high degree of homology with members of the recoverin family of Ca^{2+}-sensing proteins, particularly in the "core" regions of these proteins which contain multiple EF-hand-like domains (5). Although the KChIPs co-localize and co-immunoprecipitate with brain Kv4 α subunits, a direct association with Kv4 subunits in heart has not been demonstrated to date. Nevertheless, because the presence (and functioning) of accessory subunits of voltage-gated K$^+$ channels allows for further diversity in the properties of the expressed channels, as well as a mechanism for regulating functional cell surface expression, further studies aimed at examining KChIP expression and functioning in the mammalian myocardium are clearly warranted.

Voltage-Gated K$^+$ Channels and the Cytoskeleton

Considerable evidence has been accumulated recently, demonstrating that neurotransmitter receptors and ion channels are localized and anchored in mammalian neurons through interactions with cytoskeletal proteins (Fig. 15–4*B*), particularly members of the PSD-95/SAP-90 family of PDZ-binding proteins and α-actinin-2 (151, 197). Although the underlying molecular mechanisms are not as well understood as in the nervous system, there is also growing evidence for functional connections between the cytoskeleton, cardiac ion channels, and cardiac myocyte functioning. It has been shown, for example, that acute treatment of myocytes with cytochalasin D, which depolymerizes actin filaments, slows sodium current inactivation (128, 205). Recently, it has also been reported that sodium channel inactivation is slowed in ventricular myocytes isolated from mice with a targeted deletion in the ankyrin locus (45). Cytochalasin D treatment also reportedly alters the kinetics of Ca^{2+} transients (in rat ventricular myocytes), apparently through effects on the sarcoplasmic reticulum Ca^{2+} stores (204).

Myocardial ATP-sensitive K$^+$ channels also appear to be linked to and regulated by the cytoskeleton. Exposure to cytochalasin D, for example, accelerates the rundown of cardiac ATP-sensitive inwardly rectifying K$^+$ channels, whereas actin filament stabilizers inhibit rundown (80). Subsequent studies have suggested that cytochalasin exerts its effects by interfering with the sulfonylurea receptor-mediated regulation of the I$_{KATP}$ channels (34, 241). The rectification and the Ca^{2+} (but not Mg^{2+}) sensitivity of the inwardly rectifying (I$_{K1}$) channels in cardiac cells are also affected by treatment with cytochalasin D (132), an observation that is interpreted as suggesting that cytoskeletal interactions play a role(s) in the modulation, as well as the regulation, of myocardial ion channels. The first suggestion that voltage-gated cardiac K$^+$ channels might also be linked to the cytoskeleton was provided very recently in studies reported by Fedida and colleagues (55, 129). Using a yeast two-hybrid screen, it was shown that members of three subfamilies of voltage-gated K$^+$ channel α subunits, Kv1.5, Kv2.1, and Kv4.2, bind to α-actinin-2 (129). In addition, heterologously expressed Kv1.5 and α-actinin can be immunoprecipitated, and the functional cell surface expression of Kv1.5 channels expressed in HEK-293 cells is reduced by cytochalasin B or D (129; 55). These observations suggest that studies focused on examining the role of α-actinin-2 in controlling the properties and the functional expression of voltage-gated cardiac K$^+$ currents will be of interest. A schematic of the possible interactions between α-actinin-2 K$^+$ channels and the actin cytoskeleton is presented in Figure 15–4B. Recently, it was also suggested that GIRK channels interact with integrin (134), suggesting that K$^+$ channel expression and functioning may also be linked to the extracellular matrix. Although clearly in the very early stages, it seems reasonable to suggest that the link between the cytoskeleton (as well, perhaps, as the extracellular matrix) in the regulation of ion channel expression, localization, and functioning has been made. Further experiments aimed at exploring the role of the cytoskeleton and the extracellular matrix in regulating cardiac K$^+$ channel distribution and functioning, as well as those focused on probing the underlying molecular mechanisms mediating these actions, are clearly warranted.

MOLECULAR CORRELATES OF FUNCTIONAL VOLTAGE-GATED K$^+$ CHANNELS

The cloning of cardiac K$^+$ channel pore-forming α subunits and accessory (β, minK, MiRP1, KChIP, KChAP) subunits has made it possible to focus efforts on understanding the molecular basis of voltage-gated K$^+$ channel diversity in the mammalian heart, and considerable progress has been made in understanding the relationships between the various Kvα subunits and the functional voltage-gated K$^+$ channels expressed in cardiac cells (Table 15–2).

Molecular Genetics of Cardiac Delayed Rectifier K$^+$ Currents, I$_{Kr}$ and I$_{Ks}$

ERG1 and MiRP1 Underlie I$_{Kr}$. As noted above, ERG1 was identified as the locus of one form of long QT syndrome, LQT2 (54), and expression of ERG1 in *Xenopus* oocytes reveals voltage-gated, inwardly rectifying K$^+$-selective channels that are similar to the rapid component of delayed rectification, I$_{Kr}$, in cardiac cells (179; 201). These observations were interpreted as revealing that ERG1 is the molecular correlate of functional cardiac I$_{Kr}$ channels (179). Interestingly, however, antisense oligodeoxynucleotides (AsODNs) targeted against I$_{sK}$ (minK) attenuate I$_{Kr}$ in AT-1 (an atrial tumor line) cells (239). In addition, it has been shown that heterologously expressed human ERG1 and I$_{sK}$ co-immunoprecipitate (133). These observations suggested the interesting possibility that functional I$_{Kr}$ channels might be multimeric, comprising the protein products of ERG1 and I$_{sK}$ (133, 239). More recent work, however, has shown that ERG1 also coassembles with a homologue of minK, MiRP1, to produce I$_{Kr}$ channels, suggesting that a MiRP1 *does* play a role in the generation of cardiac I$_{Kr}$ channels (1, 136).

Alternatively processed forms of ERG1, with unique N- and C-termini, have also been cloned from mouse and human heart (112, 113, 121, 124). Based on heterologous coexpression studies, the N-terminal variants were suggested to play a role in the generation of functional I$_{Kr}$ channels (113, 121). More recent Western blot analysis of ERG1 expression in the myocardium, however, has revealed that only full-length ERG1 proteins are detected in rat, mouse, and human heart (atria and ventricles), observations interpreted as revealing that the N-terminal alternatively spliced ERG1 variants do not contribute to the formation of functional cardiac I$_{Kr}$ channels (162).

KvLQT1 and minK Underlies I$_{Ks}$. Heterologous expression of KvLQT1, the locus of mutations leading to LQT1 (218), in *Xenopus* oocytes reveals rapidly activating, non-inactivating voltage-gated K$^+$-selective currents (17, 180). Co-expression of KvLQT1 with minK, however, produces slowly activating K$^+$ currents similar to I$_{Ks}$ (17, 180). These observations, together with biochemical data demonstrating that heterologously expressed KvLQT1 and minK associate (17), have been interpreted as suggesting that minK coassembles with KvLQT1 (Fig. 15–4A) to form functional cardiac I$_{Ks}$ channels (17, 180). The fact that mutations in the transmembrane domain of minK alter the properties of the channels produced on heterologous expression minK further suggests that the transmembrane segment of minK contributes to the K$^+$-selective pore of functional cardiac I_{Ks} channels (85, 191, 193, 218). Although these results have been interpreted as revealing that minK is a structural component of I_{Ks} channels (191), direct biochemical evidence for coassembly of KvLQT1 and minK in the mammalian heart has not been provided to date, and the (KvLQT1:minK) stoichiometry of functional I_{Ks} channels is not known. In addition, the functional role of N terminal splice variants of KvLQT1, which exert a dominant negative effect on heterologously expressed full-length KvLQT1 (100), in the generation of functional cardiac I_{Ks} channels in vivo remains to be determined.

Transgenic and Targeted Gene Deletion Approaches

Kv4.2/Kv4.3 α Subunits Underlie $I_{to,f}$. Heterologous expression of three of the voltage-gated K$^+$ channel α subunits cloned from heart and brain (Table 15–2), Kv1.4 (49, 160, 170, 194, 203), Kv4.2 (15, 27, 170), and Kv4.3 (59) reveals rapidly activating, 4-AP-sensitive K$^+$ currents that qualitatively resemble cardiac transient outward K$^+$ currents. Because Kv1.4 was cloned first and from several species (49, 160, 194, 203), this subunit, either as a homomultimer (194, 203), as a heteromultimer with other Kv1.x subunits (161, 172), was considered the likely candidate for the fast cardiac transient outward K$^+$ current, now referred to as $I_{to,f}$ (Table 15–1). The finding (in rat) that the Kv4.2 message varies through the thickness of the ventricular wall, however, led Dixon and McKinnon (58) to postulate that Kv4.2, rather than Kv1.4, underlies rat ventricular $I_{to,f}$. Consistent with this hypothesis, Kv4.2 protein expression in rat heart is high, whereas Kv1.4 is barely detectable (19, 235).

Considerable experimental evidence has now been provided documenting a role for Kv α subunits of the Kv4 subfamily in the generation of cardiac $I_{to,f}$. Fiset et al. (71), for example, reported that $I_{to,f}$ is attenuated in rat ventricular myocytes exposed to antisense oligodeoxynucleotides (AsODNs) targeted against Kv4.2 or Kv4.3. Reductions in rat ventricular $I_{to,f}$ density have also been observed in cells exposed to adenoviral constructs encoding a truncated Kv4.2 subunit (Kv4.2ST) that functions as a dominant negative (102). In rat atrial myocytes, exposure to a Kv4.2 AsODN attenuates $I_{to,f}$ selectively, whereas a Kv4.3 AsODN is without effect, suggesting that Kv4.2 and Kv4.3 do not coassemble in rat atria in vivo (29). These observations also suggest a molecular explanation for the differences in the kinetic properties of rat atrial and ventricular $I_{to,f}$ (10, 33), i.e., that both Kv4.2 and Kv4.3 contribute to rat ventricular $I_{to,f}$, whereas only Kv4.2 contributes to rat atrial $I_{to,f}$ (29, 71); Nevertheless, it remains to be demonstrated directly that Kv4.2 and Kv4.3 actually associate to form heteromeric $I_{to,f}$ channels in rat ventricles in vivo.

Recently, an in vivo experimental strategy in transgenic mice was developed to test directly the hypothesis that Kv4 α subunits also underlie (mouse ventricular) $I_{to,f}$ and to examine the functional consequences of the elimination of $I_{to,f}$ (20). For this purpose, a pore mutant of Kv4.2 (Kv4.2W362F) was generated that functions as a dominant negative (20). No currents are observed on heterologous expression of Kv4.2W262F alone, and coexpression of Kv4.2W362F with wild-type Kv4.2 or Kv4.3 markedly attenuates the currents produces by the wild-type Kv4 α subunits alone (20). Importantly, coexpression of Kv4.2W362F is without effects on the currents produced by subunits of other Kv α subfamilies (20). Transgenic mice expressing this construct driven by the α-myosin heavy chain (α-MHC) promoter (to direct cardiac-specific expression of the transgene) were generated, and electrophysiological studies on ventricular myocytes randomly dispersed from these animals revealed that $I_{to,f}$ is eliminated (Fig. 15–5) and that ventricular action potential durations and QT intervals are prolonged significantly (20). Subsequent studies have revealed that $I_{to,f}$ is eliminated in all left ventricular (apex, base, and septum) cells, as well as in atrial cells and in right ventricular myocytes from the Kv4.2W362F-expressing transgenics (20, 87, 237).

The results summarized above reveal that Kv4 α subunits underlie $I_{to,f}$ in mouse and rat atrial and ventricular myocytes. Given that the properties of $I_{to,f}$ in other cells (Table 15–1) are similar, if not identical, to mouse and rat $I_{to,f}$, it seems reasonable to speculate that members of the Kv4 subfamily of α subunits also underlie $I_{to,f}$ in other species (Table 15–2). In larger animals (such as dog and human), the candidate subunit is Kv4.3 because Kv4.2 appears not to be expressed (58). Consistent with this hypothesis, it has recently been reported that $I_{to,f}$ densities are reduced in human atrial myocytes exposed to AsODNs targeted against Kv4.3 (223). Interestingly, two splice variants of Kv4.3 have been identified in human (111), as well as in rat (156, 192), heart. At the message level the longer version of Kv4.3 contains a 19 amino acid insert in the carboxy tail, and appears to more abundant in both rat and human (111, 156, 192) heart than the short form of Kv4.3. Neither the relative expression levels of the two Kv4.3 proteins nor the contributions of these subunits to the generation of functional cardiac $I_{to,f}$ channels, however, has yet been determined.

Kv1.4 Underlies $I_{to,s}$. As noted above, the transient outward K$^+$ currents in rabbit myocytes are distinct from

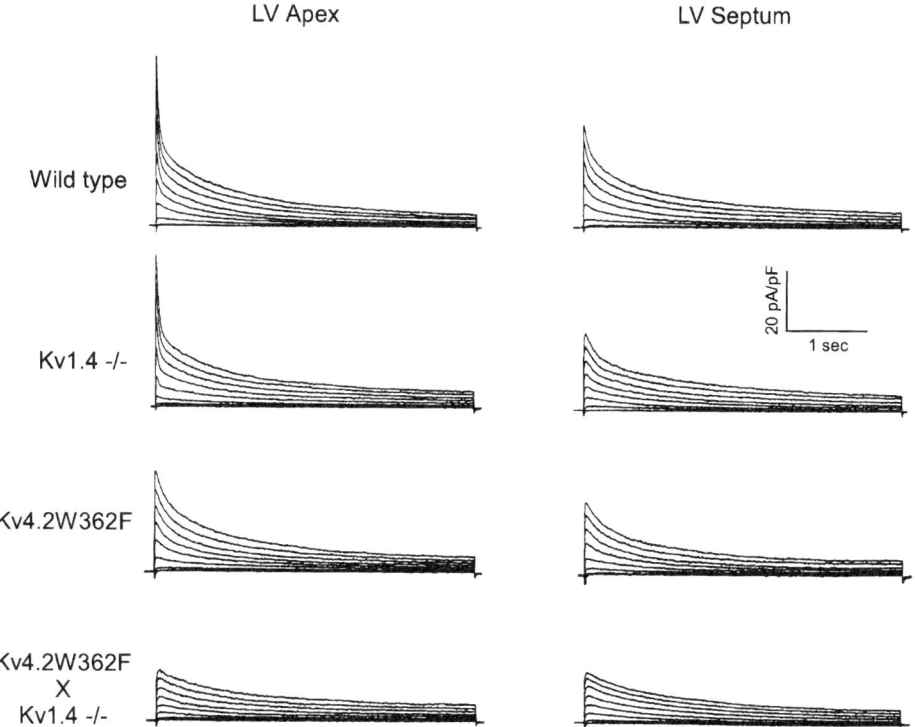

FIG. 15–5. Molecular genetic dissection of the transient outward K^+ currents $I_{to,f}$ and $I_{to,s}$ in mouse ventricular myocytes. Representative outward K^+ current waveforms recorded from adult C57BL6 mouse left ventricular (LV) apex and septum cells in response to 4.5 sec depolarizing voltage steps to −20 to +50 mV from a holding potential of −70 mV (compare with Fig. 15–2A). Records from wild-type, Kv4.2W362F-expressing, Kv1.4-/-and Kv4.2W362F × Kv1.4-/-LV cells are displayed. Expression of Kv4.2W362F results in the loss of $I_{to,f}$, whereas targeted deletion of Kv1.4 eliminates $I_{to,s}$. Both $I_{to,f}$ and $I_{to,s}$, however, are absent in cells from the Kv4.2W362F × Kv1.4-/-crossed animals, and the waveforms of the outward currents in LV apex and septum (from these animals) are indistinguishable. [Adapted from data in Guo et al. (87, 88).]

those of $I_{to,f}$ in that inactivation and recovery from steady-state inactivation are slow (46, 69, 82). The (transient K^+) currents in rabbit cells are similar to $I_{to,s}$ in mouse left ventricular septum cells (87, 236), suggesting that the currents in rabbit myocytes should also be referred to as $I_{to,s}$ (Table 15–1). The observation that the properties of rabbit $I_{to,s}$ are similar to those of heterologously expressed Kv1.4 (49, 159, 203), led to the suggestion that Kv1.4 could play a role in the generation of $I_{to,s}$ in the rabbit heart (152). Support for this hypothesis was provided in experiments focused on examining the effects of AsODNs targeted against Kv1.4 (and other Kv α subunits) on the outward K^+ currents in rabbit (and human) atrial myocytes. These experiments revealed that rabbit atrial $I_{to,s}$ is attenuated in cells exposed to the Kv1.4 AsODN, whereas human atrial $I_{to,f}$ is unaffected (223). In addition, $I_{to,s}$ is absent (87) in myocytes isolated from the left ventricular septum of mice (Fig. 15–5) with a targeted deletion in the Kv1.4 gene (Kv1.4-/-animals) (124). Taken together, these results demonstrate that the molecular correlates of mouse $I_{to,f}$ and $I_{to,s}$ are distinct and that Kv1.4 underlies $I_{to,s}$ in rabbit atrial (223) and mouse left ventricular septum (87) cells. The time- and voltage-dependent properties of the transient outward K^+ currents in ferret left ventricular epicardial and endocardial myocytes are distinct, and there are regional differences in the expression of Kv1.4 and Kv4.2/Kv4.3 (36). These observations have led to the suggestions that Kv1.4 and Kv4.2/Kv4.3 underlie $I_{to,s}$ and $I_{to,f}$ in ferret left ventricular endocardial and epicardial myocytes, respectively (36). Further experiments will be necessary to test these hypotheses directly.

In experiments completed on ventricular myocytes isolated from Kv4.2W362F-expressing transgenic animals, a "novel" rapidly activating, slowly inactivating current was reportedly evident (20). Subsequent experiments revealed that this novel current is only upregulated in left ventricular apex cells isolated from Kv4.2W362F-expressing animals; the currents in Kv4.2W362F-expressing septum cells are indistinguishable from those in wild septum cells lacking $I_{to,f}$ (87).

In addition, the properties of this novel current in Kv4.2W362F-expressing cells were shown to be similar to $I_{to,s}$ in wild-type left ventricular septum cells (Fig. 15-2), suggesting that the novel current is $I_{to,s}$ and that this current is upregulated in left ventricular apex cells in Kv4.2W362F-expressing transgenic animals. Taken together with the demonstration that Kv1.4 underlies $I_{to,s}$ in wild-type septum cells (87), these results further suggested that the presence of this current might reflect the upregulation of Kv1.4. To test this hypothesis directly, Kv4.2W362F was expressed in Kv1.4-/-mice. Electrophysiological recordings from ventricular myocytes isolated from these animals did indeed reveal that both $I_{to,f}$ and $I_{to,s}$ are eliminated (Fig. 15-5), confirming that Kv1.4 ($I_{to,s}$) is upregulated in left ventricular apex cells from Kv4.2W362F-expressing transgenic mice (87).

Molecular Correlates of Other Voltage-Gated Cardiac K⁺ Currents

Kv1.5 Underlies Human and Rat I_{Kur}. Heterologous expression of Kv1.5 in *Xenopus* oocytes reveals outward K⁺ currents with time- and voltage-dependent properties similar to the ultrarapid component of cardiac delayed rectification, I_{Kur} (Table 15-1; 33, 67, 206, 220, 221, 243, 244). These observations and the fact that the Kv1.5 message (58, 172, 194) and protein (19, 131) are abundant in heart led to the hypothesis that Kv1.5 underlies I_{Kur} (19, 67, 131, 206, 221, 244). Direct support for this hypothesis was provided in experiments demonstrating that human atrial I_{Kur} is selectively attenuated in cells exposed to AsODNs targeted against Kv1.5, whereas AsODNs against Kv1.4 were without effects (68). Rat atrial I_{Kur} is also selectively reduced following treatment with Kv1.5 AsODNs, whereas AsODNs targeted against Kv1.2, Kv.2.1, Kv4.2, Kv4.3, and KvLQT1 are without effects on rat atrial I_{Kur} (29). Although similar approaches could be exploited to test the hypothesis that Kv1.5 also underlies I_{Kp} (I_{Kur}) in guinea pig ventricular (12, 242) myocytes, as well as in other cardiac cells, it has recently been reported that Kv1.5 does not contribute to canine I_{Kur} (150). Rather, a role for Kv3.1 in the generation of canine I_{Kur} has recently been suggested (150).

Kv1.5 and Kv2.1 Contribute to Mouse $I_{K(slow)}$. A role for Kv1 α subunits in the generation of $I_{K,slow}$ in mouse ventricular myocytes was suggested by London and colleagues (123) in studies completed on transgenic mice expressing a truncated Kv1.1 α subunit, *Kv1.1N206Tag*, which functions as a dominant negative. Electrophysiological recordings from ventricular myocytes isolated from these animals revealed that $I_{K(slow)}$ is selectively attenuated (123). Detailed analysis of the outward K⁺ currents in mouse ventricular myocytes, however, suggests the presence of two components of $I_{K(slow)}$ (236). In addition, mouse ventricular $I_{K(slow)}$ (as well as I_{ss}) is blocked by TEA, suggesting a contribution from Kv α subunits of the Kv 2 subfamily. To test this hypothesis directly, a mutant Kv2.1 α subunit (Kv2.1N216) was designed to produce a truncated protein (containing the intracellular N-terminus, the S1 membrane-spanning domain, and a portion of the S1/S2 loop) that functions as a dominant negative (237). Electrophysiological recordings from ventricular myocytes isolated from Kv2.1N216FLAG-expressing transgenics revealed that $I_{K(slow)}$ is selectively reduced (237). The attenuation of $I_{K(slow)}$ is accompanied by marked action potential prolongation and, occasionally, spontaneous triggered activity (237).

Analysis of the decay phases of the outward currents in Kv2.1N216FLAG-expressing ventricular cells revealed that the density of $I_{K(slow)}$ is significantly lower than in wild-type cells. Importantly, however, and in contrast to the reported effects of *Kv1.1N206Tag* expression (124), $I_{K(slow)}$ was *not* eliminated in Kv2.1N216-expressing ventricular myocytes (237). Rather, the TEA-sensitive component of $I_{K(slow)}$ is selectively eliminated in Kv2.1N216FLAG-expressing ventricular myocytes; the component of $I_{K(slow)}$ sensitive to micromolar concentration of 4-AP remains (238). These observations are consistent with the suggestions (above) that there are two components of $I_{K(slow)}$ in mouse ventricular myocytes and that Kv2 α subunits underlie the slower, TEA-sensitive component.

Kv1.2 Underlies Rat Atrial $I_{K,DTX}$. Recent studies have shown that $I_{K(slow)}$ ($I_{K(DTX)}$) in rat atrial myocytes is selectively attenuated following exposure to AsODNs targeted against Kv1.2 (29). These observations demonstrate directly that (rat atrial) $I_{K(slow)}$ ($I_{K(DTX)}$) is a unique molecular entity, distinct from both (rat atrial) $I_{to,f}$ and I_{Kur}. As noted above, it has also been demonstrated AsODNs targeted against Kv1.5 specifically and selectively affect only I_{Kur} in rat atrial myocytes (29). The simplest interpretation of these findings is that Kv1.2 and Kv1.5 do not coassemble to form heteromultimeric K⁺ channels in rat atria in vivo.

FUNCTIONAL CONSEQUENCES OF IN VIVO ALTERATIONS IN VOLTAGE-GATED MYOCARDIAL K⁺ CHANNELS

QT Prolongation

As noted above, mutations in KvLQT1 and ERG1 are linked to inherited forms of long QT syndromes LQT1 and LQT2 (136, 176, 179, 180, 201, 234).

Electrocardiographic recordings from patients with these inherited, as well as idiopathic, Long QT syndromes are characterized by marked prolongation of QT intervals (Fig. 15–1C), and the propensity to develop cardiac arrhythmias, often leading to syncope and sudden death (176, 234). These observations suggest prominent roles for I_{Ks} and I_{Kr} in action potential repolarization in the human heart. In transgenic mice expressing an LQT2-associated mutation in ERG1 (G628S), however, QT intervals are not increased significantly compared with those measured in nontransgenic littermates (11). Although I_{Kr} is eliminated in ventricular myocytes isolated from ERG1G628S-expressing transgenics and abnormalities in the morphologies of the QRS and T waves were occasionally observed (11), the lack of effect (of ERG1G628S expression) on QT intervals suggests that I_{Kr} does not play a prominent role in (ventricular repolarization) in the mouse myocardium. Although these observations clearly demonstrate the potential limitations of using mice to study cardiac rhythm abnormalities, recent studies have documented pronounced effects on QT intervals in mice in which the functional expression of other repolarizing K^+ currents has been manipulated (20, 88, 123, 237).

In ECG recordings from *Kv1.1N260Tag*-expressing transgenics, for example, QT intervals are markedly prolonged (123). In Kv4.2W362F-expressing transgenic mice lacking functional $I_{to,f}$ channel expression, QT intervals are also significantly prolonged (Fig. 15–6) compared with wild-type, non-transgenic littermates (20), demonstrating a prominent role for $I_{to,f}$ in ventricular repolarization in the mouse. Representative telemetric ECG records obtained from wild-type,

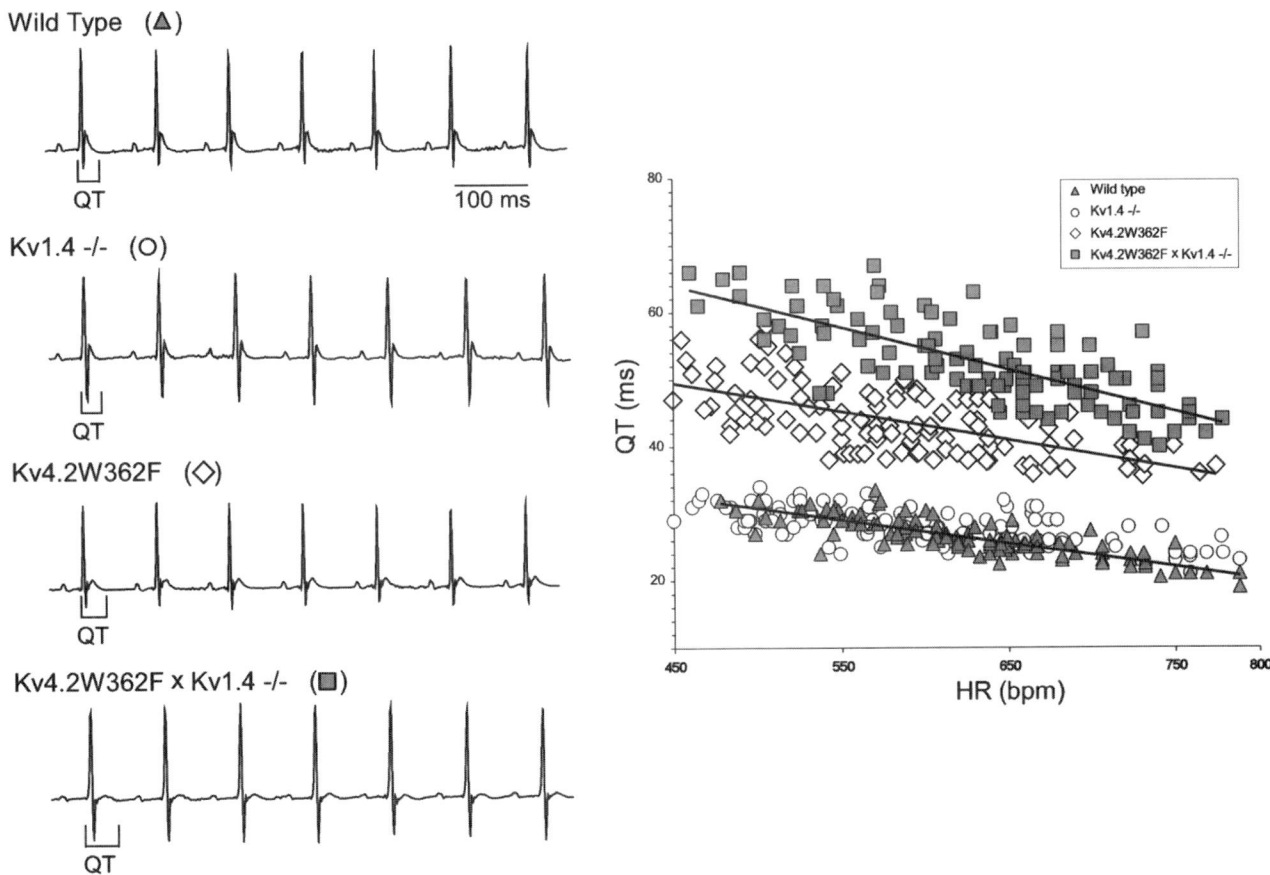

FIG. 15–6. QT prolongation in mice lacking $I_{to,f}$, $I_{to,s}$, or both $I_{to,f}$ and $I_{to,s}$. Telemetric ECG recordings were obtained from conscious adult C57BL6 mice with the phenotypes indicated. QT intervals were determined using cursors, one placed at the beginning of the QRS complex and the other placed where the T wave voltage crosses the baseline. As is evident in the *left panel*, the QT interval is markedly prolonged in Kv4.2W362F × Kv1.4-/-mice compared with wild-type Kv1.4-/-or Kv4.2W362F-expressing animals. Average QT intervals and heart rates in individual (3 min) recording episodes were determined, and each point is represented (*right panel*). The variation in the observed QT intervals with heart rate in wild-type, Kv4.2W362F-Kv1.4-/-and Kv4.2W362F × Kv1.4-/-animals are plotted in the *right panel*. As expected, QT intervals vary with heart rate and must be corrected (QTc) for differences in rates (see text). The difference between Kv4.2W362F-expressing and Kv4.2W362F × Kv1.4-/-mice is evident over a wild range of heart rates. [Records adapted from Guo et al. (87, 88).]

Kv1.4-/-, Kv4.2W362F-expressing, and Kv4.2W362F × Kv1.4-/-mice are presented in Figure 15–6. As demonstrated previously, QT intervals are significantly longer in Kv4.2W362F-expressing than in wild-type animals, whereas QT intervals in the Kv1.4-/- animals are not significantly different from controls (Figure 15–6; 88). There is a marked prolongation of the QT intervals in Kv4.2W362F × Kv1.4-/- animals when compared with wild-type, the Kv1.4-/- or Kv4.2W362F-expressing mice. In all animals, QT intervals correlate with heart rate, and the differences in QT intervals in the Kv4.2W362F × Kv1.4-/- and Kv4.2W362F-expressing mice are evident over a wide range of heart rates. When QT intervals (QTc) were corrected for heart rate (135), the differences between Kv4.2W362F × Kv1.4-/- and Kv4.2W362F transgenic animals remain highly significant (88).

In vivo telemetric recordings have also revealed marked QT prolongation in Kv2.1N216-expressing animals (237). Interestingly, however, the action potential and QT prolongation in the Kv2.1N216FLAG-expressing ventricular cells is substantially less than that observed in Kv4.2W362F-expressing mouse ventricular myocytes, which lack $I_{to,f}$ (20). These observations demonstrate that selective effects on different repolarizing K$^+$ currents will have distinct functional consequences.

Atrioventricular Block

Consistent with the absence of $I_{to,f}$ and $I_{to,s}$, action potentials recorded from Kv4.2W362F × Kv1.4-/- ventricular cells are prolonged significantly relative to action potentials in Kv4.2W362F-expressing ventricular cells (88). As noted above, the elimination of both $I_{to,f}$ and $I_{to,s}$ also results in more profound prolongation of the QT intervals compared with Kv4.2W362F-expressing transgenics (20). The increases in action potential duration seen in Kv4.2W362F × Kv1.4-/- ventricular cells and the QT prolongation in the Kv4.2W362F × Kv1.4-/- animals are also greater than those seen in either Kv1.1N206Tag-expressing mice (122) or mice expressing a dominant-negative truncated Kv2 α subunit, Kv2.1N216, in which $I_{K,slow}$ is also attenuated (238).

In addition to the pronounced effect on QT intervals, other ECG abnormalities were observed in in vivo telemetric recordings from the Kv4.2W362F × Kv1.4-/- animals (88). Mobitz type I second-degree atrioventricular block (Fig. 15–7A) and high-degree atrioventricular block with multiple sequential dropped beats, for example, were observed in ECG recordings (Fig. 15–7B) from these animals (88). Although atrioventricular block has never been seen in recordings from wild-type or in Kv1.4-/- animals, Mobitz type I second-degree atrioventricular block was observed in one (of five) Kv4.2W362F-expressing mice, 2 of 22 recording episodes (88).

Atrioventricular block has recently been reported in KvLQT1-deficient transgenic mice, suggesting a functional importance of KvLQT1 K$^+$ channels in murine atrioventricular conduction (11). Nevertheless, the molecular mechanism responsible for the development of atrioventricular block in the Kv4.2W362F × Kv1.4-/- animals remains unclear. These observations could reflect secondary effects due to loss of atrial $I_{to,f}$ and ventricular $I_{to,f}$ and $I_{to,s}$ or, alternatively, direct effects on AV nodal cells. In addition, the findings that atrioventricular block is only prominent in the Kv4.2W362F × Kv1.4-/- animals suggest that electrical remodeling (i.e., upregulation of Kv1.4 or some other subunits resulting from the absence of $I_{to,f}$ may also occur in the (atrioventricular) conducting system in Kv4.2W362F-expressing mice. The upregulation of $I_{to,s}$ in AV nodal cells, therefore is protective, and elimination of both $I_{to,f}$ and $I_{to,s}$ significantly interrupts the atrioventricular conduction. Clearly, experiments aimed at detailing the electrophysiological properties of voltage-gated K$^+$ channels, especially the $I_{to,f}$ and $I_{to,s}$ channels, in the murine atrioventricular conduction system will be of considerable interest.

Ventricular Arrhythmia/Tachycardia

Electrocardiographic recordings from *Kv1.1N206Tag*-expressing animals also revealed an increased frequency of premature ventricular beats ventricular arrhythmias (Figure 15–7C), and spontaneous ventricular tachyarrhythmias (13b, 123). Spontaneous ventricular arrhythmias are not seen, however, in the Kv4.2W362F-expressing transgenics (20, 88), although action potential durations and QT intervals are prolonged to a greater extent in the Kv4.2W362F-expressing transgenics (20) than in the *Kv1.1N206Tag*-expressing transgenics (123). Taken together, these results suggest the interesting possibility that factors, in addition prolonged ventricular repolarization, play an important role in determining the propensity to develop and to sustain arrhythmias.

Ventricular tachycardia was observed, however, in EGG recordings from one of the Kv4.2W362F × Kv1.4-/- animals (Fig. 15–7D). No evidence of ventricular arrhythmias has ever been obtained in wild-type, Kv1.4-/-, or Kv4.2W362F-expressing mice (20, 88, 122). In contrast to the effects of expression of Kv4.2W362F (and the loss of $I_{to,f}$) or the deletion of Kv1.4 (and the elimination of $I_{to,s}$) alone, therefore, elimination of both $I_{to,f}$ and $I_{to,s}$ in Kv4.2W362F × Kv1.4-/- animals has profound pathophysiological consequences. These observations suggest that the upre-

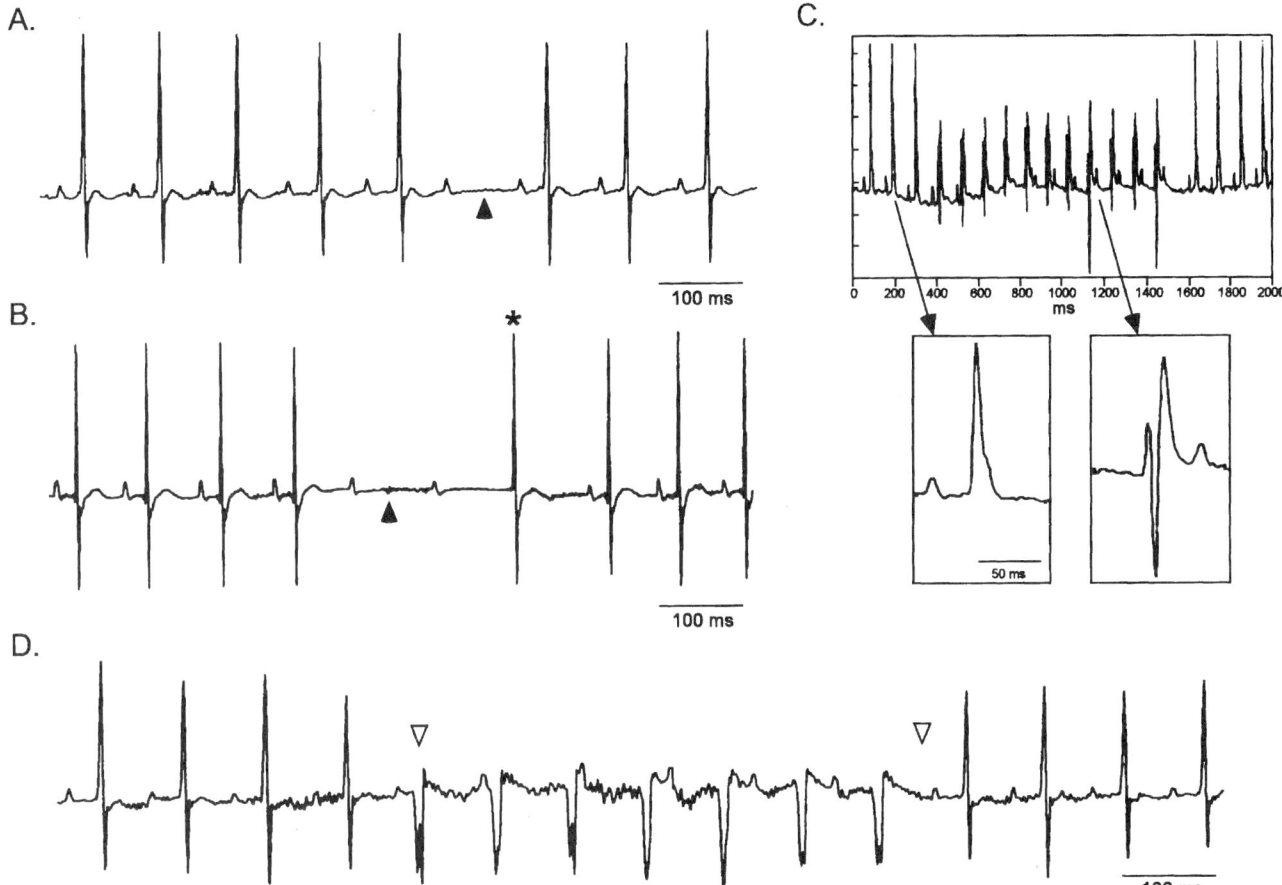

FIG. 15-7. Functional consequences of changes in repolarizing voltage-gated K⁺ currents. Atrioventricular block (*A, B*) and ventricular tachycardia (*C, D*) are evident in mice in which functional voltage-gated K⁺ channel densities have been manipulated. Recordings illustrated were from Kv4.2W362F × Kv1.4-/- (*A, B, D*) and *Kv1.1N206Tag*-(*C*) expressing animals. *A*: Recordings from a Kv4.2W362F × Kv1.4-/- mouse showing Mobitz type I second-degree atrioventricular block, and occasionally (*B*) high-degree atrioventricular block with multiple sequential dropped beats. *B*: Note that the QRS complex (*indicated by the* *) was generated by the subsidiary pacemaker. *C*: Surface EGG recording of an 11-beat run of ventricular tacchycardia in a *Kv1.1N206Tag*-expressing adult mouse. The sinus rate here was 530 beats per minute, and the rate of the ventricular tacchycardia was 570 beats per minute. *D*: Telemetric recording of a 7-beat run of ventricular tacchycardia in a Kv4.2W362F × Kv1.4-/- mouse. In both *C* and *D*, note the widened QRS complexes during nonsustained ventricular taccycardia. [Adapted from original data presented in London et al. (122; *C*) and Guo et al. (88; *A, B, D*).

gulation of Kv1.4 α subunit (and $I_{to,s}$) protects the mouse heart from the arrhythmogenic effects of loss of $I_{to,f}$ in Kv4.2W362F-expressing animals and that elimination of this upregulated $I_{to,s}$ in the Kv4.2W362F × Kv1.4-/- animals results in dramatic functional consequences.

Pathophysiology

In contrast to the marked electrophysiological consequences of expression of mutant Kv α subunits that function as dominant negatives and the resulting losses of functional voltage-gated K⁺ currents, in most cases, there appear not to be any detectable cardiac (or other) effects of these manipulations in the various lines of mice generated and studied to date (11, 20, 123, 237, 238). Heart weights, body weights, and heart to body weight ratios, for example, appear to be well within normal ranges, and no changes in the gross appearances of the heart or of isolated cardiac myocytes are evident in the *Kv1.1N206Tag*-, the Kv4.2W362F-, or the Kv2.1N216-expressing transgenic animals. Similarly, no deleterious effects have been reported in the hearts of mice with a targeted deletion of the Kv1.4 gene (122) or, more recently, of the Kv1.5 gene (124b). In transgenic mice expressing a mutant ERG1 subunit (G628S), a modest enlargement of the hearts of female animals was noted, although no pathophysiological consequences of the increased size of the heart were reported (11).

A recent report from Wickenden and colleagues (233), however, suggested profound functional consequences of cardiac specific expression of a truncated Kv4.2 α subunit (Kv4.2N). Blood pressure, for example, is elevated and contractility is enhanced in the Kv4.2N-expressing animals. In contrast to the findings on myocytes from Kv4.2W362F-expressing transgenics, $I_{to,f}$ density is reduced (*not* eliminated) and action potentials are prolonged only in a subset of ventricular myocytes isolated from young (2–3-week-old) Kv4.2N-expressing animals (233). The reason(s) for the marked heterogeneity in the functional consequences of transgene expression in Kv4.2N-expressing animals is presently unclear. Perhaps more surprising is the observation that, when the Kv4.2N-expressing transgenics age, there are profound changes in the myocardium, including hypertrophy, chamber dilation, and interstitial fibrosis (233). By 10–12 weeks of age, the Kv4.2N-expressing animals display clinical and hemodynamic features of congestive heart failure and increased incidence of sudden death (233). Electrophysiological recordings from myocytes isolated from older animals revealed marked reductions in $I_{to,f}$ and I_{K1} densities. Although these results were interpreted as suggesting that the functional consequences of manipulating voltage-gated K^+ current expression and/or action potential waveforms leads to profound changes in contractile functioning, this seems unlikely to be correct in light of the results obtained with the other transgenic animals as well as those with targeted deletions in specific Kv α subunit genes (20, 87, 88, 122, 123, 237, 238).

SUMMARY, CONCLUSIONS, AND FUTURE DIRECTIONS

Electrophysiological studies have clearly documented the expression of multiple types of voltage-gated K^+ channels in cardiac cells isolated from different species, as well as cardiac cells isolated from different regions of the heart in the same species (Table 15–1). In addition, most (mature) mammalian myocardial cells express a (stable) repertoire of voltage-gated K^+ channels that contribute importantly to shaping the waveforms of action potentials, as well as influencing automaticity and refractoriness. Molecular cloning studies have revealed an unexpected diversity of voltage-gated K^+ channel pore-forming (α) and accessory (e.g. minK, β KChIP) subunits in the myocardium, and a variety of in vitro and in vivo experimental approaches have been exploited to probe the relationship(s) between these subunits and the functional voltage-gated K^+ channels in myocardial cells. Important insights into these relationships have been provided through molecular genetics and the application of techniques that allow functional K^+ channel expression to be manipulated in vitro and in vivo, and the results of these efforts have led to the identification of the Kvα subunits contributing to the formation of most of the voltage-gated K^+ channels expressed in cardiac cells (Table 15–2). Although the roles of minK and MiRP1 in the generation of functional myocardial K^+ channels have been suggested, very little is known about the involvement and/or the functioning of these or other accessory subunits, including β subunits, KChAPs or KChIPs, as well as the various cytoskeletal elements, in the generation and the functioning of myocardial K^+ channels. Exploring the role of these proteins will certainly be an important focus of future research efforts.

Numerous studies have documented changes in the functional expression of voltage-gated K^+ channels and K^+ channel-forming α subunits in the heart during normal (fetal and postnatal) development, as well as in the damaged or diseased myocardium. Importantly, it has also been shown that electrical remodeling occurs in the mammalian heart, presumably in direct response to changes in cardiac electrical activity or cardiac output, and most of these changes can be attributed to alterations in the expression and/or the properties of voltage-gated K^+ channel/currents. Although there are numerous possible (transcriptional, translational, and post-translational) mechanisms that could be involved in regulating the expression and the properties of functional voltage-gated cardiac K^+ channels, very little is presently known about the underlying molecular mechanisms that are important in mediating the changes in channel expression evident during normal development, as well as in conjunction with myocardial damage, disease and/or electrical remodeling. Clearly, a major focus of future research will be on exploring these mechanisms in detail.

The author thanks several of the past and present members of her laboratory who have contributed importantly to the understanding of the molecular basis of functional myocardial K^+ channels diversity: Drs. Michael Apkon, Dianne M. Barry, Elias Bou-Abboud, Walter A. Boyle, Sylvain Brunet, Weinong Guo, Huilin Li, Amber L. Pond, and Haodong Xu. The author also thanks Mr. Andrew Benedict, Ms. Bridget Scheve, and Ms. Rebecca Hood for their expert technical assistance in many aspects of the research effort in her laboratory. Work in the author's laboratory cited here has been supported by grants from the National Heart, Lung and Blood Institute of the National Institutes of Health, the Monsanto/Searle/Washington University Biomedical Research Agreement, and the National Office and the Midwest Affiliate of the American Heart Association.

REFERENCES

1. Abbott, G. W., F. Sesti, I. Splawski, M. E. Lehmann, K. W. Timothy, M. T. Keating, and S. A. Goldstein. MiRP1 forms I_{Kr} potassium channels with HERG and is associated with cardiac arrhythmia. *Cell* 97:175–187, 1999.

2. Accili, E. A., J. Kiehn, Q. Yang, Z. Wang, A. M. Brown, and B. A. Wible. Separable Kv-beta subunit domains alter expression and gating of potassium channels. *J. Biol. Chem.* 272:25824–25831, 1997.
3. Accili, E. A., J. Kiehn, B. A. Wible, and A. M. Brown. Interactions among inactivating and noninactivating Kv-beta subunits, and Kv-alpha-1.2, produce potassium currents with intermediate inactivation. *J. Biol. Chem.* 272:28232–28236, 1997.
4. Amos, G. J., E. Wettwer, F. Metzger, Q. Li, H. M. Himmel, and U. Ravens. Differences between outward currents of human atrial and subepicardial ventricular myocytes. *J. Physiol, (Lond)* 491:31–50, 1996.
5. An, W. F., M. R. Bowlby, M. Betty, J. Cao, H. P. Ling, G. Mendoza, J. N. Hinson, K. I. Mattson, B. W. Strassle, J. S. Trimmer, and K. J. Rhodes. Modulation of A-type potassium channels by a family of calcium sensors. *Nature* 403:553–556, 2000.
6. Antzelevitch, C., S. Sicouri, A. Lukas, V. V. Nesterenko, D.-W Liu, and J. M. Didiego. Regional differences in the electrophysiology of ventricular cells: physiological implications. In: *Cardiac Electrophysiology: From Cell To Bedside*, edited by D. P. Zipes and J. Jalife. Philadelphia: W. B. Saunders, 1994:228–245.
7. Antzelevitch, C., W. Shimizu, G. X. Yan, S. Sicouri, J. Weissenburger, V. V. Nesterenko, A. Burashnikov, J. Di Diego, J. Saffitz, and G. P. Thomas. The M cell: its contribution to the ECG and to normal and abnormal electrical function of the heart. *J. Cardiovasc. Electrophysiol.* 10:1124–1152, 1999.
8. Anumonwo, J. M. B., L. C. Freeman, W. M Kwok, and R. S. Kass. Potassium channels in the heart: electrophysiology and pharmacological regulation. *Cardiovasc. Drug Rev.* 9:299–316, 1991.
9. Anumonwo, J. M. B., L. C. Freeman, W. M. Kwok, and R. S. Kass. Delayed rectification in single cells isolated from guinea pig sinoatrial node. *Am. J. Physiol.* 262 (*Heart Circ. Physiol.* 31):H921–H925, 1992.
10. Apkon, M., and J. M. Nerbonne. Characterization of two distinct depolarization-activated K^+ currents in isolated adult rat ventricular myocytes. *J. Gen. Physiol.* 97:973–101, 1991.
11. Babij, P., G. R. Askew, B. Nieuwenhuijsen, C. M. Su, T. R. Bridal, B. Jow, T. M. Argentieri, J. Kulik, L. J. DeGennaro, W. Spinelli, and T. J. Colatsky. Inhibition of cardiac delayed rectifier K^+ current by overexpression of the long-QT syndrome HERG G628S mutation in transgenic mice. *Circ. Res.* 83:668–678, 1998.
12. Backx, P. H. and E. Marban. Background potassium current active during the plateau of the action potential in guinea pig ventricular myocytes. *Circ. Res.* 72:890–900, 1993.
13. Bailly, P., J. P. Bénitah, M. Mouchoniere, G. Vassort, and P. Lorente. Regional alteration of the transient outward current in human left ventricular septum during compensated hypertrophy. *Circulation* 96:1266–1274, 1997.
13b. Baker, L. C., B. London, B. R. Choi, G. Koren, and G. Salama. Enhanced dispersion of repolarization and refractoriness in transgenic hearts promotes reentrant ventricular tachycardia. *Circ. Res.* 86:396–407, 2000.
14. Balati, B., A. Varro and J. G. Papp. Pharmacological modification of the dispersion of repolarization in the heart: importance of M cells. *Cardiovasc. Drug Ther.* 13:491–505, 1999.
15. Baldwin, T. J., M.-L. Tsaur, G. A. Lopez, Y. N. Jan, and L. Y. Jan. Characterization of a mammalian cDNA for an inactivating voltage-sensitive K^+ channel. *Neuron* 7:471–483, 1991.
16. Balser, J. R., P. B. Bennett, and D. M. Roden. Time-dependent outward currents in guinea pig ventricular myocytes: gating kinetics of the delayed rectifier. *J. Gen. Physiol.* 96:835–863, 1990.
17. Barhanin, J., F. Lesage, E. Guillemare, M. Fink, M. Lazdunski, and G. Romey. KvLQT1 and IsK (minK) proteins associate to form the I_{Ks} cardiac potassium current. *Nature* 384:78–80, 1996.
18. Barry, D. M. and J. M. Nerbonne. Myocardial potassium channels: electrophysiological and molecular diversity. *Annu. Rev. Physiol.* 58:363–394, 1996.
19. Barry, D. M., J. S. Trimmer, J. P. Merlie, and J. M. Nerbonne. Differential expression of voltage-gated K^+ channel subunits in adult rat heart: relationship to functional K^+ channels. *Circ. Res.* 77:361–369, 1995.
20. Barry, D. M., H. Xu, R. B. Schuessler, and J. M. Nerbonne. Functional knockout of the transient outward current, long QT syndrome and cardiac remodelling in mice expressing a dominant negative Kv4α subunit. *Circ. Res.* 83:560–567, 1998.
21. Bénitah, J. P., A. M. Gomez, P. Bailly, J. P. Da Ponte, G. Berson, C. Delgado, and P. Lorente. Heterogeneity of the early outward current in ventricular cells isolated from normal and hypertrophied rat hearts. *J. Physiol. (Lond.)* 469:111–138, 1993.
22. Benndorf, K., and B. Nilius. Properties of an early outward current in single cells of the mouse ventricle. *Gen. Physiol. Biophys.* 7:449–466, 1988.
23. Benndorf, K., F. Markwardt, and B. Nilius. Two types of transient outward currents in cardiac ventricular cells of mice. *Pflugers Arch.* 409:641–643, 1987.
24. Berul, C. I., M. A. Aronovitz, P. J. Wang, and M. E. Mendelsohn. *In vivo* cardiac electrophysiology studies in the mouse. *Circulation* 94:2641–2648, 1996.
25. Beuckelmann, D. J., M. Näbauer, and E. Erdmann. Alterations in K^+ currents in isolated human ventricular myocytes from patients with terminal heart failure. *Circ. Res.* 73:379–385, 1993.
26. Biervert, C., B. C. Schroeder, C. Kubisch, S. F. Berkoviv, P. Propping, T. J. Jentsch, and O. K. Steinlein. A potassium channel mutation in neonatal human epilepsy. *Science* 279:403–405, 1998.
27. Blair, T. A., S. L. Roberds, M. M. Tamkun, and R. P. Hartshorne. Functional characterization of RK5, a voltage-gated K^+ channel cloned from the rat cardiovascular system. *FEBS. Lett.* 295:211–213, 1991.
28. Bosch, R. F., X. R. Zeng, J. B. Gramer, K. Popovic, C. Mewis, and V. Kuhlkamp. Ionic mechanisms of electrical remodelling in human atrial fibrillation. *Cardiovasc. Res.* 44:121–131, 1999.
29. Bou-Abboud, E. and J. M. Nerbonne. Molecular correlates of the Ca^{++}-independent depolarization-activated K^+ currents in adult rat atrial myocytes. *J. Physiol. (Lond.)* 517:407–420, 1999.
29a. Bou-Abboud, E., H. Li, and J. M. Nerbonne. Molecular diversity of the repolarizing voltage-gated K^+ currents in mouse atrial myocytes. *J. Physiol., Lond.* 529:345–358, 2000.
30. Boutjdir, M., J. Y. Le Heuzey, T. Lavergne, S. Chauvaud, L. Guize, A. Carpentier, and P. Peronneau. Inhomogeneity of cellular refractoriness in human atrium: factor of arrhythmia? *Pacing Clin. Electrophysiol.* 9:1095–1100, 1986.
31. Boyden, P. A. and C. D. Jeck. Ion channel function in disease. *Cardiovasc. Res.* 29:312–318, 1995.
32. Boyle, W. A. and J. M. Nerbonne. A novel type of depolarization-activated K^+ current in isolated adult rat atrial myocytes. *Am. J. Physiol.* 260 (*Heart Circ. Physiol.* 29):H1236–H1247, 1991.
33. Boyle, W. A. and J. M. Nerbonne. Two functionally distinct 4-aminopyridine-sensitive outward K^+ currents in adult rat atrial myocytes. *J. Gen. Physiol.* 100:1047–1061, 1992.
34. Brady, P. A., A. E. Alekseev, L. A. Aleksandrova, L. A. Gomez, and A. Terzic. A disrupter of actin microfilaments impairs sulfonylurea-inhibitory gating of cardiac KATP channels. *Am. J. Physiol.* 271 (*Heart Circ. Physiol.* 40):H2710–H2716, 1996.
35. Brahmajothi, M. V., M. J. Morales, S. Liu, R. L. Rasmusson, D. L. Campbell, and H. C. Strauss. *In situ* hybridization reveals extensive diversity of K^+ channel mRNA in isolated ferret cardiac myocytes. *Circ. Res.* 78:1083–1089, 1996.
36. Brahmajothi, M. V., D. L. Campbell, R. L. Rasmusson, M. J.

Morales, J. M. Nerbonne, and H. C. Strauss. Distinct transient outward potassium current (I_{to}) phenotypes and distribution of fast-inactivating potassium channel alpha subunits in ferret left ventricular myocytes. *J. Gen. Physiol.* 113:581–600, 1999.

37. Bryant, S. M., X. P. Wan, S. J. Shipsey, and G. Hart. Regional differences in the delayed rectifier currents (I_{Kr} and I_{Ks}) contribute to the differences in action potential duration in basal left ventricular myocytes in guinea pig. *Cardiovasc. Res.* 40:322–331, 1998.

38. Busch, A. E., K. Malloy, W. J. Groh, M. D. Varnum, J. P. Adelman, and J. Maylie. The novel class III antiarrhythmics NE-10084 and NE-10133 inhibit I_{sK} channels expressed in *Xenopus* oocytes and I_{Ks} in guinea pig ventricular myocytes. *Biochem. Biophys. Res. Commun.* 202:265–270, 1994.

39. Butler, A., A. Wei, K. Baker, and L. Salkoff. A family of putative potassium channel genes in *Drosophila*. *Science* 243:943–947, 1989.

40. Campbell, D. L., R. L. Rasmusson, M. B. Comer, and H. C. Strauss. The calcium-independent transient outward potassium current in isolated ferret right ventricular myocytes. I. Basic characterization, and kinetic analysis. *J. Gen. Physiol.* 101:571–601, 1993.

41. Campbell, D. L., R. L. Rasmusson, M. B. Comer, and H. C. Strauss. The cardiac calcium-independent transient outward potassium current: kinetics, molecular properties, and role in ventricular repolarization. In: *Cardiac Electrophysiology: From Cell to Bedside*. 2nd ed., edited by D. P. Zipes and J. Jalife. Philadelphia: W. B. Saunders, 1995:83–96.

42. Castellano, A., M. D. Chiara, B. Mellströ, A. Molina, F. Monje, J. R. Naranjo, and J. Lopez-Barneo. Identification and functional characterization of a K⁺ channel α subunit with regulatory properties specific to brain. *J. Neurosci.* 17:4652–4661, 1997.

43. Castellino, R. C., M. J. Morales, H. C. Strauss, and R. L. Rasmusson. Time- and voltage-dependent modulation of a Kv1.4 channel by a β subunit (Kvβ3) cloned from ferret ventricle. *Am. J. Physiol.* 268 (*Heart Circ. Physiol.* 37):H385–H391, 1995.

44. Chandy, K. G., and G. A. Gutman. Voltage-gated K⁺ channel genes, in: *Handbook of Receptors and Channels*, edited by (R. A. North. Boca Raton, FL: CRC Press, 1995:1–71.

45. Chauhan, V. S., S. Tuvia, M. Buhusi, V. Bennett, and A. D. Grant. Abnormal cardiac Na⁺ channel properties and QT heart rate adaptative in neonatal arkyrin B knockout mice. *Circ. Res.* 86:441–447, 2000.

46. Clark, R. B., W. R. Giles, and Y. Imaizumi. Properties of the transient outward current in rabbit atrial cells. *J. Physiol. (Lond.)* 405:147–168, 1988.

47. Clark, R. B., R. A. Bouchard, E. Salinas-Stefanson, J. Sanchez-Chalupa, and W. R. Giles. Heterogeneity of action potential waveforms and potassium currents in rat ventricle. *Cardiovasc. Res.* 27:1795–1799, 1993.

48. Coetzee, W. A., Y. Amarillo, J. Chiu, A. Chow, D. Lau, T. McCormack, H. Moreno, M. S. Nadal, A. Ozaita, D. Pountney, M. Saganich, E. Vega-Saenz de Meira, and B. Rudy. Molecular diversity of K⁺ channels. *Ann. N.Y. Acad. Sci.* 868:233–285, 1999.

49. Comer, M. B., D. L. Campbell, R. L. Rasmusson, D. R. Lamson, M. J. Morales, Y. Zhang, and H. C. Strauss. Cloning and characterization of an I_{to}-like potassium channel from ferret ventricle. *Am. J. Physiol.* 267 (*Heart Circ. Physiol.* 36):H1388–H1395, 1994.

50. Coraboeuf, E. and E. Carmeliet. Existence of two transient outward currents in sheep Purkinje fibers. *Pflugers Arch.* 392:352–359, 1982.

51. Cordeiro, J. M., K. W. Spitzer, and W. R. Giles. Repolarizing K⁺ currents in rabbit heart Purkinje cells. *J. Physiol. (Lond.)* 508:811–823, 1998.

52. Covarrubias, M., A. Wei, and L. Salkoff. *Shaker, Shal, Shab*, and *Shaw* express independent K⁺ current systems. *Neuron* 7:763–773, 1991.

53. Covarrubias, M., A. Wei, L. Salkoff, and T. B. Vybas. Elimination of rapid potassium channel inactivation by phosphorylation of the inactivation gate. *Neuron* 13:1403–1412, 1994.

54. Curran, M. E., I. Splawski, K. W. Timothy, G. M. Vincent, E. D. Green, and M. T. Keating. A molecular basis for cardiac arrhythmia: *herg* mutations cause long QT syndrome. *Cell* 80:795–803, 1995.

55. Dan, P., B. Au, D. Fedida, and E. D. W. Moore. Colocalization of Kv1.5 and α-actinin-2 in HEK-293 cells, and disruption by cytochalasin D. *Biophys. J.* 78:425A, 2000.

56. Deal, K. K., S. K. England, and M. M. Tamkun. Molecular physiology of cardiac potassium channels. *Physiol. Rev.* 76:49–67, 1996.

57. Deck, K. A., and W. Trautwein. Ionic currents in cardiac excitation. *Pflugers Arch.* 280:63–80, 1964.

58. Dixon, J. E. and D. McKinnon. Quantitative analysis of mRNA expression in atrial and ventricular muscle of rats. *Circ. Res.* 75:252–260, 1994.

59. Dixon, J. E., W. S. Shi, H. S. Wang, C. McDonald, H. Yu, R. S. Wymore, I. S. Cohen, and D. McKinnon. The role of the Kv4.3 K⁺ channel in ventricular muscle. A molecular correlate for the transient outward current. *Circ. Res.* 79:659–668, 1996.

60. Drewe, J. A., S. Verma, G. Frech, and R. L. Joho. Distinct spatial and temporal expression patterns of K⁺ channel mRNAs from different subfamilies. *J. Neurosci.* 12:538–548, 1992.

61. Dudel, J., K. Peper, R. Rudel, and W. Trautwein. The dynamic chloride component of membrane current in Purkinje fibers. *Pflugers Arch.* 295:197–212, 1967.

62. England, S. K., V. N. Uebele, H. Shear, K. Kodali, P. B. Bennett, and M. M. Tamkun. Characterization of a K⁺ channel beta subunit expressed in human heart. *Proc. Natl. Acad. Sci. U.S.A.* 92:6309–6313, 1995.

63. England, S. K., V. N. Uebele, K. Kodali, P. B. Bennett, and M. M. Tamkun. A novel K⁺ channel beta subunit (hKvβ1.3) is produced via alternative mRNA splicing. *J. Biol. Chem.* 270:28531–28534, 1995.

64. Escande, D., A. Coulombe, J. F. Faivre, E. Deroubaix, and E. Corabouef. Two types of transient outward currents in adult human atrial cells. *Am. J. Physiol.* 252 (*Heart Circ. Physiol.* 21):H142–H148, 1987.

65. Faivre, J. F., T. P. G. Calmels, S. Rouanet, J. L. Javre, B. Cheval, and A. Bril. Characterization of Kv4.3 in HEK-293 cells: Comparison with the rat ventricular transient outward potassium current. *Cardiovasc. Res.* 41:188–199, 1999.

66. Fedida, D., and W. R. Giles. Regional variations in action potentials and transient outward current in myocytes isolated from rabbit left ventricle. *J. Physiol. (Lond.)* 442:191–209, 1991.

67. Fedida, D., B. Wible, Z. Wang, B. Fermini, F. Faust, S. Nattel, and A. M. Brown. Identity of a novel delayed rectifier current from human heart with a cloned K⁺ channel current. *Circ. Res.* 73:210–216, 1993.

68. Feng, J., B. Wible, G. R. Li, Z. Wang, and S. Nattel. Antisense oligonucleotides directed against Kv1.5 mRNA specifically inhibit ultrarapid delayed rectifier K⁺ current in cultured adult human atrial myocytes. *Circ. Res.* 80:572–579, 1997.

69. Fermini, B., Z. Wang, D. Duan, and S. Nattel. Differences in rate dependence of the transient outward current in rabbit and human atrium. *Am. J. Physiol.* 263 (*Heart Circ. Physiol.* 32):H1747–H1754, 1992.

70. Fink, M., F. Duprat, F. Lesage, C. Heurteux, G. Romey, J. Barhanin, and M. Lazdunski. A new K⁺ channel β subunit to specifically enhance Kv2.2 (CDRK) expression. *J. Biol. Chem.* 271:26341–26348, 1996.

71. Fiset, C., R. B. Clark, Y. Shimoni, and W. R. Giles. Shal-type

channels contribute to the Ca^{2+}-independent transient outward K$^+$ current in rat ventricle. *J. Physiol. (Lond.)* 500:51–64, 1997.

72. Fiset, C., R. B. Clark, T. S. Larsen, and W. R. Giles. A rapidly activating, sustained K$^+$ current modulates repolarization and excitation–contraction coupling in adult mouse ventricles. *J. Physiol. (Lond.)* 504:557–563, 1998.

73. Folander, K., J. S. Smith, J. Antanavage, C. Bennett, R. B. Stein, and R. Swanson. Cloning and expression of the delayed rectifier I$_{sK}$ channel from neonatal rat heart and diethylstilbestrol-primed rat uterus. *Proc. Natl. Acad. Sci. U.S.A.* 87:2975–2979, 1990.

74. Follmer, C. H. and T. J. Colatsky. Block of delayed rectifier potassium current, I$_K$, by flecainide and E-4031 in cat ventricular myocytes. *Circulation* 82:289–293, 1990.

75. Fozzard, H. A. and M. Hiraoka. The positive dynamic current and its inactivation properties in cardiac Purkinje fibres. *J. Physiol. (Lond.)* 234:569–586, 1973.

76. Freeman, L. C., and R. S. Kass. Delayed rectifier potassium channels in ventricle and sinoatrial node of guinea pig: molecular and regulatory properties. *Cardiovasc. Drugs Ther.* 7:627–635, 1993.

77. Freeman, L. C., L. M. Pacioretty, N. S. Moise, R. S. Kass, and R. F. Gilmour, Jr. Decreased density of I$_{to}$ in left ventricular myocytes from German Shepherd dogs with inherited arrhythmias. *J. Cardiovasc. Electrophysiol.* 8:872–883, 1997.

78. Furukawa, T., R. J. Myerburg, N. Furukawa, A. L. Bassett, and S. Kimura. Differences in transient outward currents of feline endocardial and epicardial myocytes. *Circ. Res.* 67:1287–1291, 1990.

79. Furukawa, T., S. Kimura, N. Furukawa, A. L. Bassett, and R. J. Myerburg. Potassium rectifier currents differ in myocytes of endocardial and epicardial origin. *Circ. Res.* 70:91–103, 1992.

80. Furukawa, T., T. Yamane, T. Terai, Y. Katayama, and M. Hiraoka. Functional linkage of the cardiac ATP-sensitive K$^+$ channel to the actin cytoskeleton. *Pflugers Arch.* 43:504–512, 1996.

81. Gadsby, D. C. Effects of β adrenergic catecholamines on membrane currents in cardiac cells. In: *Cardiac Electrophysiology: A Textbook*, edited by M. R. Rosen, M. J. Jansen, and A. L. Wit. Mt. Kisco, NY: Futura Publishing Co., 1990:857–876.

82. Giles, W. R., and Y. Imaizumi. Comparison of potassium currents in rabbit atrial and ventricular cells. *J. Physiol. (Lond.)* 405:123–145, 1988.

83. Giles, W. R., and A. C. Van Ginneken. A transient outward current in isolated cells from the crista terminalis of rabbit heart. *J. Physiol (Lond.)* 368:243–264, 1985.

84. Giles, W. R., R. B. Clark, and A. P. Braun. Ca^{2+}-independent transient outward current in mammalian heart. In: *Molecular Physiology and Pharmacology of Cardiac Ion Channels and Transporters*, edited by M. Morad, Y. Kurachi, A. Noma, and M. Hosada. Amsterdam: Kluwer, 1996:141–168.

85. Goldstein, S. A. and C. Miller. Site-specific mutations in a minimal voltage-gated K$^+$ channel alter ion selectivity and open channel block. *Neuron* 7:403–408, 1991.

86. Gomez, A. M., J.-P. Bénitah, D. Henzel, A. Vinet, P. Lorente, and C. Delgado. Modulation of electrical heterogeneity by compensated hypertrophy in rat left ventricle. *Am. J. Physiol.* 272 (*Heart Circ. Physiol.* 41):H1078–H1086, 1997.

87. Guo, W., H. Xu, B. London, and J. M. Nerbonne. Molecular basis of transient outward K$^+$ diversity in mouse ventricular myocytes. *J. Physiol. (Lond.)* 521:587–599, 1999.

88. Guo, W., H. Li, B. London, and J. M. Nerbonne. Functional consequences of elimination of I$_{to,f}$ and I$_{to,s}$: early afterdepolarizations, atrioventricular block and ventricular arrhythmias in mice lacking Kv1.4 and expressing a dominant negative Kv4 α subunit. *Circ. Res.* 87:73–79, 2000.

89. Himmel, H. M., E. Wettwer, Q. Li, and U. Ravens. Four different components contribute to outward current in rat ventricular myocytes. *Am. J. Physiol.* 277 (*Heart Cir. Physiol.* 46):H107–H1118, 1999.

90. Hiraoka, M., and S. Kawano. Calcium-sensitive and insensitive transient outward current in rabbit ventricular myocytes. *J. Physiol. (Lond.)* 410:187–212, 1989.

91. Honoré, E., B. Attali, G. Romey, C. Heurteaux, P. Ricard, F. Lesage, and M. Lazdunski. Cloning, expression, pharmacology and regulation of a delayed rectifier K$^+$ channel in mouse heart. *EMBO J.* 10:2805–2811, 1991.

92. Horie, M., S. Hayashi, and C. Kawai. Two types of delayed rectifying K$^+$ channels in atrial cells of guinea pig heart. *Jpn. J. Physiol.* 40:479–490, 1990.

93. Howarth, F. C., A. J. Levi, and J. C. Hancox. Characteristics of the delayed rectifier K current compared in myocytes isolated from the atrioventricular node and ventricle of the rabbit heart. *Pflugers Arch.* 431:713–722, 1996.

94. Hugnot, J. P., M. Salinas, F. Lesage, E. Guillemare, J. De Weile, C. Heurteaux, M. G. Mattei, and M. Lazdunski. Kv8.1, a new neuronal potassium channel subunit with specific inhibitory properties towards *Shab* and *Shaw* channels. *EMBO J.* 15:3322–3331, 1996.

95. Hume, J. R. and A. Uehara. Ionic basis of the different action potential configurations of single guinea-pig atrial and ventricular myocytes. *J. Physiol. (Lond.)* 368:525–544, 1985.

96. Inoue, M. and I. Imanaga. Masking of A-type K$^+$ channel in guinea pig cardiac cells by extracellular Ca^{++}. *Am. J. Physiol.* 264 (*Cell Physiol.* 33):C1434–C1438, 1993.

97. Iost, N., L. Virag, M. Opincariu, J. Szecsi, A. Varro, and J. G. Papp. Delayed rectifier potassium current in undiseased human ventricular myocytes. *Cardiovasc. Res.* 40:508–515, 1998.

98. Ito, H. and K. Ono. A rapidly activating delayed rectifier K$^+$ channel in rabbit sinoatrial node cells. *Am. J. Physiol.* 269 (*Heart Circ. Physiol.* 38):H443–H452, 1995.

99. Jan, L. Y., and Y. N. Jan. Structural elements involved in specific K$^+$ channel functions. *Annu. Rev. Physiol.* 54:537–555, 1992.

100. Jiang, M., J. Tseng-Crank, and G. N. Tseng. Suppression of slow delayed rectifier current by a truncated isoform of KvLQT1 cloned from normal human heart. *J. Biol. Chem.* 272:24109–24112, 1997.

101. Jing, J., T. Peretz, D. Singer-Lahat, D. Chikvashvili, W. B. Thornhill, and I. Lotan. Inactivation of a voltage-dependent K$^+$ channel by beta subunit modulation by a phosphorylation-dependent interaction between the distal C terminus of alpha subunit and cytoskeleton. *J. Biol. Chem.* 272:14021–14024, 1997.

102. Johns, D. C., H. B. Nuss, and E. Marban. Suppression of neuronal and cardiac transient outward currents by viral gene transfer of dominant-negative Kv4.2 constructs. *J. Biol. Chem.* 272:31598–31603, 1997.

103. Kääb, S., H. B. Nuss, N. Chiamvimonvat, B. O'Rourke, P. H. Pak, D. A. Kass, E. Marban, and G. F. Tomaselli. Ionic mechanism of action potential prolongation in ventricular myocytes from dogs with pacing-induced heart failure. *Circ. Res.* 78:262–273, 1996.

104. Kääb, S., J. Dixon, J. Duc, D. Ashen, M. Näbauer, D. J. Beuckelmann, G. Steinbeck, D. McKinnon, and G. F. Tomaselli. Molecular basis of transient outward potassium current down-regulation in human heart failure—a decrease in Kv4.3 mRNA correlates with a reduction in current density. *Circulation* 98:1383–1393, 1998.

105. Kamb, A., J. Tseng-Crank, and M. A. Tanouye. Multiple components of the *Drosophila Shaker* gene may contribute to potassium channel diversity. *Neuron* 1:421–430, 1988.

106. Kennedy, M. E., J. Nemeco, S. Corey, K. Wickman, and D. E. Clapham. GIRK 4 confers appropriate processing and cell sur-

face localization on G-protein-gated potassium channels. *J. Biol. Chem.* 274:2571–2582, 1999.
107. Kenyon, J. L. and W. R. Gibbons. Influence of chloride, potassium, and tetraethylammonium on the early outward current of sheep cardiac Purkinje fibers. *J. Gen. Physiol.* 73:117–138, 1979.
108. Kenyon, J. L. and W. R. Gibbons. 4-Aminopyridine and the early outward current of sheep cardiac Purkinje fibers. *J. Gen. Physiol.* 73:139–157, 1979.
109. Kodama, I., M. R. Bayett, M. R. Nikmaram, M. Yamamoto, H. Honjo, and R. Niwa. Regional differences in effects of E-4031 within the sinoatrial node. *Am. J. Physiol.* 276 (*Heart Circ. Physiol.* 45):H793–H802, 1999.
110. Konarzewska, H., G. A. Peeters, and M. C. Sanguinetti. Repolarizing K^+ currents in nonfailing human hearts: similarities between right-septal subendocardial and left epicardial ventricular myocytes. *Circulation* 92:1179–1187, 1995.
111. Kong, W., S. Po, T. Yamagishi, M. D. Ashen, G. Stetten, and G. F. Tomaselli. Isolation and characterization of the human gene encoding I_{to}: further diversity by alternative mRNA splicing. *Am. J. Physiol.* 275 (*Heart Circ. Physiol.* 44):H1963–H1970, 1998.
112. Kuperschmidt, S., D. Snyders, A. Raes, and D. Roden. A K^+ channel splice variant common in human heart lacks a C terminal domain required for expression of rapidly activating delayed rectifier current. *J. Biol. Chem.* 273:27231–27235, 1998.
113. Lees-Miller, J. P., C. Kondo, L. Wang and H. J. Duff. Electrophysiological characterization of an alternatively processed ERG K^+ channel in mouse and human hearts. *Circ. Res.* 81:719–726, 1997.
114. Lesage, F., B. Attali, M. Lazdunski, and J. Barhanin. I_{sK}, a slowly activating voltage-sensitive K^+ channel. Characterization of multiple cDNAs and gene organization in the mouse, *FEBS. Lett.* 301:168–172, 1992.
115. Levin, G., D. Chikvashvili, D. Singer-Lahat, T. Peretz, W. B. Thornhill, and I. Lotan. Phosphorylation of a K^+ channel alpha subunit modulates the inactivation conferred by a beta subunit. Involvement of cytoskeleton. *J. Biol. Chem.* 271:29321–29328, 1996.
116. Levitan, E. S. and K. Takimoto. Dynamic regulation of K^+ channel gene expression in differentiated cells. *J. Neurobiol.* 37:60–68, 1998.
117. Li, G. R., J. Feng, L. Yue, M. Carrier, and S. Nattel. Evidence for two components of delayed rectifier K^+ current in human ventricular myocytes. *Circ. Res.* 78:689–696, 1996.
118. Litovsky, S. H. and C. Antzelevitch. Transient outward current prominent in canine ventricular epicardium but not endocardium. *Circ. Res.* 72:1092–1103, 1988.
119. Liu, D.-W. and C. Antzelevitch. Characteristics of the delayed rectifier current (I_{Kr} and I_{Ks}) in canine ventricular epicardial, midmyocardial, and endocardial myocytes. *Circ. Res.* 76:351–365, 1995.
120. Liu, D.-W., G. A. Gintant, and C. Antzelevitch. Ionic basis for electrophysiological distinctions among epicardial, midmyocardial and epicardial myocytes. *Circ. Res.* 72:671–687, 1993.
121. London, B., M. C. Trudeau, K. P. Newton, A. K. Beyer, N. G. Copeland, D. J. Gilbert, N. A. Jenkins, C. A. Satler, and G. A. Robertson. Two isoforms of the mouse *ether-a-go-go-related* gene coassemble to form channels with properties similar to the rapidly activating component of the cardiac delayed rectifier K^+ current. *Circ. Res.* 81:870–878, 1997.
122. London, B., D. W. Wang, J. A. Hill, and P. B. Bennett. The transient outward current in mice lacking the potassium channel gene Kv1.4. *J. Physiol. (Lond.)* 81:870–878, 1998.
123. London, B., A. Jeron, J. Zhou, P. Buckett, X. Han, G. F. Mitchell, and G. Koren. Long QT and ventricular arrhythmias in transgenic mice expressing the N terminus and the first transmembrane segment of a voltage-gated potassium channel. *Proc. Natl. Acad. Sci., U.S.A.* 95:2926–2931, 1998.
124. London, B., E. Aydar, C. M. Lewarchik, J. S. Seibel, C. T. January, and G. A. Robertson. N- and C-terminal isoforms of HERG in the human heart. *Biophys. J.* 74:A26, 1998.
124b. London, B., W. Gno, X.-h. Pan, J. S. Lee, V. Shusterman, D. A. Logothetis, J. M. Nerbonne, and J. A. Hill. Targeted replacement of Kv1.5 in the mouse leads to loss of the 4-aminopyridine sensitive component of I_k, slow and resistance to drug-induced QT prolongation. *Circ Res.* 88: 940–946, 2001.
125. MacKinnon, R. Determination of the subunit stoichiometry of a voltage-activated potassium channel. *Nature* 350:232–235, 1991.
126. Main, M. C., S. M. Bryant, and G. Hart. Regional differences in action potential characteristics and membrane currents of guinea-pig left ventricular myocytes. *Exp. Physiol.* 83:747–761, 1998.
127. Majumder, K., M. Debiasi, Z. Wang, and B. Wible. Molecular cloning and functional expression of a novel potassium channel β subunit from human atrium. *FEBS Lett.* 361:13–16.
128. Maltsev, V. A. and A. I. Undrovinas. Cytoskeleton modulates coupling between availability and activation of cardiac sodium channel. *Am. J. Physiol.* 273 (*Heart Circ. Physiol.* 42):H1832–H1840, 1997.
129. Maruoka, N. D., B. Au, D. F. Steele, X. Zhang and D. Fedida. α-Actinin-2 couples cardiac Kv channels to the actin cytoskeleton and regulates current density. *Biophys. J.* 78:452a, 2000 (abstract).
130. Matsubara, H., E. R. Liman, P. Hess, and G. Koren. Pretranslational mechanisms determine the type of potassium channel expressed in the rat skeletal and cardiac muscles. *J. Biol. Chem.* 266:13324–13328, 1991.
131. Mays, D. J., J. M. Foose, L. H. Philipson, and M. M. Tamkun. Localization of the Kv1.5 K^+ channel protein in explanted cardiac tissue. *J. Clin. Invest.* 96:282–292, 1995.
132. Mazzanti, M., R. Assandri, A. Ferroni, and D. DiFrancesco. Cytoskeletal control of rectification and expression of four substates of cardiac inward rectifier K^+ channels. *FASEB. J.* 10: 357–361, 1996.
133. McDonald, T. V., Z. Yu, Z. Ming, E. Palma, M. B. Meyers, K. W. Wang, S. A. Goldstein, and G. I. Fishman. A minK-HERG complex regulates the cardiac potassium current $I_{(Kr)}$. *Nature* 388:289–292, 1997.
134. McPhee, J. C., X. L. Dang, N. Davidson, and H. A. Lester. Evidence for a functional interaction between integrins and G protein–activated inward rectifier K^+ channels. *J. Biol. Chem.* 273: 34696–34702, 1998.
135. Mitchell, G. F., A. Jeron, and G. Koren. Measurement of heart rate and Q-T interval in the conscious mouse. *Am. J. Physiol.* 274 (*Heart Circ. Physiol.* 43):H747–H751, 1998.
136. Mitcheson, J. S. and M. C. Sanguinetti. Biophysical properties and molecular basis of cardiac rapid and slow delayed rectifier potassium channels. *Cell. Physiol. Biochem.* 9:201–216, 1999.
137. Morales, M.J., R. C. Castellino, A. L. Crews, R. L. Rasmusson, and H. C. Strauss. A novel α subunit increases the rate of inactivation of specific voltage-gated potassium channel α subunits. *J. Biol. Chem.* 270:6272–6277, 1995.
138. Muniz, Z. M., D. N. Parcej, and J. O. Dolly. Characterization of monoclonal antibodies against voltage-dependent K^+ channels raised using α-dendrotoxin acceptors purified from bovine brain. *Biochemistry* 31:12297–12303, 1992.
139. Munk, A. A., R. A. Adjemian, J. Zhao, A. Ogbaghebriel, and A. Shrier. Electrophysiological properties of morphologically

distinct cells isolated from the rabbit atrioventricular node. *J. Physiol. (Lond.)* 493:801–818, 1996.
140. Murai, T., A. Kakizuka, T. Takumi, H. Ohkubo, and S. Nakanishi. Molecular cloning and sequence analysis of human genomic DNA encoding a novel membrane protein which exhibits slowly activating potassium channel activity. *Biochem. Biophys. Res. Commun.* 61:176–181, 1989.
141. Näbauer, M. Electrical heterogeneity in the ventricular wall and the M cell. *Cardiovasc. Res.* 40:248–250, 1998.
142. Näbauer, M and M. Kääb. Potassium channel down regulation in heart failure. *Cardiovasc. Res.* 37:324–334, 1998.
143. Näbauer, M., D. J. Beuckelmann, and E. Erdmann, Characteristics of transient outward current in human ventricular myocytes from patients with terminal heart failure. *Circ. Res.* 73: 386–394, 1993.
144. Näbauer, M., D. J. Beuckelmann, P. Überfuhr, and G. Steinbeck. Regional differences in current density and rate dependent properties of the transient outward current in subepicardial and subendocardial myocytes of human left ventricle. *Circulation* 93:168–177, 1996.
145. Näbauer, M., A. Barth, and S. Kääb. A second calcium-independent transient outward current present in human ventricular myocardium. *Circulation* 98:I-231, 1998.
146. Nagaya, N. and Papazian, D. M. Potassium channel alpha and beta subunits assemble in the endoplasmic reticulum. *J. Biol. Chem.* 272:3022–3027, 1997.
147. Nakahira, K., G. Shi, K. J. Rhodes, and J. S. Trimmer. Selective interaction of voltage-gated K$^+$ channel α subunits with β subunits. *J. Biol. Chem.* 271:7084–7089, 1996.
148. Nakayama, T. and H. Irisawa. Transient outward current carried by potassium and sodium in quiescent atrioventricular node cells of rabbits. *Circ. Res.* 57:65–73, 1985.
149. Nattel, S. Electrophysiological remodeling: are ion channels static players or dynamic movers? *J. Cardiovasc. Electrophysiol.* 10:1553–1556, 1999.
150. Nattel, S., L. Yue, and Z. Wang. Cardiac ultra rapid delayed rectifiers. A novel potassium current family of functional similarity and molecular diversity. *Cell Physiol. Biochem.* 9:217–226, 1999.
151. Nehring, R. B., E. Wishmeyer, F. Doring, R. W. Yeh, M. Sheng, and A. Karshin. Neuronal inwardly rectifying K$^+$ channels differentially coupled to PDZ proteins of the PSD-95/SAP90 family. *J. Neurosci.* 20:56–62, 2000.
152. Nerbonne, J. M. Regulation of voltage-gated K$^+$ channel expression in the developing mammalian myocardium. *J. Neurobiol.* 37:37–59, 1998.
153. Nuss, H. B. and E. Marban. Electrophysiological properties of neonatal mouse cardiac cells in primary culture. *J. Physiol. (Lond.)* 479:265–279, 1994.
154. Nuss, H. B., D. C. Johns, S. Kääb, G. F. Tomaselli, D. Kass, J. H. Lawrence, and E. Marban. Reversal of potassium channel deficiency in cells from failing hearts by adenoviral gene transfer: a prototype for gene therapy for disorders of cardiac excitability and contractility. *Gene Therapy* 3:900–912, 1996.
155. Nuss, H. B., S. Kääb, D. A. Kass, G. F. Tomaselli, and E. Marbán. Cellular basis of ventricular arrhythmias and abnormal automaticity in heart failure. *Am. J. Physiol.* 277 (*Heart Circ. Physiol.* 46):H80–H91, 1999.
156. Ohya, S., M. Tanaka, T. Oku, Y. Asai, M. Watanabe, W. R. Giles, and Y. Imaizumi. Molecular cloning and tissue distribution of an A-type K$^+$ channel α-subunit, Kv4.3 in the rat. *FEBS Lett.* 420:47–53, 1997.
157. Papazian, D. M., T. L. Schwarz, B. L. Temple, Y. N. Jan, and L. Y. Jan. Cloning of genomic and complementary DNA from *Shaker*, a putative potassium channel gene from *Drosophila Science* 237:749–753, 1987.
158. Parcej, D. N., V. E. Scott, and J. O. Dolly. Oligomeric properties of alpha-dendrotoxin-sensitive potassium ion channels purified from bovine brain. *Biochemistry* 31:11084–11088, 1992.
159. Petersen, K. R. and J. M Nerbonne. Expression environment determines K$^+$ current properties: Kv1 and Kv4 α subunit–induced K$^+$ currents in mammalian cell lines and cardiac myocytes. *Pflugers Arch.* 437:381–392, 1999.
160. Po, S., D. J. Snyders, R. Baker, M. M. Tamkun, and P. B. Bennett. Functional expression of an inactivating potassium channel cloned from human heart. *Circ. Res.* 71:732–736, 1992.
161. Po, S., S. Roberds, D. J. Snyders, M. M. Tamkun, and P. B. Bennett. Heteromultimeric assembly of human potassium channels. Molecular basis of a transient outward current? *Circ. Res.* 72:1326–1336, 1993.
162. Pond, A. L., B. K. Scheve, A. T. Benedict, K. Petrecca, D. R. Van Wagoner, A. Shrier, and J. M. Nerbonne. Expression of distinct *ERG* proteins in rat, mouse and human heart: relation to functional I$_{Kr}$ channels. *J. Biol. Chem.* 275:5997–6006, 2000.
163. Pongs, O. Molecular biology of voltage-dependent potassium channels. *Physiol. Rev.* 72:S69–S88, 1992.
164. Pong, O. Voltage-gated potassium channels from hyperexcitability to excitement. *FEBS Lett.* 452:31–35, 1999.
165. Pongs, O., N. Kecskemethy, R. Muller, I. Krah-Jentgens, A. Baumann, H. H. Kiltz, L. Canal, S. Llamazares, and A. Ferrus. *Shaker* encodes a family of putative potassium channel proteins in the nervous system. *EMBO J.* 7:1087–1096, 1988.
166. Pongs, O., T. Leicher, M. Berger, J. Roeper, R. Bahring, D. Wray, K. P. Giese, A. J. Silva, and J. F. Storm. Functional and molecular aspects of voltage-gated K$^+$ channel β subunits. *Ann. N.Y. Acad. Sci.* 868:344–355, 1999.
167. Potreau, D., J. P. Gomez, and N. Fares. Depressed transient outward current in single hypertrophied cardiomyocytes isolated from the right ventricle of ferret heart. *Cardiovasc. Res.* 30:440–448, 1996.
168. Ravens, U., E. Wettwer, A. Ohler, G. J. Amos, and T. Mewes. Electrophysiology of ion channels of the heart. *Fund. and Clin. Pharmacol.* 10:321–328, 1996.
169. Rettig, J., S. H. Heinemann, F. Wunder, C. Lorra, D. N. Parcej, J. Q. Dolly, and O. Pongs. Inactivation properties of voltage-gated K$^+$ channels altered by presence of β-subunit. *Nature* 369:289–294, 1994.
170. Roberds, S. L. and M. M. Tamkun. Cloning and tissue-specific expression of five voltage-gated potassium channel cDNAs expressed in rat heart. *Proc. Natl. Acad. Sci. U.S.A.* 88:1798–1802, 1991.
171. Roberds, S. L. and M. M. Tamkun. Developmental expression of cloned cardiac potassium channels. *FEBS Lett.* 284:152–154, 1991.
172. Roberds, S. L., K. M. Knoth, S. Po, T. A. Blair, P. B. Bennett, R. P. Hartshorne, D. J. Snyders, and M. M. Tamkun. Molecular biology of the voltage-gated potassium channels of the cardiovascular system. *J. Cardiovasc. Electrophysiol.* 4:68–80, 1993.
173. Salama, G. and B.-R. Choi. Images of action potential propagation in heart. *News Physiol. Sci.* 15:33–41, 2000.
174. Salata, J. J., N. K. Jurkiewicz, B. Jow, K. Folander, P. J. Guinoso, B. Raynor, R. Swanson, and B. Fermini. I$_K$ of rabbit ventricle is composed of two currents: evidence for I$_{ks}$. *Am. J. Physiol.* 271 (*Heart Circ, Physiol.* 40):H2477–H2489, 1996.
175. Salinas, M., F. Duprat, C. Heurteaux, J. P. Hugnot, and M. Lazdunski. New modulatory alpha subunits for mammalian *Shab* K$^+$ channels. *J. Biol. Chem.* 272:24371–24379, 1997.
176. Sanguinetti, M. C. Dysfunction of delayed rectifier potassium

176. channels in an inherited cardiac arrhythmia. *Ann. N.Y. Acad. Sci.* 868:406–413, 1999.
177. Sanguinetti, M. C. and N. K. Jurkiewicz. Two components of cardiac delayed rectifier K⁺ current. *J. Gen. Physiol.* 96:195–215, 1990.
178. Sanguinetti, M. C. and N. K. Jurkiewicz. Delayed rectifier outward K⁺ current is composed of two currents in guinea pig atrial cells. *Am. J. Physiol.* 260 (*Heart Circ, Physiol.* 29): H393–H399, 1991.
179. Sanguinetti, M. C., C. Jiang, M. E. Curran, and M. T. Keating. A mechanistic link between an inherited and an acquired cardiac arrhythmia: *HERG* encodes the I_{Kr} potassium channel. *Cell* 81:299–307, 1995.
180. Sanguinetti, M. C., M. E. Curran, A. Zou, J. Shen, P. S. Spector, D. L. Atkinson, and M. T. Keating. Coassembly of KvLQT1 and minK (IsK) proteins to form cardiac I_{Ks} potassium channel. *Nature* 384:80–83, 1996.
181. Sanguinetti, M. C., J. J. Johnson, L. G. Hammerland, P. R. Kelbaugh, R. A. Volkman, N. A. Saccomano, and A. L. Mueller. Heteropodatoxins: peptides isolated from spider venom that block Kv4.2 potassium channels. *Mol. Pharmacol.* 51:491–498, 1997.
182. Schroeder, B. J., C. Kubisch, V. Stein, and T. J. Jentsch. Moderate loss of cyclic-AMP-modulated KCNQ2/KCNQ3 K⁺ channels causes epilepsy. *Nature* 396:687–690, 1998.
183. Schwarz, T. L., B. L. Temple, D. M. Papazian, Y. N. Jan, and L. Y. Jan. Multiple potassium-channel components are produced by alternative splicing at the *Shaker* locus in *Drosophila*. *Nature* 331:137–142, 1988.
184. Sewing, S., J. Roeper, and O. Pongs. Kvβ1 subunit binding specific for *Shaker*-related potassium channel α subunits. *Neuron* 16:455–463, 1996.
185. Shi, G., K. Nakahira, S. Hammond, K. J. Rhodes, L. E. Schechter, and J. S. Trimmer. β subunits promote K⁺ channel surface expression through effects early in biosynthesis. *Neuron* 16: 843–852, 1996.
186. Shi, W., R. S. Wymore, H.-S. Wang, Z. Pan, I. S. Cohen, D. McKinnon, and J. E. Dixon. Identification of two nervous system–specific members of the erg potassium channel gene family. *J. Neurosci.* 17:9423–9432, 1997.
187. Shibasaki, T. Conductance and kinetics of delayed rectifier potassium channels in nodal cells of the rabbit heart. *J. Physiol. (Lond.)* 387:227–250, 1987.
188. Shibata, E. F., T. Drury, H. Refsum, V. Aldrete, and W. Giles. Contributions of a transient outward current to repolarization in human atrium. *Am. J. Physiol.* 257 (*Heart Circ. Physiol.* 26): H1773–H1781, 1989.
189. Sicouri, S. and C. Antzelevitch. A subpopulation of cells with unique electrophysiological properties in the deep subepicardium of the canine ventricle. The M Cell. *Circ. Res.* 68:1729–1741, 1991.
190. Snyders, D. J. Structure and function of cardiac potassium channels. *Cardiovasc. Res.* 42:377–390, 1999.
191. Tai, K.-K., and S. A. N. Goldstein. The conduction pore of a cardiac potassium channel. *Nature* 391:605–607, 1998.
192. Takimoto, K., D. Li, K. M. Hershman, P. Li, E. K. Jackson, and E. S. Levitan. Decreased expression of Kv4.2 and novel Kv4.3 K⁺ channel subunit mRNAs in ventricles of renovascular hypertensive rats. *Circ. Res.* 81:533–539, 1996.
193. Takumi, T., H. Ohkubo, and S. Nakinishi. Cloning of a membrane protein that induces a slow voltage-gated potassium current. *Science* 242:1042–1045, 1988.
194. Tamkun, M. M., K. M. Knoth, J. A. Walbridge, H. Kroemer, D. M. Roden, and D. M. Glover. Molecular cloning and characterization of two voltage-gated K⁺ channel cDNAs from human ventricle. *FASEB J.* 5:331–337, 1991.
195. Ten Eick, R. E., J. R., Houser, and A. L. Bassett. Cardiac hypertrophy and altered cellular activity of the myocardium. In: *Physiology and Pathophysiology of the Heart*, 2nd. Ed., edited by N. Speralakis. Boston: Martinus Nijhoff, 1989:573–594.
196. Ten Eick, R. E., K. Zhang, R. D. Harvey, and A. L. Bassett. Enhanced functional expression of transient outward current in hypertrophied feline myocytes. *Cardiovasc. Drugs Ther.* 7:611–619, 1993.
197. Tiffany, A.M., L. N. Manganas, E. Kim, Y. P Hseuh, M. Sheng, and J. S. Trimmer. PSD95 and SAP97 exhibit distinct mechanisms for regulating K⁺ channel surface expression and clustering. *J. Cell Biol.* 148:147–158, 2000.
198. Timpe, L. C., T. L. Schwarz, B. L. Temple, D. M. Papazian, Y. N. Jan, and L. Y. Jan. Expression of functional potassium channels from *Shaker* cDNA in *Xenopus* oocytes. *Nature* 331: 143–145, 1988.
199. Tomaselli, G. F. and E. Márban. Electrophysiological remodeling in hypertrophy and heart failure. *Cardiovasc. Res.* 42: 270–283, 1999.
200. Trimmer, J. S. Immunological identification and characterization of a delayed rectifier K⁺ channel polypeptide in rat brain. *Proc. Natl. Acad. Sci. U.S.A.* 88:10764–10768, 1991.
201. Trudeau, M. C., J. W. Warmke, B. Ganetsky, and G. A. Robertson. *H-erg*, a human inward rectifier with structural and functional homology to voltage-gated K⁺ channels. *Science* 269:92–95, 1995.
202. Tseng, G.-N. and B. F. Hoffman. Two components of transient outward current in canine ventricular myocytes. *Circ. Res.* 64: 633–647, 1989.
203. Tseng-Crank, J. C. L., G.-N. Tseng, A. Schwartz, and M. A. Tanouye, Molecular cloning and functional expression of a potassium channel cDNA isolated from a rat cardiac library. *FEBS Lett.* 268:63–68, 1990.
204. Undrovinas, A. I. and V. A. Maltsev. Cytochalasin D alters kinetics of Ca²⁺ transient in rat cardiomyocytes: an effect of altered actincytoskeleton. *J. Mol. Cell. Cardiol.* 30:1665–1670, 1998.
205. Undrovinas, A. I., G. S. Shander, and V. A. Maltsev. Cytoskeleton modulates gating of voltage-dependent sodium channel in heart. *Am. J. Physiol* 269 (*Heart Circ, Physiol.* 38):H203–H214, 1995.
206. Van Wagoner, D. R., M. Kirian, and M. Lamorgese. Phenylephrine suppresses outward K⁺ currents in rat atrial myocytes. *Am. J. Physiol.* 271 (*Heart Circ. Physiol.* 40):H937–946, 1996.
207. Van Wagoner, D. R., A. L. Pond, P. M. McCarthy, J. S. Trimmer, and J. M. Nerbonne. Outward K⁺ current densities and Kv1.5 expression are reduced in chronic human atrial fibrillation. *Circ. Res.* 80:772–781, 1997.
208. Van Wagoner, D. R., A. L. Pond, M. Lamorgese, S. S. Rossie, and J. M. Nerbonne. Atrial L-type calcium currents and human atrial fibrillation. *Circ. Res.* 85:428–436, 1999.
209. Varro, A., P. P. Nanasi, and D. A. Lathrop. Potassium currents in isolated human atrial and ventricular cardiocytes. *Acta Physiol. Scand.* 149:133–142, 1993.
210. Varro, A., B. Balati, N. Iost, J. Takacs, L. Virag, D. A. Lathrop, L. Csaba, L. Talosi, and J. G. Papp. The role of the delayed rectifier component I_{Ks} in dog ventricular muscle and Purkinje fibre repolarization. *J. Physiol. (Lond.)* 523:67–81, 2000.
211. Veldkamp, M. W., A. C. G. Van Ginneken, and L. N. Bouman. Single delayed rectifier channels in the membrane of rabbit ventricular myocytes. *Circ. Res.* 72:865–878, 1993.
212. Verkerk, A. O., M. W. Veldkamp, F. Abbate, G. Antoons, L. N. Bouman, J. H. Ravesloot, and A. C. G. Van Ginneken. Two

types of action potential configurations in single cardiac Purkinje Fibers. *Am. J. Physiol.* 277 (*Heart Circ. Physiol.* 46): H1299–H1310, 1999.

213. Volders, P. G. A., K. R. Sipido, E. Carmeliet, R. L. H. M. G. Spatjens, H. J. J. Wellens, and M. A. Vos. Repolarizing K$^+$ currents I$_{to1}$ and I$_{Ks}$ are larger in right than left canine ventricular midmyocardium. *Circulation* 99:206–210, 1999.

214. Volk, T., T. H. D. Nguyen, J. H. Schultz, and H. Ehmke. Relationship between transient outward K$^+$ current and Ca^{2+} influx in rat cardiac myocytes of endo- and epicardial origin. *J. Physiol. (Lond.)* 519:841–850, 1999.

215. Walsh, K. B., J. P. Arena, W. M. Kwok, and L. Freeman. Delayed-rectifier potassium channel activity in isolated membrane patches of guinea pig ventricular myocytes. *Am. J. Physiol.* 260 (*Heart Circ. Physiol.* 29):H1390–H1393, 1991.

216. Wang, H. S., Z. Pan, W. Shi, B. S. Brown, R. S. Wymore, I. S. Cohen, J. E. Dixon, and D. McKinnon. KCNQ2 and KCNQ3 potassium channel subunits: molecular correlates of the M-channel. *Science* 282:1890–1893, 1998.

217. Wang, K.-W., K.-K. Tai, and S. A. N. Goldstein. MinK residues line a potassium channel pore. *Neuron* 16:571–577, 1996.

218. Wang, Q., M. E. Curran, I. Splawski, T. C. Burn, J. M. Millholland, T. J. Vanray, J. Shen, K. W. Timothy, G. M. Vincent, T. Dejager, P. J. Schwartz, J. A. Toubin, A. J. Moss, D. L. Atkinson, G. M. Landes, T. D. Connors, and M. T. Keating. Positional cloning of a novel potassium channel gene: KvLQT1 mutations cause cardiac arrhythmias. *Nat. Genet.* 12:17–23, 1996.

219. Wang, Z., B. Fermini, and S. Nattel. Repolarization differences between guinea pig atrial endocardium and epicardium. *Am. J. Physiol.* 260 (*Heart Circ. Physiol.* 29):H1501–H1506, 1991.

220. Wang, Z., B. Fermini, and S. Nattel. Delayed rectifier outward current and repolarization in human atrial myocytes. *Circ. Res.* 73:276–285, 1993.

221. Wang, Z., B. Fermini, and S. Nattel. Sustained depolarization-induced outward current in human atrial myocytes. Evidence for a novel delayed rectifier K$^+$ current similar to Kv1.5 cloned channel currents. *Circ. Res.* 73:1061–1076, 1993.

222. Wang, Z., B. Fermini, and S. Nattel. Rapid and slow components of delayed rectifier current in human atrial myocytes. *Cardiovasc. Res.* 28:1540–1546, 1994.

223. Wang, Z., J. Feng, H. Shi, A. L. Pond, J. M. Nerbonne, and S. Nattel. The potential molecular basis of different physiological properties of transient outward K$^+$ current in rabbit and human atrial myocytes. *Circ. Res.* 84:551–561, 1999.

224. Warmke, J. E. and B. Ganetsky. A family of potassium channel genes related to eag in *Drosophila* and mammals. *Proc. Natl. Acad. Sci. U.S.A.* 91:3438–3442, 1994.

225. Warmke, J. E., R. Drysdale, and B. Ganetsky. A distinct potassium channel polypeptide encoded by the *Drosophila eag* locus. *Science* 252:1560–1564, 1991.

226. Wei, A., M. Covarrubias. A. Butler, K. Baker, M. Pak, and L. Salkoff. K$^+$ current diversity is produced by an extended gene family conserved in *Drosophila* and mouse. *Science* 248:599–603, 1990.

227. Wettwer, E., G. Amos, J. Gath, H.-R. Zerkowski, J.-C. Reidemeister, and U. Ravens. Transient outward current in human and rat ventricular myocytes. *Cardiovasc. Res.* 27:1662–1669, 1993.

228. Wettwer, E., G. J. Amos, H. Posival, and U. Ravens. Transient outward current in human ventricular myocytes of subepicardial and subendocardial origin. *Circ. Res.* 75:473–482, 1994.

229. Wettwer, E., H. M. Himmel, G. J. Amos, Q. Li, F. Metzger, and U. Ravens. Mechanism of block by tedisamil of transient outward current in human subepicardial myocytes. *Br. J. Pharmacol.* 125:659–666, 1998.

230. Wetzel, G. T. and T. S. Klitzner. Developmental cardiac electrophysiology: recent advances in cellular physiology. *Cardiovasc. Res.* 31:E52–E60, 1996.

231. Wible, B. A., Q. Yang, Y. A. Kuryshev, E. A. Accili, and A. M. Brown. Cloning and expression of a novel K$^+$ channel regulatory protein, KchAP. *J. Biol. Chem.* 273:11745–11751, 1998.

232. Wickenden, A. D., T. J. Jegla, R. Kaprielian, and P. H. Backx. Regional contributions of Kv1.4, Kv4.2 and Kv4.3 to transient outward K$^+$ current in rat ventricle. *Am. J. Physiol.* 276 (*Heart Circ. Physiol.* 45):H1599–H1607, 1999.

233. Wickenden, A. D., P. Lee, R. Sah, Q. Huang, G. I. Fishman, and P. H. Backx. Targeted expression of a dominant negative K(v)4.2 K$^+$ channel subunit in the mouse heart. *Circ. Res.* 85:1067–1076, 1999.

234. Wilde, A. A. M. and M. W. Veldkamp. Ion channels, the QT interval and arrhythmias. *Pacing Clin. Electrophysiol.* 20:2048–2051, 1997.

235. Xu, H., J. E. Dixon, D. M. Barry, J. S. Trimmer, J. P. Merlie, D. McKinnon, and J. M. Nerbonne. Developmental analysis reveals mismatches in the expression of K$^+$ channel α subunits and voltage-gated K$^+$ channel currents in rat ventricular myocytes. *J. Gen. Physiol.* 108:405–419, 1996.

236. Xu, H., W. Guo, and J. M. Nerbonne. Four kinetically distinct depolarization activated K$^+$ channel currents in mouse ventricular myocytes. *J. Gen. Physiol.* 113:661–678, 1999.

237. Xu, H., H. Li, D. M. Barry, and J. M. Nerbonne. Elimination of the transient outward current and action potential prolongation in atrial myocytes expressing a dominant negative Kv α subunits, Kv4.2W362F. *J. Physiol. (Lond.)* 519:11–21, 1999.

238. Xu, H., D. M. Barry, H. Li, S. Brunet, and J. M. Nerbonne. Attenuation of the slow component of delayed rectification, action potential prolongation and triggered activity in mice expressing a dominant negative Kv2 α subunit. *Circ. Res.* 85:623–633, 1999.

239. Yang, T., S. Kuperschmidt, and D. Roden. Anti-minK antisense decreases the amplitude of the cardiac delayed rectifier K$^+$ current. *Circ. Res.* 77:1246–1253, 1995.

240. Yeola, S. W. and D. J. Snyders, Electrophysiological and pharmacological correspondence between Kv4.2 current and rat cardiac transient outward current. *Cardiovasc. Res.* 33:540–547, 1997.

241. Yokoshiki, H., Y. Katsube, M. Sunugawa, T. Seki, and N. Sperelakis, Disruption of actin cytoskeleton attenuates sulfonylurea inhibition of cardiac ATP-sensitive K$^+$ channels. *Pflugers Arch.* 434:203–205, 1997.

242. Yue, D. T. and E. Marban. A novel cardiac potassium channel that is active and conductive at depolarized potentials. *Pflugers Arch.* 413:127–133, 1988.

243. Yue, L., J. Feng, G. R. Li, and S. Nattel. Transient outward and delayed rectifier currents in canine atrium: properties and role of isolation methods. *Am. J. Physiol.* 270 (*Heart Circ. Physiol.* 39):H2157–H2168, 1996.

244. Yue, L., J. Feng, G. R. Li, and S. Nattel. Characterization of an ultrarapid delayed rectifier potassium channel involved in canine atrial repolarization. *J. Physiol. (Lond.)* 496:647–662, 1996.

245. Yue, L., J. Feng, R. Gaspo, G. R. Li, Z. Wang, and S. Nattel. Ionic remodelling underlying action potential changes in a canine model of atrial fibrillation. *Circ. Res.* 81:512–525, 1997.

246. Zhou, Z., Q. Gong, B. Ye, Z. Fan, J. Makielski, G. A. Robertson, and C. T. January. Properties of HERG channels stably expressed in HEK 293 cells studied at physiological temperature. *Biophys. J.* 74:230–241, 1998.

247. Zhou, J., A. Jeron, B. London, X. Han, and G. Koren. Characterization of a slowly inactivating outward current in adult mouse ventricular myocytes. *Circ. Res.* 83:806–814, 1998.
248. Zygmunt, A. C. Intracellular calcium activates a chloride current in canine ventricular myocytes. *Am. J. Physiol.* 267 (*Heart Circ. Physiol.* 36):H1984–H1995, 1994.
249. Zygmunt, A. C. and W. R. Gibbons. Calcium-activated chloride current in rabbit ventricular myocytes. *Circ. Res.* 68:424–437, 1991.
250. Zygmunt, A. C. and W. R. Gibbons. Properties of the calcium-activated chloride current in heart. *J. Gen. Physiol.* 99:391–414, 1992.

16. Modulation of electrical properties by ions, hormones, and drugs

MASAYASU HIRAOKA | *Department of Cardiovascular Diseases, Medical Research Institute, Tokyo Medical and Dental University, Tokyo, Japan*

CHAPTER CONTENTS

Effects of Electrolytes
   Potassium ions
   Sodium ions
   Calcium and other divalent cations
   Chloride ions
Effects of pH and Physical Factors
   pH
   Temperature
   Stretch and osmotic pressure
Effects of Neurohormones and Their Receptor Stimulations
   Adrenoceptor agonists and adrenergic receptor stimulation
      β-Adrenergic agonists and β-adrenergic receptor stimulation
      α-Adrenoceptor agonists and α-adrenergic receptor stimulation
   Cholinergic agonists and cholinergic receptor stimulation
Effects of Circulatory Hormones and Autocrine/Paracrine Substances
   Thyroid hormones and thyroid states
   Insulin and diabetes mellitus
   Effects of adenosine and adenine nucleotides through purinergic receptor stimulation
     Adenosine and adenosine receptor stimulation
     External ATP and P_2 receptor stimulation
   Histamine and histamine H_2 receptor stimulation
   Angiotensin II and angiotensin receptor stimulation
   Arginine vasopressin and vasopressinergic receptor stimulation
   Endothelins
   Atrial natriuretic peptide
   Nitric oxide
Effects of Drugs
   Digitalis glucosides
   Potassium channel openers

ELECTRICAL ACTIVITY OF THE HEART is variously modulated by changes in electrolyte concentrations, hormones including neurotransmitters and paracrine/endocrine substances, as well as drugs. The changes they produce have important physiological and pathophysiological roles for the regulation of cardiac function. Studies using isolated cardiac myocytes and the patch-clamp technique have greatly advanced our understanding of the actions of these factors at the single-channel level and, at the same time, of their complex and fine-grained regulation by intracellular signaling pathways. Further advances in the molecular biology and structural clarification of ion channels have begun to yield insights into their mechanisms of action at the molecular level.

EFFECTS OF ELECTROLYTES

The electrolyte composition of the extracellular fluid has multiple effects on membrane potentials and ionic currents by a variety of mechanisms. Variation in a single ionic concentration alters the driving force and permeability of the ion as well as the channel conductance, and it sometimes influences channel gating. Each change may also affect other conductance systems, the activity of pumps, and exchange mechanisms. An altered ionic composition of the external solution may ultimately induce a shift of ionic composition of the cytoplasm. All of these factors contribute to electrical modification of the heart.

Potassium Ions

One of the most influential changes in cardiac electrical activity results from the variation in extracellular K^+ concentration ($[K^+]_o$), that occurs under various physiological and pathophysiological conditions. The effects in electrical activity depend not only on levels of $[K^+]_o$, but also on the original level and the direction and speed of the change.

Effects on resting membrane potential. In the resting state, the cardiac membrane is highly and predominantly permeable to K^+. The resting membrane potential decreases as $[K^+]_o$ is increased from the normal physiological ranges of 3.5–5.0 mM. Above 10 mM $[K^+]_o$, the relation between the resting membrane potential and $[K^+]_o$ becomes almost linear, with a slope of 60 mV/10-fold change in $[K^+]_o$ at 37°C, as predicted from the Nernst equation. With a reduction of $[K^+]_o$ below 10 mM, hyperpolarization of the membrane potential occurs with a deviation from the Nernst equation due to a relative increase in Na^+ permeability (P_{Na}) with reduced K^+ permeability (P_K). A deviation of resting potential from the Nernst equation is predicted by the Goldman-Hodgkin-Katz equation (603). The changes do not necessarily occur smoothly, but sometimes take place suddenly. For example, in Purkinje fibers, a decrease in $[K^+]_o$ below 2 mM causes a sudden and marked depolarization of resting potential to around −40 mV, and a small increase in $[K^+]_o$ induces a prompt repolarization to −80 mV (70, 290). Injection of a small depolarizing current into the cells produces immediate return to −40 mV, exhibiting two stable states of resting membrane potential (688). This behavior is brought about by the shape of the background current–voltage relation, which crosses zero current level twice at around −80 mV, and between −60 and −40 mV. Similar behavior can also be seen in single ventricular myocytes exposed to external $[K^+]_o$ of 1 mM or less (273).

The sensitivity of resting membrane potential to $[K^+]_o$ differs among cell types. Strong dependence on $[K^+]_o$ is seen in Purkinje cells (70, 579) and ventricular cells (390), with less dependence in atrial cells (30, 278), and least sensitivity in the Sinoatrial (SA) and atrioventricular (AV) node cells (300). Embryonic heart cells showing low resting potential levels are also less sensitive to $[K^+]_o$ changes and become sensitive with development, attaining a high negative value (108, 359, 510). A different sensitivity to variation of $[K^+]_o$ can be attributed largely to the types and development of background K$^+$ conductances. In Purkinje fibers (71) and ventricular cells (369), the inward rectifier K$^+$ channels (I_{K1}) play a predominant role in background conductance. Atrial cells have less developed I_{K1} channels compared to ventricular cells (202, 289), and both I_{K1} and the acetylcholine-activated K$^+$ channels ($I_{K.ACH}$) contribute to the background conductance. Nodal cells have no or little development of I_{K1} channels (481). Embryonic heart cells lack I_{K1} and neonatal cardiac cells quickly develop the current after gestation, as well as increased values of resting potential (431, 658, 695).

While the above factors contribute to determine resting membrane potential level under steady-state conditions, there are additional factors in non-steady-state conditions or during activity. It has been shown that variation of voltage clamp pulses or change in the rate of stimulation rapidly causes accumulation or depletion of K$^+$ in the restricted extracellular spaces (clefts) (29). While the cleft $[K^+]_o$ is equal to that of the bulk solution during quiescence, it increases within 1–2 minutes by a significant degree after the start of stimulation as shown by a depolarization of diastolic potentials (365). Another factor affecting resting membrane potential during activity is an operation of the electrogenic Na$^+$–K$^+$ pump (193, 210). Hyperpolarization due to electrogenic Na$^+$–K$^+$ pump activity is seen with sudden increase in the pump activity.

Effects on excitability and conduction. A mild elevation of $[K^+]_o$ (from 2.7 to 4.0 mM) sometimes increases excitability of the cells and improves conduction, resulting in increased excitability as long as the depolarization does not cause inactivation of the Na$^+$ channels (130). A further increase in $[K^+]_o$ induces membrane depolarization sufficient to inactivate the Na$^+$ channels, which reduces the maximum upstroke velocity (V_{max}) of action potentials and decreases conduction velocity (674). At 10 mM or higher $[K^+]_o$, as might occur in the ischemic myocardium, the reduction of V_{max} is much larger than that predicted from membrane depolarization (352). This extra-reduction of V_{max} is seen in ventricular cells but not in atrial cells, which can be attributed to $[K^+]_o$-dependent activation of the I_{K1} channels in the former, but not due to properties of the Na$^+$ current (I_{Na}) in the latter (681). With further elevation of $[K^+]_o$ to 20–25 mM, the cells depolarize to less than −60 mV and become inexcitable due to inactivation of I_{Na}.

Effects on automaticity. In pacemaker cells, an elevation of $[K^+]_o$ depresses the slope of slow diastolic depolarization and automatic firing. Occasionally, depression is preceded by a transient increase in automatic firing. While spontaneous activity in Purkinje fibers stops at $[K^+]_o$ of 6–8 mM or above, SA node cells usually exhibit spontaneous activity at 10–12 mM $[K^+]_o$ (115, 652). Moreover, nodal activity persists at a level of $[K^+]_o$ that would render atrial cells inexcitable. The decrease in $[K^+]_o$ from the physiological range accelerates automaticity by increasing the slope of slow diastolic depolarization due to decreased K$^+$ conductance. When $[K^+]_o$ is lowered to 2.0 mM or less, membrane potentials of Purkinje fibers and non-pacemaking cells (atrial and ventricular cells) depolarize diastolic potentials to around −60 to −40 mV and develop spontaneous activity from slow diastolic depolarization (70, 296, 338). This type of spontaneous activity resembles activity of the SA and AV node cells, but it is never seen in non-pacemaker cells under physiological conditions (abnormal automaticity; see later under Ion Channels and Cardiac Arrhythmias in Heart Disease).

Effects on action potential configurations. At moderate elevation of K$^+$ (5–10 mM), a marked shortening of action potential duration is seen in mammalian Purkinje fibers and in frog and turtle ventricular muscles (52, 278, 676). While mammalian ventricular myocytes also show shortening of action potential, the changes are much less pronounced than in Purkinje cells (97, 289), with an abbreviation of the plateau and fastened repolarization phase. This results in a triangular-shape of ventricular action potential, and forms the basis of a tall and peaked T wave (tented T wave) in the surface electrocardiogram (ECG). The shortening effects are much more prominent in ventricular than in atrial myocytes (289) because of well-developed I_{K1} channels in the former. The I_{K1} channels show increased outward current and a crossover of the current–voltage relation with elevated $[K^+]_o$; this increase occurs at voltages in the plateau phase and the final repolarization of Purkinje fibers, which have relatively smaller I_{K1} than ventricular cells (71, 97, 478). For these reasons, Purkinje fibers exhibit more sensitive shortening in action potential duration to elevated $[K^+]_o$ than ventricular cells. In contrast, atrial myocytes have a background conductance with less inward rectification than those of I_{K1}, and also two outward currents, the delayed outward K^+ current (I_K) and transient outward K^+ current (I_{to}), are prominent at the plateau phase (202, 204, 289), which accounts for a short plateau at normal $[K^+]_o$ and less sensitivity to elevated $[K^+]_o$ (Fig. 16–1).

A decrease in $[K^+]_o$ lengthens action potential duration with prolongation of the plateau phase and slowing of the final repolarization phase. This results in a decrease and flattening of the T wave in the surface ECG and may cause the appearance of a prominent U wave in the ECG because of a regional delay in repolarization. It is now evident that there are distinct cell types with different action potential configurations within the ventricular wall (epi-, end-, and midmyocardium) (10, 11). Changes in action potential duration due either to a rise or a decrease in $[K^+]_o$ are more pronounced in epicardium than in endocardium, leading to further peaked T waves, or fattened T waves, respectively, in ECG. This effect is mainly produced by different current density of I_{to} in cells from the epi- and endocardium (10, 11). With marked reduction of external K^+, depolarization of diastolic potentials to less than -60 mV and abnormal automaticity is induced. These changes are seen soon after the changes in $[K^+]_o$. When the cells are exposed to $[K^+]_o = 2.0$ mM or less, the Na^+–K^+ pump activity is also decreased, resulting in Na^+ accumulation in the cells, which develops with some time delay compared to the events due to the conductance changes. The intracellular Na^+ accumulation causes Ca^{2+} overload through the Na^+–Ca^{2+} exchange mechanism. At this stage, the cell develops delayed afterdepolarizations (DADs) and triggered activity (151, 272; under Ion Channels and Cardiac Arrhythmias).

Effects on channels. External K^+ modulates various K^+ currents. A typical example is activation of I_{K1} by increased $[K^+]_o$ with crossover (71, 369, 478). I_K is also modulated by $[K^+]_o$ without crossover (443), and its effect appears to be a direct action of external K^+ and not due to changes in intracellular ionic compositions. Activation kinetics are not altered by $[K^+]_o$ but the channel conductance is increased (580). The human *eag-related gene* (HERG) has been shown to encode the rapidly activating component of I_K (I_{kr}) in cardiac myocytes (547, 549, 636). The current shows an inward rectification at depolarized potentials due to voltage-dependent fast inactivation compared to slow activation and deactivation. Increased $[K^+]_o$ mainly slows inactivation time course to augment current amplitude (Fig. 16–2), while decreased $[K^+]_o$ reduces the current as inactivation becomes accelerated (549, 636, 665, 702).

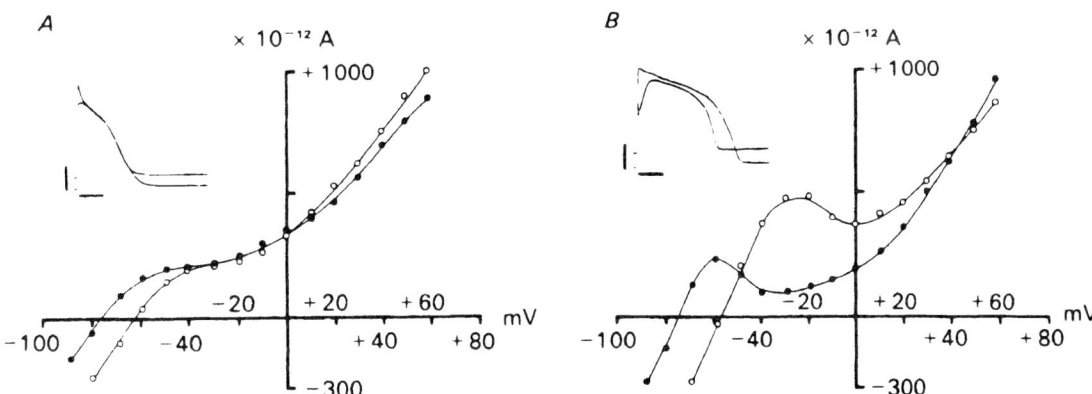

FIG. 16–1. Effects of increasing $[K^+]_o$ on action potentials and background membrane currents in atrial and ventricular myocytes. Action potentials and isochronal (5 s) current-voltage relationships at $[K^+]_o$ = 6 mM (*filled circles*) and 11 mM (*open circles*) in an atrial myocyte (A) and a ventricular myocyte (B) are shown. While action potential and the current–voltage relationship were not much changed in A with increasing $[K^+]_o$ from 6 to 11 mM, shortened action potential duration and a shift of I-V relationship with crossover were evident in B. Tetrodotoxin (3×10^{-5} M) present throughout. In each cell, the holding potential was -50 mV. Vertical calibrations for *insets in A and B* are 20 mV; horizontal calibration is 50 msec for A and 100 ms for B. [Reproduced from Figure 11 in reference (289), with permission.]

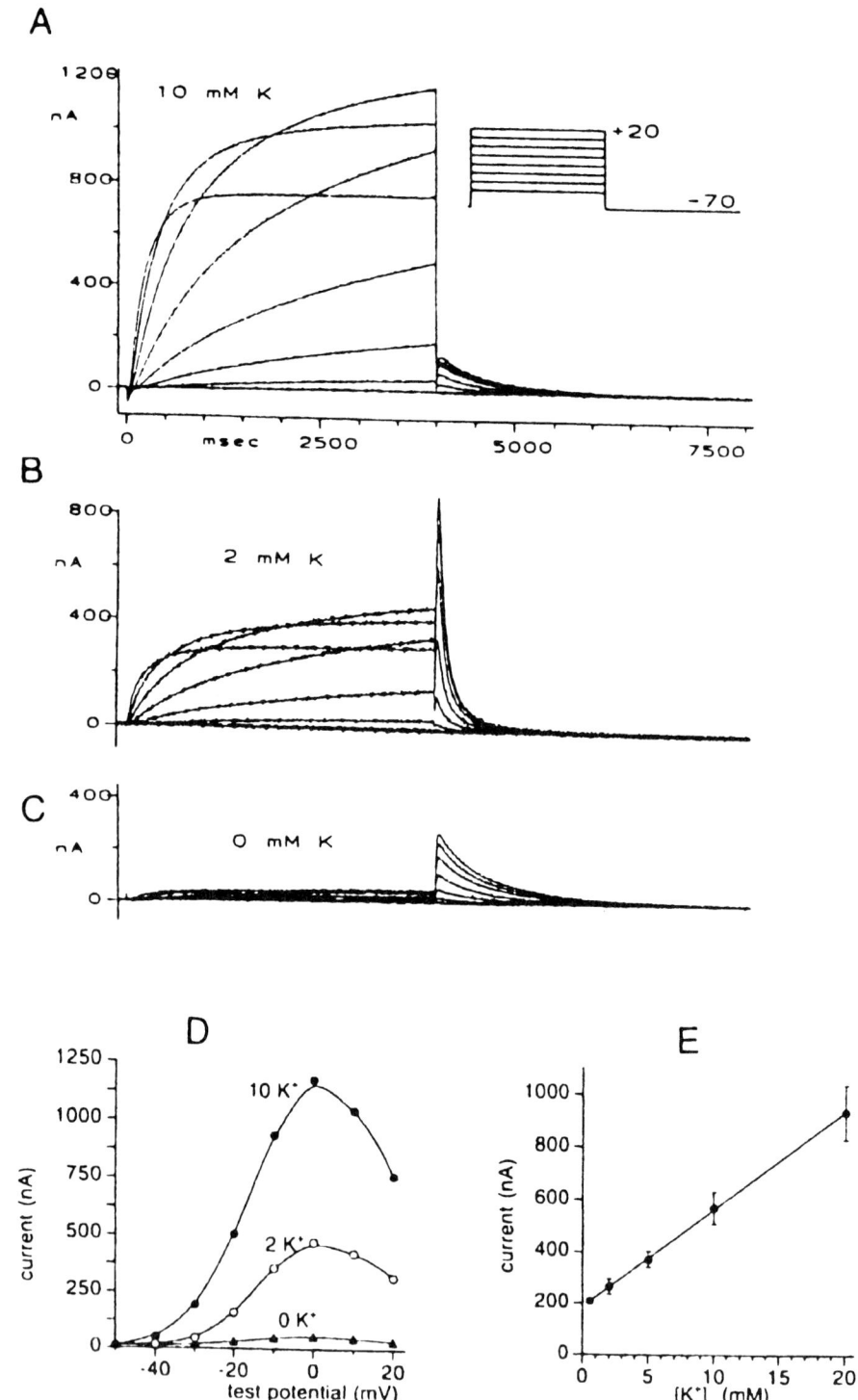

FIG. 16–2. Activation of HERG current by extracellular K$^+$ A–C: Currents elicited by 4 sec pulses to test potentials ranging from −50 to +20 mV in an oocyte bathed in modified ND96 solution containing 10 mM KCl (A) or 2 mM KCl (B) or 5 min after switching to ND96 solution with no added KCl (C). D: I-V relationship for currents shown in A–C. E: HERG current amplitude varies as a function of [K$^+$]$_o$. Currents were measured at a test potential of +20 mV (n = 4–6). The *solid line* is a linear fit to data (I_{HERG} = 189 + 37.5 [K$^+$]$_o$). Note that this relationship at lower and higher [K$^+$]$_o$ would not be expected to be a linear function of [K$^+$]$_o$. [Reproduced from Figure 4 in reference (549) with permission.]

Sodium Ions

Effects on resting membrane potential. Decrease in extracellular Na^+ concentration ($[Na^+]_o$) usually causes a moderate hyperpolarization in Purkinje cells, indicating the presence of resting Na^+ conductance. In ventricular cells, the hyperpolarization is mild, which is attributed to a small background Na^+ conductance and Na^+ regulation on I_{K1} (604). Generally, the degree of hyperpolarization depends on the background K^+ and Na^+ conductance, and the level of $[K^+]_o$ (579). The quantitative assessment of the background Na^+ conductance has revealed values of 5.0 pS/pF in atrial cells and 2.3 pS/pF in ventricular cells (355). In SA node cells, the value is three times larger than that in atrial cells (228). An increase in $[Na^+]_o$ above the normal level usually has little effect on resting membrane potential in most cardiac cells.

Effects on action potentials. $[Na^+]_o$ has marked effects on V_{max} of action potential dependent on I_{Na}. The amplitude of I_{Na} is dependent on $[Na^+]_o$ with an apparent equilibrium dissociation constant = 359 mM (474). The upstroke velocity has a close relation to the amount of I_{Na} with some non-linearity between the two parameters (577). Action potential amplitudes and overshoot are not much affected by a mild to moderate decrease in $[Na^+]_o$, because they are influenced by the inward Ca^{2+} currents, and the background and outward time-dependent K^+ currents as well. In SA node cells, V_{max} of action potentials is also dependent on $[Na^+]_o$, suggesting some contribution of I_{Na}, but the main determinant of the upstroke phase is the L-type Ca^{2+} current ($I_{Ca,L}$) (129, 300, 469).

A decrease in $[Na^+]_o$ causes marked shortening of the plateau and action potential duration (52, 473). This shortening may be caused by two factors: properties of the cardiac I_{Na} and the Na^+–Ca^{2+} exchange mechanism. It has been demonstrated that a slow or late I_{Na}, which is attributed to the window component of I_{Na} (19, 95), contributes to the action potential plateau. The measurement of cardiac I_{Na}, however, has revealed a slow decay of the current and the current flowed over a much wider range of voltages than expected from overlap between activation and inactivation curves ("window") (206, 366). In single channel recordings, reopenings or late openings of the Na^+ channels during depolarization were observed predominantly at voltages near threshold and were less frequent at depolarized voltages (366, 512). There are two types of late openings during maintained depolarization, a background type and a burst type with very rare frequencies of appearance (353). A persistent I_{Na} which has different sensitivity to tetrodotoxin (TTX) and threshold voltage for activation from the initial, rapid I_{Na}, is found in rat and embryonic chick ventricular myocytes (321, 542). Since the plateau of the action potential in Purkinje fibers starts at more negative level than that in muscle cells, the former is more sensitive to a reduction in $[Na^+]_o$, application of TTX or antiarrhythmic agents than are ventricular myocytes (19, 75, 95). Reduction of $[Na^+]_o$ affects the electrogenic Na^+–Ca^{2+} exchange mechanism which carries inward current at the plateau level (348; also see earlier, under Sodium Calcium Exchange and Cardiac Contraction). The development of an inward current during depolarization following the inactivation of $I_{Ca,L}$ can reasonably be interpreted as the current carried by the electrogenic Na^+–Ca^{2+} exchange mechanism and explain the shortened action potential duration at reduced $[Na^+]_o$ by this mechanism (147, 399, 452, 588). Because the reversal potential of the Na^+–Ca^{2+} exchange current changes dynamically during action potential from positive voltage at an early phase to negative voltage at the late repolarization phase due to changes in $[Ca^{2+}]_i$, contribution of this current to action potential repolarization depends on the level of the plateau: the Na^+–Ca^{2+} exchange current generally has a more prominent effect on the atrial action potential with a low plateau than on the ventricular one with a high plateau. Another important determinant of this current is the level of $[Na^+]_i$ and $[Na^+]_o$.

Effects on automaticity. Reduction of $[Na^+]_o$ reduces the pacemaker activity in Purkinje fibers and SA node cells (278, 300). The pacemaker current or the hyperpolarization activated inward current (I_f) is carried by Na^+ ions. This current is a main contributer to slow diastolic depolarization, at least, in Purkinje fibers (118, 120). In SA node cells, however, the explanation may be somewhat different depending on the interpretation of the contribution by either I_f (119, 120) or by the background inward Na^+ conductance (228, 301) to the formation of slow diastolic depolarization. The sustained inward current carried by Na^+ through $I_{Ca,L}$ (218) may also play a role for decreased automaticity in low $[Na^+]_o$ in SA node cells. Marked or complete reduction of $[Na^+]_o$ stops action potential generation in most cardiac preparations and inexcitability occurs at a $[Na^+]_o$ levels below 10%–20% of control (52, 113). However, cardiac preparations can generate propagated action potentials with slow upstroke velocity or slow response automaticity in the presence of external Ca^{2+} or divalent cations such as Sr^{2+} and Ba^{2+} (17, 101, 655). The excitability is produced by inward current flows through the $I_{Ca,L}$ channels. In the presence of $[Ca^{2+}]_o$, reduction of $[Na^+]_o$ can induce Ca^{2+}-overload in the cells through the Na^+–Ca^{2+} exchange mechanism, leading the development of triggered excitations based on delayed afterdepolarizations (DADs) (101).

Effects on channels. Sodium ions can modulate the

activity of other ion channels by a variety of mechanisms. External Na$^+$ and other alkali metal cations inhibit the closing of the slow inactivation gate of cardiac Na$^+$ channels (633). Na$^+$ can pass through the $I_{Ca.L}$ channels with slow activation and inactivation kinetics in the absence of external divalent cations (258, 432). An increase in [Na$^+$]$_i$ above a certain level activates a novel K$^+$ channel current (intracellular Na$^+$-activated K$^+$ channel; $I_{K.Na}$) (328). Although the initial observation indicated that the level of [Na$^+$]$_i$ required to activate the channel was above 30 mM, which is far above the physiological range, it was later found that the activation depended on the K$^+$ concentration and the activity of the Na$^+$-K$^+$ pump due to accumulation of Na$^+$ in the narrow subsarcolemmal space ("fuzzy space") (424). Intracellular Na$^+$ blocks outward current flow through several K$^+$ channels showing inward rectification, such as I_{K1}, acetylcholine-activated K$^+$ ($I_{K.ACH}$), ATP-sensitive K$^+$ (K$_{ATP}$), and $I_{K.Na}$ channels (282, 283, 434, 646, 669). The action of Na$^+$ is similar to Mg^{2+} causing open channel block of the K$^+$ outward flow in the channel pore. It is also shown that internal Na$^+$ activates $I_{K.ACH}$ by a G protein–independent mechanism (610). With decreasing [K$^+$]$_o$ less than 1 mM, I_K (mostly the rapid component; I_{kr}) is markedly decreased by reduced conductance without changes in kinetics. This decrease is not seen in the absence of [Na$^+$]$_o$, suggesting inhibitory action of external Na$^+$ on I_K in low [K$^+$]$_o$ (556). Reduction of [Na$^+$]$_o$ with replacement of other cations decreases the protein kinase A (PKA)-activated Cl$^-$ current ($I_{Cl.PKA}$), and complete removal abolishes the current (148). Inhibition of $I_{Cl.PKA}$ by Na$^+$-removal is not observed in the conditions mediated by a direct increase in intracellular cyclic AMP (cAMP) or application of phosphodiesterase inhibitors (616). Therefore, Na$^+$ may act on a process before adenylase cyclase, possibly on a process at or G protein activation but not on the channel itself.

Calcium and Other Divalent Cations

Effects on resting membrane potential. An increase in external Ca^{2+} ([Ca^{2+}]$_o$) causes hyperpolarization of resting membrane potential in Purkinje fibers and in atrial and ventricular muscles (278, 473, 675). This is caused by effects of [Ca^{2+}]$_o$ on P$_{Na}$ (674) and by results from increased internal Ca^{2+} to shift the current–voltage relation of I_{K1} in an outward direction (303). The situation is opposite for quiescent SA node cells, in which membrane depolarization was observed with increasing [Ca^{2+}]$_o$ or other divalent cations (300, 571). This response may be attributed to a lack of I_{K1} and effects of [Ca^{2+}]$_o$ on the background cation conductance in SA node cells (228, 481).

Effects on excitability and action potential generation. High [Ca^{2+}]$_o$ decreases threshold for I_{Na}-dependent excitations and low [Ca^{2+}]$_o$ increases it. Decreased excitability by high [Ca^{2+}]$_o$ is caused by the suppression of I_{Na} (576, 675). This action is ascribed to screening of negative surface charges of the membrane by Ca^{2+} and to a direct blocking action on I_{Na} (474, 576). Other divalent cations such as Co^{2+}, Mn^{2+}, Mg^{2+}, and Ba^{2+} cause similar open channel block of I_{Na} in a voltage-dependent manner. In addition, cardiac Na$^+$ channels are extremely sensitive to block by group-IIb divalent cations such as Zn^{2+} and Cd^{2+} (576, 657).

The rapid upstroke phase of the I_{Na}-mediated action potentials is composed of two phases, an initial rapid and a late slow phase. The initial rapid phase is decreased by [Na$^+$]$_o$ reduction and is sensitive to tetrodotoxin (TTX), while a late slow phase is affected by [Ca^{2+}]$_o$ in a manner competitive to [Na$^+$]$_o$ and blocked by Mn^{2+} (473, 536). A late slow phase alone can cause regenerative excitations and conducted action potentials (slow response) in reduced or absent [Na$^+$]$_o$ by $I_{Ca.L}$ (101). Slow responses are frequently associated with spontaneous activity from slow diastolic depolarization, which is produced by activation of $I_{Ca.L}$ and deactivation of I_K (296, 338). [Ca^{2+}]$_o$ is generally essential to the slow responses, but other divalent cations such as Sr^{2+} and Ba^{2+} can substitute for Ca^{2+}. While the upstroke velocity and amplitude of Ca^{2+}-mediated action potentials are dependent on [Ca^{2+}]$_o$ or divalent cation concentrations, these parameters are decreased in the coexistence of Ca^{2+} and other divalent cations compared to the presence of a single divalent cation. For example, these parameters of Sr^{2+}-mediated action potentials are decreased in the presence of [Ca^{2+}]$_o$ compared to its absence (655). This effect can be explained by anomalous mole fraction effect on $I_{Ca.L}$ (258).

Reduction of external Ca^{2+} suppresses and abolishes the Ca^{2+}-mediated action potential. Similar effects can be obtained after application of organic and inorganic Ca^{2+}-channel antagonists (358, 536). In the complete absence of [Ca^{2+}]$_o$, Na$^+$ produces slow action potential with much longer duration even when I_{Na} is completely inactivated (113, 271). This is because Na$^+$ can pass through the Ca^{2+} channel in the absence of divalent cations (258, 432). In the complete absence of both [Na$^+$]$_o$ and [Ca^{2+}]$_o$, Mn^{2+}, an inorganic Ca^{2+} channel antagonist, generates a slow action potential, since Mn^{2+} passes through Ca^{2+} channels under there conditions (488).

Effects on action potential repolarization. High [Ca^{2+}]$_o$ usually increases the plateau height, but causes either little change or shortening of action potential duration (334). The shortened action potential induces abbreviation of the QT interval on surface ECG in hypercalcemia. Apparent opposite effects on the plateau and total duration may be explained by multiple factors: A faster and larger activation of I_K due to a high starting level of the plateau, and/or an increased $[Ca^{2+}]_o$ causing high $[Ca^{2+}]_i$ shifts the current-voltage (I-V) curve of I_{K1} to the outward direction (303). Increased $[Ca^{2+}]_i$ can induce fast inactivation of the Ca^{2+} current due to Ca^{2+}-dependent inactivation (144), which may facilitate more rapid repolarization. In addition, internal Ca^{2+} can also modulate repolarization by increasing I_K, especially I_{KS} (627, 629).

Reduction of external Ca^{2+} usually produces a lowering of the plateau height with a prolongation of the total action potential duration (334). This is the basis for QT prolongation of the ECG in hypocalcemia. These effects may well be produced by the actions opposite to those in high $[Ca^{2+}]_o$ described above. Application of divalent cations having Ca^{2+} channel blocking action, such as Co^{2+}, Cd^{2+}, Ni^{2+}, Mn^{2+}, or Mg^{2+} causes effects similar to lowering $[Ca^{2+}]_o$ on the plateau and action potential duration, especially at low to moderate blocking ion concentrations (333). These cations inhibit $I_{Ca,L}$ and, at the same time, block I_K at comparable concentrations (157, 333). Inhibition of I_K (mostly I_{KS}) by Co^{2+} is caused by multiple mechanisms including the surface charge effect and voltage-independent suppression of the conductance. With partial inhibition of the current, the time course of $I_{Ca,L}$ is slowed, possibly by a reduction of the Ca^{2+}-induced inactivation, which would favor slow repolarization (721). In the complete absence of $[Ca^{2+}]_o$ and other divalent cations, especially with the addition of EDTA, a marked prolongation of action potential duration with development of abnormal automaticity can be observed (279, 550). The effects are probably produced by the Na^+ current permeating the Ca^{2+} channels.

Effects on automaticity. Changes in $[Ca^{2+}]_o$ affect automaticity of the SA node cells. High $[Ca^{2+}]_o$ increases beat frequency. Increased automaticity can be attributed to the effects of Ca^{2+} on the Ca^{2+} currents and the hyperpolarization-activated inward current (I_f) (226). Gradual activation of the T- and L-type Ca^{2+} currents accelerates the later half of slow diastolic depolarization in SA node cells (227). The diastolic $[Ca^{2+}]_i$ shows a close association with pacemaker firing rate and increased $[Ca^{2+}]_i$ accelerates pacemaker activity of SA node cells (323). Increase in $[Ca^{2+}]_i$ above certain levels or Ca^{2+}-overload in the cells leads to development of DADs carried by transient inward current (I_{TI}) and triggered activity, which constitute an important factor for the genesis of arrhythmias (101, 170, 316).

Effects on channels. The Ca^{2+}-dependent inactivation is an important determinant of the time course of $I_{Ca,L}$ during depolarization (144). This Ca^{2+}-dependent mechanism is observed with Ca^{2+} permeating the channels, with a sudden increase in Ca^{2+} release from the stores, and with a steady increase in $[Ca^{2+}]_i$ (332, 395, 415, 445, 711). The inhibiting effect of Ca^{2+} on the channels results from a decrease in channel open probability by reducing the subsequent reopenings and a shift of the gating mode toward long-lived closed states. This process seems to reflect a direct interaction between Ca^{2+} and the α_1-subunit of the L-type Ca^{2+} channel protein (112, 297). Besides Ca^{2+}-dependent inactivation, various studies have demonstrated a potentiation of $I_{Ca,L}$ by small increases in $[Ca^{2+}]_i$ (27, 220, 239, 427, 533; Fig. 16–3). Potentiation of $I_{Ca,L}$ results from increased channel open probability from increased numbers of non-blank sweeps (increased availability) as well as increased openings during non-blank sweeps. It is also associated with reduction of the longer time constant of closed time and appearance of long openings, which are abolished by protein kinase inhibitors suggesting involvement of Ca^{2+}-dependent phosphorylation (265). Involvement of Ca^{2+}/calmodn-dependent phosphorylation is also suggested in $[Ca^{2+}]_i$-dependent potentiation (8). The Ca^{2+}-dependent potentiation has been attributed to facilitation of $I_{Ca,L}$ during repeated depolarizations after a period of rest (165, 393, 637). The molecular basis of Ca^{2+}-dependent autoregulation still remains unclear, although a putative Ca^{2+}-binding EF-hand motif (112) and a nearby consensus calmodulin-binding isoleucine-glutamine ("IQ") motif (529, 598, 724) in the carboxy terminus of the cardiac type, α-subunit Ca^{2+} channels (α_{1C}) as a potential site have been suggested. Recently, Zuhlke et al. (725) and Peterson et al. (515) have demonstrated that calmodulin is a critical Ca^{2+} sensor for both inactivation and facilitation of $I_{Ca,L}$, and that the nature of the modulatory effects depends on residues within the IQ motif important for calmodulin binding (also see, earlier under Ion channels in the Heart).

Intracellular Ca^{2+} modulates I_K (I_{KS}) to increase the current amplitude independent of PKC activation but dependent on calmodulin. The I_K modulation by internal Ca^{2+} is observed at a pCa level between 8 and 6 without changing the voltage-dependent properties (627, 629). The activation may be caused by the Ca^{2+}-calmodulin complex but not mediated through phosphorylation (477). I_{KS} is formed by two molecular entities: a pore-forming subunit, *KVLQT1* and a regulatory subunit, *minK* (*KCNE1*) (25, 546). The I_{KS} current in *Xenopus* oocytes is a functional expression of the exogenous *minK* together with the endogenous *KVLQT1* in the same species. The *minK* expressed current is upregulated by treatments to increase $[Ca^{2+}]_i$ (280, 324).

The amplitude of the pacemaker current, I_f is increased by increased $[Ca^{2+}]_i$ from pCa = 10 to 7, with a shift in the activation curve to positive potential without changes in I_f kinetics (226). This action of Ca^{2+} is

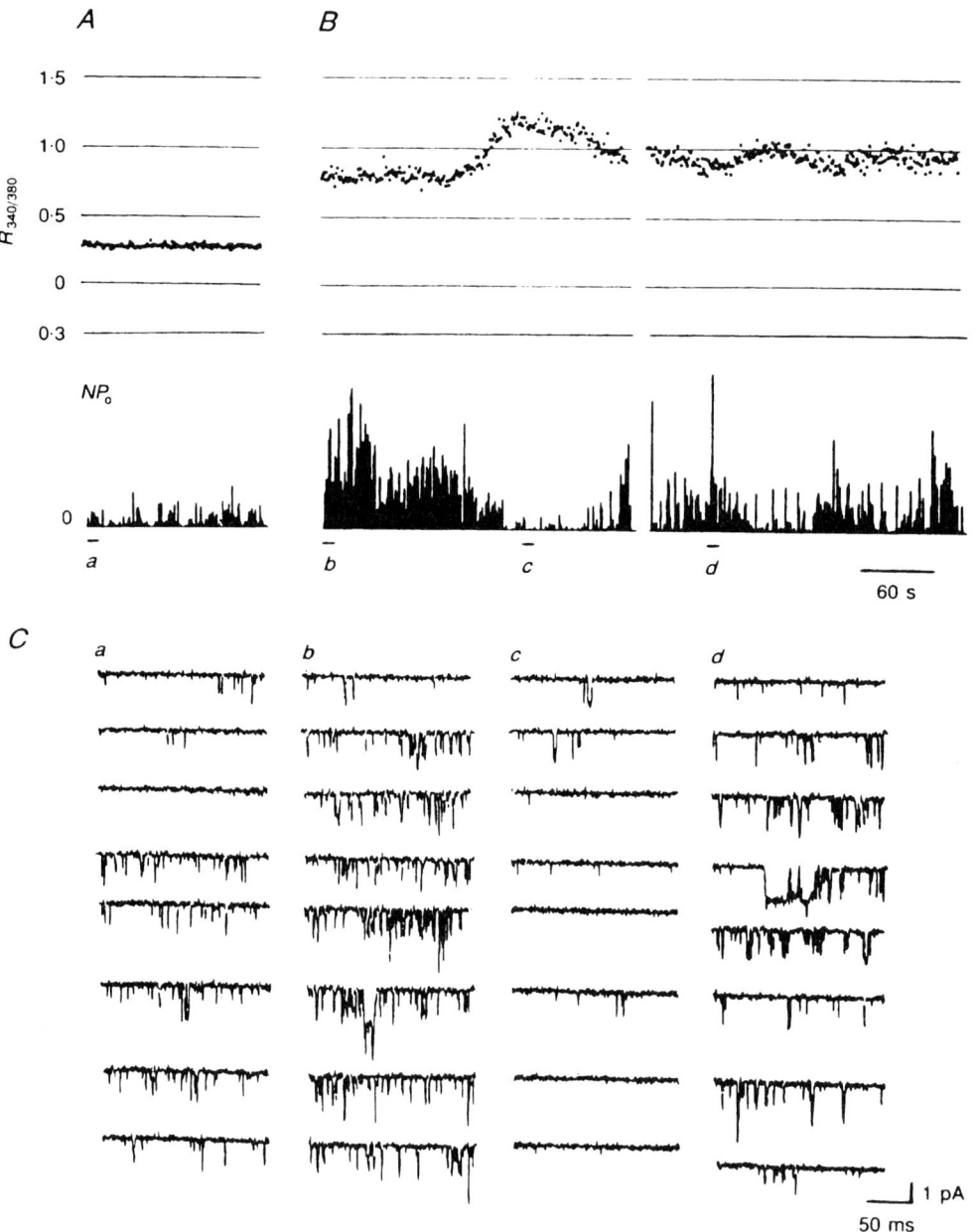

FIG. 16–3. $[Ca^{2+}]_i$ induced potentiation and inhibition in the L-type Ca^{2+} channel activity A: control; B: about 10 min after the bath solution was switched to Ca^{2+}-containing solution. *Top panels* show $R_{340/380}$ indicating $[Ca^{2+}]_i$ and *bottom panels* show NP_O of the L-type Ca^{2+} channel activity during each depolarizing pulse to 0 mV delivered at 1 Hz. C: unitary current records during the period indicated by bars in A and B. With increasing $[Ca^{2+}]_i$, channel activity was initially increased as shown in B-b and C-b. With further increase in $[Ca^{2+}]_i$ above $F_{340/380}$ ratio = 1.0, channel activity was now quickly inhibited (B-c and C-c). However, inhibitory effect was transient and with fluctuation of $[Ca^{2+}]_i$, channel activity was restored to the level which was still higher than the control B-d and C-d). [Reproduced from Figure 11 in reference (265) with permission.]

direct on the channel and is different from that of β-adrenoceptor agonist induced modulation of I_f, in which the latter mainly affects the current kinetics. This modulation of I_f by $[Ca^{2+}]_i$ may partly explain the accelerated pacemaker activity of the SA node by increased external Ca^{2+}, but concomitant changes in $I_{Ca,L}$ and I_K may mask the action on pacemaker acceleration (226). External Ca^{2+} or Mg^{2+}, on the other hand, has a weak action or no action on I_f, but Sr^{2+} and Ba^{2+} at milimolar concentrations cause voltage-dependent block of I_f (498).

The $[Ca^{2+}]_i$ activates non-selective cation channels in cultured cardiac cells (94). Similar types of channels are found in adult ventricular myocytes from guinea pig heart (150). The channels are activated by $[Ca^{2+}]_i$ at levels above 0.3 μM and the channel open probability is increased to attain the maximum value at about 10 μM $[Ca^{2+}]_i$. The increase in $[Ca^{2+}]_i$ above certain levels or the Ca^{2+}-overload in cells leads to the development of DADs and triggered activity (101, 170, 316). DADs are formed by transient inward current (I_{TI}), which is carried by some combinations of electrogenic Na^+–Ca^{2+} exchange current, Ca^{2+}-activated nonselective cation current, and Ca^{2+}-activated Cl^- current ($I_{Cl,Ca}$) (232, 335, 388, 726). The contribution of the nonselective cation current to the formation of I_{TI} may not constitute a major part, since the reversal potential of I_{TI} is not observed around 0 mV, a presumed reversal potential of the current carried by nonselective channels (16). The increase in $[Ca^{2+}]_i$ activates the Ca^{2+}-activated Cl^- current ($I_{Cl,Ca}$) in atrial and ventricular cells, and Purkinje cells, which may participate in the formation of I_{TI} (see earlier, under Ion Channels in The Heart).

Internal Ca^{2+} causes a voltage-dependent block of I_{K1}, the action similar to that of Mg^{2+}, indicating that it is one of the main mechanisms of inward rectification (433). An increase in $[Ca^{2+}]_i$ inhibits $I_{K,ATP}$ channels. Similarly, internal Mg^{2+}, Ba^{2+}, or Sr^{2+} also inhibits $I_{K,ATP}$. At the same time, Ca^{2+} and Sr^{2+} cause a quick rundown (loss of channel activity) of K_{ATP} (172, 189, 191).

External Ca^{2+} and Mg^{2+} are shown to block I_K, (mostly I_{Kr}) in SA node cells in a voltage-dependent manner, possibly through their binding in the pore of the channels (274). I_{Kr} is encoded by *HERG* (547, 549, 636), and the HERG current expressed in *Xenopus* oocytes is blocked by external Ca^{2+}, Mg^{2+}, and other divalent cations. The inhibition is caused mainly by actions on the activation process producing voltage shift and slowed activation, and by a possible reduction of the maximum conductance due to voltage-dependent block from the external side of the pore (275, 276). External Ca^{2+} hardly affects the inactivation gating in HERG current (275, 320). External divalent cations (Co^{2+}, Cd^{2+}, Zn^{2+}) block K_{ATP} by interacting with the inhibitory action of $[ATP]_i$, suggesting the modulation mechanism involving a conformational changes of the channel protein (377). External divalent cations modulate the transient outward K^+ current (I_{to}) in rat ventricular myocytes (1). Cd^{2+} shifts the activation and inactivation curves toward positive voltages with slowed activation kinetics. Similar but different concentration-dependent effects are observed among Co^{2+}, Ni^{2+}, Ca^{2+}, Cu^{2+}, and Zn^{2+}.

Effects of barium. The action of external Ba^{2+} is somewhat unique because it, not only carries the charge through the Ca^{2+} channels, but also produces slow diastolic depolarization and induces automaticity in pacemaker and non-pacemaker cells (9). The charge-carrying action can induce Ca^{2+} channel–dependent excitation with increased amplitude and duration. The pacemaker action is associated with membrane depolarization and prolongation of action potential duration suggesting decreased K^+ conductance (123, 504). Ba^{2+} depresses various types of K^+ channels, and the pacemaker action is explained by depression of I_{K1} current in a voltage- and time-dependent manner (230, 606). Block is strong at hyperpolarized voltages but becomes weaker with depolarization. During the plateau phase, the block of I_{K1} by Ba^{2+} is weak (unblocking), but upon repolarization to resting potential level the block becomes stronger with time, which causes a time-dependent decrease in the outward current of I_{K1} and, thus, produces slow diastolic depolarization (264). Sr^{2+} and Ca^{2+} exert similar voltage-dependent block of I_{K1}, but the effect is small, even at much higher concentrations (606).

Effects of magnesium. External and internal Mg^{2+} modulates cardiac ion channels in a variety of ways, and their actions often differ from those of Ca^{2+} (3). External Mg^{2+} has two major actions on channels. Mg^{2+} enters channels and reduces the current amplitude, causing open-channel block in the $I_{Ca,L}$ channel, although its effect is weak (382). Mg^{2+} is also partly responsible for the negative slope conductance of the I_{K1} channel with strong hyperpolarization (42). Second, the presence of external Mg^{2+} >10 mM produces a shift in the voltage-dependent gating parameters of the $I_{Ca,L}$ channels (3). Actions of internal Mg^{2+} are complex and the mechanisms have not been well defined. Mg^{2+} is one of the major factors causing an inward rectification of inward rectifier types of K^+ channels, I_{K1}, $I_{K,ACH}$, K_{ATP}, $I_{K,Na}$ (282, 283, 306, 433, 646, 669). The degrees of rectification are different among the four K^+ channels being most prominent for the I_{K1} channel. This is probably related to different amino acid structures in the pore regions of these channels (423, 683).

Internal Mg^{2+} has multiple actions on different cardiac ion channels. Typical examples are seen in functional modulation of K_{ATP} and $I_{Ca.L}$. K_{ATP} is fully opened in intracellular ATP-free condition in inside-out patches, but the activity decreases with time (rundown). A short exposure of Mg^{2+}-ATP to the cytoplasmic side of membranes with subsequent washout restores the channel activity. This channel recovery can only be achieved by Mg-ATP but not by Mg^{2+}-free ATP, suggesting a role of phosphorylation (490, 614). It has been shown, however, that phosphorylation by serine/threonine protein kinases seems not to be involved, but rather hydrolysis of Mg^{2+}-ATP is required (191). Furthermore, the assembly and disassembly of the actin cytoskeletal network, actions that also utilize ATP hydrolysis energy, regulate the process of rundown and reactivation of cardiac K_{ATP} (192). A different view has been presented showing that PIP_2, which inhibits various actin-binding proteins promoting polymerization of long F-actin, can itself induce the channel reactivation (260). Mg^{2+}-ADP and other nucleotide diphosphates can also stimulate and restore the K_{ATP} channel activity after rundown. These stimulating actions also require the presence of Mg^{2+} and are different from its inhibitory action (171, 643). The cardiac K_{ATP} channels are composed of two molecular elements, a pore-forming α subunit, Kir6.2, and a regulatory subunit, a cardiac type of sulfonylurea receptor (SUR2A) (18, 298, 299, 544). Stimulatory effects of Mg^{2+}-ADP are mediated through the SUR site, which has two nucleotide-binding domains, and these domains are involved in channel activation by Mg^{2+}-ADP (590, 642). The Kir6 subunit forms the ion-conducting pore and serves as the interaction site for ATP-induced inhibition (18, 642). Anionic phospholipids including PIP_2 are the critical component for the activation and maintenance of the K_{ATP} channel activity (159, 591), and these phospholipids act on the Kir6.2 subunit and change ATP sensitivity for channel inhibition (27a). Phospholipids with negative charges are required for these actions through interaction with the C-terminus of the Kir6 subunit to antagonize the ATP-induced inhibition. This modulatory mechanism is a distinction from the usual cell signaling pathway through the cleavage of phospholipids. In the presence of guanosine triphosphate (GTP), internal Mg^{2+} activates inward current through the $I_{K.ACH}$ channel via activation of G protein, while outward current is inhibited by open channel block of $I_{K.ACH}$ by Mg^{2+} (282, 372).

As to the effects of Mg^{2+} on the Ca^{2+} channels, there appear to be species differences. In frog myocytes, an increase in internal Mg^{2+} causes a relatively small decrease in $I_{Ca.L}$ of the basal condition and produces prominent decrease in the phosphorylated channels (682). In mammalian ventricular myocytes, Mg^{2+} effects are predominantly noted on the basal (nonphosphorylated) channels, and further inhibition is produced in phosphorylated channels (2). There is another indication that the inhibition of Ca^{2+} channels by $[Mg^{2+}]_i$ is modulated by $[Ca^{2+}]_i$, suggesting the competition between them at the binding site (699), and/or by a direct and phosphorylation-independent mechanism (503). Internal Mg^{2+} stimulates I_K (mostly I_{KS}) at low concentrations (<1 mM) and inhibits at high concentrations (>1 mM) (3, 141, 617, 682). These actions are not voltage dependent and appear different from β-adrenergic modulation of this current.

Chloride Ions

In cardiac muscles, intracellular Cl^- activity is higher than the level that would be expected from the passive distribution of Cl^- (28, 117). This led to the suggestion that Cl^- must be actively transported into cardiac cells (653). The Cl^- equilibrium potential (E_{Cl}) is more positive (−65 to 40 mV) than the resting membrane potential. The removal of extracellular Cl^- ($[Cl^-]_o$), however, produces only small changes in the resting membrane potential but causes dramatic changes in repolarization phase of action potential, suggesting that resting Cl^- conductance is low but may increase during depolarization (70, 290). After the introduction of the patch-clamp technique, several different types of Cl^- currents were discovered. They include the PKA-activated Cl^- current ($I_{Cl.PKA}$) (21, 248), stretch- or swelling-activated Cl^- currents ($I_{Cl.SWELL}$) (98, 229, 601, 638), Ca^{2+}-activated Cl^- current ($I_{Cl.Ca}$) (342, 596, 727, 728), the Cl^- current activated by purinergic stimulation (438), the protein kinase C (PKC)-activated Cl^- current (661, 663), and the background type Cl^- current (136, 138). The development and distributions of these Cl^- currents are tissue-, region- and species-dependent, and their functional modulations are variable (see, earlier, under Ion Channels in the Heart). Because most of these Cl^- currents are activated in the presence of agonists, stretching or swelling of membranes, and receptor stimulation in heart cells, they may contribute to action potential changes and the genesis of arrhythmias under various conditions (270, 288, 647).

$I_{Cl.PKA}$ is time-independent and outwardly rectifies under normal intracellular and extracellular Cl^- concentrations. It is stimulated by β-agonists or other means, increasing intracellular cAMP and leading to PKA activation (21, 149, 248). Activation of $I_{Cl.PKA}$ accelerates repolarization and shortens action potential duration, but has little effect on resting membrane potential (21, 247). This effect prevents excessive action potential prolongation when $I_{Ca.L}$ is stimulated. Therefore, the current activation might prevent development of arrhythmias under certain settings, but on other occasions it may provoke arrhythmias. Enhanced repolarization can perpetuate arrhythmias if a re-entrant circuit is present. When $[Cl^-]_i$ is elevated or $[Cl^-]_o$ is lowered to shift E_{Cl} closer to 0 mV, a significant depolarization of resting membrane potential and acceleration of spontaneous activity are elicited (148, 247). The current can also induce early afterdepolarizations (EADs) under conditions in which the background K^+ conductance (I_{K1}) is decreased (700). Northern blot analyses and sequencing of the transcript revealed cardiac type of *cystic fibrosis transmembrane regulator (CFTR)* as a spliced variant of epithelial *CFTR*, and thus $I_{Cl,PKA}$ is encoded by a cardiac variant of *CFTR* (284). The *CFTR* channel contains two nucleotide-binding domains (NBD), a regulatory domain and multiple consensus sites for possible PKA-dependent phosphorylation. The channel activation appears to require PKA-dependent phosphorylation as well as nucleotide binding and nucleotide hydrolysis (194, 288).

$I_{Cl,SWELL}$ can also produce nearly time-independent current with outward rectification and exhibits different electrophysiological and pharmacological properties from those of $I_{Cl,PKA}$ (98, 229, 568, 601, 638, 648). For example, at strong depolarization from high negative voltage, $I_{Cl,SWELL}$ exhibits voltage-dependent inactivation and sensitivity to Cl^- channel blockers are somewhat different between the two currents (568, 648). The activation of this current has a similar influence on membrane potentials as that of $I_{Cl,PKA}$. $I_{Cl,SWELL}$ in atrial cells is more sensitive to stretch than that in ventricular cells (601), and it is species dependent. Thus, the current may modulate atrial and SA node action potentials, and automaticity in response to stretch and, possibly, volume changes. The signaling pathway between mechanical stretch and activation of Cl^- channel is not known, but the involvement of protein phosphorylation and/or dephosphorylation is suggested. The channel protein mainly responsible for $I_{Cl,SWELL}$ was reported to be *ClC-3*, and the expressed current in the mammalian cell line was inhibited by PKC activation (139). Furthermore, both the *ClC-3*-expressed current and the native channel current from guinea pig ventricular myocytes were activated by cell swelling, and the basally activated currents were partially inhibited by endogenous PKC. The results suggested that PKC-dependent phosphorylation/dephosphorylation plays a critical role in activation of $I_{Cl,SWELL}$ (135). However, the recent study has indicated that *ClC-3* is not the swelling-activated Cl^- channel (608-a). Therefore, the molecular identification of $I_{Cl,SWELL}$ needs further clarification.

$I_{Cl,Ca}$ is activated with increased $[Ca^{2+}]_i$ induced by increased Ca^{2+} influx through the plasma membrane and release from the intracellular Ca^{2+} stores and/or a steady increase in $[Ca^{2+}]_i$ (342, 596, 727, 728) (Fig. 16-4). Thus, the current contributes to the formation of phase 1, and to action potential shortening associated with β-adrenergic stimulation, high rate of stimulation, increased intracellular cAMP, and Ca^{2+} overload in cardiac cells (269, 341, 363). The current may be involved partly in formation of I_{TI} and DADs (232, 726). The routes for Ca^{2+} influx through the membrane depend mainly on $I_{Ca,L}$ and partly on the reverse Na^+–Ca^{2+} exchange mechanism (342, 375, 596, 727). The channel responsible for carrying $I_{Cl,Ca}$ is a ligand-gated channel with $[Ca^{2+}]_i$ serving as the ligand. A single-channel study has demonstrated the existence of Cl^- channels that are activated in a $[Ca^{2+}]_i$-dependent manner. The channel activity is time independent when $[Ca^{2+}]_i$ is held constant and the channel current is blocked by anion channel blockers as for whole-cell $I_{Ca,Cl}$ (93).

EFFECTS OF pH AND PHYSICAL FACTORS

pH

Among the changes caused by pH alterations, electrical disturbances resulting from acidosis are important from the pathophysiological point of view, since intracellular pH can drop by 1.0 pH unit in the first 10 minutes of myocardial ischemia (349). Myocardial ischemia is the most frequent pathological condition leading to development of various electrical abnormalities and arrhythmias in the heart.

Effects on resting membrane potential. Both metabolic and respiratory acidosis will depolarize resting membrane potential in various cardiac preparations. When extracellular pH is decreased from 7.4 to around 6.0–6.5, the size of depolarization is generally small (less than 10 mV) (502), but occasionally a large depolarization as high as 30–40 mV is observed in Purkinje fibers (58, 385) and slow response activity appears (105). In mild to moderate acidosis, a small hyperpolarization has been transiently noted in the first few minutes (58, 553), but it is absent with more extreme acidosis (pH = 4–5). The mechanism of this depolarization can be attributed to three possible explanations: *(1)* inhibition of Na^+–K^+ ATPase and Na^+–K^+ pump activity causing extracellular K^+ accumulation, *(2)* increased $[Ca^{2+}]_i$, *(3)* decreased K^+ conductance. The first two possibilities are not likely to be the main explanation, but a suppression of K^+ currents, especially I_{K1} is the most likely explanation (501). I_{K1} is suppressed when extracellular pH is lowered, probably due to decreased $[pH]_i$ (310, 368), since reduction in $[pH]_i$ rather than $[pH]_o$ decreases single-channel conductance and channel activity. In dialyzed cells, reduc-

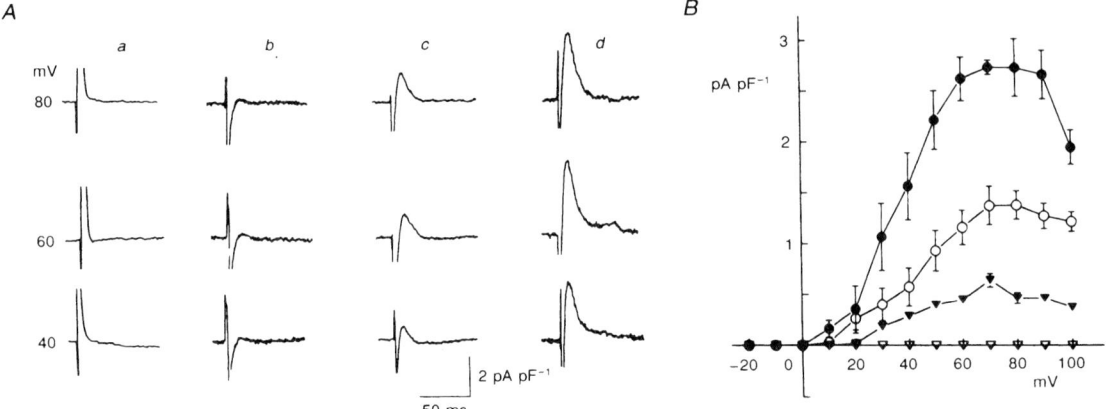

FIG. 16–4. Activation of $I_{Cl,Ca}$ in different intracellular Ca^{2+} concentrations. A: $I_{Cl,Ca}$ measured as 4,4'-ddisothiocyanatostilbene-2,2'-disulphonic acid (DIDS)-sensitive current traces at four different concentrations of Ca^{2+} in the pipette. The pipette solution contained 1 nM Ca^{2+} in a, 10 nM Ca^{2+} in b, 0.1 μM Ca^{2+} in c, and 1 μM free Ca^{2+} in d. All experiments were done in the presence of 4 mM 4-AP. Depolarizing pulses were applied from −60 mV to test potentials indicated to the left of each trace. B: current–voltage relations of $I_{Cl,Ca}$. Data represent means ± S.E.M. ●, 1 μM free Ca^{2+}; ○, 0.1 μM Ca^{2+}; ▼, 10 nM Ca^{2+}. Currents were normalized by dividing with total cell capacity. [Reproduced from Figure 6 in reference (342) with permission.]

tion of $[pH]_i$ from 7.2 to 6.0 is shown to increase I_{K1}, while further reduction of pH decreases the current (553). The reason for this increase in I_{K1} during mild acidosis is not clear, but it may be related to increased $[Ca^{2+}]_i$. This causes the transient hyperpolarization observed in some studies. In addition, internal acidosis stimulates the Na^+–H^+ exchange mechanism, which causes accumulation of $[Na^+]_i$, and then stimulates the electrogenic Na^+–K^+ pump leading to a small hyperpolarization (41).

Effects on excitability and Na^+ channels. Acidosis can alter the excitability of cardiac cells by a variety of mechanisms. Depolarization of resting membrane potential will move the membrane potential closer to threshold, leading to an increased excitability, but at the same time acidosis alters the voltage dependence of I_{Na} and shifts the threshold for the current in the positive direction (61). External and internal acidosis have variable effects on cardiac I_{Na}. Acidosis decreases the peak I_{Na}, slows activation and inactivation kinetics, and shifts voltage-dependent activation and inactivation parameters (673, 705, 717). Steady-state activation and inactivation curves shift to a positive direction with external acidosis, while internal acidosis produces a hyperpolarizing shift. These I_{Na} changes induce a reduction of the V_{max} of action potentials leading to conduction delay and failure. Increases in internal H^+ concentrations induce a rise in junctional resistance (483, 525). This factor contributes to slow impulse conduction and development of arrhythmias in acute ischemia or myocardial infarction (315; see, also earlier under Normal and Abnormal Conduction in the Heart). It is well known that acidosis can modify the action of antiarrhythmic agents on I_{Na} by multiple factors, probably due to depressed I_{Na} and depolarization of resting membrane potential as described above, and due to fractional changes in ionized and non-ionized forms of the drugs (214, 470, 677).

Effects on action potential repolarization, automaticity, and channels. The plateau height and repolarization phase of action potentials are also influenced by pH changes, especially in acidosis. Reduction of external pH has been reported either to prolong action potential duration (187) or to shorten it (84, 368). Different results may come from the multiple actions of increased external and internal H^+ concentrations on inward and outward currents responsible for the repolarization phase. Acidosis decreases the amplitude of $I_{Ca,L}$ and alkalosis increases the current amplitude (361). In addition to surface charge screening effect, increased $[H^+]_o$ strongly inhibits ion permeation through open Ca^{2+} channels and reduces channel opening (361, 517). Internal acidosis also inhibits $I_{Ca,L}$ by reducing the conductance and affecting the slow gating kinetics, and partly by an indirect effect of increased $[Ca^{2+}]_i$ (302, 325, 553). The channels are protonated at a single site with a high affinity for H^+, resulting in a subconductance state (517), and, at the same time, protons reduce the unitary flux of Ca^{2+} (361). The molecular interaction site for the modulatory effect of H^+ on Ca^{2+} channels appears to be on the P region glutametes (83). The T-type Ca^{2+} current ($I_{Ca.T}$) is also modulated by pH changes similar to $I_{Ca.L}$, with a reduction of its amplitude at low pH and an increase at high pH. In contrast to $I_{Ca.L}$, $I_{Ca.T}$ is more strongly affected by external than internal pH (644). These factors can contribute to shortening of action potential duration.

The HERG current that encodes cardiac I_{kr} is suppressed by external acidosis by multiple mechanisms: Acidosis mainly slows the current activation and accerelates deactivation time course without affecting the inactivation process at mild acidosis. Moderate to severe acidosis produces shifts in voltage dependence of activation. Acidosis also reduces the maximum conductance of the current (12, 318, 618). External acidosis inhibits other types of K^+ currents. Acidosis blocks I_{to} (698), and shifts the steady-state activation and inactivation curves to more positive potentials (608). The effects of voltage shift by increased $[H^+]_o$ are antagonized by Cd^{2+}, suggesting competition between H^+ and Cd^{2+} for a common binding site. Increased $[H^+]_i$ inhibits both I_{K1} (310, 368) and I_K (mostly I_{KS}) (553), which decreases outward currents. The above effects cause a prolongation of action potential duration. In addition, internal acidification has activated a time-independent outward K^+ current at plateau voltages (368), which might accelerate repolarization. Therefore, effects of acidosis on the plateau currents are so complex and variable that either prolongation or shortening can be anticipated depending on the cellular conditions.

Internal acidosis has induced transient inward currents (I_{TI}) similar to digitalis intoxication (368, 553). Intracellular injection of high pH (9.3–9.7) solutions produces the opposite effect. In addition, internal acidification may indirectly affect $[Ca^{2+}]_i$ and $[Na^+]_i$, and decrease the intracellular ATP levels, which may reduce the Na^+–K^+ pump activity (534). Intracellular H^+ has unique actions on K_{ATP}. An acidosis up to around pH = 6.0 stimulates K_{ATP} due to the increased probability of channel opening, probably by antagonizing ATP-induced channel inhibition (102, 104, 158), while H^+ reduces the single channel current amplitude in ATP-free conditions. Further reduction of $[pH]_i$ suppresses the channel activity by decreasing both unitary current amplitude and open-channel probability, with frequent induction of subconductance states (156).

Acidosis slows the pacing rate of the SA node preparations. External acidosis reduces both $I_{Ca.L}$ and I_K (555) and intracellular H^+ can inhibit $I_{Ca.L}$ as discussed above. External respiratory acidosis provokes DADs and I_{TI} (502). In Purkinje fibers, external acidosis induces EAD, probably due to marked depression of various K^+ currents (96).

Temperature

Changes in temperature modify ion channel functions as well as the activities of the ionic pump and exchange mechanisms. Lowering the temperature generally slows these activities, but their effects are variable among different channels. For example, temperature sensitivity is different among the Na^+ and K^+ channels from different species. For Na^+ channels, activation and inactivation kinetics behave differently with temperature changes (180, 351). When the temperature of the bath solution is lowered from 35°–37°C to 25°–27°C, a mild depolarization of the cell membrane, a slight increase in action potential amplitude, and marked prolongation of the duration are noted. A rise in temperature to around 40°C causes a minor but opposite effects on these parameters (634, 693). The most striking changes with lowering temperature in mammalian cardiac preparations are slowing the rate of repolarization and lengthening the action potential duration. Cavalie et al. (78) suggested that prolongation was caused by increased $I_{Ca.L}$ at the plateau level during hypothermia due to slowed inactivation despite a decreased peak current. Kiyosue et al. (354) concluded that I_K had the highest temperature sensitivity with an "apparent" Q_{10} (temperature coefficient) = 4.4 compared with values of 2.3 for $I_{Ca.L}$ and 1.5 for I_{K1}. I_K, therefore, was suggested to be a main factor responsible for the action potential prolongation at low temperature. Different temperature sensitivity in response to PKA-dependent phosphorylation was reported between I_K (I_{KS}) and $I_{Ca.L}$; the phosphorylation-mediated increase in I_K was nearly absent at 20°C but became prominent at 37°, whereas the phosphorylation-dependent increase in $I_{Ca.L}$ was observed at both temperatures (661). The time-independent background current, which is probably carried by the Na^+–K^+ pump, was also sensitive to the temperature in ventricular myocytes (355).

Pacemaker activity is also sensitive to temperature changes, and low temperature markedly slows the firing rate of the pacemaker cells (278, 634). Slowed automaticity may be caused by slowed current activation and depression of $I_{Ca.L}$ and I_K, as discussed above. Temperature-sensitive background current was also observed in SA node cells, suggesting the contribution of this current in slowing pacemaker activity at low temperatures (229).

Stretch and Osmotic Pressure

Mechanical loading leads to a variety of functional changes in cardiac cells including alterations in electrical activity. Since cardiac cells are subjected to dynamic movement with every beat, and chamber dilatation develops rather easily with hemodynamic overload. Mechanical stress may modulate electrical activity of the heart under physiological as well as pathological conditions. The primary mechanical transducers are generally not known, but some of the effects may be exerted through activation of mechanosensitive ion channels (379, 539a).

Effects of stretch. Mechanical stretch can increase heart rate and automaticity of the primary pacemaker of the heart (55, 300). In papillary muscle, stretch induced membrane depolarization and synchronous pacemaker activity (339). A 3–8 mV depolarization of resting membrane potential was observed in Purkinje fibers when the fibers were stretched 140% of their resting length (106). Stretch evidently lowered the threshold for excitation and decreased both the amplitude and V_{max} of action potentials with either lengthening or shortening of action potential duration (142, 339, 545). Changes in passive electrical properties also occurred under stretch (142), and it was demonstrated that stretch induced transient depolarization leading to development of abnormal automaticity (378).

The exact ionic mechanisms underlying these membrane potential changes have not been clarified, but stretch-activated channels may underlie the changes in electrical activity, forming a basis for mechanoelectric feedback (379). Activation of K^+ channels by stretch was noted in molluscan heart (593) and five different types of stretch-activated ion channels, two K^+ selective and three nonselective cation channels, were identified in cultured chick cardiac myocytes (538). It was demonstrated that stretch induces transient depolarization leading to development of abnormal automaticity, which might be caused by increased $[Ca^{2+}]_i$ mediated in part by the stretch-activated channels permeable to Na^+ and Ca^{2+} (99, 538). The nonselective cation channel sensitive to Gd^{3+} (87), was persistently activated in tachycardia-induced congestive heart failure, suggesting the involvement of this channel in the development of arrhythmias frequently encountered in this pathology (90). In SA node and atrial myocytes, the stretch-activated Cl^- current was identified, which would carry the background current and make a significant contribution to pacemaker depolarization (229) (Fig 16–5).

Effects of osmotic pressure changes. Reduction of os-

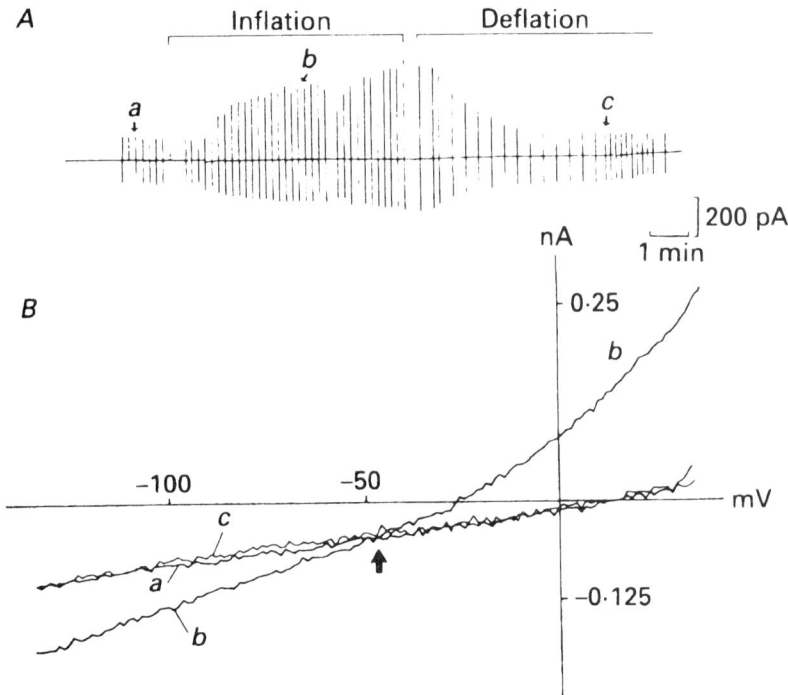

FIG. 16–5. Current changes in response to inflation and deflation of sinoatrial node cell by applying positive and negative pressure through the recording electrode. A: chart record (10 mm/min) of current changes in response to the ramp clamp. The current traces indicated by *a–c* are shown in B. The duration of inflation and deflation are indicated above the current trace. The pipette solution contained 24 mM Cl^- and the reversal potential for Cl^- (E_{Cl}) was calculated to be −49 mV. The reversal potential of the stretch-activated current was −48 mV (*arrow in B*), suggesting that the current activated in response to inflation of the cell is Cl^- elective. [Reproduced from Figure 2 in reference (229), with permission.]

motic pressure can induce swelling, which is assumed to be a similar but not equivalent stimulus as stretch on the cell membrane. The swelling-activated Cl⁻ channels ($I_{Cl,SWELL}$) have been demonstrated in various cardiac preparations, and these channels may play a role in volume regulation of cardiac cells (611). $I_{Cl,SWELL}$ is activated when the cell is immersed in hypoosmotic solution. In contrast to $I_{Cl,PKA}$, this current is not activated by phosphorylation by PKA under basal or isotonic condition, but it can be modulated by the PKA-dependent phosphorylation once it is activated by hypoosmotic solution (506, 601). The exact pathway of signaling from cell swelling to channel activation is not known. Alterations of cell volume during osmotic perturbation trigger multiple intracellular signaling events, including various second-messenger cascades, phosphorylation or dephosphorylation of target proteins, and altered gene expression (381, 541). Cell swelling has been shown to induce protein dephosphorylation, which may result from decreased kinase activity and/or increased activities of serine/threonine protein phosphatase. On the other hand, cell shrinkage can cause protein phosphorylation. In fact, cell swelling and shrinkage have been shown to induce protein dephosphorylation and phosphorylation, respectively, in various cells, including cardiac myocytes (231). $I_{Cl,SWELL}$ and its probable molecular counterpart, ClC-3, are inhibited by activation of PKC. A serine residue (serine 51) within a consensus PKC-phosphorylation site in the intracellular amino terminus of the ClC-3 channel protein is considered to be an important volume sensor of the channel (135). Another line of evidence has implicated the cytoskeleton in cell volume regulation. Cell swelling is associated with changes in F-actin conformation in a variety of cell types (450). In cultured chick cardiac myocytes, the swelling-induced changes in membrane conductance and F-actin architecture have disclosed that the dynamic disassembly and reassembly of F-actin in response to cell swelling comprise a component of the volume transduction process regulating the activation of $I_{Cl,SWELL}$ (716). $I_{Cl,SWELL}$ has been shown to be persistently activated in tachycardia-induced congestive heart failure (91). Therefore, this current may play a role in producing the abnormal electrical activity observed in this pathological condition.

Stretch can activate several K⁺ channels (345, 593). Stretch induced by hypoosmotic pressure increased I_{ks}, but not I_{kr} (526, 552). It was also demonstrated that the Na⁺–K⁺ pump current was stimulated by exposure to hypoosmolar solution (552, 680). The mechanism of this pump stimulation has not been clarified, but phosphorylation and dephosphorylation of protein kinases associated with cell swelling might be involved. The atrial $I_{K,ATP}$ was shown to be activated by pipette suction or osmotic stretch at physiological [ATP]$_i$ level (650).

EFFECTS OF NEUROHORMONES AND THEIR RECEPTOR STIMULATIONS

Adrenoceptor Agonists and Adrenergic Receptor Stimulation

Regulation by the sympathetic nervous system constitutes an important modulator of cardiac function. All regions of the heart are innervated by sympathetic nerves to varying degrees (523). The density of β-adrenoceptor in a single myocardial cell is much higher than that of $α_1$-receptors, and the effects of catecholamines during normal functioning of the heart are mediated mainly by β-adrenoceptor stimulation. For example, $α_1$-adrenoceptor stimulation–induced increase in the force of contraction amounted to only 10%–50% that induced by pure β-adrenoceptor stimulation (164, 243, 620).

β-Adrenergic Agonists and β-Adrenergic Receptor Stimulation. The β-adrenoceptor has two main subtypes ($β_1$ and $β_2$) in the heart, revealed by selective ligand binding studies, with a predominance of $β_1$ subtype in mammalian heart, while the $β_2$ subtype predominates in frog heart (236). The agonist binding to the $β_1$- and $β_2$-adrenoreceptor coupled to stimulatory G protein, G_s, induces activation of an intracellular second messenger, which modulates various cellular functions. The major effects of $β_1$- and $β_2$-adrenoceptor stimulation include increases in heart rate (chronotropic effect) and force of contraction (inotropic effect) with increased rate of relaxation and acceleration of impulse conduction (dromotropic effect) through the AV node. In addition, there is the third, $β_3$-subtype receptor, which is coupled to inhibitory G protein, G_i, (200). In contrast to $β_1$- and $β_2$-receptor stimulation, $β_3$-receptor stimulation causes myocardial depression. All three subtypes of receptors have been cloned. It is also suggested that there is a fourth type of β-receptor in the heart, but no identification of its molecular structure has been made (340).

Effects on automaticity and impulse conduction. β-adrenergic nerve stimulation and application $β_1$- and $β_2$-adrenergic agonists produce increased automaticity in dominant and latent pacemaker cells, accelerate the conduction through the AV node, and induce abnormal impulse formations in various cardiac preparations (101, 243, 278). In SA node and Purkinje fibers, accelerated automaticity is produced by increased slope of slow diastolic depolarization without changing threshold, and with no changes or only a slight increase in the maximal diastolic potential (208, 291). Latent pacemaker cells develop slow diastolic depolarization in the presence of catecholamines and β-adrenergic stimulation. Likewise, abnormal impulse formation becomes evident due to slow response automaticity in depolarized cardiac preparations in which I_{Na} is inactivated or $[Na^+]_o$ is absent, and where DADs develop and arrhythmias (101,). Conduction through the AV node is accelerated with increased upstroke velocity of action potentials in the presence of β-adrenergic agonists and nerve stimulation.

Effects on membrane potentials. β-adrenergic agonists causes a small change in resting membrane potential. Catecholamines sometimes induce a mild hyperpolarization and this is mainly due to activation of the Na$^+$–K$^+$ pump by α-adrenoceptor stimulation (see below, under α-Adrenoceptor Agonist and α-Adronergic Receptor Stimulation). Recent study has shown that isoproterenol stimulates the pump current by PKA-dependent phosphorylation, of which effect is dependent on the level of $[Ca^{2+}]_i$ (197). In other instances, β-agonists can produce depolarization and induce spontaneous excitations by activation of $I_{Cl,PKA}$ (148), but their effects may be small in ventricular tissues in physiological $[Cl^-]_i$, (700).

Both β$_1$- and β$_2$-adrenergic agonists increase plateau height, but produce little or variable effects on action potential duration. This is because β-adrenoceptor activation induces multiple effects on inward and outward currents at repolarizing voltages and the overall effects depend on the cell types, species, and conditions. Actually, isoproterenol has been shown either to prolong or shorten the action potential in the same species depending on the dominant effects either on $I_{Ca,L}$, or I_{KS} and $I_{Cl,PKA}$ (256). A part of the shortening action can be explained by the stimulation of the β$_3$-receptor subtype, which mediates cardiodepressor effects and shortening of action potential (200).

Effects on Ca^{2+} channels. A major target for β-adrenergic agonists is $I_{Ca,L}$ (243, 442, 527, 640). The agonist binding to the β-receptor or nerve stimulation induces activation of the stimulatory G protein, (G$_s$) which stimulates the catalytic site of adenylate cyclase and enhances the synthesis of cAMP in the cells. Then, increased cAMP activates PKA which phosphorylates the Ca^{2+} channel protein directly or an associated unit indirectly. β-adrenergic agonists are shown to increase peak $I_{Ca,L}$ in a dose-dependent manner with a mild (5–10 mV) shift in voltage-dependent activation and inactivation to hyperpolarizing direction (31, 63, 68, 175, 327). This increase is achieved by altering the gating properties of the $I_{Ca,L}$ channels: an increase in the available number of Ca^{2+} channels that can be activated by depolarization and an increase in the probability of channel opening without change in the single channel conductance. The increased channel open probability is produced by *(1)* increase in the proportion of sweeps with channel activity ("avilability") (or decrease in number of null-sweeps) (489, 640; Fig 16–6), *(2)* changes in gating behaviors, including prolongation of open times and shortening of closed times (63, 68), and *(3)* facilitation of long openings or "mode 2" gating (712). The question of whether these changes develop independently or through multiple processes simultaneously remains to be clarified. While Yue et al. (712) propose that graded alterations in gating time constants are the result of a new gating mode 2 during β-stimulation, the other groups (246, 266, 494, 687) suggest the involvement of multiple modulatory steps taking place simultaneously during stimulation by analysis of the channel kinetics and the effects of phosphatase inhibitors. While peak amplitude of $I_{Ca,L}$ is largely increased by β-agonists, the inactivation time course is usually not much affected in whole-cell currents despite slowed ensemble averaged currents of single-channel records (cf. ref. 489). This is probably caused by a Ca^{2+}-induced inactivation mechanism as a result of increased Ca^{2+} influx. In contrast to $I_{Ca,L}$, $I_{Ca,T}$ is usually not modulated by PKA-dependent phosphorylation.

The cardiac α subunit of the L-type Ca^{2+} channel ($α_{1C}$) has several candidate consensus sequences for PKA-dependent phosphorylation, and the cardiac β-subunit ($β_{2A}$) also has such sequences (76, 277)). The issue of whether specific consensus sequences—i.e., a single site or multiple sites of $α_{1C}$ and $β_{2A}$ subunits—are substrates for PKA-dependent phosphorylation for functional modulation has not been clarified. Several groups have reported PKA-induced potentiation of currents through Ca^{2+} channels formed by $α_{1C}$ alone in mammalian cells, although this increase was rather small or required pretreatment of the channel to PKA inhibitors in some cases. Others, however, could not reproduce these results. When expressed in *Xenopus* oocytes, currents through Ca^{2+} channels formed by $α_{1C}$ were not potentiated by PKA or PKA-activating treatment, but were reduced by PKA inhibitors, indicating an abnormally high level of the basal phosphorylation in oocytes (595). Furthermore, the potential site of functional modulation by PKA appears to be at the C-terminal domain of $α_{1C}$, but the exact site or amino acid residue is still a matter of controversy. Some studies indicated that phosphorylation of serine 1928 mediated the modulatory effect of PKA, and other studies suggested that serine 1627 and serine 1700 could be the phosphorylation sites (109, 386, 513). Involvement of PKA-dependent phosphorylation of Ca^{2+} channel $β_{2A}$ was also indicated (222).

Studies using cloned Ca^{2+} channels examined func-

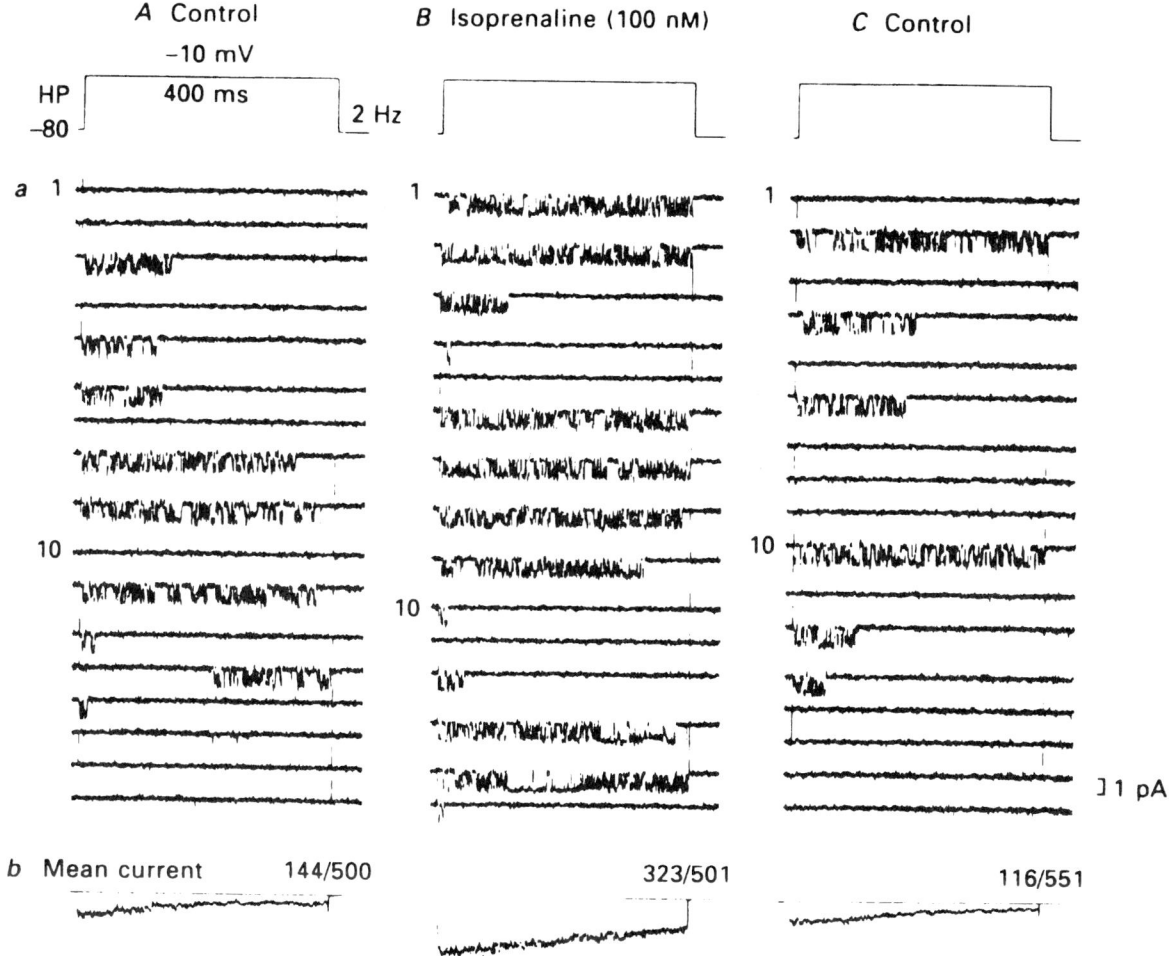

FIG. 16–6. Effect of isoprenaline on the single Ca^{2+} channel currents. A: control; B: in the presence of 100 nM isoprenaline; C: after wash-out of the drug. Depolarizing steps of 400 ms to −10 mV were applied repetitively from a holding potential (HP) of −80 mV at 2 Hz; 50 mM Ba^{2+} in the pipette. The number of steps was about 500 in each solution. a: typical current sweeps obtained after leakage current subtraction are given in the order of stimulation. Filtered at 1.5 kHz. b: the *bottom traces*: mean currents obtained by averaging the simulated openings from the total sweeps, including blank sweeps, on the same arbitrary scale. The ratio of the number of current-containing sweeps to the total number of sweeps (availability) is given above each mean current. [Reproduced from Figure 1 in reference (489), with permission.]

tional modulation have observed increased peak current at varying degrees at the macroscopic current level (267, 277, 514, 723). At the single-channel level, a similar potentiation of the current by application of 8Br-cAMP to the effects seen in native myocytes has been demonstrated with an increased number of channel openings and an increased duration of open times without changing the unitary current amplitude (267). There are, however, still certain quantitative and qualitative differences in the responses of cloned channels compared to those of native myocytes, which may be caused by differences in experimental conditions between native cells and expression systems, as well as unspecified proteins and subunit- or tissue-specificity of the channel. Gao et al. (198) have reported that channel phosphorylation and regulation are facilitated by submembrane targeting of PKA through association with an A-kinase anchoring protein called AKAP79. They suppose that the PKA-mediated regulation of the L-type Ca^{2+} channel is critically dependent on a function of AKAP79 and phosphorylation of α_{1C}.

Effects on K^+ and Cl^- channels. Not only $I_{Ca,L}$ but also I_K and $I_{Cl,PKA}$ are activated by the β_1- and β_2-adrenoceptor agonists by the same intracellular mechanism. In the presence of β-agonists, the amplitude of I_K is consistently increased with a negative shift of the activation curve, but the current kinetics are not changed (141, 662, 708). The activating action of isoproterenol and β-adrenoceptor stimulants on I_K is limited to the slow component of I_K (I_{KS}) (548). I_{KS} is composed of two molecular entities: *KVLQT1* and *minK* (25, 546). It is now known that the I_{KS} current in *Xenopus* oocytes is the functional expression of the exogenous *minK* together with the endogenous *KVLQT1* in the same species. The I_{KS} current in the oocytes is upregulated by agents that increase cellular cAMP concentrations through PKA-dependent phosphorylation (46, 324, 421). In the presence of these agents, the current amplitude is increased and shows a faster activation rate without altering voltage dependence. There are, however, no consensus phosphorylation sites for PKA on the minK protein, and, therefore, the site for modulating the currents may be on the KVLQT1 protein. The functional coupling of human $β_3$-adrenoceptor has recently been shown to up-regulate the KvLQT1/ minK channels via the stimulation of G_s proteins (336a). Activation of $I_{Cl,PKA}$ is observed in the presence but not in the absence of β-agonists associated with the cAMP-dependent process coupled to G protein involvement (21, 149, 248, 281, 292). $I_{Cl,PKA}$ in heart cells is encoded by the cardiac variant of *CFTR* (284). The CFTR channel contains two nucleotide-binding domains, a regulatory domain, and multiple consensus sites for possible PKA-dependent phosphorylation. The channel activation requires PKA-dependent phosphorylation as well as nucleotide binding and nucleotide hydrolysis (194, 288).

β-Adrenergic agonists activate $I_{K,ATP}$ in native myocytes when $[ATP]_i$ is substantially decreased. This effect is achieved through a decrease in subsarcolemmal ATP concentration rather than a direct action on the channels by phosphorylation (562). However, the channel activity of cloned cardiac K_{ATP} formed by Kir6.2, a family of inward rectifier K^+ channels, and SUR2A, a cardiac form of sulfonylurea receptor, in HEK293 cells has been activated by PKA-dependent phosphorylation (413). Functional significance of this finding in cardiac cells has to be further delineated.

Effects on Na^+ channels. There are several indications that β-adrenergic stimulation can modulate sodium channel activity through PKA-dependent phosphorylation. A reduction of I_{Na} and a shift in availability by β-adrenergic agonists are demonstrated in whole-cell (207, 497, 569) and single-channel recordings (254, 612). In contrast to these reports, stimulation of I_{Na} by β-adrenergic agonists has been described in rabbit cardiac preparations without any apparent shift of availability (435). Ono, Fozzard, and Hanck (495) have found that isoproterenol and cAMP produce shifts in the conductance and availability of I_{Na} in the hyperpolarizing direction through PKA-dependent phosphorylation with time. This result explains why the increased activity of PKA-dependent phosphorylation can either increase or decrease the amplitude of I_{Na} depending on the voltage protocols used in different experiments. In a cloned α subunit of the cardiac Na^+ channel, there are eight candidate consensus PKA phosphorylation sites at the cytosolic loop interconnecting domains I and II (76, 179, 428) and only two of these serines are the targets for PKA-dependent phosphorylation (461, 535). When cloned cardiac Na^+ channels are phosphorylated by PKA, a significant increase in peak I_{Na} is observed without any effects on kinetic parameters (186, 461, 566). No data have been presented so far as to the downregulation of channel activity by PKA-dependent phosphorylation using the cloned cardiac Na^+ channels. Recently, phosphorylation of the Na^+ channels has been implicated to induce the permeability changes accessible to Ca^{2+} ("slip-mode conductance") (551). However, there have been strong arguments against this finding (486) and, therefore, this observation needs further clarification.

Effects on channels responsible for pacemaker activity. In SA node cells, β-adrenergic agonists increase the amplitude of $I_{Ca,L}$ without shifting its voltage dependence (60, 227, 480). A consideration as to involvement of $I_{Ca,L}$ in the pacemaker depolarization is related to its activation threshold: $I_{Ca,L}$ is usually activated at voltages between -50 and -40 mV at the potential level where the slow diastolic depolarization is largely over and the upstroke phase of nodal action potential begins. Hagiwara et al. (227) have observed increased pacemaker activity by application of isoproterenol, which increases $I_{Ca,L}$, indicating the involvement of this current in pacemaker depolarization. Recently, Guo et al. (218) have demonstrated the presence of a sustained inward current, which is inhibited by dihydropyridine and stimulated by isoproterenol, at diastolic potential ranges between -70 and -50 mV in SA node cells. They conclude that the current represents a novel subtype of $I_{Ca,L}$ carried by Na^+ in the presence of divalent cations. This current component will contribute to pacemaker acceleration by β-agonists.

Although the activation range of I_f partially overlaps the voltage range of slow diastolic depolarization, application of Cs^+ at concentrations that inhibit I_f does not stop spontaneous activity completely, indicating that I_f is not a major determinant of pacemaker depolarization in SA node cells under physiological conditions (116, 649). In the presence of β-adrenergic agonists, however, the activation of I_f is shifted in a positive direction without change in the fully activated current and the rate of I_f activation is accelerated (60, 122). Therefore, I_f may become a contributing factor to accelerate the pacemaker depolarization (119, 120). While the stimulation of I_f is also coupled to G protein activation, intracellular modulation of this current seems to be controlled by cAMP directly and not through phosphorylation in SA node cells (124, 125). Pacemaker depolarization in Purkinje cells is seen at the voltage ranges, where prominent activation of I_f is observed (120). The positive shift of I_f activation is the main factor accelerating pacemaker depolarization in the presence of β-adrenergic agonists (118, 120).

In SA node cells, the decay of I_K plays an important role in the initial phase of pacemaker depolarization—i.e., near the maximum diastolic potential and its changes modulate firing rates (203, 496, 656). I_K is activated during depolarizations and decays slowly on repolarization to the level of pacemaker potential: for example, the time constant of I_K (I_{Kr}) decay is 200 msec at -60 mV in SA node cells (580). β-Adrenergic agonists increase I_K in atrial and nodal cells (60, 203, 480). The steady-state activation for I_K is consistently shifted to more negative value by isoproterenol and, therefore, the current activation is accelerated and the deactivation is slowed at comparable voltages.

Small AV node preparations or isolated single cells exhibit slow diastolic depolarization with the maximum diastolic potential between -70 and -50 mV and develop action potentials of slow upstroke velocity (237, 469, 479). The nodal cells exhibit I_{Na}, $I_{Ca.L}$, and I_K with less prominence of I_f. Therefore, the pacemaker mechanism is probably the same as that of SA node cells, with an acceleration process similar to that initiated by β-adrenoreceptor agonists. Because the slow upstroke phase of action potentials is largely dependent on $I_{Ca.L}$, an increase in this current will facilitate conduction through the AV node (237, 444, 479).

Since $I_{Ca.L}$ and I_f are activated by G protein–coupled processes (56, 442, 706), a rapid onset of chronotropic response to β-agonists is suggested to be attributable to a direct G protein and channel interaction in addition to a cAMP-mediated process. Actual contribution of the two current components coupled to a direct G protein activation to pacemaker depolarization, however, has not been demonstrated at the whole-cell level. It is also argued that a cAMP-mediated process is fast enough to describe the observed chronotropic responses with a single activation process (245). It may be possible that a major aspect of the chronotropic effect of β-adrenergic agonists can be explained by a cAMP-mediated process.

Abnormal automaticity seen in depolarized cardiac preparations is formed by $I_{Ca.L}$ and I_K (296, 338). Thus, potentiation of $I_{Ca.L}$ by β-adrenergic nerve stimulation accelerates slow response automaticity and its impulse formation. Catecholamines and β-adrenergic stimulation also induce and augment DADs, leading the appearance of triggered activity (101). Both factors contribute to development of arrhythmias under these conditions.

α-Adrenoceptor Agonists and α-Adrenergic Receptor Stimulation. α-Adrenergic receptors are divided into $α_1$- and $α_2$-subtypes based on the rank order of potency of pharmacologic agents (451). In cardiac tissues, α-adrenoceptors are mostly composed of the $α_1$-subtype as judged from pharmacological responses (164, 451, 620), but may contain the $α_2$-subtype in conducting tissues. Furthermore, there are, at least, two subtypes of $α_1$-adrenoceptors, referred as "$α_{1A}$" and "$α_{1B}$," according to pharmacological properties, that appear to be linked to different signal transduction pathways and effector systems (451). Molecular cloning of $α_1$-adrenoceptors has revealed the existence of three genes encoding distinct $α_1$-adrenoceptor subtypes, termed "$α_{1a}$, $α_{1a/d}$ or $α_{1d}$," "$α_{1b}$," and "$α_{1c}$" (176). Further evidence indicates that the gene encoding the $α_{1b}$ adrenoceptor subtype has pharmacological propeties of the classical $α_{1B}$ subtype, and the gene encoding the $α_{1c}$ adrenoceptor subtype is equivalent to pharmacologically defined $α_{1A}$ receptor subtype (449). The cloned $α_{1d}$-adrenoceptor, initially labeled $α_{1a}$ and then $α_{1a/d}$ is a novel subtype not recognized previously on the basis of pharmacological or radioligand binding studies and now is called $α_{1D}$ subtype adrenoceptor (213). Agonist binding to the $α_1$-adrenoceptors accelerates the hydrolysis of phosphoinositide, leading to production of inositol 1,4,5-triphosphate (IP_3) and diacylglycerol, which activates protein kinase C (PKC). This intracellular process induces multiple functional responses, although their exact mechanisms have not been elucidated. Modulation of cardiac functions by $α_1$-adrenoceptor stimulation includes changes in electrical and mechanical activity, metabolic alterations, and changes in gene expression/cellular hypertrophy (164, 594, 620).

Effects on membrane potentials. In rat and rabbit cardiac preparations, including atrial and ventricular cells and Purkinje fibers, $α_1$-adrenoceptor stimulation causes mild depolarization of the resting membrane potential (153, 313). $α_1$-Adrenoceptor activation prolongs action potential duration in rat, rabbit, and canine preparations but not in guinea pig cells (164, 243, 620), and it increases the force of contraction in most of the species. The effect is abolished by $α_1$-receptor antagonists but not by $α_2$-antagonists. While $α_1$-adrenoceptor stimulation prolongs the action potential in rat, rabbit, dog, and mouse, it causes shortening in guinea pig (128). Opposite effects are probably explained by different actions on I_{KS} among species by $α_1$-receptor stimulation as described below. Prolongation of the action potential by $α_1$-adrenergic stimulation is associated with abbreviation of the early notch and increase in the plateau height. The effects of α_1-stimulation are more prominent at slow heart rates than at fast rates (166, 524, 630).

In normal adult hearts, α_1-adrenoceptor agonists induce (1) no chronotropic action, (2) decreased automaticity, or (3) positive chronotropic effects, depending on preparations and species (38, 243). A part of these discrepant results may be attributed to distribution of different subtypes of α_1-receptors. For example, in 60%–70% of canine adult Purkinje fibers, decreased automaticity is observed by α_1-adrenoceptor stimulation, while the rest of the preparations respond to increased automaticity. A positive effect appears via α_{1A}-subtype activation and a negative response via the α_{1B}-subtype (110). Decreased automaticity in Purkinje cells is attributed to inhibition of Na^+–K^+ pump current with a resultant increase in $[Na^+]_i$ (714).

α_1-Adrenoceptors are implicated in the development of arrhythmias during coronary artery occlusion and reperfusion (38, 374). Adrenoceptor blockade reduces frequencies of arrhythmias and prevents development of tachycardias. DADs and triggered activity are frequently induced by α_1-adrenoceptor activation in Ca^{2+} overloaded Purkinje fibers under severe hypoxia (50, 347). During reperfusion, α_1-adrenoceptor stimulation can be expected to increase $[Na^+]_i$ by activating the Na^+–H^+ exchange, which in turn produces Ca^{2+} overload in the cells via the Na^+–Ca^{2+} exchange mechanism. This factor can aggravate the development of DADs and trigger arrhythmias, especially under the conditions of inhibited Na^+–K^+ pumping (714). Likewise, stimulation of α_1-adrenoceptors potentiates the development of digitalis cardiotoxicity and DADs (392).

Effects on Ca^{2+} channels. While measurements in multicellular preparations have demonstrated increased amplitudes of slow action potentials (453) and slow inward Ca^{2+} current (62) single-cell studies employing whole-cell recordings present no consistent increase in $I_{Ca,L}$ by α_1-adrenoceptor activation (164, 243, 620), with the exception of one study in neonatal rat ventricular myocytes (418). Although there are several reports describing increased $I_{Ca,T}$ by α_1-adrenoceptor activation (6, 639), the results are not consistent among different cell types, or the effects are transient. Furthermore, it is shown that α_1-adrenergic activation inhibits β-adrenergic stimulated $I_{Ca,L}$ (81). Recently, a transient suppression followed by a mild potentiation of $I_{Ca,L}$ by α-receptor agonists has been demonstrated by perforated patch recordings, with which the intracellular environment is disturbed very little (419, 720). Therefore, actions on the Ca^{2+} channels appear to be weak and transient, and intracellular dialysis may lose cytoplasmic key elements to modify the calcium channels in response to α_1-adrenoceptor activation.

Using the cloned cardiac Ca^{2+} channels, functional modulation by PKC activation, which is supposed to be induced by α_1-adrenergic receptor stimulation, has been demonstrated, but the results in native myocytes can not be reproduced. In the *Xenopus* oocyte expression system, PKC activation produces an initial increase in the current followed by a decrease (48). The PKC-dependent phosphorylation and PKC-induced reduction in the current depend on interaction between α_{1C} and β_{2A} subunits, while phosphorylation takes place independently in each subunit (49, 518). PKC-dependent up-regulation appears to depend on the splice variants of the amino terminus in α_{1C} (587a).

Effects on K^+ channels. There is increasing evidence that the action potential changes produced by α_1-adrenergic agonists can be attributed to the K^+ channel modulations: (1) inhibition of voltage-dependent, transient outward K^+ channel (I_{to}) (13, 166, 630), (2) reduction of a component of I_K (I_{KS}) in rat ventricular cells (14, 524), (3) block of I_{K1} in ventricular and Purkinje fibers (162, 572), and (4) activation and modulation of $I_{K,ACH}$ in atrial cells (163, 370). The action of these agonists is supposed to be mediated through activation of PKC. Inhibition of I_{to} is demonstrated in rat and rabbit ventricular myocytes, and Purkinje cells. In rat ventricle, inhibition of this current is achieved through activation of both α_{1A}- and α_{1B}-subtype receptors (666). At the single-channel level, the stimulation decreases the channel open probability with induction of burstlike openings without an increase in the numbers of blank sweeps (53; Fig. 16–7). The transduction mechanism has not been settled, or it may be different in different species, because the PKC activation seems to be involved in the inhibition in rat ventricle (13), while PKC does not mediate the response in rabbit atrial myocytes (53). The responsible channel gene for I_{to} has not been definitively determined. This may be due in part to the fact that I_{to} recorded in various experiments has some subtle differences in the time- and voltage-dependent properties depending on tissues and species of the preparations used (see 26, 105a). Several molecular correlates are proposed and they include *Kv1.4, Kv4.2,* and *Kv4.3*. The expressed currents from each gene share partial similarity to the properties of native currents in myocytes, but a single gene does not reproduce all the current features. Therefore, I_{to} may be composed of heterogeneous channel genes depending on the tissues and species. It has been shown that the human *Kv1.4* channel, which has multiple potential phosphorylation sites for PKC, is modulated by PKC activator, with an initial increase followed by a significant reduction in the expressed current amplitude (462).

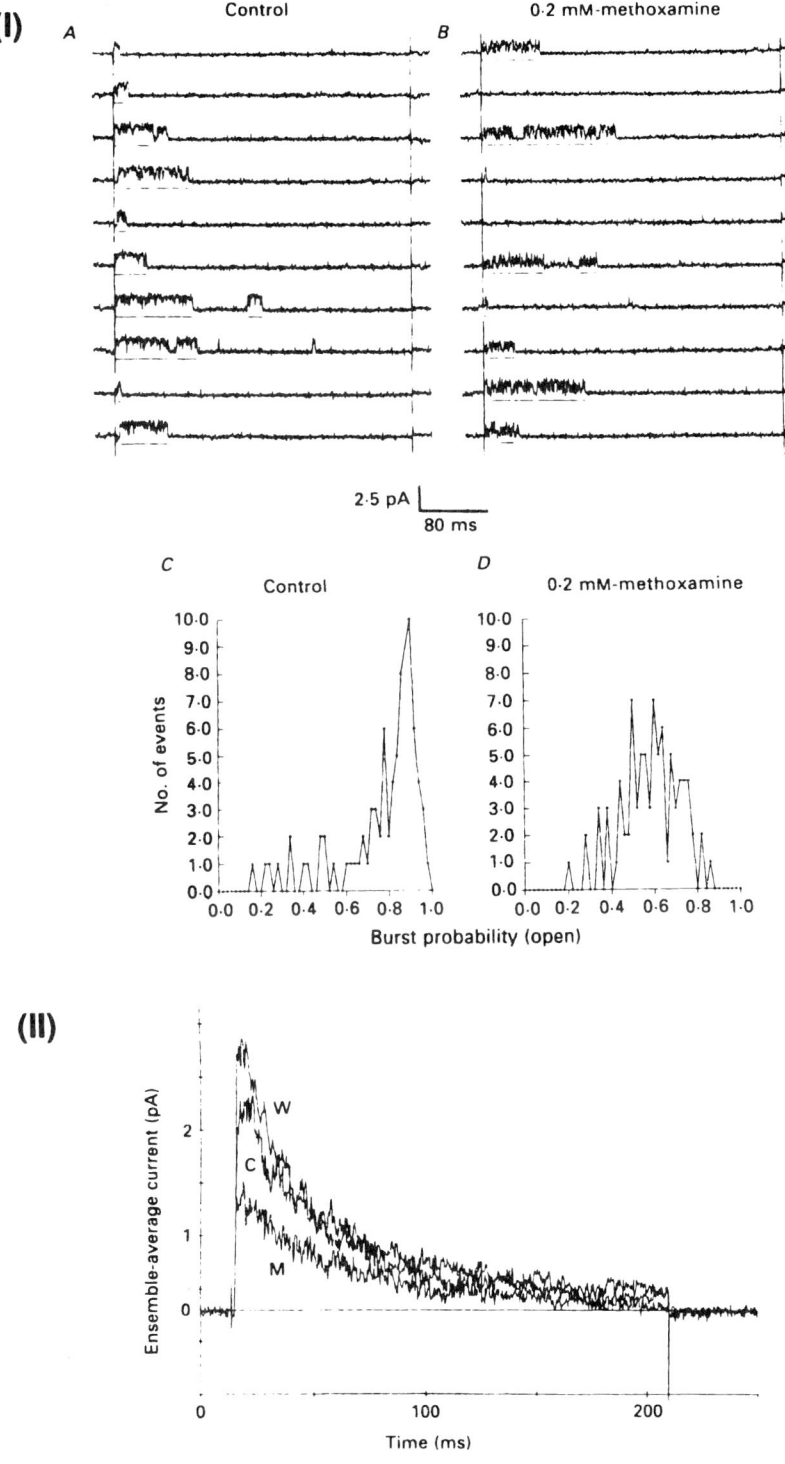

FIG. 16–7. Effects of α_1-adrenergic stimulation on I_{to} single-channel events. (I): A and B show a series of ten consecutive sweeps of single-channel openings recorded under control conditions (A) and during bath exposure of the cell to 0.2 mM methoxamine (B). I_{to} single-channel events were recorded following formation of the cell-attached seal (about 100 GΩ); the patch membrane was held at -50 mV relative to the cell resting potential. Channel openings were elicited by 350 ms depolarizing pulses (150 mV) at a rate of 0.1 Hz. To remove the capacitative and leak currents from the single-channel records, depolarizing pulses were applied at a rate of 2 Hz, and a total of ten to fifteen blank sweeps were averaged. This averaged record was then subtracted from the individual sweeps. C and D show the effect of methoxamine on the burst open probability of single I_{to} channels (same patch as A and B). The burst open probability was determined by dividing the summed durations of individual openings present with a burst by the total duration of the given burst. A total of seventy to eighty bursts were recorded under control conditions (C) and in the presence of 0.2 mM methoxamine (D). (II): Effect of methoxamine on an ensemble average of the single-channel events underlying I_{to}, from a cell-attached patch containing several channels. Groups of thirty records were averaged before (C), during application of 0.2 mM methoxamine to the bath (M), and after wash-out of methoxamine (W) from the bath. Depolarizing steps ($+200$ mV with respect to the cell resting potential; patch holding potential, -50 mV with respect to rest) were applied at a rate of 0.1Hz. [Reproduced from Figures 4 and 5 in reference (53), with permission.]

While I_K (I_{KS}) in rat ventricle is reduced (524), I_K in guinea pig ventricular myocytes is activated by α_1-adrenoceptor agonists (631, 662), which may explain opposite responses in action potential duration between the two preparations. Using the expression system of the cloned channels, the presence of PKC activators decreased the amplitude of currents expressed in oocytes from the rat or mouse *minK* gene (66, 280, 324), whereas their presence enhanced expressed current from the guinea pig *minK* gene (317, 324, 651). The I_{KS} currents expressed by the clone from the human and cat *minK* were dually modulated by activation of PKC with the time after application and concentrations of the activators used: an initial increase followed by a later decrease in the peak current, and an increase at low doses and a decrease at high doses of the activators (421). Different responses of the current to PKC activation in the cloned channels from different species may depend in part on the serine residue at position 102 on the *minK* protein.

α-Adrenergic agonists, possibly through activation of PKC, have been shown to block the I_{K1} in atrial and ventricular cells, and to modulate $I_{K.ACH}$ in atrial cells (162, 163, 309). In guinea pig atrial myocytes, $α_1$-adrenoceptor stimulation, has been shown to activate $I_{K.ACH}$ through 5-lipoxygenase metabolites of arachidonic acid (370). The ATP-sensitive K^+ channel (K_{ATP}) is activated by α-adrenergic stimulation, possibly through PKC activation (287, 309, 411, 412).

Effects on Cl⁻ channels. $α_1$-Adrenoceptor stimulation has been shown to activate a chroride conductance in guinea pig ventricular myocytes, which is mediated by PKC (660, 663, 718). It is not known whether the PKC-activated Cl⁻ current represents the different current from $I_{Cl.PKA}$, but the $I_{Cl.PKA}$ in guinea pig ventricular myocytes is inhibited by $α_1$-adrenergic agonists. This inhibitory action resembles to the action of ACh on this current, but the ACh action is exerted through antagonism with adenylate cyclase and develops upstream of adenylate cyclase (312, 491). In rabbit atrial myocytes, volume-regulated Cl⁻ current ($I_{Cl.SWELL}$) is also inhibited by $α_1$-receptor agonists in a concentration-dependent manner (137). This action is mediated by $α_{1A}$-receptor subtype activation and is PKC dependent through activation of pertussis toxin sensitive G protein.

Effects on the Na^+–K^+ pump. α-Adrenergic stimulation has been shown to activate the Na^+–K^+ pump current in atrial, ventricular, and Purkinje cells (153, 572, 714). Pump inhibition is coupled to pertussis toxin–sensitive G-protein in Purkinje cells. This action can somewhat antagonize depolarizing action of the resting potential by simultaneously blocking I_{K1} and inhibition of Na^+–H^+ exchange mechanism by α-adrenergic stimulation (572).

Cholinergic Agonists and Cholinergic Receptor Stimulation

Cholinergic nerve stimulation in the heart is produced by the agonist (acetylcholine; ACh) binding to the muscarinic receptor (mAChR), since all cardiac effects by vagal stimulation, ACh, and other cholinergic agonists are blocked by atropine. Vagal innervation and muscarinic receptors are distributed throughout the heart, although their distribution is not uniform (243, 508). So far, five mAChR subtypes (M_1 to M_5) have been identified, each subtype being encoded by a different gene (77). While cardiac mAChR subtype seems to be predominantly M_2, the existence of other subtypes has not been settled. There is some indication of the presence of M_1 subtype (196). Agonist binding to m-AChR(M_2) activates G proteins to transduce diverse cellular responses including direct activation of potassium channels in a membrane delimited fashion, inhibition of adenylate cyclase, increased phosphoinositide breakdown, and arachidonate release (86, 564).

Effects on membrane potentials. Vagal stimulation and application of cholinergic agonists produce slowing of pacemaker activity (negative chronotropic effect), reduction and shortening of atrial action potential with membrane hyperpolarization, suppression of AV node conduction (negative dromotropic effect), inhibition of contractility (negative inotropic effect), and abbreviation of β-agonist stimulated electrical and mechanical activities. These inhibitory effects do not develop in a monotonic fashion, but show complex or triphasic responses with persistent stimulation or continued exposure to the agonists (59, 243, 508). Furthermore, termination of vagal stimulation and washout of the agonist induce rebound acceleration of the activity. While the agonist-induced inhibitory effects decrease with time during prolonged exposure to ACh, which is referred as "desensitization" (51, 429), this effect is attributed in part to a decrease in inhibitory action, but it cannot explain the triphasic responses or the rebound acceleration. This raises the second explanation of stimulatory action by ACh (509; see below).

Application of ACh and cholinergic agonists caused a decrease in the amplitude and duration of atrial action potential with membrane hyperpolarization, and slowing of the pacemaker depolarization in nodal cells. These effects were assumed to be produced by increased K^+ permeability (111, 291). In ventricular tissues under basal conditions, the effects were generally least or nearly lacking in most preparations (243, 278), but shortening of action potential with hyperpolarization of diastolic potential was noted in some preparations (195, 262, 458).

Effects on K^+ channels. ACh activates a specific K^+ current, $I_{K.ACH}$ in atrial and nodal cells, which underlies a main mechanism of action potential shortening, membrane hyperpolarization, and pacemaker suppression in these cells, while the density of this channel is quite low in the ventricle. $I_{K.ACH}$ in atrial cells has similar properties to I_{K1} in the ventricle, but it displays a distinct K^+ channel current of activation, inward rectification, single channel conductance, and channel kinetics (294, 482, 540, 597). The channels open infrequently in the absence, and much more frequently in the presence, of ACh (326). The activation of $I_{K.ACH}$ is direcly coupled to the inhibitory G protein (G_i) activation sensitive to pertussis toxin (54, 371, 516; (Fig. 16–8). The main component involved in their activation appears to be the βγ subunit of G protein (309,

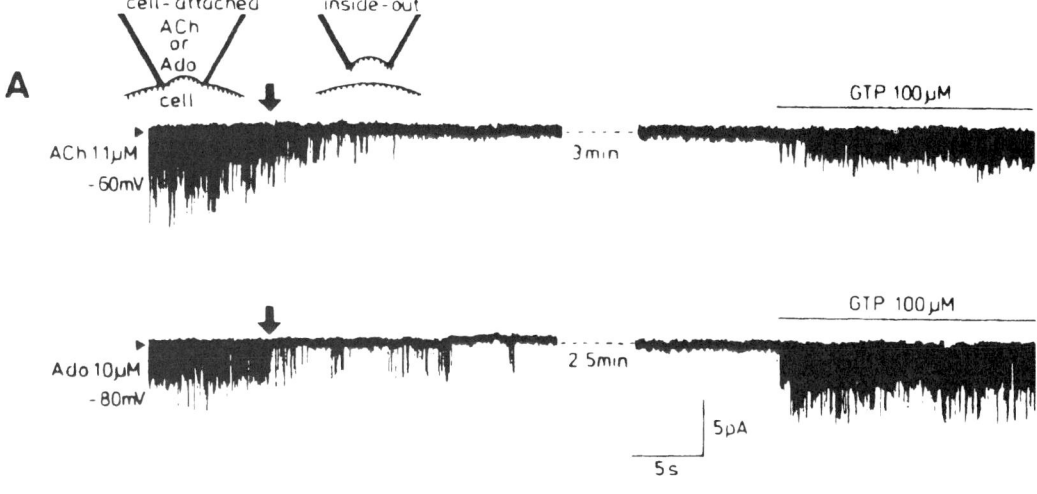

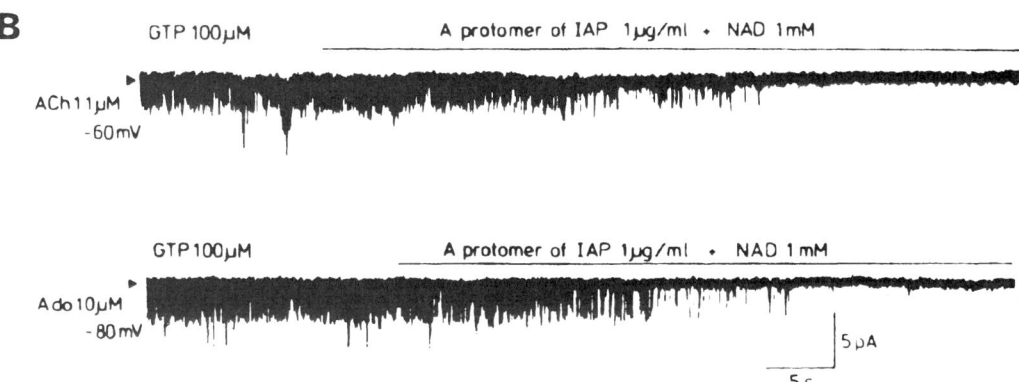

FIG. 16–8. Activation of K$^+$ channel by Ado and ACh requires intracellular GTP and blocked by IAP (islet-activating protein or pertussis toxin). A: The cells were bathed in the internal solution. The concentration of agonists and the patch membrane potential are indicated at each current trace. At the *arrow* in each trace, the patch was excised from the cell, yielding the "inside-out" patch. Activation of the channel was blocked in the "inside-out" patches. During the period shown by the *bar* above each current trace, internal solution containing GTP 100 μM was perfused. Activation of the channel resumed abruptly by addition of GTP into the bath solution. B: The same patches as those in A. With GTP 100 μM present in the intracellular side of the membrane, channels remained activated. The A (active) protomer of IAP with NAD 1 mM was added in the internal solution containing GTP during the period indicated by the bar above each trace. Channel activation was gradually blocked by IAP within 1–3 min. The blocking effect of IAP was irreversible. When the A protomer was perfused in the absence of NAD, the activation of the channel was not blocked. [Reproduced from Figure 9 in reference (371) with permission.]

422). The molecular structure of $I_{K,ACh}$ is made up of heteromultimer with the family of the inward rectifier K$^+$ channels Kir3.1 and Kir3.4 (362). The expressed channels of the $I_{K,ACh}$ clone are activated by the G protein βγ subunit (528, 686).

Not only ACh, but also somatostatin and adenosine can activate the same type of K$^+$ channel via G protein activation after binding to their specific receptors (Fig. 16–8). In the absence of extracellular agonist and cytoplasmic G protein, however, $I_{K,ACh}$ can be activated by intracellular Mg-ATP or adenosine thiotriphosphate (ATPγs; 253, 326, 505). The ATP- and ATPγs-dependent activation of $I_{K,ACh}$ are thought to be due to the (thio)phosphate transfer from ATP or ATPγs to free cytoplasmic GDP by a cellular nucleoside diphosphate kinase (NDPK), resulting in the formation of GTP or GTPγs. NDPK is contained in atrial membranes from various species (253). Under physiological conditions, NDPK can act as a GTP supply in the immediate vicinity of the G protein to ensure reliable signal transduction.

Activation of $I_{K,ACh}$ also undergoes the process of desentization causing inactivation of the channel activity (73, 373). Due to the process of desentization, the ACh actions on the heart are usually transient and fade with time (51, 429). The mechanism of desentization has not been fully clarified, but phosphorylation of the mAChR appears to be involved (225). The ACh-bound mAChR causes G protein dissociation into α- and βγ-subunits, which open $I_{K,ACh}$ (528); at the same time, βγ subunits also activate muscarinic receptor kinase, one of a family of G protein–coupled receptor kinases (225). In the presence of ACh, mAChR is quickly phosphorylated, presumably by the activated receptor kinase, and may cause uncoupling of the mAChR and G protein (225, 376). It has been suggested that G protein–coupled receptor kinase dependent phosphorylation of mAChR is responsible for the slow phase of desensitization and that a soluble intracellular factor may be responsible for rapid desentization (592). It has been shown that leukotriene C_4 is required for the rapid, ACh-mediated activation of $I_{K,ACh}$ under physiological conditions, but is not required for maintenance of the steady-state current in the presence of GTP (563). This action of leukotriene C_4, therefore, may also be responsible in part for development of desensitization.

ACh has been shown to activate $I_{K,ATP}$ via the activation of G protein with interaction to its α-subunit in guinea pig atrial myocytes (309). The action of channel activation via G protein is not strong and appears to be exerted through antagonism against the ATP-induced inhibition (311, 621). In cat atrial myocytes exposed to ACh twice, the second ACh exposure elicits a large increase in K^+ conductance due to possible activation of $I_{K,ATP}$, which is blocked by PKC inhibitors (667). However, an intracellular mechanism of this channel activation is still controversial.

Effects on Ca^{2+} channels. While it is agreed that muscarinic stimulation exerts a predominant effect to depress the stimulated $I_{Ca,L}$ by β-agonists, there is not yet complete agreement about whether ACh and cholinergic agonists affect basal, nonstimulated $I_{Ca,L}$ or not. This question has important functional implications as to the ACh actions on the modulation of the primary pacemaker mechanism in the SA node and cardiac contractility. In isolated single cell studies, most reports have described no effects of ACh on basal $I_{Ca,L}$, while, in multicellular and tissue preparations, most of the studies do find an effect on basal I_{Ca} and negative inotropic action of ACh (243). These discrepant results might be due to increased cAMP levels in certain cells by tonic stimulation of sympathetic activity or for other reasons, or due to technical problems inherent in each experimental procedure.

In the presence of β-receptor stimulation, ACh always reduces $I_{Ca,L}$ (174, 255, 465). The mechanism of this response can be explained in large part by muscarinic inhibition of adenylate cyclase activity through an inhibitory G protein (G_i) sensitive to pertussis toxin, allowing cytosolic cAMP to return toward basal levels (243, 446, 508). The stimulation of $I_{Ca,L}$ by intracellular application of cAMP or non-hydrolyzable cAMP analogues is not reduced by muscarinic agonists, indicating that the site of action by ACh is prior to cAMP production. The inhibitory effect of ACh on $I_{Ca,L}$ is prevented by pertussis toxin (465), in which cardiac substrates are G_i and G_o. G_i has been shown to antagonize the activation of adenylate cyclase by G_s. The inhibitory action of ACh on $I_{Ca,L}$ develops at concentration much lower than that on $I_{K,ACh}$ in frog atrial myocytes, and the former action cannot totally be abolished by pertussis toxin, while the latter action is completely eliminated. The pertussis toxin–resistant effect of ACh on $I_{Ca,L}$ is still mediated by G protein, since it is abolished by an inhibitor of G protein function, $GDP\beta_S$ (409). Intracellular application of non-hydrolyzable GTP analogues mimics the inhibitory effect of ACh on stimulated $I_{Ca,L}$. These data suggest that the muscarinic inhibition of $I_{Ca,L}$ is mostly due to the inhibition of adenylate cyclase (446).

Substantial evidence has been presented, however, that there is dissociation of tissue cAMP levels and effects of ACh, and that ACh can produce inhibitory actions without any detectable changes in cAMP levels (243, 446, 670). This might be attributed to the stimulation of phosphatase activity (219, 414), or to a local increase in cAMP near the sarcolemmal membrane, concentrations of which cannot be detected by the ordinary measurements. Such local increases in cAMP leading to local augmentation of $I_{Ca,L}$ by isoproterenol and inhibition by ACh have been indicated (446). There are some suggestions of a cAMP-independent pathway for the muscarinic inhibition of a $I_{Ca,L}$. Muscarinic stimulation increases cGMP levels in cardiac myocytes (201, 367, 670) and the increased cGMP is postulated to be involved in inhibition of $I_{Ca,L}$ (357, 635). This hypothesis has been supported by the findings that direct intracellular application of cGMP to frog ventricular myocytes can antagonize cAMP-dependent activation of $I_{Ca,L}$ (175, 244). This effect is attributed to stimulation of phosphodiesterane (PDE) activity (type II), since the effect can be abolished by PDE inhibitors. In mammalian ventricular myocytes, however, where predominant PDE isoform is composed of type III, cGMP is found to facilitate cAMP-dependent activation of $I_{Ca,L}$ (404, 500). Another cGMP-dependent pathway may be proposed that cGMP activation of cGMP-dependent protein kinase (PKG) can inhibit cAMP-stimulated $I_{Ca,L}$ in mamalian ventricular myocytes (448). This pathway may explain the inhibitory action by ACh on β-agonist stimulated

$I_{Ca,L}$ in both amphibian and mammalian ventricular myocytes. In relation to this hypothesis, increased guanylate cyclase activity leading to cGMP accumulation has been shown to inhibit $I_{Ca,L}$ (405, 459). A soluble guanylase cyclase activating factor is secreted from cardiac myocytes in the presence of muscarinic agonists and this factor is assumed to be nitric oxide (NO) (23). There is a suggestion that synthesis of NO may be involved in the inhibitory action of ACh (see, later, under Nitric Oxide).

Effects on other channels. Both I_K (I_{KS}) and $I_{Cl,PKA}$ stimulated by β-agonists are also inhibited by ACh. ACh has no effects or slight depression of I_K in the absence of β-adrenergic agonists (72, 262), but in the presence of isoproterenol, ACh not only reduces the amplitude of I_K but also shifts the activation curve back toward positive voltage (249, 255, 708). This ACh action is prevented either with intracellular dialysis of the non-hydrolyzable GTP analogue, Gpp(NH)p, or with application of pertussis toxin to inactivate G_i. $I_{Cl,PKA}$ activated by β-agonists is inhibited by ACh similar to $I_{Ca,L}$ (248, 499, 616), requiring (G_i activation (281, 292). I_{Na} is modulated by isoproterenol with phosphorylation-depndent manner (see, earlier, under β-Adrenergic Agonists and β-Adrenergic Receptor Stimulation). This modulatory action by β-agonists is also antagonized by cholinergic agonists through a mAChR signal transduced by a pertussis toxin–sensitive G protein (436).

Effects on automaticity and pacemaker channels. Suppression of automaticity can be exerted either by activation of $I_{K,ACH}$, inhibition of $I_{Ca,L}$, modulation of I_f or background inward current, or a combination of them. ACh reduces I_f by shifting its activation to negative potentials without changing the maximum conductance in rabbit SA node cells. The effect is opposite to the action by β-adrenergic agonists on I_f, and this action is mediated by mAChR activation through a pertussis toxin–sensitive G protein (126, 127). The ACh action on I_f, however, does not necessarily require the presence of isoproterenol. It is assumed that SA node cells have a high level of adenylate cyclase activity, which is suppressed by ACh. I_f is more sensitive to ACh than $I_{K,ACH}$ or $I_{Ca,L}$ (121) (Fig. 16–9). A high level of adenylase cyclase activity in SA node cells may be argued for reduced rate of diastolic depolarization without membrane hyperpolarization in the presence of a low concentration of ACh or when the vagal nerve is sub-

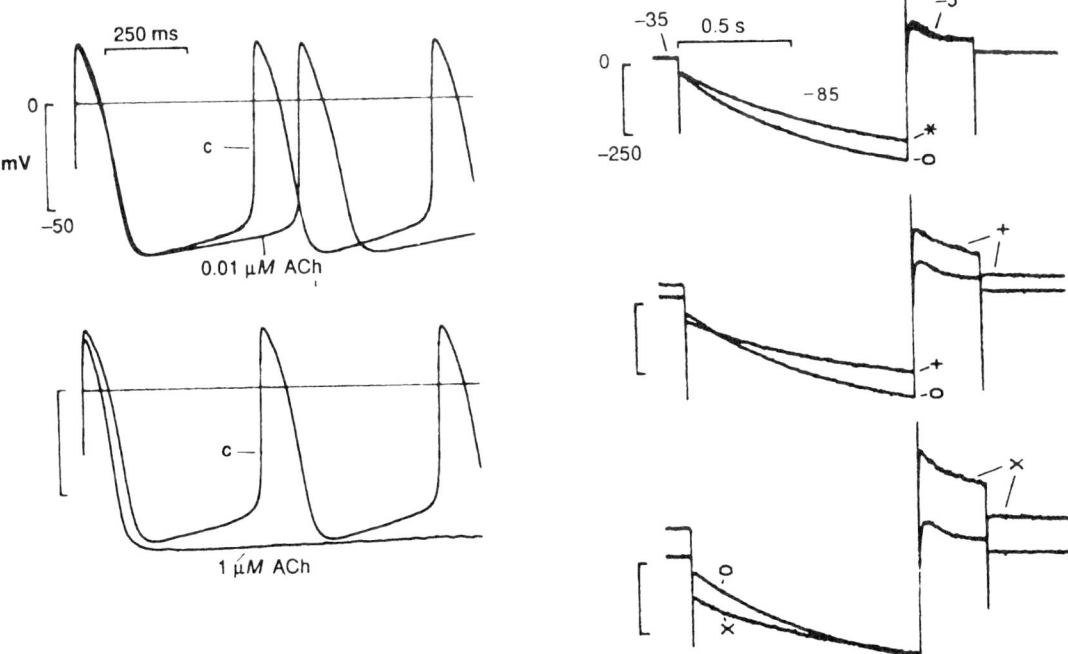

FIG. 16–9. Effects of ACh on SA node cells. *Left:* Effects of different ACh concentrations on the rate of spontaneous activity in an SA node myocyte. Activity was recorded in control Tyrode's solution (c) and during superfusion with ACh 0.01 μM (*top*) and 1 μM (*bottom*), as indicated. *Right:* Separation of the effects of ACh on I_f and $I_{K,ACH}$. Two-pulse protocols were applied every 3 sec during superfusion with various doses of ACh. The myocyte was superfused with normal Tyrode's solution (O, control) and with Tyrode's containing 0.01 (*), 0.1 (+), and 1 μM (x) ACh. In each case ACh superfusion was maintained until a steady-state effect was achieved, typically 20 sec, and was followed by an appropriate washout period. [Reproduced from Figures 1 and 3 in reference (121), with permission.]

jected to low frequency stimulation (111, 291, 581). It has further been demonstrated that hyperpolarization induced by vagal nerve stimulation is caused by decreased inward current, while externally applied ACh produces hyperpolarization by increased outward K^+ current (67). Therefore, decreased inward current seems to be a primary regulator of pacemaker activity by vagus nerve stimulation, but it does not preclude I_f as a main mechanism of pacemaking in SA node cells.

In canine Purkinje fibers, in contrast to SA node cells, ACh shifts the I_f activation to the negative direction exclusively in the presence but not in the absence of isoproterenol (80). This has been interpreted as a hierarchy of neural control of primary and subsidiary pacemakers. On the other hand, rabbit Purkinje fibers usually do not exhibit I_f, but when present, ACh reduces the time constants for the I_f activation (72). In sheep cardiac Purkinje fibers, ACh accelerates spontaneous activity to fasten the rate of diastolic depolarization and shifts the I_f activation to positive directions through activation of mACh (see below, under Stimulatory Actions of Acetylcholine). These results suggest that I_f plays an important regulatory role in subsidiary pacemakers, but there are still unsettled issues as to whether the effect is exclusively mediated through action on I_f.

Stimulatory actions of acetylcholine. In contrast to the inhibitory effects, the stimulatory action of vagal nerve or cholinergic agonists appeared at relatively higher concentrations than those of inhibitory action. The action was not blocked by β-blockers but was inhibited by atropine, indicating muscarinic response in nature (293, 509). Membrane hyperpolarization induced by ACh and other agonists was followed by rebound depolarization associated with positive inotropic effect upon washout or without preceding inhibitory action in atrial cells (211, 602, 613). In sheep Purkinje fibers, ACh increased diastolic depolarization and shifted the activation curve of I_f with prolongation of the action potential (74, 416) and washout of ACh was associated with membrane depolarization with decreased membrane current below control values (73). Two possible pathways for this stimulant action have been proposed: (*1*). Membrane depolarization and positive inotropic effect are associated with increased $[Na^+]_i$ through opening of the background Na^+ current (360, 437). This Na^+ current is resistant to TTX and is not transduced via pertussis toxin–sensitive G protein. (*2*) The other pathway involves muscarinic stimulation of phosphoinositide and phosphatidylcholine metabolism with the production of inositol phosphates. ACh and calbachol have been shown to stimulate phosphoinositide hydrolysis at higher concentrations than those required to inhibit cAMP production (57, 221) and to augment $I_{Ca,L}$ in guinea pig ventricular myocytes (196).

The stimulated phosphoinositide hydrolysis is correlated with depolarization and an increase in force of contraction (613). These two mechanisms, which are not mutually exclusive, are proposed to explain the stimulant effect (509). The stimulatory action is probably mediated through the M_1 mAChR subtype (196, 574), but involvement of the co-release of vasoactive intestinal polypeptides in the stimulatory effects (530) has not been excluded.

EFFECTS OF CIRCULATORY HORMONES AND AUTOCRINE/PARACRINE SUBSTANCES

Circulatory hormones target the heart as their effector. Humoral substances that are produced in the heart and other tissues and that presumably have their main action on organs other than the heart, may affect cardiac cells by autocrine and paracrine mechanisms. Modulation of cardiac function by these factors has not only a physiological significance but also plays important roles in pathological conditions.

Thyroid Hormones and Thyroid States

Thyroid hormone (T_3) regulates cardiac function, possibly through two aspects in acute, non-genomic actions and genomic actions. Acute actions of thyroid hormones have been shown to modulate I_{Na} (143, 240), to inhibit the inward rectifier K^+ current (543), and to stimulate the Ca^{2+} transport system in the sarcolemma (570). These acute actions on ion channels and contractile function are likely to be mediated by binding of the hormone to putative membrane receptors, since several thyroid hormone analogues have T_3-like acute effects. In genomic actions, thyroid hormone exerts its effects through multiple pathways, including modulation of expression and transcription of ion channel genes and β-adrenergic signaling pathway.

Thyroid states have significant affects on cardiac performance, since increases in heart rate, force, and velocity of contraction with concomitant hypertrophy are observed in the hyperthyroid state, while decreased heart rate and contractility are noted in the hypothyroid state (457a). Atrial tachyarrhythmias are frequently associated with hyperthyroid states in animals, as well as in humans, but they are rare in hypothyroid states. Action potentials of atrial cells showed shortened duration in hyperthyroid and increased duration in hypothyroid states, without changes in resting membrane potential and total amplitude (183). Similar results to those obtained from multicellular preparations were confirmed in isolated ventricular myocytes from guinea pigs with altered thyroid states (43, 537). The Ca^{2+} and K^+ currents were increased in hyperthyroid myocytes, and the Ca^{2+} current was decreased without changes in K^+ current in hypothyroid cells. Increased Ca^{2+} channel function by T_3 was observed in cultured chick ventricular cells (346), whereas a decrease in channel density was reported in rat ventricle (251). Injection of thyroxin into the animals two hours before cell isolation mimicked the changes in I_{Ca} in hyperthyroidism but no changes in K^+ current occurred (537).

In hyperthyroid rabbit ventricle, complex changes in action potential configurations were reported (575). Action potentials showed prolonged duration, and a prominent dome and hump at the early phase of repolarization in slow heart rate, but these changes were normalized in fast rate. These changes were attributed to increase and alteration of the transient outward K^+ current, I_{to}, with accelerated recovery from inactivation (582). Surprisingly, there were no changes in I_{to} in atrial myocytes from hyperthyroidism. More complex results were observed in rat ventricle where I_{to} was not changed in amplitude from the control in hyperthyroid states, but recovery from inactivation was speeded up in endocardial but not in epicardial myocytes (586). On the other hand, hypothyroid myocytes showed decreased amplitude of I_{to} from the control both in epicardium and in endocardium with slowed time course of the recovery. All of these results in animal models do not explain electrical abnormalities seen in patients, and further clarification is necessary.

As to a possible basis for these channel remodeling in altered thyroid status, T_3 is shown to regulate postnatal expression of transient outward K^+ channel isoforms (585, 685), and it differentially regulates the expression of different K_V channels at mRNA levels, not through the β-adrenergic signaling pathway (476). Hypothyroid status is reported to impair the early postnatal maturation of dihydropyridine receptors into junctional structure and the expression of mRNA level (684). The hyperpolarization-activated cyclic nucleotide-gated channel (HCN2) mRNA is upregulated by T_3 in rat heart, which may, in part, explain the positive chronotropic effect by this hormone (507).

Insulin and Diabetes Mellitus

Insulin plays pivotal roles for glucose metabolism and amino acid transport, in addition to many other biological activities. An insulin deficiency or impaired tissue responsiveness to insulin produces a common disease, diabetes mellitus, which is prone to produce disorders of the cardiovascular system (168). Patients with diabetes mellitus have significant alterations in myocardial function, including altered electrical activities, abnormal ECG waveforms, and an increased propensity for cardiac arrhythmias.

Insulin itself has been shown to alter ionic fluxes and membrane potentials of target cells (455). Cardiac cells respond to physiological levels of insulin with membrane hyperpolarization due to activation of the Na^+–K^+ pump (380) and other mechanisms (383), since insulin is known to regulate Na^+–K^+ ATPase activity, both acutely and chronically (155). I_{K1}, a major determinant of resting conductance, in myocytes from diabetic animals has not been affected by insulin (322, 426). Insulin is shown to stimulate $I_{Ca,L}$ in rat cardiac myocytes (20). Insulin may exert its electrical effect through indirect action on glucose metabolism. $I_{K,ATP}$ current activated by metabolic inhibition is suppressed by glucose and insulin via increased glycolysis to supply ATP (466).

In diabetic animals, a consistent finding is a prolongation of action potential duration in atrial and ventricular muscles (167, 396). The prolongation is not caused by hypothyroidism which is a frequent association in diabetes mellitus, but appears to be caused mainly by remodeling of K^+ channels. Studies using isolated myocytes from diabetic rats have confirmed the action potential prolongation and have attributed this change to decreased amplitude of I_{to} without a shift in voltage-dependent properties (322, 426, 586). Kinetics of inactivation and recovery from inactivation are either slowed (426, 584) or not changed (322). Reduced I_{to} amplitude with kinetic changes as well as decreased $I_{Ca,L}$ was also reported in chronic diabetic rats (664). Decrease in I_{to} in the ventricle is larger in epicardial than in endocardial myocytes (586). This reduces the voltage gradient during repolarization between endocardium and epicardium, which may explain frequent associations of decreased T wave amplitude in ECG of diabetic patients. The changes in action potentials and I_{to} are observed not only in chronic diabetic animals but also in short-term experimental diabetes mellitus induced by 4–6 days of streptozotocin injection (584). These changes are somewhat reversed by application of insulin to lower plasma glucose level but not completely to the control level, suggesting metabolic regulation of K^+ channel expression. Recent observations indicate that the prolongation of action potential is only seen in animal models of insulin-dependent diabetes mellitus (type I; streptozotocin-induced), but not evident in non-insulin-dependent models (type II) (583). These differences can be attributed to different behaviors of the transient and sustained components of I_{to} to insulin and metabolic alteration.

Abnormal mechanical function of the diabetic heart is mostly attributed to impaired Ca^{2+} handling (561), and its main factor is suppression of the Na^+–Ca^{2+} exchange mechanism (560). $I_{Ca,L}$ in diabetic rat myocytes is not changed from the control (641) or decreased (561), which might come from different models or stage of disorders.

Effects of Adenosine and Adenine Nucleotides Through Purinergic Receptor Stimulation

Adenosine and adenine nucleotides are present in the coronary circulation as a result of their release from tissues, including hypoxic and ischemic myocardium, aggregating platelets and damaged vessel walls (177). Adenosine and adenine nucleotides interact with specific membrane receptors in a variety of cells. The membrane receptor that have affinity to bind adenosine was first classified as the P_1 purinergic receptor and the one recognizing external ATP as agonist was the P_2 purinergic receptor (64). The adenosine receptors are now divided into four subclasses, A_1, A_{2A}, A_{2B}, and A_3, depending on either inhibition or stimulation of adenylate cyclase activity, signal transduction pathways, and pharmacology. Four different subtypes of adenosine receptors have been cloned (181, 182). The ATP receptors are now classified as two subtypes, P_{2X} and P_{2Y}. P_{2X} receptors belong to the family of transmitter-gated ion channels and P_{2Y} receptors are the family of G protein–coupled receptors.

Adenosine and Adenosine Receptor Stimulation. Adenosine has important cardiovascular actions that are mediated by activation of specific cell membrane receptors of two main subtypes, A_1- and A_2-receptors with different biochemical, physiological, and pharmacological properties (36, 492, 567, 645). Actions of adenosine A_1-receptor on the heart are mediated by the activation of a potassium current (adenosine-activated K^+ current; $I_{K.Ado}$) and inhibition of adenylate cyclase activity. Both responses are attenuated after inactivation of inhibitory G proteins by pretreatment with pertussis toxin (37, 252). Activations of A_2-receptor mediate the stimulation of adenylate cyclase activity. A universal presence and a functional manifestation of adenosine A_2-receptor in different cardiac preparations have not been confirmed, and controversial results have been reported (589, 607, 696). Activation of vascular adenosine A_2-receptor produces coronary vasodilatation and increased blood flow. A presence and role of adenosine A_3-receptor activation are suggested to be involved in ischemic preconditioning (609). Generally, the effect of adenosine receptor activation on the heart is to depress electrical and mechanical activity. Adenosine slows the rate of the SA node automaticity, induces hyperpolarization and shortening of atrial action potential, and suppresses AV nodal conduction. It antagonizes the stimulatory effects of catecholamines in both atrial and ventricular tissues.

Effects on membrane potentials and K^+ channels in basal conditions. Effects of adenosine on membrane potentials were first demonstrated to shorten action potential duration in atrial muscle but not in ventricular muscle, the actions being similar to those of ACh (242, 319). Later the mechanism was proved to be increased K^+ conductance in isolated single cells (34). The agonist binding to the A_1-receptor activates the same type of K^+ channels as $I_{K.ACH}$, and both responses are coupled to a pertussis toxin–sensitive G protein via activation of different receptors (371) (see Fig.16–8). Because of activation of $I_{K.Ado}$, adenosine causes membrane hyperpolarization and reduces the rate of slow diastolic depolarization in SA node cells. The extent of pacemaker slowing correlates with the magnitude of hyperpolarization induced by adenosine and activation of $I_{K.Ado}$ (33 37, 678). All these actions are seen in the absence of β-adrenergic agonists. Adenosine may also affect the basal I_f with a direct (cAMP-independent) mechanism in nodal cells (37, 715). In atrial cells, adenosine hyperpolarizes the membrane and shortens action potential duration by activation of $I_{K.Ado}$ (34, 371). In addition, there may be an inhibition of the basal $I_{Ca,L}$, but the degree of the $I_{Ca,L}$ depression is relatively small compared to that of the $I_{K.Ado}$ activation, playing little or no role in reduction of action potential duration and contractility (37, 79). $I_{Ca,T}$ is insensitive to adenosine.

Duration, amplitude, and V_{max} of AV node action potentials and their firing rates are decreased by adenosine in a concentration-dependent manner, and the high concentration completely abolishes action potential generation (89). In AV node cells, adenosine activates $I_{K.Ado}$, and reduces basal $I_{Ca,L}$ at concentrations greater than that required to activate $I_{K.Ado}$. It may inhibit I_f at the basal condition (37). Therefore, adenosine-induced electrical changes are uniformly seen in supraventricular tissues from various species, and the effects are mainly caused by the activation of $I_{K.Ado}$.

Membrane potentials of ventricular cells from guinea pig, rabbit, and calf, do not respond to adenosine under the basal condition because of the absence of the $I_{K.Ado}$ channels (35, 37, 304). In contrast, shortening of action potential and reduced contractility are seen in rat and ferret ventricular myocytes (37). $I_{K.Ado}$ channels in ferret ventricular myocytes are activated by A_1-adenosine receptor stimulation via G protein activation. The inhibition of basal $I_{Ca,L}$ by adenosine is also observed, which is mediated through A_1-receptor activation but not via inhibition of protein kinase A activity (520). In addition, 10–100 nM adenosine is shown to decrease the basal $I_{Ca,L}$ in guinea pig ventricular myocytes (145). The current decrease is attributed to Ca^{2+}-induced inactivation caused by Ca^{2+} release from the Ca^{2+} stores induced by IP_3. Physiological significance of the latter study, which is contradictory to previous results, needs further exploration.

Effects on stimulated channels by β-adrenergic agonists. Adenosine antagonizes the electrical and mechanical actions of catecholamines, and these actions are seen both in supraventricular and ventricular cells from almost all the species, attenuating increased cellular adenylate cyclase activity (37). $I_{Ca.L}$ and I_f in SA node cells are least sensitive to adenosine in the absence of isoproterenol but are strongly suppressed in its presence by attenuating the stimulated adenyl cyclase activity (35, 36, 285, 304). The current inhibition is achieved by decreased amplitude of $I_{Ca.L}$ without affecting the voltage dependence or the current kinetics. Decreased $I_{Ca.L}$ is produced by decreased channel availability without changing the single-channel conductance (337; Fig.16–10). In the presence of isoproterenol, the onset of activation of $I_{K.Ado}$ by adenosine precedes the attenuation of the stimulated $I_{Ca.L}$ because of a direct coupling of $I_{K.Ado}$ to receptor activation as opposed to an indirect coupling of cAMP-dependent decrease in $I_{Ca.L}$ (37). Adenosine also attenuates the catecholamine-stimulated currents, I_K and $I_{Cl.PKA}$, with the same intracellular mechanism as that of $I_{Ca.L}$ (37). Human ventricular preparations respond similarly to adenosine by attenuating the catecholamine-induced electrical and mechanical actions, but not in basal condition (47, 485). Delayed afterdepolarizations and triggered activity as well as I_{TI} induced by catecholamines are attenuated or abolished by adenosine (599), but the action of adenosine is without effects on I_{TI} induced by other means to increase cellular Ca^{2+} overload.

Effects on ATP-sensitive K^+ channels. Adenosine is shown to activate K_{ATP} via activation of inhibitory G protein, G_i, in membrane-delimited fashion (309, 311, 350), when intracellular ATP concentration is low. This action is not mediated through antagonism with increased adenylate cyclase. Adenosine and ACh appear to act through the same G protein pathway interacting with its α subunit and antagonize ATP-induced inhibition (309, 621). In contrast to these single-channel studies using inside-out patches, the activation of the channels by adenosine and A_1 receptor stimulation has not been conclusively demonstrated at the whole-cell level, since there are both supporting (408) and opposing results (37) indicating that the adenosine action is rather weak. A short ischemic episode has been shown to induce cardioprotection on subsequent long and high grades of ischemic insult, the condition called "ischemic preconditioning" (464). Since adenosine is released from ischemic myocardium, activation of K_{ATP} channels coupled to adenosine A_1-receptor stimulation

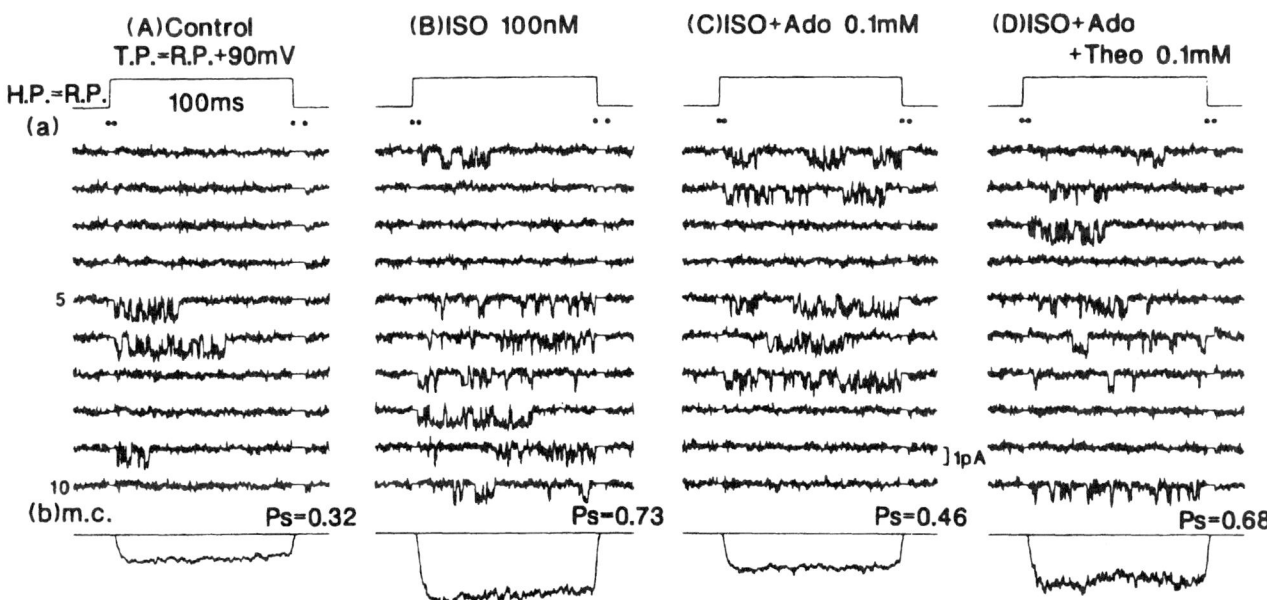

FIG. 16–10. Effect of isoproterenol (ISO), adenosine (Ado), and theophylline (Theo) on single-channel Ca^{2+} current. A: Control; B: 100 nM ISO; C: 0.1 mM Ado and ISO; D: ISO, Ado, and 0.1 mM Theo. Traces labeled *a* are ten consecutive sweeps in order of depolarization sequence. Artifacts produced by capacitive transients were erased at the intervals indicated by the *two dots*. Traces labeled *b* are mean currents (m.c.) from all traces, including blanks. Mean currents were obtained by averaging the idealized openings and are shown on a constant arbitrary scale. About 1,000 times of 100 msec depolarization steps from the resting potential (R.P.) to R.P. +90 mV were applied repetitively at 2 Hz in each solution. Cutoff frequency was 1.5 kHz. Pipette solution contained 100 mM Ba^{2+}, T.P.=test potential, H.P.=holding potential; Ps,=ratio of the number of channel currents containing sweeps to total number of sweeps. [Reproduced from Figure 1 in reference (337), with permission.]

via PKC activation has been proposed to facilitate the openings of the channels under such conditions. It is further suggested that endogenous adenosine displays a protective effect on ischemic myocardium (134, 417, 624) and that its activation of K_{ATP} will play a role in ischemic preconditioning (217, 704). However, there are several lines of evidence that do not fit or conflict with the above explanation (410, 625, see also under Potassium Channel Openers). Furthermore, various factors and signal transduction mechanisms are suggested to be involved in ischemic preconditioning under various experimental settings of different animal species (133). It has to be clarified further whether the action of adenosine is directly linked to the mechanism of ischemic preconditioning.

External ATP and P_2 Receptor Stimulation. Serum levels of ATP are normally very low because many tissues scavenge ATP from the blood very efficiently (212), but working hearts release measurable ATP into the blood. Released ATP may act locally to modulate contractility and to dilate blood vessels before it is cleared from the tissue (212, 364). ATP is also co-released from secretary granules of sympathetic or parasympathetic nerve terminals with transmitters in response to nerve stimulation (679). External ATP may play significant roles in cardiac function during pathological conditions as well, since myocardial cells suffering from ischemia and infarction, trauma and shock release large amounts of ATP into the blood and raise serum ATP levels to the micromolar range (212). External nucleotides including ATP act on cell-surface receptors known as P_2 receptors, of which several subtypes have been cloned (181, 182, 364). P_2 receptors include ligand-gated ion channels, designated P_{2x} and the G protein–coupled receptor subfamily, designated P_{2y}, each consisting of several subtypes with different physiological and pharmacological behaviors (65, 364). Because of these multiple subtypes, the effects of ATP are not uniform among different cell types and have different kinetics. Diverse effects of ATP may, in addition, be attributed in part to the fact that ATP degradation to adenosine by ectonucleotidase stimulates the A_1-adenosine receptor and thus modifies the channel functions (see above).

Effects on nonselective cation channels. Micromolar ATP activates rapid, desensitizing inward currents through stimulation of the P_2 receptor in atrial and ventricular myocytes from various species (184, 263, 511, 558, 559, 722). Once the current is activated, a second ATP application after a brief interval causes decreased response ("desensitization") and several minutes are required to effect a full recovery (Fig. 16–11). With this current activation, transient depolarization of membrane potential and increase in $[Ca^{2+}]_i$ are

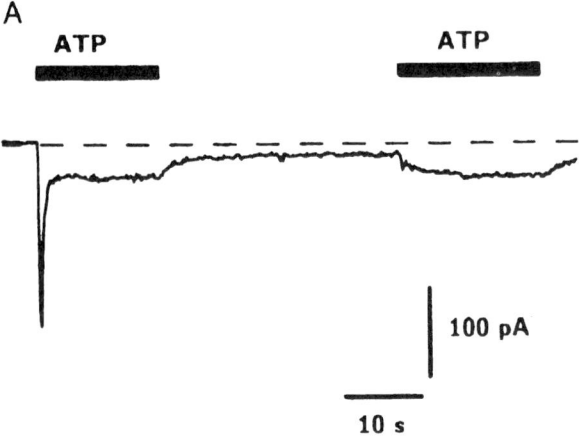

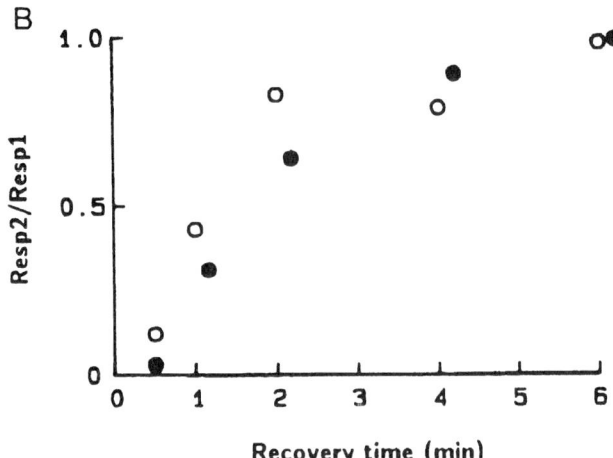

FIG. 16–11. Desensitization and resensitization of the transient component of current evoked by external ATP. *A:* Current at −130 mV during two applications of 200 μM ATP separated by 30 sec. While a transient current was lost in the second exposure to ATP due to desensitization, a maintained current response after the transient current was similarly evoked in the second exposure as in the first application. *B:* Time course of recovery from desensitization in two cells. In each trial, an initial 15-sec application of 200 μM ATP was followed by a variable recovery time, and the extent of recovery was tested with a second application of ATP. Cells were allowed to recover for 6 min between trials. *Filled circles*: cell C78E. *Open circles*: cell C79B. [Reproduced from Figure 3 in reference (184) with permission.]

observed (85, 184, 263, 558). The currents have a small unitary conductance with a linear (184) or inwardly rectifying (511) I-V relation with a reversal around 0 mV through nonselective cation channels mainly carried by Na^+. This current is antagonized by β γ-methylene ATP in bullfrog and rat myocytes (184, 559) but not in rabbit and guinea pig (263). The rank order of potency of ATP analogues cannot define the subclass of P_2 receptor, but it seems to represent the ligand-gated channel (a subtype of P_{2x}) and not coupled to G protein activation (559, 722).

Effects on K⁺ channels. The second type of current activated by external ATP is an inwardly rectifying K⁺ current (184, 185, 188, 242, 263, 329). The ATP-activated K⁺ current follows the activation of the nonselective cation current and produces relatively steady current (see Fig. 16–11). This current has a similar conductance and kinetic properties to $I_{K.Ado}$ and $I_{K.ACH}$ in atrial and nodal cells. This effect appears not due to activation of A_1 receptor by adenosine metabolized from ATP, since a non-hydrolyzable ATP analogue can also activate this K⁺ current with similar potency to ATP. It is further shown that $I_{K.Ado}$ and ATP-activated K⁺ current are regulated differently by intracellular nucleotides (188). ATP activates the same current as $I_{K.ACH}$ through activation of pertussis toxin–sensitive G protein (440) but, in addition, the continued presence of ATP rapidly inhibits the activated current with different intracellular mechanisms (439). Furthermore, external ATP is shown to activate I_K (I_{KS}) in guinea pig atrial cells through intracellular mechanisms independent of PKA, PKC, or $[Ca^{2+}]_i$ (441).

Effects on Ca²⁺ channels. The third type of channel modulation by external ATP is a stimulation of $I_{Ca.L}$ in frog (5) and rat heart (558, 559, 722), whereas both increase and decrease of $I_{Ca.L}$ are also reported in rat (557). ATP increases the amplitude of the current without shifting its voltage dependence. The receptor subtype of the $I_{Ca.L}$ stimulation appears to be P_{2y} activation through a G protein–coupled process, and this increase is partly responsible for the positive inotropic action of ATP and increased $[Ca^{2+}]_i$ (85, 364). In frog hearts, stimulation of both $I_{Ca.T}$ and $I_{Ca.L}$ has been noted (6). In ferret ventricles, however, external ATP constantly produces negative inotropic action and decreases $I_{Ca.L}$ via a pertussis toxin–insensitive G protein coupled to the P_{2y} receptor (519).

Effects on Cl⁻ channels. External ATP but not adenosine can activate Cl⁻ current with non-deactivating properties in guinea pig and rat atrial myocytes (329, 438). Activation of this Cl⁻ current follows the onset of rapid, desensitizing inward current and produces maintained current flow. The ATP-activated current in mouse heart has been shown to be the same channel current as $I_{Cl.PKA}$ which is activated through a novel intracellular signaling pathway involving the activation of PKA and PKC (140).

Histamine and Histamine H₂ Receptor Stimulation

Histamine is present in all regions of mammalian heart, with some predominance in the right atrium (see 691). Its large quantities are stored in cytoplasmic granules of mast cells. There are three types of histamine receptors, H_1, H_2, and H_3, which mediate the effects and functions both synergistically and in opposite ways (406, 691). Two of them (H_1 and H_2) have been cloned (261). Cardiac effects of histamine are mainly exerted through the H_2 receptor activation with positive chronotropic and inotropic actions, and possible arrhythmogenic actions through induction of abnormal automaticity. Released histamine may play a major role in development of arrhythmias associated with systemic allergic reactions (69). The H_1 receptor activation may mediate slowing of AV nodal conduction (negative dromotropic effect). The location of H_3-receptor is presynaptic and its modulatory role is to decrease norepinephrine release associated with adrenergic nerve activation (152).

Effects on membrane potentials. Histamine increases SA node automaticity by accelerating slow diastolic depolarization, with only slight changes in the maximum diastolic potential and threshold potential. Amplitude and duration of action potentials are not affected at all (407). Atrial automatic fibers and Purkinje fibers also respond to histamine by increased diastolic slope and firing rate with shortening of action potential duration (623, 691). Effects of histamine on normally polarized ventricular cells are not remarkable. Histamine, however, induces oscillatory activity or delayed afterdepolarization in depolarized Purkinje and muscle fibers, and it restores propagated slow action potentials (286, 460, 691). All of these effects are blocked by H_2 receptor antagonists.

Effects on membrane currents and channels. Histamine enhances $I_{Ca.L}$ dose-dependently with a threshold concentration of 10^{-8} M in mammalian ventricular myocytes (257, 403), and the maximum enhancement (about 3–4 fold) is attained at 5×10^{-6} M without changes in voltage dependence and inactivation time course. The enhancement is achieved through H_2 receptor–mediated activation of adenylate cyclase and increased cAMP via activation of the stimulatory G protein, G_s. The enhancement of $I_{Ca.L}$ can be attributed to increased automaticity in SA and AV node, increased plateau height, restoration of slow response activity, and development of Ca^{2+}-mediated abnormal automaticity. At the same time, histamine at comparable concentrations activates $I_{Cl.PKA}$ and I_K by the same G protein–coupled mechanism as $I_{Ca.L}$ (250, 281, 292, 707). Since $I_{Cl.PKA}$ and I_K carry outward repolarizing currents opposing inward Ca^{2+} current, action potential duration is either prolonged or shortened despite increased plateau height depending on the balance among the three currents. Application of histamine increased slow inward Ca^{2+} current, I_K and I_f in multicellular rabbit SA node preparations (554). Additional effects of histamine induce slowing of AV conduction, which may be mediated by the H_1 receptor (691). H_1 receptor activation may cause prolongation of action potential and increased $[Ca^{2+}]_i$ by inhibiting outward

K^+ current without affecting $I_{Ca,L}$ in atrial myocytes (709).

Angiotensin II and Angiotensin Receptor Stimulation

The renin–angiotensin cascade was originally regarded as a system regulating blood pressure in the kidney, but this system also modulates the functions of cardiac myocytes. The heart cells are not merely its target for the circulating peptide; they also produce renin and angiotensin II (ANG II) to function as an autocrine/paracrine system (22, 132)). As direct actions to the heart, ANG II has inotropic and chronotropic actions, effects on metabolism and hypertrophic growth. Cardiac ANG II binding sites in sarcolemmal membranes have two classes of high and low affinity, with high and low binding capacities, respectively (22). Recently, two major subtypes, AT_1 and AT_2 receptor subtypes, have been cloned (107, 532).

As for direct action of ANG II to the heart, positive inotropic effects have been described in various species with exceptions in guinea pig and adult rat (22). The inotropic action is dose dependent and can be blocked by ANG II receptor antagonists. ANG II increases Ca^{2+} current in Purkinje fibers (331) and $I_{Ca,L}$ in neonatal rat cardiac myocytes (4, 131). The mechanism of the $I_{Ca,L}$ increase and its link to positive inotropic action may be mediated, at least in part, by activation of PKC, since both ANG II and an activator of PKC stimulate $I_{Ca,L}$ and increase contractile frequency with enhanced phosphorylation of the same set of proteins.

ANG II has an action to stimulate I_{Na} with slowed inactivation (456) at low concentrations ($> 1\mu M$), but the higher concentrations stimulate the current (475). The I_{Na} stimulation is achieved by increased channel open probability due to decreased null sweeps. The intracellular pathway for the I_{Na} stimulation seems to be coupled to PKC activation (456, 475), but the effects of PKC activators are not consistent: phorbol ester increased current amplitude in one study (456), whereas it reduced peak amplitude of the current in another (39). In cloned cardiac Na^+ channels, however, PKC has been shown to inhibit cardiac I_{Na} with a shift in voltage-dependent inactivation (521), or to produce voltage-independent inhibition (463). Therefore, the mode and mechanism of the ANG II actions on I_{Na} have not been settled.

Chronotropic actions by ANG II seem more complex and controversial than its inotropic effects, partly because of reflex control through baroreceptor and central nervous system. ANG II increases frequency of spontaneous beating in neonatal rat myocytes with enhanced $I_{Ca,L}$ (4, 131, 531) and accelerates slow diastolic depolarization in human atrial muscles (82). On the other hand, isolated single cells from rabbit SA node respond with decreased spontaneous firing rate and action potential amplitude. These effects are attributed to inhibition of $I_{Ca,L}$ through the AT_1 receptor (223). Inhibition appears to be mediated by modulation of PKA, but not by PKC. A time-independent Cl^- current is activated by ANG II in rabbit SA node cells (40) and ventricular myocytes (457). The time course of activation is quite slow, with a half activation time of about 20 minutes that does not mimic changes in action potential repolarization after its application. The activation is internal Ca^{2+}-dependent, but details of the activation mechanism are not known. On the other hand, ANG II negatively couples to adenylate cyclase via pertussis toxin-sensitive G protein, thereby inhibiting $I_{Cl,PKA}$ activated by isoproterenol in guinea pig ventricular myocytes (487). Additional actions are to decrease I_K in SA node cells (223) and to increase I_{K1} in ventricular myocytes with undefined intracellular mechanism (457).

Not only in short-term actions, the renin–angiotensin system is implicated in regulation of cardiac function in the long term. For example, ANG II is implicated in the genesis of cardiac memory, in which T wave changes in ECG induced by ventricular pacing accumulate and persist during subsequent sinus rhythm (710). One of the factors involved is due to modulation of I_{to} by ANG II. The activation of this system may also contribute to the cellular decoupling seen in the ventricle of cardiomyopathic hamsters (114).

Arginine Vasopressin and Vasopressinergic Receptor Stimulation

Arginine vasopressin (AVP, or vasopressin) plays important roles in cardiovascular regulation, presumably through its systemic vasoconstrictor effects and neurally mediated reflexes (573). Recent evidence suggests the heart is a direct target for AVP (565). Two subtypes of the receptors, V_1 and V_2 have been identified (697).

While an intravenous application of AVP in conscious whole animals results in reduced cardiac output and increased coronary vascular resistance due to vasoconstrictor effects (259), a direct inotropic effect to the heart by AVP has also been described (565, 659). In rat cardiomyocytes, AVP is shown to increase $[Ca^{2+}]_i$ via V_1 receptor stimulation (697). As for a possible basis of the positive inotropic effect and increased $[Ca^{2+}]_i$, AVP is shown to potentiate $I_{Ca,L}$ via V_1 receptor stimulation (719). The potentiation is achieved through increased numbers of channel openings and prolonged open times without changes in single-channel conductance. An involvement of PKC activation is suggested to be the intracellular signaling pathway for this potentiation.

Endothelins

Endothelin, a 21-amino acid peptide, is a potent vasoconstrictor produced by vascular endothelial cells (701). Three isoforms of endothelin, endothelin-1 (ET-1), endothelin-2 (ET-2), and endothelin-3 (ET-3), have been identified and shown to bind to various types of tissues, eliciting a variety of physiological and pathophysiological responses (430). The diversity of biological actions by the endothelin family has been attributed to a wide distribution of ET receptors in different cells that involves at least two subtypes of ET receptors, ET_A and ET_B. In the heart, the existence of both subtypes has been demonstrated in different animals and in human (430, 454).

Endothelin exerts a prominent positive inotropic effect as well as diverse chronotropic effects in cardiac cells, which may be secondary to an endothelin-induced increase in cytosolic Ca^{2+} (307, 430). The precise mechanism(s) responsible for the Ca^{2+} increase has not been clarified, but one possibility is that endothelin increases transmembrane Ca^{2+}-influx through the Ca^{2+} channels. Direct measurements of the channel activity have revealed conflicting results: ET-1 increased the peak $I_{Ca,L}$ via pertussis toxin–insensitive G protein (384), while in human and chick ventricular myocytes, both $I_{Ca,T}$ and $I_{Ca,L}$ were enhanced through pertussis toxin–sensitive G protein (45). Either no enhancement (628), inhibition of the basal and isoproterenol-stimulated $I_{Ca,L}$ (493, 694), or no effect on the basal current and significant suppression on the isoproterenol-stimulated current (622) was demonstrated in guinea pig atrial and ventricular myocytes. In cultured neonatal rat ventricular myocytes, ET-1 increased $I_{Ca,T}$ but mildly inhibited $I_{Ca,L}$ (190; Fig. 16–12). Neither of these results can explain profound and sustained positive inotropic action by ET-1, suggesting that major Ca^{2+} supply for the ET-1 action is not through the Ca^{2+} channels. An altenative explanation for potentiation of Ca^{2+} transients in rat cardiac myocytes is implicated by action potential prolongation due to block of I_K without effect on Ca^{2+} currents (103), whereas enhanced I_K by ET-1 has been reported in guinea pig ventricular myocytes (224).

As to chronotropic action of endothelin, positive and negative effects depending on concentration have been presented in adult guinea pig and cultured rat atrial myocytes (344, 493). The mechanism of the positive chronotropic effect is not known. When the negative chronotropic effect is evident, ET-1 hyperpolarizes resting membrane potential and shortens atrial action

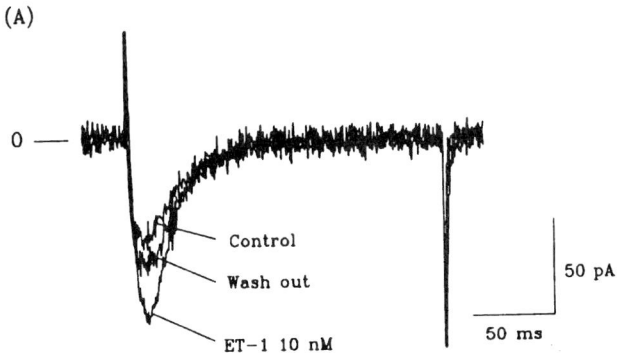

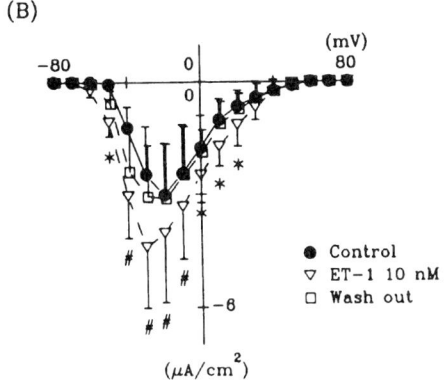

FIG. 16–12. Effect of endothelin-1 (ET-1) on the T-type Ca^{2+} current $I_{Ca,T}$. A: A series of $I_{Ca,T}$ were elicited by voltage steps to -30 mV in the control condition, 20 min after the addition of 10 nM ET-1, and 10 min after removal of ET-1, and the tracings are superimposed. B: Peak current density–voltage relations were plotted for $I_{Ca,T}$ in the control condition (closed circles), 20 min after the addition of 10 nM ET-1 (open reversed triangles), and 10 mins after the removal of ET-1 (open squares) obtained from 11 cells. *P<0.05 and # P<0.01 for the control condition vs. ET-1 and for ET-1 vs. washout of ET-1. [Reproduced from Figure 5 in reference (190) with permission.]

potential by activating $I_{K.ACH}$ and inhibiting $I_{Ca,L}$. The activating action of $I_{K.ACH}$ is shared by all three isoforms of endothelins. ET_A receptors are involved in the inhibitory action of $I_{Ca,L}$ in rabbit SA node cells (615), which is coupled to a pertussis toxin–sensitive G protein/adenylate cyclase inhibition pathway. Additionally, endothelins have been shown to inhibit $I_{Cl.PKA}$ via an ET_A receptor mediated by a pertussis toxin–sensitive G protein (314) and to block partially $I_{K.ATP}$ with undefined intracellular mechanism (356).

Atrial Natriuretic Peptide

Atrial natriuretic peptide (ANP) is one of a family of polypeptides that include ANP, brain natriuretic peptide (BNP) and C-type natriuretic peptide (CNP). ANP is synthesized and stored as a 126 amino acid prohormone (proANP) in the atria under normal conditions, and in the ventricle in the setting of hypoxia, ischemia, and heart failure. Stretch of atrial cell membrane triggers the release of ANP. Three receptors are known to modulate the action of ANP:ANPR-A and ANPR-B, and ANPR-C. ANP acts mainly via the ANPR-A receptor to initiate most of its biological activities, and the ANPR-C receptor serves primarily to remove ANP from the circulation (7, 539).

ANP has complex effects on cardiac electrophysiology, possibly due to actions at several levels: (1) directly at the cellular level, (2) on the autonomic nervous system with vagoexcitatory and sympathoinhibitory actions, and (3) to sensitize baroreceptors (88). At the level of the heart, ANP causes an increase in muscarinic receptor activity and a decrease in β_1 receptor stimulation by vagoexcitatory and sympathoinhibitory actions, mainly activating $I_{K,ACH}$ and inhibiting catecholamine-stimulated $I_{Ca,L}$. These actions will shorten action potential duration and effective refractory period and decrease both conduction velocity and slow diastolic depolarization in atrial tissues. The AV node conduction is impaired by ANP due to inhibition of $I_{Ca,L}$ as well as membrane hyperpolarization (88). These direct actions are variously modulated by complex interactions with autonomic nervous systems and baroreflex control, and by tissue basal conditions. Therefore, the firing rate of the primary pacemaker of the heart is also regulated by increased ANP secretion in a complex manner (32).

ANP has been shown to activate particular guanylate cyclase and to raise cellular cGMP concentrations (100), exhibiting a direct depressant effect on contractility of cardiac myocytes (471, 654a). In frog ventricular myocytes, ANP decreases the Ca^{2+} current that has been stimulated by β-adrenoceptor agonists but has no effects on the basal $I_{Ca,L}$ (209). The ANP-induced reduction of the stimulated I_{Ca} is assumed to be mediated by activation of cGMP-dependent phosphodiesterase (PDE II) (175, 244), but activation of PDE II in mammalian cells plays only a minor role in the $I_{Ca,L}$ decrease (404, 500). In contrast to amphibian preparations, ANP has been shown to decrease both basal and β-agonist stimulated $I_{Ca,L}$ in chick embryos (44), human atrial cells (397), and rabbit and guinea pig ventricular myocytes (600, 632). The decrease is achieved through a reduction of channel open probability without changing the conductance. Suppressive action on basal $I_{Ca,L}$ appears to be mediated by increased cGMP and activation of cGMP-dependent protein kinase (PKG).

The two studies exploring the action of ANP on I_{Na} give conflicting results. The one study found no effects in human fetal cells (44) and the other found an attenuation of I_{Na} by ANP in guinea pig ventricular myocytes with changes in ion selectivity (600). Whether these conflicting results arise from differences in species, age-dependent processes, or other reasons, has to be clarified. As for the actions on K^+ channels, ANP is shown to decreases the Ca^{2+}-independent transient outward K^+ current (I_{to}) via activation of inhibitory G_i (397) and to stimulate I_K with undefined intracellular mechanism (44).

Nitric Oxide

There is increasing evidence to support that nitric oxide plays various physiological and pathophysiological roles in many organs including the heart. NO is generated by a family of enzymes known as NO synthases (NOS), of which there are three types: neuronal NOS (nNOS or NOS1), cytokine-inducible NOS (iNOS or NOS2), and endothelial constituitive NOS (eNOS or NOS3). All three forms of are present in the heart, and NOS3 is the most prominently expressed (343). As for the effect of NO on cardiac electrical activity, most descriptions are related to its activation of guanylate cyclase. Because ACh is known as a potent activator of guanylate cyclase resulting in an increase in intracellular cGMP and activation of PKG, it may play a role in the ACh's antagonism on β-agonist stimulated inotropic and chronotropic actions (see earlier, under Cholinergic Agonists and Cholinergic Receptor Stimulation). Although a main mechanism of this ACh antagonism against the β-adrenergic agonist stimulation can be explained by attenuation of increased adenylate cyclase, part of its action may be mediated by increased gaunylate cyclase.

In cultured rat neonatal ventricular myocytes, negative chronotropic action by an ACh analogue carbachol is correlated with the activation of guanylate cyclase, and this action is reversed by inhibition of NOS, suggesting a modulatory role of NO in automaticity (23). In mammalian SA and AV node cells, inhibition of β-adrenergic-agonist–stimulated $I_{Ca,L}$ by the cholinergic agonist carbamylcholine is shown to depend on activation of NOS3 (233, 234, 235), and similar results are obtained in rat ventricular myocytes (24). These studies have confirmed no or slight effects of NO-dependent inhibition of basal $I_{Ca,L}$ in the absence of β-adrenergic agonists. In another study, ACh inhibits basal $I_{Ca,L}$, and abrupt removal of ACh induces rebound increase in the current. These effects are diminished by NOS inhibitor in feline atrial myocytes (668). The latter result may be interpreted as an indication that these preparations contain a high tonic level of adenylate cyclase activity. On the other hand, there are several reports describing no involvement of NOS in muscarinic agonist–induced inhibition of $I_{Ca,L}$ (425,

446, see 447). It is also shown that NOS inhibitors have no action on $I_{K.ACh}$ or $I_{Cl.PKA}$, the latter being activated in the presence of β-adrenergic agonists (713). Thus, the involvement of NO in the ACh-induced inhibition of $I_{Ca.L}$ remains unsettled (446), and further clarification is necessary to answer this important question. Chronotropic effects of NO donors were examined in guinea pig SA node/atrial preparations. Low concentrations of NO donors (nanomolar to micromolar) gradually increased the spontaneous rate, whereas high concentrations (milimolar) decreased it. The increase in beating rate by NO donors was produced by stimulation of I_f and SA node myocytes via the NO-cGMP pathway (464a). This may contribute to sinus tachycardia in pathological conditions associated with an increase in myocardial production of NO.

EFFECTS OF DRUGS

Digitalis Glucosides

Digitalis and its related glycoside analogues have been used to treat patients with heart failure and cardiac rhythm disturbances for many years. Despite these facts and extensive studies to clarify the mechanism of action of these drugs, there is no concrete explanation for their electrophysiological and inotropic effects. Cardiac glycosides have been known to inhibit Na^+–K^+ pump. The action is used for experimental studies of the ion-transport mechanism across cell membranes of various tissues. Inhibitory action of the Na^+–K^+ pump by digitalis compounds is implicated at least to some extent, in their electrophysiological and mechanical effects, but this action cannot give a full explanation for their mechanism of action.

Effects on membrane potential and channels in relation to positive inotropic action. It has long been recognized that when digitalis glycosides are applied to multicellular cardiac preparations, depolarization of resting membrane potential and shortening of action potentials occur (336, 692). Depolarization of resting potential can be attributed to inhibition of the outward Na^+–K^+ pump current (193, 305) and resultant accumulation of K^+ in extracellular clefts. In single ventricular myocytes where K^+ accumulation in the clefts is almost negligible, an estimate of membrane depolarization amounts to less than 1 mV, with normal $[Na^+]_i$ of about 8 mM and input resistance of approximately 20 MΩ (402), which agrees with actual measurements in guinea pig ventricular myocytes (400). The degree of depolarization may be larger in Purkinje or nodal cells, which exhibit the larger input resistance values.

Shortening of action potential duration is associated with depressed plateau height, but a transient prolongation with increased plateau is occasionally noted at low doses or in an early phase of digitalis application (336, 692). The shortened action potential duration and decreased plateau height are reflected on shortened QT intervals and ST depression in ECG of patients treated with digitalis. Studies using isolated single myocytes have confirmed similar changes observed in multicellular preparations with a transient prolongation followed by successive shortening of action potential by strophanthidin, while positive inotropic action continues to increase from the initial period (400; Fig. 16–13). Membrane currents at the time of action potential prolongation show decreased net outward current at plateau level and increased inward current at around −80 mV (401), levels consistent with inhibition of electrogenic Na^+–K^+ pump current (193, 305). Low doses of cardiac glycosides are known to stimulate Na^+–K^+ pump activity (394), which was once thought to modulate electrical and mechanical actions of digitalis at therapeutic concentrations. However single-cell studies do not support the contribution of the pump stimulation on both activities (402).

Despite the positive inotropic action of cardiac glycosides, their effects on $I_{Ca.L}$ give variable results. In single myocytes, transient activation of $I_{Ca.L}$ (173) and stimulation of both $I_{Ca.T}$ and $I_{Ca.L}$ (398) by cardiac glycosides are reported where the influence of Na^+–K^+ pump activity is minimized. However, under more physiological conditions with the presence of pump inhibition, a consistent and progressive change serves to decrease the amplitude of $I_{Ca.L}$ (173, 400, 402). Decreased $I_{Ca.L}$ is caused by accumulation of $[Ca^{2+}]_i$, leading to Ca^{2+}-induced inactivation, but not to direct suppression of the channels. Since inhibition of the Na^+–K^+ pump produces increased $[Na^+]_i$, which induces increased $[Ca^{2+}]_i$ through Na^+–Ca^{2+} exchange, and thus has a causal relation to increased positive inotropy by digitalis (389). Other currents contributing to action potential shortening are the Na^+–Ca^{2+} exchange current induced by accumulation of $[Na^+]_i$ after pump inhibition (401), and activation of $I_{K.Na}$ (424), but they may play a minor role. The currents induced by increased $[Ca^{2+}]_i$, such as Ca^{2+}-activated K^+ current or nonselective cation current, seem not to be involved in these changes. In relation to positive inotropy, a major factor can be explained by increased $[Na^+]_i$ (389), but there is a temporal dissociation between changes in $[Na^+]_i$ and contraction, where the former lags behind the latter (241). A part of this dissociation can be explained by a temporal prolongation of action potential duration, which contributes to increased contraction (391).

With much higher, toxic doses of cardiac glycosides, the frequent development of increased impulse forma-

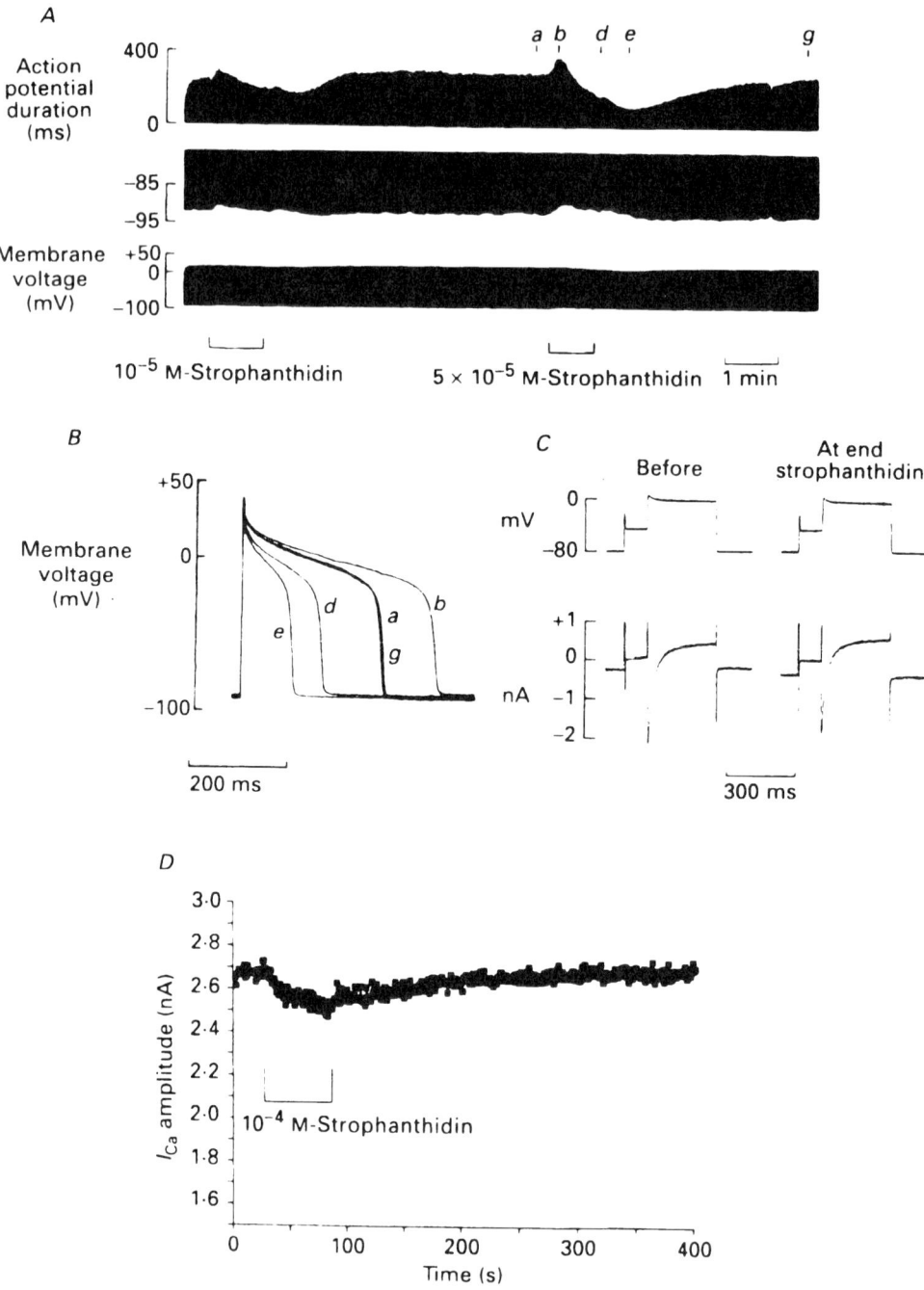

FIG. 16–13. The effect of strophanthidin on action potential and I_{Ca} when myocytes are impaled with BAPTA-filled microelectrodes to increase Ca^{2+}_i buffering. A: The effect on the action potential of exposure to two different concentrations of strophanthidin. B: individual action potentials recorded at the times indicated in A. C: I_{Ca} recorded with the two-pulse protocol before and at the end of strophanthidin exposure. D: The time course of the change in I_{Ca} during strophanthidin exposure and recovery. [Reproduced from Figure 8 in reference (400), with permission.]

tions is seen. These activities are mostly caused by DADs and I_{TI} under Ca^{2+} overload in cardiac cells (170, 335, 388). For a more complete description of this type of impulse formation, see later, under Ion Channels and Mechanisms of Arrhythmias.

Effects on membrane potentials and currents in relation to AV nodal conduction. Another important action of cardiac glycosides is to depress conduction through the AV node with little influence on conduction in atrium, ventricle, and the His-Purkinje system (626, 671). Because of this specific action, digitalis compounds are the most frequently used antiarrhythmic agent to control ventricular responses in atrial flutter and fibrillation. Parts of these actions are mediated by glycoside-induced increase in efferent vagal impulse and a reflex-induced decrease in sympathetic tone (169), and by complex and less well defined mechanism of actions on the autonomic nervous system (205). In addition, cardiac glycosides have direct membrane actions on AV node cells to delay impulse transmission. In small multicellular AV node preparations, acetylstrophanthidin decreases the amplitude and V_{max} of action potential and, at the same time, accelerates slow diastolic depolarization and spontaneous firings (672). Inhibition of $I_{Ca,L}$ is later confirmed in single AV node cells, not through direct action on the channels but through indirect blocking of the Na^+–K^+ pump leading to accumulation of $[Ca^{2+}]_i$ (238). The inhibition of $I_{Ca,L}$ causes depression of the V_{max} of action potentials and conduction velocity in the AV node since the upstroke phase of AV node cells is mainly formed by this current (469, 479). While cardiac glycosides increase $[Ca^{2+}]_i$ (389), they also increase the gap junction resistance, causing a delay in AV conduction (295). Acetylstrophanthidin also induces I_{TI} upon repolarization from depolarizing voltage steps (238, 672). The latter results indicate that cardiac glycosides increase ectopic impulse formation in this area, which may explain frequent complications in patients taking moderate to excess amounts of these drugs.

Potassium Channel Openers

The groups of agents that show diverse chemical structures exhibit actions to hyperpolarize membrane potentials of vascular smooth muscle cells and to produce vasodilation. They also affect cardiac membranes to shorten action potential duration and sometimes induce membrane hyperpolarization. Because of these actions, the drugs are supposed to increase K^+ conductance of cardiac and vascular smooth muscle cells. Common targets of these drugs are the ATP-sensitive K^+ channels (K_{ATP}) in cardiac cells (15, 154, 160, 268), and the same target channel is identified in vascular smooth muscle cells and pancreatic β cells, among other tissues (146, 522). The drugs are known as "potassium (K^+) channel openers," and they include cromakalim (a benzopyran derivative), pinacidil (a cyanoguanidine compound), nicorandil (a pyridine derivative), other compounds chemically related to any of the three, and some other unrelated compounds as well (522).

Application of the potassium channel openers to cardiac myocytes activates a time-independent current of K_{ATP} in a voltage-independent manner under high $[K^+]_o$ or symmetrical K^+ conditions on both sides of membrane (15, 154, 160, 161, 268, 467). However, the activated current under low to physiological $[K^+]_o$ = 4–5 mM shows outward-going rectification and few changes around the resting potential level. Therefore, action potential duration is markedly abbreviated by the openers, but resting potential is usually not much affected in well-polarized preparations. Another feature of the current activation is dependence on internal ATP concentrations ($[ATP]_i$): a prominent activation at low $[ATP]_i$, and least activation at high $[ATP]_i$. Furthermore, the activated current is inhibited by raising $[ATP]_i$. The current is also inhibited by application of glibenclamide and other sulfonylureas (178) and 5-hydroxydecanoate (484), blockers of K_{ATP}. At the single channel level, the potassium channel openers activate the K^+ channels with the conductance of 70–90 pS under symmetrical K^+ conditions of 150 mM without changing the current amplitude, thus increasing channel open probability (Fig. 16–14). K_{ATP} rapidly opens and closes in the bursts, and these bursts from clusters separated by long closed intervals. The potassiun channel openers do not affect fast flickerings in the bursts, but they prolong burst durations with shortened interburst intervals, actions of which are opposite those of increased $[ATP]_i$ (160, 467).

Because K_{ATP} is regulated not only by $[ATP]_i$ but also by other factors including Mg-ATP and states of the channels (387, 472, 619, 643), different potassium channel openers exhibit different profiles of the activating actions on the channels. For example, pinacidil has multiple actions, increasing the channel activity by decreasing sensitivity to $[ATP]_i$, but not in a purely antagonistic way. It reactivates the channels in the absence of $[ATP]_i$ and blocks outward current flow from inside the membrane (161). There is one type of opener that appears to exclusively antagonize the $[ATP]_i$-induced inhibition of K_{ATP} (619). Nicorandil exerts its activating action in the presence of ADP, which is unique among all potassium channel openers (578). Terzic et al. (619) propose different activating profiles among various openers, depending on the channel states, the presence and absence of nucleotide diphosphates, and antagonism with the $[ATP]_i$-induced channel inhibition.

The molecular structure of cardiac K_{ATP} is composed of heteromultimer of Kir6.2, a family of inward rectifier K^+ channels, and sulfonylurea receptor (SUR), a member of the ABC binding protein superfamily (298, 544). The ATP inhibition and the conductance properties are determined at the Kir6.2 site, and the interaction site for sulfonylurea compounds and potassium channel openers seems to be located on the SUR side (18, 298, 299, 642). It is now evident that the sensitivities to the channel opening and inhibiting agents in native K_{ATP} are different among different cell types

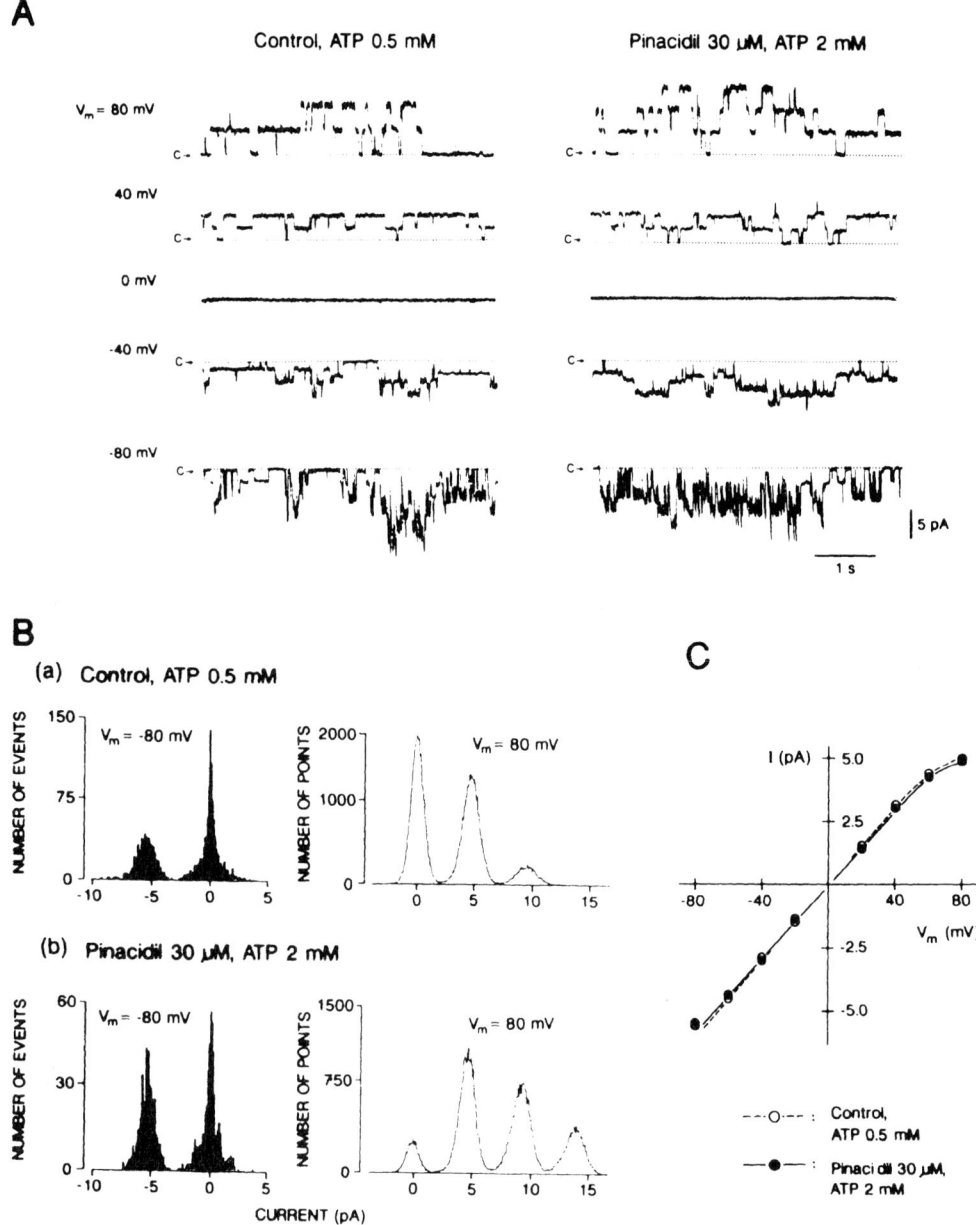

FIG. 16–14. Effects of pinacidil on activation of ATP-sensitive K$^+$ channel currents recorded from an inside-out patch membrane. A: Voltage-dependent activation. Membrane potential [V$_m$ (mV)] is indicated at the left of each trace. *Left panel* shows records taken during the control experiment with 0.5 mM ATP in the internal solution; *right panel* presents those with a solution containing 30 μM pinacidil and 2 mM ATP. The current direction is outward at positive voltages and inward at negative voltages. *B a:* Amplitude histograms (*top panel*) of the single-channel current at V$_m$ = −80 mV (*left panel*) and V$_m$ = +80 mV (*right panel*) obtained using the control solution containing 0.5 mM ATP. *B b:* Amplitude histograms (*bottom panel*) of the single-channel current at V$_m$ = 80 mV (*left panel* and V$_m$ = +80 mV (*right panel*) obtained using solution containing 30 μM pinacidil and 2 mM ATP. Note that the current amplitude of the single channel is not changed by pinacidil. C: Current–voltage relationship (I-V) and the effect of pinacidil. Pinacidil does not change the conductance of this channel current. [Reproduced from Figure 2 in reference (160), with permission.]

(619). Different sensitivities may depend on a family of structurally related but functionally distinct sulfonylurea receptors. Co-expression of the sulfonylurea receptor cloned from insulinoma cells (SUR1) and Kir6.2 exhibits the currents activated by diazoxide but not responsive to pinacidil, which has similar pharmacological and biophysical properties to those of native pancreatic K_{ATP} (298). There are two additional homologues of SUR1 termed as SUR2A and SUR2B, in which only 42 amino acid residues in the carboxyl-terminal end are different (308). SUR2A is assumed to form cardiac and skeletal muscle K_{ATP}, and SUR2B to form the vascular smooth muscle type. Functional expression of SUR2A and Kir6.2 shows the currents activated by pinacidil but not by diazoxide, similar to the properties seen in native cardiac and skeletal K_{ATP} (299, 472, 619). Co-expression of SUR2B and Kir6.2 develops the currents activated both by pinacidil and diazoxide similar to the native channels in vascular smooth muscle cells (308, 605). Furthermore, nicorandil, which can activate both cardiac and smooth muscle K_{ATP} in native channels, has much higher sensitivity to SUR2B/Kir6.2 than SUR2A/Kir6.2 (587) (Fig. 16–15). These results suggest that a main inter-

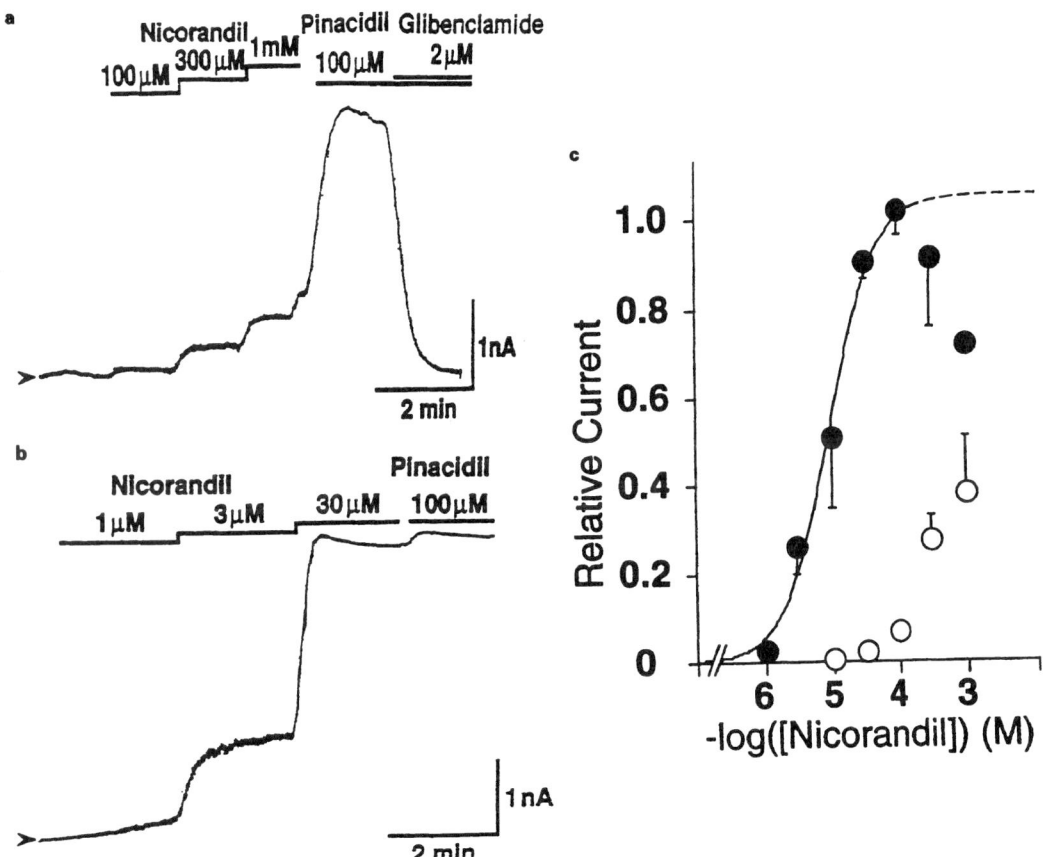

FIG. 16–15. Concentration-dependent effects of nicorandil on the SUR_{2A}/Kir6.2 and SUR_{2B}/Kir6.2 channels. Concentration-dependent effects of nicorandil on the whole-cell current of the SUR_{2A}/Kir6.2 (*a*) and SUR_{2B}/Kir6.2 channels (*b*) at −30 mV with 5.4 mM external K^+. *Arrowheads* indicate the zero current level. The perfusion protocol is indicated above. *c*: Relationship between the concentration of nicorandil and the whole-cell current of the SUR_{2A}/Kir6.2 (*open circles*) and SUR_{2B}/Kir6.2 channels (*solid circles*). The current amplitude induced by each concentration of nicorandil was normalized to the pinacidil (100 μM)-induced current in the same cell. Each symbol and vertical lines indicate the mean and SE, respectively. The number of observations at each point was 5. The line is the fit of the data with the equation,

$$\text{Relative current} = A/\{1 + (K/[\text{Nicorandil}])^{nH}\}$$

Where the relative current is the current normalized to that induced by 100 μM pinacidil in the same cell; A is the maximum relative current induced by nicorandil; and [Nicorandil], the concentration of nicorandil. The values of A, K and ^{nH} were 1.05, 9.2 μM and 1.30, respectively. [Reproduced from Figure 3 in reference (587) with permission.]

action site for nicorandil on SUR is probably located in the 42 amino acid residues at the carboxyl-terminus of SUR2B, and the site for pinacidil is in the portion proximal to this carboxyl-terminal end.

Activation of K_{ATP} by potassium channel openers shortens action potential duration and refractory period, which mimics the electrical changes developing during early ischemia. This condition may be beneficial, on the one hand, to limit the Ca^{2+}-influx during activity decreasing tension development and thereby energy (ATP) consumption. On the other hand, shortened refractory period and extracellular K^+ accumulation favor development of re-entry and serious arrhythmias (330, 689, 690). Application of K_{ATP} openers has been shown to delay the onset of ischemic contracture, to abbreviate irreversible cell injury improving mechanical recovery on reperfusion, and to limit infarct size (92, 216). The results support the notion that the openings of K_{ATP} mimic the effects of ischemic preconditioning (215, 217, 464, 703). The effects can be achieved uniformly by the openers with diverse chemical structures and different types of K_{ATP} blockers equally abolish the protective action, which provides strong support for the involvement of K_{ATP} in the cardioprotection. There are, however, numerous substances and signaling pathways that have been proposed to be involved in mediating the cardioprotective effect of ischemic preconditionig (133). Among these factors, K_{ATP} is supposed to serve as the end effector of this process (215). Furthermore, recent evidence suggests that mitochondrial K_{ATP} rather than surface membrane K_{ATP} plays an essential role as the effector for the cardioprotection (199, 420). The exact mechanism of this action is not known, and data favoring the K_{ATP} theory are dependent on the pharmacological evidence but not on direct documentation of the channel openings in the protective process. Further studies are necessary to prove the actual involvement of the K_{ATP} openings from surface or mitochondrial membranes and to define the molecular mechanism of action.

The author expresses his thanks to Dr. H. C. Hartzell, Emory University, and Dr. J. C. Makielski, University of Wisconsin, for their valuable comments and reading the manuscript. Secretarial assistance by N. Fujita is also acknowledged.

The author's works cited in this chapter are supported by grants from the Ministry of Education, Science, Sports, and Culture of Japan.

REFERENCES

1. Agus, Z. S., I. D. Dukes, and M. Morad. Divalent cations modulate the transient outward current in rat ventricular myocytes. *Am. J. Physiol.* 261 (*Cell Physiol.* 30):C310–C318, 1991.
2. Agus, Z. S., E. Kelepouris, I. Dukes, and M. Morad. Cytosolic magnesium modulates calcium channel activity in mammalian ventricular cells. *Am. J. Physiol.* 256 (*Cell Physiol.* 25):C452–C455, 1989.
3. Agus, Z. S., and M. Morad. Modulation of cardiac ion channels by magnesium. *Annu. Rev. Physiol.* 53:299–307, 1991.
4. Allen, I. S., N. M. Cohen, R. S. Dhallan, S. T. Gaa, W. J. Lederer and T. B. Rogers. Angiotensin II increases spontaneous contractile frequency and stimulates calcium current in cultured neonatal rat heart myocytes: insights into the underlying biochemical mechanism. *Circ. Res.* 62:524–534, 1988.
5. Alvarez, J. L., K. Mongo, F. Scamps, and G. Vassort. Effects of purinergic stimulation on the Ca current in single frog cardiac cells. *Pflugers Arch.* 416:189–195, 1990.
6. Alvalez, J. L. and G. Vassort. Properties of the low threshold Ca current in single frog atrial cardiomyocytes. *J. Gen. Physiol.* 100:519–545, 1992.
7. Ananda-Srivastava, M. B. and G. J. Trachte. Atrial natriuretic factor receptors and signal transduction mechanisms. *Pharmacol. Rev.* 45:455–497, 1993.
8. Anderson, M. E., A. P. Braun, H. Schulman, and B. A. Premack. Multifunctional Ca^{2+}/calmodulin-dependent protein kinase mediates Ca^{2+}-induced enhancement of the L-type Ca^{2+} current in rabbit ventricular myocytes. *Circ. Res.* 75:854–861, 1994.
9. Antoni, H. and E. Oberdisse. Elektrophysiologische Untersuchungen uber die Barium-induzierte Schrittmacher Aktivitat in der Arbeitsmuskulatur des Saugertierherzens. *Pflugers Arch.* 284:259–272, 1965.
10. Antzelevitch, C., S. Sicouri, S. H. Litovsky, A. Lukas, S. C. Krishnan, J. M. DiDiergo, G. A. Gintant, and D. W. Liu. Heterogeneity within the ventricular wall—electrophysiology and pharmacology of epicardial, endocardial, and M-cells. *Circ. Res.* 69:1427–1449, 1991.
11. Antzelevitch, C. S., A. Sicouri, V. V. Lukas, D. W. Nesterenko, W. Liu, and J. M. DiDiergo. Regional differences in the electrophysiology of ventricular cells: physiological and clinical implications. In D. P. Zipes, and J. Jalife *Cardiac Electrophysiology—From Cell to Bedside*. edited by Philadelphia: W. B. Saunders Co., 1995:228–245.
12. Anumonwo, J. M. B., J. Horta, M. Delmar, S. M. Taffet, and J. Jalife. Proton and zinc effects on HERG current. *Biophy. J.* 77:282–298, 1999.
13. Apkon, M. and J. M. Nerbonne. α-Adrenergic agonists selectively suppress voltage-dependent K^+ currents in rat ventricular myocytes. *Proc. Natl. Acad. Sci. U.S.A.* 85:8756–8760, 1988.
14. Apkon, M. and J. N. Nerbonne. Characterization of two distinct depolarization-activated K^+ currents in isolated adult rat ventricular myocytes. *J. Gen. Physiol.* 97:973–1011, 1991.
15. Arena, J. P. and R. S. Kass. Activation of ATP-sensitive K channels in heart cells by pinacidil: dependence on ATP. *Am. J. Physiol.* 257 (*Heart Circ. Physiol.* 26):H2092–H2096, 1989.
16. Arlock, P., and B. G. Katzung. Effects of sodium substrates on transient inward current and tension in guinea-pig ventricular muscle. *J. Physiol. (Lond.)* 360:105–120, 1985.
17. Aronson, R. S. and P. F. Cranefield. The electrical activity of canine Purkinje fibers in sodium-free, calcium-rich solutions. *J. Gen. Physiol.* 61:786–808, 1973.
18. Ashcroft, F. M., and F. M. Gribble. Correlating structure and function in ATP-sensitive K^+ channels. *Trends Neurosci.* 21:288–294, 1998.
19. Attwell, D., I. Cohen, D. Eisner, M. Ohba, and C. Ojeda. The steady-state TTX-sensitive ('window') sodium current in Purkinje fibres. *Pflugers Arch.* 379:137–142, 1979.
20. Aulbach, F., A. Simm, S. Maier, H. Langenfeld, U. Walter, U. Kersting, and M. Kirstein. Insulin stimulates the L-type Ca^{2+}

current in rat cardiac myocytes. *Cardiovasc. Res.* 42:113–120, 1999.
21. Bahinski, H., A. C Nairn, P. Greengard, and D. C. Gadsby. Chloride conductance regulated by cyclic AMP-dependent protein kinase in cardiac myocytes. *Nature* 340:718–721, 1989.
22. Baker, K. M., G. W. Booz, and D. E. Dostal. Cardiac actions of angiotensin II: role of an intracardiac renin-angiotensin system. *Annu. Rev. Physiol.* 54:227–241, 1992.
23. Balligand, J.-L., R. A. Kelly, P. A. Marsden, T. W. Smith, and T. Michel. Control of cardiac muscle cell function by an endogeneous nitric oxide signaling system. *Proc. Natl. Acad. Sci. U.S.A.* 90:347–351, 1993.
24. Balligand, J.-L., L. Kobzik, X. Han, D. M. Kaye, L. Belhassen, D. S. O'Hara, R. A. Kelly, W. Smith, and T. Michel. Nitric oxide-dependent parasympathetic signaling is due to activation of constitutive endothelial (type III) nitric oxide synthase in cardiac myocytes. *J. Biol. Chem.* 270:14582–14586, 1995.
25. Barhanin, J., F. Lesage, E. Guillemare, M. Fink, M. Lazdunski, and G. Romey. *KvLQT1* and *Isk (minK)* proteins associate to form the Iks cardiac potassium current. *Nature* 384:78–80, 1996.
26. Barry, D. M. and J. M. Nerbonne. Myocardial potassium channels: electrophysiological and molecular diversity. *Annu. Rev. Physiol.* 58:363–394, 1996.
27. Bates, S. E. and A. M. Gurney. Ca^{2+}-dependent block and potentiation of L-type calcium current in guinea-pig ventricular myocytes. *J. Physiol. (Lond.)* 466:345–365, 1993.
27a. Baukrowitz, T. U. Schulte, D. Oliver, S. Herlitze, T. Krauter, S. J. Tucker, J. P. Ruppersberg, and B. Falker. PIP2 and PIP as determinants for ATP inhibition of K_{ATP} channels. *Science* 282:1141–1144, 1998.
28. Baumgarten, C. M. and H. A. Fozzard. Intracellular chloride activity in mammalian ventricular muscle. *Am. J. Physiol.* 241 (*Cell Physiol.* 10):C121–C129, 1981.
29. Baumgarten, C. M., G. Isenberg, T. F. McDonald, and R. E. Ten Eick. Depletion and accumulation of potassium in the extracellular clefts of cardiac Purkinje fibres during voltage clamp hyperpolarization. Experiments in sodium-free bathing media. *J. Gen. Physiol.* 70:149–169, 1977.
30. Baumgarten, C. M., D. H. Singer, and H. A. Fozzard. Intra- and extracellular potassium activities, acetylcholine and resting potential in guinea pig atria. *Circ. Res.* 54:65–73, 1984.
31. Bean, B. P., M. C. Norwicky, and R. W. Tsien. β-Adrenergic modulation of calcium channels in frog ventricular heart cells. *Nature* 307:371–375, 1984.
32. Beaulieu, P., and C. Lambert. Peptide regulation of heart rate and interactions with autonomic nervous system. *Cardiovasc. Res.* 37:578–585, 1998.
33. Belardinelli, L., W. R. Giles, and A. West. Ionic mechanisms of adenosine actions in pacemaker cells from rabbit heart. *J. Physiol. (Lond).* 405:615–633, 1988.
34. Belardinelli, L. and G. Isenberg. Isolated atrial myocytes: Adenosine and acetylcholine increase potassium conductance. *Am. J. Physiol.* 244 (*Heart Circ. Physiol.* 13):H734–H737, 1983.
35. Belardinelli, L., and G. Isenberg. Actions of adenosine and isoproterenol on isolated mammalian ventricular myocytes. *Circ. Res.* 53:287–297, 1983.
36. Belardinelli, L., J. Linden, and R. M. Berne. The cardiac effects of adenosine. *Prog. Cardiovasc. Dis.* 22:73–97, 1989.
37. Belardinelli, L., J. C. Shryock, Y. Song, D. Wang, and M. Srinivas. Ionic basis of the electrophysiological actions of adenosine on cardiomyocytes. *FASEB J.* 9:359–365, 1995.
38. Benfey, B. G. Minireview: function of myocardial α-adrenoceptors. *Life Sci.* 46:743–757, 1990.
39. Benz, I., J. W. Herzig, and M. Kohlhardt. Opposite effects of angiotensin II and protein kinase C activator OAG on cardiac Na^+ channels. *J. Membr. Biol.* 130:183–190, 1992.
40. Bescond, J., P. Bois, J. Petit-Jacques, and J. Lenfant. Characterization of an angiotensin-II-activated chloride current in rabbit sino-atrial node cells. *J. Membr. Biol.* 140:153–161, 1994.
41. Bielen, F. V., S. Bosteels, and F. Verdonck. Consequences of CO_2 acidosis for transmembrane Na^+ transport and membrane current in rabbit cardiac Purkinje fibres. *J. Physiol. (Lond).* 427:325–345, 1990.
42. Biermans, G., J. Vereecke, and E. Carmeliet. The mechanism of the inward-rectifying K current during hyperpolarizing steps in guinea-pig ventricular myocytes. *Pflugers Arch.* 410:604–613, 1987.
43. Binah, O., I. Rubenstein, and E. Gilat. Effects of thyroid hormone on the action potential and membrane current of guinea-pig ventricular myocytes. *Pflugers Arch.* 409:214–216, 1987.
44. Bkaily, G., N. Perron, S. Wang, A. Sculptoreanu, D. Jacques, and D. Menard. Atrial natriuretic factor blocks the high-threshold Ca^{2+} current and increases K^+ current in fetal single ventricular cells. *J. Mol. Cell. Cardiol.* 25:1305–1316, 1993.
45. Bkaily, G., S. Wang, M. Bui, and D. Menard. ET-1 stimulates Ca^{2+} currents in cardiac cells. *J. Cardiovasc. Pharmacol.* 26(Suppl. 3):S293–S296, 1995.
46. Blumenthal, E. M., and L. K. Kaczmarek. Modulation by cyclic AMP of a slowly activating potassium channel expressed in *Xenopus* oocytes. *J. Neurosci.* 12:290–296, 1992.
47. Bohm, M., B. Pieske, M. Ungerer and E. Erdmann. Characterization of A1 adenosine receptors in atrial and ventricular myocardium from diseased human hearts. *Circ. Res.* 65:1201–1211, 1989.
48. Bourinet, E., F. Fournier, P. Lory, P. Charnet, and J. Nargeot. Protein kinase C regulation of cardiac calcium channels expressed in *Xenopus* oocytes. *Pflugers Arch.* 421:247–255, 1992.
49. Bouron, A., N. M. Soldatov, and H. Reuter. The beta-1 subunit is essential for modulation by protein kinase C of a human and a non-human L-type Ca^{2+} channel. *FEBS Lett.* 377:159–162, 1995.
50. Boutjdir, M., and N. El-Sheriff. α 1-Adrenoceptor regulation of delayed afterdepolarization and triggered activity in subendocardial Purkinje fibers surviving one day of myocardial infarction. *J. Mol. Cell. Cardiol.* 23:83–90, 1991.
51. Boyett, M. R. and A. Roberts. The fade of the response to acetylcholine at the rabbit isolated sino-atrial node. *J. Physiol. (Lond.)* 393:171–194, 1987.
52. Brady, A. J. and J. W. Woodbury. The sodium-potassium hypothesis as the basis of electrical activity in frog ventricle. *J. Physiol. (Lond.)* 154:385–407, 1960.
53. Braun, A. P., D. Fedida, R. B. Clark, and W. R. Giles. Intracellular mechanisms for α 1-adrenergic regulation of the transient outward current in rabbit atrial myocytes. *J. Physiol. (Lond.)* 431:689–712, 1990.
54. Breitweisscr, G. E. and G. Szabo. Uncoupling of cardiac muscarinic and β-adrenergic receptors from ion channels by a guanine nucleotide analogue. *Nature* 317:538–540, 1985.
55. Brooks, C.McC. and H. H. Lu. *The Sinoatrial Pacemaker of the Heart.* Springfield, Illinois: Thomas, 1972.
56. Brown, A. M. and L. Birnbaumer. Ionic channels and their regulation by G protein subunits. *Annu. Rev. Physiol.* 52:197–213, 1990.
57. Brown, J. H. and S. L. Brown. Agonists differentiate muscarinic receptors that inhibit cyclic AMP formation from those that stimulate phosphoinositide metabolism. *J. Biol. Chem.* 259:3777–3781, 1984.
58. Brown, R. H., I. Cohen, and D. Noble. The interactions of protons, calcium and potassium ions on cardiac Purkinje fibres. *J. Physiol. (Lond.)* 282:345–352, 1978.
59. Brown, G. L. and J. C. Eccles. The action of a single vagal volley

on the rhythm of the heart beat. *J. Physiol. (Lond.)* 82:211–240, 1934.
60. Brown, H. F., D. DiFrancesco, and S. J. Noble. How does adrenaline accelerate the heart? *Nature* 280:235–236, 1979.
61. Brown, R. H. and D. Noble. Displacement of activation thresholds in cardiac muscle by protons and calcium ions. *J. Physiol. (Lond.)* 282:333–343, 1978.
62. Bruckner, R. and H. Scholz. Effects of α-adrenoceptor stimulation with phenylephrine in the presence of propranolol on force of contraction, slow inward current and cyclic AMP content in the bovine heart. *Br. J. Pharmacol.* 82:223–232, 1984.
63. Brum, G., W. Osterrieder, and W. Trautwein. β-Adrenergic increase in the calcium conductance of cardiac myocytes studied with the patch clamp. *Pflugers Arch.* 401:111–118, 1984.
64. Burnstock, G. A basis of distinguishing two types of purinergic receptors. In *Cell Membrane Receptors for Drugs and Hormones*, edited by L. Bolis and R. W. Straub. New York: Raven Press, 1978:107–118.
65. Burnstock, G. The past, present and future of purine nucleotides as signaling molecules. *Neuropharmacology* 36:1127–1139, 1997.
66. Busch, A. E., M. P. Kavanaugh, M. D. Varnum, J. P. Adelman, and R. A. North. Regulation by second messengers of the slowly activating voltage-dependent potassium current expressed in *Xenopus* oocytes. *J. Physiol. (Lond.)* 450:491–502, 1992.
67. Bywater, R. A., G. D. Campbell, F. R. Edwards, and G. D. Hirst. Effects of vagal stimulation and applied acetylcholine on the arrested sinus venosus of the toad. *J. Physiol. (Lond.)* 425:1–27, 1990.
68. Cachelin, A. B., J. E. DePayer, S. Kokubun, and H. Reuter. Ca^{2+} channel modulation by 8-bromocyclic AMP in cultured heart cells. *Nature* 304:462–464, 1983.
69. Capurro, N. and R. Levi. The heart as a target organ of cardiac anaphylaxis in vivo and in vitro. *Circ. Res.* 36:520–528, 1975.
70. Carmeliet, E. *Chloride and Potassium Permeability in Cardiac Purkinje Fibres*. Brussels. Presses Academiques Europeenes, 1961.
71. Carmeliet, E. Introduction and removal of inward-rectification in sheep cardiac Purkinje fibres. *J. Physiol. (Lond.)* 327:285–308, 1982.
72. Carmeliet, E. and K. Mubagwa. Characterization of the acetylcholine-induced potassium current in rabbit cardiac Purkinje fibres. *J. Physiol. (Lond.)* 371:219–237, 1986.
73. Carmeliet, E. and K. Mubagwa. Desensitization of the acetylcholine-induced increase of potassium conductance in rabbit cardiac Purkinje fibres. *J. Physiol. (Lond.)* 371:239–255, 1986.
74. Carmeliet, E. and J. Ramon. Electrophysiological effects of acetylcholine in sheep cardiac Purkinje fibres. *Pflugers Arch.* 387:197–205, 1980.
75. Carmeliet, E. and T. Saikawa. Shortening of action potential and reduction of pacemaker activity by lidocaine, quinidine, and procainamide in sheep cardiac Purkinje fibers. An effect on Na or K current? *Circ. Res.* 50:257–272, 1982.
76. Catterall, W. A. Modulation of sodium and calcium channels by protein phosphorylation and G proteins. *Adv. Second Messenger Phosphoprotein Res.* 31:159–181, 1997.
77. Caulfield, M. P., and N. J. Birdsall. International Union of Pharmacology. XVII. Classification of muscarinic acetylcholine receptors. *Pharmacol. Rev.* 50:279–290, 1998.
78. Cavalie, A., T. F. McDonald, D. Pelzer, and W. Trautwein. Temperature-induced transitory and steady-state changes in the calcium current of guinea pig ventricular myocytes. *Pflugers Arch.* 405:294–296, 1985.
79. Cerbai, E., U. Klockner, and G. Isenberg. Ca-antagonistic effects of adenosine in guinea pig atrial cells. *Am. J. Physiol.* 255 (*Heart Circ. Physiol.* 24):H872–H878, 1988.
80. Chang, F., J. Gao, C. Tromba, and D. DiFrancesco. Acetylcholine reverses effects of β-agonists on pacemaker current in canine cardiac Purkinje fibers but has no direct action. *Circ. Res.* 66:633–636, 1990.
81. Chen, L., N. El-Sherif, and M. Boutjdir. α 1-Adrenergic activation inhibits β-adrenergic stimulated unitary Ca^{2+} currents in cardiac ventricular myocytes. *Circ. Res.* 79:184–193, 1996.
82. Chen, S.-A., M. S. Chang, B. N. Chiang, K. K. Cheng, and C. I. Lee. Electromechanical effects of angiotensin in human atrial tissues. *J. Mol. Cell. Cardiol.* 23:483–493, 1991.
83. Chen, X.-H., I. Bezprozvanny, and R. W. Tsien. Molecular basis of proton block of L-type Ca^{2+} channels. *J. Gen. Physiol.* 108:363–374, 1996.
84. Chesnais, J. M., E. Coraboeuf, M. P. Sauviat, and J. M. Vassort. Sensitivity to H, Li and Mg ions of the slow inward sodium current in frog atrial fibres. *J. Mol. Cell. Cardiol.* 7:627–642, 1975.
85. Christie, R., V. K. Sharma, and S. S. Sheu. Mechanism of extracellular ATP-induced increase of cytosolic Ca^{2+} concentration in isolated rat ventricular myocytes. *J. Physiol. (Lond.)* 445:365–388, 1992.
86. Clapham, D. E., and E. Neer. New roles for G-protein β γ-dimers in transmembrane signaling. *Nature* 365:403–406, 1993.
87. Clemo, H. F., and C. M. Baumgarten. Swelling-activated Gd^{3+}-sensitive current and cell volume regulation in rabbit ventricular myocytes. *J. Gen. Physiol.* 110:297–312, 1997.
88. Clemo, H. F., C. M. Baumgarten, K. A. Ellenbogen, and B. S. Stambler. Atrial natriuretic peptide and cardiac electrophysiology: autonomic and direct effects. *J. Cardiovasc. Electrophysiol.* 7:149–162, 1996.
89. Clemo, H. F. and L. Belardinelli. Effect of adenosine on atrioventricular conduction. I. Site and characterization of adenosine action in the guinea-pig atrioventricular node. *Circ. Res.* 59:427–436, 1986.
90. Clemo, H. F., B. S. Stambler, and C. M. Baumgarten. Persistent activation of a swelling-activated cation current in ventricular myocytes from dogs with tachycardia-induced congestive heart failure. *Circ. Res.* 83:147–157, 1998.
91. Clemo, H. F., B. S. Stambler, and C. M. Baumgarten. Swelling-activated chloride A current is persistently activated in ventricular myocytes from dogs with tachycardia-induced congestive heart failure. *Circ. Res.* 84:157–165, 1999.
92. Cole, W. C., C. D. McPherson, and D. Sontag. ATP-regulated K^+ channels protect the myocardium against ischemia/reperfusion damage. *Circ. Res.* 69:571–581, 1991.
93. Collier, M. L. and J. H. Hume. Unitary Co^- channels activated by cytoplasmic Ca^{2+} in canine ventricular myocytes. *Circ. Res.* 78:936–944, 1996.
94. Colquhoun, D., E. Neher, H. Reuter, and C. F. Stevens. Inward current channels activated by intracellular Ca in cultured cardiac cells. *Nature* 294:752–754, 1981.
95. Coraboeuf, E., E. Deroubaix, and A. Coulombe. Effect of tetrodotoxin on action potentials of the conducting system in the dog heart. *Am. J. Physiol.* 236 (*Heart Circ. Physiol.* 5):H561–H567, 1979.
96. Coraboeuf, E., E. Deroubaix, and A. Coulombe. Acidosis-induced abnormal repolarization and repetitive activity in isolated dog Purkinje fibres. *J. Physiol. (Paris)* 76:97–106, 1980.
97. Cordeiro, J. M., K. W. Spitzer, and W. R. Giles. Repolarizing K^+ currents in rabbit heart Purkinje cells. *J. Physiol. (Lond.)* 508:811–823, 1998.
98. Coulombe, A. and E. Coraboeuf. Large conductance chloride channels of new-born rat cardiac myocytes are activated by hypotonic media. *Pflugers Arch.* 422:143–150, 1992.
99. Craelius, W., V. Chen, and N. El-Sherif. Stretch activated ion

channels in ventricular myocytes. *Biosci. Rep.* 8:407–414, 1988.
100. Cramb, G., R. Banks, E. L. Rugg, and J. F. Aiton. Actions of atrial natriuretic peptide (ANP) on cyclic nucleotide concentrations and phosphatidylinositol turnover in ventricular myocytes. *Biochem. Biophys. Res. Commun.* 148:962–970, 1987.
101. Cranefiel, P. F. *The Conduction of the Cardiac Impulse: The Slow Response and Cardiac Arrhythmias.* Mt. Kisco, NY: Futura Publishing Co., 1975.
102. Cuevas, J., A. L. Bassett, J. S. Cameron, T. Furukawa, R. J. Myerburg, and S. Kimura. Effect of H^+ on ATP-regulated K^+ channels in feline ventricular myocytes. *Am. J. Physiol.* 261 (*Heart Circ. Physiol.* 30):H755–H761, 1991.
103. Damron, D. S., D. R. Van Wagoner, C. S. Moravec, and M. Bond. Arachidonic acid and endothelin potentiates Ca^{2+} transients in rat cardiac myocytes via inhibition of distinct K^+ channels. *J. Biol. Chem.* 268:27335–27344, 1993.
104. Davies, N. W. Modulation of ATP-sensitive K^+ channels in skeletal muscle by intracellular protons. *Nature* 343:375–377, 1990.
105. Davis, L. D., P. R. Helmer, and F. Ballantyne III. Production of slow responses in canine cardiac Purkinje fibers exposed to reduced pH. *J. Mol. Cell. Cardiol.* 8:61–76, 1976.
105a. Deal, K. K., S. K. England, and M. M. Tamkun. Molecular physiology of cardiac potassium channels. *Physiol. Rev.* 76:49–67, 1996.
106. Deck, K. A. Anderungen des Ruhepotentials und der Kabeleigenshaften von Purkinje-Faden bei der Dehnung. *Pflugers Arch.* 280:131–140, 1964.
107. de Gaspo, M., A. Husain, W. Alexander, K. J. Katt, A. T. Chiu, M. Drew, T. Goodfriend, J. W. Harding, T. Inagami, and P. B. W. M. Tommermans. A proposed update of the nomenclature of angiotensin receptors. *Hypertension* 25:924–927, 1995.
108. DeHaan, R. L. and H. Gottlieb. The electrical activity of embryonic chick heart cells isolated in tissue culture singly or in interconnected cell sheets. *J. Gen. Physiol.* 52:643–665, 1968.
109. De Jongh, K. S., B. J. Murphy, A. A. Colvin, J. W. Hell, M. Takahashi, and W. A. Catterall. Specific phosphorylation of a site in the full-length form of the alpha 1 subunit of the cardiac L-type calcium channel by adenosine 3', 5'-cyclic monophosphate-dependent protein kinase. *Biochemistry* 35:10392–10402, 1996.
110. Del Balzo, U., M. R. Rosen, G. Malfatto, L. M. Kaplan, and S. F. Steinberg. Specific α1-adrenergic receptor subtypes modulate catecholamine-induced increases and decreases in ventricular automaticity. *Circ. Res.* 67:1535–1551, 1990.
111. Del Castillo, J. and B. Katz. Production of membrane potential changes in the frog's heart by inhibitory nerve impulses. *Nature* 175:1035, 1955.
112. de Leon, M., Y. Yang, L. Jones, E. Perez-Reyes, X. Wei, T. W. Song, T. P. Snutch, and D. T. Yue. Essential Ca^{2+}-binding motif for Ca^{2+}-sensitive inactivation of L-type Ca^{2+} channels. *Science* 270:1502–1506, 1995.
113. Deleze, J. Perfusion of a strip of mammalian ventricle. Effects of K-rich and Na-deficient solutions on transmembrane potentials. *Circ. Res.* 7:461–465, 1959.
114. De Mello, W. C. Renin-angiotensin system and cell communication in the failing heart. *Hypertension* 27:1267–1272, 1996.
115. De Mello, W. C. and B. F. Hoffmann. Potassium ions and electrical activity of specialized cardiac fibers. *Am. J. Physiol.* 199:1125–1130, 1960.
116. Denyer, J. and H. Brown. Pacemaking in rabbit isolated sino-atrial node cells during Cs^+ block of the hyperpolarization-activated current, i_f. *J. Physiol. (Lond).* 429:401–409, 1990.
117. Desilets, M. and C. M. Baumgarten. K^+, Na^+ and Cl^- activities in ventricular myocytes isolated from rabbit heart. *Am. J. Physiol.* 251 (*Cell Physiol.* 20):C197–C208, 1986.
118. DiFrancesco, D. A new interpretation of the pacemaker current in calf Purkinje fibres. *J. Physiol. (Lond.)* 314:359–376, 1981.
119. DiFrancesco, D. The contribution of the 'pacemaker' current (i_f) to generation of spontaneous activity in rabbit sino-atrial node myocytes. *J. Physiol. (Lond.)* 434:23–40, 1991.
120. DiFrancesco, D. Pacemaker mechanisms in cardiac tissue. *Annu. Rev. Physiol.* 55:451–467, 1993.
121. DiFrancesco, D., P. Ducouret, and R. B. Robinson. Muscarinic modulation of cardiac rate at low acetylcholine concentrations. *Science* 243:669–671, 1989,
122. DiFrancesco, D., A. Ferroni, M. Mazzanti, and C. Tromba. Properties of the hyperpolarizing-activated current (i_f) in cells isolated from the rabbit sino-atrial node. *J. Physiol. (Lond.)* 377:61–88, 1986.
123. DiFrancesco, D., A. Ferroni, and S. Vinsentin. Barium-induced blockade of the inward rectifier in calf Purkinje fibres. *Pflugers Arch.* 402:446–453, 1984.
124. DiFrancesco, D. and M. Mangoni. Modulation of single hyperpolarization-activated channels (I_f) by cAMP in the rabbit sino-atrial node. *J. Physiol. (Lond.)* 474:473–482, 1994.
125. DiFrancesco, D. and P. Tortora. Direct activation of cardiac pacemaker channels by intracellular cyclic AMP. *Nature* 351:45–147, 1991.
126. DiFrancesco, D. and C. Tromba. Inhibition of the hyperpolarization-activated current (I_f) induced by acetylcholine in rabbit sino-atrial node myocytes. *J. Physiol. (Lond.)* 405:477–491, 1988.
127. DiFrancesco, D. and C. Tromba. Muscarinic control of the hyperpolarizing-activated current i_f in rabbit sino-atrial node myocytes. *J. Physiol. (Lond.)* 405:493–510, 1988.
128. Dirksen, R. T. and S. S. Sheu. Modulation of ventricular action potential by α1-adrenoceptors and protein kinase C. *Am. J. Physiol.* 258 (*Heart Circ. Physiol.* 27):H907–H911, 1990.
129. Doerr, T., R. Denger, and W. Trautwein. Calcium currents in single SA nodal cells of the rabbit heart studied with action potential clamp. *Pflugers Arch.* 413:599–603, 1989.
130. Dominguez, G. and H. A. Fozzard. Influence of extracellular K^+ concentration on cable properties and excitability of sheep cardiac Purkinje fibers. *Circ. Res.* 26:565–574, 1970.
131. Dosemeci, A., R. S. Dhallan, N. M. Cohen, W. J. Lederer, and T. B. Rogers. Phorbol ester increases calcium current and simulates the effects of angiotensin II on cultured neonatal rat heart myocytes. *Circ. Res.* 62:347–357, 1988.
132. Dostal, D. E. and K. M. Baker. The cardiac renin-angiotensin system. Conceptual, or a regulator of cardiac function? *Circ. Res.* 85:643–650, 1999.
133. Downey, J. M., and M. V. Cohen. Signal transduction in ischemic preconditioning. *Adv. Exp. Med. Biol.* 430:39–55, 1997.
134. Downey, J. M., G. S. Liu, and J. D. Thornton. Adenosine and the antiinfarct effects of preconditioning. *Cardiovasc. Res.* 27:3–8, 1993.
135. Duan, D., S. Cowley, B. Horowitz, and J. R. Hume. A serine residue in ClC-3 links phosphorylation-dephosphorylation to chloride channel regulation by cell volume. *J. Gen. Physiol.* 113:57–70, 1999.
136. Duan, D., B. Fermini, and S. Nattel. Sustained outward current observed after I_{to1} inactivation in rabbit atrial myocytes is a novel Cl^- current. *Am. J. Physiol.* 263 (*Heart Circ. Physiol.* 32):H1967–H1971, 1992.
137. Duan, D., B. Fermini, and S. Nattel. α-Adrenergic control of volume-regulated Cl^- currents in rabbit atrial myocytes. *Circ. Res.* 77:379–393, 1995.
138. Duan, D., and S. Nattel. Properties of single outwardly rectifying Cl^- channels in heart. *Circ. Res.* 75:789–795, 1994.

139. Duan, D., C. Winter, S. Cowley, J. R. Hume, and B. Horowitz. Molecular identification of a volume-regulated chloride channel. *Nature* 390:417–421, 1997.
140. Duan, D., L. Ye, F. Britton, L. J. Miller, J. Yamazaki, B. Horowitz, and J. R. Hume. Purinoceptor-coupled Cl⁻ channels in mouse heart: a novel, alternative pathway for CFTR regulation. *J. Physiol. (Lond.)* 521:43–56, 1999.
141. Duchatelle-Gourdon, I., H. C. Hartzell, and A. A. Lagrutta. Modulation of the delayed rectifier potassium current in frog cardiomyocytes by β-adrenergic agonists and magnesium. *J. Physiol. (Lond.)* 415:251–274, 1989.
142. Dudel, J. and W. Trautwein. Das Aktionpotential und Mechanogram des Herzmuskels unter dem Einfluss der Dehnung. *Cardiologia* 25:344–362, 1954.
143. Dudley, S. C. Jr., and C. M. Baumgarten. Bursting of cardiac sodium channels after exposure to 3,5,3'-triiodo-L-thyronine. *Circ. Res.* 73:301–313, 1993.
144. Eckert, R. and E. Chad. Inactivation of calcium channels. *Prog. Biophys. Mol. Biol.* 44:215–267, 1984.
145. Eckert, R., J. Utz, W. Trautwein, and R. M. Mentzer, Jr. Involvement of intracellular Ca^{2+} release mechanism in adenosine-induced cardiac Ca^{2+} current inhibition. *Surgery* 114:334–342, 1993.
146. Edwards, G. and A. H. Weston. The pharmacology of ATP-sensitive potassium channels. *Annu. Rev. Pharmacol. Toxicol.* 33:597–637, 1993.
147. Egan, T. M., D. Noble, S. J. Noble, T. Powell, A. J. Spindler, and V. W. Twist. Sodium-calcium exchange during the action potential in guinea-pig ventricular cells. *J. Physiol (Lond)*. 411:639–661, 1989.
148. Egan, T. M., D. Noble, S. J. Noble, T. Powell, V. W. Twist, and K. Yamaoka. On the mechanism of isoprenalin- and forskolin-induced depolarization of single guinea-pig ventricular myocytes. *J. Physiol. (Lond.)* 400:299–320, 1988.
149. Ehara, T. and K. Ishihara. Anion channels activated by adrenaline in cardiac muscle. *Nature* 347:284–286, 1990.
150. Ehara, T., A. Noma, and K. Ono. Calcium-activated nonselective cation channel in ventricular cells isolated from adult guinea-pig hearts. *J. Physiol. (Lond.)* 403:117–133, 1988.
151. Eisner, D. A. and W. J. Lederer. Inotropic and arrhythmogenic effects of potassium-depleted solutions on mammalian cardiac muscle. *J. Physiol. (Lond.)* 294:255–277, 1979.
152. Endou, M. and R. Levi. Histamine in the heart. *Eur. J. Clin. Invest.* 25 (Suppl.1):5–11, 1995.
153. Ertl, R., U. Jahnel, H. Nawrath, E. Carmeliet, and J. Vereecke. Differential electrophysiological and inotropic effects of phenylephrine in atrial and ventricular heart muscle preparations from rat. *N-S Arch. Pharmacol.* 344:574–581, 1991.
154. Escande, D., D. Thuringer, S. Le Guern, and I. Cavero. The potassium channel opener cromakalim (BRL 34915) activates ATP-dependent K^+ channels in isolated cardiac myocytes. *Biochim. Biophys. Res. Commun.* 154:620–625, 1988.
155. Ewart, H. S. and A. Klip. Hormonal regulation of the Na^+-K^+ ATPase: mechanisms underlying rapid and sustained changes in pump activity. *Am. J. Physiol.* 269 (*Cell Physiol.* 38):C295–C311, 1995.
156. Fan, Z., T. Furukawa, T. Sawanobori, J. C. Makielski, and M. Hiraoka. Cytoplasmic acidosis induces multiple conductance states in ATP-sensitive potassium channels of cardiac myocytes. *J. Membr. Biol.* 136:169–179, 1993.
157. Fan, Z. and M. Hiraoka. Depression of delayed outward K^+ current by Co^{2+} in guinea pig ventricular myocytes. *Am. J. Physiol.* 261 (*Cell Physiol.* 30):C23–C31, 1991.
158. Fan, Z. and J. C. Makielski. Intracellular H^+ and Ca^{2+} modulation of trypsin-modified ATP-sensitive K^+ channels in rabbit ventricular myocytes. *Circ. Res.* 72:715–722, 1993.
159. Fan, Z. and J. C. Makielski. Anionic phospholipids activate ATP-sensitive potassium channels. *J. Biol. Chem.* 272:5388–5395, 1997.
160. Fan, Z., K. Nakayama, and M. Hiraoka. Pinacidil activates the ATP-sensitive K^+ channel in inside-out and cell-attached patch membranes of guinea-pig ventricular myocytes. *Pflugers Arch.* 415:387–394, 1990.
161. Fan, Z., K. Nakayama, and M. Hiraoka. Multiple actions of pinacidil on adenosine triphosphate-sensitive potassium channels in guinea-pig ventricular myocytes. *J. Physiol. (Lond.)* 430:273–295, 1990.
162. Fedida, D., A. P. Braun, and W. R. Giles. α 1-Adrenoceptors reduce background K^+ current in rabbit ventricular myocytes. *J. Physiol. (Lond.)* 441:673–684, 1991.
163. Fedida, D., A. P. Braun, and W. R. Giles. Changes in the rectifying potassium currents of atrial myocytes induced by α 1-adrenoceptors in the presence and absence of acetylcholine. *Pflugers Arch.* 421:431–439, 1992.
164. Fedida, D., A. P. Braun, and W. R. Giles. α 1-Adrenoceptors in myocardium: Functional aspects and transmembrane signaling mechanisms. *Physiol. Rev.* 73:469–487, 1993.
165. Fedida, D., D. Noble, and A. J. Spindler. Mechanism of the use dependence of Ca^{2+} current in guinea-pig myocytes. *J. Physiol. (Lond.)* 405:430–460, 1988.
166. Fedida, D., Y. Shimoni, and W. R. Giles. α-Adrenergic modulation of the transient outward current in rabbit atrial myocytes. *J. Physiol. (Lond.)* 423:257–277, 1990.
167. Fein, F. S., R. S. Aronson, C. Nordin, B. Miller-Green, and E. H. Sonnenblick. Altered myocardial response to ouabain in diabetic rats: mechanisms and electrophysiology. *J. Mol. Cell. Cardiol.* 15:769–784, 1983.
168. Fein, F. S. and E. H. Sonnenblick. Diabetic cardiomyopathy. *Prog. Cardiovasc. Dis.* 27:255–270, 1985.
169. Ferguson, D. W., W. J. Berg, J. S. Sanders, P. J. Roach, J. S. Kempf, and M. G. Kienzle. Sympathoinhibitory responses to digitals glycosides in heart failure patients. Direct evidence from sympathetic neural recordings. *Circulation* 80:65–77, 1989.
170. Ferrier, G. R. Digitalis arrhythmias: role of oscillatory afterpotentials. *Prog. Cardiovasc. Dis.* 19:459–474, 1977.
171. Findlay, I. Effects of ADP upon the ATP-sensitive K^+ channel in rat ventricular myocytes. *J. Membr. Biol.* 101:83–92, 1988.
172. Findley, I. Calcium-dependent inactivation of the ATP-sensitive K^+ channel of rat ventricular myocytes. *Biochim. Biophys. Acta* 943:297–304, 1988.
173. Fischmeister, R., M. Brocas-Randolph, P. Lechene, J. A. Argibay, and G. Vassort. A dual effect of cardiac glycosides on Ca current in single cells of frog heart. *Pflugers Arch.* 406:340–342, 1986.
174. Fischmeister, R. and H. C. Hartzell. Mechanism of action of acetylcholine on calcium current in single cells from frog ventricle. *J. Physiol. (Lond.)* 376;183–202, 1986.
175. Fischmeister, R. and H. C. Hartzell. Cyclic guanosine 3': 5' monophosphate regulates the calcium current in single cells from frog ventricle. *J. Physiol. (Lond.)* 387:453–472, 1987.
176. Ford, A. P. D. W., T. J. Williams, D. R. Blue, and D. E. Clarke. α1-Adrenoceptor classification: sharpening Occam's razor. *Trends Pharmacol. Sci.* 15:167–170, 1994.
177. Forrester, T. Release of ATP from heart. *Ann. N.Y. Acad. Sci.* 603:335–351, 1990.
178. Fosset, M., J. R. de Weille, R. D. Green, H. Schmid-Antomarch, and M. Lazdunski. Antidiabetic sulphonylureas control action potential properties in heart cells via high affinity receptors that are linked to ATP-dependent K^+ channels. *J. Biol. Chem.* 263:7933–7936, 1988.
179. Fozzard, H. A., and D. A. Hanck. Structure and function of

voltage-dependent sodium channels: comparison of brain II and cardiac isoforms. *Physiol. Rev.* 76:887–926, 1996.
180. Frankenhaeuser, B. and L. E. Moore. The effect of temperature on the sodium and potassium permeability changes in myelinated nerve fibers of Xenopus laevis. *J. Physiol. (Lond.)* 169:431–437, 1963.
181. Fredholm, B. B., M. P. Abbracchio, G. Burnstock, J. W. Daly, T. K. Harden, K. A. Jacobson, P. Leef, and M. Williams. VI. Nomenclature and classification of purinoceptors. *Pharmacol. Rev.* 46:143–156, 1994.
182. Fredholm, B. B., M. P. Abbracchio, G. Burnstock, G. R. Dubyak, T. K. Harden, K. A. Jacobson, U. Schwabe, and M. Williams. Towards a revised nomenclature for P_1 and P_2 receptors. *Trends Pharmacol. Sci.* 18:79–82, 1997.
183. Freedberg, A. S., J. G. Papp, and E. M. Vaughan Williams. The effect of altered thyroid state on atrial intracellular potentials. *J. Physiol. (Lond.)* 207:357–369, 1970.
184. Friel, D. D. and B. P. Bean. Two ATP-activated conductances in bullfrog atrial cells. *J. Gen. Physiol.* 91:1–27, 1988.
185. Friel, D. D. and B. P. Bean. Dual control by ATP and acetylcholine of inwardly rectifying K^+ channels in bovine atrial cells. *Pflugers Arch.* 415:651–657, 1990.
186. Frohnwieser, B., L. Q. Chen, W. Schreibmyer, and R. G. Kallen. Modulation of the human cardiac sodium channel alpha-subunit by cAMP-dependent protein kinase and the responsible sequence domain. *J. Physiol. (Lond.)* 498:309–318, 1997.
187. Fry, C. H. and P. A. Pool-Wilson. Effects of acid-base changes on excitation-contraction coupling in guinea-pig and rabbit cardiac ventricular muscle. *J. Physiol. (Lond.)* 313:141–160, 1981.
188. Fu, C., A. Pleumsamran, U. Oh, and D. Kim. Different properties of the atrial G protein–gated K^+ channels activated by extracellular ATP and adenosine. *Am. J. Physiol.* 269 (*Heart Circ. Physiol.* 38):H1349–H1358, 1995.
189. Furukawa, T., Z. Fan, T. Sawanobori, and M. Hiraoka. Modification of the adenosine 5′-trophosphate-sensitive K^+ channel by trypsin in guinea-pig ventricular myocytes. *J. Physiol. (Lond.)* 466:707–726, 1993.
190. Furukawa, T., H. Ito, J. Nitta, M. Tsujino, S. Adachi, M. Hiroe, F. Marumo, T. Sawanobori, and M. Hiraoka. Endothelin-1 enhances calcium entry through T-type calcium channels in cultured neonatal rat ventricular myocytes. *Circ. Res.* 71:1242–1253, 1992.
191. Furukawa, T., L. Virag, N. Furukawa, T. Sawanobori, and M. Hiraoka. Mechanism for reactivation of the ATP-sensitive K^+ channel by MgATP complexes in guinea-pig ventricular myocytes. *J. Physiol. (Lond.)* 479:95–107, 1994.
192. Furukawa, T., T. Yamane, T. Terai, Y. Katayama, and M. Hiraoka. Functional linkage of the cardiac ATP-sensitive K^+ channel to the actin cytoskeleton. *Pflugers Arch.* 431:504–512, 1996.
193. Gadsby, D. C. The Na/K pump of cardiac cells. *Annu. Rev. Biophys. Bioeng.* 13:373–398, 1984.
194. Gadsby, D. C. and A. C. Nairn. Control of CFTR channel gating by phosphorylation and nucleotide hydrolysis. *Physiol. Rev.* 79:S77–S107, 1999.
195. Gadsby, D. C., A. L. Wit, and P. F. Cranefield. The effects of acetylcholine on the electrical activity of canine cardiac Purkinje fibers. *Circ. Res.* 43:29–35, 1978.
196. Gallo, M. P., G. Alloatti, C. Eva, A. Oberto, and R. C. Levi. M_1 muscarinic receptors increase calcium current and phosphoinositide turnover in guinea-pig ventricular cardiocytes. *J. Physiol. (Lond.)* 471:41–60, 1993.
197. Gao, J., I. S. Cohen, R. T. Mathias, and G. J. Baldo. Regulation of the beta-stimulation of the Na^+-K^+ pump current in guinea-pig ventricular myocytes by a cAMP-dependent PKA pathway. *J. Physiol. (Lond.)* 477:373–380, 1994.
198. Gao, T., A. Yatani, M. L. Dell'Acqua, H. Sako, S. A. Green, N. Dascal, J. D. Scott, and M. M. Hosey. cAMP-dependent regulation of cardiac L-type Ca^{2+} channels requires membrane targeting of PKA and phosphorylation of channel subunits. *Neuron* 19:185–196, 1997.
199. Garlid, K. D., P. Paucek, V. Yarov-Yaronoy, H. N. Murray, R. B. Darbenzio, A. J. D'Alonzo, N. J. Lodge, M. A. Smith, and G. J. Grover. Cardioprotective effect of diazoxide and its interaction with mitochondrial ATP-sensitive K^+ channels: possible mechanism of cardioprotection. *Circ. Res.* 81:1072–1082, 1997.
200. Gauthier, C., G. Tavernier, F. Carpentier, D. Lagin, and H. Le Marec. Functional $β_3$-adrenoceptor in the human heart. *J. Clin. Invest.* 98:556–562, 1996.
201. George, W. J., L. J. Ignarro, R. J. Paddock, L. White, and P. J. Kadowitz. Oppositional effects of acetylcholine and isoproterenol on isometric tension and cyclic nucleotide concentrations in rabbit atria. *J. Cyclic Nucleotide Res.* 1:339–347, 1975.
202. Giles, W. R. and Y. Imaizumi. Comparison of potassium currents in rabbit atrial and ventricular cells. *J. Physiol. (Lond.)* 405:123–145, 1988.
203. Giles, W. R., T. Nakajima, K. Ono, and E. F. Shibata. Modulation of the delayed rectifier K^+ current by isoprenaline in bullfrog atrial myocytes. *J. Physiol. (Lond.)* 415:233–249, 1989.
204. Giles, G. R. and A. C. G. Van Ginneken. A transient outward current in isolated cells from the crista terminalis of rabbit heart. *J. Physiol. (Lond.)* 368:243–264, 1985.
205. Gillis, R. A. and J. A. Quest. The role of the central nervous system in the cardiovascular effects of digitalis. *Pharmacol. Rev.* 31:19–97, 1980.
206. Gintant, G. A., N. B. Datyner, and I. S. Cohen. Slow inactivation of a tetrodotoxin-sensitive current in canine cardiac Purkinje fibres. *Biophys. J.* 45:509–512, 1984.
207. Gintant, G. A. and D. W. Liu. β-Adrenergic modulation of fast inward sodium current in canine myocardium: syncytial preparations versus isolated myocytes. *Circ. Res.* 70:844–850, 1992.
208. Giotti, A., F. Ledda, and P. F. Mannaioni. Effects of noradrenaline and isoprenaline, in combination with α- and β-receptor blocking substances on the action potential of cardiac Purkinje fibres. *J. Physiol. (Lond.)* 229:99–113, 1973.
209. Gisbert, M. P. and R. Fischmeister. Atrial natriuretic factor regulates the calcium current in frog isolated cardiac cells. *Circ. Res.* 62:660–667, 1988.
210. Glitsch, H. G. Electrogenic Na pumping in the heart. *Annu. Rev. Physiol.* 44:389–400, 1982.
211. Glitsch, H. G. and L. Pott. Effects of acetylcholine and parasympathetic nerve stimulation on membrane potential in quiescent guinea-pig atria. *J. Physiol. (Lond.)* 279:655–668, 1978.
212. Gordon, J. L. Extracellular ATP: effects, sources and fate. *Biochem. J.* 233:309–319, 1986.
213. Graham, R. M., Perez, D. M., J. Hwa, and M. T. Piascik. $α_1$-Adrenergic receptor subtypes. Molecular structure, function and signaling. *Circ. Res.* 78:737–749, 1996.
214. Grant, A. O., L. J. Strauss, A. G. Wallace, and H. C. Strauss. The influence of pH on the electrophysiological effects of lidocaine in guinea-pig ventricular myocardium. *Circ. Res.* 47:542–550, 1980.
215. Gross, G. J. ATP-sensitive potassium channels and myocardial preconditioning. *Basic Res. Cardiol.* 90:85–88, 1995.
216. Grover, G. L., J. R. McCullough, D. E. Henry, M. L. Condor, and P. G. Sleph. Anti-ischemic effects of the potassium channel activators pinacidil and cromakalim and the reversal of these effects with the potassium channel blocker glyburide. *J. Pharmacol. Exp. Ther.* 251:98–104, 1989.
217. Grover, G. L., P. G. Sleph, and S. Dzwonczyk. Role of ATP-

sensitive K⁺ channels in mediating preconditioning in the dog and their possible interaction with adenosine A$_1$ receptors. *Circulation* 86:1310–1316, 1992.
218. Guo, J., K. Ono, and A. Noma. A sustained inward current activated at the diastolic potential range in rabbit sino-atrial node cells. *J. Physiol. (Lond.)* 483:1–13, 1995.
219. Gupta, R. C., Neumann, J., P. Boknik, and A. M. Watanabe. M$_2$-specific muscarinic cholinergic receptor-mediated inhibition of cardiac regulatory protein phosphorylation. *Am. J. Physiol.* 266 (*Heart Circ. Physiol.* 35):H1138–H1144, 1994.
220. Gurney, A. M., P. Charnet, J. M. Pye, and J. Nargeot. Augmentation of cardiac calcium current by flash photolysis of intracellular caged-Ca^{2+} molecules. *Nature* 341:65–68, 1989.
221. Gurwitz, D. and M. Sokolovsky. Dual pathways in muscarinic receptor stimulation of phosphoinositide hydrolysis. *Biochemistry* 26:633–638, 1987.
222. Haase, H., S. Bartel, P. Karczewski, I. Morano, and E. G. Krause. In-vivo phosphorylation of the cardiac L-type calcium channel beta-subunit in response to catecholamines. *Mol. Cell. Biochem.* 163–164:99–106, 1996.
223. Habuchi, Y., L-L. Lu, J. Morikawa, and M. Yoshimura. Angiotensin II inhibition of L-type Ca^{2+} current in sinoatrial node cells of rabbits. *Am. J. Physiol.* 268 (*Heart Circ. Physiol.* 37): H1053–H1060, 1995.
224. Habuchi, Y., H. Tanaka, T. Furukawa, Y. Tsujimoto, H. Takahashi, and M. Yoshimura. Endothelin enhances delayed potassium current via phospholipase C in guinea pig ventricular myocytes. *Am. J. Physiol.* 262 (*Heart Circ. Physiol.* 31):H345–H354, 1992.
225. Haga, T., K. Haga, and K. Kameyama. G protein–coupled receptor kinases. *J. Neurochem.* 63:400–412, 1994.
226. Hagiwara, N. and H. Irisawa. Modulation by intracellular Ca^{2+} of the hyperpolarization-activated inward current in rabbit single sinoatrial node cells. *J. Physiol. (Lond.)* 409:121–141, 1989.
227. Hagiwara, N., H. Irisawa, and M. Kameyama. Contribution of two types of calcium currents to the pacemaker potentials of rabbit sino-atrial node cells. *J. Physiol. (Lond.)* 395:233–253, 1988.
228. Hagiwara, N., H. Irisawa, H. Kasanuki, and S. Hosoda. Background current in sino-atrial node cells of the rabbit heart. *J. Physiol. (Lond.)* 448:53–72, 1992.
229. Hagiwara, N., H. Masuda, M. Shoda, and H. Irisawa. Stretch-activated anion currents of rabbit cardiac myocytes. *J. Physiol. (Lond.)* 456:285–302, 1992.
230. Hagiwara, S., S. Miyazaki, W. Moody, and J. Patlak. Blocking effects of barium and hydrogen ions on the potassium current during anomalous rectification in the starfish egg. *J. Physiol. (Lond.)* 67:621–638, 1978.
231. Hall, S. K., J. Zhang, and M. Lieberman. Cyclic AMP prevents activation of a swelling-induced chloride-sensitive conductance in chick heart cell. *J. Physiol. (Lond.)* 488:359–369, 1995.
232. Han, X. and G. R. Ferrier. Ionic mechanisms of transient inward current in the absence of Na⁺-Ca^{2+} exchange in rabbit cardiac Purkinje fibres. *J. Physiol. (Lond.)* 456:19–38, 1992.
233. Han, X., L. Kobzik, J.-L. Balligand, R. A. Kelly, and T. W. Smith. Nitric oxide synthase (NOS3)-mediated cholinergic modulation of Ca^{2+} current in adult rabbit atrioventricular nodal cells. *Circ. Res.* 78:998–1008, 1996.
234. Han, X., Y. Schimoni, and W. R. Giles. An obligatory role for nitric oxide in autonomic control of mammalian heart rate. *J. Physiol. (Lond.)* 476:309–314, 1994.
235. Han, X., Y. Schimoni, and W. R. Giles. A cellular mechanism for nitric oxide–mediated cholinergic control of mammarian heart rate. *J. Gen. Physiol.* 106:45–65, 1995.
236. Hancock, A. A., A. L. DeLean, and R. J. Refkowitz. Quantitative resolution of beta-adrenergic subtypes by selective ligand binding: application of a computerized model fitting technique. *Mol. Pharmacol.* 16:1–9, 1980.
237. Hancox, J. C. and A. J. Levi. L-type calcium current in rod- and spindle-shaped myocytes isolated from rabbit atrioventricular node. *Am. J. Physiol.* 267 (*Heart Circ. Physiol.* 36): H1670–H1680, 1994.
238. Hancox, J. C. and A. J. Levi. Actions of the digitalis analogue strophanthidin on action potentials and L-type calcium current in single cells isolated from the atrioventricular node. *Br. J. Pharmacol.* 1118:1447–1454, 1996.
239. Hardley, R. W. and W. J. Lederer. Ca^{2+} and voltage inactivate Ca^{2+} channels through independent mechanisms. *J. Physiol. (Lond.)* 444:257–268, 1991.
240. Harris, D. R., W. L. Green, and W. Craelius. Acute thyroid hormone promotes slow inactivation of sodium current in neonatal cardiac myocytes. *Biochim. Biophys. Acta* 1095:175–181, 1991.
241. Harrison, S. M., E. McCall, and M. R. Boyett. The relationship between contraction and intracellular sodium in rat and guinea-pig ventricular myocytes. *J. Physiol. (Lond.)* 449:517–550, 1992.
242. Hartzell, H. C. Adenosine receptors in frog sinus venosus: slow inhibitory potentials produced by adenine compounds and acetylcholine. *J. Physiol. (Lond.)* 293:23–49, 1979.
243. Hartzell, H. C. Regulation of cardiac ion channels by catecholamines, acetylcholine and second messenger systems. *Prog. Biophys. Mol. Biol.* 52:165–247, 1988.
244. Hartzell, H. C. and R. Fischmeister. Opposite effects of cyclic GMP and cyclic AMP on Ca^{2+} current in single heart cells. *Nature* 323:273–275, 1986.
245. Hartzell, H. C. and R. Fischmeister. Direct regulation of cardiac Ca^{2+} channels by G protein: neither proven nor necessary? *Trends Pharmacol. Sci.* 13:380–385, 1992.
246. Hartzell, H. C., Y. Hirayama, and J. Petit-Jacque. Effects of protein phosphatase and kinase inhibitors on the cardiac L-type Ca current suggest two sites are phosphorylated by protein kinase A and another protein kinase. *J. Gen. Physiol.* 106:393–414, 1995.
247. Harvey, R. D., C. D. Clarck, and J. R. Hume. Chloride current in mammalian cardiac myocytes—novel mechanism for autonomic regulation of action potential duration and resting membrane potential. *J. Gen. Physiol.* 95:1077–1102, 1990.
248. Harvey, R. D. and J. R. Hume. Autonomic regulation of a chloride current in heart. *Science* 244:983–985, 1989.
249. Harvey, R. D. and J. R. Hume. Autonomic regulation of delayed rectifier K⁺ current in mammarian heart involves G protein. *Am. J. Physiol.* 257 (*Heart Circ. Physiol.* 26):H818–H823, 1989.
250. Harvey, R. D. and J. R. Hume. Histamine activates the chloride current in cardiac ventricular myocytes. *J. Cardiovasc. Electrophysiol.* 1:309–317, 1990.
251. Hawthorn, M. H., P. Gengo, X-Y. Wei, A. Rutledge, J. F. Moran, S. Gallant, and D. J. Triggle. Effect of thyroid status on β-adrenoceptors and calcium channels in rat cardiac and vascular tissue. *N-S. Arch. Pharmacol.* 337:539–544, 1988.
252. Hazeki, O. and M. Ui. Modification of islet-activating protein of receptor-mediated regulation of cyclic AMP accumulation in isolated rat heart cells. *J. Biol. Chem.* 256:2856–2862, 1981.
253. Heidebuchel, H., J. Vereecke, and E. Carmeliet. Atrial membranes contain nucleotide diphosphate kinase (NDPK) activity: its role in regulation of muscarinic K⁺ channels. *J. Cardiovasc. Electrophysiol.* 14:1721–1727, 1991.
254. Herzig, J. W. and M. Kohlhardt. Na⁺ channel blockade by cyclic AMP and other 6-aminopurines in neonatal rat heart. *J. Membr. Biol.* 119:163–170, 1991.

255. Hescheler, J., M. Kameyama, and W. Trautwein. On the mechanism of muscarinic inhibition of the cardiac Ca current. *Pflugers Arch.* 407:182–189, 1986.
256. Hescheler, J., H. Nawrath, M. Tang, and W. Trautwein. Adrenoceptor-mediated changes of excitation and contraction in ventricular heart muscle from guinea-pigs and rabbits. *J. Physiol. (Lond.)* 397:657–670, 1988.
257. Hescheler, J., M. Tang, B. Jastorff, and W. Trautwein. On the mechanism of histamine induced enhancement of the cardiac Ca^{2+} current. *Pflugers Arch.* 410:23–29, 1987.
258. Hess, P., J. B. Lansman, and R. W. Tsien. Calcium channel selectivity for divalent and monovalent cations. Voltage and concentration dependence of single channel current in ventricular heart cells. *J. Gen. Physiol.* 88:293–319, 1986.
259. Heyndrickx, G. R., D. H. Boettcher, and S. F. Vatner. Effects of angiotensin, vasopressin and methoxamine on cardiac function and blood flow distribution in conscious dogs. *Am. J. Physiol.* 231:1579–1587, 1976.
260. Hilgemann, D. W. and Ball, R. Regulation of cardiac Na^+, Ca^{2+} exchange and K_{ATP} potassium channels. *Science* 273:956–959, 1996.
261. Hill, S. J., C. R. Ganellin, H. Timmerman, J-C. Schwartz, N. P. Shankly, J. M. Young, W. Schunack, R. Levi, and H. Haas. International Union of Pharmacology. XIII. Classification of histamine receptors. *Pharmacol. Rev.* 49:252–278, 1995.
262. Hino, N. and R. Ochi. Effects of acetylcholine on membrane currents in guinea-pig papillary muscle. *J. Physiol. (Lond.)* 307: 183–197, 1980.
263. Hirano, Y., S. Abe, T. Sawanobori, and M. Hiraoka. External ATP-induced changes in $[Ca^{2+}]_i$ and membrane currents in mammalian atrial myocytes. *Am. J. Physiol.* 260 (*Cell Physiol.* 29) C673–C680, 1991.
264. Hirano, Y. and M. Hiraoka. Barium-induced automatic activity in isolated ventricular myocytes from guinea-pig hearts. *J. Physiol. (Lond.)* 359:455–472, 1988.
265. Hirano, Y. and M. Hiraoka. Dual modulation of unitary L-type Ca^{2+} channel currents by $[Ca^{2+}]_i$ in fura-2-loaded guinea-pig ventricular myocytes. *J. Physiol. (Lond.)* 480:449–463, 1994.
266. Hirano, Y., K. Suzuki, N. Yamawake, and M. Hiraoka. Multiple kinetic effects of β-adrenergic stimulation on single cardiac L-type Ca channels. *Am. J. Physiol.* 266 (*Cell Physiol.* 35): C1714–C1721, 1994.
267. Hirano, Y., T. Yoshinaga, T. Niidome, K. Katayama, and M. Hiraoka. Modulation by dihydropyridines and protein kinases of the recombinant cardiac L-type Ca channel with multiple unitary current amplitudes. *Receptors Channels* 4:93–104, 1996.
268. Hiraoka, M. and Z. Fan. Activation of ATP-sensitive outward K^+ current by nicorandil (2-nicotinamidoethyl nitrate) in isolated ventricular myocytes. *J. Pharmacol. Exp. Ther.* 250:278–285, 1989.
269. Hiraoka, M. and S. Kawano. Calcium-sensitive and insensitive transient outward current in rabbit ventricular myocytes. *J. Physiol. (Lond.)* 410:187–212, 1989.
270. Hiraoka, M., S. Kawano, Y. Hirano, and T. Furukawa. Role of chloride currents in action potential characteristics and arrhythmias. *Cardiovasc. Res.* 40:23–33, 1998.
271. Hiraoka, M. and Y. Okamoto. Two types of abnormal automaticity in canine ventricular tissues. *N-S. Arch. Pharmacol.* 317:339–344, 1981.
272. Hiraoka, M., Y. Okamoto, and T. Sano. Oscillatory afterpotentials in dog ventricular muscle fibers. *Circ. Res.* 48:510–518, 1981.
273. Hiraoka, M., A. Sunami, Z. Fan, and T. Sawanobori. Multiple ionic mechanisms of early afterdepolarizations in isolated ventricular myocytes from guine-pig hearts. *Ann. N.Y. Acad. Med.* 644:33–47, 1992.
274. Ho, W.-K., Y. E. Earm, S. H. Lee, H. F. Brown, and D. Noble. Voltage- and time-dependent block of delayed rectifier K^+ current in rabbit sino-atrial node cells by external Ca^{2+} and Mg^{2+}. *J. Physiol. (Lond.)* 494:727–742, 1996.
275. Ho, W.-K., I. Kim, C. O. Lee, and Y. E. Earm. Voltage-dependent blockade of HERG channels expressed in *Xenopus* oocytes by external Ca^{2+} and Mg^{2+}. *J. Physiol. (Lond.)* 507: 631–638, 1998.
276. Ho, W.-K., I. Kim, C. H. Lee, J. B. Youm, S. H. Lee, and Y. E. Earm. Blockade of HERG channels expressed in *Xenopus laevis* oocytes by external divalent cations. *Biophys. J.* 76:1959–1971, 1999.
277. Hofmann, F., M. Biel, and V. Flockerzi. Molecular basis for Ca^{2+} channel diversity. *Annu. Rev. Neurosci.* 17:399–418, 1994.
278. Hoffmann, B. F. and P. F. Cranefield. *Electrophysiology of the Heart.* New York: McGraw-Hill, 1960.
279. Hoffman, B. F. and E. E. Suckling. Effect of several cations on transmembrane potentials of cardiac muscle. *Am. J. Physiol.* 186:317–324, 1956.
280. Honore, E., B. Attali, G. Romey, C. Herteaux, P. Ricard, F. Lesage, M. Lazdunski, and J. Barhanin. Cloning, expression, pharmacology and regulation of a delayed rectifier K^+ channel in mouse heart. *EMBO J.* 10:2805–2811, 1991.
281. Horie, M., T.-C. Hwang, and D. C. Gadsby. Pipette GTP is essential for receptor-mediated regulation of Cl^- current in dialysed myocytes from guinea-pig ventricle. *J. Physiol. (Lond.)* 455:235–246, 1992.
282. Horie, M. and H. Irisawa. Dual effects of intracellular magnesium on muscarinic potassium channel current in single guinea-pig atrial cells. *J. Physiol. (Lond.)* 408:313–332, 1989.
283. Horie, M., H. Irisawa, and A. Noma. Voltage-dependent magnesium block of adenosine-triphosphate-sensitive potassium channel in guinea-pig ventricular cells. *J. Physiol. (Lond.)* 387: 251–272, 1987.
284. Horowitz, B, S. S. Tsung, P. Hart, P. C. Levesque, and J. R. Hume. Alternative splicing of CFTR Cl-channels in heart. *Am. J. Physiol.* 264 (*Heart Circ. Physiol.* 33):H2214–H2220, 1993.
285. Hosey, M. M., K. K. McMahon, and R. D. Green. Inhibitory adenosine receptors in the heart: characterization by ligand binding studies and effects on beta-adrenergic receptor stimulated adenylate cyclase and membrane protein phosphorylation. *J. Mol. Cell. Cardiol.* 16:931–942, 1984.
286. Houki, S. Restoration effects of histamine on action potential in potassium-depolarized guinea-pig papillary muscle. *Arch. Int. Pharmacodyn. Ther.* 206:113–120, 1973.
287. Hu, K., D. Duan, G. R. Li, and S. Nattel. Protein kinase C activates ATP-sensitive K^+ current in human and rabbit ventricular myocytes. *Circ. Res.* 78:492–498, 1996.
288. Hume, J. R., and R. D. Harvey. Chloride conductance pathways in heart. *Am. J. Physiol.* 261 (*Cell Physiol.* 30):C399–C412, 1991.
289. Hume, J. R. and A. Uehara. Ionic basis of the different action potential configurations of single guinea-pig atrial and ventricular myocytes. *J. Physiol. (Lond.)* 368:525–544, 1985.
290. Hutter, O. and D. Noble. Anion conductance of cardiac muscle. *J. Physiol. (Lond.)* 157:335–350, 1961.
291. Hutter, O. and W. Trautwein. Vagal and sympathetic effects on the pacemaker fibres in the sinus venosus of the heart. *J. Gen. Physiol.* 39:715–733, 1956.
292. Hwang, T.-C., M. Horie, A. C. Nairn, and D. C. Gadsby. Role of GTP-binding proteins in the regulation of mammalian cardiac chloride conductance. *J. Gen. Physiol.* 99:465–489, 1992.
293. Iano, T. L., M. N. Levy, and M. H. Lee. An acceleratory com-

ponent of the parasympathetic control of heart rate. *Am. J. Physiol.* 224:997–1005, 1973.

294. Iijima, T., H. Irisawa, and M. Kameyama. Membrane currents and their modification by acetylcholine in isolated single atrial cells of the guinea pig. *J. Physiol (Lond.)* 359:485–501, 1985.

295. Ikeda, N., J. Toyama, I. Kodama, and K. Yamada. The role of electrical uncoupling in the genesis of atrioventricular conduction disturbance. *J. Mol. Cell. Cardiol.* 12:800–826, 1980.

296. Imanishi, S. and B. Surawicz. Automatic activity in depolarized guinea pig ventricular myocardium. Characteristics and mechanisms. *Circ. Res.* 39:749–7559, 1976.

297. Imredy, J. P. and D. T. Yue. Mechanism of Ca^{2+}-sensitive inactivation of L-type Ca^{2+} channels. *Neuron* 12:1301–1318, 1994.

298. Inagaki, N., T. Gonoi, J. P. Clement IV, N. Namba, J. Inazawa, G. Gonzales, L. Aguilar-Bryan, S. Seino, and J. Bryan. Reconstitution of I_{KATP}: An inward rectifier subunit plus the sulfonylurea receptor. *Science* 270:1166–1170, 1995.

299. Inagaki, N., T. Gonoi, J. P. Clement IV, C.-Z. Zheng, L. Aguilar-Bryan, J. Bryan, and S. Seino. A family of sulfonylurea receptors determines the pharmacological properties of ATP-sensitive K^+ channels. *Neuron* 16:1011–1117, 1996.

300. Irisawa, H. Comparative physiology of the pacemaker mechanism. *Physiol. Rev.* 58:461–498, 1978.

301. Irisawa, H., H. F. Brown, and W. Giles. Cardiac pacemaking in the sinoatrial node. *Physiol. Rev.* 73:197–227, 1993.

302. Irisawa, H. and R. Sato. Intra- and extracellular actions of protons on the calcium current of isolated guinea pig ventricular cells. *Circ. Res.* 59:348–355, 1986.

303. Isenberg, G. Cardiac Purkinje fibres. $[Ca^{2+}]_i$ controls steady state potassium conductance. *Pflugers Arch.* 371:71–76, 1977.

304. Isenberg, G. and L. Belardinelli. Ionic basis for the antagonism between adenosine and isoproterenol on isolated mammalian ventricular myocytes. *Circ. Res.* 55:309–325, 1984.

305. Isenberg, G. and W. Trautwein. The effect of dihydro-ouabain and lithium ions on the outward current in cardiac Purkinje fibres. *Pflugers Arch.* 350:41–54, 1974.

306. Ishihara, K., T. Mitsuiye, A. Noma, and M. Takano. The Mg^{2+} block and intrinsic gating underlying inward rectification of the K^+ current in guinea-pig ventricular myocytes. *J. Physiol. (Lond.)* 419:297–320, 1989.

307. Ishikawa, T., M. Yanagisawa, S. Kimura, K. Goto, and T. Masaki. Positive inotropic action of novel vasoconstrictor peptide endothelin on guinea-pig atria. *Am. J. Physiol.* 255 (*Heart Circ. Physiol.* 24):H970–H973, 1988.

308. Isomoto, S., C. Kondo, M. Yamada, S. Matsumoto, O. Higashiguchi, Y. Horio, Y. Matsuzawa, and Y. Kurachi. A novel sulfonylurea receptor forms with BIR(Kir6.2) a smooth muscle type ATP-sensitive K^+ channel. *J. Biol. Chem.* 271:24321–24324, 1996.

309. Ito, H., R. T. Tung, T. Sugimoto, I. Kobayashi, K. Takahashi, T. Katada, M. Ui, and Y. Kurachi. On the mechanism of G protein βγ subunit activation of the muscarinic K^+ channel in guinea pig atrial cell membrane. *J. Gen. Physiol.* 99:961–983, 1992.

310. Ito, H., J. Vereecke, and E. Carmeliet. Intracellular protons inhibit inward rectifier K^+ channel of guinea pig ventricular cell membrane. *Pflugers Arch.* 422:280–286, 1992.

311. Ito, H., J. Vereecke, and E. Carmeliet. Mode of regulation by G protein of the ATP-sensitive K^+ channel in guinea-pig ventricular cell membrane. *J. Physiol. (Lond).* 478:101–108, 1994.

312. Iyadomi, I., K. Hirahara, and T. Ehara. α-Adrenergic inhibition of the β-adrenoceptor-dependent chloride current in guinea-pig ventricular myocytes. *J. Physiol. (Lond.)* 489:95–104, 1995.

313. Jahnel, U., H. Nawrath, E. Carmeliet, and J. Vereecke. Depolarization-induced influx of sodium in response to phenylephrine in rat atrial heart muscle. *J. Physiol. (Lond).* 432:621–637, 1991.

314. James, A. F., L-H. Xie, Y. Fujitani, S. Hayashi, and M. Horie. Inhibition of the cardiac protein kinase A-dependent chloride conductance by endothelin-1. *Nature* 370:297–300, 1994.

315. Janse, M. J. and A. L. Wit. Electrophysiological mechanisms of ventricular arrhythmias resulting from myocardial ischemia and infarction. *Physiol. Rev.* 69:1049–1169, 1989.

316. January, C. and H. A. Fozzard. Delayed afterdepolarizations in heart muscle: mechanism and relevance. *Pharmacol. Rev.* 40:219–227, 1988.

317. Je Zhang, Z., N. K. Jurkiewicz, K. Folander, E. Lazarides, J. J. Salata, and R. Swanson. K^+ currents expressed from the guinea pig cardiac I_{sk} protein are enhanced by activators of protein kinase C. *Proc. Natl. Acad. Sci. U.S.A.* 91:1766–1779, 1994.

318. Jo, S.-H., J. Boum, Y.-I. Kim, C. O. Lee, Y. E. Earm, and W.-K. Ho. Blockade of HERG channels expressed in *Xenopus* oocytes by external H^+. *Pflugers Arch.* 438:23–29, 1999.

319. Johnson, E. A. and M. G. McKinnon. Effect of acetylcholine and adenosine on cardiac cellular potentials. *Nature* 178:1174–1175, 1956.

320. Johnson, J. P. Jr., F. M. Mullins, and P. B. Bennett. Human *ether-a-go-go-related gene* K^+ channel gating probed with extracellular Ca^{2+}. Evidence for two distinct voltage sensors. *J. Gen. Physiol.* 113:565–580, 1999.

321. Josephson, I. R. and N. Sperelakis. Tetrodotoxin differently blocks peak and steady-state sodium channel currents in early embryonic chick ventricular myocytes. *Pflugers Arch.* 414:354–359, 1989.

322. Jourdon, P. and D. Feuvray. Calcium and potassium currents in ventricular myocytes isolated from diabetes rats. *J. Physiol. (Lond.)* 470:411–429, 1993.

323. Ju, Y. K. and D. G. Allen. Intracellular calcium and Na^+-Ca^{2+} exchange current in isolated toad pacemaker cells. *J. Physiol. (Lond.)* 508:153–166, 1998.

324. Kaczmarek, L. K., and E. M. Blumenthal. Properties and regulation of the minK potassium channel protein. *Physiol. Rev.* 77:627–641, 1997.

325. Kaibara, M. and M. Kameyama. Inhibition of the calcium channel by intracellular protons in single ventricular myocytes of the guinea-pig. *J. Physiol. (Lond.)* 403:621–640, 1988.

326. Kaibara, M., T. Nakajima, H. Irisawa, and W. Giles. Regulation of spontaneous opening of muscarinic K^+ channels in rabbit atrium. *J. Physiol. (Lond.)* 433:589–613, 1991.

327. Kameyama, M., F. Hofmann and W. Trautwein. On the mechanisms of β-adrenergic regulation of the Ca channel in the guinea-pig heart. *Pflugers Arch.* 405:285–293, 1985.

328. Kameyama, M., M. Kakei, R. Sato, T. Shibasaki, H. Matsuda, and H. Irisawa. Intracellular Na^+ activates a K^+ channel in mammalian cardiac cells. *Nature* 309:354–356, 1984.

329. Kaneda, M., K. Fukui, and K. Doi. Activation of chloride current by P_2-purinoceptors in rat ventricular myocytes. *Br. J. Pharmacol.* 111:1355–1360, 1994.

330. Kantor, P. F., W. A. Coetzee, E. Carmeliet, S. C. Denis, and L. H. Opie. Reduction of ischemic K^+ loss and arrhythmias in rat hearts. Effect of glibenclamide, a sulfonylurea. *Circ. Res.* 66:478–485, 1990.

331. Kass, R. S. and M. L. Blair. Effects of angiotensin II on membrane current in cardiac Purkinje fibers. *J. Mol. Cell. Cardiol.* 13:797–809, 1981.

332. Kass, R. S. and M. C. Sanguinetti. Inactivation of calcium channel current in the calf Purkinje fiber. Evidence for voltage- and calcium-mediated mechanisms. *J. Gen. Physiol.* 84:705–726, 1984.

333. Kass, R. S. and R. W. Tsien. Multiple effects of calcium antag-

onists on plateau currents in cardiac Purkinje fibers. *J. Gen. Physiol.* 66:169–192, 1975.
334. Kass, R. S. and R. W. Tsien. Control of action potential duration by calcium ions in cardiac Purkinje fibers. *J. Gen. Physiol.* 67:599–617, 1976.
335. Kass, R. S., R. W. Tsien and R. Weingart. Ionic basis of transient inward current induced by strophanthidin in cardiac Purkinje fibres. *J. Physiol (Lond).* 281:209–226, 1978.
336. Kassebaum, D. G. Electrophysiological effects of strophanthidin in the heart. *J. Pharmacol. Exp. Ther.* 140:329–338, 1963.
336a. Kathofer, S., W. Zhang, C. Karle, D. Thomas, W. Schoels, and J. Kiehn. Functional coupling in human β_3-adrenoceptors to the KvLQT1/ mink potassium channel. *J. Biol. Chem.* 275:26743–26747, 2000.
337. Kato, M., H. Yamaguchi and R. Ochi. Mechanism of adenosine-induced inhibition of calcium current in guinea pig ventricular cells. *Circ. Res.* 67:1134–1141, 1990.
338. Katzung, B. G. and J. A. Morgenstern. Effects of extracellular potassium on ventricular automaticity and evidence for a pacemaker current in mammalian ventricular myocardium. *Circ. Res.* 40:105–111, 1977.
339. Kaufmann, R. and U. Theophile. Automatie-fordernde Dehnungseffekte an Purkinje-faden, Papillarmuskeln und Vorhoftrabekeln von Rhesus-Affen. *Pflugers Arch.* 297:174–189, 1967.
340. Kaumann, A. J. Four β-adrenoceptor subtypes in the mammalian heart. *Trends Pharmacol Sci.* 18:70–76, 1997.
341. Kawano, S. and M. Hiraoka. Transient outward currents and action potential alterations in rabbit ventricular myocytes. *J. Mol. Cell. Cardiol.* 23:681–693, 1991.
342. Kawano, S., Y. Hirayama and M. Hiraoka. Activation mechanism of Ca^{2+}-sensitive transient outward current in rabbit ventricular myocytes. *J. Physiol. (Lond.)* 486:593–604, 1995.
343. Kelly, R. A., J.-L. Balligand, and T. W. Smith. Nitric oxide and cardiac function. *Circ. Res.* 79:363–380, 1996.
344. Kim, D. Endothelin activation of an inwardly rectifying K^+ current in atrial cells. *Circ. Res.* 69:250–255, 1991.
345. Kim, D. A mechanosensitive K^+ channel in heart cells: activation by arachidonic acid. *J. Gen. Physiol.* 100:1021–1040, 1992.
346. Kim, D., T. W. Smith, and J. D. Marsh. Effect of thyroid hormone on slow calcium channel function in cultured chick ventricular cells. *J. Clin. Invest.* 80:88–94, 1987.
347. Kimura, S., J. S. Cameron, P. L. Kozlovskis, A. L. Basset, and R. J. Myerberg. Delayed afterdepolarization and triggered activity induced in feline Purkinje fibers by α-adrenergic stimulation in the presence of elevated calcium level. *Circulation* 70:1074–1082, 1984.
348. Kimura, J., S. Miyamae, and A. Noma. Identification of sodium-calcium exchange current in single ventricular cells of guinea-pig. *J. Physiol. (Lond).* 384:199–222, 1987.
349. Kingsley, P. B., E. Y. Sako, M. Q. Yang, S. D. Zimmer, K. Ugurbi, J. E. Foker, and A. H. L. From. Ischemic contracture begins when anaerobic glycolysis stops: a ^{31}P-NMR study of isolated rat hearts. *Am. J. Physiol.* 261 (*Heart Circ. Physiol.* 30): H469–H478, 1991.
350. Kirsch, G. E., J. Codina, L. Birnbaumer, and A. M. Brown. Coupling of ATP-sensitive K^+ channels to A_1 receptors by G protein in rat ventricular myocytes. *Am. J. Physiol.* 259 (*Heart Circ. Physiol.* 28): H820–H826, 1990.
351. Kirsch, G. E. and J. S. Sykes. Temperature dependence of Na currents in rabbit and frog muscle membrane. *J. Gen. Physiol.* 89:239–251, 1987.
352. Kishida, H., B. Surawicz, and L. T. Fu. Effects of K^+ and K^+-induced polarization on $(dV/dt)_{max}$, threshold potential, and membrane input resistance in guinea pig and cat ventricular myocardium. *Circ. Res.* 44:800–814, 1979.
353. Kiyosue, T. and M. Arita. Late sodium current and its contribution to action potential configulation in guinea pig ventricular myocytes. *Circ. Res.* 64:389–397, 1989.
354. Kiyosue, T., M. Arita, H. Muramatsu, A. J. Spindler, and D. Noble. Ionic mechanisms of action potential prolongation at low temperature in guinea-pig ventricular myocytes. *J. Physiol. (Lond.)* 468:85–106, 1993.
355. Kiyosue, T., A. J. Spindler, S. J. Noble, and D. Noble. Background inward current in ventricular and atrial cells of the guinea-pig. *Proc. R. Soc. Lond. B. Biol. Sci.* 252:65–74, 1993.
356. Kobayashi, S., H. Nakaya, T. Takizawa, S. Hara, S. Kimura, T. Saito, and Y. Masuda. Endothelin-1 partially inhibits ATP-sensitive K^+ current in guinea pig ventricular cells. *J. Cardiovasc. Pharmacol.* 27:12–19, 1996.
357. Kohlhardt, M. and K. Happ. 8-Bromo-guanosine-3', 5'-monophosphate mimics the effect of acetylcholine on slow response action potential and contractile force in mammalian atrial myocardium. *J. Mol. Cell. Cardiol.* 19:573–586, 1978.
358. Kohlhardt, M., H. P. Haastert, and H. Krause. Evidence of nonspecificity of the Ca channel in mammalian myocardial fibre membranes. Substitution of Ca by Sr, Ba or Mg as charge carriers. *Pflugers Arch.* 342:125–136, 1973.
359. Kojima, M., H. Sada, and N. Sperelakis. Developmental changes in β-adrenergic and cholinergic interactions on calcium-dependent slow action potentials in rat ventricular muscles. *Br. J. Pharmacol.* 99:327–333, 1990.
360. Korth, M. and V. Kuhlkamp. Muscarinic receptor-mediated increase of intracellular Na^+-ion activity and force of contraction. *Pflugers Arch.* 403:266–272, 1985.
361. Krafte, D. E. and R. S. Kass. Hydrogen ion modulation of Ca channel current in cardiac ventricular cells. Evidence for multiple mechanisms. *J. Gen. Physiol.* 91:641–657, 1988.
362. Krapivinsky, G., E. A. Gordon, K. Wickman, B. Vellmirovic, L. Krapivinsky and D. E. Clapham. The G-protein-gated atrial K^+-channel $I_{K,ACh}$ is a heteromultimer of two inwardly rectifying K^+-channel proteins. *Nature* 374:135–141, 1995.
363. Kukushkin, N. I., R. Z. Guinullin, and E. A. Sosunov. Transient outward current and rate dependence of action potential duration in rabbit cardiac ventricular muscle. *Pflugers Arch.* 399:87–92, 1983.
364. Kunapuli, S. P. and J. L. Daniel. P_2 receptor subtypes in the cardiovascular system. *Biochem J.* 336:513–523, 1998.
365. Kunze, D. Rate dependent changes in extracellular potassium in rabbit atrium. *Circ. Res.* 41:122–127, 1977.
366. Kunze, D. L., A. E. Lacerda, D. L. Wilson, and A. M. Brown. Cardiac Na currents and the inactivating, reopening, and waiting properties of single cardiac Na channels. *J. Gen. Physiol.* 86:691–719, 1985.
367. Kuo, J. F., T. P. Lee, P. L. Reyes, K. G. Walton, T. E. Donnelly, and P. Greengard. Cyclic nucleotide-dependent protein kinases. X. An assay method for the measurement of guanosin 3', 5' monophosphate in various biological materials and a study of agents regulating its level in heart and brain. *J. Biol. Chem.* 247:16–22, 1972.
368. Kurachi, Y. The effects of intracellular protons on the electrical activity of single ventricular cells. *Pflugers Arch.* 394:264–270, 1982.
369. Kurachi, Y. Voltage-dependent activation of the inward-rectifier potassium channel in the ventricular cell membrane of guinea-pig heart. *J. Physiol. (Lond.)* 366:365–385, 1985.
370. Kurachi, Y., H. Ito, T. Sugimoto, T. Shimizu, I. Miki, and M. Ui. α-Adrenergic activation of the muscarinic K^+ channel is mediated by arachidonic acid metabolites. *Pflugers Arch.* 414:102–104, 1989.
371. Kurachi, Y., T. Nakajima, and T. Sugimoto. On the mechanism of activation of muscarinic K^+ channels by adenosine in iso-

lated atrial cells: involvement of GTP-binding proteins. *Pflugers Arch.* 407:264–274, 1986.
372. Kurachi, Y., T. Nakajima, and T. Sugimoto. Role of intracellular Mg^{2+} in the activation of muscarinic K^+ channel in cardiac atrial cell membrane. *Pflugers Arch.* 407:572–574, 1986.
373. Kurachi, Y., T. Nakajima, and T. Sugimoto. Short-term desensitization of muscarinic K^+ channel current in isolated atrial myocytes and possible role of GTP-binding proteins. *Pflugers Arch.* 410:227–233, 1987.
374. Kurtz, T., K. A. Yamada, S. D. DaTorre, and P. B. Corr. Alpha$_1$-adrenergic system and arrhythmias in ischemic heart disease. *Eur. Heart J.* 12(Suppl.F):88–98, 1991.
375. Kuruma, A., M. Hiraoka, and S. Kawano. Activation of Ca^{2+}-sensitive Cl^- current by reverse mode Na^+/Ca^{2+} exchange in rabbit ventricular myocytes. *Pflugers Arch.* 436:976–983, 1998.
376. Kwatra, M. M., E. Leung, A. C. Maan, K. K. McMahon, J. Ptasienski, R. D. Green and M. M. Hosey. Correlation of agonist-induced phosphorylation of chick heart muscarinic receptors with receptor desensitization. *J. Biol. Chem.* 262:16314–16321, 1987.
377. Kwok, W. M. and R. S. Kass. Block of cardiac ATP-sensitive K^+ channels by external divalent cations is modulated by intracellular ATP. Evidence for allosteric regulation of the channel protein. *J. Gen. Physiol.* 102:693–712, 1993.
378. Lab, M. J. Transient depolarization and action potential alterations following mechanical changes in isolated myocardium. *Cardiovasc. Res.* 14:624–637, 1980.
379. Lab, M. J. Mechanoelectrical feedback (transduction) in heart: concepts and implication. *Cardiovasc. Res.* 32:3–14, 1996.
380. LaManna, V. R. and G. F. Ferrier. Electrophysiological effects of insulin on normal and depressed cardiac tissue. *Am. J. Physiol.* 240 (*Heart Circ. Physiol.*9):H636–H644, 1981.
381. Lang, F., G. L. Busch, M. Ritter, H. Volkl, S. Waldegger, E. Gulbins, and D. Haussinger. Functional significance of cell volume regulatory mechanisms. *Physiol. Rev.* 78:247–306, 1998.
382. Lansman, J. B., P. Hess, and R. W. Tsien. Blockade of current through single calcium channels by Cd^{2+}, Mg^{2+}. Voltage and concentration dependence of calcium entry into the pore. *J. Gen. Physiol.* 88:321–347, 1986.
383. Lantz, R. C., L. J. Elsas, and R. L. DeHaan. Ouabain-resistant hyperpolarization induced by insulin in aggregates of embryonic heart cells. *Proc. Natl. Acad. Sci. U.S.A.* 77:3062–3066, 1980.
384. Lauer, M. R., M. D. Gunn, and W. T. Clusin. Endothelin activates voltage dependent Ca^{2+} current by a G protein–dependent mechanism in rabbit cardiac myocytes. *J. Physiol. (Lond.)* 448:729–747, 1992.
385. Lauer, M. R., B. F. Rusy, and L. D. Davis. H^+-induced membrane depolarization in canine cardiac Purkinje fibers. *Am. J. Physiol.* 247 (*Heart Circ. Physiol.* 16):H312–H321, 1984.
386. Leach, R. N., K. Brickley, and R. I. Norman. Cyclic AMP-dependent protein kinase phosphorylates residues in the C-terminal domain of the cardiac L-type calcium channel alpha subunit. *Biochim. Biophys. Acta* 1281:205–212, 1996.
387. Lederer, W. J. and C. G. Nichols. Nucleotide modulation of the activity of the rat heart ATP-sensitive K^+ channels in isolated membrane patches. *J. Physiol. (Lond.)* 419:193–211, 1989.
388. Lederer, W. J. and R. W. Tsien. Transient inward current underlying arrhythmogenic effects of cardiotonic steroids in Purkinje fibres. *J. Physiol (Lond).* 263:73–100, 1976.
389. Lee, C. O. 200 years of digitalis: the emerging central role of the sodium ion in the control of cardiac force. *Am. J. Physiol.* 249 (*Cell Physiol.* 18):C367–C378, 1985.
390. Lee, C. O. and H. A. Fozzard. Activities of potassium and sodium in rabbit heart muscle. *J. Gen. Physiol.* 65:694–708, 1975.
391. Lee, C. O. and A. J. Levi. The role of intracellular sodium in the control of cardiac contraction. *Ann. N.Y. Acad, Sci.* 639:408–428, 1991.
392. Lee, J. H. and M. R. Rosen. Modulation of delayed afterdepolarizations by α 1-adrenergic receptor subtypes. *Cardiovasc. Res.* 27:839–844, 1993.
393. Lee, K. S. Potentiation of the calcium-channel currents of internally perfused mammalian heart cells by repetitive depolarization. *Proc. Natl. Acad. Sci. U.S.A.* 405:3941–3945, 1987.
394. Lee, K. S. and W. Klaus. The subcellular basis for the mechanism of inotropic action of cardiac glycosides. *Pharmacol. Rev.* 23:193–261, 1971.
395. Lee, K. S., E. Marban, and R. W. Tsien. Inactivation of calcium channels in mammalian heart cells: joint dependence on membrane potential and intracellular calcium. *J. Physiol. (Lond.).* 364:395–411, 1985.
396. Legaye, F., P. Biegelman, E. Doroubaix, and E. Coraboeuf. Effect of 3-5-3'triiodothyronine treatment on cardiac action potential of streptozotocin-induced diabetic rat. *Life Sci.* 42:2269–2274, 1988.
397. Le Grand, B., E. Deroubaix, J.-P. Couetil, and E. Coraboeuf. Effects of atrionatriuretic factor on Ca^{2+} current and Ca_i-independent transient outward K^+ current in human atrial cells. *Pflugers Arch.* 421:486–491, 1992.
398. Le Grand, B., E. Deroubaix, A. Coulombe, and E. Coraboeuf. Stimulatory effect of ouabain on T- and L-type calcium currents in guinea-pig cardiac myocytes. *Am. J. Physiol.* 258 (*Heart Circ. Physiol.* 27) H1620–H1623, 1990.
399. Le Guennec, J.-V. and D. Noble. Effects of rapid changes of external Na^+ concentration at different moments during the action potential in guinea-pig myocytes. *J. Physiol. (Lond.)* 478:493–504, 1994.
400. Levi, A. J. The effect of strophanthidin on action potential, calcium current and contraction in isolated guinea-pig ventricular myocytes. *J. Physiol. (Lond.)* 443:1–23, 1991.
401. Levi, A. J. A role for Na/Ca exchange in the action potential shortening caused by strophanthidin in guinea-pig ventricular myocytes. *Cardiovasc. Res.* 27:471–481, 1993.
402. Levi, A. J., M. R. Boyett, and C. O. Lee. The cellular actions of digitalis glycosides on the heart. *Prog. Biophys. Mol. Biol.* 62:1–54, 1994.
403. Levi, R. C. and G. Alloatti. Histamine modulates calcium current in guinea pig ventricular myocytes. *J. Pharmacol. Exp. Ther.* 246:337–343, 1988.
404. Levi, R. C., G. Alloatti, and R. Fischmeister. Cyclic GMP regulates the Ca-channel current in guinea pig ventricular myocytes. *Pflugers Arch.* 413:685–687, 1989.
405. Levi, R. C., G. Alloatti, C. Penna, and M. P. Gallo. Guanylate-cyclase-mediated inhibition of cardiac I_{Ca} by carbachol and sodium nitroprusside. *Pflugers Arch.* 426:419–426, 1994.
406. Levi, R. C, D. A. A. Owen, and J. Trzeciakowski. Actions of histamine on the heart and vasculature. In *Pharmacology of Histamine Receptors*, edited by R. Ganellin and M. Parsons. London: J Wright, 1982:236–297.
407. Levi, R. C. and A. J. Pappano. Modification of the effects of histamine and norepinephrine on the sinoatrial node pacemaker by potassium and calcium. *J. Pharmacol. Exp. Ther.* 204:625–633, 1978.
408. Li, G. R., J. Feng, A. Schrier, and S. Nattel. Contribution of the ATP-sensitive potassium channels to the electrophysiological effects of adenosine in guinea-pig atrial cells. *J. Physiol. (Lond).* 484:629–642, 1995.
409. Li, Y., R. Hanf, A. S. Otero, R. Fischmeister, and G. Szabo. Differential effects of pertussis toxin on the muscarinic regu-

lation of Ca^{2+} and K$^+$ currents in frog cardiac myocytes. *J. Gen. Physiol.* 104:941–959, 1994.
410. Li, Y. and R. A. Kloner. The cardioprotective effects of ischemic "preconditioning" are not mediated by adenosine receptors in rat heart. *Circulation* 87:1642–1648, 1993.
411. Light, P. Regulation of ATP-sensitive potassium channels by protein phosphorylation. *Biochim. Biophys. Acta* 1286:65–73, 1996.
412. Light, P. E., B. G. Allen, M. P. Walsh, and R. J. French. Regulation of adenosine triphosphate-sensitive potassium channels from rabbit ventricular myocytes by protein kinase C and type 2A protein phosphatase. *Biochemistry* 34:7252–7257, 1995.
413. Lin, Y.-F., Y. N. Jan, and L. Y. Jan. Regulation of ATP-sensitive potassium channel function by protein kinase A–mediated phosphorylation in transfected HEK293 cells. *EMBO J.* 19:942–955, 2000.
414. Lindemann, J. P. and A. M. Watanabe. Muscarinic cholinergic inhibition of β-adrenergic stimulation of phospholamban phosphorylation and Ca^{2+} transport in guinea pig ventricles. *J. Biol. Chem.* 260:13122–13129, 1985.
415. Lipp, P., S. Mechmann, and L. Pott. Effects of calcium release from sarcoplasmic reticulum on membrane currents in guinea pig atrial cardioballs. *Pflugers Arch.* 410:121–131, 1987.
416. Lipsius, S. L. and W. R. Gibbons. Acetylcholine lengthens action potentials of sheep cardiac Purkinje fibers. *Am. J. Physiol.* 238 (*Heart Circ. Physiol.* 7):H237–H243, 1980.
417. Liu, G. S., J. D. Thornton, D. M. Van Winkel, A. W. H. Stanley, R. A. Olsson, and J. M. Downey. Protection against infarction afforded by preconditioning is mediated by A$_1$ adenosine receptors in rabbit heart. *Circulation* 84:350–356, 1991.
418. Liu, Q.-Y., E. Karpinski, and P. K. Pang. The L-type calcium channel current is increased by alpha-1 adrenoceptor activation in neonatal rat ventricular cells. *J. Pharmacol. Exp. Ther.* 271:935–943, 1994.
419. Liu, S. J. and R. H. Kennedy. α$_1$-Adrenergic activation of L-type Ca current in rat ventricular myocytes: perforated patch-clamp recordings. *Am. J. Physiol.* 274 (*Heart Circ. Physiol.* 41): H2203–H2207, 1998.
420. Liu, Y., T. Sato, B. O'Rourke, and E. Marban. Mitochondrial ATP-dependent potassium channels: novel effectors of cardioprotection? *Circulation* 97:2463–2469, 1998.
421. Lo, C. F., and R. Numann. Independent and exclusive modulation of cardiac delayed rectifying K$^+$ current by protein kinase C and protein kinase A. *Circ. Res.* 83:995–1002, 1998.
422. Logothetis, D. E., Y. Kurachi, J. Galper, E. J. Neer, and D. E. Clapham. The β γ subunits of GTP-binding proteins activate the muscarinic K$^+$ channels in heart. *Nature* 325:321–326, 1987.
423. Lu, Z. and R. MacKinnon. Electrostatic tuning of Mg^{2+} affinity in an inward rectifier K$^+$ channel. *Nature* 371:243–246, 1994.
424. Luk, H. N. and E. Carmeliet. Na$^+$-activated K$^+$ current in cardiac cells: rectification, open probability, block, and role in digitalis toxicity. *Pflugers Arch.* 416:766–768, 1990.
425. MacDonnel, K. L., G. F. Tibbits, and L. Diamond. cGMP elevation does not mediate muscarinic agonist-induced negative inotropy in rat ventricular cardiomyocytes. *Am. J. Physiol.* 269 (*Heart Circ. Physiol.* 38): H1905–H1912, 1995.
426. Magyar, J., Z. Rusznak, P. Szentesi, G. Szucs, and L. Kovacs. Action potentials and potassium currents in rat ventricular muscle during experimental diabetes. *J. Mol. Cell. Cardiol.* 24:841–853, 1992.
427. Marban, E. and R. W. Tsien. Enhancement of calcium current during digitalis inotropy in mammalian heart: positive feedback regulation by intracellulr calcium? *J. Physiol. (Lond.)* 329:589–614, 1982.
428. Marban, E., T. Yamagishi, and G. T. Tomaselli. Structure and function of voltage-gated sodium channels. *J. Physiol. (Lond.)* 508:647–657, 1998.
429. Martin, P., M. N. Levy, and Y. Matsuda. Fade of cardiac responses during tonic vagal stimulation. *Am. J. Physiol.* 243 (*Heart Circ. Physiol.* 12): H219–H225, 1982.
430. Masaki, T., M. Yanagisawa, and K. Goto. Physiology and pharmacology of endothelins. *Med. Res. Rev.* 12:391–421, 1992.
431. Masuda, H. and N. Sperelakis. Inwardly rectifying potassium current in rat fetal and neonatal ventricular cardiomyocytes. *Am. J. Physiol.* 265 (*Heart Circ. Physiol.* 34): H1107–H1111, 1993.
432. Matsuda, H. Sodium conductance in calcium channels of guinea-pig ventricular cells induced by removal of external calcium ions. *Pflugers Arch.* 407:465–475, 1986.
433. Matsuda, H. and J. D. S. Cruz. Voltage-dependent block by internal Ca^{2+} ions of inwardly rectifying K$^+$ channels in guinea-pig ventricular cells. *J. Physiol (Lond).* 470:295–311, 1993.
434. Matsuda, H., A. Saigusa, and H. Irisawa. Ohmic conductance through the inwardly rectifying K channel and blocking by internal Mg^{2+}. *Nature* 325:156–159, 1987.
435. Matsuda, J. J., H. Lee, and E. F. Shibata. Enhancement of rabbit cardiac sodium channels by β-adrenergic stimulation. *Circ. Res.* 70:199–207, 1992.
436. Matsuda, J. J., H. Lee and E. F. Shibata. Acetylcholine reversal of isoproterenol-stimulated sodium currents in rabbit ventricular myocytes. *Circ. Res.* 72:517–525, 1993.
437. Matsumoto, K. and A. J. Pappano. Sodium-dependent membrane current induced by carbachol in single guinea-pig ventricular myocytes. *J. Physiol. (Lond.)* 415:487–502, 1989.
438. Matsuura, H. and T. Ehara. Activation of chloride current by purinergic stimulation in guinea pig heart cells. *Circ. Res.* 70: 851–855, 1992.
439. Matsuura, H., and T. Ehara. Modulation of the muscarinic K$^+$ channel by P$_2$-purinoceptors in guinea-pig atrial myocytes. *J. Physiol. (Lond.)* 497:379–393, 1996.
440 Matsuura, H., M. Sakaguchi, Y. Tsuruhara, and T. Ehara. Activation of the muscarinic K$^+$ channel by P$_2$-purinoceptors via pertussis toxin-sensitive G protein in guinea-pig atrial cells. *J. Physiol. (Lond.)* 490:659–671, 1996.
441. Matsuura, H., Y. Tsuruhara, M. Sakaguchi, and T. Ehara. Enhancement of delayed rectifier K$^+$ current by P$_2$-purinoceptor stimulation in guinea-pig atrial cells. *J. Physiol. (Lond.)* 490: 647–658, 1996.
442. McDonald, T. F., S. Pelzer, W. Trautwein, and D. J. Pelzer. Regulation and modulation of calcium channels in cardiac, skeletal, and smooth muscle cells. *Physiol. Rev.* 74:365–507, 1994.
443. McDonald, T. F. and W. Trautwein. The potassium current underlying delayed rectification in cat ventricular muscle. *J. Physiol. (Lond.)* 274:217–246, 1978.
444. Meijler, F. L. and M. J. Janse. Morphology and electrophysiology of the mammalian atrioventricular node. *Physiol. Rev.* 68: 608–647, 1988.
445. Mentrand, D., G. Vassort, and R. Fischmeister. Calcium-mediated inactivation of the calcium conductance in cesium-loaded frog heart cells. *J. Gen. Physiol.* 83:105–131, 1984.
446. Mery, P.-F., N. Abi-Gerges, G. Vandecasteele, J. Jurevicius, T. Eschenhagen, and R. Fischmeister. Muscarinic regulation of the L-type calcium current in isolated cardiac myocytes. *Life Sci.* 60:1113–1120, 1997.
447. Mery, P.-F., L. Hove-Madsen, J.-M. Chesnais, H. C. Hartzell, and R. Fischmeister. Nitric oxide synthase does not participate in negative inotropic effect of acetylcholine in frog heart. *Am. J. Physiol.* 270 (*Heart Circ. Physiol.* 39):H1178–H1188, 1996.
448. Mery, P.-F., S. M. Lohmann, U. Walter, and R. Fischmeister. Ca^{2+} current is regulated by cyclic GMP–dependent protein ki-

nase in mammalian cardiac myocytes. *Proc. Natl. Acad. Sci. U.S.A.* 88:1197–1201, 1991.
449. Michel, M. C., B. Kenny, and D. A. Schwinn. Classification of α_1-adrenoceptor subtypes. *N-S. Arch. Pharmacol.* 352:1–10, 1995.
450. Mills, J. W., E. M. Schwiebert, and B. A. Stanton. The cytoskeleton and cell volume regulation. In: *Cellular and Molecular Physiology of Cell Volume Regulation*, edited by K. Strange. Ann Arbor, MI: CRC, 1994:241–258.
451. Minneman, K. P. α_1-Adrenergic receptor subtypes, inositol phosphates, and sources of cell Ca^{2+}. *Pharmacol. Rev.* 40:87–119, 1988.
452. Mitchell, M. R., T. Powell, D. A. Terrar, and V. W. Twist. Calcium-activated inward current and contraction in rat and guinea-pig ventricular myocytes. *J. Physiol. (Lond.)* 391:545–560, 1987.
453. Miura, Y. and J. Inui. Multiple effects of α-adrenoceptor stimulation on the action potential of the rabbit atrium. *N-S. Arch. Pharmacol.* 325:47–53, 1984.
454. Molenaar, P., G. O'Reilly, A. Sharkey, R. E. Kuc, D. P. Harding, C. Plumpton, G. A. Gresham, and A. P. Davenport. Characterization and localization of endothelin receptor subtypes in the human atrioventricular conducting system and myocardium. *Circ. Res.* 72:526–538, 1993.
455. Moore, R. D. Effects of insulin upon ion transport. *Biochim. Biophys. Acta* 737:1–49, 1983.
456. Moorman, J. R., G. E. Kirsch, A. E. Lacerda, and A. M. Brown. Angiotensin II modulates cardiac Na^+ channels in neonatal rat. *Circ. Res.* 65:1804–1809, 1989.
457. Morita, H., J. Kimura, and M. Endoh. Angiotensin II activation of a chloride current in rabbit cardiac myocytes. *J. Physiol. (Lond.)* 483; 119–130, 1995.
457a. Morkin, E., I. L. Flink, and S. Goldman. Biochemical and physiological effects of thyroid hormone on cardiac performance. *Prog. Cardiovasc. Dis.* 25:435–465, 1983.
458. Mubagwa, K. and E. Carmeliet. Effects of acetylcholine on electrophysiological properties of rabbit cardiac Purkinje fibers. *Circ. Res.* 53:740–751, 1983.
459. Mubagwa, K., T. Shirayama, M. Moreau, and A. J. Pappano. Effects of PDE inhibitors and carbachol on the L-type Ca current in guinea pig ventricular myocytes. *Am. J. Physiol.* 264 (*Heart Circ. Physiol.* 33): H1353–H1363, 1993.
460. Mugelli, A., L. Mantelli, S. Manzini, and F. Ledda. Induction by histamine of oscillatory activity in sheep Purkinje fibers and suppression by verapamil and lidocaine. *J. Cardiovasc. Pharmacol.* 2:9–15, 1980.
461. Murphy, B. J., J. Rogers, A. P. Pedichizzi, A. A. Calvin, and W. A. Catterall. cAMP-dependent phosphorylation of two sites in the alpha subunit of the cardiac sodium channel. *J. Biol. Chem.* 271:28837–28843, 1996.
462. Murray, K. T., S. A. Fahrig, K. K. Deal, S. S. Po, N. N. Hu, D. J. Snyder, M. M. Tamkun, and P. B. Bennett. Modulation of an inactivating human cardiac K^+ channel by protein kinase C. *Circ. Res.* 75:999–1005, 1994.
463. Murray, K. T., N. N. Hu, J. R. Daw, H-G. Shin, M. T. Watson, A. B. Mashburn, and A. L. George, Jr. Functional effects of protein kinase C activation on the human cardiac Na^+ channel. *Circ. Res.* 80:370–376, 1997.
464. Murry, C. E., R. B. Jennings, and K. A. Reimer. Preconditioning with ischemia: a delay of lethal cell injury in ischemic myocardium. *Circulation* 74:1124–1136, 1986.
464a Musialek, P., M. Lei, H. F. Brown, D. J. Paterson, and B. Casadei. Nitric oxide can increase heart rate by stimulating the hyperpolarization-activated inward current, $I_{(f)}$. *Circ. Res.* 81: 60–68, 1997.
465. Nakajima, T., S. Wu, H. Irisawa, and W. Giles. Mechanism of acetylcholine-induced inhibition of Ca current in bullfrog atrial myocytes. *J. Gen. Physiol.* 96:865–885, 1990.
466. Nakamura, S., T. Kiyosue, and M. Arita. Glucose reserves, 2, 4-dinitrophenol induced changes in action potentials and membrane currents of guinea pig ventricular cells via enhanced glycolysis. *Cardiovasc. Res.* 23:286–294, 1989.
467. Nakayama, K., Z. Fan, F. Marumo, and M. Hiraoka. Interrelation between pinacidil and intracellular ATP concentrations on activation of the ATP-sensitive K^+ current in guinea-pig ventricular myocytes. *Circ. Res.* 67:1124–1133, 1990.
468. Nakayama, K., Z. Fan, F. Marumo, T. Sawanobori, and M. Hiraoka. Action of nicorandil on ATP-sensitive K^+ channel in guinea-pig ventricular myocytes. *Br. J. Pharmacol.* 103:1461–1468, 1991.
469. Nakayama, T., Y. Kurachi, A. Noma, and H. Irisawa. Action potential and membrane currents of single pacemaker cells of the rabbit heart. *Pflugers Arch.* 402:248–57, 1984.
470. Nattel, S., V. Elharrar, D. P. Zilpes, and J. C. Bailey. pH dependent electrophysiological effects of quinidine and lidocaine on canine cardiac Purkinje fibers. *Circ. Res.* 48:55–61, 1981.
471. Neyses, L., and H. Vetter. Action of atrial natriuretic peptide and angiotensin II on the myocardium: studies in isolated rat ventricular cardiomyocytes. *Biochem. Biophys. Res. Commun.* 163:1435–1443, 1989.
472. Nichols, C. G. and W. J. Lederer. Adenosine triphosphate–sensitive potassium channels in the cardiovascular system. *Am. J. Physiol.* 261 (*Heart Circ. Physiol.* 30): H1675–H1686, 1991.
473. Niedergerke, R. and R. K. Orkand. The dependence of the action potential of the frog's heart on the external and intracellular sodium concentration. *J. Physiol. (Lond.)* 184:312–334, 1966.
474. Nilius, B. Calcium block of guinea-pig heart sodium channels with and without modification by the piperazinylindolem DPI 201–106. *J. Physiol. (Lond.)* 399:537–558, 1988.
475. Nilius, B., J. Tytgart, and R. Albitz. Modulation of cardiac Na channels by angiotensin II. *Biochim. Biophys. Acta* 1014:259–262, 1989.
476. Nishiyama, A., F. Kambe, K. Kamiya, H. Seo, and J. Toyama. Effects of thyroid status on expression of voltage-gated potassium channels in rat ventricle. *Cardiovasc. Res.* 40:343–351, 1998.
477. Nitta, J., T. Furukawa, F. Marumo, T. Sawanobori, and M. Hiraoka. Subcellular mechanism of Ca^{2+}-dependent enhancement of I_k in isolated membrane patches of guinea-pig ventricular myocytes. *Circ. Res.* 74:96–104, 1994.
478. Noble, D. Electrical properties of cardiac muscle attributable to inward-going (anomalous) rectification. *J. Cell. Comp. Physiol.* 66:127–136, 1965.
479. Noma, A., H. Irisawa, S. Kokubun, H. Kotake, M. Nishimura, and Y. Watanabe. Slow current system in the A-V node of the rabbit heart. *Nature* 285:228–229, 1980.
480. Noma, A., H. Kotake, and H. Irisawa. Slow inward current and its role mediating the chronotropic effect of epinephrine in the rabbit sinoatrial node. *Pflugers Arch.* 388:1–9, 1980.
481. Noma, A., T. Nakayama, Y. Kurachi, and H. Irisawa. Resting K conductance in pacemaker and non-pacemaker heart cells of the rabbit. *Jpn. J. Physiol.* 34:245–254, 1984.
482. Noma, A. and W. Trautwein. Relaxation of the ACh-induced potassium current in the rabbit sino-atrial node. *Pflugers Arch.* 377:193–200, 1978.
483. Noma, A. and N. Tsuboi. Dependence of junctional conductance on proton, calcium and magnesium ions in cardiac paired cells of guinea pig. *J. Physiol. (Lond.)* 382:193–211, 1987.
484. Notsu, T., I. Tanaka, M. Takano, and A. Noma. Blockade of the ATP-sensitive K^+ channel by 5-hydroxydecanoate in guinea

pig ventricular myocytes. *J. Pharmacol. Exp. Ther.* 260:702–708, 1992.
485. Nunain, S. O., C. Garrat, V. Paul, N. Debbas, D. E. Ward, and A. J. Camm. Effect of intravenous adenosine on human atrial and ventricular repolarisation. *Cardiovasc. Res.* 26:939–943, 1992.
486. Nuss, H. B., E. Marban, C. W. Balke, L. Goldman, R. Aggarwal, and S. R. Shrofsky. Whether "slip-mode conductance" occurs. *Science* 284:711a, 1999.
487. Obayashi, K., M. Horie, L. H. Xie, K. Tsuchiya, A. Kubota, H. Ishida, and S. Sasayama. Angiotensin II inhibits protein kinase A–dependent chloride conductance in heart via pertussis toxin–sensitive G proteins. *Circulation* 95:197–204, 1997.
488. Ochi, R. Manganese-dependent propagation potentials and their depression by electrical stimulation in guinea-pig myocardium perfused by sodium-free media. *J. Physiol. (Lond).* 263:139–156, 1976.
489. Ochi, R. and Y. Kawashima. Modulation of slow gating process of calcium channels by isoprenaline in guinea-pig ventricular cells. *J. Physiol (Lond.)* 424:184–204, 1990.
490. Ohno-Shosaku, T., B. J. Zunkler, and G. Trube. Dual effects of ATP and K^+ currents of mouse pancreatic β-cells. *Pflugers Arch.* 410:133–138, 1987.
491. Oleska, L. M., L. C. Hool, and R. D. Harvey. α_1-Adrenergic inhibition of the β-adrenergically activated Cl^- current in guinea pig ventricular myocytes. *Circ. Res.* 78:1090–1099, 1996.
492. Olsson, R. A. and J. D. Pearson. Cardiovascular purinoreceptors. *Physiol. Rev.* 70:761–845, 1990.
493. Ono, K., G. Tsujimoto, A. Sakamoto, K. Eto, T. Masaki, Y. Ozeki, and M. Satake. Endothelin-A receptor mediates cardiac inhibition by regulating calcium and potassium currents. *Nature* 370:301–304, 1994.
494. Ono, K. and H. A. Fozzard. Two phosphatase sites on the Ca^{2+} channel affecting different kinetic functions. *J. Physiol. (Lond).* 470:73–84, 1993.
495. Ono, K., H. A. Fozzard, and D. A. Hanck. Mechanism of cAMP-dependent modulation of cardiac sodium channel current kinetics. *Circ. Res.* 72:807–815, 1993.
496. Ono, K. and H. Ito. Role of rapidly activating delayed rectifier K^+ current in sinoatrial node pacemaker activity. *Am. J. Physiol.* 269 (*Heart Circ. Physiol.* 38):H453–H462, 1995.
497. Ono, K., T. Kiyosue, and M. Arita. Isoproterenol, DBcAMP, and forskolin inhibit cardiac sodium current. *Am. J. Physiol.* 256 (*Cell Physiol.* 25):C1131–C1137, 1989.
498. Ono, K., F. Maruoka, and A. Noma. Voltage-and time-dependent block of I_f by Sr^{2+} in rabbit sino-atrial node cells. *Pflugers Arch.* 427:437–443, 1994.
499. Ono, K., F. M. Tareen, A. Yoshida, and A. Noma. Synergistic action of cyclic GMP on catecholamine-induced chloride current in guinea-pig ventricular cells. *J. Physiol. (Lond.)* 453:647–661, 1992.
500. Ono, K. and W. Trautwein. Potentiation by cyclic GMP of β-adrenergic effect on Ca^{2+} current in guinea-pig ventricular cells. *J. Physiol. (Lond.)* 443:387–404, 1991.
501. Orchard, C. H. and H. E. Cingolani. Acidosis and arrhythmias in cardiac muscle. *Cardiovasc. Res.* 28:1312–1319, 1994.
502. Orchard, C. H., S. R. Houser, A. A. Kort, A. A. Bahinski, M. C. Capogrossi, and E. G. Lakatta. Acidosis facilitates spontaneous sarcoplasmic Ca^{2+} release in rat myocardium. *J. Gen. Physiol.* 90:145–165, 1987.
503. O'Rourke, B., P. H. Backx, and E. Marban. Phosphorylation-independent modulation of L-type calcium channels by magnesium-nucleotide complexes. *Science* 257:245–248, 1992.
504. Osterrieder, W., Q. F. Yang, and W. Trautwein. Effects of barium ions on the membrane currents in the rabbit S-A node. *Pflugers Arch.* 394:78–84, 1982.
505. Otero, A. S., G. E. Breitwieser, and G. Sabo. Activation of muscarinic potassium currents by ATP-γ S in atrial cells. *Science* 242:443–445, 1988.
506. Oz, M. C. and S. Sorota. Forskolin stimulates swelling-induced chloride current, not cardiac cystic fibrosis transmembrane-conductance regulator current in human cardiac myocytes. *Circ. Res.* 76:1063–1070, 1995.
507. Pachucki, J., L. A. Burmeister, and P. R. Larsen. Thyroid hormone regulates hyperpolarization-activated cyclic nucleotide-gated channel (HCN2) mRNA in the rat heart *Circ. Res.* 85:498–503, 1999.
508. Pappano, A. J. Parasympathetic control of cardiac electrical activity. In: *Cardiac Electrophysiology: From Cell to Bedside.* edited by D. P. Zipes, and J. Jalife. Philadelphia: W. B. Saunders 1990:271–277.
509. Pappano, A. J. Vagal stimulation of the heart beat: muscarinic receptor hypothesis. *J. Cardiovasc. Electrophysiol.* 2:262–273, 1991.
510. Pappano, A. J. and N. Sperelakis. Low K conductance and low resting potentials of isolated single cultured heart cells. *Am. J. Physiol.* 217:1076–1082, 1969.
511. Parker, K. E. and A. Scarpa. An ATP-activated nonselective cation channel in guinea pig ventricular myocytes. *Am. J. Physiol.* 269 (*Heart Circ. Physiol.* 38.H789–H797, 1995.
512. Patlak, J. B. and M. Oritz. Slow currents through single sodium channels of the adult rat heart. *J. Gen. Physiol.* 86:89–104, 1985.
513. Perets, T., Y. Blumenstein, E. Shistik, I. Lotan, and N. Dascal. A potential site of functional modulation by protein kinase A in the cardiac Ca^{2+} channel alpha 1C subunit. *FEBS Lett.* 384:189–192, 1996.
514. Perez-Reyes, E., W. Yang, X. Wei, and D. M. Bers. Regulation of the cloned L-type cardiac calcium channel by cyclic-AMP-dependent protein kinase. *FEBS Lett.* 342:119–123, 1994.
515. Peterson, B. Z., C. D. DeMaria, J. P. Adelman, and D. T. Yue. Calmodulin is the Ca^{2+} sensor for Ca^{2+}-dependent inactivation of L-type calcium channels. *Neuron* 22:549–558, 1999.
516. Pfaffinger, P. J., J. M. Martin, D. D. Hunter, N. M. Nathanson and B. Hille. GTP-binding proteins couple cardiac muscarinic receptors to a K channel. *Nature* 315:536–538, 1985.
517. Prod'hom, B., D. Pietrobon, and P. Hess. Interactions of protons with single open L-type calcium channels. *J. Gen. Physiol.* 94:23–42, 1989.
518. Puri, T. S., B. L. Gerhardstein, X. L. Zhao, M. B. Ladner, and M. M. Hosey. Differential effects of subunit interactions on protein kinase A- and C-mediated phosphorylation of L-type calcium channels. *Biochemistry* 36:9605–9615, 1997.
519. Qu, Y., D. L. Campbell, and H. C. Strauss. Modulation of L-type Ca^{2+} current by extracellular ATP in ferret isolated right ventricular myocytes. *J. Physiol. (Lond.)* 471:295–317, 1993.
520. Qu, Y., D. L. Campbell, A. R. Whorton, and H. C. Strauss. Modulation of basal L-type Ca^{2+} current by adenosine in ferret isolated right ventricular myocytes. *J. Physiol. (Lond.)* 471:269–293, 1993.
521. Qu, Y., J. C. Rogers, T. N. Tanada, W. A. Catterall, and T. Scheuer. Phosphorylation of S1505 in the cardiac Na^+ channel inactivation gate is required for modulation by protein kinase C. *J. Gen. Physiol.* 108:375–379, 1996.
522. Quast, U. Potassium channel openers: pharmacological and clinical aspects. *Fund. Clin. Pharmacol.* 6:279–293, 1992.
523. Randall, W. C. Selective autonomic innervation of the heart. In *Nervous Control of Cardiovascular Function*, edited by W. C. Randall. New York: Oxford University Press, 1984:46–67.
524. Ravens, U., X-L. Wang, and E. Wettwer. Alpha adrenoceptor

525. Reber, W. R. and R. Weingart. Ungulate cardiac Purkinje fibres: the influence of intracellular pH on the electrical cell-to-cell coupling. *J. Physiol. (Lond.)* 328:87–104, 1982.
526. Rees, S. A., J. L. Vandenberg, A. R. Wright, A. Yoshida, and T. Powell. Cell swelling has differential effects on the rapid and slow components of delayed rectifier potassium current in guinea pig myocytes. *J. Gen. Physiol.* 106:1151–1170, 1995.
527. Reuter, H. Calcium channel modulation by neurotransmitters, enzymes and drugs. *Nature* 301:569–574, 1983.
528. Reuveny, E., P. A. Slesinger, J. Inglese, J. M. Morales, J. A. Iniquez-Lluhi, R. J. Lefkowitz, H. R. Bourne, Y. N. Jan and L. Y. Jan Activation of the cloned muscarinic potassium channel by G protein β γ subunits. *Nature* 370:143–146, 1994.
529. Rhoads, A. R., and F. Friedberg. Sequence motifs for calmodulin recognition. *FASEB J.* 11:331–340, 1997.
530. Rigel, D. Effects of neuropeptides on heart rate in dogs: comparison of VIP, PHI, NPY, CGRP and NT. *Am. J. Physiol.* 255 (Heart Circ. Physiol. 24):H311–H317, 1988.
531. Rogers, T. B., S. T. Gaa, and I. S. Allen. Identification and characterization of functional angiotensin II receptors on cultured heart myocytes. *J. Pharmacol. Exp. Ther.* 236:638–644, 1986.
532. Rogg, H., A. Schmid and M.de Gasparo. Identification and characterization of angiotensin II receptor subtypes in rabbit ventricular myocardium. *Biochem. Biophys. Res. Commun.* 173:416–422, 1990.
533. Romanin, C., J.-O. Karlsson and H. Schindler. Activity of cardiac L-type Ca^{2+} channels is sensitive to cytoplasmic calcium. *Pflugers Arch.* 421:516–518, 1992.
534. Roos, A. and W. Boron. Intracellular pH. *Physiol. Rev.* 61:296–434, 1981.
535. Rossie, S., D. Gordon and W. A. Catterall. Identification of an intracellular domain of the sodium channel having multiple cAMP-dependent phosphorylation sites. *J. Biol. Chem.* 262:17530–17535, 1987.
536. Rougier, O., G. Vassort, D. Garnier, Y-M. Gargouil and E. Coraboeuf. Existence and role of a slow inward current during the frog atrial action potential. *Pflugers Arch.* 308:91–110, 1969.
537. Rubenstein, I. and O. Binah. Thyroid hormone modulates membrane currents in guinea pig ventricular myocytes. *N-S. Arch. Pharmacol.* 340:705–711, 1989.
538. Ruknuden, A., F. Sachs and J. O. Bustamante. Stretch-activated ion channels in tissue-cultured chick heart. *Am. J. Physiol.* 264 (Heart Circ. Physiol. 33):H960–H972, 1993.
539. Ruskoaho, H. Atrial natriuretic peptide: Synthesis, release, and metabolism. *Pharmacol. Rev.* 44:479–602, 1992.
539a. Sachs, F. Mechanical transduction by ion channels: how forces reach the channel. *Soc. Gen. Physiol. Ser.* 52:209–211, 1997.
540. Sackman, B., A. Noma and W. Trautwein. Acetylcholine activation of single muscarinic K^+ channels in isolated pacemaker cells of the mammalian heart. *Nature* 303:250–253, 1983.
541. Sadoshima, J., and S. Izumo. The cellular and molecular responses of cardiac myocytes to mechanical stress. *Annu Rev Physiol.* 59:551–571, 1997.
542. Saint, D. A., Y.-K. Ju., and P. W. Gage. A persistent sodium current in rat ventricular myocytes. *J. Physiol. (Lond.)* 453:219–231, 1992.
543. Sakaguchi, Y., G. Cui, and L. Sen. Acute effects of thyroid hormone on inward rectifier potassium channel currents in guinea pig ventricular myocytes. *Endocrinology* 137:4744–4751, 1996.
544. Sakura, H., C. Ammala, P. A. Smith, F. M. Gribble, and F. M. Ashcroft. Cloning and functional expression of the cDNA encoding a novel ATP-sensitive potassium channel subunit expressed in pancreatic β-cells, brain, heart and skeletal muscle. *FEBS Lett.* 377:338–344, 1995.
545. Sanders, R., R. J. Myerburg, H. Gelband, and A. I. Bassett. Dissimilar length–tension relations of canine ventricular muscle and false tendon: electrophysiologic alterations accompanying deformation. *J. Mol.Cell. Cardiol.* 11:209–219, 1979.
546. Sanguinetti, M. C., M. E. Curran, A. Zou, J. Shen, P. S. Spector, D. L. Atkinson, and M. T. Keating. Coassembly of K_vLQT1 and minK (Isk) proteins to form cardiac Iks potassium channel. *Nature* 384:80–83, 1996.
547. Sanguinetti, M. C. and N. K. Jurkiewicz. Two components of cardiac delayed rectifier K^+ current: differential sensitivity to block by class III antiarrhythmic agents. *J. Gen. Physiol.* 96:195–215, 1990.
548. Sanguinetti, M. C. and N. K. Jurkiewicz. Isoproterenol antagonizes prolongation of refractory period by the class III antiarrhythmic agent, E-4031 in guinea pig myocytes: mechanism of action. *Circ. Res.* 68:77–84, 1991.
549. Sanguinetti, M. C., C. Liang, M. E. Curran, and M. T. Keating. A mechanistic link between an inherited and an acquired cardiac arrhythmia: HERG encodes the I_{kr} potassium channel. *Cell* 81:299–307, 1995.
550. Sano, T. and T. Sawanobori. Abnormal automaticity in canine Purkinje fibers focally subjected to low external concentrations of calcium. *Circ. Res.* 31:158–164, 1972.
551. Santana, L. F., A. M. Gomez, and W. J. Lederer. Ca^{2+} flux through promiscuous cardiac Na^+ channels: slip-mode conductance. *Science* 279:1027–1033, 1998.
552. Sasaki, N., T. Mitsuiye, and A. Noma. Increase of the delayed rectifier K^+ and Na^+-K^+ pump currents by hypotonic solutions in guinea pig cardiac myocytes. *Circ. Res.* 75:887–895, 1994.
553. Sato, R., A. Noma, Y. Kurachi, and H. Irisawa. Effects of intracellular acidification on membrane currents in ventricular cells of the guinea pig. *Circ. Res.* 57:553–561, 1985.
554. Satoh, H. Modulation of the automaticity by histamine and cimetidine in rabbit sino-atrial node cells. *Gen. Pharmacol.* 24:1213–1222, 1993.
555. Satoh, H. and I. Seyama. On the mechanism by which changes in extracellular pH affect the electrical activity of the rabbit sino-atrial node. *J. Physiol. (Lond.)* 381:181–191, 1986.
556. Scamps, F. and E. Carmeliet. Delayed K^+ current and external K^+ in single cardiac Purkinje cells. *Am. J. Physiol.* 257 (Cell Physiol. 16):C1086–C1092, 1989.
557. Scamps, F., V. Rybin, M. Puceatu, V. Tkachuk, and G. Vassort. A Gs protein couples P_2-puringeric stimulation to cardiac Ca channels without cyclic AMP production. *J. Gen. Physiol.* 100:675–701, 1992.
558. Scamps, F. and G. Vassort. Mechanism of extracellular ATP-induced depolarization of rat ventricular myocytes. *Pflugers Arch.* 417:309–316, 1990.
559. Scamps, F., and G. Vassort. Pharmacological profile of the ATP-mediated increase in L-type calcium current amplitude and activation of a non-specific cationic current in rat ventricular cells. *Br. J. Pharmacol.* 113:982–986, 1994.
560. Schaffer, S. W., C. Ballard-Croft, S. Boerth, and S. N. Allo. Mechanisms underlying depressed Na^+/Ca^{2+} exchanger activity in the diabetic heart. *Cardiovasc. Res.* 34:129–136, 1997.
561. Schaffer, S. W., and M. Mozaffari. Abnormal mechanical function in diabetes: relation to myocardial calcium handling. *Coron. Artery Dis.* 7:109–115, 1996.
562. Schakow, T. E. and R. E. Ten Eick. Enhancement of ATP-sensitive potassium current in cat ventricular myocytes by β-adrenergic stimulation. *J. Physiol. (Lond.)* 474:131–145, 1994.
563. Scherer, R. W., C. F. Lo, and G. E. Breitwieser. Leukotriene C_4

modulation of muscarinic K⁺ current in bulfrog atrial myocytes. *J. Gen. Physiol.* 102:125–141, 1993.
564. Schimerlik, M. I. Structure and regulation of muscarinic receptors. *Annu. Rev. Physiol.* 51:217–227, 1989.
565. Schoemaker, I. E., A. L. Meuelemans, L. J. Andries, and D. L. Brutsaert. Role of endocardial endothelium in positive inotropic action of vasopressin. *Am. J. Physiol.* 259 (*Heart Circ. Physiol.* 28):H1148–H1151, 1990.
566. Schreibmayer, W., B. Frohnwieser, N. Dascal, D. Platzer, R. Spreitzer, R. G. Kallen, and H. A. Lester. β-Adrenergic modulation of currents by rat cardiac Na⁺ channels expressed in *Xenopus laevis* oocytes. *Receptors Channels* 2:339–350, 1994.
567. Schryock, J. C. and L. Belardinelli. Adenosine and adenosine receptors in the cardiovascular system: biochemistry, physiology, and pharmacology. *Am. J. Cardiol.* 79(12A):2–10, 1997.
568. Schuba, L. M., T. Ogura and T. F. McDonald. Kinetic evidence distinguishing volume-sensitive chloride current from other types in guinea-pig ventricular myocytes. *J. Physiol. (Lond.)* 491:69–80, 1996.
569. Schubert, B., A. M. J. Vandongen, G. Kirsch, and A. M. Brown. Inhibition of cardiac Na currents by isoproterenol. *Am. J. Physiol.* 258 (*Heart Circ. Physiol.* 27):H977–H982, 1990.
570. Segal, J., S. Masalha, H. Schwalb, G. Merin, J. B. Borman, and G. Uretzky. Acute effect of thyroid hormone in the rat heart: role of calcium. *J. Endocrinol.* 149:73–80, 1996.
571. Seifen, E., H. Schaer, and J. M. Marshall. Effects of calcium on the membrane potentials of single pacemaker fibers and atrial fibers in isolated rabbit atria. *Nature* 202:1223–1224, 1964.
572. Shah, A., I. S. Cohen, and M. Rosen. Stimulation of cardiac alpha receptors increases Na/K pump current and decreases G_K via a pertussis toxin-sensitive pathway. *Biophys. J.* 54:219–225, 1988.
573. Share, L. Role of vasopressin in cardiovascular regulation. *Physiol.Rev.* 68:1248–1284, 1988.
574. Sharma, V. K., H. M. Colecraft, D. X. Wang, A. I. Levey, E. V. Grigorenko, H. H. Yeh, and S.-S. Sheu. Molecular and functional identification of m_1 muscarinic acetylcholone receptors in rat ventricular myocytes. *Circ. Res.* 79:86–93, 1996.
575. Sharp, N., D. S. Neel, and R. L. Parsons. Influence of thyroid hormone levels on the electrical and mechanical properties of rabbit pappilary muscle. *J. Mol. Cell. Cardiol.* 17:119–132, 1985.
576. Sheets, M. F. and D. A. Hanck. Mechanism of extracellular divalent and trivalent cation block of the sodium current in canine cardiac Purkinje cell. *J. Physiol. (Lond.)* 454:299–320, 1992.
577. Sheets, M. F., D. A. Hanck, and H. A. Fozzard. Nonlinear relation between V_{max} and I_{Na} in canine cardiac Purkinje cells. *Circ. Res.* 63:386–398, 1988.
578. Shen, W. K., R. T. Tung, M. M. Machulda and Y. Kurachi Essential role of nucleotide diphosphates in nicorandil-mediated activation of cardiac ATP-sensitive K⁺ channels. *Circ. Res.* 69:1152–1158, 1991.
579. Sheu, S.-S., M. Korth, D. Lathrop, and H. A. Fozzard. Intra- and extracellular K⁺ and Na⁺ activities and resting membrane potential in sheep cardiac Purkinje strands. *Circ. Res.* 47:692–700, 1980.
580. Shibasaki, T. Conductance and kinetics of delayed rectifier channels in nodal cells of the rabbit heart. *J. Physiol. (Lond.)* 387:227–250, 1987.
581. Shibata, E. F. and W. R. Giles. Ionic currents which generate the spontaneous disatolic depolarization in individual cardiac pacemaker cells. *Proc. Natl. Acad. Sci. U.S.A.* 82:7796–7800, 1985.
582. Shimoni, Y., H. Banno, and R. B. Clark. Hyperthyroidism selectively modified a transient potassium current in rabbit ventricular and atrial myocytes. *J. Physiol. (Lond.)* 457:369–389, 1992.
583. Shimoni, Y., H. S. Ewart, and D. Severson. Type I and II models of diabetes produce different modifications of K⁺ currents in rat heart: role of insulin. *J. Physiol. (Lond.)* 507:485–496, 1998.
584. Shimoni, Y., L. Firek, D. Sverson, and W. Giles. Short-term diabetes alters K⁺ currents in rat ventricular myocytes. *Circ. Res.* 74:620–628, 1994.
585. Shimoni, Y., C. Fiset, R. B. Clark, J. E. Dixon, D. McKinnon, and W. R. Giles. Thyroid hormone regulates postnatal expression of transient K⁺ channel isoforms in rat ventricle. *J. Physiol. (Lond.)* 500:65–73, 1997.
586. Shimoni, Y., D. Sverson, and W. Giles. Thyroid status and diabetes modulate regional differences in potassium currents in rat ventricle. *J. Physiol. (Lond.)* 488:673–688, 1995.
587. Shindo, T., M. Yamada, S. Isomoto, Y. Horio, and Y. Kurachi. SUR2 subtype (A and B)-dependent differential activation of the cloned ATP-sensitive K⁺ channels by pinacidil and nicorandil. *Br. J. Physiol.* 124:985–991, 1998.
587a. Shistik, E., T. Ivanina, Y. Blumenstein, and N. Dascal. Crucial role of N terminus in function of cardiac L-type Ca²⁺ channel and its modulation by protein kinase C. *J. Biol. Chem.* 273:17901–17909, 1998.
588. Shouten, V. J. A. and H. E. D. J. Ter Keurs. The slow repolarization phase of the action potential in rat heart. *J. Physiol. (Lond.)* 360:13–25, 1985.
589. Shryock, J., Y. Song, D. Wang, S. P. Baker, R. A. Olsson, and L. Belardinelli. Selective A₂-adenosine receptor agonists do not alter action potential duration, twitch shortening, or cyclic AMP accumulation in guinea-pig, rat, or rabbit isolated ventricular myocytes. *Circ. Res.* 72:194–205, 1993.
590. Shyng, S., T. Ferrigni, and C. G. Nichols. Regulation of K_{ATP} channel activity by diazoxide and MgADP. Distinct functions of the two nucleotide binding folds of the sulfonylurea receptor. *J. Gen. Physiol.* 110:643–654, 1997.
591. Shyng, S. L. and C. G. Nichols. Membrane phospholipid control of nucleotide sensitivity of K_{ATP} channels. *Science* 282:1138–1141, 1998.
592. Shui, Z., M. R. Boyett, W.-J. Zang, T. Haga, and K. Kameyama. Receptor kinase–dependent desensitization of the muscarinic K⁺ current in rat atrial cells. *J. Physiol. (Lond.)* 487:359–366, 1995.
593. Sigurdson, W. J., C. E. Morris, B. L. Brezden, and D. R. Gardner. Stretch activation of a K⁺ channel in molluscan heart cells. *J. Exp. Biol.* 127:191–209, 1987.
594. Simpson, P. C. Proto-oncogenes and cardiac hypertrophy. *Annu. Rev. Physiol.* 51:189–202, 1988.
595. Singer-Lahat, D., I. Lotan, M. Biel, V. Flockerzi, F. Hofmann, and N. Dascal. Cardiac calcium channels expressed in *Xenopus* oocytes are modulated by dephosphorylation but not by cAMP-dependent phosphorylation. *Receptors Channels* 2:215–226, 1994.
596. Sipido, K. R., G. Callewaert, and E. Carmeliet. [Ca²⁺]ᵢ transients and [CA²⁺]ᵢ-dependent chloride current in single Purkinje cells from rabbit heart. *J. Physiol. (Lond.).* 468:641–667, 1993.
597. Soejima, M. and A. Noma. Mode of regulation of the ACh-sensitive K-channel by the muscarinic receptor in rabbit atrial cells. *Pflugers Arch.* 400:424–431, 1984.
598. Soldatov, N. M., R. D. Zuhlke, A. Bouron, and H. Reuter. Molecular structures involved in L-type calcium channel inactivation. Role of the carboxyl-terminal region encoded by exon 40–42 in α_{1C} subunit in the kinetics and Ca²⁺-dependent inactivation. *J. Biol. Chem.* 272:3560–3566, 1997.
599. Song, Y., S. Thedford, B. B. Lerman, and L. Belardinelli. Adenosine-sensitive afterdepolarizations and triggered activity

in guinea pig ventricular myocytes. *Circ.Res.* 70:743–753, 1992.

600. Sorbera, L. A. and M. Morad. Atrionatriuretic peptide transforms cardiac sodium channels into calcium-conducting channels. *Science* 252:449–452, 1991.

601. Sorota, S. Swelling-induced chloride-sensitive current in canine atrial cells revealed by whole-cell patch-clamp method. *Circ. Res.* 70:679–687, 1992.

602. Sorota, S., Y. Tsuji, T. Tajima, and A. J. Pappano. Pertussis toxin treatment blocks hyperpolarization by muscarinic agonists in chick atrium. *Circ. Res.* 57:748–758, 1985.

603. Sperelakis, N. Origin of the cardiac resting potential. In: *Handbook of Physiology.* Section II: *The Cardiovascular System.* edited by R. M. Berne, N. Sperelakis, and S. R. Geiger. Bethesda, MD:, American Physiological Society, 1979:187–267.

604. Spindler, A. J., S. J. Noble, D. Noble, and J. Y. LeGuennec. The effects of sodium substitution on currents determining the resting potential in guinea-pig ventricular cell. *Exp. Physiol.* 83:121–136, 1998.

605. Standen, N. B., J. M. Quayle, N. W. Davies, J. E. Brayden, Y. Huang, and M. T. Nelson. Hyperpolarizing vasodilators activate ATP-sensitive K channels in arterial smooth muscle. *Science* 245:177–180, 1989.

606. Standen, N. B. and P. R. Stanfield. A potential-and time-dependent blockade of inward rectification in frog skeletal muscle fibres by barium and strontium ions. *J. Physiol. (Lond.)* 380:169–191, 1978.

607. Stein, B., W. Schmitz, H. Scholz, and C. Seeland. Pharmacological characterization of A_2-adenosine receptors in guinea-pig ventricular cardiomyocytes. *J. Mol. Cell. Cardiol.* 26:403–414, 1994.

608. Stengl, M., E. Carmeliet, K. Mubagwa, and W. Flameng. Modulation of transient outward current by extracellular protons and Cd^{2+} in rat and human ventricular myocytes. *J. Physiol. (Lond.)* 511:827–836, 1998.

608a. Stobrawa, S. M., T. Breiderhoff, S. Takamori, D. Engel, M. Schweizer, A. A. Zdebik, M. R. Bosl, K. Ruether, H. Jahn, A. Draguhn, R. Jahn, and T. J. Jentsch. Disruption of ClC-3, a chloride channel expressed on synaptic vesicles, leads to a loss of the hippocampus. *Neuron* 29:185–196, 2001.

609. Strickler, J., K. A. Jakobson, and B. T. Liang. Direct preconditioning of cultured chick ventricular myocytes. *J. Clin. Invest.* 98:1773–1779, 1996.

610. Sui, J. L., K. W. Chan, and D. E. Logothetis. Na^+ activation of the muscarinic K^+ channel by a G-protein–independent mechanism. *J. Gen. Physiol.* 108:381–391, 1996.

611. Suleymanian, M. A. and C. M. Baumgarten. Osmotic gradient-induced water permeation across the sarcolemma of rabbit ventricular myocytes. *J. Gen. Physiol.* 107:503–514, 1996.

612. Sunami, A., Z. Fan, F. Nakamura, M. Naka, T. Tanaka, T. Sawanobori, and M. Hiraoka. The catalytic subunit of cyclic AMP-dependent protein kinase directly inhibits sodium channel activities in guinea-pig ventricular myocytes. *Pflugers Arch.* 419:415–417, 1991.

613. Tajima, T., Y. Tsuji, J. H. Brown, and A. J. Pappano. Pertussis toxin-insensitive phosphoinositide hydrolysis, membrane depolarization, and positive inotropic effect of carbachol in chick atria. *Circ. Res.* 61:436–445, 1987.

614. Takano, M., D. Qin, and A. Noma. ATP-dependent decay and recovery of K^+ channels in guinea pig cardiac myocytes. *Am. J. Physiol.* 258 (*Heart Circ. Physiol.* 27):H45–H50, 1990.

615. Tanaka, H., Y. Habuchi, T. Yamamoto, M. Nishio, J. Morikawa, and M. Yoshimura. Negative chronotropic actions of endothelin-1 on rabbit sinoatrial node pacemaker cells. *Br. J. Pharmacol.* 122:321–329, 1997.

616. Tareen, F. M., A. Yoshida, and K. Ono. Modulation of beta-adrenergic responses of chrolide and calcium currents by external cations in guinea-pig ventricular cells. *J. Physiol. (Lond).* 457:211–228, 1992.

617. Tarr, M., J. W. Trank, and K. K. Goertz. Intracellular magnesium affects I_K in single frog atrial cells. *Am. J. Physiol.* 257 (*Heart Circ. Physiol.* 26):H1663–H1669, 1989.

618. Terai, T., T. Furukawa, Y. Katayama, and M. Hiraoka. Effects of external acidosis on HERG current expressed in *Xenopus* oocytes. *J. Mol. Cell. Cardiol.* 32:11–21, 2000.

619. Terzic, A., A. Jahangir, and Y. Kurachi. Cardiac ATP-sensitive K^+ channels: regulation by intracellular nucleotides and K^+ channel opening drugs. *Am. J. Physiol.* 269 (*Cell Physiol.* 38): C525–C545, 1995.

620. Terzic, A., M. Puceat, G. Vassort, and S. M. Vogel. Cardiac α_1-adrenoceptors: an overview. *Pharmacol. Rev.* 45:147–175, 1993.

621. Terzic, A., R. T. Tung, A. Inanobe, T. Katada, and Y. Kurachi. G proteins activate ATP-sensitive K^+ channels by antagonizing the ATP-dependent gating. *Neuron* 12:885–893, 1994.

622. Thomas, G. P., S. M. Sim, and M. Karmazyn. Differential effects of endothelin-1 on basal and isoprenaline-enhanced Ca^{2+} current in guinea-pig ventricular myocytes. *J. Physiol. (Lond.)* 503:55–65, 1997.

623. Thome, U., F. Berga, U. Borchard, and D. Hafner. Electrophysiological characterization of histamine receptor subtypes in sheep cardiac Purkinje fibers. *Agents Actions* 37:30–38, 1992.

624. Thornton, J. D., G. S. Liu, R. A. Olsson, and J. M. Downey. Intravenous pretreatment with A_1-selective adenosine analogues protects the heart against infarction. *Circulation* 85:650–665, 1992.

625. Thornton, J. D., C. S. Thornton, D. L. Sterling, and J. M. Downey. Blockade of ATP-sensitive potassium channels increases infarct size but does not prevent preconditioning in rabbit hearts. *Circ. Res.* 72:44–49, 1993.

626. Toda, N. and T. C. West. The action of ouabain on the function of the atrioventricular node in rabbits. *J. Pharmacol. Exp. Ther.* 169:287–297, 1970.

627. Tohse, N. Calcium-sensitive delayed rectifier potassium current in guinea pig ventricular cells. *Am. J. Physiol.* 258 (*Heart Circ. Physiol.* 27):H1200–H1207, 1990.

628. Tohse, N., Y. Hattori, H. Nakaya, M. Endou, and M. Kanno. Inability of endothelin to increase Ca^{2+} current in guinea-pig heart cells. *Br. J. Pharmacol.* 99:437–438, 1990.

629. Tohse, N., M. Kameyama, and H. Irisawa. Intracellular Ca^{2+} and protein kinase C modulate K^+ current in guinea pig heart cells. *Am. J. Physiol.* 253 (*Heart Circ. Physiol.* 22):H1321–1324, 1987.

630. Tohse, N., H. Nakaya, Y. Hattori, M. Endou, and M. Kanno. Inhibitory effect mediated by α1-adrenoceptors on transient outward current in isolated rat ventricular cells. *Pflugers Arch.* 415:575–581, 1990.

631. Tohse, N., H. Nakaya, and M. Kanno. α_1-Adrenoceptor stimulation enhances the delayed rectifier K^+ current of guinea-pig ventricular cells through activation of protein kinase C. *Circ. Res.* 71:1441–1446, 1992.

632. Tohse, N., H. Nakaya, Y. Takeda, and M. Kanno. Cyclic GMP-mediated inhibition of L-type Ca^{2+} channel activity by human natriuretic peptide in rabbit heart cells. *Br. J. Pharmacol.* 114:1076–1082, 1995.

633. Townsend, C. and R. Horn. Effect of alkali metal cations on slow inactivation of cardiac Na^+ channels. *J. Gen. Physiol.* 110:23–33, 1997.

634. Trautwein, W. and J. Dudel. Aktionpotential und Mechanogramm des Katzen-pappillarmuskels als Funktion der Temperatur. *Pflugers Arch.* 260:104–115, 1954.

635. Trautwein, W., J. Taniguchi, and A. Norma. The effect of in-

tracellular cyclic nucleotides and calcium on the action potential and acetylcholine response of isolated cardiac cells. *Pflugers Arch.* 392:307–314, 1982.

636. Trudeau, M. C., J. W. Warmke, B. Ganetzky, and G. A. Robertson. *HERG*, a human inward rectifier in the voltage-gated potassium channel family. *Science* 269:92–95, 1995.

637. Tseng, G. N. Calcium current restitution in mammalian ventricular myocytes is modulated by intracellular calcium. *Circ. Res.* 63:468–482, 1988.

638. Tseng, G. N. Cell swelling increases membrane conductance of canine cardiac cells: evidence for a volume-sensitive Cl channel. *Am. J. Physiol.* 262 (*Cell Physiol.* 31):C1056–C1068, 1992.

639. Tseng, G. N. and P. A. Boyden. Multiple types of Ca^{2+} currents in single canine Purkinje cells. *Circ. Res.* 65:1735–1750, 1989.

640. Tsien, R. W., B. P. Bean, P. Hess, J. B. Lansman, B. Nilius, and M. C. Norwicky. Mechanisms of calcium channel modulation by β-adrenergic agents and dihydropyridine Ca agonists. *J. Mol. Cell. Cardiol.* 18:691–710, 1986.

641. Tsuchida, K., H. Watajima, and S. Otomo. Calcium current in rat diabetic ventricular myocytes. *Am. J. Physiol.* 267 (*Heart Circ. Physiol.* 36):H2280–H2289, 1994.

642. Tucker, S. J., F. M. Grible, C. Zhao, S. Trapp, and F. M. Ashcroft. Truncation of Kir6.2 produces ATP-sensitive K^+ channels in the absence of the sulfonylurea receptor. *Nature* 387:179–183, 1997.

643. Tung, R. T. and Y. Kurachi. On the mechanism of nucleotide diphosphate activation of the ATP-sensitive K^+ channel in ventricular cell of guinea-pig. *J. Physiol. (Lond.)* 437:239–256, 1991.

644. Tytgart, J., B. Nilius, and E. Carmeliet. Modulation of the T-type cardiac Ca channel by changes in proton concentration. *J. Gen. Physiol.* 96:973–990, 1990.

645. Van Calker, D., M. Muller, and B. Hamprecht. Adenosine regulates via two different types of receptors, the accumulation of cyclic AMP in cultured brain cells. *J. Neurochem.* 33:999–1005, 1979.

646. Vandenberg, C. A. Inward rectification of a potassium channel in cardiac ventricular cells depends on internal magnesium ions. *Proc. Natl. Acad. Sci. U.S.A.* 84:2560-2564, 1987.

647. Vandenberg, J. L., S. A. Rees, A. R. Wright, and T. Powell. Cell swelling and ion transport pathways in cardiac myocytes. *Cardiovasc. Res.* 1996; 32:85–97.

648. Vandenberg, J. I., A. Yoshida, K. Kirk, and T. Powell. Swelling-activated and isoprenaline-activated chloride currents in guinea pig cardiac myocytes have distinct electrophysiology and pharmacology. *J. Gen. Physiol.* 104:997–1017, 1994.

649. Van Ginneken, A. C. G. and W. R. Giles. Voltage clamp measurements of the hyperpolarization-activated current I_f in single cells from rabbit sino-atrial node. *J. Physiol. (Lond.)* 434:57–83, 1991.

650. Van Wagoner, D. R. Mechanosensitive gating of atrial ATP-sensitive potassium channels. *Circ. Res.* 72:973–983, 1993.

651. Varnum, M. D., A. E. Busch, C. T. Bond, J. Maylie, and J. P. Adelman. The min K channel underlies the cardiac potassium current I_{ks} and mediates species-specific responses to protein kinase C. *Proc. Natl. Acad. Sci. U.S.A.* 90:11528–11532, 1993.

652. Vassalle, M., K. Greenspan, S. Jomain, and B. F. Hoffmann. Effects of potassium on automaticity and conduction of canine hearts. *Am. J. Physiol.* 207:334–340, 1964.

653. Vaughan-Jones, R. D. Chloride activity and its control in skeletal and cardiac muscle. *Phil. Trans. R. Soc. Lond. B. Biol, Sci.* 299:537–548, 1982.

654. Vaughan-Jones, R. D. and M.- L. Wu. Extracellular H^+ inactivation of Na^+-H^+ exchange in the sheep cardiac Purkinje fibre. *J. Physiol. (Lond.)* 428:441–466, 1990.

654a. Vaxelaire, J.-F., S. Laurent, P. Lacolley, V. Briand, H. Schmitt, and J. B. Michel. Atrial natriuretic peptide decreases contractility of cultured chick ventricular cells. *Life Sci.* 45:41–48, 1989.

655. Vereecke, J. and E. Carmeliet. Sr action potentials in cardiac Purkinje fibres. II. Dependence of the Sr conductance on the external Sr concentration and Sr-Ca antagonism. *Pflugers Arch.* 322:73–82, 1971.

656. Verheijck, E. E., A. C. van Ginneken, J. Bourier, and L. N. Bouman. Effects of delayed rectifier current blockade by E-4031 on impulse generation in single sinoatrial nodal myocytes of the rabbit. *Circ. Res.* 76:607–615, 1995.

657. Visentin, S., A. Zaza, A. Ferroni, C. Tromba, and D. DiFrancesco. Sodium current block caused by group-IIb cations in calf Purkinje fibres and in guinea-pig ventricular myocytes. *Pflugers Arch.* 417:213–222, 1990.

658. Wahler, G. M. Developmental increase in the inwardly rectifying potassium current of rat ventricular myocytes. *Am. J. Physiol.* 262 (*Cell. Physiol.* 31):C1266–C1272, 1992.

659. Walker, B. R., M. E. Childs, and E. M. Adams. Direct cardiac effects of vasopressin: role of V_1- and V_2-vasopressinergic receptors. *Am. J. Physiol.* 255 (*Heart Circ. Physiol.* 24):H261–H265, 1988.

660. Walsh, K. B. Activation of a heart chloride conductance during stimulation of protein kinase C. *Mol. Pharmacol.* 40:342–346, 1991.

661. Walsh, K. B., T. B. Begenisich, and R. S. Kass. β-Adrenergic modulation of cardiac ion channels. Differential temperature sensitivity of potassium and calcium currents. *J. Gen. Physiol.* 93:841–854, 1989.

662. Walsh, K. B. and R. S. Kass. Regulation of a heart potassium channel by protein A and C. *Science* 242:67–69, 1988.

663. Walsh, K. B. and K. J. Long. Properties of a protein kinase C-activated chloride current in guinea pig ventricular myocytes. *Circ. Res.* 74:121–129, 1994.

664. Wang, D. W., T. Kiyosue, S. Shigematsu, and M. Arita. Abnormalities of K^+ and Ca^{2+} currents in ventricular myocytes from rats with chronic diabetes. *Am. J. Physiol.* 269 (*Heart Circ. Physiol.* 38):H1288–H1296, 1995.

665. Wang, S., M. J. Morales, S. Liu, H. C. Straus, and R. L. Rasmusson. Time, voltage and ionic concentration dependence of rectification of *h-erg* expressed in *Xenopus* oocytes. *FEBS Lett.* 389:167–173, 1996.

666. Wang, X. L., E. Wettwer, G. Gross, and U. Ravens. Reduction of cardiac outward currents by alpha$_1$-adrenoceptor stimulation: a subtype specific effect. *J. Pharmacol. Exp. Ther.* 259:783–788, 1991.

667. Wang, Y. G. and S. L. Lipsius. Acetylcholine activates a glibenclamide-sensitive K^+ current in cat atrial myocytes. *Am. J. Physiol.* 268 (*Heart Circ. Physiol.* 37):H1322–H1334, 1995.

668. Wang, Y. G., and S. L. Lipsius. Acetylcholine elicits a rebound stimulation of Ca^{2+} current mediated by pertussis toxin–sensitive G protein and cAMP-dependent protein kinase A in atrial myocytes. *Circ. Res.* 76:634–644, 1995.

669. Wang, Z., T. Kimitsuki, and A. Noma. Conductance properties of the Na^+-activated K^+ channel in guinea-pig ventricular cells. *J. Physiol. (Lond.)* 433:241–257, 1991.

670. Watanabe, A. M. and H. R. Besch. Interaction between cyclic adenosine monophosphate and cyclic guanosine monophosphate in guinea pig ventricular myocardium. *Circ. Res.* 37:309–317, 1975.

671. Watanabe, Y. and L. S. Dreifus. Electrophysiological effects of digitalis on A-V transmission. *Am. J. Physiol.* 211:1461–1466, 1966.

672. Watanabe, Y., T. Noda, and Y. Habuchi. Effect of cardiac glycosides on AV nodal impulse formation and conduction. In *Electrophysiology of the Sinoatrial and Atrioventricular Nodes.*

edited by T. Mazgalev, L. F. Dreifus, and E. L. Michelson. New York: Alan R. Liss, 1988:111–131.

673. Watson, C. L. and M. R. Gold. Effect of intracellular and extracellular acidosis on sodium current in ventricular myocytes. *Am. J. Physiol.* 268 (*Heart Circ. Physiol.* 37):H1749–H1756, 1995.

674. Weidmann, S. The effect of the cardiac membrane potential on the rapid availability of the sodium-carrying system. *J. Physiol. (Lond.)* 127:213–224, 1955.

675. Weidmann, S. Effects of calcium ions and local anesthetics on electrical properties of Purkinje fibres. *J. Physiol. (Lond.)* 129:568–582, 1955.

676. Weidmann, S. Shortening of the cardiac action potential due to a brief injection of KCl following the onset of activity. *J. Physiol. (Lond.)* 132:157–163, 1956.

677. Wendt, D. J., C. F. Starmer, and A. O. Grant. pH dependence of kinetics and steady-state block of cardiac sodium channels by lidocaine. *Am. J. Physiol.* 264 (*Heart Circ. Physiol.* 33): H1588–H1598, 1993.

678. West, G. A. and L. Belardinelli. Correlation of sinus slowing and hyperpolarization caused by adenosine in sinus node. *Pflugers Arch.* 403:75–81, 1985.

679. Westfall, D. P., K. O. Sedaa, K. Shinozuka, R. A. Bjur, and I. L. Buxton. ATP as a cotransmitter. *Ann. N.Y. Acad. Sci.* 603:300–310, 1990.

680. Whalley, D. W., L. C. Hool, R. W. Ten Eick, and H. H. Rasmussen. Effect of osmotic swelling and shrinkage on Na^+-K^+ pump activity in mammalian cardiac myocytes. *Am. J. Physiol.* 265 (*Cell Physiol.* 34):C1201–C1210, 1993.

681. Whalley, D. W., D. J. Wendt, C. F. Starmer, Y. Rudy, and A. O. Grant. Voltage-independent effects of extracellular K^+ on the Na^+ current and phase 0 of the action potential in isolated cardiac myocytes. *Circ. Res.* 75:491–502, 1994.

682. White, R. E. and H. C. Hartzell. Effects of intracellular free magnesium on calcium current in isolated cardiac myocytes. *Science* 239:778–780, 1988.

683. Wible, B. A., M. Taglialata, E. Ficker, and A. M. Brown. Gating of inwardly rectifying K^+ channels localized to a single negatively charged residue. *Nature* 371:246–249, 1994.

684. Wibo, M., O. Feron, L. Zheng, M. Maleki, F. Kolar, and T. Goodfraind. Thyroid status and postnatal changes in subsarcolemmal distribution and isoform expression of rat cardiac dihydropyridine receptors. *Cardiovasc. Res.* 37:151–159, 1998.

685. Wickenden, A. D., R. Kaprielian, T. G. Parker, O. T. Jones, and P. H. Backx. Effects of development and thyroid hormone on K^+ currents and K^+ channel gene expression in rat ventricle. *J. Physiol. (Lond.)* 504:271–286, 1997.

686. Wickman, K. D., J. A. Inigues-Lluhi, P. A. Davenport, R. Taussig, G. B. Crapivinsky, M. E. Linder, A. G. Gilman, and D. E. Clapham. Recombinant G-protein βγ subunits activate the muscarinic-gated atrial potassium channel. *Nature* 368:255–257, 1994.

687. Wiechen, K., D. T. Yue, and S. Herzig. Two distinct functional effects of protein phosphatase inhibitors on guinea-pig cardiac L-type Ca^{2+} channels. *J. Physiol. (Lond.)* 484:583–592, 1995.

688. Wiggins, J. R. and P. F. Cranefield. The effect on membrane potential and electrical activity of adding sodium to sodium-depleted cardiac Purkinje fibers. *J. Gen. Physiol.* 64:473–493, 1974.

689. Wilde, A. A. M., D. Escande, C. A. Schumacher, D. Thuringer, M. Mestre, J. W. T. Fiolet, and M. J. Janse. Potassium accumulation in the globally ischemic mammalian heart. A role for the ATP-sensitive potassium channel. *Circ. Res.* 67:835–843, 1990.

690. Wilde, A. A. M. and M. J. Janse. Electrophysiological effects of ATP-sensitive potassium channel modulation: implications for arrhythmogenesis. *Cardiovasc. Res.* 28:16–24, 1994.

691. Wolff, A. A. and R. Levi. Histamine and cardiac arrhythmias. *Circ. Res.* 58:1–16, 1986.

692. Woodbury, L. A. and H. H. Hecht. Effects of cardiac glycosides upon the electrical activity of single ventricular fibers of the frog heart, and their relation to the digitalis effect of the electrocardiogram. *Circulation* 6:172–182, 1952.

693. Woodbury, L. A., H. H. Hecht, and A. R. Christopherson. Membrane resting and action potentials of single cardiac muscle fibers of the frog ventricle. *Am. J. Physiol.* 164:307–318, 1951.

694. Xie, L.-H., M. Horie, A. F. James, M. Watanuki, and S. Sasayama. Endothelin-1 inhibits L-type Ca current enhanced by isoproterenol in guinea-pig ventricular myocytes. *Pflugers Arch.* 431:533–539, 1996.

695. Xie, L.-H., M. Takano, and A. Noma. Development of inwardly rectifying K^+ channel family in rat ventricular myocytes. *Am. J. Physiol.* 272 (*Heart Circ. Physiol.* 41):H1741–H1750, 1997.

696. Xu, D., H. Kong, and B. T. Liang. Expression and pharmacological characterization of a stimulatory subtype of adenosine receptor in fetal chick ventricular myocytes. *Circ. Res.* 70:56–65, 1992.

697. Xu, Y. J. and V. Gopalakarishnan. Vasopressin increases cytosolic free $[Ca^{2+}]$ in the neonatal rat cardiomyocyte: evidence for V_1 subtype receptors. *Circ. Res.* 69:239–245, 1991.

698. Xu, Z., and G. J. Rozanski. Proton inhibition of transient outward potassium current in rat ventricular myocytes. *J. Mol. Cell. Cardiol.* 29:481–490, 1997.

699. Yamaoka, K., and I. Seyama. Regulation of Ca channel by intracellular Ca^{2+} and Mg^{2+} in frog ventricular cells. *Pflugers Arch.* 431:305–317, 1996.

700. Yamawake, N., Y. Hirano, T. Sawanobori, and M. Hiraoka. Arrhythmogenic effects of isoproterenol-activated Cl^- current in guinea-pig ventricular myocytes. *J. Mol. Cell. Cardiol.* 24:1047–1058, 1992.

701. Yanagisawa, M., H. Kurihara, S. Kimura, Y. Tomobe, M. Kobayashi, Y. Mitsui, Y. Yazaki, K. Goto, and T. Masaki. A novel potent vasoconstrictor peptide produced by vascular endothelial cells. *Nature* 332:411–415, 1988.

702. Yang, T., D. J. Snyders, and D. M. Roden. Rapid inactivation determines the rectification and $[K^+]_0$ dependence of the rapid component of the delayed rectifier K^+ current in cardiac cells. *Circ. Res.* 80:782–789, 1997.

703. Yao, Z., I. Cavero, and G. J. Gross. Activation of cardiac K_{ATP} channels: an endogenous protective mechanism during repetitive ischemia. *Am. J. Physiol.* 264 (*Heart Circ. Physiol.* 33): H495–H504, 1993.

704. Yao, Z. and G. J. Gross. Glibenclamide antagonizes adenosine A_1 receptor-mediated cardioprotection in stunned myocardium. *Circulation* 88:235–244, 1993.

705. Yatani, A., A. M. Brown, and N. Akaike. Effect of extracellular pH on sodium current in isolated, single rat ventricular cells. *J. Membr. Biol.* 78:163–168, 1984.

706. Yatani, A., K. Okabe, J. Codina, A. Bimbaumer, and A. M. Brown. Heart rate regulation by G protein acting on the cardiac pacemaker channel. *Science* 249:1163–1166, 1990.

707. Yazawa, K. and Y. Abiko. Modulation by histamine of the delayed outward potassium current in guinea-pig ventricular myocytes. *Br. J. Pharmacol.* 109:142–147, 1993.

708. Yazawa, K. and M. Kameyama. Mechanisms of receptor-mediated modulation of the delayed outward potassium current in guinea-pig ventricular myocytes. *J. Physiol. (Lond.)* 421:135–150, 1990.

709. Yoshimoto, K., Y. Hattori, H. Houzen, M. Kanno, and K. Yasuda. Histamine H_1-receptor-mediated increase in Ca^{2+} tran-

sient without a change in the Ca^{2+} current in electrically stimulated guinea-pig atrial myocytes. *Br. J. Pharmacol.* 124:1744–1750, 1998.

710. Yu, H., D. McKinnon, J. E. Dixon, J. Gao, R. Wymore, I. S. Cohen. P. Danilo, Jr., A. Shvilkin, E. P. Anyukovsky, E. A. Sosunov, M. Hara, and M. R. Rosen. Transient outward current, I$_{to1}$ is altered in cardiac memory. *Circulation* 99:1898–1905, 1999.

711. Yue, D. T., P. H. Backx, and J. P. Imredy. Calcium-sensitive inactivation in the gating of single calcium channels. *Science* 250:1735–1738, 1990.

712. Yue, D. T., S. Herzig, and E. Marban. β-Adrenergic stimulation of calcium channels occurs by potentiation of high-activity gating modes. *Proc. Natl. Acad. Sci. U.S.A.* 87:753–757, 1990.

713. Zakharov, S. I., S. Pieramici, G. K. Kumar, N. R. Prabhakar, and R. D. Harvey. Nitric oxide synthase activity in guinea pig ventricular myocytes is not involved in muscarinic inhibition of cAMP-regulated ion channels. *Circ. Res.* 78:925–935, 1996.

714. Zaza, A., R. P. Kline, and M. R. Rosen. Effects of α-adrenergic stimulation on intracellular sodium activity and automaticity in canine Purkinje fibers. *Circ. Res.* 66:416–426, 1990.

715. Zaza, A., M. Rocchetti, and D. DiFrancesco. Modulation of the hyperpolarization-activated current (I$_f$) by adenosine in rabbit sinoatrial myocytes. *Circulation* 94:734–741, 1996.

716. Zhang, J., T. H. Larsen, and M. Lieberman. F-actin modulates swelling-activated chloride current in cultured chick cardiac myocytes. *Am. J. Physiol.* 273 (*Cell Physiol.* 42):C1215–C1224, 1997.

717. Zhang, J. and S. A. Siegelbaum. Effects of external protons on single cardiac sodium channels from guinea pig ventricular myocytes. *J. Gen. Physiol.* 98:1065–1083, 1991.

718. Zhang, K., P. L. Barrington, R. L. Martin, and R. E. Ten Eick. Protein kinase-dependent Cl$^-$ currents in feline ventricular myocytes. *Circ. Res.* 75:133–143, 1994.

719. Zhang, S., Y. Hirano, and M. Hiraoka. Arginine vasopressin-induced potentiation of unitary L-type Ca^{2+} channel current in guinea pig ventricular myocytes. *Circ. Res.* 76:592–599, 1995.

720. Zhang, S., M. Hiraoka, and Y. Hirano. Effects of α$_1$-adrenergic stimulation on L-type Ca^{2+} current in rat ventricular myocytes. *J. Mol. Cell. Cardiol.* 30:1955–1965, 1998.

721. Zhang, S., T. Sawanobori, H. Adaniya, Y. Hirano, and M. Hiraoka. Dual effects of external magnesium on action potential duration in guinea pig ventricular myocytes. *Am. J. Physiol.* 268 (*Heart Circ. Physiol.* 37):H2321–H2328, 1995.

722. Zheng, J.-S., A. Christie, M. N. Levy, and A. Scarpa. Modulation by extracellular ATP of two distinct currents in rat myocytes. *Am. J. Physiol.* 264 (*Cell Physiol.* 33):C1411–C1417, 1993.

723. Zong, X., J. Schreieck, G. Mehrke, A. Welling, A. Schuster, E. Bosse, V. Flockerzi, and F. Hofmann. On the regulation of the expressed L-type calcium channel by cAMP-dependent phosphorylation. *Pflugers Arch.* 430:340–347, 1995.

724. Zuhlke, R. D. and H. Reuter. Ca^{2+}-sensitive inactivation of L-type-Ca^{2+} channels depends on multiple cytoplasmic amino acid sequences of the α$_{1C}$ subunit. *Proc. Natl. Acad. Sci. U.S.A.* 95:3287–3294, 1998.

725. Zuhlke, R. D. G. S, Pitt, K. Deisseroth, R. W. Tsien, and H. Reuter. Calmodulin supports both inactivation and facilitation of L-type calcium channels. *Nature* 399:159–162, 1999.

726. Zygmunt, A. C. Intracellular calcium activates a chloride current in canine ventricular myocytes. *Am. J. Physiol.* 267 (*Heart Circ. Physiol.* 36): H1984–H1995, 1994.

727. Zygmunt, A. C. and W. R. Gibbons. Calcium-activated chloride current in rabbit ventricular myocytes. *Circ. Res.* 68:424–437, 1991.

728. Zygmunt, A. C. and W. R. Gibbons. Properties of calcium-activated chloride current in the heart. *J. Gen. Physiol.* 99:391–414, 1992.

17. Electrical heterogeneity in the heart: physiological, pharmacological and clinical implications

CHARLES ANTZELEVITCH
ROBERT DUMAINE | *Masonic Medical Research Laboratory, Utica, New York*

CHAPTER CONTENTS

Action Potential and Ionic Distinctions
   Methodological considerations in the assessment of electrical heterogeneity
     Transmembrane action potential recordings
     Activation recovery interval and monophasic action potential recordings
     Experimental preparations
Pharmacological Distinctions
   Epicardium versus endocardium
   M-cells versus epicardium and endocardium
   M-cells versus Purkinje cells
Molecular Distinctions
   Potassium channels
     Overview of *Shaker* type channels
     The elusive role of Kv1.5 in the ventricles (I_{Kur})
     The transient outward current (I_{to})
     The slowly activating delayed rectifier current (I_{Ks})
     The rapidly activating delayed rectifier current (I_{Kr})
   Sodium channels
   Gap junctions
   Chloride conductances
   Calcium channels
   Pumps and exchangers
     Na/Ca exchanger
     Na/K ATPase
Simulation of Action Potential Heterogeneity
Developmental Aspects
Physiological and Clinical Implications
   Transmural distribution of I_{to} and the J wave
   Phase 2 Re-entry as a Mechanism of Extrasystolic Activity
   Phase 2 Re-entry as a Trigger for VT/VF. The Brugada Syndrome
   Early Repolarization Syndrome
   Ischemia
   Role of Transmural Heterogeneity in Inscription of the Electrocardiographic T wave
   Role of Transmural Heterogeneity in Inscription of the U wave
   Role of Transmural Heterogeneity in the Long QT Syndrome
   Torsade de Pointes
   Pharmacological Therapy for LQTS: Reducing Transmural Dispersion of Repolarization
Summary

STUDIES CONDUCTED OVER THE PAST DECADE have highlighted the diversity among the myocardial cells that comprise the ventricles of the heart. The data point to regional differences in electrical properties of cells as well as to differences in the response to pharmacological agents and pathophysiological states (7, 15–19, 21, 23). Prominent among the heterogeneities thus far uncovered are electrical and pharmacologic distinctions between endocardium and epicardium of the canine, feline, rabbit, rat, and human heart (68, 69, 84, 94, 124, 125, 129, 133, 137, 243) as well as differences in the electrophysiological characteristics and pharmacological responsiveness of M-cells located in the deep structures of the canine, rabbit, guinea pig, pig and human ventricles (6, 13, 16, 24, 74, 81, 127, 132, 133, 169, 182, 193, 195–197, 200, 234, 237).

Our aim in this chapter is to review the extent to which the ventricular myocardium is electrically heterogeneous, to evaluate the ionic and molecular basis for this heterogeneity, and to examine the physiological, pharmacological, and clinical implications. Our focus is on how these cellular and ionic distinctions contribute to the inscription of the electrocardiogram and to the development of re-entrant arrhythmias, including torsade de pointes (TdP) and the Brugada syndrome.

ACTION POTENTIAL AND IONIC DISTINCTIONS

As early as 1985 the ventricles of the heart were thought to be comprised of two principal cell types: specialized conducting cells forming the His-Purkinje system and ventricular working muscle cells making up the ventricular myocardium. The ventricular myocardium was thought to be largely homogeneous with respect to electrical properties and was assumed to be homogeneous with respect to the response to drugs, hormones, and other modulators of cardiac activity. Studies from our laboratory and others conducted over the past decade have shown that the ventricular myocardium is far from homogeneous, but that it is comprised of at least three electrophysiologically and functionally distinct cell types: epicardial cells, M-cells, and endocardial cells. These three ventricular myocardial cell types differ principally with respect to phase 1 and phase 3 repolarization characteristics (Figure 17–1A). Ventricular epicardial and M-cells, but not endocardial cells, typically display a conspicuous phase 1, due to a prominent 4-aminopyridine (4-AP) sensitive transient outward current (I_{to}), giving the action potential a spike and dome or notched configuration. These regional differences in I_{to}, first suggested on the basis of action potential data (129), have now been demonstrated using whole-cell patch clamp techniques in canine (133) feline (91), rabbit (84), rat (54), and human (151, 239) ventricular myocytes.

The extent to which I_{to2}, a calcium-activated component of the transient outward current, differs among the three ventricular myocardial cell types is not known (254). I_{to2}, initially ascribed to a K^+ current, is now thought to be primarily due to the calcium-activated chloride current ($I_{Cl(Ca)}$) (254). Myocytes isolated from the epicardial region of the left ventricular wall of the rabbit show a higher density of cyclic adenosine monophosphate (cAMP)-activated chloride current (24.9 ± 12.1 uS/uF) when compared to endocardial myocytes (12.3 ± 8.5 uS/uF) (218).

In addition to transmural differences, major differences in the magnitude of the action potential notch and corresponding differences in I_{to} have been described between right and left ventricular epicardium (70). Similar interventricular differences in I_{to} have also been described for canine ventricular M-cells (228). As will be discussed later, this distinction is thought to form the basis for why the Brugada syndrome, a channelopathy-mediated form of sudden death, is a right ventricular disease.

The transmural and interventricular differences in the manifestation of I_{to} have a number of interesting consequences (11, 17–19, 70, 138, 139, 243); Table 17–1), which are discussed in more detail later, in the section on physiological and clinical IMPLICATIONS.

The M-cell is distinguished by the ability of its action potential to prolong disproportionately relative to the action potential of other ventricular myocardial cells in response to a slowing of rate and/or in response to action potential duration (APD)-prolonging agents (Fig. 17–2, 17, 24, 193). The ionic basis for these features of the M-cell include the presence of a smaller, slowly activating, delayed rectifier current (I_{Ks}) (132), but a larger late sodium current (late I_{Na}) (Fig 17–1; 79, 258). Cells isolated from the M region display an I_{Ks} tail current density of 0.92 pA/pF at −20 mV (following a 5 sec pulse to +60 mV), nearly half of the density measured in endocardial and epicardial cells (1.99 and 1.83 pA/pF, respectively) (132). Further analysis revealed that M-cells with the longest APD were largely devoid of I_{Ks}. The shorter action potential of right vs. left ventricular M-cells is due, at least in part, to a higher density of I_{Ks}. Cells from the M region display a late I_{Na} nearly twice that recorded in epicardial cells. Zygmunt and co-workers recently showed that the electrogenic sodium–calcium exchange current ($I_{Na\text{-}Ca}$) is larger in canine ventricular M-cells (257). The rapidly activating delayed rectifier (I_{Kr}) and inward rectifier (I_{K1}) currents are similar in the three transmural cell types. The data thus far available point to a smaller I_{Ks}, a larger late I_{Na} and a larger $I_{Na\text{-}Ca}$ as the basis for the longer action potential of the M-cell. It is noteworthy that transmural and apico-basal differences in the density of I_{Kr} channels have been described in the ferret heart (37). I_{Kr} and channel protein were shown to be much larger in the epicardium.

TABLE 17–1. *Consequences of a Prominent I_{to}-mediated Action Potential Notch in Epicardium but not Endocardium*

- J wave (Osborne wave) (17,243)
- Differential sensitivity to ischemia and components of ischemia (12,17,68,69)
- Differential sensitivity to drugs (10,12,17,68,124,125,131,243)
  - Neurohormones (acetylcholine and isoproterenol)
  - Transient outward current blockers
  - Calcium channel blockers
  - Sodium channel blockers
  - Potassium channel openers

Histologically, M-cells are similar to epicardial and endocardial cells. Electrophysiologically and pharmacologically, they appear to be a hybrid between Purkinje cells and ventricular cells (Table 17–2). The position of M-cells within the ventricular wall has been investigated in greatest detail in the left ventricle of the canine heart. Although transitional cells are found throughout the wall in the canine left ventricle, M-cells displaying the longest action potentials (at BCLs ≥ 2000 msec) are often localized in the deep subendocardium to midmyocardium in the anterior wall (246), deep subepicardium to midmyocardium in the lateral wall (193) and throughout the wall in the region of the right ventricular (RV) outflow tracts (14). M-cells are also present in the deep layers of endocardial structures, including papillary muscles, trabeculae, and the interventricular septum (196). Unlike Purkinje fibers, they are not found in discrete bundles or islets (196, 197).

The first description of cells with an unusually long APD and rapid V_{max} was made in a papillary muscle

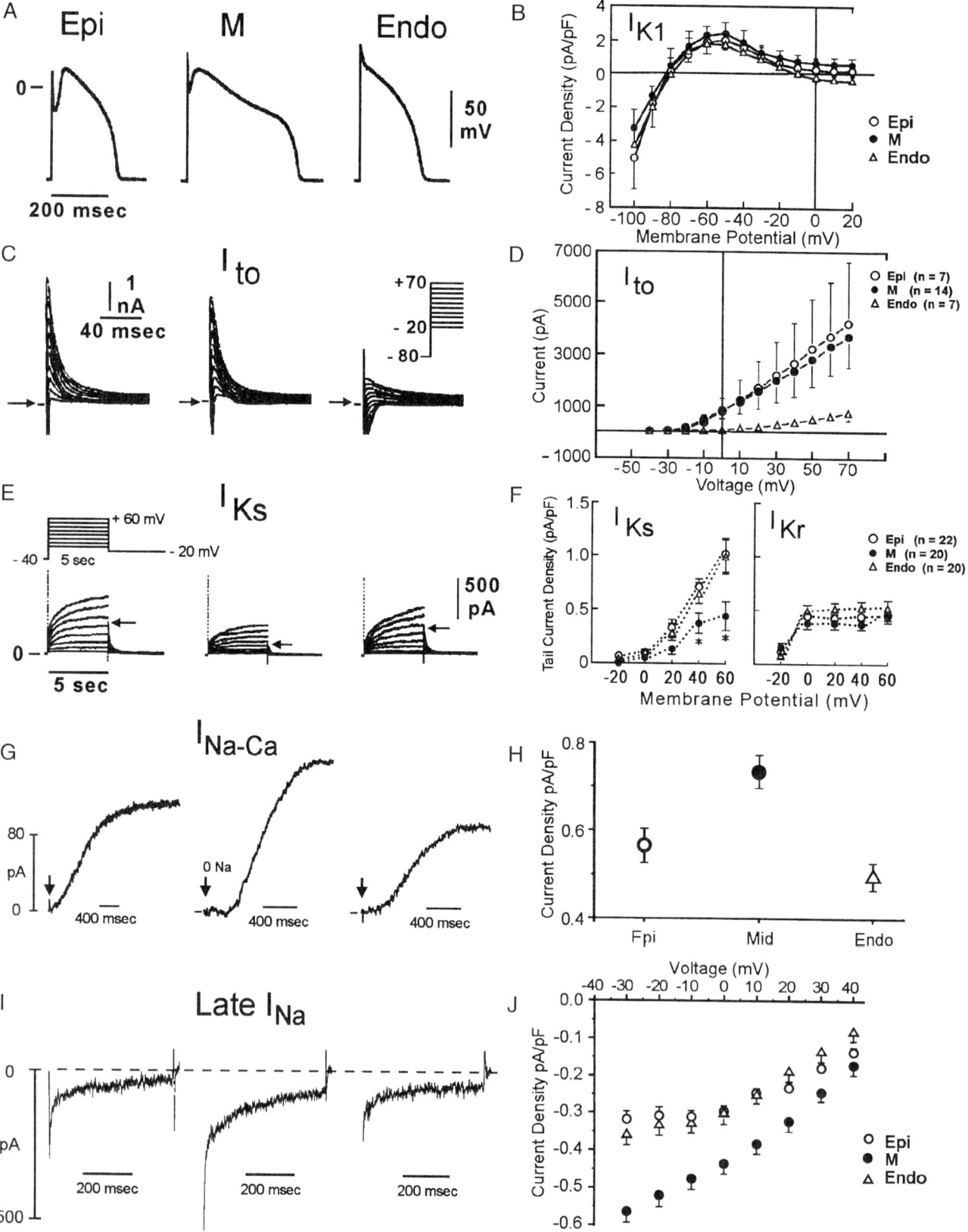

preparation (204). Figure 17–3 graphically illustrates the transmural distribution of APD$_{90}$ and tissue resistivity in the canine left ventricle (LV). M-cells with the longest action potentials are found in the deep subendocardium, and transitions in action potential duration are relatively gradual across the ventricular wall, except in the deep subepicardial region (246). A sharp increase in tissue resistivity measured in the deep subepicardium leads to reduced electrotonic interaction, thus permitting cells in this region to exhibit more of their intrinsic properties. The extent to which electrical heterogeneity is manifest across the intact ventricular wall depends on (1) the magnitude of differences in intrinsic action potential characteristics of cells spanning the wall and (2) the extent to which the cells are electrically coupled in the syncytium (227). When coupling resistance is low, intrinsic differences in APD are highly damped, but are usually perceptible over the full width of the LV wall. As coupling resistance increases, so does the ability to manifest differences of APD and other action potential parameters across the wall. In the canine ventricle, transmural heterogeneity is due to differences in intrinsic action potential characteristics as well as differences in tissue resistivity among the various transmural layers (246). A sharp increase in tissue resistivity between the M region and the epicardium is responsible for the sharp increase in APD in this region of the wall. This resistive barrier may be still more important in the lateral free wall of the left ventricle where M-cells with the longest APD are often found in the deep subepicardial to midmyocardial layers (193). Despite the relatively large increase in tissue resistivity in the deep subepicardium, conduction in this region slows only slightly, consistent with cable theory predictions. Although the basis for the abrupt rise in tissue resistivity is not fully understood, a sudden shift in the orientation of the myocardial cells in this part of the wall is thought to contribute importantly (Fig. 17–3B; 246). An abrupt shift in cell orientation in the deep subepicardium has been

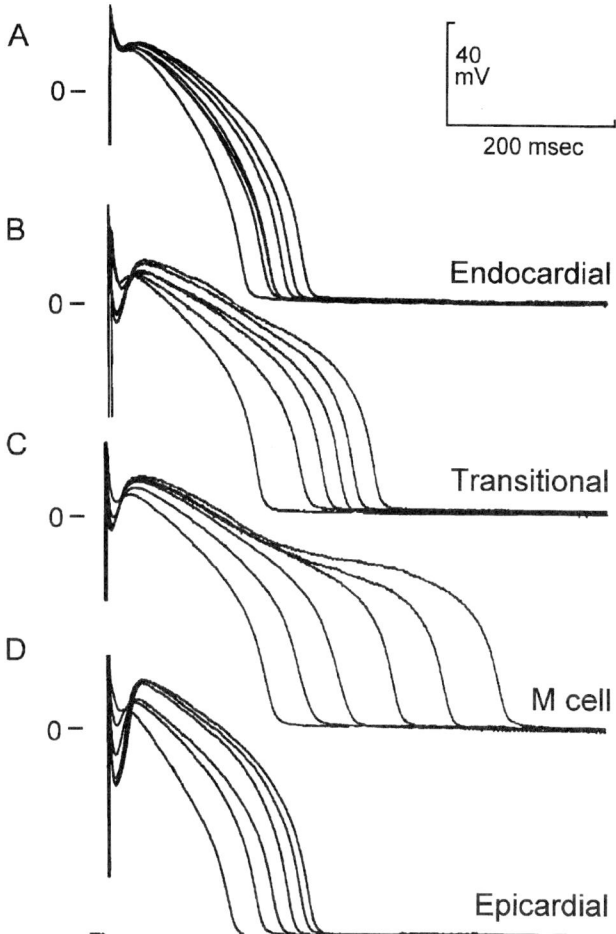

FIG. 17–2. Transmembrane activity recorded from cells isolated from the epicardial, M, and endocardial regions of the canine left ventricle at basic cycle lengths (BCL) of 300 to 5000 msec (steady-state conditions). The M-cells and transitional cells were enzymatically dissociated from the midmyocardial region. Deceleration-induced prolongation of APD in M-cells is much greater than in epicardial and endocardial cells. The spike-and-dome morphology is also more accentuated in the epicardial cell.

FIG. 17–1. A: Action potentials recorded from myocytes isolated from the epicardial (Epi), endocardial (Endo), and M regions of the canine left ventricle. B: I-V relations for I_{K1} in epicardial, endocardial, and M region myocytes. Values are mean ± S.D. C: Transient outward current (I_{to}) recorded from the three cell types (current traces recorded during depolarizing steps from a holding potential of −80 mV to test potentials ranging between −20 and +70 mV D: The average peak current–voltage relationship for I_{to} for each of the three cell types. Values are mean ± S.D. E: Voltage-dependent activation of the slowly activating component of the delayed rectifier K$^+$ current (I_{Ks}) (currents were elicited by the voltage pulse protocol shown in the inset; Na$^+$-, K$^+$- and Ca^{2+}-free solution). F: Voltage dependence of I_{Ks} (current remaining after exposure to E-4031) and I_{Kr} (E-4031-sensitive current). Values are mean ± S.E. * $p < 0.05$ compared with Epi or Endo. [From references (133, 132, 257), with permission.] G: Reverse-mode sodium–calcium exchange currents recorded in potassium- and chloride-free solutions at a voltage of −80 mV. I_{Na-Ca} was maximally activated by switching to sodium-free external solution at the time indicated by the arrow. H: Midmyocardial sodium–calcium exchanger density is 30% greater than endocardial density, calculated as the peak outward I_{Na-Ca} normalized by cell capacitance. Endocardial and epicardial densities were not significantly different. I: TTX-sensitive late sodium current. Cells were held at −80 mV and briefly pulsed to −45 mV to inactivate fast sodium current before stepping to −10 mV. J: Normalized late sodium current measured 300 msec into the test pulse was plotted as a function of test pulse potential. [Modified from reference (257) with permission.]

TABLE 17-2. *Electrophysiological Distinctions Among Epicardial, Endocardial, M-cells, and Purkinje Fibers Isolated from the Canine Heart*

	Purkinje	M	Epicardial	Endocardial
Long APD, steep APD-rate	Yes	Yes	No	No
Develop EADs in response to agents with class III actions	Yes	Yes	No	No
Develop DADs in response to digitalis, high Ca^{2+}, catecholamines	Yes	Yes	No	No
Display marked increase in APD in response to I_{Kr} blockers	Yes	Yes	No	No
Display marked increase in APD in response to I_{Ks} blockers	No	Yes	Yes	Yes
α1 Agonist-induced change in APD	↑	↓	↔	↔
$\dot{V}_{max}$	High	Intermediate	Low in surface tissues	
Phase 4 depolarization	Yes	No	No	No
Depolarize in $[K^+]_o < 2.5_mM$	Yes	No	No	No
Acceleration-induced EADs and APD prolongation in presence of I_{Kr} block	No	Yes	No	No
EADs sensitive to $[Ca^{2+}]_i$	No	Yes	No	No
Develop DADs with Bay K 8644	No	Yes	No	No
Found in bundles	Yes	No	No	No

APD = action potential duration, EAD = early afterdepolarization; DAD = delayed afterdepolarization.

TABLE 17-3. *Evidence for the M-Cells in Ventricular Myocardium of Several Mammalian Species*

Species	Recording Technique
Dog	
Myocytes (132,133)	Microelectrode
Tissue slices (24,26,169,193,196,197)	Microelectrode
Perfused wedge (20,182–184,244,246)	Microelectrode and unipolar
In Vivo—Halothane anesthesia (237)	Unipolar and MAP
—Isoflurane anesthesia (81)	Unipolar
Guinea Pig	
Tissue slices (200)	Microelectrode
Rabbit	
Tissue slices (234)	Microelectrode
Pig	
Myocytes (209)	Microelectrode
Human	
Myocytes (127)	Microelectrode
Tissue slices (74)	Patch pipette

Microelectrode = standard, floating or patch microelectrode; Unipolar = unipolar extracellular electrodes; MAP = monophasic action potential.

documented throughout the canine heart. A sharp transition in the orientation of cells is also observed in the deep subepicardium of the human left ventricle, where prolonged M-cell action potentials are first encountered (74).

The shift in the location of the M-cells from the deep subepicardium to the deep subendocardium appears to follow the transmural shift in the muscular layers that envelop the heart, as described by Streeter (211, 212), and more recently by Lukenheimer and coworkers (140).

Cells with the characteristics of M-cells have been described in the canine, guinea pig, rabbit, pig, and human ventricles (Table 17-3; 16, 24, 26, 41, 74, 81, 127, 132, 133, 169, 182–184, 187, 193, 195–197, 200, 209, 234, 237, 244, 246). Three studies have failed to discern M-cells in the ventricles of the pig, guinea pig, and rat (39, 169, 190). Another study, while clearly demonstrating the presence of M-cells in the ventricles of the canine heart in vitro, failed to delineate the unique cell type in vivo (23, 24). Methodological considerations may be responsible for these differences, as discussed below.

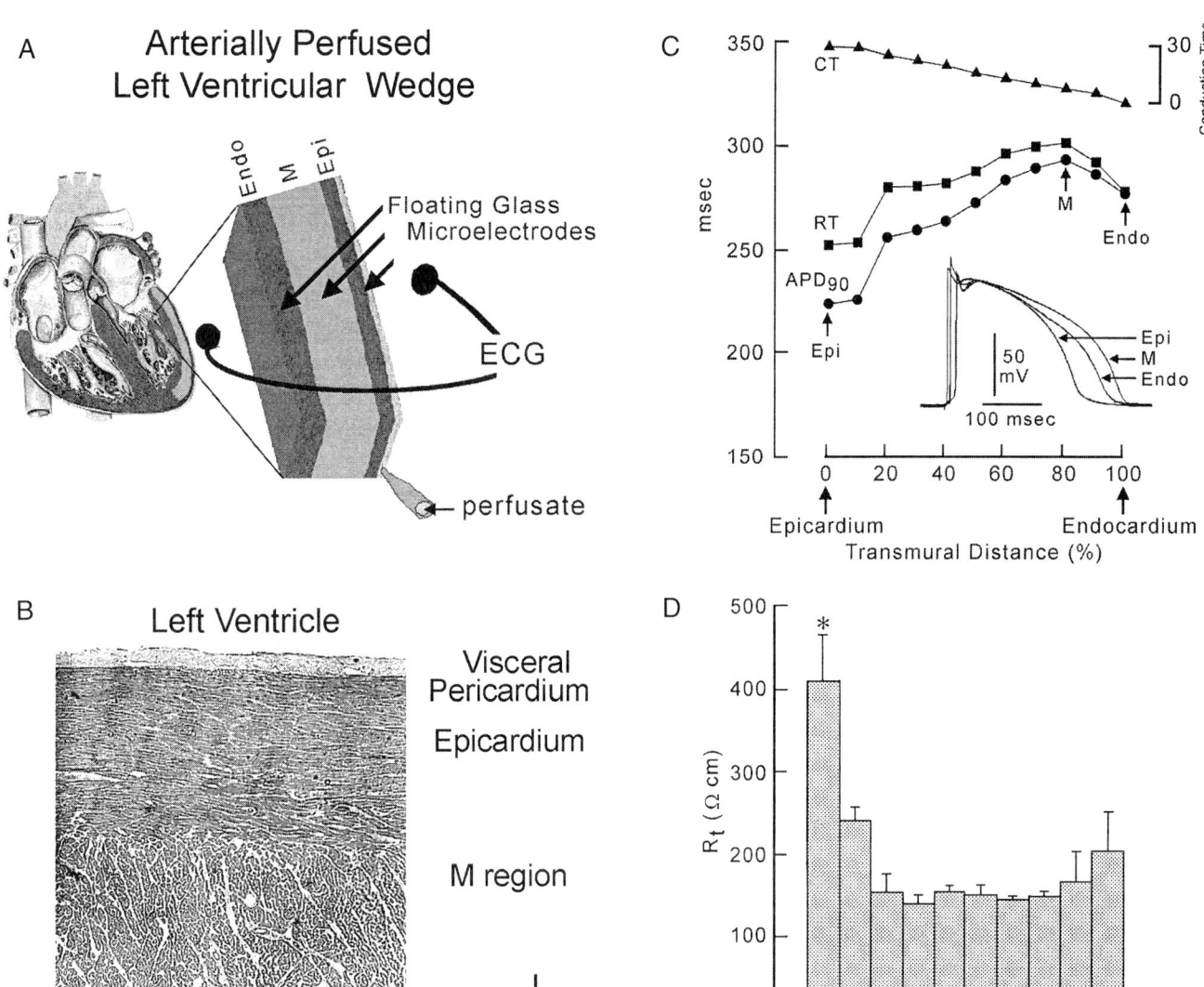

FIG. 17–3. Transmural distribution of action potential duration and tissue resistivity in the intact ventricular wall. *A:* Schematic diagram of the arterially perfused canine LV wedge preparation. The wedge is perfused with Tyrode's solution via a small native branch of the left descending coronary artery and stimulated from the endocardial surface. Transmembrane action potentials are recorded simultaneously from epicardial (Epi), M region (M), and endocardial (Endo) sites using three floating microelectrodes. A transmural ECG is recorded along the same transmural axis across the bath, registering the entire field of the wedge. *B:* Histology of a transmural slice of the left ventricular wall near the epicardial border. The region of sharp transition of cell orientation coincides with the region of high tissue resistivity depicted in *D* and the region of sharp transition of action potential duration illustrated in *C. C:* Distribution of conduction time (CT), APD_{90}, and repolarization time (RT = APD_{90} + CT) in a canine left ventricular wall wedge preparation paced at BCL of 2000 msec. A sharp transition of APD_{90} is present between epicardium and subepicardium. Epi: epicardium; M: M-cell; Endo: endocardium; RT: repolarization time; CT: conduction time. *D:* Distribution of total tissue resistivity (R_t) across the canine left ventricular wall. Transmural distances at 0% and 100% represent epicardium and endocardium, respectively. * p <0.01 compared with R_t at midwall. Tissue resistivity increases most dramatically between deep subepicardium and epicardium. Error bars represent SEM (n = 5). [From Yan et al. (246), with permission.]

Methodological Considerations in the Assessment of Electrical Heterogeneity

The extent to which transmural electrical heterogeneity is experimentally observed is based on the type of preparation studied as well as the recording techniques employed.

Transmembrane Action Potential Recordings. Regardless of the experimental preparation used, the most accurate measure of local repolarization is obtained using intracellular microelectrode techniques. Myocytes isolated from the M region of the canine LV display APDs that, on average, are 170 msec longer than those recorded from endocardium or epicardium (132, 133, 137, 193; Table 17–4). Transmural dispersion is reduced to 105 msec when recorded from slices of tissue isolated from the respective regions of the wall, and further reduced to an average of 64–67 msec when recorded from arterially perfused wedge preparations, in which the three cell types are electrotonically well coupled [at a basic cycle length (BCL) of 2000 msec; Tables 17–4 and 17–5]. APD values for each of the three ventricular cell types as well as for subendocardial Purkinje fibers recorded from the wedge using floating intracellular microelectrodes, are shown in Table 17–5. The data indicate that electrotonic interactions among the three cell types importantly abbreviate the action potential of the M-cell below its intrinsic duration and prolong the APD of epicardial and endocardial cells beyond their intrinsic values, thus reducing transmural dispersion of repolarization (20, 182).

Activation Recovery Interval and Monophasic Action Potential Recordings. Because intracellular microelectrode recordings are difficult to obtain in vivo, most studies turn to unipolar, bipolar, or monophasic action potential (MAP) electrodes. Unipolar activation recovery interval (ARI) and monophasic action potential (MAP) measurements provide a reasonable approximation of APD at local transmural sites when microelectrode recordings are not possible (81, 82). Significant transmural dispersion of repolarization is observed in the canine heart in vivo with both transmural MAP recordings (237) and with the use of unipolar electrodes to estimate the ARI (81; Table 17–4: BCL of 1400–1500 msec, young dogs (81, 82)—isoflurane or halothane anesthesia).

While unipolar electrograms provide an ARI that can be interpreted on the basis of biophysical theory (101, 161, 206, 210) and that correlates well with APD under a variety of conditions, bipolar electrograms provide a repolarization complex that is not as readily interpretable because it represents the difference in the activity of two sites. Consequently, it is difficult to make a distinction between repolarization times at the two sites, and when differences exist, they are usually obscured. Irrespective of their placement within the wall, ARI values of bipolar electrograms, measured as the interval between the negative peak of the QRS and the *latest* peak of the T wave of the differentiated electrogram, (24) can greatly underestimate transmural dispersion of repolarization and should not be used for this purpose (14).

Experimental Preparations

Isolated tissue slices. In experiments involving tissues isolated from different regions of the heart, it is important to keep the depth of the slice to under 1 mm to maintain proper oxygenation of the tissue during superfusion. This is best achieved using a dermatome. The tissue slices are usually semi-transparent. When transmural differences are studied, one should be mindful of the fact that tissues from different apico-basal regions exhibit a very different distribution of action potential characteristics (14, 197).

TABLE 17–4. *Transmural Dispersion of APD_{90}, ARI, or MAP Values Measured in Enzymatically Dissociated Myocytes, Tissue Slices, Arterially Perfused Left Ventricular Wedge Preparations and In Vivo Canine Studies*

	Control	I_{Kr} Block (d-Sotalol, 100 μM)	ATX-II (10–30 nM)
Myocytes (APD_{90}) (BCL = 2000 msec)	170 ± 51	—	—
Tissues (APD_{90}) (BCL = 2000 msec)	105 ± 45	286 ± 129	481 ± 155
Perfused Wedge (APD_{90}) (BCL = 2000 msec)	67 ± 15	87 ± 16	178 ± 44
In vivo (ARI and MAP) (BCL = 1400–1500 msec)	31 ± 5	88 ± 17	151 ± 29(81)

Values are Mean ± SD (in msec). APD_{90} = action potential duration measured at 90% repolarization measured using standard or floating microelectrodes. MAP = monophasic action potential, ARI = activation-recovery interval, BCL = basic cycle length. Dispersion of APD_{90}: difference between longest APD_{90} (usually M-cells) and shortest APD_{90} (generally epicardium). In vivo data were recorded under halothane or isoflurane anesthesia, at shorter BCLs and in some cases from smaller (younger) dogs.
Data from (14;20;23;26;81;82;132;133;169;193;194;196–198;205;237;246).

TABLE 17–5. *Action Potential Durations Measured in Arterially Perfused Canine Left Ventricular Wedge Preparations*

BCL (msec)	APD_{90} (msec)		Transmural Dispersion of APD_{90} (msec)		Transmural Dispersion of Repolarization Time (msec)	
	1000	2000	1000	2000	1000	2000
Epicardium	207 ± 20	217 ± 24	—	—	—	—
M-cell	260 ± 21	281 ± 25	51 ± 19	64 ± 25	34 ± 18	45 ± 25
Endocardium	249 ± 18	266 ± 21	—	—	—	—
Subendocardial Purkinje fiber	299 ± 17	326 ± 19	—	—	—	—

Values are Mean ± SD (in msec). APD_{90} = action potential duration measured at 90% repolarization using floating microelectrodes. BCL = basic cycle length.

From Yan et al. (246) with permission.

Isolated myocytes. Action potentials with the electrophysiological characteristics of epicardial cells, endocardial cells and M-cells are observed in isolated myocytes enzymatically dissociated from a variety of species. Recent studies reported the absence of M-cells in the ventricle of guinea pig and rat hearts (Table 17-3; 39, 190). Both studies employed cells enzymatically dissociated from the epicardial, endocardial, and midmyocardial regions of the LV wall. These studies illustrate a common methodological pitfall, namely that of cell selection. In the dog, the thickness of the epicardial layer in the LV is on the order of 500–800 μm (246); thus, when cells are enzymatically dissociated from a 1 mm slice of epicardium, one can expect the fraction to be contaminated with transitional cells and possibly M-cells to the extent of 20%–50% (132, 133). In species with smaller hearts and correspondingly thinner ventricular walls, the problem is greatly compounded in that transitional cells and M-cells, if present, will vastly outnumber the epicardial or endocardial cells. Thus, the predominant characteristics of cells in the three layers will be those of the transitional and M-cells. Thus, rather than lacking M-cells, the myocytes selected for study may be deficient in epicardial and endocardial cells. These observations highlight the difficulty of using dissociated cells to demonstrate or rule out the absence of M-cells in the heart. Ideally, such studies should be coupled with experiments designed to examine the electrophysiological and pharmacological characteristics of tissues isolated from the respective regions of the ventricular wall as well as with studies of transmural slices of the wall.

In dealing with dissociated myocytes, it is also helpful to use scattergrams or plots of individual experiments to visualize the full range of behaviors recorded from cells isolated from the different transmural regions (70, 70, 132, 133). As a consequence, differences in ionic currents and other parameters measured in isolated epicardial, M, and endocardial myocytes are likely to be underestimated. One way to circumvent this problem is to correlate the ionic current measurements with action potential characteristics (spike and dome morphology and APD-rate relations) recorded in the same cell under current clamp conditions. This approach yields much larger differences in the density of the delayed rectifier current among the three cell types than do measurements made in randomly selected cells from the epicardial, M, and endocardial fractions (132).

In vivo experiments. Dispersion of repolarization observed in vivo can vary as a function of the recording methodology, as previously discussed, as well as the anesthesia used. Transmural dispersion of repolarization is much smaller with sodium pentobarbital anesthesia than with halothane. The effect of pentobarbital to dissipate transmural heterogeneity under control conditions is still more evident in the presence of APD prolonging agents (187, 237). d-Sotalol produces a dramatic increase in transmural dispersion of repolarization under halothane, but not under sodium pentobarbital anesthesia (237). Consequently, d-sotalol-induced torsade de pointes is not observed under sodium pentobarbital anesthesia, but readily develops under halothane anesthesia. Pentobarbital totally suppresses d-sotalol-induced and ATX-II-induced TdP in the perfused wedge (187). Pentobarbital-induced block of late I_{Na} and I_{Ks} appears to underlie this action of the anesthetic (214). These findings suggest caution in the interpretation of the results of in vivo studies performed under pentobarbital anesthesia.

Recent studies also implicate α chloralose, another commonly used anesthetic, showing that the anesthetic importantly reduces transmural dispersion of repolarization via abbreviation of the APD of the M-cell with little or no change in the APD of epicardium and endocardium. This may also be due to an effect of the drug to block late I_{Na}. Similar caution may therefore need to be exercised in the interpretation and extrapolation of data obtained from studies employing α chloralose as an anesthetic.

It seems clear that differences in the anesthesia used can contribute to the failure of some studies to discern significant repolarization gradients across the canine LV wall in vivo (22–24, 31, 90) and the ability of other studies to demonstrate them consistently (81, 82, 237). A relatively small transmural dispersion of repolarization has been reported (at slow rates) in studies in vivo that have used pentobarbital or α chloralose for anesthesia (23, 24, 90, 237) vs. studies that have used other agents including isoflurane (81, 82) or halothane (237) as well as in the absence of anesthesia (187). Concordant with these findings, the development of in vivo models of TdP has met with failure when sodium pentobarbital is used for anesthesia (237) whereas TdP could be readily induced when halothane or isoflurane was employed (81, 82, 229, 237) or when no anesthesia was employed (235, 236). In the case of α chloralose anesthesia, TdP is observed when interventions in addition to I_{Kr} block are included in the protocol (α adrenergic agonists, and/or hypokalemia) (40, 48). Although transmural dispersion of repolarization can increase dramatically under halothane anesthesia, leading to TdP, it is not yet clear whether halothane and isoflurane also reduce transmural dispersion of repolarization (TDR) and thus lead to an underestimation of the transmural gradients present in the unanesthetized state or, indeed, whether they exert opposite effects due to reduced electrical coupling.

These findings explain in part the failure of earlier studies to discern the M-cell. Among the factors involved are the use of (1) relatively fast stimulation rates, (2) bipolar recording techniques to estimate ARI, or (3) sodium pentobarbital or α chloralose anesthesia, or a combination of these. One of the few early studies to infer delayed repolarization in the deep layers of the canine left ventricle was that by Burgess et al. (44), in which repolarization was estimated by local measurement of refractoriness.

PHARMACOLOGICAL DISTINCTIONS

Epicardium versus Endocardium

A consequence of a prominent I_{to}-mediated spike-and-dome morphology in epicardium but not endocardium is that the two tissues show different—in some cases opposite—responses to a wide variety of pharmacological agents (Table 17–1).

Epicardium and endocardium respond differently to both parasympathetic and sympathetic agonists. Acetylcholine (ACh) in concentrations as high as $10^{-5}\,M$ exerts essentially no effect on the action potential of canine ventricular endocardium. In contrast, ACh has been shown to either prolong or markedly abbreviate the epicardial action potential (131), providing support for claims of a direct effect of ACh in the feline and human heart in vivo (33, 165). Low concentrations (10^{-7}–$10^{-6}\,M$) cause slowing of the second upstroke, giving rise to a delay in the achievement of peak plateau. This accentuation of the epicardial action potential notch causes prolongation of action potential duration. Higher concentrations cause all-or-none repolarization and marked abbreviation of the action potential. These effects of ACh on epicardium are (1) readily reversed with atropine, (2) fail to appear when epicardium is pretreated with the transient outward current blocker 4-AP, (3) are accentuated in the presence of isoproterenol (10^{-7} to $5\times 10^{-6}\,M$; accentuated antagonism), (4) persist in the presence of propranolol, and (5) are likely due to inhibition of I_{Ca} and/or activation of $I_{K\text{-}ACh}$ (131). ACh does not influence I_{to} (150).

The differential responsiveness of epicardium and endocardium to isoproterenol is due to a diminution of the epicardial action potential notch secondary to a rebalancing of currents flowing during the early phases of the action potential. As a consequence, the epicardial action potential abbreviates more than that of endocardium in response to sympathetic stimulation. β adrenergic agonists influence all of the major currents that contribute to phase 1 and phase 3 repolarization, including I_{to}, I_{Ca}, I_K, and calcium- and cAMP-activated I_{Cl} (100, 106, 152, 218, 222, 254–256).

Dissimilar responses of epicardium and endocardium to calcium channel blockers have been reported in a number of studies. Organic Ca^{2+} channel blockers such as verapamil (170) and nifedipine (119) and inorganic inhibitors such as $MnCl_2$ (112) can cause loss of the action potential dome in canine ventricular epicardium. Exposure to Ca^{2+}-free Tyrode's solution yields similar results (112). In endocardium, calcium channel blockers cause only a slight abbreviation of the action potential (94, 118).

Sodium channel blockers produce different, and in some cases opposite, effects on canine ventricular epicardium and endocardium (124, 125). Concentrations of tetrodotoxin, propranolol, and flecainide sufficient to reduce the rate of rise of the action potential ($\dot{V}_{max}$) by approximately 40%–50% abbreviate the action potential in endocardium but prolong it in epicardium. Greater inhibition of I_{Na} leads to a marked abbreviation of the epicardial response due to loss of the action potential dome, while producing only a slight abbreviation of the action potential in endocardium. The paradoxical prolongation of the epicardial action potential is due in large part to an accentuation and widening of the action potential notch. With greater inhibition of I_{Na}, termination of phase 1 shifts to more negative potentials, at which the availability of I_{Ca} is diminished to a level where the outward currents may overwhelm the inward currents active at the end of phase 1. This results is an all-or-none repolarization at the end of phase 1, causing loss of the action potential dome and marked abbreviation of the action potential.

As discussed later, these actions of ACh and sodium channel blockers, particularly on right ventricular epicardium, facilitate the development of phase 2 re-entry, thought to be the trigger for sudden death in patients with the Brugada syndrome (see later, under Phase 2 Re-entry as a Trigger for VT/VF: The Brugada Syndrome).

As expected, epicardium and endocardium respond differently to agents that block I_{to}. In relatively low concentrations (0.5–1.0 mM) 4-AP is a fairly selective blocker of I_{to}; higher concentrations also block I_K and I_{K1} (203, 221). Low concentrations of 4-AP are effective in restoring electrical homogeneity and in abolishing arrhythmias induced by ischemia or drugs and neurohormones that cause dispersion of repolarization and phase 2 re-entry (i.e., sodium channel blockers and ACh); 10, 17, 68, 69, 137, 137). Inhibition of I_{to} by quinidine may contribute to the antiarrhythmic actions of the drug (107, 245).

Chronic exposure to amiodarone has been shown to produce very different electrophysiological effects in canine ventricular epicardium and endocardium (18, 199). Endocardial tissues excised from the hearts of dogs receiving chronic amiodarone (20–25 mg/kg/day over a 5–6 week period) show strong use dependence of $\dot{V}_{max}$ (30% ± 5.2% decrease with acceleration from a BCL of 2000–300 msec) and an action potential duration 16% longer than control. Unlike endocardium, epicardial tissues isolated from amiodarone-treated dogs are always markedly depressed (inexcitable) immediately after isolation. Tissues recovered over a period of several hours, displaying several distinct phases, including (1) conduction disturbances and (2) acceleration-induced *prolongation* of APD. Neither was seen in endocardium. As discussed below, under M-cells versus Epicardium and Endocardium, chronic amiodarone treatment also led to a major damping of the APD-rate relationship of the M-cells.

M-cells versus Epicardium and Endocardium

One of the hallmarks of the M-cell is that its action potential displays a greater prolongation in response to agents with class III actions or APD-prolonging effects (Table 17–2). I_{Kr} blockers, including d-sotalol, almokalant, E-4031, and erythromycin, produce a much greater prolongation of APD in M-cells than in epicar-

dium or endocardium (Fig. 17–4, Table 17–6). Surface epicardial and endocardial tissues isolated from the canine left ventricle show very little response. A similar preferential prolongation of the M-cell APD is seen with agents that increase calcium current, I_{Ca}, such as Bay K 8644, as well as with agents that increase late I_{Na} such as ATX-II and anthopleurin-A. An exception to this rule applies to agents that block I_{Ks}, including azimilide, quinidine, pentobarbital, amiodarone, and chromanol 293B. Chromanol 293B is the most specific of the I_{Ks} blockers. In isolated tissues, chromanol 293B produces similar percentage prolongations of APD in all three transmural cell types. The situation is more complex for drugs affecting two or more ion channels, such as quinidine, pentobarbital, amiodarone, and azimilide. In the case of quinidine, relatively low therapeutic levels of the drug (3–5 μM; 1.14–1.89 μg/ml),

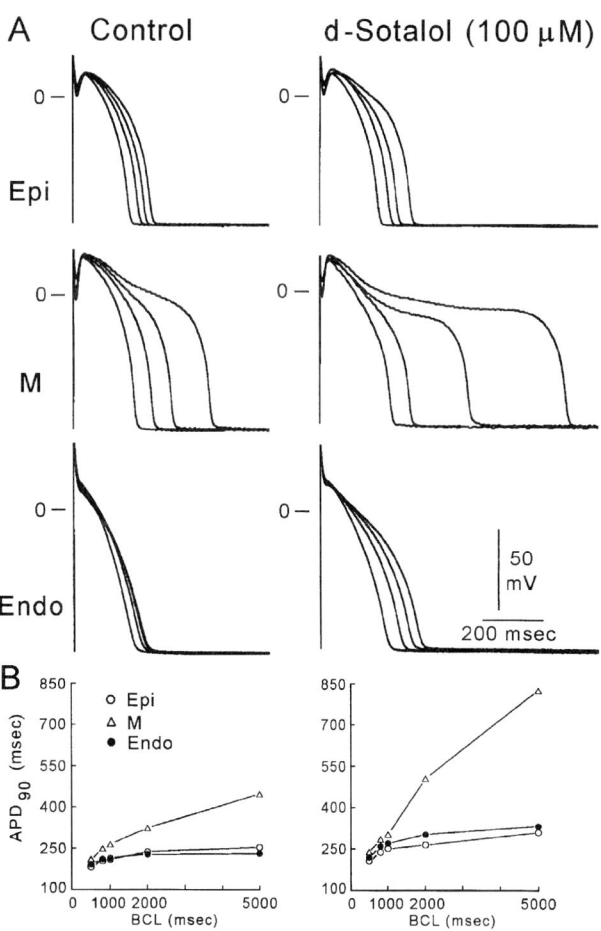

FIG. 17–4. Effect of d-sotalol, a specific I_{Kr} blocker, on transmembrane activity recorded from epicardial (Epi), endocardial (Endo), and deep subepicardial (M-cell) sites in a transmural strip of canine left ventricle. A: Each panel shows superimposed action potentials recorded at basic cycle lengths (BCL) of 300–5000 msec, before and after d-sotalol (100 μM). B: APD-rate relations. [From Sicouri et al. (198), with permission.]

TABLE 17-6. *Early Afterdepolarization (EAD)-Induced Triggered Activity and/or Prominent Action Potential Prolongation*

	Epicardium	Endocardium	M-cells
Quinidine (3.3 μM)	–	–	+++
4-Aminopyridine (2.5–5 mM)	–	–	+++
Amiloride (1–10 μM)	–	–	++
Clofilium (1 μM)	–	–	+++
Bay K 8644 (1 μM)	–	–	++
Cesium (5–10 mM)	–	–	++
Sotalol (100 μM)	–	–	+++
Erythromycin (10–100 μg/ml)	–	–	++++
E-4031 (1–5 μM)	–	–	+++
Chronic amiodarone	+	–	++
ATX-II (10–20 nM)	+	++	++++
Azimilide (5–20 μM)	+	++	+++
Chromanol 293B (10–100 μM)	+++	+++	+++

+/– Little to no response; +++++ largest response.

produce marked prolongation of the M-cell APD but not of epicardium and endocardium, consistent with a predominant effect of quinidine to block I_{Kr} at this concentration (199, 214). At higher concentrations (10–30 μM; 3.78–11.37 μg/ml), quinidine produces a further prolongation of the epicardial and endocardial action potential, consistent with an effect of the drug to block I_{Ks}, and *abbreviate* the APD of the M-cell, due to its action to suppress late I_{Na} (27). Voltage-clamp studies have shown that low concentration of quinidine (10 μM) potently block I_{Kr}, but not I_{Ks} (15.0% ± 4.6%), whereas higher concentrations (25 μM) potently block both I_{Kr} and I_{Ks} (79.8% ± 11%) (14). We hasten to point out that the dose–response relationship in these voltage-clamp experiments is markedly shifted to higher concentrations owing to the short exposure (5 min) of the myocytes to the drug. Quinidine has been shown to exert its actions to prolong APD with a biexponential time course comprised of two components with time constants of 25 and 435 min, reflecting the time course of intracellular uptake of the drug (8, 9, 64). These multiple actions of quinidine have been suggested to underlie the ability of the drug to induce TdP at low therapeutic levels, but not at high therapeutic or toxic levels (14).

Amiodarone is a potent antiarrhythmic agent used in the management of both atrial and ventricular arrhythmias. In addition to its β-blocking properties, amiodarone is known to block the sodium, potassium, and calcium channels in the heart. The high efficacy of the drug and its low incidence of proarrhythmia relative to other agents with class III actions are due to this complex pharmacology. When administered chronically (30–40 mg/kg/day orally for 30–45 days), amiodarone produces a greater prolongation of action potential duration in epicardium and endocardium, but less of an increase—or even a decrease at slow rates—in the M region, thereby reducing transmural dispersion of repolarization (Fig. 17-5; 199). Chronic amiodarone therapy also suppresses the ability of the I_{Kr} blocker, d-sotalol, to induce a marked dispersion of repolarization or early afterdepolarization activity. Thus, chronic amiodarone treatment differentially alters the cellular electrophysiology of ventricular myocardium so as to produce an important decrease in transmural dispersion of repolarization, especially under conditions in which dispersion is exaggerated. These results contribute to our understanding of the effectiveness of amio-

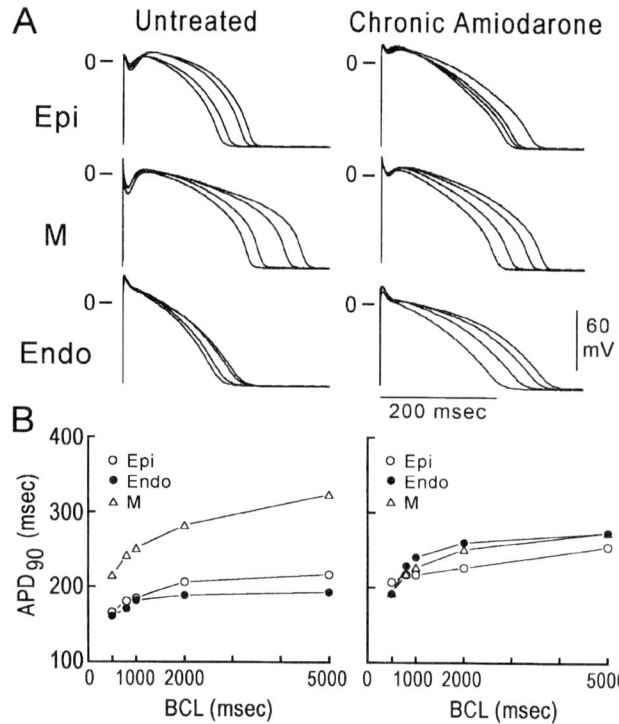

FIG. 17-5. Effects of chronic amiodarone on the rate dependence of action potential characteristics in epicardial (Epi), M, and endocardial (Endo) tissues isolated from the hearts of untreated dogs (*left*) as well as those receiving chronic amiodarone therapy (*right*). A: Transmembrane activity recorded simultaneously from Epi, M, and Endo preparations at basic cycle lengths (BCL) of 500, 800, 2000, and 5000 msec (steady-state conditions). B: Composite data from twelve untreated dogs and five amiodarone treated dogs. The graphs plot APD-rate relations for Epi (*open circles*), Endo (*closed circles*), and M (*open triangles*) of untreated (*left*) and amiodarone-treated animals (*right*). Each point represents mean ± S.D. * $p < 0.01$ amiodarone vs. control. $[K+]_o = 4$ mM. Chronic amiodarone treatment leads to much more uniform APD-rate relations in the three cell types.

darone in the treatment of life-threatening arrhythmias, as well as to our understanding of the relatively low incidence of proarrhythmia.

M-Cells versus Purkinje Cells

Purkinje cells and M-cells respond differently to α-adrenergic agonists due to predominance of α_{1a}-adrenoceptors in the former and α_{1b} adrenoceptors in the latter (42; Table 17–2). α-Agonists, including methoxamine and phenylephrine, produce a prolongation of Purkinje APD, but an abbreviation of the APD of the M-cell. Another distinction lies in the strikingly different mechanisms governing the development of early afterdepolarizations (EADs) in the two cell types. EADs induced in the M-cell are exquisitely sensitive to changes in intracellular calcium levels, whereas EADs elicited in Purkinje fibers are not. This feature of the M-cell underlies acceleration-induced EADs and action potential prolongation (41).

MOLECULAR DISTINCTIONS

The last two decades of the twentieth century were among the most exciting in the history of human biology. Major breakthroughs in genetics, molecular biology, and immunology, fueled by innovative technical advances, elevated our knowledge from the descriptive Mendelian laws of heredity and the Watson and Crick model of the DNA to practical applications involving identification and engineering of genes. Knowledge of the human brain was among the first to be advanced in studies of the genome of *Drosophila melanogaster*. It soon became evident that many of the genes found in the human brain are also expressed in the heart. The identification and heterologous expression of cardiac genes linked to ion channels, pumps, exchangers, and gap junction proteins involved in the activation and propagation of the cardiac action potential soon led to better understanding of rhythm disturbances long considered idiopathic in nature. Recent studies suggest that heterogeneities in the genetic makeup of cardiac tissues underlie transmural, apicobasal, interventricular, as well as atrioventricular differences in the expression of electrical currents in the heart. In this section we review key findings dealing with heterogeneous distribution of messenger RNA and/or gene products and assess the extent to which these may be responsible for the electrophysiological heterogeneities discussed throughout the remainder of the chapter. Our principal focus is on the distribution of mRNA and gene products in different regions of ventricular myocardium of the normal heart (Table 17–7). Chapters 15 and 19 in this book deal more extensively with the pathological consequences of altered gene expression and distribution.

Potassium Channels

Potassium channels are the most numerous and diverse family of ion channels expressed in the heart. Their propensity to pair with members of the same and/or different phylogenic branches makes their genetic linkage to cardiac current a daunting task.

Overview of Shaker Type Channels. The first voltage-gated potassium channel subunit was cloned from the *Shaker* locus in *Drosophila* (115) and it was soon discovered that *Shaker* K^+ channels are oligomeric proteins comprised of four units.(141) This family consists of four subfamily members of voltage-gated K^+ channel genes originally named *Shaker, Shab, Shaw, Shal*. (46) and now referred to as Kv1.x, Kv2.x, Kv3.x, and Kv4.x, respectively, based on the nomenclature proposed by Chandy (50). We will use this terminology in the remainder of the chapter. Within the Kv family, 11 genes have been identified at the transcriptional level in the heart: Kv1.1, Kv1.2, Kv1.3, Kv1.4, Kv1.5, Kv1.6, Kv2.1, Kv2.2, Kv3.4, Kv4.2, Kv4.3. Northern blot analysis of rat heart tissues initially revealed the presence of Kv1.1, Kv1.2, Kv1.4, Kv1.5, Kv4.2, and Kv2.1 mRNA (168). Dixon and McKinnon (72) subsequently reported the presence of only the Kv1.2, Kv1.4, Kv1.5, and Kv4.2 transcripts in the rat atria and ventricles using a ribonuclease (RNase) protection assay (RPA). Using fluorescent *in-situ* hybridization techniques, Brahmajothi et al. (35) detected a weak signal for Kv1.1 mRNA in ferret atrium and ventricles, and a much stronger signal in the Sinoatrial (SA) node (35). Atrial rat myocytes display higher levels of Kv2.1 protein than do ventricular myocytes. Kv1.5 protein density is similar in myocytes from atria and ventricles (29, 30). Kv1.2 and Kv4.2 proteins are strongly expressed in rat atrium and ventricles, with Kv4.2 being more abundant in ventricular cells and Kv1.2 and Kv2.1 preferentially expressed in atrial cells (30). The Kv1.4 proteins are poorly expressed in rat hearts (30).

In ferret heart (35), Kv1.4 mRNA is evenly distributed within the heart, and Kv1.2 has a wide distribution. Both are found in low abundance in atrial and ventricular septa. The transcript for Kv1.3 is sparse in both atria and ventricles, but more abundant in the right atrium and in atrial and ventricular septa. Kv1.6 transcript is rare but more commonly encountered in SA node. Kv2.1 is twice as abundant as Kv2.2, and both show a uniform distribution in all regions of the heart. Kv3.4 is three-fold more abundant in ventricles than in atria and all members of the Kv4 family are

TABLE 17–7. *Cardiac Localization of Genes Involved in the Formation and Propagation of the Action Potential*

Gene	Anatomical Location						Candidate Current	Species	Reference
	SA	AV	LA	RA	LV	RV			
$K_v1.1$	+++		+		+		?	Ferret	(35)
$K_v1.2$		+	+				?	Rat	(72;168)
$K_v1.3$			+	++	+	+	?	Ferret	(35)
$K_v1.4$		+	+		++ (Endo only)		I_{to} (Endo ?)	Rat, ferret	(30;72; 73;168)
$K_v1.5$			++↑↑		+↑		I_{Kur}	Rat, ferret	(29;30;85)
$K_v1.6$	++				+		?	Ferret	(35)
$K_v2.1$			++↑		+		I_{Kur} (embryonic?)	Rat, ferret	(35;242)
$K_v3.4$			+		+++		I_{to}?	Ferret	(35;36)
$K_v4.2$		++	++		+++ (Epi>>Endo)		I_{to}	Rat, Ferret	(35;72;73)
$K_v4.3$					+++		I_{to}	Human, dog, ferret rat	(30;34;35; 72;73; 111;121)
KCNE1					++↑↑Epi < Mid < Endo	+++↑↑↑	I_{Ks}	Ferret, dog	(35;166; 173)
KCNQ1					++(Ferret) +++↑↑↑(Dog) Epi> Mid< Endo	+++(Ferret), ++↑↑(Dog)	I_{Ks}	Ferret, dog	(35;166; 173)
ERG					++,↑↑Epi>	+++ (20%), ↑↑↑ Epi>	I_{Kr}	Ferret	(37)
SCN5A					+++↑↑↑		I_{Na}	All species studied (intercalated disks)	(58;87; 88)
Cx37		↑↑↑			↑↑(Endo)		Gap junction	Rabbits, dog	(225)
Cx40		↑↑↑			↑↑(Endo), ↑↑↑(PF)		Gap junction	Rabbits, dog	(114;225)
Cx42			↑↑↑ sinus venosus		↑↑↑(Epi)		Gap junction		(95;96; 114;224)
Cx43	↑↑(Hamster)		+++↑↑↑		+++↑↑↑		Gap junction	Rabbit, hamster	(63;225)
Cx45			+++↑↑↑		+++↑↑↑		Gap junction	Rabbit	(97;225)
cAMP-CFTR					Epi >>> Endo		I_{Cl}	Rabbit, guinea pig	(108;241)
α1C DHP receptor					↑↑↑ (T-tubules)		I_{Ca-L}	Rabbit, rat, guinea pig	(92;104; 217)
NCX1					↑↑↑ (T-tubules)		Na/Ca exchange	Rat	(51;89; 116;162; 163;213)
χ1 Na/K			↑↑↑	↑↑	+++↑↑↑+↑ conduction system +↑ T-tubules	++↑↑	Na/K-ATPase	Rat, rabbit, human	(122;201; 247;250)

(continued)

TABLE 17-7.—Continued

Gene	Anatomical Location						Candidate Current	Species	Reference
	SA	AV	LA	RA	LV	RV			
χ2 Na/K					+++↑↑↑ conduction system	+PM	++↑↑ Na/K-ATPase	Rat, rabbit, human	(250)6295} (181;248)
χ3 Na/K					+++↑↑↑ conduction system + PM		++↑↑ Na/K-ATPase	Rat, rabbit, human	(136;157)

SA = sinoatrial node, AV = atrioventricular node, LA and RA = left and right atrium, respectively, LV and RV = left and right ventricles, respectively, Epi = epicardium, Mid = midmyocardium, Endo = Endocardium, PF = Purkinje fibers, PM = papillary muscles. DHP = dihydropyridine. Symbols: + refers to mRNA and ↑ refers to protein detection. +++ and ↑↑↑: very abundant, easily detectable, ++ and ↑↑ abundant, detectable, + and ↑ rare, weak signal. Blank spaces denote the lack of available data.

expressed, with Kv4.2 being the most abundant. The link of some members of the Kv1 and Kv2 families to ionic current in the heart remains unclear. In the remainder of this section, we limit our discussion to genes definitively linked to known ion channels in the heart.

The Elusive Role of Kv1.5 in the Ventricles (I_{Kur}). Kv1.5 has been linked to I_{Kur}, the ultra-rapid delayed rectifier current (85, 232) found in dog atria. A similar current has yet to be found in the ventricles of the dog. Recent studies suggest that the Kv1.5 gene product may co-assemble with another protein, possibly a β subunit, which may modify its gating (65) and possibly its pharmacological properties. Brahmajothi et al. (35) described an even distribution of the Kv1.5 mRNA in ferret atria and ventricles. Kv1.5 mRNA is also found in rat ventricles, (72) where the protein product is reportedly weakly expressed (29, 30). In dog, Kv1.5 proteins are localized at the intercalated disk junctions (144, 145), suggesting a role in conduction. Interestingly, the protein diffuses from the intercalated disk to the sarcolemma of ventricular myocytes during ischemia or in cells lining the border of an infarct (144, 145). The migration of the channels is accompanied by a parallel downregulation of mRNA and proteins, suggesting transcriptional regulation of expression (93). Recent studies suggest that Kv2.1 is also involved in the expression of I_{Kur} during postnatal development of the rat heart (242).

The Transient Outward Current (I_{to}). The transmural distribution of I_{to} in the ventricles is perhaps the most striking example of electrical heterogeneity in the heart. Based on inactivation kinetics and sensitivity to 4-aminopyridine of members of the Kv1 and Kv4 families, several attempts have been made to correlate the anatomical location of these genes with the distribution of I_{to}. Dixon and McKinnon (72) first showed that the distribution of Kv4.2 parallels the gradient for I_{to} in the rat left ventricle with 8 times more mRNA in epicardium than in endocardium. The group later reported that Kv4.3 is uniformly distributed between the epicardium and the endocardium of the left ventricle in rat, and electrophysiological studies on Kv4.3 strengthened the link to I_{to} (121). Dixon et al. detected the message for Kv4.3 in canine and human left ventricles, but not for Kv4.2 (73). The distribution of Kv4.2 and Kv4.3 in rat preparations suggest that a complex formed by Kv4.2 and Kv4.3 may be responsible for I_{to}. In dog and human, however, their results suggested that KV4.3 co-assembles with another member of the *Shaker* or other family to form I_{to}. Barry et al. (30) further confirmed the expression of Kv4.2 proteins in the sarcolemma of rat ventricular myocytes.

In an elegant study conducted in the ferret heart, Brahmajothi et al. (34) combined electrophysiological and co-localization techniques to show that Kv4.2 and Kv4.3 are more abundant in the epicardium than in the endocardium, whereas Kv1.4 is observed mostly in endocardium and is absent in epicardium. On the apico-basal axis, they found that the Kv4.3 transcript was more abundant at the base of the heart in the right and left ventricular epicardium. In the same study, they report that Kv1.4 is more abundant in the apical left ventricle and septum, whereas Kv4.2 is more abundant in the epicardial region of the left ventricle. Kv4.2 mRNA distribution is more diffuse throughout the right ventricular free wall and septum. The same group reported the presence of Kv3.x subfamily members in the ferret ventricles (36). The results support the hypothesis that an heteromultimer composed of Kv4.3 and Kv4.2 forms part of I_{to} in the ferret epicardium and that Kv1.4 may contribute to formation of I_{to} in the endocardium. Interestingly, strong signals for Kv1.4 and Kv3.4 were also observed in canine hearts (73), but their contribution to I_{to} is considered unlikely on the basis of the lack of sensitivity of the current inactivation to oxidizing agents (73) and to the channel blocker tetraethylammonium (TEA). Immunoprecipitation studies may help to resolve this issue. It is important to note that co-assembly of different subunits can result in large fluctuations in drug sensitivity, as seen with KCNQ1 and KCNE1 (45, 171).

During heart failure in human, a decrease in Kv4.3 mRNA levels parallels the decreased I_{to} density (111), suggesting that Kv4.3 encodes for part of I_{to} and that it is transcriptionally regulated. The genes encoding I_{to} in larger mammals and in humans remain to be definitively determined, although most evidence points to a role for Kv4.3. Other likely co-assembling candidates from the *Shaker* family include Kv1.4 and Kv3.4, since they encode for rapidly inactivating channels and are found in the human heart (111).

The Slowly Activating Delayed Rectifier Current (I_{Ks}).

It is now well established that I_{Ks} is formed by co-assembly of the KCNE1 and KCNQ1 gene products (28, 173). In acutely dissociated cells from the ferret ventricles, KCNQ1 and KCNE1 mRNA are 34% and 70% more abundant, respectively, in right ventricle than in left ventricle. KCNE1 is also more abundant in the atria of the ferret than in the ventricles (35). Our group recently reported a similar interventricular distribution for KCNQ1 mRNA in the canine right ventricle but a 50% more abundant KCNE1 transcript in the left; protein expression paralleled the transcript distribution (166; Fig. 17–6), suggesting important regulation at the transcriptional level. Transmurally, KCNQ1 mRNA was found to be less abundant in the midmyocardium than in epicardium and endocardium of the canine left ventricle (77), consistent with the transmural distribution of I_{Ks}.

The 70 and 50 kD bands shown in Figure 17–6C likely represent the glycosylated protein expressed at the sarcolemmal surface and the unglycosylated protein trapped in the Golgi apparatus or the endoplasmic reticulum, respectively. This suggests that the expression of KCNQ1 is regulated at the transcriptional and possibly post-transcriptional levels. Another likely possibility is that the polyclonal antibody recognizes an alternative splice variant of KCNQ1 of smaller size. Such a splice variant has been identified in human (66) and shown to result in an N-terminal truncated isoform that has a dominant negative effect on the expression of normal KCNQ1 channels. Both interpretations of the results predict a smaller amplitude of I_{Ks} in the left ventricle, consistent with the electrophysiological data (228). Thus far, our group has been unable to detect the presence of mRNA or cDNA corresponding to truncated form of KCNQ1 in canine heart tissues using RT-PCR and 5′ *r*apid *a*mplification of *c*DNA *e*nds (RACE).

In contrast to KCNQ1, the distribution of KCNE1 follows an uphill gradient from epicardium to endocardium (Fig. 17–6). These results, suggest that KCNQ1 is the primary determinant of the transmural distribution of I_{Ks} in the canine left ventricle and that KCNE1 acts as a modulator of its kinetics and possibly its pharmacology. Because KCNE1 also increases the number of functional channels encoded by the human *ether-a-go-go*-related gene (HERG; 45), its distribution in the canine ventricle may influence the distribution of HERG channels.

The Rapidly Activating Delayed Rectifier Current (I_{Kr}).

In ferret heart, the ERG transcript encoding for the α subunit of I_{Kr} channels (172, 174, 223) is 20% more abundant in the right ventricle than in the left ventricle. ERG protein is found throughout the myocardium but is more abundant in the epicardium, except near the base of the heart, where it is evenly distributed across the ventricular wall (37). In the atrium, ERG is more abundant in the medial right atrium and in the region of the SA node. Concordance between protein and mRNA distribution indicates transcriptional regulation of the expression of I_{Kr}. Recent data indicate that KCNE1 is a member of a multi-gene family including KCNE2 (Mirp1)(1). *KCNE1* and *KCNE2* genes are known to modulate the function (45) and the gating (37) of HERG. It therefore remains to be determined if the distribution of these ancillary subunits share a similar pattern of expression with HERG and to what extent they may modulate the properties of I_{Kr}.

Sodium Channels

The SCN5A (hH1) gene encodes for the α subunit of the sodium channel, which conducts the tetrodotoxin (TTX)-sensitive (87, 88) fast sodium current responsible for the upstroke of the cardiac action potential. The protein is homogeneously distributed on the surface of rat atria and ventricular free wall; no transmural differences have been reported in the rat (58). Although the transmural distribution of I_{Na} is not known in the rat heart, in the canine heart I_{Na} is considerably greater in the midmyocardium than in epicardium or endocardium (79, 197). Data relative to transmural distribution of channel protein in the dog ventricle are not available. At the cellular level, sodium channel protein is generally more strongly expressed at the level of the T-tubules, along the Z-bands, with a major concentration at the intercalated disks. This subcellular distribution of the cardiac sodium channel is designed to facilitate conduction via an amplification process akin to neuronal saltatory conduction (58). To date, there

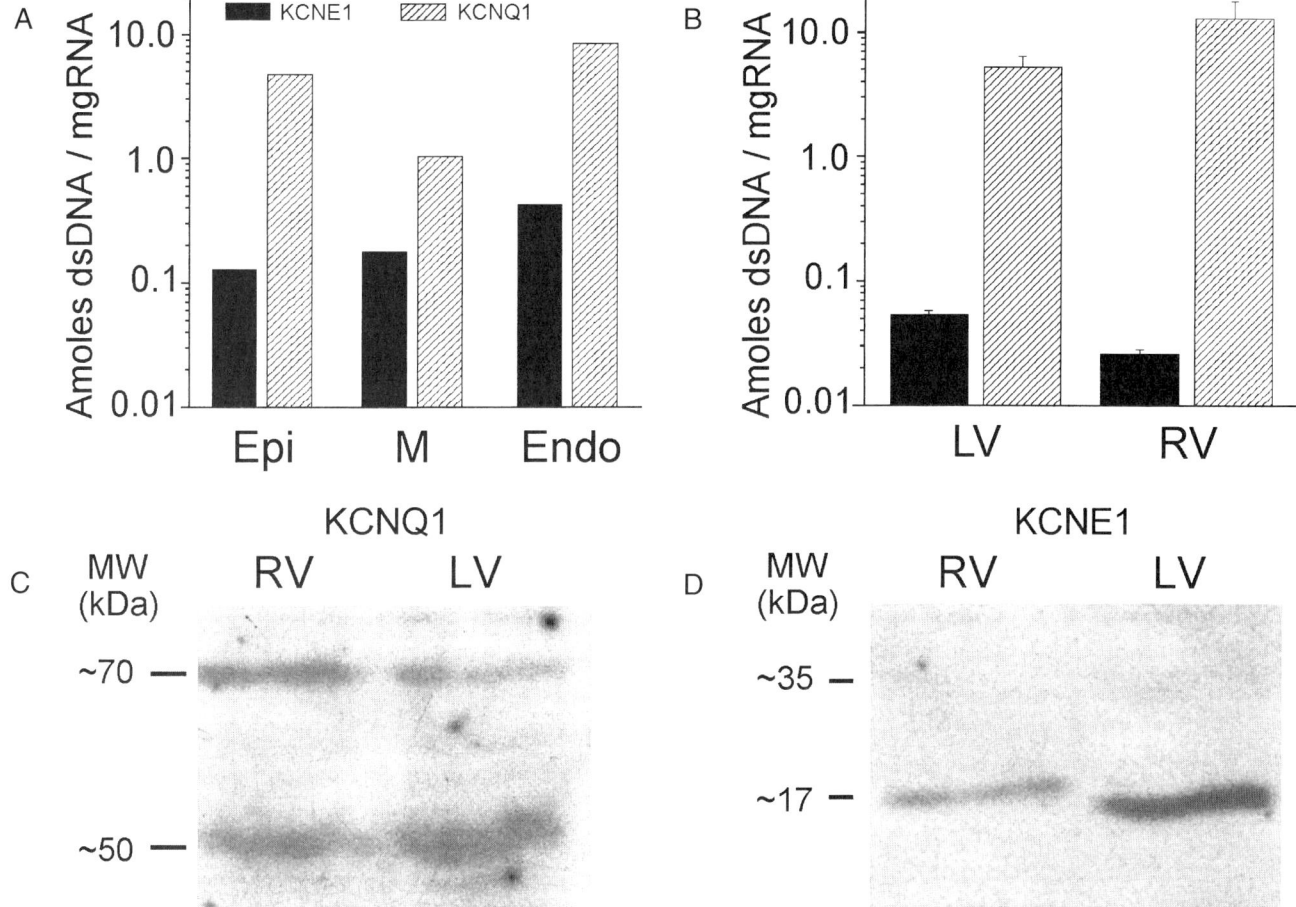

FIG. 17–6. Heterogeneous distribution of KCNE1 and KCNQ1 in canine ventricular myocardium. A: Transmural distribution of KCNE1 (filled columns) and KCNQ1 (hatched columns) mRNA as measured by competitive multiplex PCR. RNA was reverse transcribed using standard protocols and 2 μg of DNA from the epi-, mid-, and endocardium was amplified against known concentrations of an exogenous external standard (MIMIC). Data are from a pool of acutely dissociated cells from eight dogs. The concentration at which the amplitude of the two signals was equal was used to determine the amount of dsDNA presented. B: Same protocol as in A, with RNA isolated from the right (RV) and left (LV) ventricles. C: Western blot analysis of the distribution of KCNQ1 in canine right and left ventricles using polyclonal antibodies. Two bands are typically observed with a more intense signal in RV. 70 μg of protein was loaded in each well. D: Same experiment as in C with a KCNE1 antibody; the protein is more strongly expressed in LV.

have been no reports of studies that have probed for differences in regional localization of the SCN5A in the heart.

Gap Junctions

Impulse propagation in the heart depends on intercellular communication, which in turn depends on the presence of gap junctions composed of proteins referred to as *connexins* (Cx). Each connexin family displays a unique pharmacological and electrophysiological profile as well as anatomical distribution, conferring specific properties on the conductive tissues and muscle tissues of the heart. In rabbits, Cx43 and Cx45 are abundant in atrium and ventricles. In addition to Cx43, Cx40 is present in the atrium (97, 225), and Cx37 and Cx40 are preferentially localized in rabbit ventricular endocardial cells (225).

In dog, Cx40 is three-fold more abundant in Purkinje fibers than in ventricular myocardium, with mRNA levels proportional to protein expression (114). Cx42 is expressed in the sinus venosus and in the epicardial layers of the rat ventricular free wall (224). Similar levels of Cx43 and Cx44 are found in the ventricles and Purkinje fibers (114) although Cx43 appears to be absent from the AV bundle and possibly the bundle branch. Cx40 has a greater conductance than Cx43. The greater contribution of Cx40 in Purkinje fibers may explain their more rapid propagation characteristics. In hamster, coupling in the SA region is mediated by gap junctional channels formed by Cx43 (63).

Chloride Conductances

An increasing endocardial-to-epicardial gradient of mRNA for an alternatively spliced variant of cystic fibrosis transmembrane conductance regulator (CFTR) has been demonstrated in rabbit and guinea pig ventricles (108, 241). This cAMP-activated chloride conductance is activated during adrenergic stimulation (218) and is likely to contribute to the initial depolarization from the resting potential and the shortening of the ventricular action potential. The transmural distribution of cAMP-activated I_{Cl} density in the rabbit is similar to the distribution of the alternative splice variant. Myocytes isolated from the epicardial region of the rabbit left ventricular wall show a cAMP-activated chloride current density twice that of endocardial myocytes (218).

Calcium Channels

Two types of calcium channel current are generally found in the heart. A slowly inactivating, high threshold, and "long-lasting" current generated by L-type channels and a more rapid, lower threshold, transient "T"-type current. Six genes have been identified as encoding for the α1 subunit, the principal subunit of the Ca^+ channel (49, 103). The L-type is believed to be encoded by the α1C, α1D, and α1S genes owing to the sensitivity of their protein products to dihydropyridines (DHPs); 104, 113). In contrast, α1A, α1B, and α1E encode for non-DHP-sensitive channels (147, 251). The α1C gene, together with α2, β, and δ genes encode for the cardiac L-type channel.(104) In isolated adult rabbit cardiac myocytes, both the β and the full-length α1C proteins co-localize along T-tubule membranes (92). In guinea pig, the sarcolemmal L-type calcium channels are organized in clusters in the T-tubules (217). In adult rabbit ventricular cells, the L-type calcium channel, the Ryanodine receptor (RYR) and the SR triadin overlap along the T-tubules. In atrial cells, the L-type channels are also found in clusters overlapping with RYR and triadin (47). In rat, the α1D mRNA is found in lung, aorta, and atria, but not in the ventricles of the heart (219).

In all species studied, the calcium channels were found to localize adjacent to junctional sarcoplasmic reticulum, permitting a close coupling of calcium influx to trigger release of calcium from the intracellular stores. There are no studies to our knowledge that specifically probe transmural, apicobasal, or interventricular distribution of the calcium subunits.

Pumps and Exchangers

Na/Ca Exchanger. Three primary isoforms, NCX1, NCX2, and NCX3, of the sodium–calcium exchanger are now cloned (128, 154, 155). NCX1 protein predominates in the rat heart, with little expression of NCX2 and NCX3. Despite several studies showing upregulation of sodium–calcium exchanger expression in response to cardiopathologies that attend or result from increases in intracellular calcium, it is surprising that little is known about the anatomical localization of the three subunits in the normal heart. In all cell types studied, NCXs appear more abundant in the T-tubules (51, 89, 116, 162, 163, 213). During development, NCX proteins are homogenously and maximally expressed during embryogenesis and decline to adult levels after birth (120). Regulation is transcriptional and is modulated by hormonal levels. In human heart, Prestle et al. (163) found no transmural differences in the mRNA level of NCX1 across the left ventricular wall. As previously discussed, in the canine heart, reverse mode I_{Na-Ca} is nearly 30% larger in midmyocardial cells than in epicardial or endocardial cells (Fig. 17–1; 257). No data are yet available relative to the transmural distribution of NCX protein or NCX message in the canine ventricles.

Na/K ATPase. The Na^+-K^+-adenosinetriphosphatase (ATPase) plays a critical role in maintaining intracellular sodium, potassium, and calcium homeostasis in cardiac cells (80). Three isoforms of the α-subunit, α1, α2, and α3, have been described (142, 191) to have different affinities for Na^+ (110, 153) and cardiac glycosides (192, 216). The α1 subunit has a lower affinity for ouabain and a higher affinity for Na^+ than α2, and its transcript is much more abundant in the atrium than in the ventricles in the rat heart (247). The opposite relationship exists for the α2 subunit. At the protein level, the distribution of α1 is uniform in the ventricles and the conduction system; α2 protein is present in ventricular myocytes but its signal is much stronger in the conduction system, with mRNA showing similar distribution densities (249, 250). The α3 protein is also present in regions adjacent to the AV ring and in the conduction system in the rat neonate (248, 250). In the atrium, immunoreactivity for α1 is more intense in the left than in the right, and the subunit is also found in vascular endothelial tissues, along with α2. Conversely, α2 and α3 proteins are not detected in atria, a finding consistent with the lower sensitivity of atrial cells to ouabain. During development, the α3 subunit is downregulated and is gradually replaced by α2 (136, 157), while α1 remains ubiquitous in the rat heart. At the cellular level, the α1 subunit is detected in the sarcolemma, the subsarcolemmal cisternae, and more strongly in the transverse tubules proximal to other mechanisms involved in regulation of calcium homeostasis (122, 201, 202).

In human, the α1 and α3 transcripts are more abundant in the left ventricle than in the right ventricle, a distribution similar to that observed in rat left and right atria (247) and opposite that of α2 (181). In contrast with rat ventricles, α3 mRNA is a major isoform in the human ventricle. These results indicate that subunits with relatively low affinity for Na and high affinity for cardiac glycosides are more likely to be found in tissues of the conduction system, whereas subunits with relatively low affinity for digitalis and high affinity for Na+ are more ubiquitous. To the best of our knowledge, no data are available relative to the transmural, apicobasal, or transseptal distribution of Na/K-ATPase protein or message.

It seems clear that despite great strides in recent years, little is known about the contribution of heterogeneities in the transcription, translation, and expression of ion channels, carriers, and exchangers, to regional heterogeneities of electrical function in the heart.

SIMULATION OF ACTION POTENTIAL HETEROGENEITY

Recent studies by Rudy and co-workers have elegantly simulated the heterogeneity present in ventricular myocardium by varying the ratio of I_{Kr} to I_{Ks} (227). Using the Luo-Rudy (LRd) model, they demonstrated the importance of I_{Ks} density in creating dispersion of repolarization. Cells with reduced I_{Ks} (e.g., M-cells) displayed a long APD and a steep dependence of APD on rate. Accumulation of I_{Ks} activation together with an increase in sodium–calcium exchange current, I_{Na-Ca}, secondary to Na+ accumulation at fast rates, was found to underlie the steep APD-rate relation of the M-cell in the model. Using a simulation of a multicellular fiber, Viswanathan et al. showed that when cells of transmural origin are electrotonically coupled through low-resistance pathways, APD differences are reduced. The results demonstrate a strong dependence of APD heterogeneity on the degree of intercellular coupling even in the normal physiological range. Highly reduced coupling, maximizes APD heterogeneity (227).

DEVELOPMENTAL ASPECTS

At birth, ventricular myocardium is largely homogeneous. The action potential characteristics and morphology of midmyocardial cells are no different from those of epicardial or endocardial cells. The spike-and-dome morphology of the epicardial action potential is generally absent in neonates and appears over the first few months of life, reaching a plateau or quasi-steady state between 10 and 20 weeks of age in the dog (17, 109, 159; Fig. 17–7). The progressive development of the notch parallels the appearance of I_{to}. Age-related changes in the manifestation of the spike and dome have also been described in human atrial (83) and canine Purkinje (167) tissues and rat ventricular (117) cells.

Distinct M-cell behavior is usually not observed until 2–3 months of age in the dog (6) and possibly also in the pig (6, 15, 169). Rodriguez-Sinova and co-workers have shown the absence of a distinct M-cell in the left ventricle of the young pig (1–2 months of age; 169). More recent studies have described the presence of M-cells in the heart of the 4–6 month-old pig (15, 209).

Thus in the neonate, there are no M-cells, epicardial cells, or endocardial cells; the ventricular myocardium is homogeneous. The changes in ionic current density responsible for the transformation of neonatal cells into distinct adult cell types occurs over the first few weeks and months of life in the dog. It is tempting to speculate that these developmental changes in ion channel current play a role in sudden infant death syndrome (SIDS) in infants with the congenital long QT or Brugada syndromes. Recent clinical data provide support for this hypothesis (164, 180).

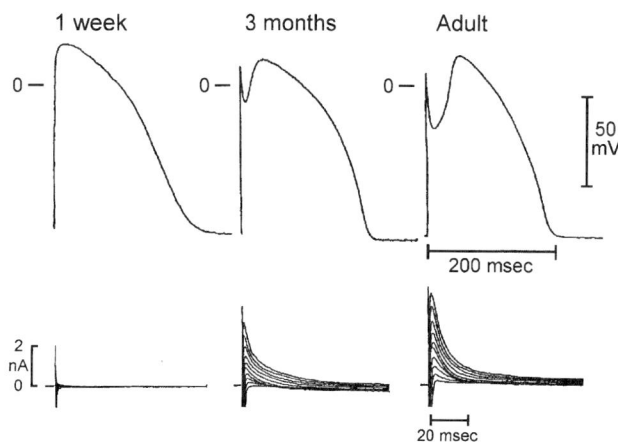

FIG. 17–7. Age-related spike-and-dome morphology and changes in I_{to} in canine ventricular epicardium. Each panel depicts transmembrane activity recorded from right ventricular epicardial tissues (*upper trace*) and transient outward current (*lower trace*) recorded from left ventricular epicardial cells isolated from a neonate (5 days of age; *A*), a young dog (3 months old; *B*), and an adult dog (*C*). BCL = 2000 msec; $[K^+]_o$ = 4 mM. The spike-and-dome configuration of the epicardial action potential and I_{to} density are absent in the neonate, relatively small in the young dog, and most prominent in the adult.

PHYSIOLOGICAL AND CLINICAL IMPLICATIONS

Transmural Distribution of I_{to} and the J Wave

The presence of a prominent action potential notch in epicardium but not endocardium gives rise to a transmural voltage gradient during ventricular activation that manifests as a late delta wave [a small secondary R wave (R') following the QRS] or what is more commonly referred to as a J wave (243) or Osborn wave. The J wave and elevated J point have been described in the ECG of animals and humans for over five decades (98) since Osborn's observation in the early 1950s (158). In humans, the appearance of a prominent J wave in the ECG is considered pathognomonic of hypothermia (55, 71, 78, 220) or hypercalcemia (123, 208). A distinct J wave is commonly observed in the ECG of some animal species including baboons and dogs, under baseline conditions and is greatly amplified under hypothermic conditions (105, 175, 238). An elevated J point is commonly encountered in humans and some animal species under normal conditions. A transmural gradient in the contribution of I_{to} is responsible for the transmural gradient in the magnitude of phase 1 and action potential notch, thought to be responsible for the inscription of the J wave or J point elevation in the ECG (18, 19, 129, 133). Direct evidence in support of the hypothesis that the J wave is caused by a transmural gradient in the magnitude of the I_{to}-mediated action potential notch derives from experiments conducted in the arterially perfused right ventricular wedge preparation (243).

Phase 2 Re-entry as a Mechanism of Extrasystolic Activity

Activation of I_{to} leads to a paradoxical prolongation of APD in canine ventricular tissues (130) and to the traditional abbreviation of APD in ventricular tissues that normally exhibit brief action potentials (e.g., rat; 117). Pathophysiological conditions (e.g., ischemia, metabolic inhibition) and some pharmacological interventions (e.g., I_{Na} or I_{Ca} blockers or I_{K-ATP} activators) cause marked abbreviation of the action potential in canine and feline ventricular cells where I_{to} is prominent.

The presence of a prominent I_{to}-mediated notch predisposes canine ventricular epicardium to all-or-none repolarization and phase 2 re-entry. Under ischemic conditions and in response to a variety of drugs, canine ventricular epicardium exhibits an all-or-none repolarization as a result of the rebalancing of currents flowing at the end of phase 1 of the action potential. Failure of the dome to develop occurs when the outward currents (principally I_{to}) overwhelm the inward currents (chiefly I_{Ca}), resulting in a remarkable (40%–70%) abbreviation of the action potential. Loss of the action potential dome is seldom homogeneous. The action potential dome is usually abolished at some epicardial sites but not others, causing a marked dispersion of repolarization within the epicardium. Conduction of the action potential dome from sites at which it is maintained to sites at which it is abolished can cause local re-excitation of the preparation. This mechanism, termed "phase 2 reentry," produces extrasystolic beats capable of initiating circus movement re-entry (138; Figs. 17–8 and 17–9) Electrical heterogeneity leads to phase 2 re-entry in canine epicardium exposed to (1) K^+ channel openers such as pinacidil (68), (2) sodium channel blockers such as flecainide (125), (3) increased $[Ca^{2+}]_o$ (69), (4) metabolic inhibition (18), and (5) simulated ischemia (138). Block of I_{to} restores electrical homogeneity and abolishes re-entrant activity in all cases.

Phase 2 Re-entry as a Trigger for VT/VF: The Brugada Syndrome

Abnormal J waves have long been linked to idiopathic ventricular fibrillation and the Brugada syndrome (3, 4, 32, 38). The Brugada syndrome is characterized by an ST segment elevation (or exaggerated J wave) in the right precordial leads, V_1 to V_3 (unrelated to ischemia, electrolyte abnormalities, or structural heart disease), a normal QT interval and a high incidence of sudden cardiac death due to ventricular tachycardia or fibrillation (VT/VF) (38). (See also Chapter 19) A right bundle branch block configuration of the ECG is observed in many cases, but not all. Recent data point to similarities between the conditions that predispose to phase 2 re-entry and those that attend the appearance of the Brugada syndrome.

Loss of the action potential dome in epicardium, but not endocardium, would be expected to generate a transmural current that manifests on the ECG as an ST segment elevation like that encountered in patients with the Brugada syndrome (18, 137, 243). Loss of the dome is caused by an outward shift in the balance of currents active during the early phases of the action potential, principally I_{to} and I_{Ca}. Autonomic neurotransmitters like ACH facilitate loss of the action potential dome (131) by suppressing I_{Ca} and/or augmenting potassium current. β-Adrenergic agonists restore the dome by augmenting I_{Ca}. Sodium channel blockers also facilitate loss of the canine right ventricular action potential dome via a negative shift in the voltage at which phase 1 begins (124, 125). These findings are consistent with clinical reports of accentuation of the ST segment elevation in patients with the Brugada syndrome following vagal maneuvers or administration of class I antiarrhythmic agents, as well as normaliza-

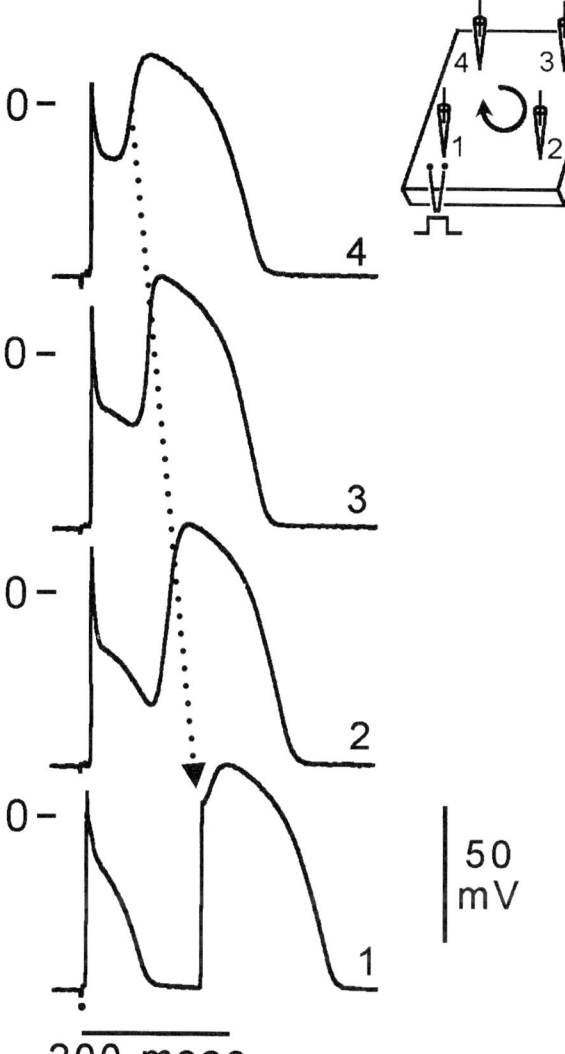

FIG. 17–8. Phase 2 re-entry. Re-entrant activity induced by exposure of a canine ventricular epicardial preparation (0.7 cm²) to simulated ischemia. Microelectrode recordings were obtained from four sites as shown in the schematic (*upper right*). After 35 min of ischemia, the action potential dome develops normally at site 4, but not at sites 1, 2, or 3. The dome then propagates in a clockwise direction reexciting sites 3, 2, and 1 with progressive delays, thus generating a closely coupled re-entrant extrasystole (156 msec) at site 1. In this example of phase 2 re-entry, propagation of the dome occurs in a direction opposite that of phase 0, a mechanism akin to reflection. BCL = 700 msec. [Modified from Lukas and Antzelevitz (138), with permission.]

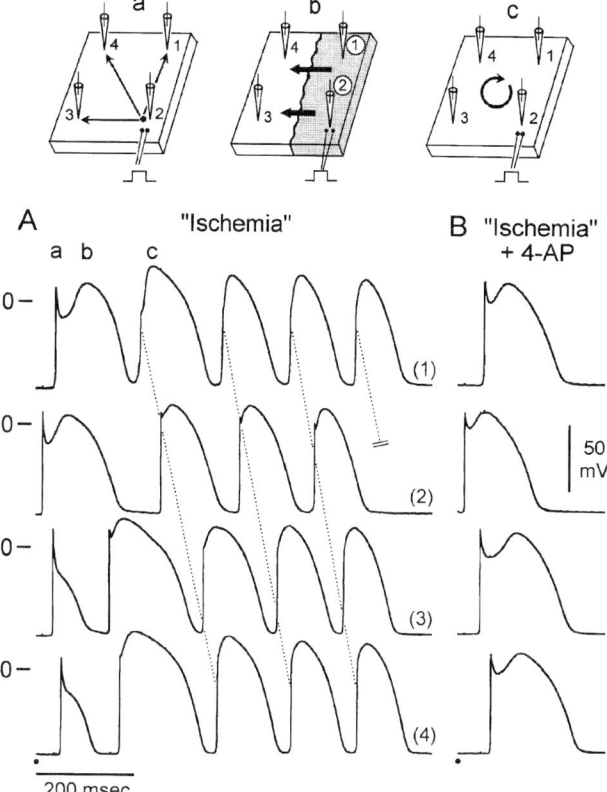

FIG. 17–9. Phase 2 re-entrant extrasystole triggers circus movement re-entry. *A:* Exposure of a relatively large canine right ventricular epicardial sheet (6.3 cm²) to simulated ischemia results in loss of the dome at sites 3 and 4 but not at sites 1 and 2 (BCL = 1100 msec). Conduction of the basic beat proceeds normally from the stimulation site (site 2; see *schematic a*). Propagation of the action potential dome from the right half of the preparation caused reexcitation of the left half via a phase 2 re-entry mechanism (see *schematic b*). The extrasystolic beat generated by phase 2 re-entry then initiates a run of tachycardia that is sustained for 4 additional cycles via typical circus movement re-entry. The proposed re-entrant path is shown in *schematic c*. Note that phase 2 re-entry provides an activation front roughly perpendicular to that of the basic beat. This type of crossfield activation has previously been shown to predispose to the development of vortex-like re-entry in isolated epicardial sheets. *B:* Recorded after addition of 1 mM 4-aminopyridine (4-AP), an inhibitor of the transient outward current. In the continued presence of ischemia, 4-AP restored the dome at all epicardial recording sites within 3 min. Thus electrical heterogeneity was restored and all re-entrant activity abolished. [Modified from Lukas and Antzelevitz (138), with permission.]

tion of the ST segment elevation following doses of β-adrenergic agents (146, 243). The appearance of an ST segment elevation only in the right precordial leads in Brugada patients is consistent with the finding that loss of the action potential dome is much more commonly encountered in right than in left canine ventricular epicardium (18, 137). The Brugada syndrome is recognized as a right ventricular disease because I_{to} density is intrinsically much greater in right ventricular epicardium, than on the left.

These observations point to a depressed right ventricular epicardial action potential dome as the basis for the ST segment elevation and to phase 2 re-entry as a trigger for episodes of ventricular tachycardia and fibrillation in patients with the Brugada syndrome and other syndromes associated with ST segment elevation. Direct evidence in support of this hypothesis was recently provided in an arterially-perfused canine right ventricular experimental model of the Brugada syndrome (Fig. 17–10; 245). The data support the hypothesis that ST segment elevation similar to that observed in patients with the Brugada syndrome results from accentuation of action potential notch or loss of the action potential dome in right ventricular epicardium, where I_{to} is most prominent. Initiation of VT/VF under these conditions occurs via phase 2 re-entry secondary to heterogeneous loss of the epicardial action potential dome (245). The VT and VF generated in these preparations is often polymorphic, resembling a very rapid form of torsade de pointes. This activity may be mechanistically related to the migrating spiral wave shown to generate a pattern resembling TdP associated with a normal or long QT interval

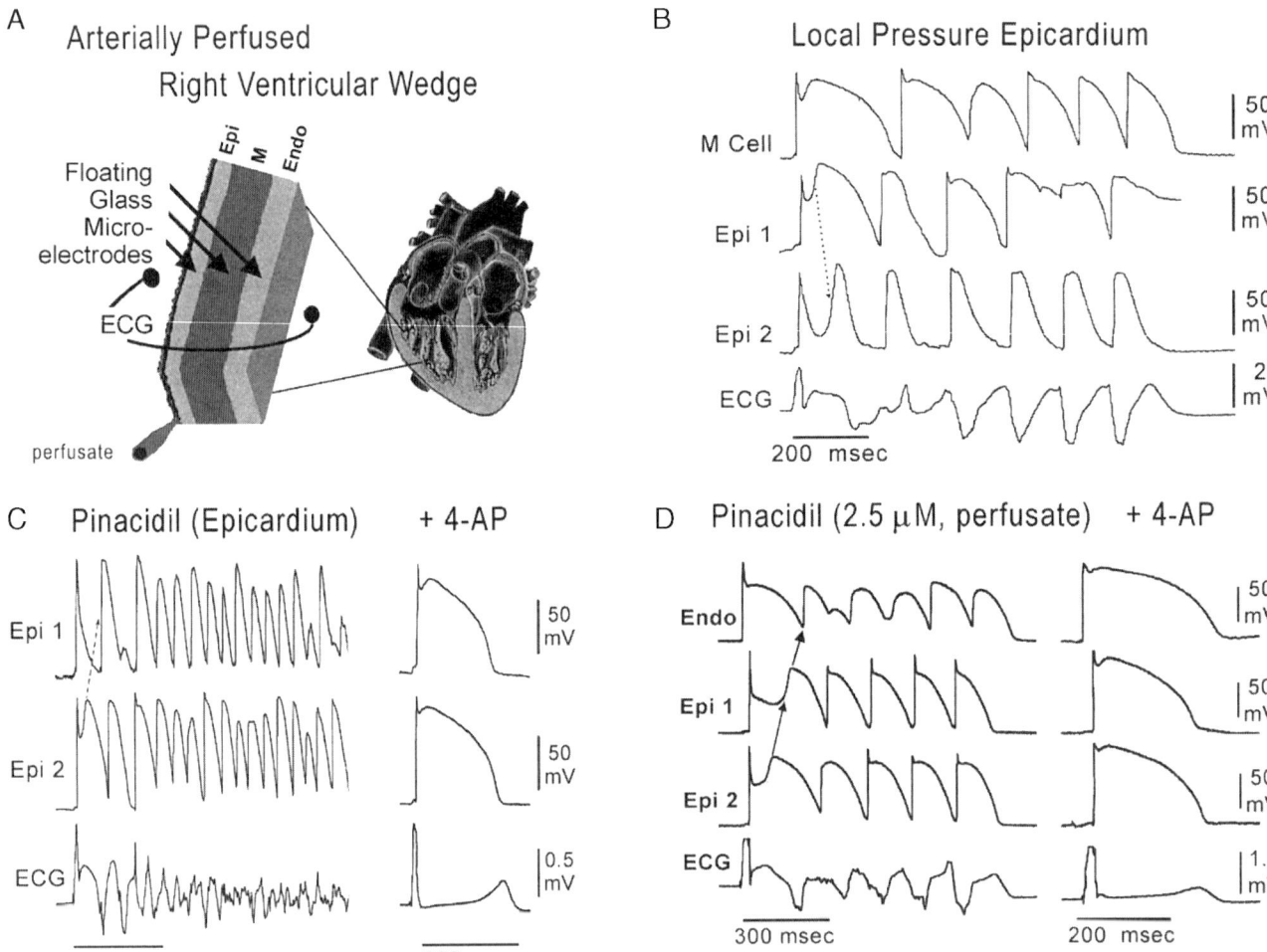

FIG. 17–10. ECG and arrhythmias with typical features of the Brugada syndrome recorded from canine right ventricular wedge preparations A: Schematic of arterially perfused right ventricular wedge preparation. B: Pressure—induced phase 2 re-entry and VT. Shown are transmembrane action potentials simultaneously recorded from two epicardial sites (Epi 1 and Epi 2) and one M region (M) site, together with a transmural ECG. Local application of pressure near Epi 2 results in loss of the action potential dome at that site but not at the Epi 1 or M sites. The dome at Epi 1 then re-excites Epi 2, giving rise to a phase 2 re-entrant extrasystole that triggers a short run of ventricular tachycardia. Note the ST segment elevation due to loss of the action potential dome in a segment of epicardium. C: Polymorphic VT/VF induced by local application of the potassium channel opener pinacidil (10 μM) to the epicardial surface of the wedge. Action potentials from two epicardial sites (Epi 1 and Epi 2) and a transmural ECG were simultaneously recorded. Loss of the dome at Epi 1 but not Epi 2 creates a marked dispersion of repolarization, giving rise to a phase 2 re-entrant extrasystole. The extrasystolic beat then triggers a long episode of ventricular fibrillation (22 sec). Right panel: Addition of 4-aminopyridine (4-AP. 2 mM), a specific I_{to} blocker, to the perfusate restored the action potential dome at Epi 1, thus reducing dispersion of repolarization and suppressing all arrhythmic activity. BCL = 2000 msec. D: Phase 2 re-entry gives rise to VT following addition of pinacidil (2.5 μM) to the coronary perfusate. Transmembrane action potentials form two epicardial sites (Epi 1 and Epi 2) and one endocardial site (Endo), as well as a transmural ECG were simultaneously recorded. Right panel: 4-AP (1 mM) markedly reduces the magnitude of the action potential notch in epicardium, thus restoring the action potential dome throughout the preparation and abolishing all arrhythmic activity. [D is from Yan and Antzelevitch (245), with permission.]

(25, 160). The proposed cellular mechanism is summarized in Figure 17–11.

Because a prominent I_{to} is pivotal to this arrhythmogenic mechanism, agents that inhibit I_{to}, including 4-aminopyridine, quinidine, and disopyramide are effective in restoring the action potential dome, thus restoring electrical homogeneity and aborting all arrhythmic activity (245). Thus class I antiarrhythmic agents that block I_{Na} but not I_{to} (procainamide and ajmaline) appear to exacerbate the Brugada syndrome, whereas those with actions to block both I_{Na} and I_{to} (quinidine and disopyramide) can exert an ameliorative effect.

The applicability of the phenomena observed in the canine heart to humans requires that action potentials in human epicardium exhibit a pronounced I_{to}-mediated spike-and-dome morphology. Several reports indicate that this is the case (151, 239). However, I_{to} reactivation is faster in human epicardium than in the dog, suggesting that electrical heterogeneity and phase 2 re-entry might occur over a much wider range of heart rates and be less influenced by heart rate in the human ventricle.

Further evidence in support of the hypothesis that the Brugada syndrome is a primary electrical disease derives from the recent demonstration by Chen et al. (52) that this syndrome is linked to a mutation in an ion channel gene (SCN5A) located on chromosome 3. Defects in SCN5A linked to the Brugada syndrome include frameshift and deletion mutations that cause failure of the channel to express (thus importantly reducing I_{Na} density) and missense mutations that shift the voltage- and time-dependence of I_{Na} activation, inactivation, or reactivation (52, 75). In the case of one missense mutation (T1620M), inactivation of I_{Na} was importantly accelerated (75), leaving I_{to} largely unopposed. Mathematical simulations confirmed that these changes could lead to all-or-none repolarization at the end of phase 1 and loss of the action potential dome, thus providing the substrate for the Brugada syndrome (Fig. 17–12). Interestingly, this change in the function of the sodium channel was observed at physiological temperatures, but not at room temperature typically used in studies of function in heterologous expression systems. These results suggest caution in the interpretation of function studies conducted at room temperature. The data also point to the possibility that patients with the Brugada syndrome may be more at risk during a febrile state.

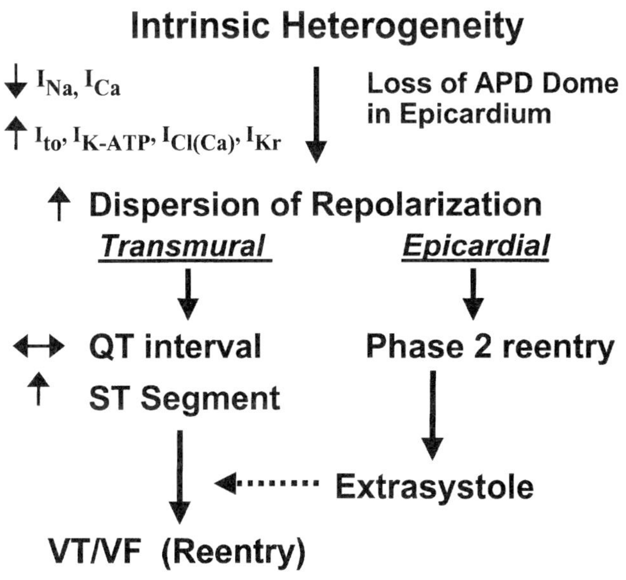

These findings implicating SCN5A are concordant with the demonstration that inhibition of the sodium channel is among the easiest means to induce ST segment elevation and phase 2 re-entry in isolated tissue preparations (124, 125). Gene mutations that diminish the density or conductance of the sodium channel are therefore prime candidates. Such mutations would also be consistent with the conduction disturbances that sometimes accompany the Brugada syndrome (143).

In addition to SCN5A, gene mutations that alter the intensity or kinetics of I_{to}, I_{Kr}, I_{K-ATP}, I_{Ca}, or $I_{Cl(Ca)}$, so as to increase the activity of the outward currents and/or diminish that of the inward currents are candidates for the Brugada syndrome. Other candidates include genes encoding for autonomic receptors. Such mutations can cause a direct modulation of ion current density and/or alter the expression of channels in the membrane (e.g., sympathetic control of I_{to}). In all cases, intrinsic heterogeneity during the early phases of the action potential would be expected to increase.

Early Repolarization Syndrome

The early repolarization syndrome (ERS), generally regarded as a benign syndrome, is characterized by an upward ST segment concavity ending in a positive T wave in leads V_2–$V_{4(5)}$. Clinical interest in ERS has been rekindled by similarities with the electrocardiographic manifestations of the highly arrhythmogenic Brugada syndrome and the potential for misdiagnosis. The benign nature of the syndrome may relate to development of a transmural voltage gradient caused by depression,

FIG. 17–11. Proposed mechanism for the Brugada syndrome. A shift in the balance of currents serves to amplify existing heterogeneities by causing loss of the action potential dome at some epicardial sites, but not endocardial sites. A vulnerable window develops as a result of the dispersion of repolarization and refractoriness within epicardium as well as across the wall. Epicardial dispersion leads to the development of phase 2 re-entry, which provides the extrasystole that captures the vulnerable window and initiates VT/VF via a circus movement re-entry mechanism.

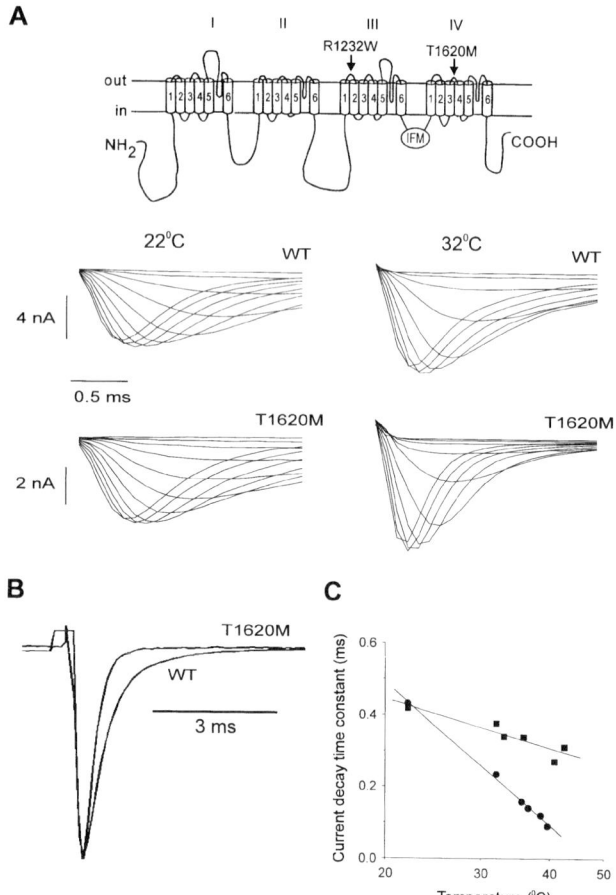

FIG. 17–12. Whole-cell current for wild-type (WT) and Brugada syndrome mutant (T1620M) in transiently transfected TSA201 cells at room temperature (22°C) and 32°C. A: The cartoon depicts the location of the missense mutations R1232W and T1620M previously described by Chen et al. (52). Current recordings obtained at different test potentials from −70 to −25 mV (32°C) and −65 to −20 (22°C) in increments of 5 mV from a holding potential of −120 mV for four representative cells. B: Current decay of T1620M at 32°C. Representative current recordings from WT and T1620M were elicited by a 20 msec depolarizing pulse to a test potential of 10 mV from a holding potential of −140 mV, normalized to the peak inward current and superimposed. C: WT decay time constant (square) is less sensitive to temperature in the physiological range. Cells were maintained at −80 mV and pulsed at 0 mV for 10 msec at temperatures between 22°C and 42°C. Current decay were fitted by a sum of two exponential functions. The fast time constant was plotted against the temperature (log scale) for WT and T1620M (filled circles). Each symbol represents a different cell. [Modified from Dumaine et al. (75), with permission.]

but not loss, of the epicardial action potential dome. Because final repolarization is not affected, a vulnerable window does not develop. In experimental models, the ECG signature of ERS can be converted to that of the Brugada syndrome, raising the possibility that ERS may not be as benign as generally thought, and that under certain conditions known to predispose to ST-segment elevation (including acute ischemia), ERS patients may be at greater risk. Further clinical and experimental data are required to test these hypotheses. The characteristics of ERS need to be more fully delineated within the framework of what has been learned about the Brugada syndrome in recent years. It is tempting to speculate that similar mechanisms may be involved in the two syndromes, but that a marked dispersion of repolarization occurs in the Brugada syndrome because of the intrinsically higher level of I_{to} in RV (V1–V3) than in septal or LV regions (V2–V5), which permits loss of the action potential dome at sites with intrinsically large I_{to}. It follows that ERS may be more likely to occur when the balance of currents in the early phases of the action potential is shifted outward (due to a decrease in inward currents or an increase in outward currents) in hearts with an intrinsically weak I_{to}. A similar shift in outward current in hearts with intrinsically prominent I_{to} might be expected to display characteristics of the Brugada syndrome rather than ERS.

Ischemia

It is noteworthy that the electrocardiographic manifestations of the Brugada syndrome are similar to those encountered during ischemia. As such, the Brugada syndrome may represent a stable (nonischemic) model of the cellular changes that occur during acute ischemic injury as well as of other syndromes associated with an ST segment elevation. The presence of an additional outward current (i.e., I_{to}) in ventricular epicardium predisposes to loss of the action dome during ischemia, leading to amplification of transmural heterogeneities and the development of phase 2 re-entry and VT/VF.

Role of Transmural Heterogeneity in Inscription of the Electrocardiographic T Wave

M-cells have been shown to play a determining role in the inscription of the electrocardiographic T wave. Data from the arterially perfused wedge have provided new insights into the cellular basis of the T wave showing that currents flowing down voltage gradients on either side of the M region are in large part responsible for the T wave (Figs. 17–13 and 17–14). (244) The interplay between these opposing currents establishes the height and width of the T wave as well as the degree to which either the ascending or descending limb of the T wave is interrupted, leading to a bifurcated or notched appearance. The voltage gradients result from more positive plateau potentials in the M region than in epicardium or endocardium, and from differences in the time-course of phase 3 of the action potential of the three predominant ventricular cell types. Under

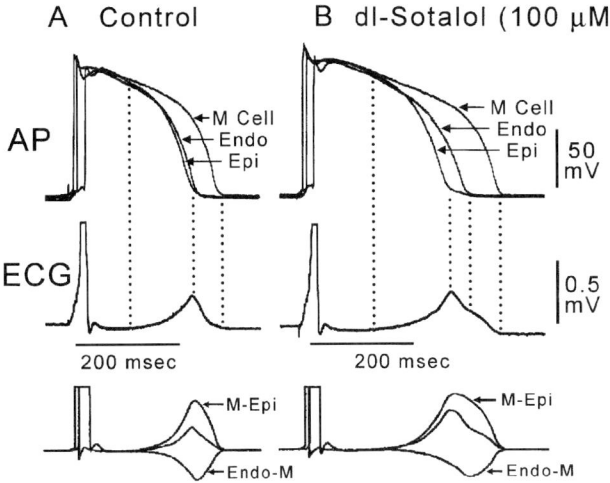
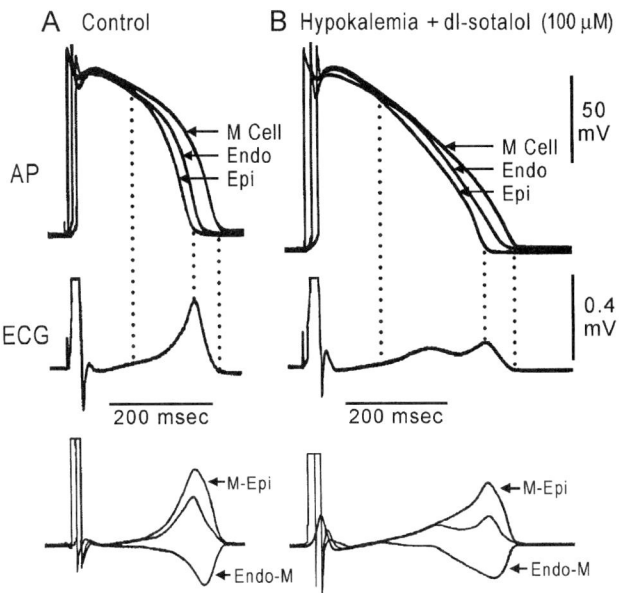

FIG. 17–13. Voltage gradients on either side of the M region are responsible for inscription of the electrocardiographic T wave. *Top:* Action potentials simultaneously recorded from endocardial, epicardial and M region sites of an arterially perfused canine left ventricular wedge preparation. *Middle:* ECG recorded across the wedge. *Bottom:* Computed voltage differences between the epicardium and M region action potentials ($\Delta V_{M\text{-}Epi}$) and between the M region and endocardium responses ($\Delta V_{Endo\text{-}M}$). If these traces are representative of the opposing voltage gradients on either side of the M region, responsible for inscription of the T wave, then the weighted sum of the two traces should yield a trace (*middle trace in bottom grouping*) resembling the ECG, which it does. The voltage gradients are weighted to account for differences in tissue resistivity between M and Epi and Endo and M regions, thus yielding the opposing currents flowing on either side of the M region. *A:* Under control conditions, the T wave begins when the plateau of epicardial action potential separates from that of the M-cell. As epicardium repolarizes, the voltage gradient between epicardium and the M region continues to grow, giving rise to the ascending limb of the T wave. The voltage gradient between the M region and the epicardium ($\Delta V_{M\text{-}Epi}$) reaches a peak when the epicardium is fully repolarized; this marks the peak of the T wave. On the other end of the ventricular wall, the endocardial plateau deviates from that of the M-cell, generating an opposing voltage gradient ($\Delta V_{Endo\text{-}M}$) and corresponding current that limits the amplitude of the T wave and contributes to the initial part of the descending limb of the T wave. The voltage gradient between the endocardium and the M region reaches a peak when the endocardium is fully repolarized. The gradient continues to decline as the M-cells repolarize. All gradients are extinguished when the longest M cells are fully repolarized. *B:* d-sotalol (100 μM) prolongs the action potential of the M-cell more than those of the epicardial and endocardial cells, thus widening the T wave and prolonging the QT interval. The greater separation of epicardial and endocardial repolarization times also gives rise to a notch in the descending limb of the T wave. Once again, the T wave begins when the plateau of epicardial action potential diverges from that of the M-cell. The same relationships as described for panel A are observed during the remainder of the T wave. The d-sotalol–induced increase in dispersion of repolarization across the wall is accompanied by a corresponding increase in the $T_{peak}\text{-}T_{end}$ interval in the pseudo-ECG. [Modified from Yan and Antzelevitch (244), with permission.]

FIG. 17–14. Transient shift of voltage gradients on either side of the M region results in T wave bifurcation. The format is the same as in Figure 17–13. All traces were simultaneously recorded form an arterially perfused left ventricular wedge preparation. *A:* Control. *B:* In the presence of hypokalemia ($[K^+]_o = 1.5$ mM), the I_{Kr} blocker dl-sotalol (100 μM) prolongs the QT interval and produces a bifurcation of the T wave, a morphology some authors refer to as T-U complex. The rate of repolarization of phase 3 of the action potential is slowed, giving rise to smaller opposing transmural currents that cross over, producing a low-amplitude bifid T wave. Initially the voltage gradient between the epicardium and M regions (M-Epi) is greater than that between endocardium and M region (Endo-M). When endocardium pulls away from the M cell, the opposing gradient (Endo-M) increases, interrupting the ascending limb of the T wave. Predominance of the M-Epi gradient is restored as the epicardial response continues to repolarize and the Epi-M gradients increases, thus resuming the ascending limb of the T wave. Full repolarization of epicardium marks the peak of the T wave. Repolarization of both endocardium and the M region contribute importantly to the descending limb. BCL = 1000 msec. [Modified from Yan and Antzelevitch (244), with permission.]

baseline and long QT conditions, the epicardial response is the earliest to repolarize, and the M-cell action potential is the last. Full repolarization of the epicardial action potential is coincident with peak of the T wave, and repolarization of the M-cells coincides with the end of the T wave. The duration of the M-cell action potential determines the duration of the QT interval under a wide variety of conditions in which the QT interval can be altered, including changes in pacing rate, prematurity, alterations in $[K^+]_o$, and exposure to APD-prolonging drugs. Under these conditions, the T_{peak}–T_{end} interval provides an index of transmural dispersion of repolarization, which may prove to be a valuable prognostic tool (7, 244), as recently reported by Lubinski et al. (135).

Previous studies have suggested that apicobasal re-

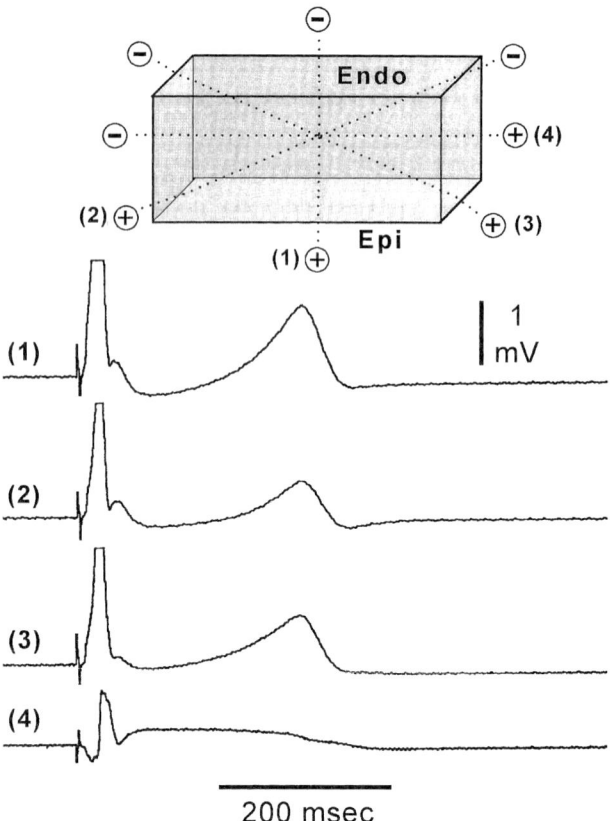

FIG. 17-15. Contribution of transmural vs. apicobasal and anterior-posterior gradients to the registration of the T wave. The four ECG traces were simultaneously recorded at 0°, 45°, −45°, and 90° (apicobasal) angles relative to the transmural axis of an arterially perfused left ventricular wedge preparation. Inscription of the T wave is largely the result of voltage gradients along the transmural axis. [Modified from Yan and Antzelevitch (244) with permission.]

polarization gradients measured along the epicardial surface may play a role in the registration of the T wave (57). In contrast, more recent studies involving the perfused wedge suggest little or no contribution principally because the ECG recorded along the apicobasal axis fails to display a T wave (Fig. 17–15; 156, 244). These findings suggest that in this part of the canine left ventricular wall (anterior, mid-apicobasal) the inscription of the T wave is largely the result of voltage gradients along the transmural axis.

Role of Transmural Heterogeneity in Inscription of the U Wave

A number of interesting theories have been advanced to explain the cellular basis for the U wave. The most popular ascribes the U wave to delayed repolarization of the His-Purkinje system (233). The small mass of the specialized conduction system is difficult to reconcile with the sometimes very large U wave deflections reported in the literature, especially in cases of acquired and congenital long QT syndrome (LQTS). It has previously been suggested that the M-cells, more abundant in mass and possessing delayed repolarization characteristics similar to those of Purkinje fibers, may be responsible for the inscription of the pathophysiological U wave. (13) More recent findings derived from the wedge clearly indicate that what many clinicians refer to as an accentuated or inverted U wave is not a U wave at all, but rather a component of the T wave whose descending or ascending limb (especially during hypokalemia) is interrupted (Fig. 17–14; 182, 244). A transient reversal in current flow across the wall due to shifting voltage gradients between epicardium and the M region and endocardium and the M region appear to underlie these phenomena. The data suggest that the "pathophysiological U wave" that develops under conditions of acquired or congenital LQTS is part of the T wave and that the various hump morphologies represent different levels of interruption of the ascending limb of the T wave, arguing for use of the term "T2" in place of "U" to describe these events, as previously suggested by Lehmann et al. (126, 244).

What then is responsible for the normal U wave, the very small but distinct deflection following the T wave? The repolarization of the His–Purkinje system as previously suggested by Watanabe and co-workers (233) remains a most plausible hypothesis. Repolarization of the Purkinje system is temporally aligned with the expected appearance of the U wave in the perfused wedge preparation (Fig. 17–16; 244). The lack of a U wave in the wedge is likely related to a low density of the Purkinje system in the dog. A test of this hypothesis awaits the availability of an experimental model displaying a prominent U wave.

Indirect support for the hypothesis derives from the recent finding that isoproterenol-induced changes in the repolarization of Purkinje fibers parallel those of the U wave. (43). In healthy humans, isoproterenol abbreviates both QT and QU intervals, whereas in LQT1 patients (defective I_{Ks}) isoproterenol remarkably prolongs the QT interval but abbreviates the QU interval (252). Experimental studies involving canine left ventricular M cell preparations and Purkinje fibers demonstrate that isoproterenol abbreviates the action potential of both cell types under normal conditions, but that under conditions mimicking LQT1 (use of chromanol 293B to block I_{Ks}) isoproterenol abbreviates the Purkinje fiber action potential, but markedly prolongs that of the M-cell (43). The isoproterenol-induced changes in Purkinje APD parallel those of the QU interval, thus providing support for the hypothesis that repolarization of the Purkinje system is responsible for the inscription of the U wave.

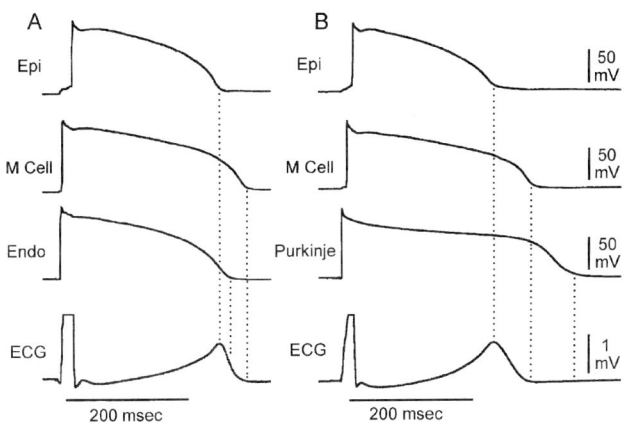

FIG. 17-16. Correlation of transmembrane and electrocardiographic activity. Transmembrane potentials and a transmural ECG recorded from two different arterially perfused canine left ventricular wedge preparations. *A:* Action potentials from epicardial (Epi), midmyocardial (M), and endocardial (Endo) sites were simultaneously recorded using floating glass microelectrodes. A transmural ECG was recorded concurrently across the bath. *B:* Action potentials from epicardium (Epi), midmyocardium (M), and subendocardial Purkinje were recorded simultaneously together with a transmural ECG. In both cases, repolarization of epicardium is coincident with the peak of the T wave of the ECG, whereas repolarization of the M-cells is coincident with the end of the T wave. The endocardial APD is intermediate (*A*). Although repolarization of the Purkinje fiber occurs after that of the M-cell (*B*), it does not register on the ECG. BCL = 2000 msec. [Modified from yan and Antzelevitch (244), with permission.]

Role of Transmural Heterogeneity in the Long QT Syndrome

The long QT syndrome (LQTS) is characterized by the appearance of long QT intervals in the ECG and atypical polymorphic ventricular tachycardias displaying features of torsade de pointes (149, 176, 253) (see also chapter 19) As previously discussed, electrical heterogeneity secondary to the presence of M-cells within the ventricular wall contributes to the manifestation of both normal and abnormal T waves in the ECG (13, 16, 18, 19, 139, 182, 244, 246). Preferential prolongation of APD in cells in the M region appears to underlie LQTS, contributing to the development of long QT intervals, abnormal T waves, and TdP. Evidence in support of these hypotheses has been advanced using the arterially perfused wedge preparation (20, 182, 183, 244, 246). The wedge model is capable of developing and sustaining a variety of arrhythmias, including TdP.

Genetic linkage studies have identified several forms of the congenital LQTS caused by mutations in ion channel genes located on chromosomes 3, 7, 11, and 21, (62, 207, 230, 231) responsible for defects in the sodium channel (*SCN5A, LQT3;* 231), the rapidly activating delayed rectifier channel (I_{Kr}) (HERG, LQT2, or KCNE2, LQT6; 1;174), and the slowly activating delayed rectifier channel (I_{Ks}) (KvLQT1, LQT1, or KCNE1, LQT5), respectively (28, 173, 207). Recent studies employing the wedge have developed experimental models to assess the contribution of electrical heterogeneity across the ventricular wall to the manifestation of the T wave under conditions of "acquired" LQTS mimicking the genetic defects that have been linked to the congenital syndrome (Fig. 17-17).

I_{Ks} block with Chromanol 293B was used to mimic LQT1, and the β-adrenergic agonist isoproterenol was used to assess β-adrenergic influence. I_{Ks} block alone produces a homogeneous prolongation of repolarization across the ventricular wall but does not induce arrhythmias. The addition of isoproterenol leads to abbreviation of epicardial and endocardial APD with little or no change in the APD of the M-cell, resulting in a marked augmentation of TDR and the development of spontaneous and stimulation-induced TdP. (183) These cellular changes generally give rise to a broad-based T wave and a long QT interval characteristic of LQT1. The development of TdP in this model is exquisitely sensitive to β-adrenergic stimulation consistent with the high sensitivity of congenital LQTS, LQT1 in particular, to sympathetic stimulation (61, 149, 176, 178, 253).

I_{Kr} block with d-sotalol was used to mimic LQT2 and the most common acquired (drug-induced) form of LQTS. In this experimental model, a greater prolongation of the M-cell action potential and slowing of phase 3 of the action potential of all three cell types results in a low-amplitude T wave, long QT interval, large transmural dispersion of repolarization, and the development of spontaneous as well as stimulation-induced TdP. The addition of hypokalemia gives rise to low-amplitude T waves with a deeply notched or bifurcated appearance, similar to those commonly seen in patients with the LQT2 syndrome (182, 244). Isoproterenol further exaggerates transmural dispersion of repolarization, thus increasing the incidence of TdP (127, 185).

Augmentation of the late I_{Na} with ATX-II was used to mimic the LQT3 syndrome (76, 182). ATX-II markedly prolongs the QT interval, delays the onset of the T wave—in some cases also widening it—and causes a sharp rise in transmural dispersion of repolarization as a result of a greater prolongation of the APD of the M-cell (Fig. 17-8F). The differential effect of ATX-II to prolong the M-cell is likely due to the presence of a larger late sodium current in the M-cell.(79) ATX-II produces a marked delay in onset of the T wave because of a relatively large effect of the drug on epicardial and endocardial APD, consistent with the late-appearing T wave pattern and long isoelectric ST

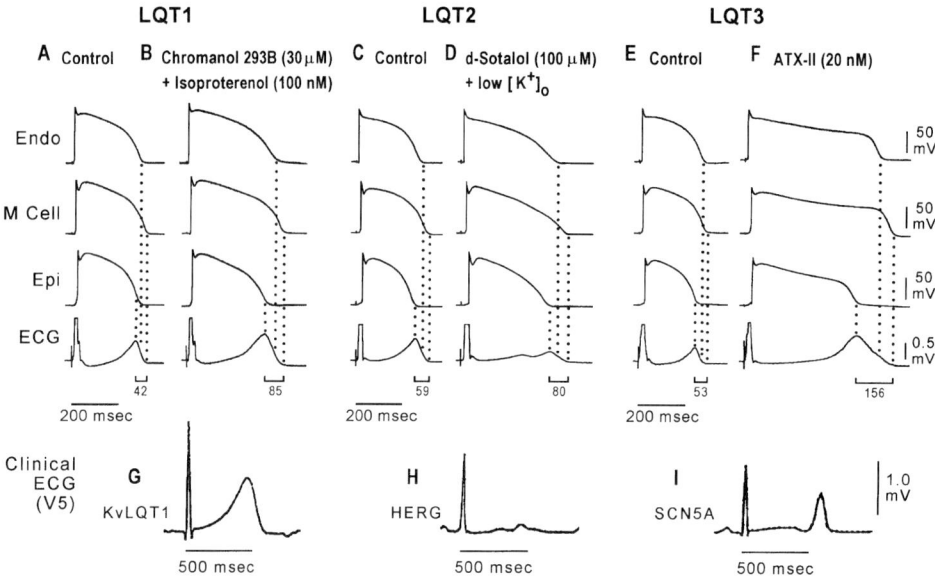

FIG. 17-17. Transmembrane action potentials and transmural electrocardiograms (ECG) in control and LQT1 (A and B), LQT2 (C and D), and LQT3 (E and F) models of LQTS (arterially perfused canine left ventricular wedge preparations), and clinical ECG (lead V_5) of patients with LQT1 (*KvLQT1* defect) (G), LQT2 (*HERG* defect) (H), and LQT3 (*SCN5A* defect) (I) syndromes. Isoproterenol + chromanol 293B—an I_{Ks} blocker, d-sotalol + low $[K^+]_o$, and ATX-II—an agent that slows inactivation of late I_{Na} are used to mimic the LQT1, LQT2 and LQT3 syndromes, respectively. A–F depict action potentials simultaneously recorded from endocardial (Endo), M, and epicardial (Epi) sites, together with a transmural ECG. BCL = 2000 msec. In all cases, the peak of the T wave in the ECG is coincident with the repolarization of the epicardial action potential, whereas the end of the T wave is coincident with the repolarization of the M-cell action potential. Repolarization of the endocardial cell is intermediate between that of the M-cell and epicardial cell. Transmural dispersion of repolarization across the ventricular wall, defined as the difference in the repolarization time between M-cells and epicardial cells, is denoted below the ECG traces. B: Isoproterenol (100 nM) in the presence of chromanol 293B (30 μM) produced a preferential prolongation of the APD of the M, resulting in an accentuated transmural dispersion of repolarization and broad-based T waves as commonly seen in LQT1 patients (G). D: d-Sotalol (100 μM) in the presence of low potassium (2 mM) gives rise to low-amplitude T waves with a notched or bifurcated appearance due to a very significant slowing of repolarization as commonly seen in LQT2 patients (H). F: ATX-II (20 nM) markedly prolongs the QT interval, widens the T wave, and causes a sharp rise in the dispersion of repolarization. ATX-II also produced a marked delay in onset of the T wave due to relatively large effects of the drug on the APD of epicardium and endocardium, consistent with the late-appearing T wave pattern observed in LQT3 patients (I). [Modified from Shimizu and Antzelevitch (182, 183), with permission.]

segment observed in patients with the LQT3 syndrome. Concordant with the clinical presentation of LQT3, the wedge model displays a steep rate dependence of the QT interval and develops TdP at slow rates. Unexpectedly, in the ATX-II model of LQT3, β-adrenergic stimulation with isoproterenol, *reduces* transmural dispersion of repolarization by abbreviating the APD of the M-cell more than that of epicardium or endocardium. Transmural dispersion of repolarization is thus reduced, as is the incidence of TdP. While the β-adrenergic blocker propranolol is protective in LQT1 and LQT2 wedge models, it exerts opposite effects in LQT3, acting to amplify transmural dispersion and to promote TdP (127, 185). Table 17–8 summarizes the distinctions in the characteristics and pharmacology of the three LQTS models. The electrocardiographic T wave patterns described are similar to those observed in patients with the respective genotype of the disease. Exceptions to these distinctive genotype-specific T wave morphologies are encountered in the wedge, as they are in the clinic.

Torsade de Pointes

The arrhythmia most commonly encountered in congenital and acquired LQTS is TdP, an atypical polymorphic ventricular tachycardia. TdP generally develops in patients receiving an I_{Kr} blocker, such as sotalol or quinidine, especially in the presence of hypokalemia and slow heart rates or long pauses. These conditions

TABLE 17-8. *Characteristics of LQT1, LQT2, and LQT3 Models of LQTS in Canine Arterially Perfused Left Ventricular Wedge Preparations*

	LQT1	LQT2	LQT3
ECG T wave pattern	Broad-based T wave	Low amplitude T wave, notched or bifurcated appearance	Late-appearing T wave
Rate dependence of QT interval	++	++	+++++
Sensitivity to catecholamines	+++++ (Sustained ↑ in TDR)	+++ (Transient ↑ in TDR)	— (↓ in TDR)
Torsade de pointes (in the clinic)	Exercise-related	Startle Alarm Clock(240)	Rest/Sleep
Effectiveness of β-blockers	+++++	+++	—
Effectiveness of Na+ channel blockers	+++	++++	+++++

TDR = transmural dispersion of repolarization.
+Small/low; +++++large/high.

are similar to those under which quinidine and d-sotalol induce EADs and triggered activity in isolated Purkinje fibers and M-cells, suggesting a role for EAD-induced triggered activity in the genesis of TdP. An EAD-induced extrasystole is believed to be responsible for the premature beat that initiates TdP, but the maintenance of the arrhythmia appears to be due to a circus movement re-entry mechanism (2, 5, 16, 16, 17, 20, 25, 67, 81, 82, 86, 160, 182, 183, 188, 189, 215, 237, 244). TdP develops spontaneously in all three wedge models and can be readily induced by introduction of a single premature beat when TDP does not occur spontaneously (Fig. 17–18). The triggering extrastimulus is most effective when applied to the site of earliest repolarization, usually on the epicardial surface.

The available data provide support for the hypothesis outlined in Fig. 17–19. The hypothesis presumes the presence of electrical heterogeneity, principally in the form of transmural dispersion of repolarization, under baseline conditions. This intrinsic heterogeneity is amplified by agents that reduce net repolarizing current via a reduction in I_{Kr} or I_{Ks} or augmentation of late I_{Ca} or late I_{Na} or by ion channel mutations that affect these currents and are responsible for the various forms of LQTS. I_{Kr} blockers and LQT2 mutations or late I_{Na} promoters and LQT3 mutations produce a preferential prolongation of the M-cell action potential. As a consequence, the QT interval prolongs and is accompanied by a dramatic increase in transmural dispersion of repolarization, which creates a vulnerable window for the development of re-entry. The reduction in net repolarizing current also predisposes to the development of EAD-induced triggered activity in M-cells and Purkinje cells, which provide the extrasystole that triggers TdP when it falls within the vulnerable period. β-

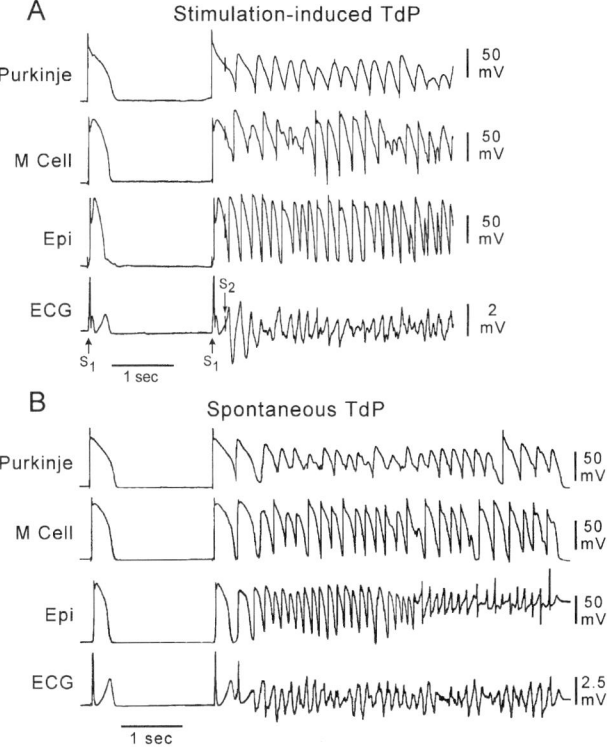

FIG. 17–18. Spontaneous and stimulation-induced polymorphic ventricular tachycardia with features of torsade de pointes (TdP). *A:* Stimulation-induced TdP in a LV wedge preparation pretreated with dl-sotalol (100 μmol/liter). S1-S1 = 2000 msec; S1-S2 = 250 msec. S2 was applied to epicardium. *B:* Spontaneous TdP in a preparation pretreated with dl-sotalol (100 μmol/liter). BCL = 2000 msec. A spontaneous premature beat with a coupling interval of 348 msec, likely originating from subendocardial Purkinje system, initiates an episode of torsade de pointes.

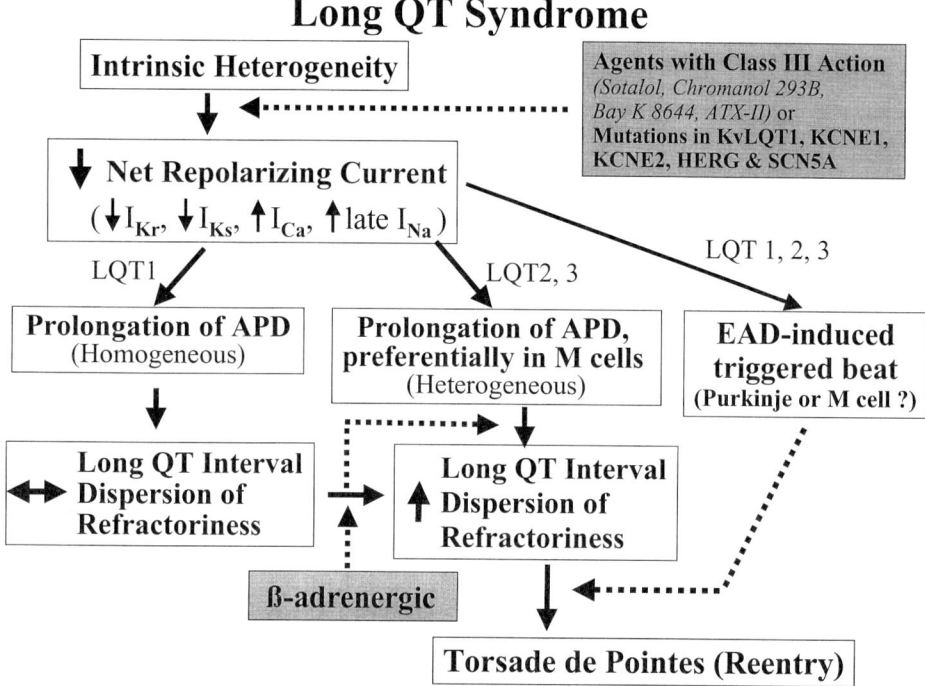

FIG. 17–19. Proposed cellular mechanism for the development of torsade de pointes in the LQT1, 2, and 3 forms of the long QT syndrome.

Adrenergic agonists further amplify transmural heterogeneity (transiently) in the case of I_{Kr} block and LQT2 but reduce it in the case of I_{Na} promoters and LQT3 (127, 185) A different picture has emerged with I_{Ks} blockers or with LQT1 mutations; I_{Ks} block leads to a *homogeneous* prolongation of APD throughout the ventricular wall, leading to a prolongation of the QT interval but with no increase in transmural dispersion of repolarization. TdP does not occur spontaneously nor can it be induced by programmed stimulation under these conditions until a β-adrenergic agonist is introduced. Isoproterenol dramatically increases transmural dispersion of repolarization and refractoriness under these conditions by abbreviating the APD of epicardium and endocardium, thus creating a vulnerable window that an EAD-induced triggered response can invade to generate TdP.

In the clinic, the onset of TdP has long been known to follow a short-long-short cycle length sequence (60, 148). Recent clinical reports indicate that a sudden moderate acceleration from an initially slow rate when followed by an intrinsic or extrinsic extrasystole holds the highest risk for the development of TdP in congenital and acquired LQTS patients (134), as well as in animal models with acquired LQTS (56, 99, 229). Similar characteristics are observed in isolated M-cell preparations as well as in wedge preparations pretreated with APD prolonging agents.

Pharmacological Therapy for LQTS: Reducing Transmural Dispersion of Repolarization

With the genotype–phenotype correlation that is emerging, it is logical to explore gene-specific therapies for the congenital form of the long QT syndrome and drug-specific therapies for the acquired forms. Schwartz and co-workers have shown that sodium channel block with mexiletine is usually more effective in abbreviating QT interval in LQT3 patients than in LQT2 patients (177, 179). Exogenously administered potassium has been reported to correct repolarization abnormalities in congenital (LQT2) and acquired LQTS patients (53, 59). Shimizu et al. recently used MAP recordings to show an improvement of repolarization abnormalities following administration of a K^+ channel opener to LQT1 patients (186). Although these clinical studies examined the effects of antiarrhythmic agents and rapid pacing on the QT interval and MAP duration, they did not evaluate the actions of these treatments on transmural dispersion of repolarization or on the relative risk for development of TdP.

A distinct advantage of studying interventions in the perfused wedge models of LQTS is that assessment of the antiarrhythmic efficacy of drugs or of pacing is possible in addition to quantification of other parameters. APD-, QT-, and transmural dispersion of repolarization-rate relations are generally much steeper in the LQT3 (ATX-II) model than in either the LQT1 (chromanol 293B) or the LQT2 (d-sotalol) model, probably because of the very slow kinetics of reactivation of late sodium current. The APD-rate relations in the LQT1, LQT2 and LQT3 models, however, are all steeper than in control (182, 183). These results suggest that, although pacemaker therapy is likely to be effective in the treatment of LQT3, its usefulness in LQT1 and LQT2 should not be discounted (102, 226). Because it produces a preferential abbreviation of the M-cell APD, pacing leads to a reversal of transmural dispersion of repolarization and suppression of EAD-induced triggered activity.

β-Blockers are widely reported to reduce the incidence of syncope and sudden cardiac death in patients with congenital LQTS (149). LQT1 and LQT2 patients appear to be well protected under β-blockade. In experimental models, therapeutic concentrations of the β-blocker propranolol completely inhibit the influence of isoproterenol to increase transmural dispersion of repolarization and to produce spontaneous as well as stimulation-induced TdP. β-Blockers have the opposite effect in LQT3.

Late sodium channel blockers like mexiletine, a class IB antiarrhythmic agent which shows rapid dissociation kinetics from the sodium channel, are known to be effective in abbreviating QT in clinical cases of LQT3, but less so in LQT1 and LQT2. Recent studies suggest that sodium channel blockers may be of therapeutic value in all three genotypes. Sodium blockers produce a preferential abbreviation of the M-cell action potential, where late I_{Na} is relatively large, thus reducing transmural dispersion of repolarization and preventing the development of spontaneous as well as stimulation-induced TdP in experimental models of LQT1, LQT2, and LQT3 (182, 183).

Nicorandil, a K$^+$ channel opener, is capable of abbreviating long QT, reducing transmural dispersion of repolarization, and preventing spontaneous and stimulation–induced TdP when LQTS is secondary to reduced I_{Ks} (LQT1) or I_{Kr} (LQT2), but not when it is due to augmented late I_{Na} (LQT3), although relatively high concentrations of nicorandil are required. Transmural dispersion is reduced by a preferential effect of the drugs to abbreviate the M-cells.

Chronic amiodarone administration produces a greater prolongation of the action potential duration in epicardium and endocardium, but less of an increase—or even a decrease—at slow rates, in the M region, thereby reducing transmural dispersion of repolarization (199). In addition, chronic amiodarone therapy

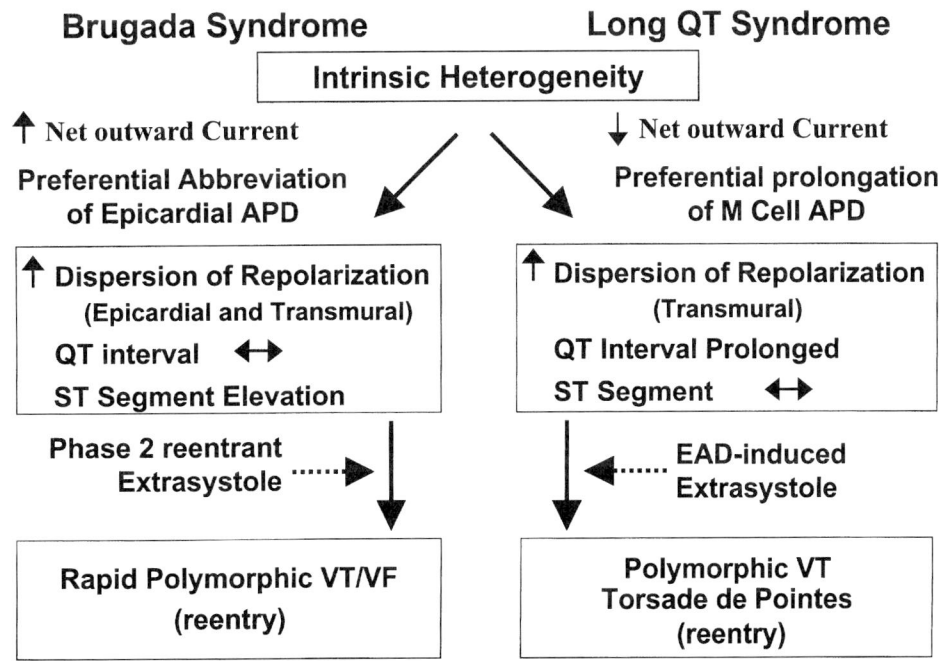

FIG. 17–20. Similarities and differences in mechanisms responsible for the development of arrhythmias in the Brugada and long QT syndromes. Amplification of intrinsic heterogeneities underlies arrhythmogenicity in both syndromes. In the case of the Brugada syndrome, an increase in net outward current amplifies the heterogeneity normally present in the early phases of the action potential, leading to accentuation of the epicardial notch and finally loss of the action potential dome, resulting in marked abbreviation of the potential at some epicardial sites. In the case of the long QT syndrome, a decrease in net outward current amplifies the heterogeneity normally present in the late phases of the action potential, by producing a preferential prolongation of the M-cell action potential.

suppresses the ability of the I_{Kr} blocker d-sotalol to induce a marked dispersion of repolarization or early afterdepolarization activity. These findings demonstrate a direct effect of chronic amiodarone to reduce transmural dispersion of repolarization, especially under conditions in which dispersion is exaggerated. The results suggest the possibility that chronic amiodarone may protect against the development of acquired LQTS.

These antiarrhythmic agents share (1) the ability to reduce or eliminate the substrate for re-entry via a reduction of transmural and other dispersions of repolarization and/or (2) the ability to suppress triggered activity responsible for the initiation of TdP.

SUMMARY

We have described a number of cellular and ionic mechanisms that contribute to electrical heterogeneity of repolarization and refractoriness in the heart, particularly across the ventricular wall (Fig. 17-20). These heterogeneities contribute prominently to the inscription of normal and abnormal waves in the electrocardiogram. Differences in pharmacology and pathophysiology of the three principal ventricular myocardial cell types serve to amplify the intrinsic electrical heterogeneities resulting in cardiac arrhythmias. Dispersion of repolarization due to abnormal *abbreviation* of APD in epicardium contributes to the development of an ST segment elevation (or accentuated J wave) and phase 2 re-entry, which in turn can precipitate VT/VF (or rapid TdP). Dispersion of repolarization within ventricular myocardium secondary to disproportionate *prolongation* of APD of the M-cell contributes to the development of a vulnerable window, long QT intervals, and notched T waves, as well as to the induction of polymorphic VT resembling torsade de pointes.

This work was supported by grants from the National Institutes of Health (HL 47678), the American Heart Association, New York State Affiliate, and the Masons of New York State and Florida.

We are grateful to Dr. Andrew Zygmunt and to Judy Hefferon for their kind assistance with the graphic illustrations.

REFERENCES

1. Abbott, G. W., F. Sesti, I. Splawski, M. E. Buck, M. H. Lehmann, K. W. Timothy, M. T. Keating, and S. A. N. Goldstein. MiRP1 forms IKr potassium channels with HERG and is associated with cardiac arrhythmia. *Cell* 97:175–187, 1999.
2. Abildskov, J. A. and R. L. Lux. The mechanism of simulated torsades de pointes in computer model of propagated excitation. *J. Cardiovasc. Electrophysiol.* 2:224–237, 1991.
3. Aizawa, Y., M. Tamura, M. Chinushi, N. Naitoh, H. Uchiyama, Y. Kusano, H. Hosono, and A. Shibata. Idiopathic ventricular fibrillation and bradycardia-dependent intraventricular block. *Am. Heart J.* 126:1473–1474, 1993.
4. Aizawa, Y., M. Tamura, M. Chinushi, S. Niwano, Y. Kusano, N. Naitoh, A. Shibata, T. Tohjoh, Y. Ueda, and K. Joho. An attempt at electrical catheter ablation of the arrhythmogenic area in idiopathic ventricular fibrillation. *Am. Heart J.* 123:257–260, 1992.
5. Akar, F. G., G. X., Yan, C., Antzelevitch, and D. S. Rosenbaum. Optical maps reveal reentrant mechanism of torsade de pointes based on topography and electrophysiology of mid-myocardial cells. Circulation 96:I-355. 1997. (Abstract)
6. Antzelevitch, C. Are M cells present in the ventricular myocardium of the pig? A question of maturity. *Cardiovasc. Res.* 36: 127–128, 1997.
7. Antzelevitch, C. The M cell. Invited Editorial Comment. *J. Cardiovasc. Pharmacol. Ther.* 2:73–76, 1997.
8. Antzelevitch, C., J. M. Davidenko, S. Sicouri, L. Cohen, A. Iodice, R. J. Goodrow, and G. A. Gintant. Electrophysiologic effects of quinidine in canine Purkinje fibers and ventricular myocardium. Slow development of the antiarrhythmic and arrhythmogenic effects of the drug. In *Recent Advances in Pharmacology and Therapeutics*, edited by M. Velasco, A. Israel, E. Romero, and H. Silva New York: Excerpta Medica, 1989:259–263.
9. Antzelevitch, C., J. M. Davidenko, S. Sicouri, L. Cohen, A. Iodice, R. J. Goodrow, and G. A. Gintant. Quinidine-induced early afterdepolarizations and triggered activity. *J. Electrophysiol.* 5: 323–338, 1989.
10. Antzelevitch, C. and J. M. Di Diego. The role of K^+ channel activators in cardiac electrophysiology and arrhythmias. *Circulation* 85:1627–1629, 1992.
11. Antzelevitch, C., J. M. Di Diego, S. Sicouri, and A. Lukas. Selective pharmacological modification of repolarizing currents. Antiarrhythmic and proarrhythmic actions of agents that influence repolarization in the heart. In: *Antiarrhythmic Drugs: Mechanisms of Antiarrhythmic and Proarrhythmic Actions*, edited by J. Breithardt. Berlin: Springer-Verlag, 1995:57–80.
12. Antzelevitch, C., S. H. Litovsky, and A. Lukas. Epicardium vs. endocardium. Electrophysiology and pharmacology. In: *Cardiac Electrophysiology, From Cell to Bedside*, edited by D. P. Zipes, and J. Jalife. Philadelphia: W. B. Saunders, 1990:386–395.
13. Antzelevitch, C., V. V. Nesterenko, and G. X. Yan. The role of M cells in acquired long QT syndrome, U waves and torsade de pointes. *J. Electrocardiol.* 28(suppl.):131–138, 1996.
14. Antzelevitch, C., W. Shimizu, G. X. Yan, S. Sicouri, J. Weissenburger, V. V. Nesterenko, A. Burashnikov, J. Di Diego, J. Saffitz, and G. P. Thomas. The M cell: its contribution to the ECG and to normal and abnormal electrical function of the heart. *J. Cardiovasc Electrophysiol.* 10:1124–1152, 1999.
16. Antzelevitch, C. and S. Sicouri. Clinical relevance of cardiac arrhythmias generated by afterdepolarizations: the role of M cells in the generation of U waves, triggered activity and torsade de pointes. *J. Am. Coll. Cardiol.* 23:259–277, 1994.
17. Antzelevitch, C., S. Sicouri, S. H. Litovsky, A. Lukas, S. C. Krishnan, J. M. Di Diego, G. A. Gintant, and D. W. Liu. Heterogeneity within the ventricular wall: electrophysiology and pharmacology of epicardial, endocardial and M cells. *Circ. Res.* 69: 1427–1449, 1991.
18. Antzelevitch, C., S. Sicouri, A. Lukas, J. M. Di Diego, V. V. Nesterenko, D. W. Liu, J. F. Roubache, A. C. Zygmunt, Z. Q. Zhang, and A. Iodice. Clinical implications of electrical heterogeneity in the heart: the electrophysiology and pharmacology of epicardial, M and endocardial cells. In: *Cardiac Arrhythmia: Mechanism, Diagnosis and Management*, edited by P. J. Podrid, and P. R. Kowey. Baltimore: William & Wilkins. 1995: 88–107.

19. Antzelevitch, C., S. Sicouri, A. Lukas, V. V. Nesterenko, D. W. Liu, and J. M. Di Diego. Regional differences in the electrophysiology of ventricular cells: physiological and clinical implications. In: *Cardiac Electrophysiology: From Cell to Bedside*, edited by D. P. Zipes and J. Jalife. Philadelphia: W. B. Saunders, 1995:228–245.

20. Antzelevitch, C., Z. Q. Sun, Z. Q. Zhang, and G. X. Yan. Cellular and ionic mechanisms underlying erythromycin-induced long QT and torsade de pointes. *J. Am. Coll. Cardiol.* 28:1836–1848, 1996.

21. Antzelevitch, C., G. X. Yan, W. Shimizu, and A. Burashnikov. Electrical heterogeneity, the ECG, and cardiac arrhythmias. In: *Cardiac Electrophysiology: From Cell to Bedside*, editeb by D. P. Zipes and J. Jalife. Philadelphia: W. B. Saunders, 1999:222–238.

22. Anyukhovsky, E. P., E. A. Sosunov, S. J. Feinmark, and M. R. Rosen. Effects of quinidine on repolarization in canine epicardium, midmyocardium, and endocardium. II. In vivo study. *Circulation* 96:4019–4026, 1997.

23. Anyukhovsky, E. P., E. A. Sosunov, R. Z. Gainullin, and M. R. Rosen. The controversial M cell. *J. Cardiovasc. Electrophysiol.* 10:244–260, 1999.

24. Anyukhovsky, E. P., E. A. Sosunov, and M. R. Rosen. Regional differences in electrophysiologic properties of epicardium, midmyocardium and endocardium: in vitro and in vivo correlations. *Circulation* 94:1981–1988, 1996.

25. Asano, Y., J. M. Davidenko, W. T. Baxter, R. A. Gray, and J. Jalife. *J. Am. Coll. Cardiol.* 29:831–842, 1997.

26. Balati, B., A. Varro, and J. G. Papp. Comparison of the cellular electrophysiological characteristics of canine left ventricular epicardium, M cells, endocardium and Purkinje fibres *Acta Physiol. Scand.* 164:181–190, 1998.

27. Balser, J. R., P. B. Bennett, L. M. Hondeghem, and D. M. Roden. Suppression of time-dependent outward current in guinea-pig ventricular myocytes. Actions of quinidine and amiodarone. *Circ.Res.* 69:519–529, 1991.

28. Barhanin, J., F. Lesage, E. Guillemare, M. Fink, M. Lazdunski, and G. Romey. KvLQT1 and IsK (minK) proteins associate to form the I_{Ks} cardiac potassium current. *Nature* 384:78–80, 1996.

29. Barry, D. M. and J. M. Nerbonne. Myocardial potassium channels: electrophysiological and molecular diversity. *Annu. Rev. Physiol.* 58:363–394, 1996.

30. Barry, D. M., J. S. Trimmer, J. P. Merlie, and J. M. Nerbonne. Differential expression of voltage-gated K$^+$ channel subunits in adult rat heart. Relation to functional K$^+$ channels? *Circ. Res.* 77:361–369, 1995.

31. Bauer, A., R. Becker, K. D. Freigang, J. C. Senges, F. Voss, A. Hansen, M. Muller, H. J. Lang, U. Gerlach, A. Busch, P. Kraft, W. Kubler, and W. Schols. Rate- and site-dependent effects of propafenone, dofetilide, and the new I(Ks)-blocking agent chromanol 293b on individual muscle layers of the intact canine heart. *Circulation* 100:2184–2190, 1999.

32. Bjerregaard, P., I. Gussak, S. I. Kotar, and J. E. Gessler. Recurrent synocope in a patient with prominent J-wave. *Am. Heart J.* 127:1426–1430, 1994.

33. Blair, R. W., T. Shimizu, and V. S. Bishop. The role of vagal afferents in the reflex control of the left ventricular refractory period in the cat. *Circ. Res.* 46:378–386, 1980.

34. Brahmajothi, M. V., D. L. Campbell, R. L. Rasmusson, M. J. Morales, J. S. Trimmer, J. M. Nerbonne, and H. C. Strauss. Distinct transient outward potassium current (Ito) phenotypes and distribution of fast-inactivating potassium channel alpha subunits in ferret left ventricular myocytes. *J. Gen. Physiol* 113:581–600, 1999.

35. Brahmajothi, M. V., M. J. Morales, R. Liu, R. L. Rasmusson, D. L. Campbell, and H. C. Strauss. In situ hybridization reveals extensive diversity of K$^+$ channel mRNA in isolated ferret cardiac myocytes. *Circ. Res.* 78:1083–1089, 1996.

36. Brahmajothi, M. V., M. J. Morales, R. L. Rasmusson, D. L. Campbell, and H. C. Strauss. Heterogeneity in K$^+$ channel transcript expression detected in isolated ferret cardiac myocytes. *Pacing Clin. Electrophysiol.* 20:388–396, 1997.

37. Brahmajothi, M. V., M. J. Morales, K. A. Reimer, and H. C. Strauss. Regional localization of ERG, the channel protein responsible for the rapid component of the delayed rectifier, K$^+$ current in the ferret heart. *Circ. Res.* 81:128–135, 1997.

38. Brugada, P. and J. Brugada. Right bundle branch block, persistent ST segment elevation and sudden cardiac death: a distinct clinical and electrocardiographic syndrome: a multicenter report. *J. Am. Coll. Cardiol.* 20:1391–1396, 1992.

39. Bryant, S. M., X. Wan, S. J. Shipsey, and G. Hart. Regional differences in the delayed rectifier current (I_{Kr} and I_{Ks}) contribute to the differences in action potential duration in basal left ventricular myocytes in guinea-pig. *Cardiovasc. Res.* 40:322–331, 1998.

40. Buchanan, L. V., G. G. Kabell, M. N. Brunden, and J. K. Gibson. Comparative assessment of ibutilide, D-sotalol, clofilium, E-4031, and UK-68,798 in a rabbit model of proarrhythmia. *J. Cardiovasc. Pharmacol.* 22:540–549, 1993.

41. Burashnikov, A. and C. Antzelevitch. Acceleration-induced action potential prolongation and early afterdepolarizations. *J. Cardiovasc. Electrophysiol.* 9:934–948, 1998.

42. Burashnikov, A. and C. Antzelevitch. Differences in the electrophysiologic response of four canine ventricular cell types to α_1-adrenergic agonists. *Cardiovasc. Res.* 43:901–908, 1999.

43. Burashnikov, A. and Antzelevitch, C. Is the Purkinje system the source of the electrocardiographic U wave? *Circulation* 100:II-386, 1999. (Abstract)

44. Burgess, M. J., L. S. Green, K. Millar, R. F. Wyatt, and J. A. Abildskov. The sequence of normal ventricular recovery. *Am. Heart J.* 84:660–669, 1972.

45. Busch, A. E., A. E. Bush, E. Ford, H. Suessbrich, H. J. Lang, R. Greger, K. Kunzelmann, B. Attali, and W. Stümer. The role of the Isk protein in the specific pharmacological properties of the IKs channel complex. *Br. J. Pharmacol.* 122:187–189, 1998.

46. Butler, A., A. G. Wei, K. Baker, and L. Salkoff. A family of putative potassium channel genes in *Drosophila*. *Science* 243:943–947, 1989.

47. Carl, S. L., K. Felix, A. H. Caswell, N. R. Brandt, W. J. Ball, Jr., P. L. Vaghy, G. Meissner, and D. G. Ferguson. Immunolocalization of sarcolemmal dihydropyridine receptor and sarcoplasmic reticular triadin and ryanodine receptor in rabbit ventricle and atrium. *J. Cell Biol.* 129:672–682, 1995.

48. Carlsson, L., O. Almgren, and G. D. Duker. Qtu-Prolongation and torsades-de-pointes induced by putative class-III antiarrhythmic agents in the rabbit—etiology and interventions. *J. Cardiovasc. Pharmacol.* 16:276–285, 1990.

49. Catterall, W. A. Structure and function of voltage-gated ion channels. *Trends Neurosci.* 16:500–506, 1993.

50. Chandy, K. G. Simplified gene nomenclature [letter]. *Nature* 352:26, 1991.

51. Chen, F., G. Mottino, T. S. Klitzner, K. D. Philipson, and J. S. Frank. Distribution of the Na$^+$/Ca^{2+} exchange protein in developing rabbit myocytes. *Am. J. Physiol* 268 (*Cell Physiol.* 35): C1126–C1132, 1995.

52. Chen, Q., G. E. Kirsch, D. Zhang, R. Brugada, J. Brugada, P. Brugada, D. Potreau, A. Moya, M. Borggrefe, G. Breithardt, M. Ortiz, Z. G. Wang, C. Antzelevitch, R. E. O'Brien, E. Schultz-Bahr, M. T. Keating, J. A. Towbin, and Q. Wang. Genetic basis and molecular mechanisms for idiopathic ventricular fibrillation. *Nature* 392:293–296, 1997.

53. Choy, A. M., C. C. Lang, D. M. Chomsky, G. H. Rayos, J. R.

Wilson, and D. M. Roden. Normalization of acquired QT prolongation in humans by intravenous potassium. *Circulation* 96: 2149–2154, 1997.

54. Clark, R. B., R. A. Bouchard, E. Salinas-Stefanon, J. Sanchez-Chapula, and W. R. Giles. Heterogeneity of action potential waveforms and potassium currents in rat ventricle. *Cardiovasc. Res.* 27:1795–1799, 1993.

55. Clements, S. D. and J. W. Hurst. Diagnostic value of ECG abnormalities observed in subjects accidentally exposed to cold. *Am. J. Cardiol.* 29:729–734, 1972.

56. Cobbe, S. M., E. P. Hoffman, A. Ritzenhoff, J. Brachmann, W. Kubler, and J. Senges. Action of sotalol on potential reentrant pathways and ventricular tachyarrhythmias in conscious dogs in the late postmyocardial infarction phase. *Circulation* 68:865–871, 1983.

57. Cohen, I. S., W. R. Giles, and D. Noble. Cellular basis for the T wave of the electrocardiogram. *Nature* 262:657–661, 1976.

58. Cohen, S. A. Immunocytochemical localization of rH1 sodium channel in adult rat heart atria and ventricle. Presence in terminal intercalated disks. *Circulation* 94:3083–3086, 1996.

59. Compton, S. J., R. L. Lux, M. R. Ramsey, K. R. Strelich, M. C. Sanguinetti, L. S. Green, M. T. Keating, and J. W. Mason. Genetically defined therapy of inherited long-QT syndrome. Correction of abnormal repolarization by potassium. *Circulation* 94: 1018–1022, 1996.

60. Coumel, P. Early afterdepolarizations and triggered activity in clinical arrhythmias. In: *Cardiac Electrophysiology: A Text Book*, edited by M. R., Rosen, M. J. Janse, and A. L. Wit. Mount Kisco, NY: Futura Publishing. 1990:387–411.

61. Crampton, R. S. Preeminence of the left stellate ganglion in the long Q-T syndrome. *Circulation* 59:769–778, 1979.

62. Curran, M. E., I. Splawski, K. W. Timothy, G. M. Vincent, E. D. Green, and M. T. Keating. A molecular basis for cardiac arrhythmia: *HERG* mutations cause long QT syndrome. *Cell* 80:795–803, 1995.

63. Daleau, P. and J. Deleze. Conduction block in Purkinje fibers by homogeneous versus localized decrease of the gap junction conductance. *Can. J Physiol Pharmacol.* 76:630–641, 1998.

64. Davidenko, J. M., L. Cohen, R. J. Goodrow, and C. Antzelevitch. Quinidine-induced action potential prolongation, early afterdepolarizations, and triggered activity in canine Purkinje fibers. Effects of stimulation rate, potassium, and magnesium. *Circulation* 79:674–686, 1989.

65. De Biasi, M., Z. G. Wang, E. Accili, B. A. Wible, and D. Fedida. Open channel block of human heart hKv1.5 by the β-subunit hKvβ1.2. *Am. J. Physiol.* 272 (*Heart Circ. Physiol.* 41):H2932–H2941, 1997.

66. Delombe, S., I. Baró, Y. Péréon, J. Bliek, R. Mohammad-Panah, H. Pollard, S. Morid, M. Mannens, A. A. M. Wilde, J. Barhanin, F. Charpentier, and D. Escande. A dominant negative isoform of the long QT syndrome 1 gene product. *J. Biol. Chem.* 273:6837–6843, 1998.

67. Derakhchan, K., R. Cardinal, S. Brunet, D. Klug, C. Pharand, T. Kus, and B. I. Sasyniuk. Polymorphic ventricular tachycardias induced by d-sotalol and phenylephrine in canine preparations of atrioventricular block: initiation in the conduction system followed by spatially unstable re-entry. *Cardiovasc. Res.* 38:617–630, 1998.

68. Di Diego, J. M. and C. Antzelevitch. Pinacidil-induced electrical heterogeneity and extrasystolic activity in canine ventricular tissues: does activation of ATP-regulated potassium current promote phase 2 reentry? *Circulation* 88:1177–1189, 1993.

69. Di Diego, J. M. and C. Antzelevitch. High [Ca^{2+}]-induced electrical heterogeneity and extrasystolic activity in isolated canine ventricular epicardium: phase 2 reentry. *Circulation* 89:1839–1850, 1994.

70. Di Diego, J. M., Z. Q. Sun, and C. Antzelevitch. I_{to} and action potential notch are smaller in left vs. right canine ventricular epicardium. *Am. J. Physiol.* 271 (*Heart Circ. Physiol.* 40):H548–H561, 1996.

71. Dillon, S. M., M. A. Allessie, P. C. Ursell, and A. L. Wit. Influences of anisotropic tissue structure on reentrant circuits in the epicardial border zone of subacute canine infarcts. *Circ. Res.* 63: 182–206, 1988.

72. Dixon, E. J. and D. McKinnon. Quantitative analysis of potassium channel mRNA in atrial and ventricular muscle of rats. *Circ. Res.* 75:252–260, 1994.

73. Dixon, E. J., W. Shi, H.-S. Wang, C. McDonald, H. Yu, R. S. Wymore, I. S. Cohen, and D. McKinnon. Role of the Kv4.3 K^+ channel in ventricular muscle. A molecular correlate for the transient outward current. *Circ. Res.* 79:659–668, 1996.

74. Drouin, E., F. Charpentier, C. Gauthier, K. Laurent, and H. Le Marec. Electrophysiological characteristics of cells spanning the left ventricular wall of human heart: evidence for the presence of M cells. *J. Am. Coll. Cardiol.* 26:185–192, 1995.

75. Dumaine, R., J. A. Towbin, P. Brugada, M. Vatta, V. V. Nesterenko, D. V. Nesterenko, R. Brugada, and C. Antzelevitch. Ionic mechanisms responsible for the electrocardiographic phenotype of the Brugada syndrome are temperature dependent. *Circ. Res.* 85:803–809, 1999.

76. Dumaine, R., Q. Wang, M. T. Keating, H. A. Hartmann, P. J. Schwartz, A. M. Brown, and G. E. Kirsch. Multiple mechanisms of Na^+ channel-linked long-QT syndrome. *Circ. Res.* 78:916–924, 1996.

77. Dumaine, R., Y. S. Wu, and C. Antzelevitch. Distribution of KvLQT1 but not minK parallels the distribution of I_{Ks} in the mid-myocardium of canine heart. *Biophys. J.* 76:A366–A366, 2000.

78. Eagle, K. Images in clinical medicine. Osborn waves of hypothermia. *N. Engl. J. Med.* 10:680, 1994.

79. Eddlestone, G. T., Zygmunt, A. C., and Antzelevitch, C. Larger late sodium current contributes to the longer action potential of the M cell in canine ventricular myocardium. *Pacing Clin. Electrophysiol.* 19:II569, 1996. (Abstract)

80. Eisner, D. A. The Na-K pump and its effectors in cardiac muscle. In: *The Heart and Cardiovascular System*, edited by H. A., Fozzard, R. B. Jennings, E. Haber, A. M. Katz, and H. E. Morgan. New York: Raven Press, 2000:863–902.

81. El-Sherif, N., E. B. Caref, H. Yin, and M. Restivo. The electrophysiological mechanism of ventricular arrhythmias in the long QT syndrome: tridimensional mapping of activation and recovery patterns. *Circ. Res.* 79:474–492, 1996.

82. El-Sherif, N., M. Chinushi, E. B. Caref, and M. Restivo. Electrophysiological mechanism of the characteristic electrocardiographic morphology of torsade de pointes tachyarrhythmias in the long-QT syndrome. Detailed analysis of ventricular tridimensional activation patterns. *Circulation* 96:4392–4399, 1997.

83. Escande, D., D. Loisance, C. Planche, and E. Coraboeuf. Age-related changes of action potential plateau shape in isolated human atrial fibers. *Am. J. Physiol.* 249 (*Heart Circ. Physiol.* 18): H843–H850, 1985.

84. Fedida, D. and W. R. Giles. Regional variations in action potentials and transient outward current in myocytes isolated from rabbit left ventricle. *J. Physiol. (Lond.)* 442:191–209, 1991.

85. Feng, J., B. A. Wible, G. R. Li, Z. G. Wang, and S. Nattel. Antisence oligodeoxynucleotides directed against Kv1.5 mRNA specifically inhibit ultrarapid delayed rectifier K^+ current in cultured adult human atrial myocytes. *Circ. Res.* 80:572–579, 1997.

86. Fontaine, G. A new look at torsades de pointes. In: *QT Prolongation and Ventricular Arrhythmias*, edited by K., Hashiba, A. J.

Moss, and P. J. Schwartz. New York: New York Academy of Science, 1992:157–177.

87. Fozzard, H. A. and D. A. Hanck. Structure and function of voltage-dependent sodium channels: comparison of brain II and cardiac isoforms. *Physiol. Rev.* 76:887–926, 1996.

88. Fozzard, H. A. and G. Lipkind. The guanidinium toxin binding site on the sodium channel. *Jpn. Heart J.* 37:683–692, 1996.

89. Frank, J. S., G. Mottino, D. Reid, R. S. Molday, and K. D. Philipson. Distribution of the Na(+)-Ca^{2+} exchange protein in mammalian cardiac myocytes: an immunofluorescence and immunocolloidal gold-labeling study. *J. Cell Biol.* 117:337–345, 1992.

90. Freigang, K. D., Becker, R., Bauer, A., Voss, F., Senges, J., and Brachmann, J. Electrophysiological properties of individual muscle layers in the in vivo canine heart. *J. Amer. Coll. Cardiol.* 27(SupplA):124A. 1996. (Abstract)

91. Furukawa, T., R. J. Myerburg, N. Furukawa, A. L. Bassett, and S. Kimura. Differences in transient outward currents of feline endocardial and epicardial myocytes. *Circ. Res.* 67:1287–1291, 1990.

92. Gao, T., T. S. Puri, B. L. Gerhardstein, A. J. Chien, R. D. Green, and M. M. Hosey. Identification and subcellular localization of the subunits of L-type calcium channels and adenylyl cyclase in cardiac myocytes. *J. Biol. Chem.* 272:19401–19407, 1997.

93. Gidh-Jain, M., B. Huang, P. Jain, and N. el Sherif. Differential expression of voltage-gated K$^+$ channel genes in left ventricular remodeled myocardium after experimental myocardial infarction. *Circ. Res* 79:669–675, 1996.

94. Gilmour, R. F., Jr. and D. P. Zipes. Different electrophysiological responses of canine endocardium and epicardium to combined hyperkalemia, hypoxia, and acidosis. *Circ. Res.* 46:814–825, 1980.

95. Gourdie, R. G., C. R. Green, and N. J. Severs. Gap junction distribution in adult mammalian myocardium revealed by an anti-peptide antibody and laser scanning confocal microscopy. *J. Cell Sci.* 99(Pt 1):41–55, 1991.

96. Gourdie, R. G., N. J. Severs, C. R. Green, S. Rothery, P. Germroth, and R. P. Thompson. The spatial distribution and relative abundance of gap-junctional connexin40 and connexin43 correlate to functional properties of components of the cardiac atrioventricular conduction system. *J. Cell Sci.* 105(Pt 4):985–991, 1993.

97. Gros, D., T. Jarry-Guichard, I. Ten Velde, A. de Maziere, M. J. van Kempen, J. Davoust, J. P. Briand, A. F. Moorman, and H. J. Jongsma. Restricted distribution of connexin40, a gap junctional protein, in mammalian heart. *Circ. Res.* 74:839–851, 1994.

98. Gussak, I., P. Bjerregaard, T. M. Egan, and B. R. Chaitman. ECG phenomenon called the J wave. History, pathophysiology, and clinical significance. *J. Electrocardiol.* 28:49–58, 1995.

99. Habbab, M. A. and N. El-Sherif. TU alternans, long QTU, and torsade de pointes: clinical and experimental observations. *Pacing Clin. Electrophysiol.* 15:916–931, 1992.

100. Harvey, R. D. and J. R. Hume. Isoproterenol activates a chloride current, not the transient outward current, in rabbit ventricular myocytes. *Am. J. Physiol.* 265 (*Cell Physiol.* 34): C1177–C1181, 1993.

101. Haws, C. W. and R. L. Lux. Correlation between in vivo transmembrane action potential durations and action-recovery intervals from electrograms. Effects of interventions that alter repolarization time. *Circulation* 81:281–288, 1990.

102. Hirao, H., W. Shimizu, T. Kurita, K. Suyama, N. Aihara, S. Kamakura, and K. Shimomura. Frequency-dependent electrophysiologic properties of ventricular repolarization in patients with congenital long QT syndrome. *J. Am. Coll. Cardiol.* 28:1269–1277, 1996.

103. Hofmann, F., M. Biel, and V. Flockerzi. Molecular basis for Ca2$^+$ channel diversity. *Annu. Rev. Neurosci.* 17:399–418, 1994.

104. Hu, H. and E. Marban. Isoform-specific inhibition of L-type calcium channels by dihydropyridines is independent of isoform-specific gating properties. *Mol. Pharmacol.* 53:902–907, 1998.

105. Hugo, N., I. C. Dormehl, and A. L. Van Gelder. A positive wave at the J-point of electrocardiograms of anaesthetized baboons. *J. Med. Primatol.* 17:347–352, 1988.

106. Hume, J. R. and R. D. Harvey. Chloride conductance pathways in heart. *Am. J. Physiol.* 261 (*Cell Physiol.* 30):C399–C412, 1991.

107. Imaizumi, Y. and W. R. Giles. Quinidine-induced inhibition of transient outward current in cardiac muscle. *Am. J. Physiol.* 253 (*Heart Circ. Physiol.* 22):H704–H708, 1987.

108. James, A. F., T. Tominaga, Y. Okada, and M. Tominaga. Distribution of cAMP-activated chloride current and CFTR mRNA in the guinea pig heart. *Circ. Res.* 79:201–207, 1996.

109. Jeck, C. D. and P. A. Boyden. Age-related appearance of outward currents may contribute to developmental differences in ventricular repolarization. *Circ. Res.* 71:1390–1403, 1992.

110. Jewell, E. A. and J. B. Lingrel. Comparison of the substrate dependence properties of the rat Na,K-ATPase alpha 1, alpha 2, and alpha 3 isoforms expressed in HeLa cells. *J Biol. Chem.* 266:16925–16930, 1991.

111. Kaab, S., J. Dixon, J. Duc, D. Ashen, M. Nabauer, D. J. Beuckelmann, G. Steinbeck, D. McKinnon, and G. F. Tomaselli. Molecular basis of transient outward potassium current down-regulation in human heart failure: a decrease in Kv4.3 mRNA correlates with a reduction in current density. *Circulation* 98:1383–1393, 1998.

112. Kamiyama, A. and Y. Saeki. Myocardial action potentials of right- and left-subepicardial muscles in the canine ventricle and effects of manganese ions. *Proc. Jpn. Acad.* 50:771–774, 1974.

113. Kamp, T. J., M. Mitas, K. L. Fields, S. Asoh, H. Chin, E. Marban, and M. Nirenberg. Transcriptional regulation of the neuronal L-type calcium channel alpha 1D subunit gene. *Cell Mol. Neurobiol.* 15:307–326, 1995.

114. Kanter, H. L., J. G. Laing, S. L. Beau, E. C. Beyer, and J. E. Saffitz. Distinct patterns of connexin expression in canine Purkinje fibers and ventricular muscle. *Circ. Res.* 72:1124–1131, 1993.

115. Kaplan, W. D. and W. E. Trout, III. The behavior of four neurological mutants of *Drosophila*. *Genetics* 61:399–409, 1969.

116. Kieval, R. S., R. J. Bloch, G. E. Lindenmayer, A. Ambesi, and W. J. Lederer. Immunofluorescence localization of the Na-Ca exchanger in heart cells. *Am. J. Physiol.* 263 (*Cell Physiol.* 32): C545–C550, 1992.

117. Kilborn, M. J. and D. Fedida. A study of the developmental changes in outward currents of rat ventricular myocytes. *J. Physiol. (Lond.)* 430:37–60, 1990.

118. Kimura, S., A. L. Bassett, T. Kohya, P. L. Kozlovskis, and R. J. Myerburg. Regional effects of verapamil on recovery of excitability and conduction time in experimental ischemia. *Circulation* 76:1146–1154, 1987.

119. Kimura, S., H. Nakaya, and M. Kanno. Electrophysiological effects of diltiazem, nifedipine and Ni^{2+} on the subepicardial muscle cells of canine heart under the condition of combined hypoxia, hyperkalemia and acidosis. *Naunyn-Schmiedebergs Arch. Pharmacol.* 324:228–232, 1983.

120. Koban, M. U., A. F. Moorman, J. Holtz, M. H. Yacoub, and K. R. Boheler. Expressional analysis of the cardiac Na-Ca ex-

changer in rat development and senescence. *Cardiovasc. Res.* 37:405–423, 1998.

121. Kong, W., S. Po, T. Yamagishi, M. D. Ashen, G. Stetten, and G. F. Tomaselli. Isolation and characterization of the human gene encoding Ito: further diversity by alternative mRNA splicing. *Am. J. Physiol.* 275 (*Heart Circ. Physiol.* 44):H1963–H1970, 1998.

122. Kossenjans, W. and M. Ashraf. Localization of sodium-potassium adenosine triphosphatase in sheep myocardium by immunoelectron microscopy. *J. Submicrosc. Cytol. Pathol.* 20:53–58, 1988.

123. Kraus, F. Ueber die wirkung des kalziums auf den kreislauf. *Deutsch. Med. Wochenschr.* 46:201–203, 1920.

124. Krishnan, S. C. and C. Antzelevitch. Sodium channel blockade produces opposite electrophysiologic effects in canine ventricular epicardium and endocardium. *Circ. Res.* 69:277–291, 1991.

125. Krishnan, S. C. and C. Antzelevitch. Flecainide-induced arrhythmia in canine ventricular epicardium: Phase 2 Reentry? *Circulation* 87:562–572, 1993.

126. Lehmann, M. H., F. Suzuki, B. S. Fromm, D. Frankovich, P. Elko, R. T. Steinman, J. Fresard, J. J. Baga, and R. T. Taggart. T-wave "humps" as a potential electrocardiographic marker of the long QT syndrome. *J. Am. Coll. Cardiol.* 24:746–754, 1994.

127. Li, G. R., J. Feng, L. Yue, and M. Carrier. Transmural heterogeneity of action potentials and Ito1 in myocytes isolated from the human right ventricle. *Am. J. Physiol.* 275 (*Heart Circ Physiol.* 44):H369–H377, 1998.

128. Li, Z., S. Matsuoka, L. V. Hryshko, D. A. Nicoll, M. M. Bersohn, E. P. Burke, R. P. Lifton, and K. D. Philipson. Cloning of the NCX2 isoform of the plasma membrane Na(+)-Ca2;+ exchanger. *J Biol. Chem.* 269:17434–17439, 1994.

129. Litovsky, S. H. and C. Antzelevitch. Transient outward current prominent in canine ventricular epicardium but not endocardium. *Circ. Res.* 62:116–126, 1988.

130. Litovsky, S. H. and C. Antzelevitch. Rate dependence of action potential duration and refractoriness in canine ventricular endocardium differs from that of epicardium: the role of the transient outward current. *J. Am. Coll. Cardiol.* 14:1053–1066, 1989.

131. Litovsky, S. H. and C. Antzelevitch. Differences in the electrophysiological response of canine ventricular subendocardium and subepicardium to acetylcholine and isoproterenol. A direct effect of acetylcholine in ventricular myocardium. *Circ. Res.* 67:615–627, 1990.

132. Liu, D. W. and C. Antzelevitch. Characteristics of the delayed rectifier current (I_{Kr} and I_{Ks}) in canine ventricular epicardial, midmyocardial and endocardial myocytes: a weaker I_{Ks} contributes to the longer action potential of the M cell. *Circ. Res.* 76:351–365, 1995.

133. Liu, D. W., G. A. Gintant, and C. Antzelevitch. Ionic bases for electrophysiological distinctions among epicardial, midmyocardial, and endocardial myocytes from the free wall of the canine left ventricle. *Circ. Res.* 72:671–687, 1993.

134. Locati, E. H., P. Maison-Blanche, P. Dejode, B. Cauchemez, and P. Coumel. Spontaneous sequences of onset of torsade de pointes in patients with acquired prolonged repolarization: quantitative analysis of Holter recordings. *J. Am. Coll. Cardiol.* 25:1564–1575, 1995.

135. Lubinski, A., E. Lewicka-Nowak, M. Kempa, A. M. Baczynska, I. Romanowska, and G. Swiatecka. New insight into repolarization abnormalities in patients with congenital long QT syndrome: the increased transmural dispersion of repolarization. *Pacing Clin. Electrophysiol.* 21:172–175, 1998.

136. Lucchesi, P. A. and K. J. Sweadner. Postnatal changes in Na,K-ATPase isoform expression in rat cardiac ventricle. Conservation of biphasic ouabain affinity. *J. Biol. Chem.* 266:9327–9331, 1991.

137. Lukas, A. and C. Antzelevitch. Differences in the electrophysiological response of canine ventricular epicardium and endocardium to ischemia: role of the transient outward current. *Circulation* 88:2903–2915, 1993.

138. Lukas, A. and C. Antzelevitch. Phase 2 reentry as a mechanism of initiation of circus movement reentry in canine epicardium exposed to simulated ischemia. The antiarrhythmic effects of 4-aminopyridine. *Cardiovasc. Res.* 32:593–603, 1996.

139. Lukas, A. and C. Antzelevitch. The contribution of K^+ currents to electrical heterogeneity across the canine ventricular wall under normal and ischemic conditions. In: *Pathophysiology of Heart Failure*, edited by N. S. Dhalla, G. N. Pierce, and V. Panagia. Boston: Academic Publishers, 1996:440–456.

140. Lunkenheimer, P. P., K. Redmann, H. H. Scheld, K.-H. Dietl, C. Cryer, K.-D. Richter, J. Merker, and W. Whimster. The heart muscle's putative "secondary structure." Functional implications of a band-like anisotropy. *Technol. Health Care* 5:53–64, 1997.

141. MacKinnon, R. Determination of the subunit stoichiometry of a voltage-activated potassium channel. *Nature* 350:232–235, 1991.

142. Martin-Vasallo, P., W. Dackowski, J. R. Emanuel, and R. Levenson. Identification of a putative isoform of the Na,K-ATPase beta subunit. Primary structure and tissue-specific expression. *J. Biol. Chem.* 264:4613–4618, 1989.

143. Matsuo, K., W. Shimizu, T. Kurita, K. Suyama, N. Aihara, S. Kamakura, and K. Shimomura. Increased dispersion of repolarization time determined by monophasic action potentials in two patients with familial idiopathic ventricular fibrillation. *J. Cardiovasc. Electrophysiol.* 9:74–83, 1998.

144. Mays, D. J., J. M. Foose, L. H. Philipson, and M. M. Tamkun. Localization of the Kv1.5 K^+ channel protein in explanted cardiac tissue. *J. Clin. Invest* 96:282–292, 1995.

145. Mays, D. J., M. M. Tamkun, and P. A. Boyden. Redistribution of the Kv1.5 K^+ channel protein on the surface of myocytes from the epicardial border zone of infarcted canine ventricle. *Cardiovasc. Pathobiol.* 2:79–87, 2000.

146. Miyazaki, T., H. Mitamura, S. Miyoshi, K. Soejima, Y. Aizawa, and S. Ogawa. Autonomic and antiarrhythmic drug modulation of ST segment elevation in patients with Brugada syndrome. *J. Am. Coll. Cardiol.* 27:1061–1070, 1996.

147. Mori, Y., G. Mikala, G. Varadi, T. Kobayashi, S. Koch, M. Wakamori, and A. Schwartz. Molecular pharmacology of voltage-dependent calcium channels. *Jpn. J. Pharmacol.* 72:83–109, 1996.

148. Moss, A. J. Long QT syndrome. In: *Cardiac Arrhythmia: Mechanisms, Diagnosis and Management*, edited by P. J. Podrid, and P. R. Kowey. Baltimore, William Wilkins. 1995:1110–1120.

149. Moss, A. J., P. J. Schwartz, R. S. Crampton, D. Tzivoni, E. H. Locati, J. W. MacCluer, W. J. Hall, L. R. Weitkamp, G. M. Vincent, A. Garson, J. L. Robinson, J. Benhorin, and S. Choi. The long QT syndrome: prospective longitudinal study of 328 families. *Circulation* 84:1136–1144, 1991.

150. Mubagwa, K. and E. Carmeliet. Effects of acetylcholine on electrophysiological properties of rabbit cardiac Purkinje fibers. *Circ. Res.* 53:740–751, 1983.

151. Nabauer, M., D. J. Beuckelmann, P. Uberfuhr, and G. Steinbeck. Regional differences in current density and rate-dependent properties of the transient outward current in subepicardial and subendocardial myocytes of human left ventricle. *Circulation* 93:168–177, 1996.

152. Nakayama, T. and H. A. Fozzard. Adrenergic modulation of

the transient outward current in isolated canine Purkinje cells. *Circ. Res.* 62:162–172, 1988.
153. Ng, Y. C. and T. Akera. Relative abundance of two molecular forms of Na$^+$,K$^+$-ATPase in the ferret heart: developmental changes and associated alterations of digitalis sensitivity. *Mol. Pharmacol.* 32:201–205, 1987.
154. Nicoll, D. A., S. Longoni, and K. D. Philipson. Molecular cloning and functional expression of the cardiac sarcolemmal Na$(+)$-Ca^{2+} exchanger. *Science* 250:562–565, 1990.
155. Nicoll, D. A., B. D. Quednau, Z. Qui, Y. R. Xia, A. J. Lusis, and K. D. Philipson. Cloning of a third mammalian Na$^+$-Ca^{2+} exchanger, NCX3. *J. Biol. Chem.* 271:24914–24921, 1996.
156. Noble, D. and I. S. Cohen. The interpretation of the T wave of the electrocardiogram. *Cardiovasc. Res.* 12:13–27, 1978.
157. Orlowski, J. and J. B. Lingrel. Tissue-specific and developmental regulation of rat Na,K-ATPase catalytic alpha isoform and beta subunit mRNAs. *J. Biol. Chem.* 263:10436–10442, 1988.
158. Osborn, J. J. Experimental hypothermia: respiratory and blood pH changes in relation to cardiac function. *Am. J. Physiol.* 175:389–398, 1953.
159. Pacioretty, L. M. and R. F. Gilmour, Jr. Developmental changes in the transient outward potassium current in canine epicardium. *Am. J. Physiol.* 268 (*Heart Circ. Physiol.* 37):H2513–H2521, 1995.
160. Pertsov, A. M., J. M. Davidenko, R. Salomonsz, W. T. Baxter, and J. Jalife. Spiral waves of excitation underlie reentrant activity in isolated cardiac muscle. *Circ. Res.* 72:631–650, 1993.
161. Plonsey, R. Action potential sources and their volume conductor fields. *Proc. IEEE* 65:601–611, 1977.
162. Porzig, H., Z. Li, D. A. Nicoll, and K. D. Philipson. Mapping of the cardiac sodium-calcium exchanger with monoclonal antibodies. *Am. J. Physiol.* 265 (*Cell Physiol.* 34):C748–C756, 1993.
163. Prestle, J., S. Dieterich, M. Preuss, U. Bieligk, and G. Hasenfuss. Heterogeneous transmural gene expression of calcium-handling proteins and natriuretic peptides in the failing human heart *Cardiovasc. Res.* 43:323–331, 1999.
164. Priori, S. G., C. Napolitano, U. Glordano, G. Collisani, and M. Memml. Brugada syndrome and sudden cardiac death in children. *Lancet* 355:808–809, 2000.
165. Prystowsky, E. N., W. M. Jackman, R. L. Rinkenberger, et al. Effect of autonomic blockade on ventricular refractoriness and atrioventricular nodal conduction in man. Evidence supporting a direct cholinergic action on ventricular muscle refractoriness. *Circ. Res.* 49:511–518, 1981.
166. Ramakers, C., Doevendans, P. A., Vos, M. A., Antzelevitch, C., and Dumaine, R. KCNQ1 and KCNE1 expression is reduced in dogs with chronic AV block. *Biophys. J.* 78:220A, 2000. (Abstract)
167. Reder, R. F., D. S. Miura, P. Danilo, and M. R. Rosen. The electrophysiological properties of normal neonatal and adult canine cardiac Purkinje fibers. *Circ. Res.* 48:658–668, 1981.
168. Roberds, S. L. and M. M. Tamkun. Cloning and tissue-specific expression of five voltage-gated potassium channel cDNAs expressed in the heart. *Proc. Natl. Acad. Sci. U.S.A.* 88:1798–1802, 1991.
169. Rodriguez-Sinovas, A., J. Cinca, A. Tapias, L. Armadans, M. Tresanchez, and J. Soler-Soler. Lack of evidence of M-cells in porcine left ventricular myocardium. *Cardiovasc. Res.* 33:307–313, 1997.
170. Saeki, Y. and A. Kamiyama. Possible mechanism of rate-dependent change of contraction in dog ventricular muscle: relation to calcium movements. In *Recent Advances in Studies on Cardiac Structure and Metabolism*, Vol. II, edited by T. Kobayashi, R. Sano, and N. S. Dhalla. Baltimore: University Park Press. 1978:131–135.
171. Salata, J. J., N. K. Jurkiewicz, J. J. Wang, and H. T. Orme. A novel benzodiazepine that activates cardiac slow delayed rectifier K+ currents. *Mol. Pharmacol.* 54:220–230, 1998.
172. Sanguinetti, M. C., M. E. Curran, P. S. Spector, and M. T. Keating. Spectrum of HERG K$^+$-channel dysfunction in an inherited cardiac arrhythmia. *Proc. Natl. Acad. Sci. U.S.A.* 93:2208–2212, 1996.
173. Sanguinetti, M. C., M. E. Curran, A. R. Zou, J. Shen, P. S. Spector, D. L. Atkinson, and M. T. Keating. Coassembly of KvLQT1 and minK (IsK) proteins to form cardiac I_{Ks} potassium channel. *Nature* 384:80–83, 1996.
174. Sanguinetti, M. C., C. Jiang, M. E. Curran, and M. T. Keating. A mechanistic link between an inherited and an acquired cardiac arrhythmia: HERG encodes the I_{Kr} potassium channel. *Cell* 81:299–307, 1995.
175. Santos, E. M. and K. C. Frederick. Electrocardiographic changes in the dog during hypothermia. *Am. Heart J.* 55:415–420, 1957.
176. Schwartz, P. J. The idiopathic long QT syndrome: progress and questions. *Am. Heart J.* 109:399–411, 1985.
177. Schwartz, P. J. The long QT syndrome. In *Clinical Approaches to Tachyarrhythmias*, edited by A. J. Camm. Armonk, NY: Futura Publishing Company, 1997:53–53.
178. Schwartz, P. J., Malteo, P. S., Moss, A. J., Priori, S. G., Wang, Q., Lehmann, M. H., Timothy, K. W., Denjoy, I. F., Haverkamp, W., Guicheney, P., Paganini, V., Scheinman, M. M., and Karnes, P. S. Gene-specific influence on the triggers for cardiac arrest in the long QT syndrome. *Circulation* 96:I-212. 1997. (Abstract)
179. Schwartz, P. J., S. G. Priori, E. H. Locati, C. Napolitano, F. Cantu, J. A. Towbin, M. T. Keating, H. Hammoude, A. M. Brown, L. S. K. Chen, and T. J. Colatsky. Long QT syndrome patients with mutations of the *SCN5A* and *HERG* genes have differential responses to Na$^+$ channel blockade and to increases in heart rate: Implications for gene-specific therapy. *Circulation* 92:3381–3386, 1995.
180. Schwartz, P. J., M. Stramba-Badiale, A. Segantini, P. Austoni, G. Bosi, R. Giorgetti, F. Grancini, E. D. Marni, F. Perticone, D. Rosti, and P. Salice. Prolongation of the QT interval and the sudden infant death syndrome *N. Engl. J. Med.* 338:1709–1714, 1998.
181. Shamraj, O. I., D. Melvin, and J. B. Lingrel. Expression of Na,K-ATPase isoforms in human heart. *Biochem. Biophys. Res. Commun.* 179:1434–1440, 1991.
182. Shimizu, W. and C. Antzelevitch. Sodium channel block with mexiletine is effective in reducing dispersion of repolarization and preventing torsade de pointes in LQT2 and LQT3 models of the long-QT syndrome. *Circulation* 96:2038–2047, 1997.
183. Shimizu, W. and C. Antzelevitch. Cellular basis for the electrocardiographic features of the LQT1 form of the long QT syndrome: Effects of β-adrenergic agonists, antagonists and sodium channel blockers on transmural dispersion of repolarization and torsade de pointes. *Circulation* 98:2314–2322, 1998.
184. Shimizu, W. and C. Antzelevitch. Cellular and ionic basis for T wave alternans under long QT conditions. *Circulation* 99:1499–1507, 1999.
185. Shimizu, W. and C. Antzelevitch. Differential response to -adrenergic agonists and antagonists in LQT1, LQT2 and LQT3 models of the long QT syndrome. *J. Am. Coll. Cardiol.* 35:778–786, 2000.
186. Shimizu, W., T. Kurita, K. Matsuo, N. Aihara, S. Kamakura, J. A. Towbin, and K. Shimomura. Improvement of repolarization abnormalities by a K$^+$ channel opener in the LQT1 form of congenital long QT syndrome. *Circulation* 97:1581–1588, 1998.

187. Shimizu, W., B. McMahon, and C. Antzelevitch. Sodium pentobarbital reduces transmural dispersion of repolarization and prevents torsade de pointes in models of acquired and congenital long QT syndromes. *J. Cardiovasc. Electrophysiol.* 10:156–164, 1999.
188. Shimizu, W., T. Ohe, T. Kurita, M. Kawade, Y. Arakaki, N. Aihara, S. Kamakura, T. Kamiya, and K. Shimomura. Effects of verapamil and propranolol on early afterdepolarizations and ventricular arrhythmias induced by epinephrine in congenital long QT syndrome. *J. Am. Coll. Cardiol.* 26:1299–1309, 1995.
189. Shimizu, W., T. Ohe, T. Kurita, H. Takaki, N. Aihara, S. Kamakura, M. Matsuhisa, and K. Shimomura. Early afterdepolarizations induced by isoproterenol in patients with congenital long QT syndrome. *Circulation* 84:1915–1923, 1991.
190. Shipsey, S. J., S. M. Bryant, and G. Hart. Effects of hypertrophy on regional action potential characteristics in the rat left ventricle: a cellular basis for T-wave inversion? *Circulation* 96:2061–2068, 1997.
191. Shull, G. E., J. Greeb, and J. B. Lingrel. Molecular cloning of three distinct forms of the Na^+,K^+-ATPase alpha-subunit from rat brain. *Biochemistry* 25:8125–8132, 1986.
192. Shyjan, A. W., V. Cena, D. C. Klein, and R. Levenson. Differential expression and enzymatic properties of the $Na^+,K(+)$-ATPase alpha 3 isoenzyme in rat pineal glands. *Proc. Natl. Acad. Sci. U.S.A* 87:1178–1182, 1990.
193. Sicouri, S. and C. Antzelevitch. A subpopulation of cells with unique electrophysiological properties in the deep subepicardium of the canine ventricle: the M cell. *Circ. Res.* 68:1729–1741, 1991.
194. Sicouri, S. and C. Antzelevitch. Afterdepolarizations and triggered activity develop in a select population of cells (M cells) in canine ventricular myocardium: the effects of acetylstrophanthidin and Bay K 8644. *Pacing Clin. Electrophysiol.* 14:1714–1720, 1991.
195. Sicouri, S. and C. Antzelevitch. Drug-induced afterdepolarizations and triggered activity occur in a discrete subpopulation of ventricular muscle cell (M cells) in the canine heart: quinidine and digitalis. *J. Cardiovasc. Electrophysiol.* 4:48–58, 1993.
196. Sicouri, S. and C. Antzelevitch. Electrophysiologic characteristics of M cells in the canine left ventricular free wall. *J. Cardiovasc. Electrophysiol.* 6:591–603, 1995.
197. Sicouri, S., J. Fish, and C. Antzelevitch. Distribution of M cells in the canine ventricle. *J. Cardiovasc. Electrophysiol.* 5:824–837, 1994.
198. Sicouri, S., S. Moro, and M. V. Elizari. d-Sotalol induces marked action potential prolongation and early afterdepolarizations in M but not epicardial or endocardial cells of the canine ventricle. *J. Cardiovasc. Pharmacol. Ther.* 2:27–38, 1997.
199. Sicouri, S., S. Moro, S. H. Litovsky, M. V. Elizari, and C. Antzelevitch. Chronic amiodarone reduces transmural dispersion of repolarization in the canine heart. *J. Cardiovasc. Electrophysiol.* 8:1269–1279, 1997.
200. Sicouri, S., M. Quist, and C. Antzelevitch. Evidence for the presence of M cells in the guinea pig ventricle. *J. Cardiovasc. Electrophysiol.* 7:503–511, 1996.
201. Slezak, J., W. Schulze, L. Okruhlicova, N. Tribulova, and P. K. Singal. Cytochemical and immunocytochemical localization of Na,K-ATPase alpha subunit isoenzymes in the rat heart. *Mol. Cell. Biochem.* 176:107–112, 1997.
202. Slezak, J., W. Schulze, Z. Stefankova, L. Okruhlicova, L. Danihel and G. Wallukat. Localization of alpha 1,2,3-subunit isoforms of Na,K-ATPase in cultured neonatal and adult rat myocardium: the immunofluorescence and immunocytochemical study. *Mol. Cell. Biochem.* 163–164:39–45, 1996.
203. Snyders, D. J. and P. P. Van Bogaert. Effects of 4-aminopyridine on inward rectifing and pacemaker currents of cardiac purkinje fibers. *Pflugers Arch.* 394:230–238, 1982.
204. Solberg, L. E., D. H. Singer, R. E. Ten Eick, and E. G. Duffin. Glass microelectrode studies on intramural papillary muscle cells. *Circ. Res.* 34:783–797, 1974.
205. Sosunov, E. A., E. P. Anyukhovsky, and M. R. Rosen. Comparison of repolarization of cells from different layers of myocardium in vitro and in vivo. *Biophys. J.* 70:A276 1996. (Abstract)
206. Spach, M. S., R. C. Barr, G. A. Serwer, J. M. Kootsey, and E. A. Johnson. Extracellular potentials related to intracellular action potentials in the dog Purkinje system. *Circ. Res.* 30:505–519, 1972.
207. Splawski, I., M. Tristani-Firouzi, M. H. Lehmann, M. C. Sanguinetti, and M. T. Keating. Mutations in the hminK gene cause long QT syndrome and suppress I_{Ks} function. *Nat. Genet.* 17:338–340, 1997.
208. Sridharan, M. R. and L. G. Horan. Electrocardiographic J wave of hypercalcemia. *Am. J. Cardiol.* 54:672–673, 1984.
209. Stankovicova, T., M. Szilard, I. De Scheerder, and K. R. Sipido. M cells and transmural heterogeneity of action potential configuration in myocytes from the left ventricular wall of the pig heart. *Cardiovasc. Res.* 45:952–960, 2000.
210. Steinhaus, B. M. Estimating cardiac transmembrane activation and recovery times from unipolar and bipolar extracellular electrograms: a simulation study. *Circ. Res.* 64:449–462, 1989.
211. Streeter, D. D. Gross morphology and fiber geometry of the heart. In: *Handbook of Physiology. Section 2: The Cardiovascular System*, edited by R. M. Berne, Baltimore: Waverly Press, 1979:61–112.
212. Streeter, D. D., H. M. Spotnitz, D. P. Patel, J. Ross, and E. H. Sonnenblick. Fiber orientation in the canine left ventricle during diastole and systole. *Circ. Res.* 24:339–347, 1969.
213. Studer, R., H. Reinecke, J. Bilger, T. Eschenhagen, M. Bohm, G. Hasenfuss, H. Just, J. Holtz, and H. Drexler. Gene expression of the cardiac $Na(+)$-Ca^{2+} exchanger in end-stage human heart failure. *Circ. Res* 75:443–453, 1994.
214. Sun, Z. Q., G. T. Eddlestone, and C. Antzelevitch. Ionic mechanisms underlying the effects of sodium pentobarbital to diminish transmural dispersion of repolarization. *Pacing Clin. Electrophysiol.* 20:11–1116, 1997. (Abstract)
215. Surawicz, B. Electrophysiologic substrate of torsade de pointes: dispersion of repolarization or early afterdepolarizations? *J. Am. Coll. Cardiol.* 14:172–184, 1989.
216. Sweadner, K. J. Isozymes of the Na^+/K^+-ATPase. *Biochim. Biophys. Acta* 988:185–220, 1989.
217. Takagishi, Y., S. Rothery, J. Issberner, A. Levi, and N. J. Severs. Spatial distribution of dihydropyridine receptors in the plasma membrane of guinea pig cardiac myocytes investigated by correlative confocal microscopy and label-fracture electron microscopy. *J. Electron. Microsc. (Tokyo)* 46:165–170, 2000.
218. Takano, M. and A. Noma. Distribution of the isoprenaline-induced chloride current in rabbit heart. *Pflugers Arch.* 420:223–226, 1992.
219. Takimoto, K., D. Li, J. M. Nerbonne, and E. S. Levitan. Distribution, splicing and glucocorticoid-induced expression of cardiac alpha 1C and alpha 1D voltage-gated Ca^{2+} channel mRNAs. *J. Mol. Cell. Cardiol.* 29:3035–3042, 1997.
220. Thompson, R., J. Rich, F. Chmelik, and W. L. Nelson. Evolutionary changes in the electrocardiogram of severe progressive hypothermia. *J. Electrocardiol.* 10:67–70, 1977.
221. Toshe, N., N. Haruaki, and M. Kanno. α 1-Adrenoceptor stimulation enhances the delayed rectifier K^+ current of guinea pig ventricular cells through the activation of protein kinase C. *Circ. Res.* 71:1441–1446, 1992.

222. Trautwein, W. and M. Kameyama. Intracellular control of calcium and potassium currents in cardiac cells. *Jpn. Heart J.* 27(Suppl 1):31–50, 1986.
223. Trudeau, M. C., J. W. Warmke, B. Ganetzky, and G. A. Robertson. HERG, a human inward rectifier in the voltage-gated potassium channel family. *Science* 269:92–95, 1995.
224. van Kempen, M. J., C. Fromaget, D. Gros, A. F. Moorman, and W. H. Lamers. Spatial distribution of connexin43, the major cardiac gap junction protein, in the developing and adult rat heart. *Circ. Res* 68:1638–1651, 1991.
225. Verheule, S., M. J. van Kempen, P. H. te Welscher, B. R. Kwak, and H. J. Jongsma. Characterization of gap junction channels in adult rabbit atrial and ventricular myocardium. *Circ. Res* 80:673–681, 1997.
226. Viskin, S., S. R. Alla, H. V. Barron, K. Heller, L. A. Saxon, I. Kitzis, G. F. Hare, M. J. Wong, M. D. Lesh, and M. M. Scheinman. Mode of onset of torsade de pointes in congenital long QT syndrome. *J. Am. Coll. Cardiol.* 28:1262–1268, 1996.
227. Viswanathan, P. C., R. M. Shaw, and Y. Rudy. Effects of I_{Kr} and I_{Ks} heterogeneity on action potential duration and its rate-dependence: a simulation study. *Circulation* 99:2466–2474, 1999.
228. Volders, P. G., K. R. Sipido, E. Carmeliet, R. L. Spatjens, H. J. Wellens, and M. A. Vos. Repolarizing K$^+$ currents ITO1 and IKs are larger in right than left canine ventricular midmyocardium. *Circulation* 99:206–210, 1999.
229. Vos, M. A., S. C. Verduyn, A. P. M. Gorgels, G. C. Lipcsei, and H. J. Wellens. Reproducible induction of early afterdepolarizations and torsade de pointes arrhythmias by d-sotalol and pacing in dogs with chronic atrioventricular block. *Circulation* 91:864–872, 1995.
230. Wang, Q., M. E. Curran, I. Splawski, T. C. Burn, J. M. Millholland, T. J. Van Raay, J. Shen, K. W. Timothy, G. M. Vincent, T. De Jager, P. J. Schwartz, J. A. Towbin, A. J. Moss, D. L. Atkinson, G. M. Landes, T. D. Connors, and M. T. Keating. Positional cloning of a novel potassium channel gene: KVLQT1 mutations cause cardiac arrhythmias. *Nat. Genet.* 12:17–23, 1996.
231. Wang, Q., J. Shen, I. Splawski, D. L. Atkinson, Z. Z. Li, J. L. Robinson, A. J. Moss, J. A. Towbin, and M. T. Keating. SCN5A mutations associated with an inherited cardiac arrhythmia, long QT syndrome. *Cell* 80:805–811, 1995.
232. Wang, Z. G., B. Fermini, and S. Nattel. Sustained depolarization-induced outward current in human atrial myocytes: evidence for a novel delayed rectifier K$^+$ current similar to Kv1.5 cloned channel currents. *Circ. Res.* 73:1061–1076, 1993.
233. Watanabe, Y. Purkinje repolarization as a possible cause of the U wave in the electrocardiogram. *Circulation* 51:1030–1037, 1975.
234. Weirich, J., Bernhardt, R., Loewen, N., Wenzel, W., and Antoni, H. Regional- and species-dependent effects of K$^+$-channel blocking agents on subendocardium and mid-wall slices of human, rabbit and guinea pig myocardium. *Pflugers Arch.* 431:R 130, 1996. (Abstract)
235. Weissenburger, J., J. M. Davy, and F. Chezalviel. Experimental models of torsades de pointes. *Fundam. Clin. Pharmacol.* 7:29–38, 1993.
236. Weissenburger, J., J. M. Davy, F. Chezalviel, O. Ertzbischoff, J. M. Poirier, F. Engel, P. Lainee, E. Penin, G. Motte, and G. Cheymol. Arrhythmogenic activities of antiarrhythmic drugs in conscious hypokalemic dogs with atrioventricular block: comparison between quinidine, lidocaine, flecainide, propranolol and sotalol. *J. Pharmacol. Exp. Ther.* 259:871–883, 1991.
237. Weissenburger, J., V. V. Nesterenko, and C. Antzelevitch. Transmural heterogeneity of ventricular repolarization under baseline and long QT conditions in the canine heart in vivo. Torsades de pointes develops with halothane but not pentobarbital anesthesia. *J. Cardiovasc. Electrophysiol.* 1:290–304, 2000.
238. West, T. C., E. L. Frederickson, and D. W. Amory. Single fiber recording of the ventricular response to induced hypothermia in the anesthetized dog. Correlation with multicellular parameters. *Circ. Res.* 7:880–888, 1959.
239. Wettwer, E., G. J. Amos, H. Posival, and U. Ravens. Transient outward current in human ventricular myocytes of subepicardial and subendocardial origin. *Circ. Res.* 75:473–482, 1994.
240. Wilde, A. A. M., R. J. E. Jongbloed, P. A. Doevendans, D. R. Düren, R. N. W. Hauer, I. M. Van Langen, J. P. Van Tintelen, H. J. M. Smeets, H. Meyer, and J. L. M. C. Geelen. Auditory stimuli as a trigger for arrhythmic events differentiate HERG-related (LQTS$_2$) patients from KVLQT1-related patients (LQTS$_1$). *J. Am. Coll. Cardiol.* 33:327–332, 1999.
241. Wong, K. R., A. E. Trezise, S. Bryant, G. Hart, and J. I. Vandenberg. Molecular and functional distributions of chloride conductances in rabbit ventricle. *Am. J. Physiol.* 277 (*Heart Circ. Physiol.* 46):H1403–H1409, 1999.
242. Xu, H., J. E. Dixon, D. M. Barry, J. S. Trimmer, J. P. Merlie, D. McKinnon, and J. M. Nerbonne. Developmental analysis reveals mismatches in the expression of K$^+$ channel alpha subunits and voltage-gated K$^+$ channel currents in rat ventricular myocytes. *J. Gen. Physiol* 108:405–419, 1996.
243. Yan, G. X. and C. Antzelevitch. Cellular basis for the electrocardiographic J wave. *Circulation* 93:372–379, 1996.
244. Yan, G. X. and C. Antzelevitch. Cellular basis for the normal T wave and the electrocardiographic manifestations of the long QT syndrome. *Circulation* 98:1928–1936, 1998.
245. Yan, G. X. and C. Antzelevitch. Cellular basis for the Brugada syndrome and other mechanisms of arrhythmogenesis associated with ST segment elevation. *Circulation* 100:1660–1666, 1999.
246. Yan, G. X., W. Shimizu, and C. Antzelevitch. Characteristics and distribution of M cells in arterially perfused canine left ventricular wedge preparations. *Circulation* 98:1921–1927, 1998.
247. Young, R. M. and J. B. Lingrel. Tissue distribution of mRNAs encoding the alpha isoforms and beta subunit of rat Na$^+$,K$^+$-ATPase. *Biochem. Biophys. Res. Commun.* 145:52–58, 1987.
248. Zahler, R., M. Brines, M. Kashgarian, E. J. Benz, Jr., and M. Gilmore-Hebert. The cardiac conduction system in the rat expresses the alpha 2 and alpha 3 isoforms of the Na$^+$,K(+)-ATPase. *Proc. Natl. Acad. Sci. U.S.A* 89:99–103, 1992.
249. Zahler, R., W. Sun, T. Ardito, M. Brines, and M. Kashgarian. The α3 isoform protein of the Na$^+$/K$^+$-ATPase is associated with the sites of neuromuscular and cardiac impulse transmission. In *The Sodium Pump: Structure, Mechanism, Hormonal Control and Its Role in Disease*, edited by E. Bamberg and W. Schoner. New York: Springer-Verlag, 2000:714–717.
250. Zahler, R., W. Sun, T. Ardito, and M. Kashgarian. Na-K-ATPase alpha-isoform expression in heart and vascular endothelia: cellular and developmental regulation. *Am. J. Physiol.* 270 (*Cell Physiol.* 39):C361–C371, 1996.
251. Zhang, J. F., A. D. Randall, P. T. Ellinor, W. A. Horne, W. A. Sather, T. Tanabe, T. L. Schwarz, and R. W. Tsien. Distinctive pharmacology and kinetics of cloned neuronal Ca^{2+} channels and their possible counterparts in mammalian CNS neurons. *Neuropharmacology* 32:1075–1088, 1993.
252. Zhang, L., S. J. Compton, C. Antzelevitch, K. W. Timothy, G. M. Vincent, and J. W. Mason. Differential response of QT and QU intervals to adrenergic stimulation in long QT patients

with IKs defects. *J. Am. Coll. Cardiol.* 33:138A, 1999. (Abstract)
253. Zipes, D. P. The long QT interval syndrome: A Rosetta stone for sympathetic related ventricular tachyarrhythmias. *Circulation* 84:1414–1419, 1991.
254. Zygmunt, A. C. Intracellular calcium activates chloride current in canine ventricular myocytes. *Am. J. Physiol.* 267 (*Heart Circ. Physiol.* 36):H1984–H1995, 1994.
255. Zygmunt, A. C. and W. R. Gibbons. Calcium-activated chloride current in rabbit ventricular myocytes. *Circ. Res.* 68:424–437, 1991.
256. Zygmunt, A. C. and W. R. Gibbons. Properties of the calcium-activated chloride current in heart. *J. Gen. Physiol.* 99:391–414, 1992.
257. Zygmunt, A. C., R. J. Goodrow, and C. Antzelevitch. I_{Na-Ca} contributes to electrical heterogeneity within the canine ventricle. *Am. J. Physiol. Heart Circ. Physiol.* 278:H1671–H1678, 2000.
258. Zygmunt, A. C., G. T. Eddlestone, G. P. Thomas, V. V. Nesterenko, C. Antzelevitch. Larger late sodium conductance in M-cells contributes to electrical heterogeneity in canine ventricle. *Am. J. Physiol. Heart Circ. Physiol.*, In press, 2001.

18. Newly cloned threshold channels

DOROTHY A. HANCK
RUTH L. MARTIN
Cardiac Electrophysiology Laboratories, University of Chicago, Chicago, Illinois

JAN TYTGAT
CHRIS ULENS
Laboratory of Toxicology, Faculty of Pharmaceutical Sciences, University of Leuven, Leuven, Belgium

CHAPTER CONTENTS

The Pacemaker Current (I_f, I_h, or HCN)
Molecular Cloning
Structure of HCN Channels
Distribution Patterns of HCN Genes
Biophysical Properties of HCN Channels
Low-Voltage Activated Calcium Channels
Molecular Cloning and Distribution
Structure
Biophysics
   Comparison of α1G, α1H, and α1I
   How voltage dependent are T-type calcium channels?
   Selectivity and block of T-type calcium channels
Summary

MANY CELL TYPES IN THE BODY are not only excitable, i.e. generate action potentials, but they exhibit rhythmic firing that is modulated by hormonal and neuronal activity. In the heart, cells of the conducting system, including the Sinoatrial (SA) and Atrioventricular (AV) nodes, as well as the His–Purkinje system fire spontaneously, i.e. without provocation from neurons. Intrinsic pacemaking is a result of the expression of hyperpolarization activated channels, which for many years were molecularly unidentified, but which are now known to be members of a gene family of at least four members as a result of cloning efforts that have recently borne fruit. In addition, rhythmicity is modulated both in the heart and in other cells by other channels active near threshold. One of the most interesting of these, the T-type calcium channel, was also elusive and only cloned in 1999. This chapter discusses the physiology, biophysics, and molecular biology of these two very important threshold channels.

THE PACEMAKER CURRENT (I_f, I_h, or HCN)

Pacemaker currents were first described in cardiac SA node cells (18, 17, 33, 142), and later in Purkinje fibers (35), ventricular (144) and atrial (148) muscle, and a variety of neurons [for review see (104)]. The newly cloned pacemaker channels give rise to currents, which are almost indistinguishable from or very similar to native pacemaker currents, termed I_f ("funny" current) in heart and I_h (hyperpolarization-activated) or I_q ("*q*ueer") in brain tissue. The family of HCN (hyperpolarization-activated, cyclic nucleotide-sensitive, cation nonselective) ion channels shares typical properties that underlie their ability to generate spontaneous oscillatory activity [for reviews see (10, 83, 114)]. First, cloned pacemaker channels activate upon hyperpolarization in a voltage range comprising the action potential threshold of the cell membrane. Second, the inward current that arises upon hyperpolarization is unselectively carried by K^+ and Na^+ ions. This depolarizing current drives the membrane potential toward the threshold of depolarization, maintaining spontaneous rhythmic activity. Third, the voltage dependence of activation is controlled by the intracellular cyclic adenosine morophosphate (cAMP) concentration through a mechanism involving direct binding of cAMP to the channel. This causes a shift of the activation curve along the voltage axis, which, in turn, determines the steepness of the pacemaker depolarization and eventually the firing frequency [for review see (37) and (104)]. The pacemaking process is also finely tuned by hormones and neurotransmitters acting through the second-messenger cAMP. In response to β-adrenergic stimulation, the intracellular cAMP concentration rises through activation of adenylyl cyclase by G_s proteins. The elevation of the intracellular cAMP shifts the voltage dependence of activation by 10 mV to more depolarized potentials, resulting in increased pacemaker current amplitudes. This mechanism is largely responsible for the increase of the heart rate in response to β-adrenergic agonists (18) and slowing of the heart rate during vagal stimulation. In this chapter, we focus on the molecular cloning of pacemaker channels, the structural determinants underlying their ability to gen-

MOLECULAR CLONING

Despite the ever-increasing number of ion channels genes from the K⁺ channel superfamily that have been discovered since the cloning of *Shaker* channels (103), attempts to clone pacemaker channels were unsuccessful until recently. The idea that the gene encoding a pacemaker channel would be related to the family of voltage-gated K⁺ channels as well as the family of cyclic nucleotide-gated (CNG) channels, contributed to the different approaches that have led to identification of the pacemaker gene family. Santoro et al. (112) used an alternative cloning strategy based on protein–protein interactions to screen a mouse cDNA library with the SH3 domain of the neural form of Src tyrosine kinase (19, 88) as bait. The deduced amino acid sequence of the isolated gene, mBCNG-1 (now termed mHCN1), revealed it to be a member of the superfamily of voltage-gated K⁺ channels, but with an unusual pore sequence, consistent with the weak K⁺-selectivity described for native pacemaker currents. The C-terminus contains a conserved cyclic nucleotide binding domain (CNBD) that is homologous to the CNBD of protein kinases (123) and CNG-channels (145). This suggested that its gating could be regulated by cyclic nucleotides, consistent with the cAMP-induced shift of the activation curve as seen with native pacemaker currents. Finally, immunohistochemical analysis indicated that mHCN1 transcripts are abundantly expressed in cortical structures, namely the neocortex, hippocampus, and cerebellum. This fits well with the presence of a pacemaker current that has been described in hippocampal pyramidal neurons (84). Functional expression of mHCN1 confirmed that this gene encodes a hyperpolarization-activated ion channel of brain that selects weakly for K⁺ over Na⁺ and is directly modulated by intracellular cAMP (113). In addition, Santoro et al. cloned partial cDNAs, representing three additional members of the pacemaker gene family (mBCNG-2, mBCNG-3, and mBCNG-4—now termed mHCN2, mHCN4, and mHCN3, respectively), while screening for full-length mHCN1 products. Two human orthologs, termed hHCN1 and hHCN2, were partially cloned following an expressed sequence tag (EST) database homology search, using the protein sequence of mHCN1 as a query. In a similar approach, Ludwig et al. (82) searched the EST database using the CNBD of CNG channels as a query sequence. This screening resulted in the isolation of three full-length coding sequences from a mouse brain cDNA library: HAC1 (corresponding to mBCNG-2), HAC2 (corresponding to mBCNG-1), and HAC3 (corresponding to mBCNG-4). HAC1 (now termed HCN2) encodes a hyperpolazition-activated cation channel that exhibits the general properties of native pacemaker channels. Given the overlap between the genes identified in the studies of Santoro et al. and Ludwig et al., a unified nomenclature has been proposed that includes all known members of this new gene family (25). According to the unifying nomenclature, the pacemaker channel genes (HCN1–4) are termed hyperpolarization-activated, cyclic-nucleotide-sensitive, cation nonselective K⁺ channels (see Table 18–1). The consensus nomenclature of the pacemaker gene family members is as follows: HCN1 corresponds to mBCNG-1 and HAC2, HCN2 corresponds to mBCNG-2 and HAC1, HCN3 corresponds to mBCNG-4 (HAC3), and HCN4 corresponds to mBCNG-3. In a third approach, Gauss et al. (48) probed a sea urchin sperm library with a DNA fragment that was amplified in a polymerase chain reaction with degenerate oligonucleotide primers based on conserved CNG channel sequences. Full-length cloning identified a fifth pacemaker gene encoding a channel polypeptide, SPIH. Functional expression of SPIH gives rise to channels with characteristics that are similar to the mammalian pacemaker channels. Using a highly conserved region from mHCN1 as a probe, Ludwig et al. (81) isolated full-length hHCN2 and hHCN4 from a human atrioventricular node cDNA library. Seifert et al. (116) isolated an identical hHCN4 clone from a thalamic-specific cDNA library, while Vaccari et al. (137) reported the isolation of an identical hHCN2 clone from human cerebellum. The HCN4 clone that was isolated from a rabbit sinoatrial (SA) node cDNA library lacks part of the N-terminal region and probably represents a partial clone (65). Cloned HCN channel homologues from rat and rabbit were obtained from brain cDNA libraries (124). The hHCN2 gene was mapped to the human chromosome 19p13.3 and contains eight exons spanning $\sim$27 kb (83), whereas the hHCN4 gene was localized on chromosome band 15q24–q25 (116).

STRUCTURE OF HCN CHANNELS

The HCN family forms a new subfamily within the K⁺ channel superfamily, most closely related to other K⁺ channels that contain a CNBD, such as *eag* K⁺ channels, CNG channels, and the plant inwardly rectifying K⁺ channels related to KAT1 (4, 119). From an evolutionary point of view, Santoro et al. (112, 114) suggested that HCN genes remained closer to the ancestral molecule that represents the genealogical link between voltage-gated K⁺ channels and CNG channels. All of the identified sequences contain the conserved motifs of a voltage-gated K$^+$ channel, including six transmembrane helices (S1–S6), a positively charged voltage sensor (S4), and a pore-forming loop between S5 and S6. Like CNG channels and *eag* K$^+$ channels, HCN channels contain a CNBD in their C-terminus. The four mammalian pacemaker channels are very closely related to one another, with a protein sequence similarity of ~60%. The homology is the highest in the central core region (transmembrane domains plus the CNBD) with a protein sequence similarity of 80%–90%. In contrast, the N- and C-termini have variable length and share only modest homology. No tissue-dependent alternative splicing events have been detected in the large number of hHCN2 clones examined, indicating that identical HCN2 channels are present in heart and brain (83). To date, no splice variants of other HCN family members have been reported.

Remarkably, the C-terminus of HCN1 contains a polyglutamine-repeat that is absent in the other pacemaker channels. In this context, it could be interesting to note that the HCN1 gene is expressed in some areas of the brain, and an increasing number of neurodegenerative disorders have been found to be caused by expanding CAG triplet repeats that code for polyglutamine (for review see ref. 109a). HCN channels also contain a serine residue in their C-terminus that lies within a consensus site for protein kinase A (PKA) phosphorylation, although this site was absent in Santoro's mBCNG-4 clone and present in Ludwig's HAC3 clone. Despite the high homology of HCN channels in the CNBD, several amino acid residues are substituted. Future mutagenesis studies will reveal whether these modest changes can account for the striking difference in cyclic-nucleotide sensitivity. At present, the possibility remains that the structural determinant for cAMP sensitivity may be localized outside of the CNBD itself (114).

Although HCN channels retain the conserved GYG-signature sequence that constitutes the main part of the selectivity filter, the channel's mixed ion-selectivity could result from nonconservative changes at key positions in the pore-forming loop. These changes include the substitution of a negatively charged amino acid residue following the GYG-triplet by a hydrophobic residue in HCN1 (alanine), a postively charged residue in HCN2 and HCN4 (arginine), and a neutral residue in HCN3 (glutamine). In addition, HCN1–4 contain a cysteine in place of a conserved threonine at −2 from the GYG-triplet and two more positively charged residues at −5 (histidine) and −9 (lysine). In view of the crystal structure that has been resolved (39), it would be plausible to suggest that these unusual substitutions could account for a loss in rigidity of the carbonyl backbone, thus allowing both K$^+$ and Na$^+$ to pass the selectivity filter. In the near future mutations at these specific sites will most likely solve the question whether the unusual substitutions in HCN channels are responsible for the channel's partial loss of K$^+$ selectivity.

The voltage-sensing S4 segment of HCN channels has a unique structure, consisting of two sequences of five positively charged residues, separated by an "in-frame" serine. The total of ten positive charges in the S4 segment is unusually high as compared to only five to seven in the S4 segment of other K$^+$ channels. In addition, the presence of a positively charged voltage sensor is somewhat surprising since HCN channels activate upon hyperpolarization. Miller and Aldrich (91) previously demonstrated that a combination of three point mutations (replacing positive charged amino acids with neutral amino acids) in the S4 segment of *Shaker* K$^+$ channels shifts, the midpoint potential of activation to extreme hyperpolarized potentials. This transforms the delayed rectifying *Shaker* K$^+$ channel into a voltage-gated inwardly rectifying K$^+$ channel. Given the high number of positively charged residues in HCN channels, this mechanism cannot account for the unusual hyperpolarization-activation of HCN channels. Recent mutagenesis results of KAT1 suggested that the hyperpolarizing shift of the activation curve for this channel is caused by an interaction of the channel's N-terminus with the S4 segment (85). However, a similar deletion of the N-terminal domain in HCN2 channels did not affect the gating of HCN channels in a similar way (24). Therefore, the coupling of S4 movement with channel gating remains poorly understood. However, the strong inward rectification might be produced by a mechanism similar to that of *HERG* channels. *HERG* channels are closed at rest and open upon depolarization. However, the rate of inactivation is faster than the rate of activation, resulting in little outward current upon depolarization. Upon hyperpolarization, the channels recover quickly from inactivation but remain open until the activation gates shut the channels off (also called deactivation).

Like voltage-gated K$^+$ channels and CNG channels, HCN channels probably function as tetramers. Because the expression pattern of the four different HCN transcripts at least partially overlaps in heart as well as in brain tissues, the possibility exists that HCN channels may form heteromultimeric complexes. The possibility that different HCN channel subunits coassemble to form heteromeric channels has been investigated using a concatenated construct encoding two connected subunits, HCN1 and HCN2 (136a). It was observed that the heteromeric channel activates only little slower than HCN1, whereas the voltage dependence of activation was more similar to HCN2. The cAMP-sensitivity of the heteromeric channels was intermediate between HCN1 and HCN2. This phenotype shows marked resemblance to the current arising from oocytes that coexpress HCN1 and HCN2 subunits and the native pacemaker current in CA1 pyramidal neurons, previously shown to express HCN1 and HCN2 (111a). These results suggest that HCN channels also function as heteromers, most likely tetramers and that heteromerization increases the functional diversity of pacemaker currents beyond the levels expected from the number of HCN channels genes and their differential distribution (136a).

DISTRIBUTION PATTERNS OF HCN GENES

Immunohistochemical analysis and in situ hybridization experiments revealed that mHCN1 shows a rather restricted distribution pattern in brain tissue, with prominent labeling in cortical structures (112, 95). In contrast, mHCN2 shows a more uniform level of expression in all brain structures, particularly in thalamic and brain stem nuclei (112, 95). In addition, Santoro et al. (113) also reported high levels of mHCN2 and mHCN4 expression in the heart. Northern blot and in situ hybridization experiments indicated that HCN2 transcripts are present in mouse heart, while HCN1 appears to be absent (82). Tissue distribution of hHCN2 and hHCN4 was investigated by Northern blot analysis and RT-PCR®, revealing that both transcripts are widespread throughout the human ventricle, atrium, and conduction tissue (83). Seifert et al. (116) also reported high expression levels of hHCN4 in heart and testis. The expression was lower in total brain, but prominent labeling was observed in the thalamus. Ishii et al. (65) reported expression of rHCN4 in rabbit heart SA node, with no significant signals in other parts of cardiac tissues, brain, or skeletal muscle. A distinct distribution pattern was revealed for mHCN3, which appears to be mainly expressed in liver, brain, lung, and kidney (112, 95). No expression of mHCN3 was detected in heart (82). Using RNase protection assays, Shi et al. (124) rather surprisingly reported that the rabbit SA node contains an abundance of HCN1 and HCN4, a detectable level of HCN2, and no HCN3 transcripts. These results show that the HCN1 isoform, thought to be expressed uniquely in brain, is expressed in rabbit SA node (18% of total mRNA) while HCN2, thought to be the most prevalent isoform in cardiac tissue, is only minimally present in rabbit SA node (0.6%). The results from Shi et al. (124) suggest HCN4 to be the dominant isoform in rabbit SA node (81%). The total expression of HCN isoforms in Purkinje fibers is only 3.9% of that expressed in SA node, with prominent levels of HCN1 (49%) and HCN4 (40%) and only low levels of HCN2 (11%). Ventricular muscle expresses only HCN2 transcripts (0.7% of the total HCN isoform expression in SA node). This tissue-dependent "isoform switching" may contribute to the wide range of I_f activation thresholds observed in cardiac tissues (124). The authors suggested that the different results obtained in their study may rely on the nonquantitative nature of methods used in previous studies.

In summary, all HCN isoforms seem to be expressed in brain tissue with a uniform distribution of HCN2, and a restricted distribution of HCN1 in cortical structures and HCN4 in thamalic neurons. In contrast, heart tissue predominantly expresses HCN2 and HCN4 in ventricle, atria, and conduction tissue. Results obtained for HCN1 seem contradictory, because only one study reported abundant expression of HCN1 in rabbit SA node.

BIOPHYSICAL PROPERTIES OF HCN CHANNELS

Upon heterologous expression, cloned pacemaker channels give rise to hyperpolarization-activated currents, unselectively carried by K^+ and Na^+, but with strikingly different gating properties and voltage-dependent kinetics. As an example, representative mHCN1 and mHCN2 current traces, obtained in our laboratory, are shown in Figure 18–1. Typically, pacemaker currents turn on with a slow time course of activation at intermediate potentials, but the rate of activation increases with increasing hyperpolarizations (Fig. 18–1A for mHCN1 and B for mHCN2). Upon repolarization, the currents deactivate in a voltage-dependent manner, generating a decaying inward tail current (Fig. 18–1C for mHCN1 and D for mHCN2). Observation of the tail current amplitudes reveals that mHCN1 activates at fewer negative membrane potentials than mHCN2. Construction of Boltzmann activation curves showed that mHCN1 activates with a $V_{1/2} = -62.58 \pm 2.48$ mV and $S = -7.56 \pm 0.94$ mV (n = 6), while mHCN2 activates with a $V_{1/2} = -93.34 \pm 2.17$ mV and $S = -5.38 \pm 0.20$ mV (n = 4). It should be noted that the voltage steps used to evoke HCN2 traces (Fig. 18–1B) may reflect physiological relevant conditions (3 sec), but do not allow the channel to reach steady-state levels of activation. Because HCN2 channels activate relatively slow, voltage pulses of 30 sec are required to fully activate the channel at intermediate membrane voltages. Under these conditions we determined a steady-state midpoint value of −75 mV, close to the threshold potential. The sigmoidal onset of activation indicates that channel activation requires a series of conformational transitions involving both closed and open states (34). However, ignoring the sigmoidal onset, the time course of activation

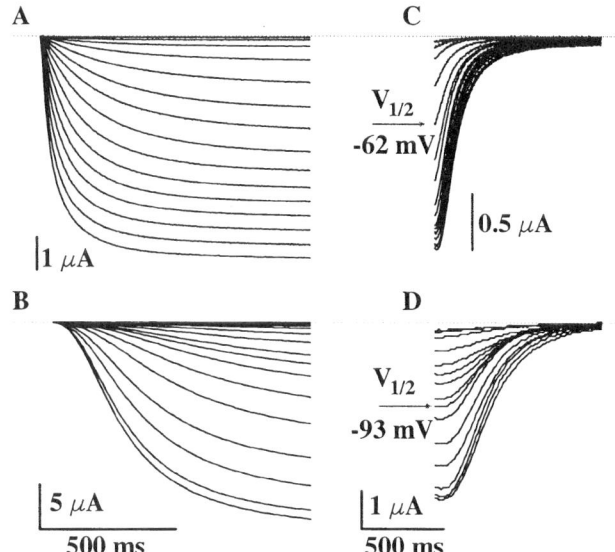

FIG. 18–1. Representative mHCN1 and mHCN2 current traces are shown in upper and lower panels, respectively. The two-microelectrode voltage-clamp technique (GeneClamp 500, Axon Instruments, USA) was used to measure hyperpolarization-activated currents evoked from *Xenopus* oocytes expressing either mHCN1 or mHCN2 cRNA (cDNA clones were a kind gift from Steven A. Siegelbaum, Columbia University, New York). Experiments were carried out using a high-potassium (HK) external solution (composition in mM: KCl 96, NaCl 2, MgCl$_2$ 1, CaCl$_2$ 1.8, HEPES 5, and pH 7.5). Currents were filtered at 200 Hz, using a 4-pole low-pass Bessel filter. To eliminate the effect of the voltage drop across the bath-grounding electrode, the bath potential was actively controlled. Capacitative and leak components were offline subtracted. For mHCN1, current traces were evoked by application of 1 sec hyperpolarizing test pulses from −45 to −115 mV in 5 mV steps from a holding potential of −40mV (*A*). The pulse interval was 3 sec. Tail currents were measured at −40 mV (*C*). For mHCN2, current traces were evoked by application of 3 sec hyperpolarizing test pulses from −60 to −130 mV in 5 mV steps from a holding potential of −40 mV (*B*). The pulse interval was 4 sec. Only the first second of the pulses is shown for comparison with mHCN1 (*A*). Both traces are plotted on the same time scale; the scale bar in *B* also applies to *A*. mHCN2 tail currents were measured at −40mV (*D*) and plotted on the same time scale as mHCN1 tail currents (*C*). The time scale bar in *D* also applies to *C*.

can be approximated by a single exponential function, although double exponential functions result in a better fit a most negative voltages (136a). It is clear from the current traces shown in Figure 18–1 that mHCN2 activates and deactivates remarkably more slowly than mHCN1. At −60 mV (approximating its $V_{1/2}$) we calculated that mHCN1 activates with a time constant of 274.02 ± 21.68 msec (n=8). At −90 mV (approximating its $V_{1/2}$) mHCN2 activates with a time constant of 4482.52 ± 1165.10 msec (n=6). This example illustrates how two cloned pacemaker channels with considerable structural homology are yet characterized by strikingly different biophysical properties. The functional data obtained in the first reports on cloned pacemaker channels are summarized in Table 18–1. In this respect, it should be noted that our $V_{1/2}$ calculated for mHCN1 is remarkably more positive than the value of −100 mV reported by Santoro et al. (113). The difference with our $V_{1/2}$ obtained in whole-cell mode can be well explained by a ~20–30 mV shift to more hyperpolarizing potentials of $V_{1/2}$ obtained in inside-out patches. A similar phenomenon has been observed for cloned pacemaker channels (82) and native pacemaker channels (38). Additionally, these differences may also depend on the expression system used (*Xenopus* oocytes or HEK293 cells) and voltage protocols applied.

Significantly, mHCN2 was shown to be strongly regulated by direct binding of cAMP to the intracellular side of the channel [$V_{1/2}$ shifted 13 mV toward more positive potentials, (82)], while mHCN1 was characterized by poor cAMP-modulation [$V_{1/2}$ shifted 1.8 mV towards more positive potentials, (112)]. The activation of HCN2 channels as well as native pacemaker channels by cAMP reveals no cooperativity [Hill coefficient 0.8; (82)] in contrast to the highly cooperative activation of CNG channels by cyclic nucleotides (49). Interestingly, the fast gating properties of mHCN1 (113) are indistinguishable from native pacemaker currents recorded from hippocampal pyramidal cells (a region where HCN1 is highly expressed), while HCN2 activates slowly (82), similar to native pacemaker currents in thalamic neurons. Alternatively, the slow gating HCN4 channel (predominantly expressed in thalamus) has been suggested to control pacemaking activity in thalamocortical neurons (116). In relation to native pacemaker currents from the heart, HCN2 and HCN4 (which are abundantly expressed in cardiac ventricle and atrial muscle as well as in conduction tissue) have been suggested to underlie the fast and slow component of the cardiac pacemaker current, respectively (83). The time course of activation for hHCN4 is intriguingly slow as compared to hHCN2 with a time constant of activation at −110 mV (approximating its $V_{1/2}$ of −109 mV) as slow as 23 ± 9 sec. However, Seifert et al. (116) elegantly demonstrated that short voltage steps do not allow complete channel activation and therefore the $V_{1/2}$ value can be seriously biased. Using long pulse durations (<60 sec), Seifert et al. (116) calculated a saturating $V_{1/2}$ of −75.2 for hHCN4, approximating the $V_{1/2}$ reported for I_h in thalamocortical neurons (20, 90, 127) and I_f in cardiac SA node (1, 36, 52). A time constant of 21.5 sec was calculated at −70 mV (approximating the calculated $V_{1/2}$ of −75.2, (116), similar to results obtained by Ludwig et al (83). Regarding the cAMP-induced shift of the activation curve for hHCN4, a 15 mV and 11 mV shift toward more positive potentials was reported by Ludwig et al. (83) and Seifert et al. (116), respectively. To

TABLE 18–1. *Comparison of Biochemical and Functional Properties of Cloned Pacemaker Channels*

	Unified Nomenclature			
	HCN1	HCN2	HCN3	HCN4
Clone (original name)	mBCNG-1 hBCNG-1* HAC2	mBCNG-2* hBCNG-2* HAC1	mBCNG-4* HAC3	mBCNG-3* HAC4* hHCN4
Amino acids	910	863	779	1203
Tissue Distribution	Brain	Brain, heart	Brain	Brain, heart
$V_{1/2}$	−100 mV†	−103 mV	n.d.	−109 mV‡ −74mV**
Time constant at $V_{1/2}$	350 ms	3740 ms	n.d	23 s‡ 21.5 s**
K_a for cAMP/Hill coefficient	n.d.	0.5 μM/0.8	n.d.	n.d.
Shift cAMP	+1.8 mV	+13 mV	n.d.	+15 mV‡ +11 mV**
P_{Na}/P_k	0.25	0.24	n.d.	0.22

* Partial cDNA sequence.   † Measured in inside-out patches.
n.d. = not determined
‡ Ludwig, A., X. Zong, J. Stieber, R. Hullin, F. Hofmann, and M. Biel. *Embo J*. 18: 2323–2329, 1999.
** Siefert, R., A. Scholten, R. Gauss, A. Mincheva, P. Lichter, and U. B. Kaupp. *Proc. Natl. Acad. Sci. U.S.A.* 96: 9391–9396, 1999.

date, no functional expression of HCN3 has been reported.

The ion-selectivity of heterologously expressed HCN channels agrees well with that of native channels, because they are fourfold more permeable to K+ than to Na+ (82, 83, 113). HCN channels are blocked by external Cs+ but not by Ba2+. Like native pacemaker currents, HCN currents are abolished upon removal of external K+ or replacement of external Cl− by large organic ions. Thus, K+ is required for the channel to carry any current, even though the inward Na+ component largely contributes to the pacemaking process under physiological conditions. Ludwig et al. (81) suggested that a multi-ion pore, similar to CNG channels (122) and Ca2+ channels (59), could account for these effects. This multi-ion HCN pore would consist of one "poly"-monovalent cation binding site in the external mouth of the channel pore, having a higher affinity for K+ and another having a higher affinity for Na+ (140). The channel's regulation by Cl− could be explained by the presence of an extracellular binding site for Cl−, related to the presence of positively charged residues in this region (81).

LOW-VOLTAGE ACTIVATED CALCIUM CHANNELS

Low-voltage activated calcium channels (T-type calcium channels) were first described in starfish eggs (54). They were discovered and first characterized in mammalian cardiac cells in 1985 (8, 98), and they were characterized in dorsal root ganglion (DRG) neurons at about the same time (21, 46, 99). They have now been described in a wide variety of both excitable and non-excitable cells, including smooth muscle (2, 67), cerebellar granule cells (109), fibroblasts (23), hippocampal neurons (2), thalamic neurons (63, 64, 66, 129) pituitary cells (58), adrenal cells (26, 42, 132), olfactory receptor cells (69), colonic myocytes (141), and sperm (6, 111), as well as neural- and neuroendocrine cell lines (89, 96). They are particularly well expressed in adult cardiac pacemaker cells (53, 78, 149) and cells of the conduction system (55, 62, 147). T channels are also found in cardiac ventricular myocytes of some species (7, 40, 136, 143). Several reviews (64, 106) and the proceedings of a meeting in 1996 devoted to T-type channels (135) summarize kinetic and pharmacological characteristics of these channels.

Because T-type calcium channels activate at significantly more negative potentials than the high-voltage activated calcium channels, and because they decay (inactivate) over tens of milliseconds during step depolarizations without a dependence on calcium, deactivate slowly (over ~100 msec), and inactivate steeply as a function of holding potential, they are well suited to modulate excitability. Evidence in support of this role has been found in cardiac pacemaker cells (53, 134, 149), and these channels have been implicated in controlling the intrinsic excitability necessary for the rhythmic brain waves (28, 64, 66). Moreover, increased levels of T-type current have been associated with absence epilepsy (50, 132), while antiepileptics decrease low-threshold calcium current in thalamic relay neurons (28).

In the cardiac pacemaking system, T-type current has been detected in feline atrial cells (149), rabbit AV node cells (55), and canine Purkinje cells (133). More compellingly, T-type current in rabbit SA nodal cells has been shown to contribute to the late phase of diastolic depolarization (53, 78), although electrophysiological evidence for T channels has not be found in adult human atrial (102) or ventricular (9) tissue.

T-type calcium channels are also good candidates for controlling calcium flux into cells. Several studies have suggested that these channels physiologically carry calcium and that this calcium can serve as a trigger for calcium release from the sarcoplasmic reticulum under some conditions (126, 147). In addition, canine bronchial smooth muscle T channels may play a role in excitation–contraction coupling (67). Also in support of the idea that these channels act as regulators of calcium, is the finding that they are often expressed in fetal or neonatal tissues, that they change their expression during development, and that they thereby influence cell growth and proliferation. T channels can be found in embryonic chick heart (16, 70), neonatal mouse ventricle (101), and neonatal rat heart (47, 77a), while they are absent in adult rat heart (87). In vascular smooth muscle cells, expression of T-type current is cell-cycle dependent, paralleling the G_1/S phase transition (73), and they have been implicated in terminal differentiation of skeletal muscle myoblasts (11).

T-type calcium channels may also play a role under a variety of pathological circumstances. For example, in vivo pathological examples of excess proliferation due to the increased expression of T-type channels may be represented by animal models of cardiac hypertrophy (43, 87, 100, 117), cardiomyopathy (118), and post-infarction (62a). Because of their kinetic characteristics, block of T channels may be cardioprotective. Using mibefradil, a selective T-channel blocker, in conjunction with a dog pacing model of atrial fibrillation, one study found that mibefradil strongly attenuated atrial fibrillation inducibility (45). Similarly, Sandmann et al. (110) found that mibefradil improved cardiac function and protected the heart against calcium overload in a rat myocardial infarction model with a permanently ligated left coronary artery. Also, Hermsmeyer (57) suggested that T-channel block would be cardioprotective if these channels were found to play a role in vascular remodeling. Finally, through calcium's role as a second messenger, T-type channels can control a significant number of biological processes including the secretion of hormones, steroids, and digestive enzymes (60).

MOLECULAR CLONING AND DISTRIBUTION

The α subunit of the T-type calcium channel was cloned by Ed Perez-Reyes and colleagues at Loyola (107). Three isoforms have been identified, α1G (94, 107), α1H (30, 105), and α1I (76). Both α1G and α1I were cloned from brain, and α1H has cloned from heart, but each has a varied distribution in brain, heart and other peripheral tissues (although at this time α1I is identified only in brain).*

Heterologous expression of α1G was first achieved in *Xenopus* oocytes, and although expression levels were modest, the gross phenotype of the currents was similar to currents reported in native neuronal cells. Expression of α1H was initially unsuccessful in oocytes, but this T-type clone expressed well from the outset in mammalian cells, and the initial report of the behavior of this clone is from HEK293 cells (30). The initial report for α1I includes both oocyte and mammalian recordings (76). Although the matter is not completely settled, it would appear that, unlike high-voltage activated calcium channels, auxiliary subunits are not required for expression and native phenotype of T channels.

Because antibodies for protein localization are only now beginning to become available, the only available data on distribution come from Northern analysis, RNAse protection assays, or in situs. An extensive study of localization of the various isoforms in brain has been carried out (131), but only limited data on the heart and cardiovascular system are available. It would appear that α1H is more abundantly expressed in heart than α1G, but both isoforms have been detected in the rodent species for which data are available (11a). Unfortunately, very few data on isoform distribution in the vascular system are available. This family of channels also appears to be evolutionarily conserved. A sequence from *Caenorhabditis elegans* is highly homologous, and T-type currents have been recorded in invertebrates, including starfish eggs (54) and mollusc (143).

It would appear that the T channels undergo alternative splicing. Three reports of splice variants for α1G are already in the literature (29, 92, 94), as is one report for α1I (93). Unpublished data are also available for α1H. Interestingly, primarily or perhaps exclusively alternative splicing results in changes in cytoplasmic linkers or C-terminal regions. One paper suggests that

---
*Since the preparation of this chapter a standardized nomenclature has been recommended for calcium channels (42a) by which α1G is Ca_v 3.1, α1H is Ca_v 3.2, and α1I is Ca_v 3.3.

there are kinetic differences between some of these channels (22a). It appears that changes in expression of channels via alternative splicing may be a major regulatory mechanism for T-type calcium channels.

It must be noted that there remains some uncertainty about whether the T current identified in the heart is generated by these T channels. Originally Snutch, who cloned the α1E isoform (Ca_v 2.3) of the high-voltage activated channel (14, 128), felt that this isoform was a good candidate for the low-voltage activated channel in brain. Recently, antisense oligonucleotides to this channel, which is also present in atria, were found to downregulate expression of T-type current in atrial myocytes (108). Therefore, it may be that the T-current in heart (and in other cells) is not generated exclusively by the new family of T-type channels despite the general enthusiasm for the concept (134).

STRUCTURE

Each of the T-channel sequences codes for proteins of >2200 amino acids with a hydropathy profile that matches the α subunit structure of high-voltage activated calcium channels and voltage-dependent sodium channels; four domains each with six membrane-spanning regions and a P loop that represents the selectivity filter. Overall amino acid similarity with other calcium channels is only about 40%, although there is strong similarity in the putative transmembrane regions and P loops both with other calcium channels and with sodium channels.

The recent determination by crystallography of a potassium selective channel for a bacterial inwardly rectifying K^+ channel (39) encourages the idea that structural predictions of channel organization can be made in relation to ion channels. For example, it is likely that the *general* motif of this first channel to be crystalized will be recapitulated for ion channels, including the T-type calcium channels: a selectivity filter near the extracellular membrane interface, helices arranged in a cone-like or teepee shape. Other features, specifically the fact that carbonyl oxygens form the selectivity filter of this class of channels, however, are likely to be specific for potassium channels. Interestingly, this is the motif of the selectivity filter that was predicted by Lipkind, Hanck, and Fozzard (80) based on the biophysical data of Heginbotham, Lu, Abramson, and MacKinnon (cf. ref. 56), i.e. only the C-end of the P loop hairpins formed the inner walls of the pore, with backbone carbonyl oxygens of the amino acids VGYGD forming the selectivity region and facing the pore.

Unfortunately, it is unlikely that direct structural determination of calcium or sodium channels will be available in the near future. The outstanding achievement of determination of a potassium selective channel was accomplished by taking advantage of two features that are not possible for calcium and sodium channels: first the fact that this was a bacterial channel allowed for isolation of large amounts of protein, and second this channel was fourfold symmetrical, and this increased the power of the analysis of the x-ray data. Therefore, although investigators can use the data from this channel to direct their thinking, it is not feasible to imagine that crystallization of the T-type channel will be forthcoming in the near future.

For calcium and sodium channels extensive data in the literature support the notion that side chain carboxyls interact with the cations as they pass through the channel (41, 61) rather than carbonyls as for the KcsA channel. Also, selectivity profiles for these channels represent very different Eisenman sequences, sodium and calcium channels being a strong field strength site and potassium channels presenting a weak field strength site. Using the crystal structure of KcsA as a starting point, Lipkind and Fozzard (79) have recently made a revised prediction of a likely organization for the filter region of voltage-gated sodium channels. Similarities between the pore regions of the high-voltage activated and low-voltage activated calcium channels and the various isoforms of sodium channel suggest there is likely to be a great deal of similarity in the motifs of all of these channels. Of course they differ in some important details (Fig. 18–2). For example, in the amino acids generally believed to form the selectivity filter, "DEKA" is the "signature" of sodium channels, while "EEEE" is common to the high-voltage activated calcium channels, and "EEDD" to the new low-voltage activated calcium channels. The difference in selectivity between high-voltage activated calcium channels and low-voltage activated channels has intrigued investigators since its discovery. Sequence differences that un-

	Domain I	*Domain III*
Na	T Q [D] C	T F [K] G
Ca(hv)	T M [E] G	T G [E] G
Ca(lv)	T L [E] G	S K [D] G

	Domain II	*Domain IV*
Na	C G [E] W	T S [A] G
Ca(hv)	T G [E] D	T G [E] A
Ca(lv)	T Q [E] D	T G [D] N

FIG. 18–2. Selectivity filters for sodium channel high-voltage activated Ca channel (hvA) and low-voltage activated Ca channel (lvA).

derlie these selectivity differences—e.g. the role of aspartate vs. glutamate in the selectivity filter—seem good candidates to contribute to these differences. A recent study in high-voltage activated calcium channels (139) identified a key role of the -1 position to the selectivity filter E in domain III that accounted for differences between α1A (Ca$_v$2.1) and α1C (Ca$_v$1.2). It seems likely that mutational experimentation will no doubt eventually lead us to understand why various calcium channels differ from one another, and why sodium channels essentially behave as a single occupancy pore at or near physiological concentrations (5), while calcium channels exhibit clear multi-ion occupancy characteristics (3, 31, 59).

The KcsA channel is, of course, not a voltage-dependent channel and so the crystal structure gives no insight into possible arrangements of the voltage sensors (S4's) or segments 1–3. The voltage-gated channels are extremely sequence conserved in their S4s. This is evident in Figure 18–3, which shows alignments of the various S4s. (Only one member of each is illustrated because other members are essentially identical in these regions.) The rat α1C channel (Ca$_v$ 1.2) is used as the example of the high-voltage activated calcium family, the rat heart sodium channel (Na$_v$ 1.5) as the example of the sodium channel family, and the *Shaker* potassium channel as the example of the voltage-gated potassium channel family (its single S4 sequence has been duplicated below each domain). There is a high degree of homology in these sequences across these very diverse voltage-gated channels, with many of the differences accounted for by extremely conservative amino acid substitutions. However, several specific homologies are worth mention. In domain I each channel type has four or five positive charges. Interestingly, it is the voltage-gated sodium channel that contains only four charges in this alignment; other channels have at least five. Domain II contains by this alignment five charges in all channels, and domain III has at least six, with a seventh at the extreme C-terminal end, which may be intracellular rather than in the membrane. In domain IV the first arginine, which in both cardiac and skeletal muscle sodium channels is associated with an inactivation-deficient muscle disease in humans (22), is not charged in the high-voltage calcium channels (serine) or *Shaker* potassium channels (alanine), but is an arginine in the new T-type channels. Also interestingly, it should be noted that some mammalian channels are not charged at the penultimate charge in domain IV. Neither the high-voltage or low-voltage calcium channels are charged at this position either. For potassium channels, these intracellularly located charges seem to be more important in setting the voltage range of gating than they are in determining voltage dependence (120). One mutagenesis study on the control of inactivation in these channels suggests an important role for the amino terminus (128a). T channels are not subject to calcium-dependent inactivation, like many of the high-voltage activated calcium channels, and they share little homology with voltage-gated sodium channels in their domain III-IV linkers.

BIOPHYSICS

Comparison of α1G, α1H, and α1I

The electrophysiologic properties of the cloned T channels are very similar to those that have been reported for T-type calcium currents found in a variety of native tissues. In Figure 18–4, examples of families of current traces are pictured for each clone (α1G, α1H, and α1I) expressed in HEK293 cells with 2 mM Ca^{2+} as the charge carrier (86). With physiological Ca^{2+}$_o$ all three channels activate near ~-60 mV, reached maximal peak inward current at ~-30 mV and have a V$_{1/2}$ of activation of ~-45 mV [see also ref. (71)]. The V$_{1/2}$ of inactivation (~-70–75 mV) is similar for all three clones. The time course of activation and decay of the currents is fastest for α1G and slowest for α1I, with α1H being somewhat slower than α1G.

```
Domain I, S4
α1H     SAV     RTV   RVL   RPL   RAIN    RVPS
α1C     kal     Raf   RVI   RPL   Rlvs    gvPS
rH1     SAl     RTf   RVI   RaL   ktIs    viPg
Sh      ail     Rvi   Rlv   Rvf   R.IF    klsr
                 ⇑     ⇑     ⇑     ⇑       ⇑

Domain II, S4
α1H     GLSVL   RTF   RLL   RVL   KLV    RFL
α1C     GiSVL   Rcy   RLL   Rif   Kit    Ryw
rH1     nLSVL   Rsf   RLL   RVf   KLa    ksw
Sh      sLaiL   Rvi   RLv   RVf   rif    kls
                 ⇑     ⇑     ⇑     ⇑      ⇑

Domain III, S4
α1H     RVL   RLL   RTL   RPL   RVIS   RAQ   GLK
α1C     kiL   RvL   RvL   RPl   RaIn   Rik   GLK
rH1     ksL   RtL   RaL   RPl   RalS   Rfe   Gmr
Sh      aiL   Rvi   Rlv   Rvf   Rif.   kls   rhsK
         ⇑     ⇑     ⇑     ⇑     ⇑      ⇑

Domain IV, S4
α1H     RIM   RVL   RIA   RVL   KLL   KMA   VGM   RAL
α1C     tff   Rlf   Rvm   Rlv   KLL   Rge   eGi   RtL
rH1     Rvi   Rla   RIg   RiL   rLi   rgA   RGa   kgi
Sh      aIl   RVi   Rlv   Rvf   rif   Kls   rhs   kgL
         ⇑     ⇑     ⇑     ⇑     ⇑     ⇑     ⇑     ⇑
```

FIG. 18–3. Alignment of S4 regions of voltage-gated ion channels.

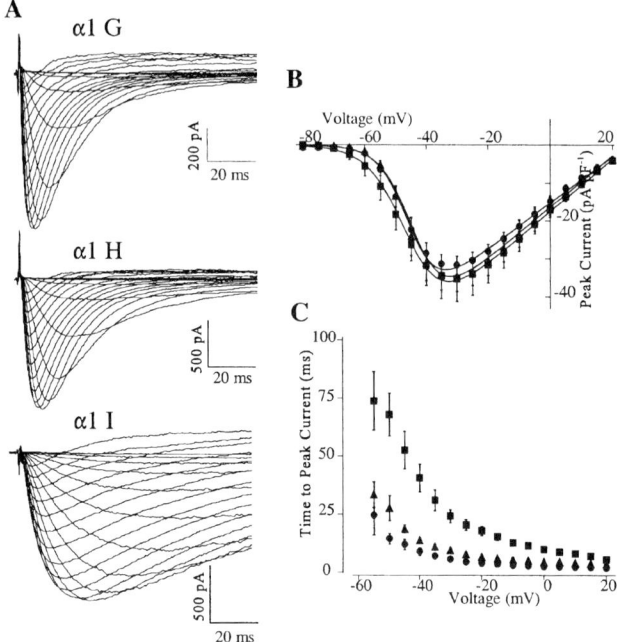

FIG. 18–4. Expression of T-type Ca currents in HEK 293 cells with 2 mM Ca^{2+}_o as the charge carrier. a) Families of current traces from representative cells expressing α1G, α1H, and α1I. Currents were recorded from a holding potential of −100 mV, stepping from −80 to +20 mV in 5 mV increments once every 5 sec. Recordings were made at 22°C. b) Current–voltage relationships from data in panel a showing peak current normalized to cell capacitance. Alpha 1G (●), Alpha 1H (▲), and Alpha 1I (■), C time to peak current plotted as a function of voltage [From Martin et al., (86), with permission]

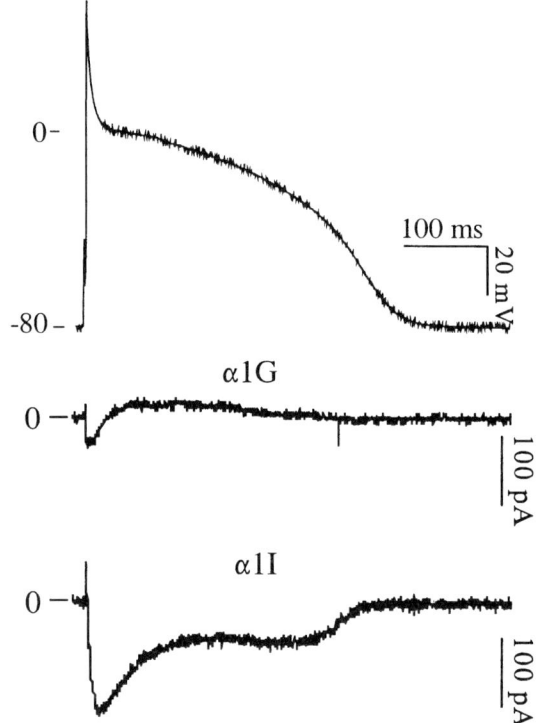

FIG. 18–5. Current response from HEK293 cells stably expressing either α1G or α1I in response to an action potential clamp. The action potential was recorded from a canine cardiac Purkinje cell (kindly provided by S. Nattel).

Because decay time constants become voltage independent at positive potentials (13, 23, 121), it is generally assumed that inactivation from the open state is voltage independent. Channels can inactivate from closed states, although they develop and recover from such inactivation slowly and with multiple time constants (71).

These kinetic characteristics make T-type channel currents active near threshold; several reports suggest they contribute to the late phase of diastolic depolarization (53, 97, 98, 149), but their slow inactivation and deactivation kinetics also suggest they could pass current during other phases of the action potential. Of course, in native cells the contribution of a given conductance must be inferred from blocking experiments. Usually for T-type calcium currents, this meant inclusion of nickel, which has multiple effects. A better method for evaluating the potential contribution of these channels is to impose an action potential clamp on a cell expressing only T channels. An example of the contribution of α1G is shown in Figure 18–5 for a cardiac Purkinje action potential, where it can be seen that the primary contribution of current is at the onset. Also shown are data for α1I. In contrast to α1G, this kinetically very slow channel contributes inward current during the entire action potential, including the repolarization phase. While α1I is, of course, not expressed in the heart, at least one splice variant of α1G exhibits greatly slowed kinetics (74), and this raises the possibility that regulation of channels can alter the role of T channels in forming action potentials.

How Voltage Dependent Are T-type Calcium Channels?

The slope factor for conductance of high-voltage activated calcium currents in cardiac cells is ~7mV (27, 68). The T-type channels commonly have a slope factor less than this. Figure 18–6 summarizes data from 44 cells expressing α1G and 48 cells expressing α1H evaluating what, if any effect, the magnitude of the current (G_{max}) has on the slope factor of conductance. Current magnitude is a prime determinant of voltage control when other factors like pipette resistance and speed of the currents are "constant," and this is reflected in the slope factor. In these experiments slope factor was modestly dependent on current magnitude,

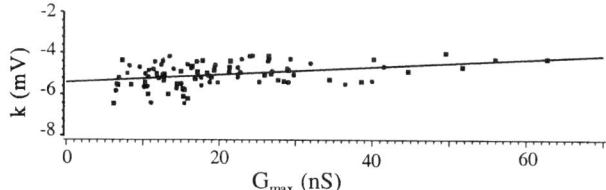

FIG. 18–6. Slope factor (k) from fits to a Boltzmann relationship (G = G_{max} / (1 + exp [(V−$V_{1/2}$)/k]) as a function of the size of the currents (G_{max}) for currents recorded in HEK293 cells expressing either α1G (■) or α1H (●).

predicting an intercept (current magnitude independent estimate of slope factor) of −5.7 mV, which was not different between α1G and α1H. Of course, clearly uncontrolled data must be excluded from such an analysis—e.g. data with conductance slope factors smaller than −4mV.

Selectivity and Block of T-Type Calcium Channels

All of the cloned voltage-gated channels share a common topological motif for the extracellular portion of their permeation paths—i.e. the P loop, a segment between the putative transmembrane segment S5 and S6, which is thought to fold back into the membrane to form the extracellular mouth of the pore and part of the ion-conducting pathway (39, 51). Despite this similarity in motif, each type of channel is characterized by high selective permeability for specific ions. Three divalent cations, Ca^{2+}, Sr^{2+}, and Ba^{2+}, pass through all known calcium channels, but with different relative conductances. Single-channel conductance of T-type calcium channels is small (usually 5–10 pS) even when divalent concentrations are raised (Fig. 18–7). Unlike high-voltage activated calcium channels, which have a higher conductance to Ba^{2+} than to Ca^{2+}, in native cells T-type channels appear to have equal conductances for Ca^{2+} and Ba^{2+}. This intriguing difference between the channel types has both fascinated and frustrated investigators. All known calcium channels, including T channels, conduct monovalents well in the absence of divalent cations, but they are virtually impermeable to monovalent ions in the presence of even quite low concentrations of divalent cations, discriminating against Na^+ and K^+ in ratios ~1000:1 and 3000:1 (125). Single-channel conductance in 60 mM Na^+ was 18 pS, whereas with 60 mM in Ba^{2+}, Ca^{2+}, or Sr^{2+}, it was ~7.2 pS.

Many divalent cations usually block current through T-type calcium channels. Nickel is the "classic" T channel blocker (53), having been repeatedly observed to block low-voltage activated calcium currents in a variety of preparations (complete by 100 μM), includ-

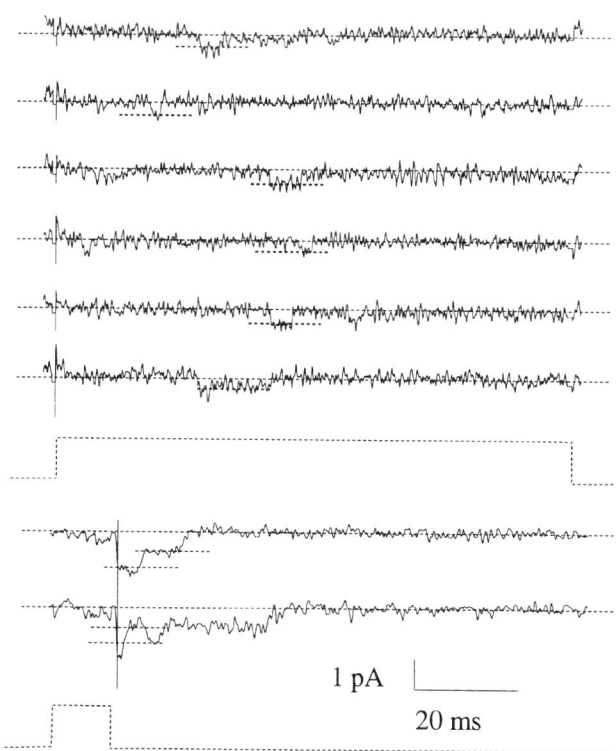

FIG. 18–7. Top panel shows representative sweeps with activity from single-channel cell attached recordings of α1H in step depolarizations from −100 mV to −20 mV. Data are shown at 10 kHz, filtered at 1kHz. Dashed lines indicate the zero current and open-channel amplitudes. Bottom panel shows sweeps with activity in the same cell when after 10 msec at 0 mV potential was changed to −100 mV. These were chosen because they showed multiple openings. To aid in comparison with data in the literature, 110 mM Ba was used as the charge carrier, and recordings were made at 22°C.

ing cardiac preparations (51, 62, 115, 149). However, there were some interesting exceptions, including at least one report in cardiac Purkinje cells (133) and many in neurons including frontal cortex (130), and thalamus (129). This discrepancy between preparations now appears to have an explanation. Of the three isoforms, α1H exhibits the highest affinity for Ni^{2+}, with an IC_{50} the range of 6–12 μM, depending on the conditions, α1I intermediate at 90–200 μM, and α1G the lowest affinity with an IC_{50} in the range of 170–250 μM (75, 77).

Other drugs and agents also block the new T channels. One new calcium channel drug, mibefradil, which was briefly marketed as Posicor, appears to be more selective for the T-type calcium channel than for other calcium channels. It behaves as a very effective antihypertensive drug, and in electrophysiological assays it has been more effective against T channels than against L-type channels by 8–50-fold (15, 44, 72). When barium is used as the charge carrier, α1G and α1H have a similar affinity for mibefradil and are 13-fold more sensitive to block than α1C (L-type calcium channels). When physiological concentrations of calcium are used, the affinity is 4.5–9 times higher (86). This relative selectivity of mibefradil for T channels draws attention to the role of T-type currents in vascular smooth muscle since this drug was a powerful antihypertensive agent.

Other drugs have also been reported to block the channels. These include ethosuximide in the millimolar range and, to some extent, isradipine and nifedipine (~15%–30% at 1 μM; 75). Modulators of high-voltage activated calcium channels, the protein kinase and protein kinase phosphorylation cascades, have less dramatic effects, if any, in native preparations. One report of arachidonic acid modulation of α1H has been published (146) and another reports cAMP modulation in NIH 3T3 cells (104a). Interestingly, another well-known type of cation channel blocker, protons, rather than blocking T-type calcium currents, dramatically shift the voltage range of activation (32), suggesting that acidosis could be potent regulator of T currents in vivo.

SUMMARY

Four different mammalian genes encoding pacemaker channels and three genes for T-type calcium channels appear to give rise to currents in a variety of native cells in which pacemaker and low threshold calcium currents have been identified. Despite their relative structural homology, HCN channels are characterized by strikingly different gating properties, voltage-dependent kinetics and sensitivity to cAMP. The T-type calcium channels have more subtle kinetic differences, but they are frequently alternatively spliced, and it is too early to know the extent to which this type of regulation affects their characteristics in various tissues. Ongoing mutagenesis studies will undoubtedly reveal the structural determinants that underlie these channel's phenotypes. The engineering of transgenic mice, with under- or over-expressed channels of these types, will perhaps shed new light on the precise role of these channels in heart, as well the other organs in which they are expressed. Now that the sequences for these two important classes of threshold channels are known, the differential expression of the genes may help in the development of therapeutic agents. For the HCN channels these include agents such as bradycardic compounds like UL-FS 49 (138) and ZD 7288 (12), which target specifically a cardiac HCN isoform. For the T-type calcium channel, second-generation mibefradil like agents are almost certainly going to be discovered. Finally, information about the genomic organization of these genes should make it possible to detect possible links between several inherited disorders of cardiac and neural pacemaking.

REFERENCES

1. Accili, E. A., G. Redaelli, and D. DiFrancesco. Differential control of the hyperpolarization-activated current (i(f)) by cAMP gating and phosphatase inhibition in rabbit sino-atrial node myocytes. *J. Physiol. (Lond.)* 500:643–51, 1997.
2. Akaike, N., H. Kanaide, T. Kuga, M. Nakamura, J. Sadoshima, and H. Tomoike. Low-voltage-activated calcium current in rat aorta smooth muscle cells in primary culture. *J. Physiol. (Lond.)* 416:141–160, 1989.
3. Almers, W. and E. W. McCleskey. Non-selective conductance in calcium channels of frog muscle: calcium selectivity in a single-file pore. *J. Physiol. (Lond.)* 353:585–608, 1984.
4. Anderson, J. A., S. S. Huprikar, L. V. Kochian, W. J. Lucas, and R. F. Gaber. Functional expression of a probable *Arabidopsis thaliana* potassium channel in *Saccharomyces cerevisiae*. *Proc. Natl. Acad. Sci. U.S.A.* 89:3736–3740, 1992.
5. Anderson, O. and R. Koeppe. Molecular determinants of channel function. *Physiol. Rev.* 72:S89–S158, 1992.
6. Arnoult, C., R. A. Cardullo, J. R. Lemos, and H. M. Florman. Activation of mouse sperm T-type Ca^{2+} channels by adhesion to the egg zona pellucida. *Proc. Natl. Acad. Sci. U.S.A.* 93:13004–13009, 1996.
7. Balke, C. W. and W. G. Wier. Modulation of L-type calcium channels by sodium ions. *Proc. Natl. Acad. Sci. U.S.A.* 89:4417–4421, 1992.
8. Bean, B. P. Two kinds of calcium channels in canine atrial cells. Differences in kinetics, selectivity, and pharmacology. *J. Gen. Physiol.* 86:1–30, 1985.
9. Beuckelmann, D. J., M. Nabauer, and E. Erdmann. Characteristics of calcium-current in isolated human ventricular myocytes from patients with terminal heart failure. *J. Mol. Cell. Cardiol.* 23:929–937, 1991.
10. Biel, M., A. Ludwig, X. Zong, and F. Hofmann. Hyperpolarization-activated cation channels: a multi-gene family. *Rev. Physiol. Biochem. Pharmacol.* 136:165–81, 1999.
11. Bijlenga, P., J. H. Liu, E. Espinos, C. A. Haenggeli, J. Fischer-Lougheed, C. R. Bader, and L. Bernheim. T-type alpha 1H Ca^{2+} channels are involved in Ca^{2+} signaling during terminal differentiation (fusion) of human myoblasts. *Proc. Natl. Acad. Sci. U.S.A.* 97:7627–7632, 2000.
11a. Bohn, G., S. Moosmang, H. Conrad, A. Ludwig, F. Hofmann, and N. Klugbauer. Expression of T- and L-type calcium channel mRNA in mrine sinoatrial node. *FEBS Lett.* 481:73–76, 2000.
12. BoSmith, R. E., I. Briggs, and N. C. Sturgess. Inhibitory actions of ZENECA ZD7288 on whole-cell hyperpolarization activated inward current (If) in guinea-pig dissociated sinoatrial node cells. *Br. J. Pharmacol.* 110:343–349, 1993.
13. Bossu, J. L. and A. Feltz. Inactivation of the low-threshold transient calcium current in rat sensory neurones: evidence for a dual process. *J. Physiol. (Lond.)* 376:341–357, 1986.
14. Bourinet, E., G. W. Zamponi, A. Stea, T. W. Soong, B. A. Lewis, L. P. Jones, D. T. Yue, and T. P. Snutch. The alpha 1E calcium channel exhibits permeation properties similar to low-voltage-activated calcium channels. *J. Neurosci.* 16:4983–4993, 1996.
15. Brogden, R. N. and A. Markham. Mibefradil. A review of its pharmacodynamic and pharmacokinetic properties, and therapeutic efficacy in the management of hypertension and angina pectoris [published erratum appears in Drugs 1998 Apr;55(4): 517]. *Drugs* 54:774–793, 1997.
16. Brotto, M. A. and T. L. Creazzo. Ca^{2+} transients in embryonic

chick heart: contributions from Ca^{2+} channels and the sarcoplasmic reticulum. *Am. J. Physiol.* 270 (*Heart Circ. Physiol.*): H518–H525, 1996.
17. Brown, H. and D. Difrancesco. Voltage-clamp investigations of membrane currents underlying pace-maker activity in rabbit sino-atrial node. *J. Physiol. (Lond.)* 308:331–351, 1980.
18. Brown, H. F., D. DiFrancesco, and S. J. Noble. How does adrenaline accelerate the heart? *Nature* 280:235–236, 1979.
19. Brugge, J. S., P. C. Cotton, A. E. Queral, J. N. Barrett, D. Nonner, and R. W. Keane. Neurones express high levels of a structurally modified, activated form of pp60c-src. *Nature* 316:554–557, 1985.
20. Budde, T., G. Biella, T. Munsch, and H. C. Pape. Lack of regulation by intracellular Ca^{2+} of the hyperpolarization-activated cation current in rat thalamic neurones. *J. Physiol. (Lond.)* 503: 79–85, 1997.
21. Carbone, E. and H. D. Lux. A low voltage-activated calcium conductance in embryonic chick sensory neurons. *Biophys. J.* 46: 413–418, 1984.
22. Chahine, M., A. L. George, Jr., M. Zhou, S. Ji, W. Sun, R. L. Barchi, and R. Horn. Sodium channel mutations in paramyotonia congenita uncouple inactivation from activation. *Neuron* 12:281–294, 1994.
22a. Chemin, J., A. Monteil, E. Rourinet, J. Nargeot, and P. Lory. Alternatively spliced α_{1G} ($Ca_V3.1$) intracellular loops promote specific T-Type Ca^{2+} channel gating properties. *Biophys. J.* 80: 1238–1250, 2001.
23. Chen, C. F. and P. Hess. Mechanism of gating of T-type calcium channels. *J. Gen. Physiol.* 96:603–630, 1990.
24. Chen, J., J. Mitcheson, and M. Sanguinetti. Structural determinants of HCN channel gating: minimal functional unit and mutational analysis of the S4 domain. *Biophys. J.* 78:1209, 2000.
25. Clapham, D. E. Not so funny anymore: pacing channels are cloned. *Neuron* 21:5–7, 1998.
26. Cohen, C. J., R. T. McCarthy, P. Q. Barrett, and H. Rasmussen. Ca channels in adrenal glomerulosa cells: K^+ and angiotensin II increase T-type Ca channel current. *Proc. Natl. Acad. Sci. U.S.A.* 85:2412–2416, 1988.
27. Cohen, N. M. and W. J. Lederer. Calcium current in isolated neonatal rat ventricular myocytes. *J. Physiol. (Lond.)* 391:169–191, 1987.
28. Coulter, D. A., J. R. Huguenard, and D. A. Prince. Differential effects of petit mal anticonvulsants and convulsants on thalamic neurones: calcium current reduction. *Br. J. Pharmacol.* 100:800–806, 1990.
29. Cribbs, L. L., J. C. Gomora, A. N. Daud, J. H. Lee, and E. Perez-Reyes. Molecular cloning and functional expression of Ca(v)3.1c, a T-type calcium channel from human brain [published erratum appears in FEBS Lett 2000 Mar 31;470(3):378]. *FEBS Lett* 466:54–58, 2000.
30. Cribbs, L. L., J. H. Lee, J. Yang, J. Satin, Y. Zhang, A. Daud, J. Barclay, M. P. Williamson, M. Fox, M. Rees, and E. Perez-Reyes. Cloning and characterization of alpha1H from human heart, a member of the T-type Ca^{2+} channel gene family. *Circ. Res.* 83: 103–109, 1998.
31. Dang, T. X. and E. W. McCleskey. Ion channel selectivity through stepwise changes in binding affinity. *J. Physiol. (Lond.)* 111:185–193, 1998.
32. Delisle, B. P. and J. Satin. pH modification of human T-type calcium channel gating. *Biophys. J.* 78:1895–1905, 2000.
33. DiFrancesco, D. Characterization of single pacemaker channels in cardiac sino-atrial node cells. *Nature* 324:470–473, 1986.
34. DiFrancesco, D. Dual allosteric modulation of pacemaker (f) channels by cAMP and voltage in rabbit SA node. *J. Physiol. (Lond.)* 515:367–376, 1999.
35. DiFrancesco, D. A new interpretation of the pace-maker current in calf Purkinje fibres. *J. Physiol. (Lond.)* 314:359–376, 1981.
36. DiFrancesco, D. The pacemaker current in the sinus node. *Eur. Heart. J.* 8 (Suppl L):19–23, 1987.
37. DiFrancesco, D. Pacemaker mechanisms in cardiac tissue. *Annu. Rev. Physiol.* 55:455–472, 1993.
38. DiFrancesco, D. and M. Mangoni. Modulation of single hyperpolarization-activated channels (i(f)) by cAMP in the rabbit sino-atrial node. *J. Physiol. (Lond.)* 474:473–482, 1994.
39. Doyle, D. A., J. Morais Cabral, R. A. Pfuetzner, A. Kuo, J. M. Gulbis, S. L. Cohen, B. T. Chait, and R. MacKinnon. The structure of the potassium channel: molecular basis of K^+ conduction and selectivity [see comments]. *Science* 280:69–77, 1998.
40. Droogmans, G. and B. Nilius. Kinetic properties of the cardiac T-type calcium channel in the guinea-pig. *J. Physiol. (Lond.)* 419:627–650, 1989.
41. Ellinor, P. T., J. Yang, W. A. Sather, J. F. Zhang, and R. W. Tsien. Ca^{2+} channel selectivity at a single locus for high-affinity Ca^{2+} interactions. *Neuron* 15:1121–1132, 1995.
42. Enyeart, J. J., B. Mlinar, and J. A. Enyeart. T-type Ca^{2+} channels are required for adrenocorticotropin-stimulated cortisol production by bovine adrenal zona fasciculata cells. *Mol. Endocrinol.* 7:1031–1040, 1993.
42a. Ertel, E. A., K. P. Campbell, M. M. Harpold, F. Hofmann, Y. Mori, E. Perez-Reyes, A. Schwartz, T. P. Snuth, T. Tanabe, L. Birnbaumer, R. W. Tsien, and W. A. Catterall. Nomenclature of voltage-gated calcium channels. *Neuron* 25:533–535, 2000.
43. Ertel, S. I. and E. A. Ertel. Low-voltage-activated T-type Ca^{2+} channels. *Trends Pharmacol. Sci.* 18:37–42, 1997.
44. Ertel, S. I., E. A. Ertel, and J. P. Clozel. T-type Ca^{2+} channels and pharmacological blockade: potential pathophysiological relevance. *Cardiovasc. Drugs. Ther.* 11:723–739, 1997.
45. Fareh, S., A. Benardeau, B. Thibault, and S. Nattel. The T-Type Ca^{2+} channel blocker mibefradil prevents the development of a substrate for atrial fibrillation by tachycardia-induced atrial remodeling in dogs. *Circ. Res.* 100:2191–2197, 1999.
46. Fedulova, S. A., P. G. Kostyuk, and N. S. Veselovsky. Two types of calcium channels in the somatic membrane of new-born rat dorsal root ganglion neurones. *J. Physiol. (Lond.)* 359:431–446, 1985.
47. Furukawa, T., H. Ito, J. Nitta, M. Tsujino, S. Adachi, M. Hiroe, F. Marumo, T. Sawanobori, and M. Hiraoka. Endothelin-1 enhances calcium entry through T-type calcium channels in cultured neonatal rat ventricular myocytes. *Circ. Res.* 71:1242–1253, 1992.
48. Gauss, R., R. Seifert, and U. B. Kaupp. Molecular identification of a hyperpolarization-activated channel in sea urchin sperm. *Nature* 393:583–587, 1998.
49. Goulding, E. H., G. R. Tibbs, and S. A. Siegelbaum. Molecular mechanism of cyclic-nucleotide-gated channel activation. *Nature* 372:369–374, 1994.
50. Grisar, T., B. Lakaye, and E. Thomas. Molecular basis of neuronal biorhythms and paroxysms. *Arch. Physiol. Biochem.* 104: 770–774, 1996.
51. Guy, H. R. and F. Conti. Pursuing the structure and function of voltage-gated channels. *Trends Neurosci.* 13:201–206, 1990.
52. Hagiwara, N. and H. Irisawa. Modulation by intracellular Ca^{2+} of the hyperpolarization-activated inward current in rabbit single sino-atrial node cells. *J. Physiol. (Lond.)* 409:121–141, 1989.
53. Hagiwara, N., H. Irisawa, and M. Kameyama. Contribution of two types of calcium currents to the pacemaker potentials of rabbit sino-atrial node cells. *J. Physiol. (Lond.)* 395:233–253, 1988.
54. Hagiwara, S., S. Ozawa, and O. Sand. Voltage clamp analysis of two inward current mechanisms in the egg cell membrane of a starfish. *J. Gen. Physiol.* 65:617–644, 1975.

55. Hancox, J. C. and A. J. Levi. L-type calcium current in rod- and spindle-shaped myocytes isolated from rabbit atrioventricular node. *Am. J. Physiol.* 267 (*Heart Circ. Physiol.*):H1670–H1680, 1994.
56. Heginbotham, L., Z. Lu, T. Abramson, and R. MacKinnon. Mutations in the K^+ channel signature sequence. *Biophys. J.* 66: 1061–1067, 1994.
57. Hermsmeyer, K. Role of T channels in cardiovascular function. *Cardiology* 89:2–9, 1998.
58. Herrington, J. and C. J. Lingle. Kinetic and pharmacological properties of low voltage-activated Ca^{2+} current in rat clonal (GH3) pituitary cells. *J. Neurophysiol.* 68:213–232, 1992.
59. Hess, P. and R. W. Tsien. Mechanism of ion permeation through calcium channels. *Nature* 309:453–456, 1984.
60. Hille, B. *Ionic Channels of Excitable Membranes*, Second Ed. *Sinauer Associates Inc.*, 1992.
61. Hille, B. Ionic selectivity of Na and K channels of nerve membranes. *In: Membranes 3* edited by G. Eisenman. New York: Marcel Dekker, 1975:255–325.
62. Hirano, Y., H. A. Fozzard, and C. T. January. Characteristics of L- and T-type Ca^{2+} currents in canine cardiac Purkinje cells. *Am. J. Physiol.* 256 (*Heart Circ. Physiol.*):H1478–H492, 1989.
62a. Huang, B, D. Qin, L. Deng, M. Boutjdir, and N. El-Sherif. Reexpression of T-type Ca^{2+} channel gene and current in post-infarction remodeled rat left ventricle. *Cardiovasc. Res.* 46:442–449, 2000.
63. Hughes, S. W., D. W. Cope, T. I. Toth, S. R. Williams, and V. Crunelli. All thalamocortical neurones possess a T-type Ca^{2+} "window" current that enables the expression of bi-stability-mediated activities. *J. Physiol. (Lond.)* 517:805–815, 1999.
64. Huguenard, J. R. Low-threshold calcium currents in central nervous system neurons. *Annu. Rev. Physiol.* 58:329–348, 1996.
65. Ishii, T. M., M. Takano, L. H. Xie, A. Noma, and H. Ohmori. Molecular characterization of the hyperpolarization-activated cation channel in rabbit heart sinoatrial node. *J. Biol. Chem.* 274:12835–12839, 1999.
66. Jahnsen, H. and R. Llinas. Voltage-dependent burst-to-tonic switching of thalamic cell activity: an in vitro study. *Arch. Ital. Biol.* 122:73–82, 1984.
67. Janssen, L. J., D. K. Walters, and J. Wattie. Regulation of $[Ca^{2+}]_i$ in canine airway smooth muscle by $Ca(2+)$-ATPase and Na^+/Ca^{2+} exchange mechanisms. *Am. J. Physiol.* 273 (*Lung Physiol.*): L322–L330, 1997.
68. Kass, R. S. and M. C. Sanguinetti. Inactivation of calcium channel current in the calf cardiac Purkinje fiber. *J. Gen. Physiol.* 84: 705–726., 1984.
69. Kawai, F. Odorants suppress T- and L-type Ca^{2+} currents in olfactory receptor cells by shifting their inactivation curves to a negative voltage. *Neurosci. Res.* 35:253–263, 1999.
70. Kawano, S. and R. L. DeHaan. Analysis of the T-type calcium channel in embryonic chick ventricular myocytes. *J. Membr. Biol.* 116:9–17, 1990.
71. Klockner, U., J. H. Lee, L. L. Cribbs, A. Daud, J. Hescheler, A. Pereverzev, E. Perez-Reyes, and T. Schneider. Comparison of the Ca^{2+} currents induced by expression of three cloned alpha1 subunits, alpha1G, alpha1H and alpha1I, of low-voltage-activated T-type Ca^{2+} channels. *Eur. J. Neurosci.* 11:4171–4178, 1999.
72. Kobrin, I., V. Charlon, E. Lindberg, and R. Pordy. Safety of mibefradil, a new once-a-day, selective T-type calcium channel antagonist. *Am. J. Cardiol.* 80:40C–46C, 1997.
73. Kuga, T., S. Kobayashi, Y. Hirakawa, H. Kanaide, and A. Takeshita. Cell cycle-dependent expression of L- and T-type Ca^{2+} currents in rat aortic smooth muscle cells in primary culture. *Circ. Res.* 79:14–19, 1996.
74. Kunze, R. S., R. L. Martin, M. C. Emerick, W. S. Agnew, and D. A. Hanck. Kinetic differences in splice variance of the alpha-1G T-type calcium channel. *Biophys. J.* 78:458A, 2000.
75. Lacinova, L., N. Klugbauer, and F. Hofmann. Regulation of the calcium channel alpha(1G) subunit by divalent cations and organic blockers *Neuropharmacology* 39:1254–1266, 2000.
76. Lee, J. H., A. N. Daud, L. L. Cribbs, A. E. Lacerda, A. Pereverzev, U. Klockner, T. Schneider, and E. Perez-Reyes. Cloning and expression of a novel member of the low voltage-activated T-type calcium channel family. *J. Neurosci.* 19:1912–1921, 1999.
77. Lee, J. H., J. C. Gomora, L. L. Cribbs, and E. Perez-Reyes. Nickel block of three cloned T-type calcium channels: low concentrations selectively block alpha1H. *Biophys. J.* 77:3034–3042, 1999.
77a. Leuranguer, V, A. Monteil, E. Bourinet, G. Dayanithi, and J. Nargeot. T-type calcium currents in rat cardiomyocytes during postnatal development: contribution to hormone secretion. *Am. J. Physiol. Heart Circ. Physiol.* 279:H2540–H2548, 2000.
78. Li, J., J. Qu, and R. D. Nathan. Ionic basis of ryanodine's negative chronotropic effect on pacemaker cells isolated from the sinoatrial node. *Am. J. Physiol.* 273:H2481–H2489, 1997.
79. Lipkind, G. M. and H. A. Fozzard. KcsA crystal structure as framework for a molecular model of the $Na(+)$ channel pore [In Process Citation]. *Biochemistry* 39:8161–8170, 2000.
80. Lipkind, G. M., D. A. Hanck, and H. A. Fozzard. A structural motif for the voltage-gated potassium channel pore. *Proc. Natl. Acad. Sci. U.S.A.* 92:9215–9219, 1995.
81. Ludwig, A., X. Zong, F. Hofmann, and M. Biel. Structure and function of cardiac pacemaker channels. *Cell. Physiol. Biochem.* 9:179–186, 1999.
82. Ludwig, A., X. Zong, M. Jeglitsch, F. Hofmann, and M. Biel. A family of hyperpolarization-activated mammalian cation channels. *Nature* 393:587–591, 1998.
83. Ludwig, A., X. Zong, J. Stieber, R. Hullin, F. Hofmann, and M. Biel. Two pacemaker channels from human heart with profoundly different activation kinetics. *Embo. J.* 18:2323–2329, 1999.
84. Maccaferri, G., M. Mangoni, A. Lazzari, and D. DiFrancesco. Properties of the hyperpolarization-activated current in rat hippocampal CA1 pyramidal cells. *J. Neurophysiol.* 69:2129–2136, 1993.
85. Marten, I. and T. Hoshi. The N-terminus of the K channel KAT1 controls its voltage-dependent gating by altering the membrane electric field. *Biophys. J.* 74:2953–2962, 1998.
86. Martin, R. L., J. H. Lee, L. L. Cribbs, E. Perez-Reyes, and D. A. Hanck. Mibefradil block of cloned T-type Ca channels. *J. Pharm. Exp. Ther.*, 295:302–308, 2000.
87. Martinez, M. L., M. P. Heredia, and C. Delgado. Expression of T-type Ca^{2+} channels in ventricular cells from hypertrophied rat hearts. *J. Mol. Cell. Cardiol.* 31:1617–1625, 1999.
88. Martinez, R., B. Mathey-Prevot, A. Bernards, and D. Baltimore. Neuronal pp60c-src contains a six-amino acid insertion relative to its non-neuronal counterpart. *Science* 237:411–415, 1987.
89. Matteson, D. R. and C. M. Armstrong. Properties of two types of calcium channels in clonal pituitary cells. *J. Gen. Physiol.* 87: 161–182, 1986.
90. McCormick, D. A. and H. C. Pape. Properties of a hyperpolarization-activated cation current and its role in rhythmic oscillation in thalamic relay neurones. *J. Physiol. (Lond.)* 431:291–318, 1990.
91. Miller, A. G. and R. W. Aldrich. Conversion of a delayed rectifier K^+ channel to a voltage-gated inward rectifier K^+ channel by three amino acid substitutions. *Neuron* 16:853–858, 1996.
92. Mittman, S., J. Guo, and W. S. Agnew. Structure and alternative splicing of the gene encoding alpha1G, a human brain T calcium channel alpha1 subunit. *Neurosci. Lett.* 274:143–146, 1999.

93. Mittman, S., J. Guo, M. C. Emerick, and W. S. Agnew. Structure and alternative splicing of the gene encoding alpha1I, a human brain T calcium channel alpha1 subunit. *Neurosci. Lett.* 269:121–124, 1999.
94. Monteil, A., J. Chemin, E. Bourinet, G. Mennessier, P. Lory, and J. Nargeot. Molecular and functional properties of the human alpha(1G) subunit that forms T-type calcium channels. *J. Biol. Chem.* 275:6090–6100, 2000.
95. Moosmang, S., M. Biel, F. Hofmann, and A. Ludwig. Differential distribution of four hyperpolarization-activated cation channels in mouse brain. *Biol. Chem.* 380:975–980, 1999.
96. Narahashi, T., A. Tsunoo, and M. Yoshii. Characterization of two types of calcium channels in mouse neuroblastoma cells. *J. Physiol. (Lond.)* 383:231–249, 1987.
97. Nilius, B. Possible functional significance of a novel type of cardiac Ca channel. *Biomed. Biochim. Acta* 45:K37–K45, 1986.
98. Nilius, B., P. Hess, J. B. Lansman, and R. W. Tsien. A novel type of cardiac calcium channel in ventricular cells. *Nature* 316:443–446, 1985.
99. Nowycky, M. C., A. P. Fox, and R. W. Tsien. Three types of neuronal calcium channel with different calcium agonist sensitivity. *Nature* 316:440–443, 1985.
100. Nuss, H. B. and S. R. Houser. T-type Ca^{2+} current is expressed in hypertrophied adult feline left ventricular myocytes. *Circ. Res.* 73:777–782, 1993.
101. Nuss, H. B. and E. Marban. Electrophysiological properties of neonatal mouse cardiac myocytes in primary culture. *J. Physiol. (Lond.)* 479:265–279, 1994.
102. Ouadid, H., J. Seguin, S. Richard, P. A. Chaptal, and J. Nargeot. Properties and modulation of Ca channels in adult human atrial cells. *J. Mol. Cell. Cardiol.* 23:41–54, 1991.
103. Papazian, D. M., T. L. Schwarz, B. L. Tempel, Y. N. Jan, and L. Y. Jan. Cloning of genomic and complementary DNA from *Shaker*, a putative potassium channel gene from *Drosophila*. *Science* 237:749–753, 1987.
104. Pape, H. C. Queer current and pacemaker: the hyperpolarization-activated cation current in neurons. *Annu. Rev. Physiol.* 58:299–327, 1996.
104a. Pemberton, K. E., L. J. Hill-Eubanks, S. V. Penelope Jones. Modulation of low-threshold T-type calcium channels by the five muscarinic receptor subtypes in NIH 3T3 cells. *Pflugers Arch.* 440:452–461, 2000.
105. Perchenet, L., A. Benardeau, and E. A. Ertel. Pharmacological properties of Ca(V)3.2, a low voltage-activated Ca^{2+} channel cloned from human heart *Naunyn-Schmiedebergs Arch. Pharmacol.* 361:590–599, 2000.
106. Perez-Reyes, E. Molecular characterization of a novel family of low voltage-activated, T-type, calcium channels. *J. Bioenerg. Biomembr.* 30:313–318, 1998.
107. Perez-Reyes, E., L. L. Cribbs, A. Daud, A. E. Lacerda, J. Barclay, M. P. Williamson, M. Fox, M. Rees, and J. H. Lee. Molecular characterization of a neuronal low-voltage-activated T-type calcium channel [see comments]. *Nature* 391:896–900, 1998.
108. Piedras-Renteria, E. S., C. C. Chen, and P. M. Best. Antisense oligonucleotides against rat brain alpha1E DNA and its atrial homologue decrease T-type calcium current in atrial myocytes. *Proc. Natl. Acad. Sci. U. S. A.* 94:14936–14941, 1997.
109. Randall, A. D. and R. W. Tsien. Contrasting biophysical and pharmacological properties of T-type and R-type calcium channels. *Neuropharmacology* 36:879–893, 1997.
109a. Ross C. A., J. D. Wood, G. Schilling, M. F. Peters, F. C. Nucifora, Jr., J. K. Cooper, A. H. Sharp, R. L. Margolis, and D. R. Borchelt. Polyglutamine pathogenesis. *Philos. Trans. R. Soc. Lond. B. Biol. Sci.* 354:1005–1011, 1999.
110. Sandmann, S., J. Y. Min, A. Meissner, and T. Unger. Effects of the calcium channel antagonist mibefradil on haemodynamic parameters and myocardial Ca(2+)-handling in infarct-induced heart failure in rats. *Cardiovasc. Res.* 44:67–80, 1999.
111. Santi, C. M., A. Darszon, and A. Hernandez-Cruz. A dihydropyridine-sensitive T-type Ca^{2+} current is the main Ca^{2+} current carrier in mouse primary spermatocytes. *Am. J. Physiol.* 271 (*Cell Physiol.*):C1583–C1593, 1996.
111a. Santoro B., S. Chen, A. Luthi, P. Pavlidis, G. P. Shumyatsky, G. R. Tibbs, S. A. Siegelbaum. Molecular and functional heterogeneity of hyperpolarization-activated pacemaker channels in the mouse CNS. *J. Neurosci.* 20:5264–5275, 2000.
112. Santoro, B., S. G. Grant, D. Bartsch, and E. R. Kandel. Interactive cloning with the SH3 domain of N-src identifies a new brain specific ion channel protein, with homology to eag and cyclic nucleotide-gated channels. *Proc. Natl. Acad. Sci. U. S. A.* 94:14815–14820, 1997.
113. Santoro, B., D. T. Liu, H. Yao, D. Bartsch, E. R. Kandel, S. A. Siegelbaum, and G. R. Tibbs. Identification of a gene encoding a hyperpolarization-activated pacemaker channel of brain. *Cell* 93:717–729, 1998.
114. Santoro, B. and G. R. Tibbs. The HCN gene family: molecular basis of the hyperpolarization-activated pacemaker channels. *Ann. N. Y. Acad. Sci.* 868:741–764, 1999.
115. Satoh, H. Role of T-type Ca^{2+} channel inhibitors in the pacemaker depolarization in rabbit sino-atrial nodal cells. *Gen. Pharmacol.* 26:581–587, 1995.
116. Seifert, R., A. Scholten, R. Gauss, A. Mincheva, P. Lichter, and U. B. Kaupp. Molecular characterization of a slowly gating human hyperpolarization-activated channel predominantly expressed in thalamus, heart, and testis. *Proc. Natl. Acad. Sci. U. S. A.* 96:9391–9396, 1999.
117. Self, D. A., K. Bian, S. K. Mishra, and K. Hermsmeyer. Stroke-prone SHR vascular muscle Ca^{2+} current amplitudes correlate with lethal increases in blood pressure. *J. Vasc. Res.* 31:359–366, 1994.
118. Sen, L. and T. W. Smith. T-type Ca^{2+} channels are abnormal in genetically determined cardiomyopathic hamster hearts. *Circ. Res.* 75:149–155, 1994.
119. Sentenac, H., N. Bonneaud, M. Minet, F. Lacroute, J. M. Salmon, F. Gaymard, and C. Grignon. Cloning and expression in yeast of a plant potassium ion transport system. *Science* 256:663–665, 1992.
120. Seoh, S. A., D. Sigg, D. M. Papazian, and F. Bezanilla. Voltage-sensing residues in the S2 and S4 segments of the *Shaker* K^+ channel. *Neuron* 16:1159–1167, 1996.
121. Serrano, J. R., E. Perez-Reyes, and S. W. Jones. State-dependent inactivation of the alpha1G T-type calcium channel. *J. Gen. Physiol.* 114:185–201, 1999.
122. Sesti, F., E. Eismann, U. B. Kaupp, M. Nizzari, and V. Torre. The multi-ion nature of the cGMP-gated channel from vertebrate rods. *J. Physiol. (Lond.)* 487:17–36, 1995.
123. Shabb, J. B., and J. D. Corbin. Cyclic nucleotide-binding domains in proteins having diverse functions. *J. Biol. Chem.* 267:5723–5726, 1992.
124. Shi, W., R. Wymore, H. Yu, J. Wu, R. T. Wymore, Z. Pan, R. B. Robinson, J. E. Dixon, D. McKinnon, and I. S. Cohen. Distribution and prevalence of hyperpolarization-activated cation channel (HCN) mRNA expression in cardiac tissues. *Circ. Res.* 85:e1–6, 1999.
125. Shuba, Y. M., V. I. Teslenko, A. N. Savchenko, and N. H. Pogorelaya. The effect of permeant ions on single calcium channel activation in mouse neuroblastoma cells: ion-channel interaction. *J. Physiol. (Lond.)* 443:25–44, 1991.
126. Sipido, K., E. Carmeliet, and F. VanDeWerf. T-type Ca^{2+} cur-

rent as a trigger for Ca^{2+} release from the sarcoplasmic reticulum in guinea-pig ventricular myocytes. *J. Physiol. (Lond.)* 508:439–452, 1998.
127. Soltesz, I., S. Lightowler, N. Leresche, D. Jassik-Gerschenfeld, C. E. Pollard, and V. Crunelli. Two inward currents and the transformation of low-frequency oscillations of rat and cat thalamocortical cells. *J. Physiol. (Lond.)* 441:175–197, 1991.
128. Soong, T. W., A. Stea, C. D. Hodson, S. J. Dubel, S. R. Vincent, and T. P. Snutch. Structure and functional expression of a member of the low voltage-activated calcium channel family. *Science* 260:1133–1136, 1993.
128a. Staes, M., K. Talavera, N. Klugbauer, J. Prenen, L. Lacinova, G. Froogmans, F. Hofmann, and B. Nilius. The amino side of the C-terminus determines fast inactivation of the T-type calcium channel α_{1G}. *J. Physiol.* 530:35–45, 2001.
129. Suzuki, S. and M. A. Rogawski. T-type calcium channels mediate the transition between tonic and phasic firing in thalamic neurons. *Proc. Natl. Acad. Sci. U. S. A.* 86:7228–7232, 1989.
130. Takahashi, K. and N. Akaike. Calcium antagonist effects on low-threshold (T-type) calcium current in rat isolated hippocampal CA1 pyramidal neurons. *J. Pharmacol. Exp. Ther.* 256:169–175, 1991.
131. Talley, E. M., L. L. Cribbs, J. H. Lee, A. Daud, E. Perez-Reyes, and D. A. Bayliss. Differential distribution of three members of a gene family encoding low voltage-activated (T-type) calcium channels. *J. Neurosci.* 19:1895–1911, 1999.
132. Tsakiridou, E., L. Bertollini, M. de Curtis, G. Avanzini, and H. C. Pape. Selective increase in T-type calcium conductance of reticular thalamic neurons in a rat model of absence epilepsy. *J. Neurosci.* 15:3110–3117, 1995.
133. Tseng, G. N. and P. A. Boyden. Multiple types of Ca^{2+} currents in single canine Purkinje cells. *Circ. Res.* 65:1735–1750, 1989.
134. Tsien, R. W. Key clockwork component cloned. *Nature* 391:839–841, 1998.
135. Tsien, R. W., J.-P. Clozel, and J. Nargeot. Low-voltage-activated T-Type calcium channels. *Proceedings from the International Electrophysiology Meeting.* Montpellier 21–22 October, 1996.
136. Tytgat, J., B. Nilius, J. Vereecke, and E. Carmeliet. The T-type Ca channel in guinea-pig ventricular myocytes is insensitive to isoproterenol. *Pflugers Arch.* 411:704–706, 1988.
136a. Ulens C. and J. Tytgat. Functional heteromerization of HCN1 and HCN2 pacemaker channels. *J. Biol. Chem.* 276:6069–6072, 2001.
137. Vaccari, T., A. Moroni, M. Rocchi, L. Gorza, M. E. Bianchi, M. Beltrame, and D. DiFrancesco. The human gene coding for HCN2, a pacemaker channel of the heart. *Biochim. Biophys. Acta.* 1446:419–425, 1999.
138. Van Bogaert, P. P. and M. Goethals. Pharmacological influence of specific bradycardic agents on the pacemaker current of sheep cardiac Purkinje fibres. A comparison between three different molecules. *Eur. Heart J.* 8 (Suppl L):35–42, 1987.
139. Williamson, A. V. and W. A. Sather. Nonglutamate pore residues in ion selection and conduction in voltage gated Ca^{2+} channels. *Biophys. J.* 77:2575–2589, 1999.
140. Wollmuth, L. P. Multiple ion binding sites in Ih channels of rod photoreceptors from tiger salamanders. *Pflugers. Arch.* 430:34–43, 1995.
141. Xiong, Z., N. Sperelakis, A. Noffsinger, and C. Fenoglio-Preiser. Ca^{2+} currents in human colonic smooth muscle cells. *Am. J. Physiol.* 269 Gastrointest:G378–G85, 1995.
142. Yanagihara, K. and H. Irisawa. Inward current activated during hyperpolarization in the rabbit sinoatrial node cell. *Pflugers. Arch.* 385:11–19, 1980.
143. Yeoman, M. S., B. L. Brezden, and P. R. Benjamin. LVA and HVA Ca(2+) currents in ventricular muscle cells of the Lymnaea heart. *J. Neurophysiol.* 82:2428–2440, 1999.
144. Yu, H., F. Chang, and I. S. Cohen. Pacemaker current exists in ventricular myocytes. *Circ. Res.* 72:232–236, 1993.
145. Zagotta, W. N. and S. A. Siegelbaum. Structure and function of cyclic nucleotide-gated channels. *Annu. Rev. Neurosci.* 19:235–263, 1996.
146. Zhang, Y., L. L. Cribbs, and J. Satin. Arachidonic acid modulation of alpha1H, a cloned human T-type calcium channel. *Am. J. Physiol.* 278:H184–H193, 2000.
147. Zhou, Z. and C. T. January. Both T- and L-type Ca^{2+} channels can contribute to excitation–contraction coupling in cardiac Purkinje cells. *Biophys. J.* 74:1830–1839, 1998.
148. Zhou, Z. and S. L. Lipsius. Properties of the pacemaker current (If) in latent pacemaker cells isolated from cat right atrium. *J. Physiol. (Lond.)* 453:503–523, 1992.
149. Zhou, Z. and S. L. Lipsius. T-type calcium current in latent pacemaker cells isolated from cat right atrium. *J. Mol. Cell. Cardiol.* 26:1211–1219, 1994.

19. Ion Channels and Cardiac Arrhythmia in Heart Disease

JONATHAN C. MAKIELSKI | Departments of Medicine and Physiology, University of Wisconsin, Madison, Madison, Wisconsin

HARRY A. FOZZARD | Department of Medicine, University of Chicago, Chicago, Illinois

CHAPTER CONTENTS

Background
   The clinical problem—tachyrhythmia in structural heart disease
   Arrhythmia and mechanisms
   Currents underlying the action potential
   The role of ion channels in arrhythmia
Electrophysiology of Acquired Heart Disease
   Human and animal models for cellular and molecular electrophysiology
   Specific cellular electrophysiological changes in acquired heart disease
Ion Channel Changes in Acquired Heart Disease
   General considerations
      Intrinsic versus extrinsic ion channel changes
      Ion current changes in disease—density, kinetics, regulation, heterogeneity
   Specific ion currents and arrhythmia
      Channels and currents
      Voltage-dependent inward currents
      Outward currents: voltage-dependent K^+ channels
      Outward currents: inwardly rectifying K^+ currents
      CL^- currents
      Hyperpolarization-induced pacemaker current I_f
      Gap Junctions
      Pumps and exchangers
      Nonspecific, background, and swell-activated currents
   Summary of electrical remodeling in acquired heart disease
The Long QT Syndrome
   Introduction
      Summary
      The clinical picture
   Arrhythmic mechanism
   Molecular mechanisms
      The genetic link
      The potassium channel culprits
      The Na channel culprit
      Other genetic causes of Long QT
   Implications for therapy
   Present status
Idiopathic Ventricular Fibrillation
Inherited Cardiomyopathy
   Introduction
   Clinical Picture
   Arrhythmic mechanisms

TACHYRHYTHMIA CAUSES OR CONTRIBUTES TO MORTALITY in more than three hundred thousand people in the United States every year (172). Structural abnormalities of the heart represent a common underlying substrate. Myerburg et al. (172) estimated the major etiologic bases for sudden cardiac death. Approximately 80% were acute and chronic coronary ischemia, 10%–15% were dilated and hypertrophy related cardiomyopathies, 5% were valvular, inflammatory, or infiltrative diseases, and a smaller percentage were ill-defined lesions such as right ventricular dysplasia and molecular abnormalities such as the congenital long QT syndrome. Although acute ischemia sometimes occurs in isolation, it is more common for acute ischemia to be superimposed upon chronic ischemic heart disease (110), failing myocardium, hypertrophied myocardium, or a diabetic heart (172). Tachyrhythmia and sudden cardiac death in the absence of ischemia also frequently occur in heart failure (261), in hypertensive hearts (67, 125), and in diabetic hearts (221). Tachyrhythmia itself may cause changes that perpetuate the arrhythmia. For example, in atrial fibrillation refractory periods shorten over time, leading to the truism that "atrial fibrillation begets atrial fibrillation" (294). This chapter reviews ion channel changes that contribute to arrhythmia in acquired heart disease including hypertrophy, heart failure, chronic ischemia (or healed infarction), diabetes, and atrial fibrillation, and also in several genetically determined heart diseases such as the long QT syndrome, idiopathic ventricular fibrillation, and hypertrophic cardiomyopathy.

BACKGROUND

The Clinical Problem—Tachyrhythmia in Structural Heart Disease

Normal heart rhythm is initiated by pacemaker depolarization in the sinus node, followed by conduction to and depolarization of the atria, then by conduction through the atrioventricular (AV) node and specialized conduction tissues, and finally depolarization of the ventricles. In the broadest sense, arrhythmia occurs whenever this normal process is interrupted. Failure of pacemaking, or block in the conduction system, can lead to bradycardia, arrhythmias not considered further in this chapter. Inappropriate tachycardias can result when depolarization is initiated outside the sinus node and conducted to the rest of the heart, usurping the normal rhythm. Other chapters provide details of the three classic mechanisms for tachyrhythmia: (1) re-entry (see Chapter 12) (2) abnormal automaticity and (3) triggered automaticity including early afterdepolarizations (see chapter 14) and delayed afterdepolarizations (see Chapter 9).

Arrythmia and Mechanisms

The mechanisms for tachyrhythmia must be considered at four levels: molecular, cellular, tissue/organ, and whole organism. At the molecular level, permeant ions, ion channels, and the molecules that regulate them underlie excitability, which is manifested at the cellular level by regenerative depolarization and repolarization—the action potential. In order for the arrhythmia to develop, the appropriate tissue substrate must be present, such as a re-entrant circuit or the appropriate coupling of automatic tissue to the rest of the heart. As detailed elsewhere (Chapter 12), the re-entrant circuit may be anatomical or it may be functional, involving heterogeneity in the electrical properties of different cells. Abnormal automaticity might be considered to be primarily a single-cell phenomenon, but to produce an arrhythmia the spontaneously active cells must be coupled to the rest of the heart—a tissue phenomenon. Finally, autonomic impulses from the central nervous system or from reflex arcs involving the hemodynamic response (see Chapter 5) are also involved. Thus, the entire organism participates in the arrhythmia.

The predominant mechanisms for arrhythmia in many heart diseases are not clear and multiple mechanisms are likely to be involved. Re-entrant mechanisms have generally been cited most prominently in acute and chronic ischemia, where the substrate for a re-entrant pathway exists in the form of a re-entrant scar (63, 196). In heart failure and hypertrophy, clear re-entrant pathways are not seen, and abnormal automaticity is suggested to play a major role (194, 261, 279). These diseased hearts do, however, also show an increased tendency to sustained re-entrant arrhythmias (159). Abnormal or enhanced automaticity may initiate arrhythmias, which are then perpetuated by re-entrant mechanisms. This chapter does not consider this issue further, but rather reviews alterations in cellular electrophysiology and ion channels that contribute to arrhythmia by all mechanisms.

Currents Underlying the Action Potential

The determinants of excitability and the normal depolarization and repolarization of the action potential in heart cells is covered in detail elsewhere in this *Handbook* (see chapter 13). The depolarization phase (phase 0) is determined mainly by the properties of the inward Na^+ current and, to a lesser extent, by the Ca^{2+} currents, except in nodal tissue and in atrial and ventricular tissue under conditions in which the Na^+ current is suppressed. In some cases residual or abnormal outward currents might influence depolarization by opposing the inward depolarizing current. In contrast, repolarization of the action potential is a more complex process, involving all ion channels present in the membrane (Fig. 19-1). An initial rapid repolarization, which may inscribe a notch (phase 1), is caused by the rapid decay of the Na^+ current combined with activation of transient outward currents carried by K^+ and Cl^- and the Na-Ca exchanger. During the action potential plateau (phase 2) membrane resistance is relatively high. Slowly decaying late residual inward currents through Na^+ and Ca^{2+} channels are balanced against voltage and time dependent activating outward (mainly K^+) currents to maintain the action potential plateau. Eventually the balance tips toward rapid repolarization (phase 3) and the inward rectifier K^+ channels provide a final assist to repolarize the membrane. The resting potential is maintained mainly by the inward rectifier K^+ channel, but multiple currents through ion channels, including the hyperpolarizing-activated pacemaker current and more slowly deactivating delayed rectifier K^+ currents, as well as currents from Na-Ca exchange and Na-K pump, can affect phase 4 depolarization and automaticity.

Two characteristics of the repolarization process must be emphasized. Firstly, repolarization must be a highly reliable process, and this may explain why multiple mechanisms for repolarization are superimposed. This multiplicity of ion channels and their currents provides an essential safety factor for repolarization. Secondly, the total membrane currents during the action potential plateau are small, as a consequence of closure of the inward rectifier channels that underlie the resting potential. Consequently, small changes in the repolarizing currents during the plateau, caused by disease or therapy, can have surprisingly large effects on the timing and pattern of repolarization.

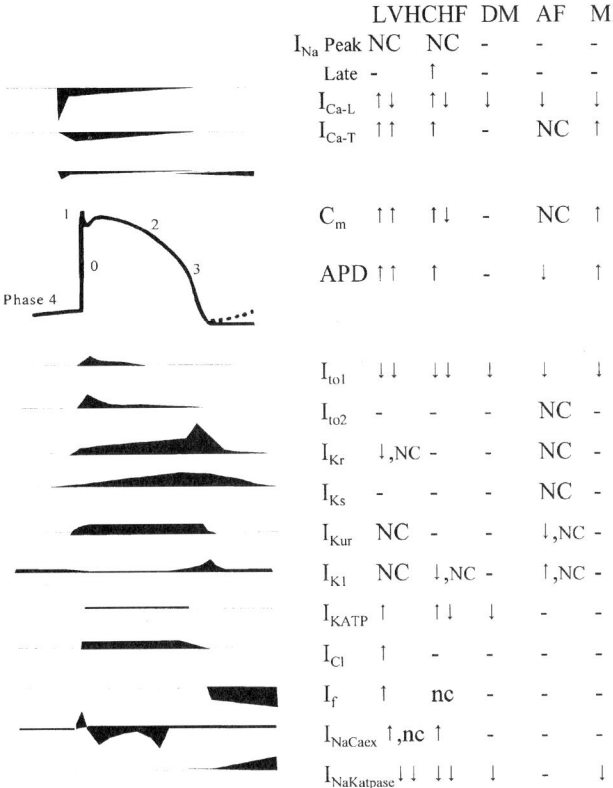

FIG. 19–1. Cardiac currents underlying the action potential and their alteration in acquired heart disease. The action potential is represented in the center, the currents are diagrammed with outward repolarized currents being upward and inward depolarizing currents as downward. The timing of each relative current amplitude in relation to the action potential is represented, but no attempt was made to represent current densities relative to other currents. Abbreviations and symbols: Nomenclature for currents is given in the text. LVH, hypertrophy; CHF, Heart failure; AF, atrial fibrillation; MI, myocardial infarction; ↑↑, consistently increased in >3 studies, ↑, usually increased in > 3 studies or increased in ≤ 3 studies; ↑↓ variably increased or decreased; NC, no change in > 3 studies; nc, no change in ≤ 3 studies; − not known. C_m, membrane capacitance as a measure of cell size; APD, action potential duration.

The Role of Ion Channels in Arrhythmia

Re-entrant arrhythmias depend upon an anatomical or functional re-entrant circuit with unidirectional block to initiate the re-entry, combined with conduction slowing and/or shortened refractory periods to sustain the arrhythmia. The determinants for re-entry must exist in a favorable combination in space and time, thus temporal and spatial heterogeneity in conduction and repolarization can favor re-entrant arrhythmias.

Depolarization of the membrane action potential by regenerative opening of Na$^+$ (or Ca^{2+}) channels, and repolarization of the action potential by the decay of these currents and the onset of K$^+$ currents is a fairly complex process. Conduction of these action potential depolarization and repolarization wavefronts in heart tissue introduces another layer of complexity. Conduction velocity for these wavefronts depends upon multiple ionic and tissue factors that can be divided conceptually into "source" and "sink," with the sink sometimes being called "loading conditions." The source for the depolarizing wavefront is the inward current and changes in Na$^+$ current (or Ca^{2+} current in nodal tissues) affect conduction directly. The "sink" is a combination of ion channel and tissue factors. The excitatory current flows through the cytoplasm of the excited cell and then through gap junctions to connected adjacent cells. The "sink" opposing excitation includes the capacitance of the connected cells, which opposes a change in membrane potential, and any outward repolarizing conductances that oppose depolarization. Thus gap junctions, tissue geometry, and the sum of membrane currents determine the spread of excitatory current. Similar considerations exist for conduction of the repolarizing wavefront. (See Chapter 12 for further discussion of impulse conduction in the heart.)

At the ion current level, decreased peak Na$^+$ current could contribute to re-entrant arrhythmias by favoring unidirectional block and/or slowing conduction, but it could also be antiarrhythmic by, for example, converting slow conduction to complete block in a re-entrant circuit. Increased plateau outward K$^+$ currents, or decreased late Na$^+$ current might contribute to re-entry by shortening refractory periods. Thus for re-entrant mechanisms, uniform lengthening of refractory periods by prolonging the action potential is generally antiarrhythmic. Under certain circumstances localized lengthening of the refractory period could cause functional unidirectional block, a substrate of re-entry. Also, any prolongation of the action potential can create the conditions for triggered automaticity by early afterdepolarizations (114). In addition, prolonging the action potential can contribute to increased intracellular Ca^{2+}, which can lead to triggered automaticity from delayed afterdepolarizations. Ca^{2+} homeostasis is altered by multiple mechansims in hypertrophy and failure and may contribute to arrhythmogenesis (194, 197).

The arrhythmic and antiarrhythmic potential for changes in peak and late inward currents and for changes in outward currents is summarized in Table 19–1. Clearly, it is difficult to state categorically that a particular change in an ion current is arrhythmogenic or antiarrhythmic. It will depend upon the tissue geometry and biological state including pre-existing tissue heterogeneity in ion currents along with possible scarring and changes in loading conditions, the time and voltage dependence of the alterations, and the balance with other ionic currents. At the cellular level,

TABLE 19–1. *Changes in Ion Currents and Arrhythmic/Antiarrhythmic Potential*

Change in Currents (Effect)	Anti-Arrhythmic Potential	Pro-Arrhythmic Potential
↓ Peak inward currents I_{Na} (↓ conduction, ↑ block)	Convert slow conduction to complete block in re-entry	Create unidirectional block or critical slowing in re-entry
↓ Late inward currents I_{Na}, I_{Ca} or ↑ late outward currents I_K (Shorten APD)	↓ triggered automaticity by ↓ QT and ↓ Ca loading	Enhance re-entry by ↓ refractory periods
↑ Late inward currents I_{Na}, I_{Ca} or ↓ late outward currents I_K (Lengthen APD)	↑ triggered automaticity by ↑ QT and ↑ Ca loading	Block re-entry by ↑ refractory periods

I_{Na} = sodium current, I_{Ca} = calcium current, I_K = potassium current, APD = action potential duration, QT = QT interval on surface electrocardiogram.

these factors interact to determine the tendency to excitation and the regulation of conduction velocity.

ELECTROPHYSIOLOGY OF ACQUIRED HEART DISEASE

Human and Animal Models for Cellular and Molecular Electrophysiology

Experimental information from human myocardial cells is increasingly available for many heart diseases because tissue can be obtained from hearts removed during cardiac transplantation. Data from nondiseased human hearts is less available, but can be obtained from donor hearts harvested but not used for transplantation, hearts harvested for valve homografts, or endocardial biopsies from patients undergoing cardiac operations. Atrial appendage tissue is also often available from surgery. Experiments on human tissue, however, remain limited by availability and especially by uncontrolled variables such as heterogeneity in the patient population with regard to disease etiology, age, and the influences of prior drug treatment. For example, treatment with Ca^{2+} channel blockers decreases Ca^{2+} current density in human atrial myocytes (138). While most relevant for human disease, in practice the data from human tissue must be augmented by experiments done in animal models of human diseases. This chapter considers hypertrophy, heart failure, atrial fibrillation, diabetes, and chronic ischemia/healed infarction as separate models of structural heart disease. It must be recognized that these models may share common features. For example, as noted below (see later, under Specific Cellular Electrophysiological Changes in Acquired Heart Disease), cellular hypertrophy also occurs variably in heart failure of different etiologies.

Animal models of hypertrophy are numerous, involving many different species and many different methods of inducing hypertrophy in either the left or right ventricle [reviewed by Hart (107)]. For ion channel studies, rat models of left ventricular hypertrophy are the most commonly studied and include rats with genetic predisposition to spontaneous hypertension or SHR (34) and rats made hypertensive by a variety of means including renal artery stenosis (Goldblatt kidney) (104), uninephrectomy with deoxycorticosterone pellet (167), acromegaly (298), 7-day isoproterenol treatment (238), phenylephrine treatment (95), hypobaric conditions (55), and abdominal aortic stenosis (224). In other species left ventricular hypertrophy models include aortic banding in cats (184), dogs (314), and guinea pigs (213). The Goldblatt (205) and perinephritic models (162) have been used in rabbits. Right ventricular hypertrophy models include pulmonary artery banding in cats (132) and ferrets (198). Ion channels have also been studied in human left ventricular hypertrophy from patients with aortic stenosis (11) and hypertrophic cardiomyopathy (234).

Multiple animal models also exist for heart failure. Many of the models for hypertrophy noted above are also models for heart failure if allowed to progress to that stage. The tachycardia-induced heart failure by pacing at rapid rates is a commonly studied model used for ion channel studies in dogs (122), rabbits (209), and pigs (171). Genetically determined heart failure is studied in the Syrian cardiomyopathic hamster (233) and in a particular strain of turkey (102). Other models include doxorubicin-induced cardiomyopathy in the rat (130) and Chagas disease cardiomyopathy in the dog (188). Because of cardiac transplantation, human tissue from failing hearts is readily available and many studies of ion channels in human heart failure are now available (26, 143, 173, 174, 187, 201, 251). Most of these studies have mixed and various etiologies, but ischemic (47) and dilated (109) cardiomyopathy have been studied separately. In addition, atrial cells are also generally available (216).

The rat streptozotocin-induced diabetes model is a standard method to create insulin dependent (type 1) diabetes (282), and a high fructose feeding rat model (237) has been used to create a high insulin model of diabetes (type 2). A genetic model of diabetes is also available in the rat (266). For atrial fibrillation, a rapid pacing model has been studied in goats (270) and dogs (312). In addition, human atrial tissue is generally readily available from surgical patients (139, 272).

Disease models using ischemia or infarction deserve special comment. Generally the left anterior descending coronary artery is occluded and ion currents in cells from various parts of the heart at different times after the occlusion are studied [see review by Pinto and Boyden (192)]. Such models exist for several species including rat (71, 72, 98, 210), dog (151, 153, 190), and cat (193) hearts. These studies in general fall into two categories: subacute and chronic. In subacute studies, predominantly in dogs, cells from the surviving epicardial layer of adjacent several day-old infarction (1, 151, 190), or nearby surviving Purkinje cells from the endocardial surface (32, 118, 191) are isolated and studied. These cells from "healing infarction" are distinctly different from more chronic models in rat (72, 98, 99, 126) cat (193, 310), or rabbit (163). In these models cells are taken weeks or months after the infarction from tissue remote from the area of infarction and likley represent hypertrophied and/or failing cells. A unique arrhythmia model is a strain of dogs with an inherited tendency to sudden death, in which a decrease in transient outward current has been described in left ventricular epicardium (87).

Dog models, such as the pacing model of heart failure (57) or chronic infarct models (151), have the advantage of having an action potential waveform and an electrophysiology closer to that of humans, as well as a rich experimental history as a model for arrhythmia. The dog model of pacing-induced heart failure has also been shown to be a model for sudden arrhythmic death (87, 189). Despite some limitations, however, rodent models, especially mice in view of the potential of transgenic animals, are likely to be important as well.

Specific Cellular Electrophysiological Changes in Acquired Heart Disease

Hypertensive cardiomyopathy represents a prototype for heart disease because the changes found in heart failure of any etiology may have cellular hypertrophy as a common component. Cellular hypertrophy is manifested as an increase in membrane surface area, which can be measured as an increase in cell capacitance. An increase in cell capacitance is universally present in models of hypertrophy (38, 44, 55, 140, 164, 193, 205, 206, 213, 238, 307), as reviewed by Hart (107), but is absent in atrial fibrillation (272, 312). Increased capacitance is variably present in heart failure. It is increased in failure from a rat chronic infarction model (210), decreased in a rat doxorubicin model (130), and unchanged in a dog pacing model (122) of heart failure. In humans with heart failure, cellular hypertrophy shown by an increase in cell capacitance was seen for both ventricular and atrial cells of human transplantation explants with heart failure of various etiologies (174, 187). In epicardial cells surviving a 5-day-old infarction in a canine model cell capacitance was increased in the absence of overt failure (151). In a more chronic 2-month feline infarction model surviving cells close to the infarction were unchanged, but more remote cells had an increased capacitance consistent with hypertrophy (193, 310), emphasizing the importance of timing and locus of study. Results of studies for hypertrophy as measured by membrane capacitance are summarized in Figure 19–1.

Action potential duration, including spatial heterogeneity of action potential duration, is a key determinant of arrhythmia. In hypertrophy the action potential duration is prolonged in all of the various animal models (3, 55, 60, 68, 89, 95, 104, 167, 205, 213, 298). In a guinea pig aortic constriction model (37) and in a rat isoproterenol model (238) of hypertrophy the action potential was prolonged in the epicardium and midmyocardium, but shortened in the endocardium. In the Syrian hamster model of heart failure, cells from the right ventricle and from the left ventricular base and apex all showed prolonged action potentials. In a study of action potentials from human heart hypertrophy, however, the action potential was prolonged by 27% in the endocardium (11); the other myocardial layers were not studied. Although absolute changes are variable from study to study, the increased transmural dispersion of refractoriness with a greater prolongation in the epicardium has been clearly demonstrated in hypertrophy (37, 162, 238). Action potentials in heart failure are modestly prolonged in most (122, 171, 209, 260) but not all (200) animal models, and they were prolonged in a human study (173). The locations of the myocytes used in these studies were not specified so the transmural distribution of repolarization is not known for heart failure. In canine epicardium bordering a 5-day-old infarction (151) the action potential was prolonged, with loss of the phase 1 notch, but action potential duration was decreased in canine Purkinje fibers cells near a 48-hour-old infarction (191). In contrast to the trend for increased action potential duration in hypertrophy, heart failure, and peri-infarction, the action potential durations in atrial fibrillation are decreased in atrial cells from a dog pacing model (312) and from humans (29, 86). In rat diabetes models the action potential duration was increased in rat left ventricle for a low insulin streptozotocin model of type I diabetes but unchanged in a high insulin high fructose model of type II diabetes (237).

ION CHANNEL CHANGES IN ACQUIRED HEART DISEASE

General Considerations

Intrinsic versus Extrinsic Ion Channel Changes. The mechanisms for ion current alterations in heart disease can be separated conceptually into (1) an intrinsic alteration in the channel density or function or (2) a normal or physiological response of the unaltered channel to extrinsic abnormal stimuli found in the disease state. In the first mechanism, the channel density, distribution, protein structure, subunit composition, or response to modulation by cell signaling pathways is altered by a process sometimes called electrical or molecular remodeling. Reports of electrophysiological remodeling in acquired diseases such as ventricular hypertrophy, chronic ischemia, heart failure, diabetes, and chronic atrial fibrillation have increased markedly. Different aspects have been reviewed by Hart (107), Boyden and Jeck (31), Näbauer and Kääb (175), Richard et al. (207), and Tomaselli and Marban (262). Remodeling may be caused by altered transcription, translation, trafficking, assembly, post-translational modification, and degradation of the ion channel subunits. Investigation of the underlying mechanisms for remodeling are just beginning.

In the second mechanism, the channel density and function are not intrinsically altered, but rather the native channel responds in a predictable way to an altered environment found in the disease, the pathophysiological state, or the effect of a treatment. The general (non-electrophysiological) remodeling that occurs involves alterations in changes in cell metabolism, signaling pathways, cytoskeleton, extraceullar matrix circulating hormones, and so on [as reviewed by Swynghedauw (252)]. These may have predictable effects on ion channels as reviewed elsewhere in this *Handbook* (see Chapter 16). In this chapter we review intrinsic alterations of ion channels in acquired heart disease and discuss the implication for arrhythmia.

Ion Current Changes in Disease—Density, Kinetics, Regulation, Heterogeneity. Many studies of ion currents in heart disease simply report peak current densities and the voltage- and time-dependent gating kinetics from myocytes under a single set of conditions. Disease states, however, may have an altered regulatory or ionic environment (for example, altered β-adrenergic regulation in heart failure) or perhaps subtle but important effects on kinetics (for example, late Na$^+$ currents). In addition, heterogeneity in the transmural or regional distribution of these changes may be important and increasing reports of transmural heterogeneity (across the wall; 38, 41, 163, 306) and regional heterogeneity (from right ventricle, left ventricle, and atria, and from base to apex) (4, 68) are available. The changes are also time dependent in the disease process and studies are beginning to address this variable (92–94). Electrical remodeling is under intensive study and the quantity and sophistication of these studies are rapidly increasing.

Specific Ion Currents and Arrhythmia

Channels and Currents. Classically, ion currents measured in native cardiac myocytes were isolated into individual components attributable to a specific channel by careful selection of the ion content of solutions, voltage clamp protocols, and pharmacological block by "specific" drugs and toxins. In many studies, particularly in older reports, these strategies may not have identified a "pure" current because of overlapping or contaminating currents unrelated to the channel of interest. With the advent of cloned ion channels and expression and electrophysiological study of these channels in heterologous systems such as *Xenopus* oocytes and immortalized noncardiac cells in culture, the "pure" channel current can be studied. Although these tools are helpful to isolate currents, they are not always easy to interpret. Expression systems are chosen for their paucity of native ion currents, but they are far from perfect. All cells have some ion channels, and contamination with endogenous currents remains a problem. A prominent example is a Ca^{2+} activated Cl$^-$ current in *Xenopus* oocytes and some cell culture systems. In addition, these artificial expression systems may not have the proper cell machinery for channel regulation and processing, nor may all the channel subunits necessary for proper currents be present. Thus, identifying the specific channel or channels underlying specific native ion currents can be difficult. Additional tools to identify specific channels are being developed, including the use of antisense DNA in cell culture (83, 178) or dominant negative strategies (120), and "knockout" of ion currents in transgenic mice (17, 149). These strategies have aided in identification of the channels underlying specific currents in human and animal hearts as reviewed by George and Roden (208).

Voltage-Dependent Inward Currents. Na$^+$ (I_{Na}), L-type Ca^{2+} (I_{Ca-L}), and T-type Ca^{2+} (I_{Ca-T}) currents, share common features of voltage- and time-dependent kinetics. During an action potential these channels activate upon membrane depolarization positive to the threshold potential and contribute to membrane depolarization. They then inactivate but continue to show a small (relative to peak) late current that sustains the action potential plateau. When the membrane repolarizes, open channels may rapidly deactivate (microsecond time scale), and inactivated channels recover more slowly (millisecond time scale) from inactivation.

Na$^+$ current—I_{Na}. I_{Na} underlies excitability in ventricular, atrial, and Purkinje cells. I_{Na} flows through the heart Na+ channel α subunit hH1. A β1 subunit can alter I_{Na} by increasing expression levels, by accelerating decay, and by shifting the midpoint of inactivation in the depolarized direction in heterologous expression systems [see reviews (42, 43, 85, 156)]. Although β1 mRNA is found in heart (111, 154), the role for this subunit in heart is not clear. More recently, a larger splice variant of the β1 subunit called β1a has been described in heart tissue (128), but its role is also undefined. In an atrial cell tumor line, altered I_{Na} kinetics and appearance of β1 were temporally correlated (137), suggesting a possible role for this subunit in vivo. β2(111) and β3(168) subunits found in brain have not yet been reported in heart.

Altered I_{Na} can be arrhythmogenic in several ways. A decrease in peak current density, whether by a decreased number of channels or a shift in inactivation that inactivates channels at the resting potential, could contribute to re-entry by slow conduction and block. Altered recovery characteristics could change postrepolarization refractoriness. Augmentation of late I_{Na} would prolong action potential duration. Although under some conditions for re-entry this is antiarrhythmic by prolonging refractory periods, prolongation of the action potential also creates proarrhythmic conditions for triggered activity by early afterdepolarizations. Increased Na+ entry because of augmented late I_{Na} could also contribute to Na overload, and by decreased Ca^{2+} extrusion by Na–Ca exchange, lead to Ca^{2+} overload. Ca^{2+} overload can be arrhythmogenic in several ways: by creating conditions for delayed afterdepolarizations and by altering function of other ion channels either directly or through Ca^{2+}-dependent phosphorylation–dephosphorylation processes.

In a canine model of atrial fibrillation peak I_{Na} (93) and mRNA message for the α subunit hH1 (313) are both decreased, where this decrease may contribute to conduction slowing. In general, peak I_{Na} has been found to be unaltered in models of other forms of acquired heart disease such as hypertrophy in rats (95, 104) and human atrium (216), and in pacing-induced canine heart failure (122), although it was increased in one report in guinea pig hypertrophy. Message for hH1 has been reported as unchanged in heart failure (121). Important subtle changes, however, such as an increase in late current might be missed if not sought carefully with long depolarizations and careful subtraction techniques. A significantly increased late I_{Na} has been shown for an ischemic dog model of failure (267) and for the dog-pacing model of heart failure (269). Studies of the Syrian hamster model of heart failure have shown variously increased late I_{Na} (113) and no change (68). A simlar late I_{Na} has been reported in humans (155) and it has been shown to be significantly greater in heart failure than in control human hearts (264). The molecular mechanisms and importance of late current in heart failure are unknown, however early afterdepolarizations were more common in the failing dog cells and could be prevented by sodium channel blocking agents (267).

L-type Ca^{2+} current—I_{Ca-L}. I_{Ca-L} activates at potentials greater than -40 mV, positive to activation of I_{Na}, and it inactivates more slowly than I_{Na}. Inactivation is partially voltage-dependent but is primarily in response to the rise in intracellular Ca^{2+}. The human L-type Ca^{2+} current consists of an α1 subunit that contains the ion-conducting pore, and several auxiliary subunits including β and α2-δ subunits [reviewed by Katz (127)]. I_{Ca-L} is heavily regulated by phosphorylation (see Chapter 14). Problems in the measurement of I_{Ca-L} include rundown, perhaps because of the dependence of current density on phosphorylation, and alterations in intracellular Ca^{2+} that may affect inactivation kinetics through Ca^{2+}-induced inactivation.

Changes in I_{Ca-L} can be arrhythmogenic by a number of mechanisms. When Na+ channels are inactivated or otherwise depressed, normal or increased I_{Ca-L} density can sustain action potential conduction and might at times underlie the slow conduction pathway in re-entrant circuits (100). Decreased I_{Ca-L} density, as found in atrial fibrillation (139, 312), may facilitate re-entry by decreasing action potential duration and therefore refractoriness. I_{Ca-L} has also been shown to carry the current for early afterdepolarizations (116) implying a role for increased I_{Ca-L} in triggered automaticity. In addition, an increase in I_{Ca-L} would also tend to prolong the action potential duration, prolonging the QT interval on the surface ECG, and facilitating triggered automaticity by early afterdepolarizations. Lastly, an increase in I_{Ca-L} might also lead to delayed afterdepolarizations by increasing cellular Ca^{2+} loading.

I_{Ca-L} density in acquired heart disease has been reported to be unchanged, increased, or decreased [reviewed by Richard (207), Balke and Shorofsky (13), and Tomaselli and Marban (262)]. In hypertrophy and heart failure models, reports of changes in current density are particularly variable. In atrial fibrillation, however, I_{Ca-L} has been shown to be uniformly decreased (29, 94, 139, 273, 312, 313) where it may contribute to the decreased refractory period [see review by Nattel (179)]. I_{Ca-L} has been most studied in various models of hypertrophy where the peak current density changes are very variable. Such variability in I_{Ca-L} density might arise from, among other considerations, the particular model of hypertrophy, the timing of measurement in the disease process, regional and transmural differences, or the phosphorylation state of the channel. Even within the same animal model (cat right ventricular hypertrophy with pulmonary banding) studied by the same investigators, however, I_{Ca-L} density has been reported to be unchanged (132) or decreased (183). In the latter report the hypertrophy was more severe, suggesting that severity or perhaps the timing of observation during the disease process may be an important variable. Interestingly, in a guinea pig model of hypertrophy Bryant et al. (37) reported an increased density in the midmyocardium and epicardium, and a decreased density in endocardium. A decrease in I_{Ca-L} in endocardium was confirmed in a cat chronic infarction model (193). The variability observed in other studies, therefore, might also arise from transmural and regional differences. This heterogeneity might also underlie dispersion of excitability and contribute to arrhythmia. In a rat aortic stenosis model of left ventricular hypertrophy, Scamps et al. (224) reported no change in unstimulated I_{Ca-L} density. After isoproterenol was applied, the maximal density of I_{Ca-L} was less in the hypertrophied cells compared with control cells. The isoproterenol-induced increase in I_{Ca-L} was 78% in hypertrophy versus 120% in control. A decrease in the isoproterenol responsiveness of I_{Ca-L} in cells isolated from patients with heart failure has also been demonstrated (187) suggesting relevance to human disease. In heart failure animal models the results for I_{Ca-L} density are variable, ranging from no change in a dog pacing model (122) to a decrease in a pig pacing model (171) and a genetic hamster model (260) and to an increase in a rat ventricular doxorubicin model (130). In subendocardial Purkinje cells and in epicardial cells surviving an infarction I_{Ca-L} was decreased (1, 32). In a study of cells from human dilated cardiomyopathy and ischemic cardiomyopathy I_{Ca-L} was increased 218% with an increased open probability, whereas Northern analysis showed no change in α1C and β subunits (227), suggesting the importance of altered channel kinetics. In diabetes I_{Ca-L} has been shown to be decreased (51, 141, 282).

With very few exceptions, most of the studies of I_{Ca-L} do not discriminate between a change in the expression of Ca^{2+} channels in the membrane, alteration of the functional effect of phosphorylation, or disruption of the adrenergic-induced phosphorylation cascade. Dihydropyridine (DHP) binding data provide an alternative approach to electrophysiology to assess the density of the channels in the membrane. In the spontaneously hypertensive rats the DHP sites increased with age and the development of hypertrophy (50, 90) but no change in I_{Ca-L} was found in the same model (34, 44). In a rat model of diabetes both DHP sites (141) and I_{Ca-L} (282) were both decreased. In cardiomyopathic hamsters DHP sites were increased (136) but in the same model I_{Ca-L} was unchanged (233) in one study and decreased (260) in another. In a cardiomyopathy model in turkeys, DHP sites first increased then decreased as failure became more severe (102) emphasizing the possible importance of the timing in the disease process. DHP sites were unchanged in human idiopathic dilated cardiomyopathy (103, 201), however they were decreased in ischemic cardiomyopathy (103) suggesting the possible role of the etiology of the disease. At this point the discrepancy between the DHP measurements and I_{Ca-L} are unresolved.

Studies that have looked at I_{Ca-L} kinetics have generally shown slowing of the decay rate (89, 129, 132, 183), and negative shifts in steady-state inactivation (193, 213), although in an infarction model I_{Ca-L} decay was accelerated (1). A negative shift in steady-state inactivation would tend to decrease I_{Ca-L} at any given holding or rest potential without having a decrease in the number of channels at the cell membrane. The slowing of the decay rate for I_{Ca-L} would tend to prolong the action potential, and contribute to Ca^{2+} loading. In summary, changes in I_{Ca-L} in acquired heart disease are common and diverse. The diversity in the findings for I_{Ca-L} probably reflects a genuine diversity in the disease model or etiology, the time dependence of the development of the changes during the disease process, and the method and conditions of measurement.

T-type Ca^{2+} current—I_{Ca-T}. The T-type Ca^{2+} current is prominent in atrial and Purkinje cells (277) and usually is present to a lesser degree in ventricular cells. This channel activates at more negative potentials than I_{Ca-L} and the density of I_{Ca-T} is generally less than that of I_{Ca-L} [see review by Vassort et al (277)]. I_{Ca-T} can be produced by expression of a novel α1 Ca^{2+} channel gene α1g and α1h (61); the role of subunits is unresolved. The physiological and pathophysiological roles of this channel in heart is uncertain, but it can participate in excitation–contraction coupling under some circumstances (241, 318) (see Chapter 18).

The role of I_{Ca-T} in causing arrhythmia is also speculative. It can participate in normal pacemaking activity (105, 277, 319) and therefore if upregulated could contribute to arrhythmogenesis through enhanced normal (phase 4) automaticity. An increase in I_{Ca-T} could also contribute to triggered automaticity by Ca^{2+} loading (delayed afterdepolarizations), or by prolonging the action potential to facilitate early afterdepolarizations. Because the voltage range for I_{Ca-T} is more negative than I_{Ca-L}, it may carry the depolarizing current for phase 3 early afterdepolarizations that occur at less positive membrane potentials (114). One reason for thinking that I_{Ca-T} may be important is that I_{Ca-T} channel density is increased in several models of hypertrophy (88, 158, 184, 297). In a hamster cardiomyopathy model I_{Ca-T} density was increased and the voltage range of activation was shifted to more negative potentials; I_{Ca-L} density was unchanged (233). In a dog pacing model of atrial fibrillation I_{Ca-T} density was not changed (312). In subendocardial Purkinje cells surviving an infarction I_{Ca-T} was decreased by more than 67% and the decay was slowed and kinetics shifted in the hyperpolarizing direction (32), but I_{Ca-T} was unchanged in surviving epicardium (1). Perhaps the recent successful cloning of this channel will lead to better tools for the study of this channel in disease.

Outward Currents: Voltage-Dependent K$^+$ Channels. Voltage-dependent K$^+$ currents can be discussed in three groups: (1) Currents with voltage-dependent activation and inactivation over the millisecond time range (the transient outward currents), (2) currents with more delayed voltage-dependent activation over tens to hundreds of milliseconds, but with very rapid inactivation that has classically been considered rectification (the delayed rectifier currents), and (3) currents that activate rapidly upon depolarization and persist (plateau and sustained currents). As with all ion currents, these potassium currents have traditionally been separated by techniques of voltage dependence and pharmacology. The identification of channel proteins underlying these potassium currents has made significant progress [see reviews by Barry and Nerbonne (16) and by Deal et al. (66)]. Nonetheless, considerable variability exists in the separation, characterization, and identification of these currents and channels.

Transient outward current—I_{to1}. I_{to1} is carried by K$^+$ channels. It activates within milliseconds upon depolarization, then inactivates over tens to hundreds of milliseconds. The specific channel clone responsible for I_{to1} differs from species to species, from tissue to tissue within the heart, and transmurally from epicardium to endocardium but all are part of the family of voltage-dependent potassium channels called Kv [see reviews (16, 66, 208)]. Kv4.2 is thought to carry I_{to1} in rat, but Kv4.2 is absent from human and dog hearts, and Kv4.3 has been suggested to carry I_{to1} in human epicardium and Kv1.4 in human endocardium (208). I_{to1} is responsible for the initial rapid repolarization or downward notch in the early phase of the action potential in epicardium. The transmural localization of I_{to1} is greatest in the epicardium where the notch is prominent, and least in the endocardium where the notch is absent (8, 145). A second type of transient outward current, I_{to2}, is activated by increases in internal Ca^{2+}, is carried by Cl$^-$ ions, and is discussed in the section on Cl$^-$ channels (see later, under Cl$^-$ Currents).

The voltage-dependent transient outward current (I_{to1}) is one of the most studied ion currents in disease states because it has generally been found to be profoundly decreased by 50% or more in nearly every animal disease model including hypertrophy (21, 44, 60, 95, 140, 144, 162, 165, 167, 198, 263, 264, 298, 307), heart failure (122, 188, 209, 210, 260), chronic infarction (4, 118, 126, 151, 210, 306), diabetes (41, 237, 266, 282, 299), and atrial fibrillation (29, 272, 312, 313). In human heart failure the decrease in I_{to1} was shown to correlate with a decrease in Kv4.3 (121) strongly suggesting that Kv4.3 underlies I_{to1} in human ventricle, and that the mechanism for the decrease in I_{to1} is a decrease in transcription. The changes in the transmural gradient for I_{to1} have recently been studied in animal models of disease. In a rat hypertrophy model (38) I_{to1} was decreased in subepicardial cells and midmyocardial cells, but unchanged in subendocardial cells. In a relatively acute (3 day) rat infarction model (306), I_{to1} was decreased more in epicardium than in endocardium. In human hearts, however, a greater decrease in I_{to1} in endocardium has generally been demonstrated, and this would enhance the transmural differences in I_{to1} normally found. In hypertrophic cells from human aortic stenosis I_{to1} was absent in the subendocardium of the right ventricular (RV) septal wall (11) but present in the atrium and the free wall, and present in the RV subendocardium from normal hearts. These data suggest that hypertrophy in humans sharply alters the regional distribution of I_{to1} and thereby increasing heterogeneity of repolarization. Nabauer and colleagues found a nearly 40% overall decrease in I_{to1} in left ventricular cells from failing hearts compared with control hearts (173). In a later human study I_{to1} was decreased 26% decrease in the epicardium (11 to 8 pA/pF), but the density was unchanged in the endocardium (2pA/pF), although with slowed recovery (174). In human right ventricle from failed explanted hearts I_{to1} was three times greater in epicardium than endocardium (143). These findings of decreased I_{to1} fit the straightforward expectation that a decrease of repolarizing currents would accompany the longer action potentials in hypertrophy and heart failure. In human atrial fibrillation Van Wagoner and colleagues (272) showed a decrease in I_{to1} of 60% or more in both left and right atrium compared to controls, consistent with changes reported in animal models of atrial fibrillation. This was somewhat unexpected because in atrial fibrillation the action potential duration is generally shortened. Consequently, changes in other ion channels must control the action potential duration in atrial fibrillation.

The mechanisms by which I_{to1} might affect the action potential are complex. Decreased I_{to1} is generally associated with a prolonged action potential duration and increased I_{to1} with shortened action potential duration both in disease states and where I_{to1} is blocked by 4-AP. Although sustained components of I_{to1} are recorded *in vivo*, the Kv4.2 and Kv4.3 channels expressed alone do not show a sustained component. If

I_{to1} decays rapidly and completely, then it would be expected to affect only the initial phase of the action potential. It could not directly affect the later repolarization; consequently, it should have little or no effect on action potential duration. Blocking I_{to} is reported to prolong action potential duration, but the agents used to block I_{to1} such as 4-AP also block delayed rectifier currents. Thus, 4-AP is not a specific tool for proving the effects of I_{to1} on action potential duration. Changes in I_{to1} do, however, alter the early action potential shape. Even if it decays completely by the time of repolarization, it could influence repolarization by altering the time- and voltage-dependent activation of other currents such as I_{Ca-L} (235). In feline myocytes block of I_{to} causes a decrease in action potential duration, but I_{to1} in this species causes prolonged action potential duration, apparently by resetting time-dependent changes of Ca^{2+} currents (257). On the other hand, decreased I_{to1} might prolong action potential duration by increasing the amplitude of the initial part of the action potential and causing increased inactivation of delayed rectifier currents.

In summary, I_{to1} density has been shown to be affected, mainly decreased, in numerous animal models of heart disease as well as in human hearts with hypertrophy, failure, and atrial fibrillation. The net effect of changes in I_{to1} on action potential duration may be indirect and depend upon the function of other ion channels. An accentuation of the transmural gradient of I_{to} density (11, 174) leading to increased heterogeneity in repolarization may be most important for arrhythmia development.

Delayed rectifier currents I_{Kr}, I_{Ks} and sustained components I_{Kur}, I_{Ksus}, and I_{Kp}. As the name "delayed" implies, the delayed rectifier K^+ currents (I_K) activate upon depolarization to a steady-state level with a voltage-dependent time course upon depolarization, contributing to termination of the action potential plateau. Also, less outward current is passed for strong depolarizations as a result of rapid partial inactivation (247) for stronger depolarizations. These currents have been divided into a rapidly activating component I_{Kr} and a slowly activating component I_{Ks} by pharmacological and kinetic dissection (219). Other components of I_K [reviewed by Barry et al. (16)] have also been identified, including persistent K^+ currents described as an ultrarapidly activating component I_{Kur} (33), a sustained component I_{Ksus} (289), and a plateau current I_{Kp} (10, 311). The literature on these currents is confusing because these components of I_K were defined and separated by different methods in previous studies as the field developed. Adding to the confusion is the natural variation of the components of I_K from species to species and region to region in the heart. The ongoing identification of the channel subunits underlying the components of I_K will help to clarify this. In heart, the expression of an ERG (*ether-a-go-go*-related gene) product, HERG in humans, yields an I_{Kr}-like current (218, 265), and the kinetics of this current more closely resemble I_{Kr} when HERG is co-expressed with a subunit called minK (161). An I_{Ks} like current is produced by co-expression of minK with a K^+ channel designated KvLQT1 (15, 217), later termed KCNQ1. The gene product Kv1.5 is thought to underlie I_{Kur} (244). It is not known whether or not separate gene products underlie the other I_K components, or whether they represent currents from those already described for I_K and I_{to}, perhaps modified by K^+ channel β subunits (77).

Mutations in HERG, KvLQT1, and minK can lead to arrhythmia in the long QT syndromes as described below (see later, under The Potassium Channel Culprits). Qualitatively similar changes in these currents in acquired heart disease could have similar arrhythmic effects. I_{Kr} and I_{Ks} have been generally little studied in disease models, and they have been difficult to detect in human tissue despite the abundance of HERG mRNA (121). These currents can be difficult to study because of problems in separating them. In the few studies reported I_K (undifferentiated but probably I_{Kr}) was decreased and activated more slowly and with deeper rectification in feline hypertrophy (133, 89). No changes in I_K were reported in hypertrophy in rat (34, 44, 55) and guinea pig (213). I_K was decreased in dog Purkinje fibers 2 days after infarction (191) and decreased in rat left ventricular endocardium and epicardium 3 days after infarction (306), although it was increased in the right ventricle in the same study. I_K was also decreased in the cat left ventricular subepicardium 2 months after infarction (310). In canine models of atrial fibrillation, I_{Kr} and I_{Ks} were separated and unchanged (312). In human cardiomyopathy, no change was found in the relatively abundant levels of HERG mRNA (121), but surprisingly little or no I_{Kr}-like or I_{Ks}-like currents were found. The presence of mRNA for HERG but the absence of HERG-like currents is unexplained. Perhaps I_{Kr} and I_{Ks} function are lost by enzymatic treatment or other processing during cell isolation.

As already noted, various persistent outward potassium plateau currents have been described. The ultrarapidly activating current I_{Kur} or sustained current I_{Ksus} were unchanged (44, 307) or decreased (162) in hypertrophy models. In a canine model of atrial fibrillation I_{Kur} was unchanged (312). In human chronic atrial fibrillation, however, I_{Ksus} was decreased about 50% in atrial cells and Kv1.5 was correspondingly downregulated (272). In human dilated atria, I_{Kur} was decreased 60% (139) compared with cells from nondilated atria.

In a dog pacing model of atrial fibrillation these currents were unchanged (312), but in human dilated atria (139) or atria from human chronic atrial fibrillation (272) these currents were decreased 60% and 53%, respectively. I_{Ksus} was decreased in a rat model of low insulin type 1 diabetes but increased in the high insulin type 2 diabetes (237). The decrease for type I diabetes was greatest for left ventricular endocardium, intermediate for left ventricular epicardium, and least for right ventricular myocardium (41).

Outward Currents: Inwardly Rectifying K$^+$ Currents. These currents have no time- and voltage-dependent gating kinetics in that they instantaneously assume their characteristic conductance at any given potential. They are, however, because of inward rectification, voltage dependent in that they more readily pass inward current at negative potentials than outward current at membrane potentials positive to the K$^+$ equilibrium potential. Some channels are strongly rectifying in that they pass very little outward current, and others are called weak rectifiers because they pass only slightly less outward current than inward current. These currents are carried by a distinct family of channels that have been cloned and have been designated Kir$_{x,y}$, where x represents the subfamily and y the particular gene product [reviewed by Nichols (181)]. A family of inwardly rectifying K$^+$ currents called TWIK, with a structure distinct from the Kir family, has been described (142), but the current, if any, carried by these channels in heart is not yet defined.

Inward rectifier I_{K1}. I_{K1} is a strongly inwardly rectifying current carried by Kir$_{2.1}$ without any known subunits. This current is largely responsible for the maintenance of the resting potential of the cell. Because I_{K1} is a strong rectifier, it passes little outward current at plateau potentials, but because of the relatively high density of these channels and the low total current during the plateau, I_{K1} could influence action potential duration. The "N-shape" of the current voltage relationship of I_{K1} makes it maximal near -40 mV and it then decreases with more positive membrane potentials; it may, therefore, play a special role during terminal or phase 3 repolarization (236). A decrease in I_{K1} would tend to prolong action potential duration, especially during the terminal phase, and could promote arrhythmia by triggered automaticity. Although not present in nodal cells, a decreased I_{K1} in subsidiary pacemakers in atria and ventricles could cause a decrease in repolarizing currents during phase 4 and enhance automaticity. An increase in I_{K1} would tend to shorten the action potential duration and decrease refractory periods, potentially promoting arrhythmia through re-entrant mechanisms. I_{K1} density tends to vary greatly from species to species, from tissue to tissue within the heart, and indeed across the ventricular wall (8). This heterogeneity, especially if it is enhanced in disease states, also contributes to arrhythmia.

In hypertrophy, I_{K1} density has been reported to be increased (89, 133), decreased (34, 162, 206), and unchanged (22, 44, 55, 213, 307); the possible role for I_{K1} to prolong action potential duration in hypertrophy is therefore unclear. I_{K1} was modestly (20%–30%) decreased in rat infarction models (4, 126, 306). In heart failure, K$^+$ channels in general tend to be downregulated (175). I_{K1} was unchanged, however, in a rabbit pacing model (209) and in a rat chronic infarction heart failure model (210). I_{K1} density in heart failure was, however, decreased in a dog pacing model (122) and also in humans with cardiomyopathy (27, 121). Interestingly, a decrease in I_{K1} in human cardiomyopathy did not correlate with a decrease in mRNA for Kir$_{2.1}$ (121), suggesting a mechanism other than decreased transcription. Inwardly rectifying channels depend upon the presence of anionic phospholipids in the membrane, especially phosphorylated phosphoinositols or PPIs (80), which interact with positively charged residues on the C-terminus of Kir channels. As noted below under ATP-sensitive K$^+$ Channel I_{KATP-} on I_{KATP}, these phospholipids may be downregulated in heart failure (81), which could account for a decrease in the current density of all inwardly rectifying currents without a downregulation of the channel protein subunits.

ATP-sensitive K$^+$ channel I_{KATP}. I_{KATP} is a weakly inwardly rectifying K$^+$ channel carried by a channel formed from a cardiac isoform of the sulfonylurea receptor SUR2B and a member of the Kir family Kir6.2 [reviewed by Aguilar-Bryan et al. (2)]. The key feature of I_{KATP} is that current is blocked by normal levels of ATP found in the cell. The role of I_{KATP} in the heart under physiological circumstances is unclear [see review by Isomoto and Kurachi (112)], but the channel opens under conditions of metabolic stress such as ischemia or acidosis leading to action potential shortening and arrhythmia (295). I_{KATP} could play a role in arrhythmogenesis in various acquired disease states where the heart is under metabolic stress or, as is quite often the case clinically, acute or chronic ischemia is imposed on the background of acquired disease such as hypertrophy and failure.

Although much studied in acute ischemia, reperfusion, and ischemic preconditioning (101), I_{KATP} has been little studied in acquired heart disease. I_{KATP} has been reported to be increased in cat LV hypertrophy (309), rat LV diabetic (242), and atria from failing human hearts (134). Trypsin increased I_{KATP} in hypertrophied rat myocytes more than in control myocytes (245). ATP sensitivity has been reported to be both decreased [IC$_{50}$ of 90 μM in control to 283 μM in hypertrophic cat ventricle (309) and IC$_{50}$ of 26 μM in control to 131 μM in failing human atria (134)], but increased in left ventricular myocytes from diabetic rat hearts (IC$_{50}$ 11 μM in control versus 5 μM in diabetes (242). ATP sensitivity of the channel, however, is quite variable as indicated by these different IC$_{50}$'s. ATP sensitivity is affected by a large number of factors (112) including other nucleotides (258), pH, and divalents (79). Like other inwardly rectifying channels, I$_{KATP}$ activity depends upon the presence of anionic phospholipids in the membrane, especially phosphorylated phosphoinositols or PPIs (80), and PPIs also decrease the sensitivity of I$_{KATP}$ to ATP (18, 239). In a dog pacing model of heart failure, I$_{KATP}$ density was found to be reduced in cells from failing left ventricle, but activity could be restored by the application of PPIs (81). The density of I$_{KATP}$ in this model was also heterogenous from cell to cell, which could contribute to arrhythmia through re-entrant mechanisms if it contributed to electrical heterogeneity.

Other inwardly rectifying K$^+$ currents I$_{KACh}$, I$_{K-Na}$. Other weak inward rectifier K$^+$ currents are less well characterized in acquired heart disease. This includes the acetylcholine activated K$^+$ channel I$_{KACh}$, which is concentrated in atrial and nodal tissue. When activated, it slows pacemaking and conduction. This current flows through a channel made up of heteromultimers of Kir3.1 and Kir3.4 (135) and the activity is coupled through G proteins to the muscarinic receptor and perhaps other receptors for activity. I$_{KACh}$ was increased in chronic human atrial fibrillation (29). Another Kir clone found in heart is Kir6.1, but it has not been definitively correlated with a current. A large conductance K$^+$ current that opens in response to increased levels (30 mM) of cytoplasmic Na$^+$, I$_{K-Na}$ or Na$^+$ activated K$^+$ channel, has been reported in guinea pig hearts (124) and implied in canine cardiac cells (222). The channel underlying this current is unknown. I$_{K-Na}$, if opened in Na$^+$ overload states, would shorten action potentials and refractory periods (152). The density and properties of I$_{K-Na}$ in acquired heart disease has not been studied.

Cl$^-$ currents I$_{Cl}$. The reversal potential for Cl$^-$ currents (I$_{Cl}$) is generally between −40 mV and −60 mV (19). Therefore, unlike the other ion channels discussed, these currents if activated would reverse direction during a normal cardiac action potential. At resting potentials I$_{Cl}$ is an inward depolarizing current; activation would enhance normal phase 4 pacemaking activity. At plateau potentials I$_{Cl}$ would be an outward repolarizing current; activation would tend to shorten action potential duration, or lower the action potential plateau (274). As reviewed by Hiraoka et al. (108), several I$_{Cl}$ have been reported in heart, all of which are not activated during the basal state or by voltage alone, but rather are opened by various agonists or by stretch. The Ca activated Cl$^-$ current I$_{Cl-Ca}$ is normally activated by the Ca^{2+} transient (320), assisting I$_{to1}$ to inscribe the notch (phase 1) in the action potential prominent in Purkinje cells, and it has also been called transient outward current 2 (I$_{to2}$). It may also play a role in generating the transient inward current associated with Ca overload and delayed afterdepolarizations (115). I$_{Cl-Ca}$ has been little studied in acquired heart disease models, but was found to be unaltered in a dog pacing model of atrial fibrillation (312). Other I$_{Cl}$ (108) are activated by stretch or swelling, protein kinase A, purinergic stimulation, and angiotensin II. These channels are not distributed uniformly in the heart, and this heterogeneity could contribute to arrhythmogenesis by re-entrant mechanisms through dispersion of refractoriness. Stretch-activated I$_{Cl}$ could clearly contribute to arrhythmogenesis during acute changes in hemodynamic load by enhancing phase 4 depolarization or by lengthening the action potential (274). One study has shown an increase in I$_{Cl}$ in rat ventricular hypertrophy (22), but alterations of I$_{Cl}$ in acquired heart disease are otherwise little studied.

Hyperpolarization-induced pacemaker current I$_f$. The pacemaker current is a nonspecific cation current (the channel is permeable to both K$^+$ and Na$^+$) that activates upon hyperpolarization and contributes to phase 4 depolarization [reviewed by (70, 182)]. The channel underlying this current in heart and nerve tissue has been cloned (150). In heart, this channel is found in greatest density in the sinus node, but it is also present in Purkinje cells (276), and atrial (106, 288) and ventricular myocytes (308). In rat models of ventricular hypertrophy I$_f$ was increased (45), and the increase was linearly related to age and β-adrenergic stimulation as well as degree of hypertrophy (46). In studies of human heart failure, I$_f$ was present in three failing hearts (47), and in a study with myocytes from both failing and nonfailing hearts a trend toward greater I$_f$ was found in the failing cells (109). If I$_f$ were increased in human disease, it would have clear implications for arrhythmia by the mechanisms of enhanced phase 4 automaticity.

Gap Junctions. Gap junctions couple cells in the myocardium by forming nonspecific cation channels called connexins [see reviews (69, 169) and Chapter 4]. Families of connexins have been cloned. Using transgenic mice, Thomas et al. (259) have shown that connexin43 mainly determines coupling in ventricles and connexin40 mainly in atria. Alterations in the density, location, and regulation of gap junctions in acquired heart disease could be arrhythmogenic through effects on conduction velocity (246). Gap junctions are modulated by internal pH, Ca^{2+}, and second messengers [see review (69)] and would be secondarily regulated by changes in these modulators found in acquired disease states such as ischemia, hypertrophy, and heart failure. Ca^{2+} overload in heart failure and hypertrophy [reviewed by Balke and Shorofsky (13)] and intracellular acidosis in hypertrophy (281) would tend to uncouple cells by lowering gap junctional conductance. Saffitz (214) has reviewed the role of gap junctions in myocardial remodeling. Gap junctions were disordered (234) in a rat model of hypertrophy, and junctional resistance between cells was increased 140% (59) in a guinea pig aortic constriction hypertrophy model. In myopathic guinea pig hearts coupling is decreased secondary to changes in the renin–angiotensin modulation of gap junctions (65), and coupling is less responsive to increase by β-adrenergic stimulation (64). Physical disruption of gap junctions has been shown in the infarct border zone in chronic canine infarction models (153), and disrupted connexin43 has been correlated with arrhythmia in this model (190). Gap junctions also were disrupted in a goat model of atrial fibrillation (270) but cellular coupling was unchanged overall.

Pumps and exchangers

NaCa exchange and I_{NaCa}. This exchanger normally expels from the cell one Ca^{2+} ion against its electrochemical gradient E_{Ca} by using the energy from admitting into the cell three Na^+ ions with the Na^+ electrochemical gradient E_{Na} [see review by Janvier and Boyett (117)]. This exchange is therefore electrogenic and has a reversal potential $E_{NaCa} = 3 E_{Na} - 2E_{Ca}$. E_{NaCa} is about -20 mV under resting conditions, but during Ca^{2+} transients or Ca^{2+} overload that increase internal Ca^{2+} E_{NaCa} is more positive, and during Na^+ overload conditions E_{NaCa} is more negative. I_{NaCa} is inward at rest (phase 4), outward transiently before the Ca^{2+} transient positively shifts E_{NaCa} to make I_{NaCa} inward again, then I_{NaCa} declines as the Ca^{2+} transient declines and E_{NaCa} shifts negatively (117). During phase 3 repolarization I_{NaCa} becomes more inward as the membrane potential moves more negative to E_{NaCa} and increases the driving force for I_{NaCa}. Clearly, depending upon the conditions, increased I_{NaCa} can be arrhythmogenic by (1) enhancing phase 4 automaticity, (2) enhancing triggered automaticity from early afterdepolarizations by prolonging action potential duration and possibly providing a depolarizing current for the early afterdepolarizations themselves, and (3) enhancing triggered automaticity by providing a depolarizing current for delayed afterdepolarizations (195). I_{NaCa} has been shown to be unchanged (167) or increased (78, 251) in rat models of hypertrophy. In a relatively acute (3d) high-altitude rat model of hypertrophy I_{NaCa} was decreased, but exchanger message and protein were unchanged (78), suggesting that activity was increased by mechanisms other than increased exchanger density. In heart failure I_{NaCa} was increased in a guinea pig aortic banding model at 4 and 8 weeks (3), in the Syrian hamster cardiomyopathy model at 120 days (68), and in a rabbit aortic insufficiency failure model (197). A decrease in both I_{NaCa} and in exchanger mRNA was found, however, in a rabbit pacing model (305). In human heart failure the exchanger activity was increased 87% and the exchanger protein itself was upregulated 160% (204, 251). In rat models of diabetes I_{NaCa} was decreased (51, 225), while no change in exchanger message was found (225).

$Na^+ K^+$ pump—Na-K-ATPase. Na–K-ATPase pumps 3 Na^+ ions out of the cell and 2 K^+ ions into the cell for every cycle, maintaining ion gradients for Na^+ and K^+, and generating an outward hyperpolarizing current under almost all ionic and membrane potential conditions during the action potential. Decreased Na–K-ATPase activity by itself would tend to lengthen the action potential duration, favoring early afterdepolarization development and it would also augment phase 4 automaticity. In addition, decreased Na–K-ATPase activity would tend to increase Ca^{2+} loading by raising intracellular Na^+ and decreasing extrusion of Ca^{2+} through the Na–Ca exchanger (favoring delayed afterdepolarizations). Enhancement of triggered automaticity by the delayed afterdepolarization mechanisms certainly occurs with decreased Na-K-ATPase activity as in digitalis toxicity (115), but digitalis tends to have either no effect or a shortening of the action potential duration, perhaps by alteration of intracellular Ca^{2+} or other indirect effects.

Na–K-ATPase is composed of an α subunit with three predominant isoforms (α1, α2, and α3) and a β subunit with two isoforms (β1 and β2), each with distinct kinetics (49, 91). In human heart the Na–K-ATPase isoforms detected were α1β1, α2β1, and α3β1, and Na^+ pump activity was 30%–50% lower in atria compared to ventricles with no differences between ventricles and septum (253, 285).

Overall Na-K-ATPase is uniformly downregulated in various human acquired heart disease and animal models of disease with the α1 subunit generally unchanged and α2 and α3 decreased. Na-K-ATPase activity was decreased in cat ventricular right ventricular hypertrophy (240), the α2 subunit decreased in rat left ventricular hypertrophy models (146, 211, 215), and α3 decreased in dog left ventricular hypertrophy model (314). In a rat chronic infarction model of heart failure Na–K-ATPase was decreased (71). In human cardiomyopathy, levels of Na–K-ATPase activity were decreased proportionally to the ejection fraction (39) but in a different study no change was found in α subunit expression (253) suggesting that the decreased activity might result from altered function rather than altered numbers of exchangers. In an exception to these trends, Na-K-ATPase activity was unchanged and the α3 isoform was increased in a dog pacing model of heart failure (14). In rat diabetes models Na-K-ATPase activity and the α2 isoform were decreased (278), and this was reversed with insulin treatment.

Nonspecific, Background, and Swell-Activated Currents.
A number of background and leak currents have been described in heart. For the most part specific ion channels have not been identified for these currents. Nonspecific cation currents conduct both K^+ and Na^+ ions and therefore have a reversal potential around 0 mV. When activated, they would have the greatest effect by depolarizing the resting potential and opposing repolarization during phase 3 of the action potential, tending to lengthen the action potential. A Ca^{2+}-activated nonspecific cation current, the transient inward current, has been described in connection with Ca^{2+} overload states and the development of delayed afterdepolarizations [reviewed by (115)]. No alterations in this current in acquired disease have been described. Swelling activation of ion channels deserves special mention because of the role this mechanism may play in arrhythmia during acute changes in hemodynamic load (250). Stretch may affect several of the ion channels and carriers already discussed, including I_{Kr} and I_{Ks}(203, 220), I_{Ca-L} (160), I_{KATP} (271), I_{Cl} (108), I_{NaCa} (296), Na-K-ATPase (220). Stretch also activates a background K^+ channel distinct from K_{ATP} (131) as well as other distinct background currents in heart (275), one of which is a nonspecific cation current. In a dog pacing model of heart failure, persistent activation of swelling-activated nonspecific cation current (56) has been reported.

Summary of Electrical Remodeling in Acquired Heart Disease

Current densities are altered in acquired heart disease, as summarized in Figure 19-1, affecting the cellular electrophysiology in a process called "electrical remodeling." I_{to1} is almost universally downregulated across all types and models of acquired heart disease, including cardiomyopathy in humans. Another slightly less consistent finding is prolongation of the action potential duration. This prolongation can be arrhythmogenic by favoring triggered automaticity, and by providing conditions for re-entry, especially if the prolongation is heterogeneous, thus promoting dispersion of refractoriness.

The changes summarized in Figure 19-1 are simply current densities in ventricle (atria for atrial fibrillation), and it is not completely clear if these current changes can account for the cellular electrophysiological changes. Changes in kinetics and changes in transmural and regional current densities need to be better described. Such changes are key to the generation of arrhythmia. Many other questions regarding ion current changes in acquired heart disease are just beginning to be addressed. What is the mechanism for alterations in current density? Is it at the level of transcription, translation, or post-translational modification, or even increased turnover? What is the underlying cause for these mechanisms? Could it be altered regulation by cell-signaling systems, especially involving alterations in Ca^{2+} signaling, in which case the altered electrophysiology could provide its own feedback on the process? Does channel function respond differently to these modulatory systems in disease? Does isoform switching occur in channel subunits, as in perhaps a recapitulation of ion current changes in development (84, 293)?

Finally, what are the differences and similarities between different diseases and the different ways of making the disease in animals and the different etiologies in humans? Are the changes species dependent? How much do the alterations in ion current density and function change during the disease process, and are these alterations in the pathogenetic pathway for the disease either causing or exacerbating the disease in a maladaptive way, or are they compensatory for the underlying process but with the unfortunate side-effect of arrhythmia?

Describing the changes and understanding the mechanisms of alterations in ion currents in acquired heart disease will be important for understanding the altered electrophysiology leading to arrhythmia, and it may also contribute to an understanding of the pathophysiology of cardiac hypertrophy and failure.

THE LONG Q-T SYNDROME

Introduction

Summary. Long QT syndrome has been recognized for a half century as a relatively rare inherited, life-threatening arrhythmia in young people. Although it has long been expected that the cause of this syndrome is a genetic abnormality of cardiac ion channels, only in the last 3-4 years has it been possible to identify the inherited ion channel mutations that underlie the long QT syndrome and its arrhythmias. Mark Keating and colleagues (62, 287) have taken advantage of a large body of scientific understanding in cardiac electrophysiology and in genetics to identify specific gene defects in affected families, and this has led to an explosion of new information about this clinical syndrome (Table 19–2). Interestingly, insight into normal ion channel function has also resulted from this work. The success story in long QT syndrome represents an exciting paradigm for the mutual interdependence of basic biological science and clinical medicine. It opens a new chapter in our effort to understand the mechanisms of potentially lethal arrhythmias.

The Clinical Picture. Prolonged QT intervals in the ECG, an indirect indicator of prolonged ventricular action potentials, characterize two long QT syndromes—acquired and inherited. Acquired long QT syndrome was first described with quinidine use for treatment of atrial fibrillation in the early post-World War II period, and the syndrome has subsequently has been associated with a variety of antiarrhythmic drugs and/or electrolyte abnormalities. The hereditary type of long QT syndrome is characterized by syncope or death from ventricular arrhythmias in young people, usually with family history of sudden death. Both acquired and hereditary types have polymorphic ventricular tachycardia (torsade de pointes) as their typical arrhythmia, further supporting the idea that they share a common arrhythmic mechanism.

Acquired long Q-T syndrome was first described as "quinidine syncope"(232). The typical clinical situation was a patient given quinidine for conversion of atrial fibrillation, who after a short QQ interval then a long one develops a polymorphic ventricular tachycardia (VT). This polymorphic VT is usually self-terminating, but may recur and degenerate into ventricular fibrillation. Quinidine is expected to prolong the QRS interval because of its block of Na^+ channels, but the arrhythmia usually occurs in the setting of normal QRS intervals but substantial prolongation of the QT interval. It also does not correlate in any obvious way with quinidine dose or blood level. Hypokalemia, perhaps because it independently prolongs the QT interval, is a predisposing factor. Subsequently, this syndrome has been seen with all of the Vaughan-Williams class IA drugs, which are known to block K^+ channels in addition to Na^+ channels, and especially with class III drugs that prolong refractoriness by more specifically blocking K^+ channels. Antihistamines and other noncardiac drugs that affect K^+ channels have also been implicated. Administration of K^+ to shorten the QT interval and acceleration of the atrial rate by β-adrenergic agonists or an electronic pacemaker will often prevent these drug-associated arrhythmic bursts. Several antiarrhythmic drugs implicated in the acquired long QT syndrome, such as amiodarone, also affect Ca^{2+} or K^+ channels and prolong the QT interval. Indeed, this proarrhythmic phenomenon has been a serious impediment in the clinical utility of several otherwise very effective antiarrhythmic, antianginal, antihistamine, and antimicrobial drugs.

Hereditary long QT syndrome is usually divided into two categories. The Jervell and Lange-Nielson autosomal recessive type is found in a small group of children with deafness, who have early death from ventricular arrhythmia. The much more common autosomal dominant Romano-Ward type is usually manifested in teenagers or young adults by syncope or death in relation to emotion or exercise, but it can also occur during sleep. This relationship to emotion and exercise led to the idea that abnormal sympathetic nerve activity was involved in triggering the arrhythmia, and a mainstay of therapy has been β-adrenergic receptor blockade. A registry of families with this syndrome has facilitated evaluation of treatment and, most importantly, laid the groundwork for genetic analysis to determine the molecular mechanisms of the arrhythmia. Thorough descriptions of these two clinical syndromes can be found elsewhere (170, 229).

Arrhythmic Mechanism

The characteristic arrhythmia in the long QT syndrome is a polymorphic VT called torsade de pointes. Important differences exist, however, between the hereditary and the acquired types in the mode of onset of the VT. Because the hallmark of this group of arrhythmias is their occurrence in the setting of delayed repolarization, judged by QT prolongation in the surface ECG leads, it is logical to consider that action potentials in all or part of the ventricles are prolonged. Prolongation of the Purkinje fiber or ventricular (par-

TABLE 19–2. *Molecular defects in Long QT Syndrome*

Linkage Group	Incidence	Gene	Channel	Current	Pathological Process
LQT-1	21%	11p15.5	KCNQ1	I_{Ks}	Dominant negative
LQT-2	19%	7q35-36	HERG	I_{Kr}	Mostly dominant negative
LQT-3	7%–8%	3p21-24	SCN5A	I_{Na}	Small noninactivating current
LQT-4	Rare	4q25-27	Unknown	Unknown	Unknown
LQT-5	Rare	21q22	KCNE1	I_{Ks}	Dominant negative

ticularly those of the M-type) action potentials by any number of mechanisms including hypokalemia, K⁺ channel block, or increased late inward currents can result in the phenomenon called early afterdepolarizations (EADs) (116). EADs are membrane depolarizations that develop during the AP plateau or during rapid repolarization as the result of recovery and reactivation of Ca^{2+} channels. EADs can occur in single cells or small groups of cells where no dispersion of recovery can exist; consequently, they represent a membrane phenomenon. If a stretch of Purkinje strand or a small region of the ventricle should manifest EADs, then that region would function like a protected pacemaker region. An alternative mechanism for EADs that has been proposed for these arrhythmias is a spatial difference in repolarization time, so that the depolarized region does not itself directly generate the action potential, but rather it supplies electrotonic current to a nearby prematurely repolarized area, bringing that area to threshold for excitation using both Na^+ and Ca^{2+} channels and a consequent re-entry process (24).

Detailed electrophysiological studies in individuals with long QT syndrome sufficient for insight into the arrhythmogenic mechanisms are not available, and there is no generally accepted animal model at this time. Two approaches to mechanism are being followed. First, ion channel gene abnormalities can in theory be produced in transgenic mice. Mice with transgene suppression of K^+ channels have been reported (148), and spontaneous or stimulated ventricular arrhythmias were seen (12). One of the problems with this approach is extrapolation of electrophysiological changes in mice to arrhythmias in humans. Second, pharmacological manipulation of ion channels can be used to imitate the delayed repolarization (199). A particularly interesting study employing this approach is that of El-Sherif and colleagues (54, 76), who used sea anemone toxin to generate a small population of non-inactivating Na^+ channels (one of the pathophysiological mechanisms in long QT synrome). The sea anemone toxins greatly prolong action potentials, especially in the middle of the myocardial wall, which has been shown by in vitro studies to have delayed repolarization (7). In the El-Sherif dog model of delayed repolarization, VT resembling torsade de pointes occurred spontaneously. Transmural mapping showed that the initiating excitation occurred at the endocardial surface (near presumed Purkinje–muscle junctions). Subsequent electrical cycles in the tachycardia resulted from excitations at nearby endocardial sites or by initiation of re-entry permitted by the extensive midmyocardial refractory period prolongation. The different sites of origin or different re-entry paths have activation fronts that resulted in progressive changes in the QRS axis ("turning of the points"), the characteristic VT of torsade de pointes.

Another example of this macrodispersion of repolarization is an imbalance between right and left sympathetic nerve activity (304), such that one region of the ventricle has greater sympathetic activation than the rest. This concept led to two related treatments for long QT syndrome: β-adrenergic blockade and ablation of the left sympathetic ganglia.

Although both acquired and hereditary types of long QT syndrome show arrhythmias that fit the EAD mechanism, a major difference between them is seen. The drug-induced type shows facilitation of triggering of the VT by bradycardia or by a long pauses following a short interval, such as can be seen in atrial fibrillation with substantial AV block. In contrast, the hereditary type often occurs during sinus tachycardia from exercise or emotion. The arrhythmia is triggered by an early extra beat, usually within the preceding T wave, rather than by a beat that occurs after a long–short pair of intervals. This clinical difference suggests that at least the initiating events may not be the same in the two syndromes.

Molecular Mechanisms

The Genetic Link. The predominant hereditary pattern for long QT syndrome with deafness is autosomal recessive, and that without deafness is autosomal dominant. However, variable patterns have been observed, and more definitive markers than the QT interval are necessary to resolve the details of the inheritance. The identification of large families with long QT syndrome has been crucial in applying genetic linkage analysis to identify specific abnormalities. Simultaneous progress in identifying the genes for ion channel proteins and other modulators of cardiac electrical excitability has revealed specific molecular defects in about half of the studied families with hereditary long QT syndrome. The variety of mutations, deletions, splice variants, and frame shifts grows daily, as more families are studied. In addition to identifying molecular abnormalities in long QT syndrome, this work has also contributed in important ways to the understanding of normal ion channels and their roles in electrogenesis. The gene abnormalities so far identified have been in K^+ and Na^+ channels, although channel abnormalities in other ion channels or in channel modulatory systems have not at all been ruled out.

The Potassium Channel Culprits

LQT1 About half of the individuals with specific gene defects identified by Wang et al. (286) had abnormalities in the delayed rectifier K^+ channel

KvLQT1, so named because the channel was first discovered by its linkage to LQT1. (The channel has subsequently been renamed KCNQ1). A subsequent study showed that 43% of individuals with identifiable defects had an abnormality in this channel (147). In the initial linkage studies, the partial sequence on chromosome 11p15.5 suggested that the abnormal gene coded for a K$^+$ channel because of homology with known voltage-dependent K$^+$ channels. The full coding sequence of this gene has been resolved (15, 218, 303) and its function as an ion channel demonstrated. The protein is normally expressed at high levels in heart, but also in kidney, pancreas, lung, placenta, and inner ear (180, 288). When the message for this protein is expressed alone in oocytes or mammalian cells, little or no current is seen. If, however, it is coexpressed with the single transmembrane-segment minK (IsK) protein (now named KCNE1), the currents resemble the slow delayed rectifier current I_{Ks}. This heteromultimeric channel shows characteristic pharmacological interactions of that current (15, 218). At least 16 different missense mutations in KCNQ1 have been identified in affected families, (212, 255, 286). In all of those studied so far, the mutated gene product fails to express any current, acting as a dominant negative. Because this defect is an autosomal dominant, the affected individuals should have one normal gene and one mutated one. The clinical syndrome therefore appears to result from partial or total loss of I_{Ks}.

With identification of more families with defects in KCNQ1, an interesting puzzle has emerged. Only a few of those with the genetic defect manifest the typical long QT syndrome, and some individuals with the gene defect even have normal QT intervals. The reasons for this are not clear. One interesting feature of KCNQ1 is that a splice variant is normally produced. The splice variant appears to act as a dominant negative to suppress the expression of I_{Ks}. Perhaps relative expression levels of the splice variant, the defective gene product, and normal KCNQ1 can result in different levels of I_{Ks} and different intensity of the manifestations. Understanding the phenomenon of asymptomatic carriers of the gene defect could provide important insight into a strategy for treatment of this type of long QT syndrome.

Of interest is that other members of this family of K$^+$ channels have also been related to disease of other systems. KCNQ2 and KCNQ3 are expressed in the central nervous system and they have been linked to an inherited form of epilepsy (302). Neither of these KCNQ channels seems to require KCNE1 (minK), suggesting that these channels may have different β subunits.

LQT2 A second linkage with long QT syndrome was established at a site in chromosome 7q35–36. Subsequently, this site has been shown to code for a human K$^+$ channel (62, 265). The channel was first cloned from heart by analogy to the *ether-a-go-go* gene in *Drosophila* (290), and it was named HERG (human *ether-a-go-go*-related gene). Defects in this gene represented 38% of the affected individuals with identified gene defects in a recent study (147). This K$^+$ channel in long QT families has multiple sequence abnormalities, including intragenic deletions, missense mutations, and a splice-donor mutation (62). The normal HERG channel expressed in oocytes demonstrated a delayed rectifier current similar to I_{Kr} (218, 265) but with different pharmacological properties (247). When HERG was expressed in mammalian cells at physiological temperatures it more closely resembled I_{Kr} kinetics and pharmacology (317). Coexpression of HERG with minK (KCNE1) altered HERG current properties (161), and minK antisense reduced current levels suggesting a role for minK or a closely related protein as a subunit of HERG. Most long QT mutations in HERG result in failure of expression by a dominant negative effect, with some channels incorrectly processed in the endoplasmic reticulum-Golgi and therefore degraded, or they form nonfunctional channels in the membrane (316). One HERG mutant has been described that simply alters the channel's kinetics.

LQT5 The gene abnormality on chromosome 21q22.1-22.2 linked with the long QT syndrome has been identified as KCNE1 (minK). This 130 amino acid protein was first cloned from rat kidney, and it has a single transmembrane segment (254). It is widely distributed, with substantial expression in the heart. When this gene was first cloned, expression of its protein product called minK was first attempted in *Xenopus* oocytes. In that system there was a very slowly developing outward K$^+$ current, as if this single transmembrane protein could assemble into a functioning channel by itself. Subsequently it was found that coexpression of KvLQT1 (KCNQ1) with KCNE1 (minK) resulted in a functional channel that resembles I_{Ks} (see above). The reason that minK message expressed alone in oocytes yielded new currents is that the oocytes contain an endogenous KCNQ1-like protein, and the combination of the endogenous KCNQ1-like protein and KCNE1 resulted in the currents (9). Several families have been found to have long QT syndrome because of mutations in KCNE1 (73, 228, 249), thereby reducing I_{Ks}. If there is a combination of mutations in both KCNQ1 and KCNE1, or a homozygous abnormality in either of the KCNE1 or the KCNQ1 genes, then the result is both long QT syndrome and deafness (Jervel and Lange-Nielson syndrome), because these proteins also compose a K$^+$ channel in the inner ear that is involved in formation of endolymph. Because of the high mortality in the Jervel and Lange-Nielson syndrome, it is important that family members be screened for abnormalities in both genes if one is found to be defective, because carriers may be symptom-free.

The Na Channel Culprit

LQT3 The long QT syndrome linkage to chromosome locus 3p21–24 (119) and the known location of the coding sequences for the cardiac Na$^+$ channel in the same segment (97) quickly led to identification of the Na$^+$ channel as one of the abnormal gene products in the long QT syndrome (287). Na$^+$ current has long been known to contribute to the action potential plateau height and duration, especially in Purkinje and ventricular M-cells. Its possible role to prolong action potentials in the long QT syndrome was suggested when a series of mutations in the skeletal muscle Na$^+$ channel were found to cause paralysis or myotonia by delay in channel inactivation (40). The first cardiac Na$^+$ channel gene abnormality was a deletion of nine nucleic acids from the domains III-IV linker, resulting in the loss of three amino acids (K1505, P1506, and Q1507) from an otherwise complete Na$^+$ channel. The domains III-IV segment was known to participate in the normal fast inactivation process (42, 85), so it was immediately expected that the KPQ deletion would alter inactivation (286). Other single amino acid alterations in the domain III S4-S5 segment (N1325S), and in domain IV (R1623Q, R1644H, D1790G) were also found to be associated with the clinical syndrome.

Introduction of these mutations in the cloned cardiac Na$^+$ channel was straightforward, and their expression in heterologous cells showed typical voltage-dependent currents. However, after rapid inactivation during prolonged depolarization, the channels showed occasional continued reopening behavior, resulting in a late current equal to about 1% of peak Na$^+$ current 20 msec after the peak (23) but lesser amounts at 240 msec after the peak (177). Single-channel studies of the three mutant channels suggested that although the continued openings may not have the same molecular kinetic mechanism (75), the end result was the same: a residual current during depolarization that was first thought to fail to inactivate, but later was shown to inactivate slowly with a time course of several hundred milliseconds (177). This late current was also shown to recover from inactivation much more slowly than peak current, resulting in an accumulation of inactivation and a reduction in late current at faster rates (177). This property is important because it may explain the shortening of prolonged QT interval with increased heart rate reported in LQT3 patients (230). A second functional defect in Na$^+$ channels is also produced by the KPQ mutation. The decay of current after initial activation is accelerated and the latency to first single-channel opening is reduced, supporting a complex kinetic effect of the mutation (48). With only a few differences, N1325S and R1664H mutants functioned much like the KPQ deletion (283, 284). Investigation of R1623Q (123), however, showed a different phenotype with a slow initial decay that could be accelerated in the presence of lidocaine. Investigations of the D1790G mutation suggested that the mechanism of the altered phenotype might involve an alteration of the interaction of the α subunit with the β1 subunit (6).

The amount of residual current that would exist during the normal action potential plateau has been difficult to predict from the voltage-clamp studies of cloned channels in heterologous cells. However, because the total ionic current is low during the plateau, even a small fraction of the peak Na$^+$ current could have a large effect on action potential duration. This behavior is a "gain of function" change, and it means that the affected individual's cardiac myocytes have one normal gene and one defective gene. This will result in a mixed population of normal and abnormal Na$^+$ channels, so that the fraction of channels with abnormal behavior can vary with factors influencing their relative expression, producing a graded severity of the disease. Nothing is known about regulation of expression of Na$^+$ channels, so it remains possible that such regulatory factors as cAMP levels might alter the membrane densities of normal and abnormal channels in a dynamic way. In the same manner, variation in the expression of repolarizing K$^+$ channels in different parts of the heart would affect the importance of the late Na$^+$ current.

Vaughan-William class I antiarrhythmic drugs target Na channels, and their blocking efficacy depends in part on the channel kinetic state ("use dependence"). Consequently, it was of obvious interest to see if these drugs could block the late current in the mutated channels. Both the inactivated state blocker lidocaine (5, 74) and the orally useful analog mexiletine (284), as well as the open state blocker flecainide (176), dramatically reduced the persistent current at doses with modest effects on the peak current during voltage-clamp study in heterologous cells. Acute administration of mexiletine in a small set of 13 persons with long QT syndrome and known gene abnormality of the Na$^+$ channel or the HERG K$^+$ channel were tested for changes in the QT interval (230). The six LQT3 patients shortened their QT interval dramatically from 535 msec to 445 msec, almost into the normal range. Seven patients with HERG defects showed small changes of borderline significance. No clinical trial of long-term administration of a local anesthetic drug has yet been reported, so the clinical efficacy of this treatment is not yet known.

Other Genetic Causes of Long QT

LQT4 The familial long QT syndrome is linked to chromosome 4q25–27, but the gene responsible for the clinical picture has not yet been identified (226). It may not be an ion channel, but rather the gene for a protein important in ion channel expression or modulation. An exciting clue has come from a *knockout* mouse (52). The Na^+ channel is known to interact with the cytoskeleton (268), and ankyrin has been copurified with the Na^+ channel. The ankyrin$_B$ gene has been localized to chromosome 4q25–27. Its knockout led to a reduced expression of Na^+ current with abnormal kinetics, suggesting that LQT-4 may be a genetic alteration in the expression and/or modulation of Na^+ channels.

LQT > 5. Only perhaps half of the families with long QT syndrome have yet been matched with one of the chromosomal abnormalities described above. Consequently, it is likely that there are other culprits yet to be found. In addition, there are other familial syndromes characterized by recurrent ventricular arrhythmias and death due to ventricular fibrillation that do not have ECG evidence of prolonged QT intervals (see later, under Idiopathic Ventricular Fibrillation). Their relationship to the sort of gene defects seen in long QT is not yet clear. Finally, the large group of individuals with acquired long QT, which appears to be an idiosyncratic reaction to drugs that target cardiac ion channels, may have polymorphisms or latent ion channel abnormalities that make them more susceptible to small changes in channel function, producing an electrical imbalance that sets the stage for torsade de pointes arrhythmia (292).

Implications for Therapy

Arrhythmias in familial long QT syndrome have been associated with two quite different clinical situations. Most are associated with physical or emotional stress and with increased heart rate. But in a smaller group of individuals the arrhythmias occur at rest or during sleep, when the heart rate is slow. Examination of the clinical setting for arrhythmias in individuals with the Na^+ channel defect (LQT3) showed that their episodes of arrhythmias are predominantly at rest. A second group of individuals with K^+ channel defects of HERG type had arrhythmias predominantly during stress (230). Increasing heart rate in the normal heart characteristically shortens the action potential and, consequently, the QT interval. In parallel with the clinical pattern, individuals with K^+ channel defects shortened their QT interval less than normal with exercise, so that deviation of the QT interval from normal was greater at higher rates. In contrast, the QT interval is excessively long at slow rates for those with the Na^+ channel defect, but it tends to normalize with exercise. The greatly slowed recovery of late Na^+ current in LQT3 may also account for the greater rate-dependent shortening in this syndrome (177). Consequently, for those with Na^+ channel abnormalities the repolarization abnormality is accentuated during slow heart rates.

Individuals clinically identified with long QT syndrome are most often female (gender ratios of 1.5–2). Furthermore, adult women have slightly longer QT intervals than men. A similar gender difference is also seen in the occurrence of acquired type of long QT syndrome. A careful longitudinal study of individuals with hereditary long QT syndrome and their near relatives (147) showed no difference in QT intervals between males and females until after the age of 15 years. Subsequently, the QT interval shortened in males, but not in females. Incidence of symptomatic cardiac events was higher in males before age 15, and then diminished. However, the somewhat lower incidence in females before age 15 continued unchanged after that age. These differences were not the result of excessive diagnostic error in females. This emphasizes that a small bias in repolarization can have a large influence on the manifestations of arrhythmias in these genetic defects.

The clinical association of arrhythmias with stress was one factor leading to use of β-adrenergic blocking drugs, which have demonstrated success in preventing episodes. The mechanism of the arrhythmogenic effect of adrenergic activity induced by emotion or exercise is not clear. Adrenergic stimulation of cAMP production results in phosphorylation of several channel types, thereby altering the action potential. The most thoroughly studied example is protein kinase A phosphorylation of L-type Ca^{2+} channels by PKA, which increases Ca^{2+} current and might be expected to lengthen the action potential. On the other hand, phosphorylation by PKA also increases K^+ currents, favoring a shorter action potential. Perhaps normally the two are in balance, but if K^+ currents are diminished, then the Ca^{2+} channel effect may predominate. A further question is if the individuals benefiting from β-blockers are the subset with the K^+ channel abnormalities where the repolarization abnormality is exaggerated at higher rates, and if those with the Na^+ channel defect are not benefited or may even be harmed.

It has long been known that increasing extracellular K^+ shortens the action potential, and its mechanism is an increase in K^+ currents (223). Compton et al. (58) have shown that the QT intervals of individuals with the HERG type of long QT syndrome were especially sensitive to intravenous administration of K^+. Such a treatment scheme is feasible and may represent a direct way to normalize the QT interval in individuals with K⁺ channel defects. However, it should not be inferred that increased serum K⁺ is a specific treatment, and additionally, long-term maintenance of elevated serum K⁺ in individuals with normal kidney function is not easily achieved with our present clinical tools. An alternative therapy might involve K⁺ channel openers to shorten the QT interval, even though they may not target the defective channels themselves.

Present Status

The identification of defective ion channel molecules responsible for the inherited long QT syndrome has had a large impact on our understanding of arrhythmias. Knowledge of the four (so far identified) ion channel proteins has allowed typing of individuals/families, markedly improving insight into clinical categories and consequently into diagnosis and treatment. It has revealed two previously unappreciated K⁺ channel proteins and provided tools to allow dissection of their normal physiological roles. Finally, it has greatly improved our attitude toward the prospect of finally understanding the molecular pathogenesis of arrhythmias. These achievements open a new window of opportunity for arrhythmia study.

Typing of individuals and families revealed that the long QT syndrome is not a homogeneous clinical entity. Those with K⁺ channel defects have a blunted response of action potential duration to frequency, and are consequently at extra risk during exercise and emotion. These individuals are likely to be the ones benefitted by β-adrenergic blockade, and they may also be treated by raising their serum K⁺. Those with Na⁺ channel defects show an exaggerated response of action potential duration to exercise and are at extra risk for arrhythmias at low heart rates. They are particularly likely to benefit from implantation of a pacemaker or by suppression of the sustained Na⁺ current with local anesthetic or other targeted drugs. Homogeneous groups can now be tested for mechanism-directed therapy. In addition, much more accurate detection of susceptible family members is now possible.

Further insight into the different manifestations of the specific gene abnormalities has recently been reported (315). In a study of 541 members of 38 families in the long QT registry, 112 had KCNQ1 defects, 72 had HERG defects, and 62 had Na⁺ channel defects. The KCNQ1 cohort showed a cumulative probability of a cardiac event (syncope, aborted cardiac arrest, sudden death) of 0.6 by age 20, with half of these by age 8. Those with the Na⁺ channel mutations developed cardiac events later and with a lower overall incidence. Those with HERG defects were intermediate. However, the cumulative probability of death during an episode was much greater for the Na⁺ channel mutation cohort, with 20% of the episodes resulting in death, most of which were first events. Further correlation of prognosis depending on the specific mutation within each large group will be important, but it will be difficult until a large enough number of individuals are typed.

The imperfect pharmacological separation of I_{Ks} and I_{Kr} is now replaced by the ability to study in heterologous systems KCNQ1 for I_{Ks} and HERG for I_{Kr}. The KCNQ1 studies have allowed us finally to understand the role of minK as a β subunit, rather than as a free-standing orphan channel. HERG has shown the fascinating kinetic problem of faster inactivation than activation, so that the physiologically relevant current is the tail current upon repolarization (243). HERG is also a major tool for investigation of the important physiological process of C-type inactivation. All of these naturally occurring mutations help to provide insights and tools for the further study of basic channel mechanisms.

In the few years since the first report of abnormal gene products in long QT syndrome, this field has moved with blinding speed. We finally have several molecular pathogenic mechanisms for a lethal arrhythmia, raising the hope that similar mechanisms may be found in drug-induced long QT syndrome, crib death (231), or even in structural heart disease. However, it should be recognized that we have not yet resolved all the questions about long QT syndrome. Here are a few: What triggers torsade de pointes or controls its maintenance at the single-cell level or in the intact heart? What terminates the VT in most episodes? Why is the arrhythmia so rare—often years without arrhythmia in the presence of the genetic abnormality? What is the role of cardiac autonomic nerve activity in pathogenesis? What are the effective long-term therapies, and when should the asymptomatic family member be treated prophylactically? Do those with acquired long QT syndrome have a genetic abnormality that makes them susceptible?

IDIOPATHIC VENTRICULAR FIBRILLATION

For some years it has been apparent that some individuals have lethal ventricular fibrillation without structural heart disease and without long QT intervals. Recently Brugada et al. (36) described a subset of these who had a characteristic ECG pattern. The ECG showed a somewhat atypical right bundle branch block pattern with elevated, domed ST segments in V_1–V_3, but with normal QT intervals. These individuals were much older than those with long QT syndrome, with an average age of 40 years. Initially, it appeared that this group was predominantly male, but as more cases are reported, the gender difference is less dramatic.

At first, this syndrome of ventricular fibrillation without structural heart disease appeared to be sporadic, but this was because of the rather small families and the high incidence of sudden death. Recently three of these families have been shown to have defects in the gene coding for the cardiac Na^+ channel (53). These include a missense mutation, a splice-donor mutation, and a frame-shift mutation. One blocks the translation of the Na^+ channel, and the others alter the sequence and produce functional change in the electrophysiological properties of the expressed channel. Clinical identification of the syndrome can be difficult, because many carriers fail to show the characteristic ECG changes. However, the changes can be provoked by the administration of Vaughan-Williams class IA Na^+ channel blocker drugs (35), as if reduction in the level of Na^+ current is responsible for the changes. Type IB drugs (e.g., lidocaine) fail to cause the ECG changes. This phenomenon should give us an important clue to the functional defect, but its mechanism remains unclear. The most exciting idea is that reduction of Na^+ current in cells with large I_{to} leads to an exaggerated notch after the initial upstroke, and even to premature repolarization by failure to trigger the opening of Ca^{2+} channels (300). Individuals with the Brugada syndrome who have survived episodes of ventricular fibrillation require implantation of intracardiac defibrillators, because recurrence without treatment, or even with treatment by β-blockade or amiodarone administration, is high.

There are a host of unanswered questions about this arrhythmia: Are they all the result of Na^+ channel defects, or are other channels involved in the pathogenesis? Are all individuals with idiopathic ventricular fibrillation without structural heart disease to be included as Brugada syndrome? What is the functional abnormality of the channel that leads to ventricular fibrillation? Why is the mean age of onset of ventricular fibrillation 40 years? Understanding why these individuals are protected until middle age could be an important clue to effective treatment without intracardiac defibrillator implantation, which is difficult to recommend at this time for asymptomatic carriers of these gene abnormalities.

INHERITED CARDIOMYOPATHY

Introduction

Cardiomyopathy is a term for dysfunction of the heart muscle cells themselves, which may be intrinsic or may result from injury to the cells from ischemia, pressure overload, etc. As prevention and improved treatment has reduced the incidence and/or lethality of the extrinsic causes of heart disease, it has become apparent that there is a large group of individuals with sudden cardiac death or heart failure because of an intrinsic defect in the myocardial cells. This intrinsic type of cardiomyopathy can be roughly divided into two large groups, those with compensatory hypertrophy (HCM) and those without hypertrophy (DCM), although this distinction is progressively less satisfactory. In the last decade the study of several large families with HCM has revealed a diverse set of gene abnormalities in several of the proteins that compose the sarcomeric contractile apparatus (28). These individuals have a high incidence of premature sudden death due to lethal arrhythmia. Less developed, but promising, is the identification of gene defects in the actin molecule in patients with DCM (166, 186). By no means can we conclude that all cardiomyopathy is the result of inherited gene abnormalities. But the explosive growth of insight into the molecular basis of cardiomyopathy makes it clear that a large fraction will turn out to be either genetically determined or more susceptible to environmental factors because of genetic changes. The sudden arrival of this knowledge of the intrinsic fundamental defect combines with the extensive understanding of normal contractile protein structure and function developed gradually over the last 50 years, setting the scene for extraordinary insight into the pathogenesis of this disease and its rational therapy.

Clinical Picture

Individuals with HCM often present with life-threatening arrhythmia, heart failure, and/or symptoms of ischemia (e.g., angina). Although they may manifest the usual arrhythmias associated with any type of heart failure, the characteristic arrhythmic problem is non-sustained or sustained VT and ventricular fibrillation. The incidence of sudden death in some families is as much as 4%–5% per year (82). Some episodes of cardiac arrest have been captured on Holter recordings, and they show initially a polymorphic VT similar to that found in the long QT syndrome. Indeed, polymorphic VT in response to programmed stimulation is a marker for those at risk for sudden death. In general the clinical course of HCM follows one of two patterns: a high incidence of sudden death in individuals after the age of 20–30 years or progressive heart failure and ischemic symptoms without premature death. The clinical course of familial dilated cardiomyopathy is usually one of insidious and progressive heart failure that is eventually refractory to usual medical management, with heart failure preceding the onset of arrhythmias. Some of these individuals with DCM have AV nodal or ventricular conduction system abnormalities that occur prior to heart failure, and sudden death can occur without heart failure.

Arrhythmic Mechanisms

In a landmark report, Watkins et al. (291) found that the prognosis in familial HCM due to β-cardiac myosin abnormality is correlated with the type of mutation in the myosin protein. In twelve families with seven different point mutations in the amino terminal half of β-cardiac myosin, four of the mutations were in one or more families large enough to calculate Kaplan-Meier survival curves. The V606M mutation was associated with long life, perhaps even a normal life span. However, the three with arginine replacements (R453C, R403N, R249N) had a high incidence of sudden death beginning around age 20 years, with 50% death by ages 40–60 years. The clinical symptomatology in those families with high and low risk mutations was not different, nor was the extent or characteristics of the hypertrophy judged by echocardiogram. The clear implication is that some mutations are associated with high incidence of lethal arrhythmia and others with no arrhythmia except those related to terminal heart failure. Further, the malignant forms are all mutations of arginine (Table 19–3).

Subsequently this relationship of lethal arrhythmia with certain mutations has been substantiated and extended (157). Other malignant mutations in β-cardiac myosin include R719W, with L908V and N256E joining the benign group. R249N and E950K show an intermediate prognosis, with sudden death still occurring, but later than in the others. Two mutations in cardiac troponin T also have a malignant course without prominent heart failure, and these mutations are remarkably of arginine (R92N and R92W). An α-tropomyosin mutation D195N is of the benign type. Insufficient outcome data are available at this time to evaluate the prognosis for other mutations in these or other sarcomeric proteins.

The correlation of premature sudden cardiac death with mutational substitution of arginine is quite a remarkable finding, and it represents a challenge to the electrophysiologist to find a mechanism. The mutations in the β-cardiac myosin cluster in the myosin head (202), but the lethal arginine mutations are widely distributed between the ATP binding pocket, the actin interaction surface, the light chain binding site, the neck, and the tail, and they are mixed with neutral mutations in no obvious pattern. Functional contractile defects in association with mutations of β-cardiac myosin are mainly characterized by slower contraction or cross-bridge cycling, and seem to be similar between the lethal and nonlethal types, and the extent of hypertrophy is similar. The troponin T mutation is distant from the myosin, and its functional effect also seems to be different—an increase in contraction speed with less hypertrophy. The tropomyosin mutation has been reported to show an increased sensitivity to Ca^{2+} activation (30). The relevant comparison between malignant and benign mutations is not simply charge. One mutation with an intermediate arrhythmia risk is glutamate to lysine, with a net increase of two positive charges. Pending more mutational correlation with prognosis, we must look for an arrhythmogenic effect of arginine replacement.

How can arginine mutations in several different sarcomeric proteins lead to lethal arrhythmias? The first thought is that the arrhythmias are some secondary consequence of the contractile defect. Several mutations with apparently the same functional effects are benign; however elegant the assays of function, they still may not discriminate the critical variable. Several general features of HCM could plausibly be related to arrhythmias. Hypertrophy by itself is a better substrate for ventricular arrhythmia by increasing the potential re-entry path length and by alteration in expression of K^+ channels and repolarization behavior. The characteristic disorganized cellular pattern and the nonuniform hypertrophy should accentuate the arrhythmic tendency. Yet none of this seems to correlate with the lethal form of HCM. The ischemic signs and symptoms in HCM are of obscure origin, but ischemia itself, through alteration in conduction and repolarization, is an arrhythmogenic process. Yet this also fails to correlate. Abnormalities of intracellular Ca^{2+} cycling play a role in some arrhythmias, and this must occur in HCM. Once again, there is no evidence of differences between the lethal and the benign forms of HCM in Ca^{2+} cycling. Energy metabolism is altered in HCM, but there is no obvious connection with the arginine residues. Fixed charges on intracellular proteins are the basis of the Donnan phenomenon, but the number of

TABLE 19–3. *Prognosis with Hypertrophic Cardiomyopathy Mutations*

	Mutation	
Gene	Normal Life Span	Shortened Life Span
b-Myosin heavy chain	Gly256Glu	Arg249Gln
	Val606Met	Arg403Gln
	Leu908Val	Arg453Cys
		Arg719Trp
		Glu930Lys
Cardiac troponinT		Arg92Gln
		Arg92Trp
α-Tropomyosin	Asp175Asn	

fixed charges is unlikely to be changed enough with only the loss of a single positive charge. The leads are few, but it must also be said that the data on electrophysiological properties of cells with these mutations are sparse.

Possible areas worthy of investigation include the fundamental electrophysiological properties of myocytes with the malignant and the benign types of mutations. There are several transgenic models recently reported. Various strategies have been used to recreate the R403Q mutation in the β-myosin heavy chain (25, 96, 248, 280), and these mice may show sudden death under stress. Two transgenic models of the troponin T defect have also been reported (185, 256), and one model of the myosin binding protein C mutation (301). Unfortunately, normal mouse heart cells are electrophysiologically quite different from the human ones, making these models difficult to interpret. Abnormal genes can be expressed transiently in primary cultures of cardiac myocytes (20). It is also possible that the abnormal genes could be expressed in embryonic stem cells and studied in the subsequently developing cardiac myocytes. Elucidation of the pathogenesis of the malignant arrhythmias in cardiomyopathy could make a valuable contribution to our understanding of basic ion channel function, as well as provide leads to the management of this lethal disease.

This work was supported by National Heart Lung and Blood Institute grants HL56441 (JCM), HL 57414 (JCM), and HL20592 (H.A.F.) from the and by the University of Wisconsin Cardiovascular Research Center and the Oscar Rennebohm Foundation. The authors thank Ms. Debra Pittz for secretarial assistance.

REFERENCES

1. Aggarwal, R. and P. A. Boyden. Diminished Ca^{2+} and Ba^{2+} currents in myocytes surviving in the epicardial border zone of the 5-day infarcted canine heart. *Circ. Res.* 77:1180–1191, 1995.
2. Aguilar-Bryan, L., J. P. Clement, G. Gonzalez, K. Kunjilwar, A. Babenko, and J. Bryan. Toward understanding the assembly and structure of KATP channels. *Physiol. Rev.* 78:227–245, 1998.
3. Ahmmed, G. U., P. H. Dong, G. Song, N. A. Ball, Y. Xu, R. A. Walsh, and N. Chiamvimonvat. Changes in Ca(2+) cycling proteins underlie cardiac action potential prolongation in a pressure-overloaded guinea pig model with cardiac hypertrophy and failure. *Circ. Res.* 86:558–570, 2000.
4. Aimond, F., J. L. Alvarez, J. M. Rauzier, P. Lorente, and G. Vassort. Ionic basis of ventricular arrhythmias in remodeled rat heart during long-term myocardial infarction. *Cardiovasc.Res.* 42:402–415, 1999.
5. An, R. H., R. Bangalore, S. Z. Rosero and R. S. Kass. Lidocaine block of LQT-3 mutant human Na^+ channels. *Circ. Res.* 79:103–108, 1996.
6. An, R. H., X. L. Wang, B. Kerem, J. Benhorin, A. Medina, M. Goldmit, and R. S. Kass. Novel LQT-3 mutation affects Na^+ channel activity through interactions between alpha- and beta1-subunits. *Circ. Res.* 83:141–146, 1998.
7. Antzelevitch, C. and S. Sicouri. Clinical relevance of cardiac arrhythmias generated by afterdepolarizations. Role of M cells in the generation of U waves, triggered activity and torsade de pointes. *J. Am. Coll. Cardiol.* 23:259–277, 1994.
8. Antzelevitch, C., S. Sicouri, S. H. Litovsky, A. Lukas, S. C. Krishnan, J. M. Di Diego, G. A. Gintant, and D. W. Liu. Heterogeneity within the ventricular wall. Electrophysiology and pharmacology of epicardial, endocardial, and M cells. *Circ. Res.* 69:1427–1449, 1991.
9. Attali, B., E. Guillemare, F. Lesage, E. Honore, G. Romey, M. Lazdunski and J. Barhanin. The protein IsK is a dual activator of K^+ and Cl^- channels. *Nature* 365:850–852, 1993.
10. Backx, P. H. and E. Marban. Background potassium current active during the plateau of the action potential in guinea pig ventricular myocytes. *Circ. Res.* 72:890–900, 1993.
11. Bailly, P., J. P. Benitah, M. Mouchoniere, G. Vassort, and P. Lorente. Regional alteration of the transient outward current in human left ventricular septum during compensated hypertrophy. *Circulation* 96:1266–1274, 1997.
12. Baker, L. C., B. London, B. R. Choi, G. Koren, and G. Salama. Enhanced dispersion of repolarization and refractoriness in transgenic mouse hearts promotes reentrant ventricular tachycardia *Circ. Res.* 86:396–407, 2000.
13. Balke, C. W. and S. R. Shorofsky. Alterations in calcium handling in cardiac hypertrophy and heart failure. *Cardiovasc. Res.* 37:290–299, 1998.
14. Barbey, O., A. Gerbi, F. Paganelli, K. Robert, S. Levy, and J. M. Maixent. Canine cardiac digitalis receptors are preserved in congestive heart failure induced by rapid ventricular pacing. *J. Recept. Signal Transduc. Res.* 17:447–458, 1997.
15. Barhanin, J., F. Lesage, E. Guillemare, M. Fink, M. Lazdunski, and G. Romey. K(V)LQT1 and lsK (minK) proteins associate to form the I(Ks) cardiac potassium current. *Nature* 384:78–80, 1996.
16. Barry, D. M. and J. M. Nerbonne. Myocardial potassium channels: electrophysiological and molecular diversity. *Annu. Rev. Physiol.* 58:363–394, 1996.
17. Barry, D. M., H. Xu, R. B. Schuessler, and J. M. Nerbonne. Functional knockout of the transient outward current, long-QT syndrome, and cardiac remodeling in mice expressing a dominant–negative Kv4 alpha subunit. *Circ. Res.* 83:560–567, 1998.
18. Baukrowitz, T., U. Schulte, D. Oliver, S. Herlitze, T. Krauter, S. J. Tucker, J. P. Ruppersberg, and B. Fakler. PIP2 and PIP as determinants for ATP inhibition of K-ATP channels. *Science* 282:1141–1144, 1998.
19. Baumgarten, C. M. and H. A. Fozzard. Intracellular chloride activity in mammalian ventricular muscle. *Amer. J. Physiol.* 241 (*Cell Physiol.* 10):C121–9, 1981.
20. Becker, K. D., K. R. Gottshall, R. Hickey, J. C. Perriard, and K. R. Chien. Point mutations in human beta cardiac myosin heavy chain have differential effects on sarcomeric structure and assembly: an ATP binding site change disrupts both thick and thin filaments, whereas hypertrophic cardiomyopathy mutations display normal assembly. *J. Cell Biol.* 137:131–140, 1997.
21. Benitah, J. P., A. M. Gomez, P. Bailly, J. P. Da Ponte, G. Berson, C. Delgado, and P. Lorente. Heterogeneity of the early outward current in ventricular cells isolated from normal and hypertrophied rat hearts. *J. Physiol.* 469:111–138, 1993.
22. Benitah, J. P., A. M. Gomez, C. Delgado, P. Lorente, and W. J. Lederer. A chloride current component induced by hypertrophy in rat ventricular myocytes. *Am. J. Physiol.* 272 (*Heart Circ. Physiol.* 41):H2500–2506, 1997.
23. Bennett, P. B., K. Yazawa, N. Makita and A. L. George, Jr. Molecular mechanism for an inherited cardiac arrhythmia. *Nature* 376:683–685, 1995.
24. Berenfeld, O. and J. Jalife. Purkinje-muscle reentry as a mecha-

nism of polymorphic ventricular arrhythmias in a 3-dimensional model of the ventricles. *Circ. Res.* 82:1063–1077, 1998.
25. Berul, C. I., M. E. Christe, M. J. Aronovitz, C. E. Seidman, Seidman, J. G., and M. E. Mendelsohn. Electrophysiological abnormalities and arrhythmias in alpha MHC mutant familial hypertrophic cardiomyopathy mice. *J. Clin. Invest.* 99:570–576, 1997.
26. Beuckelmann, D. J., M. Nabauer, and E. Erdmann. Characteristics of calcium-current in isolated human ventricular myocytes from patients with terminal heart failure. *J. Mol. Cell. Cardiol.* 23:929–937, 1991.
27. Beuckelmann, D. J., M. Nabauer, and E. Erdmann. Alterations of K^+ currents in isolated human ventricular myocytes from patients with terminal heart failure. *Circ. Res.* 73:379–385, 1993.
28. Bonne, G., L. Carrier, P. Richard, B. Hainque, and K. Schwartz. Familial hypertrophic cardiomyopathy: from mutations to functional defects. *Circ. Res.* 83:580–593, 1998.
29. Bosch, R. F., X. Zeng, J. B. Grammer, K. Popovic, C. Mewis, and V. Kuhlkamp. Ionic mechanisms of electrical remodeling in human atrial fibrillation. *Cardiovasc. Res* 44:121–131, 1999.
30. Bottinelli, R., D. A. Coviello, C. S. Redwood, M. A. Pellegrino, B. J. Maron, P. Spirito, H. Watkins, and C. Reggiani. A mutant tropomyosin that causes hypertrophic cardiomyopathy is expressed in vivo and associated with an increased calcium sensitivity. *Circ. Res.* 82:106–115, 1998.
31. Boyden, P. A. and C. D. Jeck. Ion channel function in disease. *Cardiovasc. Res.* 29:312–318, 1995.
32. Boyden, P. A. and J. M. Pinto. Reduced calcium currents in subendocardial Purkinje myocytes that survive in the 24- and 48-hour infarcted heart. *Circulation* 89:2747–2759, 1994.
33. Boyle, W. A. and J. M. Nerbonne. A novel type of depolarization-activated K^+ current in isolated adult rat atrial myocytes. *Am. J. Physiol.* 260 (*Heart Circ. Physiol.* 29):H1236–47, 1991.
34. Brooksby, P., A. J. Levi, and J. V. Jones. The electrophysiological characteristics of hypertrophied ventricular myocytes from the spontaneously hypertensive rat. *J. Hypertens.* 11:611–622, 1993.
35. Brugada, J. and P. Brugada. Further characterization of the syndrome of right bundle branch block, ST segment elevation, and sudden cardiac death. *J. Cardiovasc. Electrophysiol.* 8:325–331, 1997.
36. Brugada, P. and J. Brugada. Right bundle branch block, persistent ST segment elevation and sudden cardiac death: a distinct clinical and electrocardiographic syndrome. A multicenter report. *J. Am. Coll. Cardiol.* 20:1391–1396, 1992.
37. Bryant, S. M., S. J. Shipsey, and G. Hart. Regional differences in electrical and mechanical properties of myocytes from guinea-pig hearts with mild left ventricular hypertrophy. *Cardiovasc. Res.* 35:315–323, 1997.
38. Bryant, S. M., S. J. Shipsey, and G. Hart. Normal regional distribution of membrane current density in rat left ventricle is altered in catecholamine-induced hypertrophy. *Cardiovasc. Res.* 42:391–401, 1999.
39. Bundgaard, H. and K. Kjeldsen. Human myocardial Na,K-ATPase concentration in heart failure. *Mol. Cell. Biochem.* 163–164:277–283, 1996.
40. Cannon, S. C. Sodium channel defects in myotonia and periodic paralysis. *Annu. Rev. Neurosci.* 19:141–164, 1996.
41. Casis, O., M. Gallego, M. Iriarte, and J. A. Sanchez-Chapula. Effects of diabetic cardiomyopathy on regional electrophysiologic characteristics of rat ventricle. *Diabetologia* 43:101–109, 2000.
42. Catterall, W. A. Cellular and molecular biology of voltage-gated sodium channels. *Physiol. Rev.* 72:S15–S48, 1992.
43. Catterall, W. A. Molecular properties of sodium and calcium channels. *J. Bioenerg. Biomembr.* 28:219–230, 1996.
44. Cerbai, E., M. Barbieri, Q. Li, and A. Mugelli. Ionic basis of action potential prolongation of hypertrophied cardiac myocytes isolated from hypertensive rats of different ages. *Cardiovasc. Res.* 28:1180–1187, 1994.
45. Cerbai, E., M. Barbieri and A. Mugelli. Characterization of the hyperpolarization-activated current, I(f), in ventricular myocytes isolated from hypertensive rats. *J. Physiol. (Lond.)* 481:585–591, 1994.
46. Cerbai, E., M. Barbieri, and A. Mugelli. Occurrence and properties of the hyperpolarization-activated current If in ventricular myocytes from normotensive and hypertensive rats during aging. *Circulation* 94:1674–1681, 1996.
47. Cerbai, E., R. Pino, F. Porciatti, G. Sani, M. Toscano, M. Maccherini, G. Giunti, and A. Mugelli. Characterization of the hyperpolarization-activated current, I(f), in ventricular myocytes from human failing heart. *Circulation* 95:568–571, 1997.
48. Chandra, R., C. F. Starmer, and A. O. Grant. Multiple effects of KPQ deletion mutation on gating of human cardiac Na^+ channels expressed in mammalian cells. *Am. J. Physiol.* 274 (*Heart Circ. Physiol.* 43):H1643–H1654, 1998.
49. Charlemagne, D. and B. Swynghedauw. Myocardial phenotypic changes in Na^+, K^+ ATPase in left ventricular hypertrophy: pharmacological consequences. *Eur. Heart J.* 16 (Suppl C):20–23, 1995.
50. Chatelain, P., D. Demol, and J. Roba. Comparison of [^{3}H]nitrendipine binding to heart membranes of normotensive and spontaneously hypertensive rats. *J. Cardiovasc. Pharmacol.* 6:220–223, 1984.
51. Chattou, S., J. Diacono, and D. Feuvray. Decrease in sodium-calcium exchange and calcium currents in diabetic rat ventricular myocytes. *Acta Physiol. Scand.* 166:137–144, 1999.
52. Chauhan, V. S., S. Tuvia, M. Buhusi, V. Bennett, and A. O. Grant. Abnormal cardiac Na(+) channel properties and QT heart rate adaptation in neonatal Ankyrin(B) knockout mice. *Circ. Res.* 86:441–447, 2000.
53. Chen, Q., G. E. Kirsch, D. Zhang, R. Brugada, J. Brugada, P. Brugada, D. Potenza, A. Moya, M. Borggrefe, G. Breithardt, R. Ortiz-Lopez, Z. Wang, C. Antzelevitch, R. E. O'Brien, E. Schulze-Bahr, M. T. Keating, J. A. Towbin, and Q. Wang. Genetic basis and molecular mechanism for idiopathic ventricular fibrillation. *Nature* 392:293–296, 1998.
54. Chinushi, M., E. M. Restivo, E. B. Caref, and N. el-Sherif. Electrophysiological basis of arrhythmogenicity of QT/T alternans in the long-QT syndrome. *Circ. Res.* 83:614–628, 1998.
55. Chouabe, C., L. Espinosa, P. Megas, A. Chakir, O. Rougier, A. Freminet, and R. Bonvallet. Reduction of I(Ca,L) and I(to1) density in hypertrophied right ventricular cells by simulated high altitude in adult rats. *J. Mol. Cell. Cardiol.* 29:193–206, 1997.
56. Clemo, H. F., B. S. Stambler, and C. M. Baumgarten. Persistent activation of a swelling-activated cation current in ventricular myocytes from dogs with tachycardia-induced congestive heart failure. *Circ. Res.* 83:147–157, 1998.
57. Coleman, H. N., R. R. Taylor, P. E. Pool, G. H. Whipple, J. W. Covell, J. Ross, Jr., and E. Braunwald. Congestive heart failure following chronic tachycardia. *Am. Heart J.* 81:790–798, 1971.
58. Compton, S. J., R. L. Lux, M. R. Ramsey, K. R. Strelich, M. C. Sanguinetti, L. S. Green, M. T. Keating, and J. W. Mason. Genetically defined therapy of inherited long-QT syndrome. Correction of abnormal repolarization by potassium. *Circulation* 94:1018–1022, 1996.
59. Cooklin, M., W. R. Wallis, D. J. Sheridan, and C. H. Fry. Changes in cell-to-cell electrical coupling associated with left ventricular hypertrophy. *Circ. Res.* 80:765–771, 1997.
60. Coulombe, A., A. Momtaz, P. Richer, B. Swynghedauw, and E. Coraboeuf. Reduction of calcium-independent transient outward

potassium current density in DOCA salt hypertrophied rat ventricular myocytes. *Pflugers Arch.* 427:47–55, 1994.
61. Cribbs, L. L., J. H. Lee, J. Yang, J. Satin, Y. Zhang, A. Dav. BF, J. Barclay, M. P. Williamson, M. Fox, M. Rees, and E. Perez-Reyes. Cloning and characterization of alpha1H from human heart, a member of the T-type Ca^{2+} channel gene family. *Circ. Res.* 83:103–109, 1998.
62. Curran, M. E., I. Splawski, K. W. Timothy, G. M. Vincent, E. D. Green, and M. T. Keating. A molecular basis for cardiac arrhythmia: HERG mutations cause long QT syndrome. *Cell* 80:795–803, 1995.
63. De Bakker, J. M., F. J. van Capelle, M. J. Janse, N. M. van Hemel, R. N. Hauer, J. J. Defauw, F. E. Vermeulen, and P. F. Bakker de Wekker. Macroreentry in the infarcted human heart: the mechanism of ventricular tachycardias with a "focal" activation pattern. *J. Am. Coll. Cardiol.* 18:1005–1014, 1991.
64. De Mello, W. C. Impaired regulation of cell communication by beta-adrenergic receptor activation in the failing heart. *Hypertension* 27:265–268, 1996.
65. De Mello, W. C. Renin-angiotensin system and cell communication in the failing heart. *Hypertension* 27:1267–1272, 1996.
66. Deal, K. K., S. K. England, and M. M. Tamkun. Molecular physiology of cardiac potassium channels. *Physiol. Rev.* 76:49–67, 1996.
67. Demirovic, J. and R. J. Myerburg. Epidemiology of sudden coronary death: an overview. *Prog. Cardiovasc. Dis.* 37:39–48, 1994.
68. Deroubaix, E., D. Thuringer, A. Coulombe, J. J. Mercadier, and E. Coraboeuf. Dilation and action potential lengthening in cardiomyopathic Syrian hamster heart. *Basic Res. Cardiol.* 94:274–283, 1999.
69. Dhein, S. Gap junction channels in the cardiovascular system: pharmacological and physiological modulation. *Trends Pharmacol. Sci.* 19:229–241, 1998.
70. DiFrancesco, D. The onset and autonomic regulation of cardiac pacemaker activity: relevance of the f current. *Cardiovasc. Res.* 29:449–456, 1995.
71. Dixon, I. M., T. Hata, and N. S. Dhalla. Sarcolemmal Na(+)-K(+)-ATPase activity in congestive heart failure due to myocardial infarction. *Am. J. Physiol.* 262 (*Cell Physiol.* 31):C664–671, 1992.
72. Dixon, I. M., S. L. Lee, and N. S. Dhalla. Nitrendipine binding in congestive heart failure due to myocardial infarction. *Circ. Res.* 66:782–788, 1990.
73. Duggal, P., M. R. Vesely, D. Wattanasirichaigoon, J. Villafane, V. Kaushik and A. H. Beggs. Mutation of the gene for IsK associated with both Jervell and Lange-Nielsen and Romano-Ward forms of Long-QT syndrome. *Circulation* 97:142–146, 1998.
74. Dumaine, R. and G. E. Kirsch. Mechanism of lidocaine block of late current in long Q-T mutant Na^+ channels. *Am. J. Physiol.* 274 (*Heart Circ. Physiol.* 43):H477–H487, 1998.
75. Dumaine, R., Q. Wang, M. T. Keating, H. A. Hartmann, P. J. Schwartz, A. M. Brown, and G. E. Kirsch. Multiple mechanisms of Na^+ channel—linked long-QT syndrome. *Circ. Res.* 78:916–924, 1996.
76. El-Sherif, N., E. B. Caref, H. Yin, and M. Restivo. The electrophysiological mechanism of ventricular arrhythmias in the long QT syndrome. Tridimensional mapping of activation and recovery patterns. *Circ. Res.* 79:474–492, 1996.
77. England, S. K., V. N. Uebele, H. Shear, J. Kodali, P. B. Bennett, and M. M. Tamkun. Characterization of a voltage-gated K^+ channel beta subunit expressed in human heart. *Proc. Nat. Acad. Sci. U.S.A.* 92:6309–6313, 1995.
78. Espinosa, L., C. Chouabe, A. Morales, J. Lachuer, B. Georges, M. Fatemi, C. Terrenoire, Y. Tourneur, and R. Bonvallet. Increased sodium-calcium exchange current in right ventricular cell hypertrophy induced by simulated high altitude in adult rats. *J. Mol.Cell. Cardiol.* 32:639–653, 2000.
79. Fan, Z. and J. C. Makielski. Intracellular H^+ and Ca^{2+} modulation of trypsin-modified ATP-sensitive K^+ channels in rabbit ventricular myocytes. *Circ. Res.* 72:715–722, 1993.
80. Fan, Z. and J. C. Makielski. Anionic phospholipids activate ATP-sensitive potassium channels. *J. Biol. Chem.* 272:5388–5395, 1997.
81. Fan, Z., X.-W. Niu, R. A. Haworth, M. R. Wolff, and J. C. Makielski. ATP sensitive potassium channel activity is altered in a canine pacing congestive heart failure model. *Biophys. J.* 76: A417, 1999.(Abstract)
82. Fananapazir, L., D. McAreavey, and N. D. Epstein. *Cardiac Electrophysiology*, edited by D. P. Zipes and J. Jalife. Philadelphia: W. B. Saunders, 1995:769–779.
83. Feng, J., B. Wible, G. R. Li, Z. Wang, and S. Nattel. Antisense oligodeoxynucleotides directed against Kv1.5 mRNA specifically inhibit ultrarapid delayed rectifier K^+ current in cultured adult human atrial myocytes. *Circ. Res.* 80:572–579, 1997.
84. Fisher, D. J. Recent insights into the regulation of cardiac Ca^{2+} flux during perinatal development and in cardiac failure. *Current Opini. Cardiol.* 10:44–51, 1995.
85. Fozzard, H. A. and D. A. Hanck. Structure and function of voltage-dependent sodium channels: comparison of brain II and cardiac isoforms. *Physiol. Rev.* 76:887–926, 1996.
86. Franz, M. R., P. L. Karasik, C. Li, J. Moubarak, and M. Chavez. Electrical remodeling of the human atrium: similar effects in patients with chronic atrial fibrillation and atrial flutter. *J. Am. Coll. Cardiol.* 30:1785–1792, 1997.
87. Freeman, L. C., L. M. Pacioretty, N. S. Moise, R. S. Kass, and R. F. Gilmour, Jr. Decreased density of Ito in left ventricular myocytes from German Shepherd dogs with inherited arrhythmias. *J. Cardiovasc. Electrophysiol.* 8:872–883, 1997.
88. Furukawa, T., H. Ito, J. Nitta, M. Tsujino, S. Adachi, M. Hiroe, F. Marumo, T. Sawanobori, and M. Hiraoka. Endothelin-1 enhances calcium entry through T-type calcium channels in cultured neonatal rat ventricular myocytes. *Circ. Res.* 71:1242–1253, 1992.
89. Furukawa, T., R. J. Myerburg, N. Furukawa, S. Kimura, and A. L. Bassett. Metabolic inhibition of ICa,L and IK differs in feline left ventricular hypertrophy. *Am. J. Physiol.* 266 (*Heart Circ. Physiol.* 35):H1121–H1131, 1994.
90. Galletti, F., A. Rutledge, V. Krogh and D. J. Triggle. Age related changes in Ca^{2+} channels in spontaneously hypertensive rats. *Gen. Pharmacol.* 22:173–176, 1991.
91. Gao, J., R. T. Mathias, I. S. Cohen, and G. J. Baldo. Two functionally different Na/K pumps in cardiac ventricular myocytes. *J. Gen. Physiol.* 106:995–1030, 1995.
92. Garratt, C. J., M. Duytschaever, M. Killian, R. Dorland, F. Mast, and M. A. Allessie. Repetitive electrical remodeling by paroxysms of atrial fibrillation in the goat: no cumulative effect on inducibility or stability of atrial fibrillation. *J. Cardiovasc. Electrophysiol.* 10:1101–1108, 1999.
93. Gaspo, R., R. F. Bosch, E. Bou-Abboud, and S. Nattel. Tachycardia-induced changes in Na^+ current in a chronic dog model of atrial fibrillation. *Circ. Res.* 81:1045–1052, 1997.
94. Gaspo, R., H. Sun, S. Fareh, M. Levi, L. Yue, B. G. Allen, T. E. Hebert, and S. Nattel. Dihydropyridine and beta adrenergic receptor binding in dogs with tachycardia-induced atrial fibrillation. *Cardiovasc. Res.* 42:434–442, 1999.
95. Gaughan, J. P., C. A. Hefner, and S. R. Houser. Electrophysiological properties of neonatal rat ventricular myocytes with alpha 1-adrenergic-induced hypertrophy. *Am. J. Physiol.* 275 (*Heart Circ. Physiol.* 44):H577–H5790, 1998.
96. Geisterfer-Lowrance, A. A., M. Christe, D. A. Conner, J. S. Ingwall, F. J. Schoen, C. E. Seidman and J. G. Seidman. A mouse

model of familial hypertrophic cardiomyopathy. *Science* 272: 731–734, 1996.
97. George, A. L., Jr., T. A. Varkony, H. A. Drabkin, J. Han, J. F. Knops, W. H. Finley, G. B. Brown, D.C. Ward, and M. Haas. Assignment of the human heart tetrodotoxin-resistant voltage-gated Na$^+$ channel alpha-subunit gene (SCN5A) to band 3p21. *Cytogenet. Cell Genet.* 68:67–70, 1995.
98. Gidh-Jain, M., B. Huang, P. Jain, V. Battula, and N. el-Sherif. Reemergence of the fetal pattern of L-type calcium channel gene expression in non infarcted myocardium during left ventricular remodeling. *Biochem. Biophys. Res. Commun.* 216: 892–897, 1995.
99. Gidh-Jain, M., B. Huang, P. Jain, G. Gick, and N. el-Sherif. Alterations in cardiac gene expression during ventricular remodeling following experimental myocardial infarction. *J. Mol. Cell. Cardiol.* 30:627–637, 1998.
100. Gilmour, R. F., Jr., J. J. Heger, E. N. Prystowsky, and D. P. Zipes. Cellular electrophysiologic abnormalities of diseased human ventricular myocardium. *Am. J. Cardiol.* 51:137–144, 1983.
101. Gross, G. J. and J. A. Auchampach. Role of ATP dependent potassium channels in myocardial ischaemia. *Cardiovasc. Res.* 26:1011–1016, 1992.
102. Gruver, E. J., M. G. Glass, J. D. Marsh, and J. K. Gwathmey. An animal model of dilated cardiomyopathy: characterization of dihydropyridine receptors and contractile performance. *Am. J. Physiol.* 265 (*Heart Circ. Physiol.* 34):H1704–H1711, 1993.
103. Gruver, E. J., J. P. Morgan, B. S. Stambler, and J. K. Gwathmey. Uniformity of calcium channel number and isometric contraction in human right and left ventricular myocardium. *Basic Res. Cardiol.* 89:139–148, 1994.
104. Gulch, R. W., R. Baumann, and R. Jacob. Analysis of myocardial action potential in left ventricular hypertrophy of Goldblatt rats. *Basic Res. Cardiol.* 74:69–82, 1979.
105. Hagiwara, N., H. Irisawa, and M. Kameyama. Contribution of two types of calcium currents to the pacemaker potentials of rabbit sino-atrial node cells. *J. Physiol. (Lond)* 395:233–253, 1988.
106. Hancox, J. C. and C. Howarth. The actions of nickel on membrane currents activated by hyperpolarisation in single cells from the rabbit atrioventricular node. *Gen. Pharmacol.* 26:1727–1734, 1995.
107. Hart, G. Cellular electrophysiology in cardiac hypertrophy and failure. *Cardiovasc. Res.* 28:933–946, 1994.
108. Hiraoka, M., S. Kawano, Y. Hirano, and T. Furukawa. Role of cardiac chloride currents in changes in action potential characteristics and arrhythmias. *Cardiovasc. Res.* 40:23–33, 1998.
109. Hoppe, U. C., E. Jansen, M. Sudkamp, and D. J. Beuckelmann. Hyperpolarization-activated inward current in ventricular myocytes from normal and failing human hearts. *Circulation* 97: 55–65, 1998.
110. Hurwitz, J. L. and M. E. Josephson. Sudden cardiac death in patients with chronic coronary heart disease. *Circulation* 85: I43–I49, 1992.
111. Isom, L. L., D. S. Ragsdale, K. S. De Jongh, R. E. Westenbroek, B. F. Reber, T. Scheuer, and W. A. Catterall. Structure and function of the beta 2 subunit of brain sodium channels, a transmembrane glycoprotein with a CAM motif. *Cell* 83:433–442, 1995.
112. Isomoto, S. and Y. Kurachi. Function, regulation, pharmacology, and molecular structure of ATP-sensitive K$^+$ channels in the cardiovascular system. *J. Cardiovasc. Electrophysiol.* 8: 1431–1446, 1997.
113. Jacques, D., G. Bkaily, G. Jasmin, D. Menard, and L. Proschek. Early fetal like slow Na$^+$ current in heart cells of cardiomyopathic hamster. *Mole. Cell. Biochem.* 176:249–256, 1997.
114. January, C. T., V. Chau, and J. C. Makielski. Triggered activity in the heart: cellular mechanisms of early after-depolarizations. *Eur. Heart J.* 12(Suppl F):4–9, 1991.
115. January, C. T. and H. A. Fozzard. Delayed afterdepolarizations in heart muscle: mechanisms and relevance. *Pharmacol. Rev.* 40:219–227, 1988.
116. January, C. T. and J. M. Riddle. Early afterdepolarizations: mechanism of induction and block. A role for L-type Ca^{2+} current. *Circ. Res.* 64:977–990, 1989.
117. Janvier, N. C. and M. R. Boyett. The role of Na-Ca exchange current in the cardiac action potential. *Cardiovasc. Res.* 32:69–84, 1996.
118. Jeck, C., J. Pinto, and P. Boyden. Transient outward currents in subendocardial Purkinje myocytes surviving in the infarcted heart. *Circulation* 92:465–473, 1995.
119. Jiang, C., D. Atkinson, J. A. Towbin, I. Splawski, M. H. Lehmann, H. Li, K. Timothy, R. T. Taggart, P. J. Schwartz, G. M. Vincent, et al. Two long QT syndrome loci map to chromosomes 3 and 7 with evidence for further heterogeneity. *Nat. Genet.* 8:141–147, 1994.
120. Johns, D.C., H. B. Nuss, and E. Marban. Suppression of neuronal and cardiac transient outward currents by viral gene transfer of dominant-negative Kv4.2 constructs. *J. Biol. Chem.* 272:31598–31603, 1997.
121. Kaab, S., J. Dixon, J. Duc, D. Ashen, M. Nabauer, D. J. Beuckelmann, G. Steinbeck, D. McKinnon, and G. F. Tomaselli. Molecular basis of transient outward potassium current down-regulation in human heart failure—a decrease in KV4.3 mRNA correlates with a reduction in current density. *Circulation* 98: 1383–1393, 1998.
122. Kaab, S., H. B. Nuss, N. Chiamvimonvat, B. O'Rourke, P. H. Pak, D. A. Kass, E. Marban, and G. F. Tomaselli. Ionic mechanism of action potential prolongation in ventricular myocytes from dogs with pacing-induced heart failure. *Circ. Res.* 78: 262–273, 1996.
123. Kambouris, N. G., H. B. Nuss, D.C. Johns, G. F. Tomaselli, E. Marban, and J. R. Balser. Phenotypic characterization of a novel long-QT syndrome mutation (R1623Q) in the cardiac sodium channel. *Circulation* 97:640–644, 1998.
124. Kameyama, M., M. Kakei, R. Sato, T. Shibasaki, H. Matsuda, and H. Irisawa. Intracellular Na$^+$ activates a K$^+$ channel in mammalian cardiac cells. *Nature* 309:354–356, 1984.
125. Kaplan, N. M. Beta blockade in the primary prevention of hypertensive cardiovascular events with focus on sudden cardiac death. *Am. J. Cardiol.* 80:20J–22J, 1997.
126. Kaprielian, R., A. D. Wickenden, Z. Kassiri, T. G. Parker, P. P. Liu, and P. H. Backx. Relationship between K$^+$ channel down-regulation and [Ca^{2+}]$_i$ in rat ventricular myocytes following myocardial infarction. *J. Physiol. (Lond.)* 517(Pt 1):229–245, 1999.
127. Katz, A. M. Molecular biology of calcium channels in the cardiovascular system. *Am. J. Cardiol.* 80:17I–22I, 1997.
128. Kazen-Gillespie, K. A., D. S. Ragsdale, M. R. D'Andrea, L. N. Mattei, K. E. Rogers, and L. L. Isom. Cloning, localization, and functional expression of sodium channel beta1A subunits. *J. Biol. Chem.* 275:1079–1088, 2000.
129. Keung, E. C. Calcium current is increased in isolated adult myocytes from hypertrophied rat myocardium. *Circ. Res.* 64:753–763, 1989.
130. Keung, E. C., L. Toll, M. Ellis, and R. A. Jensen. L-type cardiac calcium channels in doxorubicin cardiomyopathy in rats morphological, biochemical, and functional correlations. *J. Clin. Invest.* 87:2108–2113, 1991.
131. Kim, D. A mechanosensitive K$^+$ channel in heart cells. Activation by arachidonic acid. *J. Gen. Physiol.* 100:1021–1040, 1992.

132. Kleiman, R. B. and S. R. Houser. Calcium currents in normal and hypertrophied isolated feline ventricular myocytes. *Am. J. Physiol.* 255 (*Heart Circ. Physiol.* 24):H1434–H1442, 1988.
133. Kleiman, R. B. and S. R. Houser. Outward currents in normal and hypertrophied feline ventricular myocytes. *Am. J. Physiol.* 256:H1450–H1461, 1989.
134. Koumi, S. I., R. L. Martin, and R. Sato. Alterations in ATP-sensitive potassium channel sensitivity to ATP in failing human hearts. *Am. J. Physiol.* 272 (*Heart Circ. Physiol.* 41):H1656–H1665, 1997.
135. Krapivinsky, G., E. A. Gordon, K. Wickman, B. Velimirovic, L. Krapivinsky, and D. E. Clapham. The G-protein-gated atrial K^+ channel IKACh is a heteromultimer of two inwardly rectifying K(+)-channel proteins. *Nature* 374:135–141, 1995.
136. Kuo, T. H., D. F. Johnson, W. Tsang, and J. Wiener. Photoaffinity labeling of the calcium channel antagonist receptor in the heart of the cardiomyopathic hamster. *Biochem. Biophys. Res. Commun.* 148:926–933, 1987.
137. Kupershmidt, S., T. Yang, and D. M. Roden. Modulation of cardiac Na^+ current phenotype by beta1-subunit expression. *Circ. Res.* 83:441–447, 1998.
138. Le Grand, B., S. Hatem, E. Deroubaix, J. P. Couetil, and E. Coraboeuf. Calcium current depression in isolated human atrial myocytes after cessation of chronic treatment with calcium antagonists. *Circ. Res.* 69:292–300, 1991.
139. Le Grand, B. L., S. Hatem, E. Deroubaix, J. P. Couetil, and E. Coraboeuf. Depressed transient outward and calcium currents in dilated human atria. *Cardiovasc. Res.* 28:548–556, 1994.
140. Lee, J. K., I. Kodama, H. Honjo, T. Anno, K. Kamiya, and J. Toyama. Stage-dependent changes in membrane currents in rats with monocrotaline-induced right ventricular hypertrophy. *Am. J. Physiol.* 272 (*Heart Circ. Physiol.* 41):H2833–H2842, 1997.
141. Lee, S. L., I. Ostadalova, F. Kolar, and N. S. Dhalla. Alterations in Ca(2+)-channels during the development of diabetic cardiomyopathy. *Mol. Cell. Biochem.* 109:173–179, 1992.
142. Lesage, F., E. Guillemare, M. Fink, F. Duprat, M. Lazdunski, G. Romey, and J. Barhanin. TWIK-1, a ubiquitous human weakly inward rectifying K^+ channel with a novel structure. *EMBO J.* 15:1004–1011, 1996.
143. Li, G. R., J. Feng, L. Yue, and M. Carrier. Transmural heterogeneity of action potentials and Ito 1 in myocytes isolated from the human right ventricle. *Am. J. Physiol.* 275 (*Heart Circ. Physiol.* 44):H369–H377, 1998.
144. Li, Q. and E. C. Keung. Effects of myocardial hypertrophy on transient outward current. *Am. J. Physiol.* 266 (*Heart Circ. Physiol.* 35):H1738–H1745, 1994.
145. Liu, D. W., G. A. Gintant, and C. Antzelevitch. Ionic bases for electrophysiological distinctions among epicardial, midmyocardial, and endocardial myocytes from the free wall of the canine left ventricle. *Circ. Res.* 72:671–687, 1993.
146. Liu, X. and E. Songu-Mize. Alterations in alpha subunit expression of cardiac Na^+,K^+-ATPase in spontaneously hypertensive rats: effect of antihypertensive therapy. *Eur. J. Pharmacol.* 327:151–156, 1997.
147. Locati, E. H., W. Zareba, A. J. Moss, P. J. Schwartz, P. J. Vincent, M. H. Lehmann, J. A. Towbin, S. G. Priori, C. Napolitano, J. L. Robinson, M. Andrews, K. Timothy, and W. J. Hall. Age- and sex-related differences in clinical manifestations in patients with congenital long-QT syndrome: findings from the International LQTS Registry. *Circulation* 97:2237–2244, 1998.
148. London, B., A. Jeron, J. Zhou, P. Buckett, X. Han, G. F. Mitchell, and G. Koren. Long QT and ventricular arrhythmias in transgenic mice expressing the N terminus and first transmembrane segment of a voltage-gated potassium channel. *Proc. Nat. Acad. Sci. U.S.A.* 95:2926–2931, 1998.
149. London, B., D. W. Wang, J. A. Hill, and P. B. Bennett. The transient outward current in mice lacking the potassium channel gene Kv1.4. *J. Physiol. (Lond.)* 509:171–182, 1998.
150. Ludwig, A., X. Zong, M. Jeglitsch, F. Hofmann, and M. Biel. A family of hyperpolarization-activated mammalian cation channels. *Nature* 393:587–591, 1998.
151. Lue, W. M. and P. A. Boyden. Abnormal electrical properties of myocytes from chronically infarcted canine heart. Alterations in V_{max} and the transient outward current. *Circulation* 85:1175–1188, 1992.
152. Luk, H. N. and E. Carmeliet. Na(+)-activated K^+ current in cardiac cells: rectification, open probability, block and role in digitalis toxicity. *Pflugers Arch.* 416:766–768, 1990.
153. Luke, R. A. and J. E. Saffitz. Remodeling of ventricular conduction pathways in healed canine infarct border zones. *J. Clin. Invest.* 87:1594–1602, 1991.
154. Makielski, J. C., J. T. Limberis, S. Y. Chang, Z. Fan, and J. W. Kyle. Coexpression of beta 1 with cardiac sodium channel alpha subunits in oocytes decreases lidocaine block. *Mol. Pharmacol.* 49:30–39, 1996.
155. Maltsev, V. A., H. N. Sabbah, R. S. D. Higgins, N. Silverman, M. Lesch, and A. I. Undrovinas. Novel, ultraslow inactivating sodium current in human ventricular cardiomyocytes. *Circulation* 98:2545–2552, 1998.
156. Marban, E., T. Yamagishi, and G. F. Tomaselli. Structure and function of voltage-gated sodium channels. *J. Physiol. (Lond.)* 508:647–657, 1998.
157. Marian, A. J. and R. Roberts. Molecular genetic basis of hypertrophic cardiomyopathy: genetic markers for sudden cardiac death. *J. Cardiovasc. Electrophysiol.* 9:88–99, 1998.
158. Martinez, M. L., M. P. Heredia and C. Delgado. Expression of T-type Ca(2+) channels in ventricular cells from hypertrophied rat hearts. *J. Mol. Cell. Cardiol.* 31:1617–1625, 1999.
159. Martins, J. B., W. Kim, and M. L. Marcus. Chronic hypertension and left ventricular hypertrophy facilitate induction of sustained ventricular tachycardia in dogs 3 hours after left circumflex coronary artery occlusion [see comments].*J. Am. Coll. Cardiol.* 14:1365–1373, 1989.
160. Matsuda, N., N. Hagiwara, M. Shoda, H. Kasanuki, and S. Hosoda. Enhancement of the L-type Ca^{2+} current by mechanical stimulation in single rabbit cardiac myocytes. *Circ. Res.* 78:650–659, 1996.
161. McDonald, T. V., Z. Yu, Z. Ming, E. Palma, M. B. Meyers, K. W. Wang, S. A. Goldstein, and G. I. Fishman. A minK-HERG complex regulates the cardiac potassium current I(Kr). *Nature* 388:289–292, 1997.
162. McIntosh, M. A., S. M. Cobbe, K. A. Kane, and A. C. Rankin. Action potential prolongation and potassium currents in left-ventricular myocytes isolated from hypertrophied rabbit hearts. *J. Mol. Cell. Cardiol.* 30:43–53, 1998.
163. McIntosh, M. A., S. M. Cobbe, and G. L. Smith. Heterogeneous changes in action potential and intracellular Ca^{2+} in left ventricular myocyte sub-types from rabbits with heart failure *Cardiovasc. Res.* 45:397–409, 2000.
164. Meszaros, J., J. J. Coutinho, S. M. Bryant, K. O. Ryder, and G. Hart. L-type calcium current in catecholamine-induced cardiac hypertrophy in the rat. *Exp. Physiol.* 82:71–83, 1997.
165. Meszaros, J., K. O. Ryder, and G. Hart. Transient outward current in catecholamine-induced cardiac hypertrophy in the rat. *Am. J. Physiol.* 271 (*Heart Circ. Physiol.* 40):H2360–H2367, 1996.
166. Michels, V. V., P. P. Moll, F. A. Miller, A. J. Tajik, J. S. Chu, D. J. Driscoll, J. C. Burnett, R. J. Rodeheffer, J. H. Chesebro and H. D. Tazelaar. The frequency of familial dilated cardiomyopathy in a series of patients with idiopathic dilated cardiomyopathy. *N. Engl. J. Med.* 326:77–82, 1992.
167. Momtaz, A., A. Coulombe, P. Richer, J. J. Mercadier, and E.

Coraboeuf. Action potential and plateau ionic currents in moderately and severely DOCA-salt hypertrophied rat hearts. *J. Mol. Cell. Cardiol.* 28:2511–2522, 1996.
168. Morgan, K., E. B. Stevens, B. Shah, P. J. Cox, A. K. Dixon, K. Lee, R. D. Pinnock, J. Hughes, P. J. Richardson, K. Mizuguchi, and A. P. Jackson. beta 3: An additional auxiliary subunit of the voltage-sensitive sodium channel that modulates channel gating with distinct kinetics. *Proc. Natl. Acad. Sci. U.S.A.* 97: 2308–2313, 2000.
169. Morley, G. E., J. F. Ek-Vitorin, S. M. Taffet, and M. Delmar. Structure of connexin43 and its regulation by pHi. *J. Cardiovasc. Electrophysiol.* 8:939–951, 1997.
170. Moss, A. J., P. J. Schwartz, R. S. Crampton, D. Tzivoni, E. H. Locati, J. MacCluer, W. J. Hall, L. Weitkamp, G. M. Vincent, and A. Garson, Jr. The long QT syndrome. Prospective longitudinal study of 328 families. *Circulation* 84:1136–1144, 1991.
171. Mukherjee, R., K. W. Hewett, and F. G. Spinale. Myocyte electrophysiological properties following the development of supraventricular tachycardia-induced cardiomyopathy. *J. Mol. Cell. Cardiol.* 27:1333–1348, 1995.
172. Myerburg, R. J., A. Interian, Jr., R. M. Mitrani, K. M. Kessler, and A. Castellanos. Frequency of sudden cardiac death and profiles of risk [see comments]. *Am. J. Cardiol.* 80:10F–19F, 1997.
173. Nabauer, M., D. J. Beuckelmann, and E. Erdmann. Characteristics of transient outward current in human ventricular myocytes from patients with terminal heart failure. *Circ. Res.* 73: 386–394, 1993.
174. Nabauer, M., D. J. Beuckelmann, P. Uberfuhr, and G. Steinbeck. Regional differences in current density and rate-dependent properties of the transient outward current in subepicardial and subendocardial myocytes of human left ventricle. *Circulation* 93:168–177, 1996.
175. Nabauer, M. and S. Kaab. Potassium channel down-regulation in heart failure. *Cardiovasc. Res.* 37:324–334, 1998.
176. Nagatomo, T., C. T. January, and J. C. Makielski. Preferential Block of Late I_{Na} in the LQT3 △KPQ Mutant by the Class IC Antiarrhythmic Flecainide. *Molecular Pharmacology* 57:101–107 2000
177. Nagatomo, T., Z. Fan, B. Ye, G. S. Tonkovich, C. T. January, J. W. Kyle, and J. C. Makielski. Temperature dependence of early and late currents in human cardiac wild-type and long QT delta KPQ Na^+ channels. *Am. J. Physiol.* 275 (Heart Circ. Physiol. 44):H2016–H2024, 1998.
178. Nakamura, T. Y., M. Artman, B. Rudy, and W. A. Coetzee. Inhibition of rat ventricular IK1 with antisense oligonucleotides targeted to Kir2.1 mRNA. *Am. J. Physiol.* 274 (Heart Circ. Physiol. 43):H892–900, 1998.
179. Nattel, S. Atrial electrophysiological remodeling caused by rapid atrial activation: underlying mechanisms and clinical relevance to atrial fibrillation. *Cardiovasc. Res* 42:298–308, 1999.
180. Neyroud, N., F. Tesson, I. Denjoy, M. Leibovici, C. Donger, J. Barhanin, S. Faure, F. Gary, P. Coumel, C. Petit, K. Schwartz and P. Guicheney. A novel mutation in the potassium channel gene KVLQT1 causes the Jervell and Lange-Nielsen cardioauditory syndrome. *Nat. Genet.* 15:186–189, 1997.
181. Nichols, C. G., E. N. Makhina, W. L. Pearson, Q. Sha, and A. N. Lopatin. Inward rectification and implications for cardiac excitability. *Circ. Res.* 78:1–7, 1996.
182. Noma, A. Ionic mechanisms of the cardiac pacemaker potential. *Jpn. Heart J.* 37:673–682, 1996.
183. Nuss, H. B. and S. R. Houser. Voltage dependence of contraction and calcium current in severely hypertrophied feline ventricular myocytes. *J. Mol. Cell. Cardiol.* 23:717–726, 1991.
184. Nuss, H. B. and S. R. Houser. T-type Ca^{2+} current is expressed in hypertrophied adult feline left ventricular myocytes. *Circ. Res.* 73:777–782, 1993.
185. Oberst, L., G. L. Zhao, J. T. Park, R. Brugada, L. H. Michael, M. L. Entman, R. Roberts, and A. J. Marian. Dominant-negative effect of a mutant cardiac troponin T on cardiac structure and function in transgenic mice. *J. Clin. Invest.* 102:1498–1505, 1998.
186. Olson, T. M., V. V. Michels, S. N. Thibodeau, Y. S. Tai, and M. T. Keating. Actin mutations in dilated cardiomyopathy, a heritable form of heart failure. *Science* 280:750–752, 1998.
187. Ouadid, H., B. Albat, and J. Nargeot. Calcium currents in diseased human cardiac cells. *J. Cardiovasc. Pharmacol.* 25:282–291, 1995.
188. Pacioretty, L. M., S. C. Barr, W. P. Han, and R. F. Gilmour, Jr. Reduction of the transient outward potassium current in a canine model of Chagas' disease. *Am. J. Physiol.* 268 (Heart Circ. Physiol. 37):H1258–H1264, 1995.
189. Pak, P. H., H. B. Nuss, R. S. Tunin, S. Kaab, G. F. Tomaselli, E. Marban, and D. A. Kass. Repolarization abnormalities, arrhythmia and sudden death in canine tachycardia-induced cardiomyopathy. *J. Am. Coll. Cardiol.* 30:576–584, 1997.
190. Peters, N. S., J. Coromilas, N. J. Severs, and A. L. Wit. Disturbed connexin43 gap junction distribution correlates with the location of reentrant circuits in the epicardial border zone of healing canine infarcts that cause ventricular tachycardia. *Circulation* 95:988–996, 1997.
191. Pinto, J. M. and P. A. Boyden. Reduced inward rectifying and increased E-4031-sensitive K^+ current density in arrhythmogenic subendocardial purkinje myocytes from the infarcted heart. *J. Cardiovasc. Electrophysiol.* 9:299–311, 1998.
192. Pinto, J. M. and P. A. Boyden. Electrical remodeling in ischemia and infarction. *Cardiovasc. Res.* 42:284–297, 1999.
193. Pinto, J. M., F. Yuan, B. J. Wasserlauf, A. L. Bassett, and R. J. Myerburg. Regional gradation of L-type calcium currents in the feline heart with a healed myocardial infarct. *J. Cardiovasc. Electrophysiol.* 8:548–560, 1997.
194. Pogwizd, S. M. Nonreentrant mechanisms underlying spontaneous ventricular arrhythmias in a model of nonischemic heart failure in rabbits. *Circulation* 92:1034–1048, 1995.
195. Pogwizd, S. M. and P. B. Corr. Biochemical and electrophysiological alterations underlying ventricular arrhythmias in the failing heart. *Eur. Heart J.* 15 (Suppl D):145–154, 1994.
196. Pogwizd, S. M., R. H. Hoyt, J. E. Saffitz, P. B. Corr, J. L. Cox, and M. E. Cain. Reentrant and focal mechanisms underlying ventricular tachycardia in the human heart. *Circulation* 86: 1872–1887, 1992.
197. Pogwizd, S. M., M. Qi, W. Yuan, A. M. Samarel, and D. M. Bers. Upregulation of $Na(+)/Ca(2+)$ exchanger expression and function in an arrhythmogenic rabbit model of heart failure. *Circ. Res.* 85:1009–1019, 1999.
198. Potreau, D., J. P. Gomez, and N. Fares. Depressed transient outward current in single hypertrophied cardiomyocytes isolated from the right ventricle of ferret heart. *Cardiovasc. Res.* 30:440–448, 1995.
199. Priori, S. G., C. Napolitano, F. Cantu, A. M. Brown, and P. J. Schwartz. Differential response to Na^+ channel blockade, beta-adrenergic stimulation, and rapid pacing in a cellular model mimicking the SCN5A and HERG defects present in the long-QT syndrome. *Circ. Res.* 78:1009–1015, 1996.
200. Pye, M. P. and S. M. Cobbe. Arrhythmogenesis in experimental models of heart failure: the role of increased load. *Cardiovasc. Res.* 32:248–257, 1996.
201. Rasmussen, R. P., W. Minobe, and M. R. Bristow. Calcium antagonist binding sites in failing and nonfailing human ventricular myocardium. *Biochem. Pharmacol.* 39:691–696, 1990.
202. Rayment, I., H. M. Holden, J. R. Sellers, L. Fananapazir, and

N. D. Epstein. Structural interpretation of the mutations in the beta-cardiac myosin that have been implicated in familial hypertrophic cardiomyopathy. *Proc. Natl. Acad. Sci. U. S. A.* 92: 3864–3868, 1995.

203. Rees, S. A., J. I. Vandenberg, A. R. Wright, A. Yoshida, and T. Powell. Cell swelling has differential effects on the rapid and slow components of delayed rectifier potassium current in guinea pig cardiac myocytes. *J. Gen. Physiol.* 106:1151–1170, 1995.

204. Reinecke, H., R. Studer, R. Vetter, J. Holtz, and H. Drexler. Cardiac Na^+/Ca^{2+} exchange activity in patients with end-stage heart failure. *Cardiovasc. Res.* 31:48–54, 1996.

205. Rials, S. J., Y. Wu, X. Xu, R. A. Filart, R. A. Marinchak, and P. R. Kowey. Regression of left ventricular hypertrophy with captopril restores normal ventricular action potential duration, dispersion of refractoriness, and vulnerability to inducible ventricular fibrillation. *Circulation* 96:1330–1336, 1997.

206. Rials, S. J., X. Xu, Y. Wu, R. A. Marinchak, and P. R. Kowey. Regression of LV hypertrophy with captopril normalizes membrane currents in rabbits. *Am. J. Physiol.* 275 (*Heart Circ. Physiol.* 44):H1216–H1224, 1998.

207. Richard, S., F. Leclercq, S. Lemaire, C. Piot, and J. Nargeot. Ca^{2+} currents in compensated hypertrophy and heart failure. *Cardiovasc. Res.* 37:300–311, 1998.

208. Roden, D. M. and A. L. George, Jr. Structure and function of cardiac sodium and potassium channels. *Am. J. Physiol.* 273 (*Heart Circ. Physiol.* 42):H511–H525, 1997.

209. Rozanski, G. J., Z. Xu, R. T. Whitney, H. Murakami, and I. H. Zucker. Electrophysiology of rabbit ventricular myocytes following sustained rapid ventricular pacing. *J. Mol. Cell. Cardiol.* 29:721–732, 1997.

210. Rozanski, G. J., Z. Xu, K. Zhang, and K. P. Patel. Altered K^+ current of ventricular myocytes in rats with chronic myocardial infarction. *Am. J. Physiol.* 274 (*Heart Circ. Physiol.* 43):H259–H265, 1998.

211. Ruiz-Opazo, N., X. H. Xiang, and V. L. Herrera. Pressure-overload deinduction of human alpha 2 Na,K-ATPase gene expression in transgenic rats. *Hypertension* 29:606–612, 1997.

212. Russell, M. W., M. Dick, F. S. Collins, and L. C. Brody. KVLQT1 mutations in three families with familial or sporadic long QT syndrome. *Hum. Mol. Genet.* 5:1319–1324, 1996.

213. Ryder, K. O., S. M. Bryant, and G. Hart. Membrane current changes in left ventricular myocytes isolated from guinea pigs after abdominal aortic coarctation. *Cardiovasc. Res.* 27:1278–1287, 1993.

214. Saffitz, J. E., R. B. Schuessler, and K. A. Yamada. Mechanisms of remodeling of gap junction distributions and the development of anatomic substrates of arrhythmias. *Cardiovasc. Res.* 42:309–317, 1999.

215. Sahin-Erdemli, I., R. M. Medford, and E. Songu-Mize. Regulation of $Na^+,K(+)$-ATPase alpha-subunit isoforms in rat tissues during hypertension. *Eur. J. Pharmacol.* 292:163–171, 1995.

216. Sakakibara, Y., J. A. Wasserstrom, T. Furukawa, H. Jia, C. E. Arentzen, R. S. Hartz, and D. H. Singer. Characterization of the sodium current in single human atrial myocytes. *Circ. Res.* 71:535–546, 1992.

217. Sanguinetti, M. C., M. E. Curran, A. Zou, J. Shen, P. S. Spector, D. L. Atkinson, and M. T. Keating. Coassembly of K(V)LQT1 and minK (IsK) proteins to form cardiac I(Ks) potassium channel. *Nature* 384:80–83, 1996.

218. Sanguinetti, M. C., C. Jiang, M. E. Curran, and M. T. Keating. A mechanistic link between an inherited and an acquired cardiac arrhythmia: HERG encodes the IKr potassium channel. *Cell* 81:299–307, 1995.

219. Sanguinetti, M. C. and N. K. Jurkiewicz. Two components of cardiac delayed rectifier K^+ current. Differential sensitivity to block by class III antiarrhythmic agents. *J. Gen. Physiol.* 96: 195–215, 1990.

220. Sasaki, N., T. Mitsuiye, Z. Wang, and A. Noma. Increase of the delayed rectifier K^+ and $Na(+)$-K^+ pump currents by hypotonic solutions in guinea pig cardiac myocytes. *Circ. Res.* 75: 887–895, 1994.

221. Sawicki, P. T., S. Kiwitt, R. Bender, and M. Berger. The value of QT interval dispersion for identification of total mortality risk in non-insulin-dependent diabetes mellitus. *J. Intern. Med.* 243:49–56, 1998.

222. Saxena, N. C., J. S. Fan, and G. N. Tseng. Effects of elevating $[Na]_i$ on membrane currents of canine ventricular myocytes: role of intracellular Ca ions. *Cardiovasc. Res.* 33:548–560, 1997.

223. Scamps, F. and E. Carmeliet. Delayed K^+ current and external K^+ in single cardiac Purkinje cells. *Am. J. Physiol.* 257 (*Cell Physiol.* 26):C1086–C1092, 1989.

224. Scamps, F., E. Mayoux, D. Charlemagne, and G. Vassort. Calcium current in single cells isolated from normal and hypertrophied rat heart. Effects of beta-adrenergic stimulation. *Circ. Res.* 67:199–208, 1990.

225. Schaffer, S. W., C. Ballard-Croft, S. Boerth, and S. N. Allo. Mechanisms underlying depressed Na^+/Ca^{2+} exchanger activity in the diabetic heart. *Cardiovasc. Res.* 34:129–136, 1997.

226. Schott, J. J., F. Charpentier, S. Peltier, P. Foley, E. Drouin, J. B. Bouhour, P. Donnelly, G. Vergnaud, L. Bachner, J. P. Moisan, et al. Mapping of a gene for long QT syndrome to chromosome 4q25–27. *Am. J. Hum. Genet.* 57:1114–1122, 1995.

227. Schroder, F., R. Handrock, D. J. Beuckelmann, S. Hirt, R. Hullin, L. Priebe, R. H. Schwinger, J. Weil, and S. Herzig. Increased availability and open probability of single L-type calcium channels from failing compared with nonfailing human ventricle. *Circulation* 98:969–976, 1998.

228. Schulze-Bahr, E., W. Haverkamp, H. Wedekind, C. Rubie, M. Hordt, M. Borggrefe, G. Assmann, G. Breithardt, and H. Funke. Autosomal recessive long-QT syndrome (Jervell Lange-Nielsen syndrome) is genetically heterogeneous. *Hum. Genet.* 100:573–576, 1997.

229. Schwartz, P. J., E. H. Locati, C. Napolitano, and S. G. Priori. The long QT syndrome. In: *Cardiac Electrophysiology*, edited by D. P. Zipes and J. Jalife. Philadelphia: W. B. Saunders, 1995: 788–811.

230. Schwartz, P. J., S. G. Priori, E. H. Locati, C. Napolitano, F. Cantu, J. A. Towbin, M. T. Keating, H. Hammoude, A. M. Brown, and L. S. Chen. Long QT syndrome patients with mutations of the SCN5A and HERG genes have differential responses to Na^+ channel blockade and to increases in heart rate. Implications for gene-specific therapy. *Circulation* 92:3381–3386, 1995.

231. Schwartz, P. J., M. Stramba-Badiale, A. Segantini, P. Austoni, G. Bosi, R. Giorgetti, F. Grancini, E. D. Marni, F. Perticone, D. Rosti, and P. Salice. Prolongation of the QT interval and the sudden infant death syndrome [see comments]. *N. Engl. J. Med.* 338:1709–1714, 1998.

232. Selzer, A. and H. W. Wray. Paroxysmal ventricular fibrillation occurring during treatment of chronic atrial arrhythmias. *Circulation* 30:17–26, 1964.

233. Sen, L. and T. W. Smith. T-type Ca^{2+} channels are abnormal in genetically determined cardiomyopathic hamster hearts. *Circ. Res.* 75:149–155, 1994.

234. Sepp, R., N. J. Severs, and R. G. Gourdie. Altered patterns of cardiac intercellular junction distribution in hypertrophic cardiomyopathy. *Heart* 76:412–417, 1996.

235. Shibata, E. F., T. Drury, H. Refsum, V. Aldrete, and W. Giles. Contributions of a transient outward current to repolarization

in human atrium. *Am. J. Physiol.* 257 (*Heart Circ. Physiol.* 26): H1773–H1781, 1989.

236. Shimoni, Y., R. B. Clark, and W. R. Giles. Role of an inwardly rectifying potassium current in rabbit ventricular action potential. *J. Physiol.* 448:709–727, 1992.

237. Shimoni, Y., H. S. Ewart, and D. Severson. Type I and II models of diabetes produce different modifications of K^+ currents in rat heart: role of insulin. *J. Physiol. (Lond.)* 507:485–496, 1998.

238. Shipsey, S. J., S. M. Bryant, and G. Hart. Effects of hypertrophy on regional action potential characteristics in the rat left ventricle: a cellular basis for T-wave inversion? *Circulation* 96: 2061–2068, 1997.

239. Shyng, S. L. and C. G. Nichols. Membrane phospholipid control of nucleotide sensitivity of K-ATP channels. *Science* 282: 1138–1141, 1998.

240. Silver, L. H. and S. R. Houser. Decreased sodium-potassium pump activity in isolated hypertrophied feline ventricular myocytes. *Life Sci.* 37:607–615, 1985.

241. Sipido, K. R., E. Carmeliet, and F. Van de Werf. T-type Ca^{2+} current as a trigger for Ca^{2+} release from the sarcoplasmic reticulum in guinea-pig ventricular myocytes. *J. Physiol.* 508: 439–451, 1998.

242. Smith, J. M. and G. M. Wahler. ATP-sensitive potassium channels are altered in ventricular myocytes from diabetic rats. *Mol. Cell. Biochem.* 158:43–51, 1996.

243. Smith, P. L., T. Baukrowitz, and G. Yellen. The inward rectification mechanism of the HERG cardiac potassium channel. *Nature* 379:833–836, 1996.

244. Snyders, D. J., M. M. Tamkun, and P. B. Bennett. A rapidly activating and slowly inactivating potassium channel cloned from human heart. Functional analysis after stable mammalian cell culture expression. *J. Gen. Physiol.* 101:513–543, 1993.

245. Sodder, V. H., L. D. Bowie, and J. S. Cameron. Trypsin alters ATP sensitivity of KATP channels in control and hypertrophied myocytes. *Eur. J. Pharmacol.* 315:115–118, 1996.

246. Spach, M. S. and J. P. Boineau. Microfibrosis produces electrical load variations due to loss of side-to-side cell connections: a major mechanism of structural heart disease arrhythmias. *Pacing Clin. Electrophysiol.* 20:397–413, 1997.

247. Spector, P. S., M. E. Curran, M. T. Keating, and M. C. Sanguinetti. Class III antiarrhythmic drugs block HERG, a human cardiac delayed rectifier K^+ channel. Open-channel block by methanesulfonanilides. *Circ. Res.* 78:499–503, 1996.

248. Spindler, M., K. W. Saupe, M. E. Christe, H. L. Sweeney, C. E., Seidman, J. G. Seidman, and J. S. Ingwall. Diastolic dysfunction and altered energetics in the alphaMHC403/+ mouse model of familial hypertrophic cardiomyopathy. *J. Clin. Invest.* 101:1775–1783, 1998.

249. Splawski, I., K. W. Timothy, G. M. Vincent, D. L. Atkinson, and M. T. Keating. Molecular basis of the long-QT syndrome associated with deafness. *N. Engl. J. Med.* 336:1562–1567, 1997.

250. Stacy, G. P., Jr., R. L. Jobe, L. K. Taylor, and D. E. Hansen. Stretch-induced depolarizations as a trigger of arrhythmias in isolated canine left ventricles. *Am. J. Physiol.* 263 (*Heart Circ. Physiol.* 32):H613–H621, 1992.

251. Studer, R., H. Reinecke, R. Vetter, J. Holtz, and H. Drexler. Expression and function of the cardiac Na^+/Ca^{2+} exchanger in postnatal development of the rat, in experimental-induced cardiac hypertrophy and in the failing human heart. *Basic Res. Cardiol.* 92 (Suppl 1):53–58, 1997.

252. Swynghedauw, B. Molecular mechanisms of myocardial remodeling. *Physiol. Rev.* 79:215–262, 1999.

253. Sylven, C., E. Jansson, P. Sotonyi, F. Waagstein, and M. Bronnegard. Na,K-ATPase receptor subunits alpha 1, alpha 2 and alpha 3 mRNA in dilated cardiomyopathy. *Biol. Pharm. Bull.* 18:907–909, 1995.

254. Takumi, T., H. Ohkubo, and S. Nakanishi. Cloning of a membrane protein that induces a slow voltage-gated potassium current. *Science* 242:1042–1045, 1988.

255. Tanaka, T., R. Nagai, H. Tomoike, S. Takata, K. Yano, Yabuta, K, N. Haneda, O. Nakano, A. Shibata, T. Sawayama, H. Kasai, Y. Yazaki, and Y. Nakamura. Four novel KVLQT1 and four novel HERG mutations in familial long-QT syndrome. *Circulation* 95:565–567, 1997.

256. Tardiff, J. C., S. M. Factor, B. D. Tompkins, T. E. Hewett, B. M., Palmer, R. L. Moore, S. Schwartz, J. Robbins, and L. A. Leinwand. A truncated cardiac troponin T molecule in transgenic mice suggests multiple cellular mechanisms for familial hypertrophic cardiomyopathy. *J. Clin. Invest.* 101:2800–2811, 1998.

257. Ten Eick, R. E., K. Zhang, R. D. Harvey, and A. L. Bassett. Enhanced functional expression of transient outward current in hypertrophied feline myocytes. *Cardiovasc. Drugs Ther.* 7 (Suppl 3):611–619, 1993.

258. Terzic, A., A. Jahangir, and Y. Kurachi. Cardiac ATP-sensitive K^+ channels: regulation by intracellular nucleotides and K^+ channel-opening drugs. *Am. J. Physiol.* 269 (*Cell Physiol.* 38): C525–C545, 1995.

259. Thomas, S. A., R. B. Schuessler, C. I. Berul, M. A. Beardslee, E. C. Beyer, M. E. Mendelsohn, and J. E. Saffitz. Disparate effects of deficient expression of connexin43 on atrial and ventricular conduction: evidence for chamber-specific molecular determinants of conduction. *Circulation* 97:686–691, 1998.

260. Thuringer, D., E. Deroubaix, A. Coulombe, E. Coraboeuf, and J. J. Mercadier. Ionic basis of the action potential prolongation in ventricular myocytes from Syrian hamsters with dilated cardiomyopathy. *Cardiovasc. Res.* 31:747–757, 1996.

261. Tomaselli, G. F., D. J. Beuckelmann, H. G. Calkins, R. D. Berger, P. D. Kessler, J. H. Lawrence, D. Kass, A. M. Feldman, and E. Marban. Sudden cardiac death in heart failure. The role of abnormal repolarization. *Circulation* 90:2534–2539, 1994.

262. Tomaselli, G. F. and E. Marban. Electrophysiological remodeling in hypertrophy and heart failure. *Cardiovasc. Res* 42:270–283, 1999.

263. Tomita, F., A. L. Bassett, R. J. Myerburg, and S. Kimura. Diminished transient outward currents in rat hypertrophied ventricular myocytes. *Circ. Res.* 75:296–303, 1994.

264. Tritthart, H., H. Luedcke, R. Bayer, H. Stierle, and R. Kaufmann. Right ventricular hypertrophy in the cat—an electrophysiological and anatomical study. *J. Mol. Cell. Cardiol.* 7: 163–174, 1975.

265. Trudeau, M. C., J. W. Warmke, B. Ganetzky, and G. A. Robertson. HERG, a human inward rectifier in the voltage-gated potassium channel family. *Science* 269:92–95, 1995.

266. Tsuchida, K. and H. Watajima. Potassium currents in ventricular myocytes from genetically diabetic rats. *Am. J. Physiol.* 273 (*Endocrinol. Metab. Gastrointest. Physiol.* 36):E695–E700, 1997.

267. Undrovinas, A. I., V. A. Maltsev, and H. N. Sabbah. Repolarization abnormalities in cardiomyocytes of dogs with chronic heart failure: role of sustained inward current. *Cell Mol. Life Sci.* 55:494–505, 1999.

268. Undrovinas, A. I., G. S. Shander, and J. C. Makielski. Cytoskeleton modulates gating of voltage-dependent sodium channel in heart. *Am. J. Physiol.* 269:H203–H214, 1995.

269. Valdivia, C. R., R. A. Haworth, J. N. Wood, and J. C. Makielski. Increased late Na^+ current from a canine heart failure model and from human heart failure. *Biophys. J.* 78:523, 2000. (Abstract)

270. Van der Velden, H. M., M. J. van Kempen, M. C. Wijffels, M.

van Zijverden, W. A. Groenewegen, M. A. Allessie, and H. J. Jongsma. Altered pattern of connexin40 distribution in persistent atrial fibrillation in the goat. *J. Cardiovasc. Electrophysiol.* 9:596–607, 1998.

271. Van Wagoner, D. R. Mechanosensitive gating of atrial ATP-sensitive potassium channels. *Circ. Res.* 72:973–983, 1993.

272. Van Wagoner, D. R., A. L. Pond, P. M. McCarthy, J. S. Trimmer, and J. M. Nerbonne. Outward K$^+$ current densities and Kv1.5 expression are reduced in chronic human atrial fibrillation. *Circ. Res.* 80:772–781, 1997.

273. Van, W. D., A. L. Pond, M. Lamorgese, S. S. Rossie, P. M. McCarthy, and J. M. Nerbonne. Atrial L-type Ca^{2+} currents and human atrial fibrillation. *Circ. Res.* 85:428–436, 1999.

274. Vandenberg, J. I., G. C. Bett, and T. Powell. Contribution of a swelling-activated chloride current to changes in the cardiac action potential. *Am. J. Physiol.* 273 (*Cell Physiol.* 42):C541–C547, 1997.

275. Vandenberg, J. I., S. A. Rees, A. R. Wright, and T. Powell. Cell swelling and ion transport pathways in cardiac myocytes. *Cardiovasc. Res.* 32:85–97, 1996.

276. Vassalle, M., H. Yu, and I. S. Cohen. The pacemaker current in cardiac Purkinje myocytes. *J. Gen. Physiol.* 106:559–578, 1995.

277. Vassort, G. and J. Alvarez. Cardiac T-type calcium current: pharmacology and roles in cardiac tissues. *J. Cardiovasc. Electrophysiol.* 5:376–393, 1994.

278. Ver, A., I. Szanto, T. Banyasz, P. Csermely, E. Vegh, and J. Somogyi. Changes in the expression of Na$^+$/K$^+$-ATPase isoenzymes in the left ventricle of diabetic rat hearts: effect of insulin treatment. *Diabetologia* 40:1255–1262, 1997.

279. Vermeulen, J. T. Mechanisms of arrhythmias in heart failure. *J. Cardiovasc. Electrophysiol.* 9:208–221, 1998.

280. Vikstrom, K. L., S. M. Factor, and L. A. Leinwand. Mice expressing mutant myosin heavy chains are a model for familial hypertrophic cardiomyopathy. *Mol. Med.* 2:556–567, 1996.

281. Wallis, W. R., C. Wu, D. J. Sheridan, and C. H. Fry. Intracellular pH and H$^+$ buffering capacity in guinea-pigs with left ventricular hypertrophy induced by constriction of the thoracic aorta. *Exp. Physiol.* 82:227–230, 1997.

282. Wang, D. W., T. Kiyosue, S. Shigematsu, and M. Arita. Abnormalities of K$^+$ and Ca^{2+} currents in ventricular myocytes from rats with chronic diabetes. *Am. J. Physiol.* 269 (*Heart Circ. Physiol.* 38):H1288–H1296, 1995.

283. Wang, D. W., K. Yazawa, A. L. George, Jr., and P. B. Bennett. Characterization of human cardiac Na$^+$ channel mutations in the congenital long QT syndrome. *Proc. Natl. Acad. Sci. U.S.A.* 93:13200–13205, 1996.

284. Wang, D. W., K. Yazawa, N. Makita, A. L. George, Jr., and P. B. Bennett. Pharmacological targeting of long QT mutant sodium channels. *J. Clin. Invest.* 99:1714–1720, 1997.

285. Wang, J., R. H. Schwinger, K. Frank, J. Muller-Ehmsen, P. Martin-Vasallo, T. A. Pressley, A. Xiang, E. Erdmann, and A. A. McDonough. Regional expression of sodium pump subunits isoforms and Na$^+$-Ca^{++} exchanger in the human heart. *J. Clin. Invest.* 98:1650–1658, 1996.

286. Wang, Q., M. E. Curran, I. Splawski, T. C. Burn, J. M. Millholland, T. J. VanRaay, J. Shen, K. W. Timothy, G. M. Vincent, T. de Jager, P. J. Schwartz, J. A. Toubin, A. J. Moss, D. L. Atkinson, G. M. Landes, T. D. Connors, and M. T. Keating. Positional cloning of a novel potassium channel gene: KVLQT1 mutations cause cardiac arrhythmias. *Nat. Genet.* 12:17–23, 1996.

287. Wang, Q., J. Shen, I. Splawski, D. Atkinson, Z. Li, J. L. Robinson, A. J. Moss, J. A. Towbin, and M. T. Keating. SCN5A mutations associated with an inherited cardiac arrhythmia, long QT syndrome. *Cell* 80:805–811, 1995.

288. Wang, Y. G. and S. L. Lipsius. A cellular mechanism contributing to postvagal tachycardia studied in isolated pacemaker cells from cat right atrium. *Circ. Res.* 79:109–114, 1996.

289. Wang, Z., B. Fermini, and S. Nattel. Sustained depolarization-induced outward current in human atrial myocytes. Evidence for a novel delayed rectifier K$^+$ current similar to Kv1.5 cloned channel currents. *Circ. Res.* 73:1061–1076, 1993.

290. Warmke, J. W. and B. Ganetzky. A family of potassium channel genes related to eag in *Drosophila* and mammals. *Proc. Natl. Acad. Sci. U.S.A.* 91:3438–3442, 1994.

291. Watkins, H., A. Rosenzweig, D. S. Hwang, T. Levi, W. McKenna, C. E. Seidman, and J. G. Seidman. Characteristics and prognostic implications of myosin missense mutations in familial hypertrophic cardiomyopathy *N. Engl. J. Med.* 326:1108–1114, 1992.

292. Wei, J., I. C.-H. Yang, A. R. Tapper, K. T. Murray, P. Viswanathan, Y. Rudy, P. B. Bennet, K. Norris, J. R. Balser, D. M. Roden, and A. L. George. KCNE1 polymorphism confers risk of drug-induced Long QT syndrome by altering kinetic properties of I_{KS} potassium channels. *Circulation* 100:I-495, 1999. (Abstract)

293. Wetzel, G. T. and T. S. Klitzner. Developmental cardiac electrophysiology recent advances in cellular physiology. *Cardiovasc. Res.* 31 (Spec No):E52–E60, 1996.

294. Wijffels, M. C., C. J. Kirchhof, R. Dorland, and M. A. Allessie. Atrial fibrillation begets atrial fibrillation. A study in awake chronically instrumented goats. *Circulation* 92:1954–1968, 1995.

295. Wilde, A. A. and M. J. Janse. Electrophysiological effects of ATP sensitive potassium channel modulation: implications for arrhythmogenesis. *Cardiovasc. Res.* 28:16–24, 1994.

296. Wright, A. R., S. A. Rees, J. I. Vandenberg, V. W. Twist, and T. Powell. Extracellular osmotic pressure modulates sodium-calcium exchange in isolated guinea-pig ventricular myocytes. *J. Physiol. (Lond.)* 488:293–301, 1995.

297. Xu, X. P. and P. M. Best. Increase in T-type calcium current in atrial myocytes from adult rats with growth hormone-secreting tumors. *Proc. Natl. Acad. Sci. U.S.A.* 87:4655–4659, 1990.

298. Xu, X. P. and P. M. Best. Decreased transient outward K$^+$ current in ventricular myocytes from acromegalic rats. *Am. J. Physiol.* 260 (*Heart Circ. Physiol.* 29):H935–H942, 1991.

299. Xu, Z., K. P. Patel, and G. J. Rozanski. Metabolic basis of decreased transient outward K$^+$ current in ventricular myocytes from diabetic rats. *Am. J. Physiol.* 271 (*Heart Circ. Physiol.* 40):H2190–H2196, 1996.

300. Yan, G. X. and C. Antzelevitch. Cellular basis for the Brugada syndrome and other mechanisms of arrhythmogenesis associated with ST-segment elevation. *Circulation* 100:1660–1666, 1999.

301. Yang, Q. L., A. Sanbe, H. Osinska, T. E. Hewett, R. Klevitsky, and J. Robbins. A mouse model of myosin binding protein C in human familial hypertrophic cardiomyopathy. *J. Clin. Invest.* 102:1292–1300, 1998.

302. Yang, W. P., P. C. Levesque, W. A. Little, M. L. Conder, P. Ramakrishnan, M. G. Neubauer and M. A. Blanar. Functional expression of two KvLQT1-related potassium channels responsible for an inherited idiopathic epilepsy. *J. Biol. Chem.* 273:19419–19423, 1998.

303. Yang, W. P., P. C. Levesque, W. A. Little, M. L. Conder, F. Y. Shalaby, and M. A. Blanar. KvLQT1, a voltage-gated potassium channel responsible for human cardiac arrhythmias. *Proc. Natl. Acad. Sci. U.S.A.* 94:4017–4021, 1997.

304. Yanowitz, F., J. B. Preston, and J. A. Abildskov. Functional distribution of right and left stellate innervation to the ventricles. Production of neurogenic electrocardiographic changes by uni-

lateral alteration of sympathetic tone. *Circ. Res.* 18:416–428, 1966.

305. Yao, A., Z. Su, A. Nonaka, I. Zubair, K. W. Spitzer, J. H. Bridge, G. Muelheims, J. J. Ross, and W. H. Barry. Abnormal myocyte Ca^{2+} homeostasis in rabbits with pacing-induced heart failure. *Am. J. Physiol.* 275 (*Heart Circ. Physiol.* 44):H1441–H14481998.

306. Yao, J. A., M. Jiang, J. S. Fan, Y. Y. Zhou, and G. N. Tseng. Heterogeneous changes in K currents in rat ventricles three days after myocardial infarction. *Cardiovasc. Res* 44:132–145, 1999.

307. Yokoshiki, H., T. Kohya, F. Tomita, N. Tohse, H. Nakaya, M. Kanno, and A. Kitabatake. Restoration of action potential duration and transient outward current by regression of left ventricular hypertrophy. *J. Mol. Cell. Cardiol.* 29:1331–1339, 1997.

308. Yu, H., F. Chang, and I. S. Cohen. Pacemaker current i(f) in adult canine cardiac ventricular myocytes. *J. Physiol.* 485:469–483, 1995.

309. Yuan, F., N. R. Brandt, J. M. Pinto, B. J. Wasserlauf, R. J. Myerburg, and A. L. Bassett. Hypertrophy decreases cardiac KATP channel responsiveness to exogenous and locally generated (glycolytic) ATP. *J. Mol. Cell. Cardiol.* 29:2837–2848, 1997.

310. Yuan, F., J. M. Pinto, Q. Li, B. J. Wasserlauf, X. Yang, A. L. Bassett, and R. J. Myerburg. Characteristics of I(K) and its response to quinidine in experimental healed myocardial infarction. *J. Cardiovasc. Electrophysiol.* 10:844–854, 1999.

311. Yue, D. T. and E. Marban. A novel cardiac potassium channel that is active and conductive at depolarized potentials. *Pflugers Arch.* 413:127–133, 1988.

312. Yue, L., J. Feng, R. Gaspo, G. R. Li, Z. Wang, and S. Nattel. Ionic remodeling underlying action potential changes in a canine model of atrial fibrillation. *Circ. Res.* 81:512–525, 1997.

313. Yue, L., P. Melnyk, R. Gaspo, Z. Wang and S. Nattel. Molecular mechanisms underlying ionic remodeling in a dog model of atrial fibrillation. *Circ. Res.* 84:776–784, 1999.

314. Zahler, R., M. Gilmore-Hebert, W. Sun, and E. J. Benz. Na, K-ATPase isoform gene expression in normal and hypertrophied dog heart. *Basic Res. Cardiol.* 91:256–266, 1996.

315. Zareba, W., A. J. Moss, P. J. Schwartz, G. M. Vincent, J. L. Robinson, S. G. Priori, J. Benhorin, E. H. Locati, J. A. Towbin, M. T. Keating, M. H. Lehmann, and W. J. Hall. Influence of the genotype on the clinical course of the Long-QT syndrome. *N. Engl. J. Med.* 339:960–965, 1998.

316. Zhou, Z., Q. Gong, M. L. Epstein, and C. T. January. HERG channel dysfunction in human long QT syndrome. Intracellular transport and functional defects. *J. Biol. Chem.* 273:21061–21066, 1998.

317. Zhou, Z., Q. Gong, B. Ye, Z. Fan, J. C. Makielski, G. A. Robertson, and C. T. January. Properties of HERG channels stably expressed in HEK 293 cells studied at physiological temperature. *Biophys. J.* 74:230–241, 1998.

318. Zhou, Z. and C. T. January. Both T- and L-type Ca^{2+} channels can contribute to excitation–contraction coupling in cardiac Purkinje cells. *Biophys. J.* 74:1830–1839, 1998.

319. Zhou, Z. and S. L. Lipsius. T-type calcium current in latent pacemaker cells isolated from cat right atrium. *J. Mol. Cell. Cardiol.* 26:1211–1219, 1994.

320. Zygmunt, A. C. and W. R. Gibbons. Properties of the calcium-activated chloride current in heart. *J. Gen. Physiol.* 99:391–414, 1992.

20. Systolic and diastolic function (mechanics) of the intact heart

JAMES W. COVELL — *University of California San Diego, School of Medicine, San Diego, California*

JOHN ROSS, JR. — *University of California San Diego, School of Medicine and Institute of Molecular Medicine, San Diego, California*

CHAPTER CONTENTS

Determinants of Systolic Function
    Changes in cardiac shape and dimensions
    Performance of the intact ventricle viewed from the perspective of isolated muscle function
    The end-systolic pressure–volume relationship
    Preload
    Afterload
    Contractility (inotropic state)
    Length-dependent activation
    Strength–interval relations
    Interaction between heart rate and β-adrenergic stimulation
    Mechanical restitution and postextrasystolic potentiation
Assessing Contractility (Inotropic State) of the Heart
    Acute changes in contractility
    Methods based on changes in ventricular volumes and dimensions in a steady state
        Stroke volume and aortic blood flow
        Ejection fraction
        Ventricular dimensions and their rate of change
    Methods derived from left ventricular pressure and the rate of change of pressure
    Comparison of indices
    Methods based on examination of ventricular function over a range of loading conditions
        The end-systolic pressure–volume (ESPV) relation
        The preload recruitable stroke work
        The relation between preload and peak dP/dt
        Venous return and cardiac output curves
    The absolute level of inotropic state
    Evaluation of ventricular function in mice and rats
Regional Function
    Regional right ventricular systolic function
    Regional left ventricular structure–function relationships
    Left ventricular structure–function relationships
    Mechanical correlates of cardiac energy consumption
Determinants of Diastolic Function
    Cardiac structural components
    Passive pressure–volume relationships
    Time-dependant properties
    Passive ventricular diastolic structure–function relationships
    Regulation of ventricular filling
    Role of the pericardium

THE PRIMARY FUNCTIONS OF THE HEART are to propel unoxygenated blood to the lungs and to deliver oxygenated blood to the peripheral tissues in accordance with their metabolic requirements. These requirements vary greatly from moment to moment; during heavy exertion an almost 20-fold increase in metabolism, as reflected in total oxygen consumption, may take place within seconds. An integrated response of the heart and the peripheral vascular bed must occur to provide this increment of oxygen and to distribute it to the appropriate tissues. In this chapter we consider the unique structure and function of the heart that allows this adaptive response. The mass of the four cardiac chambers is comprised mainly of myocytes, which make up 90% of the volume of the chamber walls but only about 10% of the cells. The cardiac chambers are comprised of a complex arrangement of myofibers and extracellular matrix, but the systolic performance of each chamber is determined by myocyte function and can be described using the same approaches applied to the study of isolated cardiac muscle. Although the function of cardiac muscle is considered in detail in other chapters in this *Handbook*, (chapters 6–11) the fundamental relationship between sarcomere length and systolic force generation and its modulation by inotropic influences form the basis for examination of function in both the intact heart and the muscle that comprises its walls.

The degree of activation during the cardiac cycle in the intact heart varies both temporally and spatially, but for purposes of this review we have elected to continue the custom of using hemodynamic parameters to separate the phases of the cardiac cycle. We will consider systole to begin at the time of atrioventricular valve closure and to end at the time of semilunar (aortic or pulmonary) valve closure, and diastole to begin at the time of semilunar valve closure and to end with atrioventricular valve closure. Others have defined the onset of diastole prior to semilunar valve closure at the onset of ventricular relaxation (36).

DETERMINANTS OF SYSTOLIC FUNCTION

Changes in Cardiac Shape and Dimensions

The shape of the cardiac chambers and the thickness and structure of the ventricular walls determine the distribution of both active and passive forces within the ventricular myocardium, as well as the length of individual sarcomeres, and hence affect the function of the chambers. In this section we focus on the shape and dimensional changes within the ventricles. There is considerably less information available concerning changes in atrial shape and volume. The shapes of normal left ventricles in most mammals are similar, and changes in diameter, volume, and wall thickness during contraction have been examined in vivo in many species by the direct application of dimension transducers or radiopaque markers to the internal or external surfaces of the heart (116, 122, 137, 173, 215, 221, 231, 262, 282), as well as by visualization of the cardiac chambers (24, 25, 51, 130a, 288). The left ventricle is the thickest and most symmetrical of the cardiac chambers and has been the most extensively studied. Ross et al. examined the dimensions of casts of hearts fixed during systole and diastole (274). In these studies in dogs, the 60% reduction in cavity volume occurring during systole was accomplished by an average 1%–4% reduction in apex-to-base length, a 26% reduction in minor axis radius, an estimated wall thickening in these studies of 28%, and a 28% reduction in mitral valve area. During systole the apex of the heart remains relatively stationary and the atrioventricular grove moves towards the apex (129). This asymmetric motion results from the unique anatomy of the heart wall and its activation sequence, and it is associated with regional differences in deformation within the left ventricular walls. During isovolumetric left ventricular contraction, the chordae tendineae tense, the mitral valve closes, and the ellipsoidal shape of the diastolic left ventricle becomes more spherical, with slight apex-to-base shortening and a small increase in the minor ventricular diameter. Studies by Rushmer, Hawthorne, Mitchell, and others were some of the first to quantitatively examine the global systolic left ventricular shape changes using radiography of implanted markers and ultrasonic dimension gauges (122, 126, 282) in conscious animals. These global shape changes are summarized in Figure 20–1 from the work of Hinds et al. (126). These changes in the left ventricular dimensions prior to ejection appear most marked when measured on the external surface of the heart (122), as illustrated by an increase in external circumference in Figure 20–1; they are accompanied by less prominent alterations in the shape of the ventricular cavity—a slight narrowing in the region of the apex, a very slight reduction of the minor equator, and a small expansion of the region just below the aortic valve (144, 282). More recent studies have indicated that the isovolumic shape change is dependant on the starting volume (229, 231), and at high end-diastolic volumes the left ventricle assumes a more ellipsoid shape during isovolumic contraction (262). Studies in closed-chest, anesthetized dogs have shown that during left ventricular ejection the minor (transverse) axis of the inner wall of the chamber shortens considerably more than the major (apex-to-base) axis by 25% vs. 8% (18, 24, 215). Similar changes occur at the inner walls of the normal left ventricle in human subjects studied by cineangiography (68, 97), and closely resemble those in casts of canine hearts described above (274). During ejection, Hinds et al. identified an asymmetric change in the long axis of the left ventricle. Early during ejection the inflow tract dimension shortened only slightly while the outflow tract dimension shortened substantially (Fig. 20–1). This shift in the long axis shortening and the large decrease in internal diameter give rise to a shift in the center of mass of the ventricular cavity and a more ellipsoid ventricular shape during ejection (126, 231). Regional variations in ejection fraction (53) and segmental ventricular shape changes have also been confirmed with echocardiography (241) and ventriculography (293). In addition to global changes in the shape of the ventricles and the cavities, the spiral orientation of myofibers in the wall of the left ventricle imposes a wringing motion on the left ventricle during contraction. Figure 20–2 is adapted from the work of Hansen et al. (117) in transplanted human hearts. Torsional deformation was defined as twisting about the ventricular long axis of the apical region with respect to the base and was maximum at end-systole (Fig. 20–2, lower panel). These torsional changes in the left ventricle during systole have now been studied extensively with radiopaque markers and magnetic resonance imaging in both humans and experimental animals (259). During ejection, a 7° to 24° counterclockwise twisting occurs about the left ventricular long axis (as viewed from apex to base). This motion varies regionally and is greatest in the apical and inferior walls. Torsional deformation occurs primarily during systole (twist) and during isovolumic relaxation (untwist) (116). In the transplanted human heart the center of intracavity volume is stable in the anterior posterior and apex base axes but shifts toward the septum during systole. The right ventricle exhibits a similar shift, leading to the hypothesis that the heart acts as a double bellows with both free walls approaching the septum (136). These changes in right and left ventricular volumes during systole occur in the setting of increasing atrial volumes, since the atrioventricular valves are closed, so that the total cardiac volume remains constant (129).

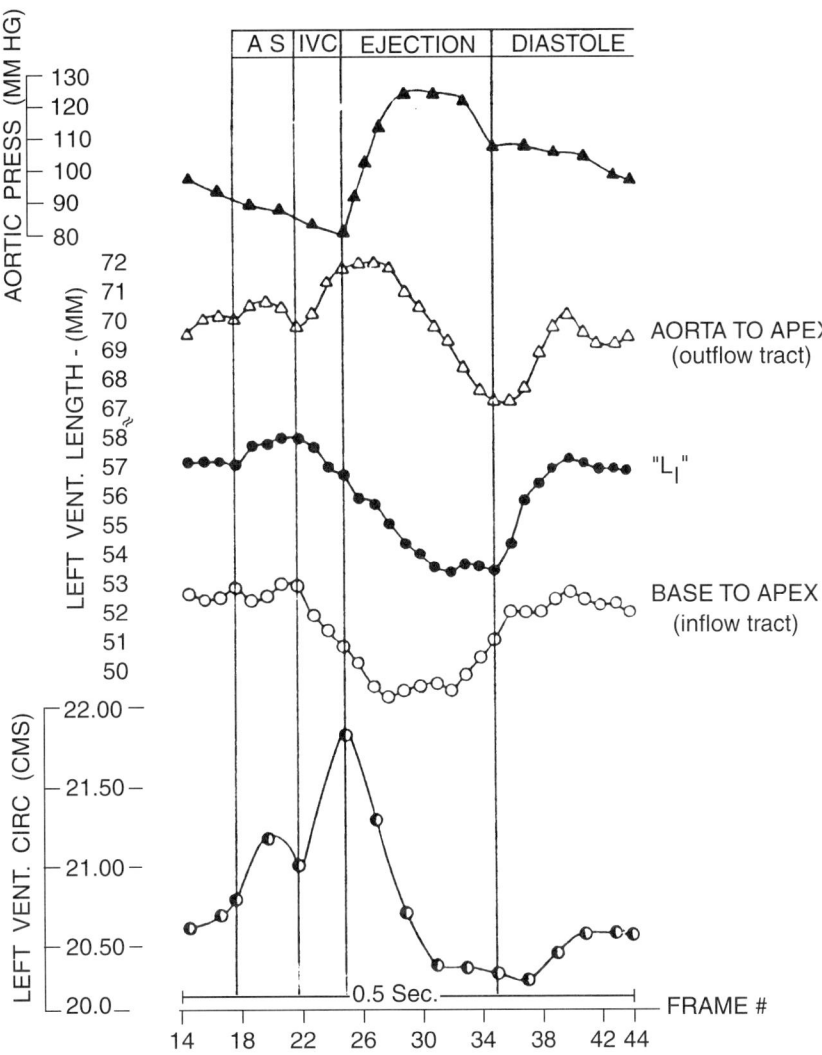

FIG. 20-1. Plot of the simultaneous changes in left ventricular circumference, base-to-apex length, circumflex-to-apex length (L_1), aorta-to-apex length during a single cardiac contraction in an awake dog. Dimensions are determined with biplane cineradiography of radiopaque markers. [Reproduced from Hinds et al. (126), with permission.]

Geometric considerations relating to a thick-walled chamber imply that as the cavity empties the inner surface must decrease proportionately more than the external surface. Thus, since muscle mass remains constant, the differences between changes in external and internal dimensions during ventricular ejection can be explained by an increase in wall thickness. Sandler and Dodge first reported between 70% and 100% left ventricular wall thickening in humans during systole using single-plane radiographic techniques (289). Wall thickening measured experimentally using implanted piezoelectric crystals or other techniques has achieved widespread use in studies of basic and clinical cardiac physiology. Most studies using implanted piezoelectric crystals have described 30%–40% total systolic wall thickening in the left ventricle (93, 299). With magnetic resonance imaging techniques, most transmural wall thickening values tend to be higher, ranging from 40% to 60% during systole (176, 246, 296). A variety of techniques, including magnetic resonance imaging, piezoelectric crystals, and radiographic tracking of transmural markers, have shown a transmural gradient in wall thickening with significantly greater wall thickening in the inner half of the ventricular wall (92, 173, 284). With some exceptions (120) most studies now indicate that wall thickening in the inner half of the left ventricle accounts for 50%–80% of the overall ventricular wall thickening (92, 108, 284, 343, 344); these results that are in good agreement with predictions from geometric models of the ventricle (71, 108). Ventricular wall thickening during systole in humans and experimental animals has seen been shown to sensi-

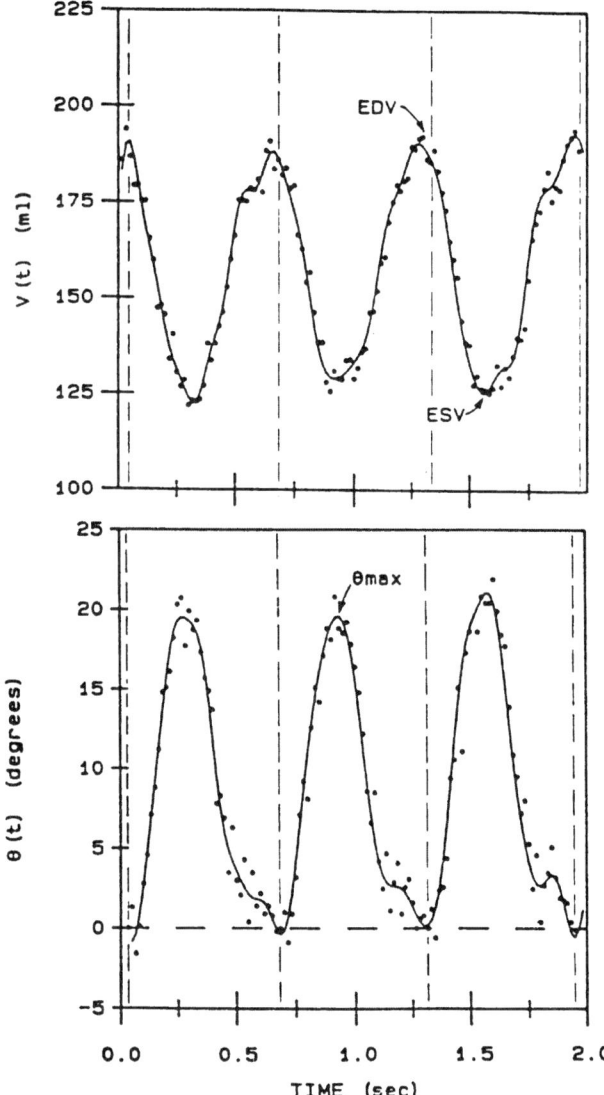

FIG. 20-2. Data obtained from surgically implanted intramyocardial markers in transplanted human hearts by Hansen et al. (117). Data shown indicate the relationship between left ventricular volume [V(t)] during four successive contractions and torsional rotation [θ(t)] of the apex with respect to the base shown as a clockwise angular rotation during systole.

tively reflect local changes in perfusion (91) and local metabolism (245).

With lesions that cause chronic pressure overload on the left ventricle (such as aortic stenosis or systemic arterial hypertension), considerable hypertrophy with increased thickness of the left ventricular wall occurs, but there may be relatively little change in the size and shape of the left ventricular cavity (so-called concentric ventricular hypertrophy); this adaptation has been well documented in experimental animals (294, 306) and in patients (67) subjected to chronic pressure overload. The myocytes show increased cross-sectional area without change in length (306). In chronic volume overload, a substantial increase in the size of the left ventricular cavity occurs, as in experimental arteriovenous fistula (183) or in patients with valvular lesions that cause chronic volume overloading (111). Left ventricular hypertrophy with increased ventricular mass occurs under these conditions, and the myocytes show an increase in cell length with some increase in cross-sectional area (183) (so-called eccentric ventricular hypertrophy). As chamber dilation occurs, there is mild lengthening of the long axis of the ventricle, but the minor equator enlarges substantially more, making the ventricle more globular (67, 111).

The shape of the right ventricle is more complex than that of the left, the outflow tract of the right ventricle being embryologically distinct from the more apical inflow region of the right ventricular free wall. The result is a complex structure, with three anatomically distinct areas (the inflow and outflow areas of the free wall and the septum) contributing to the shape of the chamber (5). The motion of the ventricular septum contributes importantly to right ventricular contraction. Indeed, early studies indicated that cardiac output is well maintained with near ablation of the right ventricular free wall (10). Thus, normal septal contraction contributes importantly to right ventricular function (290), and septal motion can be altered significantly by changes in activation sequence (66). Contraction of the right ventricular free wall is characterized by a peristalsis-like sequence originating in the inflow tract region and later extending to the outflow tract (5, 260), and during isovolumic right ventricular contraction it is possible to develop substantial intracardiac pressure gradients between the inflow and outflow regions of the right ventricle during sympathetic stimulation (5). Systolic ejection is associated with shortening of the right ventricular free wall, and the free wall myocardium frequently reaches minimum length before ventricular ejection is complete (255).

Performance of the Intact Ventricle Viewed from the Perspective of Isolated Muscle Function

The function of isolated muscle has traditionally been described in terms of the extent and velocity of muscle shortening related to initial muscle length and to the load during contraction (afterload). When the intact heart is compared to isolated muscle, volume (or diameter) is often viewed as analogous to muscle length. However, the relationship between cavity volume and sarcomere length in the wall of a cardiac chamber requires knowledge of the complex geometry of the chamber and the structure of its wall (269). In the ejecting ventricle, the stroke volume and the extent and rate of ejection may be considered analogous to the extent and velocity of shortening of isolated muscle. Using axisymmetric models of the ventricular cavity, investigators have calculated the extent and velocity of a theoretical myofiber oriented in the circumferential direction around the ventricular circumference. The rate of change of volume and an estimate of ventricular mass are then used to calculate the extent and velocity of shortening of this hypothetical "fiber." The term "fiber shortening rate" has been used to designate this variable (62, 277).

Afterload in isolated muscle is usually expressed as a stress aligned with the myofibers under study (28). In the intact heart the determination of stress is difficult. Attempts to measure stress directly in the intact heart are hampered by the effect of the gauge itself on the myocardium, and on the indirect coupling of the gauge to the myocardium. Nevertheless estimates from implanted gauges are similar to those derived from axisymmetric models and thin wall stress theory (44, 248). However, stress in the ventricles is usually estimated from axisymmetric models. Using this approach the average circumferential wall stress (force per unit cross-sectional area of wall) is related directly to the internal radius and inversely to the wall thickness. In the simplest version of the Laplace law for an ellipsoidal ventricle is: $\sigma = (Pb/h)(1 - b^2/2c^2)$ where σ = average circumferential wall stress, P = intraventricular pressure, h = wall thickness, and b and c the semiminor and semimajor axes at the endocardial surface (210). Mirsky (207) has proposed the following modification of this formula as being more accurate for circumferential midwall stress where $\sigma = (Pb/h)(1 - h/2B - B^2/2A^2)$, and A and B are, respectively, the semimajor and semiminor axes of the midwall. However, the assumptions necessary to calculate stresses from thin wall theory (axisymmetry, isotropic materials) are clearly not correct, and knowledge of the exact local geometry and material properties is necessary (363) for more appropriate estimates of stress. This is particularly true for estimates of regional and transmural stresses and under pathological circumstances in which both wall thickening and radius of curvature may change. Most geometric models of the ventricular wall predict a transmural gradient in wall stress. Most older models used to calculate stress showed that inner wall tensile stress and fiber shortening were greater then epicardial shortening and stress and fiber shortening. However, there is now clear evidence that fiber shortening is relatively constant across the wall (344). Most modern models of the left ventricle which embody estimates of residual strain, complex ventricular geometry, muscle fiber angle distribution, and anisotropic material properties also predict uniform fiber strain and tensile stress. Other stresses in these models (such as radial or cross fiber) do show transmural gradients. They are frequently compressive but this is quite model dependent. Thin wall theory does provide reasonable estimates of average transmural stress that correlate well with direct measurements of stress (44). This approach has been employed extensively to examine performance of the myocardium of the ventricular wall in the intact ventricle.

In isolated muscle there is an inverse relationship between load and extent and velocity of shortening. Similar relationships can be shown in the intact canine ventricle in which the relation between left ventricular systolic pressure and stroke volume were examined while ventricular end-diastolic volume was held constant (189, 273). The shortening characteristics and tension in the ventricular wall may be calculated during ejection from the above assumptions, and aortic pressure may be varied independent of the ventricular end-diastolic volume. This experimental design mimics that of the isolated muscle contracting under afterloaded conditions, when a force-velocity relation is determined from a constant resting muscle end- or preload, although under physiological circumstances the ventricle shortens auxotonically (against a varying afterload) rather than isotonically (against a constant afterload). With heart rate held constant, increases in stroke volume and peak flow rate occur when the aortic pressure is lowered, and the opposite effect is noted when the pressure is elevated. In variably afterloaded beats there is an inverse relation between myocardial wall stress and the velocity of circumferential fiber shortening (V_{CF}) (273). When the aortic pressure is increased to a sufficiently high level the ventricle contracts isovolumetrically, and peak ventricular systolic pressure may be used to calculate peak wall stress (analogous to P_0 of the isolated muscle). Peak stress, and the shortening velocities at all levels of afterload are altered by inotropic influences. (273) Thus, under such conditions the responses of the whole mammalian ventricle resemble the responses of isolated cardiac muscle. A more complex, servo-controlled, isolated canine left ventricular preparation has been developed in which the volume ejected by the ventricle can be regulated almost instantaneously by computer so that calculated wall forces during ejection are maintained nearly constant. This approach further refines the analogy to conditions in the isolated muscle contracting under afterloaded conditions and has permitted a more complete description of isovolumetric end—tension relations, force-velocity, force-shortening, and end—shortening relations of the whole heart (45). Figure 20–3 shows data from this study. The solid triangles indicate total estimated peak stress in an isovolumic contraction. This would correspond to total isometric stress in isolated muscle. The open symbols represent three isotonic contractions at different afterloads. Note that minimum

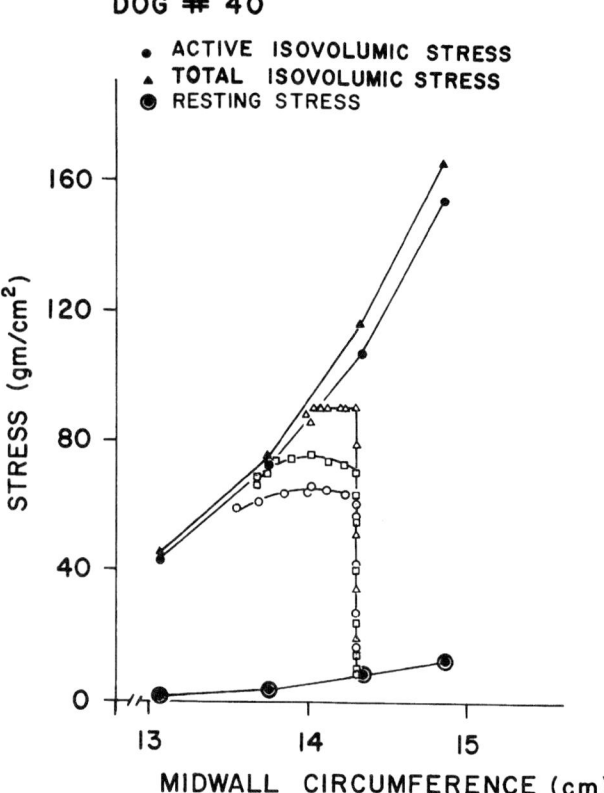

FIG. 20-3. Data from an isolated servocontrolled canine left ventricular preparation (45). *Solid symbols* show peak calculated stress in isovolumic beats. *Open symbols* depict three isotonic contractions obtained at different afterloads.

(end-systolic circumference) is achieved at approximately the peak isometric tension for that circumference. The effects of changes in afterload on the extent of shortening are also similar to that observed in isolated muscle.

The End-Systolic Pressure–Volume Relationship

Although the concept of examining the relationship between ventricular pressure and volume in a series of contractions at different loads has been used by cardiac physiologists in the past, Sagawa first observed that the ratio of pressure and volume increased progressively during systole, reached a maximum, and stabilized toward the end of ejection. This is shown in Figure 20-4 (bottom panel) (323). When the maximum ratio of instantaneous pressure to volume is examined at similar time points in variously loaded cardiac contractions these values form the linear relationship shown in Figure 20-5. The solid points are the maximum ratio of pressure to volume in each contraction, and the slope of this relationship has been termed "E_{max}" by Suga and Sagawa. Inotropic agents such as epinephrine increased the ratio of pressure to volume at all points in time and increased E_{max} without changing the volume intercept (V_d). E_{max} was thought of as a means of quantifying the inotropic state of the heart independent of loading conditions based on the concept that cardiac contraction can be modeled as a time-varying elastance (287, 322, 323). As the approach became more widely applied most investigators determined only a single slope at end-systole (E_{es}). In the isolated heart E_{max} and E_{es} are similar, but in the intact heart the two are frequently different (149). This is likely due to the load and inotropic state nonlinearities that have been observed in the end-systolic pressure–volume relationship under a variety of circumstances in the intact animal and human (8, 40, 87, 198, 212, 313). Although these difficulties have sometimes limited the use of E_{max} as a measure of contractility in the intact animal, it became clear that this approach had much broader application. For a given level of systolic and diastolic function the performance of the ventricle was bounded by the end-diastolic and end-systolic pressure–volume relationships in a directly analogous fashion to the length-tension curve of isolated cardiac muscle. The two relationships (end-systolic and end-diastolic pressure-volume relationship) provide a description of the performance of the ventricle from which a wide variety of indices of function can be derived. These include the "ventricular function curve," as defined by Sarnoff and Berglund (291) and more recently explored in the intact animal by Glower (104). In the next several sections we examine the independent effects of altering loading conditions on the performance of the intact heart. These effects may be determined from a knowledge of the two (diastolic and systolic) pressure–volume relationships.

Preload

Starling's law of the heart, which states: "The mechanical energy set free on passage from the resting to the contracted state is a function of the length of the muscle fiber, i.e., of the area of chemically active surfaces" (243) is directly reflected in the length–tension curve of isometrically contracting isolated cardiac muscle as well as in the end-systolic pressure–volume relationship. The mechanism of length–tension relation in cardiac muscle is discussed in more detail in another chapter (see chapter 11). In brief, both geometric factors (sarcomere overlap) and characteristics of the contractile proteins themselves (calcium sensitivity of troponin) are strongly length-dependent in cardiac muscle. That the latter effect, length-dependent activation, forms a significant component of preload effects has been documented not only in isolated cardiac muscle but also in the intact heart (162, 169), and it probably

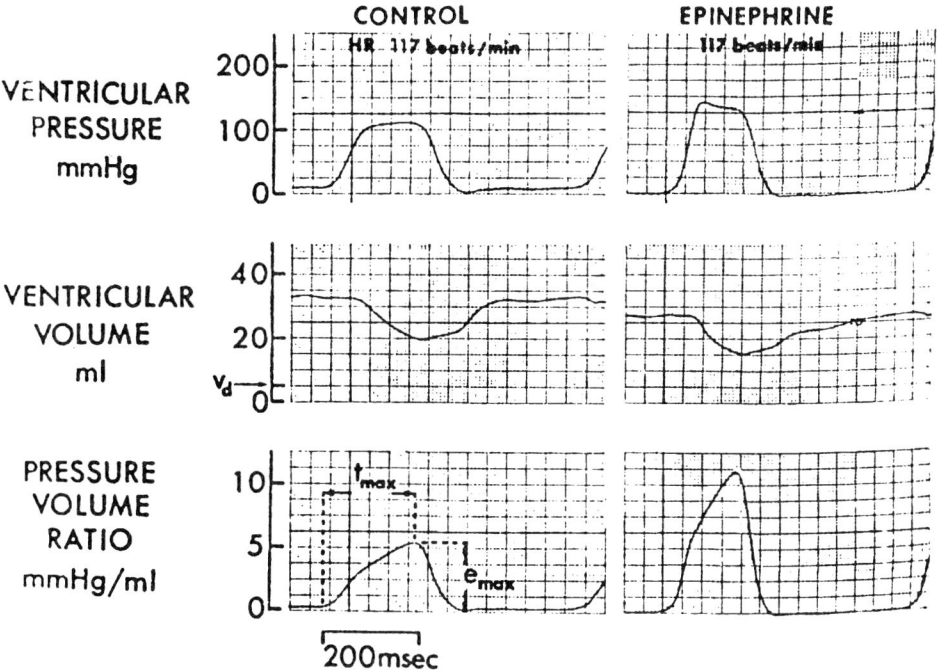

FIG. 20–4. Data from an isolated canine left ventricular preparation in which left ventricular pressure and volume are determined throughout contraction (323). Note that the ratio of pressure to volume reaches a stable maximum at end-systole.

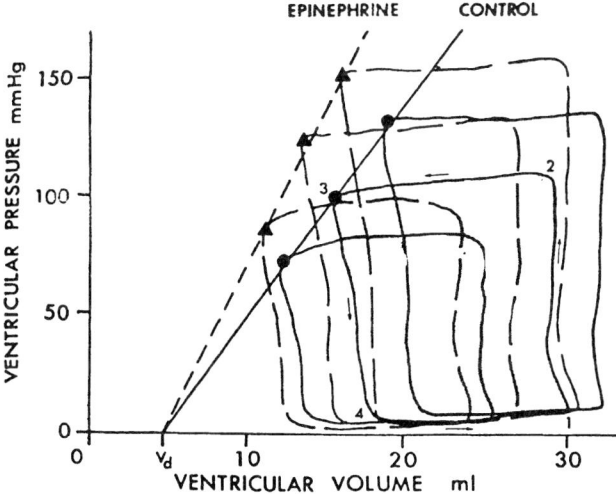

FIG. 20–5. Data from the same preparation shown in Figure 20–4, demonstrating four contractions at variable systolic pressures before and after the administration of norepinephrine. The *solid points* indicate the maximum pressure–volume ratio in each contraction. The linear relationship formed by these points has been termed "the end-systolic pressure–volume relationship." The slope of this relationship, designated E_{max} by Suga and Sagawa (322), changes with changes in inotropic state induced by norepinephrine.

constitutes the major component of the increase in contractility following increased aortic pressure in the whole heart, termed "homeometric autoregulation" or the Anrep effect (57, 338).

The capacity of the intact ventricle to vary its force of contraction on a beat-to-beat basis as a function of its initial (end-diastolic) size is one of the major principles of cardiac function and is generally referred to as the Frank-Starling relationship. Figure 20–6 shows schematically the effects of increasing preload at a constant aortic pressure. As end-diastolic volume is increased stroke volume (indicated by the horizontal arrows) is increased in proportion to the increase in end-diastolic volume. Parameters reflecting shortening of the circumference of the wall of the ventricle or of segments within the wall also increase with the increased preload when aortic pressure is held constant. If the ventricle contracts isovolumetrically, peak left ventricular systolic pressure or calculated wall stress can also be shown to be a function of preload, as reflected in the end-diastolic volume (dashed lines Fig. 20–6). These relations, both expressions of the Frank-Starling mechanism, provide the basis for function curves in the normally ejecting heart that relate ventricular end-diastolic or pressure to stroke volume and stroke work (291). With the availability of several non-invasive indices of ventricular size or volume, the func-

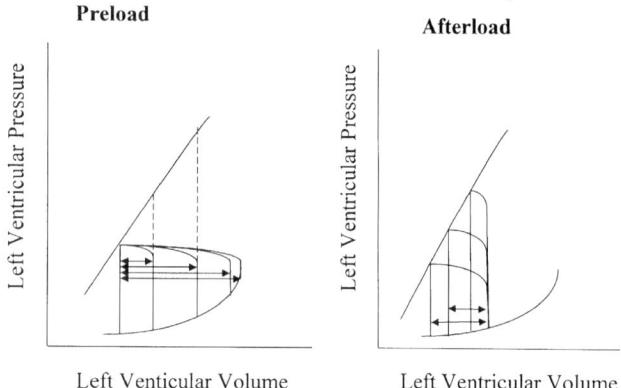

FIG. 20-6. Schematic diagram of the effects of alterations in preload and afterload on ventricular stroke volume.

tion curve approach to the examination of contractility has been revived in recent years. Measurements of left ventricular volume led to the demonstration of a linear relation between the stroke volume or stroke work and the ventricular end-diastolic volume at a given level of contractility, and alterations in myocardial contractility changed the slope of this relation. (104).

Studies using rapid cardiac fixation in the normally contracting left ventricle of the dog (274) have shown that as the diastolic sarcomere lengths at the midwall of the ventricle are increased from 1.9 to 2.2 μm, the performance of the left ventricle is progressively augmented; i.e., the ventricle operates on the ascending limb of a Starling curve. As left ventricular end-diastolic pressure is further elevated to levels exceeding 20 mm Hg, shorter sarcomeres in the endocardial and epicardial regions appear to become lengthened to near 2.2 μm (365). These studies support the concept that even at high ventricular end-diastolic pressures there is some regional recruitment of sarcomere length. Because of the nonlinear shape of the end-diastolic pressure–volume relationship, the increment in stroke volume becomes much smaller at such high end-diastolic pressures.

Using conscious dogs instrumented with a pair of ultrasonic crystals to measure left ventricular minor axis diameter Boetcher et al. (23) reported only a 3.5% increase in left ventricular end-diastolic diameter as left ventricular pressure rose from 10 mm Hg to 23 mm Hg after volume loading, with little change in stroke volume, leading the authors to conclude that the Frank-Starling was not an important controlling factor mechanism in the conscious reclining dog. In subsequent experiments in conscious reclining dogs by Lee et al. (163), in which long and short axis and wall thickness measurements were made using ultrasonic crystals to calculate left ventricular volume and wall stress during volume loading at constant mean wall stress, a stroke volume reserve of 13% was observed, associated with an increase in left ventricular end-diastolic volume of 9% and an end-diastolic pressure of 16 mm Hg. With volume plus pressure loading a 16% increase in left ventricular end-diastolic volume was noted (163). A role for the preload reserve in resting conscious dogs was also demonstrated by showing that the descending limb of function produced by pressure overload (angiotensin infusion) could be shifted upward and to the right by prior volume loading without a change in myocardial contractility, indicating that prior to volume loading the use of preload reserve was limited by the venous return (163). This effect of the preload to restore left ventricular performance in the face of increased afterload is apparent in the effect of volume loading to produce a parallel upward shift of the inverse relation between left ventricular wall stress and stroke volume produced by pressure loading, (348).

Under many conditions, the preload reserve can be considerably greater than in the supine dog at rest. The original experiments of Patterson and Starling (243), Wiggers and Katz (355), and Sarnoff and Berglund and co-workers (291) were carried out at unphysiological high heart rates, with end-diastolic volume far from maximal, allowing them to observe large changes in ventricular size with a variety of interventions including volume loading. In the standing dog, and in the upright posture in other species such as the baboon and man, heart rate is often higher and end-diastolic volume lower than in the reclining position, providing a greater preload reserve (22). During upright exercise in human subjects studied by radionuclide ventriculography (124, 252), it has been found that preload reserve is utilized during low and moderate levels of exercise, accompanied by increased stroke volume and heart rate (reflecting enhanced sympathetic tone). However, at high levels of exercise, left ventricular end-diastolic volume decreased and the stroke volume was maintained only by a decrease in end-systolic volume (124, 252).

Variations in ventricular performance occur on a beat-to-beat basis as a consequence of alterations in preload, thereby maintaining balanced outputs of the two ventricles, such as during normal respiration (105). The effects of variation in preload can be time-dependent, being influenced by the previous load and cycle length (46, 302, 303) as well as the duration of the load (172). At high diastolic volumes the diastolic pressure–volume relationship shifts to the right, allowing an increase in stroke volume at the same filling pressure (172).

While changes in the end-diastolic pressure and volume of the ventricle are useful in assessing acute directional changes in preload, under chronic conditions and in disease states sarcomere length in the intact heart is much more likely to be related to regional wall stress; however, because of differences in wall thickness and ventricular shape, end-diastolic volume may differ greatly in hearts of different size having similar wall stress. Moreover, local sarcomere lengths will also be influenced by residual stresses with in the ventricular wall. The normal effect of residual forces is to equalize wall stress across the ventricular wall (232, 270). Although it seems likely that residual stress will change with disease, there is no information available for hypertrophied hearts.

Chronically increased ventricular end-diastolic volume, as seen in volume loading secondary to an arteriovenous fistula, regurgitant valvular lesions, or in the failing heart, is an important compensatory mechanism for the maintenance of stroke volume in the intact heart. In studies of experimental arteriovenous fistula progressive increases in left ventricular end-diastolic dimensions occur over a period of several weeks after the volume overload stimulus has begun. Function in the chronically dilated left ventricle secondary to volume load is characterized by normal performance of each unit of an enlarged circumference, allowing delivery of a larger stroke volume than during the acute phase of volume loading, yet without apparent change in contractility (281). It appears that the ventricular dilatation and enhanced function that occur chronically in response to the sustained volume overloading resulting from a chronic arteriovenous fistula, or a hemodynamically similar lesion, do not involve further lengthening of sarcomeres, since diastolic sarcomeres are near maximal length (2.2 µm) after such chronic dilatation has occurred and nearly the same as during acute volume overloading (276). Rather, after the initial augmentation of stroke volume, mediated by the increased sarcomere length that occurs during the acute phase of volume overloading, elevation of preload is expressed in progressive cardiac dilatation; this is accomplished by an increase in the size, particularly the length, of myocardial cells (183), with an increase in the number of sarcomeres developing in series during the process of eccentric hypertrophy, and also perhaps by slippage between adjacent fibers and fibrils (276) a factor that may account for the rightward shift of the pressure–volume relationship.

Since the same stroke volume can be achieved with less shortening of the ventricular circumference in the chronically dilated ventricle, this volume change provides a potent compensatory mechanism to maintain stroke volume in the failing heart. This is shown in the data from a study by Komamura et al.(158) in dogs before and after the induction of tachycardia induced heart failure. Figure 20–7 shows data from the control relationship between end-diastolic volume and stroke

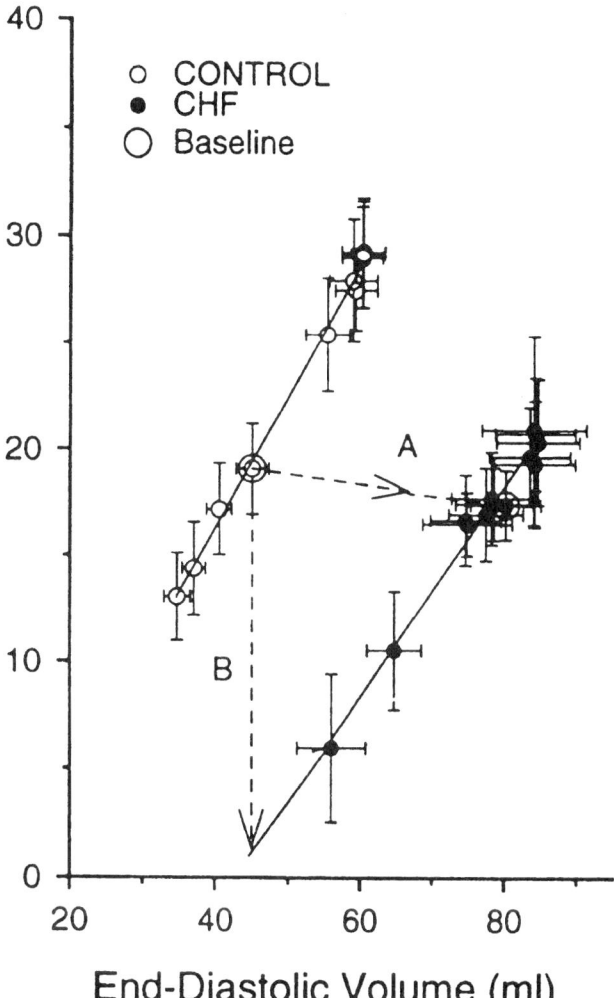

FIG. 20–7. Data from conscious animals before (*open symbols*) and after tachycardia-induced heart failure (*closed symbols*). Stroke volume is plotted on the ordinate. Note that baseline stroke volume is maintained by an increase in end-diastolic volume (158).

volume (open symbols) and following heart failure (closed symbols.) During heart failure stroke volume is relatively well maintained (dashed line A, Fig. 20–7) by an increase in end-diastolic volume that occurs as a result of both an increased end-diastolic pressure and a shift of the diastolic pressure-volume relationship to the right.

Atrial contraction contributes importantly to ventricular preload. The atrial muscle also tends to behave in accordance with Starling's law, increasing preload, resulting, within limits, in a more forceful contraction (357). When properly timed, atrial contraction serves to augment ventricular filling and preload (178, 213). This allows the mean right or left atrial pressure that exists throughout most of diastole to be relatively lower than would be the case if atrial contraction were ineffective, as in atrial fibrillation, or inappropriately timed, as in nodal rhythm or atrioventricular dissociation (29).

Afterload

"Afterload" is a term derived from studies on isolated muscle and represents the weight in addition to the preload that the muscle lifts during an isotonic contraction. In the physiology and clinical literature the term is used with much less precision and has been variously defined as aortic pressure, aortic input impedance, and a variety of parameters derived from ventricular intracavitary pressure and geometry, which are used to estimate the stress within the ventricular wall. In isolated heart preparations with end-diastolic volume controlled increases in arterial pressure reduce stroke volume and ejection fraction Figs. 20–6 and 20–8).

The arterial input impedance spectrum of the ascending aorta characterizes the hemodynamic properties of the system into which the left ventricle ejects and therefore the forces that oppose ventricular outflow; this spectrum constitutes one appropriate definition of the external load imposed on the ventricle (206). When left ventricular end-diastolic volume is controlled in the intact circulation of the dog, abrupt increases or decreases in the impedance to left ventricular ejection reciprocally alter the left ventricular stroke volume (273). However, changes in arterial input impedance do not necessarily reflect changes in ventricular performance under circumstances when ventricular wall stress is unchanged but impedance is altered (253).

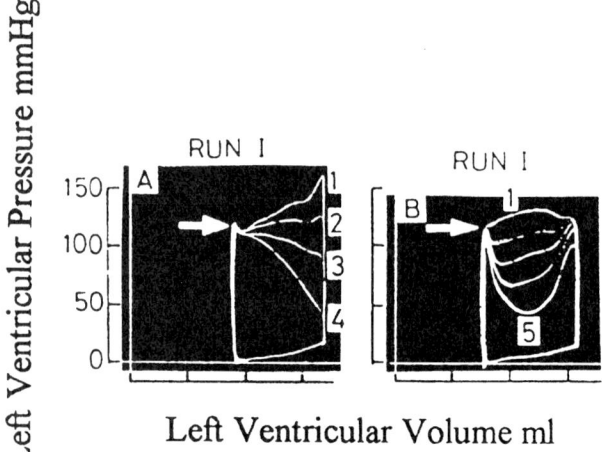

FIG. 20–8. Data from the isolated heart preparation (45). Note that in isotonic contractions there is a linear relationship between stroke volume or change in circumference (ΔL) and ventricular stress or pressure.

Thus, to evaluate the effects of afterload on ventricular performance in the intact heart, it is essential to determine the actual forces within the ventricular wall (207, 210). Such calculations require consideration of wall thickness, radii of curvature, the structure of the ventricular wall, as well as the constitutive relationship for the myocardium itself (363). Since this detailed information is usually not available, several simplifying assumptions are usually made, with the recognition that calculations will be somewhat flawed. The average circumferential force per unit length at end-diastole and end-systole, calculated from an ellipsoidal model (318), agrees well with direct measurements of mean force in the intact left ventricle made by the use of auxotonic force transducers (44). These simplified estimates of stress also are similar to the average stress across the ventricular wall estimated from more sophisticated models. Shown in Figure 20–8 are the effects of changing afterload on the performance of the intact ventricle, using the isotonically contracting isolated heart preparation in which preload, inotropic state, and contraction frequency are held constant (45). There are inverse relations between afterload and stroke volume, extent of wall shortening, and velocity of shortening (45, 189, 273). Ventricular end-systolic volume is determined by, and varies directly with, the afterload (192, 285); it is largely independent of preload and varies inversely with the inotropic state. Also, the intact, normally contracting left ventricle reaches a point at end-systole that is close to the length–active tension relation for isovolumetric contractions, regardless of the imposed afterload (327). Several investigators have imposed varying systolic loads under circumstances where end-diastolic volume and end-systolic volume can be controlled. The studies of Suga et al. (321) shown in Figure 20–9 are typical of this approach. In each panel afterload (left ventricular systolic pressure) has been allowed to vary during contraction but end-systolic and end-diastolic volumes have been held constant. In panel A the pressure at the onset of ejection is varied, and in panel B the pressure during ejection is varied. In both cases the end-systolic pressure is not altered and stroke volume is constant. These studies demonstrate that the end-diastolic and end-systolic pressure and volume determine the stroke volume not the instantaneous pressure during ejection. The low impedance to left ventricular ejection produced by *acutely* induced mitral regurgitation (335), patent ductus arteriosus, ventricular septal defect, or similar lesions results in an increased extent of shortening, an increased ejection fraction, and reduced end-systolic volumes. In the dog left ventricle that has been acutely overloaded by pressure or volume, or both, any alteration in afterload causes a reciprocal change in stroke volume (189).

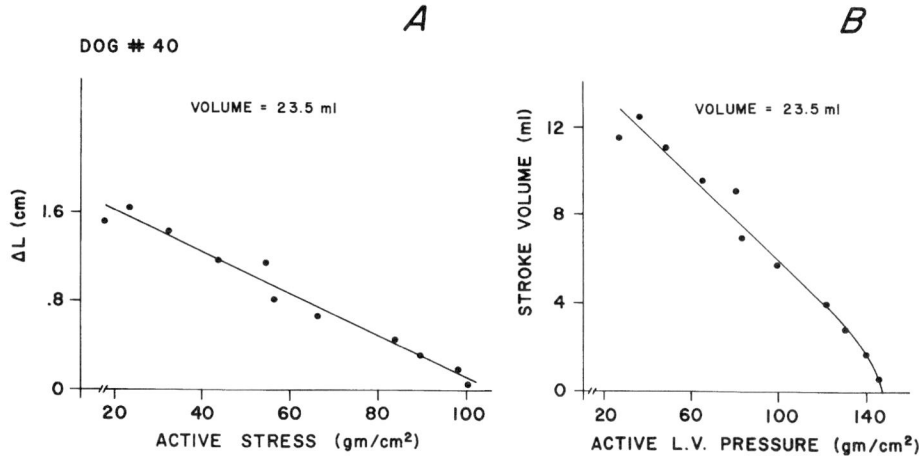

FIG. 20-9. Effects of varying the left ventricular pressure at the onset of contraction in an isolated supported canine heart preparation (A) and, in the same preparation, the pressure during ejection is varied (B). In both panels the end-systolic pressure is maintained constant and the stroke volume is largely unchanged [Reproduced by permission from Suga et al. (321), with permission].

However, rapid changes in aortic pressure have been shown to influence the course of left ventricular pressure during systole, and particularly during relaxation (59, 167). When systolic left ventricular pressure is increased during ejection, the maximum rate of pressure fall (peak negative dp/dt) is enhanced. However, later portions of the time course of left ventricular pressure fall (reflected by a slower 'time constant of relaxation, τ) (59, 90, 146) are attenuated. More recent studies on the effects of rapid pressure changes during ejection have indicated a more complex response, with different effects occurring prior to and after aortic valve closure. It remains clear, however, that abrupt changes in left ventricular pressure do not affect the portion of left ventricular pressure fall occurring after mitral valve opening and thus may have only minor effects on early ventricular filling (167).

The effects of changes in afterload in the intact circulation are much more complex. Under these circumstances increases in arterial pressure and impedance [assessed by aortic input impedance or simpler measures such as arterial elastance (148)] are accompanied by changes in ventricular volume. In animals with an intact thorax, stroke volume does not change substantially and end-diastolic volume increases when arterial pressure is acutely increased (83). The normal human heart responds to the pressor effect of infused angiotensin by maintaining or increasing stroke volume and stroke work while augmenting left ventricular end-diastolic pressure, whereas in the diseased heart the stroke volume and stroke work tend to fall (272, 277). Variations in the response to pressure loading have been observed, however, and these may be explained by differences in the adjustment of preload. Thus, when there is relative hypovolemia or a depressed myocardial contractile state, or both, a given increase in afterload can result in a reduction of stroke volume that does not occur when contractility is higher, or when inadequate venous return limits the increase in preload (163).

There has been considerable debate concerning the question of whether a descending limb of cardiac function exists in the intact left ventricle (151). No descending limb of developed wall stress or systolic pressure has been found in the isovolumetrically contracting isolated canine left ventricle until the ventricular end-diastolic pressure exceeds 60 mm Hg; developed pressure then declines by only 7.5% when diastolic ventricular pressure is further elevated to 100 mm Hg. At these extremely high end-diastolic pressures, sarcomere lengths average only 2.27–2.30 μm (219). On the basis of this and earlier work that showed that midwall sarcomere lengths did not exceed 2.27 μm at left ventricular end-diastolic pressures as high as 40 mm Hg (277), it may be postulated that the descending limb of ventricular performance, when observed in the ejecting heart, is not caused by operation of the heart on a descending limb of the sarcomere length–active tension curve; i.e., it is not due to disengagement of actin and myosin myofilaments. However, when volume loading is carried out to end-diastolic pressures exceeding 30 mm Hg after mean aortic pressure has been initially elevated, a descending limb of curves relating left ventricular end-diastolic pressure to stroke work is evident; under these circumstances, slight further increases in aortic pressure occur during volume loading, and calculated systolic wall stress (afterload) always rises as the stroke volume falls (189). Thus, in the relatively normal overloaded ventricle, the descending limb of function appears to result from reduced myocardial wall shortening due to an increased afterload at a time when the sarcomere length of the ventricle has become maximal (absent preload reserve), and not as a result of depressed cardiac performance or disengagement of sarcomeres (189, 277). A similar situation likely obtains in the failing heart, when the Frank-Starling reserve is fully utilized (158, 277).

Contractility (Inotropic State)

It was clearly shown by Patterson and Starling (243) in the heart–lung preparation that at any given level of contractility the stroke volume is a function of diastolic fiber length (of preload), and that when the heart fails (when contractility becomes depressed) a smaller than normal stroke volume is ejected from a normal or even elevated end-diastolic volume. Later, Sarnoff and Berglund (291) examined ventricular stroke work over a range of mean atrial or ventricular end-diastolic pressures and termed the resulting relation the "ventricular function curve." Plotting an index of performance against either the preload or the afterload is an extremely effective approach to assessing the performance of the heart. Examining the relationship between filling pressure and, for example, stroke work generates a family of curves since both changes in inotropic state and aortic pressure influence the result. A single curve represents principally the Frank-Starling effect, i.e., the effect of changes in preload. Displacement of the entire curve upward or downward signifies a positive or negative inotropic effect, that is, an augmentation or depression of contractility when studied at a fixed level of aortic pressure. Since the level of stroke work is pressure dependent, just as the work of isolated muscle is afterload dependent, it is the custom to plot ventricular function curves at constant aortic pressure (291, 308). More recently, investigators working in the intact circulation have used the ventricular function curve approach under conditions in which aortic pressure is not controlled. Both global (stroke volume) and regional (segment shortening) indices of performance have been used. Representative data are shown in Figure 20–10. These studies in the intact circulation demonstrate the nonlinear change in stroke work for the whole ventricle and an estimated stroke work for a region of the ventricle based on a measured segment length. When plotted against end-diastolic pressure. However, both relationships are linear functions of end-diastolic volume or segment length and are also relatively sensitive to changes in inotropic state. Later in this chapter (see below, under Assessing Inotropic State of the Heart) we consider a spectrum of approaches used in examining the contractility of the intact heart.

The term "contractility" or "myocardial contractility" and the phrase "level of inotropic state" are both used to describe the intrinsic performance of cardiac muscle. Both are thought to reflect the availability of calcium (Ca^{2+}) to the myofilament and the sensitivity of the myofilament to Ca^{2+}. The factors regulating the availability of Ca^{2+} at the myofilaments are discussed in depth in Chapter 9 and 15. In brief, following electrical stimulation, calcium entry in the myocytes increases rapidly over the first 50–100 ms at normal temperatures and heart rates (15). In the intact heart this is reflected by a gradual increase in indices of contractile state during each contraction. Figure 20–4 demonstrates this effect as a gradual increase in the slope of the end-systolic pressure–volume relationship during contraction. In the control contraction (top panel) the slope reaches a stable value between 200 and 240 msec following stimulation. When contractile state is enhanced by catecholamines the plateau is reached more quickly and maintained for a shorter period (Fig. 20–4, right-hand panel). In the intact heart the level of inotropic state is normally taken as the steady-state maximum leftward position of the end-systolic pressure–volume relationship occurring during a single twitch. Several factors importantly influence the availability of calcium at the myofilaments. These include adrenergic control of calcium entry and reuptake from the myocyte, length-dependent activation and the force-frequency relationship.

Length-Dependent Activation

The calcium dependence of force generation in cardiac muscle is influenced by muscle length. The mechanism of this length-dependent increase in force generation is thought to be a length-dependent change in the myofilament sensitivity to Ca^{2+} (19). In the intact heart this has been demonstrated as a progressive shift in the end-systolic pressure–length relationship following transfusion (169, 170). Figure 20–11 shows two sets of ventricular pressure segment length loops, one set (solid lines) before and one after (dotted lines) a steady-state increase in end-diastolic pressure. There is a leftward shift of the entire end-systolic pressure–length relationship following the sustained increase in end-diastolic pressure indicating a substantial "length-dependent" increase in contractility.

Strength-Interval Relations

In addition to the interrelated effects on cardiac performance of preload, afterload, and myocardial con-

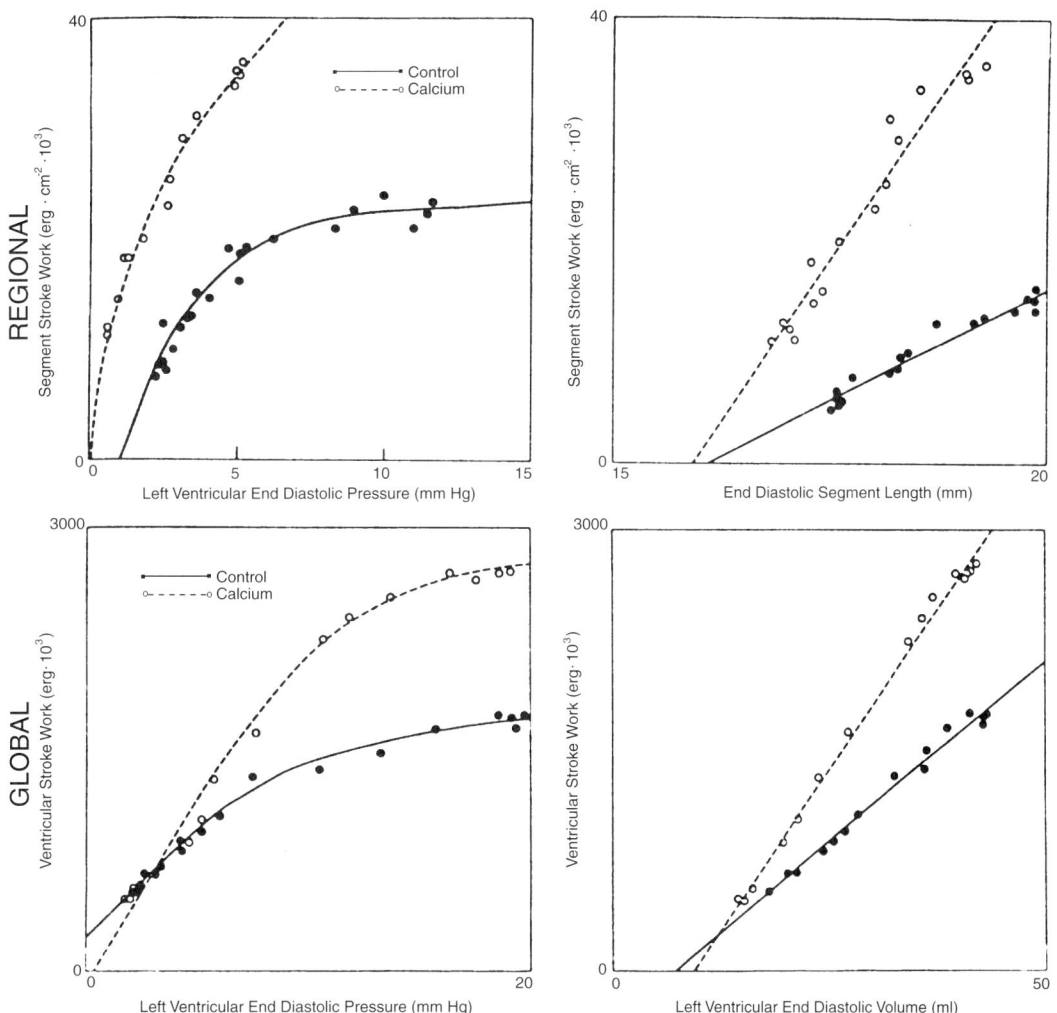

FIG. 20–10. Relationship between global and regional indices of stroke work and ventricular end-diastolic pressure or ventricular volume in conscious instrumented dogs. Changes in diastolic pressures and volumes were induced by caval occlusion. The relationships between ventricular end-diastolic pressure and segment work and stroke work are non-linear, but sensitive to the inotropic effect of calcium. The relationship ventricular between end-diastolic volume or segment work and stroke work are linear and sensitive to changes in inotropic state. [After Glower et al. (104).]

tractility, heart rate has long been known to play an important role by its action on basal myocardial contractility. This effect, often termed the force–frequency or strength-interval relation [the Bowditch staircase (26), is well known to influence myocardial contractility and relaxation (inotropic state) in isolated cardiac muscle (38, 157) and in anesthetized animals (61, 214)]. The increase in inotropic state occurring with a reduced interval between contractions is related primarily to increased Ca^{2+} availability to the myofilaments as a result of enhanced transarcolemmal Ca^{2+} influx due to increased number of action potentials, a corresponding increase in the filling of the sarcoplasmic reticulum (SR) with augmentation of subsequent Ca^{2+} transients (354), and to reduced time available for diastolic Ca^{2+} efflux via the Na^+/Ca^{2+} exchanger (15); a lag in the Na^+/K^+ ATPase pump leading to a decreased sodium gradient also appears to contribute (15). Such effects are known to be associated with increasing Ca^{2+} transients as heart rate is increased in isolated cardiac muscle obtained from relatively normal human subjects (250).

Acceleration of the frequency of contraction generally does not induce a shift of the ventricular function curve in the open-chest anesthetized dog but does increase stroke power (rate of performance of stroke work) at any given level of filling pressure (61), a finding consistent with observations in isolated cardiac

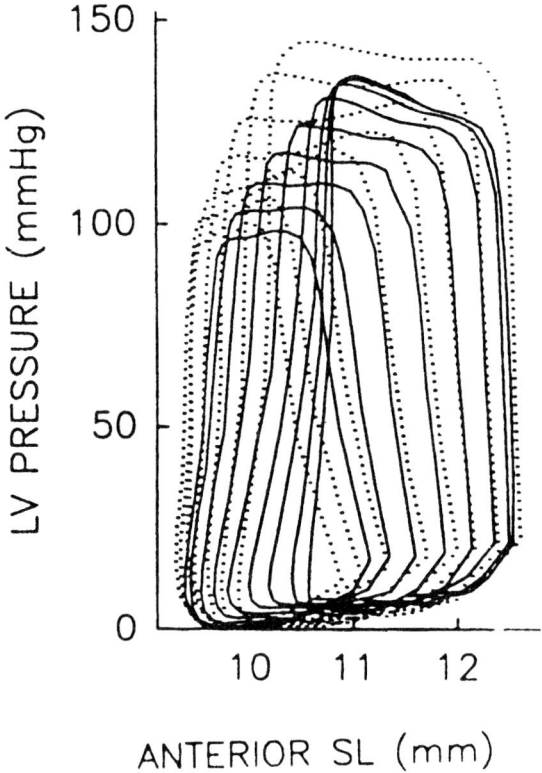

FIG. 20–11. Left ventricular pressure segment length (SL) relationships determined in the dog by caval occlusion before (*solid lines*) and after (*dotted lines*) a sustained increase in end-diastolic pressure. Following the increases in end-diastolic pressure the end-systolic pressure length points are all shifted to the left, indicating a shift in the end-systolic pressure–length relationship (170). [Reproduced with permission from Lew (170).]

muscle (30, 72) and signifies an improvement of myocardial contractility. Also, increases in contraction frequency cause a considerable increase in calculated v_{max} and a small increase in peak force in isovolumetric contractions in the anesthetized open-chest dog (61). Thus, a force "treppe" or staircase, as well as an increase in contraction velocity, occurs in the intact left ventricle. In general, the positive inotropic effect of a steady-state increase in cardiac frequency is less marked at physiological temperatures than at room temperatures and in the intact ventricle than in isolated cardiac tissue (142).

The positive inotropic effect of increasing heart rate was considered minor in conscious animals (125), although significant enhancement of contractility during rapid atrial pacing in conscious dogs was later suggested based on a sustained maximum first derivative (dP/dt) of left ventricular (LV) pressure at increased heart rates, despite a fall in left ventricular end-diastolic pressure (EDP) (LV); since left ventricular dP/dt is sensitive to preload (181, 191), a reduction in LVEDP alone would have been expected to reduce left ventricular dP/dt. More recently, progressive enhancement of the slope of the relation between left ventricular end-systolic volume and end-systolic pressure (an estimate of maximum elastance as defined in the isolated heart (323) was shown as heart rate was progressively increased by atrial pacing in conscious resting dogs (86), although the volume intercept of this relation was variable and often shifted. A positive inotropic effect of increased heart rate produced by pacing also has been demonstrated in normal human subjects (79, 307). With an irregular ventricular rate as in atrial fibrillation, cardiac performance varies from beat to beat, not only because of alterations in cardiac filling time and afterload, but also because of the influence of the strength–interval relation on contractility is manifested on a beat-to-beat basis (106).

Interaction Between Heart Rate and β-Adrenergic Stimulation

In the normal conscious human subject at rest, venous return to the heart is reflexly and metabolically stabilized so that artificially varying the heart rate between about 60 and 160 beats per min has little effect on the cardiac output, despite altered cardiac contractility (280). However, if the diastolic volume of the heart is maintained by increasing venous return as the heart rate is increased, the cardiac output will rise (336), and during exercise an increase in heart rate is highly important in enhancing the cardiac output (337).

The importance of the interaction between the heart rate, as manifested in the force-frequency relation, and β-adrenergic receptor stimulation in controlling myocardial contractility has been recognized recently (279, 279a). In conscious dogs during steady-state exercise, progressive lowering of the heart rate in steps by atrial pacing after control of the heart rate at a reduced level by a sinus node inhibitor (ULFS 49 or zatebradine, which had no direct inotropic effect) caused a progressive and marked reduction of the enhanced contractility of exercise reflected by maximum left ventricular dP/dt, despite increasing preload (Fig. 20–12), indicating the importance of increased heart rate to the positive direct myocardial inotropic effect mediated by enhanced sympathetic tone (217). In resting dogs, the relation between heart rate and maximum left ventricular dP/dt was progressively shifted upward and steepened by incremental doses of the β-adrenergic receptor agonist dobutamine (143). Thus, the effects of β-adrenergic cardiac stimulation are fully expressed only if there is a concomitant increase in heart rate. This amplification of the force–frequency effect by β-adrenergic receptor stimulation may be considered a fourth major intrinsic mechanism influencing myocar-

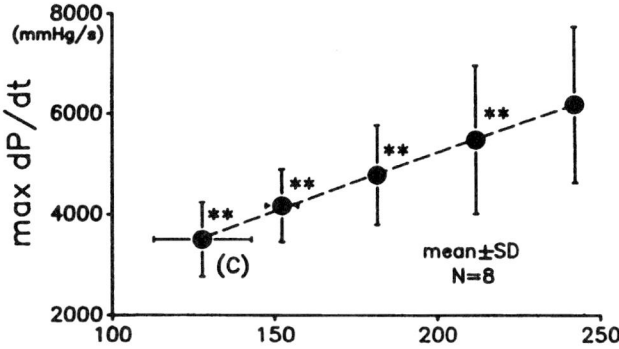

FIG. 20-12. Data from studies on the interaction of the adrenergic system and the force–frequency relationship obtained in intact dogs. The plot shows the relation between heart rate and max dP/dt (left ventricular maximum dP/dt) in conscious dogs standing at rest and during sustained exercise at several heart rates. The lowest heart rate represents the resting condition (C) and the highest heart rate, that during exercise with atrial pacing at 240 beats per minute. The intermediate heart rates show the effects of reducing the pacing rate progressively during continued exercise, with the sinus node rate controlled at a low level by zatebradine. ** = p <0.001 vs. 240 beats/min. Values are mean ± SD. [Reproduced with permission from Miura et al (217).]

dial contractility in the intact circulation (in addition to length-dependent activation, associated with increased preload, the basal force–frequency effect, and the direct positive inotropic effect of myocardial β-adrenergic receptor stimulation) (279; Fig. 20–13). Amplification of the force–frequency effect by exercise or β-adrenergic receptor agonist infusion, likely includes a further increase in intracellular Ca^{2+} availability due to phosphorylation of L-type Ca^{2+} channels by cyclic-AMP–dependent protein kinase A, leading to increased Ca^{2+} entry (332), and to phosphorylation of phospholamban causing enhanced SR Ca^{2+} reuptake, loading, and release (292); the effect on phospholamban also enhances the myocardial relaxation rate. β-Adrenergic stimulation also causes cAMP-dependent phosphorylation of troponin I with a decrease in myofilament Ca^{2+} sensitivity, and the associated off-loading of Ca^{2+} from TnI could further contribute to enhanced myocardial relaxation rate with β-adrenergic stimulation (292). Finally, Piot et al. (251) have recently shown in human atrial myocytes that increased beating frequency upregulates Ca^{2+} entry through voltage-gated Ca^{2+} channels; this process was sensitive to β-adrenergic stimulation and could be important in adrenergic amplification of the force–frequency relation.

It is likely that reduction of force–frequency amplification accompanying downregulation of the β-adrenergic receptor system is important in the reduced cardiac response to exercise after β-adrenergic blockade, as well as in experimental heart failure (73). Markedly diminished amplification the force-frequency relation is also observed in human heart failure (17) in which β-adrenergic mechanisms are impaired (33). Also, loss of amplification of the force–frequency effect during exercise as a consequence of chronotropic incompetence or heart block undoubtedly contributes to impaired cardiac responses in these conditions, since sympathetic stimulation is generally normal, and correction of impaired heart rate responses by rate-responsive pacemakers leading to amplification of the force-frequency relation may help to explain their beneficial effect on exercise performance.

Mechanical Restitution and Postextrasystolic Potentiation

In the intact ventricle, as in isolated cardiac muscle, a premature depolarization results in a reduced mechanical contraction, the magnitude of which is a function of the degree of prematurity of the extra depolarization. Mechanical restitution is the time-dependant process by which the ability of the muscle to contract returns after stimulation and is a manifestation of the force–interval relationship. Like postextrasystolic potentiation, this process is directly related to the intracellular Ca^{2+} concentration (351). Mechanical restitution has been studied in a variety of preparations ranging from isolated hearts and cardiac muscle (41, 42, 368) to intact animals (84), and its mechanism appears dependent on the rate of uptake of Ca^{2+} reuptake by the sarcoplasmic reticulum and may also relate to delayed recovery of the Ca^{2+} release channels (ryanodine receptors) (15). In the intact heart restitution of ventricular relaxation also has been shown to be a time-dependant process and is dependent on the interval between beats (256). Mechanical restitution appears to be impaired in the failing heart (257).

After a premature beat, the ensuing normally timed contraction is more forceful than normal, the degree of

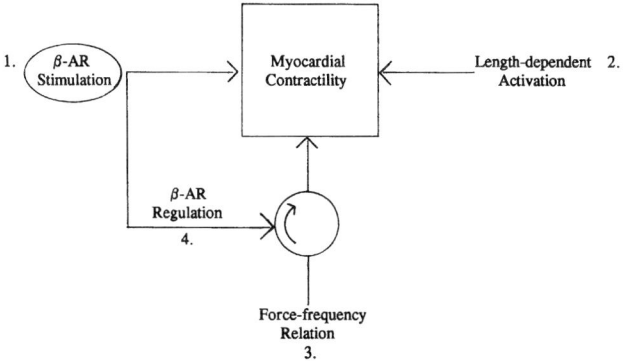

FIG. 20-13. Schematic diagram of the four major factors influencing myocardial inotropic state (279).

augmentation being greater the earlier the extra depolarization is introduced (128). This phenomenon, termed "postextrasystolic potentiation," is clearly independent of variations in diastolic filling of the ventricle, since it has been demonstrated in the isovolumetrically contracting heart (168), in isometrically contracting isolated cardiac muscle, and in the absence of a compensatory pause. When the premature beat is followed by a compensatory pause in the ejecting ventricle of the intact organism, the ventricular end-diastolic volume is augmented, and the increased preload contributes to the enhanced performance that characterizes the postextrasystolic contraction. Postextrasystolic potentiation can be produced repeatedly and result in sustained augmentation of myocardial contractility when pairs of stimuli are delivered repetitively to the intact ventricle (a condition termed "paired electrical stimulation"), the second stimulus being placed immediately after the electrical refractory period and resulting in only a minimal secondary contraction (31, 275).

ASSESSING CONTRACTILITY (INOTROPIC STATE) OF THE HEART

Intrinsic factors regulating myocardial contractility or inotropic state in the normal heart generally are recognized primarily to involve increases or decreases in the Ca^{2+} available for myofilament activation. These regulatory mechanisms include (1) neurohumoral effects particularly circulating catecholamines and local neurally mediated release of norepinephrine, (2) the strength-interval relation (one manifestation of which is the force–frequency relation in the whole heart) with a regulatory effect of β-adrenergic stimulation on the force–frequency, and (3) length-dependent activation. Changes in cardiac performance due to sudden changes in preload or afterload generally are not considered to involve changes in myocardial contractility, although the effects of preload are related in part to length-dependent activation via Ca^{2+} sensitization of the myofilaments (162, 170). Extrinsic factors also affect myocardial contractility, including pharmacologic agents (many of which affect transarcolemmal calcium efflux or Ca^{2+} uptake and release by the sarcoplasmic reticulum), hormonal, factors such as thyroid hormone and heart failure of various etiologies, which is often associated with depression of myocardial contractility (30).

Cardiac physiologists have long sought a simple and unique index of myocardial contractility that would reflect acute changes in a single subject as well as chronic changes between groups of subjects. The task of assessing inotropic state is more tractable in controlled isolated preparations of cardiac muscle and becomes progressively more complex as one approaches the intact circulation where preload, afterload, and heart rate are not controlled. For example, to determine the effects on cardiac contractility of a pharmacological agent that also acts on the arterial bed one must deal with the resultant changes in arterial pressure and secondary reflex mediated changes in heart rate and preload. The problem is further complicated when an index of the absolute level of inotropic state is required since this level may be confounded by substantial temporal variations not only in inotropic state but in loading conditions and heart rate, due to varying hormonal and neural activation. In the following sections we examine the approaches frequently taken to assessing changes in the level of inotropic state and the more difficult problem of determining the absolute level of inotropic state.

Acute Changes In Contractility

In isolated cardiac preparations the simplest approach to assessing changes in contractility is to compare isometric contractions at the same muscle length (usually L_{max}) before and after an acute intervention. The preparations used vary from isolated papillary muscles and trabeculae to isolated buffer perfused hearts. In the latter case an intracavitary balloon is usually used to control left ventricular volume and thus initial muscle length. With muscle length or volume constant, an increase in inotropic state is reflected by an increase in peak developed tension. Increases in inotropic state are also reflected by increases in the rate of tension development (presumably reflecting changes in the rate of calcium release from the sarcoplasmic reticulum) and in the rate of fall of tension reflecting changes in the dynamics of calcium uptake by the sarcoplasmic reticulum.

Methods Based on Changes in Ventricular Volumes and Dimensions in a Steady State

Left ventricular volume and dimensions can be calculated by biplane x-ray contrast left ventriculography or using the formula for an ellipsoid revolution (67–69, 288), by biplane cineradiography using implanted radiopaque markers (356), and using chronically implanted sonomicrometers in animals to measure ventricular dimensions (230). A conductance catheter positioned in the left ventricle also can be used to continuously determine left ventricular volume (9). Stroke volume, calculated by angiography as the difference between end-diastolic and end-systolic volume correlates closely with that determined by the Fick and indicator-dilution methods (68). Recently tomographic approaches using radiographic or magnetic resonance imaging techniques have been applied to the measurement of cardiac chamber volumes (129, 352); the latter approach is noninvasive and has the advantage of being able to "label" areas of myocardium using spin-label approaches (16, 37, 58). Another noninvasive approach is transthoracic echocardiography, which can be used to determine ventricular dimensions, volumes, and cardiac output using two-dimensional, M-mode, and Doppler methods (77). During the cardiac cycle the total volume of the heart (atria and ventricles) contracted within the pericardium remains constant (129). In normal human beings, the left ventricular end-diastolic volume by angiography averages 70 +20 (SD) ml/m^2 body surface area (153), whereas in normal adult rats, for example, using digital subtraction angiography this volume averages 340 ± 60 μL (236).

Stroke Volume and Aortic Blood Flow. In the conscious, resting state at a normal heart rate and arterial pressure, when the stroke volume is subnormal, and the ventricular end-diastolic pressure is abnormally elevated, myocardial contractility is probably depressed. An obvious limitation of this general approach becomes apparent when stroke volume (or stroke work) is depressed while end-diastolic pressure (or volume or both) is within the normal range or abnormally low; such findings may reflect either a depression of contractility or a reduction of preload. Disease processes may also complicate such an interpretation, as when the diastolic properties of the heart are altered by processes such as pericardial thickening, or endocardial fibrosis; in these conditions, ventricular end-diastolic pressure may be elevated without an increase of end-diastolic volume.

Although the mean and peak velocities of ejection and flow acceleration in the aorta correlate well with alterations in contractility, (224) these indices are also influenced by alterations in afterload, and to a lesser extent by changes in preload and heart rate; therefore these measures alone cannot be used as simple indices of contractility. They do, however, provide, an approach for defining directional changes in contractility. Acute enhancement of contractility maybe assumed to occur if end-diastolic pressure (or preferably volume) remains unchanged or declines, aortic pressure remains constant or rises, while the aforementioned indices (velocity of ejection, acceleration of flow) increase. With the advent of Doppler echocardiography these variables can be assessed noninvasively. Both the acceleration and peak rate of flow reflect changes in inotropic state in humans (13, 14, 283) although they remain sensitive to acute changes in preload and afterload (119, 283). Changes in intraventricular flow rates have also been observed and may be useful in detecting mechanical lesions such as outflow obstruction (7, 74, 226).

Ejection Fraction. The ratio of the stroke volume to the end-diastolic volume (the ejection fraction) is considered, largely on the basis of empirical observations, to provide a measure of myocardial contractility. It averages 0.67 ± 0.08 (± SD) in normal human subjects (153) and ranges between 0.45 and 0.70 in experimental animals, depending on the method of measurement of end-diastolic volume, the heart rate, and the condition of the animal, especially whether it is anesthetized (333). In the normal anesthetized rat, the LV ejection fraction is closely similar to that in humans, averaging 0.70 ± 0.5 (236). In the normal heart, the ejection fraction also can be predicted from the percentage decrease of the left ventricular diameter (68). Factors other than myocardial contractility that affect ventricular performance (preload, afterload, and heart rate) all influence the ejection fraction. Thus when end-diastolic volume (preload) is increased, the ejection fraction rises if afterload remains constant whereas an isolated elevation in aortic pressure reduces the ejection fraction (189). Conversely, this index may be normal in conditions such as mitral regurgitation, in which afterload is reduced even when myocardial contractility is depressed. Thus, although the ejection fraction is a useful index of contractility, it is often difficult to interpret whenever the loading conditions are altered. It is, however, more useful for assessing chronic changes in basal inotropic state, as described below.

Ventricular Dimensions and Their Rate of Change. Left ventricular dimensions can be assessed by implanted ultrasonic dimension gauges in conscious dogs (125, 337), the cineradiographically recorded motion of radiopaque markers (118, 135), and by echocardiography. The noninvasive technique of transthoracic echocardiography has now been used in many species, including the pig (73), rabbit (367), rat (56), mouse (130, 326) and human (77) to determine left ventricular diastole diameter and the extent and velocity of endocardial wall motion and wall thickening during ventricular ejection. With the placement of multiple markers for cineradiography, the extent and speed of shortening of large portions of the left ventricle can be measured (135). An index of the ejection fraction (the so-called fractional shortening, generally taken from endocardial dimensions of the mid left ventricle) is often calculated as [end diastolic length − end systolic length / end diastolic length] (236). When multiplied by π to obtain an estimate of ventricular circumference and divided by the ejection time, "VCF" (velocity of circumferential fibers) (145) is obtained. In the light of more modern studies on the complexity of the myofiber anatomy of the ventricular wall it seems difficult to relate this to a specific group of myofibers or even a theoretical "average fiber" (165). In conscious dogs, studied at a constant heart rate, the peak velocity of circumferential fiber shortening (VCF), the extent of shortening, and the VCF during ejection are relatively independent of preload but vary reciprocally with afterload; in the intact circulation VCF (and ejection fraction) remain relatively constant during acute elevations in preload because the modest increases in systolic pressure and heart size that take place result in some augmentation in wall stress and usually fortuitously offset the elevation of VCF that would have occurred with an increase in preload alone (191).

Wall stress can be related to the simultaneous extent and velocity of wall shortening in the ejecting ventricle (24, 97, 273). High-fidelity micromanometers, together with high-speed calibrated cineangiograms, from which wall motion and thickness are measured directly, are usually used; wall thickness can also be measured by echocardiography and a conductance catheter employed to measure let ventricular volume (147). As might be anticipated, both the extent and velocity of left ventricular wall shortening are reduced when afterload, as reflected in wall force, is increased acutely. This obviously limits the value of the ejection phase indices in characterizing the effects of acute interventions on changes in myocardial contractility.

Methods Derived from Left Ventricular Pressure and the Rate of Change of Pressure

Measures of the rate of change of ventricular pressure during isovolumetric ventricular contraction (so-called isovolumetric-phase indices) are sensitive to acute changes in the inotropic state (88, 197), and may be employed, often along with ventricular end-diastolic pressure, for assessing directional changes in contractility. The maximum rate of rise of ventricular pressure (peak dP/dt) is a frequently used parameter for the assessment of contractility. However, peak dP/dt cannot be reliably measured with ordinary catheter manometer systems unless special precautions are taken to prevent artifacts and the frequency response the system is carefully determined; instead, high-fidelity solid-state transducers sewn into the ventricle in experimental animals, or catheter-tip micro-manometers are now generally used, and even with the latter, artifacts due to catheter motion or entrapment during the cardiac cycle must be avoided. In most circumstances peak dP/dt is developed prior to the opening of the aortic valve (258) and, provided this occurs, peak dP/dt is largely independent of changes in afterload. If aortic valve opening occurs very early, peak dP/dt may not be fully developed (328).

Ratios of dp/dt to pressure have also been employed to examine acute changes in contractility. This approach is based (loosely) on models of contacting muscle simplified from those originally proposed by Hill. Cardiac muscle is modeled as a contractile element (CE) in series with an elastic element (SE). During an isometric contraction the velocity of the contractile element shortening is directly proportional to the ratio of rate of change of force to instantaneous force and inversely proportional to the stiffness of the elastic element (207, 360). Estimates of the SE model parameter in the intact heart are difficult and available only for the isolated supported heart (63). How the model and its parameters might change with disease is unknown. Despite these serious theoretical problems, when data derived from analysis of the isovolumetric phase are considered to be only indices of the inotropic state, rather than true measures of behavior of the CE, they can be useful for detecting changes in contractility of the intact ventricle. This approach has been applied by assessing the ratio of dp/dt to P at specific pressures and over entire isovolumic contractions (62, 189, 191).

The time to peak dP/dt also has been advocated as a measure of contractility that is insensitive to preload (3).

Comparison of Indices

The choice of an isovolumetric-phase index to determine changes in inotropic state is frequently determined by the experimental circumstances and what parameters can be measured. The various indexes described above all have different sensitivities to changes in inotropic state and loading conditions.

The effects of variations in preload, afterload, and contractility in the isolated supported heart preparation on several contractility indices are shown in Figures 20–14 and 20–15. Figure 20–15 describes the relative load sensitivity of several indexes. Note that indexes such as stroke work are relatively insensitive to changes in afterload but sensitive to alterations in preload. Ejection fraction as discussed above has an opposite pattern. These patterns of response can be used in selecting an index appropriate for the question at hand. As shown in Figure 20–14, the indexes based on the rate of change of ventricular pressure tend to be the most sensitive to alterations in inotropic state. Afterload sensitivity of these indexes is related to the timing of valve opening, and preload sensitivity remains small. The sensitivities vary somewhat with the preparation under study. For example in the conscious animal indexes derived from the ratio of dp/dt to pressure are less sensitive to changes in arterial pressure then in a more controlled preparation (150, 191). Because of their sensitivity to changes in inotropic state

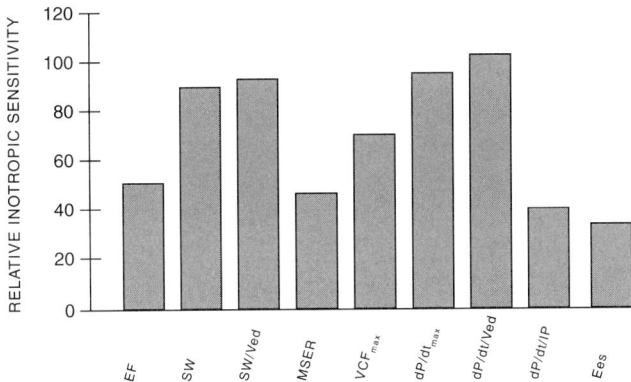

FIG. 20-14. Relative sensitivity of several indices to inotropic stimulation in an isolated canine heart preparation Ees = slope of the end-systolic pressure–volume relationship. Ef = ejection fraction, V = volume SW = stroke work; SW/Ved = stroke volume/systolic ejection period; VCF$_{max}$ = maximal value of $(-dV/dT)$/Ved; dp/dt/IP = maximum +dP/dT/ developed pressure at the time of dp/dt$_{max}$. [Reproduced from Kass et al (150), with permission.]

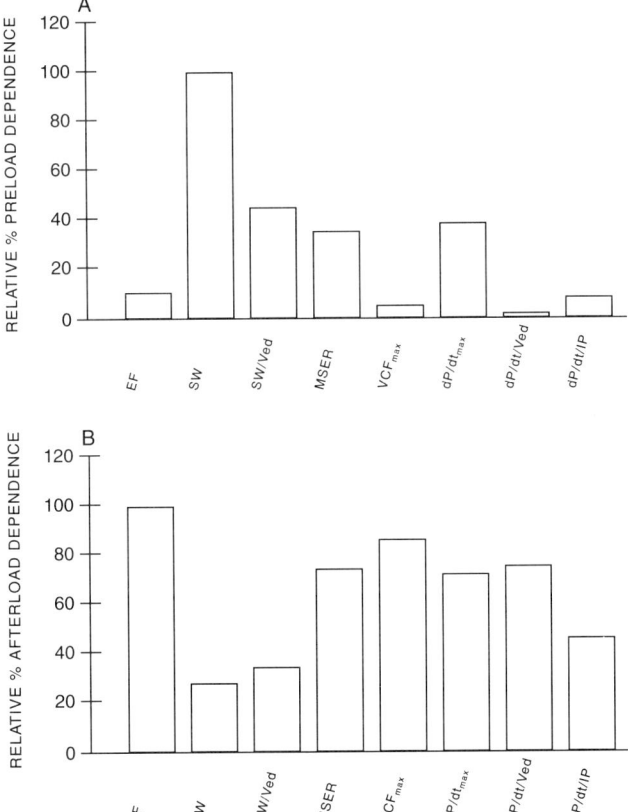

FIG. 20-15. Relative load sensitivity of several indices determined in an isolated canine heart preparation. The maximum percent change (comparing the highest and lowest load) was calculated for each index See Fig. 20-140 (150).

these dp/dt based indexes are most frequently used to reflect acute changes in inotropic state (191, 258). From a practical standpoint there does not seem to be a substantial advantage to the use of complicated measures derived from the isovolumic phase pressure tracing over the more easily obtained maximum dP/dt of the ventricle.

Methods Based on Examination of Ventricular Function over a Range of Loading Conditions

Traditionally, methods concerned with study of the heart as a pump have centered on the relation between a range of ventricular filling pressures, or diastolic volumes, both estimates of initial muscle length, and a measure of systolic function, expressed as systolic pressure, stroke output, or both. These approaches have the inherent advantage that performance is examined over a range of conditions, thus mitigating the effects of preload on the index itself. Many of the variables mentioned above for evaluation of function in single contractions have been examined during variations in ventricular filling in a wide variety of preparations (150). The end-systolic pressure-volume relationship and variations of ventricular function curve are widely used approaches to examining changes in inotropic state in open-chest animal preparations, and the intact setting. In the intact animal or in human subjects, the preload has sometimes been varied by volume infusions or pressor agents, but more commonly by partial inferior vena caval occlusion with an implanted inflatable cuff in animals (86) or inflation of a balloon catheter (147).

The End-Systolic Pressure–Volume (ESPV) Relation. The approach is not without pitfalls particularly when used in conscious animals, where changes in the volume intercept (86) and the curvelinearity of the end-systolic pressure–volume relationship (Ees) may influence the position and slope of the relationship (87, 149, 227). These relations are often used to calculate end-systolic elastance (E_{max}) (286), and they also are useful in assessing ventricular energetics (319) as well as ventriculo-arterial coupling relating a function of Ees to the effective arterial elstance (Ea) (148). Recently the use of single beat end-systolic elastance has been advocated to assess myocardial contractility (257).

The Preload Recruitable Stroke Work. As already noted, in animals a linear relation exists between left ventricular end-diastolic volume and stroke volume, and when changes in afterload are accounted for by calculating the stroke work, the slope of the end-diastolic volume-stroke work relation over a range of end-diastolic volumes (so-called preload recruitable stroke work) provides a measure of acute changes in inotropic state (104).

The Relation Between Preload and Peak dP/dt. The maximum dP/dt of the left ventricle exhibits a direct relation with the ventricular end-diastolic volume, and the slope of this relation can be used to define an acute change in myocardial contractility (181).

Venous Return and Cardiac Output Curves. In another approach in the open-chest anesthetized dog, Guyton and his associates (113) combined a venous return curve (relating venous return to mean right atrial pressure) with a cardiac output curve (relating cardiac output to mean right atrial pressure), the point of their crossover representing an equilibrium state. In this type of analysis, the position of the venous return curve is affected by factors such as blood volume and vascular resistance, and the position of the cardiac output curve is affected by myocardial contractility and afterload; all of these influences exert an effect on the net final equilibrium point relating mean right atrial pressure to cardiac output. This method of evaluating the heart and circulation is applicable in a number of a experimental conditions and is of great theoretical importance. However, while aspects of the approach such as the determination of mean systemic filling pressure can be measured in experimental animals (182), it is not useful for examining ventricular function in the conscious animal or in human beings because of the extensive surgical manipulation required.

The Absolute Level of Inotropic State

When it is necessary to compare groups of subjects or the same subjects over long periods of time, or during normal growth, or when a chronic disease (e.g. cardiac hypertrophy) alters the size, shape, or condition of the heart, the problem of assessing an altered inotropic state becomes much more difficult. Under these circumstances an estimate of the absolute level of basal inotropic state is needed.

When the ventricular end-diastolic volume is clearly elevated (i.e., > 110 ml/m2, > 2 SD above the normal mean) and the total stroke volume or cardiac index, or both, are reduced or within normal limits while heart rate and afterload remain normal, cardiac contractility may be assumed to be depressed. When heart rate, ventricular end-diastolic pressure and/or volume (as indices of ventricular preload), and aortic pressure (as an index of afterload) are constant, the stroke volume, stroke work, stroke power, peak left ventricular dP/dt, and ejection velocity all vary as a direct function of the contractile state of the myocardium. Unfortunately when comparing different groups of subjects, often it is not possible control or even measure ventricular volumes or pressures, although when some data are available they can be interpreted in view of the known sensitivities of each index to loading conditions described above. For example, an augmented maximum dP/dt or wall shortening in the presence of increased afterload or a normal or reduced ventricular end-diastolic dimension can be interpreted as augmented contractility.

Determining the absolute level of contractility is often complicated by problems of variability of the indexes used, problems of scale (comparing large and small hearts), and changes in the makeup of the myocardium.

All indexes of contractility have substantial normal variability at rest. This is probably due to a variety of factors including normal variations in autonomic tone and the resulting variation in contractility and loading conditions. Variability in the level of anesthesia, which may directly influence contractility, often complicates the evaluation of contractility at two different time points in studies where the analysis requires anesthesia or sedation. Freeman et al. compared the variability of several indexes of contractility in 6 conscious dogs at 5 different occasions over 3 weeks (Fig. 20–16). The coefficient of variation of several commonly employed indexes was 5%–7% and was increased by autonomic blockade. These data indicate that dP/dt max, VCF and ejection fraction as well as the relationship between stroke work and end diastolic volume had the least variation over the three week period. The slope of the end-systolic pressure–volume relationship had nearly a threefold greater coefficient of variation.

Cardiac output, cardiac mass, and ventricular volumes are approximately proportional to body weight and is clearly difficult to compare many normal hemodynamic variables across species and under circumstances where cardiac size is vastly different. Comparative physiologists and clinicians have usually normalized these variables to body weight or body surface area. The same approach has been taken in dealing with normal growth and development and responses to hypertrophic stimuli where there are large changes in cardiac mass, as well as in the shape of the cardiac chambers. This is a particular problem in experimental studies using rodents that continue to grow as adults; for example, left ventricular dimensions were found to correlate poorly with body weight in adult mice of various ages (326).

Indices of contractility are most often used to provide insight into myocyte contractile function. During normal growth and development and in response to injury the relative proportions of myofilaments and other constituents of the myocardium change. Under circumstances where the response of the myocardium is uniform it is often possible to normalize changes in

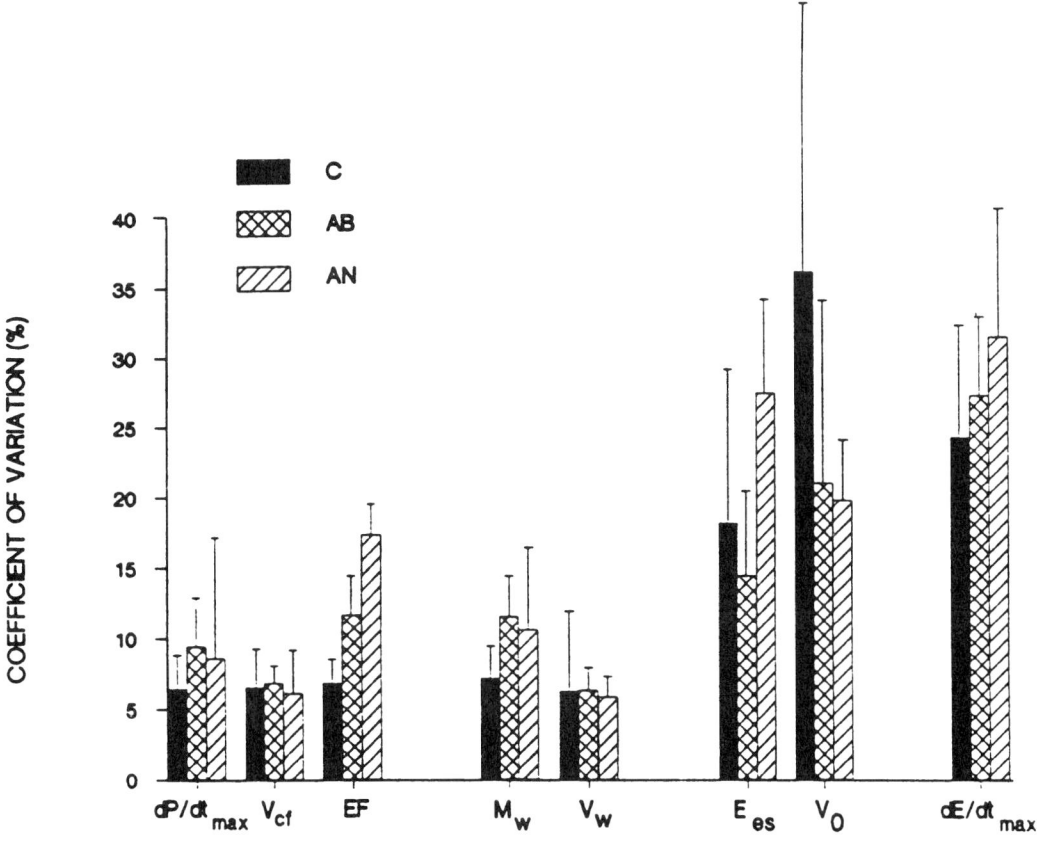

FIG. 20-16. Coefficient of variation defined as (SD/mean) × 100 for several inotropic indices determined five times over 3 weeks. C = control; AB = autonomic blockade; AN = anesthesia (85). [Reproduced by permission from Freeman et al (85).]

contractile indices by myocyte cross sectional area or by the relative proportions of myofilaments to other cellular constituents such as mitochondria (294). In ischemic heart disease where there is extensive replacement of myocardium with fibrous tissue evaluation of changes in contractile indices is more complex and estimates of regional function are usually employed (107, 171, 330).

The indices of contractility derived from isovolumetric pressure tracings must be used with caution in assessing the basal state of contractility in between groups of subjects because of variability in the resting values of these parameters. For example, the standard deviation of dP/dt/max in the conscious dog varies from 10% to 20% of the mean (64, 85, 247). Many variables derived from dP/dt show less variation over time when assessed in the same animal and may be useful in protocols where the same animal is compared over time (85). Peak dP/dt also varies among mammalian species, appearing to increase (along with increasing basal heart rate) the smaller the body weight. For example, in conscious human subjects at rest it approximates 1500–2500 (247), in the conscious standing dog the peak dP/dt averages 3000–5000 (218) whereas in the conscious mouse it is often over 10,000 mm Hg/sec (240).

In contrast, despite their limitations in detecting acute changes in contractility ejection phase indices, such as the mean velocity of wall shortening (mean VCF) and the ejection fraction appear to be useful for defining basal contractility (97, 145, 277). In human subjects the level of contractility in the basal state also may be defined from the instantaneous relation between midwall shortening velocity and wall stress throughout left ventricular ejection (97) determined by use of high-fidelity catheters and cineangiography. Normal subjects in the basal state usually exhibit circumferential shortening velocities in the minor equator in, excess of 1.4 circumferences per second at maximum wall tension (96, 97). Mean VCF, calculated from changes in dimensions and ejection time is lower but correlates well with this more complex measure (145). Mean VCF, ejection fraction, and the mean systolic ejection rate (corrected for ventricular end-diastolic volume) all successfully separate patients with normal hemodynamic function from those with clearly abnormal function (247).

During chronic pressure overloading, wall stress (afterload) generally remains normal over long periods because of the development of ventricular hypertrophy with increased wall thickness (67, 294). In chronic volume overloading, as chronic ventricular dilatation slowly occurs, sarcomere length appears not to change further and remain maximal, indicating that preload at the sarcomere level plays little role following initial dilation (276). Therefore, in contrast to the situation that applies to the assessment of acute changes in contractility, in determining absolute levels of contractility in these settings it does not appear essential to use measures of contractility that are unaffected by acute changes in preload and afterload, and indices based on the ejection phase may be used. For example, in the chronically pressure-overloaded human heart that has adapted to the change in afterload by hypertrophy, thereby returning afterload to normal, ejection phase indices may also be useful for assessing absolute contractility (277), and in dogs in which the ascending aorta is constricted and left ventricular hypertrophy develops, the percentage of circumferential fiber shortening and mean VCF at first decline and then return to normal over a period of several weeks (294).

Only when the myocardium begins to fail and contractility becomes depressed does basal performance per unit of circumference during ejection become reduced (277, 281), which may explain why the ejection phase indices appear to be more useful than those derived from isovolumetric phase pressure tracings for detecting left ventricular dysfunction in the basal state. Unlike the isovolumetric phase indices, the ejection phase indices may be more reliable because they are sensitive to afterload. Thus, when the preload reserve is fully utilized, signficant depression of myocardial contractility will result in afterload mismatch, even with a normal aortic pressure in the resting state, which is reflected in abnormal function per unit of ventricular circumference (277). In this setting, the left ventricular afterload is often increased as a consequence of chamber dilation and wall thinning associated with depressed myocardial contractility, and all of these functions appear to contribute to the ability of ejection phase measures, such as the ejection fraction or mean VCF, to detect failure of the myocardium.

Evaluation of Ventricular Function in Mice and Rats

The ability to produce animals with overexpression, ablation, or substitution of specific genes has provided investigators with a powerful new approach to understanding the function of the circulation. Although transgenic technology has been applied to larger animals these studies are most often conducted in mice and occasionally rats. However, the small size of the mouse heart (about 150 mg in a 25 g mouse) and major vessels, as well as the high resting heart rate (600 bpm) provide a challenge to investigators attempting either invasive or noninvasive assessment of cardiovascular function. The high heart rates require a transducer frequency response nearly an order of magnitude greater than in larger animals and the small vessel diameters (the thoracic aorta has an internal diameter of approximately 1mm) severely limit the response of catheter manometer systems. Miniature micromanometers are now available with adequate frequency response, although the small cavity volume of the left ventricular (~50 µL) imposes restrictions on catheter size (99, 186, 240, 268). Nevertheless micromanometer and combined micromanometer conductantace catheter systems are available (99) and can be used in the adult anesthetized mouse. Estimates of absolute ventricular volume and cardiac dimensions can be obtained with echocardiography and magnetic resonance imaging and with the conductance catheter (11, 65, 94, 130, 194, 271, 301, 325, 359). Techniques for the estimate of parallel conductance in these small catheters are still evolving and are required for the determination of absolute volume with the conductance method (98). The spatial resolution of both echocardiography and magnetic resonance imaging is steadily improving, and both have been used to detect sequential changes in ventricular dimensions in the mouse (130a), as well as to characterize hemodynamic and echocardiographic changes in murine dilated cardiomyopathy (206s). Both techniques require substantial temporal averaging to reconstruct full cardiac cycles at high heart rates.

REGIONAL FUNCTION

The ventricular walls are widely viewed as a continuous structure of directly coupled myocytes interconnected by an organized extracellular matrix (47, 316, 317). The concept that the heart consists of discrete muscle bundles arranged in a well-defined helical pathway running from apex to base was popular at the turn of the century (188, 193, 228). This concept, however, has been overshadowed in recent years by evidence of a continuous transmural distribution of myofiber directions (315, 317). This architecture of the heart walls was reviewed by Streeter in the previous edition of this *Handbook* (315). There is, however, a substantial recent body of evidence showing discontinuities of myocardial structure at both the macroscopic and microscopic levels. Caulfield and Borg (48) using scanning electron microscopy reported a connective tissue mesh surrounding loosely interconnected groups of three or more myocytes. There have been reports of connective tissue septa in several species (2, 12, 312) including man (311), other studies have shown gaps and the appearance of cleavage planes that run radially across the wall (80, 131, 132, 228, 264, 317, 353). Work from the laboratory of Smail and Hunter shows myocardium to be laminar in nature, with laminae or sheets of myocytes (on average 4 cells thick) connected by a loose collagen network which spans the cleavage planes between the sheets (134, 164, 304). Laminae in the outer third of the wall tend to be shorter and more closely coupled. The differences in orientation of laminae are particularly marked between the subendocardial regions of the anterior left ventricular and the interventricular septum of the canine heart. In the anterior left ventricle, laminae curve steeply in a basal direction as they approach the endocardium, whereas in the septum and the basal aspects of the anterior wall they approach the endocardium obliquely from the opposite direction (164).

Given the complex shape and structure of the chambers, it is not surprising that function varies substantially at different sites in the chamber walls. There is very little information on regional variations in structure and function in the two atria but substantial evidence for regional variations in function in the two ventricles.

Regional Right Ventricular Systolic Function

Right ventricular contraction is characterized by a peristalsis-like contraction sequence beginning in the inflow region and extending to an anatomically and embryologically distinct outflow tract (35, 152, 195). The right ventricular outflow tract was recognized as being anatomically and embryologically distinct from the main portion of the right ventricle by Keith (152). He showed that the bulbus cordis, which is present as a separate chamber distal to the common ventricle in all developing vertebrate embryos, becomes incorporated into the ventricles of the mammalian heart as development proceeds. Studies that investigated the sequential nature of right ventricular contraction have employed high-speed cinematography (35, 195), strain gauges sewn to the myocardium (5, 35, 203, 249, 341), or ultrasonic dimension gauges (260). Brock (35) describes rapid radiographic films taken by Prinzmetal, in which it is possible to observe the peristaltic nature of contraction passing up the infundibular portion of the right ventricle. These cinematographic observations were confirmed by March et al. (195). Thus, as contraction begins in the inflow or sinus portion of the right ventricle, the outflow tract simultaneously bulges outward concurrent with the initial systolic expansion of the pulmonary artery. The infundibular segment then contracts markedly at the end of systole and remains contracted well into diastole, finally expanding in late systole or after atrial contraction. This difference in timing of the inflow and outflow contraction can induce a pressure gradient between the inflow and outflow regions of the right ventricle (5, 239, 331). This gradient is particularly prominent during stellate ganglion stimulation.

March et al. (195) and later Armour et al. (5) also studied the sequence of contraction using Walton-Brodie strain gauges sewn to the canine right ventricular free wall at the levels of the inflow and outflow tracts. They found an average delay in the onset of outflow tract contraction of 5–43 ms compared with the inflow tract. The ability to measure local dimensions with radiography of implanted markers (203, 260) or piezoelectric dimension gauges in the thin-walled right ventricle and a knowledge of the local myofiber direction (6) has advanced our knowledge of the local structure–function relationships in the right ventricle. Raines et al. (260) found a delay in the onset of right ventricular outflow tract shortening with 68% of total inflow tract shortening occurring during this period. Associated with this delay, there was an early systolic bulge in the outflow tract cord, which was not seen in the free wall. The implication of these findings is that the lengthening of the free wall to septal dimension may be predominantly caused by septal movement toward the left ventricle. The observed early systolic expansion may be due to an actual expansion (increase in cross-sectional area) of the outflow tract. Meir et al first calculated two-dimensional finite strains in the right ventricle (203). This technique allows the calculation of the local principle strain and is thus not dependant on the orientation of the marker beads themselves. Waldman et al. recently have expanded this approach by fitting a finite element to an array of beads allowing the calculation of principle strains at any site (121, 341). These studies confirm the apex to conus sequence of the onset of shortening observed with dimension gauges and also detect considerable deformation perpendicular to the major axis of shortening. These findings imply that wall thickening in the right ventricle also be a complex process, as discussed below for the left ventricle, although the right ventricular wall is too thin to allow transmural measurements of deformation.

Regional Left Ventricular Structure–Function Relationships

In the normal heart, the ventricular shape, myocyte architecture, ventricular activation sequence, and the papillary muscle chordae tendineae system act together to produce substantial regional variations in left ventricular function. Regional variations in shortening were first detected in man by Kong et al using coronary bifurcations as surface markers during coronary angiography (159). These investigators, and later Liedke et al., using angiographic techniques showed greater shortening at the apex compared to the base of the left ventricle (175). The use of ultrasonic dimension gauges and radiography of implanted markers has allowed tracking of "material points" in the ventricular wall during the cardiac cycle, thus allowing investigators to relate the observed deformations to the local myofiber anatomy. With dimension gauges implanted at the midwall in the direction of the midwall myofibers (Fig. 20-17) shortening was found to be greatest in the apex (avg. 20%) and less at the midwall and base of the ventricle. Function in the direction of the overlying epicardial fibers was less (avg. 5%–6%) with no apex base gradient (173). Gauges implanted in the lateral and posterior walls also showed less circumferential shortening then gauges in the anterior wall. In the anterior free wall local circumferential shortening exceeded longitudinal shortening, whereas in the posterior wall longitudinal and circumferential shortening were approximately equal at all ventricular volumes (171). In the transplanted human heart, longitudinal shortening tended to be greater on the posterior wall and approximately equal to circumferential shortening at anterior locations (137). Similar results have also been obtained using finite deformation approaches (339).

Further studies with dimension gauges or specially adapted strain gauges have indicated that there is substantial local systolic myocardial shearing deformation across the left ventricular wall (78, 238). The presence of large deformations and substantial shearing makes it difficult to interpret the uniaxial data obtained from dimension gauges or other two-dimensional approaches in terms of the local structure. The presence of small amounts of in plane and transverse shear produces substantial errors in the estimate of local fiber strain using uniaxial techniques (343). Accordingly, many investigators have more recently applied the general theory of finite (large) deformations to three-dimensional deformation across the ventricular wall. This approach was first described by Waldman and co-workers (343) using three columns of transmural myocardial markers (1 mm lead beads), a technique first employed by Fenton et al. (81). Although strains are usually referred to a cardiac coordinate system first used by Meir et al. (204), strains may be calculated in any arbitrary reference system allowing the direct assessment of local myofiber strains provided the relationship between the local anatomy and the cardiac coordinate system is known. Strains may be calculated assuming homogeneous strains in a small volume of

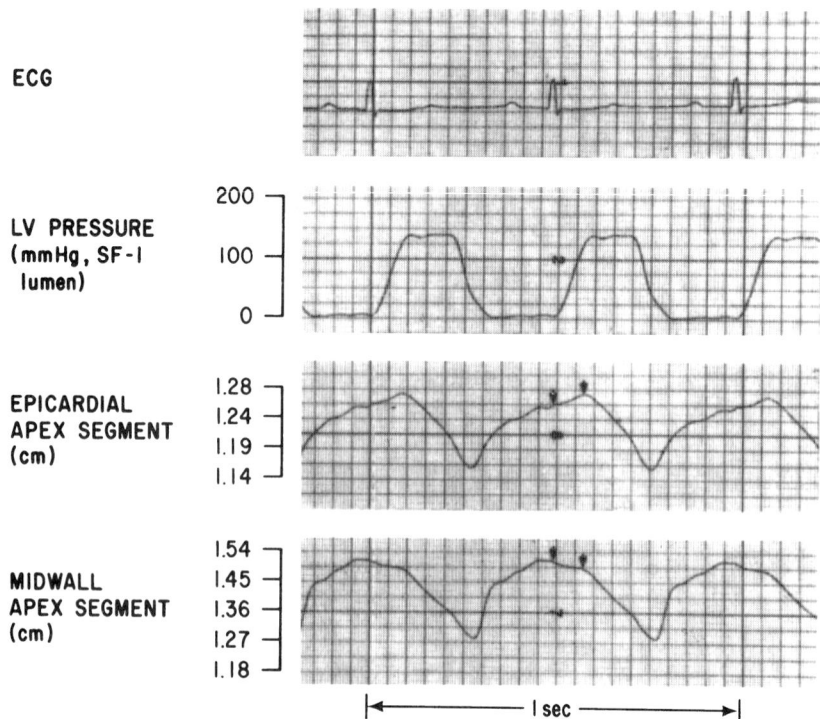

FIG. 20-17. Dimension gauge signals from an open-chest canine preparation. All three gauges are orientated in the circumferential direction. Gauges are located at three apex base levels (apex, mid, base) (173). [Reproduced by permission from Le Winter et al (173).]

myocardium, although the assumption of strain homogeneity produces potential errors in calculations of deformation as the thickness of the tetrahedra increases (70, 343). The assumption of strain homogeneity can be mitigated to some extent by fitting the bead array to a finite element that allows nonlinear transmural but no in plane gradients in strain (200). The data shown in Figure 20–18 represent normal strains in the inner third of the ventricular wall in a single systole, which has been recalculated from the study by Villarreal et al. in open-chest dogs using the finite element approach (340). At end systole, wall thickening is substantial (40%) and in plane normal strains (circumferential, E_{11}, E_{22}) are approximately equal and less than 15%. Normally one of the two transverse shear strains is large. In this case radial longitudinal shear is over 6% and the remaining shears are small. All studies using this technique as well as studies using dimension gauges and spin-labeled cardiac MRI have shown steep transmural gradients in strain (92, 165, 173, 343, 366).

Left Ventricular Structure–Function Relationships

It is clear from unidimensional measurements of regional systolic wall shortening and wall thickening that in disordered states, such as abnormal electrical activation of the left ventricle (342) or regional myocardial ischemia (278), marked abnormalities in the activation sequence or reductions in the strength of local contraction cause not only pronounced regional dysfunction but also effects on the remainder of the ventricle.

Additional insight into normal (and abnormal) left ventricular function can be obtained from three-dimensional analyses. Since the reference system for the strains in the three dimensional finite deformation approach is arbitrary it is possible to calculate deformation along any known axis. Experimental studies now indicate that shortening along the axis of the myofibers is uniform across the wall (165, 344). This supports the concept that there are not large transmural variations in load or inotropic state. Moreover, if the initial sarcomere length is known an estimate of the time course of sarcomere length in systole may be obtained. Figure 20–19 shows a different pattern of sarcomere length change during systole and diastole and a substantial sarcomere length change during isovolumic relaxation. This approach would indicate large sarcomere length changes during isovolmic relaxation and smaller changes during filling.

Although shortening along the fiber axis is relatively constant across the ventricular wall, wall thickening and transverse shear have substantial transmural gradients. Systolic wall thickening strain is near 0.1–0.2 in the anesthetized animal (78, 238, 369), much of which is due to large radial strains (0.4) in the inner wall (166, 340, 344). Simple calculations based on conservation of individual myocyte volumes lead to the conclusion that the increase in cell diameter as myocytes shorten maximally would contribute only about one-fifth of the local thickening at the inner wall (0.08), thus other mechanisms must account for the large wall thickening strains at this site. Recent descriptions of the laminar myocyte organization separated by cleavage planes (134, 164, 304) have provided a possible structural link between transmural shear and wall thickening. A consistent observation for measurements in the longitudinal-radial plane was that in the anterior left

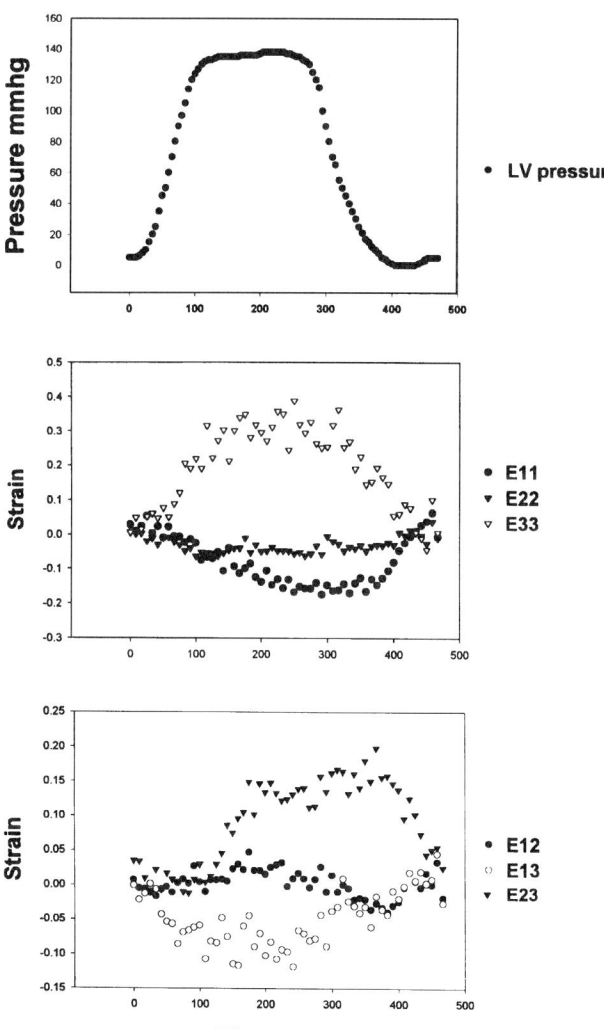

FIG. 20–18. Finite strains determined in the left ventricular free wall in an open-chest canine preparation. Data shown are from the inner half of the ventricular wall. E11 = circumferential strain; E22 = longitudinal strain; E33 = radial (wall thickening strain); E12 = circumferential longitudinal shear; E13 = circumferential radial shear; E23 = longitudinal radial shear. [Unpublished data from Villareal et al. (340).]

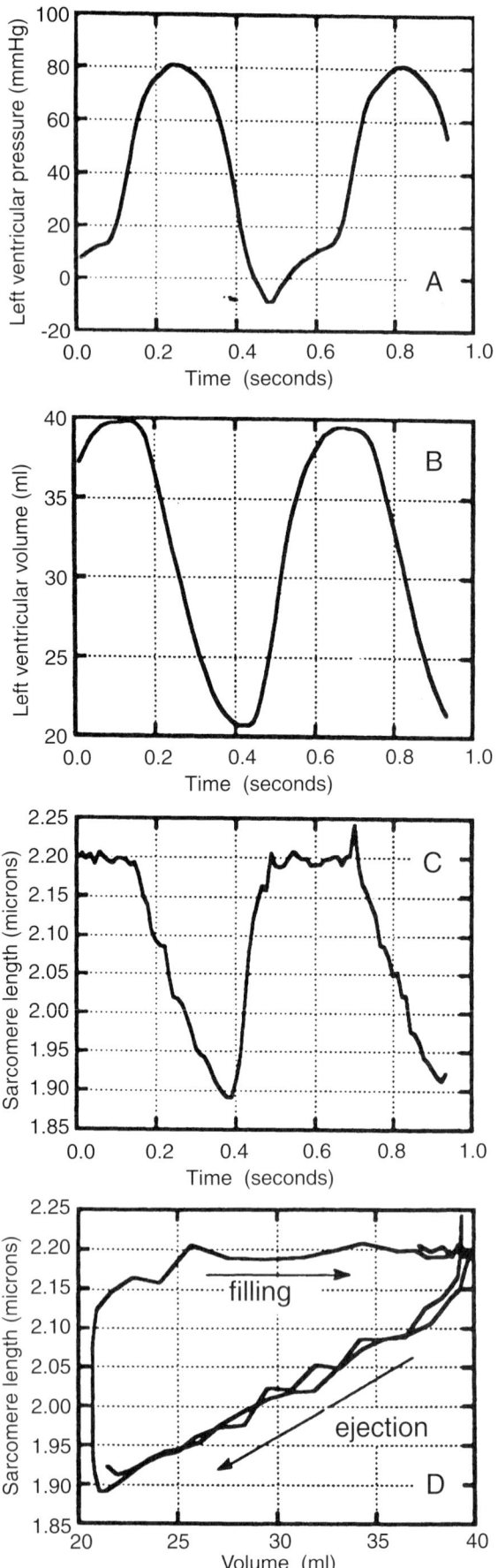

ventricular the cleavage planes approached the left ventricular endocardium obliquely from the apical direction, becoming nearly parallel with the endocardial surface (large negative angle), and in the septum the angle was positive and smaller (Fig. 20–20). Transverse shear strain was also significantly different at these two depths, positive in the anterior left ventricule, and negative in the septum.

On the septal wall both shears and cleavage plane angles are different in sign, supporting the hypothesis that wall thickening is related to the motion of these myocardial laminae. This mechanism of systolic wall thickening is supplemented to a small degree by increases in myocyte diameter as they shorten along their axis (78, 238, 340, 342–344).

Based on the above data, we propose a mechanism of systolic wall thickening operating in the inner third of the ventricular wall in Figure 20–21. On the right is a schematic longitudinal-radial section (2–3 plane) from apex to base of the left ventricular free wall with cleavage planes following characteristic curved radial patterns. The endocardium moves downward relative to the inner wall regions, giving rise to a positive E_{23} shearing deformation as measured in our cardiac coordinate system (relative upward movement of the endocardium would be a negative E_{23}). If we also assume that the myocardial laminae are stiff relative to the shearing stiffness of the space between them then they will tend to slide relative to one another, causing the endocardial surface to displace into the left ventricular cavity as it moves down in systole contributing to local wall thickening. Studies of regional mechanics in acutely ischemic myocardium demonstrated that significant systolic wall thickening changed to thinning, and this was accompanied by a marked reduction (238) or reversal of E_{23}. These results further support the idea that there is a direct link between systolic wall thickening and transmural shearing deformation.

The origin of the shearing forces which produce this deformation has not yet been defined. A first simple hypothesis relates to the fact that the left ventricular is a thick-walled chamber, the diameter of which decreases during systole. This change in global geometry results in the endocardial tissue being compressed into a smaller space. Since the tissue being compressed is laminar in nature it is likely that the

FIG. 20–19. Reconstructed sarcomere lengths (C and D) during a single cardiac cycle. Note that there are marked differences between cavity volume and sarcomere length during filling and ejection and that during isovolumic contraction there are large transitions in sarcomere length without a corresponding change in ventricular volume (B). [Reproduced from Rodriguez et al (269).]

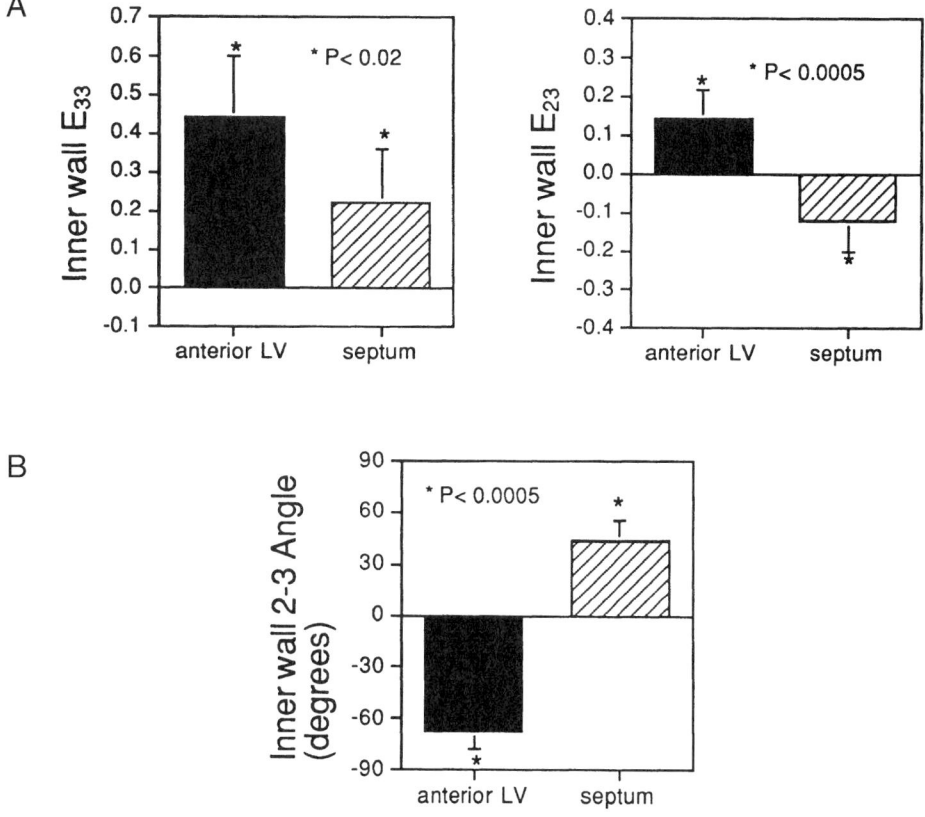

FIG. 20-20. Average end-systolic wall thickening strain (E33) and longitudinal radial shear (E23) in the subendocardium of the left ventricular free wall (*solid bars*) and septum (*hatched bars*). B shows the cleavage plane orientation at the two sites. [Reproduced from LeGrice et al. (165), with permission.]

structure will deform along lines of least resistance, i.e. the cleavage planes between the myocardial sheets. The sheets will slide relative to one another, producing a shear deformation. Regardless of the precise mechanism, correlations between three dimensional regional structure and function are beginning to provide improved understanding of the complex changes during normal ventricular systole (60a, 130b, 205a).

Mechanical Correlates of Cardiac Energy Consumption.

Cardiac oxygen consumption is directly related to the work performed during a contraction, and over the years a wide variety of mechanical correlates of ventricular oxygen consumption have been developed. These indices of myocardial oxygen consumption have been reviewed by Gibbs (100), Gibbs and Chapman in the previous addition of this *Handbook* (102), and more recently by Suga (319). The most complete direct measurements of energy consumption come from myothermic measurements in isolated cardiac muscle.

The total energy in a contraction is the sum of the initial heat, which is directly related to hydrolysis of high-energy phosphates (102), and recovery heat, which is related to the restoration of high energy phosphates by oxidative phosphorylation. There is good evidence that in well-oxygenated cardiac muscle oxygen consumption is directly comparable to total energy (52).

Studies have related ventricular oxygen consumption to heart rate (21), ventricular wall tension (109, 347), contractility (109, 310), and an additional cost associated with ejection (shortening) (34, 43). A portion of the total oxygen consumption has been ascribed to maintaining the biochemical integrity of the cell. The relative contributions of these factors to total oxygen consumption varies with the particular contraction but most estimates consider that basal oxygen consumption is approximately 1 to 2 ml/min/100g (19, 358) and thus would represent 10%–20% of total oxygen consumption. Factors comprising basal oxygen consumption remain to be fully elucidated but sarcolemmal Na^+–K^+-ATPase, and Ca^{2+}-ATPase activity has been shown to influence basal metabolism

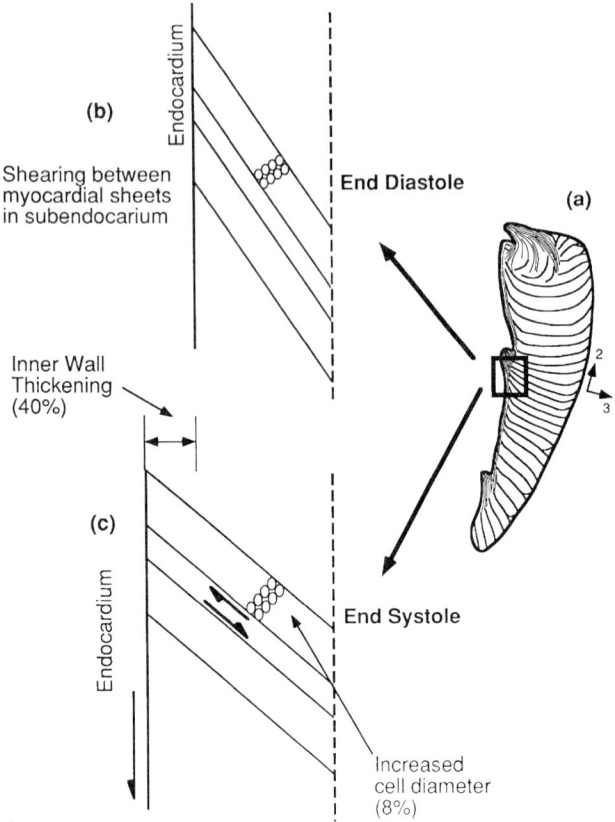

FIG. 20–21. Proposed mechanism of ventricular wall thickening. [Reproduced from LeGrice et al. (165), with permission.]

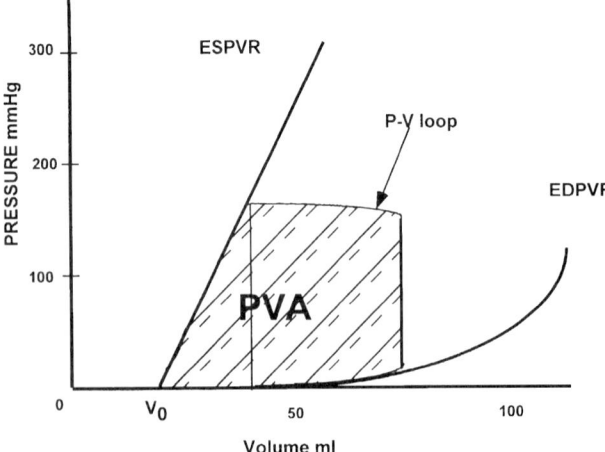

FIG. 20–22. Schematic representation of pressure–volume area (PVA). *Solid line* indicates the pressure volume trajectory of a single contraction (P-V loop) plotted in the end-systolic and end-diastolic pressure–volume framework. The area shown by the *diagonal lines* is the pressure volume area.

(185) as well as levels of Ca^{2+} (115). Under normal circumstances the relative contributions of contractility and tension have been shown to be approximately equal and to account for the majority of oxygen consumption (109). However, this balance can be affected by the relative balance the mechanical correlates (tension and contractility), which differ between contractions and in cases where inotropic state is altered pharmacologically by the agent used (22). Oxygen consumption associated with shortening has been estimated to comprise about 20% of the total (43). The energy used during active contraction may be considered as two components. A portion of the energy used during contraction is related to initiating contraction (increasing intracellular Ca^{2+} to approximately 10^{-7} mol/L). There is general agreement that this energy, termed "activation heat" or "tension-independent heat" is due to high-energy phosphate utilized to remove Ca^{2+} from the cell and to management of Na^+ released into the cell upon activation (101). The remainder of the energy during contraction may be related to cross bridge ATP hydrolysis.

A wide variety of additional hemodynamic variables have been shown to correlate with ventricular oxygen consumption, and like heart rate, tension, and contractility all these indices may be useful under certain circumstances. They include the Tension-Time Index, the pressure rate product and the triple product (systolic pressure rate product multiplied by the ejection time) and others. Rooke and Feigel compared several of the indices recently and developed another (the pressure-work index), which they showed correlated well with ventricular oxygen consumption even under circumstances where contractility changes markedly in the intact animal. In 1979 Suga and Sagawa published two manuscripts describing the relationship between the ventricular oxygen consumption and the pressure volume area. As shown in Figure 20–22 the pressure volume area (PVA) is defined as the area bounded by the isovolumic and ejection phase trajectories of the pressure volume loop and the end-systolic pressure–volume relationship (ESPVR and the end-diastolic pressure–volume relationship (EDPVR). Studies in a wide variety of preparations have shown an excellent correlation between ventricular oxygen consumption and the PVA (107, 319).

Changes in inotropic state shift the relationship between ventricular oxygen consumption and PVA upward without a change in slope. Figure 20–23 shows data from two animals following the administration of epinephrine (panel A, control, panel B following epinephrine) and calcium (panels C and D). The solid line in panels C and D represents the regression to the control data. The PV loops are shown in the inset. These data are typical of the close, highly linear relationships

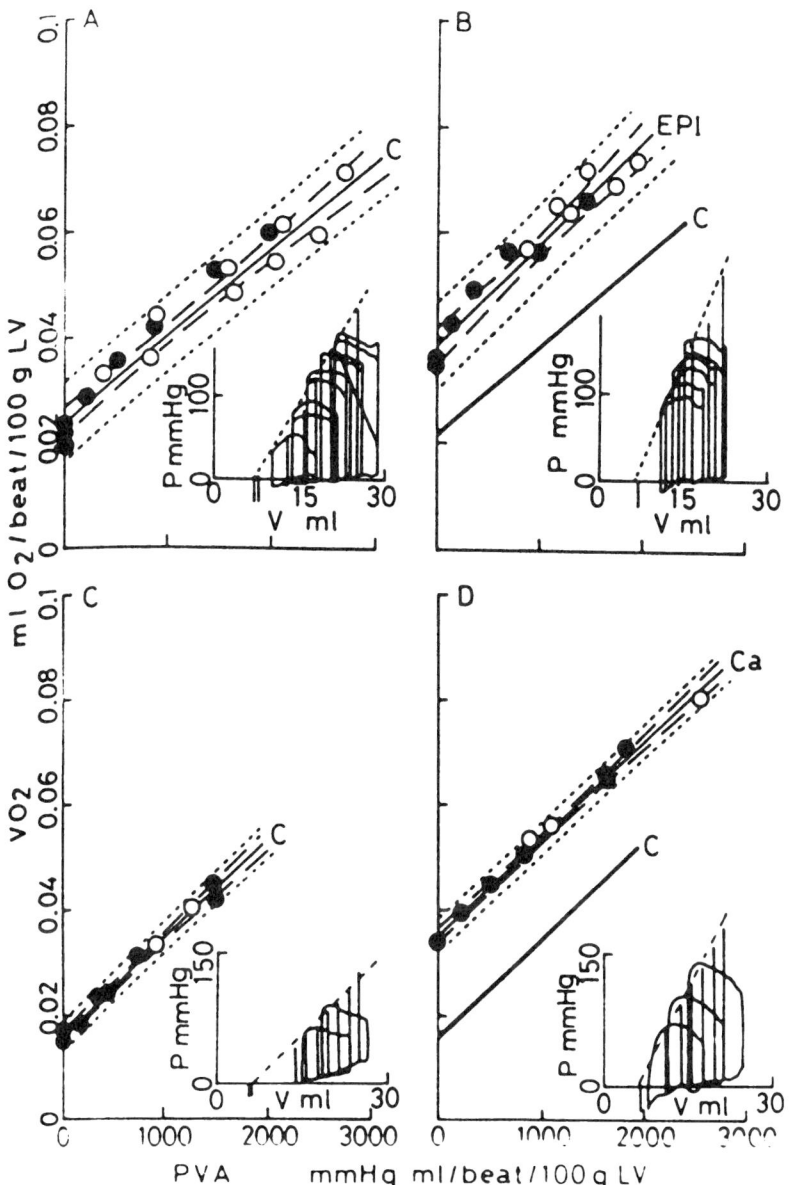

FIG. 20–23. Correlations between cardiac oxygen consumption per beat (VO_2) and PVA in control panels (A, C) and following epinephrine (B) and calcium (D). Inset shows the contractions from which the ESPVR is determined for each panel (*closed symbols* represent isovolumic beats, opening ejecting contractions). [From Suga et al. (320), with permission.]

found between oxygen consumption and PVA in several species (107).

DETERMINANTS OF DIASTOLIC FUNCTION

The properties of the myocytes are imposed upon a unique cardiac structure, the components and geometric configuration of which determine overall diastolic properties of the ventricles. Normal cardiac muscle may never be fully inactive, and several studies have shown significant energy consumption in resting cardiac muscle (60, 156). Accordingly, two traditional approaches have been employed to study diastolic function, the first assessing the properties of the cardiac chambers in the arrested (usually isolated) heart when activation of the myocardium has been prevented by hypoxia, hyperkalemia, or an agent such as 2,3-butanedione monoxime (BDM) (222, 244). In the second approach the in situ heart is examined at different time points during the cardiac cycle, so that active, passive, and time variant viscous properties contribute to the observed diastolic properties (184).

Cardiac Structural Components

Since quantitative information on ventricular structure is available primarily for the left ventricle, we focus on that chamber. The left ventricle is a thick-walled structure with a ratio of wall volume to chamber volume of roughly 2 to 1 (274). Over 90% of the wall volume is comprised of myocytes although these large cells comprise less then 10% of the total cell number (110). The large rod-shaped myocardial cells are arranged in a branching syncytium and lie with their long axis in the epicardial tangent plane. As described in detail by Streeter et al. these fibers are arranged in a "fan-like" array across the wall of the ventricle, spanning approximately 140 degrees. Four to five cell thick laminae of these fibers are arranged in radial sheets of myocardium in the inner third of the wall providing a mechanism for structural rearrangements in the wall of the ventricle during cardiac filling (165, 166). The coupling between myocytes and between groups of myocytes composing the laminae is accomplished through a highly organized system of interstitial proteins. While quantitative differences have been found, this interstitial network is conserved among species, from birds to humans. Collagen, the major structural protein of this system, is present in three principal configurations (48, 295): *intermyocyte struts*, inserting just lateral to the Z-bands, and apparently taut at all diastolic chamber volumes, probably prevent slippage between fibers in diastole, and minimize differences in end-diastolic sarcomere length; *myocyte to capillary fibers*, taut in systole, may contribute to the maintenance of capillary patency, and consist of a perimysial weave of collagen surrounding groups of three or more myocytes, forming functional units which, in turn, are only loosely connected to adjacent myocyte complexes; and the *perimysial collagen* located in the inner half of the left ventricular wall between laminae composed of sheets of myocytes 4–10 cells thick (166). It may be the perimysial collagen network that gives rise to the viscoelastic properties of the ventricle, permits the rearrangement of fibers during contraction (165, 312), and allows slippage during ventricular dilatation (48). Coiled perimysial fibers extend from the muscle-tendon junction of the papillary muscles into the ventricular wall. This crimped or coiled configuration is a common property of collagens in many tissues (95), and in the heart these fibers are taut when stretched approximately 15% (266). More recent studies (described below) have shown that these fibers "uncoil" over the normal range of diastolic pressures and thus may affect passive compliance and have a role in energy storage. In addition to these large collagenous structures, the cardiac interstitium contains a number of other fibrous and granular components (237, 267). Both the collagen bundles linking myocytes to capillaries and the perimysial weave are closely associated with elastic fibers (48). Tubular "surface cables" less than one sarcomere in length are oriented along the long axis of the myocyte in association with the glycocalyx of the cell coat and appear to have a role in preventing overextension of sarcomeres (237, 295). Isolated collagen fibrils have been identified, as well as microfibrils composed of a unique core protein coated with fibronectin (265, 267). Micro threads, some of which stain positively for fibronectin, connect the coats of adjacent myocytes, myocytes to collagen, and collagen fibers with each other, and the filamentous cell coat itself appears to be attached to the cell membrane by fine filaments up to 20 nm in length (160, 265). Cardiac interstitial collagen is comprised of types collagen I and III, and to a lesser extent, types IV and V. Type I is the primary component of left ventricular collagen and has the greatest tensile strength of the major collagenous proteins (161, 242). Proportions of type III and type I collagen vary in left ventricular tissue of different species (201). In left ventricular collagen of rats, the ratio of type III to type I collagen changes during postnatal growth and with aging. In general, the ratios of these collagens are tissue and developmental stage specific. Variation in the ratios may determine the structural and functional properties of the collagen fibril (39).

Passive Pressure–Volume Relationships

An example of the passive pressure–volume relationship of the left ventricle in an isolated canine heart is shown in Figure 20–24 (329) and shows the average left ventricular pressure–volume relationship (solid circles) as the chamber is filled, corrected for the estimated filling of the right ventricle. The overlying dashed line represents data from a single animal during filling, and the solid line represents data as volume is withdrawn from the chamber showing hysteresis. The nonlinear shape of the filling curve is typical of pressure–volume relationships of hollow organs and is similar over a wide range of mammalian species (211, 235, 269). There is a residual volume (V_0; volume at zero pressure), and the relationship is approximately exponential so that the dp/dv is a linear function of pressure (4) (see insert Figure 20–24). This slope has been used as an index of chamber stiffness. Acute changes in the passive pressure–volume relationship in a normal individual heart are rarely observed (309) and when seen experimentally are usually due to edema or changes in myocardial perfusion in isolated perfused preparations (190, 199). However, changes in the size and shape of

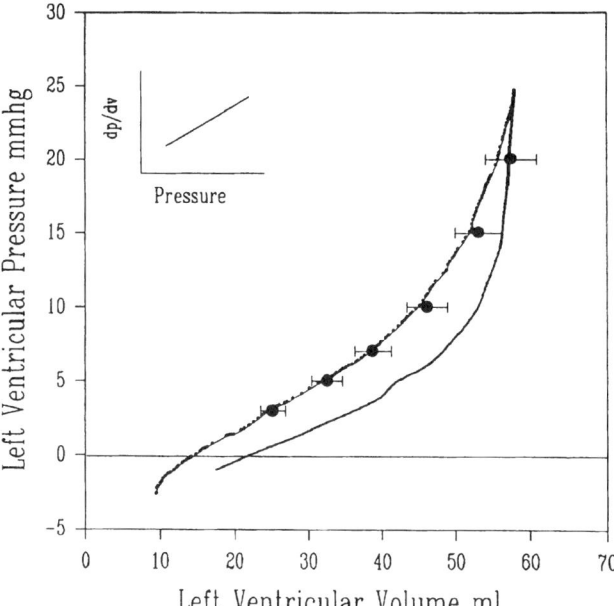

FIG. 20-24. Left ventricular pressure–volume relationship adapted from the work of Taylor et al. (329). *Dashed line* indicates the pressure–volume relationship corrected for the contribution of the right ventricle in a single animal, and the error bars indicate the SD over 8 animals. *Solid line* schematically estimates the pressure–volume relationship on deflation.

the ventricle influence both the slope and the intercept of the pressure–volume relationship, complicating the comparison of hearts from different species or from different age groups in the same species (234). This is a particularly difficult problem in humans, or in experimental studies where the mass and shape of the left ventricle is changed dramatically by disease (89, 140, 196).

Time-Dependent Properties

Muscle and other tissues are viscoelastic and viscoplastic materials (4). Thus the instantaneous relationship between pressure and volume is time, strain rate, and muscle length dependent (1, 127, 184, 187, 225). These properties of the muscular wall of the heart result in the inflation and deflation cycles of the pressure–volume relationship being significantly different (Fig. 20-24). Both creep (increasing length after application of a constant stress) and stress relaxation (decreasing stress after stretch to a fixed length) contribute to the shift in the pressure–volume relationship during the deflation cycle, and both have been demonstrated in the intact heart (139, 220). In the intact heart these properties are reflected in a significant deviation of the diastolic pressure from the static pressure–volume relationship. Figure 20-25 plots three cardiac cycles from the time of minimum diastolic pressure during each diastole to end-diastole against left ventricular diameter (254). The dashed line indicates the passive pressure–volume relationship determined from the end diastolic pressure diameter points from a number of contractions as cardiac volume is altered. Note that the pressure deviation from the passive relationship at a common diameter is greater early in the filling cycle when filling rate is highest and also is greater at the longer diastolic lengths. These properties have been demonstrated in a variety of intact preparations and in humans, and the quantitative contributions of viscous and elastic properties have been modeled (261).

Passive Ventricular Diastolic Structure–Function Relationships

The classical engineering approach to understanding cardiac structure–function relationships would be, first, to understand the material properties of the individual components and their structural relationships, and then to construct complex models to predict the behavior of the whole system. It is usually not possible to pursue this detailed approach in biological systems, and indeed the origin of resting tension in passive myocardium remains an unresolved problem (27). Most earlier studies ascribed the load-bearing properties to the stiff extracellular matrix proteins (27, 48). However, techniques to study the physiological properties of the cellular components of myocytes (75) now indicate that

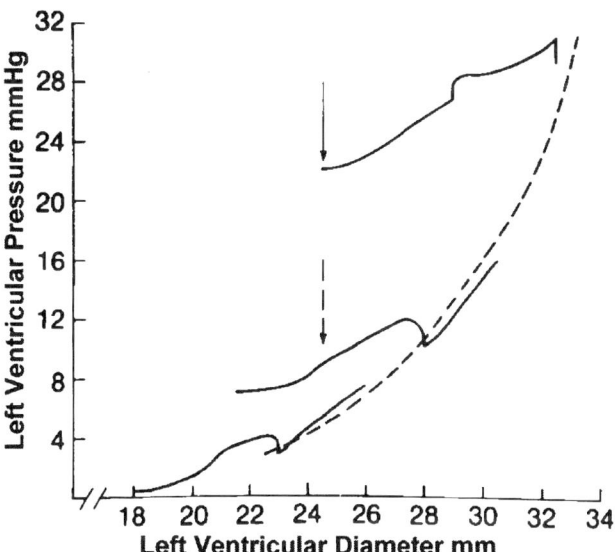

FIG. 20-25. Left ventricular pressure diameter relationships from three contractions in a conscious dog. The *dashed line* indicates the passive pressure diameter relationship determined in the same animal from the end-diastolic pressure diameter point in several contractions (254).

a portion of the resting tension originates within the myocyte. Thus, Lin et al. (180) recently found that the passive stiffness of the myofibril itself was similar to that of intact papillary muscle preparations, as well as skinned fibers, over the normal working range of sarcomere lengths (1.8 μ to 2.2 μ) (141, 154). Since in this study the passive stiffness did not change with the addition of varying concentrations of BDM, it seems likely that titin, a large polypeptide that spans the entire distance from M-line to Z-line, is the load-bearing structure. The I-band portion of titin appears to be the flexible region and to provide a functional link between the end of the thick filament and the Z-line (345). At sarcomere lengths of approximately 2.0 μ to 2.2 μ the stiffness of intact muscle deviates from that of the myofilament (180), and it seems likely that passive stiffness at these sarcomere lengths is determined by other factors such as the extracellular matrix. The dashed lines in Figure 20–26 show data from intact muscle compared to the passive tension of isolated myofilaments (180). Collagen has a stiffness module that exceeds that of titin and elastin by an order of magnitude, and this extracellular matrix component appears to dominate myocardial stiffness at sarcomere lengths above 2.2 μ. Based on these observations, the myocyte mass itself must be considered an important determinant of the diastolic properties of the ventricular wall. At normal levels of end-diastolic pressure changes in compliance have been observed without changes in the extracellular matrix in hypertrophy, and modeling studies indicate that such shifts observed in the pressure–volume curve can be explained by increased wall mass (234).

Based on ultrastructural observations in normal and diseased myocardium, it has been proposed that the extracellular matrix prevents increases in sarcomere length beyond 2.2 μ by increasing stiffness at higher filling pressures. (48, 346). The data above would support that hypothesis. Several investigators have shown that collagen concentrations or structure are altered in cardiac hypertrophy and heart failure and that this alteration is associated with changes in ventricular stiffness (32, 177, 190, 202, 349).

Recently studies in which acute changes the extracellular matrix alone have been performed. MacKenna et al. (190) and others (49, 50) have shown that reducing collagen concentration by enzymatic digestion shifts the pressure–volume relationship to the right (Fig. 20–27). In contrast to the predictions from the work on myocytes, the loss of collagen also affected filling pressure at low volumes and sarcomere lengths and thus appears to influence diastolic function over the normal working range of pressures. Further support for this concept comes from studies on the structure of the large perimysial collagen fibers. Collagen fibers (particularly type I collagen) are quite stiff, but Robinson and Factor have shown that the large perimysial fibers uncoil as the myocardium is stretched (76, 266) a property that would make the perimysial fibers less stiff than type I collagen itself and thus a potential factor in the compliance of the myocardium at lower diastolic pressures. MacKenna et al. have shown that the tortuosity of large perimysial collagen fibers decreases over the normal range of diastolic pressures, indicating that these fibers may play a role in passive stiffness at low filling pressures. A role of the extracel-

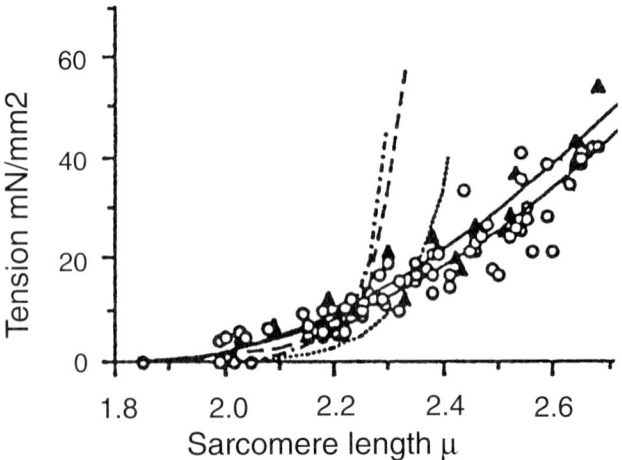

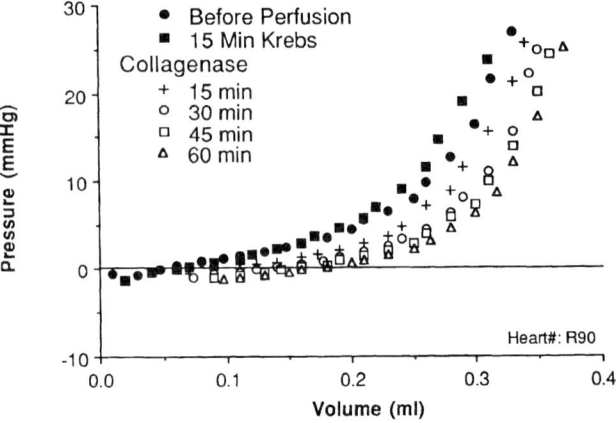

FIG. 20–26. Length–tension relationship in single cardiac myofibrils determined in relaxing solution with and without BDM (*solid lines, open and closed symbols*). The *dashed lines* indicate the sarcomere length–tension relationship in intact rabbit and rat papillary muscles and trabeculae [From Linke et al (180), with permission.]

FIG. 20–27. Pressure–volume curves in an isolated buffer perfused rat heart showing the effects of progressive infusion with collagenase. There is a shift toward greater volumes at all pressures that increases with progressive disruption of the extracellular matrix. [Reproduced with permission from MacKenna et al (190).]

lular matrix in the passive compliance of the myocardium is clear in disease states, since most chronic increases in ventricular stiffness occurring with cardiac hypertrophy or failure are accompanied by alterations in the extracellular matrix (202, 349, 350).

Additional approaches have been used to examine the relationship between the constituents of the myocardial wall contributing to the pressure–volume relationship, the simplest being to calculate the relationship between stress and strain. Measurements of strain are relatively straightforward and can be determined noninvasively in humans with a variety of techniques. Stress is much more difficult to evaluate (363), but the usual approach is to assume that thin wall stress theory can be applied to the thick walled ventricle and that the shape of the chamber can be represented by a symmetrical geometric form (usually a sphere or ellipse). These general approaches have been reviewed by Yin (363). If stress and dimension or strain (change in length/unit length) are determined, myocardial stiffness is then estimated as the local slope of these relationships (208, 209). This approach has the advantage that it tends to "normalize" for ventricles of different sizes, but it assumes that the myocardium is isotropic and homogeneous, clearly a difficult assumption for such a complex structure. A more direct approach is to place a load on isolated passive tissue and measure the local three-dimensional finite deformations. The relation between deformation and a range of stresses then can be expressed in terms of a constitutive relationship, usually taking the form of a strain–energy relationship based on those originally used by Fung in arterial wall (55) and modified by Humphries, Guccione, and others (112, 133). These approaches have the potential to explore anisotropic material properties, and most recent studies have included reasonable myofiber geometry. Most studies using this approach now indicate that myofiber stiffness is two fold greater than stiffness determined in the crossfiber direction (233, 364).

Regulation of Ventricular Filling

Flow across the mitral and tricuspid valves during diastole is governed by a wide variety of factors including atrial contraction, the compliances of the atria and the ventricles, and the pressure gradient across the valve. Flow across the mitral valve can be effectively modeled by the following relationship:

$$\Delta P = \frac{(L)dQ}{dt} + (R)Q^2$$

Where ΔP represents the atrial ventricular pressure gradient, L and R are resistive and inertial constants that are dependent on the mitral valve area, and Q is volume flow rate (205, 361). Flow across the mitral valve is thus directly (and predominantly) dependent on the pressure gradient and the mitral valve orifice size. Other factors that influence filling therefore can be interpreted in the light of how they influence the pressure gradient. Figure 20–28 shows data obtained in a chronically instrumented dog with an electromagnetic flowmeter implanted in the mitral ring. Although most early data supported the concept that mitral valve opening occurred at the moment of left atrial and left ventricular pressure crossover, the electromagnetic flow probe indicates early flow at or before the point of pressure crossover. Most recent data indicate that valve opening occurs 5–60 msec prior to pressure crossover and is associated with a change in the shape of the ventricle and the mitral annulus (334). Several lines of evidence also support their concept that the mitral valve chordae tendineae are under tension even during diastole (263, 324, 334), which would enhance early opening of the valve leaflets. Following valve opening, the very small atrioventricular pressure difference provides the driving force for the rapid increase in mitral flow rate to the maximum level observed during diastole (138). Echocardiographic studies indicate that the mitral valve leaflets reach their maximum open position approximately 25 msec before peak flow. Although atrial pressure is declining, flow into the left atrium is also large during this period, indicating that the conduit function of the atrium contributes substan-

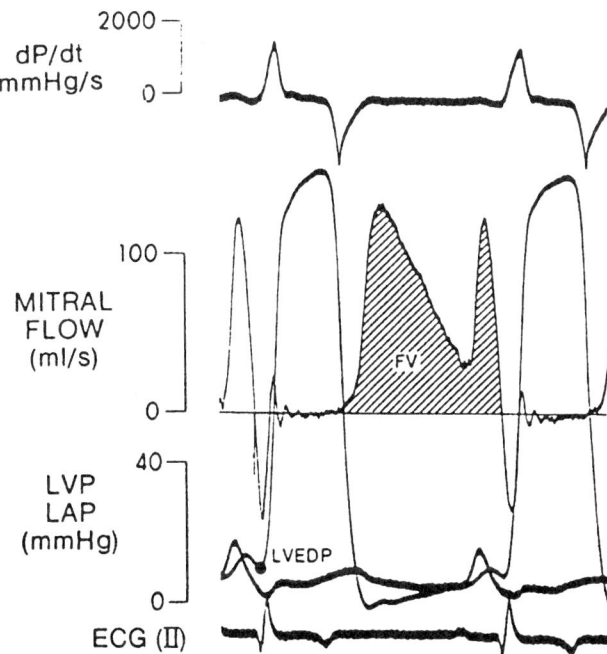

FIG. 20–28. Tracings from a conscious dog, illustrating the temporal relationships between mitral valve flow and atrial and left ventricular pressures. [Modified from Yellin et al. (361), with permission.]

tially to ventricular inflow (155). Mitral flow then rapidly decelerates as the pressure gradient falls and is maintained by inertial forces, which contribute to flow during diastasis. Echocardiographic studies indicate that the mitral leaflet motion reaches a maximum opening during this initial increase in mitral flow (the E point on the M-mode echocardiogram). As flow decelerates the valve leaflets reoppose. Large circulating vortices contribute to the reopposing of the valve leaflets at this time and during final valve closure (362). Flow then reaccelerates during atrial contraction and the mitral leaflets open more widely (the A point on the echocardiogram). Several factors contribute to mitral valve closure. In studies using radiopaque markers sewn to the valve mitral valve leaflet, valve closure followed the atrial-ventricular pressure crossover by an average of nearly 40 msec. The delay between pressure crossover and mitral valve closure was dependent on heart rate as well as factors that influenced the duration of isovolumetric contraction (334).

Other factors that influence normal left ventricular filling include the rate of isovolumetric ventricular relaxation (36), which in turn can influence the minimum ventricular pressure during early diastole (361). For example, during strenuous exercise in dogs instrumented with high-fidelity micromanometer and ultrasonic crystals for determining left ventricular volume, the time constant of relaxation (tau) decreases, the minimum left ventricular pressure falls below zero (indicating a suction effect) (223), and the pressure gradient during early ventricular filling markedly increases (54); these effects together with enhanced atrial contraction prevent a rise in the mean left atrial pressure during moderately severe exercise (54, 223). This adaptation is also dependent upon the interaction between β-adrenergic stimulation and the heart rate [amplification of the positive inotropic effect of the force-frequency relation (279)], since slowing of the sinus node rate during such exercise results in prolongation of tau with reduced filling, and upward displacement of the early portion of the left ventricular diastolic pressure–volume relation, consistent with impaired ventricular relaxation (216).

In intact human subjects Doppler echocardiographic studies of mitral valve flow (314) indicate the importance of ventricular relaxation in conditions such as ischemia, where impaired left ventricular relaxation results in reduced height of the E wave and reduced E/A ratio with slowed deceleration of the E wave fall. In contrast, increased ventricular wall stiffness in chronic hypertrophy with fibrosis can result in rapid inflow with an increased E point, followed by abnormally rapid deceleration of flow and decreased filling during atrial contraction (A wave), with increased E/A ratio (314).

Role of the Pericardium

Under normal resting conditions the pericardium has little or no effect on cardiac filling, although, during strenuous exercise and several abnormal conditions, its effect is significant. Methods for measurement of intrapericardial pressure have been controversial, and either catheters or balloons have been used (297). The pericardium was shown to influence cardiac function during exercise in normal pigs; maximal VO$_2$ and cardiac output increased after chronic pericardiectomy along with an increase in left ventricular dimension, although pericardiectomy also was associated with an increase in left ventricular mass (114).

Aside from severe exercise and disease states involving pericardial thickening or pericardial tamponade (298), the pericardium appears to limit cardiac filling under resting conditions only when acute volume overload occurs, as with fluid overload or overtransfusion. Under these circumstances, in the dog the left ventricular pressure–volume relation is displaced upward in association with elevated intrapericardial pressure (300). Administration of the arteriolar and venodilator nitroprusside after fluid overload shifted the pressure–volume relation downward, which produced large decreases in intraventricular (and pericardial) pressure without change in left ventricular volume (300). In contrast, in chronic experimental volume overload, the pericardium enlarged to accommodate the dilated heart and did not affect the ventricular diastole pressure–volume relation (174).

Experiments in dogs in which the pericardium was intact indicated that a large (50%) increase in right heart volume produced an upward shift of approximately 5 mm Hg in the left ventricular diastolic pressure–volume curve, which corresponded to the increase in intrapericardial pressure (123). Other influences can have a similar effect, including increased atrial volumes due to atrial fibrillation (179) and right ventricular infarction (305). Also, changes in left ventricular filling can alter the right ventricular pressure–volume relation through changes in intrapericardial pressure, resulting in a complex relation between pressure–volume relations in the two sides of the heart (103, 300). As noted previously, in the absence of the pericardium, ventricular interaction can occur, and the left ventricular diastolic pressure–volume relation should be corrected for the degree of right ventricular filling (329). Such ventricular interaction was shown to be of significance in determining left ventricular function in the conscious dog, particularly when changes in the volume of the right ventricle occur (230).

In human subjects in which left ventricular volume was measured by the conductance catheter method and pressure by catheter-tip micromanometry, transient obstruction of the inferior vena cava by a balloon catheter has allowed assessment of the effects of the pericardium and right ventricular filling on the left ventricle by comparing beats early after the intervention, before left heart filling is affected, to those before caval occlusion. During inferior vena caval occlusion there was a clear shift downward of the left ventricular diastolic pressure–volume relation (147).

REFERENCES

1. Abbott, B. C. and J. Lowry, Stress relaxation in muscle. *Proc. R. Soc. Lond. [Biol.]* 146:281–288, 1957.
2. Abrahams, C., J. S. Janicki, and K. T. Weber. Myocardial hypertrophy in *Macaca fascicularis*: structural remodeling of the collagen matrix. *Lab. Invest.* 56:676–683, 1987.
3. Adler, D., S. D. Nikolic, E. H. Sonnenblick, and E. L. Yellin. Time to dP/dt$_{max}$, a preload-independent index of contractility: open-chest dog study. *Basic Res. Cardiol.* 91:94–100, 1996.
4. Alexander, R. S. Viscoelastic determinants of muscle contractility and "cardiac tone." *Fed. Proc.* 21:1001–1005, 1962.
5. Armour, J. A., J. B. Pace, and W. C. Randall. Interrelationship of architecture and function of the right ventricle. *Am. J. Physiol.* 218:174–179, 1970.
6. Armour, J. A. and W. C. Randall, Structural basis for cardiac function. *Am. J. Physiol.* 252 (*Heart Circ. Physiol.* 21):1517–1523, 1987.
7. Aurigemma, G., S. Battista, D. Orsinelli, A. Sweeney, L. Pape, and H. Cuenoud. Abnormal left ventricular intracavitary flow acceleration in patients undergoing aortic valve replacement for aortic stenosis. A marker for high postoperative morbidity and mortality. *Circulation* 86:926–936, 1992.
8. Baan, J. and E. Van Der Velde. Sensitivity of left ventricular end-systolic pressure-volume relation to the type of loading intervention in dogs. *Circ. Res.* 62:1247–1258, 1988.
9. Baan, J., E. T. Van Der Velde, H. G. DeBrui, G. J. Smeenk, J. Koops, A. D. Van Dijk, D. Temmerman, J. Sender, and B. Buis. Continuous measurement of left ventricular volume in animals and human by conductance catheter. *Circulation* 70:812–823, 1984.
10. Bakos, A. C. The question of the function of the right ventricular myocardium: an experimental study. *Circ. Res.* 1:724–732, 1950.
11. Barbee, R. W., B. D. Berry, R. N. Re, and J. P. Murgo. Microsphere and dilution techniques for the determination of blood flows and volumes in conscious mice. *Am. J. Physiol.* 263 (*Renal Fluid Electrolyte Physiol.* 32):R728–R733, 1992.
12. Bashey, R. I., A. Martinez-Hernandez, and S. A. Jimenez. Isolation, characterization and localization of cardiac collagen VI: associations with other extracellular matrix components. *Circ. Res.* 70:1006–1017, 1992.
13. Bedotto, J. B., E. J. Eichhorn, and P. A. Grayburn. Effects of left ventricular preload and afterload on ascending aortic blood velocity and acceleration in coronary artery disease. *Am. J. Cardiol.* 64:856–859, 1989.
14. Bennett, E. D., S. A. Barclay, A. L. Davis, D. Mannering, and N. Mehta. Ascending aortic blood velocity and acceleration using Doppler ultrasound in the assessment of left ventricular function. *Cardiovas. Res.* 18:632–638, 1984.
15. Bers, D. M. *Excitation-Contraction Coupling and Cardiac Contractile Force*, Norwell MA: Kluwer Academic Publishers, 1991: 155–158.
16. Beyar, R., J. L. Weiss, E. P. Shapiro, W. L. Graves, W. J. Rogers, and M. L. Weisfeldt. Small apex-to-base heterogeneity in radius-to-thickness ratio by three-dimensional magnetic resonance imaging. *Am. J. Physiol.* 264 (*Heart Circ. Physiol.* 33):H133–H140, 1993.
17. Bhargava, V., R. Shabetai, R. A. Mathiasen, N. Dalton, J. J. Hunter, and J. Ross, Jr. Loss of adrenergic control of the force-frequency relation in heart failure secondary to idiopathic or ischemic cardiomyopathy. *Am. J. Cardiol.* 81:1130–1137, 1998.
18. Bishop, V. S., L. D. Horwitz, H. L. Stone, H. F. Stegall, and E. J. Engelken. Left ventricular internal diameter and cardiac function in conscious dogs. *J. Appl. Physiol.* 27:619–623, 1969.
19. Blinks, J. R. and M. Endoch. Modification of myofibrillar responsiveness to Ca^{++} as an inotropic mechanism. *Circulation* 83:III85–III98, 1986.
20. Boerth, R. C., J. W. Covell, P. E. Pool, and J. J. Ross. Increased myocardial oxygen consumption and contractile state associated with increased heart rate in dogs. *Circ. Res.* 24:725–734, 1969.
21. Boerth, R. C., J. W. Covell, S. C. Seagren, and P. E. Pool. High energy phosphate concentrations in dog myocardium during stress. *Am. J. Physiol.* 216:1103–1106, 1969.
22. Boerth, R. C., K. E. Hammermeister, and J. R. Warbasse. Comparative influence of ouabain, norepinephrine and heart rate on myocardial oxygen consumption and inotropic state in dogs. *Am. Heart J.* 96:355–362, 1978.
23. Boettcher, D. H., S. F. Vatner, G. R. Heyndrikx, and E. Braunwald. Extent of utilization of the Frank-Starling mechanisms in conscious dogs. *Am. J. Physiol.* 234 (*Heart Circ. Physiol.* 3):338, 1978.
24. Bove, A. A. and P. R. Lynch. Radiographic determination of force-velocity-length relationship in the intact dog heart. *J. Appl. Physiol.* 29:884–888, 1970.
25. Bove, A. A. and P. R. Lynch. Measurement of canine left ventricular performance by cineradiography of the heart. *Appl. Physiol.* 29:887–883, 1970.
26. Bowditch, H. P. Uber die Eigenthumlichkeiten der Reizbarkeit welche die Muskelfasern des Herzens zeigen. *Arb. Physiol. Aust. Leipzig* 6:139–176, 1871.
27. Brady, A. J. Active state in cardiac muscle. *Physiol. Rev.* 48:570–600, 1968.
28. Brady, A. J. Mechanical properties of isolated cardiac myocytes. *Physiol. Rev.* 71:413–428, 1991.
29. Braunwald, E. and C. J. Frahm. Studies on Starling's law of heart, IV. Observations on hemodynamic functions of left atrium in man. *Circulation* 24:633–642, 1961.
30. Braunwald, E., J. Ross, Jr., and E. H. Sonnenblick. *Mechanisms of Contraction of the Normal and Failing Heart*, Boston: Little, Brown, 1976.
31. Braunwald, E., E. H. Sonnenblick, P. L. Frommer, and J. Ross, Jr. Paired electric stimulation of heart: physiologic observations and clinical implications. *Adv. Intern. Med.* 13:61–96, 1967.
32. Brilla, C. G., R. Pick, L. B. Tan, J. S. Janicki, and K. T. Weber. Remodeling of the rat right and left ventricle in experimental hypertension. *Circ. Res.* 67:1355–1364, 1990.
33. Bristow, M. R., R. Ginsburg, W. Minobe, R. S. Cubicciotti, W. S. Sageman, K. Lurie, M. E. Billingham, D. C. Harrison, and E. B. Stinson. Decreased catecholamine sensitivity and β-adrenergic-receptor density in failing human hearts. *N. Engl. J. Med.* 307:205–211, 1982.
34. Britman, N. A. and H. J. Levine. Contractile element work: a major determinant of myocardial oxygen consumption. *J. Clin. Invest.* 43:1397–1408, 1964.
35. Brock, R. Control mechanisms in the outflow tract of the right ventricle in health and disease. *Guy's Hosp. Rep.* 104:356–379, 1955.
36. Brutsaert, D. L., F. E. Rademaker, and S. U. Sys. Triple control of relaxation: implications in cardiac disease. *Circulation* 69:190–196, 1984.

37. Buchalter, M. B., J. L. Weiss, W. J. Rogers, E. Z. Zerhouni, M. L. Weisfeldt, R. Beyar, and E. P. Shapiro, Noninvasive quantification of left ventricular rotational deformation in normal humans using magnetic resonance imaging myocardial tagging. *Circulation* 81:1236–1244, 1990.
38. Buckley, N. M., Z. J. Penefsky, and R. S. Litwak. Comparative force-frequency relationships in human and other mammalian ventricular myocardium. *Pflugers Arch.* 332:259–270, 1972.
39. Burgeson, R. E. New collagens, new concepts. *Annu. Rev. Cell Biol.* 4:551–577, 1988.
40. Burkhoff, D., Sugiura, S., Yue, D. T., and Sagawa, K. Contractility-dependent curvilinearity of end-systolic pressure-volume relations. *Am. J. Physiol.* 252 (*Heart Circ. Physiol.* 21): H1218–1987.
41. Burkhoff, D., D. T. Yue, M. R. Frantz, W. C. Hunter, and K. Sagawa, Mechanical restitution of isolated perfused canine left ventricles. *Am. J. Physiol.* 246 (*Heart Circ. Physiol.* 15):H8–H16, 1984.
42. Burkhoff, D., D. T. Yue, M. R. Franz, W. C. Hunter, K. Sunagawa, W. L. Maughan, and K. Sagawa. Quantitative comparison of the force-interval relationship of the canine right and left ventricles. *Circ. Res.* 54:468–473, 1984.
43. Burns, J. W. and J. W. Covell. Myocardial oxygen consumption during isotonic and isovolumic contractions in the intact heart. *Am. J. Physiol.* 223:1491–1497, 1972.
44. Burns, J. W., J. W. Covell, R. Myers, and J. Ross, Jr. Comparison of directly measured left ventricular wall stress and stress calculated from geometric reference figures. *Circulation* 28:611–621, 1971.
45. Burns, J. W., J. W. Covell, and J. Ross, Jr. Mechanics of isotonic left ventricular contractions. *Am. J. Physiol.* 224:725–732, 1973.
46. Campbell, K. B., H. Taheri, R. D. Kirkpatrick, and B. H. Slinker. Single perturbed beat vs. steady-state beats for assessing systolic function in the isolated heart. *Am. J. Physiol.* 262 (*Heart Circ. Physiol.* 31):H1631–H1639, 1992.
47. Cannon, R. O., J. W. Butany, B. M. McManus, E. Speir, A. B. Kravitz, R. Bolli, and V. J. Ferrans. Early degradation of collagen after acute myocardial infarction in the rat. *Am. J. Cardiol.* 52: 390–395, 1983.
48. Caulfield, J. B. and T. K. Borg. The collagen network of the heart. *Lab. Invest.* 40:364–372, 1979.
49. Caulfield, J. B. and P. E. Wolkowicz. Inducible collagenolytic activity in isolated, perfused rat hearts. *Am. J. Pathol.* 131:199–205, 1988.
50. Caulfield, J. B. and P. E. Wolkowicz. Myocardial connective tissue alterations. *Toxicol. Pathol.* 18:488–496, 1990.
51. Chapman, C. B., O. Baker, J. Reynolds, and F. J. Bonte. Use of biplane cinefluorography for measurement of ventricular volume. *Circulation* 18:1105–1117, 1958.
52. Chapman, J. B., C. L. Gibbs, and D. S. Loiselle. Myothermic, polarographic, and fluorometric data from mammalian muscles. *Federation Proc.* 41:176–184, 1982.
53. Chappius, F., T. Widmann, B. Guth, P. Nicod, and K. L. Peterson. Quantitative assessment of regional left ventricular function by densitometric analysis of digital-subtraction ventriculograms: correlation with myocardial systolic shortening in dogs. *Circulation* 77:457–467, 1988.
54. Cheng, C.-P., Y. Igarashi, and W. C. Little. Mechanism of augmented rate of left ventricular filling during exercise. *Am. J. Physiol.* 262 (*Heart Circ. Physiol.* 31):9–19, 1992.
55. Choung, C. J. and Y. C. Fung. Residual stress in arteries. In: *Frontiers in Biomechanics*, edited by G. W. Schmid-Schoenbein, S. L.-Y. Woo, and B. W. Zweifach. New York: Springer-Verlag, 1986:117–129.
56. Cittadini, A., H. Stromer, S. E. Katz, R. Clark, A. C. Moses, J. P. Morgan, and P. S. Douglas. Differential cardiac effects of growth hormone and insulin-like growth factor-1 in the rat. *Circulation* 93:800–809, 1996.
57. Clancy, R. L., T. P. Graham, Jr. Ross, J., E. H. Sonnenblick, and E. Braunwald. The influence of aortic pressure-induced hemometric autoregulation on myocardial performance. *Am. J. Physiol.* 214:1186–1192, 1968.
58. Clark, N., N. Reichek, P. Bergey, E. Hoffman, D. Brownson, L. Palmon, and L. Axel. Circumferential myocardial shortening in the normal human left ventricle: Assessment by magnetic resonance imaging using spatial modulation of magnetization. *Circulation* 84:67–74, 1991.
59. Cohn, P. F., A. J. Liedtke, J. Serur, E. H. Sonnenblick, and C. W. Urschel. Maximal rate of pressure fall (peak negative dP/dt) during ventricular relaxation. *Cardiovasc. Res.* 6:263–267, 1972.
60. Coleman, H. N., R. R. Taylor, P. E. Pool, G. H. Whipple, J. W. Covell, J. Ross, Jr., and E. Braunwald. Congestive heart failure following chronic tachycardia. *Am. Heart J.* 81:790–798, 1971.
60a. Costa K. D., Y. Takayama, A. D. McCulloch, and J. W. Covell. Laminar Fiber Architecture and Three-Dimensional Systolic Mechanics in Canine Ventricular Myocardium. *AJP*, 276(45): H595–H607, 1999.
61. Covell, J. W., J. Ross, Jr., R. Taylor, E. H. Sonnenblick, and E. Braunwald. Effects of increasing frequency of contraction on force-velocity relation of left ventricle. *Cardiovasc. Res.* 1:2–8, 1967.
62. Covell, J. W., J. Ross, Jr., E. H. Sonnenblick, and E. Braunwald. Comparison of force-velocity relation and ventricular function curve as measures of contractile state of intact heart. *Circulation* 19:364–372, 1966.
63. Covell, J. W., R. R. Taylor, E. H. Sonnenblick, and J. J. Ross. Series elasticity in the intact heart. Evidence for application of the Hill model for muscle to the intact left ventricle. *Pflugers Arch.* 357:225–235, 1975.
64. Davidson, D. M., J. W. Covell, C. I. Malloch, and J. Ross, Jr. Factors influencing indices of left ventricular contractility in the conscious dog. *Cardiovasc. Res.* 8:299–312, 1974.
65. De Simone, G., D. C. Wallerson, M. Volpe, and R. B. Devereux, Echocardiographic measurement of left ventricular mass and volume in normotensive and hypertensive rats. *Am. J. Hypertens.* 3:688–696, 1990.
66. Dillon, J. C., S. Chang, and H. Feigenbaum. Echocardiographic manifestations of left bundle branch block. *Circulation* 49:876 1974.
67. Dodge, H. T. and W. A. Baxley. Left ventricular volume and mass and their significance in heart disease. *Am. J. Cardiol.* 23: 528–537, 1969.
68. Dodge, H. T., R. E. Hay, and H. Sandler. An angiocardiographic method for directly determining left ventricular stroke volume in man. *Circulation Res.* 11:739–745, 1962.
69. Dodge, H. T., H. Sandler, D. W. Ballew, and Lord, Jr. The use of biplane angiocardiography for measurement of left ventricular volume in man. *Am. Heart J.* 60:762–776, 1960.
70. Douglas, A. S., W. C. Hunter, and M. C. Wiseman. Inhomogeneous deformation as a source of error in strain measurements derived from implanted markers in the canine left ventricle. *J. Biomech.* 23:331–341, 1990.
71. Dumesnil, J. G. and R. M. Shoucri. Quantitative relationships between left ventricular ejection and wall thickening and geometry. *J. Appl. Physiol.* 70:48–54, 1991.
72. Edman, K. A. P. and M. Johannsson. The contractile state of rabbit papillary muscle in relation to stimulation frequency. *J. Physiology. (Lond.)* 254:565–581, 1976.
73. Eising, G. P., H. K. Hammond, G. A. Helmer, E. Gilpin, and J. Ross, Jr. Force-frequency relations during heart failure in the pig. *Am. J. Physiol.* 267 (*Heart Circ. Physiol.* 36):H2516–H2522, 1994.

74. Elizinga, G. and N. Westerhof. The effect of an increase in inotropic state and end-diastolic volume on the pumping ability of the feline left heart. *Circ. Res.* 42:620–628, 1978.
75. Fabiato, A. and F. Fabiato. Myofilament-generated tension oscillations during partial calcium activation and activation dependence of the sarcomere length-tension relation of skinned cardiac cells. *J. Gen. Physiol.* 72:667–699, 1978.
76. Factor, S. M., M. Flomenbaum, M. J. Zhao, C. Eng, and T. F. Robinson. The effects of acutely increased ventricular cavity pressure on intrinsic myocardial connective tissue. *J. Am. Coll. Card.* 12:1582–1589, 1988.
77. Feigenbaum, H. *Echocardiography*. Philadelphia: Lea & Febriger, 1986.
78. Feigl, E. O. and D. L. Fry. Intramural myocardial shear during the cardiac cycle. *Circ. Res.* 14:536–540, 1964.
79. Feldman, M. D., J. D. Alderman, J. M. Aroesty, H. D. Royal, J. J. Ferguson, R. M. Owen, W. Grossman, and R. G. McKay. Depression of systolic and diastolic myocardial reserve during atrial pacing tachycardia in patients with dilated cardiomyopathy. *J. Clin. Invest.* 82:1661–1669, 1988.
80. Feneis, H. Das Gefuge des Herzmuskels bei Systole und Diastole. *Morphol. Jahrbuch.* 89:371, 1943.
81. Fenton, T. R., J. M. Cherry, and G. A. Klassen. Transmural myocardial deformation in the canine left ventricular wall. *Am. J. Physiol.* 235 (*Heart Circ. Physiol.* 4):H524–H530, 1978.
82. Frank, O. Zur Dynamik des Herzmuskels. *Z. Biol.* 32:370–437, 1895.
83. Freeman, G. L. Effects of increased afterload on left ventricular function in closed-chest dogs. *Am. J. Physiol.* 259 (*Heart Circ. Physiol.* 28):H619–H625, 1990.
84. Freeman, G. L. and J. T. Colston. Evaluation of left ventricular mechanical restitution in closed-chest dogs based on single beat elastance. *Circ. Res.* 67:1437–1445, 1990.
85. Freeman, G. L. and J. T. Colston. Evaluation of long-term variance of left ventricular performance indexes in closed-chest dogs. *Am. J. Physiol.* 257 (*Heart Circ. Physiol.* 26):H70–H78, 1990.
86. Freeman, G. L., W. C. Little, and R. A. O'Rouke. Influence of heart rate on left ventricular performance in conscious dogs. *Circ. Res.* 61:464, 1987.
87. Freeman, G. L., W. C. Little, and R. A. O'Rourke. The effects of vasoactive agents on the left ventricular end-systolic pressure-volume relation in closed-chest dogs. *Circulation* 74:1107, 1986.
88. Furnival, C. M., R. J. Linden, and H. M. Snow. Inotropic changes in the left ventricle: the effect of changes in heart rate, aortic pressure and end-diastolic pressure. *J. Physiol. (Lond.)* 211:359–387, 1970.
89. Gaasch, W. H. Passive elastic properties of the left ventricle. In: *Left Ventricular Diastolic Dysfunction and Heart Failure*, edited by W. H. Gaasch and M. M. LeWinter. Philadelphia: Lea & Febiger, 1994:143–149.
90. Gaasch, W. H., A. S. Blaustein, C. W. Andrias, R. P., Donahue, and B. Avitall. Myocardial relaxation, II: hemodynamic determinants of rate of left ventricular isovolumic pressure decline. *Am. J. Physiol.* 239 (*Heart Circ. Physiol.* 8):H1–H6, 1980.
91. Gallagher, K. P., R. A. Gerren, M. C. Stirling, M. Choy, R. C. Dysko, S. P. McManimon, and W. R. Dunham. The distribution of functional impairment across the lateral border of acutely ischemic myocardium. *Circ. Res.* 58:570–583, 1986.
92. Gallagher, K. P., G. Osakada, M. Matsuzaki, M. Miller, W. S. Kemper, and J. Ross, Jr. Nonuniformity of inner and outer systolic wall thickening in conscious dogs. *Am. J. Physiol.* 249 (*Heart Circ. Physiol.* 18):H241–H248, 1985.
93. Gallagher, K. P., M. C. Stirling, M. Choy, C. A. Szpunar, R. A. Gerren, M. J. Botham, and J. H. Lemmer. Dissociation between epicardial and transmural function during acute myocardial ischemia. *Circulation.* 71:1279–1291, 1985.
94. Gardin, J. M., F. M. Siri, R. N. Kitsis, J. G. Edwards, and L. A. Leinwand. Echocardiographic assessment of left ventricular mass and systolic function in mice. *Circ. Res.* 76:907–914, 1995.
95. Gathercole, L. J. and A. Keller. Crimp morphology in fiber forming tissues. *Matrix* 11:214–234, 1991.
96. Gault, J. H., J. W. Covell, E. Braunwald, and J. Ross, Jr. Left ventricular performance following correction of free aortic regurgitation. *Circulation.* 42:773–780, 1970.
97. Gault, J. H., J. J. Ross, and E. Braunwald. Contractile state of the left ventricle in man. *Circ. Res.* 22:451–463, 1968.
98. Georgakopoulos, D. and D. A. Kass. Estimation of parallel conductance by dual-frequency conductance catheter in mice. *Am. J. Physiol.* 279 (*Heart Circ Physiol.* 48):H443–H450, 2000.
99. Georgakopoulos, D. W. A. Mitner, C. Chen-Huan, B. J. Byrne, H. D. Millar, J. M. Hare, and D. A. Kass. In vivo murine left ventricular pressure-volume relations by miniaturized conductance micromanometry. *Am. J. Physiol.* 274 (*Heart Circ. Physiol.* 43):H1416–H1422, 1998.
100. Gibbs, C. L. Cardiac energetics. *Physiol. Rev.* 581:174–254, 1978.
101. Gibbs, C. L. Mechanical determinants of myocardial oxygen consumption. *Clin. Exp. Pharmacol. Physiol.* 22:1–9, 1995.
102. Gibbs, C. L. and J. B. Chapman. Cardiac Energicts. In: *Handbook of Physiology: Circulation*, Washington, D.C.: American Physiology Society, 1979:775–804.
103. Glantz, S. A. and W. W. Parmley. Factors which affect the diastolic pressure-volume curve. *Circ. Res.* 42:171–180, 1978.
104. Glower, D. D., J. A. Spratt, N. D. Snow, J. S. Kabas, J. W. Davis, C. O. Olsen, G. S. Tyson, D. C. Sabiston, and J. S. Rankin. Linearity of the Frank-Starling relationship in the intact heart: the concept of preload recruitable stroke work. *Circulation.* 71:994–1009, 1985.
105. Goldblatt, A., D. C. Harrison, G. Glick, and E. Braunwald. Studies on cardiac dimensions in intact, unanesthetized man. II. Effects of respiration. *Circ. Res.* 13:455–560, 1963.
106. Gosselink, M. A. T., P. K. Blanksma, H. J. G. M. Crijns, I. C. Van Gelder, P.-J. De Kam, H. L. Hillege, M. G. Neimeijer, K. I. Lie, and F. L. Meijler. Left ventricular beat-to-beat performance in atrial fibrillation: contribution of Frank-Starling mechanics after short rather than long RR intervals. *J. Am. Coll. Cardiol.* 26:1516–1521, 1995.
107. Goto, Y., B. K. Slinker, and M. M. LeWinter. Similar normalized E_{max} and O_2 consumption-pressure-volume area relation in rabbit and dog. *Am. J. Physiol.* 254 (*Heart Circ. Physiol.* 23):H366–H374, 1988.
108. Gould, K. L., J. W. Kennedy, M. Frimer, G. H. Pollack, and H. T. Dodge. Analysis of wall dynamics and directional components of left ventricular contraction in man. *Am. J. Cardiol.* 38:322–331, 1976.
109. Graham, T. P., J. W. Covell, E. H. Sonnenblick, J. J. Ross, and E. Braunwald. Control of myocardial oxygen consumption: relative influence of contractile state and tension development. *J. Clin. Invest.* 47:375–385, 1968.
110. Grimm, A. F. and W. V. Whitehorn. Characteristics of resting tension of myocardium and localization of ite elements. *Am. J. Physiol.* 210:1362–1368, 1966.
111. Grossman, W., D. Jones, and L. P. McLaurin. Wall stress and patterns of hypertrophy in the human left ventricle. *J. Clin. Invest.* 56:56–64, 1975.
112. Guccione, J. M., A. D. McCulloch, and L. K. Waldman. Passive material properties of intact ventricular myocardium determined from a cylindrical model. *J. Biomed. Eng.* 113:42–55, 1991.
113. Guyton, A. C., C. E. Jones, and T. G. Coleman. Cardiac output

in muscular exercise. In: *Circulatory Physiology: Cardiac Output and Its Regulation*, edited by A. C. Guyton, C. E. Jones, and T. G. Coleman. Philadelphia: W. B. Saunders, 1973:436–482.

114. Hammond, H. K., F. C. White, V. Bhargava, and R. Shabetai. Heart size and maximal cardiac-output are limited by the pericardium. *Am. J. Physiol.* 263 (*Heart Circ. Physiol.* 32): H1675–H1681, 1992.

115. Hanley, P. J., P. J. Cooper, and D. S. Loiselle. Energetic effects of caffeine in face of retarded Na^+/Ca^{2+} exchange in isolated, arrested guinea pig hearts. *Am. J. Physiol.* 267 (*Heart Circ. Physiol.* 36):H1663–H1669, 1994.

116. Hansen, D. E., G. T. Daughters, E. L. Alderman, N. B. Ingels, Jr., and D. C. Miller. Torsional deformation of the left ventricular midwall in human hearts with intramyocardial markers: regional heterogeneity and sensitivity to the inotropic effects of abrupt rate changes. *Circ. Res.* 62:941–952, 1988.

117. Hansen, D. E., G. T. Daughters, E. L. Alderman, E. B. Stinson, J. C. Baldwin, and D. C. Miller. Effect of acute human cardiac allograft rejection on left ventricular systolic torsion and diastolic recoil measured by intramyocardial markers. *Circulation.* 76:998–1008, 1987.

118. Harrison, D. C., A. Goldblatt, and E. Braunwald. Studies on cardiac dimensions in intact, unanesthetized man. I. Description of techniques and their validation. *Circ. Res.* 13:448–455, 1963.

119. Harrison, M. R., G. D. Clifton, M. R. Berk, and A. N. DeMaria. Effect of blood pressure and afterload on Doppler echocardiographic measurements of left ventricular systolic function in normal subjects. *Am. J. Cardiol.* 64:905–908, 1989.

120. Hartley, C. J., L. A. Latson, L. H. Michael, C. L. Seidel, R. M. Lewis, and M. L. Entman. Doppler measurement of myocardial thickening with a single epicardial transducer. *Am. J. Physiol.* 245 (*Heart Circ. Physiol.* 14):H1066–H1072, 1983.

121. Hashima, A. R., A. A. Young, and A. D. McCulloch. Nonhomogeneous analysis of epicardial strain distributions during acute myocardial ischemia in the dog. *J. Biomech.* 26:19–35, 1993.

122. Hawthorne, E. W. Instantaneous dimensional changes of the left ventricle in dogs. *Circ. Res.* 9:110–119, 1961.

123. Hess, O. M., V. Bhargava, J. J. Ross, and R. Shabetai. The role of the pericardium in interactions between the cardiac chambers. *Am. Heart J.* 106:1377–1385, 1983.

124. Higginbotham, M. B., K. G. Morris, S. Williams, P. A. McHale, R. E. Coleman, and F. R. Cobb. Regulation of stroke volume during submaximal and maximal upright exercise in normal man. *Circ. Res.* 58:281–291, 1986.

125. Higgins, C. B., S. F. Vatner, D. Franklin, and E. Braunwald. Extent of regulation of the heart's contractile state in the conscious dog by alteration in the frequency of contraction. *J. Clin. Invest.* 52:1187–1194, 1973.

126. Hinds, J. E., E. W. Hawthorne, C. B. Mullins, and J. H. Mitchell. Instantaneous changes in the left ventricular lengths occurring in dogs during the cardiac cycle. *Federation Proc.* 28:1351–1357, 1969.

127. Hoffman, B. F., A. L. Bassett, and H. J. Bartelstone. Some mechanical properties of isolated mammalian cardiac muscle. *Circ. Res.* 23:219–312, 1968.

128. Hoffman, B. F., E. Bindler, and E. E. Suckling. Postextrasystolic potentiation of contraction in cardiac muscle. *Am. J. Physiol.* 185:95–102, 1956.

129. Hoffman, E. A. and E. L. Ritman. Invariant total heart volume in the intact thorax. *Am. J. Physiol.* 249 (*Heart Circ. Physiol.* 18):H883–H890, 1985.

130. Hoit, B. D., S. F. Khoury, E. G. Kranias, N. Ball, and R. A. Walsh. In vivo echocardiographic detection of enhanced left ventricular function in gene-targeted mice with phospholamban deficiency.*Circ. Res.* 77:632–637, 1995.

130a. Hongo, M., T. Ryoke, J. R. Schoenfeld, J. J. Hunter, N. Dalton, R. G. Clark, D. G. Lowe, K. R. Chien, and J. Ross Jr. Effects of growth hormone on cardiac dysfunction and gene expression in genetic murine dilated cardiomyopathy. *Basic Res. Cardiol.* 95:431–441, 2000.

130b. Holmes, J. W., J. P. Nunez and J. W. Covell. Functional implications of myocardial scar structure. *AJP* 272(41):H2123–H2130, 1997.

131. Hort, W. Untersuchungen uber die Muskelfaserdehnung und das Gefuge des Myokards in der rechten Herzkammerwand des Meerschweinchens. *Vichows Arch. Pathol. Anat. Physiol. Klin. Med.* 329:649–731, 1957.

132. Hort, W. Makroskopische und mikrometrische Untersuchungen am Myokard verschieden stark gefullter linker Kammern. *Virchows Arch. Pathol. Anat. Physiol. Klin. Med.* 333:523–564, 1960.

133. Humphrey, J. D., R. K. Strumpf, and F. C. P. Yin. Determination of a constitutive relation for passive myocardium: I. A new functional form. *J. Biomed. Eng.* 112:333–339, 1990.

134. Hunter, P. J., P. M. F. Nielsen, B. H. Smaill, I. J. LeGrice, and I. W. Hunter. An anatomical heart model with applications to myocardial activation and ventricular mechanics. In:*High Performance Computing in Biomedical Research*, edited by T. C. Pilkington. Boca Raton: CRC Press, 1993:3–26.

135. Ingels, N. B., Jr., G. T. Daughters, E. B. Stinson, and E. L. Alderman. Measurement of midwall myocardial dynamics in intact man by radiography of surgically implanted markers. *Circulation* 52:859–867, 1975.

136. Ingels, N. B., Jr., G. T. Daughters, E. B. Stinson, E. L. Alderman, and D. C. Miller. Three-dimensional left ventricular midwall dynamics in the transplanted human heart. *Circulation* 81:1837–1848, 1990.

137. Ingels, N. B., Jr., D. E. Hansen, G. T. Daughters, E. B. Stinson, E. L. Alderman, and D. C. Miller. Relation between longitudinal, circumferential, and oblique shortening and torsional deformation in the left ventricle of the transplanted human heart. *Circ. Res.* 64:915–927, 1989.

138. Ishida, Y., J. S. Meisner, K. Tsujioka, J. I. Gallo, C. Yoran, R. W. Frater, and E. L. Yellin. Left ventricular filling dynamics: influence of left ventricular relaxation and left atrial pressure. *Circulation* 74:187–196, 1986.

139. Janicki, J. S. and K. T. Weber. Ejection pressure and the diastolic left ventricular pressure-volume relation. *Am. J. Physiol.* 232 (*Heart Circ. Physiol.* 1):H545–H552, 1977.

140. Janicki, J. S. and K. T. Weber. Factors influencing the diastolic pressure-volume relation of the cardiac ventricle. *Federation Proc.* 39:133–140, 1980.

141. Julian, F. J., M. R. Sollins, and R. L. Moss. Absence of a plateau in length-tension relationship of rabbit papillary muscle when internal shortening is prevented. *Nature* 26:340–342, 1976.

142. Kahn, M. L., F. Kavaler, and V. J. Fisher. Frequency-force relationships of mammalian ventricular muscle in vivo and in vitro. *Am. J. Physiol.* 230:631–636, 1976.

143. Kambayashi, M., T. Miura, B. H. Oh, H. A. Rockman, K. Murata, and J. Ross, Jr. Enhancement of force-frequency effect on myocardial contractility by adrenergic stimulation in conscious dogs. *Circulation* 86:572–580, 1992.

144. Karliner, J. S., R. J. Bouchard, and J. H. Gault. Dimensional changes of the human left ventricle prior to aortic valve opening: a cineangiographic study in patients with and without left heart disease. *Circulation.* 44:312–322, 1971.

145. Karliner, J. S., J. H. Gault, D. L. Eckberg, C. B. Mullins, and J. Ross, Jr. Mean velocity of fiber shortening: a simplified measure

of left ventricular myocardial contractility. *Circulation* 44:323–333, 1971.
146. Karliner, J. S., M. M. LeWinter, F. Mahler, R. Engler, and R. A. O'Rourke. Pharmacologic and hemodynamic influences on the rat of isovolumic left ventricular relaxation in the normal conscious dog. *J. Clin. Invest.* 60:511–521, 1977.
147. Kass, D. A. Clinical evaluation of left heart function by conductance catheter technique. *Eur. Heart J.* 13:57–64, 1992.
148. Kass, D. A. and R. P. Kelly. Ventriculo-arteral coupling: concepts, assumptions, and applications. *Ann. Biomed. Eng.* 20: 41–62, 1992.
149. Kass, D. A. and W. L. Maughan. From 'Emax' to pressure-volume relations: a broader view. *Circulation* 77:1203–1212, 1988.
150. Kass, D. A., W. L. Maughan, Z. M. Guo, A. Kono, K. Sunagawa, and K. Sagawa. Comparative influence of load versus inotropic states on indexes of ventricular contractility: experimental and theoretical analysis based on pressure-volume relationships. *Circulation* 76:1422–1436, 1987.
151. Katz, A. M. The descending limb of the Starling curve and the failing heart (Editorial). *Circulation* 32:871–875, 1965.
151a. Karlon, J. W., A. M. McCulloch, J. W. Covell, J. J. Hunter, and J. H. Omens. Regional dysfunction correlates with myofiber disarray in transgenic mice with ventricular expression of ras. *AJP* 278:H898–H906, 2000.
152. Keith, A. Fate of the bulbus cordis in the human heart. *Lancet* 2:1267–1273, 1924.
153. Kennedy, J. W., W. A. Baxley, M. M. Figley, H. T. Dodge, and J. R. Blackman. Quantitative angiocardiography. I. The normal left ventricle in man. *Circulation* 34:272–278, 1966.
154. Kentish, J. C., H. E. D. J. ter Keurs, L. Ricciardi, J. J. J. Bucx, and M. I. M. Noble. Comparison between the sarcomere length-force relations of intact and skinned trabeculae from rat right ventricle. *Circ. Res.* 58:755–768, 1986.
155. Keren, G., J. Sherez, R. Megidish, B. Levitt, and S. Laniado. Pulmonary venous flow pattern—its relationship to cardiac dynamics. A pulsed Doppler echocardiographic study. *Circulation* 71:1105–1112, 1985.
156. Klocke, F. J., E. Braunwald, and J. J. Ross. Oxygen cost of electrical activation of the heart. *Circ. Res.* 18:357–365, 1966.
157. Koch-Weser, J. and J. R. Blinks. The influence of the interval between beats on myocardial contractility. *Pharmacol. Rev.* 15: 601–652, 1963.
158. Komamura, K., R. P. Shannon, T. Ihara, Y. T. Shen, I. Mirsky, S. P. Bishop, and S. F. Vatner. Exhaustion of Frank-Starling mechanism in conscious dogs with heart failure. *Am. J. Physiol.* 265 (*Heart Circ. Physiol.* 34):H1119–H1131, 1993.
159. Kong, Y., J. J. Morris, and H. D. McIntosh. Assessment of regional myocardial performance from biplane coronary cineangiograms. *Am. J. Cardiol.* 27:529–537, 1971.
160. Koteliansky, V. E., V. P. Shirinsky, G. N. Gneushev, and M. A. Chernousov. The role of actin-binding proteins vinculin, filamin, and fibronectin in intracellular and intercellular linkages in cardiac muscle. *Adv. Myocardiol.* 5:215–221, 1985.
161. Kwan, K. M. and S. L.-Y. Woo. A structural model to describe the nonlinear stress strain behavior for parallel-fibered collagenous tissues. *no journal*. 111:361–363, 1989.
162. Lakatta, E. G. Starling's law of the heart is explained by an intimate interaction of muscle length and myofilament calcium activation. *J. Am. Coll. Card.* 10:1157–1164, 1987.
163. Lee, J. D., T. Tajimi, J. Patritti, and J. Ross, Jr. Preload reserve and mechanisms of afterload mismatch in the normal conscious dog. *Am. J. Physiol.* 250 (*Heart Circ. Physiol.* 19):H464, 1986.
164. LeGrice, I. J., B. H. Smaill, L. Z. Chai, S. G. Edgar, J. B. Gavin, and P. J. Hunter. Laminar structure of the heart: ventricular myocyte arrangement and connective tissue architecture in the dog. *Am. J. Physiol.* 269 (*Heart Circ. Physiol.* 38):H571, 1995.
165. LeGrice, I. J., Y. Takayama, and J. W. Covell. Transverse shear along myocardial cleavage planes provides a mechanism for normal systolic wall thickening. *Circ. Res.* 77:182–193, 1995.
166. LeGrice, I. J., Y. Takayama, J. W. Holmes, and J. W. Covell. Impaired subendocardial function in tachycardia induced cardiac failure. *Am. J. Physiol.* 268 (*Heart Circ. Physiol.* 37): H1788–H1794, 1995.
167. Leite-Moreira, A. F. and T. C. Gillebert. Nonuniform course of left ventricular pressure fall and its regulation by load and contractile state. *Circulation* 90:2481–2491, 1994.
168. Lendrum, B., H. Feinberg, E. Boyd, and L. N. Katz. Rhythm effects on contractility of beating isovolumic left ventricle. *Am. J. Physiol.* 199:1115–1120, 1960.
169. Lew, W. Y. Time-dependent increase in the left ventricular contractility following acute volume loading in the dog. *Circ. Res.* 63:635–647, 1988.
170. Lew, W. Y. Mechanisms of volume-induced increase in left ventricular contractility. *Am. J. Physiol.* 265 (*Heart Circ. Physiol.* 34):H1778–H1786, 1993.
171. Lew, W. Y. and M. M. LeWinter. Regional comparison of midwall segment and area shortening in the canine left ventricle. *Circ. Res.* 58:678–691, 1986.
172. LeWinter, M. M., R. Engler, and R. S. Pavelec. Time-dependent shifts of the left ventricular diastolic filling relationship in conscious dogs. *Circ. Res.* 45:641–653, 1979.
173. LeWinter, M. M., R. S. Kent, J. M. Kroener, T. E. Carew, and J. W. Covell. Regional differences in myocardial performance in the left ventricle of the dog. *Circ. Res.* 37:191–199, 1975.
174. LeWinter, M. M. and R. Pavelec. Influence of the pericardium on left ventricular end-diastolic pressure-segment length relations during early and late stages of experimental chronic volume overloads in dogs. *Circ. Res.* 50:501–509, 1982.
175. Liedtke, J. A., J. H. Gault, D. M. Leman, and M. S. Blumenthal. Geometry of left ventricular contraction in the systolic click syndrome. *Circulation* 47:27–35, 1973.
176. Lima, J. A. C., R. Jeremy, W. Guier, S. Bouton, E. A. Zerhouni, E. McVeigh, M. B. Buchalter, M. L. Weisfeldt, E. P. Shapiro, and J. L. Weiss. Accurate systolic wall thickening by nuclear magnetic resonance imaging with tissue tagging: correlation with sonomicrometers in normal and ischemic myocardium. *J. Am. Coll. Cardiol.* 21:1741–1751, 1993.
177. Limoto, D. S., J. W. Covell, and E. Harper. Increase in cross-linking of type I and type III collagens associated with volume overload hypertrophy. *Circ. Res.* 63:399–408, 1988.
178. Linden, R. J. and J. H. Mitchell. Relationship between left ventricular diastolic pressure and myocardial segment length and observations on contribution of atrial systole. *Circ. Res.* 8: 1092–1099, 1960.
179. Linderer, T., K. Chatterjee, W. W. Parmlee, R. E. Sievers, S. A. Glantz, and J. V. Tyberg. Influence of atrial systole on the Frank-Starling relation and the end-diastolic pressure-diameter relation of the left ventricle. *Circulation* 67:1045–10536, 1983.
180. Linke, W. A., V. I. Popov, and G. H. Pollack. Passive and active tension in single cardiac myofibrils. *Biophys. J.* 67:782–792, 1994.
181. Little, W. C. The left ventricular dP/dt_{max} end-diastolic volume relation in closed-chest dogs. *Circ. Res.* 56:808–815, 1985.
182. Litwin, S. E., T. E. Raya, S. Daugherty, and S. Goldman. Peripheral circulatory control of cardiac output in diabetic rats. *Am. J. Physiol.* 261 (*Heart Circ. Physiol.* 30):H836–H842, 1991.
183. Liu, Z., D. R. Hilbelink, W. B. Crockett, and A. M. Gerdes. Regional changes in hemodynamics and cardiac myocyte size

in rats with aortocaval fistulas. 1. Developing and established hypertrophy. *Circ. Res.* 69:52–58, 1991.
184. Loeffler, L. and K. Sagawa. A one-dimensional viscoelastic model of cat heart muscle studied by small length perturbations during isometric contraction. *Circ. Res.* 36:498–512, 1975.
185. Loiselle, D. S. Cardiac basal and activation metabolisms. In: *Cardiac Energetics Basic Mechanisms and Clinical Implications*, edited by R. Jacob and H. Just. Darmstadt: Verlag, 37–50, 1987.
186. Lorenz, J. N. and J. Robbins. Measurement of intraventricular pressure and cardiac performance in the intact closed-chest anesthetized mouse. *Am J. Physiol.* 272 (*Heart Circ. Physiol.* 41): H1137–H1146 1997.
187. Ludin, G. Mechanical properties of cardiac muscle. *Acta. Physiol. Scand.* 7:1–85, 1944.
188. MacCallum, J. B. On the muscular architecture and growth of the ventricles of the heart. *Johns Hopkins Hosp. Rep.* 9:307–335, 1900.
189. MacGregor, D. C., J. W. Covell, F. Mahler, R. B. Dilley, and J. Ross, Jr. Relations between afterload, stroke volume, and the descending limb of Starling's curve. *Am. J. Physiol.* 227:884–890, 1974.
190. MacKenna, D. A., J. H. Omens, A. D. McCulloch, and J. W. Covell. Contribution of collagen matrix to passive left ventricular mechanics in isolated rat hearts. *Am. J. Physiol.* 266 (*Heart Circ. Physiol.* 35):H1007–H1018, 1994.
191. Mahler, F., J. W. Covell, R. A. O'Rouke, and J. Ross, Jr. Effects of acute changes in loading and inotropic state on left ventricular performance and contractility measures in the conscious dog. *Am. J. Cardiol.* 35:626–634, 1975.
192. Mahler, F., J. W. Covell, and J. Ross, Jr. Systolic pressure-diameter relations in the normal conscious dog. *Cardiovasc. Res.* 9:447–455, 1975.
193. Mall, F. P. On the muscular architecture of the ventricles of the human heart. *Am. J. Anat.* 11:211–266, 1911.
194. Manning, W. J., J. Y. Wei, S. E. Katz, S. E. Litwin, and P. S. Douglas. In vivo assessment of LV mass in mice using high-frequency cardiac ultrasound: necropsy validation. *Am. J. Physiol.* 266 (*Heart Circ. Physiol.* 35):H1672–H1675, 1994.
195. March, H. W., J. K. Ross, and R. R. Lower. Observations on the behavior of the right ventricular outflow tract, with reference to its developmental origins. *Am. J. Med.* 32:835–845, 1962.
196. Maruyama, Y., K. Ashikawa, S. Isoyama, H. Kanatsuka, E. Ion-Oka, and T. Takishima. Mechanical interactions between four heart chambers with and without the pericardium in canine hearts. *Circ. Res.* 50:86–100, 1982.
197. Mason, D. T. Usefulness and limitations of the rate of rise of intraventricular pressure (dp/dt) in the evaluation of myocardial contractility in man. *Am. J. Cardiol.* 23:516–527, 1969.
198. Maughan, W. L., K. Sunagawa, D. Burkhoff, and K. Sagawa. Effect of arterial impedance changes on the end-systolic pressure-volume relation. *Circ. Res.* 54:595, 1984.
199. May-Newman, K., J. H. Omens, R. S. Pavelec, and A. D. McCulloch. Three-dimensional transmural mechanical interaction between the coronary vasculature and passive myocardium in the dog. *Circ. Res.* 74:1166–1178, 1994.
200. McCulloch, A. D. and J. H. Omens. Non-homogeneous analysis of three-dimensional transmural finite deformation in canine ventricular myocardium. *J. Biomech.* 24:539–548, 1991.
201. Medugorac, I. Myocardial collagen in different forms of hypertrophy in the rat. *Res. Exp. Med. (Berl).* 177:201–211, 1980.
202. Medugorac, I. Characterization of intramuscular collagen in mammalian left ventricle. *Basic Res. Cardiol.* 77:589–598, 1982.
203. Meier, G. D., A. A. Bove, W. P. Santamore, and P. R. Lynch. Contractile function in canine right ventricle. *Am. J. Physiol.* 239 (*Heart Circ. Physiol.* 8):H794–H804, 1980.
204. Meier, G. D., M. C. Ziskin, W. P. Santamore, and A. A. Bove. Kinematics of the beating heart. *IEEE Trans. Biomed. Eng.* 27: 319–329, 1980.
205. Meisner, J. S., O. E. Pajaro, and E. L. Yellin. Investigation of left ventricular filling dynamics: development of a model. *Einstein Q. J. Biol. Med.* 4:47–57, 1986.
205a. Mazhari, R., J. H. Omens, J. Covell and A. D. McCulloch. Structural basis of regional dysfunction in acutely ischemic myocardium. *Cardiovasc. Res.* 284–293, 2000.
206. Milnor, W. R. Arterial impedance as ventricular afterload. *Circ. Res.* 36:565–570, 1975.
206a. Minamisawa, S., M. Hoshijima, G. Chu, C. A. Ward, K. Frank, Y. Gu, M. E. Martone, Y. Wang, J. Ross, Jr., E. G. Kranias, W. R. Giles, and K. R. Chien. Chronic phospholamban-sarcoplasmic reticulum calcium ATPase interaction is the critical calcium cycling defect in dilated cardiomyopathy. *Cell* 99: 313–322, 1999.
207. Mirsky, I. Left ventricular stresses in the intact human heart. *Biophysics* 9:189–208, 1969.
208. Mirsky, I. Basic terminology and formulae for left ventricular wall stress. In:*Cardiac Mechanics: Physiological, Clinical and Mathematical Considerations*, edited by I. Mirsky, D. Ghista, and H. Sandler. New York: Wiley, 1974:3–10.
209. Mirsky, I. Assessment of diastolic function: suggested methods and future considerations. *Circulation* 69:836–841, 1984.
210. Mirsky, I. and W. W. Parmley. Force-velocity studies in isolated and intact heart muscle. In: *Cardiac Mechanics: Physiological, Clinical and Mathematical Considerations*, edited by I. Mirksy, D. Ghista, and H. Sandler. New York: Wiley, 1974:87–112.
211. Mirsky, I., J. M. Pfeffer, M. A. Pfeffer, and E. Braunwald. The contractile state as the major determinant in the evolution of left ventricular dysfunction in the spontaneously hypertensive rat. *Circ. Res.* 53:767–778, 1983.
212. Mirsky, I., T. Tajimi, and K. L. Peterson. The development of the entire end-systolic pressure-volume and ejection-fraction-afterload relations: a new concept of systolic myocardial stiffness. *Circulation* 76:343 1987.
213. Mitchell, J. H., J. P. Gilmore, and S. J. Sarnoff. The transport function of the atrium. Factors influencing the relation between mean left atrial pressure and left ventricular end-diastolic pressure. *Am. J. Cardiol.* 9:237–247, 1962.
214. Mitchell, J. H., A. G. Wallace, and N. S. Skinner, Jr. Intrinsic effects of heart rate on left ventricular performance. *Am. J. Physiol.* 205:41–48, 1963.
215. Mitchell, J. H., K. Wildenthal, and C. B. Mullins. Geometrical studies of the left ventricle utilizing biplane cinefluorography. *Federation Proc.* 28:1343, 1969.
216. Miura, T., S. Miyazaki, B. D. Guth, C. Indolfi, and J. J. Ross. Heart rate and force-frequency effects on diastolic function of the left ventricle in exercising dogs. *Circulation* 89:2361–2368, 1994.
217. Miura, T., S. Miyazaki, B. D. Guth, M. Kambayashi, and J. Ross, Jr. Influence of the force-frequency relation on left ventricular function during exercise in conscious dogs. *Circulation* 86:563–571, 1992.
218. Miyazaki, S., B. D. Guth, T. Miura, C. Indolfi, R. Schulz, and J. J. Ross. Changes of left ventricular diastolic function in exercising dogs without and with ischemia. *Circulation* 81:1058–1070, 1990.
219. Monroe, R. G., W. J. Gamble, C. G. LaFarge, A. E. Kumar, and F. J. Manasek. Left ventricular performance at high end-diastolic pressures in isolated, perfused dog hearts. *Circ. Res.* 26:85–99, 1970.

220. Monroe, R. G., G. LaFarge, W. J. Gamble, A. Rosenthal, and S. Honda. Left ventricular pressure-volume relations and performance as affected by sudden increases in developed pressure. *Circ. Res.* 22:333–344, 1968.

221. Moon, M. R., N. B. Ingels, Jr., G. T. Daughters, E. B. Stinson, D. E. Hansen, and C. Miller. Alterations in left ventricular twist mechanics with inotropic stimulation and volume loading in human subjects. *Circulation* 89:142–150, 1994.

222. Mulieri, L. A., G. Hasenfuss, F. Ittleman, E. M. Blanchard, and N. R. Alpert. Protection of human left ventricular myocardium from cutting injury with 2,3-butanedione monoxime. *Circ. Res.* 65:1441–1444, 1989.

223. Myazaki, S., Y. Goto, B. D. Guth, T. Miura, C. Indolfi, and J. J. Ross. Changes in regional myocardial function and external work in exercising dogs with ischemia. *Am. J. Physiol.* 264 (*Heart Circ. Physiol.* 33):H110–H116, 1993.

224. Noble, M. I. M., I. T. Gabe, D. Trenchard, and A. Guz. Blood pressure and flow in the ascending aorta of conscious dogs. *Cardiovasc. Res.* 1:9–20, 1967.

225. Noble, M. I. M., E. N. C. Milne, R. J. Goerke, E. Carlsson, R. J. Domenick, K. B. Saunders, and J. I. E. Hoffman. Left ventricular filling and diastolic pressure-volume relations in the conscious dog. *Circ. Res.* 24:269–283, 1969.

226. Noble, M. I. M., D. Trenchard, and A. Guz. Left ventricular ejection in conscious dogs: measurement and significance of the maximum acceleration of blood from the left ventricle. *Circ. Res.* 19:139–147, 1966.

227. Noda, T., C. P. Cheng, P. P. DeTombe, and W. C. Little. Curvilinearity of LV end-systolic pressure-volume and dP/dt max-end-diastolic volume relations. *Am. J. Physiol.* 265 (*Heart Circ. Physiol.* 34):H910–H917, 1993.

228. Olivetti, G., J. M. Capasso, E. H. Sonnenblick, and P. Anversa. Side-to-side slippage of myocytes participates in ventricular wall remodeling acutely after myocardial infarction in rats. *Circ. Res.* 67:23–34, 1990.

229. Olsen, C. O., J. S. Rankin, C. E. Arentzen, W. S. Ring, P. A. McHale, and R. W. Anderson. The deformational characteristics of the left ventricle in the conscious dog. *Circ. Res.* 49:843–855, 1981.

230. Olsen, C. O., G. S. Tyson, G. W. Maier, J. A. Spratt, J. W. Davis, and J. S. Rankin. Dynamic ventricular interaction in the conscious dog. *Circ. Res.* 51:85–104, 1983.

231. Olsen, C. O., P. VanTrigt, and J. S. Rankin. Dynamic geometry of the intact left ventricle. *Federation Proc.* 40:2023–2030, 1981.

232. Omens, J. H. and Y. C. Fung. Residual strain in rat left ventricle. *Circ. Res.* 66:37–45, 1990.

233. Omens, J. H., K. D. May, and A. D. McCulloch. Transmural distribution of three-dimensional strain in the isolated arrested canine left ventricle. *Am. J. Physiol.* 261 (*Heart Circ. Physiol.* 30):H918–H928, 1991.

234. Omens, J. H., D. E. Milkes, and J. W. Covell. Effects of pressure overload on the passive mechanics of the rat left ventricle. *Ann. Biomed. Eng.* 23:152–163, 1995.

235. Omens, J. H., H. A. Rockman, and J. W. Covell. Passive ventricular mechanics in the tight-skin mouse. *Am. J. Physiol.* 266 (*Heart Circ. Physiol.* 35):H1007–H1018, 1994.

236. Ono, S., V. Bhargava, L. Mao, G. Hagan, H. A. Rockman, and J. J. Ross. In vivo assessment of left ventricular remodelling after myocardial infarction by digital video contrast angiography in the rat. *Cardiovasc. Res.* 28:349–357, 1984.

237. Orenstein, J., D. Hogan, and S. Bloom. Surface cables of cardiac myocytes. *J. Cell. Mol. Cardiol.* 12:771–780, 1980.

238. Osakada, G., S. Sasayama, C. Kawai, A. Hirakawa, W. S. Kemper, D. Franklin, and J. Ross, Jr. The analysis of left ventricular wall thickness and shear by an ultrasonic triangulation technique in the dog. *Circ. Res.* 47:173–181, 1980.

239. Pace, J. B., W. F. Keefe, J. A. Armour, and W. C. Randall. Influence of sympathetic nerve stimulation on right ventricular outflow-tract pressures in anesthetized dogs. *Circ. Res.* 24:397–407, 1969.

240. Palakodeti, V., S. Oh, B.-H. Oh, L. Mao, and J. J. Ross. The force-frequency effect is a powerful determinant of myocardial contractility in the mouse. *Circulation* 94:I-309 1996.

241. Parisi, A. F., P. F. Moynihan, E. D. Folland, and C. L. Feldman. Quantitative detection of regional left ventricular contraction abnormalities by two dimensional echocardiography. II. Accuracy in coronary artery disease. *Circulation* 63:761–767, 1981.

242. Parry, D. A. D. The molecular and fibrillar structure of collagen and its relationship to mechanical properties of connective tissue. *Biophys. Chem.* 29:195–209, 1988.

243. Patterson, W. W. and E. H. Starling. On mechanical factors which determine output of ventricles. *Physioly.* 48:357–379, 1914.

244. Perreault, C. L., L. A. Mulieri, N. R. Alpert, B. J. Ransil, P. D. Allen, and J. P. Morgan. Cellular basis of negative inotropic effect of 2,3-butanedione monoxime in human myocardium. *Am. J. Physiol.* 263 (*Heart Circ. Physiol.* 32):H503–H510, 1992.

245. Perrone-Filardi, P., S. L. Bacharach, V. Dilsizian, S. Maurea, J. A. Frank, and R. O. Bonow. Regional left ventricular wall thickening. Relation to regional uptake of ^{18}Fluorodeoxyglucose and ^{201}Tl in patients with chronic coronary artery disease and left ventricular dysfunction. *Circulation* 86:1125–1137, 1982.

246. Peshock, R. M., R. Rokey, C. M. Malloy, P. McNamee, L. M. Buja, R. W. Parkey, and J. T. Willerson. Assessment of myocardial systolic wall thickening using nuclear magnetic resonance imaging. *J. Am. Coll. Cardiol.* 14:653–659, 1989.

247. Peterson, K. L., D. Sklovan, P. Ludbrook, J. B. Uther, and J. Ross, Jr. Comparison of isovolumic and ejection phase indices of myocardial performance in man. *Circulation* 49:1088–1101, 1974.

248. Piene, H. and J. W. Covell. A force-length-time relationship describes the mechanics of canine left ventricular wall segments during auxotonic contractions. *Circ. Res.* 49:70–79, 1981.

249. Piene, H. and J. W. Covell. Local auxotonic systolic force and work in canine right ventricular free wall. *Am. J. Physiol.* 244 (*Heart Circ. Physiol.* 13):H186–H193, 1983.

250. Pieske, B., B. Kretschmann, M. Meyer, C. Holubarsch, J. Weirich, H. Posival, K. Minami, H. Just, and G. Hasenfuss. Alterations in intracellular calcium handling associated with the inverse force-frequency relation in human dilated cardiomyopathy. *Circulation* 92:1069–1178, 1995.

251. Piot, C., S. Lemaire, B. Albat, J. Sequin, J. Narjeot, and S. Richard. High frequency-induced upregulation of human cardiac calcium currents. *Circulation* 93:120–128, 1996.

252. Plotnick, G. D., L. C. Becker, M. L. Risher, G. Gerstenblith, D. G. Renlund, J. L. Fleg, M. L. Weisfeldt, and E. G. Lakatta. Use of the Frank-Starling mechanism during submaximal versus maximal upright exercise. *Am. J. Physiol.* 251 (*Heart Circ. Physiol.* 20):H1101–H1105, 1988.

253. Pouleur, H., J. W. Covell, and J. J. Ross. Effects of alterations in aortic input impedance on force-velocity-length relationship in the intact canine heart. *Circ. Res.* 45:126–135, 1979.

254. Pouleur, H., J. S. Karliner, M. M. LeWinter, and J. W. Covell. Diastolic viscous properties of the intact canine left ventricle. *Circ. Res.* 45:410–419, 1979.

255. Pouleur, H., J. Lefevre, H. VanMechelen, and A. A. Charlier. Free-wall shortening and relaxation during ejection in the canine right ventricle. *Am. J. Physiol.* 239 (*Heart Circ. Physiol.* 8):H601–H113, 1980.

256. Prabhu, S. D. and G. L. Freeman. Kinetics of restitution of left ventricular relaxation. *Circ. Res.* 70:29–38, 1992.
257. Prabhu, S. D. and G. L. Freeman. Effect of tachycardia heart failure on the restitution of left ventricular function in closed-chest dogs. *Circulation* 91:176–185, 1995.
258. Quinones, M. A., W. H. Gaasch, and J. K. Alexander. Influence of acute changes in preload, afterload, contractile state and heart rate on ejection and isovolumic indices of myocardial contractility in man. *Circulation* 53:293–302, 1976.
259. Rademakers, F. E., M. B. Buchalter, W. J. Rogers, E. A. Zerhouni, M. L. Weisfeldt, J. L. Weiss, and E. P. Shapiro. Dissasocation between left ventricular untwisting and filling. *Circulation* 85:1572–1581, 1992.
260. Raines, R. A., M. M. LeWinter, and J. W. Covell. Regional shortening patterns in canine right ventricle. *Am. J. Physiol.* 231:1395–1400, 1976.
261. Rankin, J. S., E. C. Arentzen, P. A. McHale, D. Ling, and R. W. Anderson. Viscoelastic properties of the diastolic left ventricle in the conscious dog. *Circ. Res.* 41:37–45, 1977.
262. Rankin, J. S., P. A. McHale, C. E. Arentzen, D. Ling, J. C. Greenfield, and R. W. Anderson. The three-dimensional dynamic geometry of the left ventricle in the conscious dog. *Circulation* 39:304–313, 1976.
263. Rayhill, S. C., G. T. Daughters, L. J. Castro, M. A. Niczyporuk, M. R. Moon, N. B. Ingels, M. L. Stadius, G. C. Derby, A. F. Bolger, and D. C. Miller. Dynamics of normal and ischemic canine papillary muscles. *Circ. Res.* 74:1179–1187, 1994.
264. Robb, J. S. and R. C. Robb. The normal heart. Anatomy and physiology of the structural units. *Am. Heart J.* 23:455–467, 1942.
265. Robinson, T. F., S. M. Factor, J. M. Capasso, B. A. Wittenberg, O. O. Blumenfeld, and S. Seifter. Morphology, composition, and function of struts between cardiac myocytes of rat and hamster. *Cell Tissue Res.* 249:247–255, 1987.
266. Robinson, T. F., M. A. Geraci, E. H. Sonnenblick, and S. M. Factor. Coiled perimysial fibers of papillary muscle in rat heart: morphology, distribution, and changes in configuration. *Circ. Res.* 63:577–592, 1988.
267. Robinson, T. F. and S. Winegrad. A variety of intercellular connections in heart muscle. *J. Mol. Cell. Cardiol.* 13:185–195, 1981.
268. Rockman, H. A., S. Ono, R. S. Ross, L. R. Jones, M. Karimi, V. Bhargava, J. Ross Jr., and K. R. Chien. Molecular and physiological alterations in murine ventricular dysfunction. *Proc. Natl. Acad. Sci. U.S.A.* 91:2694–2698, 1994.
269. Rodriguez, E. K., W. C. Hunter, M. J. Royce, M. K. Leppo, A. S. Douglas, and H. F. Weisman. A method to reconstruct myocardial sarcomere lengths and orientations at transmural sites in beating canine hearts. *Am. J. Physiol.* 263 (*Heart Circ. Physiol.* 32):H293–H306, 1992.
270. Rodriguez, E. K., J. H. Omens, and A. D. McCulloch. Effect of residual stress on transmural sarcomere length distribution in rat left ventricle. *Am. J. Physiol.* 264 (*Heart Circ. Physiol.* 33): H1048–H1056, 1993.
271. Rose, S. E., S. J. Wilson, F. O. Zelaya, S. Crozier, and D. M. Doddrell. High resolution high field rodent cardiac imaging with flow enhancement supression. *Magn. Reson. Imaging* 12:1183–1190, 1994.
272. Ross, J. Jr., and E. Braunwald. The study of left ventricular function in man by increasing resistance to ventricular ejection with angiotensin. *Circulation* 29:739–749, 1964.
273. Ross, J. Jr., J. W. Covell, E. H. Sonnenblick, and E. Braunwald. Contractile state of the heart characterized by force-velocity relations in variably afterloaded and isovolumic beats. *Circ. Res.* 18:149–163, 1966.
274. Ross, J. Jr., E. H. Sonnenblick, J. W. Covell, G. Kaiser, and D. Spiro. The architecture of the heart in systole and diastole: technique of rapid fixation and analysis of left ventricular geometry. *Circ. Res.* 21:409–421, 1967.
275. Ross, J. Jr., E. H. Sonnenblick, G. A. Kaiser, P. L. Frommer, and E. Braunwald. Electroaugmentation of ventricular performance and oxygen consumption by repetitive application of paired electrical stimuli. *Circ. Res.* 16:332–342, 1965.
276. Ross, J. Jr., E. H. Sonnenblick, R. R. Taylor, and J. W. Covell. Diastolic geometry and sarcomere length in the chronically dilated canine left ventricle. *Circ. Res.* 28:49–61, 1971.
277. Ross, Jr. Afterload mismatch and preload reserve. A conceptual framework for the analysis of ventricular function. *Prog. Cardiac. Dis.* 18:255–264, 1976.
278. Ross, J. Jr., Mechanical consequences of regional myocardial ischemia. In: *The Heart and Cardiovascular System: Scientific Foundations*, edited by H. A. Fozzard, A. Haber, R. B. Jennings, A. M. Katz, and H. E. Morgan. New York: Raven Press, 1991:1997–2020.
279. Ross, J. Jr., T. Miura, M. Kamabayashi, G. P. Eising, and K.-H. Ryu. Adrenergic control of the force-frequency relation. *Circulation* 92:2327–2332, 1995.
279a. Ross J Jr., Adrenergic regulation of the force-frequency effect. In: *Heart Rate as a Determinant of Cardiac Function-Basic Mechanisms and Clinical Significance.* Hasenfuss, G. and H. Just (ed). Steinkopff, Darmstadt: Springer publishing group, pp 155–165, 2000.
280. Ross, J. Jr., J. W. Linhart, and E. Braunwald. Effects of changing heart rate by electrical stimulation of the right atrium in man: studies at rest, during muscular exercise, and with isoproterenol. *Circulation* 32:549–558, 1965.
281. Ross, J. Jr., and W. H. McCullagh. The nature of enhanced performance of the dilated left ventricle during chronic volume overloading. *Circ. Res.* 30:549–556, 1972.
282. Rushmer, R. F., D. L. Franklin, and R. M. Ellis. Left ventricular dimensions recorded by senocardiometry. *Circ. Res.* 4:684–688, 1956.
283. Sabbah, H. N., F. Khaja, J. F. Brymer, T. M. McFarland, D. E. Albert, J. E. Snyder, S. Goldstein, and P. D. Stein. Noninvasive evaluation of left ventricular performance based on peak aortic blood acceleration measured with a continuous-wave Doppler velocity meter. *Circulation* 4:323–329, 1986.
284. Sabbah, H. N., M. Marzilli, and P. D. Stein. The relative role of subendocardium and subepicardium in left ventricular mechanics. *Am. J. Physiol.* 240 (*Heart Circ. Physiol.* 9):H920–H926, 1981.
285. Sagawa, K. Analysis of the ventricular pumping capacity as a function of input and output pressure loads. In: *Physical Bases of Circulatory Transport: Regulation and Exchange*, edited by E. B. Reeve and A. C. Guyton. Philadelphia: W. B. Saunders, 149, 1967.
286. Sagawa, K. The ventricular pressure-volume diagram revisited. *Circ. Res.* 43:677–687, 1978.
287. Sagawa, K., H. Suga, A. A. Shoukas, and K. M. Bakalar. End-systolic pressure-volume ratio: a new index of contractility. *Am. J. Cardiol.* 40:748 1979.
288. Sandler, H. and E. Alderman. Determination of the left ventricular size and shape. *Circ. Res.* 34:1–8, 1974.
289. Sandler, H. and H. T. Dodge. Left ventricular tension and stress in man. *Circulation* 13:91 1963.
290. Santamore, W. P., P. R. Lynch, J. L. Heckman, A. A. Bove, and G. D. Meier. Left ventricular effects on right ventricular developed pressure. *J. Appl. Physiol.* 41:925–930, 1976.
291. Sarnoff, S. J. and E. Berglund. Ventricular function. I. Starling's law of the heart studied by means of simultaneous right and left ventricular function cures in the dog. *Circulation* 9:706–718, 1954.

292. Sasaki, T., M. Inui, T. Kimura, and M. Tada. Molecular mechanism of regulation of Ca^{2+} pump ATPase by phospholamban in cardiac sarcoplasmic reticulum. *J. Biol. Chem.* 267:1674–1679, 1992.
293. Sasayama, S., H. Nonogi, and C. Kawm. Assessment of left ventricular function using an angiographic method. *Jpn. Circ. J.* 46:1127–1137, 1982.
294. Sasayama, S., J. J. Ross, D. Franklin, C. M. Bloor, S. Bishop, and R. B. Dilley. Adaptations of the left ventricle to chronic pressure overload. *Circ. Res.* 38:172–178, 1976.
295. Sato, S., M. Ashraf, R. W. Millard, H. Fujinara, and A. Schwartz. Connective tissue changes in early ischemia of porcine myocardium: An ultrastructural study. *J. Cell. Mol. Cardiol.* 15:261–275, 1983.
296. Sechtem, U., B. A. Sommerhoff, W. Markiewicz, R. D. White, M. D. Cheitlin, and C. B. Higgins. Regional left ventricular wall thickening by magnetic resonance imaging: evaluation in normal persons and patients with global and regional dysfunction. *Am. J. Cardiol.* 59:145–151, 1987.
297. Shabetai, R. Pericardial and cardiac pressure. *Circulation* 77:1–5, 1988.
298. Shabetai, R. Diseases in the pericardium. In: *The Heart*, edited by R. C. Schlant and R. W. Alexander. New York: McGraw-Hill, 1994:1647–1674.
299. Sheehan, F. H., M. P. Feneley, N. P. DePruijn, J. S. Rankin, J. W. Davis, E. L. Bolson, P. S. Glass, and F. M. Clements. Quantitative analysis of regional wall thickening by transesophageal echocardiography. *J. Thorac. Cardiovasc. Surg.* 103:347–354, 1992.
300. Shirato, K., R. Shabetai, V. Bhargava, D. Franklin, and J. J. Ross. Alteration of the left ventricular diastolic pressure-segment length relation produced by the pericardium: effects of cardiac distension and afterload reduction in conscious dogs. *Circulation* 57:1191–1198, 1978.
301. Siri, F. M., L. A. Jelicks, L. A. Leinwand, and J. M. Gardin. Gated magnetic resonance imaging of normal and hypertrophied murine hearts. *Am. J. Physiol.* 272 (*Heart Circ. Physiol.* 41):H2394–H2402, 1997.
302. Slinker, B. K. and S. A. Glantz. Beat-to-beat regulation of left ventricular function in the intact cardiovascular system. *Am. J. Physiol.* 256 (*Renal Fluid Electrolyte Physiol.* 25):R962–R975, 1989.
303. Slinker, B. K., S. G. Shroff, R. D. Kirkpatrick, and K. B. Campbell. Left ventricular function depends on previous beat ejection but no previous beat pressure load. *Circ. Res.* 69:1051–1057, 1991.
304. Smaill, B. and P. Hunter. Structure and function of the diastolic heart: material properties of passive myocardium. In: *Theory of Heart: Biomechanics, Biophysics, and Nonlinear Dynamics of Cardiac Function*, edited by L. Glass, P. Hunter, and A. McCulloch. New York: Springer-Verlag, 1991:1–29.
305. Smiseth, O. A., M. A. Frais, I. Kingma, E. R. Smith, and J. V. Tyberg. Assessment of pericardial constraint in dogs. *Circulation* 71:158–164, 1985.
306. Smith, S. H., M. McCaslin, C. Sreenan, and S. P. Bishop. Regional myocyte size in two-kidney, one clip renal hypertension. *J. Mol. Cell. Cardiol.* 20:1035–1042, 1988.
307. Sonnenblick, E. H., E. Braunwald, J. F. Williams, Jr., and G. Glick. Effects of exercise on myocardial force-velocity relations in intact unanesthetized man: relative role of changes in heart rate, sympathetic activity, and ventricular dimensions. *J. Clin. Invest.* 44:2051–2062, 1965.
308. Sonnenblick, E. H. and S. E. Downing. Afterload as a primary determinant of ventricular performance. *Am. J. Physiol.* 204:604–610, 1963.
309. Sonnenblick, E. H., J. Ross, Jr., J. W. Covell, and E. Braunwald. Alterations in resting length-tension relations of cardiac muscle induced by changes in contractile force. *Circ. Res.* 19:980–988, 1966.
310. Sonnenblick, E. H., J. J. Ross, J. W. Covell, G. A. Kaiser, and E. Braunwald. Velocity of contraction as a determinant of myocardial oxygen consumption. *Am. J. Physiol.* 209:919–927, 1965.
311. Spach, M. and P. C. Dolber. Relating extracellular potentials and their derivatives to anisotropic propagation at a microscopic level in human cardiac muscle. Evidence for electrical uncoupling of side-to-side fiber connections with increasing age. *Circ. Res.* 58:356–371, 1986.
312. Spotnitz, H. M., W. D. Spotnitz, T. S. Cottrell, D. Spiro, and E. H. Sonnenblick. Cellular basis for volume related wall thickness changes in the rat ventricle. *J. Mol. Cell. Cardiol.* 6:317–331, 1974.
313. Spratt, J. A., G. S. Tyson, D. D. Glower, J. W. David, L. H. Muhibaier, C. O. Olson, and J. S. Rankin. The end-systolic pressure-volume relationship in conscious dogs. *Circulation* 75:1295 1987.
314. Stoddard, M. F., A. C. Pearson, M. J. Kern, J. Ratcliff, D. G. Mrosek, and A. J. Labovitz. Left ventricular diastolic function: comparison of pulsed Doppler echocardiographic and hemodynaimc indexes in subjects with and without coronary artery disease. *J. Am. Coll. Cardiol.* 13:327–336, 1989.
315. Streeter, D. D., Jr. Gross morphology and fiber geometry of the heart. In:*Handbook of Physiology. Section 2: The Cardiovascular System*, edited by R. M. Berne, N. Sperelakis, and S. R. Geiger. Baltimore: American Physiological Society, 1979:61–112.
316. Streeter, D. D., Jr. and D. L. Bassett. An engineering analysis of myocardial fiber orientation in pig's left ventricle in systole. *Anat. Rec.* 155:503–511, 1966.
317. Streeter, D. D., Jr., H. M. Spotnitz, D. P. Patel, J. Ross, Jr. and E. H. Sonnenblick. Fiber orientation in the canine left ventricle during diastole and systole. *Circ. Res.* 24:339–347, 1969.
318. Streeter, D. D., Jr., R. X. Vaishnav, D. J. Patel, H. N. Spotnitz, J. Ross, Jr., and E. H. Sonnenblick. Stress distribution in the canine left ventricle during diastole and systole. *Biophys. J.* 10:345–363, 1970.
319. Suga, H. Ventricular energetics. *Physiol. Rev.* 70:247–277, 1990.
320. Suga, H., R. Hisano, Y. Goto, O. Yamada, and Y. Igarashi. Effect of positive inotropic agents on the relation between oxygen consumption and systolic pressure volume area in canine left ventricle. *Circ. Res.* 53:306–318, 1983.
321. Suga, H., A. Kitabatake, and K. Sagawa. End-systolic pressure determines stroke volume from fixed end-diastolic volume in the isolated canine left ventricle under a constant contractile state. *Circ. Res.* 44:238–249, 1979.
322. Suga, H. and K. Sagawa. Instantaneous pressure-volume relationships and their ratio in the excised, supported canine left ventricle. *Circulation* 35:117 1974.
323. Suga, H., K. Sagawa, and A. A. Shoukas. Load independence of the instantaneous pressure-volume ratio of the canine left ventricle and effects of epinephrine and heart rate on the ratio. *Circ. Res.* 314–322, 1973.
324. Takayama, Y., J. W. Holmes, I. J. LeGrice, and J. W. Covell. Enhanced regional deformation at the anterior papillary muscle insertion site after chordal transection. *Circulation* 1995.
325. Tanaka, N., N. Dalton, L. Mao, H. A. Rockman, K. L. Peterson, K. R. Gottshall, J. J. Hunter, K. R. Chien, and J. Ross, Jr. Transthoracic echocardiography in models of cardiac disease in the mouse. *Circulation* 94:1109–1117, 1996.
327. Taylor, R. R., J. W. Covell, and J. Ross, Jr. Volume-tension di-

agrams of ejecting and isovolumic contractions in left ventricle. *Am. J. Physiol.* 216:1097–1102, 1969.
328. Taylor, R. R., J. W. Covell, and J. J. Ross. Influence of thyroid state on left ventricular tension-elocity relations in the intact, sedated dog. *J. Clin. Invest.* 48:775–784, 1969.
329. Taylor, R. R., J. W. Covell, E. H. Sonnenblick, and J. J. Ross. Dependence of ventricular distensibility on filling the opposite ventricle. *Am. J. Physiol.* 213:711–718, 1967.
330. Theroux, P., D. Franklin, J. Ross, Jr., and W. S. Kemper. Regional myocardial function during acute coronary artery occlusion and its modification by pharmacologic agents in the dog. *Circ. Res.* 35:896–908, 1974.
331. Tobin, J. R., P. E. Blundell, R. G. Goodrich, and H. J. C. Swan. Induced pressure gradients across infundibular zone of right ventricle in normal dogs. *Circ. Res.* 15:162–173, 1965.
332. Trautwein, W. and J. Heschler. Regulation of cardiac L-type calcium current by phosphorylation and G proteins. *Annu. Rev. Physiol.* 52:257–274, 1990.
333. Tsakiris, A. G., D. E. Donald, R. E. Sturm, and E. H. Wood, Volume, ejection fraction, and internal dimensions of left ventricle determined by biplane videometry. *Federation Proc.* 28:1358–1367, 1969.
334. Tsakiris, A. G., D. A. Gordon, R. Padiyar, and D. Frechette. Relation of mitral valve opening and closure to left atrial and ventriular pressures in the intact dog. *Am. J. Physiol.* 234 (*Heart Circ. Physiol.* 3):H146–H151, 1978.
335. Urschel, D. W., J. W. Covell, E. H. Sonnenblick, J. Ross, Jr., and E. Braunwald. Myocardial mechanics in aortic and mitral valvular regurgitation: the concept of instantaneous impedance as a determinant of the performance of the infarct heart. *J. Clin. Invest.* 47:867–883, 1968.
336. Vatner, S. F., D. H. Boettcher, G. R. Heyndrickx, and R. J. McRitchie. Reduced baroreflex sensitivity with volume loading in conscious dogs. *Circ. Res.* 37:236–242, 1975.
337. Vatner, S. F., D. Franklin, C. B. Higgins, T. Patrick, and E. Braunwald. Left ventricular response to severe exertion in untethered dogs. *J. Clin. Invest.* 51:3052–3060, 1972.
338. Vatner, S. F., R. G. Monroe, and R. J. McRitchie. Effects of anesthesia, tachycardia, and autonomic blockade on the Anrep effect in intact dogs. *Am. J. Physiol.* 226:1450–1456, 1974.
339. Villarreal, F. J. and W. Y. W. Lew. Finite strains in anterior and posterior wall of canine left ventricle. *Am. J. Physiol.* 259 (*Heart Circ. Physiol.* 28):H1409–H1418, 1990.
340. Villarreal, F. J., W. Y. W. Lew, L. K. Waldman, and J. W. Covell. Transmural myocardial deformation in the ischemic canine left ventricle. *Circ. Res.* 68:368–381, 1991.
341. Waldman, L. K., J. J. Allen, R. S. Pavelec, and A. D. McCulloch. Distributed mechanics of the right ventricle: effects of varying preload. *J. Biomech.* 1996.
342. Waldman, L. K. and J. W. Covell. Effects of ventricular pacing on finite deformation in canine left ventricles. *Am. J. Physiol.* 252 (*Heart Circ. Physiol.* 21):H1023–H1030, 1987.
343. Waldman, L. K., Y. Fung, and J. W. Covell. Transmural myocardial deformation in the canine left ventricle: normal in vivo three-dimensional finite strains. *Circ. Res.* 57:152–163, 1985.
344. Waldman, L. K., D. Nosan, F. J. Villarreal, and J. W. Covell. Relation between transmural deformation and local myofiber direction in canine left ventricle. *Circ. Res.* 63:550–562, 1988.
345. Wang, K., R. McCarter, J. Wright, J. Beverly, and R. Ramirez-Mitchel. Viscoelasticity of the sarcomere matrix skeletal muscles. The titin-myosin composite filament is a dual-stage molecular spring. *Biophys. J.* 64:1161–1177, 1993.
346. Weber, K. T. Cardiac interstitium in health and disease: the fibrillar collagen network. *J. Am. Coll. Cardiol.* 13:1637–1652, 1989.
347. Weber, K. T. and J. S. Janicki. Myocardial oxygen consumption. The role of wall force and shortening. *Am. J. Physiol.* 233 (*Heart Circ. Physiol.* 2):H421–H430, 1977.
348. Weber, K. T., J. S. Janicki, W. C. Hunter, S. Shroff, E. S. Pearlman, and A. P. Fishman. The contractile behavior of the heart and its functional coupling to the circulation. *Prog. Cardiac Dis.* 24:375–400, 1985.
349. Weber, K. T., J. S. Janicki, S. G. Shroff, R. Pick, R. M. Chen, and R. I. Bashey. Collagen remodeling of the pressure-overloaded, hypertrophied nonhuman primate myocardium. *Circ. Res.* 62:757–765, 1988.
350. Weber, K. T., R. Pick, M. A. Silver, G. W. Moe, J. S. Janicki, I. H. Zucker, and P. W. Armstrong. Fibrillar collagen and remodeling of dilated canine left ventricle. *Circ. Res.* 82:1387–1401, 1990.
351. Weir, W. G. and D. T. Yue. Intracellular calcium transients underlying the short-term force-interval relationship in ferret ventricular myocardium. *J. Physiol. (Lond.)* 376:507–530, 1986.
352. Weiss, J. L. Echocardiography as an aid in understanding the electrocardiographic changes of left ventricular hypertrophy, ischemia, and infarction. *Ann. N.Y. Acad. Sci.* 601:61–66, 1990.
353. Weitz, G. Uber das unterschiedliche Verhalten der Lage der Herzmuskelfasern in kontrahiertem und dilatierem Zustand. *Med. Klin. Munich* 46:1031–1032, 1951.
354. Wier, W. G. and D. T. Yue. Intracellular calcium transients underlying the short-term force-interval relation in ferret ventricular myocardium. *J. Physiol. (Lond.)* 376:507–530, 1986.
355. Wiggers, C. J. and L. N. Katz. The contour of the ventricular volume curves under different conditions. *Am. J. Physiol.* 58:439–475, 1922.
356. Wildenthal, K. and J. H. Mitchell. Dimensional analysis of the left ventricle in unanesthetized dogs. *J. Appl. Physiol.* 27:115–119, 1969.
357. Williams, J. R., Jr., E. H. Sonnenblick, and E. Braunwald. Determinants of atrial contractile force in the intact heart. *Am. J. Physiol.* 209:1061–1068, 1965.
358. Yaku, H., B. S. Slinker, T. Mochizuki, B. H. Lorell, and M. LeWinter. Use of 2,3-butanedione monoxime to estimate nonmechanical VO_2 in rabbit hearts. *Am. J. Physiol.* 265 (*Heart Circ. Physiol.* 34):H834–H842, 1993.
359. Yang, X., Y. Liu, N. Rhaleb, N. Kurihara, H. E. Kim, and O. A. Carretero. Echocardiographic assessment of cardiac function in conscious and anesthetized mice. *Am. J. Physiol.* 277 (*Heart Circ. Physiol.* 46):H1967–H1974, 1999.
360. Yeatman, L. A., Jr. W. W. Parmley, C. W. Urschel, and E. H. Sonnenblick. Dynamics of contractile elements in isometric contractions of cardiac muscle. *Am. J. Physiol.* 220:534–542, 1971.
361. Yellin, E. L., S. Nikolic, and R. W. M. Frater. Left ventricular filling dynamics and diastolic function. *Prog. Cardiovasc. Dis.* 32:247–271, 1990.
362. Yellin, E. L., C. Peskin, C. Yoran, M. Koenigsberg, M. Matsumoto, S. Laniado, D. McQueen, D. Shore, and R. W. Frater. Mechanisms of mitral valve motion during diastole. *Am. J. Physiol.* 241 (*Heart Circ. Physiol.* 10):H389–H400, 1981.
363. Yin, F. C. P. Ventricular wall stress. *Circ. Res.* 49:829–842, 1981.
364. Yin, F. C. P., R. K. Strumpf, P. H. Chew, and S. L. Seger. Quantification of the mechanical properties of noncontracting canine myocardium under simultaneous biaxial loading. *J. Biomech.* 20:577–589, 1987.
365. Yoran, C., J. W. Covell, and J. Ross, Jr. Structural basis for the ascending limb of left ventricular function. *Circ. Res.* 32:297–303, 1973.
366. Young, A. A., H. Imai, C. Chang, and L. Axel. Two-

dimensional left ventricular deformation during systole using magnetic resonance imaging with spatial modulation of magnetization. *Circulation* 89:740–752, 1994.

367. Young, M. S., N. M. Magid, D. C. Wallerson, R. S. Goldweit, R. B. Devereux, and J. N. Cater. Echocardiographic left ventricular mass measurement in small animals: anatomic validation in normal and aortic regurgitant rabbits. *Am. J. Noninvas. Cardiol.* 4:145–154, 1990.

368. Yue, D. T., D. Burkhoff, M. R. Franz, W. C. Hunter, and K. Sagawa. Postextrasystolic potentiation of the isolated canine left ventricle: relationship to mechanical restitution. *Circ. Res.* 56:340–350, 1985.

369. Zhu, W., M. L. Myers, C. J. Hartley, R. Roberts, and R. Bolli. Validation of a single crystal for measurements of transmural and epicardial thickening. *Am. J. Physiol.* 251 (*Heart Circ. Physiol.* 20):H1045–H1055, 1986.

21. A modern view of heart failure: practical applications of cardiovascular physiology

ARNOLD M. KATZ | *Cardiology Division, University of Connecticut Health Center, Farmington, Connecticut*

CHAPTER CONTENTS

Paradigmatic Shifts
Definition of Heart Failure
The Paradigm of Organ Physiology: The Failing Heart as a
    Defective Pump
  Backward and forward failure
  Systolic and diastolic dysfunction
  Right and left heart failure
  The neurohumoral response in heart failure
  Crossovers between functional and proliferative signaling
  Coupling between the failing heart and the circulation: pressure–
    volume loops
  Architectural changes in the failing heart
The Paradigm of Biochemistry and Biophysics: The Failing Heart
    as a Weakly Contracting, Incompletely Relaxing Muscle
  Inotropic and lusitropic abnormalities
  Energy starvation
    The phosphocreatine shuttle
    Reduced oxygen delivery
    Mitochondrial changes
    Consequences of decreased ATP levels
  Molecular alterations and architectural changes
The Paradigm of Gene Expression: The Failing Heart as an
    Abnormal Molecular Structure
  Adaptive and maladaptive hypertrophy
  Cardiac myocyte phenotypes
  Shape changes in the cells of the overloaded heart
  Myocardial cell death
Summary and Conclusions

HEART FAILURE, NOW A LEADING CAUSE OF HOSPITALIZATION in the United States (31) was, until the 1990s, viewed as a disorder in which depressed contractility and slowed relaxation impair the emptying and filling of a diseased heart. It is not surprising, therefore, that strategies to manage this condition had focused on the hemodynamic consequences of the pump dysfunction, and on the biochemical abnormalities that depress contractility and slow relaxation in diseased cardiac myocytes (49). However, it is now clear that heart failure is a progressive condition in which most patients die within five years from the time of diagnosis (33). For this reason, optimal treatment must not only improve symptoms, but also seek to prolong survival.

The importance of prognosis as a goal of therapy in heart failure became apparent when a number of clinical trials demonstrated that drugs that improve symptoms over the short term often have adverse effects on long-term prognosis, and vice versa (for reviews, see references 14, 18, 35, 50, 51, 53, 61, 62, 74, 77, 88). These counterintuitive findings are changing the way that we view this condition by shifting emphasis away from the hemodynamic abnormalities caused by impaired pumping of the diseased heart, and the contraction and relaxation abnormalities in failing myocardial cells. Instead, the focus of heart failure research has turned to abnormalities of the failing heart itself.

The remarkable advances in our understanding of heart failure over the past 30 years can be viewed as a series of paradigmatic shifts (48, 56), first from organ physiology (impaired pumping) to cell biochemistry (contraction and relaxation abnormalities), and more recently to the role of altered gene expression in causing the progressive deterioration of the failing heart.

PARADIGMATIC SHIFTS

During the first half of the twentieth century, heart failure was viewed primarily as a clinical syndrome, caused by impaired ventricular ejection, in which salt and water retention by the kidneys led to dyspnea and anasarca. The importance of cellular changes in the failing heart was not recognized until the late 1960s, when it was shown conclusively that myocardial contractility was impaired in animals with heart failure (86). This demonstration, which drew attention to the contractile and energetic abnormalities in the failing cardiac myocytes, led to a shift from the paradigm of organ physiology to the paradigm of cell biochemistry and biophysics. Within a decade, there was general recognition of the importance of abnormal calcium fluxes in causing the depressed contractility of failing cardiac myocytes (46), and by the early 1980s, it had become apparent that impaired relaxation also played an important pathogenic role in the pump dysfunction seen in patients with heart failure (85).

New understanding of the roles of calcium and cyclic adenosine monophosphate (c-AMP) in determining the contractile performance of the heart made it possible to develop powerful drugs to increase myocardial contractility (7). These inotropic agents, all of which led to short-term symptomatic and hemodynamic improvement, had been used widely, but not universally, to provide effective long-term treatment for this condition. It was not until the early 1990s that data from an appropriately designed survival trial of inotropic therapy first appeared (73); this trial, like several others that followed, demonstrated that powerful inotropic drugs, while of short-term benefit in improving pump function, worsen long-term prognosis (14, 16, 18, 35, 53, 61, 62, 69, 74, 77, 88). More recently, β-adrenergic blockade, which causes a transient worsening of heart failure, has been found to improve long-term prognosis (see below). These and other findings require revision of the traditional definition of this clinical syndrome as a hemodynamic disorder; such definitions, which focus only on pump dysfunction, are so incomplete as to be misleading.

The problems that arise when heart failure is viewed simply as disordered pump function are also seen in the findings of clinical trials of vasodilators, another class of drugs initially thought to provide rational treatment by unloading the failing heart (20). As predicted by the paradigms of organ physiology and cell biochemistry, reducing peripheral resistance provides short-term relief of the symptoms caused when a failing left ventricle ejects against an excessive overload. However, like the clinical response to inotropes, short-term and long-term effects of vasodilators are often very different. Not only do most classes of vasodilator fail to improve long-term prognosis (13), several actually accelerate the deterioration of the failing heart and worsen survival (Table 21–1). These apparently counterintuitive findings, like those with the inotropes, illustrate the misconceptions that can arise when heart failure is defined simply as a clinical syndrome caused by a weakened cardiac pump, rather than a condition in which progressive degeneration of the myocardium shortens survival.

DEFINITION OF HEART FAILURE

It is clear that any clinically useful definition of this condition must highlight the molecular abnormalities responsible for the poor prognosis and deterioration of the failing heart, as well as the impaired pump and

TABLE 21–1. *Counterintuitive Findings in Clinical Trials for the Treatment of Heart Failure*

Drugs that Transiently Improve Symptoms but Worsen Prognosis
    Phosphodiesterase inhibitors (amrinone, milrinone, pimobendan, vesnarinone)
    β-adrenergic agonists (dobutamine, xamoterol)
    α-adrenergic agonists (prazocin)
    Dopaminergic agonists (ibopamine)
    Flosequinan
    Prostacyclin (flolan)
    Short-acting calcium channel blockers (diltiazem, nifedipine)
    Moxonidine

Drugs that Transiently Worsen Symptoms but Improve Prognosis
    Converting enzyme inhibitors
    β-adrenergic blockers

myocyte performance To be useful, therefore, the definition must expand our view beyond the traditional focus on impaired pump function and depressed myocardial contractility to include the molecular changes that destroy the failing heart. According to one such definition (53), heart failure is *a clinical syndrome in which heart disease reduces cardiac output, increases venous pressures, and is accompanied by molecular abnormalities that cause progressive deterioration of the failing heart and premature myocardial cell death.*

THE PARADIGM OF ORGAN PHYSIOLOGY: THE FAILING HEART AS A DEFECTIVE PUMP

Abnormal pumping by the failing heart is often classified in terms of the associated hemodynamic abnormalities (Table 21–2). However, because blood flows in a circle, and because a heart that fills poorly cannot eject a normal stroke volume, and a heart that empties poorly cannot fill normally, these classifications are less useful than is often assumed.

Backward and Forward Failure

The hemodynamic consequences of heart failure are conceptually simple because, like any pump, the heart has only two ways to fail: inadequate emptying of the venous reservoirs (backward failure) and reduced ejection of blood under pressure into the aorta and pulmonary artery (forward failure). Causes of backward failure of the left heart include mitral stenosis, where narrowing of the mitral valve orifice reduces blood flow into a normal left ventricle, and hypertrophic cardiomyopathy, where left ventricular cavity obliteration caused by inappropriate myocardial growth impairs diastolic filling. Forward failure of the left heart can oc-

TABLE 21–2. *Classifications of Heart Failure Based on Abnormal Pump Function*

Forward and Backward Failure

Site of failure	Type of failure	Major hemodynamic consequence
Right heart	Forward	Reduced ejection into pulmonary artery—low cardiac output
Right heart	Backward	Increased systemic venous pressure
Left heart	Forward	Reduced ejection into aorta—low cardiac output
Left heart	Backward	Increased pulmonary venous pressure

Systolic and Diastolic Dysfunction

Systolic Dysfunction—Eccentric hypertrophy, increased cavity volume

    Global: Dilated cardiomyopathies, viral or toxic myocarditis, chronic volume overload

    Regional: Myocardial infarction

Diastolic Dysfunction—Concentric hypertrophy, reduced cavity volume

    Hypertrophic cardiomyopathy, hypertensive heart disease, chronic pressure overload

[Modified from Katz (54).]

cur when a mechanical obstruction inhibits ejection, as in aortic stenosis, when weakness of the left ventricle reduces systolic shortening, as occurs with myocarditis, or when the ventricle is scarred after a large myocardial infarction. An obvious limitation to the usefulness of the concepts of forward and backward failure is that ejection is a major determinant of filling in the subsequent cardiac cycle, and filling is a major determinant of ejection. This is simply because a heart that empties poorly retains an excessive residual (end-systolic) volume that reduces filling during the subsequent diastole, while a heart that does not fill adequately cannot eject a normal stroke volume. For these reasons, backward and forward failure invariably coexist.

Neurohumoral responses, such as vasoconstriction and salt and water retention, modify the hemodynamic patterns of backward and forward failure. Although the major hemodynamic abnormalities caused by impaired left ventricular ejection (forward failure) are a fall in blood pressure and in cardiac output, the extent to which either is reduced is determined not only by the heart, but also by the neurohumoral response to impaired ejection. Most important is the extent of peripheral vasoconstriction, which maintains blood pressure when left ventricular performance is impaired, albeit at the expense of reduced ejection. The result is that the reduction of cardiac output in patients with heart failure is usually greater than the fall in arterial blood pressure. Exceptions include such conditions as systemic arteriovenous fistula and beriberi heart disease, where chronically reduced peripheral resistance maintains a high cardiac output; these conditions, which are rare, represent examples of "high output failure." The neurohumoral response, by causing salt and water retention, increases ventricular diastolic pressures (backward failure) in most patients with heart failure.

It is customary to equate forward failure with depressed contractility (decreased inotropy), and backward failure with impaired relaxation (decreased lusitropy). However, the link between these biochemical abnormalities and altered hemodynamics is tenuous, because the neurohumoral response and alterations in the architecture of the hypertrophied heart, rather than depressed contractility and relaxation, are the major determinants of the extent of forward and backward failure. Arterial vasoconstriction, for example, worsens forward failure by reducing cardiac output, while fluid retention by the kidneys increases venous pressure and so worsens backward failure. Concentric hypertrophy of the pressure-overloaded left ventricle in the hypertensive patient, while facilitating ejection, impairs filling and so increases the severity of backward failure. Conversely, dilatation (remodeling) of the left ventricle in a patient with a dilated cardiomyopathy increases systolic wall tension (according to the Law of Laplace), and so worsens forward failure. For these reasons, the severity of either forward or backward failure, as evaluated in terms of reduced cardiac output and increased venous pressure, generally provides little information as to whether the primary hemodynamic abnormality is impaired relaxation or depressed contractility.

Therapy is also a major determinant of the extent of forward and backward failure in the patient with heart failure. Vasodilator therapy, which reduces the afterload on a failing left ventricle, improves ejection and so can alleviate the symptoms of forward failure without directly affecting either inotropy or lusitropy. Even more dramatic are the effects of diuretics, which by depleting vascular volume can relieve backward failure (increased venous pressure) while at the same time worsening forward failure (low cardiac output). For these reasons, the hemodynamic distinction between forward and backward failure is useful mainly in evaluating the immediate hemodynamic consequences of specific structural abnormalities in a failing heart. This distinction is quite useful in explaining signs and symptoms, but it provides little information about etiology and pathophysiology in the patient with chronic heart disease.

Systolic and Diastolic Dysfunction

A more useful categorization than that based on the concepts of forward and backward failure is the distinction between systolic and diastolic dysfunction (Table 21–2). These terms are most appropriately defined according to ventricular architecture: *systolic dysfunction* describes a ventricle whose output is limited by impaired emptying, whereas *diastolic dysfunction* describes a ventricle in which filling is limited. Systolic dysfunction in a patient with left ventricular failure is therefore present when the left ventricle is dilated (eccentric hypertrophy), whereas in diastolic dysfunction, cavity size is reduced in a noncompliant, thick-walled left ventricle (concentric hypertrophy).

Systolic and diastolic dysfunction are sometimes equated with forward and backward failure, respectively. However this is incorrect because, as already noted, a ventricle that does not empty normally cannot fill normally, and vice versa. For this reason, systolic and diastolic dysfunction cannot be distinguished by measurements of such hemodynamic variables as filling pressures and cardiac output. Instead, this distinction requires that the architecture of the failing ventricle be determined, for example by echocardiography or a radionuclear study.

Systolic dysfunction, which occurs when a dilated ventricle fails to eject its contents, is readily quantified by the reduction in *ejection fraction*, the ratio between the stroke volume and end-diastolic volume. Because stroke volume is also reduced in patients with diastolic dysfunction, the diagnosis of systolic dysfunction depends in large part on increased ventricular cavity size. Diastolic dysfunction, which usually occurs when hypertrophy reduces cavity volume, is associated with a normal, or even an increased, ejection fraction. Ventricular filling pressures are increased by both systolic and diastolic dysfunction. In the latter, ventricular diastolic pressure is elevated because of reduced cavity size, whereas in patients with systolic dysfunction, an abnormally high end-systolic (residual) volume is responsible for the increased filling pressures.

Systolic and diastolic dysfunction result from different pathophysiological processes. Diastolic dysfunction is most commonly seen in patients with left ventricular hypertrophy secondary to chronic hypertension or aortic stenosis, or more rarely when hypertrophy is primary, as in a familial hypertrophic cardiomyopathy. Systolic dysfunction, which is caused by diseases that weaken or damage the myocardium, can be manifest as a uniform depression of ventricular wall motion in such conditions as myocarditis or a dilated cardiomyopathy, while regional wall motion abnormalities are usually seen when coronary artery occlusion has caused a myocardial infarction.

Right and Left Heart Failure

The distinction between right and left heart failure (Table 21–2) is especially useful in patients with congenital and valvular heart disease, where the primary abnormality usually involves predominantly either the right or left side of the heart. Left heart failure is most prevalent in developed countries, where the major etiologies are coronary and hypertensive heart disease; even in patients with dilated cardiomyopathies, the clinical picture is generally dominated by signs and symptoms of left heart failure. Right heart failure, which is much less common, occurs most often in congenital heart disease and cor pulmonale; the latter can be caused by chronic lung disease, multiple pulmonary emboli, or primary pulmonary hypertension. Right heart failure can come to dominate the picture in patients with advanced left heart failure, when chronically elevated pulmonary venous pressure leads to vasoconstriction and proliferative changes in the pulmonary arterioles. In these patients, the increased pulmonary arterial resistance, by reducing pulmonary blood flow, "protects" against pulmonary congestion, albeit by replacing the clinical picture of left heart failure with that of right heart failure (100).

The Neurohumoral Response in Heart Failure

A fall in cardiac output evokes a powerful neurohumoral response, the most important component of which is a hemodynamic defense reaction characterized by vasoconstriction, salt and water retention, and adrenergic stimulation of the heart (20, 29, 53, 71); Table 21–3). Whereas all provide valuable support for the circulation in patients with a transient decrease in cardiac output, they can become harmful when sustained in the patient with heart failure. Differences between the short-term and long-term consequences of these neurohumoral responses illustrate an important dichotomy. As pointed out by Harris (29), these differences probably arose because the neurohumoral response in heart failure evolved as a short-term adaptive mechanism that operates during exercise and hemorrhage, rather than a mechanism to provide long-term compensation for a chronic illness like heart failure.

The neurohumoral response that operates in heart failure includes α-adrenergic stimulation which causes vasoconstriction, several mechanisms that act on the kidneys to increase circulating blood volume by causing salt and water retention, and β-adrenergic stimulation that increases heart rate and stroke volume. Whereas all help to maintain blood pressure and cardiac output following such short-term insults as cardiogenic shock or hemorrhage, in the patient with chronic heart failure they are generally deleterious and worsen the long-term disability (Table 21–3). Adverse effects occur when vasoconstriction (increased afterload) exacerbates the low output state in patients with heart failure (80). Salt and water retention, by increas-

TABLE 21–3. *Compensatory Mechanisms Initiated by Low Cardiac Output**

Mechanism	Short-Term, Adaptive	Long-Term, Maladaptive
HEMODYNAMIC		
Salt and water retention	↑ Preload	Edema, Anasarca
	Maintain cardiac output	Pulmonary Congestion
Vasoconstriction	↑ Afterload	↓ Cardiac Output
	Maintain blood pressure	↑ Cardiac Energy Demand
	Maintain cardiac output	Cardiac Necrosis
Increased cardiac adrenergic drive	↑ Contractility ⎫	↑ Cytosolic Calcium
	↑ Relaxation ⎬ Maintain cardiac output	↑ Cardiac Energy Demand
	↑ Heart Rate ⎭	Cardiac Necrosis
		Arrhythmias, Sudden Death
INFLAMMATORY	"ANTI-OTHER"	"ANTI-SELF"
Macrophages, cytokines, free radicals, etc.	Antimicrobial	Cardiac cachexia
	Attack foreign bodies	Cardiac apoptosis, necrosis
GROWTH	**ADAPTIVE HYPERTROPHY**	**MALADAPTIVE HYPERTROPHY**
Proliferative (transcriptional) signaling	↑ Sarcomere Number	Remodeling
	Maintain cardiac output	↑ Energy demand
	↓ Load, ↓ Energy demand	Cardiac necrosis, apoptosis

*These compensatory mechanisms, when evoked to meet a short-term challenge, generate an adaptive response. When sustained, as in heart failure, these same mechanisms give rise to maladaptive responses that further reduce cardiac output and accelerate cell death. Initial responses are shown in **bold** type, secondary responses are in normal type. [Modified from Katz (53).]

ing filling pressures (preload), causes the failing heart to dilate and worsens the manifestations of backward failure (29). β-Adrenergic stimulation, along with the increased afterload and ventricular dilatation, increases the energy demands of the failing heart, in which the balance between energy production and energy utilization is already precarious (37: see below under Energy Starvation). These responses have additional maladaptive effects that occur because most of the chemical transmitters, like α- and β-adrenergic agonists and angiotensin II, that mediate the functional responses also stimulate proliferative responses that contribute to maladaptive hypertrophy. A cytokine-mediated inflammatory response also appears to damage the failing heart, and may be responsible for the skeletal muscle myopathy in heart failure (61).

Vasodilators, by dilating arteriolar resistance vessels, increase cardiac output and unload the ventricle so as to provide short-term symptomatic improvement in patients with left ventricular failure. However, adverse long-term effects are seen with most classes of vasodilators, including calcium channel blockers, phosphodiesterase inhibitors, prostacyclin, dopaminergic agents and probably α-adrenergic blockers [for review see (14, 18, 35, 53, 61, 62, 74, 77)]. The mechanisms responsible for these deleterious effects are not fully understood and may vary from one drug to another; one major cause may be related to proliferative effects of the neurohumoral responses initiated by an overly rapid or excessive fall in blood pressure (see below, under The Paradigm of Gene Expression).

Diuretics, which reduce the expanded blood volume caused when the kidneys retain salt and water, improve the symptoms of backward failure caused by increased venous pressures. However, excessive reduction in blood volume can impair perfusion of such vital organs as the kidney and liver, so that over-diuresis can lead to renal and hepatic failure, especially in end-stage heart failure. The ability of diuretics to reduce preload also decreases ventricular end-diastolic volume. Although this might be expected to reduce the work of the heart (according to the Frank-Starling relationship), this is generally of minor importance because failing hearts usually operate on a flattened Starling curve. The more important consequence of reduced left ventricular diastolic volume is to decrease wall stress (according to the Law of Laplace). Because wall stress is a major determinant of cardiac energy requirements, the ability of diuretics to decrease diastolic volume reduces energy expenditure by the failing heart.

β-Adrenergic blockade also has both harmful and beneficial effects. Use of these agents for the treatment of chronic heart failure had, until recently, been resisted by most cardiologists because their negative inotropic, lusitropic, and chronotropic effects cause an immediate fall in cardiac output. Furthermore, β-adrenergic stimulation has obvious short-term benefits in acute heart failure, such as can occur following myocardial infarction. It is now clear, however, that the adverse effects of β-blockers in chronic heart failure are generally transient (28) and can be minimized by careful titration of these drugs. More important is solid evidence that long-term administration of β-blockers is of considerable benefit in prolonging survival of patients with heart failure (12, 57, 66, 72). The beneficial responses to these drugs may reflect their ability to decrease the inotropic and chronotropic effects of β-adrenergic stimulation, which would benefit the failing heart by reducing energy expenditure (45), as well as their ability to blunt the arrhythmogenic effects of cAMP (59, 76). There is growing evidence that an even more important long-term beneficial effect of β-blockade derives from their ability to inhibit ventricular remodeling. This reflects a crossover between the obvious inhibition of such functional responses as the increased contractility and heart rate, and a more slowly developing inhibition of proliferative signals that cause a maladaptive growth response in the failing heart.

Crossover Between Functional and Proliferative Signaling

One mechanism that may explain why neurohumoral blockade prolongs survival and improves symptoms in patients with heart failure is inhibition of neurohumoral signals that, in addition to activating adaptive functional responses that maintain blood pressure and cardiac output, also evoke more slowly developing maladaptive proliferative responses that damage the failing heart. One example of a crossover between functional and proliferative signaling occurs after sympathetic activation. Although β-adrenergic agonists and phosphodiesterase inhibitors, both of which increase AMP levels, cause short-term increases in heart rate, contractility, and relaxation that improve pump function in patients with heart failure, they also cause arrhythmias and stimulate proliferative responses that cause progressive dilatation (remodeling) and apoptosis [for review, see 53, 54]. This crossover can explain the long-term clinical benefits of β-blockers, which although they initially worsen the hemodynamic abnormalities, improve prognosis and slow progressive dilatation (remodeling). Crossover between functional and proliferative signaling can also explain the long-term benefits angiotensin-coverting enzyme of (ACE) inhibitors, which have an important antiproliferative effect that reflects the role of angiotensin II to regulate gene expression. The beneficial long-term response to ACE inhibitors, which reduces mortality caused by heart failure progression, is quite different from the response to vasodilators that act directly on arteriolar smooth muscle, many of which significantly *worsen* prognosis (Table 21–1). These and other clinical observations indicate that a major long-term problem in heart failure is initiated by the neurohumoral response that, even though the short-term functional effect is to improve hemodynamics, also activates long-term proliferative responses that worsen prognosis.

Coupling Between the Failing Heart and the Circulation: Pressure–Volume Loops

The interplay between inotropic and lusitropic abnormalities in the failing myocardium and the circulatory variables of preload and afterload can be understood by examining the pressure–volume loops generated during the cardiac cycle (Fig. 21–1A). Each loop is constrained between two "limits" that define the state of the ventricle at the beginning and end of ventricular systole (47, 54). The end-systolic limit is the *end-systolic pressure–volume relationship*, which like a Starling curve, describes the ability of the ventricle to perform work at different ventricular volumes (the inotropic state of the heart). The actual point along this relationship at which systole ends in a given cardiac cycle is determined by the afterload, which is determined largely by aortic impedance. The other limit, which describes the ability of the ventricle to fill at end-diastole, is the *end-diastolic pressure volume relationship* (the lusitropic properties of the heart). The end-diastolic point along this curve is the preload, which is determined by venous return and end-systolic volume.

Both the end-systolic and end-diastolic pressure–volume relationships are usually abnormal in heart failure. Decreased contractility, which causes a downward shift in the end-systolic pressure–volume relationship, can be viewed as a depressed Starling curve (Fig. 21–1B). The end-diastolic pressure–volume relationship is usually shifted upward (decreased compliance or increased stiffness) by a decrease in lusitropy (Fig. 21–1C). In most patients with heart failure, both pressure–volume relationships are abnormal. More important, however, are shifts in these curves caused by abnormal patterns of hypertrophy.

Architectural Changes in the Failing Heart

Changes in the size, shape, and thickness of the failing ventricle modify the pressure–volume loops obtained in patients with heart failure (44). Cardiac hypertrophy

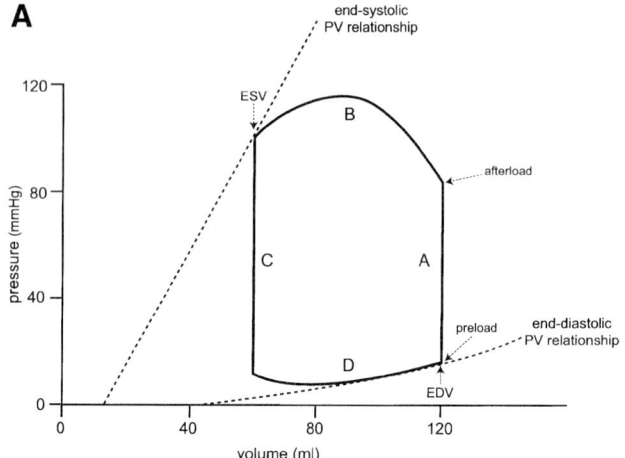

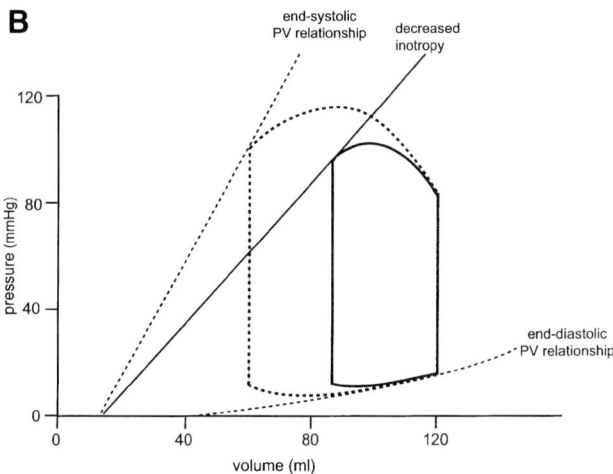

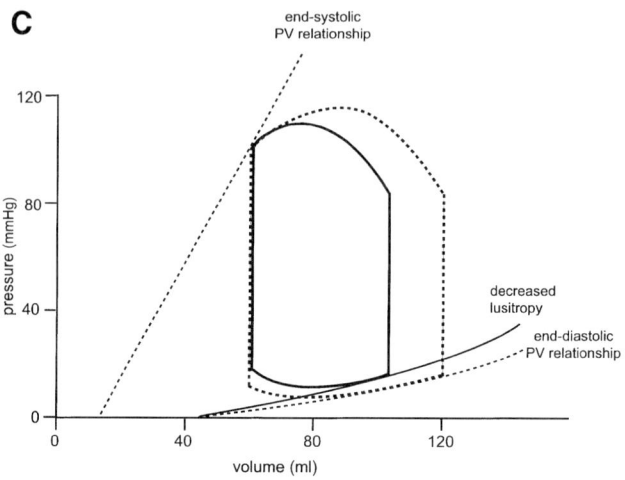

FIG. 21-1. Left ventricular pressure-volume loops. *A:* Preload, which is generated during diastole by the venous return and atrial systole, determines the point along the end-diastolic pressure–volume relationship (the lusitropic state) at which systole begins. After the onset of ventricular systole, the mitral valve closes and wall stress continues to increase during isovolumic contraction (A), which ends when the aortic valve opens and the ventricle meets its afterload, the aortic pressure. Aortic pressure rises and falls during ejection (B), when volume decreases. Systole ends when ventricular pressure and volume reach the end-systolic pressure–volume relationship that describes the inotropic state of the ventricle. After aortic valve closure removes the afterload (aortic pressure) from the ventricular cavity, blood can neither enter nor leave the ventricle; as a result, relaxation begins under isovolumic conditions (C). When left ventricular pressure falls below that in the left atrium, the mitral valve opens and blood flows from the atrium into the ventricle during the filling phase (D). The cycle ends when ventricular pressure and volume reach the end-diastolic pressure–volume relationship and the next cycle begins. *B:* A negative inotropic intervention shifts the end-systolic pressure–volume relationship to the right and downward (*solid curves*); if afterload remains constant, stroke volume will be reduced. (The control loop and end-systolic and end-diastolic pressure–volume relationships are shown as dashed lines.) *C:* A negative lusitropic intervention shifts the end-diastolic PV relationship to the left and upward (*solid curves*); if afterload remains constant, stroke volume is reduced. (From reference 54).

not only increases the mass of the heart, but depending on the underlying abnormality of cardiac function, has important effects on both ventricular architecture [see The Paradigm of Gene Expression and energetics (see below)]. Where heart failure is caused by an abnormally high afterload, as in aortic stenosis or hypertension, the hypertrophic response to the elevated systolic wall stress increases wall thickness with little or no increase, and often a decrease, in ventricular volume, This growth pattern, called *concentric hypertrophy*, is a major cause of diastolic dysfunction. In patients in whom heart failure is caused by a volume overload, such as aortic or mitral insufficiency, the left ventricle must dilate to accommodate the regurgitant volume. Other causes of left ventricular dilatation are a large myocardial infarction, which causes a regional wall motion abnormality, and the dilated cardiomyopathies, in which the depressed wall motion is global. By increasing wall stress, according to the Law of Laplace, dilatation adds to diastolic stretch, which initiates a pattern of left ventricular hypertrophy that increases diastolic volume. This growth response, called *eccentric hypertrophy*, is an important cause of systolic dysfunction.

The patterns of left ventricular hypertrophy described above have different effects on the pressure–volume loop. Dilatation of the ventricular cavity in eccentric hypertrophy shifts the entire pressure–volume loop to the right (see Fig. 21-3). This increases wall stress, which, along with the depressed myocardial contractility commonly seen in these patients, reduces the ability of the dilated ventricle to eject. This situation is generally exacerbated by progressive dilatation ("remodeling"). Concentric hypertrophy, on the other hand, reduces diastolic compliance (increases stiffness), which impairs filling and reduces cavity volume so as to shift the pressure–volume loop to the left (see Fig. 21-3). The basis for these different growth responses is discussed below under The Paradigm of Gene Expression.

THE PARADIGM OF BIOCHEMISTRY AND BIOPHYSICS: THE FAILING HEART AS A WEAKLY CONTRACTING, INCOMPLETELY RELAXING MUSCLE

Cardiac myocyte contraction and relaxation are impaired in virtually every patient with heart failure. These abnormalities in cell function can either be primary, where the disease process involves the myocardium itself, or secondary to changes initiated by chronic overloading of previously normal heart muscle. Biochemical abnormalities can affect many systems in the failing heart, including (1) the metabolic pathways that generate high-energy phosphates by oxidizing fats and carbohydrates, (2) the ion pumps and ion channels which participate in the calcium cycles that control contraction and relaxation, and (3) the contractile proteins responsible for the work of the heart. Abnormalities are also found in non-myocytes; for example, altered collagen synthesis in fibroblasts modifies the extracellular matrix secreted by these cells (97). From a functional standpoint, the most important of these biochemical and biophysical abnormalities are those that impair cardiac contraction and relaxation.

Inotropic and Lusitropic Abnormalities

Reduced myocardial contractility and relaxation that is delayed or incomplete, commonly both, contribute to the hemodynamic abnormalities in most patients with heart failure. A major cause of the depressed mechanical performance of the failing heart is slowing of virtually all of the calcium fluxes responsible for contraction, relaxation, and excitation–contraction coupling. These fluxes can be viewed as two "calcium cycles" (54): an *extracellular cycle* in which calcium moves between the extracellular space and the cytosol, and an *intracellular cycle* involving calcium fluxes between the sarcoplasmic reticulum, the cytosol, and the myofilaments (Fig. 21-2). The intracellular calcium cycle provides most of the calcium that activates contraction in adult mammalian cardiac myocytes, where the major role of the extracellular calcium cycle is to "trigger" calcium release from intracellular stores in the sarcoplasmic reticulum.

The calcium fluxes shown in Figure 21-2 can be slowed in the failing heart by two different mechanisms. The first is initiated by a state of energy starvation caused by an imbalance between the increased energy demands and impaired energy production in the failing cardiac myocytes. Because adenosine triphosphate (ATP) provides the substrate for the myosin cross-bridges when the heart contracts, and for the ion pumps that relax the heart, energy starvation might be expected to affect both inotropy and lusitropy directly. However, as discussed below, the most important effects of a decline in ATP levels on contraction and relaxation are due to attenuation of allosteric effects of the nucleotide and reduction in the free energy released during ATP hydrolysis.

Molecular changes in the proteins and membrane structures responsible for excitation-contraction coupling, contraction, and relaxation represent the second mechanism that contributes to the inotropic and lusitropic abnormalities in the failing heart. These changes in molecular composition involve such key structures as the contractile proteins and sarcoplasmic reticulum membrane, and they are caused in part when the growth stimuli that initiate hypertrophy of the overloaded heart also favor expression of the fetal phenotype. Increased expression of the low ATPase fetal isoform of the myosin heavy chain, for example, reduces myocardial contractility, while decreased density of sarcoplasmic reticulum calcium pump ATPase molecules, which is also a reversion to the fetal phenotype, impairs relaxation by slowing calcium removal from the cytosol during diastole.

Energy-Starvation

High-energy phosphate contents are reduced in overloaded or failing animal hearts and failing human hearts [for review, see 53], due both to impaired oxidative metabolism [for review see (5)] and reduced glycolytic activity (19, 42). The latter is a serious problem because of a special role of glycolytic ATP, which explains why glycolytic inhibition is especially harmful in causing diastolic dysfunction in the failing heart (3, 17, 40). Phosphocreatine content is generally more depressed than that of ATP, largely because phosphocreatine buffers ATP concentration when the rate of energy utilization exceeds that of energy production. Phosphocreatine also participates in a "shuttle" that transfers energy from the mitochondria, where high-energy phosphates are generated, to the cytosol, where they are consumed.

The Phosphocreatine Shuttle. The rate-limiting step in supplying high-energy phosphate to the contractile proteins and ion pumps is not, as might be expected, the delivery of ATP to these energy-consuming cytosolic structures. Instead, diffusion of adenosine diphosphate (ADP) back to the mitochondria is rate-limiting because of the very low cytosolic ADP concentration, which is about 100-fold lower than the ATP concentration (36, 78). To circumvent problems that could arise because of the extremely slow diffusion of these

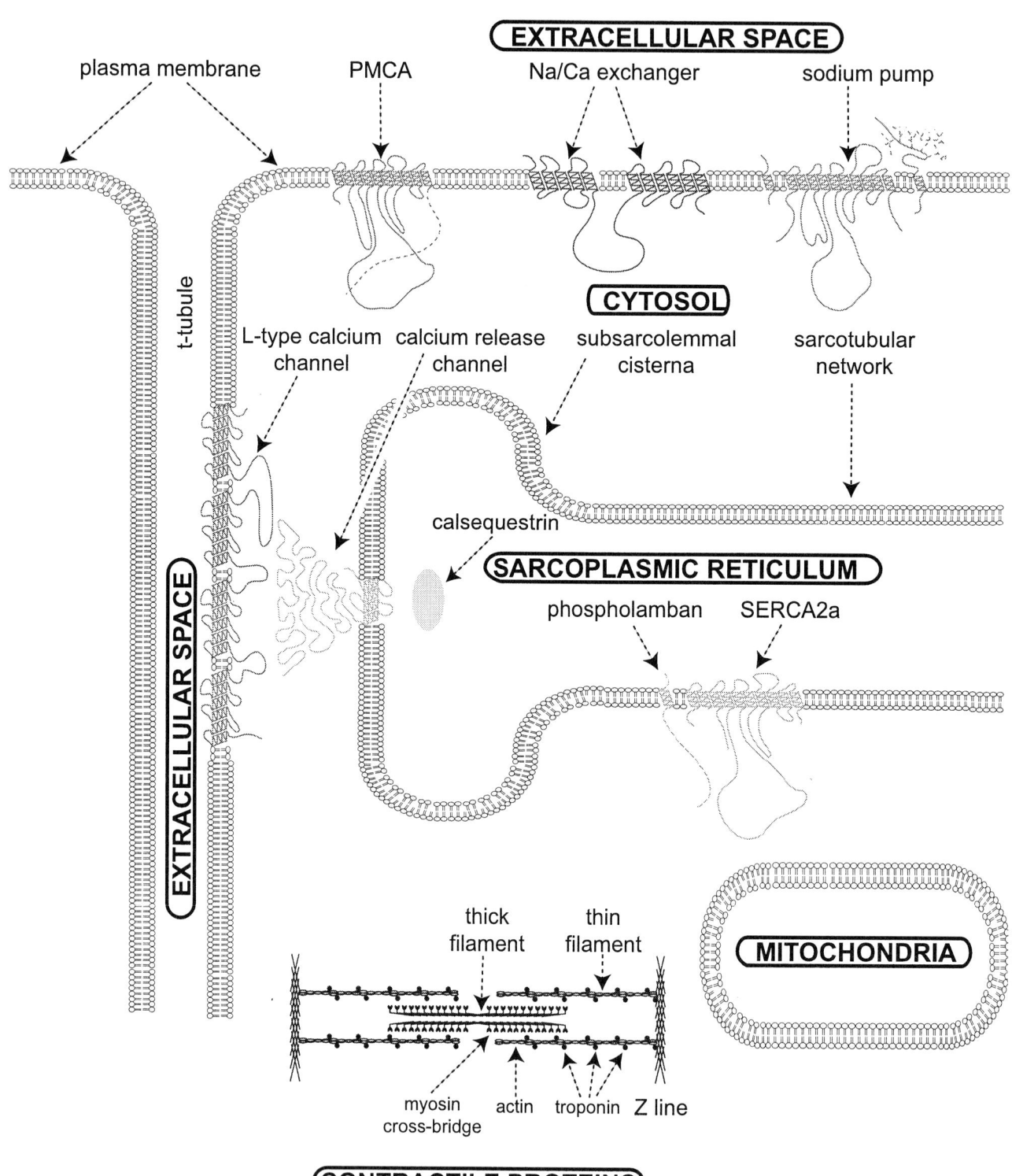

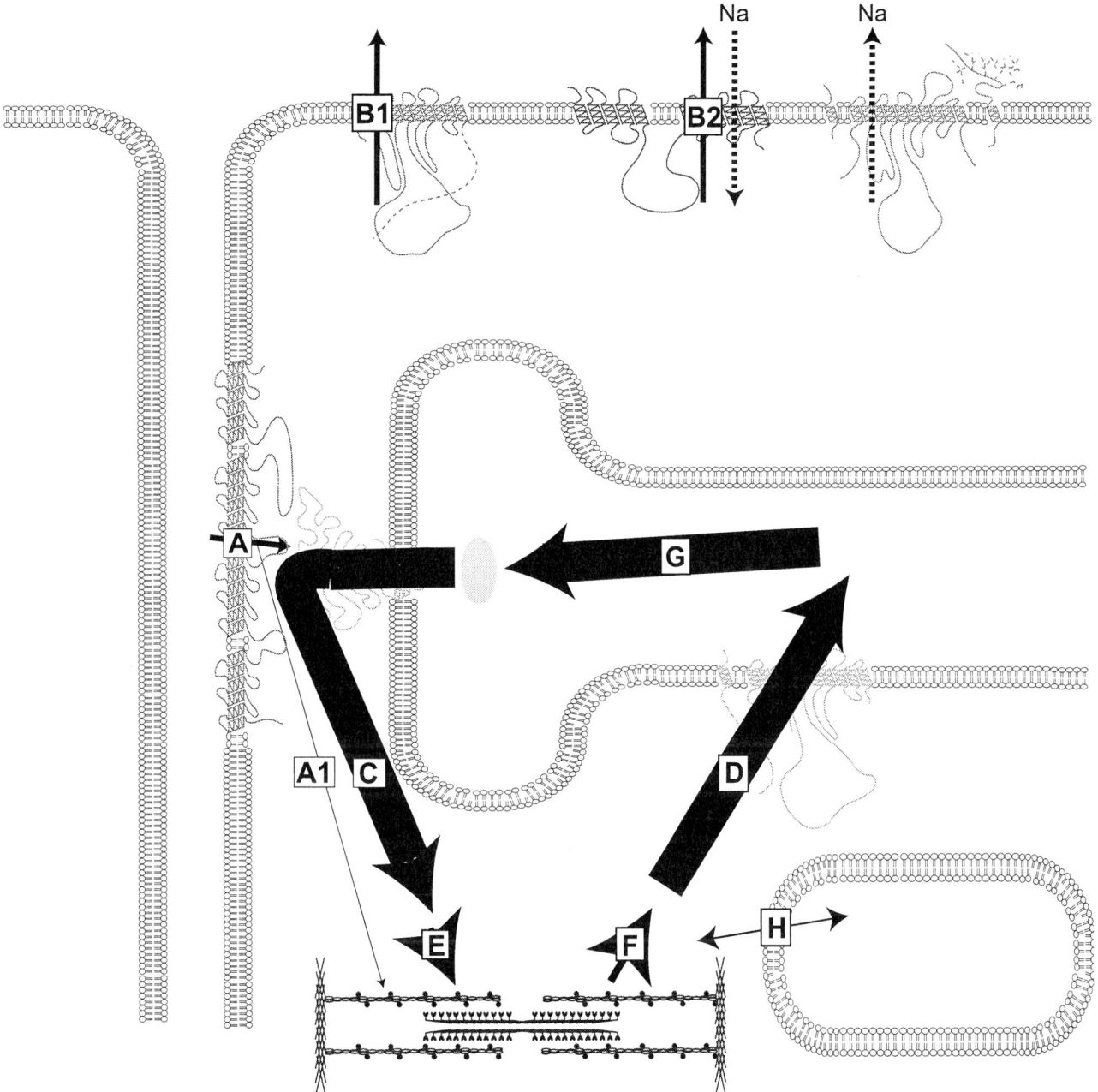

FIG. 21–2. Schematic diagram showing key structures (*Left*) and calcium fluxes (*Right*) that control cardiac excitation-contraction coupling and relaxation in the heart. *Left:* the calcium "pools" are in bold capital letters. *Right:* which shows the calcium fluxes between these pools, the thickness of the arrows indicates the magnitude of the calcium fluxes, while their vertical orientations describe their "energetics": downward arrows represent passive calcium fluxes and upward arrows represent energy-dependent active calcium transport. Most of the calcium that enters the cell from the extracellular fluid via L-type calcium channels (*arrow A*) triggers calcium release from the sarcoplasmic reticulum; only a small portion directly activates the contractile proteins (*arrow A1*). Calcium is actively transported back into the extracellular fluid by the plasma membrane calcium pump ATPase (PMCA, *arrow B1*), and the Na/Ca exchanger (*arrow B2*); the sodium that enters the cell in exchange for calcium via the latter is pumped out of the cytosol by the sodium pump (*dashed lines*). Two calcium fluxes are regulated by the sarcoplasmic reticulum: calcium efflux from the subsarcolemmal cisternae via calcium release channels (*arrow C*) and calcium uptake into the sarcotubular network by the sarco(endo)plasmic reticulum calcium pump ATPase (*arrow D*). Calcium diffuses within the sarcoplasmic reticulum from the sarcotubular network to the subsarcolemmal cisternae (*arrow G*), where it is stored in a complex with calsequestrin and other calcium-binding proteins. Calcium binding to (*arrow E*) and dissociation from (*arrow F*) high-affinity calcium-binding sites of troponin C activate and inhibit the interactions of the contractile proteins. Calcium movements into and out of mitochondria (*arrow H*) buffer cytosolic calcium concentration. The extracellular calcium cycle consists of *arrows A, B1,* and *B2*, while the intracellular cycle involves *arrows C, E, F, D,* and *G*. [From reference (54).]

small amounts of ADP, creatine (which is present in the cytosol at much higher concentrations) not ADP, serves as the high-energy phosphate receptor in a system called the "phosphocreatine shuttle" (39). This shuttle depends on reactions that are catalyzed by *creatine phosphokinase*, an enzyme that transfers high-energy phosphate in the cytosol from phosphocreatine to ADP according to the overall reaction:

$$\text{phosphocreatine} + \text{ADP} \leftrightarrow \text{ATP} + \text{creatine}.$$

Conversely, creatine provides the acceptor for the high-energy phosphates generated in the mitochondria when a similar reaction, catalyzed by mitochondrial creatine phosphokinase, regenerates phosphocreatine using the high-energy phosphate in ATP generated by oxidative phosphorylation. These reactions allow phosphocreatine to transfer high-energy phosphate generated in the mitochondria to the contractile proteins and other energy-consuming systems in the cytosol. Slowing of the phosphocreatine shuttle contributes to the state of energy starvation seen in the failing heart.

Reduced Oxygen Delivery. Several abnormalities impair high-energy phosphate production in the failing heart by reducing oxygen delivery to the mitochondria [for review see (53)]. Diffusion of substrates, notably oxygen, is impaired by increased intercapillary distance and decreased density of transverse capillary profiles. Hypertrophy also decreases nutrient coronary flow (63, 96, 98) in part by increasing the length of the small arteries that penetrate the ventricular wall from their origins as branches of the large epicardial coronary arteries. The resulting imbalance between energy production and consumption is especially marked in the relatively underperfused subendocardial regions of the thick-walled hypertrophied left ventricle (34), where a combination of high wall stress and reduced perfusion can lead to a state of energy starvation so severe as to cause myocyte necrosis.

Mitochondrial Changes. Loss of mitochondria, due in part to mitochondrial DNA deletions, probably plays a major role in decreasing high-energy phosphate production in end-stage heart failure (68, 79, 89). Decreased total creatine phosphokinase activity, by slowing ADP rephosphorylation via the phosphocreatine shuttle, may also play a major role in exacerbating a state of energy starvation in the failing heart (38, 67). Some compensation for these abnormalities is achieved by an isoform switch in the hypertrophied heart that replaces the M isoform of creatine phosphokinase with the B isoform (38, 65, 67). Because the affinity of the B isoform of this enzyme for ADP is higher than that of the M isoform, this molecular response facilitates ADP rephosphorylation by the phosphocreatine shuttle. In spite of this adaptive isoform switch, however, decreased phosphocreatine levels and loss of mitochondria slow ADP phosphorylation, and so probably play an important role in limiting energy production in failing cardiac myocytes (37).

Consequences of Decreased ATP Levels. Although ATP levels are low, lack of substrate ATP does not deprive substrate-binding sites on the contractile proteins and ion pumps of their energy source, and so cannot cause the initial impairment of inotropy and lusitropy. This is because the normal cytosolic ATP concentration is 5–10 μM, whereas the substrate-binding sites of most ATP-hydrolyzing systems are saturated at ATP concentrations less than 1 μM. For this reason, except in the dying heart, ATP concentrations do not fall to levels below those needed to saturate known energy-consuming reactions.

High ATP concentrations have allosteric effects that accelerate ion pumps, ion exchangers, and passive ion fluxes through membrane channels. Reduction in these allosteric effects can reduce inotropy and lusitropy in the ischemic heart by slowing both the intracellular and extracellular calcium cycles, while attenuation of the allosteric effect that dissociates actin and myosin may contribute to the ability of a modest fall of ATP concentration to increase diastolic stiffness. A minor fall in ATP concentration can increase intracellular sodium concentration because an allosteric effect of ATP stimulates the sodium pump. However, sodium pump inhibition, by increasing cytosolic sodium concentration, reduces calcium efflux via the Na/Ca exchanger; this has both a positive inotropic and a negative lusitropic effect.

The most important consequence of ATP depletion is probably a decrease in the free energy of ATP hydrolysis, called $-\Delta G$, which is the amount of energy that can be made available by hydrolysis of the terminal phosphate of ATP. Even a 15%–25% reduction in $-\Delta G$, from ~60 kJ/mol in the normal heart to between 45 and 50 kJ/mol, can impair ATP-dependent reactions (43, 92), which reflects the heart's surprisingly small free energy reserve. For this reason, the slight fall in the ATP/ADP ratio in the ischemic heart, which is due mainly to an increase in ADP concentration, appears able to reduce the free energy of ATP hydrolysis to levels that can slow both the calcium pump of the sarcoplasmic reticulum (92) and cross-bridge cycling (91, 93).

Molecular Alterations and Architectural Changes

Molecular abnormalities in the failing heart, along with energy starvation, can modify virtually all of the calcium fluxes shown in Figure 21–2. These molecular abnormalities, which involve most of the structures that mediate both the intracellular and extracellular calcium cycles, represent a major cause of the depressed inotropy and lusitropy in the patient with heart failure. These molecular changes are initiated by the same proliferative stimuli that initiate hypertrophy, so that in addition to causing enlargement of cardiac myocytes, the proliferative signal transduction systems activated in the overloaded heart slow the interactions between the myofibrillar proteins and reduce the densities of the ion pumps and channels that participate in excitation–contraction coupling and relaxation.

THE PARADIGM OF GENE EXPRESSION: THE FAILING HEART AS AN ABNORMAL MOLECULAR STRUCTURE

The most recently recognized of the paradigms that describe the abnormalities in the failing heart describes the many architectural and molecular changes that occur as the result of abnormal proliferative signaling. This paradigm of abnormal gene expression appears to hold the key to explaining both the poor prognosis in heart failure and the apparently counterintuitive findings of many clinical trials of therapy.

In considering the effects of proliferative stimuli on the heart, it is important to appreciate the limited growth potential of adult cardiac myocytes. These terminally differentiated cells have lost most, if not all, of their ability to divide, so that they can respond to proliferative stimuli only by becoming larger. This differs markedly from the mitotic response of the less differentiated embryonic cardiac myocytes, and of the connective tissue cells in the adult heart.

As long as the differentiated myocytes of the normal adult heart are not stimulated to grow, these cells function for the lifetime of the organism. In the human heart, for example, cardiac myocytes generally live upwards of 80–90 years. Although aging is accompanied by the slow death of cardiac myocytes, hypertrophy of the surviving cells in most elderly patients provides adequate compensation for this cell loss as long as the heart is not overloaded or damaged. However, because the aged heart contains a reduced number of moderately hypertrophied cells, it is poorly equipped to meet the challenge caused by a hemodynamic overload or disease. These considerations probably explain the marked increase in the prevalence of heart failure in the elderly (31).

The inability of terminally differentiated cardiac myocytes to divide has important consequences when the heart is overloaded or damaged. This is because activation of proliferative signaling, instead of causing cell division, initiates a maladaptive growth response that, while causing myocytes to enlarge, appears to shorten their survival. Thus, like the other responses to a fall in cardiac output listed in Table 21–3, the proliferative response of the overloaded adult heart has both adaptive and maladaptive consequences. Like the functional signals evoked by neurohumoral stimulation (see above, under The Neurohuman Responses in Heart Failure), proliferative signaling stimulates a growth response whose short-term effects are adaptive, but whose long-term effects are maladaptive.

Adaptive and Maladaptive Hypertrophy

The dichotomy between the adaptive short-term and maladaptive long-term effects of the compensatory responses to a fall in cardiac output, which has already been highlighted in terms of the paradigms of organ physiology and cell biochemistry (Table 21–3), is seen in the hypertrophic response of the adult mammalian heart. Although the mechanisms responsible for this dichotomy are only now coming into focus, the fact that hypertrophy could be both adaptive and maladaptive was known to the great clinician-scientists of the nineteenth century [for a review of this history, see (52)].

Two observations, made in the 1960's, indicated that the major problem in heart failure is not only the defective pump (the paradigm of organ physiology) and weakened muscle (the paradigm of cell biochemistry and biophysics), but also molecular abnormalities within the heart muscle (the paradigm of gene expression and molecular biology). In 1962, Alpert and Gordon (1) reported that myofibrillar adenosine triphosphatase activity, a measure of the intrinsic rate of energy liberation by the cardiac contractile proteins, is depressed in preparations purified from patients with congestive heart failure. At about the same time, Meerson (64) observed that hypertrophy could be both adaptive and maladaptive (Table 21–4). Meerson constricted the aortae of dogs and rabbits and found that development of left ventricular hypertrophy alleviated

TABLE 21–4. *Three Stages in the Response to a Sudden Increase in Afterload*

STAGE I "Transient Breakdown" (days)
  Acute heart failure, pulmonary congestion, low cardiac output
  Acute left ventricular dilatation, early hypertrophy

STAGE II "Stable Hyperfunction" (weeks)
  Resolved pulmonary congestion, increased cardiac output
  Established hypertrophy

STAGE III "Exhaustion and Progressive Cardiosclerosis" (months)
  Progressive left ventricular dilatation and failure
  Further hypertrophy, cell death, fibrosis

[Based on Meerson (64).]

the acute heart failure seen immediately after imposition of the pressure overload. However, subsequent maladaptive changes led to progressive deterioration of the hypertrophied heart that eventually caused the animals to die of heart failure.

The hypertrophic response to pressure overload, by increasing wall thickness and reducing cavity size, initially returns the elevated systolic wall stress to normal levels (26, 32, 82). Because hypertrophy virtually normalizes systolic wall stress, factors other than sustained wall stress play a major role in determining the poor long-term prognosis in heart failure.

A growing number of studies, both clinical and molecular, support the view that changes in myocardial structure and composition play a key role in determining the poor prognosis in patients with heart failure. Perhaps the most convincing evidence that heart failure is not simply a clinical syndrome caused by weakness of the heart muscle is found in the counterintuitive results of a number of long-term clinical trials, where drugs that improve the disordered circulatory dynamics (organ physiology) or depressed myocardial contractility (cell biochemistry) often worsen prognosis, whereas drugs whose immediate effects worsen hemodynamics or weaken the heart can have beneficial long-term effects (Table 21–1).

Cardiac Myocyte Phenotypes

The normal human heart contains many different cardiac myocyte phenotypes (Table 21–5); these appear not only during embryonic development, but are also found in different regions within the adult heart. Most important in terms of the pathophysiology of heart failure is the appearance of different abnormal phenotypes in response to different types and duration of hemodynamic overloading. Table 21–5 is by no means a comprehensive overview of these phenotypic patterns. Normal cardiac development, for example, is not a simple transition from the fetal to the adult phenotype, but instead proceeds by a series of changes in both overall structure and molecular composition that follow different sequences in various regions of the embryonic heart.

A number of distinct cardiac myocyte phenotypes can be identified in hypertrophied adult human hearts. One of these, seen in exercise-induced hypertrophy (the "athlete's heart"), can be viewed as a physiological growth response, whereas the others represent abnormal cardiac growth patterns. The signal transduction systems that initiate and control each of these growth patterns are not yet well understood, although there is evidence that different growth signals can generate different morphological phenotypes (99). In the case of physiological hypertrophy, where both inotropy and

TABLE 21–5. *Examples of Different Cardiac Myocyte Phenotypes*

Normal Embryonic Phenotypes

Normal Adult Phenotypes
   Working myocardial cells
      Atrial myocardium
      Ventricular myocardium
   Specialized cells
      Nodal cells
      His-Purkinje cells

Physiological Hypertrophy Phenotype
   The "athlete's heart": exercise-induced hypertrophy

Pathological Phenotypes
   Concentric hypertrophy
      Early or mild pressure overload (e.g. aortic stenosis, hypertension)
   Eccentric hypertrophy
      Early or mild volume overload (e.g. aortic and mitral insufficiency)
      Diffuse myocardial damage (e.g. viral or toxic myocarditis)
      Localized myocardial damage (myocardial Infarction)
      Decompensated hypertrophy, remodeling: end-stage heart failure

Familial Cardiomyopathies:
   Hypertrophic cardiomyopathies
   Dilated cardiomyopathies

[From reference (53).]

lusitropy are increased (60, 75), the growth stimulus is probably initiated by the brief periods of intense adrenergic stimulation accompanied by increased preload and reduced afterload that occur during training.

Concentric hypertrophy in compensated pressure overload, which, as discussed below, is characterized mainly by increased fiber diameter, differs from eccentric hypertrophy in compensated volume overload, in which both fiber diameter and length are increased. This may reflect the importance of increased systolic wall stress in concentric hypertrophy and increased diastolic stretch in eccentric hypertrophy. Phenotypic differences also exist in different forms of eccentric hypertrophy. The phenotype in compensated volume overload, where ventricular dilatation represents a necessary compensation for the increased stroke volume caused by a valve leak, differs from the phenotype in hearts with idiopathic dilated cardiomyopathies where, although the ventricular cavity is also dilated, stroke volume is reduced. Shortening of myocyte survival associated with these abnormal phenotypes indicates that pathological hypertrophy is associated with maladaptive changes that lead to myocardial cell death. One exception appears to be the eccentric right ventricular hypertrophy in congenital atrial septal defect (100), where the shunt causes a volume overload on the right ventricle; these patients can live to a very old age if they do not develop pulmonary hypertension. In general, prognosis is poorer in patients with systolic dysfunction than in those with diastolic dysfunction (95), which indicates that different phenotypes are associated with different rates of myocardial cell death (4, 8, 25, 27, 55, 87).

Re-expression of the slow (β) myosin heavy chain isoform in the failing heart (see above, under Molecular Alterations and Architectural Changes) is an example of a reversion to the fetal phenotype that accompanies the hypertrophic response to chronic overload (for review see 9, 53, 90). The phenotypic changes in the failing heart, however, are much more than a simple reversion to a fetal patterns noted above, and the myocytes generated in exercise-induced physiological hypertrophy (the "athlete's heart") differ from those seen in pressure overload–induced hypertrophy. In the latter, which is an example of pathologic hypertrophy, both myosin ATPase activity and sarcoplasmic reticulum calcium transport are reduced, whereas both are increased in physiologic hypertrophy. Differences between pressure- and volume-overloaded hearts are also seen in the messenger RNAs that encode both signaling and structural proteins (11).

The significance of the many molecular changes identified in failing hearts is not well understood. Findings are often controversial because of technical problems, the fact that mRNA and protein levels do not always change in the same way, differences between species and between different heart failure models, the age of the animals studied, and the time after an intervention that causes the heart to fail. The availability of explanted human hearts, obtained at the time of heart transplantation, has added to this knowledge, but most human tissue has come from end-stage heart failure. For these reasons, the molecular changes that occur in the failing human heart are not fully understood. A tentative summary of some of these changes is provided in Table 21–6.

Shape Changes in the Cells of the Overloaded Heart

The different growth responses initiated by different types of hemodynamic overload (Fig. 21–3) are seen in the changes of myocardial cell length and cross-sectional area in concentric and eccentric hypertrophy. Early reports suggested that the number of fiber layers remains constant during remodeling of the left ventricle, which implies that the progressive chamber enlargement is due to the radial rearrangement of a constant number of muscle fibers ("fiber slippage") rather than fiber elongation (58). However, more recent studies of the failing human left ventricle have found myocyte length to be increased in both end-stage ischemic cardiomyopathy (6) and decompensated eccentric hypertrophy (23). Fiber slippage probably plays a major role in acute ventricular dilatation, such as occurs immediately after a large myocardial infarction (70), but the slower dilatation (remodeling) of a damaged ventricle appears to be caused by a combination of myocyte elongation and myocyte death (21). Although there are reports of myocyte hyperplasia in the failing human heart (41), proliferation of these terminally differentiated cells is limited and so is unlikely to play an important role in the long-term compensation to a chronic overload.

Studies of myocytes isolated from normal and diseased human hearts provide elegant support for the view that different loading abnormalities, by eliciting morphologically different growth responses, generate different cardiac myocyte phenotypes. In non-dilated, hypertrophied hypertensive hearts, myocyte size is increased largely by a greater cross-sectional area (22). Cell length, which appears to increase only minimally in these hearts, has been found to be almost 50% greater in myocytes isolated from dilated, failing hearts

TABLE 21–6. *Molecular Alterations in the Failing Human Heart*

Protein	Human Heart Failure
CONTRACTILE PROTEINS	
Myosin heavy chain	Reversion to fetal phenotype
Myosin light chains	Reversion to fetal phenotype
Actin	No change
Troponin I	Reversion to fetal phenotype
Troponin T	? Reversion to fetal phenotype
Troponin C	No change
Tropomyosin	No change
SARCOPLASMIC RETICULUM PROTEINS	
Calcium pump ATPase (SERCA)	Probably decreased
Phospholamban	Probably decreased
Calcium release channel (ryanodine receptor)	Probably decreased
Calsequestrin	Normal
Calreticulin	Normal
PLASMA MEMBRANE PROTEINS	
L-type calcium channels	?Increased channel opening
Na/Ca exchanger	Increased
Sodium pump	Re-expression of fetal isoforms

[From reference (53).]

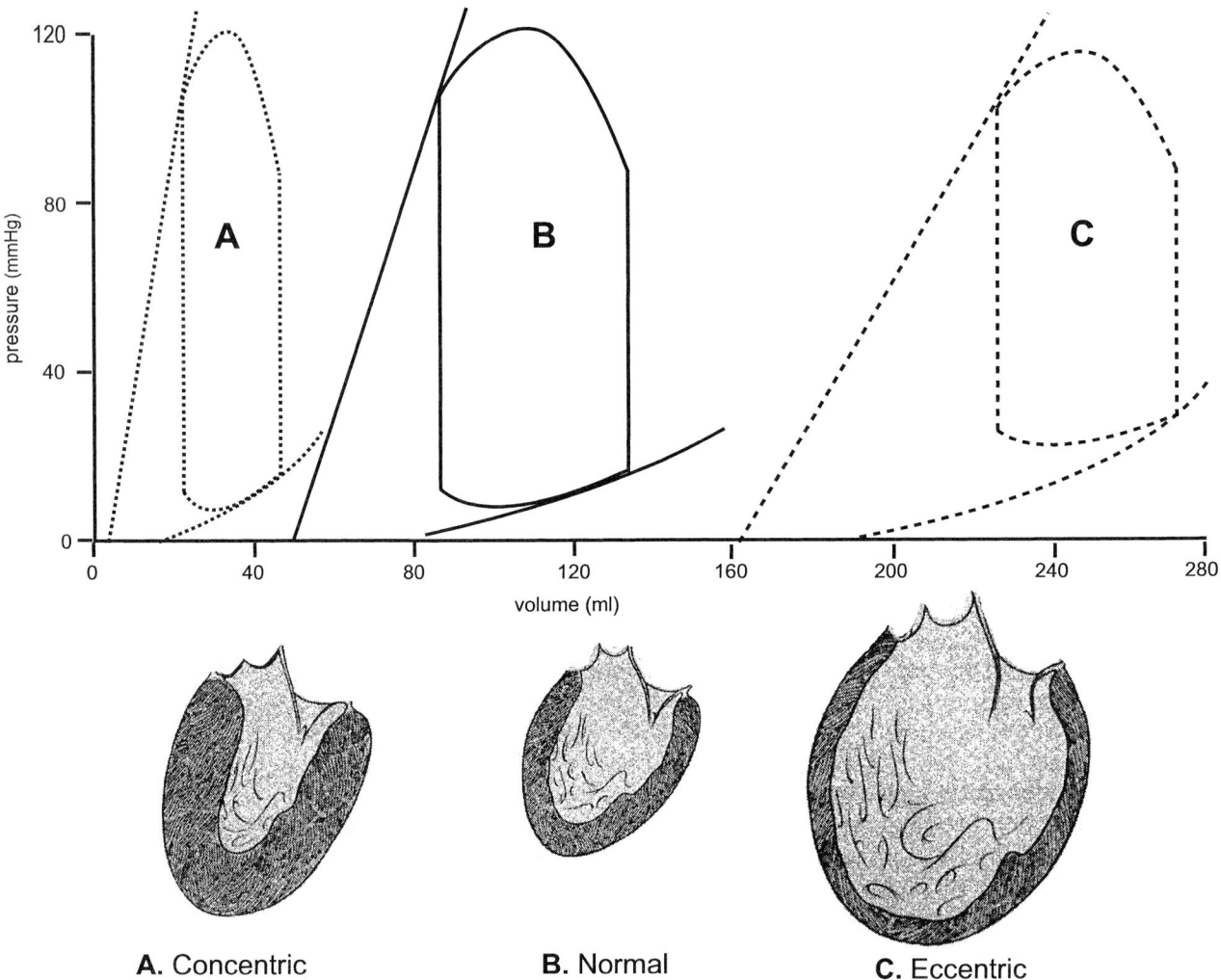

FIG. 21–3. Effects of changing cardiac phenotype (*below*) on the pressure–volume loop (*above*). *A:* Concentric hypertrophy; *B:* normal; *C.* eccentric hypertrophy. Note that the major cause of reduced stroke volume is not a decrease in contractility (the end-systolic pressure volume relationship), but instead, architectural changes in the ventricle. [From reference (54).]

in patients following myocardial infarction (23, 24) and with dilated cardiomyopathies (23).

A possible mechanism for the different hypertrophied myocyte phenotypes in compensated pressure and volume overload is that increased systolic wall stress initiates concentric hypertrophy by causing new sarcomeres to be added mainly in parallel, in the eccentrically hypertrophied ventricle, diastolic stretch causes new sarcomeric units to be added in series. This explanation implies that cardiac myocyte thickening and elongation are controlled by different signaling pathways. Experimental support for this view is found in a recent report that cardiotrophin-1, one of the family of cytokines, induces a pattern of cardiac hypertrophy in cultured neonatal cardiac myocytes where sarcomeres are added in series (99). This paper provides evidence that this growth stimulus, which utilizes a tyrosine kinase-catalyzed phosphorylation, induces cell elongation (eccentric hypertrophy), whereas the growth stimuli activated by α-adrenergic agonists lead to a more uniform increase in myocyte size (concentric hypertrophy). It is not yet clear, however, whether similar signaling systems control the appearance of these different phenotypes in the adult heart.

The discovery that different growth signals can generate different cardiac myocyte phenotypes has important therapeutic implications. It might become possible, for example, to find drugs that activate a growth-promoting signal transduction system that increases cell diameter (concentric hypertrophy) while inhibiting systems that cause cells to elongate (eccentric hypertrophy). The resulting increase in cell thickness without cell elongation could inhibit remodeling. Surprisingly, the findings of several experimental studies and clinical trials in patients with heart failure indicates that such drugs already exist! This is evidenced, for example, by the ability of both β-adrenergic blockers (28, 81), and converting enzyme inhibitors (81, 84) to inhibit remodeling. For this reason, new knowledge of the molecular signals that initiate and maintain these different growth responses may hold the key not only to understanding differences between adaptive and maladaptive cardiac hypertrophy, but may also lead to the development of drugs able to prevent the progressive, and generally lethal, remodeling of the failing heart. Regulation of the proliferative signaling responsible for these phenotypic changes may therefore provide a key to preventing the transition from adaptive to maladaptive hypertrophy.

Myocardial Cell Death

Both necrosis and apoptosis appear to be responsible for cardiac myocyte death in the failing heart. Possible causes of necrosis include membrane damage and calcium overload [for review see (53)], while many parallels between the factors that stimulate mitosis and apoptosis support the view that proliferative signals which stimulate the failing heart to hypertrophy also cause programed cell death (94).

Apoptosis is not only a natural phenomenon, it is essential in organs made up of proliferating cells, where surviving cells divide and their progeny take over for their lost cousins. However, a cell that dies in an organ made up of terminally differentiated cells cannot be replaced, which is especially damaging in the heart, where overload-induced myocyte loss increases the burden on the surviving myocytes. This establishes a vicious cycle in which cell death increases overload, which accelerates cell death, which increases overload etc. The importance of apoptosis in the failing heart is not clear, as this field is changing rapidly (30). Evidence that many published estimates greatly overestimate the number of apoptotic cells in failing hearts (10, 53) has given rise to a controversy regarding the importance of programed cell death in the failing heart that has not yet been resolved (2, 83).

SUMMARY AND CONCLUSIONS

This chapter highlights the fact that heart failure, while manifest clinically as a disorder of cardiac pumping, is also a cellular and molecular disorder that drastically shortens clinical survival. Although therapy that alleviates the circulatory abnormalities caused by the failing cardiac pump has improved dramatically, it is only recently that the focus in treating this condition has shifted to the more ominous problem of prognosis.

Efforts to improve pump performance, while of short-term benefit to these patients, often have harmful long-term effects, while several classes of drugs that transiently worsen symptoms improve long-term survival (Table 21–1). Although the mechanisms responsible for these differences between the short-term and long-term effects are not yet fully understood, it has become clear that efforts to treat heart failure by alleviating the hemodynamic abnormalities can worsen the bleak prognosis in this condition. This illustrates the fallacy of defining heart failure simply as a clinical syndrome where reduced cardiac pumping is caused by impaired myocardial contraction and relaxation; instead, heart failure must be viewed as a progressive syndrome in which patients die prematurely as the result of abnormalities in the hypertrophied myocardium.

Effective ways to alleviate maladaptive aspects of the hypertrophic response to overload offer considerable promise for improving prognosis in the patient with heart failure. The hypertrophic response, whether caused by abnormal hemodynamic overloading or myocardial damage, initially normalizes fiber stress and so is adaptive. When sustained, however, this proliferative response leads to deleterious architectural changes in the heart, notably remodeling, and shortens myocardial cell survival. For this reason, this maladaptive growth response can be viewed as a "cardiomyopathy of overload" (50). Features of the proliferative response of the overloaded heart that could accelerate myocardial deterioration include alterations in cardiac myocyte phenotype that lead to the progressive dilatation, which weakens the heart and increases cardiac energy expenditure. Mitochondrial DNA abnormalities also contribute to a state of energy starvation in the failing heart. The ability of proliferative signal transduction to stimulate apoptosis (programmed cell death) may also play an important role in the poor prognosis in this condition.

It is remarkable that much of the progress in treating heart failure over the past decade has been made by what appears to have been serendipity! Yet much has been learned since 1986, when it was first demonstrated that *any* treatment can improve prognosis in heart failure (15). Recent clinical trials indicate that drugs that improve prognosis in heart failure act not only by reducing energy expenditure, but also by modifying proliferative stimuli that can cause cardiac myocyte elongation and apoptosis. This suggests that new knowledge of the signal transduction systems that control cell growth may provide additional means to slow, or even eliminate, the maladaptive growth responses responsible for the poor prognosis in patients with heart failure.

REFERENCES

1. Alpert, N. R., and M. S. Gordon. Myofibrillar adenosine triphosphatase activity in congestive heart failure. *Am. J. Physiol.* 202:940–946, 1962.
2. Anversa, P. Myocyte death in the pathological heart. *Circ. Res.* 86:121–124, 2000.
3. Apstein, C. S., F. N. Gravino and C. C. Haudenschild. Determinants of a protective effect of glucose and insulin on the ischemic myocardium: Effects on contractile function, diastolic compliance, metabolism and ultrastructure during ischemia and reperfusion. *Circ. Res.* 52:515–526, 1983.
4. Baig, M. K., J. H. Goldman, A. L. P. Caforio, A. S. Coonar, P. J. Keeling, and W. J. McKenna. Familial dilated cardiomyopathy: cardiac abnormalities are common in asymptomatic relatives and may represent early disease. *J. Am. Coll. Cardiol.* 31:195–201, 1998.
5. Barger, P. M., and D. P. Kelly. Fatty acid utilization in the hypertrophied and failing heart: molecular regulatory mechanisms. *Am. J. Med. Sci.* 318:36–42, 1999.
6. Beltrami, C. A., N. Finato, M. Rocco, G. A. Feruglio, C. Puricelli, E. Cigola, F. Quaini, E. H. Sonnenblick, G. Olivetti, and P. Anversa. Structural basis for end-stage failure in ischemic cardiomyopathy in humans. *Circulation* 89:151–163, 1994.
7. Benotti, J. R., W. Grossman, E. Braunwald, D. D. Dovolos, and A. A. Alousi. Hemodynamic assessment of amrinone: a new inotropic agent. *N. Engl. J. Med.* 299:1373–1377, 1978.
8. Bonne, G., L. Carrier, P. Richard, B. Hainque, and K. Schwartz. Familial hypertrophic cardiomyopathy. From mutations to functional defects. *Circ. Res.* 83:580–593, 1998.
9. Bugaisky, L., M. Gupta, M. G. Gupta, and R. Zak. Cellular and molecular mechanisms of hypertrophy In: *The Heart and Cardiovascular System*, Second Ed., edited by H. Fozzard, E. Haber, A. Katz, R. Jennings, and H. E. Morgan. New York: Raven Press. 1992:1621–1640.
10. Buja, L. M., and M. L. Entman. Models of myocardial cell injury and cell death in ischemic heart disease. *Circulation* 98:1355–1357, 1998.
11. Calderone, A., N. Takahashi, N. J. Izzo, Jr., C. M. Thaik, and W. S. Colucci. Pressure- and volume-induced left ventricular hypertrophies are associated with distinct myocyte phenotypes and differential induction of peptide growth factor mRNAs. *Circulation* 92:2385–2390, 1995.
12. CIBIS-II Investigators and Committees The cardiac insufficiency bisoprolol study II (CIBIS-II): a randomised trial. *Lancet* 353:9–13, 1999.
13. Cohn, J. N. Introduction. The Vasodilator-Heart Failure Trials (V-HeFT). Mechanistic studies from the VA cooperative studies. *Circulation* 87(Suppl VI):VI-1–VI-4, 1993.
14. Cohn, J. N. Treatment of heart failure. *N. Engl. J. Med.* 335:490–498, 1996.
15. Cohn, J. N., D. G. Archibald, S. Ziesche, J. A. Franciosa, W. E. Harston, F. E. Tristani, W. B. Dunkman, W. Jacobs, G. S. Francis, F. R. Cobb, P. M. Shah, R. Saunders, R. D. Fletcher, H. S. Loeb, V. C. Hughes, and B. Baker. Effect of vasodilator therapy on mortality in chronic congestive heart failure. Results of a Veterans Administration cooperative study(V-HeFT). *N. Engl. J. Med.* 314:1547–1552, 1986.
16. Cohn, J. N., S. O. Goldstein, B. H. Greenberg, B. H. Lorell, R. C. Bourge, B. E. Jaski, S. O. Gottlieb, F. McGrew 3rd, D. L. DeMets, and B. G. White. A dose-dependent increase in mortality with vesnarinone among patients with severe heart failure. Vesnarinone Trial Investigators. *N. Engl. J. Med.* 339:1810–1816, 1998.
17. Cunningham, M. L., C. S. Apstein, E. O. Weinberg, W. M. Vogel, and B. H. Lorell. Influence of glucose and insulin on the exaggerated diastolic and systolic dysfunction of hypertrophied rat hearts during hypoxia. *Circ. Res.* 66:406–415, 1990.
18. Eichhorn, E. J., and M. R. Bristow. Medial therapy can improve the biological properties of the chronically failing heart. *Circulation* 94:2285–2296, 1996.
19. Eichhorn, E. J., B. Hatfield, L. Marcoux and R. C. Risser. Functional importance of myocardial relaxation in patients with congestive heart failure. *J. Cardiac Failure* 1:45–56, 1994.
20. Francis, G. S., S. R. Goldsmith, T. B. Levine, M. T. Olivari, and J. N. Cohn. The neurohumoral axis in congestive heart failure. *Ann. Intern. Med.* 101:370–377, 1984.
21. Gerdes, A. M., and J. M. Capasso. Editorial Review: structural remodeling and mechanical dysfunction of cardiac myocytes in heart failure. *J. Mol. Cell. Cardiol.* 27:849–856, 1995.
22. Gerdes, A. M., S. E. Kellerman, K. B. Malec, and D. D. Schocken. Transverse shape characteristics of cardiac myocytes from rats and humans. *Cardioscience* 5:31–36, 1994.
23. Gerdes A. M., S. E. Kellerman, J. A. Moore, K. E. Muffy, L. C. Clark, P. Y. Reeves, K. B. Malec, P. P. McKeown, and D. D. Schocken. Structural remodeling of cardiac myocytes in patients with ischemic cardiomyopathy. *Circulation* 85:426–430, 1992.
24. Gerdes A. M., S. E. Kellerman, and D. D. Schocken. Implications of cardiomyocyte remodeling in heart dysfunction. In: *The Failing Heart*, edited by N. S. Dhalla, R. E. Beamish, N. Takeda, and M. Nagano. Philadelphia: Lippincott-Raven, 1995:197–205.
25. Graham, R. M., and W. A. Owens. Pathogenesis of inherited forms of dilated cardiomyopathy. *N. Engl. J. Med.* 341:1759–1762, 1999.
26. Grossman, W., D. Jones, and L. P. McLaurin. Wall stress and patterns of hypertrophy in the human left ventricle. *J. Clin. Invest.* 56:56–64, 1975.
27. Grünig, E., J. A. Tasman, H. Kücherer, W. Franz, W. Kübler, and H. A. Katus. Frequency and phenotypes of familial dilated cardiomyopathy. *J. Am. Coll. Cardiol.* 31:186–194, 1998.
28. Hall, S. A., C. G. Cigarroa, L. Marcoux, R. C. Risser, P. A. Grayburn, and E. J. Eichhorn. Time course of improvement in left ventricular function, mass and geometry in patients with congestive heart failure treated with beta-adrenergic blockade. *J. Am. Coll. Cardiol.* 25:1154–1161, 1995.
29. Harris, P. Evolution and the cardiac patient. *Cardiovasc. Res.* 17:313–319, 373–378, 437–445, 1983.
30. Haunstetter, A., and S. Izumo. Apoptosis. basic mechanisms and implications for cardiovascular disease. *Circ. Res.* 82:1111–1129, 1998.
31. Hennen, J., H. M. Krumholz, and M. J. Radford. Twenty most frequent DRG groups among Medicare inpatients age 65 or older in Connecticut hospitals, fiscal years 1991, 1992, and 1993. *Conn. Med.* 59:11–15, 1995.
32. Hood, W. P., Jr., C. E. Rackley, and E. L. Rolett. Wall stress in the normal and hypertrophied human left ventricle. *Am. J. Cardiol.* 22:5550–558, 1968.
33. Ho, K. K. L., K. M. Anderson, W. B. Kannel, W. Grossman, and D. Levy. Survival after the onset of congestive heart failure in Framingham heart study subjects. *Circulation* 88:107–115, 1993.
34. Hoffman, J. E. I. Transmural myocardial perfusion. *Prog. Cardiovasc. Dis.* 29:429–464, 1987.
35. Hosenpud, J. D., and B. H. Greenberg, Editors. *Congestive Heart Failure*, 2nd Ed. Baltimore. Lippincott Williams and Wilkins, 2000.

36. Illingworth, J. A., W. Christopher, L. Ford, K. Kobayashi, and J. R. Williamson. Regulation of myocardial energy metabolism. In: *Recent Advances in Studies on Cardiac Structure and Metabolism*, edited by P-E. Roy and P. Harris, 1975:271–290, vol. 8.
37. Ingwall, J. S. Is cardiac failure a consequence of decreased energy reserve. *Circulation* 87(Suppl VII):VII-58–VII-62, 1993.
38. Ingwall, J. S., M. F. Kramer, M. A. Fifer, B. H. Lorell, R. Shemin, W. Grossman, and P. D. Allen. The creatine kinase sytem in normal and depressed human myocardium. *N. Engl. J. Med.* 313:1050–1054, 1985.
39. Jacobus W. E. Respiratory control and the integration of heart high-energy metabolism by mitochondrial creatine kinase. *Annu. Rev. Physiol.* 47:707–725, 1985.
40. Kagaya Y., E. O. Weinberg, N. Ito, T. Mochizuki, W. H. Barry, and B. H. Lorell. Glycolytic inhibition: effects on diastolic relaxation and intracellular calcium handling in hypertrophied rat ventricular myocytes. *J. Clin. Invest.* 95:2766–2776, 1995.
41. Kajstura, J., X. Zhang, K. Reiss, E. Szoke, P. Li, C. Lagrasta, W. Cheng, et al. Myocyte cellular hyperplasia and myocyte cellular hypertrophy contribute to chronic ventricular remodeling in coronary artery narrowing-induced cardiomyopathy in rats. *Circ. Res.* 74:383–400, 1994.
42. Kalsi, K. K., R. T. Smolenski, R. D. Pritchart, A. Khagani, A. M. Seymour, and M. H. Yacoub. Energetics and function of the failing human heart with dilated or hypertrophic cardiomyopathy. *Eur. J. Clin. Invest.* 29:469–477, 1999.
43. Kammermeier, H., P. Schmidt, and E. Jüngling. Free energy change of ATP-hydrolysis: a causal factor of early hypoxic failure of the myocardium? *J. Mol. Cell. Cardiol.* 14:267–277, 1982.
44. Kass, D. A. Evaluation of left-ventricular systolic function. *Heart Failure* 4:198–205, 1988.
45. Katz, A. M. Biochemical "defect" in the hypertrophied and failing heart: deleterious or compensatory? *Circulation* 47:1076–1079, 1973.
46. Katz, A. M. Congestive heart failure: role of altered myocardial cellular control. *N. Engl. J. Med.* 293:1184–1191, 1975.
47. Katz, A. M. Influence of altered inotropy and lusitropy on ventricular pressure-volume loops. *J. Am. Coll. Cardiol.* 11:438–445, 1988.
48. Katz, A. M. Molecular biology in cardiology, a paradigmatic shift. *J. Mol. Cell. Cardiol.* 20:355–366, 1988.
49. Katz, A. M. Changing strategies in the management of heart failure. *J. Am. Coll. Cardiol.* 13:513–523, 1989.
50. Katz, A. M. Cardiomyopathy of overload. A major determinant of prognosis in congestive heart failure. *N. Engl. J. Med.* 322:100–110, 1990.
51. Katz, A. M. Cardiomyopathy of overload. An unnatural growth response in the hypertrophied heart. *Ann. Intern. Med.* 121:363–371, 1994.
52. Katz, A. M. Evolving concepts of heart failure: cooling furnace, malfunctioning pump, enlarging muscle. *J. Cardiac Failure.* 3:319–334, 1997; 4:67–81, 1998.
53. Katz, A. M. *Heart Failure: Pathophysiology, Molecular Biology, Clinical Management.* Philadelphia: Lippincott Williams and Wilkins, 2000.
54. Katz, A. M. *Physiology of the Heart*, Third Ed. Philadelphia: Lippincott Williams and Wilkins, 2001.
55. Keeling, P. J., Y. Gang, G. Smith, H. Seo, S. E. Bent, V. Murday, A. L. P. Caforio, and W. J. McKenna. Familial dilated cardiomyopathy in the United Kingdom. *Br. Heart J.* 73:417–421, 1995.
56. Kuhn, T. S. *The Structure of Scientific Revolutions*, 2nd Ed. Chicago: The University of Chicago Press, 1970.
57. LeChat, P., M. Packer, S. Chalon, M. Cucherat, T. Arab, and J-P. Boissel. Clinical effects of β-adrenergic blockade in chronic heart failure. *Circulation* 98:1184–1191, 1998.
58. Linzbach, A. J. Heart failure from the point of view of quantitative anatomy. *Am. J. Cardiol.* 5:370–382, 1960.
59. Lubbe, W. F., T. Podzweit, P. S. Daries, and L. H. Opie. The role of cyclic adenosine monophosphate in adrenergic effects on ventricular vulnerability to fibrillation in the isolated perfused heart. *J. Clin. Invest.* 61:1260–1269, 1978.
60. Malhotra, A., S. Penpargkul, T. Schaible, and J. Scheuer. Contractile proteins and sarcoplasmic reticulum in physiologic cardiac hypertrophy. *Am. J. Physiol.* 241 (*Heart Circ. Physiol.* 10): H263–H267, 1981.
61. Mann, D. L. Mechanisms of heart failure. *Circulation* 100:999–1008, 1999.
62. McCall, D., and S. H. Rahimtoola, Eds. *Heart Failure.* New York: Chapman & Hall, 1995.
63. Marcus, M. L., D. B. Doty, L. F. Hiratzka, C. B. Wright, and C. L. Eastham. Decreased coronary reserve: a mechanism for angina pectoris in patients with aortic stenosis and normal coronary arteries. *N. Engl. J. Med.* 307:1362–1366, 1982.
64. Meerson, F. Z. On the mechanism of compensatory hyperfunction and insufficiency of the heart. *Cor et Vasa* 3:161–177, 1961.
65. Meerson, F. Z., and M. P. Javick. Isozyme pattern and activity of myocardial creatine phosphokinase under heart adaptation to chronic overload. *Basic Res. Cardiol.* 77:349–358, 1982.
66. Merit-HF Study Group. Effect of metoprolol CR/XL in chronic heart failure: Metoprolol CR/XL randomized intervention trial in congestive heart failure (MERIT-HF) *Lancet* 353:2001–2007, 1999.
67. Neubauer, S., M. Horn, A. Naumann, R. Tian, M. Laser, J. Friedrich, P. Gaudron, K. Schnackerz, J. S. Ingwall, and G. Errl. Impairment of energy metabolism in intact residual myocardium of rat hearts with chronic myocardial infarction. *J. Clin. Invest.* 95:1092–1100, 1995.
68. Obayashi, T. K., S. Hattori, S. Sugiyama, M. Taneka, T. Tanaka, S. Itoyama, et al. Point mutations in mitochondrial DNA in patients with hypertrophic cardiomyopathy. *Am. Heart J.* 124:1263–1269, 1992.
69. O.Connor, C. M., W. A. Gattis B. F. Uretsky K. F. Adams, Jr., S. E. McNulty, S. H. Grossman, W. J. McKenna, F. Zannad, K. Swedberg, M. Gheorghiade, and R. M. Califf, for the FIRST Investigators. Continuous intravenous dobutamine is associated with an increased risk of death in patients with advanced heart failure: insights from the Flolan International Randomized Survival Trial (FIRST). *Am. Heart. J.* 138:78–86, 1999.
70. Olivetti, G., J. M. Capasso, E. H. Sonnenblick, and P. Anversa. Side-to-side slippage of myocytes participates in ventricular wall remodeling acutely after myocardial infarction in rats. *Circ. Res.* 67:23–34, 1990.
71. Packer, M. The neurohumoral hypothesis: a theory to explain the mechanism of disease progression in heart failure. *J. Am. Coll. Cardiol.* 20:248–254, 1992.
72. Packer, M., M. R. Bristow, J. N. Cohn, W. S. Colucci, M. B. Fowler, E. M. Gilbert, and N. H. Shusterman for the US Carvedilol Heart Failure Study Group. *N. Engl. J. Med.* 334:1349–1355, 1996.
73. Packer, M., J. R. Carver, R. J. Rodeheffer, R. J. Ivanhoe, R. DiBianco, S. M. Zeldis, G. H. Hendrix, W. J. Bommer, El-kayam, M. L. Kukin, G. I. Mallis, J. A. Sollano, J. Shannon, P. K. Tandon, and D. L. DeMets. Effect of oral milrinone on mortality in severe heart failure. *N. Engl. J. Med.* 325:1468–1475, 1991.
74. Packer, M., and J. N. Cohn. Consensus recommendations for the management of heart failure *Am. J. Cardiol.* 83(Suppl 2a):1A–38A, 1999.
75. Penpargkul, S., D. I. Repke, A. M., Katz, and J. Scheuer Effect of physical training on calcium transport by rat cardiac sarcoplasmic reticulum. *Circ. Res.* 40:134–138, 1977.

76. Podzuweit, T., W. F., Lubbe, and L. H. Opie Cyclic adenosine monophosphate, ventricular fibrillation, and antiarrhythmic drugs. *Lancet* 1:341–342, 1976.
77. Poole-Wilson, P. A., W. S. Colucci, B. M. Massie, K. Chatterjee, A. S. Coats, Editors. *Heart Failure. Scientific Principles and Clinical Practice*. New York: Churchill Livingstone, 1997.
78. Rauch, B., B. Schultze, and H. P. Schultheiss. Alteration of the cytosolic-mitochondrial distribution of high-energy phosphates during global myocardial ischemia may contribute to early contractile failure. *Circ. Res.* 75:760–769, 1994.
79. Remes, A. M., I. E. Hassinen, M. J. Ikäheimo, R. Herva, J. Hirvonen, and K. J. Peuhkurinen. Mitochondrial DNA deletions in dilated cardiomyopathy: a clinical study employing endomyocardial sampling. *J. Am. Coll. Cardiol.* 23:935–942, 1993.
80. Ross, J., Jr. Afterload mismatch and preload reserve: a conceptual framework for the analysis of ventricular function. *Prog. Cardiovasc. Dis.* 18:255–264, 1976.
81. Sabbah, H. N., H. Shimoyama, T. Kono, R. C. Gupta, V. G. Sharov, G. Scicli, T. B. Levine, and S. Goldstein. Effect of long-term monotherapy with enalapril, metoprolol, and digoxin on the progression of left ventricular dysfunction and dilatation in dogs with reduced ejection fraction. *Circulation* 89:2852–2859, 1994.
82. Sandler, H., and H. T. Dodge. Left ventricular tension and stress in man. *Circ. Res.* 13:91–104, 1963.
83. Schaper, J., A. Elsässer, and S. Kostin. The role of cell death in heart failure. *Circ. Res.* 85:867–869, 1999.
84. Schieffer, B., A. Wirger, M. Meybrunn, S. Seitz, J. Holtz, U. N. Riede, H. Drexler. Comparative effects of chronic angiotensin-converting enzyme inhibition and angiotensin type 1 receptor blockade on cardiac remodeling after myocardial infarction in the rat. *Circulation* 89:2273–2282, 1994.
85. Smith, V-E., M. L. Weisfeldt, and A. M. Katz. Relaxation and diastolic properties of the heart. In *The Heart and Cardiovascular System*, edited by H. Fozzard, E. Haber, A. Katz, R. Jennings, and H. E. Morgan. New York: Raven Press, 1986:803–818.
86. Spann, J. F., Jr., R. A. Bucino, E. H. Sonnenblick, and E. Braunwald. Contractile state of cardiac muscle obtained from cats with experimentally produced ventricular hypertrophy and heart failure. *Circ. Res.* 21341–21354, 1967.
87. Spirito, P., C. E. Seidman, W. J. McKenna, and B. J. Maron. The management of hypertrophic cardiomyopathy. *N. Engl. J. Med.* 336:775–785, 1997.
88. Stevenson, L. W., B. M. Massie, and G. S. Francis. Optimizing therapy for complex or refractory heart failure: a management problem. *Am. Heart J.* 135:S293–S309, 1998.
89. Suomalainen, A., A. Paetau, H. Leinonen, A. Majander, L. Peltonen, and H. Somer. Inherited idiopathic dilated cardiomyopathy with multiple deletions of mitochondrial DNA. *Lancet* 340:1319–1320, 1992.
90. Swynghedauw, B. Molecular mechanisms of myocardial remodeling. *Physiol. Rev.* 79:215–262, 1999.
91. Tian, R., M. E. Christe, M. Spindler, J. .C. A. Hopkins, J. M. Halow, S. A. Camacho, and J. S. Ingwall. Role of MgADP in the development of diastolic dysfunction in the intact beating rat heart. *J. Clin. Invest.* 99:745–751, 1997.
92. Tian, R. and J. S. Ingwall. Energetic basis for reduced contractile reserve in isolated rat hearts. *Am. J. Physiol.* 270 (*Heart Circ. Physiol.* 39):H1207–H1216, 1996.
93. Tian, R., L. Nascimben, J. S. Ingwall, and B. H. Lorell. Failure to maintain a low ADP concentration impairs diastolic function in hypertrophied rat hearts. *Circulation* 96:1313–1319, 1997.
94. Ucker, D. S., Death by suicide: one way to go in mammalian development? *New Biologist* 3:103–109, 1991.
95. Vasan, R. S., E. J. Benjamin, J. C. Evans, M. G. Larson, C. K. Reiss, and D. Levy. Prognosis of diastolic heart failure: Framingham Heart Study. (abstract) *Circulation* 92:(Suppl I)1–665, 1996.
96. Wangler, R. D., K. G. Peters, M. L. Marcus, and R. J. Tomanek. Effects of duration and severity of arterial hypertension and cardiac hypertrophy on coronary vasodilator rserve. *Circ. Res.* 51:10–18, 1982.
97. Weber, K. T., J. S. Janicki, S. G. Schroff, R. Pick, R. M. Chen, and R. I. Bashey. Collagen remodeling of the pressure-overloaded, hypertrophied nonhuman primate myocardium. *Circ. Res.* 62:757–65, 1988.
98. Wicker, P., R. C. Tarazi, and K. Kobayashi. Coronary blood flow during the development and regression of left ventricular hypertrophy in renovascular hypertensive rats. *Am. J. Cardiol.* 51:1744–1749, 1983.
99. Wollert, K. C., T. Taga, M. Saito, M. Narazaki, T. Kishimoto, C. C. Glembotski, A. B. Vernallis, J. K. Heath, D. Pennica, W. I. Wood, K. R. Chien. Corticotrophin-1 activates a distinct form of cardiac muscle cell hypertrophy. Assembly of sarcomeric units in series via gp130/leukemia inhibitory factor receptor-dependent pathways. *J. Biol. Chem.* 271:9535–9545, 1996.
100. Wood, P. *Diseases of the Heart*, 2nd Ed. London: Routledge. 1956.

Index

Page numbers followed by f and t indicate figures and tables, respectively.

A-band, 36, 40f, 41f, 241f
Acetylcholine
   cellular responsiveness to, 662
   effects on automaticity and pacemaker channels, 619–20, 619f
   effects on chloride channels, 619
   effects on L-type channels, 618–19
   effects on membrane potentials, 616
   potassium channel activation by, 560–61, 616–18, 617f, 720
   stimulatory actions, 620
Acidosis
   in contraction regulation, 439–40
   electrophysiological effects, 541, 605–7
Actin, 36
   atomic structure, 255f, 256
   in contraction regulation, 426
   domains, 266–67, 267f
   isoform expression, 426
   modulatory proteins associated with, 265f, 266
   tropomyosin interactions, 266, 267, 267f
α-Actinin-2 potassium channel, 577f, 579
Actin-myosin crossbridges. See Crossbridge cycling
Action potential, 531–43. See also Afterdepolarization
   activation recovery interval, 660, 660t
   calcium influx during, 345–46, 345f, 347f, 551
   currents underlying, 710, 711f
   depolarization, 494–98, 495f–497f, 710
   digitalis effects, 629–30, 630f
   in dorsal vagal nucleus, 219, 220f
   duration
      by cell type, 536–38, 537f–538f, 659t, 661t
      transient outward current and, 717–18
      transmural dispersion, 660, 660t, 661t
   on electrocardiogram, 569f, 570–71
   fundamental principles, 531–32
   generation, calcium effects, 600
   genes involved in, cardiac localization, 666t–667t
   heterogeneity
      by cell type, 536–38, 537f–538f, 654–62, 656f–657f, 658t, 659f, 661t
      developmental aspects, 671–72, 671f
      methodological considerations, 660–62, 660t, 661t
      simulation, 671
   histamine effects, 625–26
   insulin effects, 621
   interactive processes, 532, 534f
   ionic basis, 532–36, 534f–535f
   ionic concentration effects, 540–41, 541f
   in isolated myocytes, 661
   in isolated tissue slices, 660–61
   Luo-Rudy model, 532, 533f
   maximal upstroke velocity, 459, 531
      in anisotropic cellular network, 469–70, 471–72, 473f
      in cell chain, 468, 468f
      effects of depolarization, 494–95, 496f
      effects of resistive discontinuities, 464f, 465f, 466–67, 467f
      effects of superfusate fluid, 473–74, 474f, 476, 477f
      recovery from activation, 497, 497f
   monophasic, 660, 660t
   Na^{2+}-Ca^{2+} exchanger during, 350–54, 352f–354f
   normal, 532–34, 534f–535f
   notch, 655, 655t
   pacing effects
      fast, 536, 536f
      slow, 537–38, 538f
   pathological, ischemia-induced, 541–42, 542f
   phases, 569f, 570–71, 710
   potassium effects, 596–97, 597f
   premature, 534–36, 535f–536f
   prolongation
      drug-induced, 663–64, 663f, 664t
      in long QT syndrome, 538–40, 539f, 540f
   rate adaptation, 536, 536f
   repolarization
      abnormal, 538–40, 539f, 540f
      calcium effects, 600–601
      currents underlying, 710
      early, electrical heterogeneity, 674–76
      pH effects, 606–7
      safety factor for, 710
      transmural dispersion of, anesthesia and, 661–62
   sodium effects, 540–41, 541f, 552, 553f, 599
   stretch effects, 608
   temperature effects, 607
   thyroid state effects, 621
   transmembrane recordings, 660, 660t, 661t
   in vivo, 661–62
   waveforms, 569f
Activation heat, 768
Actomyosin, 255f, 256
Actomyosin ATPase, 243, 245
Adenosine
   effects on ATP-sensitive potassium channels, 623–24
   effects on channels stimulated by β-adrenergic agonists, 623, 623f
   effects on membrane potentials and potassium channels in basal conditions, 622–23
   potassium channel activation by, 617
Adenosine A1 receptor, in calveolae, 156
Adenosine diphosphate (ADP), 251–52, 259–60
Adenosine monophosphate, cyclic. See Cyclic adenosine monophosphate (cAMP)
Adenosine receptors, 622
Adenosine thiotriphosphate, potassium channel activation by, 617
Adenosine triphosphate (ATP)
   binding, 249
   binding mutants, 312f, 313–14
   caged, 249f
   cleavage, 249–50
   effects on calcium channels, 625
   effects on chloride channels, 625
   in heart failure, 796
   hydrolysis
      calcium-dependent, 304–5, 306
         adult vs. neonatal, 307
         calcium uptake and, 305
         cardiac vs. skeletal, 306
         effect of phospholamban on, 317–18
         steps, 306–7
      in crossbridge cycle, 259
         cardiac vs. skeletal, 245
         energetics, 244–45
         rate, 242–44, 243f
         reversibility, 244
         steps, 249–50
   products, accumulation of, 440–41
   potassium channel sensitive to, 542, 561, 562f, 625, 719–20
      activation, 618, 631, 632f
      adenosine effects, 623–24
      sensitivities, 631, 633
      purinergic receptor stimulation and, 624–25, 624f

805

Adenosine triphosphate (ATP) receptors, 622
Adenoviral transfection, of Na^{2+}-Ca^{2+} exchange proteins, 407
ADP (adenosine diphosphate), 251–52, 259–60
α-Adrenergic agonists
  calcium sensitivity of tension and, 441
  effects on calcium channels, 614
  effects on chloride channels, 616
  effects on M-cells vs. Purkinje cells, 658t, 665
  effects on Na^+–K^+ pump, 616
  effects on potassium channels, 614–16, 615f
  effects on resting membrane potential, 613–14
β-Adrenergic agonists
  adenosine effects, 623, 623f
  calcium sensitivity of tension and, 441
  chronotropic effect, 609
  crossbridge cycling rate and, 445
  dromotropic effect, 609
  effects on automaticity and conduction, 609–10
  effects on calcium channels, 550, 550f, 610–11, 611f
  effects on chloride channels, 611–12
  effects on pacemaker channels, 612–13
  effects on potassium channels, 611–12
  effects on resting membrane potential, 610
  effects on sodium channels, 612
  in heart failure, 790, 790t, 791
  heart rate and, 754–55, 755f
  inotropic effects, 609
  shortening velocity and, 444
β-Adrenergic blocking agents
  for heart failure, 787, 791
  for long QT syndrome, 682, 727
Adrenergic receptors
  α-subtypes, 613
  β-subtypes, 609
Adriamycin cardiomyopathy, Ca^{2+}-ATPase activity and, 308
Affective behavior, cardiorespiratory changes during, 230–31
Afterdepolarization
  delayed, calcium-dependent, 603
  early, 538–40, 539f, 540f
    in M-cells vs. Purkinje cells, 658t, 665
    mechanism for, 724
    triggered activity induced by, 681–82, 682f, 683f
Afterload
  defined, 750
  effect on contractility indices, 758, 759f
  sudden increase in, 797t
  systolic function and, 748f, 750–52, 750f–751f
Afterload mismatch, 762
Aging of heart, 93–105
  as adaptation vs. disease, 94
  cardiac hypertrophy and, 94, 100–102, 101f

coronary arterial and capillary tree and, 102–5, 103f–104f
myocyte number and, 94, 97–100, 98f
ventricular remodeling and, 94–97, 95f
Airway input to cardiac vagal motoneurons, 224, 226
Airway receptors, upper, 226–27
Alcohol, gap junction channel sensitivity to, 198
Aldehyde fixation, in electron microscopy, 63
4-Aminopyridine, cellular responsiveness to, 663, 664t
Amiodarone, chronic
  cellular responsiveness to, 663, 664–65, 664f, 664t
  for long QT syndrome, 683
Amorphin, in Z-band, 50
AMP, cyclic. See Cyclic adenosine monophosphate (cAMP)
Anatomic reentry, 504–7, 505f–506f
Anchorin, 15
Anemia, hypochromic, myocyte hypertrophy in, 112–13
Anesthesia, in vivo electrophysiologic recordings and, 661–62
Angiotensin II
  chronotropic effects, 626
  inotropic effects, 626
Angiotensin receptors, subtypes, 626
Angiotensin-converting enzyme inhibitors, for heart failure, 791
Animal models
  for heart disease, 712–13
  mice. See Mice
  rats, 762
Anisotropic conduction
  arrhythmias and, 179
  bathing solution and, 476, 477f
  in cellular network, 469–72, 472f, 473f
  at macroscopic level, 469
  properties, 178
  structural determinants, 461–63, 462f, 462t, 463f, 463t
  unidirectional block, 502–4, 503f, 504f
Anisotropic media, spiral waves in, 515–16
Anisotropic properties of cardiac tissue, 178, 179
Anisotropic reentry, 518
Ankyrin, Na^{2+}-Ca^{2+} exchanger and, 403
Annexin V, in Z-band, 50
Anoxia, electrophysiological effect, 541
ANP. See Atrial natriuretic peptide
Anrep effect, 747
Anti-α-actinin, 49
Antiarrhythmic agents, for long QT syndrome, 682–83
Antiarrhythmic peptides, gap junction channel sensitivity to, 200
Antibody labeling. See Immunocytochemistry
Anti-desmin antibodies, 15
Antisense oligonucleotides, Na^{2+}-Ca^{2+} exchange and, 407
Aortic banding, papillary muscle

hypertrophy from, myocyte adaptations and, 111–12, 111f
Aortic blood flow, as index of contractility, 757
Aortic pressure, 750
Apoptosis, myocyte loss by, 99–100
Aquaporin-1, 153, 154
Arachidonic acid, gap junction channel sensitivity to, 198
Arginine vasopressin, cardiac effects, 626–27
Arrhythmias. See also Heart disease; specific arrhythmia
  delayed rectifier currents in, 718–19
  gap junctions in, 720–21
  in heart disease, 709–31
  inwardly rectifying K^+ currents in, 719–20
  ion channels in, 711–12, 712t
  ischemic cardiomyopathy and, 129
  L-type calcium channels and, 715
  mechanisms, 710
  Na^{2+}-Ca^{2+} exchanger and, 721
  Na^+–K^+ ATPase and, 721–22
  pacemaker current in, 720
  sodium channels and, 714–15
  transient outward current and, 717–18
  T-type calcium channels and, 716–17
Arteries
  of aging heart, 103
  cardiac hypertrophy and, 116
  in cardiac muscle, 12
  to cardiac vagal motoneurons
    baroreceptor, 221–22
    chemoreceptor, 224, 225f, 226f
  morphometric analysis, 85–86, 86f
Arterioles
  of aging heart, 103–4, 104f
  cardiac hypertrophy and, 116–17
  in cardiac muscle, 12
Atomic force microscopy, 65
ATP. See Adenosine triphosphate (ATP)
ATPase(s)
  F-type, 303
  P-type, 303–4, 308–9, 309f
  V-type, 303
Atrial activation, 479–82, 479f, 481f
Atrial cells
  calveolae and granules in, relationship between, 154, 154f
  potassium sensitivity, 596
Atrial contraction, 774
  preload and, 749–50
Atrial fibrillation
  animal models, 712
  electrophysiologic changes, 713
Atrial muscle, conduction velocity, 456t
Atrial natriuretic peptide
  in calveolae, 154–55, 155f
  cardiac effects, 627–28
Atrioventricular block, potassium channels and, 584, 585f
Atrioventricular junctional area, 482–90
  atrial components, 482, 483f
  compact node. See Atrioventricular node

electrophysiological studies, 484, 485f
structure, 482–84, 483f
Atrioventricular nodal conduction delay
causes, 487–90, 489f, 490f
cycle-length dependence, 489, 490f
Atrioventricular nodal reentry, 487
Atrioventricular node
activation, 484–87, 486f
β-adrenergic effects, 613
anatomy, 483–84
cells, 484, 485f
conduction, 456t, 487–88, 488f
dead-end pathways, 486, 489–90
digitalis effects, 630–31
dual pathways, 486–87
electrophysiological studies, 484
ATX-II, cellular responsiveness to, 663, 664t
Automaticity
acetylcholine effects, 619–20, 619f
β-adrenergic effects, 609–10
calcium effects, 601
pH effects, 607
potassium effects, 596
sodium effects, 599
stretch effects, 608
temperature effects, 608
Autonomic nerve fibers, in cardiac muscle, 12
AV node. See Atrioventricular node

Bachmann's bundle
conduction velocity, 456t
left atrial activation via, 482
Barium, cardiac effects, 603
Barrier-free path (BFP), 157
Basket weave (bw) lattice pattern, in Z-band, 44f, 50–51, 55f, 56f
Bay K 8644, cellular responsiveness to, 663, 664t
Belousov-Zhabotinsky reaction, spiral waves in, 509–10, 510f
B-fibers
cardiac vagus. See Cardiac vagal motoneurons, B-fiber
cervical vagus, stimulation, 214, 215f
Blood vessels. See Coronary vasculature; *specific type*
Boltzmann relationships, in gap junction channels, 189, 190f, 193t
Bowditch staircase, 752–54
Bradycardia-dependent block, 495–96, 496f
Brain
HCN channels in, 696, 697t
T-type calcium channel in, 699
Brugada syndrome
gene mutations, 674, 676f
mechanism, 674, 676f
ST segment elevation, 672–74, 675f, 676f
vs. long QT syndrome, 684f
Bundle branch
conduction velocity, 490

left, 490, 491f
right, 493
Bundle of His, 483–84

Ca^{2+}. See Calcium
Ca^{2+}-ATPase gene. See Phospholamban–Ca^{2+}-ATPase system; Sarcolemmal Ca^{2+}-ATPase; Sarcoplasmic reticulum Ca^{2+}-ATPase
chromosomal mapping, 323
structure, 322–24, 323f
transcriptional regulation, 324
Cable properties of cardiac tissue, 178
Caged compounds, for crossbridge cycle analysis, 249, 249f, 433
Calcineurin, activation, 280
Calcium
binding
Ca^{2+}-ATPase, 305, 310–11, 310f, 312f, 313
cooperativity in, 436
sites
in myocytes, 336–40, 337f–338f, 339t
in Na^+-Ca^{2+} exchanger, 401
troponin C, 427
caged, 249f
chloride channel activated by, 605, 605f
cytosolic buffering, 336–40
during calcium transient, 341–42, 342f, 342t
competitive factors, 341
fast, 337–38, 338f, 339t
slow, 338–39, 338f, 339t
effects on action potential generation, 600
effects on action potential repolarization, 600–601
effects on automaticity, 601
effects on channels, 601–3, 602f
effects on crossbridge kinetics, 258, 259
effects on excitability, 600
effects on pacemaker channels, 601, 603, 698
effects on resting membrane potential, 600
gap junction channel gating by, 196–97
in heart failure, 793, 794f–795f
intracellular
refilling depleted stores, 375, 375f
rest-dependent decline, 373–75, 374f
transport, 355–64. See also Calcium transport
myofilament response to, 265
overload, arrhythmias and, 715
requirements, for contractile activation, 340–41, 341f
sensitivity, in contraction regulation, 429, 435–45
slow wave propagation of, gap junctions and, 186–88, 187f, Plate 7

transport. See Calcium transport
uptake, ATP hydrolysis and, 304–5, 306
adult vs. neonatal, 307
cardiac vs. skeletal, 306
coupling ratio between, 305
phospholamban effects, 317–18
Calcium affinity, Ca^{2+}-ATPase, mutants, 312f
Calcium channel(s), 548–51
in action potential, 345–46, 345f, 347f, 551
α-adrenergic effects, 614
angiotensin II effects, 626
ATP effects, 625
currents, 498, 532, 533f, 540, 540f
digitalis effects, 629–30, 630f
dihydropyridine sensitive, 670
endothelin effect, 627, 627f
gap junction channels as, 186–88, 187f, Plate 7
genes, 667t, 670
inactivation, 344–45, 344f, 345f
L-type, 343, 343f, 344, 715
acetylcholine effects, 618–19
β-adrenergic effects, 550, 550f, 610–11, 611f
arrhythmias and, 715
calcium-dependent modulation, 601, 602f
in heart disease, 715–16
S4 segment, 701, 701f
selectivity profile, 700, 700f
subunits, 548, 549f, 550
magnesium effects, 604
pH effects, 607
regulation, 346–47
ryanodine receptor, 359–61, 361t
sodium effects, 600
temperature effects, 607–8
thyroid state and, 620–21
transient inward current, 341–42, 342f, 342t, 722
T-type, 343, 343f, 344, 551, 698–704
arrhythmias and, 716–17
biophysics, 701–4, 702f–703f
blockade, 703
distribution, 699
in heart disease, 716–17
molecular cloning, 699
role of, 698–99
S4 segment, 701, 701f
selectivity, 700, 700f, 703, 703f
structure, 700–701, 700f–701f
voltage dependence, 702, 702f
Calcium channel blockers
cellular responsiveness to, 662
mechanism of action, 551, 552f
Calcium release channel
gene, chromosomal locations, 323, 324
sarcoplasmic reticulum, 359–61, 361t
Calcium transport
during action potential, 345–46, 345f, 347f, 551
during contraction, 369–72, 370f–371f, 370t

Calcium transport (*continued*)
  cytosolic volume conventions, 336, 337t
  in heart failure, 793, 794f–795f
  intracellular, 355–64
  mitochondrial, 361–64, 362f, 363f
  recycling from mitochondria back to sarcoplasmic reticulum, 369
  during relaxation
    developmental differences, 368–69
    relative contributions of transporters, 364–67, 364f, 365f, 367f
    species differences, 368, 368t
    temperature differences, 368, 368t
  sarcolemmal, 342–55. *See also* Calcium channel(s); Na^{2+}-Ca^{2+} exchange
  sarcoplasmic reticulum Ca^{2+}-ATPase
    electrogenicity, 305
    measurement, 356–59, 358f, 359f
    model for, 314–15
    regulation, 355–56, 355f
    steps, 306–7, 306f
    systems, 335–36, 336f
Calcium-calmodulin–dependent protein kinase phosphorylation
  of phospholamban, 317
  of SERCA2a, 307
Calcium-dependent conduction, 498
Calcium-induced calcium release
  in Luo-Rudy ventricular cell model, 532, 533f
  through reverse Na^{2+}-Ca^{2+} exchange, 391–92
Calcium-magnesium binding sites, calcium buffering at, 338–39, 338f, 339t
Calcium-pumping ATPase. *See* Ca^{2+}-ATPase gene; Phospholamban–Ca^{2+}-ATPase system; Sarcolemmal Ca^{2+}-ATPase; Sarcoplasmic reticulum Ca^{2+}-ATPase
Calcium-sodium exchange. *See* Na^{2+}-Ca^{2+} exchange
Calsequestrin gene, chromosomal locations, 323, 324
Calveolae, 145–63
  adenosine A1 receptor in, 156
  aquaporin-1 in, 153, 154
  atrial, atrial granules and, 154, 154f
  atrial natriuretic peptide in, 154–55, 155f
  closure, 149
  cytoskeleton-associated proteins and, 156
  endothelial nitric oxide synthase in, 155
  extracellular matrix and, 156
  in hypertonic solutions
    cell volume and, 149–50, 150f–151f
    neck surface density and diameter and, 150–52, 152f
  macromolecule uptake by, 148–49, 148f
  monocarboxylate transporter in, 156
  morphometric studies, 145f–148f, 146–48

  neuregulin binding in, 156
  opening, 149
  paradoxical closure, 150
  paradoxical swelling
    aquaporin-1 in, 153
    in hypertonic solutions, 149–50, 150f–151f
  as plasma membrane microdomains, 157–58
  protein kinase C isoforms in, 155–56
  proteins
    analysis techniques, 157
    artifact issues, 161–63
    calveolin as, 158–61. *See also* Calveolin
  sphingolipid/cholesterol rafts and, 156–57
  T-cadherin and, 163
  ultrastructure, 13, 17f, 145
Calveolar necks, surface density, in hypertonic solutions, 150–52, 152f
Calveolin
  biochemistry, 158–59
  cycling, 160
  function, 159–61
  isoforms, 159
  muscle, 159
Calveolin-3
  aquaporin-1 co-localization with, 153, 154
  endothelium-derived nitric oxide synthase co-localization with, 155
  specificity, 159
Calx-α and Calx-β motifs, 398
cAMP. *See* Cyclic adenosine monophosphate (cAMP)
Capillaries
  of aging heart, 102–3, 103f, 104–5
  cardiac hypertrophy and, 114–16, 116f, 117
  in cardiac muscle, 12
  ischemic cardiomyopathy and, 128–29
  morphometric analysis, 84–85
  numerical density, 92
  postnatal adaptations, 91–93, 93f
Capillary domain model, 85
Capillary-to-myocyte ratio, 92, 93
CapZ protein, 49
Cardiac. *See also* Coronary; Heart
Cardiac action potential. *See* Action potential
Cardiac arrhythmias. *See* Arrhythmias
Cardiac conduction. *See* Conduction
Cardiac hypertrophy, 105–17. *See also* Cardiomyopathy, hypertrophic; Myocytes, hypertrophy
  aging-associated, 94, 100–102, 101f
  Ca^{2+}-ATPase activity and, 307–8
  coronary arterial and capillary tree and, 114–17, 116f
  in heart failure, 791–93
    adaptive and maladaptive, 790f, 797–98, 797t

    myocyte phenotype and, 798–99, 798t
    myocyte size, shape and number and, 107–13, 110f–112f, Plate 3
    myocyte volume composition and, 113–14
    physiologic, 107, 798
    troponin I phosphorylation in, 279–80
Cardiac injury, Na^{2+}-Ca^{2+} exchange abnormalities, 409
Cardiac muscle. *See also* Cardiac tissue
  autonomic nerve fibers, 12
  blood vessels, 12
  collagen weave, 9f–16f, 12–13
  crossbridge cycle, 245, 252
  extracellular matrix, 12–14
  fasciae adherentes, 5
  fibroblasts, 12, 19f
  interior supporting network, 14–15, 33–35
  intermediate filaments, 5, 14–15, 27f–30f
  junctional conductance, 195–96
  microtubules, 5, 8f, 14, 20f–27f
  mitochondria, 5, 6f, 8f, 32f, 35, 37f
  muscle proteins, 36, 48, 421–29
  myofilament bundles, 5, 30f–42f, 35–36, 48
  nebulette, 35, 49
  sarcolemmal associations, 15, 33
  sarcomere, 35–36, 48
  structure, 27f
  thick filament. *See* Thick filament
  thin filament. *See* Thin filament
  titin filaments, 33–34
  ultrastructure, 3–66, 302f
    developmental constraints, 5
    force vectors and, 5
    imaging and analysis, 61–66
    key words related to, 4
    mechanical vectors and, 4–5
    shape vectors and, 4, 5
    species comparisons, 5
    summary, 51, 61
  water-channel proteins, 152–53
  Z-band lattice, 48–51, 60f. *See also* Z-band
Cardiac output
  curves
    venous return and, 760
  exercise effects, 231–32
  in heart failure, 788, 788t
  low, compensatory mechanisms initiated by, 790t
Cardiac sarcoplasmic reticulum, 302–3, 305–6. *See also* Sarcoplasmic reticulum
Cardiac tissue. *See also* Cardiac muscle
  anisotropic properties, 178, 179
  bidomain behavior, 474–76, 475f–477f
  cable properties, 178
  connectivity of cells, 461, 462t, 471
  discontinuous, interaction between active membrane properties and, 467

gap junction organization, 178–80, 179f
resistivities, 458, 458t, 657, 659f
space constants, 458, 458t
structure, anisotropic conduction and, 461–63, 462f, 462t, 463f, 463t
Cardiac vagal motoneurons
airway inputs, 224, 226
arterial chemoreceptor inputs, 224, 225f, 226f
baroreceptor input, 221–22
B-fiber
baroreceptor influence on, 221–22
extrinsic control of, 227
hyperpolarization, during inspiration, 222–23, 223f
localization, 217, 219f
physiological properties, 221
respiratory influence on, 222
role of, 232
stimulation, 214, 215f
biophysical properties, 219–20, 220f
cardiac receptors and, 227
C-fiber
localization, 217, 219f
physiological properties, 221
role of, 232–33
stimulation, 214, 215f
chronotropic actions, 213–14, 215f
physiological mapping, 217–18, 218f, 219f
physiological properties, 220–21, 220f
pulmonary C-fibers and, 226
pulmonary inputs
rapidly adapting, 226
slowly adapting, 224, 226
reflex inputs
central modifications, 229–31
CNS organization, 226f, 227
interactions between, 227–28
respiratory influences on, 232
role of nucleus tractus solitarii, 231–32
respiratory influences on, 222, 222f
respiratory patterning in, 222–24, 223f
somata location, 214–15, 216f, 217f
upper airway receptors and, 226–27
Cardiomyopathy, 729–31
adriamycin, Ca^{2+}-ATPase activity and, 308
animal models, 712
clinical picture, 729–30
diabetic, troponin I phosphorylation in, 279
dilated, clinical manifestations, 729–30
diphtheria, gap junction abnormalities in, 202, Plate 8
hypertrophic
arrhythmic mechanisms, 730–31, 730t
clinical manifestations, 729, 730
β-MHC gene mutation in, 423–24
tropomyosin gene mutations in, 428–29
troponin T isoform expression in, 428

ischemic, 117–29
arrhythmias and, 129
coronary capillary tree and, 128–29
gap junction abnormalities in, 201–2
myocyte cell loss and, 121–24, 123f–124f
myocyte hyperplasia and, 126–28, 127f, Plates 4–5
myocyte hypertrophy and, 124–26, 125f
myocyte volume composition and, 128
ventricular function and, 121–24
ventricular remodeling and, 118–21, 119f, 121f
Cardiovascular disease. See Heart disease
Catecholamines, cardiac effects, 609–13. See also β-Adrenergic agonists
Cell(s)
electrical heterogeneity. See Electrical heterogeneity
partial uncoupling, reversal of unidirectional conduction block from, 502, Plate 11
volume regulation, 608–9
Cell bundles, formation, 462
C-fibers
cardiac vagal. See Cardiac vagal motoneurons, C-fiber
pulmonary, 226
Chagas' disease, gap junction abnormalities in, 200–201, 201f
Chloride channels
acetylcholine effects, 619
α-adrenergic effects, 616
β-adrenergic effects, 611–12
ATP effects, 625
calcium-activated, 605, 605f
cAMP-activated, 667t, 670
in heart disease, 720
PKA-activated, 604–5
sodium effects, 600
stretch-activated, 608, 608f
swelling-activated, 605, 608–9
Chloride ions, 604–5
Cholesterol, calveolin binding of, 160
Cholesterol/sphingolipid rafts, calveolae as, 156–57, 158
Cholinergic agonists
effects on automaticity and pacemaker channels, 619–20, 619f
effects on chloride channels, 619
effects on L-type channels, 618–19
effects on membrane potentials, 616
potassium channel activation by, 560–61, 616–18, 617f, 720
stimulatory actions, 620
Chromanol 293B, cellular responsiveness to, 663, 664t
Chronotropic actions
of β-adrenergic agonists, 609
of angiotensin II, 626
of endothelins, 627, 627f
of vagal efferent fibers, 213–14, 215f
Circumferential fiber shortening
left ventricle, 764, 764f

velocity of, as index of contractility, 745, 757–58, 761
Circus movement reentry. See Reentry
Collagen
deposition, ischemic cardiomyopathy and, 124
in diastole, 770
in passive compliance of myocardium, 772–73, 772f
Collagen bundles, 9f–20f, 12
Collagen fibrils
cross-banding, 9f, 12f, 13
granules along, 13, 16f
Collagen microthreads, 9f, 13, 16f
Collagen struts, 12
Collagen weave, 9f–16f, 12–13
Colloidal gold stain, 64
Concentric hypertrophy
in heart failure, 787–89, 788t, 792, 798–99, 799, 800f
ventricular, 744
Conduction
β-adrenergic effects, 609–10
anisotropic. See Anisotropic conduction
and bidomain behavior of cardiac tissue, 474–76, 475f–477f
calcium-dependent, 498
continuous cable model, 457–59, 457f, 458f
discontinuous
active membrane properties and, 467
in cell chain, 467–68, 468f, 470f
in cell strand, 468–69, 471f
conduction slowing and, 498–99
gap junctions and, 182
from high- to low-impedance region, 464–65, 465f
with periodically spaced resistive obstacles, 465–67, 466f, 467f
with sealed end, 463–64, 464f
structural determinants, 461–63, 462f, 462t, 463f, 463t
extracellular resistance and, 472–74, 473f, 474f
gap junction distribution and, 179
gap junction effects on, 178, 179, 180, 181f, 182
liminal area concept, 460–61, 461f
mechanisms, 457–76
one-dimensional, 458–59, 458f
potassium effects, 494–98, 495f–497f, 596
saltatory, 467
schematic representation, 456f
supernormal, 494, 495f
two-dimensional, 180, 181f, 459–61, 459f–461f
velocity
in cell chain, 467–68, 468f
in continuous structure, 459
effects of resistive discontinuities, 465, 466f
effects of superfusate fluid, 473–74, 474f
extracellular resistance and, 472–73
longitudinal vs. transverse, 456t, 469–

Conduction (*continued*)
73, 472f, 473f. *See also* Anisotropic conduction
wavefront curvature and, 459–61, 459f–461f
virtual electrode effect, 475, 475f, 476f
Conduction block
during phase 4 depolarization, 495–96, 496f
role of calcium inward current, 498
unidirectional, 499–504
in anisotropic tissue, 502–4, 503f, 504f
asymmetrical, 500–501, 501f
at current-to-load mismatch sites, 501–2, 502f, Plate 11
dependence on bidomain behavior, 504
dependence on resistive tissue barriers, 502–4, 503f, 504f
dependence on tissue geometry, 501–2, 502f
in initiation of reentrant excitation, 505
at isthmus, 504, 504f
from propagation with refractory tail, 499–501, 501f
in wake of preceding excitation, 499, 500f
Conduction disorders
effects of resting membrane potential and inhibition of Na+ channels, 494–98, 495f–497f
and safety factor of propagation, 493–94, 494f
Connexin(s)
antibodies, gap junction channel sensitivity to, 200
and connexon topology, 173–74, 174f, 184, Plate 6
distribution, 175–77, 175f, 175t, 461–62, 463t, 669–70
genomic organization, 173, 174f
heterologous pairings, 195
life cycle, 182–84, 183f
multiple, selective pressure for, 177–78
phosphorylation, 184
regulation, 184–85
structure, 171f, 172–73
transcriptional regulation, 185–86
ubiquitin incorporation into, 184
Connexin multigene family, 174f
Connexin32, pH sensitivity of, 197–98
Connexin37, 175, 177, 178, 193t, 194, 667t
Connexin40, 175, 177, 178, 179f
in exogenous systems, 193t, 194
expression, 462, 463t, 667t, 670
knockout phenotype, 202–3, 203f
transcriptional regulation, 185–86
Connexin42, 667t, 670
Connexin43, 175, 176f, 177, 178, 179f
arrhythmias and, 182
in exogenous systems, 192–94, 193t
expression, 461, 462, 463t, 667t, 669, 670

knockout phenotype, 202
life cycle, 182, 183f, 184
pairing with connexin40, 195
pairing with connexin45, 195
phosphorylation, 198–200, 199f
regulation, 184–85
transcriptional regulation, 185
Connexin45, 175, 177, 178, 179f
in exogenous systems, 193t, 194
expression, 462, 463t, 667t, 669
pH sensitivity, 197, 198f
transcriptional regulation, 185–86
Connexin46, 177
Connexin50, 177, 193t, 194–95
Connexons
formation, 184
movement, 184
topology, 173–74, 174f, Plate 6
Contractile properties of myocardium
assessment, 429–35
calcium sensitivity, 421, 429, 435–45
force-velocity relationship, 430–31, 431f, 432f
isometric tension and, 429–30, 435–42
power vs. load curves, 431–32, 432f
regulation, 435–45
tension redevelopment, 433–35, 434f
tension transients, 249, 432–35, 433f
tension–pCa relationship, 429, 435–37
Contractile proteins, 36, 48, 421–29. *See also specific protein*
Contractility
β-adrenergic stimulation and, 754–55, 755f
age-related changes, 96
assessment, 756–62
absolute level, 760–62, 761f
acute changes, 756
comparison of indices, 758–59, 759f
left ventricular pressure and, 758
in mice and rats, 762
ventricular dimensions/volumes in steady state, 756–58
ventricular function over range of loading conditions, 759–60
factors influencing, 755, 755f, 756
in heart failure, 792f, 793
length-dependent activation, 752, 754f
strength-interval relations and, 752–54
systolic function and, 752, 753f
Contraction. *See also* Crossbridge cycling; Relaxation
activation
calcium requirements, 340–41, 341f
calcium supply, 369–73, 370f–371f, 370t, 373f
cooperativity and, 435–36, 444–45
effects on velocity of shortening, 442–44, 442f, 443f
kinetics, 444–45
excitation and, coupling between, 335, 360–61
force-frequency relationships, 376–77, 377f, 753
isovolumic, peak stress in, 745–46, 746f

maximal velocity, 246, 247f, 430–31, 431f, 432f, 442–44, 443f, 444f
regulation, 420–46
by ATP hydrolysis products, 440–41
by contractile and regulatory proteins, 421–29
by inotropic agonists, 441, 444
by myocardial acidosis, 439–40
by myocardial cell length, 437–39
by PKA-dependent phosphorylation, 274, 276
by stimulus frequency, 437
tension-pCa relationship, 435–37
by thick filament accessory proteins, 441–42
by velocity of shortening, 442–44, 442f, 443f
sliding filament mechanism, 240–42, 241f
tension development and relaxation, 444–45
twitch
rest-decay, 374f, 375
rest-potentiation, 374f, 375–76
Contrast manipulation, 65
Corbular structures, in sarcoplasmic reticulum, 303
Coronary heart disease. *See* Heart disease
Coronary vasculature
aging and, 102–5, 103f–104f
cardiac hypertrophy and, 114–17, 116f
in cardiac muscle, 12
morphometric analysis, 84–86, 86f
random distribution test, 86
rarefaction, 104, 116
Costamere, 15
Counterstaining, in electron microscopy, 63
C-protein. *See* Myosin binding protein C
Creatine kinase, in M-band, 48
Creatine phosphokinase, in heart failure, 796
Crista terminalis
conduction velocity, 456t
connectivity of cells, 462t
right atrial activation via, 480–81, 481f
Cromakalim, 631
Crossbridge cycling, 240–60. *See also* Contraction
binding states, 244–45, 266f, 270–71, 426–27, 437
in cardiac muscle, 245, 252
chemical pathway, 246, 247f
cooperative unit size and, 268, 269, 270, 435–36
in diastole and systole, 266f, 270–71
energy transduction, 246–49, 246f–248f
force-velocity relationships, 246, 247f, 430–31, 431f, 432f, 442–44, 443f, 444f
load-dependence, 247–48, 248f
in muscle, 245–52
muscle mechanics in, 246–49, 246f–248f

INDEX 811

myofilament protein phosphorylation
  in, 259, 264–92
power vs. load curves, 431–32, 432f
protein isoform switching in, 259
rate
  acidosis and, 440
  β-adrenergic stimulation and, 445
  calcium and, 258, 259
  protein kinase C-dependent
    phosphorylation and, 274, 276
  recent progress related to, 257–58
  regulation, 242, 258–59
    dual, 258–59
    kinetic, 258, 444–45
    phosphorylation and protein isoform
      switching, 259
    steric blocking model, 258, 426
  shortening velocity and, 430–32, 431f–432f
  sinusoidal analysis, 251–52
  sliding filament model, 240–42, 241f
  steps
    ADP dissociation, 251–52
    ATP binding and detachment, 249
    ATP cleavage, 249–50
    energetics, 244–45
    force generation, 250–51, 250f
    phosphate dissociation, 250–51, 250f
    rates, 242–44, 243f
    structural models, 256–57
  summary, 259–60
  tension redevelopment, 433–35, 434f
  tension transients, 249, 432–35, 433f
  transient kinetics
    following rapid length reductions,
      432–33, 433f
    using caged compounds, 249, 249f,
      433
  in vitro motility assay, 252–54
Crossbridge interconnections, between
  thick and thin filaments, 40f,
  41f
Cross-field stimulation, spiral wave
  initiation by, 511–12, 512f
Cryofixation, 63–64
Cryosubstitution, 63–64
Current threshold, electrode radius and,
  460–61, 461f
Curvature
  defined, 459
  wavefront
    conduction block and, 504
    conduction velocity and, 459–61,
      459f–461f
Cyclic adenosine monophosphate (cAMP)
  chloride channel activated by, 667t,
    670
  effects on pacemaker current, 693
  protein kinase phosphorylation
    dependence on, 317
Cycling
  crossbridge. See Crossbridge cycling
  structural dynamics of, 4
Cystic fibrosis transmembrane
  conductance regulator (CFTR),
  cAMP-, 667t, 670

Cytochalasin D, and potassium channels,
  577f, 578–79
Cytochemistry, 64–65
  antibody labeling in. See
    Immunocytochemistry
Cytoskeleton
  in cell volume regulation, 609
  Na^{2+}-Ca^{2+} exchanger interactions, 403
  potassium channels and, 577f, 578–79
  proteins associated with, calveolae and,
    156
  sarcolemmal associations, 15, 33
Cytosolic calcium buffering, 336–40
  during calcium transient, 341–42, 342f,
    342t
  competitive factors, 341
  fast, 337–38, 338f, 339t
  slow, 338–39, 338f, 339t
Cytosolic volume
  conversion factors, 336, 337t
  defined, 339–40

Death, sudden, animal models, 713
Defense reaction, central modulation of,
  230–31, 230f
Depolarization, 494–98, 495f–497f. See
  also Action potential;
  Afterdepolarization
Desmin, 15
Desmosomes, 5
Detergent-insoluble glycolipid-rich (DIG)
  domains, calveolae as, 156–57,
  158
Diabetes mellitus
  animal models, 712
  cardiac effects, 621–22
  cardiomyopathy in, troponin I
    phosphorylation in, 279
  electrophysiologic changes, 713
  troponin T isoform expression in, 428
Diastole
  collagen in, 770
  crossbridge cycling in, 265–66, 266f,
    270–71
  interstitial proteins in, 770
  myofilament proteins in, 265–66, 265f,
    266f, 772
  thick filament proteins in, 265f, 269–70
  thin filament proteins in, 266–69, 267f,
    268f
  thin filament states in, 266f, 270–71
Diastolic function
  cardiac structural components, 770
  determinants, 769–75
  in heart failure, 787–89, 788t, 792,
    798–99
  passive ventricular structure-function
    relationships, 771–73, 772f
  pressure–volume relationships, 770–71,
    771f
  role of pericardium, 774–75
  time-dependent properties, 771, 771f
  ventricular filling regulation, 773–74,
    773f
Dieldrin, gap junction channel sensitivity
  to, 200

DIG (detergent-insoluble glycolipid-rich)
  domains, calveolae as, 156–57,
  158
Digitalis
  AV nodal conduction effects, 630–31
  inotropic effects, 392–93, 629–30, 630f
Dihydropyridine receptor, 667t, 670
Diphtheria cardiomyopathy, gap junction
  abnormalities in, 202, Plate 8
Diuretics, for heart failure, 790
DNA synthesis, in myocyte, 90, 94, 100,
  126
  cardiac hypertrophy and, 108, 109
  ischemic cardiomyopathy and, 127,
    Plates 4–5
Doppler effect, 515, 516f
Dorsal vagal nucleus
  biophysical properties, 219–20, 220f
  cardiac vagal motoneurons in, 214–15,
    216f
  CNS pathways impinging on, 227, 227t
$DP/dt_{(peak)}$ (maximum rate of rise of
  ventricular pressure), 758, 760,
  761
Drug(s)
  action potential prolongation caused
    by, 663–64, 663f, 664t
  long QT syndrome caused by, 723
  sensitivity to
    M-cells vs. endocardial and
      epicardial cells, 663–65, 663f,
      664f, 664t
    M-cells vs. Purkinje cells, 658t, 665
DTX-sensitive potassium channel, 570t,
  574
Dual voltage-clamp technique, 188
Duty ratio, 248
DV/dt_{max}. See Action potential, maximal
  upstroke velocity
Dyad structure, in sarcoplasmic
  reticulum, 303
Dystroglycan, calveolae and, 156
Dystrophin
  calveolae and, 156
  in myofibril-sarcolemmal association,
    33

E~P formation, 305
E-4031, cellular responsiveness to, 663,
  664t
Eag (ether-a-go-go) gene subfamily, 575t,
  576. See also ERG (*eag*-related)
  genes
Eccentric hypertrophy
  in heart failure, 787–89, 788t, 792,
    798–99, 799, 800f
  ventricular, 744
Ejection fraction, as index of contractility,
  757, 761
Electrical current, in cable, 457–58, 457f
Electrical heterogeneity
  action potential and ionic distinctions,
    536–38, 654–62
  in Brugada syndrome, 672–74, 675f,
    676f
  developmental aspects, 671–72, 671f

Electrical heterogeneity (*continued*)
  in early repolarization syndrome, 674–76
    in inscription of T wave, 676–78, 677f, 678f
    in inscription of U wave, 678–79, 678f
  in ischemia, 676
  in long QT syndrome, 679–81, 680f, 681t
  molecular distinctions, 665–71
  pharmacologic distinctions, 662–65
  physiological and clinical implications, 672–83
  simulation, 671
  in torsades de pointes, 681–82, 682f, 683f
Electrical remodeling, in heart disease, 711f, 714, 722
Electrical resistance, extracellular space, 472–74, 473f, 474f
Electrocardiogram, action potential on, 569f, 570–71
Electrolytes, cardiac effects, 595–607. *See also specific electrolyte*
Electron(s)
  backscattered, 62
  transmitted, 62
Electron energy loss spectroscopy, 62
Electron microscopy
  advances in, 61
  cytochemical analysis, 64–65
  image enhancement techniques, 65
  image processing and analysis, 65–66
  scanning, 62
  specimen preparation
    low-temperature, 63–64
    room temperature, 62–63
  transmission, 61–62
ELK (*eag*-like) genes, 576
Embedding, in electron microscopy, 63
End-diastolic pressure, left ventricular, in heart failure, 791, 792f
End-diastolic pressure–stroke volume relation, 747–48
End-diastolic pressure–stroke work relation, 752, 753f
End-diastolic volume, left ventricular, 757
End-diastolic volume–stroke work relation, 759–60
Endocardial cells
  action potential distinctions, 655, 656f–657f, 658t, 659f, 661t
  action potential duration, 536–38, 537f–538f, 659t, 661t
  drug sensitivity
    vs. epicardial cells, 655t, 662–63
    vs. M-cells, 663–65, 663f, 664f, 664t
  ionic distinctions, 656f–657f
  tissue resistivity, 657, 659f
Endoplasmic reticulum. *See also* Sarcoplasmic reticulum
  smooth, in pressure overload hypertrophy, 113–14
  structure, 302
Endosarcomeric lattice, 14

Endothelial nitric oxide synthase, in calveolae, 155
Endothelins
  chronotropic effect, 627, 627f
  inotropic effects, 627, 627f
End-systolic pressure, left ventricle, in heart failure, 791, 792f
End-systolic pressure–volume relation, 746, 747f, 759
Energy dispersive spectroscopy, 62
Energy starvation, in heart failure, 793, 796
Energy transduction, during crossbridge cycling, 246–49, 246f–248f
Energy transfer studies, of Ca^{2+}-ATPase, 311
Environmental scanning electron microscopy, 62
Enzymatic dissociation of muscle cells, 81, Plate 2
Epicardial cells
  action potential distinctions, 655, 656f–657f, 658t, 659f, 661t
  action potential duration, 536–38, 537f–538f, 659t, 661t
  action potential notch, 655, 655t
  drug sensitivity
    vs. endocardial cells, 655t, 662–63
    vs. M-cells, 663–65, 663f, 664f, 664t
  ionic distinctions, 656f–657f
  tissue resistivity, 657, 659f
ERG (*eag*-related) genes, 575t, 576, 666t, 668, 718
  activation, by extracellular potassium, 597, 598f
ERG1 gene, 579
Erythromycin, cellular responsiveness to, 663, 664t
Eu-actinin, in Z-band, 50
Exchanger inhibitory peptide (XIP), 350, 400–401, 403–4
Excitability
  calcium effects, 600
  pH effects, 606
  potassium effects, 596
Excitation
  during phase 4 depolarization, 495–96, 496f
  reentrant. *See* Reentry
  supernormal, 494, 495f
Excitation-contraction coupling, 335, 360–61. *See also* Contraction
Exercise
  cardiorespiratory changes during, 231–32
  physiologic hypertrophy caused by, 107, 798
Extracellular matrix, 12–14
  calveolae and, 156
  collagen weave, 9f–16f, 12–13
  composition, 12
  in passive compliance, 772–73, 772f
  transverse tubular system, 13–14, 18f–20f
Extracellular space, electrical resistance, 472–74, 473f, 474f

F-actin, 426, 609
Fasciae adherentes, 5
Fascicles, formation, 462
Ferritin
  antibody labeling with, 64
  calveolar uptake of, 149
Fetus
  heart of, 86–87
  Na^{2+}-Ca^{2+} exchange, 408
  troponin T isoforms, 281, 427–28
Fiber branching, conduction slowing and, 499
Fibroblasts, in cardiac muscle, 12, 19f
Fibrosis
  age-related, 94, 95f
  definition, 117–18
  ischemic cardiomyopathy and, 122, 123f
  myocyte loss and, 99
Figure-8 reentry, 508
Filament sliding, crossbridges and, 240–42, 241f. *See also* Crossbridge cycling
Fine deformation theory, 764
Fixation
  in electron microscopy
    chemical, 61, 62–63, 64
    embedding after, 63
  by rapid freezing. *See* Cryofixation
Flecainide, cellular responsiveness to, 662
Fluorescence recovery after photobleaching (FRAP), 157
Fluorescent energy transfer studies, of Ca^{2+}-ATPase, 311
Force generation, in crossbridge cycle, 250–51, 250f
Force vectors, cardiac ultrastructure and, 5
Force-frequency relationships, in contraction-relaxation cycle, 376–77, 377f, 753
Force-velocity relationships, in crossbridge cycle, 246, 247f, 430–31, 431f, 432f, 442–44, 443f, 444f
Formaldehyde fixation, 64
Frank-Starling relationship, 747–48, 748f
Freeze substitution, 63–64
Freeze-etching, 62, 64
Freeze-fracturing, 62, 64
Freezing
  jet, 63
  plunge, 63
  slam, 63
F-type ATPase, 303

G proteins
  ACh regulation, 616–18, 617f
  calveolin regulation, 159–60
G-actin, 426
Gamma-filamin/ABP-L, in Z-band, 50
Gap junction(s), 169–204
  abnormalities, disease states associated with, 200–202, Plate 8

developmental differentiation, 170, 171f
distribution, 13, 461–62, 463t, 669–70
effects on conduction, 178, 179, 180, 181f, 182
fuzzy appearance, 172
in heart disease, 720–21
history of research, 170
internalized, 184
knockout murine models, 202–4, 203f
life cycle, 182–84, 183f
organization, 178–80, 179f
projection images, 171f, 172–73
proteins, 170–78. *See also* Connexin(s)
regulation, 184–85
sinus node, 478
transcriptional regulation, 185–86
in two-dimensional cardiac conduction model, 180, 181f
ultrastructural features, 5, 27f, 170–72, 171f
Gap junction channel(s)
biophysical properties, 188–89
as calcium channel, 186–88, 187f, Plate 7
functional properties, 177–78, 186–200, 187f–188f
gating of, 177, 196–200
by calcium, 196–97
by lipophilic molecules, 198
by phosphorylation, 198–200, 199f
by protons, 197–98, 198f
by transjunctional voltage, 189–92, 190f–192f, 193t
as potassium channel, 186
properties, in cardiovascular cells, 195–96
as second messenger channels, 186–88, 187f–188f
Gap junctional resistance, conduction velocity and, 498–99
Genetically modified mice. *See* Transgenic mice model
Giant excised patch technique, 389
Glutaraldehyde fixation, in electron microscopy, 63
Glycyrrhetinic acid, gap junction channel sensitivity to, 200
Gold, antibody labeling with, 64
GPI-anchored proteins, in calveolae, 161–63
GTPase activity of G proteins
ACh regulation, 616–18, 617f
calveolin regulation, 159–60
Guanylate cyclase
ANP activation, 628
nitric oxide activation, 628

Halothane, gap junction channel sensitivity to, 198
HCN (hyperpolarization-activated, cyclic-nucleotide-sensitive) channels
biophysical properties, 696–98, 696f, 697t
distribution patterns, 695–96

nomenclature, 694, 697t
structure, 694–95
Heart disease. *See also* Arrhythmias
action potential current abnormalities in, 710, 711f
cellular changes, 713
chloride currents in, 720
delayed rectifier currents in, 718–19
electrophysiology, 712–13
gap junctions in, 720–21
human and animal models, 712–13
inwardly rectifying K$^+$ currents in, 719–20
ion channel changes, 713–22
electrical remodeling and, 711f, 714, 722
intrinsic vs. extrinsic, 713–14
L-type calcium channels in, 715–16
Na^{2+}-Ca^{2+} exchanger in, 721
Na$^+$-K$^+$ ATPase in, 721–22
pacemaker current in, 720
swell-activated currents in, 722
tachyrhythmia in, 709–10
transient inward current in, 722
transient outward current in, 717–18
T-type calcium channels and, 716–17
Heart failure, 786–802
β-adrenergic stimulation in, 790, 790t, 791
animal models, 712
architectural changes, 791–93, 796–801, 798t, 799t, 800f
ATP depletion in, 796
backward, 787–88, 788t
Ca^{2+}-ATPase activity and, 308
calcium fluxes in, 793, 794f–795f
cardiac hypertrophy in, 791–93
adaptive and maladaptive, 790f, 797–98, 797t
concentric, 787–89, 788t, 792, 798–99, 799, 800f
eccentric, 787–89, 788t, 792, 798–99, 799, 800f
myocyte phenotype and, 798–99, 798t
cardiac output in, 788, 788t
classifications, 787, 788t
defined, 787
diastolic dysfunction, 787–89, 788t, 792, 798–99
digitalis effects, 393
electrophysiologic changes, 713
energy starvation in, 793, 796
forward, 787–88, 788t
hemodynamic consequences, 780t, 787–88, 788t, 789–90
inotropic abnormalities, 792f, 793
left, 788t, 789
lusitropic abnormalities, 792f, 793
mitochondrial changes, 796
molecular alterations, 791–93, 796–801, 798t, 799t, 800f
myocardial cell death in, 801
myocyte mitotic division in, 110, 110f, Plate 3
myocyte phenotypes in, 798–99, 798t

myocyte shape changes in, 799–800, 800f
myosin light chain abnormalities, 425–26
Na^{2+}-Ca^{2+} exchange abnormalities in, 409–10
neurohumoral response, 789–90, 790t
paradigms
biochemistry and biophysics, 793–97
gene expression, 797–801
organ physiology, 787–93
shifts in, 786–87
phosphocreatine shuttle in, 793, 796
pressure-volume loops in, 791–93, 792f, 800f
proliferative signaling in
functional signaling and, crossover between, 791
hypertrophic response to, 790f, 797–98, 797t
reduced oxygen delivery in, 796
right, 788t, 789
salt retention in, 789–90, 790t
stroke volume in, 749, 749f
systolic dysfunction, 787–89, 788t, 792, 798–99
treatment
β-adrenergic blockade, 787, 791
β-adrenergic stimulation, 791
angiotensin-converting enzyme inhibitors, 791
counterintuitive findings, 787, 787t
diuretics, 790
vasodilators, 787, 790
troponin I phosphorylation in, 279–80
troponin T isoform expression in, 427–28
vasoconstriction in, 789, 790t
water retention in, 789–90, 790t
Heart rate. *See also* Chronotropic actions
β-adrenergic stimulation and, 754–55, 755f
exercise effects, 231–32
inotropic effects, 754
reflex inputs in control of
central modifications, 229–31
CNS organization, 226f, 227
interactions between, 227–28
respiratory influences on, 232
role of nucleus tractus solitarii, 231–32
vagal effects, 213–14, 215f. *See also* Cardiac vagal motoneurons
Heart rhythm, disorders of. *See* Arrhythmias
Heart weight, 97
Hemichannels. *See* Connexons
Heptanol, gap junction channel sensitivity to, 198
HERG (human *eag*-related gene), 575t, 576, 597, 598f, 666t, 668, 718
His bundle, 483–84
Histamine
cardiac effects, 625–26
receptors, 625
Homeometric autoregulation, 747

Horseradish peroxidase, calveolar uptake of, 148, 148f, 149
Human *eag*-related gene (HERG), 575t, 576, 597, 598f, 666t, 668, 718
Hyperkalemia, electrophysiological effect, 541
Hypertrophic cardiomyopathy. *See* Cardiomyopathy, hypertrophic
Hypertrophy. *See* Cardiac hypertrophy; Concentric hypertrophy; Eccentric hypertrophy; Myocytes, hypertrophy; Pressure overload hypertrophy; Volume overload hypertrophy
Hypochromic anemia, myocyte hypertrophy in, 112–13
Hypothalamic defense area, 230, 230f, 231

I-band, 36, 42f, 241f
Image averaging, 65
Image processing and analysis, 65–66
Imaging techniques, 61–66. *See also specific technique, e.g.,* Electron microscopy
Immunocytochemistry, 64–65
Impulse propagation. *See* Conduction
Inotropic state. *See* Contractility
Inotropic stimulation
  in contraction regulation, 441, 444
  effect on contractility indices, 758, 759f
Insulin, cardiac effects, 621–22
Integrin(s)
  distribution, 33
  in myofibril-sarcolemmal association, 15, 33
  β1-subunit, 33
Interatrial band. *See* Bachmann's bundle
Intercalated disk
  gap junctions at, 170–72, 171f
  role of, 5
  ultrastructural features, 5, 6f, 27f
Intermediate filaments, 5, 14–15, 27f–30f
Intermediate junctions, 5, 33
Interstitial fibrosis
  age-related, 94, 95f
  definition, 118
  ischemic cardiomyopathy and, 122, 123f
  myocyte loss and, 99
Ion channels. *See also specific channel*
  calcium effects, 601–3, 602f
  in heart disease, 713–22
    electrical remodeling and, 711f, 714, 722
    intrinsic vs. extrinsic, 713–14
  pH effects, 606, 607
  potassium effects, 597, 598f
  sodium effects, 599–600
  voltage-gated, schematic overview, 549f
Ionic basis of action potential, 532–36, 534f–535f
Ionic concentrations, effects on action potential, 540–41, 541f
Ionic currents, 458, 458f, 531

Ionic distinctions in ventricular myocardium, 536–38, 654–62
Ischemia
  action potential abnormalities, 541–42, 542f
  animal models, 712–13
  electrical heterogeneity, 676
Ischemic cardiomyopathy. *See* Cardiomyopathy, ischemic
Ischemic heart disease, gap junction abnormalities in, 202
Ischemic necrosis, myocyte loss by, 99
Ischemic preconditioning, cardioprotective effects, 634
Isometric tension, determinants, 429–30, 437–42
Isoproterenol, cellular responsiveness to, 662
Isovolumetric-phase indices of contractility, 758, 761
Isovolumic stress, 745–46, 746f

J wave, transmural distribution of I_{to} and, 672
Jervell and Lange-Nielsen syndrome, 723
Junctional channels. *See* Gap junction channel(s)
Junctional conductance, 190f–192f, 193t

K^+. *See* Potassium
KB-R7943, Na^{2+}-Ca^{2+} exchange inhibition by, 404–5
KCNE1 gene, 577, 577f, 579–80, 666t, 668, 669f, 725
KCNQ1 gene, 575t, 576–77, 577f, 579–80, 666t, 668, 669f
KCNQ2/KCNQ3 gene, 577
Koch's triangle, 482, 483f
KPQ deletion mutant channel, in long QT syndrome, 552, 553f, 556–57, 556f, 726
Krogh's cylinder model, 85
Kv1 *(Shaker)* gene, 575t, 576, 665, 666t
Kv1.5 gene, 666
Kv2 *(Shab)* gene, 575t, 576, 665, 666t
Kv3 *(Shaw)* gene, 575t, 576, 665, 666t
Kv4 *(Shal)* gene, 575t, 576, 665, 666t
Kv5.x–Kv9.x genes, 575t, 576
KvLQT1. *See* KCNQ1

LC_2. *See* Myosin light chain 2
Lead citrate, for counterstaining, 63
Leading circle reentry, 508–9
Left heart failure, 788t
Length-tension relationship, 437–39, 746–47
Licorice, gap junction channel sensitivity to, 200
Lidocaine, sodium channel blockage by, 554
Light microscopy, 77–78, 80
Liminal area concept, 460–61, 461f
Linear cable theory, 457–59, 457f, 458f
Lipophilic molecules, gap junction channel sensitivity to, 198
Load curves, 432f

Local anesthetics, sodium channel blockage by, 554, 555–56
Long QT syndrome
  action potential prolongation in, 538–40, 539f, 540f
  arrhythmic mechanism, 723–24
  clinical picture, 723
  drug-induced, 723
  molecular defects, 722–23, 723t
  molecular mechanisms, 724–27
  pharmacologic therapy, 682–83, 727–28
  potassium channel gene mutations, 575t, 576–77, 577f, 579–80, 582–84, 583f, 724–26
  present status, 728
  sodium channel gene mutation, 552, 553f, 556–57, 556f, 726
  transmural heterogeneity in, experimental models, 679–81, 680f, 681t
  vs. Brugada syndrome, 684f
Longitudinal fiber shortening, left ventricle, 764
Luo-Rudy ventricular cell model, 532, 533f
Lusitropic abnormalities, in heart failure, 792f, 793
Lymph vessels, in cardiac muscle, 12

Magnesium, cardiac effects, 603–4
M-band
  M-lines in, 36
  protein constituents in, 48
  thick filament anchoring at, 36, 41f, 42f
M-cells
  action potential distinctions, 654–62, 656f–657f, 658t, 659f, 661t
  action potential duration, 536–38, 537f–538f, 659t, 661t
  developmental aspects, 671–72
  drug sensitivity
    vs. endocardial and epicardial cells, 663–65, 663f, 664f, 664t
    vs. Purkinje cells, 658t, 665
  evidence for, 658, 658t
  in inscription of T wave, 676–78, 677f, 678f
  ionic distinctions, 655, 656f–657f
  position, 655
  tissue resistivity, 657, 659f
Mechanical restitution, 755
Mechanical vectors, cardiac ultrastructure and, 4–5
Membrane current, in cable, 458, 458f
Membrane potential. *See also* Action potential
  acetylcholine effects, 616
  adenosine effects, 622–23
  α-adrenergic effects, 613–14
  β-adrenergic effects, 610
  calcium effects, 600
  effects on conduction, 494–98, 495f–497f
  histamine effects, 625

pH effects, 605–6
potassium effects, 595–96
sodium effects, 599
Men
  myocyte hypertrophy in, aging and, 101f
  myocyte number in, aging and, 98f
Meromyosin, heavy, 269
Metal staining, in electron microscopy, 61–62, 63
Mexiletine
  for long QT syndrome, 682
  sodium channel blockage by, 554
Mg-ATP, potassium channel activation by, 617
Mibefradil, T-type calcium channel blockade by, 703
Mice
  phospholamban gene targeting, 322
  transgenic
    Na^{2+}-Ca^{2+} exchanger overexpression, 406–7
    phosphorylation effects, 276, 284
    ventricular function, 762
Microtubules, in cardiac muscle, 5, 8f, 14, 20f–26f
Minimal subunit potassium channel (minK, MiRP1). See KCNE1
Mitochondria
  calcium transport, 361–64, 362f, 363f
  cardiac hypertrophy and, 113
  in cardiac muscle, 5, 6f, 8f, 32f, 35, 37f
  heart failure and, 796
  ischemic cardiomyopathy and, 128
  postnatal development, 91
Mitotic division
  cardiac hypertrophy and, 109
  in heart failure, 110, 110f, Plate 3
  ischemic cardiomyopathy and, 127–28, 127f, Plates 4–5
Mitotic index, myocyte, in heart failure, 110f
Mitral valve
  closure, 773
  flow, 772–73, 772f
M-line, 241f
Molecular alterations, in heart failure, 791–93, 796–801, 798t, 799t, 800f
Molecular distinctions, electrical heterogeneity, 665–71
Monocarboxylate transporter (MCT-1), in calveolae, 156
Morphometric analysis
  of coronary vasculature, 84–86, 86f
  definition, 76
  electron microscopy for, 65, 77–78, 79–80
  in ischemic cardiomyopathy, 117–29
  light microscopy for, 77–78, 80
  of myocyte
    by confocal microscopic procedures, 81–84, 82f–84f
    by enzymatic dissociation, 81, Plate 2
    methodological considerations, 80–81

  by in situ procedures, 76–80, 77f, 78f, 82f–84f
  of pressure and volume overload hypertrophy, 105–17
M-protein, 48
Muscarinic receptors, 616
Muscle
  cardiac. See Cardiac muscle
  crossbridge cycle in, 245–52
  skeletal
    thin filament in, 35
    Z-band lattice pattern in, 51, 59f
Muscle fiber, ultrastructure, 240, 241f
MyBP-C. See Myosin binding protein C
Myocardial acidosis
  in contraction regulation, 439–40
  electrophysiological effects, 541, 605–7
Myocardial contractility. See Contractile properties of myocardium; Contractility
Myocardial contraction. See Contraction
Myocardial growth
  aging-associated, 94, 100–102, 101f
  analysis. See Morphometric analysis
  during early postnatal period, 86–88, 89f
  pathological. See Cardiac hypertrophy
  physiological, 86–93, 89f, 93f
Myocardial hibernation, gap junction abnormalities in, 202
Myocardial infarction
  animal models, 712–13
  border zones, connectivity of cells, 462t
  electrophysiologic changes, 713
  gap junction abnormalities, 201
  size
    myocyte volume and, 125, 125f
    ventricular function and, 122
Myocardial ischemia
  action potential abnormalities, 541–42, 542f
  animal models, 712–13
  electrical heterogeneity, 676
Myocardial oxygen consumption, mechanical correlates of, 767–69, 768f–769f
Myocardial remodeling. See Ventricular remodeling
Myocardial stunning, calcium sensitivity abnormalities in, 440–41
Myocytes
  calcium binding sites, 336–40, 337f–338f, 339t
  calcium slow wave propagation, 187–88, 187f, Plate 7
  calcium transport. See Calcium transport
  calveolae in. See Calveolae
  DNA synthesis, 90, 94, 100, 126
    cardiac hypertrophy and, 108, 109
    ischemic cardiomyopathy and, 127, Plates 4–5
  electrical heterogeneity. See Electrical heterogeneity
  hyperplasia, ischemic cardiomyopathy and, 126–28, 127f, Plates 4–5

  hypertrophy, 107–13, 110f–112f, Plate 3. See also Cardiac hypertrophy
    aging and, 100–102, 101f
    in hypochromic anemia, 112–13
    in ischemic cardiomyopathy, 124–26, 125f
    pulmonary artery banding and, 112, 112f
    reactive, 101f
  isolation
    by enzymatic dissociation, 81, Plate 2
    three-dimensional optical reconstruction after, 81–84, 82f–84f
  length
    aging and, 101
    calcium sensitivity of tension and, 437–39
    morphometric analysis, 78–79
  loss
    age-related, 94, 97–100, 98f
    in heart failure, 801
    ischemic cardiomyopathy and, 121–24, 123f–124f
    mechanisms, 99, 102–3
    reactive hypertrophy in response to, 100–102, 101f
  mitotic division
    cardiac hypertrophy and, 109
    in heart failure, 110, 110f, Plate 3
    ischemic cardiomyopathy and, 127–28, 127f, Plates 4–5
  multinucleated, postnatal changes in, 90
  mural slippage, ischemic cardiomyopathy and, 119–20, 119f
  number
    aggregate, 84
    aging and, 94, 97–100, 98f
    cardiac hypertrophy and, 107
    morphometric analysis, 76–78, 77f, 78f
    postnatal changes, 89–90, 89f
    transmural, 80
  patterned cell cultures, optical imaging of, 180, 182
  phenotypes, in heart failure, 798–99, 798t
  ploidy formation, cardiac hypertrophy and, 108–9
  postnatal adaptations
    cytoplasmic, 90–91
    in size and number, 89–90, 89f
  shape, 5
    cardiac hypertrophy and, 107–8
    in heart failure, 799–800, 800f
    ischemic cardiomyopathy and, 120–21
  size
    aging and, 100–102, 101f
    cardiac hypertrophy and, 107–8
    ischemic cardiomyopathy and, 120–21
    morphometric analysis, 78–79
    postnatal changes in, 89, 89f

Myocytes (*continued*)
  triggered propagated contractions, 187–88, 188f
  volume
    confocal microscopic measurements, 81–84, 82f–84f
    Coulter counter estimation, 81
    infarct size and, 125, 125f
  volume composition
    cardiac hypertrophy and, 113–14
    ischemic cardiomyopathy and, 128
    water-channel proteins, 152–53
Myocyte-to-capillary ratio, 92, 93
Myofibrils
  α3-integrin association with, 33
  ischemic cardiomyopathy and, 128
  postnatal development, 90–91
Myofilament bundles, 5, 30f–42f, 35–36, 48
Myofilament proteins. *See also specific protein*
  in diastole, 265–66, 265f, 266f, 772
  isoform switching, 259
  modulation, as physiological regulatory device, 264–65
  phosphorylation, 259, 264–92
  in systole, 265f, 266, 266f
Myomesin, in M-band, 48
Myosin, 36, 421–26
  cleavage, 422
  crossbridges. *See also* Crossbridge cycling
    activation of reserve, 264
    in diastole and systole, 265f, 269–70
    filament sliding and, 240–42, 241f
  head, 240, 241f, 422
  isolated
    elementary mechanical transitions in, 252–53, 253f
    force output, 253–54
  modulatory proteins associated with, 265f, 266
  non-muscle, 257
  orientation, 421–22
  structure, 421
Myosin ATPase, 242–43
Myosin binding protein C, 429
  calcium sensitivity of tension and, 441
  in diastolic/systolic transition, 270
  functional domains, 289–91
  location, 265f, 270, 289
  phosphorylation
    contraction regulation and, 441–42
    sites, 291–92
  primary structure, 289, 290
Myosin heavy chain, 422–24
Myosin light chain, 424–26
Myosin light chain 1, 269, 425–26
Myosin light chain 2, 424–25
  calcium sensitivity of tension and, 441
  in crossbridge cycle regulation, 287–89
  in diastolic/systolic transition, 270
  functional domains, 285
  isoforms, 424
  metal binding to, 285–86
  in modulation of striated muscle contraction, 286–87, 424
  phosphorylation, 424–25
  primary structure, 285
Myosin light chain kinase
  phosphorylation, of myosin light chain 2, 284, 289, 424–25
Myosin RLC. *See* Myosin light chain 2
Myosin S1
  atomic structure, 254, 255f, 422–23, 423f
  ATP hydrolysis reaction on, 242–43, 243f
  binding curves, 270
  X-ray analysis, 269–70
Myosin S1 ATPase, 245
Myosin step size, 240
Myosin V1, 257, 422
Myosin V2, 422
Myosin V3, 422
Myotendinous junction, skeletal, 33

Na^+. *See* Sodium
Na^{2+}-Ba^{2+} exchange, 396
Na^{2+}-Ca^{2+} exchange
  current, 533, 533f
  developmental changes, 408
  digitalis effects, 392–93
  in heart disease, 721
  historical review, 388–410
  insulin effects, 622
  KB-R7943 inhibition, 404–5
  kinetic properties, 407–8
  molecular biology, 397–99
  pathophysiologic alterations, 409–10
  peptide inhibition, 403–4
  pharmacology, 403–6
  reverse, 391–92
  species differences, 408–9
  transgenic mice model, 406–7
  transport properties, 394–97
Na^{2+}-Ca^{2+} exchanger
  alternative splicing, 398–99
  calcium binding site, 401
  calcium-dependent regulation, 399–400
  Calx-α and Calx-β motifs, 398
  cardiac, 388–410
    during action potential, 350–54, 352f–354f
    adenoviral transfection, 407
    antisense oligonucleotide studies, 407
    characterization, 347–49, 348f–350f
    cloning, 349–50, 351f, 388–89
    exchanger density, 396
    immunolocalization, 393–94
    ion selectivity, 396
    overexpression, 406–7
    physiological role, 350, 389–91
    prototypical (NCX1.1), 397
    regulation, 391
    during relaxation, 364–67, 364f, 365f, 367f
    stoichiometry, 347–48, 394–95
    structure, 349–50, 351f
    temperature dependence, 396–97
    topology, 397–98
    transport mechanism, 395
    turnover rates, 395–96
  cytoskeletal interactions, 403
  distribution, 13
  NCKX family, 394–95
  NCX family, 397, 667t, 670
  regulation
    ionic, 399–401
    by pH, 402–3
    by phosphorylation, 401–2
    by PIP_2, 402
  sodium-dependent inactivation, 399
  superfamily, 397
  XIP region, 350, 400–401, 403–4
Na^{2+}-Sr^{2+} exchange, 396
Na^+-K^+ ATPase
  α-adrenergic effects, 616
  current, 533–34, 533f
  in heart disease, 721–22
  isoforms, 670–71
Nebulette, 35, 49
Nebulin
  in thin filament, 35
  in Z-band, 49
Nebulin-titin lattice, 14
Neonate, cardiac muscle of, 307
Nerve fibers, autonomic, in cardiac muscle, 12
Neuregulin, 156
Neurohumoral response, in heart failure, 789–90, 790t
Nickel, T-type calcium channel blockade by, 703
Nicorandil, 631, 633–34, 633f
  for long QT syndrome, 682–83
Nitric oxide, cardiac effects, 628–29
Nitric oxide synthase
  endothelium-derived, calveolin3 co-localization with, 155
  types, 628
N-lines, 36, 39f
Nucleus ambiguus
  biophysical properties, 220
  cardiac vagal motoneurons in, 215, 216f, 217f
  CNS pathways impinging on, 227, 227t
Nucleus tractus solitarii
  afferent innervation, 227–28
  arterial chemoreceptor inputs, 228–29
  baroreceptor inputs, 228, 229f, 230f
  in reflex adjustments, 231–32

Octanol, gap junction channel sensitivity to, 198
Optical microscopy
  confocal, 65, 81–84, 82f–84f
  indications, 61
Optical traps, in study of isolated myosin, 252–53, 253f
Osborn wave, transmural distribution of I_{to} and, 672
Osmium tetroxide fixation
  advantages, 63
  in transmission electron microscopy, 61
Osmotic pressure change, electrophysiological effects, 608–9

Overstretch phenomenon, 34
Oxygen
  consumption, mechanical correlates of, 767–69, 768f–769f
  delivery, in heart failure, 796
  diffusion distance, 85
    aging effects, 102, 103f
    postnatal development effects, 92–93, 93f
Oxygenation potential, age-related reduction, 103f

P light chain. See Myosin light chain 2
P wave, 569f, 570, 571
Pacemaker cells, sinus node
  electrophysiological studies, 477–78
  sites, 478–79
Pacemaker channels
  acetylcholine effects, 619–20, 629f
  β-adrenergic effects, 612–13
  calcium effects, 601, 603, 698
  cAMP effects, 693
  cloned. See HCN channels
  in heart disease, 720
  molecular cloning, 693–94
Pacing effects
  fast, 536, 536f
  slow, 537–38, 538f
Papillary muscle hypertrophy, from aortic banding, 111–12, 111f
Paradoxical calveolar closure and swelling, 150
Patch-clamp technique, 188–89
Pericardium, diastolic role, 774–75
Peroxidase, antibody labeling with, 64
pH
  calcium sensitivity of tension and, 437
  effects on action potential repolarization, 606–7
  effects on automaticity, 607
  effects on channels, 606, 607
  effects on excitability, 606
  effects on Na^{2+}-Ca^{2+} exchanger, 402–3
  effects on resting membrane potential, 605–6
  gap junction channel sensitivity to, 197–98, 198f
Phorbol 12-myristate 13-acetate, 155
Phosphatase-1, 317
Phosphate
  burst, 243
  caged, 249f
  dissociation, in crossbridge cycle, 250–51, 250f, 259
Phosphatidylinositol-4,5-biphosphate, Na^{2+}-Ca^{2+} exchanger regulation by, 402
Phosphocreatine shuttle, in heart failure, 793, 796
Phospholamban, 315–22
  Ca^{2+}-ATPase interactions. See Phospholamban–Ca^{2+}-ATPase system
  Ca^{2+}-ATPase-interaction sites in, 321f, Plate 9
  function, 316f, 317–18

  gene
    chromosomal location, 323
    structure, 324
    targeting in mice, 322
    transcriptional regulation, 324
  phosphorylation, 307, 317
    Ca^{2+}-ATPase activity and, 307, 317–18, 320–21, 321f
  structure, 315–17, 316f
Phospholamban–Ca^{2+}-ATPase system
  Ca^{2+}-ATPase-interaction sites, 319–20, 321f, Plate 9
  molecular mechanism, 320–21, 321f
  phospholamban-interaction site, 318–19, 319f, 320f
  physiological relevance, 321–22
Phosphoprotein phosphatase, 317
Pinacidil, 631, 632f, 634
Plasma membrane
  methods for studying, 157
  proteins
    in heart failure, 799t
    movement, 157–58
  sphingolipid/cholesterol rafts in, 156–57
Plasma membrane Ca^{2+}-ATPase. See Sarcolemmal Ca^{2+}-ATPase
Playing dead response, 231
PMCA family of Ca^{2+}-ATPase. See Sarcolemmal Ca^{2+}-ATPase
Polypeptides, gap junction channel sensitivity to, 200
Postextrasystolic potentiation, 755–56
Potassium
  effects on action potential configurations, 596–97, 597f
  effects on automaticity, 596
  effects on channels, 541, 597, 598f
  effects on conduction, 494–98, 495f–497f, 596
  effects on excitability, 596
  effects on resting membrane potential, 595–96
  for long QT syndrome, 682, 727–28
Potassium channel(s), 557–61, 568–86
  accessory subunits, 577–78, 577f
  ACh-activated, 560–61, 616–18, 617f, 720
  α-actinin-2, 577f, 579
  adenosine effects, 622–23
  adenosine-activated, 617
  α-adrenergic effects, 614–16, 615f
  β-adrenergic effects, 611–12
  associated proteins, 577f, 578
  ATP-sensitive, 542, 561, 562f, 625, 719–20
    activation, 618, 631, 632f
    adenosine effects, 623–24
    sensitivities, 631, 633
  atrioventricular block and, 584, 585f
  barium effects, 603
  calcium effects, 603
  cellular/regional heterogeneity, 574, 665–68
  clustering, 471
  currents, 532–33, 533f, 535, 535f

  cytoskeleton and, 577f, 578–79
  delayed rectifier current, 559–60, 559f, 570t, 572f, 573–74, 718
    in heart disease, 718–19
    molecular genetics, 579–80
    rapid, 570t, 573, 574, 579, 668
    with rapid activation and slow inactivation, 570t, 572f, 573–74
    slow, 570t, 573, 574, 577f, 579–80, 668
    ultra-rapid, 570t, 573, 666
  DTX-sensitive, 570t, 574
  eag (ether-a-go-go) gene subfamily, 575t, 576
  ELK (*eag*-like) genes, 576
  endothelin effect, 627
  ERG (*eag*-related) genes, 575t, 576, 666t, 668, 718
    activation, by extracellular potassium, 597, 598f
  ERG1, 579
  gap junction channels as, 186
  HCN
    biophysical properties, 696–98, 696f, 697t
    distribution patterns, 695–96
    nomenclature, 694, 697t
    structure, 694–95
  interacting proteins, 578
  inward rectifier, 557, 560–61, 561f–562f
    cardiac, 560, 561f, 719
    in heart disease, 719–20
  KCNE1, 577, 577f, 579–80, 666t, 668, 669f, 725
  KCNQ1, 575t, 666t, 668, 669f
  KCNQ1subfamily, 575t, 576–77, 577f, 579–80
  KCNQ2/KCNQ3, 577
  Kvα subunits, 574–76, 575t, 576f, 580–82, 581f, 666t
    Kv1 (*Shaker*), 575t, 576, 665, 666t
    Kv1.5, 666
    Kv2 (*Shab*), 575t, 576, 665, 666t
    Kv3 (*Shaw*), 575t, 576, 665, 666t
    Kv4 (*Shal*), 575t, 576, 665, 666t
    Kv5.x–Kv9.x, 575t, 576
    overview, 665–66
  Kvβ subunits, 577–78, 577f
  magnesium effects, 603–4
  minimal subunit. See KCNE1
  molecular determinants, 665–68, 666t–667t
  pH effects, 607
  pore-forming α subunits, 574–77, 575t, 576f
  QT prolongation and, 582–84, 583f, 724–26
  sodium effects, 600
  sodium-activated, 720
  stretch-activated, 608, 609
  temperature effects, 607
  thyroid state and, 620–21
  transgenic and targeted gene deletion approaches, 580–82, 581f

Potassium channel(s) (continued)
  transient outward current, 557–59, 558f, 570t, 571–73, 572f, 717
    with fast inactivation, 570t, 571, 572f, 574, 580, 581f
    in heart disease, 717–18
    interventricular differences, 655
    J wave and, 672
    molecular genetics, 580–82, 581f, 666–68
    with slow inactivation, 570t, 571–73, 572f, 574, 580–82, 581f
    transmural distribution, 655, 672
    ventricular arrhythmia/tachycardia and, 584–85, 585f
  voltage-gated, 557–60, 558f–559f
    electrophysiological diversity, 569–74, 570t
    in-vivo alterations, functional consequences, 582–86
    molecular correlates, 579–82
    molecular determinants, 574–79
Potassium channel openers
  ATP-sensitive potassium channel activation by, 631, 632f
  cardiac effects, 631–34
  cardioprotective effects, 634
  for long QT syndrome, 682
  sulfonylurea co-expression, 633–34, 633f
Power curves, 431–32, 432f
PR interval, 569f, 571
Preload
  atrial contraction and, 749–50
  effect on contractility indices, 758, 759f
  peak dP/dt and, 760
  systolic function and, 746–50, 748f–749f
Preload recruitable stroke work, as index of contractility, 759–60
Preload reserve, 748
Premature action potential, 534–36, 535f–536f
Pressure overload hypertrophy
  capillary adaptations and, 115, 116f
  clinical manifestations, 105
  morphometric analysis, 105–17
  myocyte volume composition and, 113–14
  ventricular remodeling in, 106–7, 111–12, 111f–112f, 744
Pressure-volume area, ventricular oxygen consumption and, 768–69, 768f–769f
Pressure-volume loops, in heart failure, 791–93, 792f, 800f
Projection density maps, of gap junctions, 171f, 172–73
Propranolol
  cellular responsiveness to, 662
  for long QT syndrome, 682
Protein kinase(s), mechanism of activity, 317
Protein kinase A
  chloride channels activated by, 604–5
  phosphorylation by
    Na^{2+}-Ca^{2+} exchanger, 401–2
    troponin I, 273–76
    in regulation of phospholamban–Ca^{2+}-ATPase system, 320–21, 321f
Protein kinase C
  isoforms, in calveolae, 155–56
  phosphorylation by
    crossbridge cycling rate and, 274, 276
    myosin light chain 2, 284, 289
    Na^{2+}-Ca^{2+} exchanger, 401
    phospholamban, 317
    troponin I, 275–79
    troponin T, 283
Proteins. See also specific protein
  calveolar
    analysis techniques, 157
    artifact issues, 161–63
    calveolin as, 158–61
    gap junction, 170–78
    muscle, 36, 48, 421–29
    myofilament. See Myofilament proteins
    phosphorylation, cardiac myofilament modulation by, 259
    plasma membrane, 157–58, 799t
    skeletal, 34, 156
    water-channel, 152–53
P-type ATPase, 303–4, 308–9, 309f
Pulmonary artery banding, right ventricle hypertrophy from
  capillary adaptations, 115, 116f
  myocyte adaptations, 112, 112f
Pulmonary receptors
  rapidly adapting, 226
  slowly adapting, 224, 226
Purinergic receptor stimulation, external ATP and, 624–25, 624f
Purkinje cells, potassium sensitivity, 596
Purkinje fibers
  acetylcholine effects, 620
  cable properties, 170
  conduction velocity, 456t
  relationship between conduction time and maximal upstroke velocity, 494–95, 496f
  supernormal conduction, 494, 495f
Purkinje–ventricular muscle junction
  conduction across, 491, 492f
  structure, 491–92, 493f

QRS complex, 569f, 570, 571
QT interval, 569f, 571
  prolongation of. See Long QT syndrome
Quinidine
  cellular responsiveness to, 664, 664t
  long QT syndrome caused by, 723

Random reentry, 508
Rat model, contractility assessment, 762
Reentry, 497, 498, 502, 504
  anatomic, 504–7, 505f–506f
  anisotropic, 518
  atrioventricular nodal, 487
  figure-8, 508
  functional, 507–9, 508f–509f
  leading circle, 508–9
  phase 2
    electrical heterogeneity and, 672–74, 675f, 676f
    as mechanism of extrasystolic activity, 672, 673f
    as trigger for ventricular tachycardia/fibrillation, 672–74, 675f, 676f
  random, 508
  spiral wave, 509–17, 510f–513f, 516f–517f. See also Spiral waves
  transition from functional to anatomic, 517–18, 517f
Refractory period, 497–98
  heterogeneity, spiral wave drift from, 515, 516f
Regulatory light chain. See Myosin light chain 2
Relaxation. See also Contraction
  calcium transport during
    developmental differences, 368–69
    relative contributions of transporters, 364–67, 364f, 365f, 367f
    species differences, 368, 368t
    temperature differences, 368, 368t
Replacement fibrosis
  age-related, 94, 95f
  definition, 117–18
  ischemic cardiomyopathy and, 122, 123f
  myocyte loss and, 99
Respiratory influences, on cardiac vagal motoneurons, 222, 222f
Respiratory patterning, in cardiac vagal motoneurons, 222–24, 223f
Restitution dependence, in anatomic reentry, 507
Reversal potential, 531–32
Right heart failure, 788t
Romano-Ward syndrome, 723
Ryanodine receptor calcium channel, 359–61, 361t

Safety factor
  for action potential repolarization, 710
  of propagation, 493–94, 494f
Saltatory conduction, 467
Sarcolemma
  associations, 15, 33
  calcium transport, 342–55. See also Calcium channel(s); Na^{2+}-Ca^{2+} exchange
  calveolae of. See Calveolae
  cell membrane, 13
  surface area, 79
Sarcolemmal Ca^{2+}-ATPase, 302
  kinetic properties, 354–55, 355t
  role in calcium removal, 390
Sarcomere
  banding patterns, 36
  filament arrays, 36, 40f–42f
  length
    during contraction-relaxation cycle, 765, 766f
    definition, 36
    I-band width and, 36

morphometric analysis, 79
myofilament response to, 265
myofilament proteins. See Myofilament proteins
organization, 4
structure, 30f–42f, 35–36, 48
titin filaments, 33–34
Sarcoplasmic reticulum
  calcium content
    frequency dependence, 376–77, 377f
    measurements, 359, 360t
    rest-dependent decline, 373–75, 374f
  calcium pumping function. See Sarcoplasmic reticulum Ca^{2+}-ATPase
  calcium release
    during contraction
      fraction of, 372–73, 373f
      vs. calcium influx, 369–72, 370f–371f, 370t
      reverse Na^{2+}-Ca^{2+} exchange as trigger for, 391–92
    cardiac
      components, 303
      isolation and characterization, 303
      reconstitution, 303
      vs. skeletal, 302–3, 305–6
    functions, 301–2
    in heart failure, 799t
    phospholamban of. See Phospholamban
    structure, 302–3, 302f
    transverse tubule junction with, 302, 302f, 303
Sarcoplasmic reticulum Ca^{2+}-ATPase, 301–24. See also Phospholamban
  ATP binding mutants, 312f, 313–14
  ATP hydrolysis, 306–7, 306f
  calcium affinity, 318
    mutants, 312f, 313
  calcium binding
    fluorescent probes of, 310–11, 310f
    mutants, 312f, 313
    stoichiometry, 305
  calcium transport
    electrogenicity, 305
    measurement, 356–59, 358f, 359f
    model for, 314–15
    steps, 306–7, 306f
  calcium uptake, 304–5, 306
  in cardiac hypertrophy, 307–8
  cardiac vs. skeletal, 305–6
  chemical modifications, 310–12, 310f
  chimeric, 315
  conformational change, 307
  conformational change mutants, 314
  coupling ratio, 305
  fluorescent energy transfer studies, 311
  function, 303–15, 304–6
  mechanism of activity, 306–7, 306f
  mutagenesis, site-directed, 312–15, 312f
  phospholamban-interaction site, 318–19, 319f, 320f, 321f, Plate 9. See also Phospholamban–Ca^{2+}-ATPase system
  phosphorylation mutants, 312f, 313–14
  PMCA family of, 36

reaction cycle, 306–7, 306f
regulation, 307–8, 315–22, 355–56, 355f
rotational diffusion studies, 311
SERCA family, 36
spectroscopic studies, 311–12
structure, 302f
  primary sequences, 308
  secondary model, 308–9, 309f
  three-dimensional reconstruction, 309–10, 309f
thapsigargin inhibition of, 304–5
uncoupling mutant, 314
x-ray diffraction studies, 312
Sarcoplasmic reticulum calcium release channel, 359–61, 361t
Saturation-transfer electron paramagnetic resonance (ST-EPR), 311
Scanning electron microscopy, 62
Scanning probe microscopy, 65
Scanning tunneling microscope, 65
SCN5A gene, 666t, 668–69, 674, 676f
Scroll wave, 517
Segmental fibrosis
  definition, 117
  ischemic cardiomyopathy and, 122, 123f
SERCA family of Ca^{2+}-ATPase, 36
  phospholamban-interaction site, 318–19, 319f, 320f
  thapsigargin inhibition of, 304–5
SERCA isoform chimeras, 315
SERCA1 gene, 308
  chromosomal mapping, 323
  gene analysis, 322–23, 323f
  three-dimensional structure, 309–10, 309f
SERCA2 gene
  chromosomal mapping, 323
  gene analysis, 323, 323f
SERCA2a gene, 308
  phosphorylation
    Ca^{2+}-ATPase activity and, 307
    by Ca^{2+}-/calmodulin-dependent protein kinase, 307
SERCA2b gene, 308
SERCA3 gene, 308
Shape vectors, cardiac ultrastructure and, 4, 5
Single particle tracking, 157
Sinoatrial node
  acetylcholine effects, 619–20, 619f
  β-adrenergic effects, 612–13
Sinus arrhythmia
  sympathetic component, 224
  vagal mediation in, 223–24
Sinus node
  cellular structure, 476–77
  conduction, 478–79, 478f
  connective tissue, 477
  gap junctions, 478
  interaction with atrial cells, 478
  pacemaker cells
    electrophysiological studies, 477–78
    sites, 478–79
Sinusoidal analysis, of crossbridge cycle, 251–52

Skelemin, 15
Skeletal muscle
  thin filament in, 35
  Z-band lattice pattern in, 51, 59f
Skeletal proteins
  calveolae and, 156
  redundancies in, 34
Sliding filaments, crossbridges and, 240–42, 241f. See also Crossbridge cycling
Small square (ss) lattice pattern, in Z-band, 44f, 50–51, 56f, 58f
Sodium
  effects on action potential, 540–41, 541f, 599
  effects on automaticity, 599
  effects on channels, 599–600
  effects on chloride channels, 625
  effects on resting membrane potential, 599
  elevation, causes, 540
  potassium channel activation by, 720
  retention, in heart failure, 789–90, 790t
Sodium channel(s), 551–57
  acetylcholine effects, 619
  in action potential, 540–41, 541f, 552, 553f
  β-adrenergic effects, 612
  angiotensin II effects, 626
  arrhythmias and, 715
  clustering, 471
  currents, 532, 533f, 714–15
  gating, 553–54
  gene mutation
    in idiopathic ventricular fibrillation, 729
    in long QT syndrome, 552, 553f, 556–57, 556f, 726
  in heart disease, 715
  inactivation, 554
  inhibition, conduction effects, 494–98, 495f–497f
  local anesthetic effects, 554, 555–56
  molecular pharmacology, 555–56
  pH effects, 606
  primary structure, 555
  S4 segment, 701, 701f
  selectivity profile, 700, 700f
  slip-mode conductance, digitalis effects, 393
  α-subunit, 555, 714–15
    KPQ deletion mutation, 552, 553f, 556–57, 556f
    SCN5A gene, 666t, 668–69, 674, 676f
  β-subunit, 555, 715
  temperature effects, 607
  tetrodotoxin-sensitive, 668–69
Sodium channel blockers
  cellular responsiveness to, 662–63
  for long QT syndrome, 682
Sodium inward current
  in anisotropic cellular network, 470, 473f
  effects of resistive discontinuities, 464f, 465f, 467

820 INDEX

Sodium-calcium exchange. See Na^{2+}-Ca^{2+} exchange
Somatostatin, potassium channel activation by, 617
Sotalol, cellular responsiveness to, 663, 663f, 664t
Space constant of the voltage decay (λ)
 in atrioventricular node, 487
 in heart, 458, 458t
 in one-dimensional cable, 457
 in two-dimensional tissue, 458
Spectrin, 15
Spectroscopy
 of Ca^{2+}-ATPase, 311–12
 energy dispersive, 62
Sphingolipid/cholesterol rafts, calveolae as, 156–57, 158
Spiral waves, 509–17, 510f–513f, 516f–517f
 anchoring, 517–18, 517f
 in anisotropic and microscopically discontinuous media, 515–16
 in Belousov-Zhabotinsky reaction, 509–10, 510f
 breakup and multiplication, 514–15
 drift, 515, 516f
 dynamics, 513–15
 initiation, 510–13, 511f–513f
 meandering, 513–14, 513f
 in three dimensions, 517
 in ventricular muscle, 510, 510f
ST segment elevation, in Brugada syndrome, 672–74, 675f, 676f
Staining, in electron microscopy, 61–62, 63, 64
Stereology, 65, 76
Steric blocking model of crossbridge cycle, 258, 426
Strength-interval relation, inotropic state and, 753
Stretch, mechanical, electrophysiological effects, 608, 608f
Stroke volume
 afterload and, 748f, 750, 750f
 in heart failure, 749, 749f
 as index of contractility, 757
 preload and, 747, 748f
Stroke volume–end-diastolic pressure relation, 747–48
Stroke work, preload recruitable, as index of contractility, 759–60
Stroke work–end-diastolic pressure relation, 752, 753f
Stroke work–end-diastolic volume relation, 759–60
Sudden death, animal models, 713
Sulfonylurea, co-expression, with potassium channel openers, 633–34, 633f
Swell-activated chloride channel, 605, 608–9
Swell-activated currents, in heart disease, 722
Systole
 crossbridge cycling in, 266, 266f, 270–71
 myofilament proteins in, 265f, 266, 266f
 thick filament proteins in, 265f, 269–70
 thin filament proteins in, 266–69, 267f, 268f
 thin filament states in, 266f, 270–71
Systolic function
 afterload and, 748f, 750–52, 750f–751f
 cardiac shape/dimensions and, 742–44, 743f–744f
 contractility and, 752, 753f
 determinants, 742–56
 end-systolic pressure–volume relationship, 746, 747f, 759
 in heart failure, 787–89, 788t, 792, 798–99
 interaction between heart rate and β-adrenergic stimulation, 754–55, 755f
 isolated muscle function perspective, 744–46, 746f
 length-dependent activation and, 752, 754f
 mechanical restitution and, 755–56
 postextrasystolic potentiation and, 755–56
 preload and, 746–50, 748f–749f
 strength-interval relations and, 752–54

T tubules, 13–14, 18f–20f, 302, 302f, 303
T wave, 569f, 570, 571
 inscription of, transmural heterogeneity in, 676–78, 677f, 678f
 potassium sensitivity, 597
Talin, in myofibril-sarcolemmal association, 33
Temperature, electrophysiological effects, 607–8
Tension, isometric, determinants, 429–30, 437–42
Tension cost, of energy transduction, 246
Tetrodotoxin, cellular responsiveness to, 662
Thapsigargin, Ca^{2+}-ATPase inhibition by, 304–5
Thick filament, 241f
 interdigitation of, 36, 40f, 41f
 myosin in. See Myosin
 ordering of, 36, 41f, 42f
 proteins, 265f, 269–70, 441–42
 schematic representation, 421f
 titin in, 34
Thin filament, 241f
 actin in. See Actin
 cooperative binding to, 436
 interdigitation of, 36, 40f, 41f
 length, regulation of, 35
 proteins, 266–69, 267f, 268f
 schematic representation, 421f
 states, in diastole and systole, 266f, 270–71
 tropomyosin in. See Tropomyosin
 in Z-band lattice, 49
 Z-filament cross-connection of, 49
Three-dimensional reconstruction
 of isolated myocyte, 81–84, 82f–84f
 technique for, 65–66
 of Z-band, 51, 59f–60f, Plate 1
Thyroid hormones, cardiac effects, 620, 621
Time-resolved phosphorescence anisotropy (TPA), 311
Titin
 binding properties, 34
 myosin and, 34
 in thick filament, 34
Titin filaments, in cardiac muscle, 33–34
Titin-nebulin lattice, 14
Torsades de pointes
 electrical heterogeneity in, 681–82, 682f, 683f
 in long QT syndrome, 723–24
Transgenic mice model
 Na^{2+}-Ca^{2+} exchanger overexpression, 406–7
 phosphorylation effects, 276, 284
 ventricular function, 762
Transient entrainment, in anatomic reentry, 505
Transient inward current, 341–42, 342f, 342t, 722
Transient outward current (I_{to}). See Potassium channel(s), transient outward current
Transmembrane potential, in cable, 458, 458f
Transmembrane recordings, action potential, 660, 660t, 661t
Transmission electron microscopy, 61–62
Transverse tubules, 13–14, 18f–20f, 302, 302f, 303
Triad structure, in sarcoplasmic reticulum, 302
Tropomyosin, 36, 428–29
 actin interactions, 266, 267, 267f
 in contraction-relaxation cycle, 267–68
 cooperative unit size and, 283–84, 436
 function, 283–84
 gene mutations, 428–29
 isoform expression, 283, 284, 428
 movement on thin filament, 267, 267f
 phosphorylation, 284–85
 in steric blocking model of crossbridge cycle, 258
 structure, 267, 267f
 thin filament state and, 266f, 270–71
 transgenic studies, 284, 428
 troponin T interactions, 268f, 283
Troponin
 in contraction regulation, 426–28
 phosphorylation of, in crossbridge cycle, 259
 subunits, 426
 thin filament state and, 266f, 270–71
Troponin C
 calcium binding sites, 427
 calcium sensitivity of tension and, 439–40
 in diastolic/systolic transition, 268, 268f
 isoforms, 427

Troponin I, 427
  calcium sensitivity of tension and, 439
  C-terminal domain, 273
  in diastolic/systolic transition, 268f, 269
  inhibitory region, 272–73
  near NH$_2$-terminal region, 272
  NH$_2$-terminal extension, 271–72
  phosphorylation
    in heart failure, 279–80
    by protein kinase A, 275–76
    by protein kinase C, 278–79
    in reduced calcium sensitivity, 427
    sites, 268f, 271–73
  primary structure, 271
  protein kinase A sites, 273–75
  protein kinase C sites, 275–78
Troponin T
  in diastolic/systolic transition, 268f, 269
  functional domains, 268f, 280–82
  isoform expression, 281, 427–28
  phosphorylation sites, 282–83
  primary structure, 280

U wave, inscription of, transmural heterogeneity in, 678–79, 678f
Ubiquitin, 184
Uranyl staining, in electron microscopy, 63

Vagal efferent fibers, cardiac. See Cardiac vagal motoneurons
Vasculature. See Coronary vasculature
Vasoconstriction, in heart failure, 789, 790t
Vasodilators, for heart failure, 787, 790
Vasopressin, cardiac effects, 626–27
Veins, in cardiac muscle, 12
Velocity of circumferential fiber shortening, as index of contractility, 745, 757–58, 761
Velocity of shortening
  contraction activation effects, 442–44, 442f, 443f
  crossbridge cycling and, 430–32, 431f–432f
Venous return, cardiac output curves and, 760
Ventricle(s)
  activation, 490–93, 492f, Plate 10
  conduction velocity, 456t
  developmental aspects, 671–72
  diastolic structure-function relationships, passive, 771–73, 772f
  dilation, in ischemic cardiomyopathy, 118
  end-diastolic pressure
    length relationships, 752, 754f
    stroke volume and, 747–48
    stroke work and, 752, 753f
  end-diastolic volume, in heart failure, 749, 749f
  filling, in diastole, 773–74, 773f

function
  infarct size and, 122
  ischemic cardiomyopathy and, 121–24
  over range of loading conditions, 759–60
  regional variations, 762–69
hypertrophy. See Ventricular hypertrophy
ionic distinctions, 536–38, 654–62
laminar structure, 462–63, 463f, 763
left
  activation, 492–93, Plate 10
  collagen in, 770
  connectivity of cells, 461, 462f, 462t
  dimensions
    as index of contractility, 756
    measurement, 756
    systolic function and, 742–44, 743f–744f
  ejection fraction, 757, 761
  end-diastolic pressure, in heart failure, 791, 792f
  end-diastolic volume, 757
  end-systolic pressure, in heart failure, 791, 792f
  fine strains in, 764–65, 765f
  postnatal development, 88, 89f
  pressure, contractility and, 758
  pressure–volume relationship
    in diastole, 771, 771f
    passive, 770–71, 771f
  shortening, regional variations, 763–64, 764f
  structure-function relationships
    regional, 763–65, 764f–765f
    three-dimensional analysis, 765–67, 766f–767f
  wall stress, 745–46, 746f
  wall thickening, 765–66, 767f
myocyte number, aging and, 97, 98f
oxygen consumption, mechanical correlates of, 767–69, 768f–769f
pressure, maximum rate of rise, 758, 760, 761
remodeling. See Ventricular remodeling
right
  activation, 493, Plate 10
  dimensions, systolic function and, 744
  hypertrophy
    after myocardial infarction, 126
    ischemic cardiomyopathy and, 126
    from pulmonary artery banding, 112, 112f, 115, 116f
  postnatal development, 88
  prenatal preponderance, 87
  systolic function, regional, 763
spiral waves in, 510, 510f
stress measurements, 745–46, 746f
Ventricular action potential. See Action potential
Ventricular cell
  Luo-Rudy model, 532, 533f

morphometric analysis, 76–80, 77f, 78f, 82f–84f
potassium sensitivity, 596
tissue resistivity, 657, 659f
Ventricular chamber
  dimensions
    in steady state, 756–58
    during systole, 742–44, 743f–744f
  volume, ischemic cardiomyopathy and, 121, 121f
Ventricular fibrillation
  idiopathic, 728–29
  phase 2 reentry as trigger for, 672–74, 675f, 676f
  potassium channels and, 584–85, 585f
Ventricular hypertrophy
  animal models, 712
  concentric, 744
  eccentric, 744
  electrophysiologic changes, 713
  pressure overload, 106–7, 111–12, 111f–112f, 744
  volume overload, 106–7, 112–13, 744
Ventricular remodeling
  aging and, 94–97, 95f
  cardiac hypertrophy and, 106–7
  ischemic cardiomyopathy and, 118–21, 119f, 121f
  postnatal, 86–87, 88, 89f
  prenatal, 87–88
Ventricular tachycardia
  phase 2 reentry as trigger for, 672–74, 675f, 676f
  polymorphic. See Torsades de pointes
  potassium channels and, 584–85, 585f
V_{max}. See Contraction, maximal velocity
Volume overload hypertrophy
  capillary adaptations and, 115
  clinical manifestations, 105
  morphometric analysis, 105–17
  myocyte volume composition and, 113
  ventricular remodeling in, 106–7, 112–13, 744
V-type ATPase, 303

Wall, ventricular
  stress, 745–46, 746f
  thickening, 765–66, 767f
Water retention, in heart failure, 789–90, 790t
Water-channel proteins, in cardiac muscle, 152–53
Wavefront collision, 464, 464f
Wavefront curvature
  conduction block and, 504
  conduction velocity and, 459–61, 459f–461f
Wavefront dispersion, 464–65, 465f
Wavefront propagation
  from high- to low-impedance region, 464–65, 465f
  toward resistive discontinuity, 463–64, 464f
Wenckebach phenomenon, abnormal, 488, 489f

Wheat germ agglutin, calveolar uptake of, 149
Women, myocyte number in, aging and, 98f, 99

XIP (exchanger inhibitory peptide), 350, 400–401, 403–4
X-ray diffraction studies, of Ca^{2+}-ATPase, 312
X-ray emission, in scanning electron microscopy, 62

Z-band, 35–36, 39f, 43f
α-actinin in, 48, 49
centering of, 36
contractile and elastic components in relation to, 44f–47f, 48–49, 52f, 54f–55f
functional states, 44f, 50–51, 54f–60f
gravity effects, 50
intermediate filament linkage with, 15
lattice patterns in, 44f, 50–51, 54f–60f
perturbed states, 50, 52f–54f
protein composition, 49–50
three-dimensional reconstruction, 51, 59f–60f, Plate 1
titin filament linkage with, 34, 49
width, 36
abnormalities, 50, 52f–54f
regulation, 50
Z-crystals/rods, 50, 51, 52f–54f
Zeugmatin, in Z-band, 50
Z-line, 241f

QP 111.4
111.4
H25
2002